steno- narrow, compressed, contracted
stenocoriasis (contraction of the pupil of the eye)
stenopeic (having a narrow slit or opening)

sub-, sup- under, below
subarachonoid (under arachnoid)
subcutaneous (under skin)

super- above, beyond, extreme
supermedial (above the middle)
supernumerary (an extreme number)

supra- above, upon
suprarenal (above kidney)
suprascapular (on upper part of the scapula)

sym-, syn- together, with
symphysis (growing together)
synapsis (joining together)

tachy- swift, rapid
tachycardia (rapid action of the heart)

trans- across, through, beyond
transection (cut across)
transduodenal (through the duodenum)

ultra- beyond, in excess
ultraligation (ligation of vessel beyond point of origin)
ultrasonic (sound waves above the human ear's audibility limit)

SUFFIXES

-able, ible ability to, capable of
viable (capable of living)

-al, -ar pertaining to
labial (pertaining to the lip or lips)
ocular (pertaining to the eye)

-algia a painful condition
neuralgia (pain that affects nerves)

-ary pertaining to, connected with
ciliary (resembling a hairlike structure)
ovary (connected with the ovum)

-ate action or state
degenerate (to decline in condition)
hemolysate (product of hemolysis)

-cle, -cula, -cule, -culum, -culus diminutive
cerebellum (little brain)
molecule (small physical unit)
pedicle (small footlike part)

-ectasia, -ectasis a dilated or distended state
bronchiectasis (dilatation of the bronchi)
lymphectasia (distention with lymph)

-ectomy cutting out
appendectomy (excision of the appendix)

-esthesia condition of sensation
somatesthesia (somatic sense)

-form shape, structure
multiform (occurring in many shapes)
ossiform (resembling the structure of bones)

-fugal moving away from, driving away
centrifugal (moving away from a center)
febrifugal (relieving fever)

-gen, genic producing, produced by
allergen (allergy producing)
carcinogenic (cancer-producing agent)

-gram a record, writing
electrocardiogram (the graphic record of an electrocardiograph)
mammogram (an x-ray film of breast tissue)

-ia state, condition
amblyopia (dimness of vision)
septicemia (poisoning of the blood)

-ic pertaining to
manic (affected with madness)
orchidic (pertaining to the testes)

-ile pertaining to, characteristic of
febrile (pertaining to fever)
infantile (characteristic of infants)

-ion process, action
flexion (act of bending)
hydration (the act of combining with water)

-ism condition, state
astigmatism (defect of vision due to corneal irregularity)
rheumatism (inflammation, typically of muscles and joints)

-itis inflammation
appendicitis (inflammation of the appendix)
carditis (inflammation of the heart muscles)

-ity state
disparity (inequality)
hyperacidity (state characterized by the presence of excess acid)

-logy a collected body of knowledge
biology (the branch of knowledge that deals with living organisms)
pathology (the study of characteristics, causes, and effects of disease)

-lysis disintegration, dissolution
cytolysis (cell destruction)
hemolysis (the dissolution of red blood cells)

-odyne, -odynia pain, referring to/location of pain
gastrodynia (stomach pain)
odontodynia (toothache)

-oid resembling, like
epidermoid (resembling epidermis)
thyroid (shaped like a shield)

-ole, -olus diminutive
centriole (a small center)
malleolus (a small hammer)

-or agent
donor (one who donates)
levator (an agent that elevates)

-penia a deficiency
leukopenia (deficiency of white blood cells)
thrombocytopenia (deficiency of thrombocytes)

-phagia, -phagy ingestion of, consumption of, practice of eating of a substance
geophagy (eating earthy substances)
lipophagia (ingestion of fat by cells)

-plegia a paralyzed state
esophagoplegia (paralysis of the esophagus)
hemiplegia (paralysis of one side of the body)

-poiesis formation of, production of
cholanopoiesis (production of bile acids)
hematopoiesis (formation of red blood cells)

-ptosis downward displacement, prolapse
enteroptosis (downward displacement of the intestine)
hepatoptosis (displacement of the liver)

-rrhagia a breaking forth, bursting, fluid discharge
lymphorrhagia (a flow of lymph)
tracheorrhagia (bleeding from the trachea)

-rrhaphy a suturing in place
cysticorrhaphy (suturing the bladder)
gastrorrhaphy (surgical suture of the stomach)

-rrhea flow
diarrhea (abnormally frequent intestinal evacuations)
laryngorrhea (excessive mucus flow whenever the voice is used)

-tomy cut into, incision into
phlebotomy (incision of a vein)
tracheotomy (cutting into the trachea)

-sis (-asis, -esis, -osis) state or process
dermatosis (a skin disease)
hematemesis (vomiting blood)

Pathophysiology

CONCEPTS OF
ALTERED
HEALTH STATES

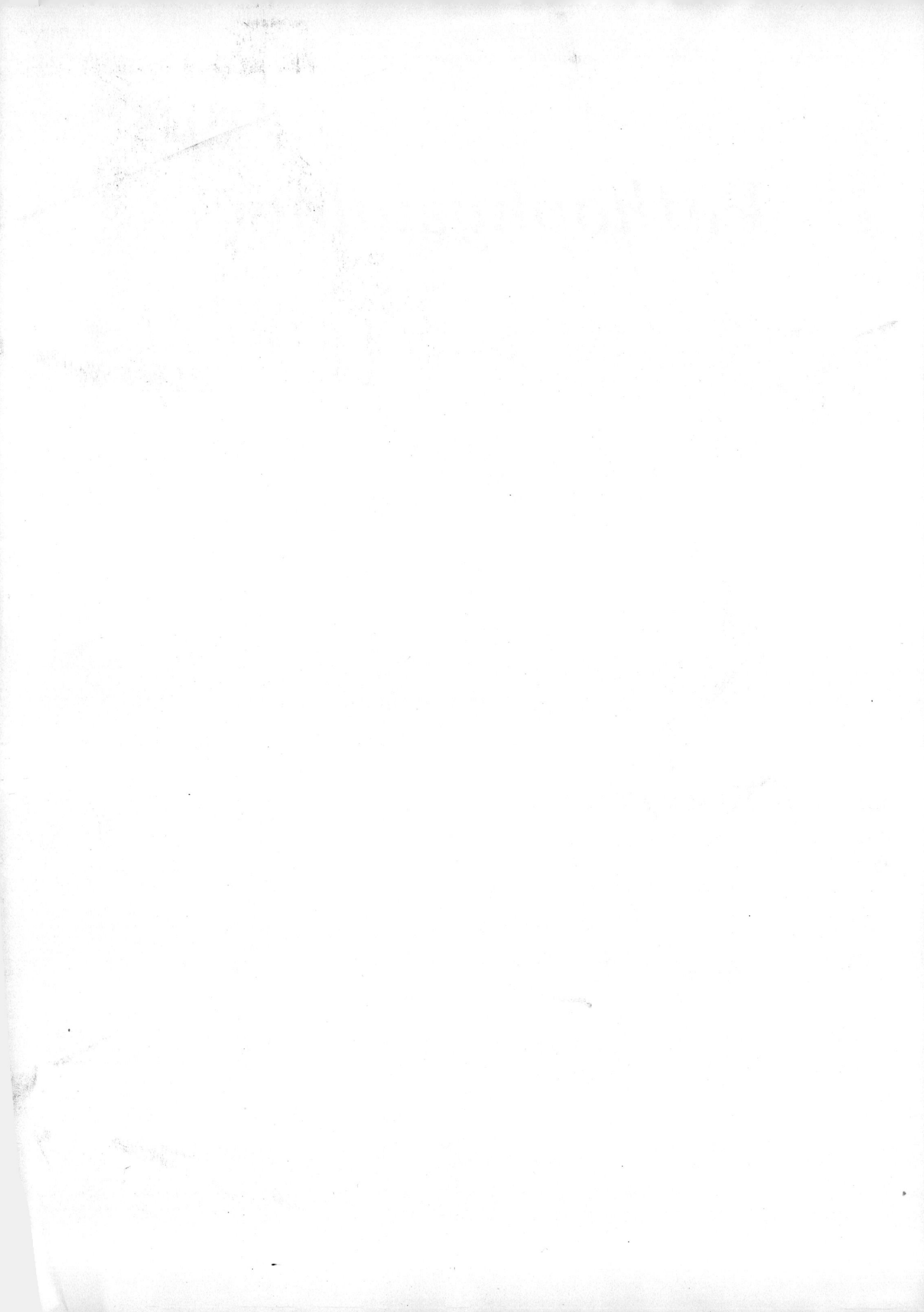

FIFTH EDITION

Pathophysiology

CONCEPTS OF ALTERED HEALTH STATES

Carol Mattson Porth

R.N., M.S.N., Ph.D. (Physiology)
Professor Emeritus, School of Nursing
University of Wisconsin—Milwaukee
Milwaukee, Wisconsin

With 28 Contributors

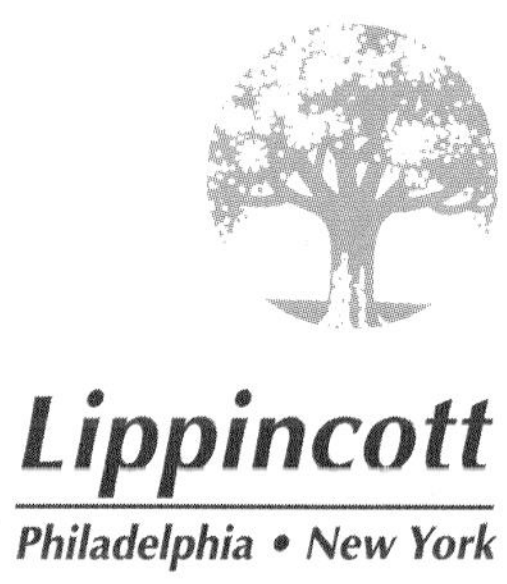

Lippincott
Philadelphia • New York

Acquisitions Editor: Lisa Stead
Assistant Editor: Claudia Vaughn
Project Editor: Tom Gibbons
Senior Production Manager: Helen Ewan
Senior Production Coordinator: Nannette Winski
Assistant Art Director: Kathy Kelley-Luedtke
Indexer: Maria Coughlin

A list of illustrations borrowed from Lippincott-Raven publications is found at the back of the book.

5th Edition

Library of Congress Cataloging in Publications Data

Porth, Carol.
Pathophysiology:concepts of altered health states/Carol Mattson Porth; with 28 contributors. —5th ed.
p. cm.
Includes bibliographical references and index.
ISBN 0-397-55413-3 (cloth:alk. paper)
1. Physiology, Pathological. 2. Nursing. I. Title.
[DNLM: 1. Disease—nurses' instruction. 2. Pathology—nurses' instruction. 3. Physiology—nurses' instruction. QZ 4 P851p 1998]
RB113.P67 1998
616.07—dc21
DNLM/DLC
for Library of Congress 97–49116
CIP

Care has been taken to confirm the accuracy of the information presented and to describe generally accepted practices. However, the authors, editors, and publisher are not responsible for errors or omissions or for any consequences from application of the information in this book and make no warranty, express or implied, with respect to the contents of the publication.

The authors, editors and publisher have exerted every effort to ensure that drug selection and dosage set forth in this text are in accordance with current recommendations and practice at the time of publication. However, in view of ongoing research, changes in government regulations, and the constant flow of information relating to drug therapy and drug reactions, the reader is urged to check the package insert for each drug for any change in indications and dosage and for added warnings and precautions. This is particularly important when the recommended agent is a new or infrequently employed drug.

Some drugs and medical devices presented in this publication have Food and Drug Administration (FDA) clearance for limited use in restricted research settings. It is the responsibility of the health care provider to ascertain the FDA status of each drug or device planned for use in their clinical practice.

9 8 7 6 5 4 3

Learning without thought is labor lost.

CONFUCIUS

This book is dedicated to the students,
past and present,
for whom this book was written.

CONTRIBUTORS

Debra Bancroft, R.N., M.S.N., N.P.
Nurse Practitioner
Rheumatic Disease Center
Milwaukee, Wisconsin

Marion E. Broome, R.N., Ph.D., F.A.A.N
Professor and Research Chair, Nursing of Children
Acting Dean, Center for Nursing Research
University of Wisconsin—Milwaukee and The Children's Hospital of Wisconsin
Milwaukee, Wisconsin

Edward W. Carroll, M.S., Ph.D.
Clinical/Laboratory Supervisor, Department of Basic Health Sciences
Marquette University, College of Health Sciences
Milwaukee, Wisconsin

Kathryn Ann Caudell, R.N., Ph.D.
Assistant Professor, Adult Health Section
University of New Mexico, College of Nursing
Albuquerque, New Mexico

Elizabeth Corwin, B.S.N., Ph.D., C.R.N.P.
Assisstant Professor, Physiology
Coordinator, Family Nurse Practitioner Program
Pennsylvania State University, School of Nursing
University Park, Pennsylvania

Robin Curtis, Ph.D.
Adjunct Professor
Department of Cellular Biology and Anatomy
Department of Physical Medicine and Rehabilitation
Department of Neurosurgery
The Medical College of Wisconsin—Milwaukee, Department of Basic Sciences
Marquette University, College of Health Sciences
Milwaukee, Wisconsin

Sheila Curtis, R.N., M.S.
Senior Lecturer
University of Wisconsin—Milwaukee, School of Nursing
Milwaukee, Wisconsin

Susan E. Dietz, R.N., M.S.
Chief, Training and Technical Support Systems Branch
Division of HIV/AIDS Prevention
Centers for Disease Control and Prevention
Atlanta, Georgia

William Michael Dunne, Jr., Ph.D.
Division Head, Microbiology
Henry Ford Health System
Detroit, Michigan
Associate Professor
Case Western Reserve, Department of Pathology
Cleveland, Ohio

Susan Gallagher-Lepak, R.N., M.S.N., Ph.D.
Psychology Staff
Curative Rehabilitation Services
Milwaukee, Wisconsin

Kathryn J. Gaspard, Ph.D.
Senior Lecturer, Health Restoration Department
University of Wisconsin—Milwaukee, School of Nursing
Milwaukee, Wisconsin

Kathleen Gunta, R.N., M.S.N., O.N.C.
Clinical Nurse Specialist, Orthopaedics
St. Luke's Medical Center
Milwaukee, Wisconsin

Safak Guven, M.D.
Senior Endocrinology Fellow, Endocrinology, Metabolism and Nutrition
Medical College of Wisconsin
Milwaukee, Wisconsin

Mary Kay Jiricka, R.N., M.S.N., C.S., C.C.R.N.,
Clinical Nurse Specialist
St. Luke's Medical Center
Milwaukee, Wisconsin

Camille J. Kolotylo, R.N., M.Sc.N.
Doctoral Student, School of Nursing
University of Wisconsin—Milwaukee
Milwaukee, Wisconsin

Julie A. Kuenzi, R.N., M.S.N., C.D.E.
Diabetes Care Center Manager
Diabetes Nurse Specialist
Medical College of Wisconsin and Froedtert Memorial Lutheran Hospital
Milwaukee, Wisconsin

Judy Wright Lott, R.N.C., D.S.N., N.N.P.
Associate Professor, Parent Child Health
University of Cincinnati, College of Nursing
Cincinnati, Ohio

Sylvia Eichner McDonald, M.D., R.N., C.R.R.N.
Rehabilitation Clinical Nurse Specialist
Mercy Medical Center
Oshkosh, Wisconsin

Patricia L. Mehring, R.N.C., M.S.N., O.G.N.P.
Obstetrics and Gynecology Nurse Practitioner
Women Care
Waukesha, Wisconsin
Department of Foundations
University of Wisconsin—Milwaukee, School of Nursing
Milwaukee, Wisconsin

Janice Smith Pigg, B.S.N., R.N., M.S.
Nurse Consultant—Rheumatology
Smith-Pigg Consultants
Cedarburg, Wisconsin

Janice Kuiper Pikna, M.S.N., R.N., C.S.
Clinical Nurse Specialist, Gerontology
Froedtert Memorial Lutheran Hospital, Senior Health Program
Milwaukee, Wisconsin

Joan Pleuss, M.S., R.D., C.D.E.
Senior Research Dietitian
Clinical Research Center
Medical College of Wisconsin, Froedtert Memorial Lutheran Hospital
Milwaukee, Wisconsin

Marianne Sigda, R.N.C., M.N., N.N.P.
Neonatal Nurse Practitioner
Emory University, Nell Hudson Woodroff School of Nursing
Atlanta, Georgia

Gladys Simandl, R.N., Ph.D.
Associate Professor
Columbia College of Nursing
Milwaukee, Wisconsin

Cynthia V. Sommer, Ph.D., M.T.(A.S.C.P.)
Associate Professor, Department of Biological Sciences
University of Wisconsin—Milwaukee
Milwaukee, Wisconsin

Stephanie Stewart, R.N., Ph.D.
Director, Undergraduate Program
University of Wisconsin—Oshkosh, College of Nursing
Oshkosh, Wisconsin

Nancie Urban, R.N., M.S.N.
Director, Clinical Practice and Research
Wisconsin Heart Group, S.C.
Milwaukee, Wisconsin

Jill White, R.N., Ph.D.
Assistant Professor, Health Restoration Department
University of Wisconsin—Milwaukee, College of Nursing
Milwaukee, Wisconsin

REVIEWERS

Patricia Bowne, M.S., Ph.D.
Chair, Natural Sciences, Mathematics and Technology Division
Alverno College
Milwaukee, Wisconsin

Judith D. Bryan, R.N., B.S.N., M.S.N., Ed.D.
Assistant Professor
University of Indianapolis, School of Nursing
Indianapolis, Indiana

Mary Pat Kunert, R.N., Ph.D.
Assistant Professor
University of Marquette College of Nursing
Milwaukee, Wisconsin

Patricia J. Nefsey, B.S., M.S., R.D., Ph.D.
Assistant Professor
University of Connecticut—Storrs, School of Nursing
Storrs, Connecticut

Catherine Paradiso, R.N., M.S.N.
Clinical Nurse Specialist
Mobile Health Unit Coordinator
Staten Island, New York

Patricia K. Taylor Porthier, R.N., M.S.
Assistant Professor of Nursing
Loma Linda University, School of Nursing
Loma Linda, California

Virginia A. Rahr, R.N., M.S.N., Ed.D.
Associate Professor
University of Texas—Galveston, School of Nursing
Galveston, Texas

Kathy Rodgers, R.N., M.S.N., C.N.S., C.C.R.N., C.E.N.
Advanced Clinical Educator, Critical Care
St. Elizabeth Hospital
Beaumont, Texas

Mary C. Shoemaker, R.N., Ph.D.
Saint Francis Medical Center, College of Nursing
Peoria, Illinois

Elizabeth Wilkerson, B.S.N., M.S.N., Ph.D.
Professor
California State University—Fresno, Department of Nursing
Fresno, California

PREFACE

As the 20th century draws to a close, we are reminded of the phenomenal advances that have occurred in understanding and treating disease. Yet, despite these advances, we are also reminded that illness and disease continue to occur and impact the physiologic as well as social, psychological, and economic well-being of individuals, their families, the community, and the world at large.

As a nurse-physiologist, my major emphasis in the fifth edition of *Pathophysiology: Concepts of Altered Health States,* as in previous editions, is to relate normal body functioning to the physiologic changes that participate in disease production and occur as a result of disease, as well as the body's remarkable ability to compensate for these changes. The beauty of physiology is that it integrates all of the aspects of the individual cells and organs of the human body into a total functional whole that can be used to explain both the physical and psychological aspects of altered health. Indeed, it has been my philosophy to share the beauty of the human body and to emphasize that in disease as in health, there is more "going right" in the body than is "going wrong." This book is an extension of my career and, as such, of my philosophy. It is my hope that readers will learn to appreciate the marvelous potential of the body, incorporating it into their own philosophy and ultimately sharing it with their clients.

One of the strengths of the book is that it is a book to grow with. Although intended as a course textbook for students, it is also designed to serve as a reference book that students can take with them and use in their practice once the course is finished. Although the book was written with undergraduate students in mind, it is also appropriate for graduate students in nurse practitioner and clinical nurse specialist programs and for students in other health care disciplines.

Those who are familiar with the previous edition will find many changes. Probably the most readily apparent is the use of full color in the design and illustrations. This was done with the intent of adding visual appeal as well as enhancing conceptual learning. As the process of adding color to the many illustrations in the book progressed, it became apparent that in addition to motivating reader interest, the use of color provided a mechanism for linking text content with illustration content. With this in mind, both the selection of illustrations and the addition of color have been done with the intent of providing a visually appealing book as well as one that would assist the reader in understanding and appreciating the sometimes complex content of the text.

Also new to this edition are lists of suffixes, prefixes, and normal laboratory values; a glossary; and historical vignettes. The suffixes and prefixes are readily accessible, appearing on the inside front cover and facing page of the book. The glossary at the end of the book provides a comprehensive support for the reader; it is followed by laboratory values. As a point of interest, brief historical vignettes introduce each unit, forming the bridge that links our history to the present.

The pedagogical tools for this edition have been arranged differently from the last editions. The objectives have been placed at the beginning of each major section in the chapter. The purpose behind this was twofold: to focus the reader's attention as he or she moves from section to section and to allow faculty to select sections of a chapter for student assignments. Summary statements remain as in the previous edition.

As in other editions, every attempt has been made to develop a text that is current, accurate, and presented in a logical manner. The content has been arranged so that concepts build on one another. Words are defined as content is presented. Concepts from physiology, biochemistry, physics, and other sciences are reviewed as deemed appropriate. A conceptual model that integrates the developmental and preventive aspects of health has been used. Selection of content was based on common health problems, including the special needs of children and elderly persons.

The writing of this book has been a meaningful endeavor for the authors. It was accomplished through an extensive review of the literature and through the use of critiques provided by students, faculty, and content specialists. As this vast amount of information was processed, inaccuracies or omissions may have occurred. Readers are encouraged to contact us about such errors. Such feedback is essential to the continual development of the book.

ACKNOWLEDGMENTS

As in previous editions, many persons contributed to the development of this edition.

The contributing authors deserve a special mention, for they worked long hours to supply essential content. To have put a book of this magnitude together without their help would have been impossible. Laura Burke, Mark LaRoccha, and Linda Hurwitz were not able to contribute to this edition. Their contributions to the previous edition greatly facilitated the preparation of this edition.

Several other persons deserve special recognition. Georgianne Heymann, RN, BSN, prepared the list of suffixes and prefixes, the short historical vignettes that appear at the beginning of each unit, and the glossary. She also assisted in editing the manuscript. As with previous editions, she provided not only excellent editorial assistance but also encouragement and support when the tasks associated with manuscript preparation became most frustrating. Kathryn Gaspard, PhD, Mary Pat Kunert, RN, PhD, Patricia Bowne, PhD, and Milena Sigatore, RN, MSN, read and provided valuable input for various parts of the book. In addition, a number of persons who reviewed the text for the publisher, but who were unknown to the author, made valuable comments and are to be commended.

In terms of illustrations, many of you will recognize the excellent illustrations that Carole Hilmer, medical illustrator, prepared for previous editions of the book. Although they are now in color, the detail and accuracy of these illustrations would not have been possible without her excellent work. I would also like to acknowledge the contributions of other authors who have shared their illustrations and photos. I particularly want to thank the other Lippincott authors whose citations appear in the back of the book.

I would also like to recognize the efforts of the editorial and production staff at Lippincott-Raven that were directed by Lisa Stead, Acquisitions Editor. I particularly want to thank Claudia Vaughn for her day-to-day performance of all the tasks and communication that go into producing a book of this size and complexity; Susan Hermansen for orchestrating the addition of color into the illustrations for the book; and Tom Gibbons for managing the editing and production of the book.

And last, but not least, I would like to acknowledge my family, my friends, and my colleagues for their patience, their understanding, and their encouragement through the entire process.

CONTENTS

CHAPTER 9
Disorders of White Blood Cells and Lymphoid Tissues 151
Kathryn Ann Caudell

UNIT III
Immunity and Inflammation 165

CHAPTER 10
Mechanisms of Infectious Disease 167
W. Michael Dunne, Jr.

CHAPTER 11
Immunity and Inflammation 189
Cynthia Sommers

CHAPTER 12
Alterations in the Immune Response 213
Carol Mattson Porth and W. Michael Dunne, Jr.

CHAPTER 13

Acquired Immunodeficiency Syndrome 235

Susan E. Dietz

UNIT IV

Integumentary Function 249

CHAPTER 14

Control of Integumentary Function 251

Gladys Simandl

CHAPTER 15

Alterations in Skin Function and Integrity 259

Gladys Simandl

UNIT V

Circulatory Function 301

CHAPTER 16

Control of the Circulation 303

CHAPTER 17

Alterations in Blood Flow in the Systemic Circulation 335

Alterations in Cell Function and Growth

With its elegant structure and astonishing range of functions, the living cell is an object of wonder. It is the basic unit of all living organisms. There are more than 300 trillion cells in the human body, and every second of every day, more than 10 million die and are replaced.

In 1665, these impressive structures were named. While examining a thin slice of cork, Robert Hooke (1635–1703), an English scientist and pioneer microscopist, noted that it was made up of tiny boxlike units. The units reminded him of the small enclosures in which monks lived, and he named the microscopic spaces "cells," from the Latin word cells, meaning "small enclosures."

Although Hooke, as well as other scientists, intently studied microscopic life, few guessed the significance of cells. That would be delayed until microscopes were advanced enough to yield more detailed information. It was with the work of Anton van Leeuwenhoek (1632–1723), a Dutch biologist and microscopist, that the mysteries and importance of the cell were revealed. He ground a single lens to such perfection that he was able to produce a microscope with great resolving power—one that was capable of magnifying a specimen from approximately 50 to 300 times in diameter. Van Leeuwenhoek's work, which included constructing an aquatic microscope that he used to study red blood cells and their flow through the body, was responsible for helping scientists investigate human tissues in ways that once they only dreamed of.

UNIT I

CHAPTER 1

Cell and Tissue Characteristics

Carol M. Porth and Edward W. Carroll

To understand the functioning of the human body in health and disease, it is necessary to understand how the individual cells of the body are structured and how they function. The *cell* is the smallest functional unit that an organism can be divided into and still retain the characteristics necessary for life. Cells are organized into larger functional units called *tissues*. Tissues combine to form body structures and organs. Although the cells of different tissues and organs vary in structure and function, certain characteristics are common to all cells. Cells are remarkably similar in their ability to exchange materials with their immediate environment, obtaining energy from organic nutrients, synthesizing complex molecules, and replicating themselves. It is at the level of the cell that most disease processes initiate their effects. Some diseases affect the cells of a single organ, others affect the cells of a particular tissue type, and still others affect the cells of the entire organism. This chapter discusses the functional components of the cell, integration of cell function and growth, movement across the cell membrane and membrane potentials, and tissue types.

Functional Components of the Cell

After you have completed this section of the chapter, you should be able to meet the following objectives:

- List the components of the cell protoplasm
- State why the nucleus is called the "control center" of the cell

- Explain the associations among DNA, genes, and chromosomes
- Name the three types of RNA and cite their functions
- List the components of the cytoplasm and state their functions
- State four functions of the cell membrane

Although diverse in their organization, all eucaryotic cells have common structures that perform unique functions. When seen under a light microscope, three major components of the cell become evident: the nucleus, the cytoplasm, and the cell membrane (Figs. 1-1 and 1-2).

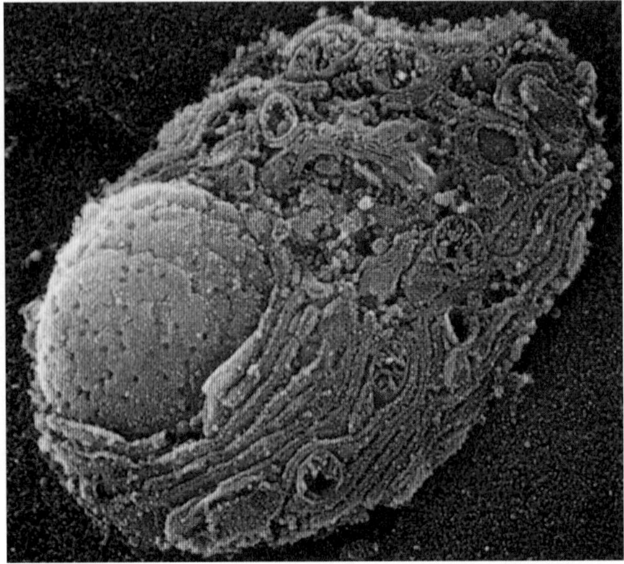

FIGURE 1-2
Nucleus and cytoplasmic membrane systems of a chondrocyte revealed in three dimensions by scanning electron microscope (×12,000).

Protoplasm

The internal components that make up the cells of living organisms are collectively referred to as *protoplasm*. Protoplasm is composed of water, proteins, lipids, carbohydrates, and electrolytes. Water makes up 70% to 85% of the cell's protoplasm. The second most abundant constituents (10% to 20%) of protoplasm are the cell proteins, which form cell structures, and the enzymes necessary for cellular reactions. Proteins can also be found complexed to other compounds such as nucleoproteins, glycoproteins, and lipoproteins. Lipids constitute 2% to 3% of most cells. The most important lipids are the phospholipids and cholesterol, which are mainly insoluble in water; they combine with proteins to form the cell membrane and the membranous barriers that separate different cell compartments. Some cells also contain large amounts of triglycerides. In the so-called fat cells, triglycerides can constitute up to 95% of the total cell mass. The fat stored in these cells represents stored energy, which can be mobilized and used wherever it is needed in the body. Only small amounts of carbohydrates are found in the cell, and these are used primarily for fuel. The major intracellular electrolytes are potassium, magnesium, phosphate, sulfate, and bicarbonate. There are also smaller quantities of sodium, chloride, and calcium. These electrolytes facilitate the generation and transmission of electrochemical impulses in nerve and muscle cells. Intracellular electrolytes participate in reactions that are necessary for cellular metabolism.

The Nucleus

The nucleus of the cell appears as a rounded or elongated structure, usually located in the center of the cell (see Fig 1-2). It is enclosed in a nuclear membrane and contains chromatin and one or more nucleoli. All eucaryotic cells have at least one nucleus; some typically have two or more nuclei (which contrasts with procaryotic cells of bacteria, which lack a nucleus and nuclear membrane.)

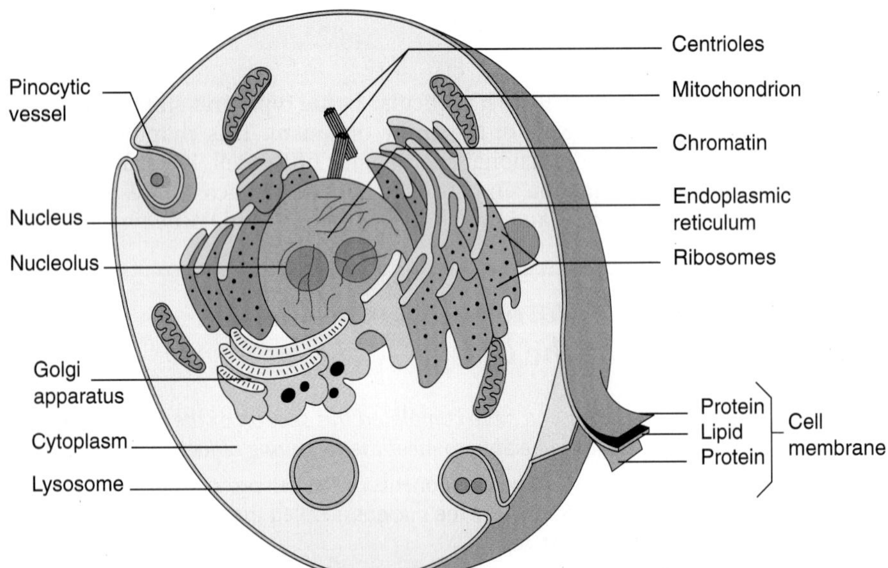

FIGURE 1-1
Composite cell designed to show in one cell all of the various components of the nucleus and cytoplasm.

The nucleus is the control center for the cell. It contains deoxyribonucleic acid (DNA) that is essential to the cell because its genes contain the information necessary for the synthesis of the various proteins that the cell must produce to stay alive. These proteins include enzymes that are used to synthesize other substances, including carbohydrates and lipids, made by the cell. The genes also represent the individual units of inheritance that transmit information from one generation to another.

Each DNA molecule is made up of two extremely long double-stranded helical chains containing variable sequences of four nitrogenous bases (see Chapter 3). These bases form the genetic code. Within the nucleus, each double-stranded DNA molecule is periodically coiled about basic proteins called *histones*, forming regularly spaced spherical structures called *nucleosomes* that are similar to beads on a string (Fig. 1-3). The string of beads is further wound into filaments that make up the

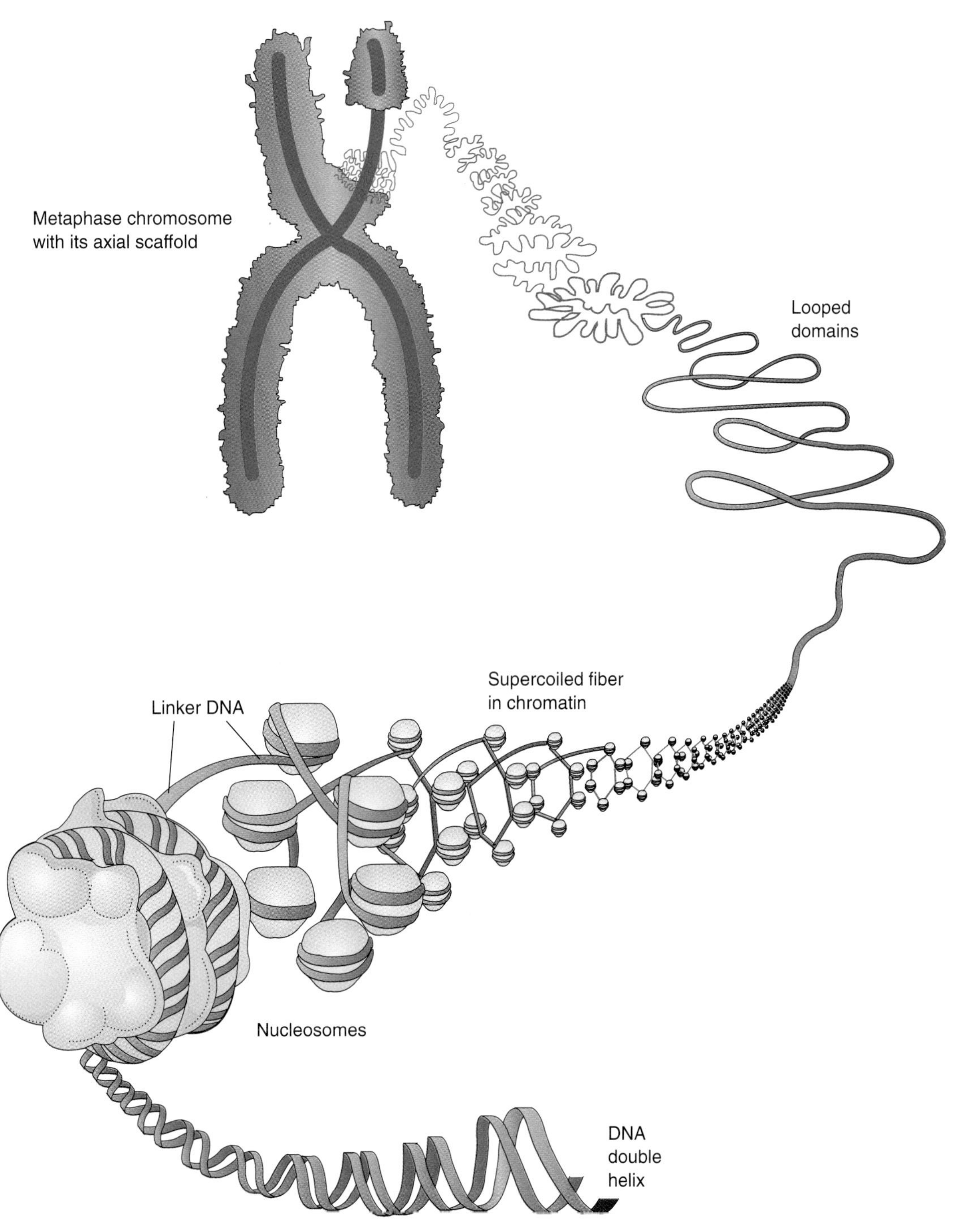

FIGURE 1-3
Increasing orders of DNA compaction in chromatin and mitotic chromosomes.

structure of chromatin. Further coiling produces structures known as *chromosomes*, which are visible during cell division. Although each DNA molecule contains a great many genetic instructions, it is not made up entirely of genes. Stretches of meaningless DNA can lie between one gene and the next and sometimes reside within the gene sequence itself. The amino acid sequence of the gene that is interpreted is called an *exon*, and the interspersed meaningless portion is called an *intron*. In cells that are about to divide, the DNA must be replicated before mitosis or cell division occurs. In the process of replication, complimentary pairs of DNA are generated such that each daughter cells receives an identical set of genes.

Although chromosomes are condensed and can be recognized when the cell is dividing at mitosis, they are not recognizable at other times. They nevertheless persist in a partly condensed and partly extended state, including sections of DNA that are actively being transcribed. In the mature or nondividing cell, darkly stained granules represent inactive regions of chromosomal material called *heterochromatin*. Regions of active genes called *euchromatin* do not stain or are lightly stained. The intensity of nuclear staining can be used as a guide to cell activity. A more active cell contains greater amounts of euchromatin. The complex structure of DNA and DNA-associated proteins dispersed in the nuclear matrix is called *chromatin*. Chromatin is also the site of ribonucleic acid (RNA) synthesis. There are three kinds of RNA: messenger RNA (mRNA), which copies and carries the DNA instructions for protein synthesis to the cytoplasm; ribosomal RNA (rRNA), which moves to the cytoplasm where it becomes the site of protein synthesis; and transfer RNA (tRNA), which also moves into the cytoplasm, where it transports amino acids to the elongating protein as it is being synthesized. The nucleus also contains one or more darkly stained round bodies called a *nucleolus*. Ribosomal RNA is transcribed exclusively in the nucleoli. Nucleoli contain regions from several chromosomes, each with part of the genetic code that is needed for the synthesis of rRNA. Cells that are actively synthesizing proteins can be recognized because their nucleoli are large and prominent and the nucleus as a whole is euchromatic.

The nuclear contents are surrounded by a doubled membrane called the *nuclear envelope* or *nuclear membrane*. This structure has many circular *pores*, where the two membranes fuse to form a gap filled with a thin protein diaphragm. Evidence suggests that many classes of molecules, including fluids, electrolytes, RNA, some proteins, and perhaps some hormones, can move in both directions across the nuclear pores. The nuclear pore structure apparently regulates which molecules pass from the cytoplasm to the nucleus and vice versa.

The Cytoplasm and Its Organelles

The cytoplasm surrounds the nucleus, and it is in the cytoplasm that the work of the cell takes place. The cytoplasm is essentially a colloidal solution that contains water, electrolytes, suspended proteins, neutral fats, and glycogen molecules. Although they do not contribute to the cell's function, pigments may also accumulate in the cytoplasm. Some pigments, such as melanin, which gives skin its color, are normal constituents of the cell. Bilirubin is a normal major pigment of bile. Excess accumulation of bilirubin within cells is abnormal; it is evidenced clinically by a yellowish discoloration of the skin and sclera, a condition called *jaundice*.

Embedded in the cytoplasm are the *organelles*, which are inner organs of the cell. These include the ribosomes, endoplasmic reticulum (ER), Golgi complex, mitochondria, lysosomes, microtubules, and filaments.

Ribosomes

The ribosomes serve as sites of protein synthesis in the cell. They are small particles of nucleoproteins (rRNA and proteins) that can be found attached to the wall of the ER or as free ribosomes (Fig. 1-4). The free ribosomes are scattered singly in the cytoplasm or joined to form functional units called *polyribosomes*. The free ribosomes are involved in the synthesis of proteins, such as intracellular enzymes, that are used mainly within the cytoplasm of the cell. The ribosomes that are attached to the ER synthesize proteins that are destined for incorporation into cell membranes or exportation from the cell.

Endoplasmic Reticulum

The ER is an extensive system of paired membranes and flat vesicles that connects various parts of the inner cell (see Fig. 1-4). The fluid-filled space, called the matrix, between the paired ER membrane layers is con-

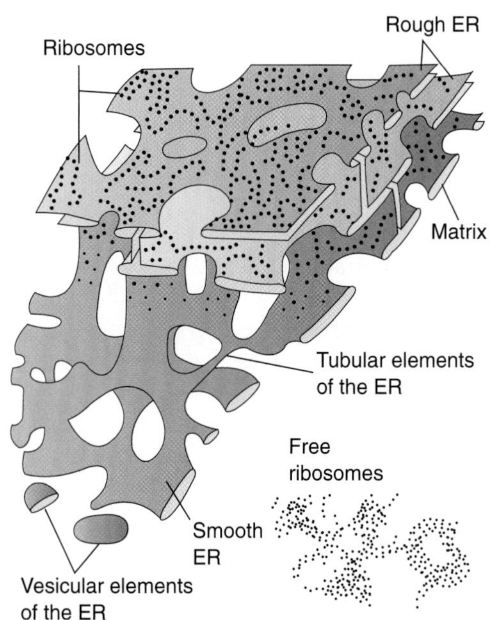

FIGURE 1-4
Three-dimensional view of the rough endoplasmic reticulum (ER) with its attached ribosomal RNA and the smooth endoplasmic reticulum.

nected with the space between the two membranes of the double-layered nuclear membrane, the cell membrane, and various cytoplasmic organelles. It functions as a tubular communication system through which substances can be transported from one part of the cell to another. The large surface area and multiple enzyme systems attached to the ER membranes also provide the machinery for a major share of the metabolic functions of the cell.

There are two types of ER: rough and smooth. The rough ER is studded with ribosomes. The ribosomes of the rough ER synthesize proteins for cell membranes, lysomosomal enzymes, and all the proteins that are exported from the cell. The rough ER segregates these proteins from other components of the cytoplasm and modifies their structure for a specific function. For example, the synthesis of digestive enzymes by the acinar cells in the pancreas and production of plasma protein by liver cells take place in the rough ER. All cells require rough ER for the synthesis of lysosomal enzymes.

The smooth ER is free of ribosomes and is continuous with the rough ER. The smooth ER does not participate in protein synthesis; it instead contains enzymes involved in the synthesis of lipid molecules, regulation of intracellular calcium, and metabolism and detoxification of certain hormones and drugs. It is the site of lipid, lipoprotein, and steroid hormone synthesis. The sarcoplasmic reticulum of skeletal and cardiac muscle cells is a form of smooth ER. Calcium ions needed for muscle contraction are stored and released from cisternae located in the sarcoplasmic reticulum of these cells.

In the liver, the smooth ER is involved in glycogen storage and metabolism of lipid-soluble drugs. An interesting form of adaptation occurs in the smooth ER of the liver cells responsible for metabolizing certain drugs such as phenobarbital. Repeated administration of phenobarbital leads to a state of increased tolerance to the drug, such that the same dose no longer produces the same degree of sedation. This response has been traced to increased drug metabolism resulting from increased synthesis of drug-metabolizing enzymes by the smooth ER of these cells. This enzyme system is sometimes called the *microsomal system* because the ER can be fragmented in the laboratory; when this is done, small vesicles called *microsomes* are formed. The microsomal enzyme system responsible for metabolizing phenobarbital has a crossover effect that influences the metabolism of other drugs that use the same metabolic pathway.

Golgi Complex

The Golgi apparatus, sometimes referred to as the Golgi complex, consists of stacks of thin, flat vesicle–covered membranous sacs. These Golgi bodies are found near the nucleus and function in association with the ER. Substances produced in the ER are carried to the Golgi complex in small, membrane-covered transfer vesicles. Many cells synthesize proteins that are larger than the active product. Insulin, for example, is synthesized as a larger, inactive proinsulin molecule that is cut apart to produce a smaller, active insulin molecule within the Golgi complex of the beta cells of the pancreas. The Golgi complex modifies these substances and packages them into secretory granules or vesicles. Enzymes destined for export from the cell are packaged in secretory vesicles; after an appropriate signal, the secretory vesicles move out of the Golgi complex into the cytoplasm and fuse to the inner side of the membrane, where they release their contents into the extracellular fluid. Figure 1-5 is a diagram of the synthesis and movement of a hormone through the ER and Golgi complex. In addition to its function in producing secretory granules, the Golgi complex is thought to produce some of the larger carbohydrate molecules that combine with proteins in the rough ER to form glycoproteins. The Golgi apparatus also forms the acrosomal cap on the head of the sperm.

Lysosomes and Peroxisomes

The lysosomes can be viewed as the digestive system of the cell. They consist of small membrane-enclosed sacs that contain hydrolytic enzymes capable of breaking down worn-out cell parts so they can be recycled. They also break down foreign substances such as bacteria that have been taken into the cell. All of the lysosomal enzymes are acid hydrolases, which mean that they require an acid environment; the lysosomes provide this environment by maintaining a pH of about 5 in their interior. The pH of the cytoplasm is about 7.2; this protects other cell structures. Like many other organelles, lysosomes have a unique surrounding membrane that can be pinched off to form vesicles that are used for transport of materials in the cytoplasm.

Lysosomal enzymes are synthesized in the rough ER and then transported to the Golgi apparatus, where they are biochemically modified and packed as lysosomes. Unlike other organelles, there is a wide diversity in the sizes and functions of the lysosomes. This diversity is determined by the type of enzyme packaged in the lyso-

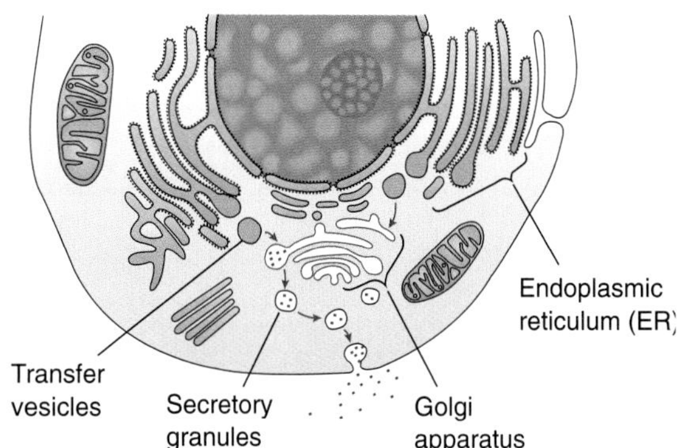

FIGURE 1-5
Hormone synthesis and secretion. In hormone secretion, the hormone is synthesized by the ribosomes attached to the rough endoplasmic reticulum. It moves from the rough ER to the Golgi complex, where it is stored in the form of secretory granules. These leave the Golgi complex and are stored within the cytoplasm until released from the cell in response to an appropriate signal.

some by the Golgi complex. Lysosomes that contain hydrolytic enzymes and that have not entered into the digestive process are called *primary lysosomes. Secondary lysosomes* are those in which the hydrolytic enzymes have been activated and the chemical degradation process has begun. They form when primary lysosomes fuse with material that needs to be digested. Secondary lysosomes can be formed in one of two ways: heterophagy or autophagy (Fig. 1-6). *Heterophagocytosis* refers to the uptake of material from outside the cell. External materials are taken into the cell by an infolding of the cell membrane to form a surrounding phagocytic vesicle or *phagosome.* Primary lysosomes fuse with phagosomes to form secondary lysosomes. Heterophagocytosis is most common in phagocytic white blood cells such as neutrophils and macrophages. *Autophagocytosis* involves the removal of individual cell organelles, such as mitochondria or ER, that have been damaged and must be removed if the cell's normal function is to continue. It is most pronounced in cells undergoing atrophy.

Although the enzymes in the secondary lysosomes are capable of breaking down most proteins, carbohydrates, and lipids to their basic constituents that diffuse through the lysosomal membrane into the cytoplasm, some materials remain undigested. These undigested materials may remain in the cytoplasm as *residual bodies* or be extruded from the cell. In some long-lived cells, such as neurons and heart muscle cells, large quantities of residual bodies accumulate as lipofuscin or age pigment. Other indigestible pigments, such as inhaled carbon particles in the lung and tattoo pigments in the skin, also accumulate and persist in residual bodies of macrophages for decades.

Lysosomes play an important role in the normal metabolism of certain substances in the body. In some inherited diseases known as *lysosomal storage diseases,* a specific lysosomal enzyme is absent or inactive, in which case the digestion of certain cellular substances (*e.g.,* cerebrosides, gangliosides, sphingomyelin) does not occur. As a result, these substances accumulate in the cell. In Tay-Sachs disease, an autosomal recessive disorder, hexosaminidase A, which is the lysosomal enzyme needed for degrading the GM_2 ganglioside found in nerve cell membranes, is deficient. Although the GM_2 ganglioside accumulates in many tissues (*e.g.,* heart, liver, spleen), its accumulation in the nervous system and retina of the eye causes the most damage. Infants born with the disorder are normal at birth but soon begin to develop motor and mental deterioration and blindness as the GM_2 gangliosides accumulate in the nervous system. The course of the disease is rapid and relentless, and death usually occurs in the second or third year of life.

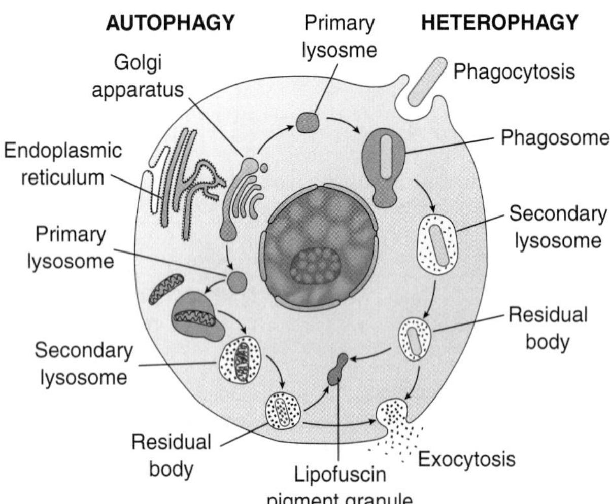

FIGURE 1-6
The process of autophagy and heterophagy, showing the primary and secondary lysosomes, residual bodies, extrusion of residual body contents from the cell, and lipofuscin-containing residual bodies.

Even smaller than the lysosomes, spherical, membrane-bound organelles, called *peroxisomes,* contain a special enzyme that degrades peroxides (*e.g.,* hydrogen peroxide). The peroxisomes function in the control of free radicals (see Chapter 2). Unless degraded, these highly unstable chemical compounds would otherwise damage other cytoplasmic molecules. For example, catalase degrades toxic hydrogen peroxide molecules to water. Peroxisomes also contain the enzymes needed for breaking down very long chain fatty acids, which are ineffectively degraded by mitochondrial enzymes. In liver cells, enzymes of peroxisomes are involved in the formation of the bile acids. In a condition called *adrenoleukodystrophy,* the most common peroxisomal disorder, impaired β-oxidation of fatty acids results in dementia and adrenal failure due to accumulation of fatty acids in the brain, spinal cord, and adrenal gland.

Mitochondria

The mitochondria are literally the "power plants" of the cell, because it is here that the organic compounds are transformed into energy that is easily accessible to the cell. Energy is not made here but is extracted from organic compounds. Mitochondria contain the enzymes needed for capturing most of the energy in foodstuffs and converting it into cellular energy. This multistep process is generally referred to as *cellular respiration* because it requires oxygen. Much of this energy is stored in the high-energy phosphate bonds of compounds such as adenosine triphosphate (ATP), which powers the various cellular activities (Fig. 1-7). Energy that is not used or stored as ATP is dissipated as heat used to maintain body temperature.

The mitochondria are located close to the site of energy consumption in the cell (*e.g.,* near the myofibrils in muscle cells). The number of mitochondria in a given cell type is largely determined by the type of activity the cell performs and the amount of energy needed to perform this activity. For example, a large increase in mitochondria has been observed in resting skeletal muscle that has been repeatedly stimulated to contract.

Mitochondria are encased in double membranes. An outer membrane encloses the periphery of the mitochon-

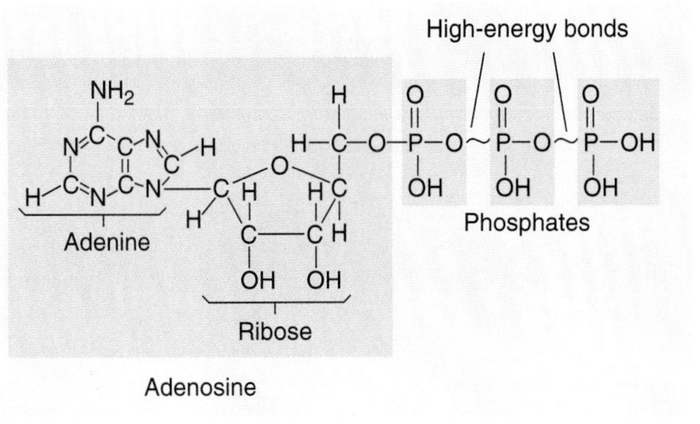

FIGURE 1-7
Structure of the adenosine triphosphate (ATP) molecule.

dria, and an inner membrane is enfolded to form the cristae, which aid in the production and temporary storage of ATP (Fig. 1-8). The inner and outer membranes form two spaces. The outer space is located between the two membranes, and the inner space is enclosed by the inner membrane. The inner space, which is filled with an amorphous matrix, is called the *matrix space.* Nutrients are broken down and processed by enzymes, some of which are dissolved in the mitochondrial matrix while others form part of the crista membrane.

Mitochondria contain both DNA and RNA and are self-replicating. The DNA found in the mitochondria is distinct from the chromosomal DNA found in the cell nucleus. Mitochondrial DNA, known as the "other human genome," is a double-stranded, circular molecule that encodes the rRNA and tRNA required for intramitochrondial synthesis of proteins needed for the energy-generating function of the mitochondria. Although mitochondrial DNA directs the synthesis of 13 of the proteins required for mitochondrial function, the DNA of the nucleus encodes the structural proteins of the mitochondria and other proteins needed to carry out cellular respiration.

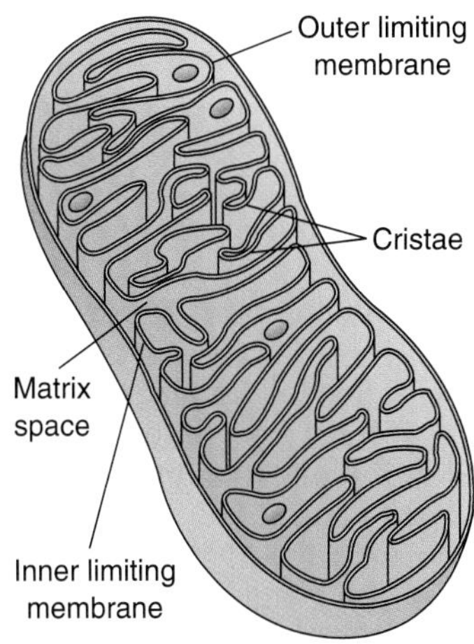

FIGURE 1-8
Mitochondrion. The inner membrane forms transverse folds called cristae, where the enzymes needed for the final step in adenosine triphosphate (ATP) production (i.e., oxidative phosphorylation) are located.

Mitochondrial DNA is inherited matrilineally (*i.e.,* from the mother). Mutations have been found in each of the mitochondrial genes, and an understanding of the role of mitochondrial DNA in certain diseases is beginning to emerge. Almost all tissues in the body depend to some extent on oxidative metabolism and can therefore be affected by mitochondrial DNA mutations.

Cytoskeleton

In addition to its organelles, the cytoplasm contains a network of microtubules, microfilaments, intermediate filaments, and thick filaments. Because they control cell shape and movement, these structures are a major component of the structural elements called the *cytoskeleton.*

Microtubules. The microtubules are slender tubular structures composed of globular proteins called *tubulin.* Microtubules function in a number of ways, including development and maintenance of cell form; participation in intracellular transport mechanisms, including axoplasmic transport in neurons and melanin dispersion in pigment cells of the skin; and formation of the basic structure for several complex cytoplasmic organelles, including the centrioles, basal bodies, cilia, and flagella. The *centrioles* are cylindrical structures composed of highly organized microtubules. In dividing cells, they form the mitotic spindle that aids in the separation and movement of the chromosomes. *Cilia* and *flagella* are hairlike processes extending from the cell membrane that are capable of sweeping and flailing movements, which can move surrounding fluids or move the cell through fluid media (Fig. 1-9). They contain a highly organized core of microtubules anchored to a basal body that is similar to a centriole in structure. Cilia are found on the wet surface of the epithelial lining of certain body cavities or passages such as the upper respiratory system. Flagella are tail-like structures that provide motility for sperm.

Abnormalities of the cytoskeletal system may contribute to alterations in cell mobility and function. For example, proper functioning of the microtubules is essential for various stages of leukocyte migration. In certain disease conditions, such as diabetes mellitus, alterations in leukocyte mobility and migration may interfere with the chemotaxis and phagocytosis of the inflammatory response and predispose toward the development of bacterial infection.

Microtubules can be rapidly assembled and disassembled according to the needs of the cell. The assembly of microtubules is halted by the action of the plant alkaloid *colchicine.* This compound stops cell mitosis by interfering with formation of the mitotic spindle and is used for cytogenetic (chromosome) studies. It is also used as a drug for treating gout. It is thought that the drug's ability to reduce the inflammatory reaction associated with this condition stems from its ability to interfere with microtubular function of white blood cells and their migration into the area.

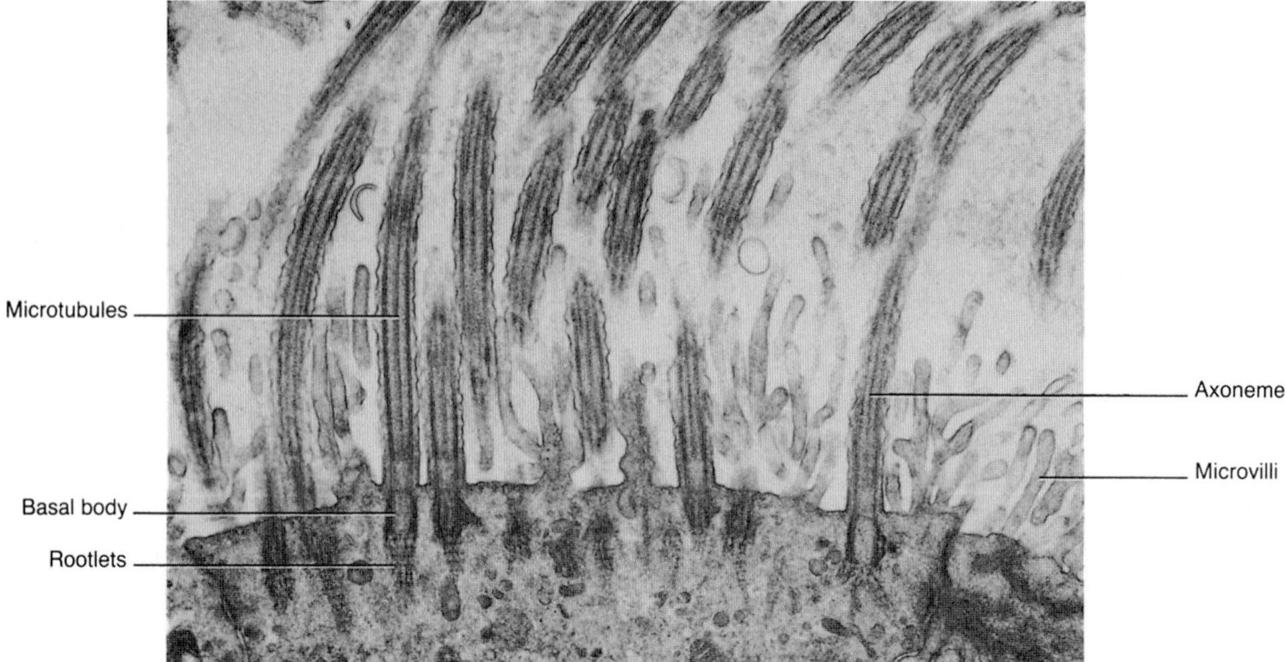

FIGURE 1-9
Electron micrograph showing ciliated cells of the bronchus. Cilia in an oblique or longitudinal section may be compared with microvilli cut in a similar plane. (From Sturgess J. [1982]. In P. Quinton, P. Martinez [Eds.]. *Fluid and electrolyte abnormalities in exocrine glands in cystic fibrosis.* San Francisco: San Francisco Press)

Filaments. The filaments are thin, threadlike cytoplasmic structures. There are three classes of filaments: microfilaments, which are equivalent to the thin actin filaments in muscle; intermediate filaments, which are a heterogeneous group of filaments with diameter sizes between the thick and thin filaments; and thick myosin filaments, which are present in muscle cells, but may also exist temporarily in other cells.

Muscle contraction depends on the interaction between the thin actin filaments and thick myosin filaments. Microfilaments are present in the superficial zone of the cytoplasm in almost all cells. Contractile activities involving the microfilaments and associated thick myosin filaments contribute to associated movement of the cytoplasm and cell membrane during endocytosis and exocytosis. Microfilaments are also present in the microvilli of the intestine. The intermediate filaments aid in supporting and maintaining the asymmetric shape of cells. Examples of intermediate filaments are the keratin filaments that are found anchored to the cell membrane of epidermal keratinocytes of the skin and the glial filaments that are found in astrocytes and other glial cells of the nervous system.

Cell Membrane

The cell is enclosed in a thin membrane that separates the intracellular contents from the extracellular environment. To differentiate it from the other cell membranes, such as the mitochondrial or nuclear membranes, the cell membrane is often called the *plasma membrane.* In many respects, the plasma membrane is one of the most important parts of the cell. It acts as a semipermeable structure that separates the intracellular and extracellular environments, provides receptors for hormones and other biologically active substances, participates in the electrical events that occur in nerve and muscle cells, and aids in the regulation of cell growth and proliferation. It is also thought that the cell membrane may play an important role in the behavior of cancer cells, which is discussed in Chapter 5.

The cell membrane consists of an organized arrangement of lipids, carbohydrates, and proteins (Fig. 1-10). The main structural component of the membrane is its lipid bilayer. It is a bimolecular layer that consists primarily of phospholipids, together with glycolipids and cholesterol. The lipids form a bilayer structure that is essentially impermeable to all but lipid-soluble substances. About 75% of the lipids are phospholipids, each with a hydrophilic (water-soluble) head and a hydrophobic (water-insoluble) tails. The phospholipid molecules along with the glycolipids are aligned such that their hydrophilic heads face the water on each side of the membrane and their tails are in the middle of the membrane. The hydrophilic heads retain water and help cells adhere to one another. At normal body temperature, the viscosity at the lipid component of the membrane is equivalent to that of olive oil. The presence of cholesterol stiffens the membrane.

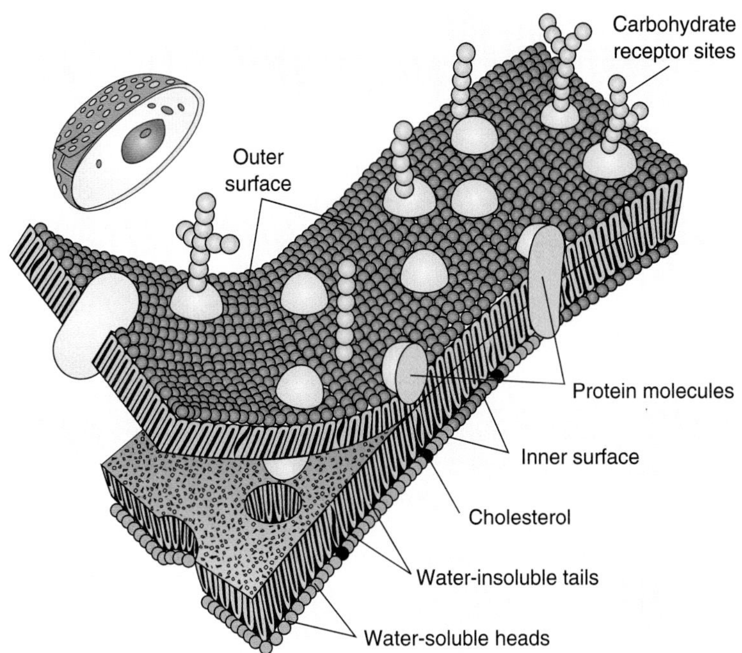

FIGURE 1-10
Cell membrane. The right end is intact, but the left end has been split along the plane of the lipid tails.

A second major component of the cell membrane is its protein molecules. Globular proteins embedded in this lipid bilayer participate in the transport of lipid-insoluble particles through the plasma membrane. Some of the globular proteins move within the membrane structure and act as carriers; some are attached to either side of the membrane; and others pass directly through the membrane and communicate with the inside and the outside of the cell. Many of these proteins function in the transport of nutrients such as glucose across the cell membrane; other proteins form ion channels that allow for the exchange of electrolytes such as sodium and potassium.

The cell surface is surrounded by a fuzzy-looking layer called the *cell coat*, or *glycocalyx*. This layer is made up of long, complex carbohydrate chains that are attached to protein molecules that penetrate the outside half of the membrane (*i.e.*, glycoproteins) and outward facing membrane lipids (*i.e.*, glycolipids) and carbohydrate-binding proteins called lectins. The cell coat participates in cell-to-cell recognition and adhesion, and it contains tissue transplant antigens that label cells as self or nonself. The ABO blood group antigens are contained in the cell coat of red blood cells. There is an intimate relationship between the cell membrane and the cell coat. If the cell coat is enzymatically removed, the cell remains viable and can generate a new cell coat, but damage to the cell membrane usually results in cell death.

In summary, the cell is a remarkably autonomous structure that functions in a manner strikingly similar to that of the total organism. The nucleus controls cell function and is the mastermind of the cell. It contains the DNA, which provides the information necessary for the synthesis of the various proteins that the cell must produce to stay alive and to transmit information from one generation to another.

The cytoplasm contains the cell's organelles and the enzymes necessary for glycolysis. The ribosomes serve as sites for protein synthesis in the cell. The ER functions as a tubular communication system through which substances can be transported from one part of the cell to another and as the site of protein (rough ER), carbohydrate, and lipid (smooth ER) synthesis. The Golgi complex modifies materials synthesized in the ER and packages them into secretory granules for transport within the cell or for export from the cell. The lysosomes, which can be viewed as the digestive system of the cell, contain hydrolytic enzymes that digest worn-out cell parts and foreign materials. They are membranous structures that are formed in the Golgi complex from hydrolytic enzymes that are synthesized in the rough ER. The mitochondria serve as power plants for the cell as they transform food energy into ATP, which is used to power cell activities. Mitochondria contain their own extrachromosomal DNA, which is used in the synthesis of mitochondrial RNAs and proteins used in oxidative metabolism. The microtubules are slender, stiff, tubular structures that influence cell shape, provide a means of moving organelles through the cytoplasm, and affect movement of the cilia and of chromosomes during cell division. Several types of threadlike filaments, including the actin and myosin filaments, participate in muscle contraction.

The plasma membrane is a lipid bilayer that surrounds the cell and separates it from its surrounding external environment. The cell surface is surrounded by a fuzzy-looking layer called the cell coat or glycocalyx, which contains tissue antigens and participates in cell-to-cell recognition and adhesion.

Integration of Cell Function and Replication

After you have completed this section of the chapter, you should be able to meet the following objectives:

- Trace the pathway for cell communication, beginning at the receptor and ending with effector response, and explain why the process is often referred to as signal transduction
- Describe the function of G proteins in signal transduction
- List three classifications of growth factors
- Describe the five phases of the cell cycle
- Compare the processes involved in aerobic and anaerobic metabolism

Cell Communication

Cells in multicellular organisms need to communicate with one another to coordinate their function and control their growth. Cells communicate with each other by means of chemical messenger systems. Within some tissues, messengers move from cell to cell through gap junctions without entering the extracellular fluid. In other tissues, cells communicate by chemical messengers secreted into the extracellular fluid. Many types of chemical messengers bind to receptors on or near the cell surface. These chemical messengers are sometimes called *first messengers* because, by one means or another, their external signal is converted into internal signals carried by a second chemical called a *second messenger*. It is the second messenger that triggers the intracellular changes that produce the desired physiologic effect. Some lipid-soluble chemical messengers move through the membrane and bind to cytoplasmic or nuclear receptors as a means of exerting their physiologic effects.

The three basic types of intercellular communication mediated by messengers in the extracellular fluid are hormonal communication, paracrine and autocrine communication, and neural communication. Endocrine signaling relies on hormones that are carried in the bloodstream to cells throughout the body. With paracrine signaling, the chemical mediators are rapidly metabolized and act mainly on nearby cells. In autocrine signaling, a cell releases a chemical into the extracellular fluid that affects its own activity. Synaptic signaling occurs in the nervous system, where neurotransmitters act only on adjacent nerve cells through special contact areas called synapses. In some parts of the body, the same chemical messenger can function as a neurotransmitter, a paracrine mediator, and a hormone secreted by neurons into the bloodstream.

Neurotransmitters, protein and peptide hormones, and other chemical messengers do not exert their effects by entering cells. Their messages are converted (*i.e.*, transduced) by cell membrane proteins into signals within the cell, a process often referred to as *signal transduction*. Many of the molecules involved in signal transduction are proteins. One of the unique properties of proteins that allows them to function in this way is their ability to change their shape or conformation, thereby changing their function and consequently the functions of the cell. These conformational changes are often accomplished through enzymes called *protein kinases* that catalyze the phosphorylation of amino acids in the protein structure.

Cell Receptors

Each cell type in the body contains a distinctive set of receptor proteins that enable it to respond to a complementary set of signaling molecules in a specific, preprogrammed way. These receptors, which span the cell membrane, relay information to a series of intracellular intermediates that eventually pass the signal on to its final destination. Many of the receptors for chemical messengers have been isolated and characterized. These proteins are not static components of the cell membrane; rather, they increase or decrease in number according to the needs of the cell. When excess amounts of a chemical messenger are present, the number of active receptors decreases in a process called *down-regulation*, and when there is a deficiency of the messenger, the number of active receptors increases through *up-regulation*.

G Proteins and Signal Transduction

G proteins constitute the on-off switch for signal transduction. Although there are numerous intercellular messengers, many of them rely on a class of molecules called *G proteins* to convert external signals (first messengers) into internal signals (second messengers), which then induce biochemical changes within the cell that lead to the desired physiologic effects. G proteins are so named because they bind to guanine nucleotides such as guanine diphosphate (GDP) and guanine triphosphate (GTP).

Signal transduction relies on a series of orchestrated biochemical events (Fig. 1-11). All signal transduction systems have a receptor component that functions as a signal discriminator by recognizing a specific first messenger. After a first messenger binds to a receptor, conformational changes occur in the receptor, which activates the G protein. The activated G protein acts on other membrane-bound intermediates called effectors. Often, the effector is an enzyme that converts an inactive precursor molecule into a second messenger, which diffuses into the cytoplasm and carries the signal beyond the cell membrane. A number of members of the G protein family have been identified. At least one subset of G proteins is present in all cells; it regulates signal transmission by the second messenger 3',5'-cyclic adenosine monophosphate (cAMP).

Although there are differences between the G proteins, all share a number of features. All are located on the cytoplasmic layer of the cell membrane, and all involve what is called the *GTPase cycle*, which functions as the on-off switch for G-protein activity. GTPase is an

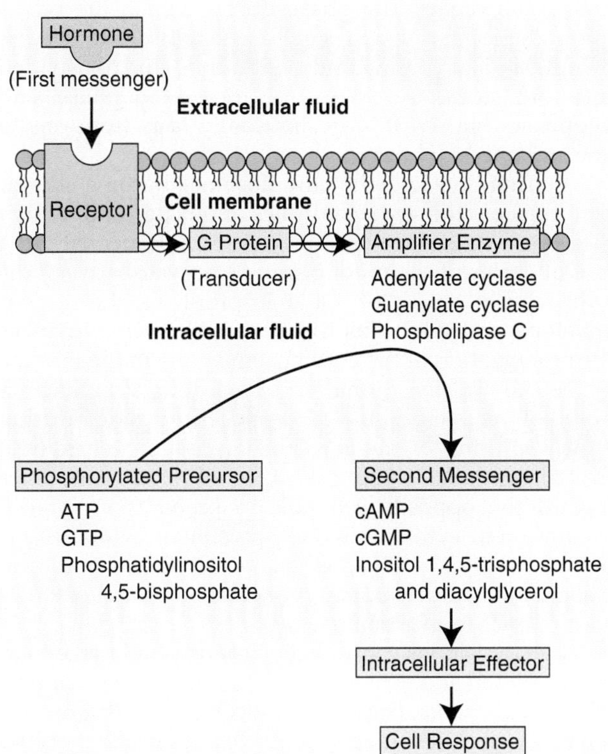

FIGURE 1-11
Signal transduction pattern common to several second messenger systems. A protein or peptide hormone is the first messenger to a membrane receptor, stimulating or inhibiting a membrane-bound enzyme by means of a G protein. The amplifier enzyme catalyzes the production of a second messenger from a phosphorylated precursor. The second messenger then activates an internal effector, which leads to the cell response. (Redrawn from Rhoades R.A., Tanner G.A. [1996]. *Medical physiology.* Boston: Little, Brown)

enzyme that converts GTP with its three phosphate groups to GDP with its two phosphate groups. In the inactive state, G proteins contain tightly bound GDP. When a receptor coupled to a G protein is activated, the G protein releases the GDP and binds GTP; this causes the G protein to dissociate from the receptor and to activate the effector. During the process of signal transduction, GTPase converts bound GTP to GDP, thereby returning the G protein to it resting state and switching the signal off. Certain bacterial toxins can bind to the G proteins, causing inhibition or stimulation. One such toxin, the toxin of *Vibrio cholerae,* binds and activates the stimulatory G protein that is linked to the cAMP system that controls the secretion of fluid into the intestine. In response to the cholera toxin, these cells overproduce fluid, leading to severe diarrhea and life-threatening depletion of extracellular fluid volume.

Second Messenger Systems

Many chemical messengers mediate their effects through G protein activated second messengers. A common second messenger is cAMP. It is activated by the enzyme adenyl cyclase, which generates cAMP by transferring phosphate groups from ATP to other proteins. This transfer alters the configuration and function of these proteins. Such changes eventually produce the cell response to the first messenger, whether it is secretion, muscle contraction or relaxation, or a change in metabolism. In some cases, it is the opening of an ion channel involving calcium or potassium influx.

Messenger-Mediated Control of Nuclear Function

Although many chemical messengers act through second messengers in effecting changes in cytoplasmic structures in the cell, some messengers such as thyroid hormone and steroid hormones move across the lipid layer of the cell membrane and are carried to the cell nucleus, where they influence DNA activity. Many of these hormones bind to a cytoplasmic receptor and are then carried to the nucleus. Binding of the receptor-hormone complex to DNA increases transcription of mRNA. The mRNAs are translated in the ribosomes, with the production of increased amounts of proteins that alter cell function.

Growth Factors

Growth factors are polypeptides and proteins. They are important factors in cell replacement and cell growth. These growth factors can be divided into three groups: factors that foster the multiplication and development of various cell types such as nerve growth factor and epidermal growth factor; lymphokines and cytokines, which are important in the regulation of the immune system (see Chapter 11); and colony-stimulating factors, which regulate the proliferation and maturation of white and red blood cells (see Chapter 6).

Like other cell messengers, many of the growth factors bind to their receptors, many of which are involved in activating second messengers that lead to changes in cell function or DNA replication. Most growth factors also influence a great number of other cells functions, and many initiate cell migration, differentiation, and tissue remodeling and may be involved in various stages of wound healing. Much of our current knowledge about growth factors comes from the discovery of oncogenes, the genes that influence cancer formation (see Chapter 5).

The Cell Cycle and Cell Division

The life of a cell is called the cell cycle. It is divided into five phases: G_0, G_1, S, G_2, and M. G_0 is the stage during interphase when the cell is performing routine functions and is not preparing for cell division. G_1 is the stage during which the cell is starting to prepare for mitosis through DNA and protein synthesis and an increase in organelle and cytoskeletal elements. The S phase is the synthesis phase, during which DNA replication occurs and the centrioles are beginning to replicate. G_2 is the premitotic phase and is similar to G_1 in terms of RNA and protein synthesis. The M phase is the phase during which cell mitosis occurs. Nondividing cells, such as

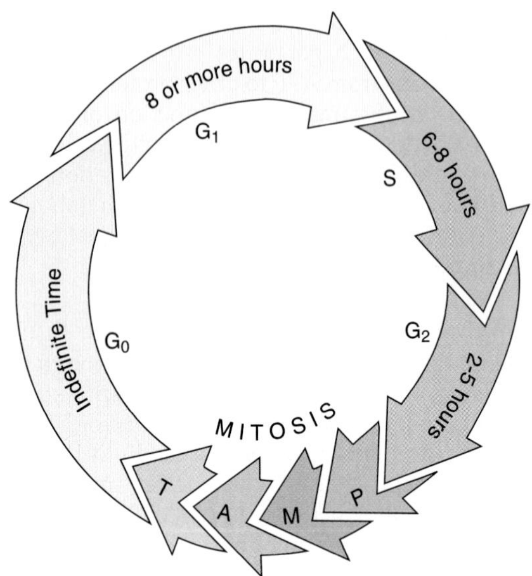

FIGURE 1-12
Cell cycle. G_0, normal cell functions, nondividing cell; G_1, cell growth; S, DNA replication; G_2, protein synthesis; M, mitosis, which lasts for 1 to 3 hours and is followed by cytokinesis.

mature nerve cells or cells not preparing for mitosis, are said to be in the G_0 phase of the cell cycle (Fig. 1-12).

Cell Division

Cell division, or *mitosis,* is the process during which a parent cell divides and each daughter cell receives a chromosomal karyotype identical to the parent cell. It is the process by which somatic or body cells effect growth and tissue repair. The phase during which the cell is not undergoing division is called *interphase*. The process of mitosis is dynamic and continuous and is divided into four stages: prophase, metaphase, anaphase, and telophase (Fig. 1-13). Mitosis usually lasts from one to one and one-half hours.

During *prophase,* the chromosomes become shorter and thicker, the two centrioles replicate, and a pair moves to each side of the cell. Simultaneously, the microtubules of the mitotic spindle appear between the two pairs of centrioles. Later in prophase, the nuclear envelope and nucleolus disappear. *Metaphase* involves the organization of the chromosome pairs in the midline of the cell and the formation of a mitotic spindle composed of the microtubules. *Anaphase* is the period during which splitting of the chromosome pairs occurs, with the microtubules pulling each set of 46 chromosomes toward the opposite cell pole in preparation for cell separation or cytokinesis. Cell division or cytokinesis is completed after *telophase*, when the mitotic spindles vanish and a new nuclear membrane develops and encloses each of the sets of chromosomes.

Cell division is controlled by changes in intracellular concentration and activity of a group of intracellular proteins called *cyclins*. These proteins complex with a protein kinase enzyme, resulting in activation of a number of substrate proteins involved in DNA synthesis and mitosis.

Cell Metabolism and Energy Sources

Energy is defined as the ability to do work. Cells use oxygen and the breakdown products of the foods we eat to produce the energy needed for muscle contrac-

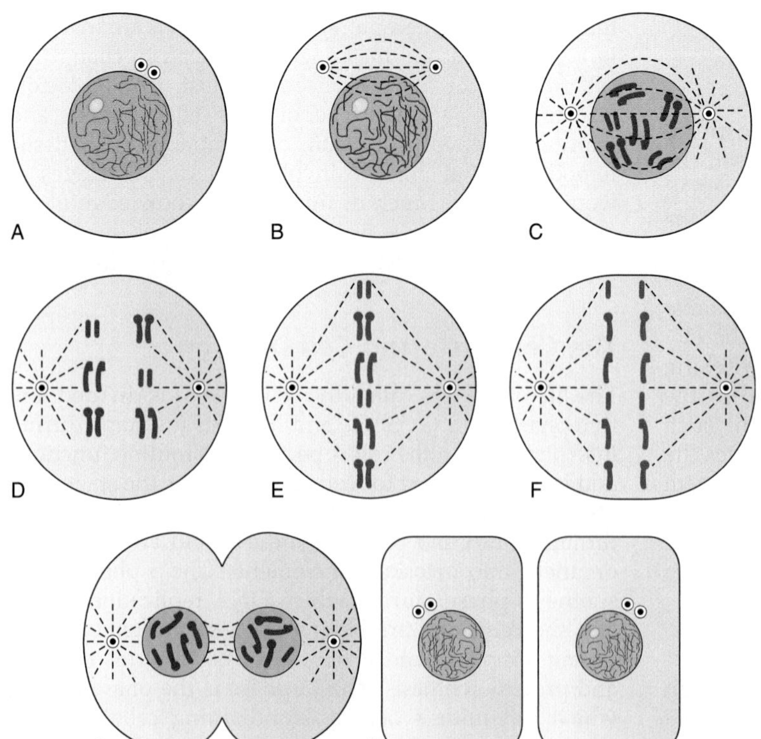

FIGURE 1-13
Cell mitosis. *A* and *H* represent the nondividing cell; *B*, *C*, and *D* represent prophase; *E* represents anaphase; and *G* represents telophase.

tion, transport of ions and molecules, and the synthesis of enzymes, hormones, and other macromolecules. *Energy metabolism* refers to the processes by which fats, proteins, and carbohydrates from the foods we eat are converted into energy or complex energy sources within the cell. There are two phases of metabolism: catabolism and anabolism. *Catabolism* consists of breaking down stored nutrients and body tissues to produce energy. *Anabolism* is a constructive process in which more complex molecules are formed from simpler ones.

The special carrier for cellular energy is ATP. The ATP molecule consists of adenosine, a nitrogenous base; ribose, a five-carbon sugar; and three phosphate groups (see Fig. 1-8). The phosphate groups are attached by two high-energy bonds. Large amounts of free energy are released when ATP is hydrolyzed to form adenosine diphosphate (ADP), an adenosine molecule that contains two phosphate groups. The free energy liberated from the hydrolysis of ATP is used to drive reactions that require free energy, such as muscle contraction. Energy from foodstuffs is used to convert ADP back to ATP. ATP is often referred to as the "energy currency" of the cell; energy can be "saved or spent" using ATP as an exchange currency.

There are two sites of energy production in the cell: the anaerobic (*i.e.,* without oxygen) glycolytic pathway, which is located in the cytoplasm, and the aerobic (*i.e.,* with oxygen) pathways in the mitochondria. The glycolytic pathway serves as the prelude to the aerobic pathways.

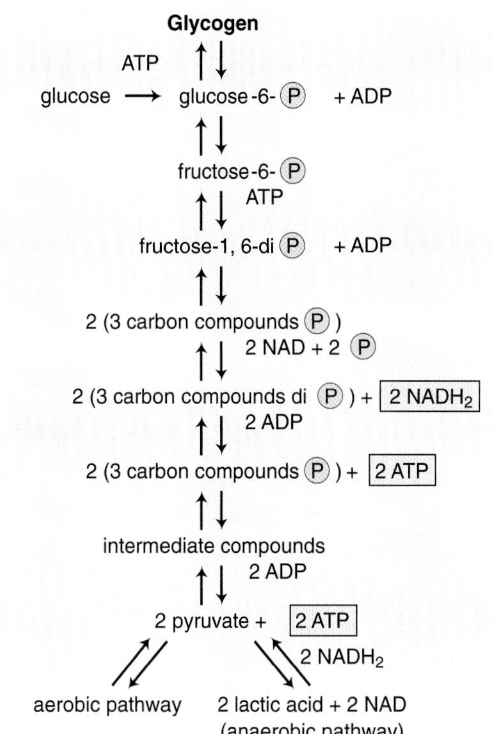

FIGURE 1-14
Glycolytic pathway.

Anaerobic Metabolism

Glycolysis is the process by which energy is liberated from glucose (Fig. 1-14). Glycolysis is an important energy provider for cells that lack mitochondria, the cell organelle in which aerobic metabolism occurs. The process also provides energy in situations when delivery of oxygen to the cell is delayed or impaired. The process involves a sequence of reactions that converts glucose to pyruvate, with the concomitant production of ATP from ADP. The net gain of energy from the glycolysis of one molecule of glucose is two ATP molecules. Although relatively inefficient in terms of energy yield, the glycolytic pathway is important during periods of decreased oxygen delivery, as occurs in skeletal muscle during the first few minutes of exercise.

Glycolysis requires the presence of nicotinamide-adenine dinucleotide (NAD^+), a hydrogen carrier. The end-products of glycolysis are pyruvate and NADH. When oxygen is present, pyruvate moves into the aerobic mitochondrial pathway, and NADH subsequently enters into oxidative chemical reactions that remove the hydrogen atoms. The transfer of hydrogen from NADH during the oxidative reactions allows the glycolytic process to continue by facilitating the regeneration of NAD^+. Under anaerobic conditions, such as cardiac arrest or circulatory shock, most pyruvate is converted to lactic acid, which diffuses out of the cells into the extracellular fluid. The conversion of pyruvate to lactic acid is reversible, and after the oxygen supply has been restored, lactic acid is converted back to pyruvate or used to synthesize glucose.

Heart muscle cells are particularly efficient in converting lactic acid to pyruvic acid and use this as a fuel source. This is a particularly important source of fuel for the heart during heavy exercise when the skeletal muscles are producing large amounts of lactic acid and releasing it into the bloodstream. The liver removes lactic acid from the bloodstream and converts it to glucose in a process called *gluconeogenesis*. This glucose is released into the bloodstream to be used again by the muscles or by the central nervous system. This recycling of lactic acid is referred to as the *Cori cycle*.

Aerobic Metabolism

Aerobic metabolism occurs in the cell's mitochondria and involves the citric acid cycle and oxidative phosphorylation. It is here that hydrogen and carbon molecules from the fats, proteins, and carbohydrates in our diet are broken down and combined with molecular oxygen to form carbon dioxide and water as energy is released. Unlike lactic acid, which is an end-product of anaerobic metabolism, carbon dioxide and water are relatively harmless and easily eliminated from the body. In a 24-hour period, oxidative metabolism supplies the body with 300 to 500 ml of water.

The citric acid cycle, sometimes called the *tricarboxylic acid* or *Krebs cycle*, provides the final common pathway for the metabolism of nutrients (Fig. 1-15). In

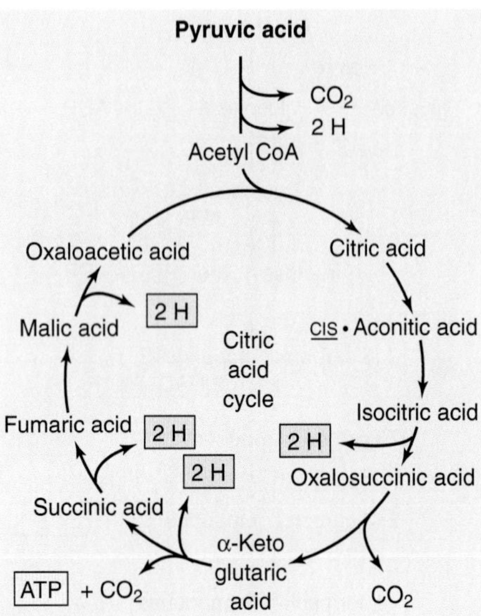

FIGURE 1-15
Citric acid cycle.

the citric acid cycle, an activated two-carbon molecule of acetyl coenzyme A (acetyl-CoA) condenses with a four-carbon molecule of oxaloacetic acid and moves through a series of enzyme-mediated steps in which hydrogen and carbon dioxide are formed. As hydrogen is generated, it combines with one of two special carriers, NAD^+ or flavin adenine dinucleotide (FAD), as a means of transfer to the electron transport system. The carbon dioxide molecule that is formed is carried to the lungs and exhaled. In the citric acid cycle, each of the two pyruvate molecules that were formed in the cytoplasm from one molecule of glucose yields another molecule of ATP along with two molecules of carbon dioxide and eight hydrogen atoms. These hydrogen molecules are transferred to the electron transport system on the inner mitochondrial membrane for oxidation. In addition to pyruvate from the glycolysis of glucose, products of amino acid and fatty acid degradation enter the citric acid cycle.

Oxidative metabolism, which supplies 90% of the body's energy needs, is the process whereby hydrogen that is generated during the citric acid cycle combines with oxygen to form ATP and water. It is accomplished by a series of enzymatically catalyzed reactions that split each hydrogen atom into a hydrogen ion and an electron. During the process of ionization, the electrons that are removed from the hydrogen atoms enter an electron transport chain that is conducted on the inner membrane of the mitochondrion. This electron transport chain consists of electron acceptors that can be reversibly reduced or oxidized by accepting or giving up electrons. Each electron is shuttled from one acceptor to another until it reaches the end of the chain, where its final two electrons are used to reduce elemental oxygen, which combines with the hydrogen ions to form water. As the electrons move along the electron transport chain, large amounts of energy are released. This energy is used to convert ADP to ATP. Because the formation of ATP involves the addition of a high-energy phosphate bond to ADP, the process is sometimes called *oxidative phosphorylation*. Cyanide causes death by poisoning the enzymes needed for one of the final steps in the oxidative phosphorylation sequence.

In summary, cells communicate by means of chemical messengers. Many chemical messengers bind to specific receptors on the cell surface and exert their effects through internal second messengers that are activated by the G protein signal transduction system. Cell division, or mitosis, is the process during which a parent cell divides into two daughter cells, with each receiving an identical pair of chromosomes. The process of mitosis is dynamic and continuous and is divided into four stages: prophase, metaphase, anaphase, and telophase.

Cellular energy metabolism is the process whereby the carbohydrates, fats, and proteins from the foods we eat are broken down and converted into energy that is stored in the form of ATP's high-energy bonds. There are two sites of energy metabolism in cells: the mitochondria and the cytoplasmic matrix. The most efficient of these pathways are the aerobic pathways located in the mitochondria. These pathways require oxygen and produce carbon dioxide and water as end-products. The glycolytic pathway, which is located in the cytoplasm, involves the breakdown of glucose to form ATP. It requires the presence of NAD±_as a hydrogen acceptor. The end-products of glycolysis are pyruvate and NADH (hydrogen atoms attached to NAD±). When oxygen is not available, NADH transfers its hydrogen atoms to pyruvate with the resultant formation of lactic acid.

Movement Across the Cell Membranes and Membrane Potentials

After you have completed this section of the chapter, you should be able to meet the following objectives:

- Describe the mechanism of membrane transport associated with diffusion, osmosis, endocytosis, and exocytosis and compare with active transport mechanisms
- Describe the function of ion channels
- Describe the origin of the membrane potential
- Explain the relationship between membrane permeability and membrane potential

Movement Across the Cell Membrane

The unique properties of the cell's membrane are responsible for differences in the composition of intracellular and extracellular fluids. However, a constant movement of molecules and ions across the cell membrane is required to maintain the functions of the cell. Movement through the cell membrane occurs in essentially two ways: passively or actively. In passive processes, substances move across the membrane without an expenditure of energy; active transport involves an expenditure of energy. The cell membrane is also capable of engulfing a particle, forming a membrane-coated vesicle, and then moving the membrane-coated vesicle into the cell in a process called *endocytosis* or out of the cell by *exocytosis*.

Passive Movement

The passive movement of ions across the cell membrane is directly influenced by chemical or electrical gradients. Differences in the number of particles on either side of the membrane creates a chemical gradient and provides the basis for passive movement. Electrical gradients are generated by electrically charged particles or ions. Chemical and electrical gradients often are linked and are called *electrochemical gradients*.

Diffusion. *Diffusion* refers to the process by which molecules and other particles in a solution become widely dispersed and reach a uniform concentration as a result of energy created by their spontaneous kinetic movements (Fig. 1-16). In the case of ions, diffusion is affected by energy supplied by their electrical charge. Molecules of gases in other substances move from an area of higher to an area of lower concentration as they diffuse and become evenly distributed across the cell membrane. Lipid-soluble molecules such as oxygen, carbon dioxide, alcohol, and fatty acids become dissolved in the lipid matrix of the cell membrane and diffuse through the membrane in the same manner that diffusion occurs in water. Other substances diffuse through minute pores of the cell membrane. The rate of movement depends on the amount of substance available for diffusion, the velocity of the kinetic movement of the particles, and the number of openings in the cell membrane through which the particles can move. Temperature changes the motion of the particles; the greater the temperature, the greater is the thermal motion of the molecules. Thus, diffusion increases in direct proportion to the increased temperature.

Osmosis. Most cell membranes are semipermeable in that they are permeable to water but not all solute particles. Water moves through a semipermeable membrane along a concentration gradient, moving from an area of higher to one of lower concentration (see Fig. 1-16). This process is called *osmosis*, and the pressure water generates as it moves through the membrane is called *osmotic pressure*. Osmosis is regulated by the concentration of nondiffusible particles on either side of the membrane. For example, when different concentrations of particles exist on the two sides of a semipermeable membrane, water moves from the side with fewer particles and higher concentration of water to the side with the greater number of particles and lower concentration of water. The movement of water continues until the concentration of solute particles on both sides of the membrane are equally diluted or until the hydrostatic pressure created by the movement of water opposes its flow.

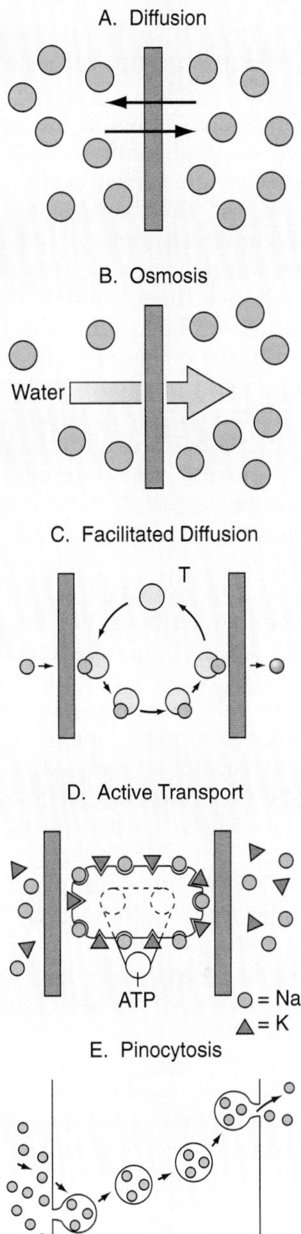

FIGURE 1-16
Mechanisms of membrane transport. (**A**) Diffusion, in which particles move to become equally distributed across the membrane. (**B**) The osmotically active particles regulate the flow of water. (**C**) Facilitated diffusion uses a carrier system. (**D**) In active transport, selected molecules are transported across the membrane using the energy-driven (ATP) pump. (**E**) The membrane forms a vesicle that engulfs the particle and transports it across the membrane, where it is released. This is called pinocytosis.

Facilitated Diffusion. Facilitated diffusion involves a carrier system (see Fig. 1-16). Some substances, such as glucose, cannot pass through the cell membrane because they are not lipid-soluble or are too large to pass through the membrane's pores. These substances combine with a special lipid-soluble carrier at the membrane's outer surface, are carried across the membrane attached to the carrier, and then released. In facilitated diffusion, a substance can move only from an area of higher concentration to an area of lower concentration. The rate at which a substance moves across the membrane as a result of facilitated diffusion depends on the difference in concentration between the two sides of the membrane, the amount of carrier that is available for transport, and the rapidity with which the carrier can bind and release the substance. It is thought that insulin, which increases glucose transport, may increase the amount of carrier present or the rate at which the reactions between glucose and the carrier take place.

Active Transport and Cotransport

The process of diffusion describes the movement of substances from an area of higher concentration to one of lower concentration, resulting in a equal distribution across the cell membrane. In some instances, however, different concentrations of a substance are needed in the intracellular and extracellular fluids. For example, the intracellular functioning of the cell requires a much higher concentration of potassium than is present in the extracellular fluid while maintaining a much lower concentration of sodium than in the extracellular fluid. In these situations, energy is required to pump the ions "uphill" or against the concentration gradient. When cells use energy to move ions against an electrical or chemical gradient, the process is called *active transport*.

The active transport system that has been studied in the greatest detail is the sodium-potassium pump, or Na^+/K^+ ATPase (see Fig. 1-16). The Na^+/K^+ ATPase pump moves sodium from the inside to the outside of the cell, where its concentration is about 14 times greater than inside, and returns potassium to the inside, where its concentration is about 35 times greater than it is outside the cell. The energy used to pump sodium out of cell and pump potassium into the cell is obtained by splitting and releasing energy from the high-energy phosphate bond in ATP by the enzyme ATPase. Were it not for the activity of the sodium-potassium pump, the osmotically active sodium particles would accumulate within the cell, causing cellular swelling due to an accompanying influx of water (see Chapter 2).

There are two types of active transport systems: primary active transport and secondary active transport. In *primary active transport*, the source of energy (*e.g.*, ATP) is directly used in the transport of a substance. *Secondary active transport* mechanisms harness the energy derived from primary active transport of one substance, usually sodium, for cotransport of a second substance. For example, when sodium is actively transported out of a cell by primary active transport, a large concentration difference develops (*i.e.*, high concentration on the outside and low on the inside). This concentration gradient represents a large storehouse of energy because sodium is always attempting to diffuse into the cell. Similar to facilitated diffusion, secondary transport mechanisms use membrane carrier proteins. These proteins have two binding sites, one for sodium and the other for the substance undergoing secondary transport. Secondary transport systems are classified into two groups: *cotransport* or *symport* systems, in which the sodium ion and solute are transported in the same direction, and *countertransport* or *antiport* systems, in which sodium and the solute are transported in the opposite direction (Fig. 1-17). Examples of cotransport mechanisms are the sodium-coupled transport of glucose and amino acids in the small intestine and kidney.

Endocytosis and Exocytosis

Endocytosis is the process by which cells engulf materials from their surroundings. It includes pinocytosis and phagocytosis. *Pinocytosis* involves the ingestion of small amounts of extracellular fluid and dissolved particles by engulfing them into small membrane-surrounded vesicles for movement into the cytoplasm; it is important in the transport of proteins and strong solutions of electrolytes (see Fig. 1-16).

Phagocytosis literally means *cell eating* and can be compared with pinocytosis, which means *cell drinking*. It involves the engulfment and subsequent killing or

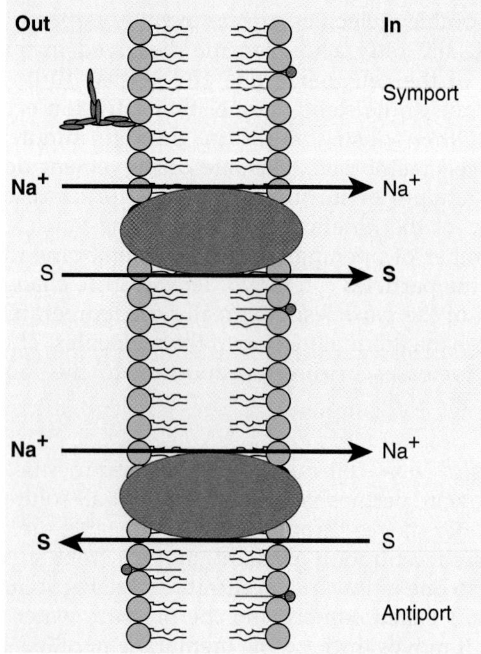

FIGURE 1-17
Secondary active transport systems. Symport or cotransport (**top**) carries the transported solute (**s**) in the same direction as the Na^+ ion. Antiport or counter-transport carries the solute and Na^+ in the opposite direction. (Rhoades R.A., Tanner G.A. [1996]. *Medical physiology.* Boston: Little Brown)

degradation of microorganisms and other particulate matter. During phagocytosis, a particle comes in contact with the cell surface and is surrounded on all sides by the cell membrane, forming a phagocytic vesicle or phagosome. Once formed, the phagosome breaks away from the cell membrane and moves into the cytoplasm, where it eventually fuses with a lysosome allowing the ingested material to be degraded by lysosomal enzymes. Certain types of cells, such as macrophages and polymorphonuclear leukocytes (neutrophils), are specialized for taking in and disposing of invading organisms, damaged cells, and unneeded extracellular constituents (see Chapter 11). Receptor-mediated endocytosis involves the binding of substances such as low-density lipoproteins to a receptor on the cell surface. Binding of the ligand (*i.e.*, a substance with a high affinity for a receptor) to the receptor normally causes widely distributed receptors to accumulate in clarthrin-coated pits. An aggregation of special proteins on the cytoplasmic side of the pit forms a dome that causes the coated pit to invaginate and pinch off, forming a clathrin-coated vesicle that carries the ligand and its receptor into the cell.

Exocytosis is the mechanism for the secretion of intracellular substances into the extracellular spaces. It is the reverse of endocytosis in that a secretory granule fuses to the inner side of the cell membrane and an opening occurs to the outside of the cell surface. This opening allows the contents of the granule to be released into the extracellular fluid. Exocytosis is important in removing cellular debris and releasing substances, such as hormones, that have been synthesized in the cell.

During endocytosis, portions of the cell membrane become an endocytotic vesicle; during exocytosis the membrane is returned to the cell surface. In this way, cell membranes can be conserved and reused.

Ion Channels

The electrical charge on small ions such as Na^+ and K^+ makes it difficult for these ions to move across the lipid layer of the cell membrane. However, fast movement of these ions is required for many types of cell functions such as nerve activity. This is accomplished by *facilitated diffusion through selective ion channels*. Ion channels are intrinsic proteins that span the width of membrane and are normally composed of several polypeptide or protein subunits that form a gating system. Specific stimuli cause the protein subunits to undergo conformational changes to form an open channel or gate through which the ions can move (Fig. 1-18). In this way ions do not need to cross the lipid soluble portion of the membrane but can remain in the aqueous solution that fills the ion channel. Specific interactions between the ions and the sides of the channel can produce an extremely rapid rate of ion movement. For example, the ion channel can become negatively charged, facilitating the rapid movement of positively charged ions. Ion channels are highly selective; some channels only allow for passage sodium ions, and others are selective for potassium, calcium, or chloride ions.

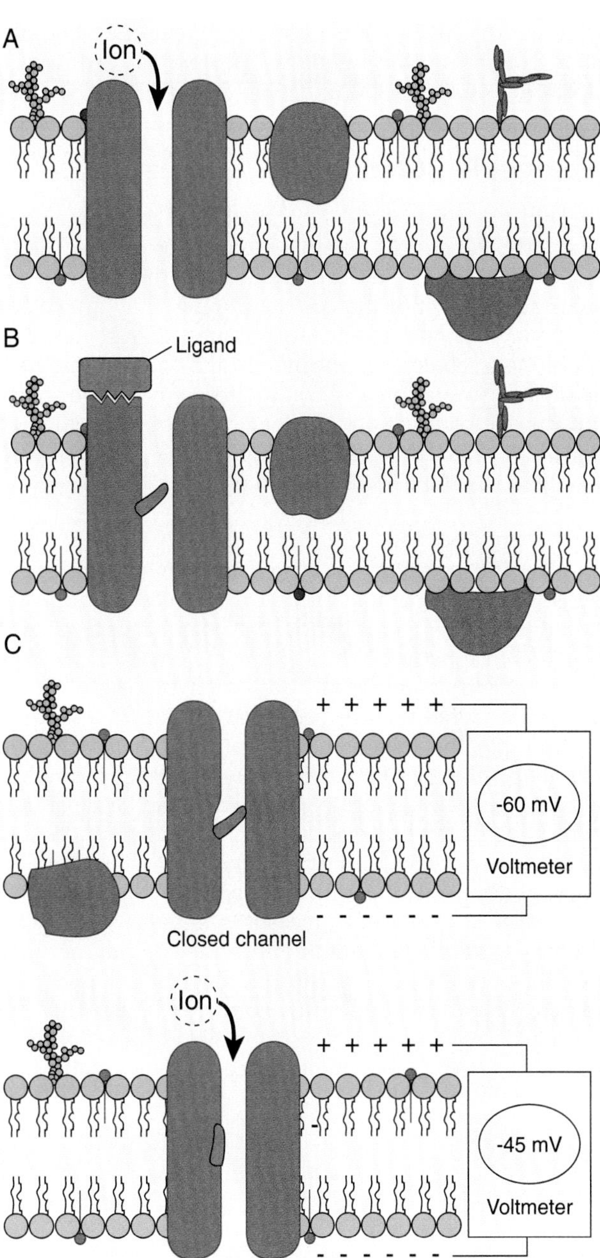

FIGURE 1-18
Ion channels. **(A)** Nongated ion channel remains open, permitting free movement of ions across the membrane. **(B)** Ligand-gated channel is controlled by ligand binding to the receptor. **(C)** Voltage-gated channel is controlled by a change in membrane potential. (Rhoades R.A., Tanner G.A. [1996]. *Medical physiology.* Boston: Little Brown)

Ion channels can be classified into two groups according to the stimuli that cause their gates to open and close. *Voltage-gated channels* have electrically operated gates that open when the membrane potential changes beyond a certain point (discussed in the next section). *Ligand-gated channels* have chemically operated gates that respond to specific receptor-bound ligands such as the neurotransmitter acetylcholine. Ligand-gated channels often involve G protein activation of a second messenger system.

Membrane Potentials

The human body runs on a system of self-generated electricity. Electrical potentials exist across the membranes of most cells in the body. Because these potentials occur at the level of the cell membrane, they are called *membrane potentials*. In excitable tissues, such as nerve or muscle cells, changes in the membrane potential are necessary for generation and conduction of nerve impulses and muscle contraction. In other types of cells, such as glandular cells, changes in the membrane potential contribute to hormone secretion and other functions.

Electrical Potentials

An electrical potential, measured in volts (V), describes the ability of separated electrical charges of opposite polarity (+ and −) to do work. The potential difference is the difference between the separated charges. The terms *potential difference* and *voltage* are synonymous. Voltage is always measured with respect to two points in a system. For example, the voltage in a car battery (6 or 12 V) is the potential difference between the two battery terminals. Because the total amount of charge that can be separated by a biologic membrane is small, the potential differences are small and are measured in *millivolts* (1/1000 of a volt). The voltage or potential difference between the inside and the outside of a cell can be measured in the laboratory by inserting a very fine electrode into the cell and another into the extracellular fluid surrounding the cell and connecting the two electrodes to a voltmeter (Fig. 1-19). The movement of charge between two points is called *current;* it occurs when a potential difference has been established and a connection is made such that the charged particles are able to move between the two points.

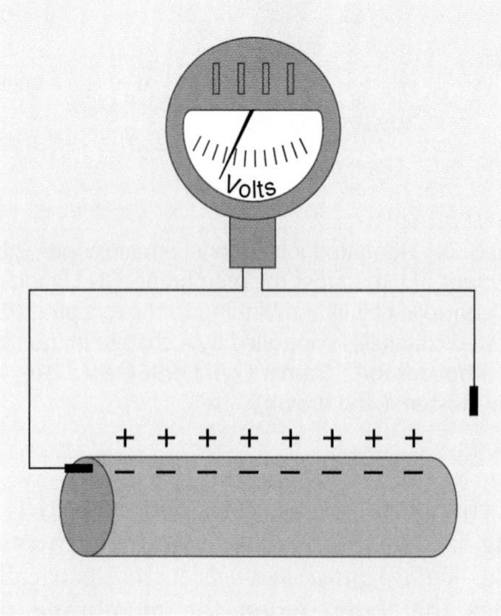

FIGURE 1-19 Alignment of charge along the cell membrane. The electrical potential is negative on the inside of the cell membrane in relation to the outside.

Extracellular and intracellular fluids are electrolyte solutions containing about 150 to 160 mmol/L of positively charged ions and an equal concentration of negatively charged ions; these are the *current-carrying ions* responsible for generating and conducting membrane potentials. Generally, there is a small excess of positively charged ions outside the cell membrane. This is represented as positive charges on the outside of the membrane and equal numbers of negative charges on the inside. Because of the extreme thinness of the cell membrane, these ions accumulate on either side of the membrane, contributing to the establishment of a membrane potential.

Diffusion Potentials

A diffusion potential describes the voltage that is generated by ions that diffuse across the membrane. Two conditions are necessary for a membrane potential to occur as a result of diffusion: the membrane must be selectively permeable, allowing a single type of ion to diffuse through membrane pores, and the concentration of the diffusible ion must be greater on one side of the membrane than on the other. In the resting or unexcited state, when the membrane is highly permeable to potassium, the concentration of potassium ions inside of the cell is about 35 times that on the outside of the cell. Because of the large concentration gradient from inside to outside, there is a strong tendency for the potassium ions to diffuse outward. As they do so, they carry their positive charges with them, and the inside becomes negative in relation to the outside. This new potential difference repels further outward movement of the positively charged potassium ions. The same phenomenon occurs during an action potential, when the membrane is highly permeable to sodium. The sodium ions move to the inside of the membrane, creating a membrane potential of the opposite polarity. An *equilibrium potential* is one in which there is no net movement of ions because the diffusion and electrical forces are exactly balanced. The following equation, known as the *Nernst equation,* can be used to calculate the equilibrium potential (electromotive force [EMF] in millivolts [mV]) of an univalent ion at a body temperature of 37° C.

$$\text{EMF (mV)} = -61 \times \log_{10}\left[\frac{\text{ion concentration inside}}{\text{ion concentration outside}}\right]$$

For example, if the concentration of an ion inside the membrane was 100 mmol/L and the concentration outside was 10 mmol/L, the equilibrium potential (mV) for that ion would be $-61 \log_{10}$ (100/10 = 10, and the $\log_{10}$ of 10 is 1). It would take 61 mV of charge inside of the membrane to balance the diffusion potential created by the concentration difference across the membrane for this ion.

If the membrane were permeable only to potassium and there was no pumping of ions across the membrane, the equilibrium potential for the potassium ion, using normal intracellular (140 mmol/L) and extracellular (4 mmol/L) concentrations, would be −94 mV (−61 × $\log_{10}$ 140 mmol/L/4 mmol/L). This value approximates the −70 mV to − 90 mV resting membrane potential for nerve fibers that has been measured in laboratory studies. Likewise, the equilibrium potential for sodium (intracellular 14 mmol/L and extracellular 140 mmol/L) would be about +61 mV (−61 × $\log_{10}$ 14 mmol/L/140 mmol/L) during the fraction of a second that occurs at the peak of the action potential when the membrane is much more permeable to the sodium ion than to the potassium ion. This value is similar to the +45 mV value that has been measured experimentally in nerve fibers. When the membrane is permeable to several different ions, the diffusion potential reflects the sum of the diffusion potentials for the different ions.

Variations in Membrane Potentials

The membrane potential can be altered by changes in membrane permeability. Calcium ions decrease membrane permeability to sodium ions. If there are not enough calcium ions available, the permeability of the membrane to sodium increases, and as a result, membrane excitability increases—sometimes to the extent that spontaneous muscle movements (tetany) occur. *Local anesthetic agents* (*e.g.*, procaine, cocaine) act directly on neural membranes to decrease their permeability to sodium.

In summary, movement of materials across the cell's membrane is essential for survival of the cell. Diffusion is a process by which substances such as ions move from areas of greater concentration to areas of lesser concentrations in an attempt to reach a uniform distribution. Osmosis refers to the diffusion of water molecules through a semipermeable membrane along a concentration gradient. In facilitated diffusion, molecules that normally cannot pass through the cell's membranes can do so with the assistance of a carrier molecule. Diffusion of water molecules by osmosis or ions by facilitated diffusion do not require an expenditure of energy by the cell and are therefore passive in nature. Another type of transport, called active transport, requires the cell to expend energy in moving ions against a concentration gradient. There are two types of active transport, primary and secondary; both require carrier proteins. The Na^+/K^+ ATPase pump is the best known type of active transport.

Endocytosis is a process by which cells engulf materials from the surrounding medium. Small particles are ingested by a process called pinocytosis; larger particles are engulfed by a process called phagocytosis. Some particles require bonding with a ligand, and the process is called receptor-mediated endocytosis. Exocytosis involves the removal of large particles from the cell and is essentially the reverse of endocytosis.

Ion channels are intrinsic proteins that span the width of membrane and are normally composed of several polypeptide or protein subunits that form a gating system. Many ions can diffuse through the cell membrane only if there are conformation changes in the membrane proteins that comprise the ion channel. Two types of ion channels exist: voltage-gated channels and ligand-gated channels, which often require G protein activation of a second messenger.

Electrical potentials (negative on the inside and positive on the outside) exist across the membranes of most cells in the body. These electrical potentials result from the selective permeability of the cell membrane to Na±_and K±, the presence of nondiffusible anions inside the cell membrane, and the activity of the sodium-potassium membrane pump, which extrudes Na±_from the inside of the membrane and returns K±_to the inside. In the resting state, there is no net flow of electrically charged ions across the cell membranes in excitable tissues.

Body Tissues

After you have finished this section of the chapter, you should be able to meet the following objectives:

- Explain the process of cell differentiation in terms of development of organ systems in the embryo and the continued regeneration of tissues in postnatal life
- Explain the function of stem cells
- Describe the characteristics of the four different tissue types
- Explain the function of the intercellular adhesions and junctions
- Characterize the composition and functions of the extracellular matrix

In the preceding sections, we discussed the individual cell, its metabolic processes, and mechanisms of communication and replication. Although cells are similar, their structure and function vary according to the special needs of the body. For example, muscle cells must be able to perform different functions than skin cells or nerve cells. Groups of cells that are closely associated in structure and perform common or similar functions are called tissues. There are four categories of tissue: epithelium, connective tissue, muscle, and nerve. These tissues do not exist in isolated units, but in association with each other and in variable proportions, forming different structures and organs. This section provides a brief overview of the cells in each of these four tissue types, the structures that hold these cells together, and the extracellular matrix in which they live.

Cell Differentiation

After conception, the fertilized ovum divides and subdivides and ultimately forms about 200 different cell types. The formation of different types of cells and the disposition of these cells into tissue types is called *cell differentiation,* a process that is controlled by a system that switches genes on and off. Embryonic cells must become different to develop into all of the various organ systems, and they must remain different after the signal that initiated cell diversification has disappeared. The process of cell differentiation is controlled by cell memory, which is maintained through regulatory proteins contained within the individual members of a particular cell type. Cell differentiation also involves the sequential activation of multiple genes and their protein products. This means that, after differentiation has occurred, the tissue type does not revert to an earlier stage of differentiation. The process of cell differentiation normally moves forward, producing cells that are more specialized than their predecessors. Usually, highly differentiated cell types, such as skeletal muscle and nervous tissue, lose their ability to undergo cell division.

Although most cells proceed through differentiation into specialized cell types, many tissues contain a few cells, called *stem cells*, that apparently are only partially differentiated. These stem cells are still capable of cell division and serve as a reserve source for continued production of specialized cells throughout the life of the organism. They are the major source of cells that make regeneration possible in some tissues. Stem cells have varying abilities to differentiate. Some tissues such as skeletal muscle tissue lack undifferentiated cells and have limited regenerative capacity. Stem cells of the hematopoietic (blood) system have the greatest potential for differentiation. These cells can potentially reconstitute the entire blood-producing and immune systems. They are the major ingredient in bone marrow transplants. Other stem cells, such as those that replenish the

TABLE 1-1

Classification of Tissue Types

Tissue Type	Location
Epithelial Tissue	
Covering and lining of body surfaces	
Simple epithelium	
Squamous	Lining of blood vessels, body cavities, alveoli of lungs
Cuboidal	Collecting tubules of kidney; covering of ovaries
Columnar	Lining of intestine and gallbladder
Stratified epithelium	
Squamous keritanized	Skin
Squamous nonkeritanized	Mucous membranes of mouth, esophagus, and vagina
Cuboidal	Ducts of sweat glands
Columnar	Large ducts of salivary and mammary glands; also found in conjunctiva
Transitional	Bladder, ureters, renal pelvis
Pseudostratified	Tracheal and respiratory passages
Glandular	
Endocrine	Pituitary gland, thyroid gland, adrenal, and other glands
Exocrine	Sweat glands and glands in gastrointestinal tract
Neuroepithelium	Olfactory mucosa, retina, tongue
Reproductive epithelium	Seminiferous tubules of testis; cortical portion of ovary
Connective Tissue	
Embryonic connective tissue	
Mesenchymal	Embryonic mesoderm
Mucous	Umbilical cord (Wharton's jelly)
Adult connective tissue	
Loose or areolar	Subcutaneous areas
Dense regular	Tendons and ligaments
Dense irregular	Dermis of skin
Adipose	Fat pads, subcutaneous layers
Reticular	Framework of lymphoid organs, bone marrow, liver
Specialized connective tissue	
Bone	Long bones, flat bones
Cartilage	Tracheal rings, external ear, articular surfaces
Hematopoietic	Blood cells, myeloid tissue (bone marrow)
Muscle Tissue	
Skeletal	Skeletal muscles
Cardiac	Heart muscles
Smooth	Gastrointestinal tract, blood vessels, bronchi, bladder, and others
Nervous Tissue	
Neurons	Central and peripheral neurons and nerve fibers
Supporting cells	Glial and ependymal cells in central nervous system; Schwann and satelitte cells in peripheral nervous system

mucosal surface of the gastrointestinal tract, are less general but can still differentiate several times. Cancer cells are thought to originate from undifferentiated stem cells (see Chapter 5).

Embryonic Origin of Tissue Types

All of the approximately 200 different types of body cells can be classified under four basic or primary tissue types: epithelial, connective, muscle, and nervous (Table 1-1). These basic tissue types are often described in terms of their embryonic origin. The embryo is essentially a three-layered tubular structure (Fig. 1-20). The outer layer of the tube is called the *ectoderm;* the middle layer is *mesoderm;* and the inner layer the *endoderm.* All of the adult body tissues originate from these three cellular layers. Epithelium has its origin in all three embryonic layers, connective tissue and muscle develop mainly from the mesoderm, and nervous tissue develops from the ectoderm.

Epithelial Tissue

Origin and Characteristics

Epithelial tissue forms sheets that cover the body's outer surface, line the internal surfaces, and form the glandular tissue. Underneath all types of epithelial tissue is a small amount of extracellular matrix, called the basement membrane. The basement membrane consists of the basal lamina and an underlying reticular layer. The terms basal lamina and basement membrane are often used interchangeably. Epithelial cells have strong intracellular protein filaments (*i.e.,* cytoskeleton) that are important in transmitting mechanical stresses from one cell to another.

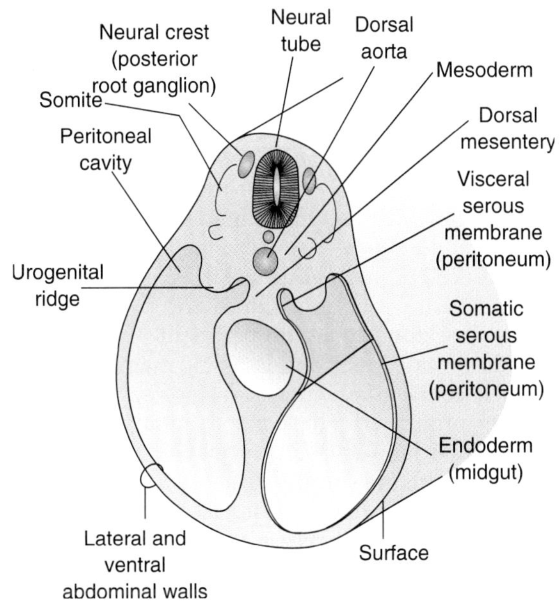

FIGURE 1-20
Cross section of a human embryo illustrating the development of the somatic and visceral structures.

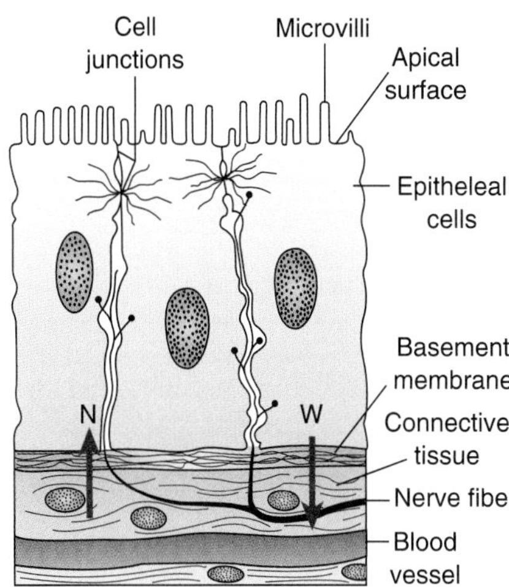

FIGURE 1-21
Typical arrangement of epithelial cells in relation to underlying tissues and blood supply. Epithelial tissue has no blood supply of its own but relies on the blood vessels in the underlying connective tissue for nutrition (**N**) and elimination of wastes (**W**).

The cells of epithelial tissue are tightly bound together by specialized junctions. These specialized junctions enable these cells to form barriers to the movement of water, solutes, and cells from one body compartment to the next. Epithelial tissue is avascular (*i.e.,* without blood vessels) and must therefore receive oxygen and nutrients from the capillaries of the connective tissue on which the epithelial tissue rests (Fig. 1-21). Epithelial tissue may contain nerve endings. To survive, epithelial tissue must be kept moist. Even the seemingly dry skin epithelium is kept moist by a nonvitalized, waterproof layer of superficial skin cells filled with intermediate-diameter filaments of tough protein called *keratin,* which prevents evaporation of moisture from the deeper living cells.

Epithelia are derived from all three embryonic layers. Most of the epithelium of the skin, mouth, nose, and anus are derived from the ectoderm. The linings of the respiratory tract, the gastrointestinal tract, and the glands of the digestive tract are of endodermal origin. The endothelial lining of blood vessels originates from the mesoderm. Many types of epithelial tissue retain the ability to differentiate and undergo rapid proliferation as a means of replacing injured tissue.

Types of Epithelial Cells

The three types of epithelial tissues are classified according to the shape of the cells and the number of layers that are present: *simple, stratified,* and *pseudostratified.* The terms *squamous* (thin and flat), *cuboidal* (cube shaped), and *columnar* (resembling a column) refer to the cell shapes (Fig. 1-22).

Simple epithelium contains a single layer of cells, all of which rest on the basement membrane. Simple squamous epithelium is adapted for filtration; it is found lining the blood vessels, lymph nodes, and alveoli of the lungs. The single layer of squamous epithelium that lines the inside of the heart and blood vessels is known as the *endothelium.* A similar type of layer, called the *mesothelium,* is found in the serous membranes that line

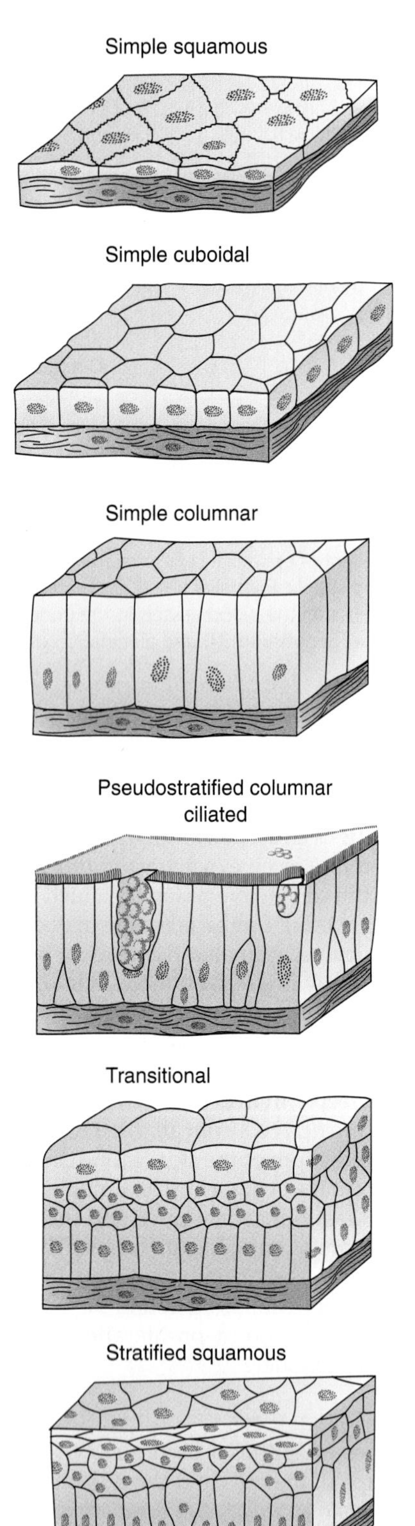

FIGURE 1-22
Representation of the various epithelial tissue types.

the pleural, pericardial, and peritoneal cavities. *Simple cuboidal epithelium* is found on the surface of the ovary and in the thyroid. *Simple columnar epithelium* lines the intestine. One form of simple columnar epithelium has hairlike projections called *cilia*, often with specialized mucus-secreting cells called *goblet* cells.

Stratified epithelium contains more than one layer of cells, with only the deepest layer resting on the basement membrane. It is designed to protect the body surface. *Stratified squamous keratinized epithelium* makes up the epidermis of the skin. *Keratin* is a tough, fibrous protein in the form of filaments within the outer cells of skin epithelium. Stratified squamous keratinized epithelium is made up of many layers; the layers closest to the underlying tissues are cuboidal or columnar. The cells become more irregular and thinner as they move closer to the surface. The outermost cells become totally filled with keratin and die, to be sloughed off and replaced by the deeper cells. Stratified squamous nonkeratinized epithelium is found on wet surfaces such as the mouth and tongue. Stratified cuboidal and columnar epithelia are found in the ducts of salivary glands and the larger ducts of the mammary glands. *Pseudostratified epithelium* is a form of stratified epithelium in which all of the cells are in contact with the underlying intercellular matrix, but some do not extend to the surface. Pseudostratified columnar ciliated epithelium with goblet cells forms the lining of most of the upper respiratory tract. All of the tall cells reaching the surface of this type of epithelium are ciliated cells or mucus-producing goblet cells. The basal cells that do not reach the surface serve as stem cells for the ciliated cells and goblet cells. *Transitional epithelium* is a stratified epithelium characterized by cells that can change shape and become thinner when the tissue is stretched. Such tissue can be stretched without pulling the superficial cells apart. Transitional epithelium is well adapted for the lining of organs that are constantly changing their volume, such as the urinary bladder.

Glandular epithelial tissue is formed by cells specialized to produce a fluid secretion. This process is usually accompanied by the intracellular synthesis of macromolecules. The chemical nature of these macromolecules is variable. The macromolecules typically are stored in the cells in small membrane-bound vesicles called secretory granules. For example, glandular epithelia can synthesize, store, and secrete proteins (*e.g.*, insulin), lipids (*e.g.*, adrenocortical hormones, secretions of the sebaceous glands), and complexes of carbohydrates and proteins (*e.g.*, saliva). Less common are secretions, such as those produced by the sweat glands, which required minimal synthetic activity.

All glandular cells arise from the covering epithelia by means of cell proliferation and invasion of the adjacent connective tissue, and all produce and expel their contents into an extracellular compartment. *Exocrine glands*, such as the sweat glands and lactating mammary glands, retain their connection with the surface epithelium from which they originated. This connection takes the form of epithelial lined tubular ducts through which their secretion pass to reach the surface of the tissue where they are located. Exocrine glands are often classified according to the way secretory products are released by their cells. In *holocrine* type cells (*e.g.*, sebaceous glands) the glandular cell ruptures, releasing its entire contents into the duct system. New generations of cells are replaced by mitosis of basal cells. *Merocrine* or eccrine type glands (*e.g.*, salivary glands, exocrine glands of the pancreas) release their glandular products by exocytosis; in *apocrine* secretions (*e.g.*, mammary gland, certain sweat glands), the apical portion of the cell along with small portions of the cytoplasm are pinched off the glandular cells. The *endocrine glands* are epithelial structures that have had their connection with the surface obliterated during development. These glands are ductless and produce secretions (*i.e.*, hormones) that move directly into the bloodstream.

Connective Tissue

Origin and Characteristics

Connective tissue is the most abundant tissue in the body. As its name indicates, it connects and holds tissues together. The capsules that surround organs of the body are composed of connective tissue. Bone, adipose tissue, and cartilage are specialized types of connective tissue that function to support the soft tissues of the body and store fat. Connective tissue is unique in that its cells produce the extracellular matrix that supports and holds tissues together. Connective tissue has a role in tissue nutrition. It is in proximity to blood vessels; the connective tissue matrix serves as the medium through which nutrients and metabolic wastes are exchanged.

Most connective tissue is derived from the embryonic mesoderm, but some is derived from the neural crest, a derivative of the ectoderm. During embryonic development, mesodermal cells migrate from their site of origin and then surround and penetrate the developing organ. These cells are called *mesenchymal cells*, and the tissue they form is called *mesenchyme*. Tissues derived from embryonic mesenchymal cells include bone, cartilage, and adipose (fat) cells. In addition to providing the source or origin of most connective tissues, mesenchyme develops into other structures such as blood cells and blood vessels. Connective tissue cells include fibroblasts, chondroblasts, osteoblasts, hematopoietic stem cells, blood cells, macrophages, mast cells, and adipocytes. The matrix of the umbilical cord is composed of a second type of embryonic mesoderm called *mucous connective tissue*.

Adult connective tissue can be divided into four types: loose or areolar, reticular, adipose, and dense connective tissue, which can be subdivided into irregular and regular connective tissue. Specialized connective tissue types such as blood and blood-forming tissues are discussed in Chapter 6, and cartilage and bone are discussed in Chapter 44.

Loose Connective Tissue

Loose connective tissue, also known as areolar tissue, is soft and pliable and contains large amounts of intercellular substance (Fig. 1-23). It fills spaces between muscle sheaths and forms a layer that encases blood and lymphatic vessels. Loose connective tissue supports the epithelial tissues and provides the means by which these tissues are nourished. In an organ containing functioning epithelial tissue and supporting connective tissue, the term *parenchymal tissue* is used to describe the

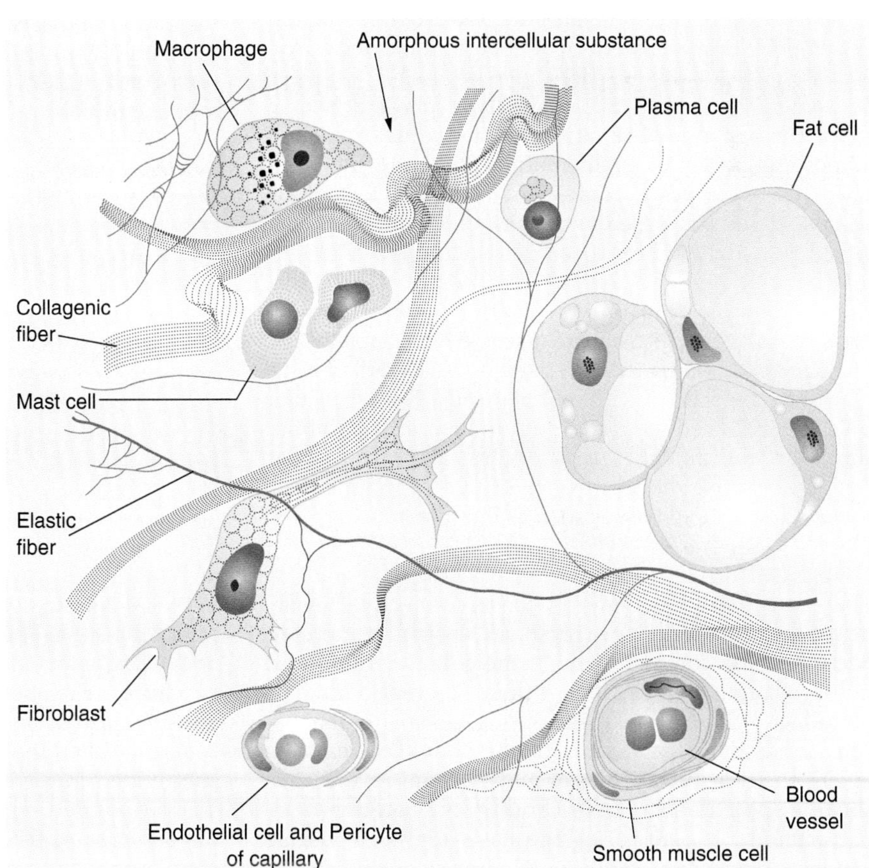

FIGURE 1-23 Diagrammatic representation of cells that may be seen in loose connective tissue. The cells lie in an intercellular matrix that is bathed in tissue fluid that originates in capillaries.

functioning epithelium in contradistinction to the connective tissue framework or stroma. Cells of loose connective tissue include fibroblasts, mast cells, adipose or fat cells, macrophages, plasma cells, and leukocytes. Loose connective tissue cells secrete substances that form the extracellular matrix that supports and connects body cells.

Fibroblasts are the most abundant of these cells. They are responsible for the synthesis of the fibrous and gel-like substance that fills the intercellular spaces of the body and for the production of collagen, elastic, and reticular fibers. The *basal lamina* is a special type of intercellular matrix that is present where connective tissue comes in contact with the tissue it supports. The basal lamina is only visible with an electron microscope. The basal lamina is produced by the epithelial cells. In many locations, reticular fibers, produced by the connective tissue cells, are associated with the basal lamina. Together the basal lamina and the reticular layer form the basement membrane seen by light microscopy. A basement membrane is found along the interface between connective tissue and muscle fibers, on Schwann cells of the peripheral nervous system, on the basal surface of endothelial cells, and on fat cells. These basement membranes bond cells to the underlying or surrounding connective tissues, serve as selective filters for particles that pass between connective tissue and other cells, and contribute to cell regeneration and repair.

Adipose tissue is a special form of connective tissue in which adipocytes predominate. Adipocytes do not generate an extracellular matrix but maintain a large intracellular space. Adipocytes store large quantities of triglycerides and are the largest repository of energy in the body. Adipose tissue helps fill up spaces between tissues and helps to keep organs in place. Subcutaneous layers of fat help to shape the body. Because fat is a poor conductor of heat, adipose tissue serves as thermal insulation for the body. There are two types of adipose tissue. Unilocular (white) adipose tissue composed of cells in which the fat is contained in a single, large droplet in the cytoplasm. Multilocular (brown) adipose tissue is composed of cells that contain multiple droplets of fat and numerous mitochondria. These two types of fat are discussed in Chapter 54.

Reticular tissue is characterized by a network of reticular fibers associated with reticular cells. These reticular cells are believed to retain multipotential capabilities similar to undifferentiated mesenchymal cells. Reticular tissues comprise the framework of the liver, bone marrow, and lymphoid tissues such as the spleen.

Dense Connective Tissue

There are two categories of dense connective tissue: dense irregular and dense regular. Dense irregular connective tissue consists of the same components found in loose connective tissue, but there is a predominance of collagen fibers and fewer cells. Dense irregular tissue is found in the dermis of the skin (*i.e.*, reticular layer), the fibrous capsules of many organs, the fibrous sheaths of cartilage (*i.e.*, perichondrium), and bone (*i.e.*, periosteum). It also forms the basis for most fasciae that invest muscles and organs. Dense regular connective tissues are rich in collagen fibers and form the tendons and aponeuroses that join muscles to bone or other muscles and the ligaments that join bones to bone. Tendons and ligaments are white fibers because of an abundance of collagen. Ligaments such as the ligamentum flava of the vertebral column and the true vocal folds are referred to as yellow fibers because of the abundance of elastic fibers.

Muscle Tissue

There are three types of muscle tissue: *skeletal, cardiac,* and *smooth*. Skeletal and cardiac muscles are striated muscles. The actin and myosin filaments are arranged in large parallel arrays in bundles, giving the muscle fibers a striped or striated appearance when they are viewed through a microscope.

Skeletal muscle is the largest tissue in the body, accounting for 40% to 45% of the total body weight. Most skeletal muscles are attached to bones, and their contractions are responsible for movements of the skeleton. It differs from cardiac and smooth muscle in that it is innervated by the somatic rather than the autonomic nervous system. Cardiac muscle, found in the myocardium, is designed to pump blood continuously. It has inherent properties of automaticity, rhythmicity, and conductivity. The pumping action of the heart is controlled by impulses originating in the cardiac conduction system and is modified by bloodborne neural mediators and impulses from the autonomic nervous system. Smooth muscle is found in many organs, including the walls of blood vessels, the iris of the eye, and in tubes that connect many internal organs, such as the ureters and bile ducts. Neither skeletal nor cardiac muscle is able to undergo the mitotic activity needed to replace injured cells. Smooth muscle, however, may proliferate and undergo mitotic activity. Some increases in smooth muscle are physiologic, as occurs in the uterus during pregnancy. Other increases, such as the increase in smooth muscle that occurs in the arteries of persons with chronic hypertension, are pathologic.

Although the three types of muscle tissue differ significantly in structure, contractile properties, and control mechanisms, they have many similarities. In the following section, the structural properties of skeletal muscle are presented as the prototype of muscle tissue. Smooth muscle and the ways in which it differs from skeletal muscle are discussed. Cardiac muscle is described in Chapter 16.

Skeletal Muscle

Muscle tissue is highly specialized for contractility and producing movement of internal and external body structures. Skeletal muscles such as the biceps brachii are surrounded by a dense, irregular connective tissue covering called the *epimysium* (Fig. 1-24). Each muscle is subdivided into smaller bundles called *fascicles,* which are surrounded by a connective tissue covering called the *perimysium*. The number of fascicles and their size varies among muscles. Fascicles consist of numerous elongated structures called muscle fibers, each of which is surrounded by connective tissue called the *endomysium*. The cytoplasm of the muscle fiber (*i.e.*, sarcoplasm) is contained within the sarcolemma, which represents the cell membrane. Skeletal muscles are syncytial or multinucleated structures, which means that there are no true cell boundaries with a skeletal muscle fiber.

Embedded in the sarcoplasm are the contractile elements, *actin* and *myosin*. The thin, lighter-staining myofilaments (*i.e.*, actin) and the thicker, darker-staining myofilaments (*i.e.*, myosin) are arranged in parallel bundles (*i.e.*, myofibrils) throughout the sarcoplasm. Each myofibril consists of regularly repeating units along the length of the myofibril; each of these units is called a *sarcomere* (Fig. 1-25). The sarcomeres are the structural and functional units of cardiac and skeletal muscle. A sarcomere extends from one Z line to another Z line. Within the sarcomere are alternating light and dark bands. The dark band contains mainly myosin filaments, with some overlap with actin filaments. The lighter I band contains only actin filaments and straddles the Z band; it takes two sarcomeres to make a complete I band. The H zone is found in the middle of the A band and represents the region where only myosin filaments are found. In the center of the H zone is a thin, dark band called the M band or line that is produced by linkages between the myosin filaments. The Z bands consist of short elements that interconnect and provide the thin actin filaments from two adjoining sarcomeres with an anchoring point.

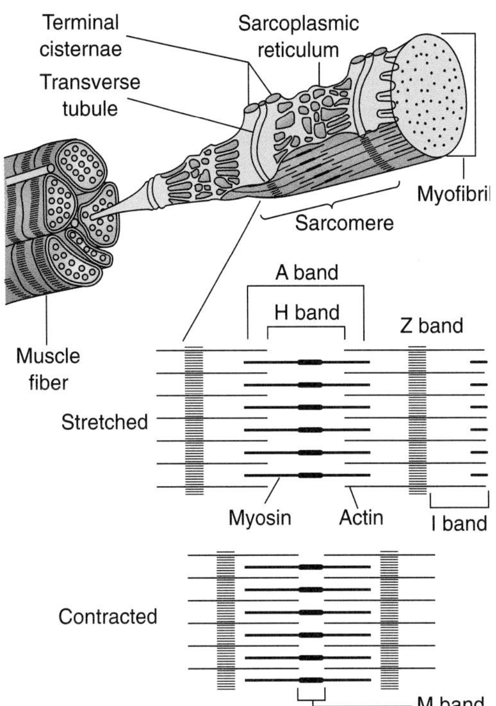

FIGURE 1-25
Muscle fiber, structures of the myofibril, and the relation between actin and myosin filaments when the muscle is stretched or contracted.

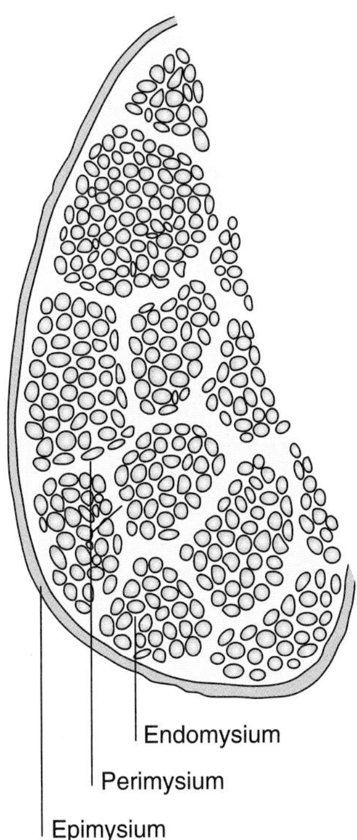

FIGURE 1-24
Connective tissue components of skeletal muscle (transerve section).

The *sarcoplasmic reticulum*, which is comparable to the smooth ER, is composed of longitudinal tubules that run parallel to the muscle fiber and surround each myofibril. The sarcoplasmic reticulum ends in enlarged, saclike regions called the *lateral sacs*, or *terminal cisternae*. The lateral sacs store calcium to be released during muscle contraction. A second system of tubules consists of the *transverse*, or *T-tubules*, which run perpendicular to the muscle fiber. The hollow part or lumen of the transverse tubule is continuous with the extracellular fluid compartment, and the membrane of the T-tubule is able to propagate action potentials, which are rapidly conducted over the surface of the muscle fiber and into the sarcoplasmic reticulum. As the action potential moves through the lateral sacs, the sacs release calcium, which initiates muscle contraction. The membrane of the sarcoplasmic reticulum also has an active transport mechanism for pumping the calcium ions back into the reticulum as a means of removing them from the vicinity of the actin and myosin interactions on termination of muscle contraction.

During muscle contraction, the thick myosin and thin actin filaments slide over each other, causing shortening of the muscle fiber, although the length of the individual thick and thin filaments remains unchanged. The structures that produce the sliding of the filaments are the myosin heads that form cross-bridges with the thin actin filaments (Fig. 1-26). When activated by ATP,

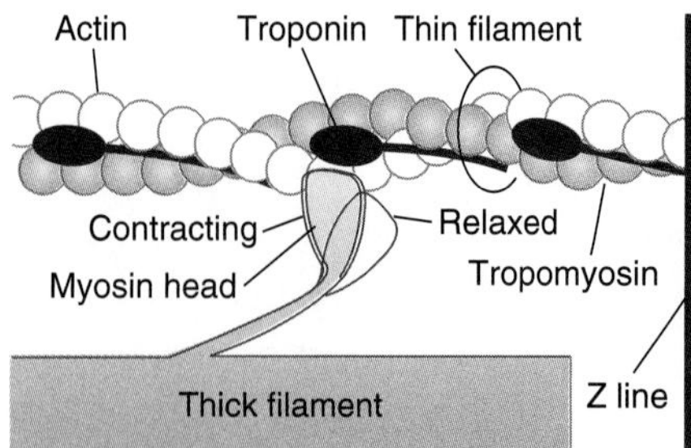

FIGURE 1-26
Molecular structure of the thin actin filament and the thicker myosin filament of striated muscle. The thin filament is a double-stranded helix of actin molecules with tropomyosin and troponin molecules lying along the grooves of the actin strands. During muscle contraction, the ATP-activated heads of the thick myosin filament swivel into position, much like the oars on a boat, form a cross-bridge with a reactive site on tropomyosin, and then pull the actin filament forward. During muscle relaxation, the troponin molecules cover the reactive sites on tropomyosin.

the cross-bridges swivel in a fixed arc, much like the oars of a boat, as they become attached to the actin filament. During contraction, each cross-bridge undergoes its own cycle of movement, forming a bridge attachment and releasing it, and moving to another site where the same sequence of movement occurs. This has the effect of pulling the thin and thick filaments past each other.

Myosin is the chief constituent of the thick filament; it consists of a thin tail, which provides the structural backbone for the filament, and a globular head. Each globular head contains a binding site able to bind to a complementary site on the actin molecule. In addition to the binding site for actin, each myosin head has a separate active site that catalyzes the breakdown of ATP to provide the energy needed to activate the myosin head so it can form a cross-bridge with actin. After contraction, myosin also binds ATP as a means of breaking the linkage between actin and myosin. The myosin molecules are bundled together side by side in the thick filaments such that one half have their heads toward one end of the filament and their tails toward the other end, while the other half are arranged in the opposite manner.

The thin filaments are composed mainly of actin, a globular protein that is lined up in two rows that coil around each other to form a long helical strand. Associated with each actin filament are two regulatory proteins, tropomyosin and troponin (see Fig. 1-26). *Tropomyosin,* which lies in grooves of the actin strand, provides the site for attachment of the globular heads of the myosin filament. In the noncontractile state, *troponin* covers the tropomyosin binding sites and prevents formation of cross-bridges between the actin and myosin. During an action potential, calcium ions that are released from the sarcoplasmic reticulum diffuse to the adjacent myofibrils, where they bind to troponin. The binding of calcium to troponin uncovers the tropomyosin binding sites such that the myosin heads can attach and form cross-bridges. Energy from ATP is used to break the actin and myosin cross-bridges and terminate muscle contraction. After breaking of the linkage between actin and myosin, the concentration of calcium around the myofibrils decreases as calcium is actively transported into the sarcoplasmic reticulum by a membrane pump that uses energy derived from ATP.

Smooth Muscle

Smooth muscle is often called *involuntary muscle* because its activity arises spontaneously or through activity of the autonomic nervous system. Smooth muscle contraction usually tends to be slower and more sustained than skeletal or cardiac muscle contraction. Smooth muscle cells are spindle shaped and considerably smaller than skeletal muscle fibers. Each smooth muscle cell has one centrally positioned nucleus. There are no Z or M lines in smooth muscle fibers, and the cross-striations are absent because the bundles of filaments are not parallel but crisscross obliquely through the cell. Instead, the actin filaments are attached to structures called *dense bodies*. Some of the dense bodies are attached to the cell membrane, and others are dispersed in the cell and linked together by structural proteins (Fig. 1-27).

The lack of Z lines and regular overlapping of the contractile elements provides a greater range of tension development. This is important in hollow organs that undergo changes in volume, with consequent changes in the length of the smooth muscle fibers in their walls. Even with distention of a hollow organ, the smooth muscle fiber retains some ability to develop tension, whereas such distention would have stretched skeletal muscle beyond the area where the thick and thin filaments overlap. Smooth muscle is generally arranged in sheets or bundles. In hollow organs, such as the intestines, the bundles are organized into a two-layered muscularis externa consisting of an outer, longitudinal layer and an inner, circular layer. A thinner muscularis mucosa often lies between the muscularis externa and the endothelium. In blood vessels, the bundles are arranged in a circular or helical manner around the vessel wall. Smooth muscle differs from skeletal muscle in the way its cross-bridges are formed. In smooth muscle, calcium binds to a cytoplasmic protein, called *calmodulin*. The calcium-calmodulin complex binds to and activates the myosin-containing thick filaments, which interact with actin. The sarcoplasmic reticulum is less well developed in smooth muscle than in skeletal muscle, and there are no transverse tubules connected to the cell membrane. Smooth muscle relies on the entrance of extracellular calcium across the cell membrane and the release of calcium from the sarcoplasmic reticulum for muscle contraction. This dependence on movement of extracellular calcium across the cell membrane during muscle contraction is the basis for the action of calcium-blocking drugs that are used in treatment of cardiovascular disease.

Smooth muscle may be divided into two broad categories according to the mode of activation: multiunit and single-unit smooth muscle. In *multiunit* smooth muscle, each unit operates almost independently of the others and is often innervated by a single nerve, such as occurs in skeletal muscle. It has little or no inherent activity and

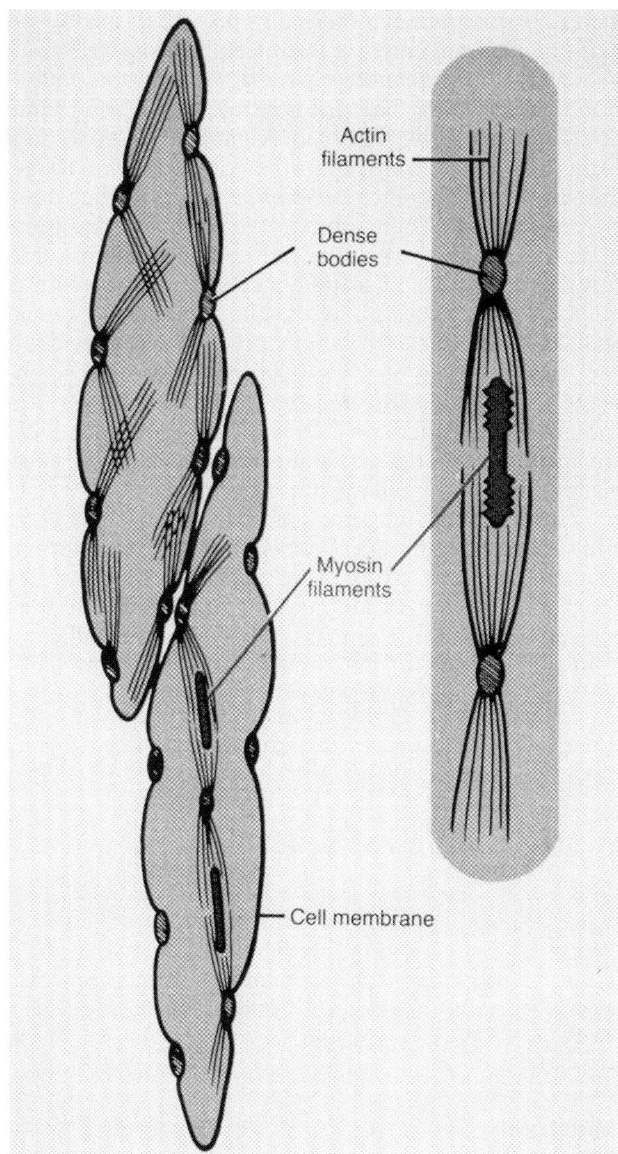

FIGURE 1-27
Physical structure of smooth muscle. Upper left-hand diagram show dense bodies. The right-hand drawing illustrates the relation of actin and myosin filaments to dense body. (Redrawn from Guyton A.C., Hall J.E. [1996]. *Textbook of medical physiology* [9th ed.]. Philadelphia; W.B. Saunders)

depends on the autonomic nervous system for its activation. Smooth muscle of this type is found in the iris, in the walls of the vas deferens, and attached to hairs in the skin. The fibers in single-unit smooth muscle are in close contact with each other and are able to contract spontaneously in the absence of nerve or hormonal stimulation. Normally, a large number of muscle fibers contract synchronously, hence the term *single-unit* smooth muscle. Some single-unit smooth muscle, such as that found in the gastrointestinal tract, is self-excitable. This is usually associated with a basic slow wave rhythm that is transmitted from cell to cell by nexus (*i.e.,* gap junctions) formed by the fusion of adjacent cell membranes. The cause of this slow wave is unknown. The intensity of contraction increases with the frequency of the action potential. Certain hormones, other agents, and local factors can modify smooth muscle activity by depolarizing or hyperpolarizing the membrane. The smooth muscle of the uterus and small-diameter blood vessels is also single-unit smooth muscle.

Nerve Tissue

Nerve tissue is distributed throughout the body as an integrated communication system. Anatomically, the nervous system is divided into the central nervous system (CNS), which consists of the brain and spinal cord, and the peripheral nervous system (PNS), composed of nerve fibers and ganglia that exist outside the CNS. Nerve cells develop from the embryonic ectoderm. Nerve cells are highly differentiated and therefore incapable of regeneration in postnatal life. The embryonic development of the nervous system and the structure and function of the nervous system is discussed more fully in Chapter 37.

Structurally, nerve tissue consists of two cell types: nerve cells or neurons and glial or supporting cells. Most nerve cells consist of three parts: the soma or cell body, dendrites, and axon. The cytoplasm-filled dendrites, which are multiple, elongated processes, receive and carry stimuli from the environment, from sensory epithelial cells, and from other neurons to the cell. The axon, which is a single cytoplasm-filled process, is specialized for generating and conducting nerve impulses away from the cell body to other nerve cells, muscle cells, and glandular cells.

Neurons can be classified as afferent and efferent neurons according to their function. Afferent or sensory neurons carry information toward the CNS; they are involved in the reception of sensory information from the external environment and from within the body. Efferent or motor neurons carry information away from the CNS; they are needed for control of muscle fibers and endocrine and exocrine glands.

Communication between neurons and effector organs such as muscle cells occurs at specialized structures called synapses, where chemical messengers (*i.e.,* neurotransmitters) alter the membrane potential as a means of conducting impulses from one nerve to another or from a neuron to a effector cell. There are also electrical synapses in which nerve cells are linked through gap junctions that permit the passage of ions from cell to another.

The neuroglia (*glia* means glue) are cells that support neurons, form myelin, and have trophic and phagocytic functions. There four types of neuroglia in the CNS: astrocytes, oligodendrocytes, microglia, and ependymal cells. Astrocytes are the most abundant of the neuroglia. They have numerous long process that surround and ensheathe blood vessels in the CNS. They provide structural support for the neurons and their extensions form a sealed barrier that protects the CNS. The oligodendrocytes provide myelination of neuronal processes in the CNS. The microglia are phagocytic cells that represent the mononuclear phagocytic system in the nervous system. The ependymal cells line the cavities of the brain and spinal cord and are in contact with the cerebrospinal fluid. In the PNS, supporting cells consist of the Schwann and satellite cells. The Schwann cells provide myelination of the axons and dendrites, and the satellite cells enclose and protect the dorsal root ganglia and autonomic ganglion cells.

Cell Junctions and Cell-to-Cell Adhesion

Cell junctions occur at many points in cell-to-cell contact, but they are particularly plentiful and important in epithelial tissue. There are at least three types of intercellular junctions: continuous tight junctions, adhering junctions, and gap junctions (Fig. 1-28). Often, the cells in epithelial tissue are joined by all three types of junctions. *Continuous tight* or *occluding junctions* (*i.e.*, zona occludens), which are found only in epithelial tissue, actually seal the surface membranes of adjacent cells together. This type of intercellular junction prevents materials such as macromolecules present in the intestinal contents from entering the intercellular space.

Adhering junctions represent a site of strong adhesion between cells. The primary role of adhering junctions appears to be that of preventing cell separation. Adhering junctions are not restricted to epithelial tissue; they provide adherence between adjacent cardiac muscle cells as well. There are two types of adhering junctions: continuous, beltlike adhesive junctions (*i.e.*, zonula adherens) and scattered, spotlike adhesive junctions, called *desmosomes* (*i.e.*, macula adherens). A special feature of the adhesion belt junction is that it provides a site for anchorage of microfilaments to the cell membrane. In epithelial desmosomes, bundles of keratin-containing intermediate filaments (*i.e.*, tonofilaments) are anchored to the desmosome attachment on the cytoplasmic area of the cell membrane.

Gap junctions, or *nexus junctions*, involve the close adherence of adjoining cell membranes with the formation of channels that link the cytoplasm of the two cells. Gap junctions are not unique to epithelial tissue; they play an essential role in many types of cell-to-cell communication. Because they are low-resistance channels, gap junctions are important in cell-to-cell conduction of

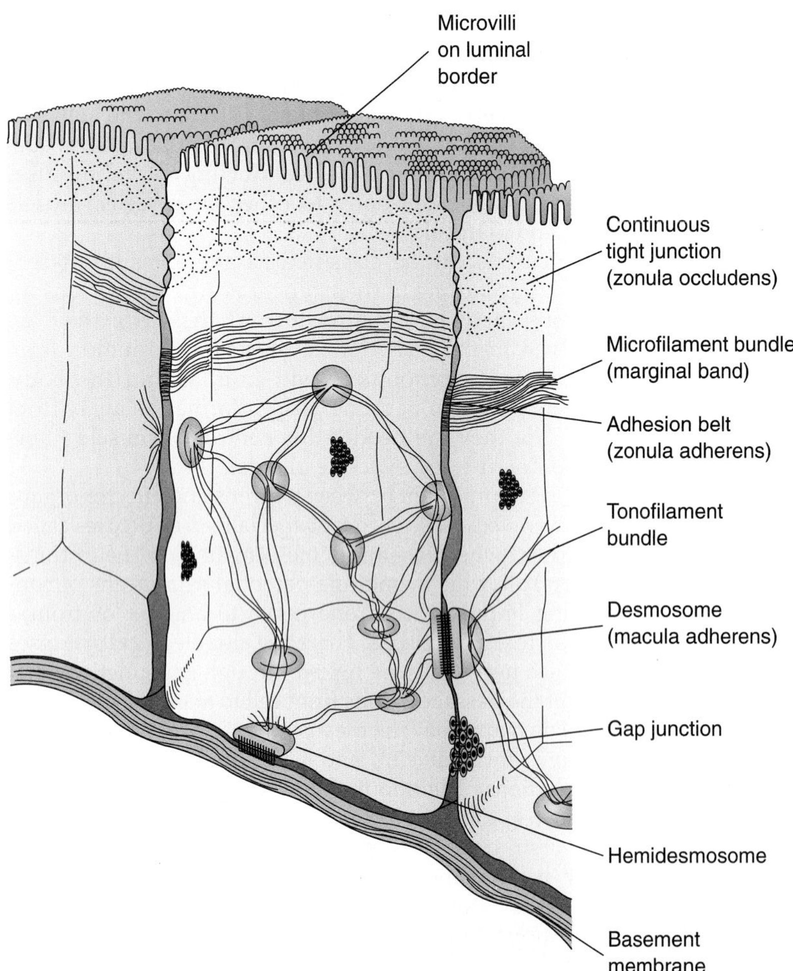

FIGURE 1-28 The chief types of intercellular junctions found in epithelial tissue.

electrical signals such as between cells in sheets of smooth muscle or between adjacent cardiac muscle cells, where they function as electrical synapses. These multiple communication channels also enable ions and small molecules to pass directly from one cell to another.

Hemidesmosomes are another type of junction. They are found at the base of epithelial cells and help attach the epithelial cell to the underlying connective tissue. They resemble one half of a desmosome; hence, their name.

Extracellular Matrix

Tissues are not made up solely of cells. A large part of their volume is made up of extracellular matrix. This matrix is composed of variety of proteins and polysaccharides (*i.e.,* a molecule made up of many sugars). These proteins and polysaccharides are secreted locally and are organized into a supporting meshwork in close association with the cells that produced them. The amount of tissue and composition of matrix varies with the different tissues and their function. In bone, for example, the matrix is more plentiful than the cells that surround it; in the brain, the cells are much more abundant and the matrix is only a minor constituent.

Two main classes of extracellular macromolecules make up the extracellular matrix. The first is composed of polysaccharide chains of a class called *glycoaminoglycans* (GAGs), which are usually found linked to protein in the form of proteoglycans. The second type consists of the fibrous proteins (*i.e.,* collagen and elastin) and the fibrous adhesive proteins (*i.e.,* fibronectin and laminin) that are found in the basement membrane. The members of each of these two classes of extracellular macromolecules come in a variety of shapes and sizes. The GAG and proteoglycan molecules in connective tissue form a highly hydrated gel-like substance, or tissue gel, in which the fibrous proteins are embedded. The polysaccharide gel resists compressive forces, the collagen fibers strengthen and help organize the matrix, the rubber-like elastin adds resilience, and the adhesive proteins help cells attach to the appropriate part of the matrix. The polysaccharides in the tissue gel are highly hydrophilic, and they form gels even at low concentrations. They also tend to accumulate a negative charge that attracts cations such as sodium, which are osmotically active, causing large amounts of water to be sucked into the matrix. This creates a swelling pressure, or turgor, that enables the matrix to withstand extensive compressive forces. This is in contrast to collagen, which resists stretching forces. For example, the cartilage matrix that lines the knee joint can support pressures of hundreds of atmospheres by this mechanism.

The amount of GAG and proteoglycan molecules in connective tissue usually constitutes less than 10% by weight of fibrous tissue. Because they form a hydrated gel, the molecules fill most of the extracellular space, providing mechanical support to the tissues while ensuring rapid diffusion of water and electrolytes and the migration of cells. One of the GAGs, hyaluronan or hyaluronic acid, is thought to play an important role as a space filler during embryonic development. It creates a cell-free space into which cells subsequently migrate. When cell migration and organ development are complete, the excess hyaluronan is degraded by the enzyme hyaluronidase. Hyaluronan is also important in directing the cell replacement that occurs during wound repair.

There are three types of fibers in the extracellular space: collagen, elastin, and reticular fibers. *Collagen* is the most common protein in the body; it is a tough, nonliving, white fiber that serves as the structural framework for skin, ligaments, tendons, and numerous other structures. *Elastin* acts like a rubber band; it can be stretched and then return to its original form. Elastin fibers are abundant in structures that are subjected to frequent stretching, such as the aorta and some ligaments. *Reticular fibers* are extremely thin fibers that create a flexible network in organs that are subjected to changes in form or volume, such as the spleen, liver, uterus, or intestinal muscle layer.

In summary, body cells are organized into four basic tissue types: epithelial, connective, muscle, and nervous. The epithelium covers and lines the body surfaces and forms the functional components of glandular structures. Epithelial tissue is classified into three types according to the shape of the cells and the number of layers that are present: simple, stratified, and pseudostratified. The cells in epithelial tissue are held together by three types of intercellular junctions: tight, adhering, and gap. They are attached to the underlying tissue by hemidesmosomes. Connective tissue supports and connects body structures; it forms the bones and skeletal system, the joint structures, the blood cells, and the intercellular substances. Adult connective tissue can be divided into four types: loose or areolar, reticular, adipose, and dense (regular and irregular).

Muscle tissue is a specialized tissue that is designed for contractility. There are three types of muscle tissue: skeletal, cardiac, and smooth. Actin and myosin filaments interact to produce muscle shortening, a process activated by the presence of calcium. In skeletal muscle, calcium is released from the sarcoplasmic reticulum in response to an action potential. Smooth muscle is often referred to as involuntary muscle because it contracts spontaneously or through activity of the autonomic nervous system. It differs from skeletal muscle in that it has a less well-defined sarcoplasmic reticulum and depends on entry of extracellular calcium ions for muscle contraction.

Nervous tissue is designed for communication purposes and includes the neurons, the supporting neural structures, and the ependymal cells that line the ventricles of the brain and the spinal canal.

The extracellular matrix is made up of a variety of proteins and polysaccharides. These proteins and polysaccharides are secreted locally and are organized into a supporting meshwork in close association with the cells that produced them. The amount of tissue and composition of matrix varies with the different tissues and their function. Extracellular fibers include collagen fibers, which comprise tendons and ligaments; elastic fibers found in large arteries and some ligaments; and thin reticular fibers, which are plentiful in organs that are subject to a change in volume (*e.g.*, spleen and liver).

BIBLIOGRAPHY

Alberts B., Bray D., Lewis J., Raff M., Roberts K., Watson J. (1994). *Molecular Biology of the Cell* (3rd ed.). New York: Garland Publishing.

Brown A.M., Birnbaumer L. (1989). Ion channels and G proteins. *Hospital Practice* 24 (7), 189–204.

Cormack D.H. (1993). *Essential histology* (pp. 2–120). Philadelphia: J.B. Lippincott.

Cotran S.L., Kumar R.S., Robbins S.L. (1994). *Robbins' pathologic basis of disease* (4th ed., pp. 28, 100, 110). Philadelphia: W.B. Saunders.

Glover D.M., Gonzalez C., Raff J.W. (1993). The centrosome. *Scientific American* 268 (6), 62–68.

Guyton A. (1996). *Medical physiology* (9th ed., pp. 11–24). Philadelphia: W.B. Saunders.

Johns D.R. (1995). Mitochondrial DNA and disease. *New England Jounal of Medicine* 33 (10), 638.

Nasmyth K. (1996). Viewpoint: Putting the cell cycle in order. *Science* 274, 1643–1645.

Oakley B.R., Oakley C.E. (1995). Tubulin and microtubules. *Scientific American* 272 (1), 58–67.

Ross M.H., Romrell L.J, Kaye G.I. (1995). *Histology: A text and atlas* (Chapters 2–5, 10). Baltimore: Williams and Wilkins.

Rothman J.E., Orci L. (1996). Budding vesicles in living cells. *Scientific American*. 274 (3), 70–75.

Sharon N., Lis H. (1993). Carbohydrates in cell recognition. *Scientific American* 268 (1), 82–88.

Stevens A., Lowe J. (1997). *Histology* (Chapters 2–6). New York: Gower Medical Publishing.

CHAPTER 2

Cellular Adaptation, Injury, and Death and Wound Healing

When confronted with stresses that tend to disrupt its normal structure and function, the cell undergoes adaptive changes that permit survival and maintenance of function. It is only when the stress is overwhelming or adaptation is ineffective that cell injury and death occur. This chapter focuses on cellular adaptation, cell injury and death, and wound healing.

Cellular Adaptation

After you have completed this section of the chapter, you should be able to meet the following objectives:

- Cite the general purpose of changes in cell structure and function that occur as the result of normal adaptive processes
- Describe cell changes that occur with atrophy, hypertrophy, hyperplasia, metaplasia, and dysplasia and state general conditions under which the changes occur

Cells adapt to changes in the internal environment, just as the total organism adapts to changes in the external environment. Cells may adapt by undergoing changes in size, number, and type. These changes, occurring singly or in combination, may lead to atrophy, hypertrophy, hyperplasia, metaplasia, and dysplasia (Fig. 2-1). Whether adaptive cellular changes are normal or abnormal depends on whether the response was mediated by an appropriate stimulus. Normal adaptive responses occur in response to need and an appropriate stimulus. After the need has been removed, the adaptive response ceases.

Atrophy

When confronted with a decrease in work demands or adverse environmental conditions, most cells are able to revert to a smaller size and a lower and more efficient level of functioning that is compatible with survival. This decrease in cell size is called *atrophy*. Cell size, particularly in muscle tissue, is related to work load. As the work load of a cell diminishes, oxygen consumption and protein synthesis decrease. Cells that are atrophied reduce their oxygen consumption and other cellular functions by decreasing the number and size of their organelles and other structures. There are fewer mitochondria, myofilaments, and endoplasmic reticulum structures. When a sufficient number of cells are involved, the entire tissue or muscle atrophies.[1]

The general causes of atrophy can be grouped into five categories: disuse, denervation, lack of endocrine stimulation, decreased nutrition, and ischemia or a decrease in blood flow. Disuse atrophy occurs when there is a reduction in skeletal muscle use. An extreme example of disuse atrophy is seen in the muscles of

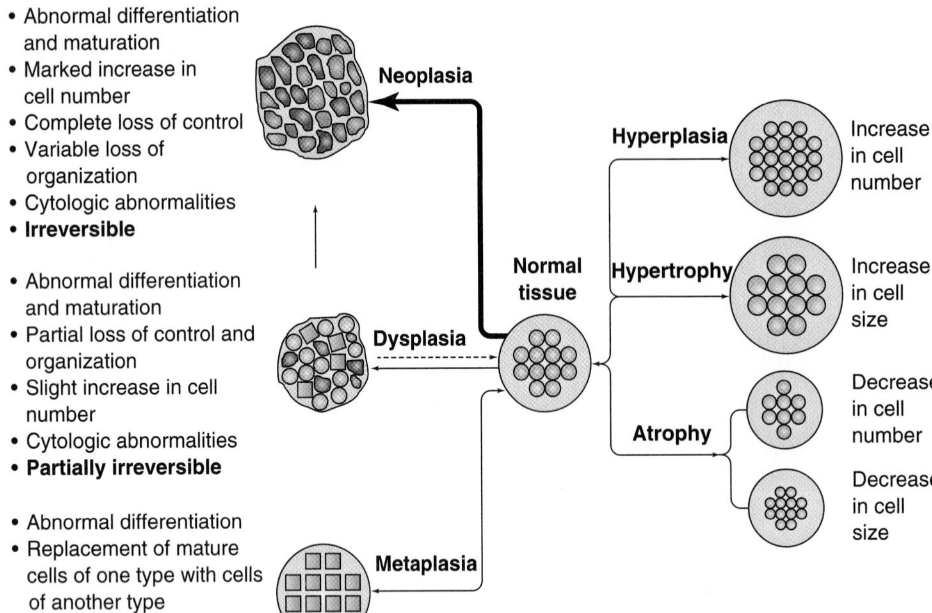

Figure 2-1 Abnormalities of cell growth and maturation. (Chandrasoma P., Taylor C.R. [1995]. *Concise pathology* [2nd ed.]. Norwalk, CT: Appleton and Lange)

extremities that have been encased in plaster casts. Because atrophy is adaptive and reversible, muscle size is restored after the cast is removed and muscle use is resumed. Denervation atrophy is a form of disuse atrophy that occurs in the muscles of paralyzed limbs. A lack of endocrine stimulation also produces a form of disuse atrophy. In women, the loss of estrogen stimulation during menopause results in atrophic changes in the reproductive organs. With malnutrition and decreased blood flow, cells decrease their size and energy requirements as a means of survival.

In some cases, atrophy is accompanied by the presence of a yellow-brown intracellular pigment called *lipofuscin*. This form of atrophy is referred to as *brown atrophy*. The discoloration represents the accumulation of indigestible residues resulting from destruction of cell components (*e.g.*, mitochondria, endoplasmic reticulum). The accumulation of lipofuscin increases with age, and it is sometimes referred to as the wear-and-tear pigment. It is seen more commonly in heart, nerve, and liver cells than in other types of tissue. Lipofuscin is not injurious to cell structure or function.

Hypertrophy

Hypertrophy represents an increase in cell size and with it an increase in the amount of functioning tissue mass. It results from an increased work load imposed on an organ or body part and is commonly seen in cardiac and skeletal muscle tissue, which cannot adapt to an increase in work load through mitotic division and formation of more cells. Hypertrophy involves an increase in the functional components of the cell that allows it to achieve an equilibrium between demand and functional capacity. For example, as muscle cells hypertrophy, additional actin and myosin filaments, cell enzymes, and adenosine triphosphate (ATP) are synthesized.

Hypertrophy may occur as the result of normal physiologic or abnormal pathologic conditions. The increase in muscle mass associated with exercise is an example of physiologic hypertrophy. Pathologic hypertrophy occurs as the result of disease conditions and may be adaptive or compensatory. Examples of adaptive hypertrophy are the thickening of the urinary bladder from long-continued obstruction of urinary outflow and the myocardial hypertrophy that results from valvular heart disease or hypertension. Compensatory hypertrophy is the enlargement of a remaining organ or tissue after a portion has been surgically removed or rendered inactive. For instance, if one kidney is removed, the remaining kidney enlarges to compensate for the loss.

The precise signal for hypertrophy is unknown. It may be related to ATP depletion, stretching of muscle fibers, activation of cell degradation products, or hormonal factors.[1] Whatever the mechanism, a limit is eventually reached beyond which further enlargement of the tissue mass is no longer able to compensate for the increased work demands. The limiting factors for continued hypertrophy may be related to limitations in blood flow. In hypertension, for example, the increased work load required to pump blood against an elevated arterial pressure results in a progressive increase in left ventricular muscle mass. Eventually, the heart is no longer able to maintain sufficient blood flow to compensate for the increased burden, and heart failure ensues.

Hyperplasia

Hyperplasia refers to an increase in the number of cells in an organ or tissue. It occurs in tissues with cells that are capable of mitotic division, such as the epidermis, intestinal epithelium, and glandular tissue. Nerve cells and skeletal and cardiac muscle do not divide and therefore have no capacity for hyperplastic growth. There is evidence that hyperplasia involves activation of genes controlling cell proliferation and the use of polypeptide growth hormones. As with other normal adaptive cellular responses, hyperplasia is a controlled process that occurs in response to an appropriate stimulus and ceases after the stimulus has been removed.

The stimuli that induce hyperplasia may be physiologic or nonphysiologic. There are two common types of physiologic hyperplasia: hormonal and compensatory. Breast and uterine enlargement during pregnancy are examples of a physiologic hyperplasia that results from estrogen stimulation. The regeneration the liver that occurs after partial hepatectomy (*i.e.*, partial removal of the liver) is an example of compensatory hyperplasia. Nonphysiologic hyperplasia occurs in response to abnormal hormonal stimulation of target cells. Excessive estrogen production can cause endometrial hyperplasia and abnormal menstrual bleeding. Although hypertrophy and hyperplasia are two distinct processes, they may occur together and are often triggered by the same mechanism.[1] For example, the pregnant uterus undergoes hypertrophy and hyperplasia as the result of estrogen stimulation. Hyperplasia is also an important response of connective tissue in wound healing, during which proliferating fibroblasts and blood vessels contribute to wound repair.

Metaplasia

Metaplasia represents the conversion from one adult cell type to another adult cell type. Metaplasia is thought to involve the reprogramming of undifferentiated or stem cells present in the tissue undergoing the metaplastic changes.

Metaplasia usually occurs in response to chronic irritation and inflammation and allows for substitution of cells that are better able to survive under circumstances in which a more fragile cell type might succumb. However, the conversion of cell types never oversteps the boundaries of the primary groups of tissue (*e.g.*, one type of epithelial cell may be converted to another type of epithelial cell but not to a connective tissue cell). An example of metaplasia is the adaptive substitution of stratified squamous epithelial cells for the ciliated columnar epithelial cells in the trachea and large airways of a habitual cigarette smoker. A vitamin A deficiency also induces squamous metaplasia of the respiratory tract. Although the squamous epithelium is better able to survive in these situations, the protective function that the ciliated epithelium provides for the respiratory tract is lost. Continued exposure to the influences that cause metaplasia may predispose to cancerous transformation of the metaplastic epithelium.

Dysplasia

Dysplasia is characterized by deranged cell growth of a specific tissue that results in cells that vary in size, shape, and appearance. Minor degrees of dysplasia are associated with chronic irritation or inflammation. The pattern is most frequently encountered in metaplastic squamous epithelium of the respiratory tract and uterine cervix. Although dysplasia is abnormal, it is adaptive in that it is potentially reversible after the irritating cause has been found and removed. Dysplasia is strongly implicated as a precursor of cancer. In cancer of respiratory tract and cancer of uterine cervix, dysplastic changes have been found adjacent to the foci of cancerous transformation. Through the use of the Papanicolaou (Pap) smear, it has been documented that cancer of uterine cervix develops in a series of incremental epithelial changes ranging from severe dysplasia to invasive cancer. However, dysplasia is an adaptive process and as such does not necessarily lead to cancer. In many cases, the dysplastic cells will revert to their former structure and function.

In summary, cells adapt to changes in their environment and in their work demands by changing their size, number, and characteristics. When confronted with a decrease in work demands or adverse environmental conditions, cells *atrophy* or reduce their size and revert to a lower and more efficient level of functioning. *Hypertrophy* represents an increase in tissue size brought about by an increase in cell size and functional components within the cell. An increase in the number of cells in an organ or tissue that is still capable of mitotic division is called *hyperplasia.*

Metaplasia occurs in response to chronic irritation and represents the substitution of cells of a type that are better able to survive under circumstances in which a more fragile cell type might succumb. *Dysplasia* is characterized by deranged cell growth of a specific tissue that results in cells that vary in size, shape, and appearance. It is a precursor of cancer. These adaptive changes are consistent with the needs of the cell and occur in response to an appropriate stimulus. The changes are usually reversed after the stimulus has been withdrawn.

Cell Injury and Death

After you have completed this section of the chapter, you should be able to meet the following objectives:

- Describe three types of reversible cell changes that can occur with cell injury and those that result from inborn errors of metabolism

- Define *free radical* and relate free radical formation to cell injury and death
- Describe cell changes that occur with hypoxic cell injury
- Describe the mechanism of electrical injury, and thermal injury
- Explain how injurious effects of biologic agents differ from those produced by physical and chemical agents
- Differentiate between the effects of ionizing and nonionizing radiation in terms of their ability to cause cell injury
- State how nutritional imbalances contribute to cell injury
- Differentiate cell death associated with necrosis and apoptosis
- Cite the reasons for the changes that occur with the wet and dry forms of gangrene
- Compare the outcomes of intracellular accumulations from various systemic disorders

Cells can be injured in many ways. The extent to which any injurious agent can cause cell injury and death depends in large measure on the intensity and duration of the injury and the type of cell that is involved. When cells are injured or the need to adapt becomes overwhelming, degenerative changes begin to appear.

Degeneration is a process in which cellular deterioration occurs along with changes in the chemical structure and microscopic appearance of the cell. Degeneration can follow many paths that eventually lead to cell changes, some of which are reversible and others irreversible. Irreversible changes consist of necrosis (*i.e.*, cell death) and tissue dissolution. Whether a specific stress causes irreversible or reversible cell injury depends on the severity of the insult and on many cellular characteristics, including their particular vulnerability, blood supply, nutritional status, and previous reserves and state of functioning. Cell degeneration and cell death are ongoing processes, and in the healthy state, they are balanced by cell renewal.

Causes of Cell Injury

Cell damage can occur in many ways. For purposes of discussion, the ways by which cells are injured have been grouped into five categories: injury from physical agents, radiation injury, chemical injury, injury from biologic agents, and injury from nutritional imbalances.

Injury From Physical Agents

Physical agents responsible for cell and tissue injury include mechanical forces, extremes of temperature, and electrical forces.

Mechanical Forces. Injury due to mechanical forces occurs as the result of body impact with another object. The body or the mass can be in motion, or as sometimes happens, both can be in motion at the time of impact. These types of injuries split and tear tissue, fracture bones, injure blood vessels, and disrupt blood flow.

Extremes of Temperature. Extremes of heat and cold cause damage to the cell, its organelles, and its enzyme systems. Exposure to low-intensity heat (43° to 46°C), such as occurs with partial-thickness burns and severe heat stroke, causes cell injury by inducing vascular injury, accelerating cell metabolism, inactivating temperature-sensitive enzymes, and disrupting the cell membrane. With more intense heat, coagulation of blood vessels and tissue proteins occurs. Exposure to cold induces vasoconstriction by direct action on blood vessels and through reflex activity of the sympathetic nervous system. The resultant decrease in blood flow may lead to hypoxic tissue injury, depending on the degree and duration of cold exposure. Injury from freezing is probably a combination of ice crystal formation and vasoconstriction. The decreased blood flow leads to capillary stasis and arteriolar and capillary thrombosis. Edema results from increased capillary permeability.

Electrical Injuries. Electrical injuries can affect the body through extensive tissue injury and disruption of neural and cardiac impulses. The effect of electricity on the body is mainly determined by its voltage, the type of current (*i.e.*, direct or alternating), its amperage, the resistance of the intervening tissue, the pathway of the current, and the duration of exposure.[2,3]

Lightening and high-voltage wires that carry several thousand volts produce the most severe damage.[2] Alternating current (AC) is usually more dangerous than direct current (DC), because it causes violent muscle contractions, preventing release of the electrical source and sometimes resulting in fractures and dislocations. In electrical injuries, the body acts as a conductor of the electrical current; the current enters the body from an electrical source such as an exposed wire and passes through the body and exits to another conductor, such as the moisture on the ground or a piece of metal the person is holding. The pathway that a current takes is critical, because the electrical energy disrupts impulses in excitable tissues. Current flow through the brain may interrupt impulses from respiratory centers in the brain stem, and current flow through the chest may cause fatal cardiac arrhythmias.

In electrical circuits, resistance to the flow of current transforms electrical energy into heat. This is why the elements in electrical heating devices are made of highly resistive metals. Much of the tissue damage produced by electrical injuries is caused by heat production in tissues that have the highest electrical resistance. Resistance to electrical current varies from the greatest to the least in bone, fat, tendons, skin, muscles, blood, and nerves. The most severe tissue injury usually occurs at the skin sites where the current enters and leaves the body. After electricity has penetrated the skin, it passes rapidly through the body along the lines of least resistance—through body fluids and nerves. Degeneration of vessel walls may occur, and thrombi may form as current flows along the blood vessels. This can cause extensive muscle and deep tissue injury. Thick, dry skin is more resistant to the flow of electricity than thin, wet skin. It is generally believed that the greater the skin resistance, the greater is the amount of local skin burn; the less the resistance, the greater is the deep and systemic effects.

Radiation Injury

Electromagnetic radiation comprises a wide spectrum of wave-propagated energy, ranging from ionizing gamma rays to radiofrequency waves (Fig. 2-2).[2,4] A photon is a particle of radiation energy. Radiation energy above the ultraviolet range is called *ionizing radiation* because the photons have enough energy to knock electrons off atoms and molecules. Radiation energy at frequencies below that of visible light is often referred to as *nonionizing radiation.* Ultraviolet radiation represents the portion of the spectrum of electromagnetic radiation just above the visible range. It contains increasingly energetic rays that are powerful enough to disrupt intracellular bonds and cause sunburn (discussed in Chapter 15).

Ionizing Radiation. Ionizing radiation affects cells by causing ionization of molecules and atoms within the cells by directly hitting the target molecules or by producing free radicals that interact with critical cell components. It can immediately kill cells, interrupt cell replication, or cause a variety of mutations, which may or may not be lethal. The cell's initial response to radiation exposure is characterized by swelling, disruption of the mitochondria and other organelles, alterations in the cell membrane, and marked changes in the nucleus. Because of the effect on deoxyribonucleic acid DNA synthesis and interference with the mitotic process, rapidly dividing cells such as those of the bone marrow and gastrointestinal epithelium are more susceptible to radiation injury than nondividing cells. Because cancer cells are rapidly proliferating cells, radiation therapy is often used in treating cancer (see Chapter 5).

Dose-dependent vascular changes occur in all irradiated tissues. During the immediate postirradiation period, only vessel dilatation takes place (*e.g.,* the initial erythema of the skin after radiotherapy). Later or with higher levels of radiation, destructive changes occur in small blood vessels such as the capillaries and venules.

At relatively low doses, normal cells and cancer cells are able to repair radiation damage. If, however, cell recovery is not complete at the time of the next exposure, there may be additional damage. The importance of cell repair in protecting against radiation injury is evidenced by the vulnerability of persons who lack enzymes to repair ultraviolet-induced defects in DNA replication. In a genetic disorder called *xeroderma pigmentosum,* an enzyme needed to repair sunlight-induced defects in DNA replication is lacking, predisposing the affected person to skin cancer at a very early age.

Nonionizing Radiation. Nonionizing radiation includes infrared light, ultrasound, microwaves, and laser energy. Unlike ionizing radiation, which can directly break chemical bonds, nonionizing radiation exerts its effects by causing vibrations and rotations of atoms and molecules. All of this vibrational and rotational energy is eventually converted to thermal energy. Low-frequency nonionizing radiation is used widely in radar, television, industrial operations (*e.g,* heating, welding, melting of metals, processing of wood and plastic), household appliances (*e.g.,* microwave ovens), and medical applications (*e.g.,* diathermy). Isolated cases of skin burns and thermal injury to deeper tissues have occurred in industrial settings and from improperly used household microwave ovens. Injury from these sources is mainly thermal and, because of the deep penetration of the infrared or microwave rays, tends to involve subcutaneous and dermal injury.

Chemical Injury

Chemicals capable of damaging cells are everywhere around us. Air and water pollution yield chemicals capable of tissue injury, as does tobacco smoke and chemicals contained in foods. Some of the most damaging chemicals exist in our environment, including gases such as carbon monoxide, insecticides, and trace metals such as lead.

Chemical agents can injure the cell membrane and other cell structures, block enzymatic pathways, coagulate cell proteins, and disrupt the osmotic and ionic

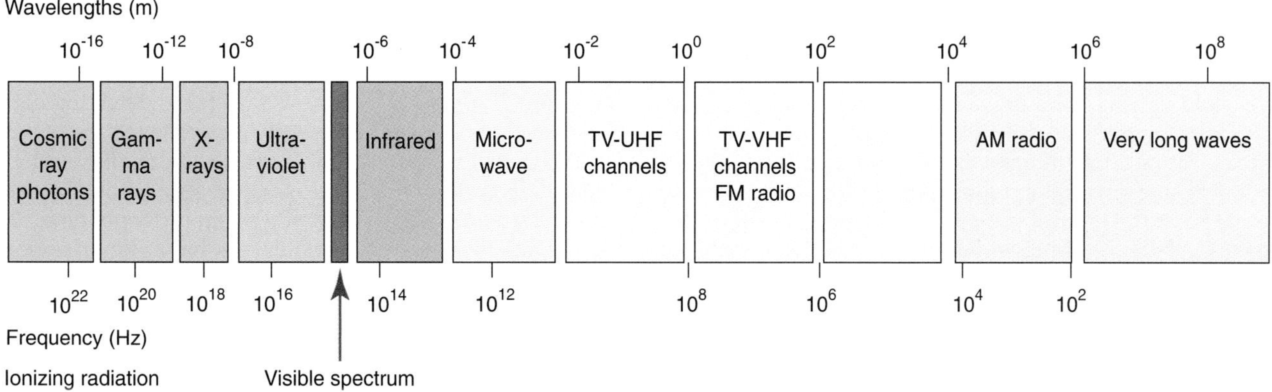

Figure 2-2
Spectrum of electromagnetic radiation.

balance of the cell. Corrosive substances such as strong acids and bases destroy cells as the substances come into contact with the body. Other chemicals may injure cells in the process of metabolism or elimination. Carbon tetrachloride (CCl_4), for example, causes little damage until it is metabolized by liver enzymes to a highly reactive free radical ($CCl_3\cdot$). Carbon tetrachloride is extremely toxic to liver cells. Still other types of chemicals are selective in their sites of action.

Drugs. Many drugs–alcohol, prescription drugs, over-the-counter drugs, and street drugs–are capable of directly or indirectly damaging tissues. Ethyl alcohol can harm the gastric mucosa, liver (see Chapter 32), the developing fetus (see Chapter 4), and other organs. Antineoplastic and immunosuppressant drugs can directly injure cells. Other drugs produce metabolic end products that are toxic to cells. Acetaminophen, a commonly used analgesic drug, is detoxified in the liver, where small amounts of the drug are converted to a highly toxic metabolite. This metabolite is detoxified by interaction with a substance (*i.e.*, glutathione) normally present in the liver. When large amounts of the drug are ingested, toxic metabolites accumulate, causing massive liver necrosis, usually 3 to 5 days after ingestion of a toxic dose.

Lead Toxicity. Lead is a particularly toxic metal. Small amounts accumulate to reach toxic levels. There are innumerable sources of lead in the environment, including flaking paint, lead-contaminated dust and soil, lead-contaminated root vegetables, lead water pipes or soldered joints, pottery glazes, and newsprint.[1] Adults often encounter lead through occupational exposure. Lead and other metal smelter workers, miners, welders, storage battery workers, and pottery makers are particularly at risk.[5,6] Children are exposed to lead through ingestion of peeling lead paint, by breathing dust from lead paint (*e.g.*, during remodeling), or from playing in contaminated soil. There has been a substantial decline in blood lead levels of the entire population since the removal of lead from gasoline and removal of lead from soldered food cans.[7] However, high lead blood levels continue to be a problem, particularly among children. In the Third National Health and Nutrition Examination Survey (NHANES III, 1988 to 1991), blood lead levels were highest in 1- to 2-year-old children and lowest in 12- to 19-year-old youths.[7] The prevalence of elevated blood lead levels is higher for children living in more urbanized areas. By race or ethnicity, non-Hispanic black children residing in central cities with a population of 1 million or more have the highest proportion of elevated blood lead levels. A high percentage of Mexican-American children living in the most urbanized areas also had elevated lead levels.[8]

Lead is absorbed through the gastrointestinal tract or through the lungs into the blood. Urban adults have a daily intake of about 100 to 150 μg of which about 10% is absorbed. A deficiency in calcium, iron, or zinc increases lead absorption. In children, most lead is absorbed through the lungs. Although children may have the same or a lower intake of lead, about 50% of lead is absorbed.[1] Lead crosses the placenta, exposing the fetus to levels of lead that are comparable to those of the mother. Lead is stored in bone and eliminated by the kidneys. About 85% of absorbed lead is stored in bone (and teeth of young children); 5% to 10% remains in the blood; and the remainder accumulates in soft tissue deposits. Although the half-life of lead is hours to days, bone deposits serve a repository from which blood levels are maintained. In a sense, bone protects other tissues, but the slow turnover maintains blood levels for months to years.

Lead poisons enzymes by binding to sulfhydryl groups and denaturing proteins. It also binds to transfer RNA (tRNA) and causes derangement of second messenger systems in the nervous system. Major targets are red blood cells, the nervous system, the gastrointestinal tract, and the kidneys. Lead causes a microcytic, hypochromic, and mild hemolytic anemia with basophilic stippling.

Lead toxicity is characterized in the nervous system by demyelination of cerebral and cerebellar white matter and death of cortical cells. When this occurs in early childhood, it can affect neurobehavioral development and result in lower intelligence and poorer classroom performance.[9] Peripheral demyelinating neuropathy may occur in adults. The most serious manifestation of lead poisoning is acute encephalopathy. It is manifested by persistent vomiting, ataxia, seizures, papilledema, impaired consciousness, and coma. Acute encephalopathy may manifest suddenly, or it may be preceded by other signs of lead toxicity such as behavioral changes or abdominal complaints.

The gastrointestinal tract is the main source of symptoms in the adult. This is characterized by "lead colic," a severe and poorly localized form of acute abdominal pain. A lead line formed by precipitated lead sulfite may appear along the gingival margins. The lead line is seldom seen in children.

The kidneys are affected less than the blood, but a chronic tubulointerstitial nephritis may develop. It is characterized by glycosuria, aminoaciduria, and phosphaturia (*i.e.*, Fanconi's syndrome) from altered tubular transport mechanisms.

Lead damages an enzyme needed for heme synthesis in red blood cells; this results in an increase in erythrocyte protoporphyrin (EP). Screening for lead toxicity involves use of capillary blood obtained from a finger stick to measure free EP levels. The EP test is useful in detecting high lead levels but does not usually detect levels below 20 to 25 μg/dL. This test also reflects the effects of iron deficiency, a condition that increases lead absorption.[10] A safe blood level of lead is still uncertain. At one time, 25 μg/dL was considered safe. Surveys have shown abnormally low IQ levels in children with levels as low as 10 to 15 μg; in 1991, the safe level was lowered to 10 μg/dL.[10]

Diagnosis of lead toxicity is often delayed. Anemia may provide the first clues to the disorder. Laboratory tests are necessary to establish a diagnosis. Measurement of lead levels in venous blood is usually employed. Treatment involves removal of the lead source and, in cases of severe toxicity, administration of a chelating agent. Asymptomatic children with blood levels of 45 to 69 μg/dL are usually treated. A public health team should evaluate the source of lead, because meticulous removal is needed.

Injury From Biologic Agents

Biologic agents differ from other injurious agents in that they are able to replicate and can continue to produce their injurious effects. These agents range from submicroscopic viruses to the larger parasites. Biologic agents injure cells by diverse mechanisms. Viruses enter the cell and become incorporated into its DNA synthetic machinery. Certain bacteria elaborate exotoxins that interfere with cellular production of ATP. Other bacteria, such as the gram-negative bacilli, release endotoxins that cause cell injury and increased capillary permeability. Other microorganisms produce their effects through inflammatory or immune mechanisms. Infectious processes are discussed in Chapter 10.

Injury From Nutritional Imbalances

Nutritional excesses and nutritional deficiencies predispose cells to injury. Obesity and diets high in saturated fats are thought to predispose persons to atherosclerosis. The body requires more than 60 organic and inorganic substances in amounts ranging from micrograms to grams. These nutrients include minerals, vitamins, certain fatty acids, and specific amino acids. Dietary deficiencies can occur in the form of starvation, in which there is a deficiency of all nutrients and vitamins, or because of a selective deficiency of a single nutrient or vitamin. Iron-deficiency anemia, scurvy, beriberi, and pellagra are examples of injury caused by the lack of specific vitamins or minerals. The protein and calorie deficiencies that occur with starvation cause widespread tissue damage.

Mechanisms of Cell Injury

The mechanisms by which injurious agent cause cell injury and death are complex. Some agents, such as heat, produce direct cell injury; other factors, such as genetic derangements, produce their effects indirectly through metabolic disturbances and altered immune responses. There seem to be at least three major mechanisms whereby most injurious agents exert their effects: free radical formation, hypoxia and ATP depletion, and disruption of intracellular calcium homeostasis.

Free Radical Injury

Many injurious agents exert their damaging effects through a reactive chemical species called a *free radical*.[11–13] Free radical injury is rapidly emerging as a final common pathway for tissue damage by many injurious agents.

In most atoms, the outer electron orbits are filled with paired electrons moving in opposite directions to balance their spin. A free radical is a highly reactive chemical species arising from an atom that has one or more unpaired electrons in its outer orbit. In this state, the radical is highly unstable and can enter into reactions with cellular constituents, particularly key molecules in cell membranes and nucleic acids. Moreover, free radicals can establish chain reactions, sometimes thousands of events long, as the molecules they react with form free radicals. Chain reactions may branch, causing even greater damage. Uncontrolled free radical production causes damage to cell membranes, cross-linking of cell proteins, inactivation of enzyme systems, or damage to the nucleic acids that make up DNA.

Free radical formation is a byproduct of many normal cellular reactions within the body, including energy generation, breakdown of lipids and proteins, and inflammatory processes. For example, free radical generation is the main mechanism for killing microbes in phagocytic white blood cells. Oxygen, with its two unpaired outer electrons, is the most frequent source of free radicals. During the course of normal cell metabolism, cells process energy-producing oxygen into water; in some reactions, a superoxide radical is formed. Lipid oxidation (*i.e.*, peroxidation) is another source of free radicals. In this case, an oxygen free radical combines with free fatty acids to form water and a carbon-centered free radical. Carbon-centered free radicals form branching reactions that oxidize cholesterol, alter proteins, and impair the function of critical cell enzymes and receptors.

Exogenous sources of free radicals include tobacco smoke, certain pollutants and organic solvents, hyperoxic environments, pesticides, and radiation. Some of these compounds and certain medications are metabolized to free radical intermediates that cause oxidative damage to target tissues.

Under normal conditions, most cells have chemical mechanisms that protect them from the injurious effects of free radicals. These mechanisms commonly break down when the cell is deprived of oxygen or exposed to certain chemical agents, radiation, or other injurious agents. Free radical formation is a particular threat to tissues in which the blood flow has been interrupted and then restored. During the period of interrupted flow, the intracellular mechanisms that control free radicals are inactivated or damaged. When blood flow is restored, the cell is suddenly confronted with an excess of free radicals that it cannot control.

Scientists continue to investigate the use of free radical scavengers to protect against cell injury during periods when protective cellular mechanisms are impaired. Defenses against free radicals include vitamin E, vitamin C, and β-carotene.[12] Vitamin E is the major lipid-soluble antioxidant present in all cellular membranes. Vitamin C is an important water-soluble cytosolic chain-breaking antioxidant; it acts directly with superoxide and singlet oxygen radicals. β-Carotene, a pigment found in most plants, reacts with singlet oxygen and can also function as an antioxidant.

Hypoxic Cell Injury

Hypoxia deprives the cell of oxygen and interrupts oxidative metabolism and the generation of ATP. The actual time necessary to produce irreversible cell damage depends on the degree of oxygen deprivation and the metabolic needs of the cell. Well-differentiated cells such as those in the heart, brain, and kidney require large amounts of oxygen to provide energy for their special functions. Brain cells, for example, begin to undergo permanent damage after 4 to 6 minutes of oxygen deprivation. A thin margin can exist between the time involved in reversible and irreversible cell damage. One study found that the epithelial cells of the proximal tubule of the kidney in the rat could survive 20 but not 30 minutes of ischemia.[14]

Hypoxia can result from an inadequate amount of oxygen in the air, respiratory disease, ischemia (*i.e.*, decreased blood flow due to circulatory disorders), anemia, edema, or inability of the cells to use oxygen. Ischemia is characterized by impaired oxygen delivery and impaired removal of metabolic end products such as lactic acid. In contrast to pure hypoxia, which affects the oxygen content of the blood and affects all of the cells in the body, ischemia commonly affects blood flow through small numbers of blood vessels and produces local tissue injury. In cases of edema, the distance for diffusion of oxygen may become a limiting factor. In hypermetabolic states, the cells may require more oxygen than can be supplied by normal respiratory function and oxygen transport. Hypoxia also serves as the ultimate cause of cell death in other injuries. For example, toxins from certain microorganisms interfere with cellular use of oxygen, and a physical agent such as cold causes severe vasoconstriction and impairs blood flow.

Hypoxia causes a power failure within the cell, with widespread effects on the cell's functional and structural components. As oxygen tension within the cell falls, oxidative metabolism ceases, and the cell reverts to anaerobic metabolism, using the cell's limited glycogen stores in an attempt to maintain vital cell functions. Cellular pH falls as lactic acid accumulates within the cell. This reduction in pH can have profound effects on intracellular structures. The nuclear chromatin clumps, and myelin figures, which derive from destructive changes in cell membranes and intracellular structures, are seen within the cytoplasm and extracellular spaces.

One of the earliest effects of reduced ATP is acute cellular swelling caused by failure of the energy-dependent sodium-potassium membrane pump, which extrudes sodium from and returns potassium to the cell. With impaired function of this pump, intracellular potassium levels decrease, and sodium and water accumulate within the cell. The movement of fluid and ions into the cell is associated with dilatation of the endoplasmic reticulum, increased membrane permeability, and decreased mitochondrial function.[1]

To this point, the cellular changes are reversible if oxygenation is restored. If the oxygen supply is not restored, however, there is a continued loss of essential enzymes, proteins, and ribonucleic acid through the hyperpermeable membrane of the cell. Injury to the lysosomal membranes results in leakage of destructive lysosomal enzymes into the cytoplasm of the cell and enzymatic digestion of cell components. Leakage of intracellular enzymes through the permeable cell membrane into the extracellular fluid is used as an important clinical indicator of cell injury and death. These enzymes enter the blood and can be measured by laboratory tests. For example, heart muscle liberates glutamic-oxaloacetic transaminase (GOT), creatine phosphokinase (CPK), and lactate dehydrogenase (LDH) when injured. Because different types of tissue have different enzymes, elevated levels of specific enzymes provide information about the location of tissue injury due to hypoxia.

Impaired Calcium Homeostasis

Calcium functions as a messenger for release of many intracellular enzymes. Normally, intracellular calcium levels are kept at an extremely low level compared with extracellular levels. These low intracellular levels are maintained by energy-dependent membrane-associated calcium-magnesium ATPase exchange systems.[1] Ischemia and certain toxins lead to an increase in cytosolic calcium because of increased influx across the cell membrane and the release of calcium stored in the mitochondria and endoplasmic reticulum. The increased calcium level activates a number of enzymes with potentially damaging effects. The enzymes include the phospholipases responsible for damaging the cell membrane, proteases that damage the cell skeleton and membrane proteins, ATPases that break down ATP and hasten its depletion, and endonucleases that fragment chromatin. Although it is known that injured cells accumulate calcium, it is unknown whether this is the ultimate cause of irreversible cell injury.

Reversible Cell Injury

Reversible cell injury, although impairing cell function, does not result in cell death. Two patterns of reversible cell injury can be observed under the microscope: cellular swelling and fatty change. Cellular swelling occurs with impairment of the energy-dependent sodium-potassium membrane pump, usually as the result of hypoxic cell injury.

Fatty changes are linked to intracellular accumulation of fat. When fatty changes occur, small vacuoles of fat disperse throughout the cytoplasm. The process is usually more ominous than cloudy swelling, and although it is reversible, it usually indicates severe injury. These fatty changes may occur because normal cells are presented with an increased fat load or because injured cells are unable to metabolize the fat properly. In obese persons, fatty infiltrates often occur within and between the cells of the liver and heart because of an increased fat load. Pathways for fat metabolism may be impaired during cell injury, and fat may accumulate within the cell as production exceeds use and export. The liver, where most fats are synthesized and metabolized, is particularly susceptible to fatty change, but fatty changes may also occur in the kidney, the heart, and other organs.

Cell Death

Within each cell line, the control of cell number is regulated by a balance of cell proliferation and cell death. Cell death can involve apoptosis or necrosis. Apoptotic cell death involves controlled cell destruction and is involved in normal cell deletion and renewal. For example, blood cells that undergo constant renewal from progenitor cells in the bone marrow are removed by apoptotic cell death. Necrotic cell death is a pathologic form of cell death resulting from cell injury. It is characterized by cell swelling, rupture of the cell membrane, and inflammation.

Apoptosis

Apoptosis, from Greek *apo* for "apart" and *ptosis* for "fallen," means fallen apart. Apoptotic cell death, which is equated with cell suicide, eliminates cells that are worn out, have been produced in excess, have developed improperly, or have genetic damage. In normal cell turnover, this process provides the space needed for cell replacement. The process, which was first described in 1972, has become one of the most vigorously investigated processes in biology.[15] Apoptosis is thought to be involved in several physiologic and pathologic processes. Current research is focusing on the genetic control mechanisms in an attempt to understand the pathogenesis of many disease states such as cancer and autoimmune disease. Evidence indicates that apoptosis may be involved in the death of $CD4^+$ helper T cells in persons with acquired immunodeficiency disease (AIDS).[15] Apoptotic cell death is characterized by controlled autodigestion of cell components. Cells appear to initiate their own death through the activation of endogenous enzymes. This results in cell shrinkage brought about by disruption of the cytoskeleton, condensation of the cytoplasmic organelles, disruption and clumping of nuclear DNA, and a distinctive wrinkling of the cell membrane.[1] As the cell shrinks, the nucleus breaks into spheres, and the cell eventually divides into membrane-covered fragments. During the process, membrane signals changes occur, signaling surrounding phagocytic cells to engulf the apoptotic cell and complete the degradation process (Fig. 2-3).

Apoptosis is thought to be responsible for several normal physiologic processes, including programed destruction of cells during embryonic development, hormone-dependent involution of tissues, death of immune cells, cell death by cytotoxic T cells, and cell death in proliferating cell populations. During embryogenesis, the development of a number of organs such as the heart, which begins as a single pulsating tube and is gradually modified to become a four-chambered pump, apoptotic cell death allows the next stage of organ development. The control of immune cell numbers and destruction of autoreactive T cells in the thymus have been credited to apoptosis. Cytotoxic T cells and natural killer cells are thought to destroy target cells by inducing apoptotic cell death. Apoptotic cell death occurs in the hormone-dependent involution of endometrial cells during the menstrual cycle and in the regression of breast tissue after weaning from breast feeding.

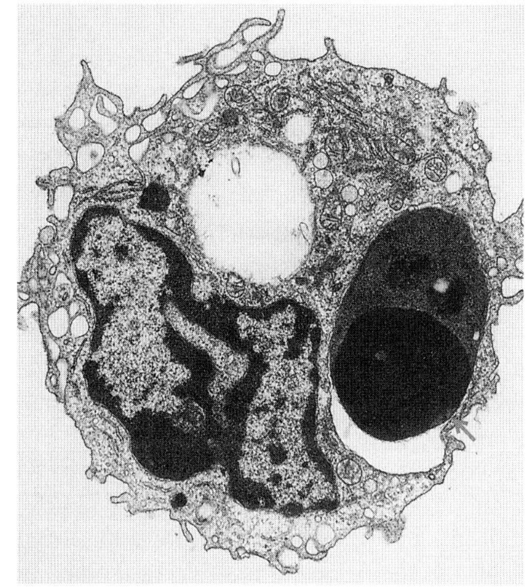

Figure 2-3
Exposure of phosphatidylserine on the surface of an apoptotic lymphhocyte triggers specific recognition and removal by macrophages. (Fadock V.A., Voelker D.R., Campbell P.A., et al [1992]. *Journal of Immunology* 148: 2207–2211)

Apoptosis appears to be linked to several pathologic events. For example, suppression of apoptosis may a determinant in the growth of cancers. Apoptosis is also thought to be involved in the cell death associated with certain viral infections, such as hepatitis B and C, and in cell death caused by a variety of injurious agents, such as mild thermal injury and radiation injury. Apoptosis may also be involved in neurodegenerative disorders such as Alzheimer's disease, Parkinson's disease, and amyotrophic lateral sclerosis (ALS). The loss of cells in these disorders does not induce inflammation; although the initiating event is unknown, apoptosis appears to be the mechanism of cell death.[16]

Several mechanisms appear to be involved in initiating cell death by apoptosis. As in the case of endometrial changes that occur during the menstrual cycle, the process can be triggered by the addition or withdrawal of hormones. Certain oncogenes and suppressor genes involved in the development of cancer seem to play an active role in stimulation or suppression of apoptosis. Injured cells may induce apoptotic cell death through increased cytoplasmic calcium, which leads to activation of nuclear enzymes that break down DNA. In some instances, gene transcription and protein synthesis, the events that produce new cells, may be the initiating factors. In other cases, cell surface signaling or receptor activation appears to be the influencing force.

Necrosis

Necrosis refers to cell death in an organ or tissue that is still part of a living person. Necrosis differs from apoptosis in that it involves unregulated enzymatic digestion of cell components, loss of cell membrane integrity with uncontrolled release of the products of cell death into the intracellular space, and incitation of the inflammatory response. Apoptosis functions in removing cells so they can be replaced by new cells, but necrosis often interferes with cell replacement and tissue regeneration.

With necrotic cell death, there are marked changes in the appearance of the cytoplasmic contents and the nucleus. These changes are often not visible, even under the microscope, for hours after cell death. The dissolution of the necrotic cell or tissue can follow several paths. The cell can undergo liquefaction (*i.e.*, liquefaction necrosis); it can be transformed to a gray, firm mass (*i.e.*, coagulation necrosis); or it can be converted to a cheesy material by infiltration of fatlike substances (*i.e.*, caseous necrosis). *Liquefaction necrosis* occurs when some of the cells die but their catalytic enzymes are not destroyed. An example of liquefaction necrosis is the softening of the center of an abscess with discharge of its contents. During *coagulation necrosis*, acidosis develops and denatures the enzymatic and structural proteins of the cell. This type of necrosis is characteristic of hypoxic injury and is seen in infarcted areas. *Infarction* (*i.e.*, tissue death) occurs when an artery supplying an organ or part of the body becomes occluded and no other source of blood supply exists. As a rule, the infarct's shape is conical and corresponds to the distribution of the artery and its branches. An artery may be occluded by an embolus, a thrombus, disease of the arterial wall, or pressure from outside the vessel. *Caseous necrosis* (*i.e.*, soft, cheeselike center) is a distinctive form of coagulation necrosis. It is most commonly associated with tubercular lesions and is thought to result from immune mechanisms.

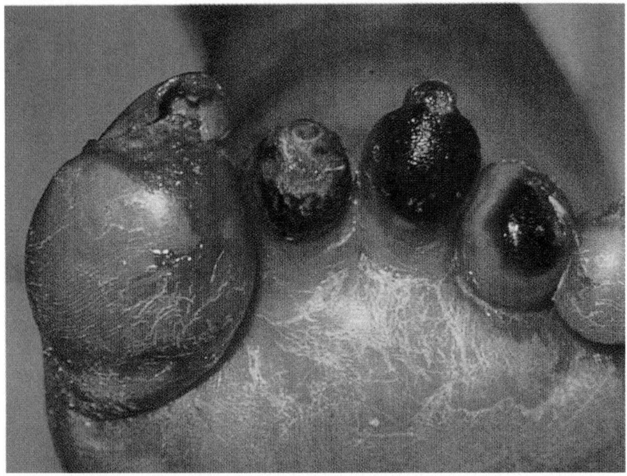

Figure 2-4
Gangrenous toes. (Biomedical Communications Group, Southern Illinois University School of Medicine, Springfield, IL)

Gangrene

The term *gangrene* is applied when a considerable mass of tissue undergoes necrosis. Gangrene may be classified as dry or moist. In dry gangrene, the part becomes dry and shrinks, the skin wrinkles, and its color changes to dark brown or black. The spread of dry gangrene is slow, and its symptoms are not as marked as those of wet gangrene. The irritation caused by the dead tissue produces a line of inflammatory reaction (*i.e.*, line of demarcation) between the dead tissue of the gangrenous area and the healthy tissue (Fig. 2-4). Dry gangrene usually results from interference with arterial blood supply to a part without interference with venous return and is a form of coagulation necrosis.

In moist or wet gangrene, the area is cold, swollen, and pulseless. The skin is moist, black, and under tension. Blebs form on the surface, liquefaction occurs, and a foul odor is caused by bacterial action. There is no line of demarcation between the normal and diseased tissues, and the spread of tissue damage is rapid. Systemic symptoms are usually severe, and death may occur unless the condition can be arrested. Moist or wet gangrene primarily results from interference with the venous return from the part. Bacterial invasion plays an important role in the development of wet gangrene and is responsible for many of its prominent symptoms. Dry gangrene is confined almost exclusively to the extremities, but moist gangrene may affect the internal organs or the extremities. If bacteria invade the necrotic tissue, dry gangrene may be converted to wet gangrene.

Gas gangrene is a special type of gangrene that results from infection of devitalized tissues by one of several *Clostridium* bacteria. The anaerobic and spore-forming organisms are widespread in nature, particularly in soil; gas gangrene is prone to occur in trauma and compound fractures in which dirt and debris are embedded. Some species have been isolated in the stomach, gallbladder, intestine, vagina, and skin of healthy persons. The bacteria produce toxins that dissolve the cell membranes, causing death of muscle cells, massive spreading edema, hemolysis of red blood cells, hemolytic anemia, hemoglobinuria, and renal toxicity.[17] Characteristic of this disorder are the bubbles of hydrogen sulfide gas that form in the muscle. Gas gangrene is a serious and potentially fatal disease. Because the organism is anaerobic, oxygen is sometimes administered in a hyperbaric chamber.

Intracellular Accumulations

Under certain conditions, various substances may accumulate in normal and abnormal cells. Intracellular accumulation can be grouped into three categories: normal cellular constituents, such as lipids, proteins, and carbohydrates, which are present in large amounts; abnormal substances, such as those resulting from inborn errors of metabolism; and products of excessive intracellular synthesis. The previously described fatty changes are an example of intracellular accumulation of a normal cell constituent. The intracellular accumulation of abnormal substances can result from genetic disorders that disrupt the metabolism of selected substances. A normal enzyme may be replaced with an abnormal one, resulting in the formation of a substance that cannot be used or eliminated from the cell, or an enzyme may be missing, so that an intermediate product accumulates within the cell. For example, there are at least 10 inborn errors of glycogen metabolism, most of which lead to the accumulation of intracellular glycogen stores. In the most common form of this disorder, von Gierke's disease, large amounts of glycogen accumulate in the liver and kidneys because of a deficiency of the enzyme glucose phosphatase. Without this enzyme, glucose-6-phosphate, stored in the form of glycogen, cannot be broken down to form glucose that can be used by the cell or released into the bloodstream. In a similar manner, other enzyme defects lead to the accumulation of other substances.

Pigments are colored substances that may accumulate within cells. They can be endogenous (*i.e.*, arising from within the body) or exogenous (*i.e.*, arising from outside the body). Icterus, also called jaundice, is a yellow discoloration of tissue caused by the retention of bilirubin, an endogenous bile pigment. This condition may result from increased bilirubin production from red blood cell destruction, obstruction of bile passage into the intestine, or toxic diseases that affect the liver's ability to remove bilirubin from the blood. One of the most common exogenous pigments is carbon in the form of coal dust. In coal miners or persons exposed to heavily polluted environments, the accumulation of carbon dust blackens the lung tissue and may cause serious lung disease. The formation of a blue lead line along the margins of the gum is one of the diagnostic features of lead poisoning.

Whatever the nature or cause of the abnormal accumulation, it implies storage of some substance by a cell. If the accumulation results from a correctable systemic disorder, such as hyperbilirubinemia that causes jaundice, the accumulation is reversible. If the disorder cannot be corrected, as often occurs in many inborn errors of metabolism, the cells become overloaded, causing cell injury and death.

In summary, cell injury can be caused by a number of agents. The injury may produce sublethal and reversible cellular damage or may lead to irreversible cell injury and death. Partially reduced oxygen species called free radicals are important mediators of cell injury in many pathologic conditions. They are an important cause of cell injury in hypoxia and after exposure to radiation and certain chemical agents. Lack of oxygen underlies the pathogenesis of cell injury in hypoxia and ischemia. Hypoxia can result from inadequate oxygen in the air, cardiorespiratory disease, anemia, or the inability of the cells to use oxygen. Among the physical agents that generate cell injury are mechanical forces that produce tissue trauma, extremes of temperature, electricity, and radiation. Chemical agents can cause cell injury through several mechanisms; they can block enzymatic pathways, cause coagulation of tissues, or disrupt the osmotic or ionic balance of the cell. Biologic agents differ from other injurious agents in that they are able to replicate and continue to produce injury. Among the nutritional factors that contribute to cell injury are excesses and deficiencies of nutrients, vitamins, and minerals. Cell death can involve two mechanisms: apoptosis or necrosis. Apoptosis involves controlled cell destruction and is the means by which the body removes and replaces cells that have been produced in excess, developed improperly, have genetic damage, or are worn out. Necrosis refers to cell death that is characterized by cell swelling, rupture of the cell membrane, and inflammation.

Under some circumstances, normal cells may accumulate abnormal amounts of various substances. If the accumulation reflects a correctable systemic disorder, such as hyperbilirubinemia that causes jaundice, the accumulation is reversible. If the disorder cannot be corrected, as often occurs in many inborn errors of metabolism, the cells become overloaded, causing cell injury and death.

Tissue Repair and Wound Healing

After you have completed this section of the chapter, you should be able to meet the following objectives:

- Define *parenchymal* and *stromal* as they relate to the tissues of an organ
- Compare labile, stable, and permanent cell types in terms of their capacity for regeneration
- Describe healing by primary and secondary intention
- Trace the wound-healing process through the inflammatory, proliferative, and remodeling phases
- Explain the effect of malnutrition; ischemia and oxygen deprivation; impaired immune and inflammatory responses; and infection, wound separation, and foreign bodies on wound healing
- Discuss the effect of age on wound healing

Body organs and structures contain two types of tissues: parenchymal and stromal. The parenchymal (*i.e.*, from the Greek for anything poured in) tissues contain the functioning cells of an organ or body part (*e.g.*, hepatocytes, renal tubular cells). The stromal tissues (*i.e.*, from the Greek for something laid out to lie on) consist of the supporting connective tissues, blood vessels, and nerve fibers.

Injured tissues are repaired by regeneration of parenchymal cells or by connective tissue repair in which scar tissue is substituted for the parenchymal cells of the injured tissue. The primary objective of the healing process is to fill the gap created by tissue destruction and to restore the structural continuity of the injured part. When regeneration cannot occur, healing by replacement with a connective scar tissue provides the means for maintaining this continuity. Although scar tissue fills the gap created by tissue death, it does not repair the structure with functioning parenchymal cells. Because the regenerative capabilities of most tissues are limited, wound healing usually involves some connective tissue repair.

Considerable research has contributed to the understanding of chemical mediators and growth factors that orchestrate the healing process.[18,19] These chemical mediators and growth factors are released in an orderly manner from many of the cells that participate in the healing process. Some growth factors act as chemoattractants, enhancing the migration of white blood cells and fibroblasts to the wound site, and others act as mitogens, causing increased proliferation of cells that participate in the healing process. For example, platelet-derived growth factor, which is released from activated platelets, attracts white blood cells and acts as a growth factor for blood vessels and fibroblasts. Many of the cytokines (see Chapter 11) are growth factors.

Regeneration

Regeneration involves replacement of the injured tissue with cells of the same parenchymal type, leaving little or no evidence of the previous injury. The ability to regenerate varies with the tissue and cell type. Body cells are divided into three types according to their ability to undergo regeneration: labile, stable, or permanent cells.[1]

Labile cells continue to divide and replicate throughout life, replacing cells that are continually being destroyed. Labile cells can be found in tissues that have a daily turnover of cells. They include the surface epithelial cells of the skin, the oral cavity, vagina, and cervix; the columnar epithelium of the gastrointestinal tract, uterus, and fallopian tubes; the transitional epithelium of the urinary tract; and bone marrow cells.

Stable cells normally stop dividing when growth ceases. These cells are capable, however, of undergoing regeneration when confronted with an appropriate stimulus. For stable cells to regenerate and restore tissues to their original state, the supporting stromal framework must be present. When this framework has been destroyed, the replacement of tissues is haphazard. The hepatocytes of the liver are one form of stable cell, and the importance of the supporting framework to regeneration is evidenced by two forms of liver disease. In some types of viral hepatitis, for example, there is selective destruction of the parenchymal liver cells, although the cells of the supporting tissue remain unharmed. After the disease has subsided, the injured cells regenerate, and liver function returns to normal. In cirrhosis of the liver, fibrous bands of tissue form and replace the normal supporting tissues of the liver, causing disordered replacement of liver cells and disturbance of liver function.

Permanent or fixed cells cannot undergo mitotic division. The fixed cells include nerve cells, skeletal cells, and cardiac muscle cells. These cells cannot regenerate; once destroyed, they are replaced with fibrous scar tissue that lacks the functional characteristics of the destroyed tissue. For example, the scar tissue that develops in the heart after a heart attack cannot conduct impulses nor can it contract to pump blood.

Connective Tissue Repair

Connective tissue replacement is an important process in the repair of tissue. It allows replacement of nonregenerated parenchymal cells by a connective tissue scar. Depending on the extent of tissue loss, wound closure and healing occur by *primary* or *secondary intention* (see Fig. 2-5). A sutured surgical incision is an example of healing by primary intention. Larger wounds (*e.g.*, burns and large surface wounds) that have a greater loss of tissue and contamination, heal by secondary intention. Healing by secondary intention is slower than healing by primary intention and results in the formation of larger amounts of scar tissue. A wound that might otherwise have healed by primary intention may become infected and heal by secondary intention.

Wound healing is commonly divided into three phases: the inflammatory phase, the proliferative phase, and the maturational or remodeling phase.[19–21] In wounds healing by primary intention, the duration of the phases is

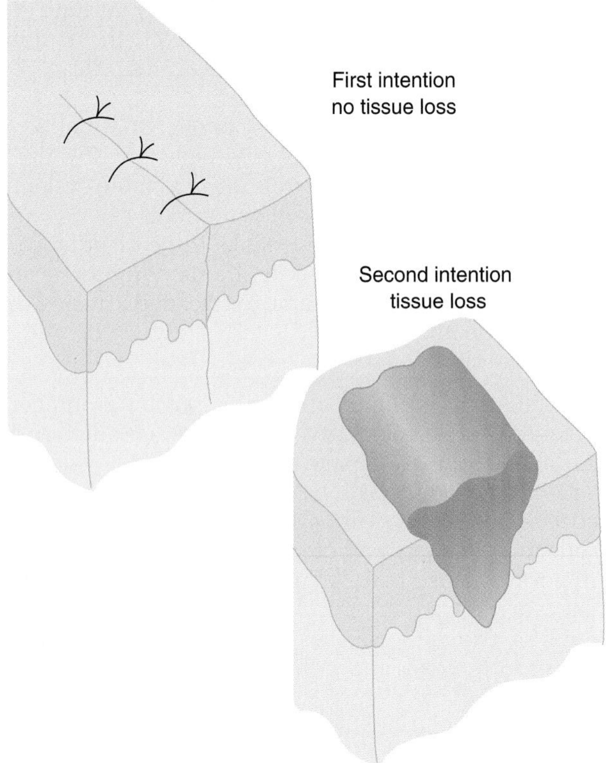

Figure 2-5
Healing by primary and secondary intention.

fairly predictable. In wounds healing by secondary intention, the process depends on the extent of injury and the healing environment.

Inflammatory Phase

The inflammatory phase of wound healing begins at the time of injury and is a critical period because it prepares the wound environment for healing. It includes hemostasis (Chapter 17) and the vascular and cellular phases of inflammation (Chapter 13). Hemostatic processes are activated immediately at the time of injury. There is constriction of injured blood vessel and initiation of blood clotting by way of platelet activation and aggregation. After a brief period of constriction, these same vessels dilate and capillaries increase their permeability, allowing plasma and blood components to leak into the injured area. In small surface wounds, the clot loses fluid and becomes a hard, desiccated scab that protects the area.

The cellular phase of inflammation follows and is evidenced by the migration of phagocytic white blood cells that digest and remove invading organisms, fibrin, extracellular debris, and other foreign matter. The polymorphonuclear cells (PMNs) are the first cells to arrive and are usually gone by day 3 or 4. They ingest bacteria and cellular debris. About 24 hours after arrival of the PMNs, a larger and less specific phagocytic cell, called a *macrophage*, enters the wound area and remains for an extended period. This cell, arising from blood monocytes, is an essential cell in the healing process. Its functions include phagocytosis and release of growth factors that stimulate epithelial cell growth, angiogenesis (*i.e.*, growth of new blood vessels), and attraction of fibroblasts. When a large defect occurs in deeper tissues, PMNs and macrophages are required to remove the debris and facilitate wound closure. Although a wound may heal in the absence of PMNs, it cannot heal in the absence of macrophages.

Proliferative Phase

The proliferative phase of healing usually begins within 2 to 3 days of injury and may last as long as 3 weeks in wounds healing by primary intention. The primary processes during this time focus on the building of new tissue to fill the wound space. The key cell during this phase is the fibroblast. The fibroblast is a connective tissue cell that synthesizes and secretes collagen and other intercellular elements needed for wound healing. Fibroblasts also produce a family of growth factors that induce new blood vessel formation (*i.e.*, angiogenesis) and endothelial cell proliferation and migration.

As early as 24 to 48 hours after injury, fibroblasts and vascular endothelial cells begin proliferating to form a specialized type of soft, pink granular tissue, called *granulation tissue*, that serves as the foundation for scar tissue development (Fig. 2-6). This tissue is fragile and bleeds easily because of the numerous, newly developed capillary buds. Wounds that heal by secondary intention have more necrotic debris and exudate that must be removed, and they involve larger amounts of granulation tissue. The newly formed blood vessels are leaky and allow plasma proteins and white blood cells to leak into the tissues. At about the same time, epithelial cells at the margin of the wound begin to regenerate and move toward the center of the wound, forming a new surface layer that is similar to that destroyed by the injury. In wounds that heal by primary intention, these epidermal cells proliferate and seal the wound within 24 to 48 hours.[23] When a scab has formed on the wound, the epithelial cells migrate between it and the underlying viable tissue; when a significant portion of the wound has been covered with epithelial tissue, the scab lifts off. At times, excessive granulation tissue, sometimes referred to as "proud flesh," may form and extend above the edges of wound, preventing reepithelialization from taking place. Surgical removal or chemical cauterization of the defect allows healing to proceed.

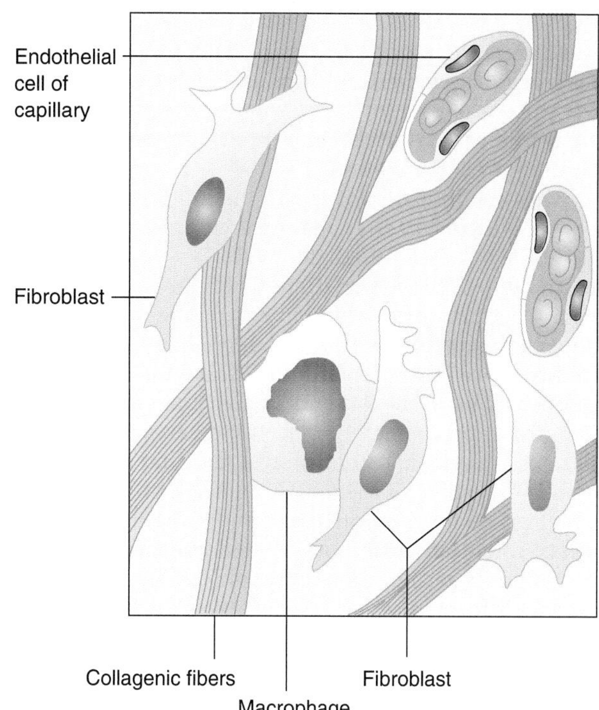

Figure 2-6
Cells involved in the development of granulation tissue.

As the proliferative phase progresses, there is continued accumulation of collagen and proliferation of fibroblasts. Collagen synthesis reaches a peak within 5 to 7 days and continues for several weeks, depending on wound size. By the second week, the white blood cells have largely left the area, the edema has diminished, and the wound begins to blanch as the small blood vessels become thrombosed and degenerate.

Remodeling Phase

The third phase of wound healing, the remodeling process, begins approximately 3 weeks after injury and can continue for 6 months to 2 years, depending on the extent of the wound. As the term implies, there is continued remodeling of scar tissue by simultaneous synthesis of collagen by fibroblasts and lysis by collagenase enzymes. As a result of these two processes, the architecture of the scar becomes reoriented to increase the tensile strength of the wound.

Most wounds do not regain the full tensile strength of unwounded skin after healing is completed. Carefully sutured wounds immediately after surgery have approximately 70% of the strength of unwounded skin, largely because of the placement of the sutures. This allows persons to move about freely after surgery without fear of wound separation. When the sutures are removed, usually at the end of the first week, wound strength is approximately 10%. It increases rapidly over the next 4 weeks and then slows, reaching a plateau of about 70% to 80% of the tensile strength of unwounded skin at the end of 3 months.[1] An injury that heals by secondary intention undergoes wound contraction during the proliferative and remodeling phases. As a result, the scar that is formed is considerably smaller than the original wound. Cosmetically, this may be desirable because it reduces the size of the visible defect. However, contraction of scar tissue over joints and other body structures tends to limit movement and cause deformities. As a result of loss of elasticity, scar tissue that is stretched fails to return to its original length.

An abnormality in healing by scar tissue repair is *keloid* formation. Keloids are tumorlike masses caused by excess production of scar tissue. The tendency to develop keloids is more common in African Americans and seems to have a genetic basis.

Factors That Affect Wound Healing

Many local and systemic factors influence wound healing. Although science has found a few ways to hasten the normal process of wound repair, there are many factors that impair healing. Among the causes of impaired wound healing are malnutrition; impaired blood flow and oxygen delivery; impaired inflammatory and immune responses; infection, wound separation, and foreign bodies; and age effects.

Malnutrition

Successful wound healing depends in part on adequate nutritional stores of proteins, carbohydrates, fats, vitamins, and minerals. It is well recognized that malnutrition slows the healing process, causing wounds to heal inadequately or incompletely.[24,25]

Protein deficiencies prolong the inflammatory phase of healing and impair fibroblast proliferation, collagen, and protein matrix synthesis, angiogenesis, and wound remodeling. Carbohydrates are needed as an energy source for white blood cells. Carbohydrates also have a protein-sparing effect and help to prevent the use of amino acids for fuel when they are needed for the healing process. Fats are essential constituents of cell membranes and are needed for the synthesis of new cells.

Although all vitamins are essential cofactors for daily functions of the body, vitamins A and C play an essential role in the healing process. Vitamin C is needed for collagen synthesis. In vitamin C deficiency, improper sequencing of amino acids occurs, proper linking of amino acids does not take place, the byproducts of collagen synthesis are not removed from the cell, new wounds do not heal properly, and old wounds may fall apart. Administration of vitamin C rapidly restores the healing process to normal. Vitamin A functions in stimulating and supporting epithelialization, capillary formation, and collagen synthesis. Vitamin A has also been shown to counteract the antiinflammatory effects of corticosteroid drugs and can be used to reverse these effects in persons who are on chronic steroid therapy. The B vitamins are important cofactors in enzymatic reactions that contribute to the wound-healing process. All are water soluble, and with the exception of vitamin B_{12}, which is stored in the liver, almost all must be replaced daily. Vitamin K plays an indirect role in wound healing by preventing bleeding disorders that contribute to hematoma formation and subsequent infection.

The role of minerals in wound healing is less clearly defined. The macrominerals, including sodium, potassium, calcium, and phosphorus, as well as the microminerals such as copper and zinc, must be present for normal cell function. Zinc is a cofactor in a variety of enzyme systems responsible for cell proliferation. In animal studies, zinc has been found to aid in reepithelialization.

Blood Flow and Oxygen Delivery

For healing to occur, wounds must have adequate blood flow to supply the necessary nutrients and to remove the resulting waste, local toxins, bacteria, and other debris. Impaired wound healing due to poor blood flow may occur as a result of wound conditions (*e.g.*, swelling) or preexisting health problems. Arterial disease and venous pathology are well-documented causes of impaired wound healing. In situations of trauma, a decrease in blood volume may cause a reduction in blood flow to injured tissues.

Molecular oxygen is required for collagen synthesis. It has been shown that even a temporary lack of oxygen can result in the formation of less stable collagen.[26,27] Wounds in ischemic tissue become infected more frequently than wounds in well-vascularized tissue. PMNs and macrophages require oxygen for destruction of microorganisms that have invaded the area. Although these cells can accomplish phagocytosis in a relatively anoxic environment, they cannot digest bacteria.

Impaired Inflammatory and Immune Responses

Inflammatory and immune mechanisms function in wound healing. Inflammation is essential to the first phase of wound healing, and immune mechanisms prevent infections that impair wound healing. Among the conditions that impair inflammation and immune function are disorders of phagocytic function, diabetes mellitus, and therapeutic administration of corticosteroid drugs.

Phagocytic disorders may be divided into extrinsic and intrinsic defects. Extrinsic disorders are those that impair attraction of phagocytic cells to the wound site, prepare bacteria and foreign agents for engulfment by the phagocytic cells (*i.e.*, opsonization), or cause suppression in the total number of phagocytic cells (*e.g.*, immunosuppressive agents). Intrinsic phagocytic disorders are the result of enzymatic deficiencies within the metabolic pathway for destroying the ingested bacteria by the phagocytic cell. The intrinsic phagocytic disorders include chronic granulomatous disease (see Chapter 12), an X-linked inherited disease in which there is a deficiency of myeloperoxidase and nicotinamide-adenine dinucleotide peroxidase (NADPH)-dependent oxidase enzyme. Deficiencies of these compounds prevent generation of hydrogen superoxide and hydrogen peroxide needed for killing bacteria.

Wound healing is a problem in persons with diabetes mellitus, particularly those who have poorly controlled blood glucose levels. Studies have shown delayed wound healing, poor collagen formation, and poor tensile strength in diabetic animals. Of particular importance is the effect of hyperglycemia on phagocytic function. Neutrophils, for example, have diminished chemotaxic and phagocytic function, including engulfment and intracellular killing of bacteria when exposed to altered glucose levels. Small blood vessel disease is also common among persons with diabetes, impairing the delivery of inflammatory cells, oxygen, and nutrients to the wound site.

The therapeutic administration of adrenal corticosteroids decreases the inflammatory process and delays healing. These hormones decrease capillary permeability during the early stages of inflammation, impair the phagocytic property of the leukocytes, and inhibit fibroblast proliferation and function.

Infection, Wound Separation, and Foreign Bodies

Wound contamination, wound separation, and foreign bodies delay wound healing. Infection impairs all dimensions of wound healing. It prolongs the inflammatory phase, impairs the formation of granulation tissue, and inhibits proliferation of fibroblasts and deposition of collagen fibers. All wounds are contaminated at the time of injury. Although body defenses can handle the invasion of microorganisms at the time of wounding, badly contaminated wounds can overwhelm host defenses. Trauma and existing impairment of host defenses also can contribute to the development of wound infections.

Approximation of the wound edges (*i.e.*, suturing of an incision type of wound) greatly enhances healing and prevents infection. Epithelialization of a wound with closely approximated edges occurs within 1 to 2 days. Large, gapping wounds tend to heal more slowly, because it is often impossible to effect wound closure with this type of wound. Foreign bodies tend to invite bacterial contamination and delay healing. Fragments of wood, steel, glass, and other compounds may have entered the wound at the site of injury and can be difficult to locate when the wound is treated. Sutures are also foreign bodies, and although needed for the closure of surgical wounds, they are an impediment to healing. This is why sutures are removed as soon as possible after surgery. Wound infections are of special concern in persons with implantation of foreign bodies such as orthopedic devices (*e.g.*, pins, stabilization devices), cardiac pacemakers, and shunt catheters. These infections are difficult to treat and may require removal of device.

Effect of Age

The effects of immaturity and aging affect healing. The rate of skin replacement slows with aging.

Wound Healing in Neonates and Children. Wound healing in the pediatric population follows a course similar to that in the adult population.[28] The child has greater capacity for repair than the adult but may lack the reserves needed to ensure proper healing. Such lack is evidenced by an easily upset electrolyte balance, sudden elevation or lowering of temperature, and rapid spread of infection. The neonate and small child may have an immature immune system with no antigenic experience with organisms that contaminate wounds. The younger the child, the more likely is the development of immune depression.

Successful wound healing also depends on adequate nutrition. Children need sufficient calories to maintain growth and wound healing. The premature infant is often born with immature organ systems and minimal energy stores but high metabolic requirements—a condition that predisposes to impaired wound healing.

Wound Healing in Aged Persons. The rate of cell replacement is slowed in normal aging skin and in epithelialization of open wounds.[29] The skin is more fragile and easily wounded. There is a gradual decline in immune function in the elderly. Multiple illnesses, circulatory problems, and nutritional deficits compound the wound-healing process.

In summary, the ability of tissues to repair damage due to injury depends on the body's ability to replace the parenchymal cells and to organize them as they were originally. Regeneration describes the process by which tissue is replaced with cells of a similar type and function. Healing by regeneration is limited to tissue with cells that are able to divide and to replace the injured cells. Body cells are divided into types according to their ability to regenerate: labile cells, such as the epithelial cells of the skin and gastrointestinal tract, which continue to regenerate throughout life; stable cells, such as those in the liver, which normally do not divide but which are capable of regeneration when confronted with an appropriate stimulus; and permanent or fixed cells, such as nerve cells, which are unable to regenerate. Scar tissue repair involves the substitution of fibrous connective tissue for injured tissue that cannot be repaired by regeneration.

Tissue injury is followed almost immediately by bleeding into the area and the development of a blood clot that contains fibrin and blood cells. Within several hours, the surface of the clot loses fluid and becomes a hard, dehydrated scab that protects the area. At about the same time, inflammatory cells enter the injured area and begin to break down and remove the inflammatory debris.

REFERENCES

1. Cotran R.S., Kumar V., Robbins S.L. (1994). *Robbins pathologic basis of disease* (6th ed., pp. 5, 6–15, 17–21, 46, 48, 85–80, 390–392). Philadelphia: W.B. Saunders.
2. Chandrasoma D., Taylor C.R. (1995). *Concise pathology* (2nd ed. pp. 158–172). Norwalk, CT: Appleton & Lange.
3. Goodwin C.W. Electrical injury. In Bennett J.C., Plum F. (1996). *Cecil textbook of medicine* (20th ed., pp. 64–67). Philadelphia, W.B. Saunders.
4. Upton A.C. Radiation injury. In Bennett J.C., Plum F. (1996). *Cecil textbook of medicine* (20th ed. pp. 59–64). Philadelphia: W.B. Saunders.
5. Landrigan P.J., Todd A.C. (1994). Lead poisoning. *West Journal of Medicine* 161, 153–156.
6. Rubin E., Farber J.L. (1994) *Pathology* (2nd ed., pp. 310–312). Philadelphia: J.B. Lippincott.
7. Brody D.J., Pirkle J.L, Kramer R.A. (1994). Blood lead levels in the US population: Phase I of the Third National Health and Nutrition Examination Survey (NHANES III, 1988–1991). *JAMA* 272, 277.
8. Pirkle J.L., Brody D.J., Gunter E.W. (1994). The decline in blood lead levels in the United States: The National Health and Nutrition Examination Surveys (NHANES). *JAMA* 272, 284.
9. Piomelli S. Lead poisoning. In Behrman R.E., Kliegman R.M., Arvin A.M. (1996). *Nelson textbook of pediatrics* (15th ed., pp. 2010-2013). Philadelphia: W.B. Saunders.
10. Centers for Disease Control. *Preventing Lead Poisoning in Young Children: A Statement by the Centers for Disease Control*. Atlanta: U.S. Department of Health and Human Services, Public Health Service, 1991.
11. Sinclair A.J., Barnett H., Lunec J. (1990). Free radicals and antioxidant systems in health and disease. *British Journal of Hospital Medicine* 43 (2), 334–344.
12. Machlin L.J., Bendich A. (1987). Free radical tissue damage: Protective role of antioxidant nutrients. *FASEB Journal* 1, 441–445.
13. Kerr M.E., Bender C.M., Monti E.J. (1996). An introduction to oxygen free radicals. *Heart Lung* 25, 200–209.
14. Vogt M.T., Farber E. (1968). On the molecular pathology of ischemic renal cell death: Reversible and irreversible cellular and mitochondrial metabolic alterations. *American Journal of Pathology* 53, 1.
15. Cohen J.J. (1993). Apoptosis: The physiologic pathway of cell death. *Hospital Practice* 28 (2), 35–43.
16. Thompson C.B. (1995). Apoptosis in the pathogenesis and treatment of disease. *Science* 267, 1456–1462.
17. Corry M., Montoya L. (1990). Gas gangrene: Certain diagnosis or certain death. *Critical Care Nursing* 9 (10), 30–38.
18. Pessa M.E., Bland K.I., Copeland E.M. III. (1987). Growth factors and determinants of wound repair. *Journal of Surgical Research* 42, 207–217.
19. Sporn M.B., Roberts A.B. (1986). Peptide growth factors and inflammation, tissue repair, and cancer. *Journal of Clinical Investigation* 78, 329–332.
20. Norris S.O., Provo B., Stotts N.A. (1990). Physiology of wound healing and risk factors that impede the healing process. *Clinical Issues in Critical Care Nursing* 1, 545–552.
21. Flynn M.B. (1994). Wound management of the traumatically injured patient. *Critical Care Nursing Clinics of North America* 6 (3), 491–499.
22. Flynn M.B. (1996). Wound healing and critical illness. *Critical Care Clinics of North America* 8 (2), 115–124.
23. Orgill D., Deming H.R. (1988). Current concepts and approaches to healing. *Critical Care Medicine* 16, 899–908.
24. Albina J.E. (1995). Nutrition and wound healing. *Journal of Parenteral and Enteral Nutrition* 18 (4), 367–376
25. Stotts N.A., Washington D. (1990). Nutrition: A critical component of wound healing. *Clinical Issues in Critical Care Nursing* 1, 585–592.
26. Whitney J.D. (1989). Physiologic effects of tissue oxygenation on wound healing. *Heart and Lung* 18, 466–474.
27. Whitney J.D. (1990). The influence of tissue oxygenation and perfusion on wound healing. *Clinical Issues in Critical Care Nursing* 1, 578–584.
28. Garvin G. (1990). Wound healing in pediatrics. *Nursing Clinics of North America* 25, 181–191.
29. Jones P., Millman A. (1990). Wound healing and the aged patient. *Nursing Clinics of North America* 25, 263–277.

ADDITIONAL READINGS

Bagley S.M. (1996). Nutritional needs of the acutely ill with acute wounds. *Critical Care Clinics of North America* 8 (2), 159–168.

Brown G.L., Nanney L.B., Griffen J. (1989). Enhancement of wound healing by topical treatment with epidermal growth factor. *New England Journal of Medicine* 321, 76–79.

Cooper D.M. (1990). Optimizing wound healing. *Nursing Clinics of North America* 25, 165–171.

Duke R.C., Ojius D.M., Young D. (1996). Cell suicide in health and disease. *Scientific American* 276, 80–87.

Meyer J.S. (1996). Diabetes and wound healing. *Critical Care Clinics of North America* 8 (2), 195–201.

Pierce G.F., Mustoe T.A. (1995). Pharmacologic enhancement of wound healing. *Annual Review of Medicine* 46, 467–481.

Young M.E. (1988). Malnutrition and wound healing. *Heart and Lung* 17, 6067.

CHAPTER 3

Genetic Control of Cell Function and Inheritance

Edward W. Carroll

The word *gene* is defined as the *fundamental unit of information storage*. This information is stored within the structure of *deoxyribonucleic acid (DNA)*, an extremely stable macromolecule within the nucleus of each cell. Because of the stable structure of DNA, the genetic information is able to survive the many processes of reduction division to form the gametes (*i.e.*, ovum and sperm), fertilization, and the many mitotic cell divisions involved in the formation of a new organism from the single-celled fertilized ovum called the *zygote*. Genes determine the types of proteins and enzymes that are made by the cell and thereby control inheritance and the day-to-day function of all the cells in the body. For example, genes control the type and quantity of hormones that a cell produces, the antigens and receptors that are present on the cell membrane, and the synthesis of enzymes needed for metabolism. Of the estimated 50,000 to 100,000 genes that humans possess, more than 5000 have been identified and over 2300 have been localized to a particular chromosome. With few exceptions, each gene provides the instructions for the synthesis of a single protein. This chapter includes discussions of genetic regulation of cell function, chromosomal structure, patterns of inheritance, and gene technology.

Genetic Control of Cell Function

After you have completed this section of the chapter, you should be able to meet the following objectives:

- Describe the structure of a gene
- Explain the mechanisms whereby genes control cell function and another generation
- Describe the concept of induction and repression in terms of gene function
- Define gene locus and allele
- Describe the pathogenesis of gene mutation
- Explain how gene expressivity and penetrance determine the effects of a mutant gene that codes for the production of an essential enzyme

The genetic information needed for protein synthesis is encoded within the DNA contained in the cell nucleus. A second type of nucleic acid, *ribonucleic acid* (RNA), is involved in the actual synthesis of cellular enzymes and proteins. Cells contain several types of RNA: messenger RNA, transfer RNA, and ribosomal RNA. *Messenger RNA* contains the transcribed instructions for protein synthesis obtained from the DNA molecule and carries them into the cytoplasm. Transcription is followed by translation, the synthesis of proteins according to the instructions carried by messenger RNA. *Ribosomal RNA* provides the machinery needed for protein synthesis. *Transfer RNA* reads the instructions and delivers the appropriate amino acids to the ribosome, where they are incorporated into the protein being synthesized.

The mechanism for genetic control of cell function is illustrated in Figure 3–1. The nuclei of all the cells in an organism contain the same accumulation of genes derived from the gametes of the two parents. This means that liver cells contain the same genetic information as skin and muscle cells. For this to be true, the molecular code must be duplicated before each succeeding cell division, or mitosis. Theoretically, although not yet achieved in humans, any of the highly differentiated cells of an organism could be used to produce a complete, genetically identical organism, or clone. Each particular tissue uses only some of the information stored in the genetic code. Although information required for the function of other types of tissues is still present, it is repressed.

In addition to nuclear DNA, a portion of the DNA of a cell resides in the mitochondria. The mitochondrial DNA is inherited from the mother by her offspring (*i.e.*, matrilineal inheritance). Several genetic disorders are attributed to defects in mitochondrial DNA. Leber's hereditary optic neuropathy was the first human disease attributed to mutation in mitochondrial DNA.

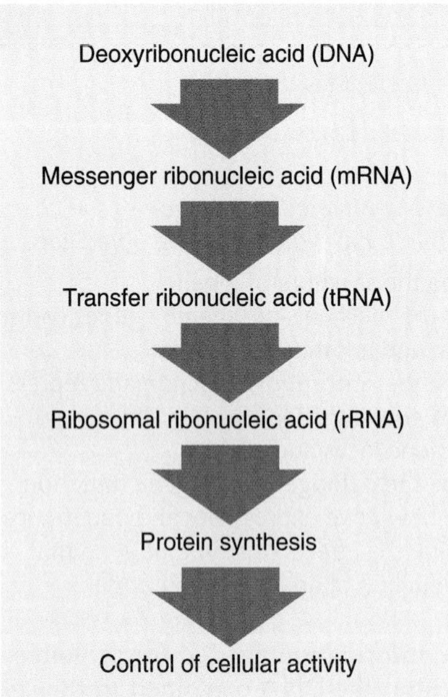

Figure 3-1
DNA-directed control of cellular activity through synthesis of cellular proteins. Messenger RNA carries the transcribed message, which directs protein synthesis, from the nucleus to the cytoplasm. Transfer RNA selects the appropriate amino acids and carries them to ribosomal RNA where assembly of the proteins takes place.

Gene Structure

The structure that stores the genetic information within the nucleus is a long, double-stranded, helical molecule of DNA. The DNA molecule is composed of nucleotides, which consist of phosphoric acid, a five-carbon sugar called *deoxyribose*, and one of four nitrogenous bases. The nitrogenous bases carry the genetic information. These four bases can be divided into two groups: the purine bases, *adenine* and *guanine*, which have two nitrogen ring structures, and the pyrimidine bases, *thymine* and *cytosine*, which have one ring. Alternating groups of sugar and phosphoric acid form the backbone of the molecule, with the paired bases projecting inward from the sides of the sugar molecule. The entire chain is like a spiral staircase, with the paired bases representing the steps (Fig. 3–2). There is a precise complementary pairing of purine and pyrimidine bases in the double-stranded DNA molecule. Adenine is paired with thymine, and guanine is paired with cytosine. Each nucleotide in a pair is on one strand of the DNA molecule, with the bases of the pairs bound together by hydrogen bonds that are relatively stable under normal conditions. Enzymes called DNA heicases separate the two strands so that the genetic information can be duplicated or transcribed.

A gene can be regarded as being represented by several hundred to almost a million base pairs; the size is proportional to the protein product it encodes. Of the two DNA strands, only one is used in transcribing the information for the cell's polypeptide-building machinery. If the genetic information of one strand is meaningful, the complementary code of the other strand will not make sense and will be ignored. Both strands, however, are involved in DNA duplication. Before cell division, the two strands of the helix separate and a complementary molecule is organized next to each original strand. Two strands become four strands. During cell division, the newly duplicated double-stranded molecules are separated and placed in each daughter cell by the mechanics of mitosis. As a result, each of the daughter cells again contains the meaningful strand and the complementary strand joined in the form of a double helix. Replication of DNA has been termed *semiconservative* because each new daughter molecule contains one parental strand.

The DNA molecule is combined with several types of protein and small amounts of RNA into a complex known as *chromatin*. Chromatin is the more readily stainable portion of the cell nucleus. Some of these proteins form binding sites for repressor molecules and hormones that regulate genetic transcription. Other proteins may block genetic transcription by preventing access of nucleotides to the surface of the DNA molecule. A specific group of proteins called *histones* are thought to control the folding of the DNA strands.

Genetic Code

The four bases, guanine, adenine, cytosine, and thymine (uracil is substituted for thymine in RNA), make up the

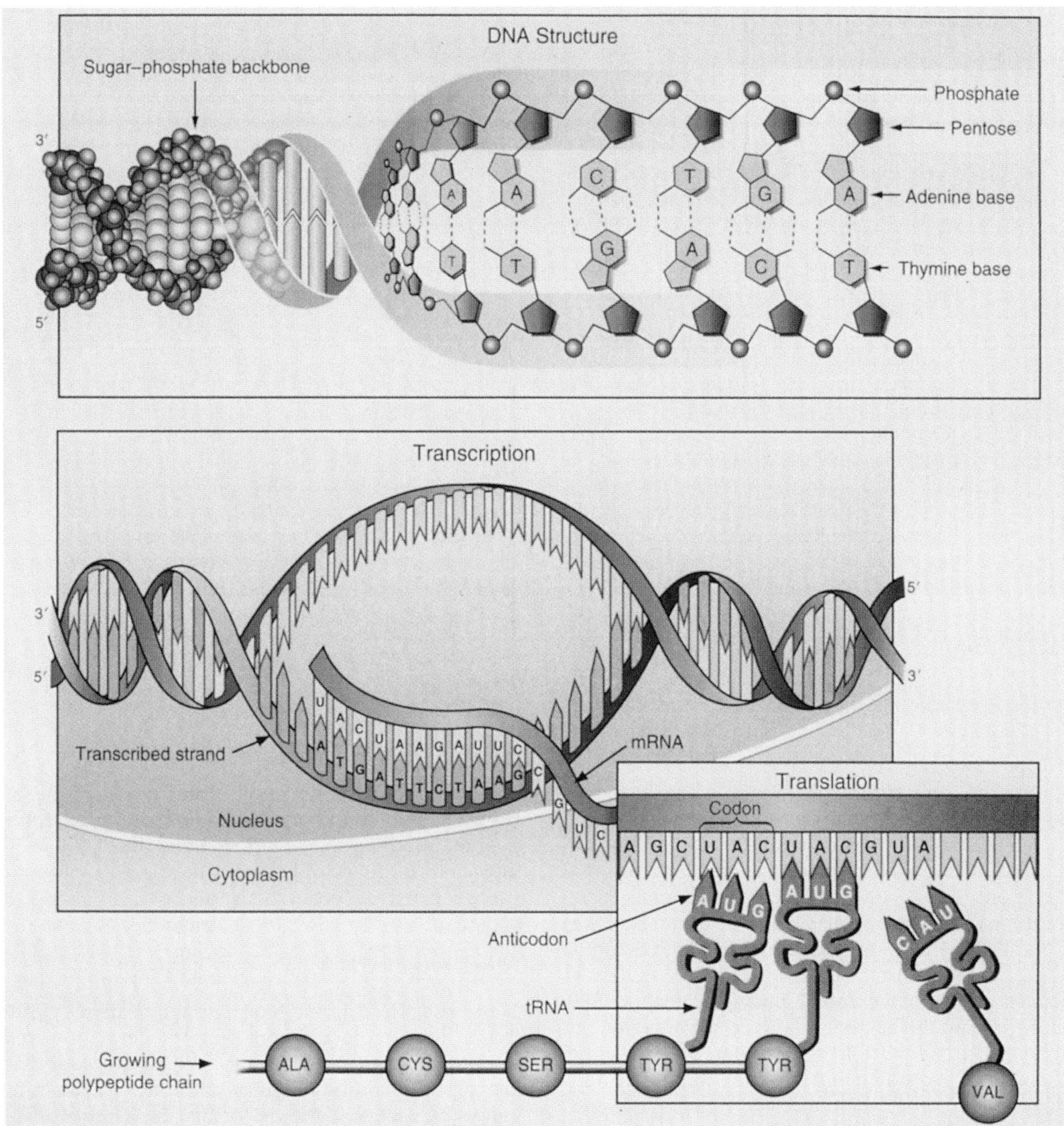

Figure 3-2
The DNA double helix and the flow of genetic information. The top panel shows the sequence of four bases (guanine, adenine, thymine, and cytosine, in orange), which determines the specificity of genetic information. The bases face inward from the sugar-phosphate backbone and form pairs (*dashed lines*) with complementary bases on the opposing strand. In the larger bottom panel, transcription in the nucleus creates a complementary nucleic acid copy (mRNA, in red) from one of the DNA strands in the double helix. The mRNA leaves the nucleus and associates with ribosomes in the cytoplasm, where it is translated into protein (*smaller bottom panel*). Special transfer RNAs (tRNA, in purple) align the corresponding amino acids (blue) along the mRNA, using the three-base genetic code to transform the nucleic acid sequence into a protein sequence. (Rosenthal N. [1994]. DNA and the genetic code. *New England Journal of Medicine* 331 [1], 40)

alphabet of the genetic code. A sequence of three of these bases constitutes the fundamental triplet code used in transmitting the genetic information needed for protein synthesis; this triplet code is called a *codon* (Table 3–1). An example is the nucleotide sequence GCU (*i.e.*, guanine, cytosine, and uracil), which is the triplet RNA code for the amino acid alanine. The genetic code is a universal language used by almost all living cells (*i.e.*, the code

TABLE 3-1
Triplet Codes for Amino Acids

Amino Acid	RNA Codons					
Alanine	GCU	GCC	GCA	GCG		
Arginine	CGU	CGC	CGA	CGG	AGA	AGG
Asparagine	AAU	AAC				
Aspartic acid	GAU	GAC				
Cysteine	UGU	UGC				
Glutamic acid	GAA	GAG				
Glutamine	CAA	CAG				
Glycine	GGU	GGC	GGA	GGG		
Histidine	CAU	CAC				
Isoleucine	AUU	AUC	AUA			
Leucine	CUU	CUC	CUA	CUG	UUA	UUG
Lysine	AAA	AAG				
Methionine	AUG					
Phenylalanine	UUU	UUC				
Proline	CCU	CCC	CCA	CCG		
Serine	UCU	UCC	UCA	UCG	AGC	AGU
Threonine	ACU	ACC	ACA	ACG		
Tryptophan	UGG					
Tyrosine	UAU	UAC				
Valine	GUU	GUC	GUA	GUG		
Start (CI)	AUG					
Stop (CT)	UAA	UAG	UGA			

(Guyton A. [1996]. *Textbook of medical physiology* [9th ed., p. 31]. Philadelphia: W.B. Saunders)

for the amino acid tryptophan is the same in a bacterium, a plant, and a human being). There are also stop codes, which signal the end of a protein molecule. Mathematically, the four bases can be arranged in 64 different combinations ($4 \times 4 \times 4 = 64$). Sixty-one triplets correspond to particular amino acids, and three are stop signals. Because there are only 20 amino acids that can be used in protein synthesis in humans, there may be several codes for the same amino acid. The genetic code therefore is said to be redundant or degenerate. For example, AUG is a part of the initiation or start signal and the codon for the amino acid methionine. Codons that specify the same amino acid are called synonyms. Synonyms usually have the same first two bases but differ in the third base.

Protein Synthesis

Although DNA determines the type of biochemical product that the cell synthesizes, the transmission and decoding of information needed for protein synthesis are carried out by RNA, the formation of which is directed by DNA. The general structure of RNA differs from DNA in three respects: RNA is a single rather than a double-stranded molecule; the sugar in each nucleotide of RNA is ribose instead of deoxyribose; and the pyrimidine base thymine in DNA is replaced by uracil in RNA. There are three types of RNA: messenger RNA (mRNA), transfer RNA (tRNA), and ribosomal RNA (rRNA). All three types are synthesized in the nucleus by RNA polymerase enzymes that take directions from DNA. Because the ribose sugars found in RNA are more susceptible to degradation than the sugars in DNA, the types of RNA molecules in the cytoplasm can be altered rapidly in response to extracellular signals.

Messenger RNA

Messenger RNA is the template for protein synthesis. It is a long molecule containing several hundred to several thousand nucleotides, which are codons that are exactly complementary to code words on the genes. Messenger RNA is formed by a process called *transcription*, in which the weak hydrogen bonds of the DNA are broken so that free RNA nucleotides can pair with their exposed DNA counterparts on the meaningful strand of the DNA molecule. As with the base pairing of the DNA strands, complementary RNA bases pair with the DNA bases; uracil, which replaces thymine in RNA, pairs with adenine.

During transcription, a specialized nuclear enzyme, called *RNA polymerase*, recognizes the beginning or start sequence of a gene, attaches to the double-stranded DNA, and proceeds to copy the meaningful strand into a single strand of RNA as it travels along the length of the gene. Upon reaching the stop signal, the enzyme leaves the gene and releases the RNA strand. The RNA strand is processed. Processing involves the addition of certain nucleic acids at the ends of the RNA strand and cutting and splicing of certain internal sequences. Splicing often involves the removal of stretches of RNA. Because of the splicing process, matured mRNA differs in sequence from the original DNA template. RNA sequences that are retained are called *exons*, and those that are excised are called *introns*. The functions of the introns are unknown. They are thought to be involved in the activation or deactivation of genes during various stages of development.

Splicing permits a cell to produce different mRNA molecules from a single gene by splicing segments of the initial RNA differently. For example, in a muscle cell, the original tropomyosin RNA transcriptase is spliced in as many as 10 different ways, yielding distinctly different protein products. This permits different proteins to be expressed from a single gene and compresses the amount of DNA that must be contained in the genome.

Transfer RNA

Transfer RNA carries amino acids in the activated form to protein molecules as they are being synthesized in the ribosomes. It is clover shaped and contains about 80 nucleotides, making it the smallest RNA molecule. There are at least 20 different types of tRNA, each of which recognizes and binds to only one type of amino acid. Each tRNA has two recognition sites: one for the mRNA codon and a second for the amino acid itself. Each type of tRNA carries its own specific amino acid to the ribosomes, where protein synthesis is taking place; there it recognizes the appropriate codon on the mRNA and delivers the amino acid to the newly forming protein molecule.

Ribosomal RNA

The ribosome is the physical structure in the cytoplasm where protein synthesis takes place. Ribosomal RNA constitutes 60% of the ribosome, with the remainder of the ribosome composed of structural proteins and enzymes needed for protein synthesis. As with the other types of RNA, rRNA is synthesized in the nucleus. Unlike other RNAs, ribosomal RNA is produced in specialized nuclear structure called the nucleolus. Nucleoli are formed from long DNA loops of several chromosomes, each contributing an rRNA gene. Once formed, the rRNA combines with ribosomal proteins in the nucleus and is then transported into the cytoplasm. During protein synthesis, most ribosomes become attached to the endoplasmic reticulum. There is no specificity of ribosomes for synthesis of a particular protein; a particular mRNA can direct protein synthesis in any ribosome.

Proteins are made from a standard set of amino acids, which are joined end to end to form the long polypeptide chains of protein molecules. Each polypeptide chain may have as many as 100 to more than 300 amino acids in it. The process of protein synthesis is called *translation*, because the genetic code is translated into the production language needed for protein assembly. In addition to rRNA, translation requires the coordinated actions of mRNA and tRNA. Each of the 20 different tRNA molecules transports its specific amino acid to the ribosome for incorporation into the developing protein molecule. Messenger RNA provides the information needed for placing the amino acids in their proper order for each specific type of protein. During protein synthesis, mRNA comes in contact with and passes through the ribosome, reading the directions for protein synthesis in much the same way that a tape is read as it passes through a tape player. As mRNA passes through the ribosome, tRNA delivers the appropriate amino acids for attachment to the growing polypeptide chain. The long mRNA molecule usually travels through and directs protein synthesis in more than one ribosome at a time. After the first part of the mRNA is read by the first ribosome, it moves on to a second and a third; as a result, ribosomes that are actively involved in protein synthesis are often found in clusters called *polyribosomes*. The process of protein synthesis is depicted in Figure 3–2.

Regulation of Gene Expression

Although all cells contain the same genes, not all genes are active all of the time, nor are the same genes active in all cell types. On the contrary, only a small, select group of genes is active in directing protein synthesis in the cell, and this group varies from one cell type to another. For different types of cells to develop in the various organs and tissues of the body as a result of cell differentiation, the protein synthesis in some cells must be different from that in others. To adapt to an ever-changing environment, certain cells may need to produce varying amounts and types of proteins. Certain enzymes, such as carbonic anhydrase, are synthesized by all cells for the fundamental metabolic processes on which life depends.

The degree to which a gene or particular group of genes is active is referred to as *gene expression*. A phenomenon termed *induction* is an important process whereby gene expression is increased. Except in early embryonic development, induction is produced by some external influence. Gene *repression* is the process whereby a regulatory gene acts to reduce or prevent gene expression. Some genes are normally dormant and can be activated by inducer substances, and other genes are naturally active and can be inhibited by repressor substances. Genetic mechanisms for the control of protein synthesis are better understood in microorganisms than in humans. It can be assumed, however, that many of the same principles apply.

The mechanism that has been most extensively studied is the one by which the synthesis of particular proteins can be turned on and off. In the bacterium *Escherichia coli* grown in a nutrient medium containing the disaccharide lactose, the enzyme galactosidase can be isolated. It catalyzes the splitting of lactose into a molecule of glucose and a molecule of galactose; this is necessary if lactose is to be metabolized by *E. coli*. However, if the *E. coli* is grown in a medium that does not contain lactose, very little of the enzyme is produced. From these and other studies, it is theorized that the synthesis of a particular protein, such as galactosidase, requires a series of reactions, each of which is catalyzed by a specific enzyme.

There are probably at least two types of genes that control protein synthesis: structural genes that specify the amino acid sequence of a polypeptide chain and regulator genes that serve a regulatory function without stipulating the structure of protein molecules. The regulation of protein synthesis is controlled by a sequence of genes, called an *operon,* located on adjacent sites on the same chromosome (Fig. 3–3). An operon consists of a set of structural genes that code for enzymes used in the synthesis of a particular product and a promoter site that binds RNA polymerase and initiates transcription of the structural genes. The function of the operon is further regulated by an activator operator and a repressor operator, which induce or repress the function of the promoter. The activator and repressor sites commonly monitor levels of the synthesized product and regulate the activity of the operon in a negative feedback manner; whenever product levels decrease, the function of the operon is activated, and, when levels increase, its function is repressed. Regulatory genes located elsewhere in the genetic complex can exert control over an operon through activator or repressor substances. Not all genes are subject to induction and repression.

Gene Mutations

Rarely, accidental errors in duplication of DNA occur. These errors are called *mutations*. Mutations result from the substitution of one base pair for another, the loss or addition of one or more base pairs, or rearrangements of base pairs. Many of these mutations occur spontaneously; others are caused by environmental agents, chemicals, and radiation. Mutations may arise in somatic cells or in germ cells. Only those DNA changes that occur in germ cells can be inherited. A somatic mutation affects a cell line that differentiates into one or more of the many tissues of the body and is not transmissible to the next generation. Somatic mutations that do not have an impact on the health or functioning of a person are called *polymorphisms*. Occasionally, a person is born with one brown eye and one blue eye as a result of a somatic mutation. The change or loss of gene information is just as likely to affect the fundamental processes of cell function or organ differentiation. Such somatic mutations in the early embryonic period can result in embryonic death or congenital malformations. Somatic mutations are important causes of cancer and other tumors in which cell differentiation and growth get out of hand. Each year hundreds of thousands of random changes occur in the DNA molecule due to environmental events or metabolic accidents. Fortunately, fewer than 1 in 1000 base pair changes result in serious mutations. Most of these defects are corrected by DNA repair mechanisms. Several mechanisms exist, and each depends on specific enzymes such as DNA repair nuclease. Fishermen, farmers, and others who are excessively exposed to the ultraviolet radiation of sunlight have an increased risk of developing skin cancer resulting from potential radiation damage to the genetic structure of the skin-forming cells.

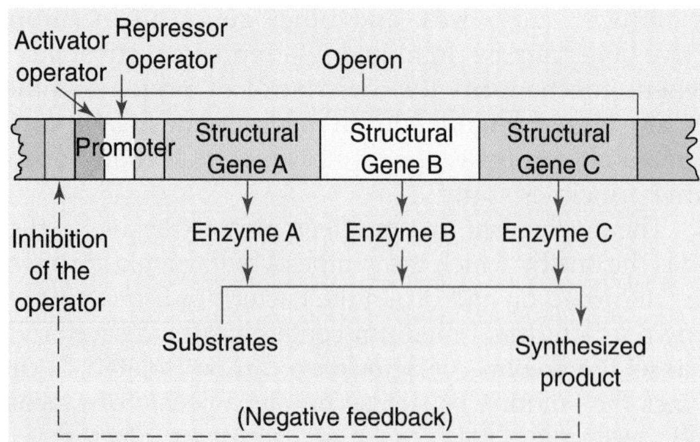

Figure 3-3
Function of the operon to control biosynthesis. The synthesized product exerts negative feedback to inhibit function of the operon, in this way automatically controlling the concentration of the product itself. (Guyton A. [1996]. *Medical physiology* [9th ed.]. Philadelphia: W.B. Saunders)

In summary, genes are the fundamental unit of information storage in the cell. They determine the types of proteins and enzymes made by the cell and therefore control inheritance and day-to-day cell function. Genes store information in the form of a stable macromolecule called DNA. Genes transmit information in the form of a triplet code, which uses the nitrogenous bases of the four nucleotides (i.e., adenine, guanine, thymine [or uracil in RNA], and cytosine) of which the DNA molecule is composed. The transfer of stored information into production of cell products is accomplished through a second type of macromolecule called RNA. Messenger RNA transcribes the instructions for product synthesis from the DNA molecule and carries it into the cell's cytoplasm, where ribosomal RNA uses the information to direct product synthesis. Transfer RNA acts as a carrier system for delivering the appropriate amino acids to the ribosomes, where the synthesis of cell products occurs. Although all cells contain the same genes, only a small, select group of genes is active in a given cell type. In all cells, some genetic information is repressed whereas other information is expressed. Gene mutations represent accidental errors in duplication, rearrangements, or deletion of parts of the genetic code. Fortunately, most mutations are repaired by DNA repair mechanisms in the cell.

Chromosomes

After you have completed this section of the chapter, you should be able to meet the following objectives:

- Define the terms autosomes, chromatin, meiosis, and mitosis

- List the steps in constructing a karyotype using cytogenetic studies
- Explain the significance of the Barr body

Most genetic information of a cell is organized, stored, and retrieved in the form of small cellular structures called *chromosomes*. Although the chromosomes are visible only in dividing cells, they retain their integrity between cell divisions. The chromosomes are arranged in pairs; one member of the pair is inherited from the father, the other from the mother. Each species has a characteristic number of chromosomes. There are 46 single or 23 pairs of human chromosomes. Of the 23 pairs of human chromosomes, there are 22 pairs called the *autosomes* that are alike in males and females. Each of the 22 pairs of autosomes has the same appearance in all individuals, and each has been given a numeric designation for classification purposes (Fig. 3–4).

The sex chromosomes constitute the 23rd pair of chromosomes. There are two sex chromosomes that determine the sex of a person. All males have an X and Y chromosome (*i.e.*, an X chromosome from the mother and a Y chromosome from the father), and all females have two X chromosomes (*i.e.*, one from each parent). It is believed that, of the two X chromosomes in the female, only one is active in controlling the expression of genetic traits. Both X chromosomes are involved, however, in transmission to the offspring. In the female, the active X chromosome is invisible, but the inactive X chromosome can be demonstrated on appropriate nuclear staining as the *chromatin mass* or *Barr body* in epithelial cells or as the drumstick body in the chromatin of neutrophils. The genetic sex of a child can be determined by microscopic study of cell or tissue samples. The total number of X chromosomes is equal to the number of Barr bodies plus one (*i.e.*, an inactive plus an active X chromosome). For example, the cells of a normal female have one Barr body and therefore a total of two X chromosomes. A male has no Barr bodies. In the female, whether the X chromosome derived from the mother or that derived from the father is active is determined within a few days after conception; the selection is random for each postmitotic cell line. This is called the Lyon principle, after Mary Lyon, the British geneticist who developed it.

Cell Division

There are two types of cell division—mitosis (see Chapter 1) and meiosis. *Meiosis* is limited to replicating germ cells and only takes place once in a cell line. It results in the formation of gametes or reproductive cells (*i.e.*, ovum and sperm), each of which has only a single set of 23 chromosomes.

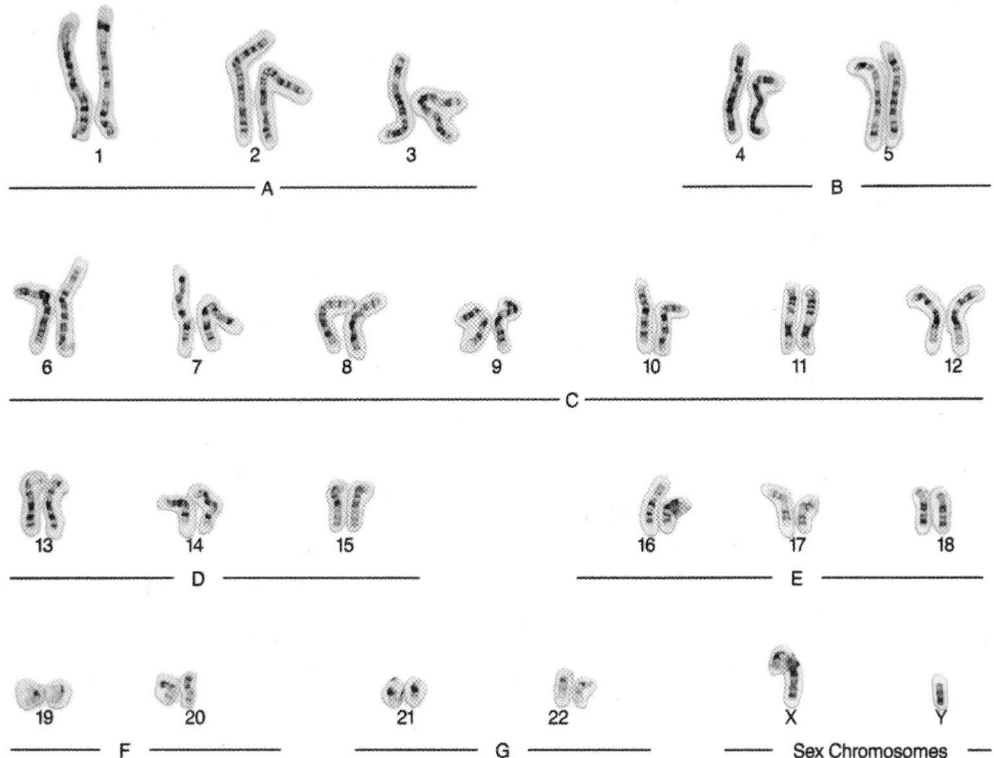

Figure 3-4
Karyotype of normal human boy. (Courtesy of the Prenatal Diagnostic and Imaging Center, Sacramento, CA. Frederick W. Hansen, MD, Medical Director)

Meiosis is typically divided into two distinct phases: meiotic divisions I and II. Similar to mitosis, cells about to undergo first meiotic division replicate their DNA during interphase. During metaphase I, homologous chromosomes pair up, forming a synapsis or tetrad (2 chromatids per chromosome), sometimes referred to as the *bivalents*. The X and Y chromosomes do not form bivalents, nor are bivalents formed during mitotic division. While in metaphase I, an interchange of chromatid segments can occur; this process is called *crossing over* (Fig. 3–5). Crossing over allows for new combinations of genes, increasing genetic variability. After telophase I, each of the two daughter cells contains one member of each homologous pair of chromosomes and a sex chromosome (23 double-stranded chromosomes). No DNA synthesis occurs before meiotic division II. During anaphase II, the 23 double-stranded chromosomes (2 chromatids) of each of the two daughter cells from meiosis I divide at their centromeres. Each subsequent daughter cell receives 23 single-stranded chromatids. A total of four daughter cells are formed by a meiotic division of one cell (Fig. 3–6).

Meiosis, which only occurs in the gamete-producing cells found in either testes or ovaries, has a different outcome in males and females. In males, meiosis (spermatogenesis) results in four viable daughter cells called spermatids which differentiate into sperm cells. In females, gamete formation or oogenesis is quite different. After the first meiotic division of a primary oocyte, a secondary oocyte and another structure called a polar body are formed. This small polar body contains little or no cytoplasm, but it may undergo the second meiotic division resulting in two polar bodies (Fig. 3–7). The secondary oocyte undergoes its second meiotic division producing one mature oocyte and another polar body. There are four viable end products from spermatogenesis and only one from oogenesis.

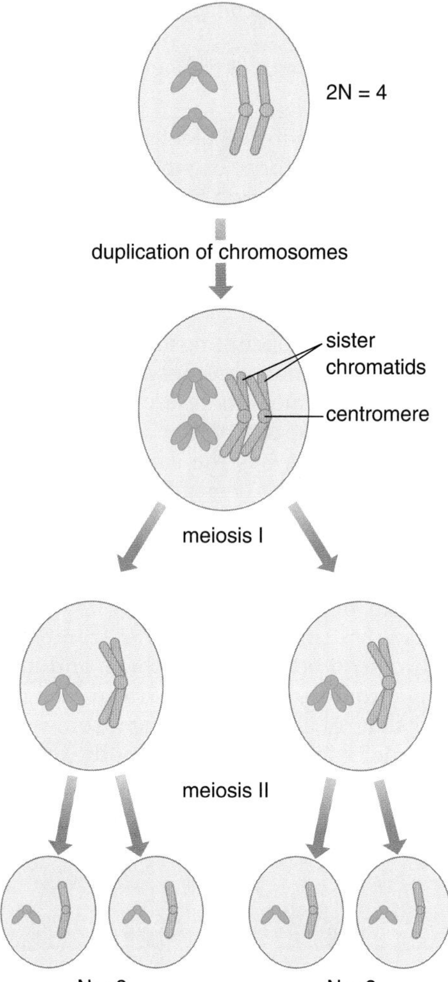

Figure 3-6
Separation of chromosomes at the time of meiosis.

Chromosome Structure

Cytogenetics is the study of the structure and numeric characteristics of the cell's chromosomes. Chromosome studies can be done on any tissue or cell that grows and divides in culture. The lymphocytes from venous blood are frequently used for this purpose. After the cells have been cultured, a drug called *colchicine* is used to arrest mitosis in metaphase. A chromosome spread is prepared by fixing and spreading the chromosomes on a slide and using a staining technique to demonstrate chromosomal banding patterns so they can be identified. The chromosomes are photographed, and the photomicrograph of each chromosome is cut out and arranged in pairs according to a standard classification system. The completed picture is called a *karyotype*, and the procedure for preparing the picture is called *karyotyping*. The uniform system of chromosome classification was originally formulated at the 1971 Paris Chromosome Conference and was later revised to describe the chromosomes as seen in more elongated prophase and prometaphase preparation.

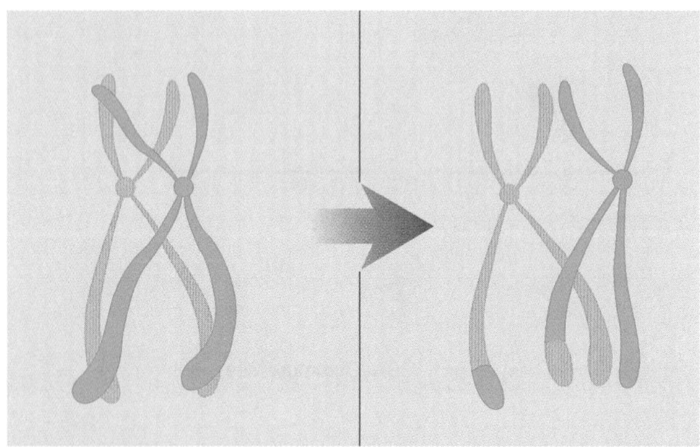

Figure 3-5
Crossing over of DNA at the time of meiosis.

In the metaphase spread, each chromosome takes the form of chromatids to form an X or "wishbone" configuration. Human chromosomes are divided into three types according to centromere (*i.e.*, central constriction) position (Fig. 3–8). If the centromere is in the center and the arms are of approximately the same length, the chromosome is said to be *metacentric;* if it is off center and the arms are of clearly different lengths, it is *submetacentric;* and if it is near one end, it is *acrocentric.* The short arm of the chromosome is designated as "p" for petite, and the long arm is designated as "q" for no other reason than it is the next letter of the alphabet. Arms of the chromosome are indicated by the chromosome number followed by the p or q designation. Chromosomes 13, 14, 15, 21, and 22 have small

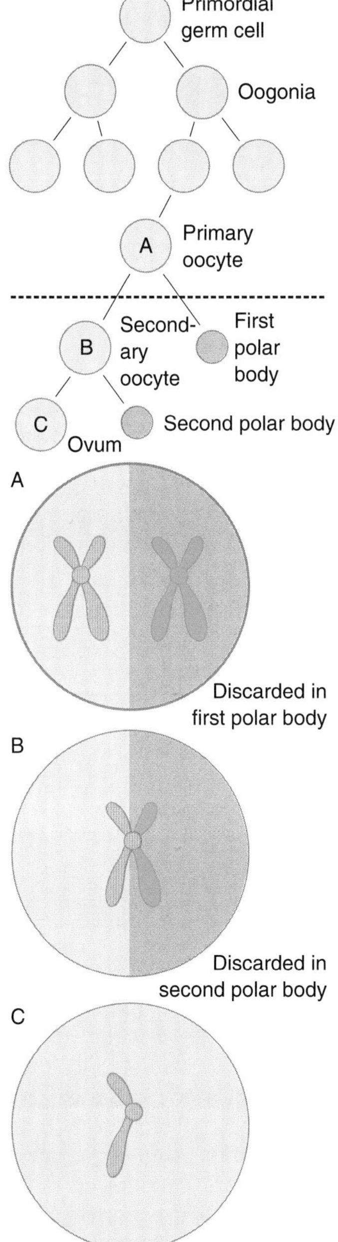

Figure 3-7
Essential stages of meiosis in a female, with discarding of the first and second polar bodies and formation of the ovum with the haploid number of chromosomes. The *dotted line* indicates reduction division.

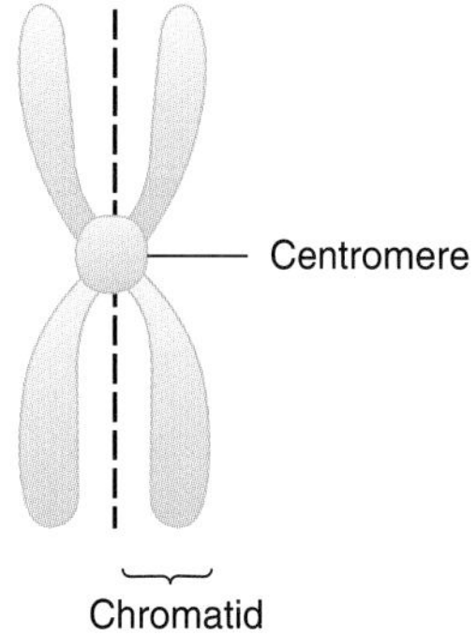

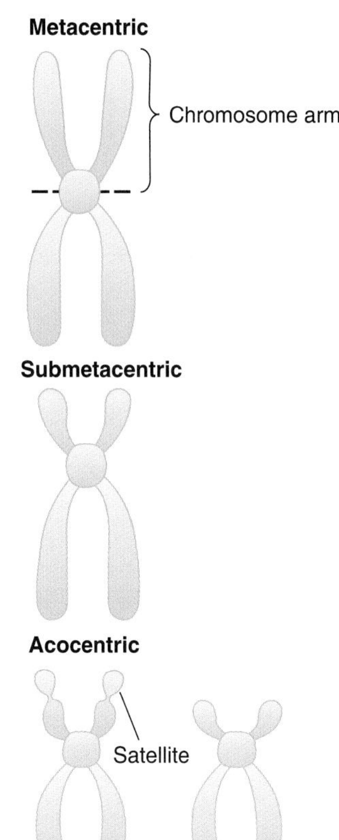

Figure 3-8
Three basic shapes and the component parts of human metaphase chromosomes. The relative size of the satellite on the acrocentric is exaggerated for visibility.

masses of chromatin called *satellites* attached to their short arms by narrow stalks. At the ends of each chromosome are special DNA sequences called telomeres. Telomeres allow the end of the DNA molecule to be replicated completely.

The banding patterns of a chromosome are used in describing the position of a gene. The regions on a chromosome are numbered from the centromere outward. The regions are further divided into bands and subbands, which are also numbered (Fig. 3–9). These numbers are used in designating the position of a gene on a chromosome. For example, Xp22.2 refers to subband 2, band 2, region 2 of the short arm (p) of the X chromosome.

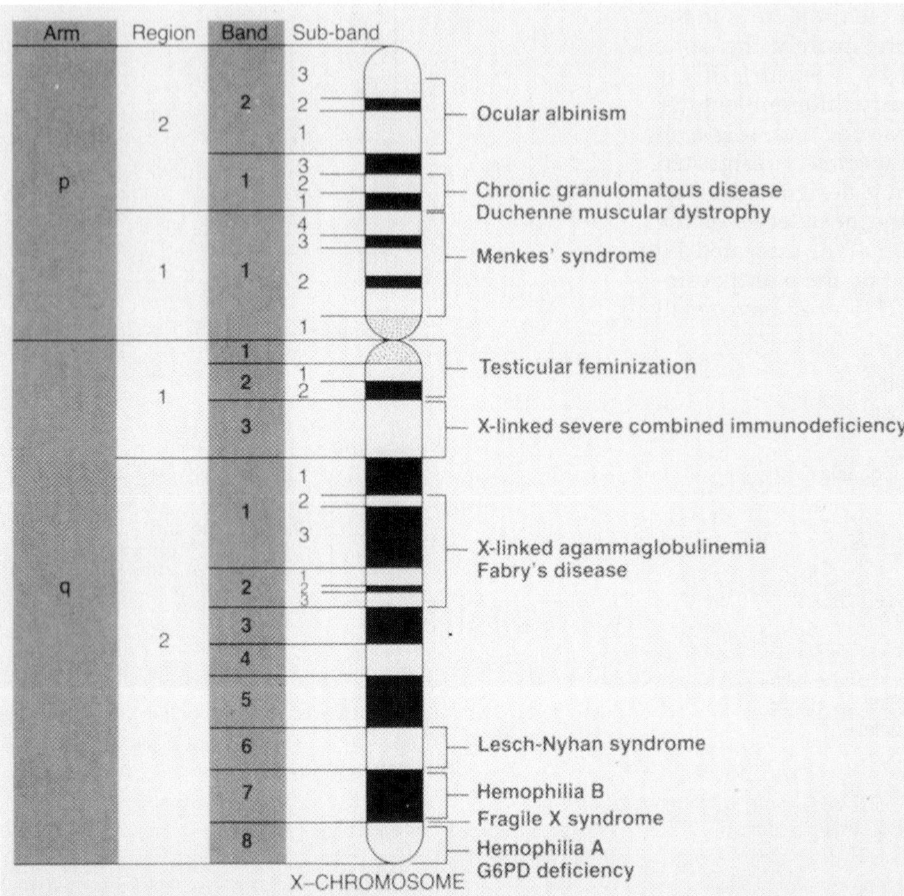

Figure 3-9 Details of a banded karyotype of the X chromosome. Notice the nomenclature of arms, regions, bands, and subbands. On the right side, the approximate locations of some errors that cause disease are indicated. (Cotran R.S., Kumar V., Robbins S.L. [1994]. *Robbins pathologic basis of disease* [5th ed.]. Philadelphia: W.B. Saunders)

In summary, the genetic information in a cell is organized, stored, and retrieved in the form of small cellular structures called chromosomes. There are 46 chromosomes arranged in 23 pairs. Twenty-two of these pairs are autosomes. The 23rd pair are the sex chromosomes, which determine the sex of a person. There are two kinds of cell division—meiosis and mitosis. Meiosis is limited to replicating germ cells and results in the formation of gametes or reproductive cells (ovum and sperm) each of which has only a single set of 23 chromosomes. Mitotic division occurs in somatic cells and results in the formation of 23 pairs of chromosomes. A karyotype is a photograph of a person's chromosomes. It is prepared by special laboratory techniques in which body cells are cultured, fixed, stained to demonstrate identifiable banding patterns, and photographed.

Patterns of Inheritance

After you have completed this section of the chapter, you should be able to meet the following objectives:

- Construct a hypothetical pedigree for a recessive and dominant trait according to Mendel's law
- Contrast genotype and phenotype
- Define the terms allele, locus, expressivity and penetrance

The characteristics that are inherited from a person's parents are inscribed in gene pairs located along the length of the chromosomes. Alternate forms of the same gene are possible (*i.e.,* one inherited from the mother and the other from the father), and each may produce a different aspect of a trait.

Definitions

Genetics has its own set of definitions. The *genotype* of a person is the genetic information stored in the base sequence triplet code. The *phenotype* refers to the recognizable traits, physical or biochemical, associated with a specific genotype. In many instances, the genotype is not evident by available detection methods. More than one genotype may have the same phenotype. Some brown-eyed persons are carriers of the code for blue eyes, and other brown-eyed persons are not. Phenotypically, these two types of brown-eyed persons are the same, but genotypically they are different.

When it comes to a genetic disorder, not all persons with a mutant gene are affected to the same extent. *Expressivity* refers to the expression of the gene in the phenotype, which can range from mild to severe. *Penetrance* means the ability of a gene to express its function. Seventy-five percent penetrance means that only 75% of the persons of a particular genotype will demonstrate a recognizable phenotype. Syndactyly and blue sclera are genetic mutations that often do not exhibit 100% penetrance.

The position of a gene on a chromosome is called its *locus*, and alternate forms of a gene at the same locus are called *alleles*. When only one pair of genes is involved in the transmission of information, the term *single-gene trait* is used. Single-gene traits follow the mendelian laws of inheritance. *Polygenic* inheritance involves multiple genes at different loci, with each gene exerting a small additive effect in determining a trait. Most human traits are determined by multiple pairs of genes, many with alternate codes, accounting for some of the dissimilar forms that occur with certain genetic disorders. Polygenic traits are predictable, but less so than single-gene traits.

Multifactorial inheritance is somewhat similar to polygenic inheritance in that multiple alleles at different loci affect the outcome; the difference is that multifactorial inheritance includes environmental effects on the genes. Many other gene-gene interactions are known, these include *epistasis*, in which one gene masks the phenotypic effects of another nonallelic gene; *multiple alleles*, in which more than one allele affects the same trait (*e.g.*, ABO blood types); *complementary genes*, in which each gene is mutually dependent on the other; and *collaborative genes*, in which two different genes influencing the same trait interact to produce a phenotype neither gene alone could produce.

Another type of inheritance pattern called *genomic imprinting* or *parenteral imprinting* has been described. In this type of inheritance, the phenotypic expression of the trait depends on whether the gene is inherited from the male or from the female.

Mendel's Laws

The main feature of inheritance is predictability: given certain conditions, the likelihood of the occurrence or recurrence of a specific trait is remarkably predictable. The units of inheritance are the genes, and the pattern of single-gene expression can be predicted using Mendel's laws, with some modification as the result of knowledge accumulated since 1865, the date of Mendel's publication.

Mendel discovered the basic pattern of inheritance by conducting carefully planned experiments with simple garden peas. From his experiments with wrinkled and round peas and other phenotypic traits in peas, Mendel proposed that inherited traits are transmitted from parents to offspring by means of independently inherited factors—now known as genes—and that these factors are transmitted as recessive and dominant traits. Mendel labeled dominant factors (his round peas) "A" and recessive factors (his wrinkled peas) "a." Geneticists continue to use capital letters to designate dominant traits and lower-case letters to identify recessive traits. The possible combinations that can occur with transmission of single-gene dominant and recessive traits can be described by constructing a figure called a *Punnet square* using capital and lower-case letters (Fig. 3–10).

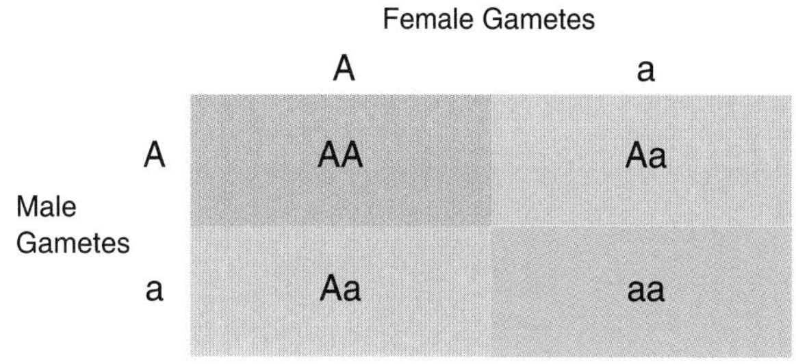

Figure 3-10
Possible combinations that can occur with transmission of a single-gene trait.

The observable traits are inherited by the offspring from the parents. During maturation, the primordial germ cells (*i.e.*, sperm and ovum) of both parents undergo meiosis, or reduction division, in which the number of chromosomes is divided in half (from 46 to 23). At this time, the two alleles from a gene locus separate so that each germ cell receives only one allele from each pair (*i.e.*, Mendel's first law). According to Mendel's second law, the alleles from the different gene loci segregate independently and recombine in a random fashion in the zygote formed by the union of the two germ cells. Persons in whom the two alleles of a given pair are the same (AA or aa) are called *homozygotes*. *Heterozygotes* have different (Aa) alleles at a gene locus. A *recessive trait* is one that is expressed only in a homozygous pairing; a *dominant trait* is one that is expressed in a homozygous or a heterozygous pairing. All persons with a dominant allele manifest that trait. A *carrier* is a person who is heterozygous for a recessive trait and does not manifest the trait. For example, if the genes for blond hair were determined to be recessive and those for brunette hair were dominant, then only persons with a genotype with two alleles for blond hair would be blond, and all persons with one or two brunette alleles would have dark hair.

Pedigree

A pedigree is a graphic method for portraying a family history of an inherited trait. It is constructed from a carefully obtained family history and is useful for tracing the pattern of inheritance for a particular trait.

In summary, inheritance represents the likelihood of the occurrence or recurrence of a specific genetic trait. The genotype refers to information stored in the genetic code of a person. The phenotype represents the recognizable traits, physical and biochemical, associated with the genotype. Expressivity refers to the expression of a gene in the phenotype, and penetrance is the ability of a gene to express its function. The point on the DNA molecule that controls the inheritance of a particular trait is called a gene locus. Alternate codes at one gene locus are called alleles. The alleles at a gene locus may be recessive or dominant traits. A recessive trait is one that is expressed only when there is homozygous pairing of the alleles. A dominant trait is expressed with homozygous or heterozygous pairing of the alleles. A pedigree is a graphic method for portraying a family history of an inherited trait.

Gene Technology

After you have completed this section of the chapter, you should be able to meet the following objectives:

- Define genomic mapping
- Briefly describe the methods used in linkage studies, dosage studies, and hybridization studies

Genomic Mapping

The genome is the gene complement of an organism. Genomic mapping is the assignment of genes to specific chromosomes or parts of the chromosome. The Human Genome Project, which started in 1990, is an international project to identify and localize all 50,000 to 100,000 genes in the human genome. The national effort toward genomic mapping is jointly coordinated by the National Institutes of Health and the Department of Energy. Organizers of the U.S. Human Genome Project hope to have the completed map by the year 2005. It is also anticipated that the project will reveal the chemical basis for as many as 4000 genetic diseases. It is expected to provide tests for screening and diagnosing genetic disorders and provide the basis for new treatments.

There are two types of genomic maps: genetic maps and physical maps. Genetic maps are like highway maps. They use linkage studies (*e.g.*, dosage, hybridization) to estimate the distances between chromosomal landmarks (*i.e.*, gene markers). Physical maps are similar to a surveyor's map. They measure the actual physical distance between chromosomal elements in biochemical units, the smallest being the nucleotide base.

Genetic maps and physical maps have been refined over the decades. The earliest mapping efforts localized genes on the X chromosome. The initial assignment of a gene to a particular chromosome was made in 1911 for the color blindness gene that was inherited from the mother (*i.e.*, followed the X-linked pattern of inheritance). In 1968, the specific location of the Duffy blood group on the long arm of chromosome 1 was determined. The locations of more than 2300 expressed human genes have been mapped to a specific chromosome and most of them to a specific region on the chromosome. However, genetic mapping is proceeding so rapidly that these numbers are constantly being updated. Documentation of gene assignments to specific human chromosomes is updated almost daily in the *Online Mendelian Inheritance in Man (OMIM)*, an encyclopedia of expressed gene loci, and in the Genome Data Base, the central database for mapped genes and international repository for most mapping information. A number of methods have been used for developing genetic maps. The most important ones used are family linkage studies, gene dosage methods, and hybridization studies. Often, the specific assignment of a gene is made possible by the use of information from several mapping techniques.

Linkage Studies

Linkage studies assume that genes occur in a linear array along the chromosomes. During meiosis, the paired chromosomes of the diploid germ cell exchange genetic material in a phenomenon called *crossing over* (see Fig. 3–5). This exchange involves not single, but large blocks of genes, each accounting for a sizable fraction of the chromosome. Although the point at which one block separates from another occurs in a random fashion, the closer together two genes are on the same chromosome, the greater the chance is that they will be passed on together to the offspring. When two inherited traits occur together at a rate significantly greater than would occur by chance, they are said to be *linked.*

There are several methods of using the crossing over and recombination of genes to map a particular gene. In one method, any gene that is already assigned to a chromosome can be used as a marker to assign other linked genes. For example, it was found that an extra-long chromosome 1 and the Duffy blood group were inherited as a dominant trait, placing the position of the blood group gene close to the extra material on chromosome 1. Color blindness has been linked to classic hemophilia A (*i.e.*, lack of factor VIII) in some pedigrees; hemophilia A has been linked to glucose 6-phosphate dehydrogenase deficiency in others; and color blindness has been linked to glucose 6-phosphate dehydrogenase deficiency in still others. Because the gene for color blindness is known to be located on the X chromosome, all three genes must be located in a small section of the X chromosome. Linkage analysis can be used clinically to identify affected persons in a family with a known genetic defect. Males, because they have one X and one Y chromosome, are said to be *hemizygous* for sex-linked traits. Females can be homozygous (normal or mutant) or heterozygous for sex-linked traits. Heterozygous females are known as carriers for X-linked defects.

Two autosomal recessive disorders successfully diagnosed prenatally by linkage studies using amniocentesis are congenital adrenal hyperplasia (due to 21-hydroxylase deficiency) which is linked to an immune response gene (HLA type). Postnatally, linkage studies have been used in diagnosing hemochromatosis, which is closely linked to another HLA type (see Chapter 11). Persons with this disorder are unable to metabolize iron, and it accumulates in the liver and other organs. It cannot be diagnosed by conventional means until irreversible damage has been done. Given a family history of the disorder, HLA typing can determine if the gene is present; if present, dietary restriction of iron intake may be used to prevent organ damage.

Dosage Studies

Dosage studies involve measuring enzyme activity. Autosomal genes are normally arranged in pairs, and normally both are expressed. If both alleles are present and both are expressed, the activity of the enzyme should be 100%. If one member of the gene pair is missing, only 50% of the enzyme activity is present, reflecting the activity of the remaining normal allele.

Hybridization Studies

One of the biologic discoveries in recent years is that two somatic cells from different species, when grown together in the same culture, occasionally fuse together to form new hybrid cell. Two types of hybridization methods are used in genomic studies: somatic cell hybridization and in situ hybridization.

Somatic cell hybridization involves the fusion of human somatic cells with those of a different species (typically, the mouse) to yield a cell containing the chromosomes of both species. Because these hybrid cells are unstable, they begin to lose chromosomes of both species during subsequent cell divisions. This makes it possible to obtain cells with different partial combinations of human chromosomes. By studying the enzymes that these cells produce, it is possible to determine that an enzyme is only produced when a certain chromosome is present; the coding for that enzyme must be located on that chromosome. In situ hybridization involves the use of a specific sequence of DNA or RNA to locate genes that do not express themselves in cell culture. DNA and RNA can be chemically tagged with radioactive or fluorescent markers. These chemically tagged DNA or RNA sequences are used as probes to determine gene location. The probe is added to a chromosome spread after the DNA strands have been separated. If the probe matches the complementary DNA of a chromosome segment, it hybridizes and remains at the precise location (hence the term in situ) on a chromosome. The radioactive or fluorescent markers are used to determine the location of the probe.

Recombinant DNA Technology

During the past several decades, genetic engineering has provided the methods for manipulating nucleic acids and recombining genes (recombinant DNA) into hybrid molecules that can be inserted into unicellular organisms and reproduced many times over. Each hybrid molecule gives rise to a genetically identical population, called a *clone*, that reflects its common ancestor.

The techniques of gene isolation and cloning rely on the fact that the genes of all organisms, from bacteria through mammals are based on similar molecular organization. Gene cloning requires cutting a DNA molecule apart, modifying and reassembling its fragments, and producing copies of the modified DNA, its mRNA, and its gene product. The DNA molecule is cut apart through the use of a bacterial enzyme, called a *restriction enzyme*, that binds to DNA wherever a particular short sequence of base pairs is found and cleaves the molecule at a specific nucleotide site. In this way, a long DNA molecule can be broken down into smaller discrete fragments with the intent that one of the fragments contains the gene of interest. More than 100 restriction enzymes are commercially available that will cut DNA at different recognition sites.

The selected gene fragment is replicated through insertion into a unicellular organism, such as a bacterium. To do this, a cloning vector such as a bacterial virus or a small DNA circle that is found in most bacteria, called a *plasmid*, is used. Viral and plasmid vectors replicate autonomously in the host bacterial cell. In the process of gene cloning, a bacterial vector and the DNA fragment are mixed together and joined by a special enzyme called a *DNA ligase*. The recombinant vectors are introduced into a suitable culture of bacteria, and the bacteria are allowed to replicate and express the recombinant vector gene. Sometimes, mRNA taken from a tissue that expresses a high level of the gene is used to produce a complementary DNA molecule that can be used in the cloning process. Because the fragments of the entire DNA molecule are used in the cloning process, additional steps are taken to identify and separate the clone that contains the gene of interest.

In terms of biologic research and technology, cloning makes it possible to identify the DNA sequence in a gene and produce the protein product encoded by a gene. The specific nucleotide sequence of a cloned DNA fragment can often be identified by analyzing the amino acid sequence and mRNA codons of its protein product. It is also possible to synthesize short sequences of base pairs that can be radioactively labeled and used to identify their complementary sequence. In this way, it is possible to identify normal and abnormal gene structures. Proteins that formerly were only available in small amounts can now be made in large quantities once their respective genes have been isolated. For example, genes encoding for insulin and growth hormone have been cloned to produce these hormones for pharmacologic use. Although quite different from inserting genetic material into a unicellular organism such as bacteria, techniques are available for inserting genes into the genome of intact multicellular plants and animals. However, the introduction of the cloned gene into the multicellular organism can only influence the few cells that acquire the gene. An answer to this problem would be the insertion of the gene into a sperm or ovum, and after fertilization, the gene would be replicated in all of the differentiating cell types. Even so, techniques for cell insertion are limited. Not only are moral and ethical issues involved, but these techniques cannot direct the inserted DNA to attach to a particular chromosome, nor can they supplant an existing gene by knocking it out of its place.

DNA Fingerprinting

The technique of DNA fingerprinting is based in part on those used in recombinant DNA technology and those originally used in medical genetics that detect slight variations in the genomes of different individuals. Using restrictive endonucleases, DNA is cleaved at specific regions. The DNA fragments are separated according to size by electrophoresis (*i.e.,* Southern blot) and transferred to a nylon membrane. The fragments are then broken apart and subsequently annealed with a series of radioactive probes specific for regions within each fragment. Autoradiography reveals the DNA fragments on the membrane. When used in forensic pathology, this procedure is undertaken on specimens from the suspect and the forensic specimen. The banding patterns are then analyzed to see if they match. With conventional methods of analysis of blood and serum enzymes, there is a 1 in 100 to 1000 chance that the two specimens match because of chance. With DNA fingerprinting, these odds are 1 in 100,000 to 1 million.

In summary, the genome is the gene complement of an organism. Genomic mapping is a method used to assign genes to particular chromosomes or parts of a chromosome. The most important ones used are family linkage studies, gene dosage methods, and hybridization studies. Often the specific assignment of a gene is made possible by the use of information from several mapping techniques. Linkage studies assign a chromosome location to genes based on their close association with other genes of known location. Recombinant DNA studies involve the extraction of specific types of messenger RNA used in synthesis of complementary DNA strands. The complementary DNA strands, labeled with a radioisotope, bind with the genes for which they are complementary and are used as gene probes. Now underway is an international project to identify and localize all 50,000 to 100,000 genes in the human genome. Genetic engineering has provided the methods for manipulating nucleic acids and recombining genes (recombinant DNA) into hybrid molecules that can be inserted into unicellular organisms and reproduced many times over. As a result, proteins that formerly were only available in small amounts can now be made in large quantities once their respective genes have been isolated. DNA fingerprinting, which relies on recombinant DNA technologies and those of genetic mapping, is often employed in forensic investigations.

BIBLIOGRAPHY

Alberts B., Bray D., Lewis J, Raff M., Roberts K., Watson J.D. (1994). *Molecular biology of the cell.* (3rd ed., pp.379–380, 242–251). New York: Garland Publishing.

Cassel C.K., Levison D. (1995). The human genome project: Who's looking out for ELSI [editorial]? *Hospital Practice* 30 (4), 11–14.

Gelehter T.D., Collins F.S. (1990). *Principles of Medical Genetics.* Baltimore: Williams and Wilkins.

Guyton A. (1996). *Textbook of medical physiology* (9th ed., pp. 27–38). Philadelphia: W.B. Saunders.

International Committee on Human Cytogenic Nomenclature. (1981). An international system for human cytogenetic nomenclature—high resolution banding. *Birth Defects* 17 (5), 1–32.

Johns D.R. (1995). Mitochondrial DNA and disease. *New England Journal of Medicine* 333 (10), 638—644.

Karf B. (1995). Molecular diagnosis (part I). *New England Journal of Medicine* 332 (18), 1218–1220.

Rosenthal N. (1994). DNA and the genetic code. *New England Journal of Medicine* 331 (1), 39–41.

Sadler R.W. (1995). *Langman's medical embryology* (7th ed., pp. 3–22, 50–51).

Sapienza C. (1990). Parenteral imprinting of genes. *Scientific American* 263 (4), 52–60.

Shapiro L.J. The molecular basis of genetic disorders. In Behrman R.E., Kliegman R.M., Nelson W., Vaughan V.C. III. (1996). *Nelson textbook of pediatrics* (15th ed., pp. 299–312). Philadelphia: W.B. Saunders.

Stine G.J. (1989). *The new human genetics.* Dubuque, IA: W.C. Brown Publishers.

Thompson M., McGinnes R.R., Willard H.F. (1991). *Genetics in medicine.* Philadelphia: W.B. Saunders.

White R., Lalouel J. (1988). Chromosomal mapping with DNA markers. *Scientific American* 258 (2), 40–49.

CHAPTER 4

Genetic and Congenital Disorders

Genetic and congenital defects are important at all levels of health care, because they affect all age groups and can involve almost any of the body tissues and organs. Congenital defects, sometimes called *birth defects*, develop during prenatal life and are usually apparent at birth or shortly thereafter. Spina bifida and cleft lip, for example, are apparent at birth, but other malformations, such as kidney and heart defects, may be present at birth but may not become apparent until they begin to produce symptoms. Not all genetic disorders are congenital, and many are not apparent until later in life.

Congenital defects may be caused by genetic factors (*i.e.*, single-gene or multifactorial inheritance or chromosomal aberrations), or they may be caused by environmental factors that occurred during embryonic or fetal development (*i.e.*, maternal disease, infections, or drugs taken during pregnancy). In rare cases, congenital defects may be the result of intrauterine factors such as crowding, fetal positioning, or entanglement of fetal parts with the amnion. Birth defects occur in 1 of every 14 live births[1] and are associated with approximately 30% of all admissions to pediatric hospitals. A large prospective study showed that African Americans have higher overall rates of minor birth defects such as polydactyly and supernumerary nipples and that whites have higher rates of major malformations.[2] Native Americans have the highest rate of fetal alcohol syndrome.[2] This chapter provides an overview of genetic and congenital disorders and is divided into three parts: genetic and chromosomal disorders; disorders caused by environmental agents; and diagnosis and counseling.

Genetic and Chromosomal Disorders

After you have completed this section of the chapter, you should be able to meet the following objectives:

- Define congenital defect
- Describe three types of single-gene disorders
- Contrast disorders due to multifactorial inheritance to those caused by single-gene inheritance
- Describe two chromosomal abnormalities that demonstrate aneuploidy
- Describe three patterns of chromosomal breakage and rearrangement
- Relate maternal age and occurrence of Down syndrome

Genetic disorders involve a permanent change (or mutation) in the genome. A genetic disorder can involve a single-gene trait, multifactorial inheritance, or a chromosome disorder.

Single-gene Disorders

Single-gene disorders are caused by a single defective or mutant gene. The defective gene may be present on only one member of a gene pair (matched with a normal gene) or in both members of the pair. Single-gene defects follow the mendelian patterns of inheritance (see Chapter 3) and are often called mendelian disorders. At last count, there were more than 6500 single-gene disorders[3]; of these, 933 disorders have been mapped to a specific chromosome.

The genes on each chromosome are arranged in pairs and in strict order, with each gene occupying a specific location or locus. The two members of a gene pair, one inherited from the mother and the other from the father, are called *alleles*. If both members of a gene pair are identical (*i.e.*, code the exact same gene product), the person is *homozygous* and if both members are different, the person is *heterozygous*. The genetic composition of a person is called a *genotype*, whereas the *phenotype* is the observable expression of a genotype in terms of morphologic, biochemical, or molecular traits. If the trait is only expressed in the heterozygote, it is said to be *dominant;* if it is only expressed in the homozygote, it is *recessive*.

Although gene expression usually follows a dominant or recessive pattern, it is possible for both alleles (members) of a gene pair to be fully expressed in the heterozygote, a condition called *codominance*. Many genes have only one normal version, called a *"wild type"* allele. Other genes have more than one normal allele (alternate forms) at the same locus. This is called *polymorphism*. Blood group inheritance (*e.g.*, AO, BO, AB) is an example of codominance and polymorphism.

A single mutant gene may be expressed in many different parts of the body. Marfan's syndrome is a defect in connective tissue that has widespread effects involving skeletal, eye, and cardiovascular structures. In other single-gene disorders, the same defect can be caused by mutations at several different loci. Childhood deafness can result from 16 different types of autosomal recessive mutations.

Single-gene disorders are characterized by their patterns of transmission, which are usually obtained through a family genetic history. The patterns of inheritance depend on whether the phenotype is dominant or recessive, and whether the gene is located on an autosomal or sex chromosome. The most common types of single-gene disorders are autosomal dominant, autosomal

TABLE 4-1 Some Disorders of Mendelian or Single-Gene Inheritance and Their Significance

Disorder	Significance
Autosomal Dominant	
Achondroplasia	Short-limb dwarfism
Adult polycystic kidney disease	Kidney failure
Huntington's chorea	Neurodegenerative disorder
Familial hypercholesterolemia	Premature atherosclerosis
Marfan's syndrome	Connective tissue disorder with abnormalities if skeletal, ocular, cardiovascular systems
Neurofibromatosis (NF)	Neurogenic tumors: fibromatous skin tumors, pigmented skin lesions, and ocular nodules in NF-1; bilateral acoustic neuromas in NF-2.
Osteogenesis imperfecta	Molecular defects of collagen
Spherocytosis	Disorder of red blood cells
von Willebrand's disease	Bleeding disorder
Autosomal Recessive	
Color blindness	Color blindness
Cystic fibrosis	Disorder of membrane transport of ions in exocrine glands causing lung and pancreatic disease
Glycogen storage diseases	Excess accumulation of glycogen in the liver and hypoglycemia (von Glerke's disease); glycogen accumulation in striated muscle in myopathic forms
Oculocutaneous albinism	Hypopigmentation of skin, hair, eyes as result of inability to synthesize melanin
Phenylketonuria (PKU)	Lack of phenylalanine hydroxylase with hyperphenylaninemia and impaired brain development
Sickle cell disease	Red blood cell defect
Tay-Sachs disease	Deficiency of hexosaminidase A; severe mental and physical deterioration beginning in infancy
X-Linked Recessive	
Bruton-type hypogammaglobulinemia	Immunodeficiency
Hemophilia A	Bleeding disorder
Duchenne's dystrophy	Muscular dystrophy
Fragile X syndrome	Mental retardation

recessive, and X-linked (on the female chromosome). Occasionally, a gene for an X-linked dominant disorder, such as color blindness, is present in the father and mother, resulting in an X-linked recessive disorder. Disorders of the Y, or male, chromosome are rare. Table 4–1 lists some of the common single-gene disorders and their significance. Many of these disorders are described in other parts of this book.

Disorders of Autosomal Inheritance

The autosomes are represented on 22 homologous pairs of autosomal chromosomes. Disorders of autosomal inheritance include autosomal dominant and autosomal recessive traits. Among the approximate 4500 single-gene disorders, more than half are autosomal dominant. Autosomal recessive phenotypes are less common, accounting for about one third of single-gene disorders.[4]

Autosomal Dominant Disorders. In autosomal dominant disorders, a single mutant allele from an affected parent is transmitted to an offspring regardless of sex. The affected parent has a 50% chance of transmitting the disorder to each offspring (Fig. 4–1). The unaffected relatives of the parent or unaffected siblings of the offspring do not transmit the disorder. In many conditions, the age of onset is delayed, and the signs and symptoms of the disorder do not appear until later in life, as in Huntington's chorea (see Chapter 38).

Autosomal dominant disorders may also manifest as a new mutation. Whether the mutation is passed on to the next generation depends on the affected person's reproductive capacity. Many new autosomal dominant mutations are accompanied by reduced reproductive capacity; therefore, the defect is not perpetuated in future generations. If an autosomal defect is accompanied by a total inability to reproduce, essentially all new cases of the disorder will be due to new mutations. If the defect does not affect reproductive capacity, it is more likely to be inherited.

Although there is a 50% chance of inheriting a dominant genetic disorder, there can be wide variation in gene penetration and expression. When a person inherits a dominant mutant gene but fails to express it, the trait is described as having *reduced penetrance*. Penetrance is expressed in mathematical terms; a 50% penetrance indicates that a person who inherits the defective gene has a 50% chance of expressing the disorder. The person who has a mutant gene but does not express it is an important exception to the rule that unaffected persons do not transmit an autosomal dominant trait. These persons can transmit the gene to their descendants and so produce a skipped generation. Autosomal dominant disorders can also display *variable expressivity*, meaning that they can be expressed differently among individuals. Polydactyly or supernumerary digits, for example, may be expressed in the fingers or the toes.

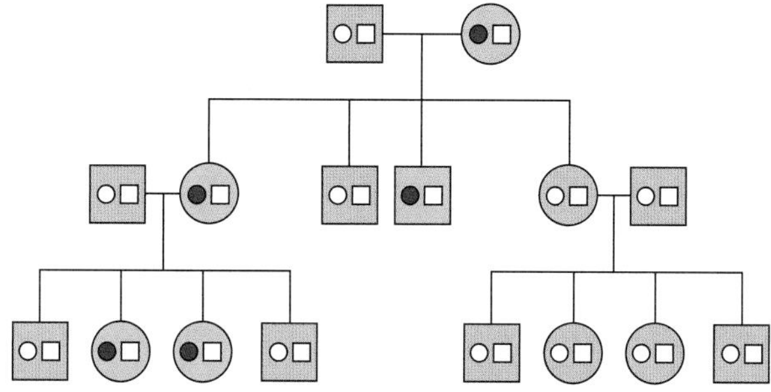

Figure 4-1
Simple pedigree for inheritance of an autosomal dominant trait. The small colored circle represents the mutant gene. An affected parent with an autosomal dominant trait has a 50% chance of passing the mutant gene on to each child regardless of sex.

The gene products of autosomal dominant disorders are usually regulatory proteins involved in complex metabolic pathways, abnormal membrane-bound transport systems, or key structural proteins such as collagen.

Marfan's syndrome is a connective tissue disorder that is manifested by changes in the skeleton, eyes, and cardiovascular system. There is a wide range of variation in expression of the disorder. Persons may have abnormalities of one or all three systems. The skeletal deformities, which are the most obvious features of the disorder, include a long thin body with exceptionally long extremities and long, tapering fingers (called *arachnodactyly* or *spider fingers*), hyperextensible joints, and a variety of spinal deformities including kyphoscoliosis. Chest deformity, pectus excavatum (*i.e.*, deeply depressed sternum), or pigeon chest deformity, is often present. The most common eye disorder is bilateral dislocation of the lens due to weakness of the suspensory ligaments. Myopia and predisposition to retinal detachment (see Chapter 42) are also common, the result of increased optic globe length due to altered connective tissue support of ocular structures. However, the most life-threatening aspects of the disorder are the cardiovascular defects, which include mitral valve prolapse, progressive dilation of the aortic valve ring, and weakness of aorta and other arteries. Dissection and rupture of the aorta often lead to premature death (see Chapter 18). The average age of death in persons with Marfan's syndrome is 30 to 40 years.

Neurofibromatosis (*NF*) is a condition involving neurogenic tumors that arise from Schwann cells and other elements of the peripheral nervous system.[5,6] It is a relatively common disorder with a frequency of 1 in 3000. Approximately 50% of cases have a family history of autosomal dominant transmission, and the remaining 50% appear to represent a new mutation. There are at least two genetically and clinically distinct forms of the disorder. Type 1 neurofibromatosis (NF-1), also known as *von Recklinghausen's disease*, and type 2 bilateral acoustic neurofibromatosis (NF-2). The gene for NF-1 has been mapped to chromosome 17, and the gene for NF-2 has been mapped to chromosome 22.

NF-1, which accounts for more than 90% of cases, is characterized by multiple hyperpigmented macular skin lesions, neurofibromatosis, and small, pigmented, tumor-like nodules (also called *Lisch* nodules) of the iris. The hyperpigmented skin lesions, known as *café-au-lait* spots, are large, flat lesions (usually 15 mm or more in diameter) of uniform light brown color in whites and darker brown in African Americans, with sharply demarcated edges (Fig. 4–2). Although small single lesions may be found in normal children, larger lesions or six or more spots larger than 1.5 cm in diameter suggest NF-1. The skin pigmentations become more evident with age as the melanosomes in the epidermal cells accumulate melanin. The Lisch nodules, which are specific for NF-1, are usually present after 6 years of age. They do not present any clinical problem but are useful in establishing a diagnosis.

The neurofibromas are of three types: cutaneous, subcutaneous, and plexiform. The cutaneous neurofibromas manifest as soft pedunculated lesions that project from the skin. They are the most common type, are often not apparent until puberty, and are present in greatest density over the trunk (Fig. 4–3). The subcutaneous neurofibromas become apparent toward the end of the first decade of life. When large numbers occur near the vertebral column, they may cause erosion of the spinal column with eventual spinal cord compression. The plexiform lesions are congenital and enlarge steadily with age. They are disfiguring multilobular masses that involve the subcutaneous tissue, are often hyperpigmented, and contain numerous tortuous thickened nerves.

In addition to the neurofibromatosis, persons with NF-1 have a variety of other associated lesions, the most common being skeletal lesions such as scoliosis and erosive bone defects. Persons with NF-1 are also at increased risk for developing other nervous system tumors such as meningiomas, optic gliomas, and pheochromocytomas.

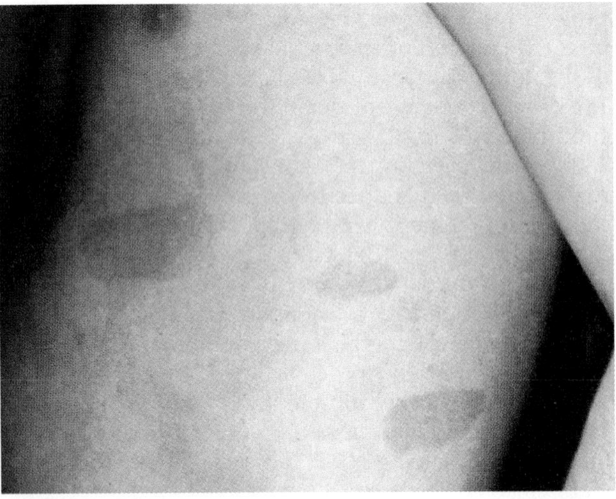

Figure 4-2
Neurofibromatosis with early café-au-lait spots in a 5-year-old child. (Owen Laboratories, Inc.)

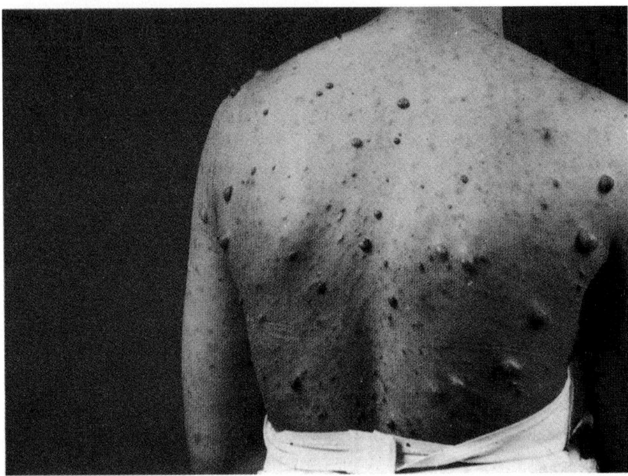

Figure 4-3
Neurofibromatosis on the back. (Reed and Carnick Pharmaceuticals)

NF-2 is characterized by tumors of the acoustic nerves. Most often the disorder is asymptomatic through the first 15 years of life. The most frequent symptoms are headaches, hearing loss, and tinnitus (*i.e.*, ringing in the ears). There may be associated intracranial and spinal meningiomas. The condition is made worse by pregnancy, and oral contraceptives may increase the growth and symptoms of tumors. Persons with the disorder should be warned that severe disorientation may occur during diving or swimming underwater and drowning may result. Surgery may be indicated for debulking or removal of the tumors.

Autosomal Recessive Disorders. Autosomal recessive disorders are manifested only when both members of the gene pair are affected. In this case, both parents may be unaffected but are carriers of the defective gene. Autosomal recessive disorders affect both sexes. The occurrence risk in each pregnancy is one in four for an affected child, two in four for a carrier child, and one in four for a normal (noncarrier, unaffected) homozygous child (Fig. 4–4).

With autosomal recessive disorders, the expression of the gene tends to be more uniform than with autosomal dominant disorders; the age of onset is frequently early in life; and in many cases, enzyme proteins are affected by the mutation. These enzyme defects may result in any of the following: deficiency of a metabolic end product, production of harmful intermediates or toxic byproducts of metabolism, or accumulation of destructive substances within the cell. Two examples of autosomal recessive disorders that are not covered elsewhere in the book are phenylketonuria and Tay-Sachs disease.

Phenylketonuria (PKU) is a genetically inherited enzyme defect. It is characterized by a deficiency of phenylalanine hydroxylase, the enzyme needed for conversion

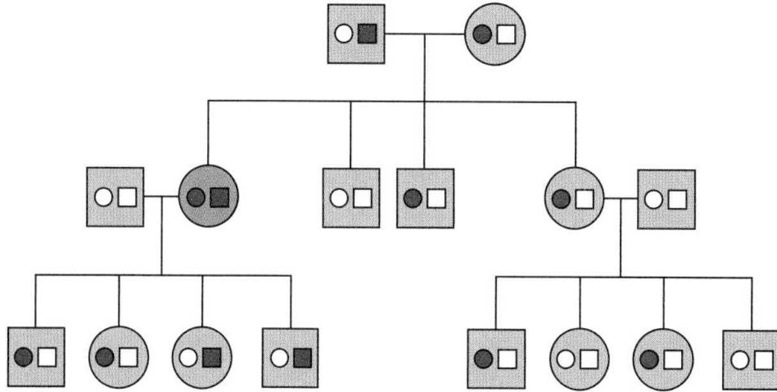

Figure 4-4
Simple pedigree for inheritance of an autosomal recessive trait. The small colored circle and square represent a mutant gene. When both parents are carriers of a mutant gene, there is a 25% chance of having an affected child, a 50% chance of a carrier child, and a 25% chance of a nonaffected or noncarrier child, regardless of sex. All children (100%) of an affected parent are carriers.

of phenylalanine to tyrosine, and as a result of this deficiency, toxic levels of phenylalanine accumulate in the blood. Like other inborn errors of metabolism, PKU is inherited as a recessive trait and is manifested only in the homozygote. It is possible to identify carriers of the trait by subjecting them to a phenylalanine test in which a large dose of phenylalanine is administered orally and the rate at which it disappears from the bloodstream is measured. PKU occurs once in approximately 10,000 births, and damage to the developing brain almost always results when high concentrations of phenylalanine and other metabolites persist in the blood. Newborn infants are routinely screened for abnormal levels of serum phenylalanine. Infants with the disorder are treated with a special diet that restricts phenylalanine intake. Dietary treatment must be started early in neonatal life to prevent brain damage.

Tay-Sachs disease is caused by an accumulation of ganglioside GM_2 (a glycolipid) in body tissues due to an enzyme deficiency (hexosaminidase A), resulting in gangliosidosis. Although gangliosides accumulate in many tissues, involvement of the central and autonomic nervous system and retina are produce the most prominent effects. The disease is particularly prevalent among eastern European (Ashkenazi) Jews. Infants with Tay-Sachs appear normal at birth but begin to manifest neurologic signs at about 6 months of age. These neurologic manifestations eventually lead to muscle flaccidity, dementia, and finally death at about 2 to 3 years of age. Although there is no cure for the disease, analysis of the blood serum for a deficiency of hexosaminidase A allows accurate identification of the genetic carriers for the disease.

Disorders of Sex-linked Inheritance

Sex-linked disorders are almost always associated with the X, or female, chromosome, and the inheritance pattern is predominantly recessive. Because of a normal paired gene, heterozygous females rarely experience the effects of a defective gene. The common pattern of inheritance is one in which an unaffected mother carries one normal and one mutant allele on the X chromosome. This means that she has a 50% chance of transmitting the defective gene to her sons and that her female children have a 50% chance of being carriers of the mutant gene. When the affected male procreates, he transmits the defective gene to all of his daughters, who become carriers of the mutant gene. Because the genes of the Y chromosome are unaffected, the affected male does not transmit the defect to any of his sons and they will not be carriers or transmit the disorder to their children. X-linked recessive disorders include glucose-6-phosphate dehydrogenase deficiency (see Chapter 8), hemophilia A (see Chapter 7), and Bruton's hypogammaglobulinemia (see Chapter 12).

The *fragile X syndrome* is an X-linked disorder associated with a fragile site on the X chromosome where the chromatin fails to condense during mitosis. It has a frequency of 1 in 1500 male births and is a common cause of mental retardation. Males with the disorder also have coarse facial features and macroorchidism. The basic defect responsible for this syndrome is unknown. The disorder cannot be categorized as a pure dominant or recessive trait because female carriers may or may not be retarded and may or may not reveal the fragile site on their chromosomes.

Disorders of Multifactorial Inheritance

Multifactorial inheritance disorders (also called polygenic disorders) are caused by multiple genes and, in many cases, environmental factors. The exact number of genes contributing to multifactorial traits is not known, and these traits do not follow a clear-cut pattern of inheritance as do single-gene disorders. Multifactorial inheritance has been described as a threshold phenomenon in which the factors contributing to the trait might be compared to water filling a glass.[7] Using this analogy, one might say that expression of the disorder occurs when the glass overflows. Disorders of multifactorial inheritance can be expressed during fetal life and be present at birth, or they may be expressed later in life. Congenital disorders that are thought to arise through multifactorial inheritance include anencephaly, cleft lip or palate, clubfoot, congenital dislocation of the hip, congenital heart disease, hydrocephalus, myelomeningocele, pyloric stenosis, and urinary tract malformation. Environmental factors are thought to play a greater role in disorders of multifactorial inheritance that develop in adult life, such as coronary artery disease, diabetes mellitus, hypertension, cancer, and the common psychiatric disorders such as manic-depressive psychoses and schizophrenia.

Although multifactorial traits cannot be predicted with the same degree of accuracy as the mendelian single-gene mutations, characteristic patterns exist. First, multifactorial congenital malformations tend to involve a single organ or tissue derived from the same embryonic developmental field. Second, the risk of recurrence in future pregnancies is for the same or a similar defect.

This means that parents of a child with cleft palate defect have an increased risk of having another child with a cleft palate, but not with spina bifida. Third, the increased risk (compared with the general population) among first-degree relatives of the affected person is 2% to 5%, and among second-degree relatives, it is about one half that amount. The risk increases with increasing incidence of the defect among relatives. This means that the risk is greatly increased when a second child with the defect is born to a couple. The risk also increases with severity of the disorder and when the defect occurs in the sex not generally affected by the disorder.

Chromosomal Disorders

Chromosome disorders form a major category of genetic disease, accounting for a large proportion of reproductive wastage (early gestational abortions), congenital malformations, and mental retardation. Specific chromosomal abnormalities can be linked to more than 60 identifiable syndromes that are present in 0.7% of all live births, 2% of all pregnancies in women older than 35 years of age, and 50% of all first-term abortions.[4]

During cell division (*i.e.*, mitosis) in nongerm cells, the chromosomes replicate so that each cell receives a full diploid number. In germ cells, a different form of division (*i.e.*, meiosis) takes place. During meiosis, the double sets of 22 autosomes and the 2 sex chromosomes (normal diploid number) become reduced to single sets (haploid number) in each gamete. At the time of conception, the haploid number in the ovum and that in the sperm join and restore the diploid number of chromosomes. Chromosomal defects usually develop because of defective movement during meiosis or because of breakage of a chromosome with loss or translocation of genetic material.

Chromosome abnormalities are commonly described according to shorthand description of the karyotype. In this system the total number of chromosomes is given first, followed by the sex chromosome complement, and then the description of any abnormality. For example, a male with trisomy 21 is designated 47,XY,+21.

Alterations in Chromosome Duplication

Mosaicism is the presence in one individual of two or more cell lines characterized by distinctive karyotypes. This defect results from an accident during chromosomal duplication. Sometimes, mosaicism consists of an abnormal karyotype and a normal one, in which case the physical deformities caused by the abnormal cell line are usually less severe.

Alterations in Chromosome Number

A change in chromosome number is called *aneuploidy*. Among the causes of aneuploidy is failure of the chromosomes to separate during oogenesis or spermatogenesis. This can occur in the autosomes or the sex chromosomes and is called *nondisjunction*. Nondisjunction gives rise to germ cells that have an even number of chromosomes (22 or 24). The products of conception formed from this even number of chromosomes have an uneven number of chromosomes, 45 or 47. *Monosomy* refers to the presence of only one member of a chromosome pair. The defects associated with monosomy of the autosomes are severe and usually cause abortion. Monosomy of the X chromosome (45,X/O), or Turner's syndrome, causes less severe defects. *Polysomy*, or the presence of more than two chromosomes to a set, occurs when a germ cell containing more than 23 chromosomes is involved in conception. This defect has been described for the autosomes and the sex chromosomes. Trisomies of chromosomes 8, 13, 18, and 21 are the more common forms of polysomy of the autosomes. There are several forms of polysomy of the sex chromosomes in which extra X or Y chromosomes are present.

Trisomy 21. Trisomy 21, or Down syndrome, is the most common form of chromosome disorder. There are 300,000 persons with Down syndrome in the United States; as many as 10,000 infants are born each year with the disorder.[7,8] Ninety percent of cases are caused by trisomy 21 due to nondisjunction; the remaining cases are caused by translocations (usually 14/21). The condition is accompanied by various levels of mental retardation.

The risk of having a baby with Down syndrome is greater in women who are 35 years of age or older at the time of delivery. Although the reason for the correlation between maternal age and nondisjunction is unknown, it is thought to reflect some aspect of aging of the oocyte. Although males continue to produce sperm throughout their reproductive life, females are born with all the oocytes they will ever have. These oocytes may change as a result of the aging process. With increasing age, there is a greater chance of a woman having been exposed to damaging environmental agents such as drugs, chemicals, and radiation. Although 95% of Down syndrome cases result from trisomy 21, other chromosomal aberrations can be involved, the most frequent being the Robertsonian translocation. Unlike trisomy 21, the Robertsonian translocation shows no relation to maternal age but has a relatively high recurrence risk in families when a parent, particularly the mother, is a carrier.

The physical features of a child with Down syndrome are distinctive, and therefore the condition is usually apparent at birth. These features include a small and rather square head. There is upward slanting of the eyes; small, low-set, and malformed ears; a fat pad at the back of the neck; an open mouth; and a large, protruding tongue (Fig. 4–5). The child's hands are usually short and stubby, with fingers that curl inward, and there is usually only a single palmar (*i.e.*, simian) crease. Hypotonia and joint laxity are also present in infants and young children. There are often accompanying congenital heart defects and an increased risk of gastrointestinal malformations. About 1% of persons with trisomy 21 Down syndrome have mosaicism (*i.e.*, cell populations with normal and trisomy 21); these persons may be less severely affected. Of particular concern is the much greater risk of for development of acute leukemia among children with Down syndrome—10 to 20 times

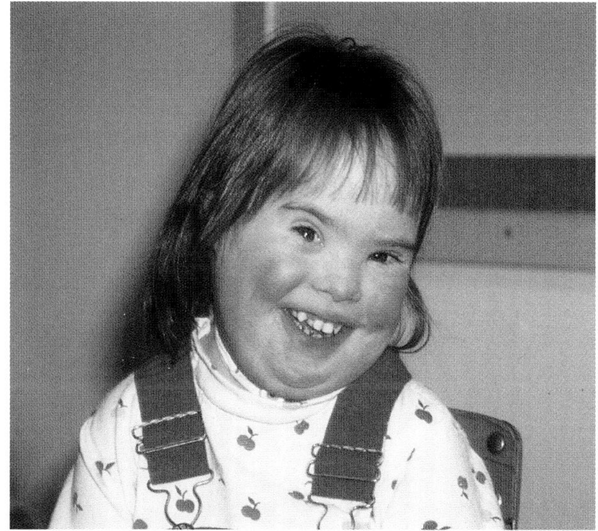

Figure 4-5
A child with Down syndrome. (Courtesy of March of Dimes Birth Defects Foundation, White Plains, NY)

greater than other children.[9] With increased life expectancy due to improved health care, it has been found that there is an increased risk of Alzheimer's disease among older persons with Down syndrome.

Monosomy X. Monosomy X, or Turner's syndrome, describes a monosomy of the X chromosome (45,X/0) with gonadal agenesis, or absence of the ovaries. This disorder affects about 1 of every 1500 to 2500 live births, and as many as 15% of spontaneous miscarriages have a 45,X/0 karyotype.[9] There are variations in the syndrome, with abnormalities ranging from essentially none to webbing of the neck with redundant skin folds, nonpitting edema of the hands and feet, and congenital heart defects, particularly coarctation of the aorta. There may also be abnormalities in kidney development (*i.e.,* abnormal location, abnormal vascular supply, or double collecting system).

Characteristically, the female with Turner's syndrome is short in stature, but her body proportions are normal. She does not menstruate and shows no signs of secondary sex characteristics. When a mosaic cell line (*i.e.,* 45,X/O and 46,X/X or 45,X/0 and 46,X/Y) is present, the manifestations associated with the chromosomal defect tend to be less severe.

Administration of female sex hormones (*i.e.,* estrogens) is used to promote development of secondary sexual characteristics and to produce additional skeletal growth in women with Turner's syndrome. Growth hormone may also be used to increase skeletal growth. Although women with Turner's syndrome are infertile, successful pregnancies have been achieved using in vitro fertilization.[10]

Polysomy X. Polysomy X, or Klinefelter's syndrome, is characterized by an X-chromatin–positive (47,X/X/Y) male and is associated with testicular dysgenesis.[11] In rare cases, there may be more than one extra X chromosome (*e.g.,* 47,X/X/X/Y). Paternal nondisjunction occurs at the first meiotic division accounts for a little more than one half the cases with the father donating the extra X chromosome. Most of the remaining cases result from nondisjunction during the first maternal meiotic division.[8] The incidence of Klinefelter's syndrome is about 1 case in 850 live births. The condition may not be detected in the newborn. The infant usually has normal male genitalia, with a small penis and small, firm testicles. Hypogonadism during puberty usually leads to a tall stature with abnormal body proportions in which the lower part of the body is longer than the upper part. Later in life, the body build may become heavy with a female distribution of subcutaneous fat and variable degrees of breast enlargement. There may be deficient secondary male sex characteristics, such as a voice that remains feminine in pitch and sparse beard and pubic hair. There may be sexual dysfunction, along with complete infertility and impotence. Personality problems may occur, but the intellect is usually normal. Replacement hormone therapy with testosterone is used to treat the disorder.

Alterations in Chromosome Structure

Aberrations in chromosome structure occur when there is a break in one or more of the chromosomes followed by rearrangement or deletion of the chromosome parts. Among the factors believed to cause chromosome breakage are exposure to radiation sources, such as x-rays; influence of certain chemicals; extreme changes in the cellular environment; and viral infections.

Several patterns of chromosome breakage and rearrangement can occur (Fig. 4–6). There can be a *deletion* of the broken portion of the chromosome. When one chromosome is involved, the broken parts may be *inverted. Isochromosome formation* occurs when the centromere, or central portion, of the chromosome separates horizontally instead of vertically. *Ring formation* results when deletion is followed by uniting of the chromatids to form a ring. *Translocation* occurs when there are simultaneous breaks in two chromosomes from different pairs with exchange of chromosome parts. With a balanced reciprocal translocation, no genetic information is lost; therefore, persons with translocations are generally normal. These persons are, however, translocation carriers and may have normal and abnormal children. A special form of translocation called a *centric fusion* or *Robertsonian translocation* involves two acrocentric chromosomes in which the centromere is near the end. Typically, the break occurs near the centromere affecting the short arm in one chromosome and the long arm in the other. Transfer of the chromosome fragments leads to one long and one extremely short chromosome (see Fig. 4–6). The short fragments are commonly lost. In this case, the person has only 45 chromosomes, but the amount of genetic material that is lost is so small that it often goes unnoticed. Difficulty, however, arises during meiosis; the result is gametes with an unbalanced number of chromosomes. A rare form of Down syndrome can

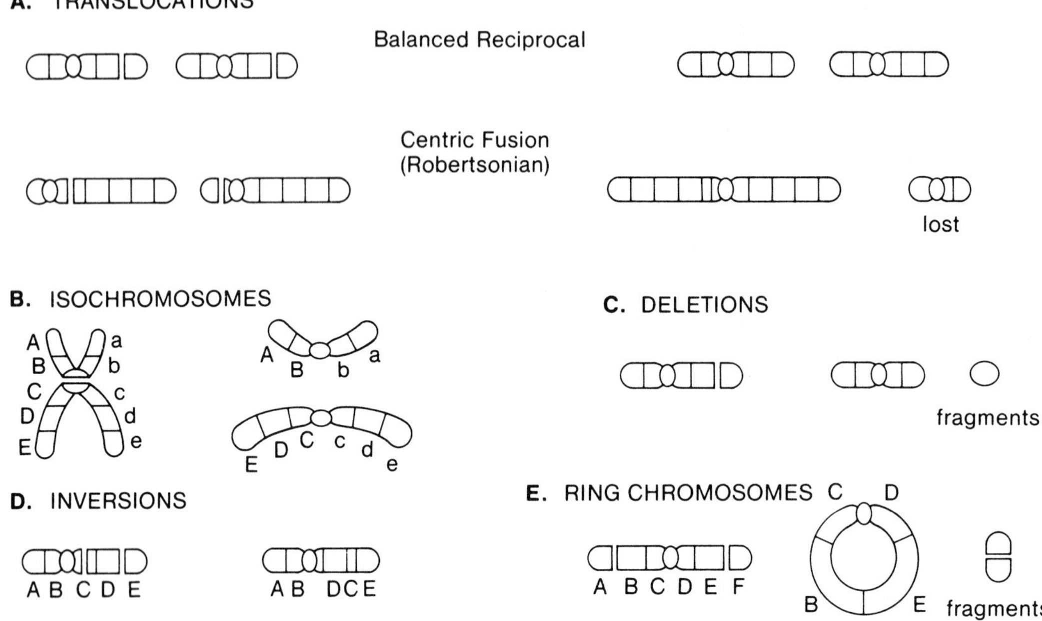

Figure 4-6
Rearrangement after breaks in chromosome structures. (Cotran R.S., Ramzi V., Robbins S. L. [1994]. *Pathologic basis of disease.* [5th ed., p. 154]. Philadelphia: W.B. Saunders)

occur in the offspring of persons in whom there has been a translocation involving the long arm of chromosome 21q and the long arm of one of the acrocentric chromosomes (most often 14 or 22). The translocation adds to the normal long arm of chromosome 21; therefore, the person with this type of Down syndrome has 46 chromosomes, but essentially a trisomy of 21q.[4]

The manifestations of aberrations in chromosome structure depend to a great extent on the amount of genetic material that is lost. Many cells suffering unrestored breaks are eliminated within the next few mitoses because of deficiencies that may in themselves be fatal. This is beneficial, because it prevents the damaged cells from becoming a permanent part of the organism or, if it occurs in the gametes, from giving rise to grossly defective zygotes. Some altered chromosomes, such as those that occur with translocations, are passed on to the next generation.

In summary, genetic and congenital disorders affect all age groups and all body structures. Genetic disorders can affect a single gene (mendelian inheritance) or several genes (polygenic inheritance). Chromosome disorders result from a change in chromosome number or structure. A change in chromosome number is called aneuploidy. Monosomy involves the presence of only one member of a chromosome pair; it is seen in Turner's syndrome, in which there is monosomy of the X chromosome. Polysomy refers to the presence of more than two chromosomes in a set. Klinefelter's syndrome involves polysomy of the X chromosome. Trisomy 21 (*i.e.*, Down syndrome) is the most common form of chromosome disorder. Alterations in chromosome structure involve deletion or addition of genetic material, which may involve a translocation of genetic material from one chromosome pair to another.

Disorders Due to Environmental Influences

After you have completed this section of the chapter, you should be able to meet the following objectives:

- Cite the most susceptible period of intrauterine life for development of defects due to environmental agents
- State the cautions that should be observed when considering use of drugs during pregnancy
- Describe the effects of alcohol and cocaine abuse on fetal development and birth outcomes
- List four infectious agents that cause congenital defects
- List types of information that are usually considered when doing assessment of genetic risk
- Cite examples of fetal information that can be obtained with use of ultrasound, amniocentesis, chorionic villus sampling, percutaneous blood sampling

The developing embryo is subject to many nongenetic influences. After conception, development is influenced by the environmental factors that the embryo shares with the mother. The physiologic status of the mother—her hormone balance, her general state of health, her nutritional status, and the drugs she takes—undoubtedly influences the development of the unborn child. For example, diabetes mellitus is associated with increased risk of congenital anomalies. Smoking is associated with lower than normal neonatal weight. Alcohol, in the context of chronic alcoholism, is known to cause fetal abnormalities. Some agents cause early abortion. Measles and other infectious agents cause congenital malformations. Other agents, such as radiation, can cause chromosomal and genetic defects and produce developmental disorders.

Period of Vulnerability

The embryo's development is most easily disturbed during the period when differentiation and development of the organs are taking place. This time interval, which is often referred to as the period of *organogenesis*, extends from day 15 to day 60 after conception. Environmental influences during the first 2 weeks after fertilization may interfere with implantation and result in abortion or early resorption of the products of conception. Each organ has a critical period during which it is highly susceptible to environmental derangements (Fig. 4–7). Often, the effect is expressed at the biochemical level just before the organ begins to develop. The same agent may affect different organ systems that are developing at the same time.

Teratogenic Agents

A teratogenic agent is an environmental agent that produces abnormalities during embryonic or fetal development. It is important to remember that, in this case, the environment is that of the embryo and fetus. Maternal disease or altered metabolic state can also affect the environment of the embryo or fetus. For discussion purposes, teratogenic agents have been divided into three groups: irradiation, drugs and chemical substances, and infectious agents.

Chart 4–1 lists commonly identified agents in each of these groups. Theoretically, environmental agents can cause birth defects in three ways: by direct exposure of the pregnant woman and the embryo or fetus to the agent; through exposure of the soon-to-be-pregnant woman with an agent that has a slow clearance rate such that a teratogenic dose is retained during early pregnancy; or as a result of mutagenic effects of an environmental agent that occur before pregnancy causing permanent damage to a woman's (or a man's) reproductive cells.

Irradiation

Heavy doses of ionizing radiation have been shown to cause microcephaly, skeletal malformations, and

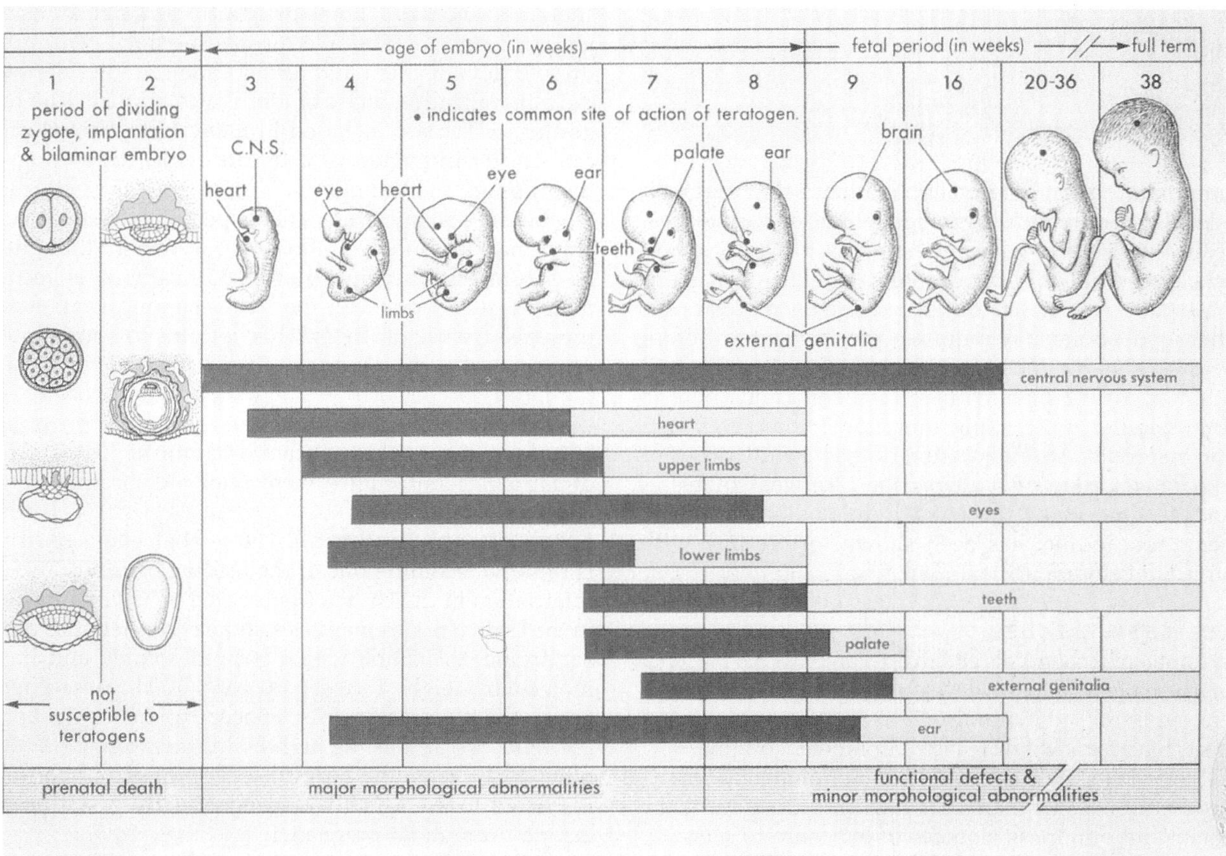

Figure 4-7
Critical periods in human development. (K.L. Moore. [1988]. *The developing human* [4th ed., p. 145]. Philadelphia: W.B. Saunders)

CHART 4-1
*Teratogenic Agents**

Irradiation

Drugs and Chemical Substances

Alcohol
Anticoagulants
- Warfarin

Anticonvulsants
Cancer drugs
- Aminopterin
- Methotrexate
- 6-Mercaptopurine

Isotretinoin (Accutane)
Progestins and oral contraceptive drugs
Propylthiouracil
Tetracycline
Thalidomide

Infectious Agents

Viruses
- Cytomegalovirus
- Herpes simplex virus
- Measles (rubella)
- Mumps
- Chickenpox

Nonviral factors
- Syphillis
- Toxoplasmosis

*Not inclusive.

mental retardation. There is no evidence that diagnostic levels of radiation cause congenital abnormalities. Because the question of safety remains, however, many agencies require that the day of a woman's last menstrual period be noted on all radiologic requisitions. Other institutions may require a pregnancy test before any extensive diagnostic x-ray studies are performed. Radiation is teratogenic and mutagenic, and there is the possibility of effecting inheritable changes in genetic materials. Administration of therapeutic doses of radioactive iodine (^{131}I) during the 13th week of gestation, the time when the fetal thyroid is beginning to concentrate iodine, has been shown to interfere with thyroid development.

Chemicals and Drugs

Environmental chemicals and drugs can cross the placenta and cause damage to the developing embryo and fetus. It has been estimated that only 2% to 3% of developmental defects have a known drug or environmental origin.

Some of the best-documented environmental teratogens are the organic mercurials, which cause neurologic deficits and blindness. Sources of exposure to mercury include contaminated food (fish) and water. The precise mechanism by which chemicals and drugs exert their teratogenic effects is largely unknown. They may produce cytotoxic (cell killing), antimetabolic, or growth-inhibiting properties. Often their effects depend on the time of exposure (in terms of embryonic and fetal development) and extent of exposure (dosage). Drugs top the list of chemical teratogens, probably because they are regularly used at elevated doses. Although the placenta is virtually impermeable to compounds of molecular weight greater than 1000, most drugs have a molecular weight of less than 500.[12] Lipid-soluble drugs tend to cross the placenta more readily and enter the fetal circulation. Equilibration of a drug between the mother and the fetus ranges from 2 minutes to 2 hours. Fetal serum levels are generally 30% to 75% of the concentration in the mother's serum.[12]

A number of drugs are suspected of being teratogens, but only a few have been identified with certainty. Perhaps the best known of these drugs is thalidomide, which has been shown to give rise to a full range of malformations, including phocomelia (*i.e.*, short, flipper-like appendages) of all four extremities. Other drugs known to cause fetal abnormalities are the antimetabolites used in the treatment of cancer, the anticoagulant drug warfarin, several of the anticonvulsant drugs, isotretinoin (*i.e.*, derivative of vitamin A) used in the treatment of cystic acne, ethyl alcohol, and cocaine. Megadoses of vitamin A have also been associated with congenital abnormalities. Although the exact teratogenic dose is unknown, it is recommended that doses greater than 10,000 should be avoided.[13] Some drugs affect a single developing structure; for example, propylthiouracil can impair thyroid development and tetracycline can interfere with the mineralization phase of tooth development. The progestins, which are included in many birth control pills, can cause virilization of a female fetus, depending on their dosage and timing.

Because many drugs are suspected of causing fetal abnormalities, and even those that were once thought to be safe are now being viewed critically, it is recommended that women in their childbearing years avoid unnecessary use of drugs. This pertains to nonpregnant women and pregnant ones because many developmental defects occur early in pregnancy. As happened with thalidomide, the damage to the embryo often occurs before pregnancy is suspected or confirmed. Two drugs of particular importance are alcohol and cocaine.

Fetal Alcohol Syndrome. The fetal alcohol syndrome is rapidly becoming one of the leading causes of mental retardation in the United States. One of 750 infants born in the United States manifests some characteristics of the syndrome.[14] Alcohol, which is lipid soluble and has a molecular weight between 600 and 1000, passes freely across the placental barrier; concentrations of alcohol in the fetus are at least as high as in the mother.[14] Unlike other teratogens, the harmful effects of alcohol are not restricted to the sensitive period of early gestation but extend throughout pregnancy.

Alcohol has widely variable effects on fetal development, ranging from minor abnormalities to a unique constellation of anomalies that has been termed the *fetal alcohol syndrome* (FAS). Criteria for defining FAS were standardized by the Fetal Alcohol Study Group of the Research Society on Alcoholism in 1980,[15] and modifications were proposed in 1989 by Sokol and Clarren.[16] The proposed criteria are prenatal or postnatal growth retardation (*i.e.,* weight or length below the 10th percentile); central nervous system involvement, including neurologic abnormalities, developmental delays, behavioral dysfunction, intellectual impairment, and skull and brain malformation; and a characteristic face with short palpebral fissures (*i.e.,* eye openings), a thin upper lip, and an elongated, flattened midface and philtrum (*i.e.,* the groove in the middle of the upper lip). The facial features of FAS may not be as apparent in the newborn but become more prominent as the infant develops (Fig. 4–8). As the children grow into adulthood the facial features become more subtle, making diagnosis of FAS in older individuals more difficult.[17] Each of these defects can vary in severity, probably reflecting the timing of alcohol consumption in terms of the period of fetal development, amount of alcohol consumed, and hereditary and environmental influences. Sokol and Clarren suggested that the term *alcohol-related birth defects* be used to describe the anatomic and functional abnormalities associated with prenatal alcohol exposure.[16]

The mechanisms whereby alcohol exerts its teratogenic effects are unclear. Evidence suggest that effects of alcohol observed in children with FAS are related to the timing of alcohol consumption and peak alcohol dose. Several mechanisms have been proposed including the direct effects of alcohol or its metabolite acetaldehyde on the developing fetus, the interaction of alcohol with prostaglandins involved in wide range of biologic activities related to normal fetal growth and development, or to the effects of alcohol on placental blood flow.[18] In studies using pregnant monkeys, alcohol administration produced transient but marked collapse of the umbilical cord, causing severe hypoxia and acidosis in the fetus.[19] If this phenomenon occurs in humans, it could explain the teratogenicity of alcohol. Even in late gestation, the unborn child could be at risk for alcohol-induced hypoxia.

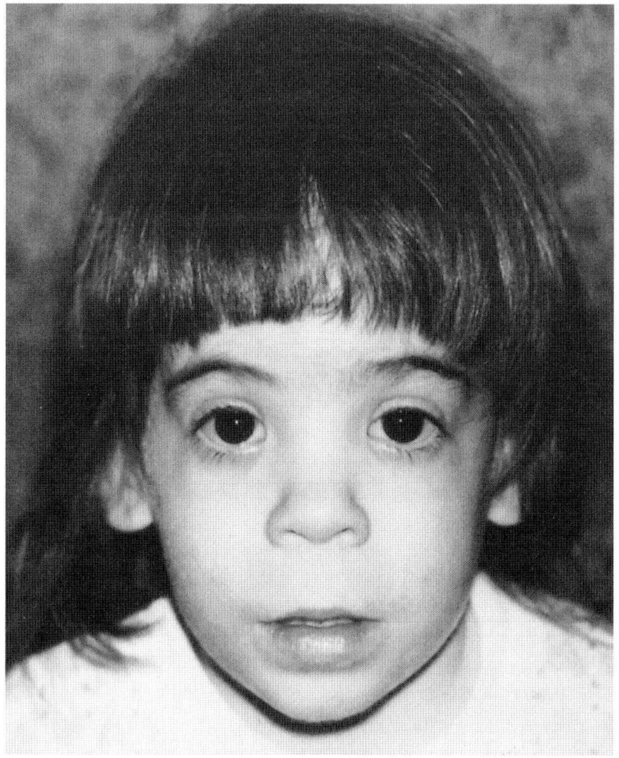

Figure 4-8
Child with fetal alcohol syndrome. (Clarren S.K., Smith D.W. [1978]. The fetal alcohol syndrome. *New England Journal of Medicine.* 298, 1065)

The amount of alcohol that can be safely consumed during pregnancy is also unknown. Animal studies suggest that the fetotoxic effects of alcohol are dose dependent rather than threshold dependent. Studies suggest that even three drinks per day may be associated with a lower IQ at age 4.[20] However, it may be that the time during which alcohol is consumed is equally important. Even small amounts of alcohol consumed during critical periods of fetal development may be teratogenic. For example, if alcohol is consumed during the period of organogenesis a variety of skeletal and organ defects may result. When alcohol is consumed later in gestation when the brain is undergoing rapid development, there may be behavior and cognitive disorders in absence of physical abnormalities. Chronic alcohol consumption throughout pregnancy may result in variety of effects ranging from physical abnormalities to growth retardation and compromised central nervous system functioning. Evidence suggests that short-lived high concentrations of alcohol such as those that occur with binge drinking may be particularly significant with abnormalities being unique to the period of exposure. Recommendations of the U.S. Surgeon General is that women abstain completely from alcohol during pregnancy.[21]

Cocaine Babies. Of concern is the increasing use of cocaine by pregnant women. From 10% to 45% of women cared for at urban teaching hospitals take cocaine during their pregnancies. [22] Determining exposure of infants to maternal cocaine use is often difficult. In utero exposure is often ascertained by testing maternal urine for cocaine and its metabolites and by interviewing the mother. Urine testing only provides evidence of recent cocaine use and information from an interview may be inaccurate. Urine testing of infants only provides evidence of recent exposure to cocaine.

Among the effects of cocaine use during pregnancy is a decrease in uteroplacental blood flow, maternal hypertension, stimulation of uterine contractions, and fetal vasoconstriction. The decrease in uteroplacental blood flow is associated with an increase in preterm births, lower birth weight, and delivery of small for gestational age infants.[23,24] Maternal hypertension may increase the risk of abruptio placentae, particularly if it is accompanied by a decrease in uteroplacental blood flow.[23] Fetal vasoconstriction has been suggested as the cause of fetal anomalies, particularly limb reduction defects and urogenital tract defects such as hydronephrosis, hypospadias and undescended testicles, and ambiguous genitalia.[23,25] Exposure of the fetus to cocaine may also lead to destructive lesions of the brain including cerebral infarction and intracranial hemorrhage. Sudden infant death syndrome (SIDS) has also been more common in babies of mothers who have used cocaine during their pregnancy.[26]

Other reported effects of maternal cocaine use on the infant are small head size, altered neonatal behavior patterns, and impaired neonatal brain stem auditory system development.[27] One study reported that 39% of 28 cocaine-exposed babies exhibited cerebral infarctions as documented on cranial ultrasound at birth.[28] Although the immediate effects of maternal cocaine use on infant behavior are being reported, the long-term effects are largely unknown. Unfortunately, cocaine addiction often affects the behavior of the pregnant woman to the extent that the need to procure larger amounts of the drug overwhelms all other considerations of maternal and fetal well-being; other factors such as malnutrition, use of other drugs and teratogens, and lack of prenatal care may also contribute to fetal disorders.

Folic Acid Deficiency. Although most birth defect are related to exposure to a teratogenic agent, deficiencies of nutrients and vitamins may also be a factor. Folic acid deficiency has been implicated in the development of neural tube defects (*e.g.*, anencephaly, spina bifida, encephalocele). Studies have shown a reduction in neural tube defects when folic acid was taken before conception and continued during the first trimester of pregnancy.[31] The Public Health Service recently recommended that all women of childbearing age should take 0.4 mg of folic acid daily. It has been suggested that this recommendation may help to prevent as many as 50% of neural tube defects.[32] These recommendation are particularly important for women who have previously had an affected pregnancy; for couples with a close relative with the disorder, and for women with diabetes mellitus and those on anticonvulsant drugs who are at increased risk for having babies with birth defects.

Infectious Agents

Many microorganisms cross the placenta and enter the fetal circulation, often producing multiple malformations. The acronym TORCH stands for *t*oxoplasmosis, *o*ther, *r*ubella, *c*ytomegalovirus, and *h*erpes, which are the agents most frequently implicated in fetal anomalies.[29,30] "Other" stands for type B hepatitis virus, coxsackie virus B, mumps, poliovirus, rubeola, varicella, listeria, gonorrhea, streptococcus, and syphilis. Of these, hepatitis B poses the greatest threat to mother and infant. The TORCH screening test examines the infant's serum for the presence of antibodies to these agents. These infections tend to cause similar clinical manifestations, including microcephaly, hydrocephaly, defects of the eye, and hearing problems. Cytomegalovirus may cause mental retardation, and rubella virus may cause congenital heart defects.

Toxoplasmosis is a protozoal infection that can be contracted by eating raw or poorly cooked meat. The domestic cat also seems to carry the organism, excreting the protozoa in its stools. It has been suggested that pregnant women should avoid contact with the excrement from the family cat. *Rubella* (*i.e.*, German measles) is a commonly recognized viral teratogen. About 15% to 20% of babies born to women who have had rubella during the first trimester have abnormalities.[30] The epidemiology of the *cytomegalovirus* is largely unknown. Some babies are severely affected at birth, and others, although having evidence of the infection, have no symptoms. In some symptom-free babies, brain damage becomes evident over a span of several years. There is also evidence that some babies contract the infection during the first year of life and in some of them the infection leads to retardation a year or two later. *Herpes simplex 2* is considered to be a genital infection and is usually transmitted through sexual contact. The infant acquires this infection in utero or in passage through the birth canal.

In summary, a teratogenic agent is one that produces abnormalities during embryonic or fetal life. It is during the early part of pregnancy (15 to 60 days after conception) that environmental agents are most apt to produce their deleterious effects on the developing embryo. A number of environmental agents can be damaging to the unborn child, including radiation, drugs and chemicals, and infectious agents. The fetal alcohol syndrome is a recently recognized risk for infants of women who regularly consume alcohol during pregnancy. Of recent concern is the use of cocaine by pregnant women. Because many drugs have the potential for causing fetal abnormalities, often at an early stage of pregnancy, it is recommended that women of childbearing age avoid unnecessary use of drugs. It has also been shown folic acid deficiency can contribute to neural tube defects. The acronym TORCH stands for toxoplasmosis, other, rubella, cytomegalovirus, and herpes, which are the infectious agents most frequently implicated in fetal anomalies."Other" stands for type B hepatitis virus, coxsackie virus B, mumps, poliovirus, rubeola, varicella, listeria, gonorrhea, streptococcus, and syphilis.

Diagnosis and Counseling

After you have completed this section of the chapter, you should be able to meet the following objectives:

- Describe the process of genetic assessment
- Cite the rationale for prenatal diagnosis
- Describe methods used in arriving at a prenatal diagnosis including ultrasonography, amniocentesis, chorionic villus sampling, percutaneous umbilical fetal blood sampling, and laboratory methods to determine the biochemical and genetic makeup of the fetus

The birth of a defective child is a traumatic event in any parent's life. Usually two issues must be resolved. The first deals with the immediate and future care of the affected child, and the second with the possibility of future children in the family having a similar defect. Genetic assessment and counseling can help to determine whether the defect was inherited and the risk of recurrence. Prenatal diagnosis provides a means of determining whether the unborn child has certain types of abnormalities.

Genetic Assessment

Effective genetic counseling involves accurate diagnosis and communication of the findings and of the risks of recurrence, to the parents and other family members who need such information. Counseling may be provided after the birth of an affected child, or it may be offered to persons at risk for having defective children (*i.e.*, siblings of persons with birth defects). A team of trained counselors can help the family to understand the problem and can support their decisions about having more children.

Assessment of genetic risk and prognosis is usually directed by a clinical geneticist, often with the aid of laboratory and clinical specialists. A detailed family history (*i.e.*, pedigree), a pregnancy history, and detailed accounts of the birth process and postnatal health and development are included. A careful physical examination of the affected child and often of the parents and siblings is usually needed. Laboratory work, including chromosomal analysis and biochemical studies, often precedes a definitive diagnosis.

The creases and dermal ridges on the palms and soles are examined in a genetic study called *dermatoglyphic analysis*. This is of value because the dermal ridges are formed by 16 weeks of gestation and any abnormalities document the time during which the developmental defect occurred. Dermatoglyphic analysis includes examination of the patterns of the arches on the fingertips, the flexion creases of the fifth finger, and the arch pattern of the base of the great toe.

Prenatal Diagnosis

Prenatal diagnosis should begin with measures to identify pregnancies in which there is a recognizable risk of diagnosable fetal disorder.[33] The use of a questionnaire to elicit genetic information is currently recommended by the American College of Obstetricians and Gynecologists before prenatal diagnosis is undertaken.[34]

The purpose of prenatal diagnosis is not just to detect fetal abnormalities. Rather, it has the following objectives: to provide parents with information needed to make an informed choice at having a child with an abnormality; to provide reassurance and reduce anxiety among high-risk groups; to allow parents at risk for having a child with a specific defect, who might otherwise forgo having a children, to begin pregnancy with the assurance that knowledge about the presence or absence of the disorder in the fetus can be confirmed by testing.

Among the methods used for fetal diagnosis are ultrasonography, amniocentesis, chorionic villus sampling, percutaneous umbilical fetal blood sampling, and laboratory methods to determine the biochemical and genetic makeup of the fetus. Sampling of maternal serum levels of alpha-fetoprotein (AFP) is used as a screening test. Termination of pregnancy is only indicated in a small number of cases; in the rest, the fetus is normal and the procedure provides reassurance for the parents. Prenatal diagnosis can also provide the information needed for prescribing prenatal treatment for the fetus. For example, if congenital adrenal hyperplasia is diagnosed, the mother can be treated with adrenal cortical hormones to prevent masculinization of a female fetus.

Maternal Serum Markers

AFP is a major fetal plasma protein and has a structure similar to the albumin that is found in postnatal life. AFP is made initially by the yolk sac and later by the liver. It peaks at about 12 to 14 weeks in the fetus and falls thereafter.[35] AFP is found in the amniotic fluid at about one hundredth the concentration found in fetal serum. AFP reaches the maternal bloodstream and can be measured by laboratory methods. The normal maternal serum AFP level rises from 13 weeks and peaks at 32 weeks gestation. In pregnancies where the fetus has a neural tube defect (*i.e.*, anencephaly and open spina bifida) or certain other malformations such as an anterior abdominal wall defect, maternal and amniotic levels of AFP are elevated because open neural tube and ventral wall defects are associated with exposed fetal membrane and blood vessel surfaces that the increases the AFP in the amniotic fluid and maternal blood. Screening of maternal blood samples is usually done between weeks 16 and 18 of gestation.[33] If the AFP level is elevated, a second serum sample is taken and ultrasound studies are advised to check for a missed abortion or multiple pregnancy, both of which produce elevated AFP levels. When a second maternal blood sample is found to contain elevated levels of AFP, more extensive ultrasound and amniocentesis are advised.

Although neural tube defects have been associated with elevated levels of AFP, decreased levels have been associated with Down syndrome. The single maternal serum marker that yields the highest detection rate for Down syndrome is an elevated level of human chorionic gonadotropin. The combined use of three maternal serum markers, decreased AFP and unconjugated estriol and elevated human gonadotropin, between 16 and 20 weeks of pregnancy has been shown shown to detect as many as 60% of Down syndrome pregnancies.[33] The use of ultrasound to verify fetal age can reduce the number of false-positive tests with this screening method.

Ultrasound

Ultrasound is a noninvasive diagnostic method that uses reflections of high-frequency sound waves to visualize soft tissue structures. Since its introduction in 1958, it has been used during pregnancy to determine number of fetuses, fetal size, fetal position, amount of amniotic fluid that is present, and placental location. it is also possible to assess fetal movement, breathing movements, and heart pattern. Improved resolution and real-time units have enhanced the ability of ultrasound scanners to detect congenital anomalies. With this more sophisticated equipment, it is possible to obtain information such as measurements of hourly urine output in a high-risk fetus. Ultrasound makes possible the in utero diagnosis of hydrocephalus, spina bifida, facial defects, congenital heart defects, congenital diaphragmatic hernias, disorders of the gastrointestinal tract, and skeletal anomalies. Cardiovascular abnormalities are the most commonly missed malformation. A four-chamber view of the fetal heart improves the detection of cardiac malformations. Intrauterine diagnosis of congenital abnormalities permits planning of surgical correction shortly after birth, preterm delivery for early correction, selection of cesarean section to reduce fetal injury, and in some cases, in utero therapy. When a congenital abnormality is suspected, a diagnosis made using ultrasound can generally be obtained by weeks 16 to 18 of gestation.

Amniocentesis

Amniocentesis involves the withdrawal of a sample of amniotic fluid from the pregnant uterus by means of a needle inserted through the abdominal wall (Fig. 4–9). The procedure is useful in women older than 35 years of age who have an increased risk of giving birth to a baby with Down syndrome; in parents who have another child with chromosomal abnormalities; and in situations in which parent is known to be a carrier of an inherited disease. Ultrasound is used to gain additional information and to guide the placement of the amniocentesis needle. The amniotic fluid and cells that have been shed by the fetus are studied. Usually, a determination of fetal status can be made by the 16th to 17th week of pregnancy. For chromosomal analysis, the fetal cells are grown in culture and the result is available in 10–14 days. The amniotic fluid can also be tested using various biochemical tests.

Early amniocentesis (before 15 weeks) can be done. However, its safety has not been established. The volume of fluid removed in relation to total amniotic fluid is greater, which may have an effect on fetal loss and fetal lung function.

Chorionic Villus Sampling

Sampling of the chorionic villi is performed at 8 to 12 weeks of gestation. The chorionic villi are the site of exchange of nutrients between the maternal blood and the embryo—the chorionic sac encloses the early amniotic sac and fetus and the villi are the primitive blood vessels that develop into the placenta. The biopsy is taken through the cervix using a catheter and gentle suctioning under ultrasound guidance. Sometimes an abdominal approach is needed if the transcervical approach is inadequate or if a sample is required after the 12th week of gestation. The tissue that is obtained can be used for fetal chromosome studies, DNA analysis, and biochemical

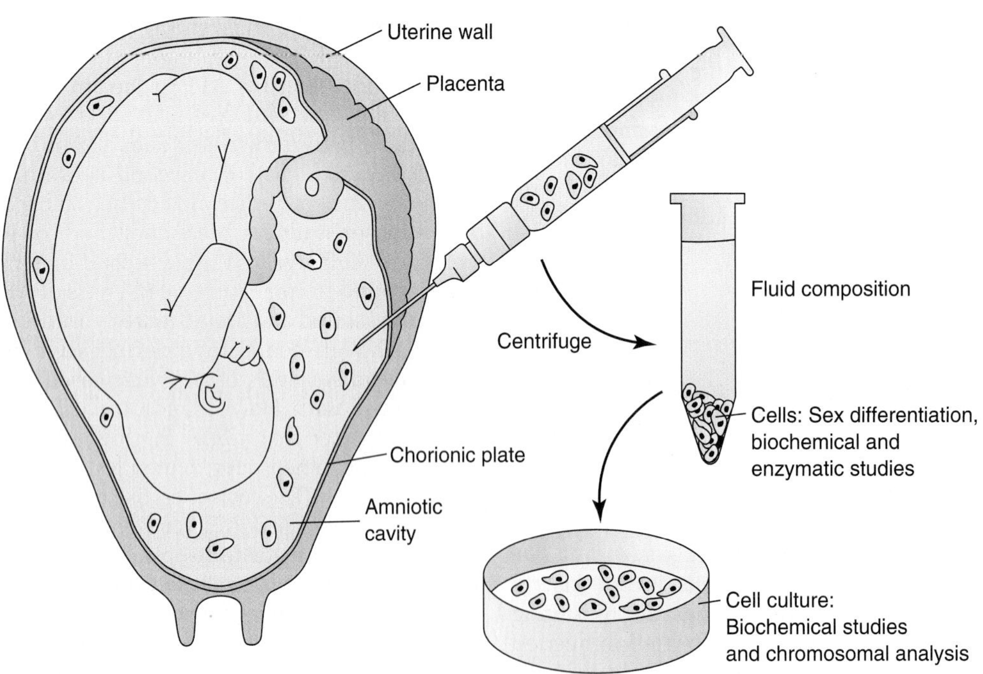

Figure 4-9
Amniocentesis. A needle is inserted into the uterus through the abdominal wall, and a sample of amniotic fluid is withdrawn for chromosomal and biochemical studies. (Department of Health, Education and Welfare. [1977]. *What are the facts about genetic disease?* Washington, DC: DHEW)

studies. The fetal tissue does not have to be cultured, and fetal chromosome analysis can be made available in 24 hours. DNA analysis and biochemical tests can be completed in 1 to 2 weeks. Limb-reduction defects have been reported with increased frequency when chorionic villus sampling is performed between 56 and 66 days of gestation.[35]

Percutaneous Umbilical Blood Sampling

Percutaneous fetal blood sampling involves the transcutaneous insertion of a needle through the uterine wall and into the umbilical artery. It is performed under ultrasound guidance and can be done anytime after 16 weeks of gestation. It is used for prenatal diagnosis of hemoglobinopathies, coagulation disorders, metabolic and cytogenic disorders, and immunodeficiencies. Fetal infections such as rubella and toxoplasmosis can be detected through measurement of IgM antibodies or direct blood cultures. Results from cytogenic studies are usually available within 48 to 72 hours. Because the procedure carries a greater risk of pregnancy loss than amniocentesis, it usually reserved for situations in which rapid cytogenic analysis is needed or in which diagnostic information cannot be obtained by other methods.

Fetal Biopsy

Fetal biopsy is done with a fetoscope under ultrasound guidance. It is used to detect certain genetic skin defects that cannot be diagnosed with DNA analysis. It may also be done to obtain muscle tissue for use in diagnosis of Duchenne muscular dystrophy.

Cytogenic and Biochemical Analyses

Amniocentesis and chorionic villus sampling yield cells that can be used for cytogenetic and DNA analyses. Biochemical analyses can be used to detect abnormal levels of fetal proteins (AFP) and abnormal biochemical products in the maternal blood and in specimens of amniotic fluid and fetal blood.

Cytogenetic studies are used for fetal karyotyping to determine the chromosome makeup of the fetus. It is done to detect abnormalities of chromosome number and structure. Karyotyping also reveals the sex of the fetus. This may be useful when an inherited defect is known to affect only one sex.

DNA analysis is done on cells extracted from the amniotic fluid or obtained by chorionic villus sampling. It is done to detect genetic defects such as inborn errors of metabolism. The defect may be established through direct demonstration of the molecular defect or through methods that break the DNA into fragments so that the fragments may be studied to determine the presence of an abnormal gene. Direct demonstration of the molecular defect is done by growing the amniotic fluid cells in culture and measuring the enzymes that the cultured cells produce. Many of the enzymes are expressed in the chorionic villi; this permits earlier prenatal diagnosis because the cells do not need to be subjected to prior culture. DNA studies are used to detect genetic defects that cause inborn errors of metabolism such as Tay-Sachs disease, glycogen storage diseases, and familial hypercholesterolemia. Prenatal diagnoses are possible for more than 70 inborn errors of metabolism.

In summary, genetic and prenatal diagnosis and counseling are done in an effort to determine the risk of having a child with a genetic or chromosomal disorder. They often involve a detailed family history (*i.e.*, pedigree), examination of any affected and other family members, and laboratory studies including chromosomal analysis and biochemical studies. They are usually done by a genetic counselor and a specially prepared team of health care professionals. Ultrasound and amniocentesis can be used to screen for congenital defects. Ultrasound is used for determination of fetal size and position and for the presence of structural anomalies. Amniocentesis and chorionic villus sampling are used to obtain specimens for cytogenetic and biochemical studies. They are used in the prenatal diagnosis of more than 60 genetic disorders.

REFERENCES

1. *Birth defects*. (1992). White Plains, NY: March of Dimes.
2. Chavez G.F., Cordero J.F., Becerra J.E. (1988). Leading major congenital malformations among minority groups in the United States, 1981–6. *Morbidity and Mortality Weekly Reports* (SS-3), 17–24.
3. McKusick V.A. (1994). *Mendelian inheritance in man: Catalogs of autosomal dominant, autosomal recessive, and X-linked phenotypes*. Baltimore: Johns Hopkins University Press.
4. Thompson M.W., McInnes R.R., Willard H.F. (1991). *Thompson & Thompson genetics in medicine* (5th ed., pp. 59–66, 201, 411–425). Philadelphia: W.B. Saunders.
5. Oski F.A. (Ed.). (1994). *Principles and practices of pediatrics* (2nd ed., pp. 2128–2133). Philadelphia: J.B. Lippincott.
6. Behrman R.E., Kliegman R.M., Arvin A.M. (Eds.). (1996). *Nelson textbook of pediatrics* (15th ed., pp. 1705–1707). Philadelphia: W.B. Saunders.
7. Riccardi V.M. (1977). *The genetic approach to human disease* (pp. 92, 500). New York: Oxford University Press.
8. Hayes A., Batshaw M.L. (1993). Down syndrome. *Pediatric Clinics of North America* 40 (3), 523–535.
9. Cotran, Ramzi, Robbins. (1994). *Robbins pathologic basis of disease* (5th ed, pp. 152–161). Philadelphia, W.B. Saunders.
10. Saenger P. (1996). Turner's syndrome. *New England Journal of Medicine* 335 (23), 1749–1754.
11. Rubin E., Farber J.L. (1994) *Pathology* (2nd ed., p. 222). Philadelphia: J.B. Lippincott.
12. Hill, L.M. (1984). Effects of drugs and chemicals on the fetus and newborn (first of two parts). *Mayo Clinic Proceedings* 59, 7–16.
13. Oakley G.P., Erickson J.D. (1995). Vitamin A and birth defects. *New England Journal of Medicine* 333 (21), 1414–1415.
14. Able E.L., Sokol R.J. (1991). A revised conservative estimate of the incidence of FAS and its economic impact. *Alcohol Clinical and Experimental Research* 14, 645–47.
15. Rosett H.L. (1980). A clinical perspective of the fetal alcohol syndrome. *Alcohol, Clinical and Experimental Research* 4, 118.
16. Sokol R.J., Clarren S.K. (1980). Guidelines for use of terminology describing the impact of prenatal alcohol on the

offspring. *Alcohol, Clinical and Experimental Research* 13, 587–589.
17. Lewis D.D., Woods S.E. (1994). Fetal alcohol syndrome. *American Family Physician* 50 (5), 1025–1032.
18. Schenker S., Becker H.G., Randall C.L., Phillips D.K., Baskin G.S., Henderson G.I. (1990). Fetal alcohol syndrome: Current status of pathogenesis. *Alcohol Clinical and Experimental Research* 14, 635–647.
19. Mukherjee A.B., Hodgen G.D. (1982). Maternal alcohol exposure induces transient impairment of umbilical circulation and fetal hypoxia in monkeys. *Science* 218, 200.
20. Ernhart C.B., Bowden D.M., Astley S.J. (1987). Alcohol teratogenicity in the human: A detailed assessment of specificity, critical period, and threshold. *American Journal of Obstetrics and Gynecology* 156, 33–39.
21. Surgeon General's advisory on alcohol and pregnancy. (1981). *FDA Drug Bulletin* 2, 10–6.
22. Volpe J.J. (1992). Effect of cocaine use on the fetus. *New England Journal of Medicine* 327 (6), 399–407.
23. MacGregor S.N., Keith L.G., Chasnoff I.J., Rosner M.A., Chisnum G.M., Shaw P., Minogue J.P. (1987). Cocaine use during pregnancy: Adverse outcome. *American Journal of Obstetrics and Gynecology* 157 (3), 686.
24. Chasnoff I.J., Griffith D.R. (1989). Cocaine: Clinical studies of pregnancy and the newborn. *Annals of the New York Academy of Sciences* 562, 260.
25. Chasnoff I.J., Chisum G.M., Kaplan W.E. (1988). Maternal cocaine use and genitourinary malformations. *Teratology* 37, 201.
26. Riley J.B., Brodsky N.L., Porat R. (1988). Risk of SIDS in infants with *in utero* cocaine exposure: A prospective study [abstract]. *Pediatric Research* 23, 454A.
27. Shih B., Cone-Wesson B., Reddix B., Wu P.Y.K. (1988). Effects of maternal cocaine abuse on the neonatal auditory system [abstract]. *Pediatric Research* 23, 264A.
28. Dixon S.D., Bejar R. (1988). Brain lesions in cocaine and methamphetamine-exposed neonates [abstract]. *Pediatric Research* 23, 405A.
29. DeVore N.E., Jackson V.M., Piening S.L. (1983). TORCH infections. *American Journal of Nursing* 83, 1660.
30. Seaver L.H., Hoyme H. (1992). Teratology in pediatric practice. *Pediatric Clinics of North America* 39 (1), 111–134.
31. Committee on Genetics. (1993). Folic acid for the prevention of neural tube defects. *Pediatrics* 92 (5), 493–94.
32. Centers for Disease Control. (1992). Recommendations for use of folic acid to reduce the number of cases of spina bifida and other neural tube defects. *Morbidity and Mortality Reports* 41, 1–8.
33. D'Alton M.E., DeCherney A.H. (1993). Prenatal diagnosis. *New England Journal of Medicine* 328 (2), 114–120.
34. Antenatal diagnosis of genetic disorders. Technical bulletin no. 108. (1987). Washington, DC: American College of Obstetricians and Gynecologists, pp. 1–8
35. Workshop Report. (1993). Report of National Institute of Child Health and Human Development Workshop on Chorionic Villus Sampling and Limb and Other Defects. *American Journal of Obstetrics and Gynecology* 169 (1), 1–6.

ADDITIONAL READINGS

Buehler B., Delimont D., van Waes M., et al. (1990). Prenatal prediction of fetal hydantoin syndrome. *New England Journal of Medicine* 322, 1567–1572.

Cunningham F.G., Gilstrap L.C. (1991). Maternal alpha-fetoprotein screening. *New England Journal of Medicine* 325, 55–57.

D'Alton M.E. (1994). Prenatal diagnostic procedures. *Seminars in Perinatology* 18 (3), 140–162.

Langlois S. (1992). Genetic diagnosis based on molecular analysis. *Pediatric Clinics of North America* 39, 91–105.

Lemons P.K., Brock M.J. (1990). Prenatal diagnosis and congenital disease: Role of the clinical nurse specialist. *Neonatal Network* 9 (3), 15–22.

Little B.B., Snell L.M., Rosenfeld C.R., et al. (1990). Failure to recognize fetal alcohol syndrome in newborn infants. *American Journal of Diseases of Children* 144, 1142–1146.

Shapiro L.R. (1992). The fragile X-syndrome—a peculiar pattern of inheritance. *New England Journal of Medicine* 325, 1736–1738.

Sokol R.J., Martier S.S., Ager J.W. (1989). The T-ACE questions: Practical prenatal detection of risk drinking. *American Journal of Obstetrics and Gynecology* 160, 863–870.

Streissguth A.P., Aase J.M., Clarren S.K., et al. (1991). Fetal alcohol syndrome in adolescents and adults. *Journal of the American Medical Association* 265, 1961–1967.

Volpe J.J. (1992). Effect of cocaine use on the fetus. *New England Journal of Medicine* 327, 399–407.

CHAPTER 5

Alterations in Cell Differentiation: Neoplasia

Kathryn Ann Caudell

Cancer is the second leading cause of death in the United States after cardiovascular disease. The disease affects all age groups, causing more death among children 3 to 15 years of age than any other disease. The American Cancer Society has estimated that 1.36 million Americans developed cancer in 1996, and that one in two males and one in three females will develop cancer during their lifetime. Approximately 555,000 Americans die each year from neoplastic diseases.[1] It is estimated that as age-adjusted cancer mortality rates increase and heart disease mortality decreases, cancer will become the leading cause of death in a few decades.[2] Trends in cancer survival demonstrate that relative 5-year survival rates have improved since the early 1960s. It is estimated that approximately 58% of persons who develop cancer each year will be alive 5 years later.

Concepts of Cell Growth

On completion of this section of the chapter, you should be able to do the following:

- Define neoplasm and explain how neoplastic growth differs from the normal adaptive changes seen in atrophy, hypertrophy, and hyperplasia
- Distinguish between cell proliferation and differentiation
- Describe the five phases of the cell cycle
- Characterize the properties of stem cells

Cancers result from altered cell differentiation and growth. The resulting tissue is called neoplasia. The term *neoplasm* comes from a Greek word meaning new formation. Unlike the tissue growth that occurs with hypertrophy and hyperplasia, the growth of a neoplasm is uncoordinated and relatively autonomous in that it lacks normal regulatory controls over cell growth and division. Neoplasms tend to increase in size and continue to grow after the stimulus has ceased or the needs of the organism have been met.

Cancer is not a single disease. The term describes almost all forms of malignant neoplasia. Cancer can originate in almost any organ, with the prostate being the most common site in men and the breast in women (Fig. 5–1). The ability of cancer to be cured varies considerably

CANCER INCIDENCE AND DEATHS BY SITE AND SEX-1996 ESTIMATES			
CANCER INCIDENCE BY SITE AND SEX		CANCER DEATHS BY SITE AND SEX	
MALES	FEMALES	MALES	FEMALES
PROSTATE 317,100	BREAST 184,300	LUNG 94,400	LUNG 64,300
LUNG 98,900	COLON & RECTUM 65,900	PROSTATE 41,400	BREAST 44,300
COLON & RECTUM 67,600	LUNG 78,100	COLON & RECTUM 27,400	COLON & RECTUM 27,500
BLADDER 38,300	UTERUS 49,700	PANCREAS 13,600	PANCREAS 14,200
LYMPHOMA 33,900	LYMPHOMA 26,300	LYMPHOMA 13,250	OVARY 14,800
ORAL 20,100	OVARY 26,700	LEUKEMIA 11,600	UTERUS 10,900
MELANOMA OF THE SKIN 21,800	MELANOMA OF THE SKIN 16,500	STOMACH 8,300	LYMPHOMA 11,560
KIDNEY 18,500	PANCREAS 13,900	ESOPHAGUS 8,500	LEUKEMIA 9,400
LEUKEMIA 15,300	BLADDER 14,600	LIVER 8,400	LIVER 6,800
STOMACH 14,000	LEUKEMIA 12,300	BRAIN 7,200	BRAIN 6,100
PANCREAS 12,400	KIDNEY 12,100	KIDNEY 7,300	STOMACH 5,700
LARYNX 9,200	ORAL 9,390	BLADDER 7,800	MULTIPLE MYELOMA 5,100
ALL SITES 764,300	ALL SITES 594,850	ALL SITES 292,300	ALL SITES 262,440

FIGURE 5-1
Cancer incidence and deaths (1996 estimates) by site and sex. (Developed from Parker S. L., Tong T., Bolden S., et al. (1996). Cancer statistics, 1996. *CA Cancer Journal for Clinicians* 46 (1), 5–27)

and depends on the type of cancer and the extent of the disease at diagnosis. Cancers such as acute lymphocytic leukemia, Hodgkin's disease, testicular cancer, and osteosarcoma, which only a few decades ago had poor prognoses, are today cured in many cases. However, lung cancer, which is the leading cause of death in men and women in the United States, is resistant to therapy, and although some progress has been made in its treatment, mortality remains high. This chapter is divided into five sections: concepts of cell growth and differentiation, characteristics of benign and malignant neoplasms, carcinogenesis and causes of cancer, diagnosis and treatment, and childhood cancers. Specific types of cancer are discussed elsewhere in this book.

Cell growth involves cell proliferation and differentiation. Proliferation of cell division is an inherent adaptive mechanism for replacing body cells when old cells die or additional cells are needed. Differentiation is the process of specialization whereby new cells develop the structure and function of the cells they replace. The size of cell populations is regulated by a balance of cellular signals that stimulate or inhibit proliferation and differentiation. If these cellular functions are disturbed in a particular tissue, abnormal increases in the cell population may occur. Defects in these two processes underlie the nature of neoplasia.

The Cell Cycle

The cell cycle is the interval between each cell division. It regulates the duplication of genetic information and appropriately aligns the duplicated chromosomes to be received by the daughter cells. Pauses or checkpoints in the cell cycle determine the accuracy with which deoxyribonucleic acid (DNA) is duplicated. These checkpoints allow any defects to be edited and repaired, thereby ensuring that the daughter cells receive the full complement of genetic information, identical to that of the parent cell.[3]

The cell cycle is divided into four distinct phases referred to as G_1, S, G_2, and M (Fig. 5–2). G_1 (gap 1), is the postmitotic phase during which DNA synthesis ceases while RNA and protein synthesis and cell growth take place. During the S phase, DNA synthesis occurs, giving rise to two separate sets of chromosomes, one for each daughter cell. G_2 (gap 2) is the premitotic phase and is similar to G_1 in that DNA synthesis ceases while RNA and protein synthesis continues. The M phase is the phase of cellular division or mitosis. Mammalian cells that are not actively dividing are quiescent and reside in a resting phase, the G_0 phase. In response to extracellular nutrients, growth factors, hormones, and other signals such as blood loss or tissue injury that call for cell renewal, these quiescent cells reenter the cell cycle.[4–6]

Cells of the body divide at different rates. Neurons and skeletal muscle cells do not divide. Liver cells usually divide once every 1 to 2 years, and some gastrointestinal epithelial cells divide two or more times daily to regenerate the lining of the gastrointestinal tract.[4] The duration of the phases of the cell cycle depends on the cell type, the frequency with which the cells divide, and host characteristics such as the presence of appropriate growth factors. Very rapidly dividing cells can complete the cell cycle in less than 8 hours, while others can take longer than 1 year. Most variability occurs in the G_0 and G_1 phases. The duration of the S phase (10 to 20 hours), the G_2 phase (2 to 10 hours), and the M phase (0.5 to 1 hour) appears to be relatively constant.

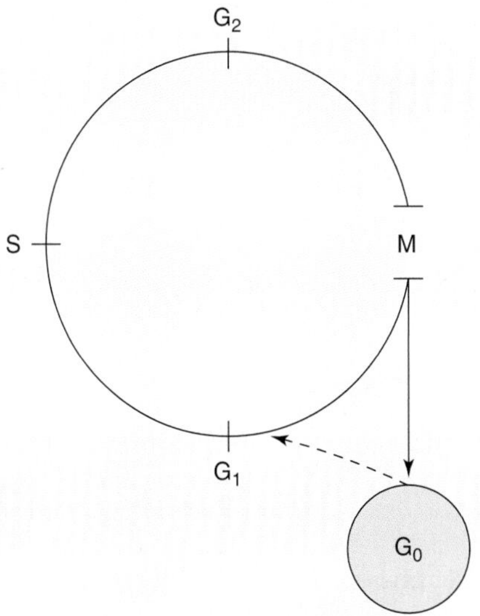

FIGURE 5-2
Phases of the cell cycle. The cycle represents the interval from the midpoint of mitosis to the subsequent end point in mitosis in a daughter cell. G_1 is the postmitotic phase during which RNA and protein synthesis is increased and cell growth occurs. G_0 is the resting or dormant phase of the cell cycle. The S phase represents synthesis of nucleic acids with chromosome replication in preparation for cell mitosis. During G_2, RNA and protein synthesis occurs, as in G_1.

Cell Proliferation

The term proliferation refers to the process by which cells divide and reproduce. In normal tissue, cell proliferation is regulated so that the number of cells actively dividing is equivalent to the number dying or being shed. In humans, there are two major categories of cells: gametes and somatic cells. The gametes are haploid, having only one set of chromosomes from one parent, and are designed specifically for sexual fusion. Gametes consist of the egg or ovum and the sperm. After fusion, a diploid cell containing both sets of chromosomes is formed. This cell is the somatic cell that goes on to form the rest of the body.

In terms of cell proliferation, the 200 or more cell types of the body can be divided into three large groups: the well-differentiated neurons and cells of skeletal and cardiac muscle that are unable to divide and reproduce; the parent, or progenitor cells, that continue to divide and reproduce, such as blood cells, skin cells, and liver cells; and the undifferentiated stem cells that can be triggered to enter the cell cycle and produce large numbers of progenitor cells when the need arises. The rates of reproduction of these cells vary greatly. White blood cells and cells that line the gastrointestinal tract live several days and must be replaced constantly. In most tissues, the rate of cell reproduction is greatly increased when tissue is injured or lost. Bleeding, for example, stimulates the rapid reproduction of the blood-forming cells of the bone marrow. In some types of tissue, the genetic program for cell replication is normally repressed, but it can be resumed under certain conditions. The liver, as an example, has extensive regenerative capabilities under certain conditions.

Cell Differentiation

Cell differentiation is the process whereby proliferating cells are transformed into different and more specialized cell types. This process leads to a fully differentiated, adult cell that has achieved its specific set of structural, functional, and life expectancy characteristics. For example, a red blood cell is programmed to develop into a concave disk that functions as a vehicle for oxygen transport and lives approximately 120 days.

All of the different cell types of the body originate from a single cell—the fertilized ovum. As the embryonic cells increase in number, they engage in an orderly process of differentiation that is necessary for the development of all the various organs of the body. The process of differentiation is regulated by a combination of internal programming that involves the expression of specific genes and external stimuli provided by neighboring cells, the proximity to the maternal circulation, and a variety of growth factors, nutrients, oxygen, and ions.[7]

What makes the cells of one organ different from those of another organ is the type of gene that is expressed. Although all cells have the same complement of genes, only a small number of these genes are expressed in postnatal life. When cells, such as those of the developing embryo, differentiate and give rise to committed cells of a particular tissue type, the appropriate genes are maintained in an active state while the remainder are inactive. Normally, the rate of cell reproduction and the process of cell differentiation are precisely controlled in prenatal and postnatal life so that both of these mechanisms cease after the appropriate numbers and types of cells are formed.

The process of differentiation occurs in orderly steps; with each progressive step, increased specialization is exchanged for a loss of ability to develop different cell characteristics and different cell lines. The more highly specialized a cell becomes, the more likely it is to lose its ability to undergo mitosis. Neurons, which are the most highly specialized cells in the body, lose their ability to divide and reproduce after development of the nervous system is complete. More importantly, there are no reserve or parent cells to direct their replacement. However, these cell types have appropriate numbers of cells generated in the embryo such that loss of a certain percentage of cells does not affect the total cell population. Although these cells never divide and are not replaced if lost, they exist in sufficient numbers to carry out their specific functions. In other less specialized tissues, such as the skin and mucosal lining, cell renewal continues throughout life.

Even in the continuously renewing cell populations, highly specialized cells are similarly unable to divide. An alternative mechanism provides for their replacement. There are progenitor cells of the same lineage that have not yet differentiated to the extent that they have lost their ability to divide. These cells are sufficiently differentiated that their daughter cells are limited to the same cell line, but they are insufficiently differentiated to preclude the potential for active proliferation. As a result, these parent or progenitor cells are able to provide large numbers of replacement cells. The progenitor cells, however, have limited capacity for self-renewal, and they become restricted to producing a single type of cell.

Another type of cell, called a stem cell, remains incompletely differentiated throughout life. Stem cells are reserve cells that remain quiescent until there is a need for cell replenishment, in which case they divide, producing other stem cells and cells that can carry out the functions of the differentiated cell (Fig. 5–3). There are several types of stem cells, some of which include the muscle satellite cell, the epidermal stem cell, the spermatogonium, and the basal cell of the olfactory epithelium. These stem cells are unipotent in that they give rise to only one type of differentiated cell. Oligopotent stem cells can produce a small number of cells, and pluripotent stem cells, such as those involved in hematopoiesis, give rise to numerous cell types.[4] Stem cells are the primary cellular component of bone marrow transplantation, in which the stem cells in the transplanted marrow reestablish the recipient's blood production and immune system. Peripheral blood stem cell transplantation is a new transplantation procedure that bypasses the need for bone marrow infusion and infuses stem cells that have been pheresed from the circulation.

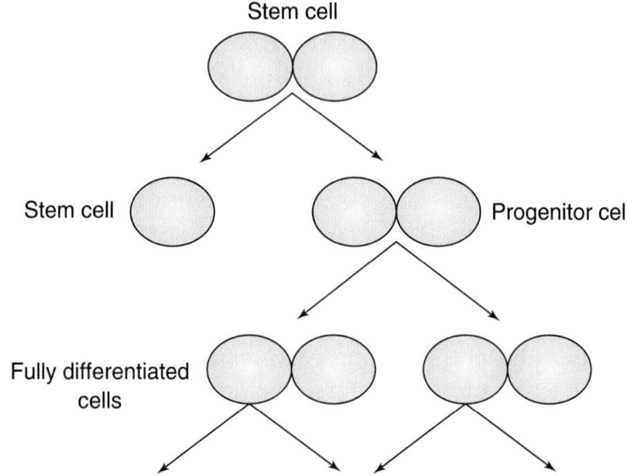

FIGURE 5-3
Mechanism of cell replacement.

In summary, the term neoplasm refers to an abnormal mass of tissue in which the growth exceeds and is uncoordinated with that of the normal tissues. Unlike normal cellular adaptive processes such as hypertrophy and hyperplasia, neoplasms do not obey the laws of normal cell growth. They serve no useful purpose, they do not occur in response to an appropriate stimulus, and they continue to grow at the expense of the host.

Cell proliferation is the process whereby cells divide and bear offspring; it is normally regulated so that the number of cells that are actively dividing is equal to the number dying or being shed.

The process of cell growth and division is called the cell cycle. It is divided into four phases: G_1, the postmitotic phase during which DNA synthesis ceases while RNA and protein synthesis and cell growth take place; S, the phase during which DNA synthesis occurs, giving rise to two separate sets of chromosomes; G_2, the premitotic phase during which RNA and protein synthesis continues; and M, the phase of cell mitosis or cell division. The G_0 phase is a resting or quiescent phase in which cells reside.

Cell differentiation is the process whereby cells are transformed into different and more specialized cell types as they proliferate. It determines the structure, function, and life span of a cell. There are three types of cells: well-differentiated cells that are no longer able to divide, progenitor or parent cells that continue to divide and bear offspring, and undifferentiated stem cells that can be recruited to become progenitor cells when the need arises. As a cell line becomes more differentiated, it becomes more highly specialized in its function and less able to divide.

Characteristics of Benign and Malignant Neoplasms

On completion of this section of the chapter, you should be able to do the following:

- Cite the method used for naming benign and malignant neoplasms
- State at least six ways in which benign and malignant neoplasms differ
- Relate the properties of cell differentiation to the development of a cancer cell line and the behavior of the tumor
- Trace the pathway for hematologic spread of a metastatic cancer cell
- Use the concepts of growth fraction and doubling time to explain the growth of cancerous tissue
- Describe the general effects of cancer on body systems

Neoplasms are composed of two types of tissue: parenchymal tissue and the stroma or supporting tissue. The parenchymal cells represent the functional components of an organ. The supporting tissue consists of the connective tissue, blood vessels, and lymph structures. The parenchymal cells of a tumor determine its behavior and are the component for which a tumor is named. The

TABLE 5-1

Names of Selected Benign and Malignant Tumors According to Tissue Types

Tissue Type	Benign Tumors	Malignant Tumors
Epithelial		
Surface	Papilloma	Squamous cell carcinoma
Glandular	Adenoma	Adenocarcinoma
Connective		
Fibrous	Fibroma	Fibrosarcoma
Adipose	Lipoma	Liposarcoma
Cartilage	Chondroma	Chondrosarcoma
Bone	Osteoma	Osetosarcoma
Blood vessels	Hemangioma	Hemangiosarcoma
Lymph vessels	Lymphangioma	Lymphoangiosarcoma
Lymph tissue		Lymphosarcoma
Muscle		
Smooth	Leiomyoma	Leiomyosarcoma
Striated	Rhabodomyoma	Rhabdomyosarcoma
Neural Tissue		
Nerve cell	Neuroma	Neuroblastoma
Glial tissue	Glioma (benign)	Glioblastoma, astrocytoma, medulloblastoma, oligodendroglioma
Nerve sheaths	Neurilemmoma	Neurilemmal sarcoma
Meninges	Meningioma	Meningeal sarcoma
Hematologic		
Granulocytic		Myelocytic leukemia
Erythrocytic		Erythrocytic leukemia
Plasma cells		Multiple myeloma
Lymphocytic		Lymphocytic leukemia or lymphoma
Monocytic		Monocytic leukemia
Endothelial Tissue		
Blood vessels	Hemangioma	Hemangiosarcoma
Lymph vessels	Lymphangioma	Lymphangiosarcoma
Endothelial lining		Ewing's sarcoma

supporting tissue carries the blood vessels and provides support for tumor survival and growth.

Terminology

By definition, a tumor is a swelling that can be caused by a number of conditions, including inflammation and trauma. Although they are not synonymous, the terms *tumor* and *neoplasms* are often used interchangeably. Neoplasms that contain cells that are clustered together in a single mass are considered to be benign. These tumors usually do not cause death unless their location or size interferes with vital functions. Neoplasms that have the ability to break loose, enter the circulatory or lymphatic systems, and form secondary tumors at other sites that are malignant. Malignant neoplasms usually cause suffering and death if untreated or uncontrolled.

Tumors are usually named by adding the suffix *-oma* to the parenchymal tissue type from which the growth originated. A benign tumor of glandular epithelial tissue is called an adenoma, and a benign tumor of bone tissue is called an osteoma. The term *carcinoma* is used to designate a malignant tumor of epithelial tissue origin. In the case of a malignant adenoma, the term adenocarcinoma is used. Malignant tumors of mesenchymal origin are called sarcomas (*e.g.*, osteosarcoma). Papillomas are benign microscopic or macroscopic, fingerlike projections that grow on any surface. A polyp is growth that projects from a mucosal surface, such as the intestine. Although the term usually implies a benign neoplasm, some malignant tumors also appear as polyps.[8] Oncology is the study of tumors and their treatment. Table 5–1 lists the names of selected benign and malignant tumors according to tissue types.

Benign and malignant neoplasms are generally differentiated by their cell characteristics, manner of growth, rate of growth, potential for metastasizing or spreading to other parts of the body, ability to produce generalized effects, tendency to cause tissue destruction, and capacity to cause death. The characteristics of benign and malignant neoplasms are summarized in Table 5–2.

Benign Neoplasms

Benign tumors are characterized by a slow, progressive rate of growth that may come to a standstill or regress, an expansive manner of growth, the presence of a well-defined fibrous capsule, and failure to metastasize to distant sites. Benign tumors are composed of well-differentiated cells that resemble the cells of the tissue of origin. For example, the cells of a uterine leiomyoma resemble uterine smooth muscle cells. For unknown reasons, benign tumors seem to have lost the ability to suppress the genetic program for cell replication but retain the program for normal cell differentiation. Benign tumors grow by expansion and are enclosed in a fibrous capsule. This pattern is in sharp contrast to malignant neoplasms, which grow by infiltrating the surrounding tissue (Fig. 5–4). The capsule is responsible for a sharp line of demarcation between the benign tumor and the adjacent tissues, a factor that facilitates surgical removal. The formation of the capsule is thought to represent the reaction of the surrounding tissues to the tumor.[7]

TABLE 5-2

Characteristics of Benign and Malignant Neoplasms

Characteristics	Benign	Malignant
Cell characteristics	Well-differentiated cells that resemble normal cells of the tissue from which the tumor originated	Cells are undifferentiated and often bear little resemblance to the normal cells of the tissue from which they arose
Mode of growth	Tumor grows by expansion and does not infiltrate the surrounding tissues; usually encapsulated	Grows at the periphery and sends out processes that infiltrate and destroy the surrounding tissues
Rate of growth	Rate of growth is usually slow	Rate of growth is variable and depends on level of differentiation; the more anaplastic the tumor, the more rapid the rate of growth
Metastasis	Does not spread by metastasis	Gains access to the blood and lymph channels and metastasizes to other areas of the body
General effects	Is usually a localized phenomenon that does not cause generalized effects unless its location interferes with vital functions	Often causes generalized effects such as anemia, weakness, and weight loss
Tissue destruction	Does not usually cause tissue damage unless its location interferes with blood flow	Often causes extensive tissue damage as the tumor outgrows its blood supply or encroaches on blood flow to the area; may also produce substances that cause cell damage
Ability to cause death	Does not usually cause death unless its location interferes with vital functions	Usually causes death unless growth can be controlled

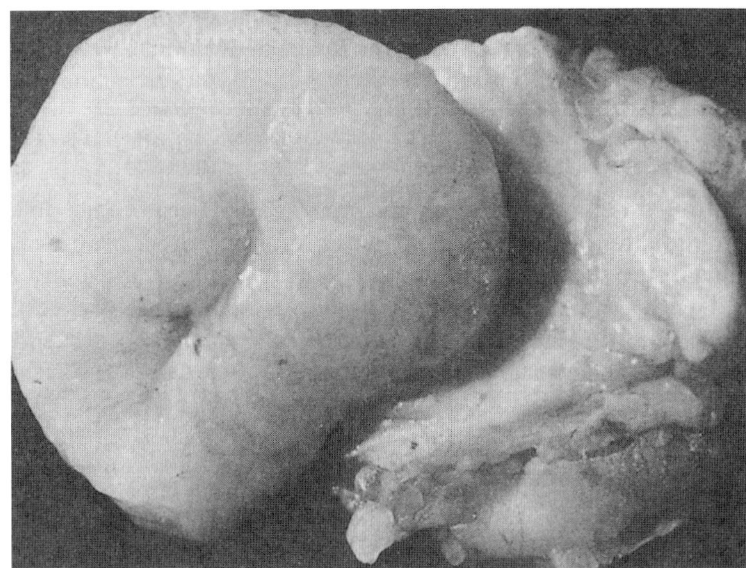

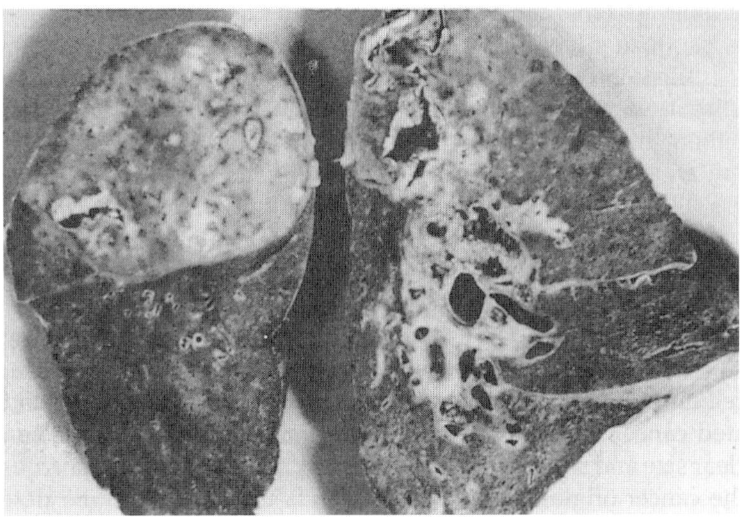

FIGURE 5-4
Photograph of a benign encapsulated fibroadenoma of the breast at the top and a bronchogenic carcinoma of the lung at the bottom. The fibroadenoma has sharply defined edges, but the bronchogenic carcinoma is diffuse and infiltrates the surrounding tissues.

Benign tumors do not undergo degenerative changes as readily as malignant tumors, and they do not usually cause death unless by their location they interfere with vital functions. For instance, a benign tumor growing in the cranial cavity can eventually cause death by compressing brain structures. Benign tumors can also cause disturbances in the function of adjacent or distant structures by producing pressure on tissues, blood vessels, or nerves. Some benign tumors are also known for their ability to cause alterations in body function through elaboration of hormones.

Malignant Neoplasms

Malignant neoplasms tend to grow rapidly, spread widely, and kill regardless of their original location. Because of their rapid rate of growth, malignant tumors tend to compress blood vessels and outgrow their blood supply, causing ischemia and tissue necrosis; to rob normal tissues of essential nutrients; and to liberate enzymes and toxins that destroy tumor tissue and normal tissue. The destructive nature of malignant tumors is related to their lack of cell differentiation, cell characteristics, rate of growth, and ability to spread and metastasize.

There are two categories of cancer—solid tumors and hematologic cancers. Solid tumors initially are confined to a specific tissue or organ. As the growth of a solid tumor progresses, cells are shed from the original tumor mass and travel through the blood and lymph systems to produce metastasis in distant sites. Hematologic cancers involve the blood-forming cells that naturally migrate to the blood and lymph systems, thereby making them disseminated diseases from the beginning.

Cancer Cell Characteristics

In tissues capable of regeneration, replacement cells are usually derived from progenitor or undifferentiated stem cells. The process of cell differentiation involves changes in gene expression such that each step in the process is accomplished by expression of genes that produce more specialized cell functions. Expression of certain genes is accomplished by gene regulatory proteins that when bound to DNA can facilitate or inhibit transcription of adjacent genes. Combinations of these regulatory proteins generate a large number of different cells. Within this regulatory protein group exist proteins called master gene-encoded regulatory proteins, which exhibit decisive coordinating effects in controlling large sets of genes. These master proteins have the ability to affect the production of many proteins in cells, thereby facilitating cellular differentiation.

When a stem cell divides, one daughter cell retains the stem cell characteristics, and the other daughter cell becomes a progenitor daughter cell that leads to an irreversible terminal differentiation. The progeny of each progenitor cell continues along the same genetic program, with the differentiating cells undergoing multiple mitotic divisions in the process of becoming a mature cell type and with each generation of cells becoming more specialized. In this way, a single stem cell can give rise to the many cells needed for normal tissue repair or blood cell responses. When the dividing cells become fully differentiated, they are no longer capable of mitosis. In the immune system, for example, appropriately stimulated B lymphocytes become progressively more differentiated as they undergo successive mitotic divisions, until they become mature plasma cells that can no longer divide but are capable of releasing large amounts of membrane-bound antibody.

Cancer cells, unlike normal cells, fail to undergo normal cell proliferation and differentiation. It is thought that cancer cells develop from mutations that occur during the differentiation process (Fig. 5–5). When the mutation occurs early in the process, the resulting tumor is poorly differentiated and highly malignant; when it occurs later in the process, more fully differentiated and less malignant tumors result.

The term *anaplasia* is used to describe the lack of cell differentiation in cancerous tissue. Undifferentiated cancer cells are altered in appearance and in nuclear size and shape from the cells in the tissue from which the cancer originated. In descending the scale of differentiation, enzymes and specialized pathways of metabolism are lost and cells undergo functional simplification.[8] Highly anaplastic cancer cells, whatever their tissue origin, begin to resemble each other more than they do their tissue of origin. For example, when examined under the microscope, cancerous tissue that originates in the liver does not have the appearance of normal liver tissue. Some cancers display only slight anaplasia, and others display marked anaplasia.

Because cancer cells lack differentiation, they do not function properly, nor do they die within the time frame than normal cells do. In some types of leukemia, for example, the lymphocytes do not follow the normal developmental process. They do not differentiate fully, acquire the ability to destroy bacteria, or die on schedule. Instead, these long-lived, defective cells continue to grow, crowding the normally developing blood cells and thereby affecting the development of other cell lineages such as the erythrocytes, platelets, and other white blood cells. This results in reduced numbers of mature, effectively functioning cells, producing white blood cells that cannot effectively fight infection, erythrocytes that cannot effectively transport oxygen to tissues, or platelets that cannot participate in the clotting system.

Alterations in cell differentiation are also accompanied by changes in cell characteristics and cell function

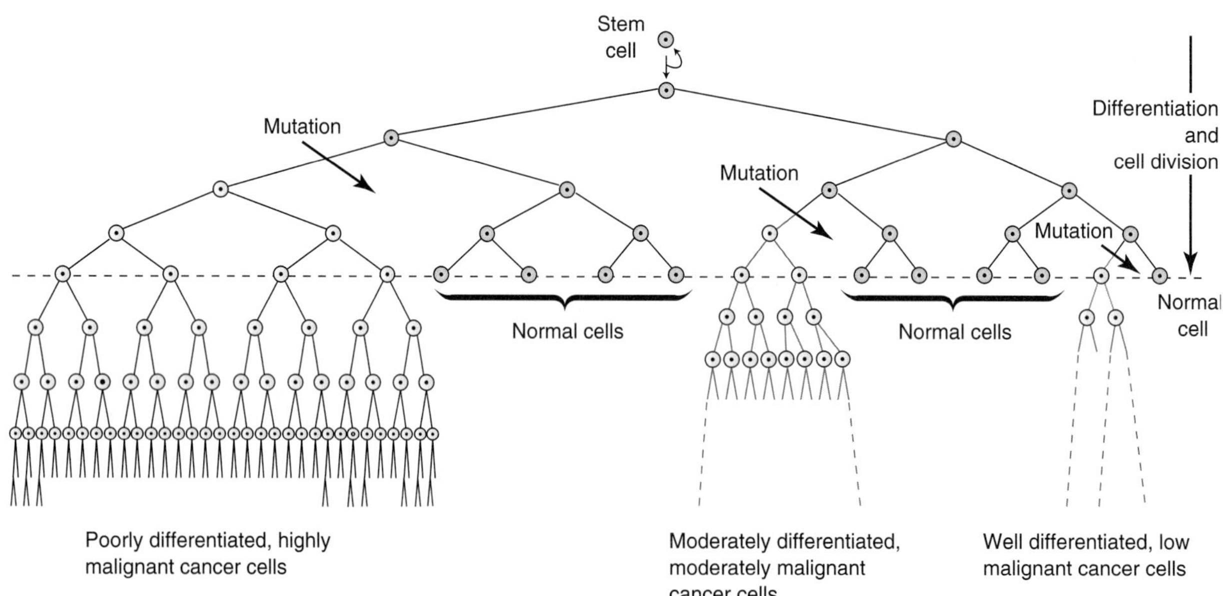

FIGURE 5-5
Mutation of a cancer cell line. (Prescott D. M., Flexer A. S. [1986]. *Cancer, the misguided cell.* Sunderland, MA: Sinauer Associates)

that distinguish cancer cells from their fully differentiated normal counterparts. These changes include alterations in contact inhibition; loss of cohesiveness and adhesion; impaired cell-to-cell communication; expression of altered tissue antigens; and elaboration of degradative enzymes that participate in invasion and metastatic spread.

Contact inhibition is the cessation of growth after a cell comes in contact with another cell. Contact inhibition usually switches off cell growth by blocking the synthesis of DNA, RNA, and protein. In wound healing, contact inhibition causes fibrous tissue growth to cease at the point where the edges of the wound come together. Cancer cells, however, tend to grow rampantly, without regard for other tissue. The reduced tendency of cancer cells to stick together (*i.e.,* cohesiveness and adhesiveness) permits shedding of the tumor's surface cells; these cells appear in the surrounding body fluids or secretions and can often be detected using the Papanicolaou (Pap) test. Impaired cell-to-cell communication may interfere with formation of intercellular connections and responsiveness to membrane-derived signals.

Cancer cells express a number of cell surface molecules or antigens that are immunologically identified as foreign. These *tissue antigens* are coded by the genes of a cell. Many transformed cancer cells revert to earlier stages of gene expression and produce antigens that are immunologically distinct from the antigens that are expressed by cells of the well-differentiated tissue from which the cancer originated. Some cancers express fetal antigens that are not produced by comparable cells in the adult. Tumor antigens may be used clinically as markers to indicate the presence or progressive growth of a cancer. Most cancers synthesize and secrete enzymes (*i.e.,* proteases and glycosidases) that break down proteins involved in assuring intracellular organization and cell-to-cell cohesion. The degradation of the extracellular matrix by these enzymes facilitates invasiveness of the tumor. The production of degradative enzymes such as fibrinolysins contributes to the breakdown of the intercellular matrix, which leads to changes in the organization of the cell's cytoskeleton and affects cell-to-cell adhesion, cellular migration, and cellular communication. Cancers of nonendocrine tissues may assume hormone synthesis to produce so-called ectopic hormones (to be discusses under paraneoplastic syndrome).

Invasion and Metastasis

Cancer spreads by direct invasion and extension, seeding of cancer cells within body cavities, and metastatic spread through the blood or lymph pathways. Unlike benign tumors, which grow by expansion and are usually surrounded by a capsule, malignant cancers grow by extensive infiltration and invasion of the surrounding tissues. The word *cancer* is derived from the Latin word meaning crablike, because cancerous growth spreads by sending crablike projections into the surrounding tissues. The lack of a sharp line of demarcation separating them from the surrounding tissue makes the complete surgical removal of malignant tumors more difficult than removal of benign tumors. *Seeding* of cancer cells into body cavities occurs when a tumor erodes into these spaces. Most often, the peritoneal cavity is involved, but other spaces such as the pleural cavity, pericardial cavity, and joint spaces may be involved. Seeding into the peritoneal cavity is particularly common with ovarian cancers.

The term *metastasis* is used to describe the development of a secondary tumor in a location distant from the primary tumor. Metastatic tumors retain many of the characteristics of the primary tumor from which they were derived. Because of this, it is usually possible to determine the site of the primary tumor from the cellular characteristics of the metastatic tumor.

Some tumors tend to metastasize early in their developmental course, but others do not metastasize until later. Occasionally, the metastatic tumor is far advanced before the primary tumor becomes clinically detectable. Malignant tumors of the kidney, for example, may go completely undetected and be asymptomatic even when a metastatic lesion is found in the lung.

Metastasis occurs by way of the lymph channels (*i.e.,* lymphatic spread) and blood vessels (*i.e.,* hematogenic spread). In many types of cancer, the first evidence of disseminated disease is the presence of tumor cells in the lymph nodes that drain the tumor area. When metastasis occurs by way of the lymphatic channels, the tumor cells lodge first in the regional lymph nodes that received drainage from the tumor site. Once in the lymph node, the cells may die because of the lack of a proper environment, grow into a discernible mass, or remain dormant for unknown reasons. Because the lymphatic channels empty into the venous system, cancer cells that survive may eventually break loose and gain access to the venous system.

With hematologic spread, the blood-borne cancer cells typically follow the venous flow that drains the site of the neoplasm. Before entering the general circulation, venous blood from the gastrointestinal tract, pancreas, and spleen is routed through the portal vein to the liver. The liver is therefore a common site for metastatic spread for cancers that originate in these organs. Although the site of hematologic spread is generally related to vascular drainage of the primary tumor, some tumors metastasize to distant and unrelated sites. As tumor growth progresses, malignant cells evolve and change their metastatic propensity and site preference. These metastatic cells increase their responsiveness to growth signals at distant sites by overexpressing certain growth factor receptors. They also exhibit decreased responsiveness to tissue-of-origin growth signals. Another explanation for the occurrence of metastatic site preference involves the responsiveness of metastatic cells to cytokines (*i.e.,* protein hormones synthesized and secreted from a number of cell types) released by tissue cells at the metastasis site.[9] For example, transferrin, a growth-promoting substance isolated from lung tissue, has been found to stimulate the growth of extremely malignant cells that typically metastasize to the lungs. Other organs that are preferential sites for metastasis contain their own specific sets of cytokines.[10]

Examples of cancer cells preferentially metastasizing to distant sites include prostatic cancer spread to bone, bronchiogenic cancer spread to the adrenal glands and brain, and neuroblastoma spread to the liver and bones. Even among tumors that arise in the lung and metastasize to the brain, different tumors selectively metastasize to distinct sites within the brain.[11] Certain organs such as the heart, skin, and skeletal muscle are rarely a site of metastasis despite ample blood flow capable of transporting metastatic cells to these tissues.

The selective nature of hematologic spread indicates that metastasis is a finely orchestrated multistep process, and only a small select clone of cancer cells have the right combination of gene products to perform all of the steps needed for establishment of a secondary tumor. It has been estimated that fewer than 1 in 10,000 tumor cells that leave a primary tumor survives to start a secondary tumor.[12] To metastasize, a cancer cell must be able to break loose from the primary tumor, invade the surrounding extracellular matrix, gain access to a blood vessel, survive its passage in the blood stream, emerge from the blood stream at a favorable location, invade the surrounding tissue, and begin to grow (Fig. 5–6).

Considerable evidence suggests that cancer cells capable of metastasis secrete enzymes that break down the surrounding extracellular matrix, allowing them to move through the degraded matrix and gain access to a blood vessel. Once in the circulation, the tumor cells are vulnerable to destruction by host immune cells. Some tumor cells gain protection from the antitumor host cells by aggregating and adhering to circulating blood components, particularly platelets, to form tumor emboli. Tumor cells that survive their travel in the circulation must be able to halt their passage by adhering to the vessel wall. Tumor cells express various cell surface attachment factors such as laminin receptors that facilitate their anchoring to laminin in the basement membranes. After attachment, the tumor cells then secrete proteolytic enzymes such as type IV collagenase that degrade the basement membrane and facilitate the migration of the tumor cells through the membrane into the interstitial area where they subsequently establish growth of a secondary tumor.

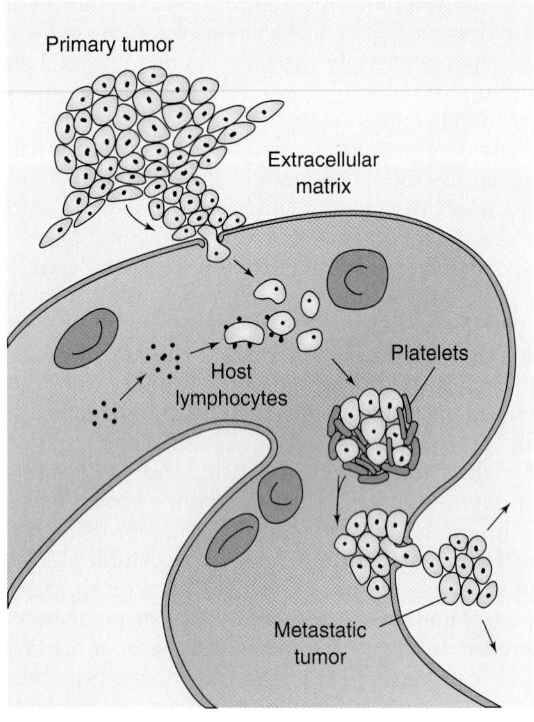

FIGURE 5-6

Mechanism of hematogenic metastasis. (Adapted from Kumar V., et al. [1992]. *Basic pathology* [6th ed., p. 196]. Philadelphia: W.B. Saunders)

Once in the target tissue, the process of tumor development depends on the establishment of blood vessels and specific growth factors that promote proliferation of the tumor cells. Tumor cells secrete tumor-angiogenesis factor, which enables development of new blood vessels within the tumor, a process called *angiogenesis.*

The selective nature of metastasis raises the question about whether there are tumor genes that elicit or inhibit metastasis as their major function. If such genes were found to exist, their presence could be used to predict the likelihood of cancer metastasis and provide information that could be used in designing treatment protocols. No single gene marker has yet been associated with metastasis of cancer cells. However, there has been interest in a tumor suppressor gene (*NM23*). In a series of human breast cancers, the *NM23* levels were highest in tumors that had spread to three or fewer nodes. However, in a study investigating colon cancer metastasis, this gene was not found to suppress metastasis. Because of these controversial findings, it may be that the *NM23* tumor suppressor gene is tissue specific, suppressing breast tumors but not colon tumors.[8]

Tumor Growth

The rate of tissue growth in normal and cancerous tissue depends on three factors: the number of cells that are actively dividing or moving through the cell cycle, the duration of the cell cycle, and the number of cells that are being lost compared with the number of new cells being developed. One of the reasons cancerous tumors often seem to grow so rapidly relates to the size of the cell pool that is actively engaged in cycling. It has been shown that the cell cycle time of cancerous tissue cells is not necessarily shorter than that of normal cells; rather, cancer cells do not die on schedule. The growth factors that allow cells to enter the G_0 phase when they are not needed for cell replacement is lacking. A greater percentage of cells are actively engaged in cycling than occurs in normal tissue.

The ratio of dividing cells to resting cells in a tissue mass is called the *growth fraction.* The doubling time (T_D) is the length of time it takes for the total mass of cells in a tumor to double. As the growth fraction increases, the doubling time decreases. When normal tissues reach their adult size, an equilibrium between cell birth and cell death is reached. Cancer cells, however, continue to divide until limitations in blood supply and nutrients inhibit their growth. As this happens, the doubling time for cancer cells decreases. If tumor growth is plotted against time on a semilogarithmic scale, the initial growth rate is exponential and then tends to decrease or flatten out over time. This characterization of tumor growth is called the *gompertzian model*.[6]

The rate of tumor growth is not necessarily constant and is influenced by factors such as hormones and blood supply. Menopause and pregnancy may cause a proliferation of tumor cells that had been previously static. Although it is generally thought that benign tumors grow slow and cancerous tumors grow fast and erratic, it is important to keep in mind that there are variables that can cause growth rates to vary or stray from typical growth characteristics.[8]

It is also thought that the degree of differentiation of a tumor is correlated with its growth rate. For example, undifferentiated tumors grow more rapidly than the more differentiated benign tumors. Although this is generally true, some malignant tumors apparently dormant for a number of years suddenly begin to proliferate rapidly, causing death in a short time.[8]

Experimentally, it is possible to determine the growth rate by calculating the proportion of dividing cells in the S phase and comparing this number with the total proportion of cells in that phase. Tumor growth is determined by measuring tumor volume as a function of time. Although it may seem reasonable that the T_D of tumors could be calculated by knowing the growth fraction and cell cycle phase durations, a number of cells are lost during the growth of a tumor, perhaps from necrosis, metastases, or differentiation. For this reason, the T_D of tumors is slower than one would expect.[6]

A tumor is generally undetectable until it has doubled 30 times and contains more than a billion (10^9) cells. At this point, it is about 1 cm in diameter (Fig. 5–7). After 35 doublings, the mass contains more than a trillion (10^{12}) cells, which is a sufficient number to kill the host.

Cancer in situ is a localized preinvasive lesion. Depending on its location, this type of lesion can usually be removed surgically or treated so that the changes of recurrence are small. For example, cancer in situ of the cervix is essentially 100% curable.

General Effects

There is probably not a single body function left unaffected by the presence of cancer (Table 5–3). Because tumor cells replace normal functioning parenchymal tissue, the initial manifestations of cancer usually reflect the primary site of involvement. For example, cancer of the lung initially produces impairment of respiratory function; as the tumor grows and metastasizes, other body structures become affected.

Cancer disrupts tissue integrity. As cancers grow, they compress and erode blood vessels, causing ulceration and necrosis along with frank bleeding and sometimes with hemorrhage. One of the early warning signals of colorectal cancer is blood in the stool. Cancer cells may also produce enzymes and metabolic toxins that are destructive to the surrounding tissues. Usually, tissue damaged by cancerous growth does not heal normally. Instead, the damaged area persists and often continues to grow. A sore that does not heal is a second warning signal of cancer. Cancer has no regard for normal anatomic boundaries; as it grows, it invades and

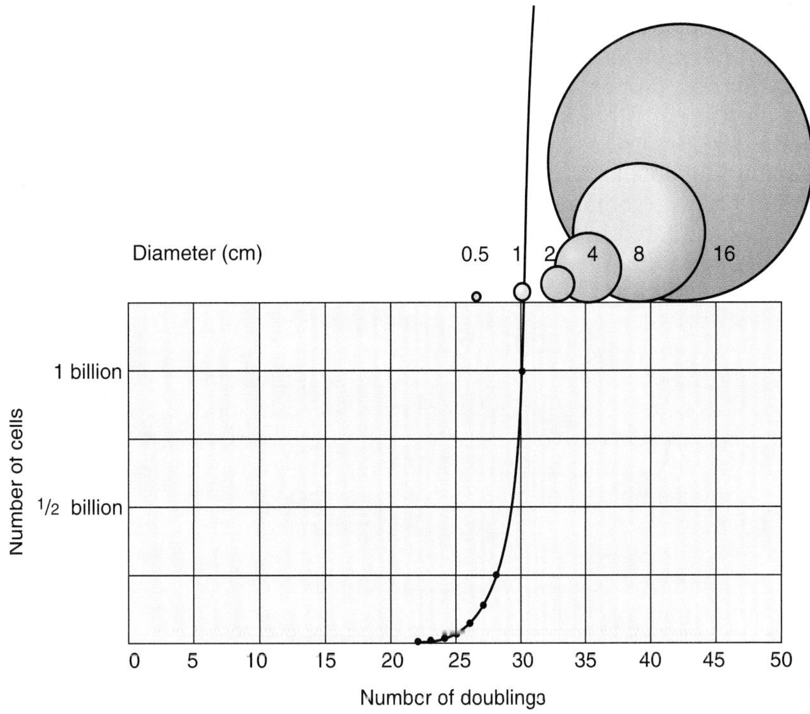

FIGURE 5-7
Growth curve of a hypothetical tumor on arithmetic coordinates. Notice the number of doubling times before the tumor reaches an appreciable size. (Adapted from Collins V. P., et al. [1956]. Observations of growth rates of human tumors. *American Journal of Roentgenology, Radiation Therapy, and Nuclear Medicine* 76, 988)

TABLE 5-3

General Effects on Body Function Associated with Cancer Growth

Overall Effect	Related Tumor Action
Altered function of the involved tissue	Destruction and replacement of parenchymal tissue by neoplastic growth
Bleeding and hemorrhage	Compression of blood vessels, with ischemia and necrosis of tissue; or tumor may outgrow its blood supply
Ulceration, necrosis, and infection of tumor area	Ischemia associated with rapid growth, with subsequent bacterial invasion
Obstruction of hollow viscera or communication pathways	Expansive growth of tumor with compression and invasion of tissues
Effusion in serous cavities	Impaired lymph flow from the serous cavity or erosion of tumor into the cavity
Increased risk of vascular thrombosis	Abnormal production of coagulation factors by the tumor, obstruction of venous channels, and immobility
Anemia	Bleeding and depression of red blood cell production
Bone destruction	Metastatic invasion of bony structures
Hypercalcemia	Destruction of bone due to metastasis or production by the tumor or parathyroid-like hormone
Pain	Liberation of pain mediators by the tumor, compression, or ischemia of structures
Cachexia, weakness, wasting of tissues	Catabolic effect of the tumor on body metabolism along with selective trapping of nutrients by rapidly growing tumor cells
Inappropriate hormone production (e.g., ADH or ACTH secretion by cancers such as bronchogenic carcinoma)	Production by the tumor of hormones or hormone-like substances that are not regulated by normal feedback mechanisms

compresses adjacent structures. Abdominal cancer, for example, often compresses the viscera and causes bowel obstruction. Cancer may obstruct lymph flow and penetrate serous cavities, causing pleural effusion and ascites. In its late stages, cancer often causes pain (see Chapter 38). Pain is probably one of the most dreaded aspects of cancer. Pain management is one of the major treatment concerns for persons with incurable cancers.

Abnormalities in a person's energy, carbohydrate, lipid, and protein regulation are common manifestations during progressive tumor growth. Many cancers are associated with weight loss and wasting of body fat and lean protein, a condition called cancer *cachexia.* Although anorexia, reduced food intake, and abnormalities of taste are common in persons with cancer and are often accentuated by treatment methods, the extent of weight loss and protein wasting cannot be explained in terms of diminished food intake alone. There is also a disparity between the size of the tumor and the severity of cachexia that supports the existence of other mediators in the development of cachexia. Cachexia is thought to be the result of tumor-derived or host-derived factors that cause anorexia directly by acting on satiety centers in the hypothalamus or indirectly by injuring tissues that subsequently release anorexigenic substances.

Cachectin was the first identified cytokine associated with wasting. Cachectin was later found to be identical to tumor necrosis factor (TNF), a cytokine secreted primarily from macrophages in response to tumor cell growth or gram-negative bacterial infections.[13] TNF causes anorexia by suppressing satiety centers and by suppressing the synthesis of lipoprotein lipase, an enzyme that facilitates the release of fatty acids from lipoproteins so they can be used by tissues. TNF is an endogenous pyrogen that induces fever by its actions on cells in the hypothalamic regulatory regions of the brain. TNF also induces a number of inflammatory responses, activates the coagulation system, suppresses bone marrow stem cell division, acts on hepatocytes to increase the synthesis of specific serum proteins in response to inflammatory stimuli,[14] and mediates endotoxic shock secondary to trauma, burns, and sepsis. The role of TNF and its full impact on cancer cachexia are uncertain. It has been suggested by some that the hormone may be an endogenous antineoplastic agent.[15] Interleukin-1, another cytokine secreted from macrophages, shares with TNF the ability to initiate cachexia.[14]

In addition to signs and symptoms at the sites of primary and metastatic disease, cancer can produce manifestations in sites that are not directly affected by the disease. Such manifestations are collectively referred to as *paraneoplastic syndromes.* Some of these manifestations are caused by the elaboration of hormones by cancer cells, and others result from the production of circulating factors that produce nonmetastatic hematopoietic, neurologic, and dermatologic syndromes. For example, cancers may produce procoagulation factors that contribute to an increased risk of venous thrombosis. It is estimated that about 7% of persons with cancer are affected by these syndromes. The three most common endocrine syndromes associated with cancer are the syndrome of inappropriate antidiuretic hormone (SIADH) secretion (see Chapter 26), Cushing's syndrome due to ectopic adrenocorticotropic hormone (ACTH, now called corticotropin) production (see Chapter XX), and hypercalcemia (see Chapter 26). Hypercalcemia of malignancy does not appear to be related to parathyroid hormone (PTH) but to parathyroid hormone–related protein (PTHrP), which shares several biologic actions with PTH. It can also be caused by osteolytic processes induced by cancer such as multiple myeloma or bony metastases from other cancers. The paraneoplastic syndromes may be the earliest indication that a person has cancer; they may also signal early recurrence of the disease in previously treated persons. In some persons with cancer, a paraneoplastic syndrome such as hypercalcemia can be disabling and even life threatening.[8]

In summary, neoplasms may be benign or malignant. Benign and malignant tumors differ in terms of cell characteristics, manner of growth, rate of growth, potential for metastasis, ability to produce generalized effects, tendency to cause tissue destruction, and capacity to cause death. The growth of a benign tumor is restricted to the site of origin, and the tumor will not usually cause death unless it interferes with vital functions. Cancer or malignant neoplasms, however, grow wildly and without organization, spread to distant parts of the body, and cause death unless its growth is inhibited or stopped by treatment.

There are two types of cancer: solid tumors and hematologic tumors. Solid tumors are initially confined to a specific organ or tissue, but hematologic cancers are disseminated from the onset. Cancer is a disorder of cell proliferation and differentiation. Cancer cells are often poorly differentiated in comparison to normal cells, they display abnormal membrane characteristics, have abnormal antigens, produce abnormal biochemical products, and have abnormal karyotypes. All cancers result from nonlethal genetic changes that transform a normal cell into a cancer cell. The spread of cancer occurs by three pathways: direct invasion and extension; seeding of cancer cells within body cavities; and metastatic spread through the blood or lymph pathways. Only a small clone of cancer cells is capable of metastasis. To metastasize, a cancer cell must be able to break loose from the primary tumor, invade the surrounding extracellular matrix, gain access to a blood vessel, survive its passage in the blood stream, emerge from the bloodstream at a favorable location, invade the surrounding tissue, and begin to grow.

Cancer disrupts tissue integrity. Cancers also produce chemical mediators called cytokines such as tissue necrosis factor that produce weight loss and tissue wasting. Paraneoplastic syndromes describe the ability of neoplasms to elaboration hormones and other chemical messengers produce nonmetastatic endocrine, hematopoietic, neurologic, and dermatologic syndromes.

Carcinogenesis and Causes of Cancer

On completion of this section of the chapter, you should be able to do the following:

- Describe the role of proto-oncogenes and anti-oncogenes in the transformation of a normal life line to a cancer cell line
- Name the steps in the transformation of normal cells to cancer cells by the carcinogens
- State how lifestyle can contribute to the cancer risk through increased exposure to carcinogenic agents
- Relate the function of the immune system to prevention of cancer

Because cancer is not a single disease, it is reasonable to assume that it does not have a single cause. More likely, cancer occurs because of interactions between multiple risk factors or repeated exposure to a single carcinogenic (cancer-producing) agent. Among the risk factors that have been linked to cancer are heredity, chemical and environmental carcinogens, cancer-causing viruses, and immunologic defects. All cancers result from nonlethal genetic changes that transform a normal cell into a cancerous cell.

Oncogenesis

The term *oncogenesis* refers to a genetic mechanism whereby normal cells are transformed into cancer cells. Two kinds of genes control normal cell growth and replication: growth-promoting regulatory genes called *proto-oncogenes* and growth-inhibiting regulatory genes called *anti-oncogenes*. These genes have been implicated as principal targets of genetic damage that occurs during the development of a cancer cell.[16,17] Such genetic damage may be acquired by the action of chemicals, radiation, or viruses, or it may be inherited in the germ line. Most cancers are probably multifactoral in origin, with several factors acting in concert or sequentially to produce the multiple genetic abnormalities that are characteristic of cancer cells.

Oncogenes are mutations of normal growth-regulating genes. The oncogene theory dates to 1911, when Francis Peyton Rous discovered a virus that causes sarcomas in chickens. Over the years, various oncogenic viruses have been identified that can produce cancerous transformations in laboratory cell cultures and animals. As the research with virus-induced cell transformation progressed, it was discovered that normal cells contain DNA sequences similar to the viral genes that cause cancerous transformation of laboratory cells. These DNA sequences, called proto-oncogenes, have essential roles in regulating the growth and proliferation of normal cells. Proto-oncogene products may act as growth factors, as receptors for growth factors, or as second messengers that transmit growth factor signals. The involvement of these genes in the cancer process is due to a somatic mutation that takes place in a specific target tissue, converting its proto-oncogenes into oncogenes.

Another discovery identified a different class of genes, the cancer-suppressor genes or anti-oncogenes. These tumor-suppressing genes inhibit the proliferation of cells in a tumor. When this type of gene is inactivated, a genetic signal that normally inhibits proliferation is removed, thereby causing the cell to begin unregulated growth. Several human tumor suppressor genes have been identified.[18] Of particular interest in this group is the *P53* gene, located on the short arm of chromosome 17. This gene codes for a protein that is pivotal in growth regulation functioning as a suppressor of tumor growth. Its mutation has been implicated in the development of astrocytoma, breast cancer, small-cell lung cancer and colorectal cancer.[17] The *P53* tumor suppressor gene has been found to be altered at some point in the development of approximately one half of human cancers.[19]

Another newly discovered suppressor gene is *FHIT*, located in a fragile region on the short arm of chromosome 3. The fragile characteristic of its location has led researchers to suggest it may be particularly susceptible to mutation by carcinogens such as those contained in tobacco smoke. It has been found to be completely or partially absent in a number of cancers, including colon, breast, and lung.[20]

There have been numerous distinctions discovered between the proto-oncogenes and the tumor suppressor genes. The mutations that cause proto-oncogenes to change to oncogenes are thought to occur in the structural gene or the regulatory gene that results in overproduction of the normal protein product. The cell acquires a new function that often is a continuous or some abnormal signal for unregulated cellular proliferation. These mutations exhibit a dominant inheritance pattern in that one defective gene and one normal allele are inherited. Fetuses that inherit this mutation usually do not survive to term. In contrast, the mutation that affects tumor suppressor genes exhibits a recessive inheritance pattern and usually occurs in both inherited genes. Individuals who inherit this type of mutation usually are at high risk for developing cancers that demonstrate a common tissue or cell type preference.[17]

Normally, proto-oncogenes are specifically turned on for only a brief period in the cell cycle. When their oncogenes or their products are altered by mutation, they may operate continuously, causing unregulated cell growth. Significantly, it appears that the acquisition of a single oncogene is not sufficient to transform normal cells into cancer cells. Instead, cancerous transformation appears to require the activation of many independently mutated genes.

The transformation of normal cells to cancer cells by carcinogenic agents is a multistep process that can be divided into three stages: initiation, promotion, and progression. *Initiation* involves the exposure of cells to appropriate doses of a carcinogenic agent that makes them susceptible to malignant transformation. The carcinogenic agents can be chemical, physical or biologic, and produce irreversible changes in the genome of a previously normal cell. Because the effects of initiating agents are irreversible, multiple divided doses may achieve the same effects as single exposures of the same comparable dose or small amounts of highly carcinogenic substances. The most susceptible cells for mutagenic alterations in the genome are the cells that are actively synthesizing DNA.[21]

Promotion involves the induction of unregulated accelerated growth in already initiated cells by various chemicals and growth factors. Promotion is reversible if the promoter substance is removed. Cells that have been irreversibly initiated may be promoted even after long latency periods. The latency period varies with the type of agent, the dosage, and the characteristics of the target cells. Many chemical carcinogens are called complete carcinogens because they can initiate and promote neoplastic transformation. *Progression* is the process whereby tumor cells acquire malignant phenotypic changes that allow invasiveness, metastatic competence, a tendency for autonomous growth, and increased karyotypic instability.[21]

Carcinogenic agents can be divided into two categories: direct-reacting agents, which do not require activation in the body to become carcinogenic, and indirect-reacting agents, called *procarcinogens*, which become active only after metabolic conversion. The carcinogenicity of some chemicals is augmented by agents that by themselves have little or no cancer-causing ability. These agents are called *promoters*. It is believed that promoting agents exert their effect by changing the expression of genetic material within a cell, increasing DNA synthesis, enhancing gene amplification (*i.e.*, number of gene copies that are made), and altering intercellular communication. Some hormones, for example, may alter the endocrine balance and act as promoters. Several carcinogenic agents may act together or with other types of carcinogenic influences such as viruses or radiation to produce cancer.[8]

Direct- and indirect-acting agents form highly reactive species (*i.e.*, electrophiles and free radicals) that bind with the nucleophilic residues on DNA, RNA, or cellular proteins. The action of these reactive species tends to cause cell mutation or alteration in synthesis of cell enzymes and structural proteins in a manner that alters cell replication and interferes with cell regulatory controls. Antioxidants such as vitamins A, C, and E inhibit the formation of free radicals and may thus inhibit the damaging effects of carcinogens on DNA. The direct-acting agents generally are weak carcinogens and, depending on the dose and duration of exposure, may cause cancer. Among these direct-acting agents are the alkylating drugs used in the treatment of cancer.

The indirect-acting procarcinogens require metabolic conversion to active carcinogens. Among the most potent of the procarcinogens are the polycyclic hydrocarbons. The polycyclic hydrocarbons are of particular interest because they are produced in the combustion of tobacco and are present in cigarette smoke.

They are also produced from animal fat in the process of broiling meats and are present in smoked meats and fish. Another class of procarcinogens are the aromatic amines and azo dyes. The carcinogenicity of these agents is exerted mainly in the liver, where the metabolic process that activates the procarcinogen occurs. An exception is beta-naphthylamine, which is broken down in the urine and causes bladder cancer. It has been responsible for a 50-fold increase in bladder cancer in workers exposed to aniline dye and rubber industries. Some of the azo dyes have been developed into food colors, which are federally regulated in the United States. Aflatoxin B_1 is a naturally occurring carcinogen produced by some strains of *Aspergillus*, a mold that grows in improperly stored grains and nuts. It may also be found in peanuts and peanut butter. There is a high correlation between dietary levels of this food contaminant and liver cancer in some parts of Africa and the Far East. Hepatitis B is also endemic in these areas, and it has been suggested it may contribute to carcinogenic effects of aflatoxin B_1.[8]

Heredity

A hereditary predisposition for approximately 50 types of cancer has been observed in families. Breast cancer, for example, occurs more frequently in women whose grandmothers, mothers, aunts, and sisters also have experienced a breast malignancy. The genetic predisposition for development of cancer has been documented for a number of cancerous and precancerous lesions that follow mendelian inheritance patterns. Cancer is found in approximately 10% of persons having one affected first-degree relative, in approximately 15% of persons having two affected family members, and in 30% of persons having three affected family members. The risk increases to approximately 50% in women 65 years of age who have multiple family members with breast cancer. Two oncogenes called *BRCA1* (breast carcinoma 1) and *BRCA2* (breast carcinoma 2) have been implicated in a genetic susceptibility to breast cancer. Li-Fraumeni syndrome, an autosomal dominant inherited disorder (*i.e.*, mutation in the *P53* tumor suppressor gene), places women at high risk for developing breast cancer in their twenties and thirties and of developing other cancers, including sarcomas, leukemia, and brain tumors.[7]

Several cancers exhibit an autosomal dominant inheritance pattern. In about 40% of cases, retinoblastoma is inherited as an autosomal dominant trait; the remaining cases are nonhereditary. The penetrance of the genetic trait is high; in carriers of the dominant retinoblastoma gene, the penetrance for this gene is 95% for at least one tumor, and the affected person may be unilaterally or bilaterally affected.[22] Familial adenomatous polyposis (FAP) of the colon also follows an autosomal dominant inheritance pattern. Individuals who inherit this gene may develop hundreds of adenomatous polyps, some of which inevitably become malignant.[8,18] Retinoblastoma and heritable forms of cancer are discussed further in the section on childhood cancers.

Carcinogens

A carcinogen is an agent capable of causing cancer. The role of environmental agents in causation of cancer was first noticed in 1775 by Sir Percivall Pott, who related the high incidence of scrotal cancer in chimney sweeps to their exposure to coal soot. In 1915, Yamagiwa and Ichikawa conducted the first experiments in which a chemical agent was used to produce cancer. These investigators found that a cancerous growth developed when they painted a rabbit's ear with coal tar. Coal tar has since been found to contain potent polycyclic aromatic hydrocarbons. Since then, many carcinogenic agents have been identified. It has been estimated that 80% to 85% of human cancers are associated with exposure to environmental or chemical agents (Chart 5–1).[23]

Chemical Carcinogens. More than 6 million chemicals have been identified. It is estimated that fewer than 1000 of these have been extensively examined for their carcinogenic potential.[24] Some have been found to cause cancers in animals, and others are known to cause cancers in humans. These agents include natural (*e.g.*, aflatoxin B_1) and artificial products (*e.g.*, vinyl chloride).

Approximately 2% to 4% of cancer deaths are associated with an exposure to an occupational hazard. Those substances identified as having carcinogenic capabilities were found to be closely associated with abnormal clustering of certain cancers. For example,

CHART **5-1**
Chemical and Environmental Agents Known to be Carcinogenic in Humans

Polycyclic Hydrocarbons
Soots, tars, and oils
Cigarette smoke

Industrial Agents
Aniline and azo dyes
Arsenic compounds
Asbestos
β-Naphthylamine
Benzene
Benzopyrene
Carbon tetrachloride
Insecticides, fungicides
Nickel and chromium compounds
Polychlorinated biphenyls
Vinyl chloride

Food and Drugs
Smoked foods
Nitrosamines
Aflatoxin B_1
Diethylstibestrol
Estrogens
Anticancer drugs (e.g., alkylating agents, cyclophosphamide, chlorambucil, nitrosourea)

occupational exposure to asbestos fibers is significantly related to increased risks of developing several cancers, including lung, laryngeal, and gastrointestinal cancers and mesothelioma. Increased incidences of leukemia are associated with benzene exposure.[7]

Herbicide exposure, particularly that of the phenoxy herbicides, has been associated with an increased incidence of non-Hodgkin's lymphoma among farmers. Other studies have discovered a relation between this class of herbicides and soft tissue sarcomas and cancers of the colon, lung, nasal passages, prostate, ovary, leukemia, and multiple myeloma. However, definitive studies are too few to demonstrate exposure-risk correlations.

Many cancers are associated with lifestyle risk factors, such as smoking, dietary factors, and alcohol consumption. Cigarette smoke contains procarcinogens and promoters. It is directly associated with lung and laryngeal cancer[25] and has been linked with cancers of the esophagus, pancreas, kidney, uterine cervix, and bladder.[26] Chewing tobacco or tobacco products increases the risk of cancers of the oral cavity and esophagus. It has been estimated that 30% of current cancer deaths in the United States are related to tobacco. Not only is the smoker at risk, but others passively exposed to cigarette smoke are also at risk. Environmental tobacco smoke has been classified as a "group A" carcinogen based on the Environmental Protection Agency's system of carcinogen classification. It is also estimated that between 20% and 60% of the deaths each year occurring from nonsmoking-related lung cancers may be caused by environmental tobacco smoke.[27]

There is strong evidence that certain elements in the diet contribute to cancer risk. For example, benzo[*a*]pyrene and other polycyclic hydrocarbons may be produced when meat and fish are charcoal broiled or smoked or when foods are fried in fat that has been reused multiple times. Nitrosamines, which are powerful carcinogens, may be formed from nitrites that are derived from nitrates that have been added to vegetables and foods as a preservative. Formation of these nitrosamines may be inhibited by the presence of antioxidants such as vitamin C in the stomach.

Cancer of the colon has been associated with high dietary intake of fat, protein, and beef and low intake of dietary fiber. The carcinogenic factors associated with a high fat diet have yet to be confirmed. However, some studies have shown a relation between high levels of fecally excreted bile acids and colon cancer. A high fat diet increases the flow of primary bile acids. These acids are converted to secondary bile acids such as lithocholic acid and deoxycholic acid in the presence of anaerobic bacteria in the colon. These acids are thought to be tumor promoters rather than initiators.[7,23]

Alcohol modifies the metabolism of carcinogens in the liver and esophagus.[23] It is believed to influence the transport of carcinogens, increasing the contact between an externally induced carcinogen and the stem cells that line the upper oral cavity and esophagus. The carcinogenic effect of cigarette smoke can be enhanced by concomitant consumption of alcohol; persons who smoke and drink considerable amounts of alcohol are at increased risk for development of cancer of the oral cavity and esophagus.

The effects of carcinogenic agents are usually dose dependent—the larger the dose or the longer the duration of exposure, the greater is the risk that cancer will develop. Some chemical carcinogens may act in concert with other carcinogenic influences such as viruses or radiation to induce neoplasia. There is usually a delay ranging from 5 to 30 years from the time of chemical carcinogen exposure to the development of overt cancer. This is unfortunate, because many persons may have been exposed to the agent and its carcinogenic effects before the association is recognized. This occurred, for example, with the use of diethylstilbestrol, which was widely used in the United States from the mid-1940s to 1970 to prevent miscarriages. It was not until the late 1960s that many cases of vaginal adenosis and adenocarcinoma in young women were found to be the result of their exposure in utero to diethylstilbestrol.[28]

Radiation. The effects of *ionizing radiation* in the contribution of carcinogenesis has been well documented in atomic bomb survivors, patients diagnostically exposed, industrial workers, and scientists and physicians who were exposed during employment. Malignant epitheliomas of the skin and leukemia were significantly elevated in these populations.[7] Between 1950 and 1970, the death rate from leukemia alone in the most heavily exposed population groups of the atomic bomb survivors in Hiroshima and Nagasaki was 147 per 100,000 persons, 30 times the expected rate.[29]

The type of cancer that developed depended on the dose of radiation, the sex of the person, and the age at which exposure occurred. For instance, approximately 25 to 30 years after total body or trunk irradiation, there were increased incidences of leukemia and cancers of the breast, lung, stomach, thyroid, salivary gland, gastrointestinal system, and lymphoid tissues. The age of the individual is related to the length of time between exposure and the onset of cancer. Children exposed to ionizing radiation in utero have an increased risk for developing leukemias and childhood tumors, particularly 2 to 3 years after birth. This latency period for leukemia extends to 5 to 10 years if the child was exposed after birth and 20 years for certain solid tumors.[7] For example, the latency period for the development of thyroid cancer in infants and small children who received radiation to the head and neck to decrease the size of the tonsils or thymus was as long as 35 years after exposure.

The association between sunlight and the development of skin cancer has been reported for longer than 100 years. William Dubreuilh, a French dermatologist, published in 1907 epidemiologic data that implicated sunlight as a cause for skin cancer. *Ultraviolet radiation* emits low-energy rays that do not deeply penetrate the skin. However, the skin absorbs most of the rays, which leads to excited energy states of the nucleic acid bases and results in photochemical reactions between DNA bases.[7] As with other carcinogens, the effects of radiation are usually additive, and there is usually a long delay between the time of exposure and the time that cancer can be detected. This is true of skin cancer, which is caused by overexposure to the sun and usually takes many years to develop.

The evidence supporting the role of ultraviolet radiation in the cause of skin cancer includes skin cancer that develops primarily on the areas of skin more frequently exposed to sunlight (*e.g.*, the head, neck, arms, hands, legs), an incidence that is higher in light-complexioned individuals who lack the ultraviolet filtering skin pigment melanin, and the intensity of ultraviolet exposure that is directly related to the incidence of skin cancer, as evidenced by higher rates occurring in Australia and the American Southwest.[7] There are also studies that suggest intense, episodic exposure to sunlight, particularly during childhood is more important, particularly in the development of melanoma, than prolonged, low-intensity exposure.[30]

Radon is a radioactive gas that is formed from the decay of radium-236 and is found in soil and rocks. Different geographic areas contain various amounts. Studies have found that persons exposed to high amounts (approaching 3000 picocuries [pCi]/L of air) of the gas, such as miners, have higher incidences of bronchogenic carcinoma. Residential home monitoring began in some communities across the country in the 1980s. Lung cancer risk estimates from radon exposure in residential homes were based on extrapolations from the miner exposure data. One study in the late 1980s examined exposure levels in 400 women diagnosed with lung cancer. The investigation found that lung cancer risk increased for women exposed to radon levels of 2 pCi/L, but the results were not statistically significant.[31] Most homes in the United States contain radon levels below 2 pCi/L.[7]

Oncogenic Viruses

It has been suspected for some time that viruses play an important role in the development of certain forms of cancer, particularly leukemia and lymphoma. Ellermann in 1908 and Rous in 1911 were the first to describe the transmissibility of avian leukemia and sarcoma, respectively. Because these initial studies were carried out in birds, the interest in the findings remained isolated to avian research. Subsequent studies discovered that in rabbits, squamous cell carcinomas would develop from benign papillomas, lesions that were caused by the papillomavirus. Interest in the field of viral oncology, particularly in human populations, has burgeoned with the discovery of reverse transcriptase, the development of recombinant DNA technology, and more recently with the discovery of oncogenes and tumor-suppressor genes.[32]

An oncogenic virus is one that can induce cancer. Viruses, which are small particles containing genetic (DNA or RNA) material, enter a host cell and become incorporated into its chromosomal DNA or take control of the cell's machinery for the purpose of producing viral proteins. A large number of DNA and RNA viruses (*i.e.*, retroviruses) have been shown to be oncogenic in animals. However, only a few viruses have been linked to cancer in humans.[8,23] Among the recognized oncogenic viruses in humans are the human T-cell leukemia virus-I (HTLV-I), human papillomavirus (HPV), Epstein-Barr virus (EBV), and hepatitis B virus (HBV).[7] Herpes simplex II has been also been associated with cervical cancer, but the evidence supporting its role as a carcinogenic influence is less clear.

Although there are a number of retroviruses (RNA viruses) that cause cancer in animals, there is only one known human retrovirus that is associated with cancer. HTLV-I is associated with a form of T-cell leukemia that is endemic in certain parts of Japan, some areas of the Caribbean, and Africa, and it is found sporadically elsewhere, including the United States and Europe. Like the human immunodeficiency virus (HIV), HTLV-I is attracted to the $CD4^+$ T cells, and this subset of T cells is therefore the major target for cancerous transformation. The virus requires transmission of infected T cells by way of sexual intercourse, infected blood, or breast milk. Adult T-cell leukemia (ATL) develops in about 2% to 5% of persons seropositive for HTLV-I and is an aggressive cancer, with a median survival of 3 to 4 months from the time of diagnosis. Evidence suggests that the HTLV-I virus has a direct effect in causing cancer, because infants who are born in areas with high incidence rates but move to another part of the world exhibit the same likelihood of developing ATL. In vitro studies also have found that the virus is capable of transforming T cells contained in normal human umbilical cord blood to immortalized precancerous cells.

A second type of HTLV virus, HTLV-II, has been isolated from individuals with an unusual form of hairy cell leukemia. Hairy cell leukemia normally is the result of alterations in the B-lymphocyte lineage. However, the HTLV-II variant involves the T-lymphocyte lineage.[8,32]

Three DNA viruses have been implicated in human cancers: HPV, EBV, and HBV. The transforming DNA viruses form stable associations with the human genome using genes that allow them to complete their replication cycle and be expressed in transformed cells. There is strong evidence to suggest that the DNA viruses act in concert with other factors to cause cancer.

There are more than 60 genetically different types of HPVs. Some types (*i.e.*, types 1, 2, 4, and 7) have been shown to cause benign squamous papillomas (*i.e.*, warts). HPVs have also been implicated in squamous cell carcinoma of the cervix and the anogenital region. HPV type 16 and 18 have been found in 75% to 100% of squamous cell carcinomas of the cervix and presumed precursors (*i.e.*, severe cervical dysplasia and carcinoma in situ).

EBV is a member of the herpesvirus family. It has been implicated in the pathogenesis of four human cancers: Burkitt's lymphoma, nasopharyngeal cancer, B-cell lymphomas in immunosuppressed individuals such as those with AIDS, and in some cases of Hodgkin's lymphoma.[7] Burkitt's lymphoma, a tumor of B lymphocytes, is endemic in parts of East Africa and occurs sporadically in other areas worldwide. In persons with normal immune function, the EBV-driven B-cell proliferation is readily controlled and the person becomes asymptomatic or develops a self-limited episode of infectious mononucleosis (see Chapter 9). In regions of the world where Burkitt's lymphoma is endemic, concurrent malaria or other infections cause impaired immune function, allowing sustained B-lymphocyte proliferation. Incidence rates for nasopharyngeal cancer are high in some areas of China, particularly in southern China and in the Cantonese population in Singapore. EBV genomes have been found in almost all of the nasopharyngeal tumor specimens in these areas.

HBV is the etiologic agent in the development of hepatitis B, cirrhosis, and hepatocellular carcinoma (HCC). Epidemiologic data strongly support the role of HBV in the development of human HCC. There is a significant correlation between elevated incidence rates of HCC worldwide and the prevalence of HBV carriers. Other etiologic factors may also contribute to the development of liver cancer. Ingestion of aflatoxin and infec-

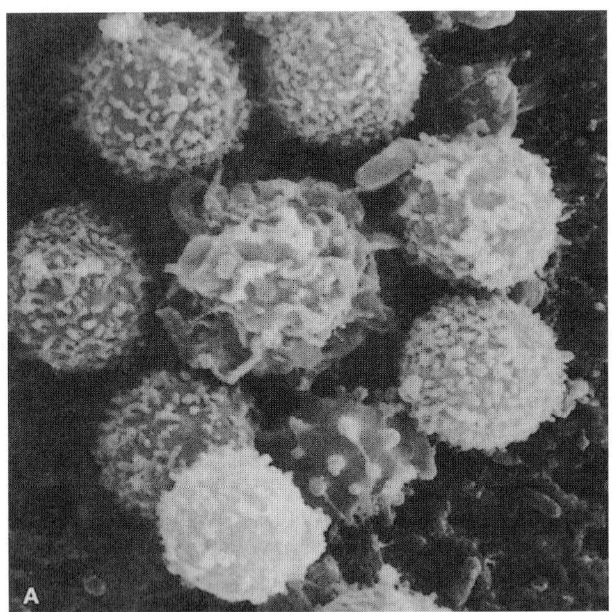

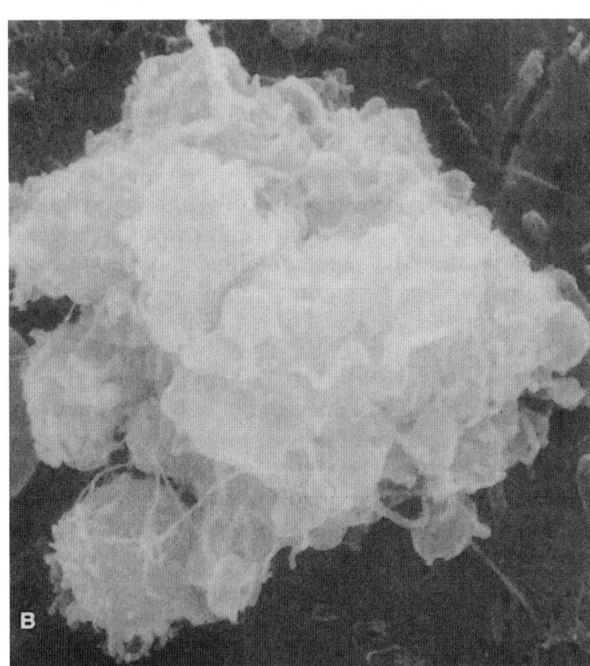

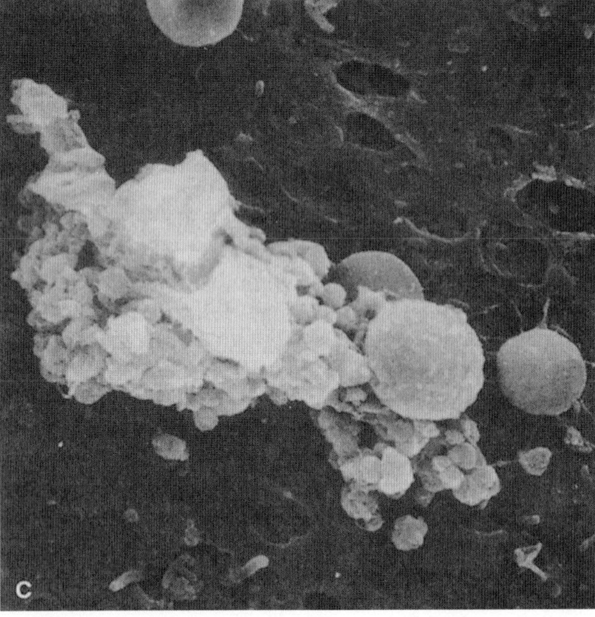

FIGURE 5-8
Scanning electron micrographs show the combination of a cancer cell and lymphocytes removed from the same patient and studied in the laboratory. (**A**) The lymphocytes surround the cancer cell (60 min). (**B**) Lymphocytes attack the cancer cell (150 min). (**C**) The integrity of the cancer cell has been destroyed (240 min). (Courtesy of Kenneth Siegesmund, Ph.D., and Burton A. Waisbren, Sr., M.D., Anatomy Department, The Medical College of Wisconsin)

tion with hepatitis C virus (HCV) have also been implicated. The precise mechanism by which HBV induces HCC has not been determined, although it has been suggested that HCC is the result of prolonged HBV-induced liver damage and regeneration. A number of countries endemic for HBV infections have begun widespread vaccinations against the virus. It will be interesting to observe if these vaccinations lower the incidence of HCC.[7,32]

Immunologic Defects

There is growing evidence for the immune system's participation in resistance against the progression and spread of cancer. The central concept, known as the immune surveillance hypothesis, which was first proposed by Paul Ehrlich in 1909, postulates that the immune system plays a central role in resistance against the development of tumors.[33] In addition to cancer-host interactions as a mechanism of cancer development, immunologic mechanisms provide a means for the detection, classification, and prognostic evaluation of cancers and as a potential method of treatment. *Immunotherapy* (discussed in a later section) is a cancer treatment modality designed to heighten the patient's general immune responses to increase tumor destruction.

It has been suggested that the development of cancer might be associated with impairment or decline in the surveillance capacity of the immune system. For example, increases in cancer incidence have been observed in persons with immunodeficiency diseases and in persons with organ transplants who are receiving immunosuppressant drugs. The incidence of cancer is also increased in the elderly, in whom there is a known decrease in immune activity. The association of Kaposi's sarcoma with AIDS further emphasizes the role of the immune system in preventing malignant cell proliferation.[34]

It has been shown that most tumor cells have molecular configurations that can be specifically recognized by immune T cells or by antibodies and hence are called tumor antigens.[35] The most relevant tumor antigens fall into two categories: unique tumor-specific antigens found only on tumor cells and tumor-associated antigens found on tumor cells and on normal cells. Quantitative and qualitative differences permit the use of these tumor-associated antigens to distinguish cancer cells from normal cells.[34]

Virtually all of the components of immune system have the potential for eradicating cancer cells, including T lymphocytes, B lymphocytes and antibodies, macrophages, and natural killer (NK) cells (see Chapter 11). The T-cell response is undoubtedly one of the most important host responses for controlling the growth of antigenic tumor cells; it is responsible for direct killing of tumor cells and for activation of other components of the immune system. The T-cell immunity to cancer cells reflects the function of two subsets of T cells: the CD4 helper T cells and CD8 cytotoxic T cells. Figure 5–8 illustrates the function of T-cell immunity in the lysis of cancer cells. The finding of tumor-reactive antibodies in the serum of persons with cancer supports the role of the B cell as a member of the immune surveillance team. Antibodies can destroy cancer cells through complement-mediated mechanisms or through antibody-dependent cellular cytotoxicity, in which the antibody binds the cancer cell to another effector cell such as the NK cell that does the actual killing of the cancer cell. NK cells do not require antigen recognition and can lyse a wide variety of target cells. The cytotoxic activity of NK cells can be augmented by the lymphokines, interleukin-2 (IL-2), and interferon, and NK activity can be amplified by immune T-cell responses.[36] Macrophages are important in tumor immunity as antigen-presenting cells to initiate the immune response and as potential effector cells to participate in tumor cell lysis.

In summary, because cancer is not a single disease, it is reasonable to assume that it does not have a single cause. Multiple factors probably interact at the genetic level to transform normal cells into cancer cells. This transformation process is called oncogenesis. Two kinds of genes control normal cell growth and replication: growth-promoting regulatory genes (i.e., proto-oncogenes) and growth-inhibiting regulatory genes (i.e., anti-oncogenes). These genes are implicated as principal targets of genetic damage that occurs during the development a cancer cell. Such genetic damage may be acquired by the action of chemicals (i.e., chemical carcinogens), radiation, or viruses, or it may be inherited in the cell line.

Diagnosis and Treatment

On completion of this section of the chapter, you should be able to do the following:

- Describe methods used in detection and diagnosis of cancer, including the Papanicolaou smear, tissue biopsy, tumor markers, and polymerase chain reaction
- Compare methods used in grading and staging cancers
- Explain the mechanism by which radiation exerts its beneficial effects in the treatment of cancer
- Describe the adverse effects of radiation therapy
- Compare the action of cell cycle–specific and cell cycle–independent chemotherapeutic drugs
- Describe the three mechanisms whereby biotherapy exerts its effects
- Describe four uses of gene therapy in the treatment of cancer

Diagnostic Methods

The methods used in the diagnosis and staging of cancer are determined largely by the location and type of cancer suspected. A number of diagnostic procedures are used in diagnosis of cancer, including x-ray studies;

endoscopic examinations; urine and stool tests; blood tests for tumor markers; bone marrow aspirations; ultrasound imaging; magnetic resonance imaging (MRI); and computed tomography (CT scan). Four diagnostic methods are discussed in this chapter: the Pap smear, tissue biopsy, tumor markers, and the polymerase chain reaction (PCR).

The Pap Smear

The Pap smear is an example of the type of test called *exfoliative cytology*. It consists of microscopic examination of a properly prepared slide by a cytotechnologist or pathologist for the purpose of detecting the presence of abnormal cells. The usefulness of exfoliative cytology relies on the fact that the cancer cells lack the cohesive properties and intercellular junctions that are characteristic of normal tissue; without these characteristics, cancer cells tend to exfoliate and become mixed with secretions surrounding the tumor growth. The American Cancer Society recommends that the test be done annually to detect cervical cancer in women who are or have been sexually active and who have reached age 18. After three consecutive normal findings, the test may be performed less frequently at the discretion of the physician.[37] Exfoliative cytology can also be performed on other body secretions, including nipple drainage, pleural or peritoneal fluid, and gastric washings.

Biopsy

Tissue biopsy is the removal of a tissue specimen for microscopic study. Biopsies are obtained in a number of ways, including needle aspiration (*i.e.*, fine, percutaneous, or core needle); by endoscopic methods, such as bronchoscopy or cystoscopy, which involve the passage of a scope through an orifice and into the involved structure; or by laparoscopic methods. In some instances, a surgical incision is made from which biopsy specimens are obtained. Excisional biopsies are those in which all of the tumor is removed. The tumors are usually small, solid, palpable masses. If the tumor is too large to be completely removed, a wedge of tissue from the mass can be excised for examination. Tissue diagnosis is of critical importance in designing the treatment plan should cancer cells be found.[38]

Tumor Markers

Tumor markers are antigens that are expressed on the surface of tumor cells or substances released from normal cells in response to the presence of tumor. Some substances such as hormones and enzymes are produced normally by the tissue involved but become overexpressed as a result of cancer. Other tumor markers, such as oncofetal proteins, are produced during fetal development and are induced to reappear later in life as a result of benign and malignant neoplasms. Tumor markers are used for screening, for diagnosis, for establishing prognosis, for monitoring treatment, and for detecting recurrent disease.[34]

As diagnostic tools, tumor markers have limitations. The value of a marker depends on its sensitivity, specificity, proportionality, and feasibility.[39] Sensitivity implies that the marker is apparent early in the development of the tumor and has few false-negative results. Specificity indicates that the marker is specific for the specific cancer and is not elevated in other disease conditions (*i.e.*, has few false-positive results). Proportionality means that the level of marker accurately reflects the growth of the tumor, such that higher levels reflect a larger growth. Feasibility implies that the methods are readily available, easy to use, and that the cost is not prohibitive. Nearly all markers can be elevated in benign conditions, and most are not elevated in the early stages of malignancy. Hence, tumor markers have limited value as screening tests. Extremely elevated levels of a tumor marker can indicate a poor prognosis or the need for more aggressive treatment. Perhaps the greatest value of tumor markers is in monitoring therapy in persons with widespread cancer. Nearly all markers show an association with the clinical course of the disease. The levels of most markers decline with successful treatment and increase with recurrence of the tumor.

The markers that have been most useful in practice have been human chorionic gonadotropin (hCG), CA 125, prostate-specific antigen (PSA), prostatic acid phosphatase (PAP), α-fetoprotein (AFP), and carcinoembryonic antigen (CEA). HCG is a hormone normally produced by the placenta. It is used as a marker for diagnosing, prescribing treatment, and following the disease course in persons with high-risk gestational trophoblastic tumors. PSA and PAP are used as markers in prostate cancer, and CA 125 is used as a marker in ovarian cancer.

Some cancers express oncofetal antigens, which are differentiation antigens normally presented only during embryonal development.[34] The two that have proven the most useful as tumor markers are AFP and CEA. AFP is synthesized by the fetal liver, yolk sac, and gastrointestinal tract and is the major serum protein in the fetus. Elevated levels are encountered in persons with primary liver cancers and have also been observed in some testicular, ovarian, pancreatic, and stomach cancers. CEA is normally produced by embryonic tissue in the gut, pancreas, and liver and is elaborated by a number of different cancers. Depending on the serum level adopted for significant elevation, CEA is elevated in approximately 60% to 90% of colorectal carcinomas, 50% to 80% of pancreatic cancers, and 25% to 50% of gastric and breast tumors.[8] As with most other tumor markers, elevated levels of CEA and AFP are found in other noncancerous conditions, and elevated levels of both depend on tumor size so that neither is useful as an early test for cancer.

Polymerase Chain Reaction

PCR is a highly sensitive in vitro technique designed to identify specific circulating tumor cells and micrometastases in leukemias, lymphomas, melanoma, neuroblastoma, and a variety of carcinomas. Tumor-specific abnormalities contained in the DNA of tumor cells are amplified, which allow identification of these abnormalities among cell populations containing only a few tumor cells (see Chapter 10). The PCR technique is so sensitive that one tumor cell can be identified within a million to a billion normal cells.[40]

Although PCR has been found to be superior to conventional techniques in detecting circulating tumor cells and micrometastasis, several limitations are associated with this technique. Because of the extreme sensitivity of the test, there is a tendency for false-positive results to occur if certain precautions are not taken to prevent contamination of the samples. Inhibitor substances are contained in some tissues, and fluids can also decrease the sensitivity. Most tumor cells that reach the bloodstream are destroyed by mechanical or immunologic mechanisms, thereby reducing the number of cells in the peripheral circulation. The number of tumor cells identified in blood obtained from peripheral sites may not be reflective of the extent of circulating cells.

More research is needed to determine the extent of this technique's application to the field of oncology. Perhaps patients with low tumor burdens can be given systemic therapy at an earlier stage, when better results could be achieved. PCR may also improve preoperative staging in patients with certain epithelial cancers that could lead to more conservative and less disfiguring surgeries.

Staging and Grading of Tumors

The two basic methods for classifying cancers are grading according to the histologic or cellular characteristics of the tumor and staging according to the clinical spread of the disease. Both methods are used to determine the course of the disease and to aid in selecting an appropriate treatment or management plan. Grading of tumors involves the microscopic examination of cancer cells to determine their level of differentiation and the number of mitoses. Cancers are classified as grades I, II, III, and IV, with increasing anaplasia or lack of differentiation. Staging of cancers uses methods to determine the progress and spread of the disease. Surgery may be used to determine tumor size and lymph node involvement.

The clinical staging of cancer is intended to provide a means by which information related to the progress of the disease, the methods and success of treatment modalities, and the prognosis can be communicated to others. The TNM system, which has evolved from the work of the International Union Against Cancer (IUAC) and the American Joint Committee on Cancer Staging and End Stage Reporting (AJCCS), is used by many cancer facilities. This system, which is briefly described in Chart 5–2, classifies the disease into stages using three tumor components: T stands for the extent of the primary tumor, N refers to the involvement of the regional lymph nodes, and M describes the extent of the metastatic involvement. The time of staging is indicated as cTNM, clinical-diagnostic staging; pTNM, postsurgical resection-pathologic staging; sTNM, surgical-evaluative staging; rTNM, retreatment staging; and aTNM, autopsy staging.[41]

CHART 5-2
TNM Classification System

T (tumor)

Tx	Tumor cannot be adequately assessed
T0	No evidence of primary tumor
Tis	Carcinoma in situ
T1–4	Progressive increase in tumor size or involvement

N (nodes)

Nx	Regional lymph nodes cannot be assessed
N0	No evidence of regional node metastasis
N 1–3	Increasing involvement of regional lymph nodes

M (metastasis)

Mx	Not assessed
M0	No distant metastasis
M1	Distant metastasis present, specify sites

Cancer Treatment

The goals of treatment methods fall into three categories: curative, control, and palliative. The most common modalities are surgery, radiation, chemotherapy, hormonal therapy, and biotherapy. The treatment of cancer involves the use of a carefully planned program that combines the benefits of multiple treatment modalities and the expertise of an interdisciplinary team of specialists including medical, surgical and radiation oncologists, clinical nurse specialists, nurse practitioners, pharmacists, and a variety of ancillary personnel.

Surgery

It is estimated that 90% of all cancer patients will undergo a surgical procedure during the course of their management.[42] Surgery is used for diagnosis, the staging of cancer, tumor removal, and palliation (*i.e.*, relief of symptoms) when a cure cannot be achieved. The type of surgery to be used is determined by the extent of the disease, the location and structures involved, the tumor growth rate and invasiveness, the surgical risk of the patient, and the quality of life the patient will experience after the surgery. If the tumor is small and has well-defined margins, the entire tumor often can be removed. If, however, the tumor is large or involves vital tissues, surgical removal may be difficult if not impossible.

Surgical techniques consist of a number of approaches to cancer care. For example, surgery can be the primary, curative treatment for cancers that are locally or regionally contained, have not metastasized, or have not invaded major organs. It is also used as a component of adjuvant therapy when used in addition to chemotherapy or radiation therapy in other types of cancers. Surgical techniques may also used to control oncologic emergencies such as gastrointestinal hemorrhages. Another approach includes using surgical techniques for prophylaxis in families that have a high genetically confirmed risk for developing cancer. For instance, colectomy may be suggested for families that have familial adenomatous polyposis coli. Prophylactic mastectomy may also be encouraged for women who are at very high risk for developing breast cancer.[38]

Surgical techniques have expanded to include electrosurgery, cryosurgery, chemosurgery, cytoreductive surgery, and laser surgery. Electrosurgery uses the cutting and coagulating effects of high-frequency current applied by needle, blade, or electrodes. Once considered a palliative type of procedure, it is now being used as an alternative treatment for certain cancers of the skin, oral cavity, and rectum. Cryosurgery involves the instillation of liquid nitrogen into the tumor through a probe. It is used in treating cancers of the oral cavity, brain, and prostate. Chemosurgery is used in skin cancers. It involves the use of a corrosive paste in combination with multiple frozen sections to ensure complete removal of the tumor. Laser surgery uses a laser beam to resect a tumor. It has been used effectively in retinal and vocal cord surgery.

Cooperative efforts among cancer centers throughout the world have helped to standardize and improve surgical procedures, determine which cancers benefit from surgical intervention, and establish in what order surgical and other treatment modalities should be used. Increased emphasis has also been placed on the development of surgical techniques, such as limb-salvage surgery, which is used in the treatment of osteogenic sarcoma to preserve functional abilities while permitting complete removal of the tumor.

Discovery of Ionizing Radiation

Ionizing radiation was discovered by Marie and Pierre Curie and by Wilhelm Conrad Roentgen just before the turn of the century. Development of the first cathode-ray tube followed during the 1920s, along with quantitative methods for measuring radiation dosage. The first use of radium to treat cancer occurred 1 to 2 years after development of the cathode-ray tube. During this same period, Claude Regauc (Foundation Curie in Paris) was able to demonstrate that fractionated, small, sublethal doses of radiation could permanently halt spermatogenesis, but no single lethal dose could do so without causing severe damage to the surrounding tissues. This observation linked external irradiation to the treatment of cancer. Another advance in radiation therapy was the development of radioactive cobalt. Since then, advances in technology have resulted in the sophisticated equipment that produces high-voltage x-ray and electron beams capable of delivering a therapeutic dose of radiation to the tumor with limited morbidity to surrounding tissues.

Radiation Therapy

More than 50% of patients with cancer receive radiation therapy, alone or in combination with other forms of treatment. Radiation can be used alone as the primary method of treatment for Hodgkin's disease and for early-stage breast, laryngeal, prostate, vaginal, and uterine cervix cancers. If radiation is used as the primary treatment for cure, the duration of treatment is usually longer and the dose is higher than in palliative treatment modalities. Radiation therapy is also used as an adjuvant treatment with surgery administered presurgically or postsurgically, with chemotherapy, or with chemotherapy and surgery. In patients with acute lymphocytic leukemia in which the primary treatment is chemotherapy, radiation is used to treat sanctuary sites such as the central nervous system, because it has been found to enhance the ability of chemotherapy to cross the blood-brain barrier. It is used as a palliative treatment to reduce symptoms in approximately 50% of patients with advanced cancers who receive radiation therapy. It is effective in reducing the pain associated with bone metastasis and, in some cases, improves mobility. Radiation is also used to treat several oncologic emergencies such as superior vena cava syndrome, spinal cord compression, bronchial obstruction, and hemorrhage.[43]

Mechanism of Action. Ionizing radiation is radiation that is capable of ejecting one or more electrons from an atom. Ionizing radiation causes significant biologic effects with small amounts of localized energy that is powerful enough to break chemical bonds. It affects cells by direct ionization of molecules or, more commonly, by indirect ionization. Indirect ionization produced by x-rays and gamma rays causes cellular damage when they are absorbed into tissue and give up their energy by producing fast-moving electrons. These electrons interact with free or loosely bonded electrons of the absorber cells and subsequently produce free radicals that interact with critical cell components (see Chapter 2).[44] It can immediately kill cells, delay or halt cell cycle progression, or at dose levels commonly used in radiation therapy, can cause damage within the nucleus resulting in cell death after replication. Cell damage may be sublethal, in which case a single break in the strand of DNA can repair itself if there is time before the next radiation insult. Double-strand breaks in DNA are generally believed to be the primary damage that leads to radiation death in cells. The result of unrepaired DNA is that cells may continue to function until they undergo cell mitosis, at which time the genetic damage from the irradiation may result in death of the cell. The clinical significance is that the rapidly proliferating and poorly differentiated cells of a cancerous tumor are more likely to be injured by radiation therapy than are the slower proliferating cells of normal tissue. To some extent, however, radiation is injurious to all rapidly proliferating cells, including those of the bone marrow and the mucosal lining of the gastrointestinal tract. In addition to its lethal effects, radiation also produces sublethal injury. Recovery from sublethal doses of radiation occurs in the interval between the first dose of radiation and subsequent doses. This is why large total doses of radiation can be tolerated when they are divided into multiple smaller fractionated doses. Normal tissue is usually able to recover from radiation damage more readily than cancerous tissue.

Radiation, Sensitivity, and Responsiveness. The term radiosensitivity describes the inherent properties of a tumor that determine its responsiveness to radiation. It varies widely among the different types of cancers and is thought to vary as a function of their position in the cell cycle. Fast-growing cells, for example, that have cell cycle durations of 9 or 10 hours typically are more radiosensitive in mitosis (M) or late in the G_2 phase. More slowly growing cells that have longer S phases are more radioresistant.[44] Acute lymphocytic leukemia and lymphoma are highly radiosensitive cancers, but rhabdomyosarcomas and melanomas are much less so.

The radiation dose that is chosen for treatment of a particular cancer is determined by factors such as the radiosensitivity of the tumor type, size of the tumor, and more importantly, the tolerance of the surrounding tissues. Dose-response curves, which express the extent of lethal tissue injury in relation to the dose of radiation, are determined by number of cells that survive graded, fractional doses of radiation. With the use of fractionated doses, it is likely that the cancer cells will be dividing and in the vulnerable period of the cell cycle. This dose also allows time for normal tissues to repair the radiation damage. Studies are being conducted to find ways to increase the radiosensitivity of tumors by altering their DNA in a manner that makes it more sensitive to radiation or less able to repair radiation damage.

Radiation responsiveness describes the manner in which a radiosensitive tumor responds to irradiation. One of the major determinants of radiation responsiveness is tumor oxygenation, because oxygen is a rich source of free radicals that form and destroy essential cell components during irradiation. Many rapidly growing tumors outgrow their blood supply and become deprived of oxygen. The hypoxic cells of these tumors are more resistant to radiation than normal or well-oxygenated tumor cells. Methods of ensuring adequate oxygen delivery, such as adequate hemoglobin levels, are important. Agents that act as radiosensitizers are being investigated. These agents increase the production of free radicals during radiation in a manner similar to oxygen.

Administration. Ionizing radiation includes two distinct forms: electromagnetic waves and fast-moving, high-energy particles. Electromagnetic radiation consists of x-rays and gamma rays, both of which are similar in nature, but differ in the way they are made. X-rays are produced by electrical devices that accelerate electrons to high energy levels and abruptly stops them at a target. Gamma rays are emitted from the spontaneous decay of radioactive isotopes such as cobalt and cesium. The electromagnetic radiation is energetic and extremely penetrating. Particulate radiation used in radiotherapy includes electrons, protons, alpha particles, neutrons, negative pi-mesons, and heavy ions These particles are accelerated by electrical magnetic fields in linear accelerators and cyclotrons.[44]

Several types of equipment and beams can be used for administering radiation therapy. Large radiotherapy centers have a selection suitable to the treatment of almost any malignancy in any part of the body. Therapy can be delivered by external beam radiation machines that have sources of radiation located some distance from the patient (sometimes called teletherapy) or by short-distance therapy (brachytherapy) in which a sealed radioactive source is placed close to or directly in the tumor site. Radioisotopes with a short half-life may be injected or given by mouth as a palliative or curative treatment for some forms of cancer.

External beam radiation machines deliver a penetrating radiation dose, depending on the energy or voltage rating that is used. The higher the energy, the greater is the depth of penetration. The early forms of radiation therapy used x-ray machines with energy from 100 to 250 kV. These machines delivered low-penetrance rays that exerted their maximum tumor dose within 1 to 2 cm of the skin surface. They are now used only in treating superficial skin lesions or tumors located near the skin surface. The newer megavoltage machines produce x-rays by allowing high-energy electrons to be accelerated by microwaves. These x-rays are much more penetrating and allow treatment from a number of directions (*i.e.*, cross firing). This allows delivery of curative doses of radiation without causing extensive damage to skin or other tissues. The megavoltage rays also spare bone structures more than lower-energy x-rays. Various beam-modifying wedges, rotational techniques, and other specific approaches are used to increase the radiation damage to the tumor site while sparing the normal surrounding tissues. Cobalt-60 machines deliver gamma rays that are comparable to megavolt x-rays. They were once the most common type of equipment used, but because the radiation source is a radioactive isotope, it is undergoing decay and needs to be replaced every 5 to 6 years to avoid lengthy treatment times. As the name implies, linear accelerators produce megavoltage electromagnetic wave radiation by accelerating electrons in a straight line. Linear accelerators have distinct advantages, including the speed with which treatment can be given. This reduces the time the patient must spend in awkward and uncomfortable positions. Some linear accelerators are also equipped to produce particulate radiation. With particulate radiation, most of the energy is expended at a certain depth, sparing surrounding tissues.

Brachytherapy involves the insertion of sealed radioactive sources into a body cavity (intracavitary) or directly into body tissues (interstitial). Radiation sources are sealed within applicators of almost any size or shape. Most commonly, they are packed into needles, beads, seeds, ribbons, or catheters, which are then implanted directly into the tumor. Removable devices make it possible to insert a radioactive material into a tumor area for a period (1 or 2 days to 1 week) and remove it. The radioactive sources used most commonly for this purpose are cesium-137, iridium-192, and iodine-125. Cancers of the cervix and uterus are often treated with removable cesium insertions or iridium implants. Radioactive materials with a relatively short half-life, such as gold-198, radium-226, iodine-125, or palladium-103, are commonly encapsulated and used in permanent implants. This type of treatment is used for oral, bladder, and prostate cancers.

Unsealed internal radiation sources are injected intravenously, administered by mouth, or instilled into a body cavity. Iodine-131, which is given orally, is used in the treatment of thyroid cancer. Gold-198 and phosphorus-32 are instilled directly into body cavities to control effusions (*i.e.*, collections of fluid within a serous cavity).

Internal radiation sources are a source of radiation exposure as long as a sealed implant remains in the body or an unsealed implant or injected radioisotope emanates rays of radiant energy. It is essential that the type of ray that is being emitted and the half-life of the radioisotope be considered when care is provided for a person receiving internal radiation. Some radioisotopes, such as phosphorus-32, produce only beta rays, which do not create a radiation hazard because of the limited range of beta radiation. Others, such as cesium implants, pose a radiation hazard because they emit gamma rays. Institutions that practice nuclear medicine must be licensed by the Atomic Energy Commission and have a radiation safety officer, who is responsible for establishing policies and maintaining radiation safety within the institution.

Adverse Effects. Radiation cannot distinguish between malignant cells and the rapidly proliferating cells of normal tissue. During radiation treatment, injury to normal cells can produce adverse effects. Radiation effects are dose and fractionation dependent. Tissues that are most frequently affected are the skin, the mucosal lining of the gastrointestinal tract, and the bone marrow. Anorexia, nausea, emesis, and diarrhea are common depending on the site of treatment. These can usually be controlled by medication and dietary measures. Other systemic signs include fatigue, profuse perspiration, and chills. These effects are temporary and reversible.

Irradiation also causes bone marrow depression, which subsequently affects the blood count and predisposes the individual to infection and bleeding. The first cells to decrease in number are the leukocytes, then the thrombocytes (platelets), and finally the red blood cells. Frequent blood cell counts are used during radiation therapy to monitor bone marrow function.

External beam radiation must first penetrate the skin; depending on the total dose and type of radiation used, reactions of the skin may develop. With moderate doses of radiation to the skin, the hair falls out spontaneously or when being combed after the 10th to the 14th day; with larger doses, erythema develops (much like a sunburn), and skin may turn brown; and at higher doses, patches of dry or moist desquamation may develop. Fortunately, epithelialization takes place after the treatments have been stopped. Mucositis, desquamation of the oral and pharyngeal mucous membranes, which may sometimes be severe, may occur as a predictable side effect in persons receiving head and neck irradiation. The most severe effect is dry mouth because the parotid gland is within the treatment field.

Chemotherapy

In the past 4 decades, cancer chemotherapy has evolved as a major treatment modality. More than 30 different chemotherapeutic drugs are used alone or in various combinations. Administering higher doses of multiple drugs may be used as a strategy to achieve cure or optimal palliation; however, the adverse drug interactions and side effects can be unpredictable and intense. Chemotherapeutic drugs may be the primary form of treatment, or they may be used as adjuncts to other treatments. Chemotherapy is the primary treatment for most hematologic and some solid tumors, including choriocarcinoma, testicular cancer, acute and chronic leukemia, Burkitt's lymphoma, Hodgkin's disease, and multiple myeloma.

Cancer chemotherapeutic drugs exert their effects through several mechanisms. At the cellular level, they exert their lethal action by creating adverse conditions that prevent cell growth and replication. These mechanisms include disrupting production of essential enzymes; inhibiting DNA, RNA, and protein synthesis; and preventing cell mitosis.[6,45]

For most chemotherapy drugs, the relation between tumor cell survival and drug dose is exponential, with the number of cells surviving being proportional to drug dose and the number of cells at risk for exposure being proportional to destructive action of the drug. Chemotherapeutic drugs are most effective in treating tumors that have a high growth fraction because of their ability to kill rapidly dividing cells. Exponential killing implies that a proportion or percentage of tumor cells are killed, rather than an absolute number. This proportion is a constant percentage of the total number of cells. For this reason, multiple courses of treatment are needed if the tumor is to be eradicated.[6]

The anticancer drugs may be classified as cell cycle specific or cell cycle nonspecific. Drugs are cell cycle specific if they exert their action during a specific phase of the cell cycle. For example, methotrexate, an antimetabolite, acts by interfering with DNA synthesis and thereby interrupts the S phase of the cell cycle. Drugs that are cell cycle nonspecific affect cancer cells through all the phases of the cell cycle. The alkylating agents, which are cell cycle nonspecific, act by disrupting DNA when the cells are in the resting state and when they are dividing. The site of action of various cancer drugs varies. Chemotherapeutic drugs that have similar structures and effects on cell function are generally grouped together, and these drugs usually have similar toxic effects and side effects. Because they differ in their mechanisms of action, combinations of cell cycle–specific and cell cycle–nonspecific agents are often used to treat cancer.

Combination chemotherapy has been found to be more effective than treatment with a single drug. With this method, several drugs with different mechanisms of action, metabolic pathways, times of onset of action and recovery, side effects, and onset of side effects are used. Drugs used in combinations are individually effective against the tumor and synergistic with each other. The regimens for combination therapy are often referred to by acronyms. Two well-known combinations are MOPP (mechlorethamine, Oncovin (vincristine), procarbazine, and prednisone), used in the treatment of Hodgkin's disease, and CMF (cyclophosphamide, methotrexate, and 5-fluorouracil), used in the treatment of breast cancer. The maximum possible drug doses are usually used to ensure the maximum cell killing. Routes of administration and dosage schedules are carefully designed to ensure optimal delivery of the active forms of the drugs to a tumor during the sensitive phase of the cell cycle.

Several new chemotherapy drugs have recently become available. The taxanes, derived from the *Taxus* (yew) plant bark, exert their effect in the M phase to inhibit mitosis. These drugs are used primarily to treat refractory ovarian and breast cancers, and are under investigation in the treatment of other solid tumors and lung cancers.[45] Liposomal therapy, in which chemotherapy drugs are encapsulated by coated liposomes, has been found to distribute more of the chemotherapy to desired site with fewer toxic effects than the administration of the chemotherapy alone. This therapy has been approved for use to treat AIDS-related Kaposi's sarcoma, ovarian, and breast cancer.[46,47]

Many of these drugs are administered intravenously. Venous access devices are often used for persons with poor venous access and those who require frequent or continuous intravenous therapy. Devices can be used for home administration of chemotherapy drugs, blood sampling, and administration of blood components. These systems use an implanted venous catheter with vascular access ports. In some cases, the drugs are administered by continuous infusion using a special ambulatory infusion pump that allows the person to remain at home and maintain daily activities.[48]

Adverse Effects. Because cancer cells are derived from normal cells, they retain many of normal cells' properties. Chemotherapeutic drugs affect the neoplastic cells and the rapidly proliferating cells of normal tissue. The nadir (*i.e.*, lowest point) is the point of maximal toxicity for a given adverse effect of a drug and is stated in the time it takes to reach that point. The nadir for leukopenia with thiotepa, for example, occurs at 14 days after initiation of treatment. Because many toxic effects of chemotherapeutic drugs persist for some time after the drug is discontinued, the nadir times and recovery rates are useful guides in evaluating the effects of cancer therapy.

Anorexia, nausea, and vomiting are common problems associated with cancer chemotherapy. The severity of the vomiting is related to the emetic potential of the particular drug. These symptoms can occur within minutes or hours of drug administration and are thought to result from stimulation of the chemoreceptor trigger zone (*i.e.*, vomiting center) in the medullary lateral reticular formation. The chemoreceptor trigger zone responds to levels of chemicals circulating in the blood.[49] The symptoms usually subside within 24 to 48 hours and often can be relieved by antiemetics.[50] Newly developed antiemetics, such as ondansetron and granisetron, that block the serotonin 5-HT_3 receptors have facilitated the use of highly emetic chemotherapy drugs by more effectively reducing the nausea and vomiting incurred by these drug.[51]

Diarrhea is another problem associated with cancer chemotherapy. Chemotherapy can cause a temporary lactose intolerance or an increase in gastric motility. Pharmacologic and dietary interventions are helpful in reducing the severity of diarrhea. For example, Lomotil and Immodium are frequently prescribed, and patients should be advised to eat low-residue, small, frequent meals; avoid spicy or greasy foods; drink 2 to 3 quarts of uncarbonated beverages daily; avoid extreme temperatures in foods or beverages; and use nutritional supplements when necessary.[49]

Some drugs cause stomatitis and damage to the rapidly proliferating cells of the gastrointestinal tract mucosal lining. Most chemotherapeutic drugs suppress bone marrow function and formation of blood cells, leading to anemia, leukopenia, and thrombocytopenia. With severe granulocytopenia, there is risk of developing serious infections. Fatigue is one of the most prevalent problems experienced by cancer patients and is estimated to occur in 96% of individuals receiving chemotherapy. The cause is multifactoral and poorly understood.[52] Hair loss results from impaired proliferation of the hair follicles and is a side effect of a number of cancer drugs; it is usually temporary, and the hair tends to regrow when treatment is stopped. The rapidly proliferating structures of the reproductive system are particularly sensitive to the action of the cancer drugs. Women may experience changes in menstrual flow or have amenorrhea. Men may develop decreased sperm count (*i.e.*, oligospermia) or absence of sperm (*i.e.*, azoospermia). Many chemotherapeutic agents may also have teratogenic or mutagenic effects leading to fetal abnormalities.

Chemotherapy drugs are toxic to all cells. The mutagenic, carcinogenic, and teratogenic potential of these drugs has been strongly supported by animal and human studies. Because of these potential risks, special care is required when handling or administering the drugs. Drugs, drug containers, and administration equipment require special disposal as hazardous waste. Several organizations including the Occupational Safety and Health Administration (OSHA), the Oncology Nursing Society (ONS), and American Society of Healthsystem Pharmacists have developed special guidelines for the safe handling and disposal of antineoplastic drugs and for accidental spills and exposure.[53,54]

Epidemiologic studies have shown an increased risk of second malignancies such as acute nonlymphocytic leukemia after long-term use of alkylating agents[55,56] and semustine[57] for treatment of various forms of cancer. These second malignancies are thought to result from direct cellular changes produced by the drug or from suppression of the immune response.

Hormone Therapy

Hormone therapy consists of administration of hormones or hormone-blocking drugs. It is used for cancers that are responsive to or dependent on hormones for growth. The actions of hormones depend on the presence of specific receptors in the tumor. Among the tumors known to be responsive to hormonal manipulations are those of the breast, prostate, adrenal gland, and uterine endometrium. Hormones commonly used for cancer treatment include estrogens (*e.g.*, diethylstilbestrol, estradiol), androgens (*e.g.*, testosterone), and progestins (*e.g.*, hydroxyprogesterone). Hormone therapy also involves use of the adrenal corticosteroid hormones such as prednisone, dexamethasone, and methylprednisolone. These compounds inhibit mitosis and are cytotoxic to cells of lymphocytic origin. Hormones are cell cycle nonspecific and are thought to alter the synthesis of RNA and proteins by binding to receptor sites. Hormone-blocking drugs include the antiestrogen drugs tamoxifen and leuprolide (*i.e.*, gonadotropin-releasing hormone analog that blocks estrogens and androgens) and the antiadrenal drug aminoglutethimide. The side effects of hormonal treatment are directly related to the normal action of the hormones. Because dosages of these drugs are usually higher than those that normally occur in the body, the normal actions of the hormone are accentuated.[45]

Biotherapy

Biotherapy involves the use of biologic response modifiers (BRMs) that change the person's own biologic response to cancer. The BRMs are products normally produced in the body that serve as regulators and messengers of normal cellular function. Although biotherapy relies heavily on immune mechanisms, it is not limited to them. Three major mechanisms by which biotherapy exerts its effects are modification of host responses, direct destruction of cancer cells by suppressing tumor growth or killing the tumor cell, and modification of tumor cell biology.

Immunotherapy techniques include active and passive immunotherapy. The active immunotherapy involves nonspecific techniques such as the use of bacille Calmette-Guérin (BCG) and levamisole, and specific techniques such as purified or recombinant antigens. Passive immunotherapy is divided into nonspecific techniques such as lymphokine-activated killer (LAK) cells and cytokine therapy, specific techniques such as antibody therapy, and combined techniques that include LAK cells and antibodies. Active immunotherapy focuses on stimulating immune response. BCG is an attenuated strain of the bacterium that causes bovine tuberculosis. BCG acts as a nonspecific stimulant of the immune system. A second method involves the use of vaccines made from the patient's own tumor (autologous) or from pooled tumor-associated antigens (allogeneic) that have been obtained from a number of tumors. Active immunotherapy has been studied as treatment for melanoma, renal cell carcinoma, and leukemia.[34]

Adoptive immunotherapy is a technique that uses lymphokine-activated NK cells or tumor-specific T-cell immunity as a means of eradicating cancer cells. Originally, only LAK cells were used. These NK cells are grown in culture supported by IL-2. Because NK cells are nonspecific in their function, LAK cells attack normal and tumor cells. The technique of adoptive therapy has been expanded to the production of tumor-specific T cells. These cells are derived from a person's own *tumor-infiltrating lymphocytes* (TIL cells) that have been expanded in the laboratory so that a large amount of cells are available for reinfusion. Because the TIL cells are tumor specific, they do not attack normal host cells.

Four types of biologic response modifiers are being used or investigated: interferon therapy, interleukin therapy, monoclonal antibodies, and hematopoietic growth factors. Some agents, such as the interferons, have more than one biologic action that include antiviral, immunomodulatory, and antiproliferative actions. The *interferons* are endogenous polypeptides that are synthesized by a number of cells in response to a variety of cellular or viral stimuli. The three major types of interferons are alpha (α), beta (β), and gamma (γ), each group differing in terms of their cell surface receptors. The exact physiologic roles of each of the interferons remain unclear. They appear to inhibit viral replication and may be involved in inhibiting tumor protein synthesis and in prolonging the cell cycle and increasing the percentage of cells in the G_0 phase. Interferons stimulate NK cells and killer T cells. Interferon-γ has been approved for the treatment of hairy cell leukemia, AIDS-related Kaposi's sarcoma, chronic myelogenous leukemia, condylomata acuminate (genital warts), and as adjuvant therapy for patients that are high-risk for recurrent melanoma.[58] Its use with other cancers, including renal cell carcinoma, colorectal cancer, cutaneous T-cell lymphoma, and multiple myeloma, is being investigated. Research is focusing on combining interferons with other forms of cancer therapy and establishing optimal doses and treatment protocols.

The *interleukins* consist of 17 identified interleukins (ILs), and only one, IL-2, has been approved by the Federal Drug Administration in the treatment of metastatic renal cell carcinoma. IL-1, IL-3, IL-4, IL-6, IL-11, and IL-12 are under investigation in clinical trials. IL-2 has been found to reduce tumor size in a minority of patients with metastatic renal cancer and melanoma.[59]

Monoclonal antibodies (MoAbs) are highly specific antibodies derived from cloned cells or hybridomas. Scientists were able to produce large quantities of these MoAbs that were specific for tumor cells. Two MoAbs have been approved: muromonab-CD3 (OKT-3), which targets the CD3 receptor of human T cells for the treatment of acute allograft rejection in renal transplant patients, and satumomab pendetide, which is used in the detection of colorectal and ovarian cancers.[60]

Hematopoietic growth factors are growth and maturation factors that include the colony-stimulating factors (CSFs). The CSFs consist of factors that control the production of neutrophils, monocytes or macrophages, erythropoietin, and thrombopoietin.[61]

Bone Marrow and Peripheral Blood Stem Cell Transplantation

Bone marrow transplantation (BMT) and peripheral blood stem cell transplantation (PBSCT) are two treatment approaches for individuals with inherited disorders, immunodeficiencies, leukemias, certain solid tumors, and other cancers previously thought to be incurable. BMT techniques include *allogeneic BMT,* in which the recipient receives the bone marrow from another person who is human leukocyte antigen- (HLA-) matched; *syngeneic BMT,* in which the donor is an identical twin; and *autologous BMT,* in which the recipient's bone marrow is harvested and reinfused after treatment.

The first allogeneic BMT was successfully performed in 1968 to treat advanced leukemia. Since then, advancements in BMT such as supportive measures including platelet administration, graft-versus-host disease pretreatment and prophylaxis, and hematopoietic growth factors have increased survival for a number of patients. Allogeneic transplantation is used primarily to treat all types of leukemia but also has been used in a limited fashion to treat multiple myeloma. Autologous BMT is considered when a HLA-matched donor is not available. Auto-BMTs are used for certain hematologic malignancies such as Hodgkin's and non-Hodgkin's lymphomas, for solid tumors such as metastatic or highly aggressive breast cancer, neuroblastoma, and testicular cancer. The primary goal of auto-BMT is to administer high-dose chemotherapy to achieve the maximum tumoricidal effect while providing a hematologic rescue to decrease the potentially fatal hematologic side effects.[62]

PBSCT, an alternative to BMT, uses the patient's peripheral blood stem cells to repopulate the bone marrow after extensive high-dose chemotherapy. It is a treatment option when there may be bone marrow abnormalities such as metastases or hypocellularity. PBSCT has been found to be more advantageous than BMT for a number of reasons. Stem cells can be harvested through pheresis techniques, which are less invasive and do not require general anesthesia. PBSCT is an outpatient procedure that is easier and safer for the patients and costs approximately one half that of BMT. The period of aplasia after high-dose chemotherapy is shorter, thereby reducing the risks associated with granulocytopenia, the number of transfusions the patients require, and the intensive supportive care needed during BMT. Graft-versus-host disease is eliminated because patients receive their own stem cells. Despite the apparent advantages this technique has to offer, some disadvantages exist. Fewer pluripotent stem cells are contained in the peripheral blood; therefore, multiple leukapheresis sessions are necessary to harvest sufficient numbers of stem cells. There may also be the risk of infusing malignant cells, although this risk is less than in auto BMT. Although there is uncertainty surrounding the number and types of cells harvested during the leukapheresis procedures and the most ideal time during the course of the disease to perform PBSCT, it represents an exciting alternative to BMT. Research is being undertaken to investigate the efficacy of PBSCT in fetal therapy, sequential PBSCTs in patients with residual disease, treatments involving combinations of PBSCT and auto-BMT, and the use of growth factors for cell mobilization to improve the quantity of cells harvested at one pheresis session.[63]

Gene therapy, a rapidly evolving treatment modality, is defined as the alteration of an individual's genetic material to fight or prevent disease.[64] The process by which one or more genes are inserted into a cell's genome is called gene transfer. There are two major applications of gene transfer. Gene therapy involves inserting genes into the patient's genome, a technique called somatic cell gene therapy, to correct an error or manipulate a particular cell's biologic behavior. Gene therapy is based on Boveri's somatic mutation theory of cancer development, which proposes that malignancies result from an imbalance in the normal chromosome structure that is essential for normal growth and development. Germ-line gene therapy, which has not been approved by the Food and Drug Administration and the National Institutes of Health, attempts to genetically manipulate the ova and sperm to pass genetic changes to future generations.[65] *Gene marking* is the process whereby labeled genes are inserted into cells for future identification. This process can facilitate the determination of sources of relapse after auto-BMT.

Genes are transferred by chemical or physical techniques, including calcium phosphate coprecipitation, microinjection, receptor-mediated DNA transfer, and liposomal membrane fusion or by retroviral vectors in which human genes are inserted into the genome of the virus. The virus attaches to the target cells and empties its genetic material into the cell, and by reverse transcriptase, the new gene is inserted into the DNA of the patient's cell. Current uses of gene therapy to correct a genetic error include the insertion of the adenosine deaminase (ADA) gene in children with severe combined immunodeficiency disease (SCID) who lack this gene and the insertion of *KRAS* and *P53* genes into lung cancer cells. Several techniques that have been used to add a new function to cells, one of which involves inserting the multidrug resistance 1 (*MDR1*) gene to bone marrow stem cells in an attempt to increase their resistance to chemotherapy. Other cancers in which gene therapy is being investigated include malignant melanoma, brain tumors such as glioblastoma and neuroblastoma, acute myelogenous and chronic myelogenous leukemia, and breast cancer.[66]

In summary, the methods used in the diagnosis of cancer vary with the type of cancer and its location. Because many cancers are curable if diagnosed early, health care practices designed to promote early detection are important. These practices include breast self-examination by women, testicular self-examination by men, and consulting a physician when any of the early warning signals of cancer are noticed. Pap smear and tissue biopsies are used to detect the presence of cancer cells and in diagnosis. There are two basic methods of classifying tumors: grading according to the histologic or tissue characteristics and clinical staging according to spread of the disease. Histologic studies are done in the laboratory using cells or tissue specimens. The TNM system for clinical staging of cancer uses tumor size, lymph node involvement, and presence of metastasis.

Treatment plans that use more than one type of therapy, often in combination, are providing cures for a number of cancers that a few decades ago had a poor prognosis and are increasing the life expectancy of persons with other types of cancer. Surgical procedures are more precise as a result of improved diagnostic equipment and new techniques such as laser surgery. Radiation equipment and radioactive sources permit greater and more controlled destruction of cancer cells while causing less damage to normal tissues. Successes with immunotherapy techniques offer hope that the body's own defenses can be used in fighting cancer. BMT and PBSCT allow a greater tumoricidal effect while replenishing the pluripotent stem cells. Gene therapy, although investigational, may provide a foundation for the development of more effective treatments in the future.

Childhood Cancers

On completion of this section of the chapter, you should be able to do the following:

- Cite the early warning signs of cancer in children
- Discuss possible concerns of adult survivors of childhood cancer

In the United States, cancer is the second leading cause of death due to disease in children 1 to 15 years of age. Between 1974 and 1991, children younger than 14 years of age had a 1% average yearly increase in the incidence of all malignant neoplasms, with a 1.6% average increase in the incidence of acute lymphocytic leukemia and a more than 2% increase for astroglial tumors, rhabdomyosarcomas, germ cell tumors, and osteosarcomas.[67] The spectrum of cancers that affect children differs markedly from those that affect adults. Although most adult cancers are of epithelial cell origin (*e.g.*, lung cancer, breast cancer, colorectal cancers), childhood cancers usually involve the hematopoietic system, nervous system, or connective tissue. Chart 5–3 lists the most common forms of solid childhood cancers.

As with adult cancers, there is probably no one cause of childhood cancer. However, many forms of childhood cancer repeat within families and may result from polygenic or single-gene inheritance, chromosomal aberrations (*e.g.*, translocations, deletions, insertions, inversions, duplications), exposure to mutagenic environmental agents, or a combination of these factors (see Chapter 4). If one child develops cancer, the risk of cancer in siblings is approximately twice that of the general population, and if two children in the same family develop the disease, the risk is even greater.

Heritable forms of cancer tend to have an earlier age of onset, a higher frequency of multifocal lesions within a single organ, and bilateral involvement of paired organs or multiple primary tumors. The two-hit hypothesis has been used as one explanation of heritable cancers.[36] The first "hit" or mutation occurs prezygotically (*i.e.*, in germ cells before conception) and is present in the genetic material of all somatic cells. Cancer subsequently develops in one or several somatic cell lines that undergo a second mutation.

Children with heritable disorders are at increased risk for developing certain forms of cancer. For example, Down syndrome is associated with increased risk of leukemia; primary immunodeficiency disorders (see Chapter 15) are associated with lymphoma, leukemia, and brain cancer; and xeroderma pigmentosum is associated with basal and squamous cell carcinoma, and melanoma.

CHART 5-3
Common Solid Tumors of Childhood

Brain and nervous system tumors
- Medulloblastoma
- Glioma

Neuroblastoma
Wilms' tumor
Rhabdomyosarcoma and embryonal sarcoma
Retinoblastoma
Osteosarcoma
Ewing's sarcoma

Diagnosis and Treatment

The early diagnosis of childhood cancers is often overlooked because the signs and symptoms are often similar to those of common childhood diseases and because cancer occurs less frequently in children than in adults. Symptoms of prolonged fever, unexplained weight loss, and growing masses (especially in association with weight loss) should be viewed as warning signs of cancer in children. Diagnosis of childhood cancers involves many of the same methods that are used in adults. Accurate disease staging is especially beneficial in childhood cancers, in which the potential benefits of treatment must be carefully weighed against potential long-term effects.

The treatment of childhood cancers is complex, intensive, prolonged, and continuously evolving. Improved therapy and supportive care have led to progressive increases in survival. Among white children, the 5-year survival rate for all cancer sites is 70%; for acute lymphocytic leukemia, 78%, for acute myeloid leukemia, 28%; for bone cancer, 64%; for neuroblastoma, 61%; for brain and central nervous system (CNS) cancers, 60%; for Wilms' tumor, 92%; for Hodgkin's disease, 92%; and for non-Hodgkin's lymphoma, 69%.[1]

Adult Survivors of Childhood Cancer

With improvement in treatment methods, the number of children who survive childhood cancer is continuing to increase.[68,69] Unfortunately, therapy may produce late sequelae, such as impaired growth, neurologic dysfunction, hormonal dysfunction, cardiomyopathy, pulmonary fibrosis, and risk of second malignancies. Although cures for large numbers of children have only been possible since the 1970s, much is already known about the potential for delayed effects.

Children reaching adulthood after cancer therapy may have reduced physical stature because of the therapy they received, particularly radiation, which retards the growth of normal tissues along with that of cancer tissue. The younger the age and the higher the radiation dose, the greater is the deviation from normal growth. There is also concern that CNS radiation as a prophylactic measure in childhood leukemia has an effect on cognition and learning. Children younger than 6 years at the time of radiation and those receiving the highest radiation doses are most likely to have subsequent cognitive difficulties.

Delayed sexual maturation in boys and girls can result from irradiation of the gonads. Delayed sexual maturation is also related to treatment of children with alkylating agents. Cranial irradiation may result in premature menarche in girls, with subsequent early closure of the epiphysis and a reduction in final growth achieved. Data related to fertility and health of the offspring of childhood cancer survivors are just becoming available.

Vital organs such as the heart and lungs may be affected by cancer treatment. Children who received anthracyclines (*i.e.*, doxorubicin or daunorubicin) may be at risk for developing cardiomyopathy and congestive heart failure. Pulmonary irradiation may cause lung dysfunction and restrictive lung disease. Drugs such as bleomycin, methotrexate, and bisulfan can also cause lung pathology.

For survivors of childhood cancers, the risk of second cancers is reported to be 3% to 12%. There is a special risk of second cancers in children with the retinoblastoma gene. Because of this risk, children who have been treated for cancer should be followed routinely.

In summary, although most adult cancers are of epithelial cell origin, most childhood cancers usually involve the hematopoietic system, nervous system, or connective tissue. Heritable forms of cancer tend to have an earlier age of onset, a higher frequency of multifocal lesions within a single organ, and bilateral involvement of paired organs or multiple primary tumors. The early diagnosis of childhood cancers is often overlooked because the signs and symptoms are often similar to those of other childhood diseases. With improved treatment methods, the number of children who survive childhood cancer is continuing to increase. As these children approach adulthood, there is continued concern that the lifesaving therapy they received during childhood may produce late sequelae, such as impaired growth, neurologic dysfunction, hormonal dysfunction, cardiomyopathy, pulmonary fibrosis, and risk of second malignancies.

REFERENCES

1. Parker S.L., Tong T., Bolden S., et al. (1996). Cancer statistics, 1996. *CA Cancer Journal for Clinicians* 46 (1), 5–27.
2. Li F.P. (1996). Hereditary cancer susceptibility. *Cancer* 78 (3), 553–557.
3. Murakami M.S., Strobel M.C., Vande Woude G.F. (1995). Cell cycle, regulation, oncogenes, and antineoplastic drugs. In Mendelsohn J., Howley P.M., Israel M.A., Liotta L.A. (Eds.). *The molecular basis of cancer* (pp. 3–17). Philadelphia: W.B. Saunders.
4. Alberts B., Bray D., Lewis J., et al. (1989). Cell growth and division. *Molecular biology of the cell* (pp. 727–790). New York: Garland Publishing.
5. Sorrentino V. (1996). The cell cycle. In Pusztai L., Lewis C.E., Yap E. (Eds.). *Cell proliferation in cancer: Regulatory mechanisms of neoplastic cell growth* (pp. 26–44). Oxford: Oxford University Press.
6. Buick R.N. (1994). Cellular basis of chemotherapy. In Dorr R.T., Von Hoff D.D. (Eds.). *Cancer chemotherapy handbook* (pp. 3–14). Norwalk: Appleton & Lange.
7. Ruddon R.W. (Ed.). (1995). *Cancer biology* (pp. 3–18, 19–60, 141–276). New York: Oxford University Press.
8. Cotran R.S., Kumar V., Robbins S.L. (1994). Neoplasia. In *Pathologic basis of disease.* (5th ed., pp. 241–303). Philadelphia: W.B. Saunders.
9. Roitt I, Brostoff J., Male D. (eds.) (1996). Cell cooperation in the antibody response. In *Immunology* (4th ed., pp. 8.8–8.11). London: Mosby.
10. Nicolson G.L. (1993). Physiology in medicine: Growth mechanisms and cancer progression. *Hospital Practice* 28 (2), 43–53.
11. Zetter B.R. (1990). The cellular basis of site specific tumor metastasis. *New England Journal of Medicine* 322, 605–612.
12. Liotta L.A. (1992). Cancer cell invasion and metastasis. *Scientific American* 266 (2), 54–63.
13. Beutler B. (1993). Cytokines and cancer cachexia. *Hospital Practice* 28 (4), 45–52.
14. Abbas A.K., Lichtman A.H., Pober J.S. (Eds.). (1995). Cytokines. In *Cellular and molecular immunology.* Philadelphia: W.B. Saunders.
15. Rothstein J.L., et al. (1986). Tumor necrosis factor: A potent effector molecule for tumor cell killing by activated macrophages. *Proceedings of the National Academy of Sciences of the United States of America* 83, 8318.
16. Caudell K.A., Cuaron L.J., Gallucci B.B. (1996). Cancer biology: Molecular and cellular aspects. In McCorkle, R., Grant, M., Frank-Stromborg M., Baird S.B. (Eds.). *Cancer*

nursing: A comprehensive textbook (2nd ed., pp. 150–170). Philadelphia: W.B. Saunders.

17. Levine A.J. (1996). Tumor suppressor genes. In Pusztai L., Lewis C.E., Yap E. (Eds.). *Cell proliferation in cancer: Regulatory mechanisms of neoplastic cell growth* (pp. 86–104). Oxford: Oxford University Press.
18. Loescher L.J. (1995). Genetics in cancer prediction, screening, and counseling: Part 1, Genetics in cancer prediction and screening. *Oncology Nursing Forum* 22 (2), 10–19.
19. Li F.P. (1996). Hereditary cancer susceptibility. *Cancer* 78 (3), 553–557.
20. Pennisi E. (1996). New gene forges link between fragile site and many cancers. *Science* 272, 649.
21. Pusztai L., Cooper K. (1996). Introduction: Cell proliferation and carcinogenesis. In Pusztai L., Lewis C.E., Yap E. (Eds.). *Cell proliferation in cancer: Regulatory mechanisms of neoplastic cell growth* (pp. 3–24), Oxford: Oxford University Press.
22. Knudson A.G. (1974). Heredity and human cancer. *American Journal of Pathology* 77 (1), 77.
23. McMillan S. (1992). Carcinogenesis. *Seminars in Oncology Nursing* 8 (1), 10–19.
24. Stellman J.M., Stellman S.D. (1996). Cancer and the Workplace. *CA: Cancer Journal for Clinicians* 46 (2), 70–92.
25. Frank-Stromberg M., Heusinkveld K.B., Rohan K. (1996). Evaluating cancer risks and preventive oncology. In McCorkle R., Grant M., Frank-Stromborg M., Baird S.B. (Eds.). *Cancer nursing: A comprehensive textbook* (2nd ed., pp. 213–264). Philadelphia: W.B. Saunders.
26. Weisburger J.H., Horn C.L. (1991). The causes of cancer. In Holleb A.I., Fink D.J., Murphy G.P. *American Cancer Society textbook of clinical oncology* (pp. 80–98). Atlanta: American Cancer Society.
27. Bartecchi C.E., MacKenzie T.D., Schrier R. (1994). The human costs of tobacco use. *New England Journal of Medicine* 330 (13), 907–912.
28. Poskanzer D.C., Herbst A. (1977). Epidemiology of vaginal adenosis and adenocarcinoma associated with exposure to stilbestrol in utero. *Cancer* 39 (4), 1792.
29. Jablon S., Kato H. (1972). Studies of the mortality of A-bomb survivors: 5. Radiation dose and mortality, 1950–1970. *Radiation Research* 50, 649.
30. Marks R. (1996). Prevention and control of melanoma: The public health approach. *CA Cancer Journal for Clinicians* 46 (4), 199–216.
31. Schoenberg J., Klotz J. (1989). A case-control study of radon and lung cancer among New Jersey women. *New Jersey State Department of Health Technical Report, Phase I.* Trenton, NJ: New Jersey Department of Health.
32. Howley P.M. (1996). Viral carcinogenesis. In Pusztai L., Lewis C.E., Yap E. (Eds.). *Cell proliferation in cancer: Regulatory mechanisms of neoplastic cell growth* (pp. 38–58). Oxford: Oxford University Press.
33. Burnett F.M. (1967). Immunologic aspects of malignant disease. *Lancet* 1, 1171.
34. Beverley P. (1996). Tumor Immunology. In Roitt I., Brostoff J., Male D. (Eds.). *Immunology* (4th ed., pp. 20.1–20.8), London: Mosby.
35. Haberman R.B. (1991). Principles of tumor immunology. In Holleb A.I., Fink D.J., Murphy G.P. *American Cancer Society textbook of clinical oncology* (pp. 69–79). Atlanta: American Cancer Society.
36. Stites D.P., Terr A.I. (1991). *Basic and clinical immunology* (7th ed.). San Mateo, CA: Appleton & Lange.
37. American Cancer Society. (1993). *American Cancer Society facts and figures: 1993.* Atlanta: American Cancer Society.
38. Weintraub F.N., Neumark D.E. (1996). Surgical Oncology. In McCorkle R., Grant M., Frank-Stromborg M., Baird S.B. (Eds.). *Cancer nursing: A comprehensive textbook* (2nd ed., pp. 315–330). Philadelphia: W.B. Saunders.
39. Collins M.C. (1990). Tumor markers and screening tools in cancer detection. *Nursing Clinics of North America* 25, 283–290.
40. Ghossein R.A., Rosai J. (1996). Polymerase chain reaction in the detection of micrometastases and circulating tumor cells. *Cancer* 78 (1), 10–16.
41. Beahrs O.H., Myers M.H. (Eds.). (1983). *Manual for staging of cancer* (2nd ed., p. 6). Philadelphia: J.B. Lippincott.
42. Daly J.M., Wanebo J., DeCosse J.J. (1993). Principles of surgical oncology. In Calabresi P., Schein P.S. (Eds.). *Medical oncology basic principles and clinical management of cancer* (2nd ed.). Philadelphia: W.B. Saunders.
43. Hilderley L.J., Dow K.H. (1996). Radiation oncology. In McCorkle R., Grant M., Frank-Stromborg M., Baird S.B. (Eds.). *Cancer nursing: A comprehensive textbook* (2nd ed., pp. 331–358). Philadelphia: W.B. Saunders.
44. Hall E.J., Cox J.D. (1994). Physical and biologic basis of radiation therapy. In J.D. Cox (Ed.). *Moss' radiation oncology: Rationale, technique, results* (7th ed., pp. 3–66). St. Louis: Mosby.
45. Guy J.L., Ingram B.A. (1996). Medical oncology: The agents. In McCorkle R., Grant M., Frank-Stromborg M., Baird S.B. (Eds.). *Cancer nursing: A comprehensive textbook* (2nd ed., pp. 359–394). Philadelphia: W.B. Saunders.
46. Bogner J.R., Kronawitter U., Rolinski B. et al. (1994). Liposomal doxorubicin in the treatment of advanced AIDS-related Kaposi's sarcoma. *Journal of Acquired Immune Deficiency Syndrome* 7, 463–468.
47. Uziely B., Jeffers S., Isacson R., et al. (1995). Liposomal doxorubicin: Antitumor activity and unique toxicities during two complementary phase I studies. *Journal of Clinical Oncology* 13, 1777–1785.
48. Martin V.R., Walker R.E., Goodman M (1996). Delivery of cancer chemotherapy. In McCorkle R., Grant M., Frank-Stromborg M., Baird S.B. (Eds.). *Cancer nursing: A comprehensive textbook* (2nd ed., pp. 395–433). Philadelphia: W.B. Saunders.
49. Grant M., Ropka M.E. (1996). Alterations in nutrition. In McCorkle R., Grant M., Frank-Stromborg M., Baird S.B. (Eds.). *Cancer nursing: A comprehensive textbook* (2nd ed., pp. 919–943). Philadelphia: W.B. Saunders.
50. Gralla R.J. (1992). Antiemetic drugs for chemotherapeutic support. *Cancer* (Suppl) 70 (4), 1003–1006.
51. Krakoff I.H. (1996). Systemic treatment of cancer. *CA Cancer Journal of Clinicians* 46 (3), 134–141.
52. Irvine D., Vincent L., Graydon J., Bubela N., Thompson L. (1994). The prevalence and correlates of fatigue in patients receiving treatment with chemotherapy and radiotherapy. *Cancer Nursing* 17, 367–378.
53. U.S. Department of Labor. Office of Occupational Medicine, Occupational Safety and Health Administration (OSHA). (1986). *Work practice guidelines for personnel dealing with cytotoxic (antineoplastic) drugs,* Publication no. 8-1.1. Washington, DC: U.S. Department of Labor.
54. Oncology Nursing Society. (1988). *Cancer chemotherapy guideline: Module I, II, III, IV.* Pittsburgh: Oncology Nursing Press.
55. Pederson-Bjergaard J., Larson S.O. (1982). Incidence of acute nonlymphocytic leukemia, preleukemia and acute myeloproliferative syndrome up to 10 years after treatment of Hodgkin's disease. *New England Journal of Medicine* 307, 964.
56. Coltman C.A., Jr., Dixon D.O. (1982). Second malignancies complicating Hodgkin's disease: A Southwest Oncology Group 10 year follow-up. *Cancer Treatment Reports* 66, 1023.
57. Boise J.D., Greene M.H., Killen J.Y., et al. (1983). Leukemia and preleukemia after adjuvant treatment of gastrointestinal cancer with semustine. *New England Journal of Medicine* 309, 1079.

58. Skalla K. (1996). The interferons. *Seminars in Oncology Nursing* 12 (2), 97–105.
59. Royal R.E., Steinberg S.M., Krouse R.S., et al. (1996). Correlates of response to IL-2 therapy in patients treated for metastatic renal cancer and melanoma. *The Cancer Journal* 2 (2), 91–98.
60. Farrell M.M. (1996). Biotherapy and the oncology nurse. *Seminars in Oncology Nursing* 12 (2), 82–88.
61. Wujick D. (1995). Hematopoietic growth factors. In Rieger P.T. (Ed.) *Biotherapy: A comprehensive overview* (pp. 113–133). Boston: Jones & Barlett.
62. Whedon M.B. (1995). Bone marrow transplantation nursing: Into the twenty-first century. In Buchse P.C., Whedon M.B. (Eds.), *Bone marrow transplantation: Administrative and clinical strategies* (pp. 1–18). Boston: Jones & Bartlett.
63. King C.R. (1995). Peripheral stem cell transplantation: Past, present, and future. In Buchsel P.C., Whedon M.B. (Eds.). *Bone marrow transplantation: Administrative and clinical strategies* (pp. 187–212). Boston: Jones & Bartlett.
64. Cancer Facts. (1993). *Questions and answers about gene therapy*. Washington, DC: National Cancer Institute.
65. Robinson K.D., Abernathy E., Conrad K.J. (1996). Gene therapy of cancer. *Seminars in Oncology Nursing* 12 (2), 142–151.
66. Wheeler V.S. (1995). Gene therapy: Current strategies and future applications. *Oncology Nursing Forum* 22 (2), Supplement, 20–26.
67. Gurney J.G., Davis S., Severson R.K., et al. (1996). Trends in cancer incidence among children in the U.S. *Cancer* 78 (3), 532–541.
68. Meadows A.T. (1991). Follow-up and care of childhood cancer survivors. *Hospital Practice* 15, 99–108.
69. Carter M., Thompson E.I., Simone J.V. (1991). The survivors of childhood cancer. *Nursing Clinics of North America* 38, 505–526.

ADDITIONAL READINGS

Appelbaum J.W. (1992). The role of the immune system in the pathogenesis of cancer. *Seminars in Oncology Nursing* 9 (1), 51–62.

Bates S.E. (1991). Clinical application of serum tumor markers. *Annals of Internal Medicine* 115 (8), 623–638.

Bingham B. (1985). Hazards to health care workers from antineoplastic drugs. *New England Journal of Medicine* 313, 1220–1221.

Cole J.S., Grube J. (1992). Progress and prospects for human cancer vaccines. *Journal of the National Cancer Institute* 24 (1), 18–21.

Cordon-Cardo C. (1995). Mutation of cell cycle regulators. Biological and clinical implications for human neoplasia. *American Journal of Pathology* 147 (3), 545–560.

DeLast C.A., Lampkin B.C. (1992). Long-term survivors of childhood cancer: Evaluation and identification of sequelae of treatment. *CA: A Cancer Journal for Clinicians* 42 (5), 263–282.

Dudjak L.A. (1992). Cancer metastasis. *Seminars in Oncology Nursing* 8 (1), 40–50.

Greenberg P.D., Riddel S.R. (1992). Tumor specific T-cell immunity: Ready for prime time? *Journal of the National Cancer Institute* 14, 105961.

Harris C.C., Hollstein M. (1993). Clinical implications of the p53 tumor-suppressor gene. *The New England Journal of Medicine* 329 (18), 1318–1326.

Hartwell L.H., Kastan M.B. (1994). Cell cycle control and cancer. *Science* 266, 1821–1828.

Lind J. (1991). Tumor cell growth and cell kinetics. *Seminars in Oncology Nursing* 3 (1), 15–22.

Peters L.J. (1996). Radiation therapy tolerance limits. *Cancer* 77 (11), 2379–2385.

Rieger P.T. (Ed.). (1996). Biotherapy: Present accomplishments and future projections. *Seminars in Oncology Nursing* 12 (2), 81–170.

Rosenberg S.A. (1995). The development of new cancer therapies based on the molecular identification of cancer regression antigens. *The Cancer Journal from Scientific American* 1 (2), 90–100.

Wheelock L.D., Summers B.L.Y. (1996). New chemotherapy agents in cancer care. *Oncology Nursing Updates* 3 (4), 1–12.

Woods N.F. (1996). Cancer risk controversies: Women's exposure to exogenous ovarian hormones. *Oncology Nursing Updates* 3 (1), 1–16

UNIT II

Hematopoietic Function

From ancient times, the importance of blood as a determinant of health was recognized. Its life-affecting powers are well described in the written treatises of Greek physician Galen (AD 130–200). Galen, who reigned as the foremost medical authority for nearly 1500 years, believed that an individual stayed healthy as long as four body fluids—blood, phlegm, yellow bile, and black bile—remained in the right proportion. He also believed that the four humors determined one's basic temperament. Whether an individual was sanguine, sluggish and dull, quick to anger, or melancholy was determined by the degree to which one or another of the humors predominated. The most desirable personality type was achieved when blood was thought to predominate, yielding a warm and cheerful person.

The workings of blood were traced by Galen from its creation, which he believed took place in the liver, throughout the body. He came to believe that disease manifested itself if any one of the fluids was in excess or deficient and was carried in the blood. The theory led to bloodletting—the drawing of blood from the vein of a sick person so the disease could flow out with the blood. For many centuries, bloodletting was the standard treatment for a myriad of ills.

CHAPTER 6

Blood Cells and the Hematopoietic System

Kathryn J. Gaspard

Blood consists of blood cells (*i.e.*, red blood cells, thrombocytes or platelets, and white blood cells) and the plasma in which the cells are suspended. Blood cells have a relatively short life span and must be continually replaced. The generation of blood cells takes place in the hematopoietic (from the Greek *haima* for blood and *poiesis* for making) system. The hematopoietic system encompasses all of the blood cells and their precursors, the bone marrow where blood cells have their origin, and the lymphoid tissues where blood cells circulate as they develop and mature.

Composition of Blood and Formation of Blood Cells

After you have completed this section of the chapter, you should be able to meet the following objectives:

- Describe the composition of plasma
- Name the formed elements of blood and cite their function and life span
- Trace the process of hematopoiesis from stem cell to mature blood cell

When blood is removed from the circulatory system, it clots. The clot contains the blood cells and fibrin strands formed from the conversion of the plasma protein fibrinogen. It is surrounded by a yellow liquid called *serum*.

Blood that is kept from clotting by the addition of an anticoagulant (*e.g.*, heparin, citrate) and then centrifuged separates into layers (Fig. 6–1). The lower layer (about 42% to 47% of the whole blood volume) contains the erythrocytes, or red blood cells, and is referred to as the hematocrit. The intermediate layer (about 1%) containing the leukocytes is white or gray and is called the buffy layer. Above the leukocytes is a thin layer of platelets that are not discernible to the naked eye. The translucent, yellowish fluid that forms on the top of the cells is the plasma, which comprises about 55% of the total volume.

Plasma

The plasma component of blood carries the cells that transport gases, aid in body defenses, and prevent blood loss. It transports nutrients that are absorbed from the gastrointestinal tract to body cells and delivers the waste products from cellular metabolism to the kidney for elimination; it transports hormones and permits the exchange of chemical messengers; it facilitates the exchange of body heat; and it participates in electrolyte and acid-base balance and the osmotic regulation of body fluids. Plasma is 90% to 91% water by weight, 6.5% to 8% proteins by weight, and 2% other small molecular substances (Table 6–1).

Plasma Proteins

The plasma proteins are the most abundant solutes in plasma. Most proteins are formed in the liver and serve a variety of functions. The major types are albumin, globulins, and fibrinogen. Albumin is the most abundant and makes up about 54% of the plasma proteins. It does not diffuse through the vascular endothelium and therefore contributes to plasma osmotic pressure and the maintenance of blood volume. Albumin also serves as a carrier for certain substances and acts as a blood buffer. Three types of globulins comprise about 38% of plasma proteins. The alpha globulins transport bilirubin and steroids, the beta globulins transport iron and copper, and the gamma globulins, synthesized by lymphocytes, contain the antibodies

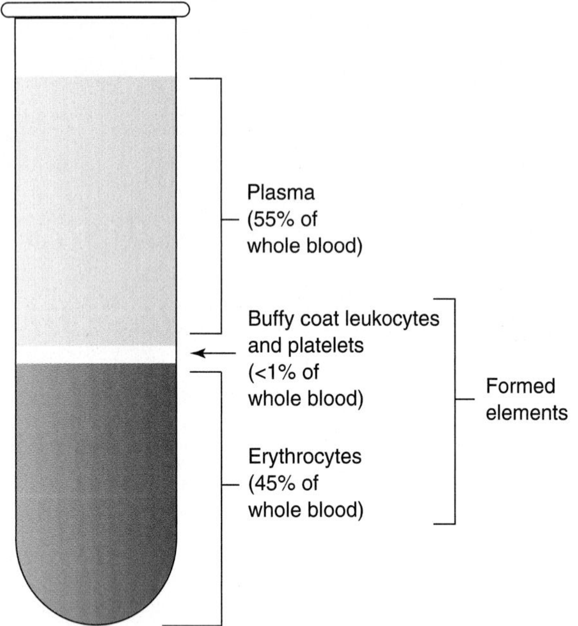

Figure 6-1
Layering of blood components in an anticoagulated and centrifuged blood sample.

released by plasma cells. Fibrinogen makes up about 7% of the plasma proteins and is converted to fibrin in the clotting process. The remaining 1% of circulating proteins are hormones, enzymes, complement, and carriers for lipids.

Blood Cells

The blood cells or formed elements are not all true cells and most survive for only a few days in the circulation. They do not divide but are renewed by the process of hematopoiesis in the bone marrow. Blood cells include the erythrocytes or red blood cells, the leukocytes or white blood cells, and platelets (Table 6–2).

Erythrocytes

The erythrocytes, or red blood cells, are the most numerous of the formed elements. They are small, biconcave disks with a large surface area and can easily deform in small capillaries. They contain the oxygen-carrying protein, hemoglobin, that functions in the transport of oxygen. The erythrocytes are derived from the myeloid stem cell and live about 120 days in the circulation (see Chapter 8).

Leukocytes

The leukocytes, or white blood cells, constitute only 1% of the total blood volume. They originate in the bone marrow and circulate throughout the lymphoid tissues of the body. There they function in the inflammatory and immune processes. They include the granulocytes, the monocytes, and the lymphocytes (Fig. 6–2).

Granulocytes. The granulocytes are all phagocytic cells and are identifiable because of their cytoplasmic granules. These white blood cells are spherical and have distinctive multilobar nuclei. The granulocytes are divided into three types (neutrophils, eosinophils, and basophils) according to the staining properties of the granules. Functionally all granulocytes are phagocytes.

Neutrophils. The *neutrophils,* which constitute 50% to 60% of the total number of white blood cells, have granules that are neutral and hence do not stain with an acidic or a basic dye. These granules contain degrading enzymes that are used in destroying foreign substances and correspond to lysosomes found in other cells (see Chapter 1). Because these white cells have nuclei that are divided into three to five lobes, they are often called *polymorphonuclear leukocytes* (PMNs).

The neutrophils have a brief existence between their formation in the bone marrow and their subsequent phagocytic and microbial activity in the tissue sites of inflammation. They are primarily responsible for maintaining normal host defenses against invading bacteria, fungi, cell remains, and a variety of foreign substances. The cytoplasm of mature neutrophils contains fine granules. Enzymes and oxidizing agents associated with these granules are capable of degrading a variety of natural and synthetic substances, including complex polysaccharides, proteins, and lipids. These enzymes are important in maintaining normal host defenses and in mediating inflammation.

The neutrophils are the first cells to arrive at the site of inflammation, usually appearing within 90 minutes

TABLE 6-1
Plasma Components

Plasma	Percentage of Plasma Volume	Description
Water	50–55	
Proteins	6–8	
Albumin		54% Plasma proteins
Globulins		38% Plasma proteins
Fibrinogen		07% Plasma proteins
Other substances	1–2	Hormones, enzymes, carbohydrates, fats, amino acids, gases, electrolytes, excretory products

TABLE 6-2
Blood Cell Counts

Blood Cells	Number of cells/μL	Percentage of White Boood Cells
Red blood cell count	$4.2–5.4 \times 10^6$, $3.6–5.0 \times 10^{6*}$	
White blood cell count	$4.40–11.3 \times 10^3$	
Differential count		
Granulocytes		
Neutrophils		
Segs		47–63
Bands		0–4
Eosinophils		0–3
Basophils		0–2
Lymphocytes		24–40
Monocytes		4–9
Platelet Count	$150–400 \times 10^3$	

*First value is for women and the second for men.

of injury. The neutrophil count increases greatly during the inflammatory process. When this happens, immature forms of neutrophils are released from the bone marrow. These immature cells are often called *bands* or *stabs* because of the horseshoe shape of their nuclei. They represent a storage pool of neutrophil precursors. After being released from the bone marrow, circulating neutrophils have a short life span and therefore must be constantly replaced if their numbers are to remain adequate.

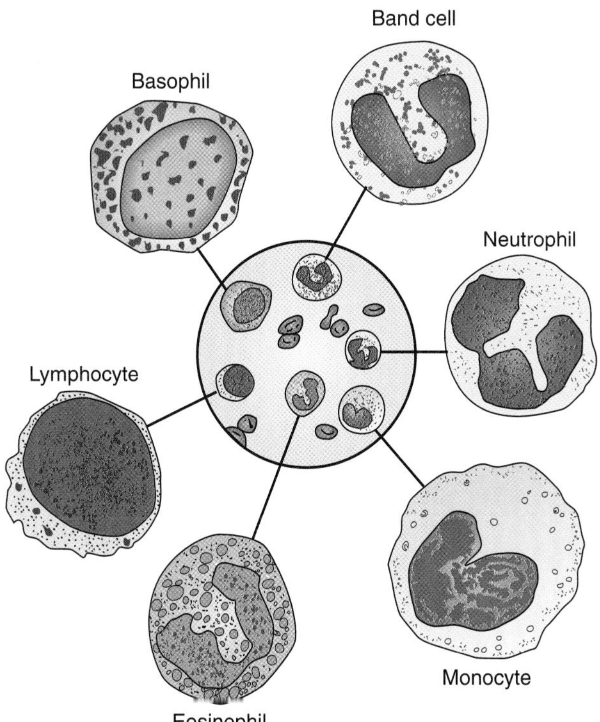

Figure 6-2
White blood cells.

The neutrophils have their origin in the myeloblasts that are found in the bone marrow (Fig. 6–3). The myeloblasts are the committed precursors of the granulocyte pathway and do not normally appear in the peripheral circulation. When they are present, it suggests a disorder of blood cell proliferation and differentiation. The myeloblasts differentiate into promyelocytes and then myelocytes. Generally, a cell is not called a myelocyte until it has at least 12 granules. The myelocytes mature to become metamyelocytes (Greek *meta* for beyond), at which point they lose their capacity for mitosis. Subsequent development of the neutrophil involves reduction in size, with transformation from an indented to an oval to a horseshoe-shaped nucleus (*i.e.*, band cell) and then to a mature cell with a segmented nucleus. These mature neutrophils are often referred to as *segs* because of their segmented nucleus. Development from stem cell to mature neutrophil takes about 2 weeks. It is at this point the neutrophil enters the bloodstream.

After release from the marrow, the neutrophils spend only about 10 hours in the circulation before moving into the tissues. Their survival in the tissues lasts about 1 to 3 days. They die in the tissues in discharging their phagocytic function or die of senescence. The pool of circulating neutrophils (*i.e.*, those that appear in the blood count) are in rapid equilibrium with a similar-sized pool of cells marginating along the walls of small blood vessels. These are the neutrophils that respond to chemotactic factors and migrate into the tissues toward the offending agent. Epinephrine, exercise, stress, and corticosteroid drug therapy can cause rapid increases in the circulating neutrophil count by shifting cells from the marginating to the circulating pool. Endotoxins or microbes have the opposite effect, producing a transient decrease in neutrophils by attracting neutrophils into the tissues.

Eosinophils. The cytoplasmic granules of the *eosinophils* stain red with the acidic dye eosin. These leukocytes constitute 1% to 3% of the total number of white blood cells

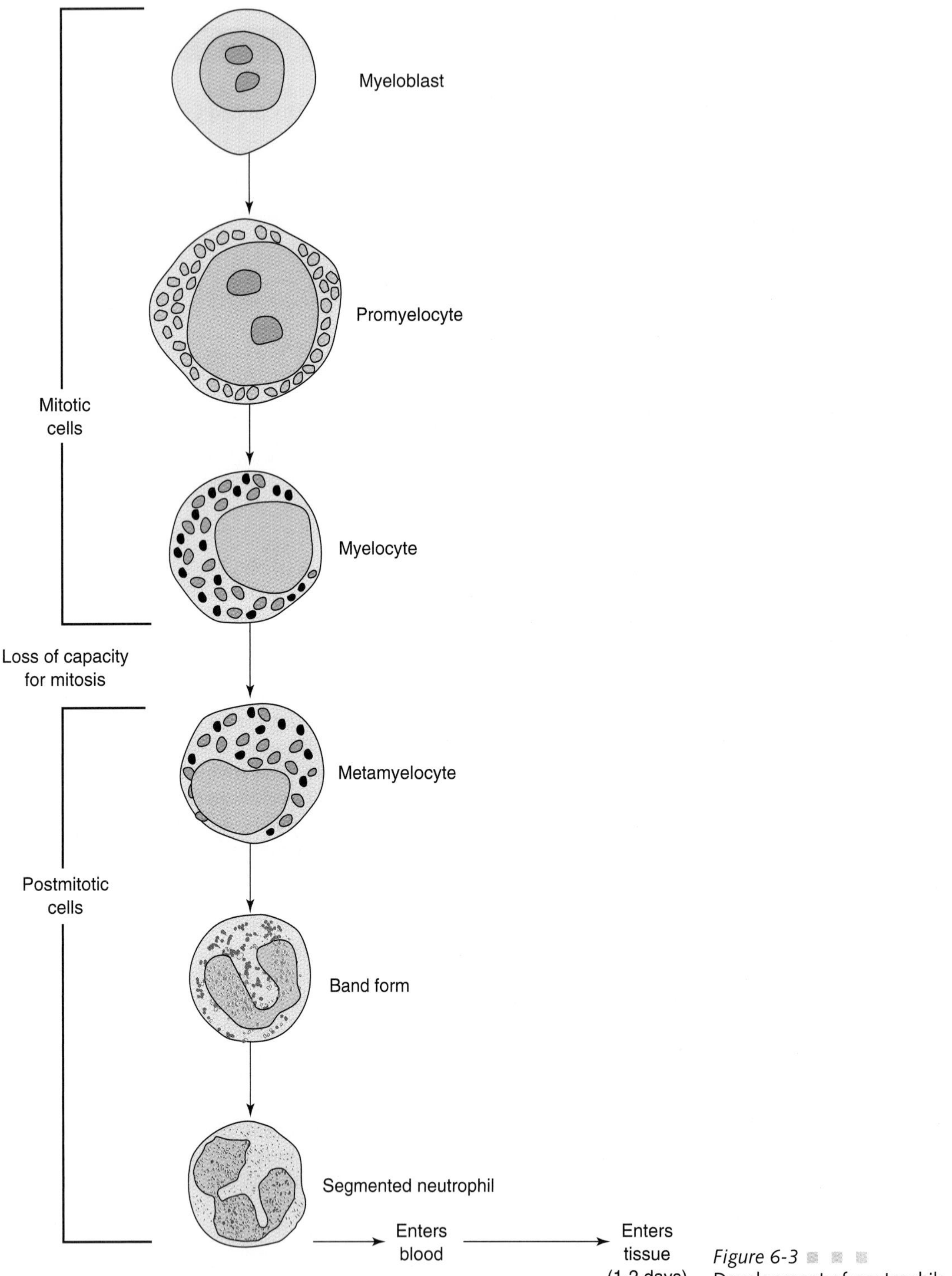

Figure 6-3 Development of neutrophils.

and increase in number during allergic reactions and parasitic infections. It is thought that they release enzymes that detoxify the agents or chemical mediators associated with allergic reactions and assist in terminating the response.

Basophils. The granules of the *basophils* stain blue with a basic dye. These cells constitute only about 0.3% to 0.5% of the white blood cells. The granules in the basophils contain heparin an anticoagulant and histamine a vasodilator. The basophils share properties of mast cells and are thought to be involved in allergic and stress responses.

Lymphocytes. The lymphocytes constitute 20% to 30% of the white blood cell count. There are two types of lymphocytes: B lymphocytes and T lymphocytes. The lymphocytes play an important role in the immune response. They move between blood and lymph tissue, where they may be stored for hours or years. Their function in the lymph nodes or spleen is to defend against foreign microbes in the immune response (see Chapter 11). The B lymphocytes differentiate to form antibody-producing plasma cells and are involved in humoral-mediated immunity. The T lymphocytes are involved in cell-mediated immunity.

Monocytes and Macrophages. Monocytes are the largest of the white blood cells and constitute about 3% to 8% of the total leukocyte count. The circulating life span of the monocyte is about 1 to 3 days, three to four times longer than that of the granulocytes. These cells survive for months to years in the tissues. The monocytes, which are phagocytic cells, are often referred to as *macrophages* when they enter the tissues. The monocytes engulf larger and greater quantities of foreign material than the neutrophils. These leukocytes play an important role in chronic inflammation and are also involved in the immune response by activating lymphocytes and by presenting antigen to T cells. When the monocyte leaves the vascular system and enters the tissues, it functions as a macrophage with specific activity. The macrophages are known as *histiocytes* in loose connective tissue, *microglial cells* in the brain, and *Kupffer cells* in the liver. Some macrophages function in the alveoli. They can also proliferate to form a capsule, enclosing foreign material that cannot be digested.

Thrombocytes

Thrombocytes or platelets are circulating cell fragments of the large megakaryocytes that are derived from the myeloid stem cell. They function to form a platelet plug to control bleeding after injury to a vessel wall (see Chapter 7). Their cytoplasmic granules release mediators required for hemostasis. Thrombocytes have no nucleus, cannot replicate, and if not used, they last about 8 to 9 days in the circulation before they are removed by the phagocytic cells of the spleen.

Hematopoiesis

The generation of blood cells begins in the endothelial cells of the developing blood vessels during the fifth week of gestation and then continues in the liver and spleen. After birth, this function is gradually taken over by the bone marrow. The marrow is a network of connective tissue containing immature blood cells. At sites where the marrow is hematopoietically active, it produces so many erythrocytes that it has a red color, hence the name *red bone marrow*. Fat cells are also present in bone marrow, but they are inactive in terms of blood cell generation. Marrow that is made up predominately of fat cells is called *yellow bone marrow*. During active skeletal growth, red marrow is gradually replaced by yellow marrow in most of the long bones. In adults, red marrow is largely restricted to the flat bones of the pelvis, ribs, and sternum. As a person ages, the cellularity of the marrow declines. When the demand for red cell replacement increases, as in hemolytic anemia, there can be resubstitution of red marrow for yellow marrow. Some hematopoiesis may also be generated in the spleen and the liver.

Blood Cell Precursors

The blood-forming population of bone marrow is made up of three types of cells: self-renewing stem cells, differentiated progenitor (parent) cells, and functional mature blood cells. All of the blood cell precursors of the erythrocyte (*i.e.*, red cell), myelocyte (*i.e.*, granulocyte or monocyte), lymphocyte (*i.e.*, T-lymphocyte and B-lymphocyte), and megakaryocyte (*i.e.*, platelet) series are derived from a small population of primitive cells called the *pluripotent stem cells* (Fig. 6–4). Their lifelong potential for proliferation and self-renewal makes them an indispensable and lifesaving source of reserve cells for the entire hematopoietic system. Several levels of differentiation lead to the development of committed unipotential cells, which are the progenitor for each of the blood cell types. The progenitor cells lose their capacity for self-renewal but retain the potential to differentiate in response to lineage-specific growth factors. They develop into the precursor cells that give rise to mature erythrocytes, monocytes, megakaryocytes, or lymphocytes.

Disorders of hematopoietic stem cells include aplastic anemia, the myelogenous leukemias, and myeloproliferative disorders. In some cases, bone marrow transplantation replenishes the recipient with a normal population of pluripotent stem cells. The stem cells are derived from a histocompatible donor or the patient's own bone marrow harvested before chemotherapy treatment. Umbilical cord blood is used as a source of stem cells to treat children. Methods of collecting and propagating stem cells from peripheral blood are being investigated as an alternative to bone marrow transplantation.

Regulation of Hematopoiesis

Under normal conditions, the numbers and total mass for each type of circulating blood cell remain relatively constant. The blood cells are produced in different numbers according to needs and regulatory factors. This regulation of blood cells is thought to be at least partially controlled by hormone-like growth factors called *cytokines*. The cytokines are a family of glycoproteins that stimulate the proliferation, differentiation, and functional activation of the various blood cell precursors in bone marrow. They are produced by many blood cells and the capillary endothelium and act locally in the bone marrow.

Some cytokines are colony-stimulating factors (CSF) that were named for their ability to promote growth of blood cell colonies in culture. There are at least four lineage-specific CSFs that act on committed

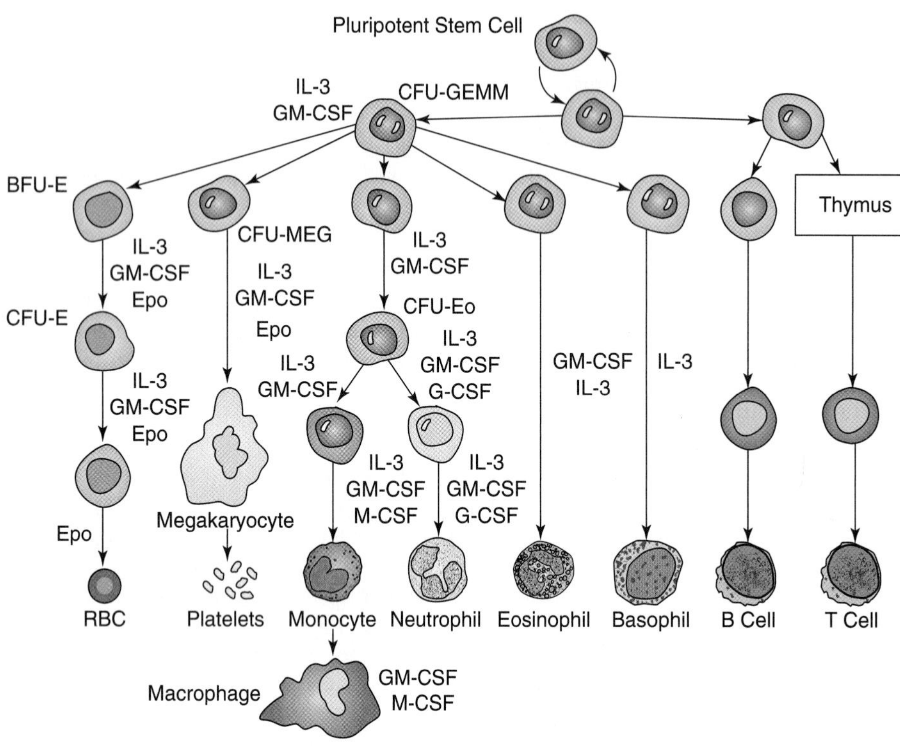

Figure 6-4 Stem cell maturation. BFU, burst-forming unit; CFU, colony-forming unit; CSF, colony-stimulating factor; GM, granulocyte-macrophage; GEMM, granulocyte-erythrocyte-macrophage-megakaryocyte; Epo, erythropoietin; IL-3, interleukin-3. [Developed by Dr. David H. Johnson.] (Hays, K. [1990]. Physiology of normal bone marrow. *Seminars in Oncology Nursing*, 6[1], 3-8)

progenitor cells: erythropoietin, granulocyte colony-stimulating factor (G-CSF), monocyte-macrophage colony-stimulating factor (M-CSF), and thrombopoietin. There are also nonspecific cytokines that support the proliferation of the earlier hematopoietic precursors: granulocyte-monocyte colony-stimulating factor (GM-CSF) and interleukin-3, also known as multi-CSF. Although the CSFs act at different points in the proliferation and differentiation pathway, their functions overlap. Other cytokines, such as interleukins 1, 4, 5, 6, and 7 and interferon, act synergistically to support the functions of the CSFs (see Chapter 11).

The genes for some hematopoietic growth factors have been cloned and their recombinant proteins have been generated for use in a wide range of clinical diseases. These include bone marrow failure caused by chemotherapy or aplastic anemia, the anemia of kidney failure, hematopoietic neoplasms, infectious diseases such as acquired immune deficiency syndrome (AIDS), congenital and myeloproliferative disorders, and some solid tumors. Growth factors are used to accelerate cell proliferation after bone marrow engraftment. Many of these uses are still investigational.

In summary, blood is composed of plasma, plasma proteins, formed elements or blood cells, and substances such as hormones, enzymes, electrolytes, and byproducts of cellular waste. The blood cells consist of erythrocytes or red blood cells, leukocytes or white blood cells, and thrombocytes or platelets. Blood cells are generated from pluripotent stem cells located in the bone marrow. Blood cell production is regulated by chemical messengers called cytokines and growth factors.

Diagnostic Tests

After you have completed this section of the chapter, you should be able to meet the following objectives:

- Cite information gained from a complete blood count
- State the purpose of the erythrocyte sedimentation rate
- Describe the procedure used in bone marrow aspiration

Blood specimens can be obtained through skin puncture (capillary blood), venipuncture, arterial puncture, or bone marrow aspiration.

Blood Count

Tests of the hematologic system provide information regarding the number of blood cells and their structural and functional characteristics. A complete blood count (CBC) is a commonly performed screening test that determines the number of red blood cells, white blood cells, and platelets per unit of blood. The white cell differential count is the determination of the relative proportion (%) of individual white cell types. Measurement of hemoglobin, hematocrit, mean corpuscular volume (MCV), mean corpuscular hemoglobin concentration (MCHC), and mean cell hemoglobin (MCH) are usually included in the CBC. Inspection of the blood smear identifies morphologic abnormalities such as a change in size, shape, or color of cells. Specific tests of red blood cell function are found in Chapter 8 and of white blood cell function in Chapter 11.

Erythrocyte Sedimentation Rate

The erythrocyte sedimentation rate (ESR) is a screening test for monitoring the fluctuations in the clinical course of a disease. In anticoagulated blood, red blood cells aggregate and sediment to the bottom of a tube. The rate of fall of the aggregates is accelerated in the presence of fibrinogen and other plasma proteins that are often increased in inflammatory diseases. The ESR is the distance in millimeters that a red cell column travels in 1 hour. Normal values are 1 to 13 mm/hour for men and 1 to 20 mm/hour for women.

Bone Marrow Aspiration and Biopsy

Tests of bone marrow function are done on samples obtained using bone marrow aspiration or bone marrow biopsy. *Bone marrow aspiration* is performed with a special needle inserted into the bone marrow cavity, and a sample of marrow is withdrawn. Usually, the posterior iliac crest is used in all persons older than 12 to 18 months of age. Other sites include the anterior iliac crest, sternum, and spinous processes T10 through L4. The sternum is not commonly used in children, because the cavity is too shallow and because there is danger of mediastinal and cardiac perforation. Because aspiration disturbs the marrow architecture, this technique is used primarily to determine the type of cells present and their relative numbers. Stained smears of bone marrow aspirates are usually subjected to several studies: determination of the erythroid to myeloid cell count (*i.e.,* normal ratio is 1:3); differential cell count, search for abnormal cells, evaluation of iron stores in reticulum cells, and special stains and immunochemical studies.

Bone marrow biopsy is done with a special biopsy needle inserted into the posterior iliac crest. Biopsy removes an actual sample of bone marrow tissue and allows study of the architecture of the tissue. It is used to determine the marrow to fat ratio and the presence of fibrosis, plasma cells, and granulomas and cancer cells.

The major hazard of these procedures is the slight risk of hemorrhage. This risk is increased in persons with a reduced platelet count.

In summary, diagnostic tests of the blood include complete blood count that is used to describe the number and characteristics of the erythrocytes, leukocytes, and platelets. The erythrocyte sedimentation rate is used to detect inflammation. Bone marrow aspiration is used to determine the function of the bone marrow in generating blood cells.

BIBLIOGRAPHY

Beck W.S. (Ed.). (1991). *Hematology* (5th ed.). Cambridge, MA: MIT Press.

Ganong W.F. (1993). *Review of medical physiology* (16th ed., p. 469). Norwalk, CT: Appleton & Lange.

Glaspy J. (1993). Biologic response modifiers useful in hematology. In Bick R.L. (Ed.). *Hematology: Clinical and laboratory practice* (pp. 157–160). St. Louis: Mosby.

Golde D.W. (1991). The stem cell. *Scientific American* 265, 86.

Golde D.W. (1990). Overview of myeloid growth factors. *Seminars in Hematology* 27 (Suppl 3), 1.

Guyton A.C., Hall J.E. (1996). *Textbook of medical physiology* (9th ed.). Philadelphia: W.B.Saunders.

Jagannath S., Barlogie B., Tricot G. (1993). Hematopoietic stem cell transplantation. *Hospital Practice* 28, 79.

Kessinger A. (1995). Circulating stem cells—waxing hematopoietic. *New England Journal of Medicine* 333, 315.

Robinson S.H., Reich P.R. (Eds.). (1993). *Hematology: Pathophysiological basis for clinical practice* (3rd ed.). Boston: Little, Brown and Co.

Spangrude G.J. (1994). Biological and clinical aspects of hematopoietic stem cells. *Annual Review of Medicine* 45, 93.

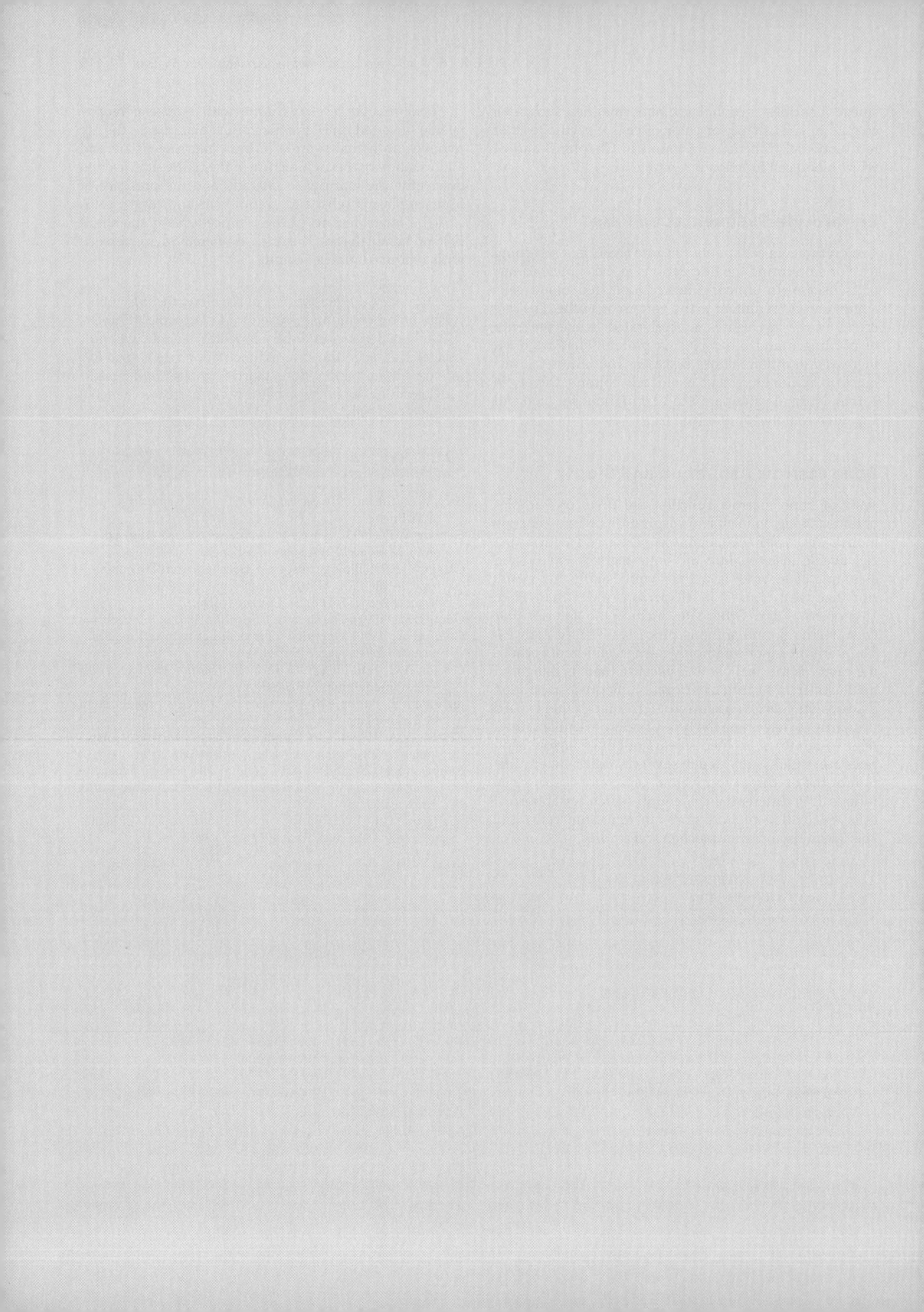

CHAPTER 7

Alterations in Hemostasis

Kathryn J. Gaspard

The term *hemostasis* refers to the stoppage of blood flow. The normal process of hemostasis is regulated by a complex array of activators and inhibitors that maintain blood fluidity and prevent blood loss from vessels. Hemostasis is normal when it seals a blood vessel to prevent blood loss and hemorrhage. It is abnormal when it causes inappropriate blood clotting or when clotting is insufficient to stop the flow of blood from the vascular compartment. Disorders of hemostasis fall into two main categories: the inappropriate formation of clots within the vascular system (*i.e.*, thrombosis) and the failure of blood to clot in response to an appropriate stimulus (*i.e.*, bleeding).

Mechanisms of Hemostasis

After you have completed this section of the chapter, you should be able to meet the following objectives:

- State the five stages of hemostasis
- Describe the formation of the platelet plug
- State the purpose of coagulation
- State the function of clot retraction
- Trace the process of fibrinolysis

Hemostasis is divided into five stages: vessel spasm, formation of the platelet plug, blood coagulation or development of an insoluble fibrin clot, clot retraction, and clot dissolution. These steps are summarized in Chart 7–1.

Vessel Spasm

Vessel spasm is initiated by endothelial injury and caused by local and humoral mechanisms. A spasm constricts the vessel and reduces blood flow. It is a transient event that usually lasts less than 1 minute. Thromboxane A_2, released from the platelets and cells, contributes to vasoconstriction.

Formation of the Platelet Plug

The platelet plug, the second line of defense, is initiated as platelets come in contact with the vessel wall. Platelets, also called thrombocytes, are large fragments from the cytoplasm of bone marrow stem cells called the megakaryocytes. They are enclosed in a membrane but have no nucleus and cannot reproduce. Their cytoplasmic granules release mediators for hemostasis. The life span of a platelet is only 8 to 9 days. Platelet production presumably is controlled by a substance called thrombopoietin that causes proliferation and maturation of megakaryocytes.[1] The source of thrombopoietin may be other platelets, liver, kidney, or muscle. It appears that its production and release are regulated

CHART 7-1
Steps in Hemostasis

Vessel spasm
Formation of the platelet plug
Platelet adherence to the vessel wall
Platelet aggregation to form the platelet plug
Blood coagulation
Activation of the intrinsic or extrinsic coagulation pathway
Conversion of fibrinogen to fibrin
Clot retraction
Clot dissolution (fibrinolysis)

by the number of platelets in the circulation. The newly formed platelets that are released from the bone marrow spend up to 8 hours in the spleen before they are released into the blood.

Formation of the platelet plug also involves a small protein molecule called *von Willebrand factor*. This factor is produced by the endothelial cells of blood vessels and circulates in the blood as a carrier protein for coagulation factor VIII.

Formation of a platelet plug involves adhesion and aggregation of platelets (Fig. 7–1*A*). Platelets are attracted to a damaged vessel wall, become activated, and change from smooth disks to spiny spheres, exposing receptors on their surfaces. Adhesion to the vessel subendothelial layer occurs when the platelet receptor binds to von Willebrand factor at the injury site, bridging the platelet to exposed collagen. The process of adhesion is controlled by local hormones and substances released by platelet granules. Aggregation occurs as platelets become attached to one another, forming a meshwork. Adenosine diphosphate, thrombin, and thromboxane A_2 (a prostaglandin), released by the platelets, induce the aggregation process.

The coagulation factors become activated on the platelet surface to finally convert fibrinogen to fibrin, thereby stabilizing the platelet plug (see Fig. 7–1*B*). Defective platelet plug formation causes bleeding in persons who are deficient in platelet receptor sites or von Willebrand factor. In addition to sealing vascular breaks, platelets play an almost continuous role in maintaining normal vascular integrity. They may supply growth factors for the endothelial cells and arterial smooth muscle cells. Persons with platelet deficiency have increased capillary permeability and develop small skin hemorrhages from the slightest trauma or change in blood pressure.

Blood Coagulation

Blood coagulation is the process by which fibrin strands create a meshwork that cements blood components together (Fig. 7–2). It results from activation of the intrinsic or the extrinsic coagulation pathways (Fig. 7–3). The intrinsic pathway, which is a relatively slow process, occurs in the vascular system; the extrinsic pathway, which is a much faster process, occurs in the tissues. The terminal steps in both pathways are the same: the activation of factor X and thrombin-induced formation of fibrin, the material that stabilizes a clot. Both pathways are needed for normal hemostasis, and many interrelations exist between them. Bleeding, when it occurs because of defects in the extrinsic system, usually is not as severe as that which results from defects in the intrinsic pathway. Both systems are activated when blood passes out of the vascular system. The intrinsic system is activated as blood comes in contact with collagen in the injured vessel wall; the extrinsic system is activated when blood is exposed to tissue extracts.

The purpose of the coagulation process is to form an insoluble fibrin clot. This process is controlled by many substances that promote clotting (*i.e.*, procoagulation factors) or inhibit it (*i.e.*, anticoagulation factors). Each of the procoagulation factors, identified by Roman numerals, performs a specific step in the coagulation process. The action of one coagulation factor is designed to acti-

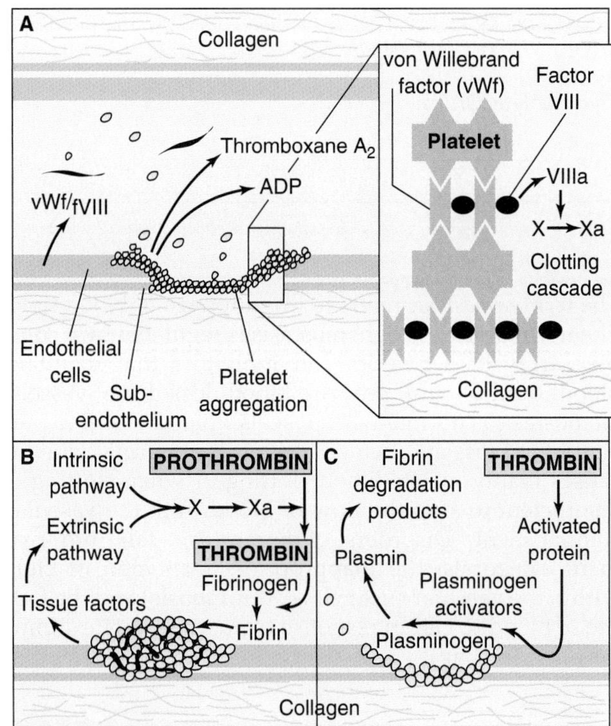

Figure 7-1
(**A** The platelet plug occurs seconds after vessel injury. Von Willebrand's factor, released from the endothelial cells, binds to platelet receptors, causing *adhesion* of platelets to the exposed collagen. Platelet *aggregation* is induced by release of thromboxane A_2 and adenosine diphosphate. (**B**) Coagulation factors, activated on the platelet surface, lead to the formation of thrombin and fibrin, which stabilize the platelet plug. (**C**) Control of the coagulation process and clot dissolution are governed by thrombin and plasminogen activators. Thrombin activates protein C, which stimulates the release of plasminogen activators. The plasminogen activators in turn promote the formation of plasmin, which digests the fibrin strands.

vate the next factor in the sequence (*i.e.*, cascade effect). Because most of the inactive procoagulation factors are present in the blood at all times, the multistep process ensures that a massive episode of intravascular clotting does not occur by chance. It also means that abnormalities of the clotting process occur when one or more of the factors are deficient or when conditions lead to inappropriate activation of any of the steps.

Calcium (factor IV) is required in all but the first two steps of the clotting process. The body usually has sufficient amounts of calcium for these reactions. Inactivation of the calcium ion prevents blood from clotting when removed from the body. The addition of citrate to blood stored for transfusion purposes prevents clotting by chelating ionic calcium. Another chelator, EDTA, is often added to blood samples used for analysis in the clinical laboratory.

Coagulation is also regulated by several natural anticoagulants. Antithrombin III inactivates coagulation factors and neutralizes thrombin, the last enzyme in the pathway for the conversion of fibrinogen to fibrin. When complexed with naturally occurring heparin, its action is accelerated and provides protection against uncontrolled thrombus formation on the endothelial surface. Protein C, on combining with its receptor, thrombomodulin, inhibits thrombin and several coagulation factors. Protein S accelerates the action of protein

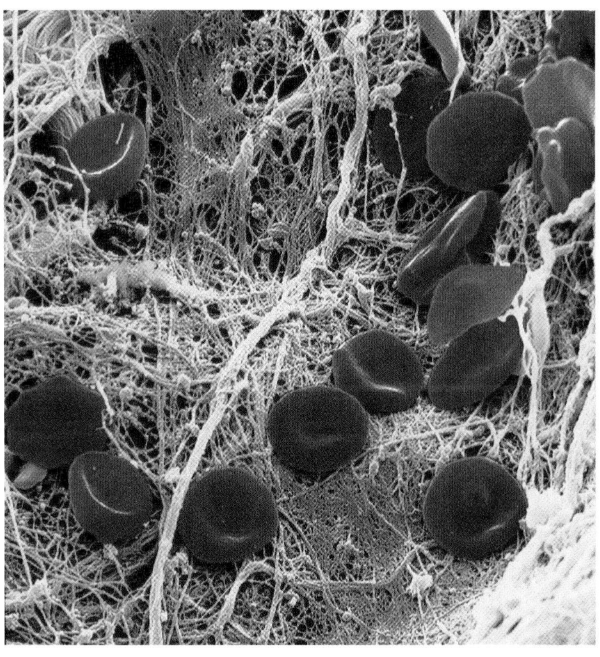

Figure 7-2
Scanning electron micrograph of a blood clot (×3600). The fibrous bridges that form a meshwork between red blood cells are fibrin fibers. (© Oliver Meckes, Science Source/ Photo Researchers)

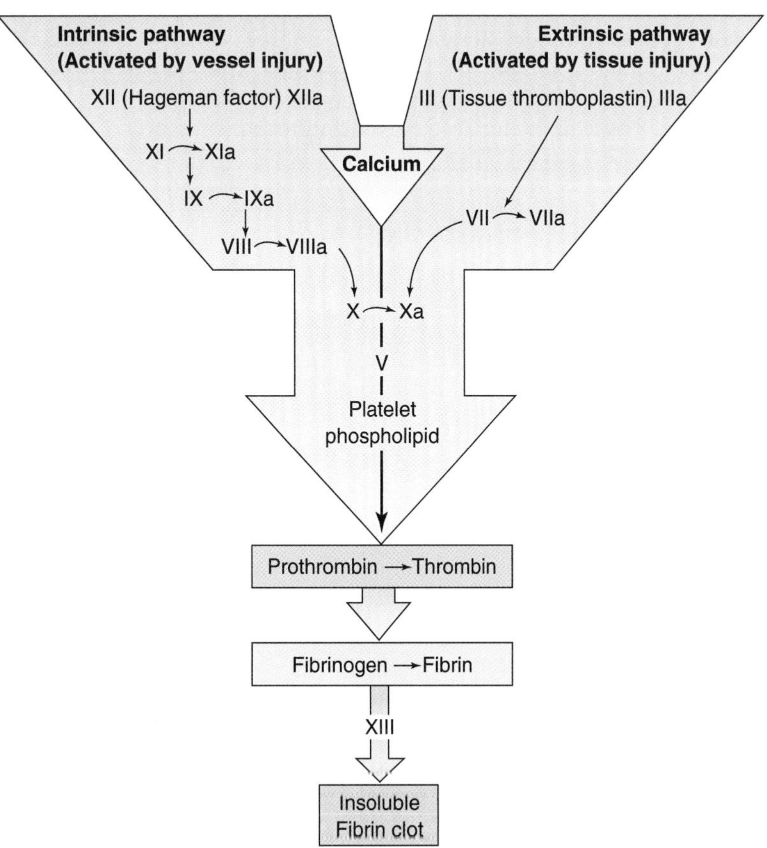

Figure 7-3
Intrinsic and extrinsic coagulation pathways. The terminal steps in both pathways are the same. Calcium, factors X and V, and platelet phospholipids combine to form prothrombin activator, which then converts prothrombin to thrombin. This interaction causes conversion of fibrinogen into the fibrin strands that create the insoluble blood clot.

C. Deficiencies of antithrombin III, protein C, or protein S result in hypercoagulable states and an increased risk for thromboembolism.[2]

Clot Retraction

After the clot has formed, clot retraction, which requires large numbers of platelets, contributes to hemostasis by squeezing serum from the clot and joining the edges of the broken vessel.

Clot Dissolution

The dissolution of a blood clot begins shortly after its formation; this allows blood flow to be reestablished and permanent tissue repair to take place (see Fig. 7–1C). The process by which a blood clot dissolves is called *fibrinolysis.* As with clot formation, clot dissolution requires a sequence of steps controlled by activators and inhibitors (Fig. 7–4). *Plasminogen,* the proenzyme for the fibrinolytic process, normally is present in the blood in its inactive form. It is converted to its active form, *plasmin,* by plasminogen activators formed in the vascular endothelium, liver, and kidneys. The plasmin formed from plasminogen digests the fibrin strands of the clot and certain clotting factors, such as fibrinogen, factor V, and factor VIII. Circulating plasmin is rapidly inactivated by α_2-plasmin inhibitor, which limits fibrinolysis to the local clot and prevents it from occurring in the entire circulation.

Two naturally occurring plasminogen activators are tissue-type plasminogen activator (t-PA) and urokinase-type plasminogen activator.[1] The liver, plasma, and vascular endothelium are the major sources of physiologic activators. These activators are released in response to a number of stimuli, including vasoactive drugs, venous occlusion, elevated body temperature, and exercise. The activators are unstable and rapidly inactivated by inhibitors synthesized by the endothelium and the liver. For this reason, chronic liver disease may cause altered fibrinolytic activity. A major inhibitor, plasminogen activator inhibitor-1 (PAI-1), in high concentrations has been associated with deep vein thrombosis and myocardial infarction.[3]

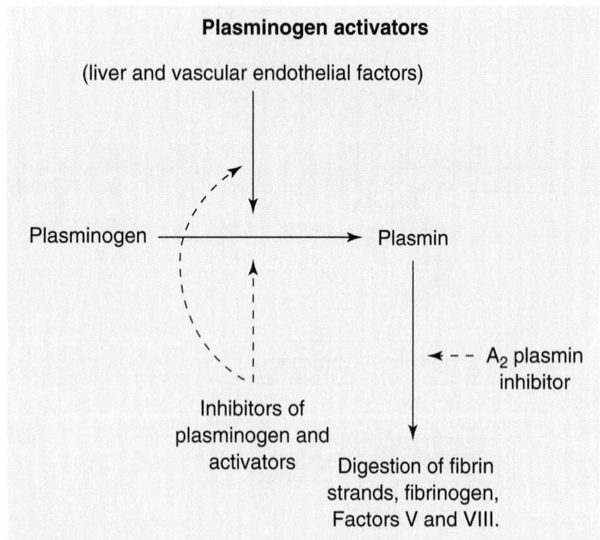

Figure 7-4
Fibrinolytic system and its modifiers. The *solid lines* indicate activation, and the *broken lines* indicate inactivation.

In summary, hemostasis is designed to maintain the integrity of the vascular compartment. The process is divided into five phases: vessel spasm, which constricts the size of the vessel and reduces blood flow; platelet adherence and formation of the platelet plug; formation of the fibrin clot, which cements the platelet plug together; clot retraction, which pulls the edges of the injured vessel together; and clot dissolution, which involves the action of plasmin that dissolves the clot and allows blood flow to be reestablished and tissue healing to take place. Blood coagulation requires the stepwise activation of coagulation factors, carefully controlled by activators and inhibitors.

Hypercoagulability States

After you have completed this section of the chapter, you should be able to meet the following objectives:

- Compare normal and abnormal clotting
- State the causes and effects of increased platelet function
- State two conditions that contribute to increased clotting activity

There are two general forms of hypercoagulability states or thrombosis: conditions that create increased platelet function and conditions that cause accelerated activity of the coagulation system. Thrombosis represents hemostasis in an exaggerated form. Arterial thrombi are composed of platelet aggregates, and venous thrombi may be platelet aggregates and fibrin complexes that result from excess coagulation. Chart 7–2 summarizes conditions commonly associated with hypercoagulability states.

Increased Platelet Function

The causes of increased platelet function are disturbances in flow and endothelial damage and increased sensitivity of platelets to factors that cause adhesiveness and aggregation. Atherosclerotic plaques disturb flow, cause endothelial damage, and promote platelet adherence. Platelets that adhere to the vessel wall release growth factors that cause proliferation of smooth muscle and thereby contribute to the development of atherosclerosis. Smoking, elevated levels of blood lipids and cholesterol, hemodynamic stress, diabetes mellitus, and immune mechanisms may cause vessel damage, platelet

CHART 7-2
Conditions Associated with Hypercoagulability States

Increased Platelet Function

Atherosclerosis
Diabetes mellitus
Smoking
Elevated blood lipid and cholesterol levels
Increased platelet levels

Accelerated Activity of the Clotting System

Pregnancy and the puerperium
Use of oral contraceptives
Postsurgical state
Immobility
Congestive heart failure
Malignant diseases

adherence, and eventually, thrombosis. Cancer and some diseases are associated with high platelet counts and the potential for thrombosis. The term *thrombosis* is used to describe elevation in platelet count above 1,000,000/mm^3. This occurs in some malignancies and inflammation and after splenectomy. Myeloproliferative disorders produce excess platelets that may predispose to thrombosis or, paradoxically, bleeding when the rapidly produced platelets are defective.

Increased Clotting Activity

Factors that increase the activation of the coagulation system are stasis of blood flow and alterations in the coagulation components of the blood (*i.e.,* an increase in procoagulation factors or a decrease in anticoagulation factors). Stasis causes the accumulation of activated clotting factors and platelets and prevents their interactions with inhibitors. Slow and disturbed flow is a common cause of venous thrombosis in the immobilized or postsurgical patient. Heart failure also contributes to venous congestion and thrombosis. Elevated levels of estrogen increase coagulation factors. The incidence of stroke, thromboemboli, and myocardial infarction is greater in women who use oral contraceptives, particularly after age 35, and in heavy smokers.[4] Clotting factors are also increased during normal pregnancy; these changes, along with limited activity during the puerperium (immediate postpartum period), predispose to venous thrombosis. Hypercoagulability is common in cancer and sepsis. Many tumor cells are thought to release tissue factor molecules, which along with the increased immobility and sepsis seen in patients with malignant disease, contribute to thrombosis in these patients. A reduction in anticoagulants such as antithrombin III, protein C, and protein S predisposes to venous thrombosis.[2] Deficiencies of these inhibitor proteins are uncommon inherited defects.

Another cause of increased venous and arterial clotting is a condition known as the *antiphospholipid syndrome*. The syndrome is caused by the development of antiphospholipid antibodies and recurrent thrombosis of vessels of any size. Women with the disorder have a history of recurrent pregnancy losses due to ischemia and thrombosis of placental vessels. Diagnosis is based on two positive test results for lupus anticoagulant or high IgG or IgM anticardiolipin antibodies tested at least 12 weeks apart. Persons with the disorder have a history of having one or more of the following: deep venous thrombosis; arterial thrombosis, including stroke, myocardial infarction, or gangrene; recurrent fetal loss; or thrombocytopenia.[5] Exactly how antiphospholipid antibodies relate to thrombosis is unclear. One suggested mechanism is that the antibodies inhibit prostacylin production by endothelial cells, with a consequent increase in platelet aggregation. Another is that the antibodies inhibit the activation of protein C. Because protein C counteracts clotting, inhibition of its activation would favor thrombosis.[5] Treatment focuses on removal or reduction in factors that predispose to thrombosis, including advice to stop smoking and counseling against use of estrogen-containing oral contraceptives by women. Prolonged prophylactic therapy to reduce thrombus formation is recommended. Some studies suggest that daily aspirin is as effective as oral anticoagulants.[5]

In summary, hypercoagulability causes excessive clotting and contributes to thrombus formation. It results from conditions that create increased platelet function or conditions that cause accelerated activity of the coagulation system. Increased platelet function usually results from disorders such as atherosclerosis that damage the vessel endothelium and disturb blood flow or from conditions such as smoking that cause increased sensitivity of platelets to factors that promote adhesiveness and aggregation. Factors that cause accelerated activity of the coagulation system include the stasis of blood flow, resulting in an accumulation of coagulation factors, and alterations in the components of the coagulation system (*i.e.,* an increase in procoagulation factors or a decrease in anticoagulation factors).

Bleeding Disorders

After you have completed this section of the chapter, you should be able to meet the following objectives:

- State the mechanisms of drug-induced thrombocytopenia and idiopathic thrombocytopenia and the differing features in terms of onset and resolution of the disorders
- Describe the manifestations of thrombocytopenia
- Describe the role of vitamin K in coagulation
- State three common defects of coagulation factors and the causes of each

- Differentiate between the mechanisms of bleeding in hemophilia A and von Willebrand disease
- Describe the physiologic basis of acute disseminated intravascular coagulation
- Describe the effect of vascular disorders on hemostasis

Bleeding disorders or impairment of blood coagulation can result from defects in any of the factors that contribute to hemostasis. Defects are associated with platelets, coagulation factors, and vascular integrity.

Platelet Defects

Bleeding can occur as a result of a decrease in the number of circulating platelets (*i.e.*, thrombocytopenia) or impaired platelet function (*i.e.*, thrombocytopathia). The depletion of platelets must be relatively severe (10,000 to 20,000/μL, compared with the normal values of 150,000 to 400,000/μL) before hemorrhagic tendencies or spontaneous bleeding become evident. Bleeding that results from platelet deficiency is characterized by petechiae (*i.e.*, pinpoint purplish red spots) and purpura (*i.e.*, purple areas of bruising) on the arms and thighs. Bleeding from mucous membranes of the nose, mouth, gastrointestinal tract, and vagina is characteristic. Bleeding of the intracranial vessels is a rare danger with severe platelet depletion.

Thrombocytopenia

Platelets are produced by cells in the bone marrow and then stored in the spleen before being released into the circulation. Consequently, a decrease in the number of circulating platelets, a condition called *thrombocytopenia*, can result from a decrease in platelet production by the bone marrow, an increased pooling of platelets in the spleen, or decreased platelet survival by immune destruction or nonimmune mechanisms.

Loss of bone marrow function in aplastic anemia (see Chapter 8) or replacement of bone marrow by malignant cells, such as occurs in leukemia, results in decreased production of platelets. Infection with human immunodeficiency virus (HIV) suppresses the production of megakaryocytes. Radiation therapy and drugs such as those used in the treatment of cancer may depress bone marrow function and reduce platelet production.

There may be normal production of platelets but excessive pooling of platelets in the spleen. The spleen normally sequesters about 30% to 40% of the platelets. When the spleen is enlarged (*i.e.*, splenomegaly), however, as many as 80% of the platelets can be sequestered in the spleen. Splenomegaly occurs in cirrhosis with portal hypertension and in lymphomas.

Premature destruction of platelets occurs by a variety of immune mechanisms (e.g., antibodies produced against the platelet). In acute disseminated intravascular clotting (DIC) or thrombotic thrombocytopenic purpura (TTP), excessive platelet consumption leads to a deficiency.

Drug-Induced Thrombocytopenia. Some drugs, such as quinine, quinidine, and certain sulfa-containing antibiotics, induce thrombocytopenia. These drugs act as a hapten (see Chapter 11) and induce antigen-antibody response and formation of immune complexes that cause platelet destruction by complement-mediated lysis. In persons with drug-associated thrombocytopenia, there is a rapid fall in platelet count within 2 to 3 days of resuming a drug or 7 or more days (*i.e.*, the time needed to develop an immune response) after starting a drug for the first time. The platelet count rises rapidly after the drug is discontinued. The anticoagulant drug heparin has been increasingly implicated in thrombocytopenia and paradoxically in thrombosis. The complications typically occur 5 days after start of therapy and result from heparin-dependent antiplatelet antibodies that cause platelet aggregation and their removal from the circulation. The antibodies often bind to vessel walls, causing injury and thrombosis. A new, low-molecular-weight heparin has been shown to be effective in reducing the incidence of heparin-induced complications (see the Anticoagulant Drugs section).[6]

Idiopathic Thrombocytopenic Purpura. Idiopathic thrombocytopenic purpura, an autoimmune disorder, results in platelet antibody formation and excess destruction of platelets. The antibody binds to two identified membrane glycoproteins while in the circulation. The platelets are destroyed in the spleen, because the antibody made them more susceptible to phagocytosis. In children, acute idiopathic thrombocytopenic purpura commonly follows a viral infection and is a self-limited disorder. In contrast, the adult form seldom follows an infection and usually is chronic. It is a disease of young people, with a peak incidence between the ages of 20 and 50, and is seen twice as often in women as in men. It may be associated with other immune disorders such as acquired immunodeficiency syndrome (AIDS) or systemic lupus erythematosus. The condition occasionally presents precipitously with signs of bleeding, often into the skin (*i.e.*, purpura and petechiae) or oral mucosa. The patient commonly has a history of bruising, bleeding from gums, epistaxis (*i.e.*, nosebleeds), and abnormal menstrual bleeding. Because the spleen is the site of platelet destruction, splenic enlargement may occur. Diagnosis usually is based on severe thrombocytopenia (platelet counts less than 20,000/μL), splenomegaly, and exclusion of other causes. Tests for the platelet antibody are available but lack specificity (*e.g.*, they react with platelet antibodies from other sources). Treatment includes the use of corticosteroid drugs, immune globulin, and splenectomy. Use of high-dose dexamethasone, given in cycles over 1 month, has proven to be effective in patients who relapse.[7]

Thrombotic Thrombocytopenic Purpura. Thrombotic thrombocytopenic purpura (TTP) is a combination of thrombocytopenia, hemolytic anemia, fever, and signs of vascular occlusion. The onset is abrupt, and the outcome may be fatal. Widespread vascular occlusions consist of thrombi in arterioles and capillaries of many organs. Erythrocytes become fragmented as they circulate through the partly occluded vessels and cause the hemolytic anemia. TTP is probably caused by widespread endothelial damage that releases mediators resulting in platelet aggregation. The disorder is similar to DIC but does not involve the clotting system. Treatment for TTP includes plasma exchange or transfusion of normal plasma alone.

Thrombocytopathia

Impaired platelet function may result from inherited disorders of adhesion (*e.g.*, von Willebrand disease) or acquired defects caused by drugs, disease, or extracorporeal circulation.

Use of aspirin and nonsteroidal antiinflammatory drugs (NSAIDs) are the most common acquired causes of platelet impairment. These drugs inhibit platelet cyclooxygenase activity and consequently the synthesis of thromboxane A_2 required for platelet aggregation. The effect of aspirin on platelet aggregation lasts for the life of the platelet—usually about 8 to 9 days. The effect of nonsteroidal antiinflammatory drugs is reversible in about 6 hours.[8] Aspirin commonly is used to prevent formation of arterial thrombi. A 1989 report indicated a 44% reduction in risk of myocardial infarction in persons older than 50 years who had taken low doses of aspirin.[9] Chart 7–3 lists other drugs that impair platelet function. Defective platelet function is also common in uremia, presumably because of unexcreted waste products. Cardiopulmonary bypass also causes platelet defects and destruction.

CHART 7-3
Drugs That May Predispose to Bleeding

Interference with Platelet Production or Function

Acetazolamide
Alcohol
Antimetabolite and anticancer drugs
Antibiotics such as penicillin and the cephalosporins
Aspirin and salicylates
Carbamazepine
Clofibrate
Colchicine
Dextran
Dipyridamole
Thiazide diuretics
Gold salts
Heparin
Nonsteroidal antiinflammatory drugs
Quinine derivatives (quinidine and hydroxychloroquine)
Sulfinpyrazone
Sulfonamides

Interference with Coagulation Factors

Amiodarone
Anabolic steroids
Coumadin
Heparin

Decrease in Vitamin K Levels

Antibiotics
Clofibrate

Coagulation Defects

Impairment of blood coagulation can result from deficiencies of one or more of the known clotting factors. Deficiencies can arise because of defective synthesis, inherited disease, or increased consumption of the clotting factors. Bleeding that results from clotting factor deficiency typically occurs after injury or trauma. Large bruises, hematomas, or prolonged bleeding into the gastrointestinal or urinary tracts or joints are common.

Impaired Synthesis

Coagulation factors V, VII, IX, X, XI, and XII; prothrombin; and fibrinogen are synthesized in the liver. In liver disease, synthesis of these clotting factors is reduced, and bleeding may result. Of the coagulation factors synthesized in the liver, factors VII, IX, and X and prothrombin require the presence of vitamin K for normal activity. In vitamin K deficiency, the liver produces the clotting factor but in an inactive form. Vitamin K is a fat-soluble vitamin that is continuously being synthesized by intestinal bacteria. This means that a deficiency in vitamin K is not likely to occur unless intestinal synthesis is interrupted or absorption of the vitamin is impaired. Vitamin K deficiency can occur in the newborn infant before the establishment of the intestinal flora; it can also occur as a result of treatment with broad-spectrum antibiotics that destroy intestinal flora. Because vitamin K is a fat-soluble vitamin, its absorption requires bile salts. Vitamin K deficiency may result from impaired fat absorption caused by liver or gallbladder disease.

Hereditary Disorders

Hereditary defects have been reported for each of the clotting factors, but most are rare diseases. The most common bleeding disorders involve the factor VIII–von Willebrand complex. The disorders are hemophilia A, which affects 1 in 10,000 males, and von Willebrand disease, which occurs in 1 in 10,000 persons.[10] Factor IX deficiency (*i.e.*, hemophilia B) occurs in about 1 in 50,000 persons and is genetically and clinically similar to hemophilia A.

Hemophilia A. Circulating factor VIII is part of a complex molecule, bound to von Willebrand factor. Factor VIII coagulant protein is the functional portion produced by the liver and endothelial cells. Von Willebrand factor, synthesized by the endothelium and megakaryocytes, binds and stabilizes factor VIII in the circulation by preventing proteolysis. It is also required for platelet adhesion.

Hemophilia A, which is factor VIII deficiency, is an X-linked recessive disorder that primarily affects males. Although, it is a hereditary disorder, there is no family history of the disorder in about one third of newly diagnosed cases, suggesting that it has arisen as a new mutation.[10] About 90% of persons with hemophilia produce insufficient quantities of the factor and 10% produce a defective form. The percentage of normal factor VIII activity in the circulation depends on the genetic defect and varies with the severity of hemophilia (*i.e.*, 5% to 25% in mild hemophilia, 1% to 4% in moderate hemophilia, and 1% or less in severe forms of hemophilia).[11] In mild or moderate forms of the disease, bleeding usually does not occur unless there is a local lesion or trauma. The mild disorder may not be detected in childhood. In severe hemophilia, bleeding usually occurs in childhood (*e.g.*, it may be noticed at the time of circumcision) and is spontaneous and severe. Characteristically, bleeding occurs in soft tissues, the gastrointestinal tract, and the hip, knee, elbow, and ankle joints. Joint bleeding usually begins when a child begins to walk. Often, a target joint is prone to repeated bleeding. The bleeding causes inflammation of the synovium and without proper treatment is followed by fibrosis and contractures and is a major cause of disability.

Minimizing injury and preventing bleeding are primary concerns. However, an important chronic complication of treatment is the development of hepatitis C and the increased risk for hepatocellular carcinoma. In hemophilia patients older than 7 to 8 years of age, 60% to 95% have hepatitis C infection.[12]

Factor VIII replacement therapy is initiated when bleeding occurs or as prophylaxis with repeated bleeding episodes. The purpose is to limit the extent of tissue damage. *Cryoprecipitate*, prepared from fresh-frozen plasma, contains factor VIII. Its use is no longer recommended unless prepared from the father of the child with hemophilia. Highly purified factor VIII and factor IX concentrates are the usual replacement products for persons with severe hemophilia. Before blood was tested for infectious diseases, these products were prepared from multiple donor samples and carried a high risk of exposure to viruses for hepatitis and AIDS. Pasteurized or monoclonal antibody-purified concentrates have reduced the transmission of hepatitis viruses and HIV. The lyophilized concentrates make self-administration convenient.

As the quality and safety of clotting factors have risen, so has the cost, which sometimes restricts its use. Factor VIII produced by recombinant DNA technology is now available. Because it is not derived from human plasma, recombinant factor VIII does not have the potential for transmitting HIV, hepatitis B and C, or other viruses. Although there are many advantages of recombinant factor VIII, the cost may be prohibitive. There is also the question of whether the recombinant product will incite a higher incidence of antibodies to factor VIII than plasma-derived concentrates.[11] The newer recombinant products and continuous infusion pumps may allow prevention rather than therapy for hemorrhage.

The cloning of the factor VIII gene and progress in gene delivery systems have led to hope that hemophilia A may be cured by gene therapy.[11] Carrier detection and prenatal diagnosis can now be done by analysis of direct gene mutation or DNA linkage studies. Prenatal amniocentesis of chorionic villus samples is used to predict complications and determine therapy. It may eventually be used to select patients for gene addition.[13]

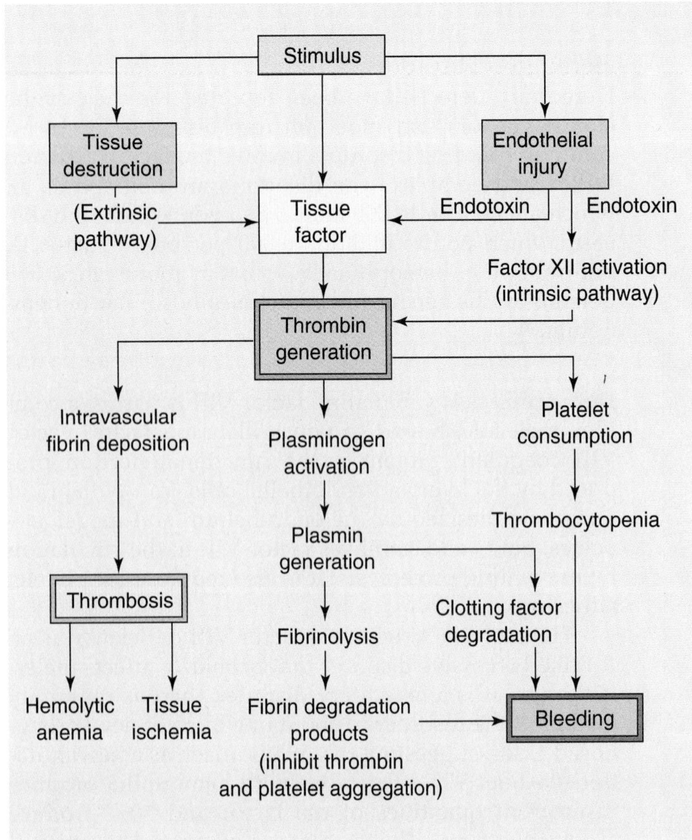

Figure 7-5
Pathophysiology of disseminated intravascular coagulation

Von Willebrand Disease. Von Willebrand disease, which typically is diagnosed in adulthood, is the most common hereditary bleeding disorder. Transmitted as an autosomal trait, it is caused by a deficiency of or defect in von Willebrand factor. This deficiency results in reduced platelet adhesion. There are many variants of the disease, and manifestations range from mild to severe. Because von Willebrand factor carries factor VIII, its deficiency may also be accompanied by reduced levels of factor VIII and results in defective clot formation. Symptoms include bruising, excessive menstrual flow, and bleeding from the nose, mouth, and gastrointestinal tract. Many persons with the disorder are diagnosed when surgery or dental extraction results in prolonged bleeding.[14]

In severe cases, cryoprecipitate or factor VIII products that contain von Willebrand factor are infused to replace the deficient clotting factors. Many persons can now be treated with desmopressin acetate (DDAVP), a synthetic analogue of the hormone vasopressin, which stimulates the endothelial cells to release von Willebrand factor and plasminogen activator. DDAVP can also be used to treat mild hemophilia A and platelet dysfunction caused by uremia, heart bypass, and the effects of aspirin.[15]

Disseminated Intravascular Coagulation

DIC is a paradox in the hemostatic sequence in which blood coagulation, clot dissolution, and bleeding all take place at the same time. The condition begins with massive activation of the coagulation sequence that overwhelms the normal anticoagulant control mechanisms (Fig. 7–5). The microthrombi that result cause vessel occlusion and tissue ischemia. Clot formation consumes all available coagulation proteins and platelets, and severe hemorrhage results. The fibrinolytic system is activated, releasing products of fibrin degradation, which act as natural anticoagulants and contribute to further bleeding.

DIC is not a primary disorder; it occurs as a complication in various disease conditions. The coagulation process can be initiated by activation of the extrinsic pathway, through liberation of tissue factors, or the intrinsic pathway, through extensive endothelial damage caused by viruses, infections, and immune mechanisms or stasis of blood. Release of endotoxins may be the common mediating trigger. Endotoxins generate or release tissue factor from endothelial cells or directly activate factor XII.[16] Obstetric disorders that involve necrotic placental or fetal tissue commonly are associated with DIC. Other inciting clinical conditions include massive trauma, burns, sepsis, shock, meningococcemia, and malignant disease. Chart 7–4 summarizes the conditions associated with DIC.

Although the coagulation and formation of microemboli initiate the events that occur in DIC, its acute manifestations usually are more directly related to the bleeding problems that occur. The bleeding may be present as petechiae, purpura, oozing from puncture sites, or severe hemorrhage. Cardiovascular shock is a common complication. Uncontrolled postpartum bleeding may indicate DIC. Microemboli may obstruct blood vessels and cause tissue hypoxia and necrotic damage to organ structures, such as the kidneys, heart, lungs, and brain. As a result, common clinical signs may be due to renal, circulatory, or respiratory failure or convulsions and coma. A form of hemolytic anemia may develop as red cells are damaged as they pass through vessels partially blocked by thrombus.

The treatment of DIC is directed toward managing the primary disease, replacing clotting components, and preventing further activation of clotting mechanisms. Transfusions of fresh-frozen plasma, platelets, or fibrinogen-containing cryoprecipitate may correct the clotting factor deficiency. Heparin may be given to decrease blood coagulation, thereby interrupting the clotting process. Heparin therapy is controversial, however, and the risk of hemorrhage may limit its use to severe cases. It typically is given as a continuous intravenous infusion that can be interrupted promptly if bleeding is accentuated.

CHART 7-4
Conditions That Have Been Associated With DIC

Obstetric Conditions
Abruptio placenta
Dead fetus syndrome
Preeclampsia and eclampsia
Amniotic fluid embolism

Cancers
Metastatic cancer
Leukemia

Infections
Acute bacterial infections (*e.g.*, meningococcal meningitis)
Acute viral infections
Rickettsial infections (*e.g.*, Rockey Mountain spotted fever)
Parasitic infection (*e.g.*, malaria)

Shock
Septic shock
Severe hypovolemic shock

Trauma or Surgery
Burns
Massive trauma
Surgery involving extracorporeal circulation
Snake bite
Heatstroke

Hematologic Conditions
Blood transfusion reactions

Vascular Disorders

Bleeding from small blood vessels may result from vascular disorders. These disorders may occur because of structurally weak vessel walls or because of vessels damaged by inflammation or immune responses. Among the vascular disorders that cause bleeding are hemorrhagic telangiectasia, an uncommon autosomal dominant disorder characterized by thin-walled, dilated capillaries and arterioles; vitamin C deficiency (*i.e.,* scurvy), resulting in poor collagen synthesis and failure of the endothelial cells to be cemented together properly causing a fragile wall; Cushing's disease, causing protein wasting and loss of vessel tissue support because of excess cortisol; and senile purpura (*i.e.,* bruising in elderly persons) caused by the aging process. Vascular defects also occur in the course of DIC as a result of the presence of the microthrombi and corticosteroid therapy.

Vascular disorders are characterized by easy bruising and the spontaneous appearance of petechiae and purpura of the skin and mucous membranes. In persons with bleeding disorders caused by vascular defects, the platelet count and other tests for coagulation factors are normal.

In summary, bleeding disorders or impairment of blood coagulation can result from defects in any of the factors that contribute to hemostasis: platelets, coagulation factors, or vascular integrity. The number of circulating platelets can be decreased (i.e., thrombocytopenia) or platelet function can be impaired (i.e., thrombocytopathia). Impairment of blood coagulation can result from deficiencies of one or more of the known clotting factors. Deficiencies can arise because of defective synthesis (i.e., liver disease or vitamin K deficiency), inherited diseases (i.e., hemophilia or von Willebrand disease), or increased consumption of the clotting factors (DIC). Bleeding may also occur from structurally weak vessels that result from impaired synthesis of vessel wall components (i.e., vitamin C deficiency, excessive cortisol levels as in Cushing's disease, or the aging process) or that have been damaged by genetic mechanisms (i.e., hemorrhagic telangiectasis) or the presence of microthrombi.

Effects of Drugs on Hemostasis

After you have completed this section of the chapter, you should be able to meet the following objectives:

- State the mechanism by which aspirin, warfarin, and heparin alter blood clotting
- State the mechanism and use of thrombolytic drugs

A number of drugs serve to enhance or impair hemostasis. Oral contraceptives and corticosteroids are associated with an increase in coagulation factors. Drugs that impair platelet production and function and those that interfere with coagulation are summarized in Chart 7–3.

Anticoagulant Drugs

Therapeutic agents commonly are used to prevent thrombus formation. Antiplatelet drugs, particularly aspirin, are used to prevent arterial thrombi. In low doses, aspirin increases survival after myocardial infarction, decreases the incidence of stroke, and assists in maintaining the patency of bypass grafts.[17]

The anticoagulant drugs warfarin and heparin are used to prevent venous thrombi and thromboembolic disease, such as deep vein thrombosis and pulmonary embolism. They are also used in the treatment of ischemic heart disease and the prevention of emboli due to atrial fibrillation, valvular heart disease, and other cardiac disorders.[18] Warfarin acts by decreasing prothrombin and other procoagulation factors. It alters vitamin K such that it reduces its availability to participate in synthesis of the vitamin K–dependent coagulation factors in the liver. Warfarin's maximum effect takes 36 to 72 hours because of preformed clotting factors that remain in the circulation. It is given orally and interacts with many drugs. The major adverse effect is bleeding, which can be reversed with vitamin K.

Heparin is naturally formed in large quantities in mast cells and in the basophilic cells of the blood. Pharmacologic preparations of heparin are extracted from animal tissues. Heparin must be injected because it is not absorbed in the gastrointestinal tract. It binds to antithrombin III, causing a conformational change that increases the ability of antithrombin III to inactivate thrombin. As a result, clotting factors are inactivated, and the formation of fibrin is suppressed. The effect of heparin is immediate and is reversed with protamine sulfate. Low-molecular-weight heparin (LMWH), prepared from natural heparin, is now increasingly used to reduce the complications of heparin therapy (*i.e.,* thrombocytopenia and thrombosis). The lower-molecular-weight product permits greater inhibition of factor Xa and thereby reduces thrombus formation. It has lower binding affinity for endothelial cells and plasma proteins such as platelet factor IV and von Willebrand factor and thereby reduces platelet activation. LMWH has a longer half-life than standard heparin, allowing for once-daily dosing with greater bioavailability. In one study, patients treated with LMWH had reduced platelet antibody formation and lower incidence of thrombocytopenia and thrombosis than those treated with standard heparin.[6]

Thrombolytic Drugs

Thrombolytic drugs convert plasminogen to plasmin and therefore cause lysis of an existing clot. They are used to treat acute coronary occlusion, deep vein thrombosis, and pulmonary embolism. Streptokinase, a protein elaborated by certain β-hemolytic streptococci, is inexpensive and widely used but may cause hypersensitivity reactions in persons previously infected with *Streptococcus.* Urokinase, prepared from human kidney cells, is also effective but costly. An alternative fibrinolytic drug, t-PA, is produced by DNA recombinant techniques and identical to the natural tissue plasminogen activator. t-PA is localized to the clot, binding more avidly to the fibrin than streptokinase. It is used early in acute myocardial infarction to limit damage and preserve left ventricular function.[19] Anisoylated plasminogen streptokinase activator complex (antistreplase), is a conjugate of streptokinase that is inactive until the anisoyl group is activated, which gradually occurs after it is injected. The drug is concentrated at the site of the thrombus and is activated locally. It can be injected as a bolus and provide continuing thrombolytic activity.

Results from multicenter trials investigating the use of streptokinase and t-PA in the treatment of acute ischemic stroke are problematic. High mortality rates resulted from treatment, but survivors had improved function.[20]

In summary, a number of drugs serve to enhance or impair hemostasis. Oral contraceptives and corticosteroids are associated with an increase in coagulation factors. Therapeutic agents commonly are used to prevent thrombus formation. *Antiplatelet* drugs, particularly aspirin, are used to prevent arterial thrombi. The anticoagulant drugs warfarin and heparin are used to prevent venous thrombi (*e.g.*, deep vein thrombosis) and emboli. Thrombolytic drugs convert plasminogen to plasmin and therefore cause lysis of an existing clot. They frequently are used to treat acute coronary occlusion.

REFERENCES

1. Kaushansky K. (1996). Thrombopoietin and platelet development. *Western Journal of Medicine* 164, 209.
2. Alving B.M. (1993). The hypercoagulable states. *Hospital Practice* 28 (2), 109–121.
3. Rosenberg R.D. (1991). Hemorrhagic disorders: 1. Protein interactions in the clotting mechanism. In Beck W.S. (Ed.). *Hematology* (5th ed., p. 540). Cambridge, MA: MIT Press.
4. Goldfien A. (1995). The gonadal hormones and inhibitors. In Katzung B.G. (Ed.). *Basic and clinical pharmacology* (6th ed., p. 623). Norwalk, CT: Appleton & Lange.
5. Harris E.N. (1994). Diagnosis and management of antiphospholipid syndrome. *Hospital Practice* 29 (4), 65–76.
6. Warkentin T.E., Levine M.N., Hirsh J. et al. (1995). Heparin-induced thrombocytopenia in patients treated with low-molecular-weight heparin or unfractionated heparin. *New England Journal of Medicine* 332, 1330.
7. Andersen J. (1994). Response of resistant idiopathic thrombocytopenic purpura to pulsed high-dose dexamethasone therapy. *New England Journal of Medicine* 330, 1560.
8. Kuter D.J. (1991). Hemorrhagic disorders: 2. Platelets. In Beck W.S. (Ed.). *Hematology* (5th ed., p. 571). Cambridge, MA: MIT Press.
9. Steering Committee Physicians' Health Study Research Group. (1989). Final report on the aspirin content of the ongoing physicians' health study. *New England Journal of Medicine* 321, 129.
10. Kuter D.J., Rosenberg R.D. (1991). Hemorrhagic disorders: 2. Disorders of hemostasis. In Beck W.S. (Ed.). *Hematology* (5th ed., p. 588). Cambridge, MA: MIT Press.
11. Hoyer L.W. (1994). Hemophilia A. *New England Journal of Medicine* 330 (1), 38–47.
12. Troisi C.L., Hallinger F.B., Hoots W.K., et al. (1993). A multicenter study of viral hepatitis in a United States hemophilic population. *Blood* 81, 412.
13. Jenkins P.V., Collins P.W., Goldman E. et al. (1994). Analysis of intron 22 inversions at the factor VIII gene in severe hemophilia A: Implications for genetic counseling. *Blood* 84, 2197.
14. Rapaport S.I. (1987). *Introduction to hematology* (2nd ed., pp. 510, 528). Philadelphia: J.B. Lippincott.
15. Aledort L.M. (1989). New approaches to management of bleeding disorders. *Hospital Practice* 24, 207.
16. Seligsohn U. (1995). Disseminated intravascular coagulation. In Buetler E., Lichtman M.A., Coller B.S., Kipps T.J. (Eds.). *William's hematology* (5th ed., p. 1497). New York: McGraw-Hill.
17. Patrono C. (1994). Aspirin as an antiplatelet drug. *New England Journal of Medicine* 330 (8), 1287–1294.
18. Berkman S.A. (1992). Current concepts in anticoagulation. *Hospital Practice* 27, 187.
19. Simoons M.L. (1989). Thrombolytic therapy in acute myocardial infarction. *Annual Review of Medicine* 40, 181.
20. The Multicenter Acute Stroke Trial—Europe Study Group. (1996). Thrombolytic therapy with streptokinase in acute ischemic stroke. *New England Journal of Medicine* 335, 145.

ADDITIONAL READINGS

Aledort L.M. (1992). Prophylaxis: The next hemophilia treatment (editorial comment). *Journal of Internal Medicine* 232, 1.

Alving B.M. (1993). The hypercoagulable states. *Hospital Practice* 28, 109.

Astor R.H. (1995). Heparin-induced thrombocytopenia and thrombosis. *New England Journal of Medicine* 332 (30), 1374–1376.

Benedict C.R., Mueller S., Anderson H.V., Willerson J.T. (1992). Thrombolytic therapy: A state of the art review. *Hospital Practice* 27, 61.

Bennett J.S. (1992). Mechanisms of platelet adhesion and aggregation: An update. *Hospital Practice* 27, 124.

Berkman S.A. (1992). Current concepts in anticoagulation. *Hospital Practice* 27 (2), 187.

Bloom A.L. (1991). Von Willebrand factor: Clinical features of inherited and acquired disorders. *Mayo Clinic Proceedings* 66, 743.

Broze G.J. (1992). Why do hemophiliacs bleed? *Hospital Practice* 27 (3), 71–86.

Bray G.L., Gomperts E.D., Courter S., et al. (1994) A multicenter study of recombinant factor VIII (Recombinate): Safety, efficacy, and inhibitor risk in previously untreated patients with hemophilia A. *Blood* 83, 2428.

DiMichele D. (1996). Hemophilia 1996. In Buchanan G.R. (Ed.). *The Pediatric Clinics of North America* 43, 709.

George J.M., El-Harake M.A.. Raskob G.E. (1994). Chronic idiopathic thrombocytopenic purpura. *New England Journal of Medicine* 331, 1207–1212.

Hirsh J. (1991). Heparin. *New England Journal of Medicine* 324 (22), 1565–1573.

Kurachi K., Yao S., Furukawa M., Kurachi S. (1992). Deficiencies in factors IX and VIII: What is now known. *Hospital Practice* 27, 41.

Roberts H.R., Lozier J.N. (1992). New perspectives on the coagulation cascade. *Hospital Practice* 27, 97.

Rose E.H., Aledort L.M. (1991). Nasal spray desmopressin (DDAVP) for mild hemophilia A and von Willebrand disease. *Annals of Internal Medicine* 14, 563.

Scott J.P., Montgomery R.R. (1993). Therapy of von Willebrand disease. *Seminars in Thrombosis and Hemostasis* 19,37.

Waters A.H. (1992). Autoimmune thrombocytopenia: clinical aspects. *Seminars in Hematology* 29,18.

CHAPTER 8

The Red Blood Cell and Alterations in Oxygen Transport

Kathryn J. Gaspard

Although the lungs provide the means for gas exchange between the external and internal environment, it is the hemoglobin in the red blood cells that transports oxygen to the tissues. The red blood cells also function as carriers of carbon dioxide and participate in acid-base balance. The function of the red blood cells, in terms of oxygen transport, is discussed in Chapter 26, and acid-base balance is covered in Chapter 30. This chapter focuses on the red blood cell, anemia, and polycythemia.

The Red Blood Cell

After you have completed this section of the chapter, you should be able to meet the following objectives:

- Trace the development of a red blood cell from erythroblast to erythrocyte
- Discuss the function of iron in the formation of hemoglobin
- Describe the formation, transport, and elimination of bilirubin
- Explain the function of the enzyme glucose-6-phosphate dehydrogenase in the red blood cell
- State the meaning of the red blood cell count, percentage of reticulocytes, hemoglobin, hematocrit, mean corpuscular volume, and mean corpuscular hemoglobin concentration as it relates to the diagnosis of anemia

The mature red blood cell, the erythrocyte, is a nonnucleated, biconcave disk (Fig. 8–1). This shape increases the surface area available for diffusion of oxygen and allows the cell to change in volume and shape without rupturing its membrane. A cytoskeleton of proteins attached to the lipid bilayer provides this unique shape and flexibility. The biconcave form presents the plasma with a surface 20 to 30 times greater than if the red blood cell were an absolute sphere. The erythrocytes, 500 to 1000 times more numerous than other blood cells, are the most common type of blood cell.

The function of the red blood cell, facilitated by the hemoglobin molecule, is to transport oxygen to the tissues. Hemoglobin also binds some carbon dioxide and carries it from the tissues to the lungs. The hemoglobin molecule is composed of two pairs of structurally different polypeptide chains controlled by genes (Fig. 8–2). Alterations in these genes result in abnormal hemoglobins. Each of the four polypeptide chains is attached to a heme unit, which surrounds an atom of iron that binds oxygen. Four molecules of oxygen can be carried by one hemoglobin molecule.

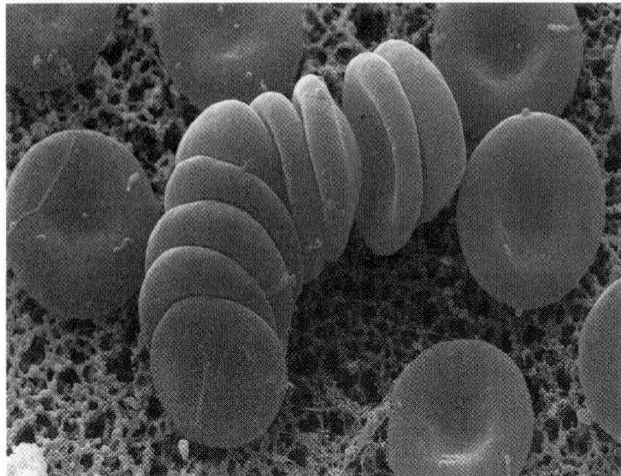

Figure 8-1
Scanning micrograph of normal red blood cells shows their normal concave appearance (×3000). (© Andrew Syred, Science Photo Lab, Science Source/Photo Researchers)

The two major types of normal hemoglobin are *adult hemoglobin* (HbA) and *fetal hemoglobin* (HbF). HbA consists of a pair of α chains and a pair of β chains. HbF is the predominant hemoglobin in the fetus from the third through the ninth month of gestation. It has a pair of γ chains substituted for the β chains. Because of this chain substitution, HbF has a high affinity for oxygen. This facilitates the transfer of oxygen across the placenta. HbF is replaced within 6 months of birth with HbA.

The rate at which hemoglobin is synthesized depends on the availability of iron for heme synthesis. The lack of iron results in relatively small amounts of hemoglobin in the red blood cells. The amount of iron in the body is about 35 to 50 mg per 1 kg of body weight for males and less for females. Body iron is found in several compartments. Most iron (80%) is complexed to heme in hemoglobin, with small amounts found in myoglobin and plasma. About 20% is stored in the bone marrow, liver, spleen, and other organs. Iron in the hemoglobin compartment is recycled. When red blood cells age and are destroyed in the spleen, macrophages store the iron to be released and returned to the bone marrow for incorporation into new cells.

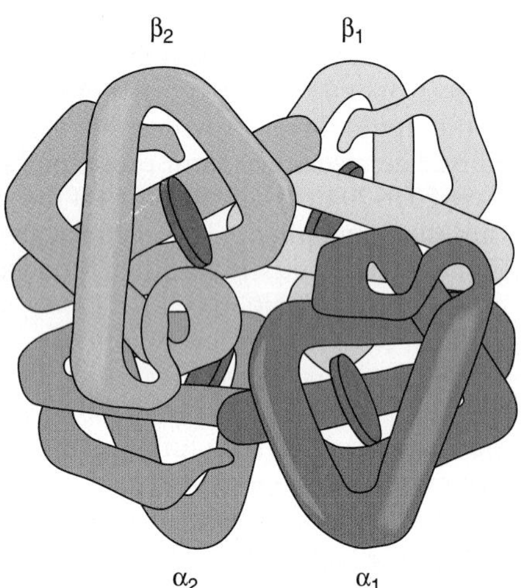

Figure 8-2
Structure of the hemoglobin molecule, showing the four subunits.

Dietary iron also helps to maintain body stores. Iron, principally derived from meat, is absorbed in the small intestine, especially the duodenum. When body stores are diminished or erythropoiesis is stimulated, absorption is increased. In iron overload, excretion of iron is accelerated. Normally, some iron is sequestered in the intestinal epithelial cells and is shed in the feces. The remainder enters the circulation and is loosely bound to a beta-globulin called *transferrin*. From plasma, iron can be deposited in tissues such as liver and bone marrow. The storage form of iron in the liver is ferritin, a protein-iron complex, that can easily return to the circulation. This form can also be measured in serum and provides an index of body iron stores. Transferrin can also deliver iron to the developing red cell in bone marrow by binding to membrane receptors. The iron is internalized into the cytoplasm, where the mitochondria use it in heme synthesis.

Red Cell Production, Metabolism, and Regulation

Erythropoiesis is the production of red blood cells. After birth, red cells are produced in the red bone marrow. Until age 5, almost all bones produce red cells to meet growth needs. After this period, bone marrow activity gradually declines; after age 20, red cell production takes place mainly in the membranous bones of the vertebrae, sternum, ribs, and pelvis. With this reduction in activity, the red bone marrow is replaced with fatty yellow bone marrow.

The red cells are derived from the erythroblasts, which are continuously being formed from the pluripotent stem cells in the bone marrow (Fig. 8–3). In developing into a mature red cell, the red cell precursors move through a series of divisions, each producing a smaller cell. Hemoglobin synthesis begins at the erythroblast stage and continues until the cell becomes an erythrocyte. During its transformation from normoblast to reticulocyte, the red blood cell accumulates hemoglobin as the nucleus condenses and is finally lost. The period from stem cell to emergence of the reticulocyte in the circulation normally takes about 1 week. Maturation of reticulocyte to erythrocyte takes about 24 to 48 hours. During this process, the red cell loses its mitochondria and ribosomes, along with its ability to produce hemoglobin and engage in oxidative metabolism. Most maturing red cells enter the blood as reticulocytes. About 1% of red blood cells are generated from bone marrow each day, and the

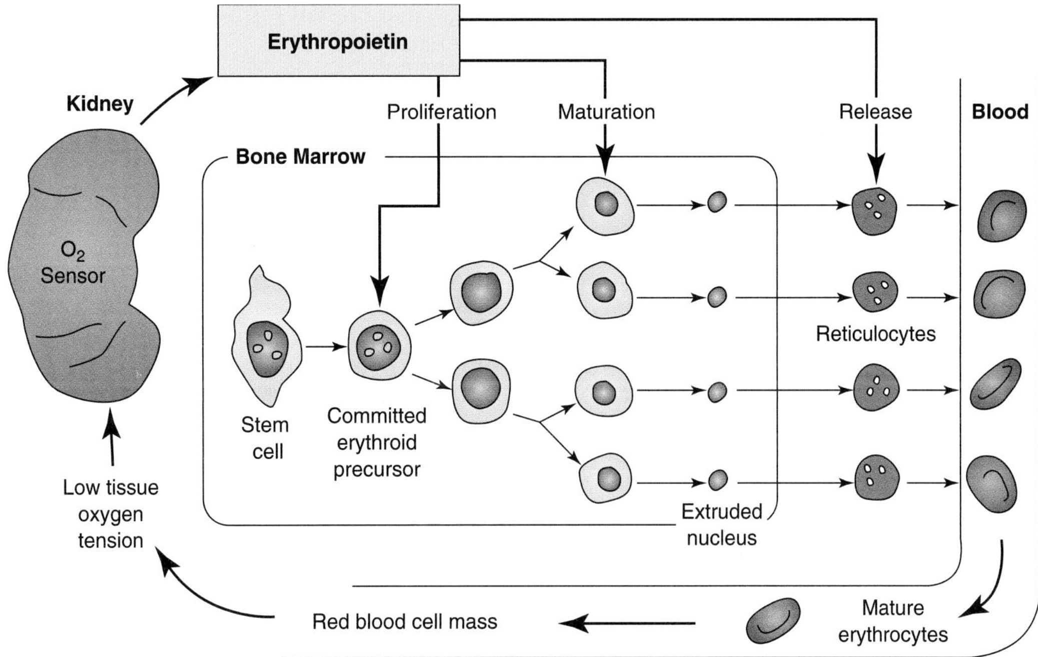

Figure 8-3
Red blood cell development.

reticulocyte count therefore serves as an index of the erythropoietic activity of the bone marrow.

The red blood cell, which lacks mitochondria, relies on glucose and the glycolytic pathway for its metabolic needs. The enzyme-mediated anaerobic metabolism of glucose generates the adenosine triphosphate (ATP) needed for normal membrane function and ion transport. The depletion of glucose or the functional deficiency of one of the glycolytic enzymes leads to the premature death of the red blood cell. An offshoot of the glycolytic pathway provides a large amount of 2,3-diphosphoglycerate (2,3-DPG), which binds to the hemoglobin molecule and reduces the affinity of hemoglobin for oxygen. This facilitates the release of oxygen at the tissue level, particularly in cases of hypoxia and anemia.

Two additional pathways prevent the oxidation of hemoglobin by environmental oxidants such as peroxide and superoxide. The methemoglobin reductase pathway prevents the oxidation of hemoglobin to methemoglobin, a nonfunctional molecule with reduced oxygen-carrying capacity. The pentose phosphate pathway depends on the enzyme glucose-6-phosphate dehydrogenase (G6PD). In the presence of environmental oxidants, G6PD activity prevents oxidative denaturation of hemoglobin, with resultant red cell injury and lysis.

Erythropoiesis is governed for the most part by tissue oxygen needs. *Hypoxia* is the main *stimulus* for red cell production but does not act directly on the bone marrow. Instead, oxygen is sensed by the kidneys, which then produce the hormone *erythropoietin*. Erythropoietin, a glycoprotein with a molecular weight of about 34,000, is produced primarily by the interstitial and endothelial cells that line the peritubular capillaries. About 5% to 10% of erythropoietin is released by the liver and other tissues.

Erythropoietin takes several days to effect this release of red blood cells from the bone marrow, and only after 5 or more days does red blood cell production reach a maximum. Erythropoietin acts in the bone marrow by binding to receptors on committed stem cells. It functions on many levels to promote hemoglobin synthesis, increase production of membrane proteins, and cause differentiation of erythroblasts. Because red blood cells are released into the blood as reticulocytes, the percentage of these cells is higher when there is a marked increase in red blood cell production. In some severe anemias, for example, the reticulocytes may account for as much as 30% of the total red cell count. In some situations, red cell production is so accelerated that numerous erythroblasts appear in the blood. Human erythropoietin can be produced by deoxyribonucleic acid (DNA)–recombinant technology. It is used for the management of anemia in cases of chronic renal failure, for anemias induced by chemotherapy for malignancies, and in the treatment of human immunodeficiency virus–infected patients treated with zidovudine.

Red Cell Destruction

Mature red blood cells have a life span of about 4 months, or 120 days. As the red blood cell ages, a number of changes occur. The metabolic activities within the cell decrease, enzyme activity falls off, and ATP, potassium, and membrane lipids decrease. The rate of red cell destruction (1% per day) normally is equal to red cell production, but in conditions such as hemolytic anemia, the cell's life span may be shorter.

The destruction of red blood cells is accomplished by a group of large phagocytic cells found in the spleen, liver, bone marrow, and lymph nodes. These phagocytic cells recognize old and defective red cells and then ingest and destroy them in a series of enzymatic reactions. During these reactions, the amino acids from the globulin chains and iron from the heme units are salvaged and reused. The bulk of the heme unit is converted to bilirubin, the pigment of bile, which is insoluble in plasma and attaches to the plasma proteins for transport. Bilirubin is removed from the blood by the liver and conjugated with glucuronide to render it water soluble so that it can be excreted in the bile. The plasma-insoluble form of bilirubin is referred to as unconjugated bilirubin; the water-soluble form is referred to as conjugated bilirubin. Serum levels of conjugated and unconjugated bilirubin can be measured in the laboratory and are reported as direct and indirect, respectively.

If red cell destruction and consequent bilirubin production are excessive, unconjugated bilirubin accumulates in the blood. This results in a yellow discoloration of the skin, called *jaundice* (see Chapter 33).

When red blood cell destruction takes place in the circulation, as in hemolytic anemia, the hemoglobin remains in the plasma. The plasma contains a hemoglobin-binding protein called haptoglobin. Other plasma proteins, such as albumin, can also bind hemoglobin. With extensive intravascular destruction of red blood cells, hemoglobin levels may exceed the hemoglobin-binding capacity of haptoglobin. When this happens, free hemoglobin appears in the blood (*i.e.*, hemoglobinemia) and is excreted in the urine (*i.e.*, hemoglobinuria). Because excessive red blood cell destruction can occur in hemolytic transfusion reactions, urine samples are tested for free hemoglobin after a transfusion reaction.

Laboratory Tests

Red blood cells can be studied by means of a sample of blood (Table 8–1). In the laboratory, automated blood cell counters rapidly provide accurate measurements of red cell content and cell indices. The *red blood cell count* measures the *total number* of red blood cells in 1 mm^3 of blood. The *percentage of reticulocytes* (normally about 1%) provides an index of the rate of red cell production. The *hemoglobin* (grams per 100 ml of blood) measures the *hemoglobin content* of the blood. The major components of blood are the red cell mass and plasma volume. The *hematocrit* measures the volume of red cell mass in 100 ml of plasma volume. To determine the hematocrit, a sample of blood is placed in a glass tube, which is then centrifuged to separate the cells and the plasma. The hematocrit may be deceptive, because it varies with the quantity of extracellular fluid, rising with dehydration and falling with overexpansion of extracellular fluid volume.

Red cell indices are used to differentiate types of anemias by size or color of red cells. The *mean corpuscular volume* (MCV) reflects the volume or size of the red cells. The MCV falls in microcytic (small cell) anemia and rises in macrocytic (large cell) anemia. Some anemias are normocytic (*i.e.*, cells are of normal size or MCV). The *mean corpuscular hemoglobin concentration* (MCHC) is the concentration of hemoglobin in each cell. Anemias are described as normochromic (normal color or MCHC) or hypochromic (decreased color or MCHC). Mean cell hemoglobin (MCH) refers to the mass of the red cell and is less useful in classifying anemias.

A stained blood smear provides information about the size, color, and shape of red cells and the presence of immature or abnormal cells. If blood smear results are abnormal, examination of the bone marrow may be

TABLE 8-1

Standard Laboratory Values for Red Blood Cells

Test	Normal Values	Significance
Red blood cell count (RBC)		
Men	4.2–5.4 × $10^6/\mu L$)	Number of red cells in the blood
Women	3.6–5.0 × $10^6/\mu L$	
Reticulocytes	1.0%–1.5% of total RBC	Rate of red cell production
Hemoglobin		
Men	14–16.5 g/dL	Hemoglobin content of the blood
Women	12–15 g/dL	
Hematocrit		
Men	40%–50%	Volume of cells in 100 mL of blood
Women	37%–47%	
Mean corpuscular volume	85–100 fL/red cells	Size of the red cell
Mean corpuscular hemoglobin concentration	31–35 g/dL	Concentration of hemoglobin in the red cell
Mean cell hemoglobin	27–34 pg/cell	Red cell mass

important. Marrow commonly is aspirated with a special needle from the posterior iliac crest or the sternum. The aspirate is stained and observed for number and maturity of cells and abnormal types.

In summary, the red blood cell provides the means for transporting oxygen from the lungs to the tissues. Red cells develop from stem cells in the bone marrow and are released as reticulocytes into the blood, where they become mature erythrocytes. The life span of a red blood cell is about 120 days. Red cell destruction normally occurs in the spleen, liver, bone marrow, and lymph nodes. In the process of destruction, the heme portion of the hemoglobin molecule is converted to bilirubin. Bilirubin, which is insoluble in plasma, attaches to plasma proteins for transport in the blood. It is removed from the blood by the liver and conjugated to a water-soluble form so that it can be excreted in the bile.

Anemia

After you have completed this section of the chapter, you should be able to meet the following objectives:

- Describe the manifestations of anemia and their mechanisms
- Explain the difference between intravascular and extravascular hemolysis
- Compare the hemoglobinopathies associated with sickle cell anemia and thalassemia
- Explain the cause of sickling in sickle cell anemia
- Cite common causes of iron-deficiency anemia in infancy, adolescence, and adulthood
- Describe the relation between vitamin B_{12} deficiency and megaloblastic anemia
- List three causes of aplastic anemia
- Compare characteristics of the red blood cells in acute blood loss, hereditary spherocytosis, sickle cell anemia, iron-deficiency anemia, and aplastic anemia

Anemia is defined as an abnormally low number of circulating red blood cells or hemoglobin level, or both, resulting in diminished oxygen-carrying capacity. Anemia usually results from excessive loss (*i.e.*, bleeding) or destruction (*i.e.*, hemolysis) of red blood cells or from deficient red blood cell production because of a lack of nutritional elements or bone marrow failure.

Manifestations

Anemia is not a disease; it is an indication of some disease process or alteration in body function. The manifestations of anemia can be grouped into three categories: impaired oxygen transport, alterations in red cell structure, and signs and symptoms associated with the pathologic process that is causing the anemia. The manifestations of anemia also depend on its severity, the rapidity of its development, and the patient's age, health status, and compensatory mechanisms. With rapid blood loss, circulatory shock and circulatory collapse may occur. Because the body adapts to slowly developing anemia, the loss of red cell mass may reach 50% without the occurrence of signs and symptoms.[1]

In anemia, the oxygen-carrying capacity of hemoglobin is reduced, causing tissue hypoxia. Tissue hypoxia can give rise to angina, night cramps, fatigue, weakness, and dyspnea. The redistribution of the blood from cutaneous tissues or a lack of hemoglobin causes pallor of the skin, mucous membranes, conjunctiva, and nail beds. Tachycardia and palpitations may occur as the body tries to compensate with an increase in cardiac output. A flow-type systolic murmur may result from changes in blood viscosity. Ventricular hypertrophy and high-output heart failure may develop in patients with severe anemia or in elderly persons, even at hemoglobin levels of 10 g/dl.[2] Erythropoietin activity is accelerated and may be recognized by diffuse bone pain and sternal tenderness. The production of 2,3-DPG is a compensatory mechanism that reduces the hemoglobin affinity for oxygen, as evidenced by a shift to the right in the oxygen-hemoglobin saturation curve; this causes more oxygen to be released to the tissues rather than remaining bound to hemoglobin. In addition to the common anemic manifestations, hemolytic anemias are accompanied by jaundice caused by increased blood levels of bilirubin. In aplastic anemia, petechiae and purpura (*i.e.*, red spots caused by small-vessel bleeding) are the result of reduced platelet function.

Blood Loss Anemia

With anemia caused by bleeding, iron and other components of the erythrocyte are lost from the body. Blood loss may be acute or chronic. Acute blood loss carries a risk of hypovolemia and shock rather than anemia (see Chapter 20). The red cells are normal in size and color. A fall in the red blood cell count, hematocrit, and hemoglobin results from hemodilution caused by movement of fluid into the vascular compartment. The hypoxia that results from blood loss stimulates red cell production by the bone marrow. If the bleeding is controlled and sufficient iron stores are available, the red cell concentration returns to normal within 3 to 4 weeks. Chronic blood loss does not affect blood volume but instead leads to iron-deficiency anemia when iron stores are depleted. Because of compensatory mechanisms, patients are commonly asymptomatic until the hemoglobin level is less than 8 g/dL. The red cells that are produced have too little hemoglobin, giving rise to microcytic hypochromic anemia.

Hemolytic Anemia

Hemolytic anemia is characterized by the premature destruction of red cells, with retention in the body of iron and the other products of red cell destruction. Almost all types of hemolytic anemia are distinguished by normocytic and normochromic red cells. Because of the red blood cell's shortened life span, the bone marrow usually is hyperactive, resulting in an increase in the number of reticulocytes in the circulating blood. As with other types of anemias, the patient experiences easy fatigability, dyspnea, and other signs and symptoms of impaired oxygen transport. The patient may have mild jaundice. In hemolytic anemia, red cell breakdown can occur within the vascular compartment, or it can result from phagocytosis by the reticuloendothelial system. Intravascular hemolysis is manifested by hemoglobinemia and hemoglobinuria.

The cause of hemolytic anemia can be intrinsic or extrinsic to the red blood cell. Intrinsic causes include defects of the red cell membrane, the various hemoglobinopathies, and inherited enzyme defects. Acquired forms of hemolytic anemia are caused by agents extrinsic to the red blood cell, such as drugs, bacterial and other toxins, antibodies, and physical trauma. Although all these factors can cause premature and accelerated destruction of red cells, they cannot all be treated in the same way. Some respond to splenectomy, others respond to treatment with corticosteroid hormones, and still others do not resolve until the primary disorder is corrected.

Inherited Disorders of the Red Cell Membrane

Hereditary spherocytosis, transmitted as an autosomal dominant trait, is the most common inherited disorder of the red cell membrane. The disorder is a deficiency of membrane proteins (i.e., spectrin and ankyrin) that leads to gradual loss of the membrane surface during the life span of the red blood cell, resulting in a tight sphere instead of a concave disk. Although the spherical cell retains its ability to transport oxygen, it is poorly deformable and susceptible to destruction as it passes through the venous sinuses of the splenic circulation. Clinical signs are variable but typically include mild anemia, jaundice, splenomegaly, and bilirubin gallstones. A life-threatening aplastic crisis may occur when a sudden disruption of red cell production (in most cases from a viral infection) causes a rapid drop in hematocrit and the hemoglobin level. The disorder usually is treated with splenectomy to reduce red cell destruction.

Hemoglobinopathies

Abnormalities in hemoglobin structure can lead to accelerated red cell destruction. Two main types of hemoglobinopathies can cause red cell hemolysis: the abnormal substitution of an amino acid in the hemoglobin molecule, as in sickle cell anemia, and the defective synthesis of one of the polypeptide chains that form the globin portion of hemoglobin, as in the thalassemias.

Sickle Cell Anemia. Sickle cell disease affects about 50,000 (0.1% to 0.2%) black Americans. About 9% of black Americans carry the trait.[3] Sickle cell anemia results from a defect in the β chain of the hemoglobin molecule, with an abnormal substitution of a single amino acid, valine, for glutamic acid. Sickle hemoglobin (HbS) is transmitted by recessive inheritance and can manifest as sickle cell trait (i.e., heterozygote) or sickle cell disease (i.e., homozygote). In the heterozygote, only about 40% of the hemoglobin is HbS, but in the homozygote, almost all the hemoglobin is HbS. Variations in proportions exist, and the concentration of HbS correlates with the risk of sickling.

In the homozygote, the HbS becomes sickled when deoxygenated or at an oxygen tension of about 40 mm Hg.[4] The deoxygenated hemoglobin aggregates and polymerizes, causing a semisolid gel that changes the shape and deformability of the cell (Fig. 8–4). After repeated episodes of deoxygenation, the cells remain permanently sickled. These deformed red cells obstruct blood flow in the microcirculation, causing tissue hypoxia. The person with sickle cell trait who has less HbS has little tendency to sickle except during severe hypoxia and is virtually asymptomatic. Fetal hemoglobin (HbF) does not interact with HbS or sickle; therefore, most children with sickle cell anemia do not begin to experience the effects of the sickling until sometime after 4 to 6 months of age, when the HbF has been replaced by HbS. The factors associated with sickling and consequent vaso-occlusive crisis include exertion; infection; illnesses that may cause hypoxia, acidosis, or dehydration; or even such trivial incidents as reduced oxygen tension induced by sleep.

Hardly an organ is spared in sickle cell anemia. Affected persons develop severe hemolytic anemia, painful crises, organ damage, and chronic hyperbilirubinemia. A painful crisis results from vessel occlusion and can occur suddenly in almost any part of the body. The frequency ranges from daily to yearly. Common sites obstructed by sickled cells include the abdomen, chest, and joints. Infarctions caused by sluggish blood flow may cause chronic damage to the liver, spleen, heart, kidneys, retina and other organs. *Acute chest*

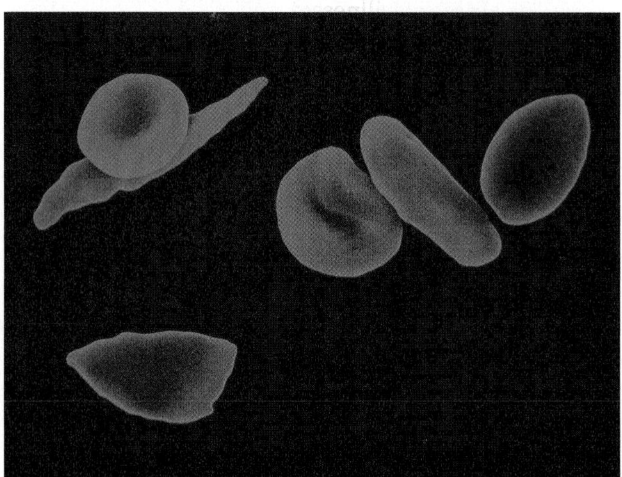

Figure 8-4
Photograph of a sickled cell and a normal red blood cell. (© Dr. Gopal Murti, Science Photo Library, Science Source/Photo Researchers)

syndrome is an atypical pneumonia resulting from pulmonary infarction. The most serious complication is stroke resulting from cerebral occlusion. Stroke associated with a painful crisis occurs in children 1 to 15 years of age and may recur in two thirds of those afflicted. The hyperbilirubinemia that results from the breakdown products of hemoglobin often leads to jaundice and the production of pigment stones in the gallbladder. Children may experience growth retardation and reduced spleen function with frequent infections.

The spleen is especially susceptible to damage by sickle cell hemoglobin. Splenic injury begins as early as 3 to 6 months of age with intense congestion and is usually asymptomatic.[5] The congestion causes functional asplenia and predisposes the person to life-treatening infections by encapsulated organisms such as *Streptococcus pneumoniae, Haemophilus influenzae* type b, and *Klebsiella sp.* Neonates and small children have not had time to develop antibodies to these organisms and rely on the spleen for their removal. In the absence of specific antibody to the polysaccharide capsular antigens of these organisms, splenic activity is essential for removing these organisms when they enter the blood. One study showed that 28% of children with sickle cell disease were functionally asplenic at 1 year, 58% at 2 years, and 94% at 5 years.[6]

Most children with sickle cell disease are at risk for fulminant septicemia and death during the first 3 years of life, when bacteremia from encapsulated organisms occurs commonly even in normal children. Neonatal screening and early diagnosis of sickle cell disease has facilitated prophylactic administration of penicillin. Prophylactic penicillin should be begun before 3 months of age and continued until at least 5 years of age. Routine immunizations, including *H. influenza* vaccine and pneumococcal vaccine, should be administered at 2 and 5 years of age.[5] Parents and caregivers need to be - educated regarding the manifestations of sickle cell complications and the importance of early medical evaluation of all febrile illnesses and other complications. There is no known cure or therapeutic regimen that prevents the problems associated with sickle cell anemia, and treatment includes pain control and management of complications. The patient is advised to avoid situations that precipitate sickling episodes, such as infections, cold exposure, severe physical exertion, acidosis, and dehydration. Infections are aggressively treated, and blood transfusions may be warranted in a crisis or given chronically in severe disease.

A promising treatment using hydroxyurea allows synthesis of more HbF and less HbS, thereby decreasing sickling. Hydroxyurea administered to adults reduced painful crises, but the long-term effects on organ damage are unknown.[7] Studies of this treatment for children are ongoing. Bone marrow transplantation has been tried with good results but remains experimental and carries the risk of graft-versus-host disease.[8] In the United States, neonatal diagnosis of sickle cell disease is made on the basis of clinical findings and hemoglobin solubility results, which are confirmed by hemoglobin electrophoresis. Prenatal diagnosis is done by the analysis of fetal DNA obtained by amniocentesis.[9]

In the United States, screening programs have been implemented to detect newborns with sickle cell disease and other hemoglobinopathies. Cord blood samples are subjected to electrophoresis to separate the HbF from the small amount of HbA and HbS. Other hemoglobins may be detected and quantified by further laboratory evaluation. Many states mandate neonatal screening of all newborns, regardless of ethnic origin. Ideally, the effective screening program also includes expert genetic counseling and education about pregnancy options.

Thalassemias. In contrast to sickle cell anemia, the thalassemias result from absent or defective synthesis of the α or the β chains of hemoglobin. The β-thalassemias represent a defect in β-chain synthesis, and the α-thalassemias represent a defect in α-chain synthesis. The defect is inherited as a mendelian trait, and a person may be heterozygous for the trait and have a mild form of the disease or be homozygous and have the severe form of the disease. Like sickle cell anemia, the thalassemias occur with high degree of frequency in certain populations. The β-thalassemias, sometimes called *Cooley's anemia* or *Mediterranean anemia,* are most common in the Mediterranean populations of southern Italy and Greece, and the α-thalassemias are most common among Asians. Both α- and β-thalassemias are common in Africans and black Americans.

Two factors contribute to the anemia that occurs in thalassemia: reduced hemoglobin synthesis and an imbalance in globin chain production. In α- and β-thalassemia, defective globin chain production leads to deficient hemoglobin production and the development of a hypochromic microcytic anemia. The unaffected type of chain continues to be synthesized, accumulates in the red cell, and contributes to red cell destruction and anemia. In β-thalassemia, the excess α chains are denatured to form precipitates (*i.e.,* Heinz bodies) within the bone marrow red cell precursors. These Heinz bodies impair DNA synthesis and cause damage to the red cell membrane. Severely affected red cell precursors are destroyed in the bone marrow, and those that escape intramedullary death are at increased risk of destruction in the spleen.

The clinical manifestations of β-thalassemias are based on the severity of the anemia. The presence of one normal gene in heterozygous persons usually results in sufficient normal hemoglobin synthesis to prevent severe anemia. Persons who are homozygous for the trait have severe transfusion-dependent anemia. Severe growth retardation affects children with the disorder. Increased hematopoiesis in response to erythropoietin causes bone marrow expansion and increases iron absorption, and splenomegaly and hepatomegaly result from increased red cell destruction. Bone marrow expansion leads to thinning of the cortical bone, with new bone formation evident on the maxilla and frontal bones of the face (*i.e.*, chipmunk facies). The long bones, ribs, and vertebrae may become vulnerable to fracture. Frequent transfusions prevent most of these complications and enable the patient to survive to the second or third decade.[10] Excess iron stores, which accumulate from increased dietary absorption and repeated transfusions, are deposited in the myocardium, liver, and pancreas and induce organ injury and congestive heart failure. Bone marrow transplantation is a potential cure for some patients.

Synthesis of the α-globin chains of hemoglobin is controlled by two pairs of genes; hence, α-thalassemia shows great variations in severity. Silent carriers have deletion of a single α-globin gene and are asymptomatic. The most severe form of α-thalassemia occurs in infants in whom all four α-globin genes are deleted. Such a defect results in a hemoglobin molecule (Hb Bart's) that is formed exclusively from the chains of HbF. Hb Bart's, which has an extremely high oxygen affinity, cannot release oxygen in the tissues. Affected infants suffer from severe hypoxia and are stillborn or die shortly after birth. Deletion of three of the four α-chain genes leads to unstable aggregates of β chains called *hemoglobin H* (HbH). The β chains are more soluble than the α chains, and their accumulation is less toxic to the red cells, so that senescent, rather than precursor, red cells are affected. Most persons with HbH have only mild to moderate hemolytic anemia, and manifestations of ineffective erythropoiesis (*i.e.*, bone marrow expansion and iron overload) are absent.

Inherited Enzyme Defects

The most common inherited enzyme defect that results in hemolytic anemia is a deficiency of G6PD. The gene that determines this enzyme is located on the X chromosome, and the defect is expressed only in males and homozygous females. There are many genetic variants of this disorder. The African variant has been found in 10% of black Americans.[3] The disorder makes red cells more vulnerable to oxidants and causes direct oxidation of hemoglobin to methemoglobin and the denaturing of the hemoglobin molecule to form *Heinz bodies.* Hemolysis usually occurs as the damaged red blood cells move through the narrow vessels of the spleen, causing hemoglobinemia, hemoglobinuria, and jaundice. In blacks, the defect is mildly expressed and is not associated with chronic hemolytic anemia unless triggered by oxidant drugs, acidosis, or infection.

The antimalarial drugs primaquine and quinacrine, the sulfonamides, nitrofurantoin, aspirin, phenacetin, and other drugs cause hemolysis. Free radicals generated by phagocytes during infections also are possible triggers. A more severe deficiency of G6PD is found in people of Mediterranean descent (e.g., Sardinians, Sephardic Jews, Arabs). In some of these persons, chronic hemolysis occurs in the absence of exposure to oxidants. The disorder can be diagnosed through the use of a G6PD assay or screening test.

Acquired Hemolytic Anemias

Several acquired factors exogenous to the red blood cell produce hemolysis by direct membrane destruction or by antibody-mediated lysis. Various drugs, chemicals, toxins, venoms, and infections such as malaria destroy red cell membranes. Hemolysis can also be caused by mechanical factors such as prosthetic heart valves, vasculitis, and severe burns. Obstructions in the microcirculation as in disseminated intravascular coagulation, thrombotic thrombocytopenic purpura, and renal disease may traumatize the red cells by changes in turbulence and pressure gradients.

Many hemolytic anemias are immune mediated, caused by antibodies that destroy the red cell. Autoantibodies may be produced by a person in response to drugs and disease. Alloantibodies come from an exogenous source and are responsible for transfusion reactions and hemolytic disease of the newborn.

The autoantibodies that cause red cell destruction are of two types: warm-reacting antibodies of the immunoglobulin G (IgG) type, which are maximally active at 37°C, and cold-reacting antibodies of the immunoglobulin M (IgM) type, which are optimally active at or near 4°C. The warm-reacting antibodies cause no morphologic or metabolic alteration in the red cell. Instead, they react with antigens on the red cell membrane, causing destructive changes that lead to spherocytosis, with subsequent phagocytic destruction in the spleen or reticuloendothelial system. They lack specificity for the ABO antigens but may react with the Rh antigens. The hemolytic reactions associated with the warm-reacting antibodies have varied causes; about 60% are idiopathic, 25% to 30% are drug induced, and most of the remainder are related to cancers of the lymphoproliferative system (e.g., chronic lymphocytic leukemia, lymphoma) or collagen diseases (e.g., systemic lupus erythematosus).[11] The antihypertensive drug α-methyldopa produces almost 70% of drug-induced hemolysis, and penicillin accounts for about 23%.[12] The cold-reacting antibodies activate complement. Chronic hemolytic anemia caused by cold-reacting antibodies occurs with lymphoproliferative disorders and as an idiopathic disorder of unknown cause. The hemolytic process occurs in distal body parts, where the temperature may fall below 30° C. Vascular obstruction by red cells results in pallor, cyanosis of the body parts exposed to cold temperatures, and Raynaud's phenomenon (see Chapter 17). Hemolytic anemia caused by cold-reacting antibodies develops in only a few persons.

The Coombs' test, or antiglobulin test, is used to diagnose immune hemolytic anemias. It detects the presence of antibody or complement on the surface of the red cell. The direct antiglobulin test (DAT) detects the antibody on red blood cells. In this test, red cells that have been washed free of serum are mixed with antihuman globulin reagent. The red cells agglutinate if the reagent binds to and bridges the antibody or complement on adjacent red cells. The DAT result is positive in cases of autoimmune hemolytic anemia, erythroblastosis fetalis (*i.e.*, Rh disease of the newborn), transfusion reactions, and drug-induced hemolysis. The indirect antiglobulin test (IAT) detects antibody in the serum, and the result is positive for specific antibodies. It is used for antibody detection and crossmatching before transfusion.

Anemias of Deficient Red Cell Production

Anemia may result from the decreased production of erythrocytes by the bone marrow. A deficiency of nutrients for hemoglobin synthesis (iron) or DNA synthesis (cobalamin or folic acid) may reduce red cell production by the bone marrow. A deficiency of red cells also results when the marrow itself fails or is replaced by nonfunctional tissue.

Iron-Deficiency Anemia

Iron deficiency is a common worldwide cause of anemia affecting persons of all ages. The anemia results from dietary deficiency, loss of iron through bleeding, or increased demands. Because iron is a component of heme, the lack leads to a decrease in hemoglobin synthesis and consequent impairment of oxygen delivery.

Body iron is repeatedly used. When red cells become senescent and are broken down, their iron is released and reused in the production of new red cells. Despite this efficiency, small amounts of iron are lost in the feces and need to be replaced by dietary uptake. Iron balance is maintained by the absorption of 0.5 to 1.5 mg daily to replace the 1 mg lost in the feces. The average Western diet contains about 10 to 15 mg of iron, of which 5% to 10% is absorbed.[13] The absorbed iron is more than sufficient to supply the needs of most individuals but may be barely adequate in females and young children. Dietary deficiency of iron is not common except in certain populations. Most iron is derived from meat, and when meat is not available, as for deprived populations, or is not a dietary constituent, as for vegetarians, iron deficiency may occur. The usual reason for iron deficiency in adults is chronic blood loss because iron cannot be recycled to the pool. In men and postmenopausal women, blood loss may occur from gastrointestinal bleeding because of peptic ulcer, intestinal polyps, hemorrhoids, or cancer. Excessive aspirin intake may cause undetected gastrointestinal bleeding. In women, menstruation may account for an average of 22 mg of iron lost per month or 0.7 to 2.0 mg of iron per day, causing a deficiency.[14] Although cessation of menstruation spares iron loss in the pregnant woman, iron requirements increase at this time, and deficiency is common. The expansion of the mother's blood volume requires about 480 mg of additional iron, and the growing fetus requires about 390 mg, averaging about 3.6 mg of iron daily. In the postnatal period, lactation requires about 30 mg of iron monthly.[15]

A child's growth places extra demands on the body. Blood volume increases, with a greater need for iron. Iron requirements are proportionally higher in infancy (3 to 24 months) than at any other age, although they are also increased in childhood and adolescence. In infancy, the two main causes of iron-deficiency anemia are low iron levels at birth because of maternal deficiency and a diet consisting mainly of cow's milk, which is low in absorbable iron. Thirty percent of infants in low-income populations are reported to be anemic.[16]

Iron deficiency is characterized by a low hemoglobin and hematocrit, decreased iron stores and low serum iron and ferritin. The red cells are decreased in number and are microcytic, hypochromic, and often malformed (*i.e.*, poikilocytosis). The laboratory values indicate reduced MCHC and MCV. Membrane changes may predispose to hemolysis, causing further loss of red cells.

The signs and symptoms of iron-deficiency anemia are related to impaired oxygen transport and lack of hemoglobin. Depending on the severity of the anemia, fatigability, palpitations, dyspnea, angina, and tachycardia may occur. Epithelial atrophy is common and results in waxy pallor, brittle hair and nails, smooth tongue, sores in the corners of the mouth, and sometimes in dysphagia and decreased acid secretion. A poorly understood symptom that sometimes is seen is pica, the bizarre compulsive eating of ice, dirt, or other abnormal substances.

The treatment of iron-deficiency anemia is directed toward controlling chronic blood loss, increasing dietary intake of iron, and administering supplemental iron. Ferrous sulfate, which is the usual oral replacement therapy, replenishes iron stores in several months. Parenteral iron may be given if oral forms are not tolerated or ineffective. Special care is required when administering an iron preparation (*e.g.*, Imferon) intramuscularly; it must be injected deeply by pulling the skin to one side before inserting the needle (*i.e.*, Z-track) to prevent leakage into the tissues, with subsequent skin discoloration.

Megaloblastic Anemias

Megaloblastic anemias are caused by abnormal nucleic acid synthesis that results in enlarged red cells (MCV >100) and deficient nuclear maturation. Cobalamin (vitamin B_{12}) and folic acid deficiencies are the most common megaloblastic anemias. (One form of megaloblastic anemia, unresponsive to vitamin B_{12} or folic acid therapy, is not discussed here.) Because megaloblastic anemias develop slowly, there are often few symptoms until the anemia is far advanced.

Cobalamin (Vitamin B_{12})–Deficiency Anemia. Vitamin B_{12} is essential for the synthesis of DNA. When it is deficient, nuclear maturation and cell division, especially of the rapidly proliferating red cells, fail to occur. When vitamin B_{12} is deficient, the red cells that are produced are abnormally large because of excess RNA production of hemoglobin and structural protein. They have flimsy membranes and are oval rather than biconcave. These oddly shaped cells have a short life span that can be measured in weeks rather than months. The MCV is elevated, and the MCHC is normal.

An important cause of vitamin B_{12} deficiency is pernicious anemia, resulting from diminished intestinal absorption of B_{12}. The absorption of vitamin B_{12} in the intestine requires the presence of *intrinsic factor,* which is produced by the gastric mucosa. Intrinsic factor binds to vitamin B_{12} in food, protects it from the enzymatic actions of the gut, and facilitates its absorption. As discussed in Chapter 32, the immune-mediated chronic atrophic gastritis is a disorder that destroys the gastric mucosa and produces antibodies that interfere with the action of intrinsic factor. The loss of intrinsic factor leads to pernicious anemia.

Neurologic changes accompany the disorder and are caused by deranged methylation of myelin protein. Demyelination of the dorsal and lateral columns of the spinal cord causes symmetric paresthesias of the feet and fingers, causes a loss of vibratory and position sense, and eventually progresses to spastic ataxia. Lifelong treatment consisting of intramuscular injections of vitamin B_{12} reverses the anemia and improves the neurologic changes.

Folic Acid–Deficiency Anemia. Folic acid is also required for red cell maturation, and its deficiency produces the same type of red cell changes that occur in vitamin B_{12}–deficiency anemia (*i.e.,* increased MCV and normal MCHC). Symptoms are also similar, but the neurologic manifestations are not present.

Folic acid is readily absorbed from the intestine. It is found in vegetables (particularly the green leafy types), fruits, cereals, and meats. Much of the vitamin, however, is lost in cooking. The most common causes of folic acid deficiency are malnutrition or dietary lack, especially in association with alcoholism, and malabsorption syndromes such as sprue or other intestinal disorders. Because pregnancy increases the need for folic acid 5- to 10-fold, a deficiency can occur. Studies also show an association between folate deficiency and neural tube defects, which suggests routine supplementation of 1 mg folate daily in pregnancy.[17] Poor dietary habits, anorexia, and nausea are other reasons for folic acid deficiency during pregnancy. In neoplastic disease, tumor cells compete for folate, and deficiency is common. Some drugs used to treat seizure disorders (*e.g.,* primidone, phenytoin, phenobarbital) and triamterene, a diuretic, predispose to a deficiency by interfering with folic acid absorption. Methotrexate, a folic acid analogue used in the treatment of cancer, impairs the action of folic acid by blocking its conversion to the active form.

Aplastic Anemia

Aplastic anemia (*i.e.,* bone marrow depression) describes a primary condition of bone marrow stem cells that results in a reduction of all three hematopoietic cell lines—red blood cells, white blood cells, and platelets—with fatty replacement of bone marrow. Pure red cell aplasia, in which only the red cells are affected, rarely occurs.

Anemia results from the failure of the marrow to replace senescent red cells that are destroyed and leave the circulation, although the cells that remain are of normal size and color. At the same time, because the leukocytes, particularly the neutrophils, and the thrombocytes have a short life span, a deficiency of these cells usually is apparent before the anemia becomes severe.

The onset of aplastic anemia may be insidious, or it may strike with suddenness and great severity. It can occur at any age. The initial presenting symptoms include weakness, fatigability, and pallor caused by anemia. Petechiae (*i.e.,* small punctate skin hemorrhages) and ecchymoses (*i.e.,* bruises) often occur on the skin, and bleeding from the nose, gums, vagina, or gastrointestinal tract may occur because of decreased platelet levels. The decrease in the number of neutrophils increases susceptibility to infection.

Among the causes of aplastic anemia are exposure to high doses of radiation, chemicals, and toxins that suppress hematopoiesis directly or through immune mechanisms. Identified toxic agents include benzene, the antibiotic chloramphenicol, and the alkylating agents and antimetabolites used in the treatment of cancer (see Chapter 5). Aplastic anemia caused by exposure to chemical agents may be an idiosyncratic reaction, because it affects only certain susceptible persons. It typically occurs weeks after a drug is initiated. Such reactions often are severe and sometimes irreversible and fatal. Aplastic anemia can develop in the course of many infections and has been reported most often as a complication of viral hepatitis, mononucleosis, and other viral illnesses, including acquired immunodeficiency syndrome (AIDS). In two thirds of cases, the cause is unknown, and these are called *idiopathic aplastic anemia.*

Therapy for aplastic anemia in the young and severely affected includes bone marrow transplantation. Histocompatible donors supply stem cells to replace the patient's destroyed marrow cells. Graft-versus-host disease and infections are major risks of the procedure, yet up to 70% survival is reported.[18] Immunosuppressive therapy with lymphocyte immune globulin (*i.e.,* antithymocyte globulin) prevents suppression of proliferating stem cells, producing remission in 50% of patients.[18] Patients with aplastic anemia should avoid the offending agents and be treated with antibiotics for infection. Red cell transfusions to correct the anemia and platelets and corticosteroid therapy to minimize bleeding may also be required. Bone marrow depression often results from cancer treatment. Chemotherapy and irradiation commonly cause anemia and deficiency of platelets and leukocytes as a result of bone marrow depression.

Chronic Disease Anemias

Chronic renal failure almost always results in a normocytic, normochromic anemia, primarily because of a deficiency of erythropoietin. Uremic toxins also interfere with the actions of erythropoietin and red cell production. They also cause hemolysis and bleeding tendencies, which contribute to the anemia. Until recently, dialysis and red cell transfusions constituted the only therapy. Recombinant erythropoietin injected several times each week for 10 or more weeks dramatically elevates the hemoglobin level and hematocrit to a range of 32% to 38% and eliminates the need for transfusions.[19] Oral iron is usually required for a good response. Anemia often occurs as a complication of chronic infections, inflammation, and cancer. Common disorders include AIDS, osteomyelitis, rheumatoid arthritis, and Hodgkin's disease. It is theorized that the short life span, deficient red cell production, and low serum iron are caused by actions of macrophages and lymphocytes in response to cell injury. Macrophages sequester iron in the spleen and contribute to red cell destruction, and the lymphocytes release cytokines that suppress erythropoietin production and action.[20] The mild to moderate anemia is usually reversed when the underlying disease is treated.

In summary, anemia describes a condition in which the red cell mass is decreased. It is not a disease but a manifestation of some disease process or alteration in body function. Anemia typically is caused by the excessive loss of red cells (i.e., blood loss or destruction) or by impaired production. The manifestations of anemia include those associated with impaired oxygen transport, alterations in red blood cell structure, and the signs and symptoms of the underlying process causing the anemia.

Transfusion Therapy

After you have completed this section of the chapter, you should be able to meet the following objectives:

- Differentiate red cell antigens from antibodies in persons with type A, B, AB, or O blood
- Explain the determination of the Rh factor
- List the signs and symptoms of a blood transfusion reaction

Anemias of various causes are treated with transfusions of whole blood or red blood cells only when oxygen delivery to the tissues is compromised, as evidenced by measures of oxygen transport and use, hemoglobin, and hematocrit.[21] Acute massive blood loss usually is replaced with whole blood transfusion. Most anemias, however, are treated with transfusions of red cell concentrates, which supply only the blood component that is deficient. Since the 1960s, devices that mechanically separate a unit of blood into its constituents provide red cell components, platelets, fresh-frozen plasma, cryoprecipitate, and clotting factor concentrates. In this way, a unit of blood can be used efficiently for several recipients to correct specific deficiencies.

Several red cell components that are used for transfusion are prepared and stored under specific conditions and have unique uses, as described in Table 8–2. These red cell components are derived principally from voluntary blood donors.

The use of *autologous* donation and transfusion has been advocated. Autologous transfusion refers to the procedure of receiving one's own blood—usually to replenish a surgical loss—thereby eliminating the risk of blood-borne disease or transfusion reaction. Up to 10% of red cell transfusions could be provided by the recipient.[22] Autologous blood can be provided by several means: predeposit, hemodilution, and intraoperative salvage. A patient who is anticipating elective plastic or orthopedic surgery may predeposit blood (*i.e.*, have the blood collected up to 6 weeks in advance and stored) for later transfusion during the surgery. Hemodilution involves phlebotomy before surgery with transfusion of the patient's blood at the completion of surgery. The procedure requires the use of fluid infusions to maintain blood volume and is limited to open heart surgery. Intraoperative blood salvage is the collection of blood shed from the operative site for reinfusion into the patient. Semiautomated devices are used to collect, anticoagulate, wash, and resuspend red cells for reinfusion during many procedures, including vascular, cardiac, and orthopedic surgery.[21]

Before red cells or whole blood from a volunteer donor source is transfused, a series of procedures are required to ensure a successful transfusion. Donor and recipient samples are typed to determine ABO and Rh groups and screened for unexpected red cell antibodies. Donor samples are also tested for blood-borne diseases, such as hepatitis B and hepatitis C, human immunodeficiency virus types 1 and 2, human T-cell lymphocytic virus (HTLV-I), and syphilis. The crossmatch is performed by incubating the donor cells with the recipient's serum and observing for agglutination. If none appears, the donor and recipient blood types are compatible.

ABO Blood Groups

ABO compatibility is essential for effective transfusion therapy and requires knowledge of ABO antigens and antibodies. There are four major ABO blood groups as determined by the presence or absence of two red cell antigens (A and B). Persons who have neither A nor B antigens are classified as having type O blood; those with A antigens are classified as having type A blood; those with B antigens, as having type B blood; and those with A and B antigens, as having type AB blood (Table 8–3). The ABO blood groups are genetically determined. The type O gene is apparently functionless in production of a red cell antigen. Each of the other genes is expressed by the presence of a strong antigen on the surface of the red cell. Six genotypes, or gene combinations, result in four phenotypes, or blood type expressions. ABO antibodies predictably develop in the serum of persons whose red cells lack the corresponding antigen. Persons with type A antigens on their red cells develop type B antibodies; persons with type B antigens develop type A antibodies in their serum; persons with type O blood develop type A and type B antibodies; and persons with type AB blood develop neither A nor B antibodies. The ABO antibodies usually are not present at birth but begin to develop at 3 to 6 months of age and reach maximum levels between the ages of 5 and 10 years.[23]

TABLE 8-2 Red Blood Cell Components Used in Transfusion Therapy

Component	Preparation	Use	Limitations
Whole blood	Drawn from donor Anticoagulant-preservative solutions added, usually citrate-phosphate-dextrose (CPDA-1) adenine; stored at 1°–6°C until expiration, up to 35 days	Replacement of blood volume and oxygen-carrying capacity lost in massive bleeding	Contains few viable platelets or granulocytes and is dificient in coagulation factors V and VIII; may cause hypervolemia, febrile and allergic reactions and infectious disease (*i.e.*, hepatitis and AIDS)
Red blood cells	Removal of two thirds of plasma by centrifugation; additive solution contains adenine and dextrose to extend shelf life up to 42 days and maintain ATP levels	Standard transfusion to increase oxygen-carrying capacity in chronic anemia and slow hemorrhage; reduce danger of hypervolemia	Contains no viable platelets or granulocytes; risk of reactions and infectious disease
Leukocyte-poor red blood cells	Removal of 70%–90% of leukocytes, platelets, and debris by centrifugation or filtration	Reduces risk of nonhemolytic febrile reactions in susceptible persons	Preparation may reduce red cell mass to 70%; 24-hr outdate and infectious disease risk
Washed red blood cells	Red cells are washed in normal saline solution and centrifuged several times to remove plasma and constituents.	Reduces risk of febrile and allergic reactions	Loss of red cell mass, 24-hr outdate, costly preparation, and infectious disease risk
Frozen red blood cells	Red cells are mixed with glycerol to prevent ice crystals from forming and rupturing the cell membrane; cells must be thawed, deglycerolized, and washed before transfusing.	Reduces risk of severe febrile reactions; preserves rare and autologous (self-donated) units for transfusion up to 10 yr	Costly and lengthy preparation; loss of red cell mass, 24-hr outdate, and infectious disease risk

ATP, adenosine triphosphate.
(Data from Reynolds A., Steckler D. [1986]. *Practical aspects of blood administration* [pp. 43–93]. Arlington, VA: American Association of Blood Banks; and Widmann, F.K. [Ed.][1985]. *Technical manual* [9th ed., pp. 35–58]. Arlington, VA: American Association of Blood Banks)

RH Types

The D antigen of the Rh system is also important in transfusion compatibility and is routinely tested. The Rh type is coded by three gene pairs: C, c, D, d, and E, e. Each allele, with the exception of d, codes for a specific antigen. The D antigen is the most immunogenic. Persons who express the D antigen are designated Rh positive, and those who do not express the D antigen are Rh negative. Unlike serum antibodies for the ABO blood types, which develop spontaneously after birth, Rh antibodies develop after exposure to one or more of the Rh antigens. About 50% to 75% of Rh-negative persons develop the antibody to D antigen if they are exposed to Rh-positive blood.[12] Because it takes several weeks to produce antibodies, a reaction may be delayed and usually is mild. If subsequent transfusions of Rh-positive blood are given to a person who has become sensitized, the person may have a severe, immediate reaction.

TABLE 8-3 ABO System for Blood Typing

Genotype	Red Cell Antigens	Blood Type	Serum Antibodies
OO	None	O	AB
AO	A	A	B
AA	A	A	B
BO	B	B	A
BB	B	B	A
AB	AB	AB	None

Blood Transfusion Reactions

The seriousness of blood transfusion reactions prompts the need for extreme caution when blood is administered. Because most transfusion reactions result from clerical errors or misidentification, care should be taken to correctly identify the recipient and the transfusion source.[21] The recipient's vital signs should be monitored before and during the transfusion, and careful observation for signs of transfusion reaction is imperative. The most feared and lethal transfusion reaction is the destruction of donor red cells by reaction with antibody in the recipient's serum. This immediate hemolytic reaction usually is caused by ABO incompatibility. The signs and symptoms of such a reaction include sensation of heat along the vein where the blood is being infused, flushing of the face, urticaria, headache, pain in the lumbar area, chills, fever, constricting pain in the chest, cramping pain in the abdomen, nausea, vomiting, tachycardia, hypotension, and dyspnea. If any of these adverse effects occur, the transfusion should be stopped immediately. Access to a vein should be maintained, because it may be necessary to administer intravenous medications and take blood samples. The blood must be saved for studies to determine the cause of the reaction.

Hemoglobin that is released from the hemolyzed donor cells is filtered in the glomeruli of the kidneys. Two possible complications of a blood transfusion reaction are oliguria and renal shutdown because of the adverse effects of the filtered hemoglobin on renal tubular flow. The urine should be examined for the presence of hemoglobin, urobilinogen, and red blood cells.

A febrile reaction, the most common transfusion reaction, occurs in about 2% of transfusions.[21] Recipient antibodies directed against the donor's white cells or platelets cause chills and fever. Antipyretics are used to treat this reaction. Future febrile reactions may be avoided by the use of leukocyte-poor blood.

Allergic reactions are caused by patient antibodies against donor proteins, particularly immunoglobulin A. Urticaria and itching occur and can be relieved with antihistamines. Susceptible persons may be transfused with washed red cells to prevent reactions. Delayed hemolytic reactions may occur more than 10 days after transfusion and are caused by undetected antibodies in the recipient's serum. The reaction is accompanied by a fall in hematocrit and jaundice, but most recipients are asymptomatic.

In summary, transfusion therapy provides the means for replacement of red blood cells and other blood components. Red blood cells contain surface antigens, and reciprocal antibodies are found in the serum. Four major ABO blood types are determined by the presence or absence of two red cell antigens: A and B. The D antigen determines the Rh-positive type; absence of the D antigen determines the Rh-negative type. ABO and Rh types must be determined in recipient and donor blood before transfusion to ensure compatibility.

Polycythemia

After you have completed this section of the chapter, you should be able to meet the following objectives:

- Define the term polycythemia
- Compare polycythemia vera and secondary polycythemia

Polycythemia is an abnormally high total red blood cell mass. It is categorized as relative, primary, or secondary. In *relative polycythemia,* the hematocrit rises because of a loss of plasma volume without a corresponding decrease in red cells. This may occur with water deprivation or excess use of diuretics. *Primary polycythemia,* or *polycythemia vera,* is a proliferative disease of the pluripotent cells of the bone marrow characterized by an absolute increase in total red blood cell mass accompanied by elevated white cell and platelet counts. It most commonly is seen in men between the ages of 40 and 60 years. *Secondary polycythemia* results from an increase in the level of erythropoietin, commonly as a compensatory response to hypoxia. This elevation is related to living at high altitudes, chronic heart and lung disease, and smoking, all of which are causes of hypoxia.

In polycythemia vera, the signs and symptoms are related to increased blood viscosity, hypermetabolism, and an increase in the red cell count, hemoglobin level, and hematocrit. The increased blood volume gives rise to hypertension. The patient may complain of headache, inability to concentrate, and some difficulty in hearing because of decreased cerebral blood flow. There is a plethoric appearance or dusky redness—even cyanosis—particularly of the lips, fingernails, and mucous membranes. Because of the concentration of blood cells, the person may experience itching and pain in the fingers or toes, and the hypermetabolism may induce night sweats and weight loss. With the increased blood viscosity and stagnation of blood flow, thrombosis and hemorrhage are possible complications and are associated with manifestations of anginal pain, deep vein thrombosis, or cerebral insufficiency with transient ischemic attacks.

Relative polycythemia is corrected by increasing the vascular fluid volume. Treatment of secondary polycythemia focuses on relieving hypoxia. For example, continuous low-flow oxygen therapy can be used to correct the severe hypoxia that occurs in some persons with chronic obstructive lung disease. This form of treatment is thought to relieve the pulmonary hypertension and polycythemia and to delay the onset of cor pulmonale. The goal of treatment in primary polycythemia is to reduce blood viscosity. This can be done by withdrawing blood by means of periodic phlebotomy to reduce red cell volume. Control of platelet and white cell counts is accomplished by suppressing bone marrow function with chemotherapy or radiation therapy.

In summary, polycythemia describes a condition in which the red blood cell mass is increased. It may be relative, with the red cell mass increased because of a loss of vascular fluid; primary, with proliferative changes in the bone marrow; or secondary, with elevated erythropoietin levels caused by hypoxia.

Age-Related Changes in Red Blood Cells

After you have completed this section of the chapter, you should be able to meet the following objectives:

- Cite the function of hemoglobin F in the neonate and describe the red blood cell changes that occur during the early neonatal period
- Cite the factors that predispose to hyperbilirubinemia in the infant
- Describe the pathogenesis of hemolytic disease of the newborn
- Compare conjugated and unconjugated bilirubin in terms of production of encephalopathy in the neonate
- Explain the action of phototherapy in the treatment of hyperbilirubinemia in the neonate
- State the changes in the red blood cells that occur with aging

Red Cell Changes in the Neonate

At birth, changes in the red blood cell indices reflect the transition to extrauterine life and the need to transport oxygen from the lungs (Table 8–4). Hemoglobin concentrations at birth are high, reflecting the high synthetic activity in utero to provide adequate oxygen delivery.[24] Toward the end of the first postnatal week, hemoglobin concentration begins to decline, gradually falling to a minimum value at about age 2 months. The red cell count, hematocrit, and MCV likewise fall. The factors responsible for the decline include reduced red cell production and plasma dilution caused by increased blood volume with growth. Neonatal red cells also have a shorter life span of 50 to 70 days and are thought to be more fragile than those of older persons. During the early neonatal period, there is also a switch from HbF to HbA. The amount of HbF in term infants varies from 53% to 95% and decreases by about 3% per week after birth.[25] At 6 months of age, HbF usually accounts for less than 2% of total hemoglobin. The switch to HbA provides greater unloading of oxygen to the tissues, because HbA has a lower affinity for oxygen compared with HbF. Infants who are small for gestational age or born to diabetic or smoking mothers or who experienced hypoxia in utero have higher total hemoglobin levels, higher HbF levels, and a delayed switch to HbA.

A *physiologic anemia of the newborn* develops at about age 2 months. It seldom produces symptoms and cannot be altered by nutritional supplements. *Anemia of prematurity*, an exaggerated physiologic response in low-birth-weight infants, is thought to result from a poor erythropoietin response. The hemoglobin level rapidly declines after birth to a low of 7 to 10 g/dl at about 6 weeks of age. Signs and symptoms include apnea, poor weight gain, pallor, decreased activity, and tachycardia. In infants born before 33 weeks gestation or those with hematocrits below 33%, the clinical features are more evident. One study suggests that the protein content of breast milk may not be sufficient for hematopoiesis in the premature infant. Protein supplementation significantly elevates the hemoglobin concentrations between the ages of 4 and 10 weeks.[24]

Anemia at birth, characterized by pallor, congestive heart failure, or shock, usually is caused by hemolytic disease of the newborn. Bleeding from the umbilical cord, internal hemorrhage, congenital hemolytic disease, or frequent blood sampling are other possible causes of anemia. The severity of symptoms and presence of coexisting disease may warrant red cell transfusion.

Hyperbilirubinemia in the Neonate

Hyperbilirubinemia, an increased level of serum bilirubin, is a common cause of jaundice in the neonate. A benign, self-limited condition, it most often is related to

TABLE 8-4 Red Cell Values for Term Infants

AGE	RBC $\times 10^6/\mu L$ MEAN ±SD	Hb (g/dL) MEAN ±SD	Hct (%) MEAN ±SD	MCV (fl) MEAN ±SD
Days				
1	5.14 ±0.7	19.3 ±2.2	61 ±7.4	119 ± 9.4
4	5.00 ±0.6	18.6 ±2.1	57 ±8.1	114 ± 7.5
7	4.86 ±0.6	17.9 ±2.5	56 ±9.4	118 ±11.2
Weeks				
1–2	4.80 ±0.8	17.3 ±2.3	54 ±8.3	112 ±19.0
3–4	4.00 ±0.6	14.2 ±2.1	43 ±5.7	105 ±7.5
8–9	3.40 ±0.5	10.7 ±0.9	31 ±2.5	93 ±12.0
11–12	3.70 ±0.3	11.3 ±0.9	33 ±3.3	88 ± 7.9

Hb, hemoglobin; Hct, hematocrit; MCV, mean corpuscular volume.
(Adapted from Matoth Y., Zaizor R., Varsano I. [1971]. Postnatal changes in some red cell parameters. *Acta Paediatrica Scandinavica 60*, 317)

the developmental state of the neonate. Fewer cases of hyperbilirubinemia are pathologic and may lead to kernicterus and serious brain damage.

In the first week of life, about 60% of term and 80% of preterm neonates are jaundiced.[26] This *physiologic jaundice* appears in term infants on the second or third day of life, and bilirubin levels peak at less than 12 mg/dl. This complication probably is related to the increased fetal red cell breakdown and the inability of the immature liver to conjugate bilirubin. Premature infants exhibit a similar rise in serum bilirubin level, perhaps because of poor hepatic uptake and reduced albumin binding of bilirubin. The rise is slower, appearing at day 3 or 4, and peak levels of bilirubin are higher (>15 mg/dl). Most neonatal jaundice resolves within 1 week and is untreated.

When jaundice appears at atypical times (*i.e.*, at birth or after 1 week), the cause is sought to prevent exaggerated hyperbilirubinemia and its toxic consequences. Many factors cause elevated bilirubin levels in the neonate: breast-feeding, hemolytic disease of the newborn, hypoxia, infections, acidosis, and albumin-binding drugs (*e.g.*, furosemide, hydrocortisone, gentamicin, digoxin).[27] Bowel or biliary obstruction and liver disease are less common causes. Associated risk factors include prematurity, Asian ancestry, and maternal diabetes. *Breast milk jaundice* occurs in about 1 in 200 breast-fed babies.[26] These neonates develop significant levels of unconjugated bilirubin 4 to 7 days after birth and reach maximum levels in the third week of life. This type of jaundice disappears if breast-feeding is discontinued. Nursing can be resumed in 3 to 4 days without any hyperbilirubinemia ensuing. It is thought that the breast milk contains fatty acids that inhibit bilirubin conjugation in the neonatal liver. A factor in milk is also thought to increase the absorption of bilirubin in the duodenum.

Hyperbilirubinemia places the neonate at risk of developing a neurologic syndrome called *kernicterus*. This condition is caused by the accumulation of unconjugated bilirubin in brain cells. Unconjugated bilirubin is lipid-soluble, crosses the permeable blood-brain barrier of the neonate, and is deposited in cells of the basal ganglia to cause brain damage. Symptoms may appear 2 to 7 days after birth or later in the neonatal period. Lethargy, poor feeding, and short-term behavioral changes may be evident in mildly affected infants. Severe manifestations include rigidity, tremors, ataxia, and hearing loss. Extreme cases cause seizures and death. Most survivors are seriously damaged and by age 3 exhibit involuntary muscle spasm, seizures, mental retardation, and deafness. The potential for developing kernicterus is related to the level of unconjugated bilirubin in the serum, regardless of cause, and predisposing factors such as gestational age and weight. Signs and symptoms of kernicterus in term infants occur at indirect bilirubin levels of 25 to 30 mg/dl; less mature or ill infants are susceptible at lower levels.[28] Infants at risk for developing kernicterus are those with clinically apparent jaundice in the first 24 hours; an increase in total serum bilirubin of more than 5 mg/dl per day; a total bilirubin concentration higher than 12 mg/dl in term or 14 mg/dl in preterm infants; direct serum bilirubin levels higher than 1 mg/dl; and visible jaundice lasting for more than 1 week in term infants or 2 weeks in premature infants.[26]

Hyperbilirubinemia in the neonate is treated with phototherapy or exchange transfusion. Phototherapy is more commonly used to treat jaundiced infants and reduce the risk of kernicterus. Exposure to fluorescent light in the blue range of the visible spectrum (420- to 470-nm wavelength) reduces bilirubin levels. Bilirubin in the skin absorbs the light energy and is converted to a structural isomer that is more water soluble and can be excreted in the stool and urine. Effective treatment depends on the area of skin exposed and the infant's ability to metabolize and excrete bilirubin. Frequent monitoring of bilirubin levels, body temperature, and hydration is critical to the infant's care. Exchange transfusion is considered when signs of kernicterus are evident or hyperbilirubinemia is sustained or rising and unresponsive to phototherapy.

Hemolytic Disease of the Newborn

Erythroblastosis fetalis, or hemolytic disease of the newborn, occurs in Rh-positive infants of Rh-negative mothers who have been sensitized. The mother can produce anti-Rh antibodies from pregnancies in which the infants are Rh positive or by blood transfusions of Rh-positive blood. The Rh-negative mother usually becomes sensitized during the first few days after delivery, when fetal Rh-positive red cells from the placental site are released into the maternal circulation. Because the antibodies take several weeks to develop, the first Rh-positive infant of an Rh-negative mother usually is not affected. Infants with Rh-negative blood have no antigens on their red cells to react with the maternal antibodies and are not affected.

After an Rh-negative mother has been sensitized, the Rh antibodies from her blood are transferred to subsequent babies through the placental circulation. These antibodies react with the red cell antigens of the Rh-positive infant, causing agglutination and hemolysis. This leads to severe anemia with compensatory hyperplasia and enlargement of the blood-forming organs, including the spleen and liver, in the fetus. Liver function may be impaired, with decreased production of albumin causing massive edema, called *hydrops fetalis*. If blood levels of unconjugated bilirubin are abnormally high because of red cell hemolysis, there is danger of the infant's developing kernicterus. Only 10% of infants so affected survive.[29]

Three advances have served to decrease the threat to infants born to Rh-negative mothers: prevention of sensitization, intrauterine transfusion to the affected fetus, and exchange transfusion. The injection of *Rh immune globulin* (*i.e.*, gamma-globulin–containing Rh antibody) prevents sensitization in Rh-negative mothers who have given birth to Rh-positive infants if administered within 72 hours of delivery, abortion, genetic amniocentesis, or fetal-maternal bleeding. After sensitization has developed, the immune globulin is of no value. Since 1968, the year Rh immune globulin was introduced, the incidence of sensitization of Rh-negative women has dropped by more than 80%.[30] Early prenatal care and screening of maternal blood continue to be important in reducing immunization. Efforts to improve therapy are aimed at production of monoclonal anti-D, the Rh antibody.

In the past, about 20% of erythroblastotic fetuses died in utero. It is now possible to increase the chance of survival of such infants by studying the amniotic fluid to determine the bilirubin concentration, which reflects the severity of the disease. If the fetus is erythroblastotic, intrauterine transfusions of red cells are given into the fetus's peritoneal cavity or by the more difficult direct intravascular technique.[29] Exchange transfusions are administered after birth. In this technique, 10 to 20 ml of the infant's blood is removed and replaced with an equal amount of type O Rh-negative blood. This procedure is repeated until twice the blood volume of the infant has been exchanged. The exchange transfusion removes 85% to 90% of the hemolyzed red cells and about 25% of the total bilirubin, treating the anemia and hyperbilirubinemia.[29]

Red Cell Changes With Aging

Aging is associated with red cell changes. Bone marrow cellularity declines with age, from about 50% cellularity at age 65 to about 30% at age 75. The decline may reflect osteoporosis rather than a decrease in hematopoietic cells.[31]

Hemoglobin levels decline after middle age. In studies of men older than 60, mean hemoglobin levels ranged from 15.3 to 12.4 g/dl, with the lowest levels found in the oldest persons. The decline is less in women, with mean levels ranging from 13.8 to 11.7 mg/dl.[31] In most asymptomatic elderly persons, lower hemoglobin levels result from iron deficiency and anemia of chronic disease. Orally administered iron is poorly used in older adults, despite normal iron absorption. Underlying neoplasms also may contribute to anemia in this population.

In summary, hemoglobin concentrations at birth are high, reflecting the in utero need for oxygen delivery; toward the end of the first postnatal week, these levels begins to decline, gradually falling to a minimum value at about 2 months of age. During the early neonatal period, there is a shift from fetal to adult hemoglobin. Many babies develop physiologic jaundice due to hyperbilirubinemia during the first week of life, probably related to increased red cell breakdown and the inability of the infant's liver to conjugate bilirubin. The term kernicterus describes elevated levels of lipid-soluble, unconjugated bilirubin, which can be toxic to brain cells. Depending on severity, it is treated with phototherapy or exchange transfusions (or both). Hemolytic disease of the newborn occurs in Rh-positive infants of Rh-negative mothers who have been sensitized. It involves hemolysis of infant red cell in response to maternal Rh antibodies that have crossed the placenta. Administration of Rh immune globulin to the mother within 72 hours of delivery of an Rh-positive infant, abortion, or amniocentesis prevents sensitization. Aging is associated with red cell changes. Bone marrow cellularity decreases and there is a decrease in hemoglobin.

REFERENCES

1. Beck W.S. (1991). Erythropoiesis and introduction to the anemias. In Beck W.S. (Ed.). *Hematology* (5th ed., pp. 27, 29). Cambridge, MA: MIT Press.
2. Hillman R.S., Finch C.A. (1985). *Red cell manual* (5th ed., p. 33). Philadelphia: F.A. Davis.
3. Chandrasoma P., Taylor C.R. (1991). *Concise pathology* (p. 394). East Norwalk, CT: Appleton & Lange.
4. Beutler E. (1995). The sickle cell diseases and related disorders. In Beutler E., Lichtman A., Coller B.S., Kipps T.J. (Eds.). *William's hematology* (5th ed., p. 616). New York: McGraw-Hill.
5. Lane P. (1996). Sickle cell disease. In Buchanan G.R. (Ed.). *Pediatric Clinics of North America* (vol. 43, pp. 639–666). Philadelphia: W.B. Saunders.
6. Brown A.K., Sleeper L.A., Miller S.T., et al. (1994). Reference values and hematologic changes from birth to 5 years in patients with sickle cell disease. *Archives of Pediatric and Adolescent Medicine* 148, 796.
7. Charache S., Terrin M.L., Moore R.D. et al. (1995). Effect of hydroxyurea on the frequency of painful crises in sickle cell anemia. *New England Journal of Medicine* 332, 1317.
8. Walters M.C. Patience M., Leisenring W., et al. (1996). Bone marrow transplantation for sickle cell disease. *New England Journal of Medicine* 335, 369.
9. Cotran R.S., Kumar V., Robbins S.L. (Eds.). (1994). *Robbin's pathologic basis of disease* (5th ed. p. 595). Philadelphia: W.B. Saunders.
10. Nathan D.G. (1991). The thalassemias. In Beck W.S. (Ed.). *Hematology* (5th ed., p. 213). Cambridge, MA: MIT Press.
11. Churchill W.H., Jr., Jandl J.H. (1991). Hemolytic anemias II. Immunohemolytic anemias. In Beck W.S. (Ed.). *Hematology* (5th ed., p. 246). Cambridge, MA: MIT Press.
12. Committee on Technical Manual, Widmann F.K. (Ed.). (1985). *Technical manual* (9th ed., pp. 260, 128). Arlington, VA: American Association of Blood Banks.
13. Bubley G.J., Lange R.F. (1993). Microcytic anemias. In Robinson S.H., Reich P.R. (Eds.). *Hematology, pathophysiological basis for clinical practice* (3rd ed. p. 35). Boston: Little, Brown.
14. Beck W.S. (1991). Hypochromic anemias I. Iron deficiency and excess. In Beck W.S. (Ed.). *Hematology* (5th ed., p. 135). Cambridge, MA: MIT Press.
15. Fairbanks V.F., Beutler E. (1995). Iron deficiency. In Beutler E., Lichtman M.A., Coller B.S., Kipps T.J. (Eds.). *William's hematology* (5th ed. p.490) New York: McGraw-Hill.
16. Lane M., Johnson C.L. (1981). Prevalence of iron deficiency. In Oski F.A., Pearson H.A. (Eds.). *Iron nutrition revisited—infancy, childhood, adolescence: Report of the Eighty-Second Ross Conference on Pediatric Research* (pp. 31–46). Columbus, OH: Ross Laboratories.
17. Babior B.M. (1995). The megaloblastic anemias. In Beutler E., Lichtman M.A., Coller B.S., Kipps T.J. (Eds.). *William's hematology* (5th ed., p. 471). New York: McGraw-Hill.

18. Beck W.S. (1991). Normocytic anemias. In Beck W.S. (Ed.). *Hematology* (5th ed., pp. 72, 78). Cambridge, MA: MIT Press.
19. Caro J., Erslev A.J. (1995) Anemia of chronic renal failure. In Beutler E., Lichtman M.A., Coller B.S., Kipps T.J. (Eds.). *William's hematology* (5th ed., p. 456). New York: McGraw-Hill.
20. Erslev A.J. (1995). Anemia of chronic disease. In Beutler E., Lichtman M.A., Coller B.S., Kipps T.J. (Eds.). *William's hematology* (5th ed., p. 518). New York: McGraw-Hill.
21. Huestis D.W., Bove J.R., Case J. (1988). *Practical blood transfusion* (4th ed., pp. 211, 226, 254, 259). Boston: Little, Brown.
22. Toy P.T.C.Y., Strauss R.G., Stehling L., et al. (1987). Predeposited autologous blood for elective surgery. *New England Journal of Medicine* 316, 517.
23. Pittiglio D.H. (Ed.). (1983). *Modern blood banking and transfusion practices* (pp. 91–92). Philadelphia: F.A. Davis.
24. Brown M.S. (1988). Physiologic anemia of infancy: Nutritional factors and abnormal states. In Stockman J.A., Pochedly C. (Eds.). *Developmental and neonatal hematology* (pp. 252, 274). New York: Raven Press.
25. Segel G.B. (1995). Hematology of the newborn. In Beutler E., Lichtman M.A., Coller B.S., Kipps T.J. (Eds.). *William's hematology* (5th ed., p. 59). New York: McGraw-Hill.
26. Kliegman R.M. (1996). The fetus and neonatal infant. In Behrman R.E., Kliegman R.M., Nelson W.E., Vaughan V.C. (Eds.). (1996). *Nelson textbook of pediatrics* (15th ed., pp. 493–499). Philadelphia: W.B. Saunders.
27. Hazinski M.F. (1992). *Nursing care of the critically ill child* (2nd ed., p. 739). St. Louis: Mosby–Year Book.
28. Cashore W.J. (1994). Neonatal hyperbilirubinemia. In Oski F.A., DeAngelis C.D., Feigin R.D., Warshaw J.B. (Eds.). *Principles and practice of pediatrics* (2nd ed., p. 447–445). Philadelphia: J.B. Lippincott.
29. Bowman J.M. (1988). Alloimmune hemolytic disease of the neonate. In Stockman J.A., Pochedly C. (Eds.). *Developmental and neonatal hematology* (pp. 226, 232, 233). New York: Raven Press.
30. Bowman J.M. (1988). The prevention of Rh immunization. *Transfusion Medicine Reviews* 2, 129.
31. Williams W.J. (1995). Hematology in the aged. In Beutler E., Lichtman M.A., Coller B.S., Kipps T.J. (Eds.). *William's hematology* (5th ed., p. 73). New York: McGraw-Hill.

ADDITIONAL READINGS

Agency for Health Care Policy and Research. (1993) *Sickle cell disease: Screening, diagnosis, management, and counseling in newborns and infants.* Rockville, MD: Agency for Health Care Policy and Research, AHCPR Pub. No. 93–0562, 93–0563, and 93–0564.

Arese P., DeFlora A. (1990). Denaturation of normal and abnormal erythrocytes: II Pathophysiology of hemolysis in glucose-6-phosphate dehydrogenase deficiency. *Seminars in Hematology* 27, 1.

Boyd H.K., Lappin T.R.J. (1991). Erythropoietin deficiency in the anemia of chronic disorders. *European Journal of Haematology* 46, 198.

Brugger W., Heimfeld S., Berenson R.J., Mertelsmann R., Kanz L. (1995). Reconstitution of hematopoiesis after high-dose chemotherapy by autologous progenitor cells generated ex vivo. *New England Journal of Medicine* 333, 283.

Castro O., Brambilla D.J., Thorington B., et al. (1994). The acute chest syndrome in sickle cell disease: Incidence and risk factors. *Blood* 84, 643.

Duggan D.B. (1992). Anemia in the hospitalized patient. *Hospital Practice* 27, 125.

Embury S.H. (1996). New treatments of sickle cell disease. *Western Journal of Medicine* 164, 444.

Kazazian H.H. (1990). The thalassemia syndromes: Molecular basis and prenatal diagnosis in 1990. *Seminars in Hematology* 27, 209.

Luban N.L.C. (1993). The new and the old molecular diagnostics and hemolytic disease of the newborn. *New England Journal of Medicine* 329, 658.

McManus M.L., Churchwell K.B., Strange K. (1995). Regulation of cell volume in health and disease. *New England Journal of Medicine* 333, 1260.

Weatherall D.J. (1992). Bone marrow transplantation for thalassemia and other inherited disorders of hemoglobin. *Blood* 80, 1379.

CHAPTER 9

Disorders of White Blood Cells and Lymphoid Tissues

Kathryn Ann Caudell

The white blood cells protect the body against invasion by foreign agents. They include phagocytic cells (*i.e.,* granulocytes and monocytes), which mediate innate immune responses, and the lymphocytes (*i.e.,* B cells and T cells), which are involved in acquired immunity. Disorders of white blood cells fall into two broad categories: deficiency disorders and proliferative disorders. This chapter focuses on disorders of white blood cell deficiency, infectious mononucleosis a self-limiting benign lymphoproliferative disorder, the leukemias and myeloproliferative disorders, malignant lymphomas, and multiple myeloma. The origin and differentiation of the white blood cells were discussed in Chapter 6. The lymphoid system is presented in Chapter 11.

Hematopoietic and Lymphoid Tissues

After you have completed this section of the chapter, you should be able to meet the following objectives:

- List the cells and tissues of the hematopoietic system
- Trace the development of the different blood cells from their origin in the pluripotent bone marrow stem cell to their circulation in the blood stream

The hematopoietic system encompasses all the blood cells, their precursors, and their derivatives: red blood cells, thrombocytes or platelets, and white blood cells. It includes the *myeloid* or bone marrow tissue in which the white blood cells are formed, and the *lymphoid* tissues of the lymph nodes, thymus, and spleen, in which the white blood cells circulate and mature. The development of different cell lineages depends on cellular interactions and exposure to cytokines.

White Blood Cells

The white blood cells include granulocytes (*i.e.,* neutrophils, eosinophils, and basophils), the monocyte and macrophage lineage, and lymphocytes. Granulocytes and monocytes are derived from the myeloid stem cell in the bone marrow and circulate in the blood. T cells and B cells originate in bone marrow and migrate between blood and lymph. T lymphocytes mature in the thymus, and B cells mature in the bone marrow, the mammalian equivalent of the avian bursa of Fabricius.[1] Another population of lymphocytes includes the large granular lymphocytes, or natural killer cells, which do not share characteristics of the T lymphocytes or the B lymphocytes, but they do have the ability to lyse target cells.[2]

The Bone Marrow and Hematopoiesis

The entire hematopoietic system, in all its complexity, arises from a small number of stem cells that differentiate to form blood cells and replenish bone marrow by a process of self-renewal. All the hematopoietic precursors, including the erythroid (red blood cell), myelocyte (granulocyte and monocyte), lymphocyte (T cell and B cell), and megakaryocyte (platelet) series, are derived from a small population of cells called the *pluripotent stem cells*. These cells are capable of providing progenitor cells (*i.e.*, parent cells) for lymphopoiesis and myelopoiesis, processes by which lymphoid and myeloid blood cells are made, respectively. Several levels of differentiation lead to the development of committed unipotent cells, which are the progenitors for each of the blood cell types. The progenitor cells lose their capacity for self-renewal but retain the potential to differentiate into erythrocytes, monocytes, megakaryocytes, or lymphocytes. This regulation of blood cells is thought to be at least partially controlled by protein hormone messengers, called *cytokines*, that regulate the function of other cells, in this case the blood cell precursors.[3,4]

The colony-stimulating factors (CSFs) are a family of glycoproteins that support hematopoietic colony formation. Several of the CSFs influence the growth and development of many cell lines and are known as multilineage CSFs. Interleukin-3 acts on the most immature marrow progenitor cells, promoting the development of cells that can differentiate into a number of cell types. Stem cell factor (also called *c-kit* ligand), mediates the activation of stem cells and stimulates their differentiation into various cell lineages. There are several lineage-specific CSFs: erythropoietin, granulocyte CSF (G-CSF), monocyte-macrophage CSF, and interleukins. Although the CSFs act at different points in the proliferation and differentiation pathway, their functions overlap. Other cytokines, such as interleukin-1, interleukin-4, interleukin-6, and interferon, act synergistically to support the functions of the CSFs (see Chapter 11).[5]

The identification and characterization of the various cytokines and growth factors have led to their use in treating a wide range of diseases, including bone marrow failure, hematopoietic neoplasms, infectious diseases, congenital and myeloproliferative disorders. Many of these uses are investigational.

Lymphoid Tissues

The body's lymphatic system, which consists of the lymphatic vessels, lymph nodes, spleen, and thymus, is made up of lymphoid tissue (see Chapter 11). Lymph is body fluid that originates as excess fluid from the capillaries. It is returned to the vascular compartment and the right side of the heart through lymphatic vessels.

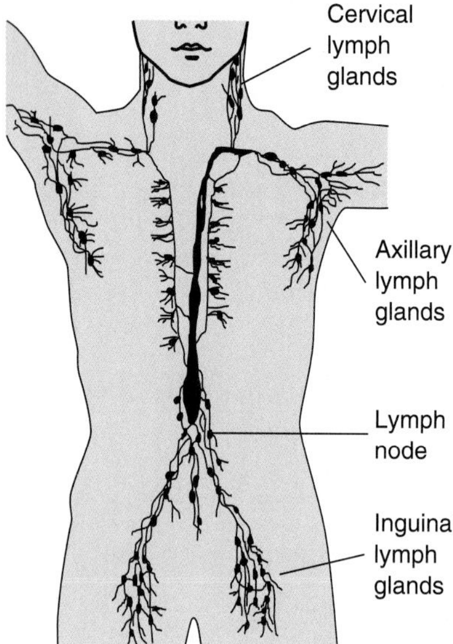

Figure 9-1
Location of a portion of the lymph nodes in the human body. (*What you need to know about Hodgkin's disease.* [1981]. Washington, DC: Department of Health and Human Services)

The lymph nodes, which are situated along the lymphatic channels, filter the lymph before it is returned to the circulation (Fig. 9–1). Lymph enters a lymph node through afferent lymphatic channels, percolates through a labyrinthine system of minute channels lined with endothelial and phagocytic cells, and then emerges through efferent lymphatic vessels. A number of efferent vessels join to form collecting trunks. Each collecting trunk drains a definite area of the body. By filtering bacteria and other particulate matter, the lymph nodes serve as a secondary line of defense even when clinical disease is not present. In the event of malignant neoplasm development, cancer cells are filtered and retained by the lymph nodes for a period before being disseminated to other parts of the body. Because of their contribution to the development of the immune system, lymph nodes are relatively large at birth and progressively atrophy throughout life.

Disorders of White Blood Cell Deficiency

After you have completed this section of the chapter, you should be able to meet the following objectives:

- Define the terms leukopenia, neutropenia, granulocytopenia, and aplastic anemia
- Cite two general causes of neutropenia
- Describe the mechanism of symptom production in neutropenia

The number of leukocytes, or white blood cells, in the peripheral circulation normally ranges from 5000 to 10,000/μl of blood. About 50% to 70% of the leukocytes are granulocytes (50% to 70% neutrophils, 1% to 4% eosinophils, and 0.4% basophils), 20% to 30% are lymphocytes, and 2% to 8% are monocytes. The term *leukopenia* describes an absolute decrease in white blood cell numbers. The disorder may affect any of the specific types of white blood cells, but most often it affects the neutrophils, which are the predominant type of granulocyte.

Neutropenia

Neutropenia, also called *granulocytopenia,* refers specifically to a decrease in neutrophils. It commonly is defined as a circulating neutrophil count of less than 1500 cells/μl. Agranulocytosis, which denotes a severe granulocytopenia, is characterized by a circulating neutrophil count of less than 200 cells/μl.[6]

Neutropenia can be acquired or congenital. It usually is the result of one or more of the following: a decrease in the production of neutrophils (*i.e.,* granulopoiesis) by the bone marrow; impairment of release from the bone marrow; increased destruction of neutrophils leading to depletion of neutrophil numbers contained in bone marrow storage pools; and abnormal distribution of neutrophils leading to a pseudoneutropenia.[6] The causes of neutropenia are summarized in Table 9-1.

Acquired Neutropenia

Granulopoiesis is impaired due to complication of certain procedures such as chemotherapy and irradiation or disease conditions such as aplastic anemia systemic lupus erythematosus, rheumatoid arthritis, or infectious mononucleosis, which interfere with the formation of all blood cells. Infectious processes by viruses or bacteria may drain neutrophils from the blood faster than they can be replaced, thereby depleting the neutrophil storage pool in the bone marrow.[6] Overgrowth of neoplastic cells in cases of nonmyelocytic leukemia and lymphoma may also suppress the function of neutrophil precursors. Because of the neutrophil's short life span of about 1 day in the peripheral blood, neutropenia occurs rapidly when granulopoiesis is impaired. Under these conditions, neutropenia usually is accompanied by thrombocytopenia (*i.e.,* platelet deficiency).

In *aplastic anemia,* all of the myeloid stem cells are affected, resulting in anemia, thrombocytopenia, and agranulocytosis. Autoimmune disorders or idiosyncratic drug reactions may cause increased and premature destruction of neutrophils. In splenomegaly, neutrophils may be trapped in the spleen along with other blood cells. In Felty's syndrome, a variant of rheumatoid arthritis, there is increased destruction of neutrophils in the spleen. Most cases of neutropenia are drug related. Chemotherapeutic drugs used in the treatment of cancer (*e.g.,* alkylating agents, antimetabolites) cause predictable dose-dependent suppression of bone marrow function.

The term *idiosyncratic* is used to describe drug reactions that are different from the effects obtained in most persons and that cannot be explained in terms of allergy. A number of drugs, such as chloramphenicol (an antibiotic), phenothiazine tranquilizers, sulfonamides, propylthiouracil (used in treatment of hyperthyroidism), and phenylbutazone (used in the treatment of arthritis), may cause idiosyncratic depression of bone marrow function. Some drugs, such as hydantoin derivatives and primidone (used in the treatment of seizure disorders), can cause intramedullary destruction of granulocytes and thereby impair production. Many idiosyncratic cases of drug-induced neutropenia are thought to be caused by immunologic mechanisms, with the drug or its metabolites acting as antigens (*i.e.,* haptens) to incite the

TABLE 9-1

Causes of Neutropenia

Cause	Mechanism
Accelerated removal (*e.g.,* inflammation and infection)	Removal of neutrophils from the circulation exceeds production
Drug-induced granulocytopenia	
Defective production	
Cytotoxic drugs used in cancer therapy	Predictable damage to precursor cells, usually dose dependent
Phenothiazine, thiouracil, chloramphenicol, phenylbutazone, and others	Idiosyncratic depression of bone marrow function
Hydantoinates, primidone, and others	Intramedullary destruction of granulocytes
Immune destruction	Immunologic mechanisms with cytolysis or leukoagglutination
Aminopyrine, and others	
Periodic or cyclic neutropenia (occurs during infancy and later)	Unknown
Neoplasms involving bone marrow (*e.g.,* leukemias and lymphomas)	Overgrowth of neoplastic cells, which crowd out granulopoietic precursors
Idiopathic neutropenia that occurs in the absence of other disease or provoking influence	Autoimmune reaction
Felty's syndrome	Intrasplenic destruction of neutrophils

production of antibodies reactive against the neutrophils. Neutrophils possess human leukocyte antigens (HLA) and other antigens specific to a given leukocyte line. Antibodies to these specific antigens have been identified in some cases of drug-induced neutropenia.[6]

Congenital Neutropenia

Periodic or cyclic neutropenia is a genetic disorder (*i.e.,* autosomal dominant with various expression) that begins in infancy and persists for decades. It is characterized by periodic neutropenia that develops every 21 to 30 days and lasts about 3 to 6 days. Although the cause is undetermined, it is thought to result from impaired feedback regulation of granulocyte production and release. Another congenital autosomal dominant agranulocytosis of the Kostmann type causes severe neutropenia while preserving the erythroid and megakaryocyte cell lineages. The total white blood cell count may be within normal limits, but the neutrophil count is less than 200/μl. Monocyte and eosinophil levels may be elevated.[6] Transient neutropenia occurs in neonates whose mothers have hypertension. It usually lasts from 1 to 60 hours but can persist for 3 to 30 days. This type of neutropenia, which is associated with increased risk of nosocomial infection, is thought to result from transiently reduced neutrophil production.[7]

Manifestations and Treatment

Because the neutrophil is essential to the cellular phase of inflammation, infections are common in persons with neutropenia, and extreme caution is needed to protect them from exposure to infectious organisms. Infections that may go unnoticed in a person with a normal neutrophil count can prove fatal in a person with neutropenia.

The clinical features of neutropenia usually stem from severe infections that are characteristic of the disorder. These infections commonly are caused by organisms that colonize the skin and the gastrointestinal tract. However, the most common site of serious infection is the respiratory tract. Bacteria, fungi, and protozoa frequently colonize upper and lower respiratory tracts. The signs and symptoms initially include malaise, chills, and fever, followed by extreme weakness and fatigue. The white blood cell count often is reduced to 1000/μl and, in certain cases, may fall to 200 to 300/μl. Ulcerative necrotizing lesions of the mouth are common in neutropenia. Ulcerations of the skin, vagina, and gastrointestinal tract may also occur.[8]

Antibiotics are used to treat infections in those situations in which neutrophil destruction can be controlled or the neutropoietic function of the bone marrow can be recovered. CSFs such as G-CSF and granulocyte-macrophage CSF (GM-CSF) are being used more commonly to stimulate the maturation and differentiation of the polymorphonuclear cell lineage. Treatment with these biologic response modifiers has reduced the period of neutropenia and the risk of developing potentially fatal septicemia.

In summary. neutropenia, a marked reduction in the number of circulating neutrophils, is one of the major disorders of the white blood cells. It can be acquired or congenital in nature and result from a combination of mechanisms. Severe neutropenia can occur as a complication of lymphoproliferative diseases, in which neoplastic cells crowd out neutrophil precursor cells, or of radiation therapy or treatment with cytotoxic drugs, which destroy neutrophil precursor cells. Neutropenia may also be encountered as an idiosyncratic reaction to various drugs. Because the neutrophil is essential to the cellular stage of inflammation, severe and often life-threatening infections are common in persons with neutropenia.

Infectious Mononucleosis

After you have completed this section of the chapter, you should be able to meet the following objectives:

- Name the virus that causes infectious mononucleosis and describe how it is spread
- Describe the pathogenesis and manifestations of infectious mononucleosis
- List the signs and symptoms of infectious mononucleosis

Infectious mononucleosis is a self-limiting lymphoproliferative disorder caused by the Epstein-Barr virus (EBV). One of the herpesviruses, EBV, is ubiquitous in all human populations. Infectious mononucleosis is most prevalent in adolescents and young adults in the upper socioeconomic classes in developed countries. This is probably because the disease, which is relatively asymptomatic when it occurs during childhood, confers complete immunity to the virus. In upper socioeconomic families, exposure to the virus may be delayed until late adolescence or early adulthood. In such persons, the mode of infection, size of the viral pool, and physiologic and immunologic condition of the host may determine whether or not the infection occurs.

Infectious mononucleosis has been called the "kissing disease," and evidence suggests that exposure to EBV-contaminated saliva is one of the main modes of transfer. The virus undergoes a replicative cycle in the oropharyngeal epithelium and then invades the blood by selectively infecting B cells, a cell population that has specific surface receptors for the virus. It is shed from the oropharynx for as long as 18 months after primary infection; thereafter, it may be spread intermittently by persons who are EBV seropositive despite the absence of clinical disease.[9] Immunosuppressed persons shed the virus more frequently. Asymptomatic shedding of EBV by healthy persons accounts for most of the spread of infectious mononucleosis, despite the fact that it is not a highly contagious disease.

Pathogenesis

Infectious mononucleosis is characterized by fever, generalized lymphadenopathy, sore throat (*i.e.,* pharyngitis), and the appearance in the blood of atypical lymphocytes. In the course of infection, EBV invades the B cells of oropharyngeal lymphoid tissues. Replication of the virus ensues, with the subsequent death of the B cells and release of the virus into the blood, causing the febrile reaction and specific immunologic responses. Concurrent with the febrile reaction, antiviral antibodies (*i.e.*, immunoglobulin M and immunoglobulin G) appear, and the virus disappears from the blood. Other virus-determined antibodies develop, including the well-known *heterophil* (*i.e.*, the Paul-Bunnel antibody) that is used in the diagnosis of infectious mononucleosis.

Although infectious B cells and free virions disappear from the blood, some EBV-transformed B cells remain in the circulation with the genome of the virus integrated into their genetic structure. These B cells display virus-directed membrane antigens. These B-cell antigens stimulate production of cytotoxic ($CD8^+$) and suppressor ($CD4^+$) T cells. Together, the suppressor-cytotoxic ($CD8^+$) T cells are the atypical lymphocytes seen in the blood of patients with infectious mononucleosis. The proliferation of atypical lymphocytes throughout the body is responsible for the lymphadenopathy and hepatosplenomegaly. The progressive increase in the number of EBV-specific antibodies and cytotoxic ($CD8^+$) T cells eventually brings the disease under control and eliminates the latently infected B cells.[9]

Manifestations

The onset of infectious mononucleosis usually is insidious. The incubation period lasts between 4 to 8 weeks. A prodromal period follows, which lasts for several days and is characterized by malaise, anorexia, and chills. The prodromal period precedes the onset of fever, pharyngitis, and lymphadenopathy. Occasionally, the disorder comes on abruptly with a high fever. Most persons seek medical attention for severe pharyngitis, which is usually the most severe for 5 to 7 days and persists for 7 to 14 days. Severe toxic pharyngotonsillitis may cause airway obstruction.

Lymphadenopathy affects 90% of patients, who have symmetrically enlarged and often tender lymph nodes. Its duration is variable but seldom exceeds 3 weeks. Hepatitis and splenomegaly are common manifestations of infectious mononucleosis and are thought to be immune mediated. Hepatitis is characterized by hepatomegaly, nausea, anorexia, and jaundice. Although discomforting, it usually is a benign condition that resolves without causing permanent liver damage. The spleen may be enlarged two to three times its normal size, and rupture of the spleen is an infrequent complication. A rash that resembles rubella develops in 10% to 15% of cases.[9] Treatment with amoxicillin or ampicillin frequently produces skin eruptions.[10] The reason for this is unknown. Fewer than 1% of cases, mostly in the adult age group, develop complications of the central nervous system (CNS). These complications include cranial nerve palsies, encephalitis, meningitis, transverse myelitis, and Guillain-Barré syndrome.

The peripheral blood usually shows an increase in the number of leukocytes, with a white blood cell count between 12,000 and 18,000/µl, 95% of which are lymphocytes. The rise in white blood cells begins during the first week; rises even higher during the second week of the infection, and then returns to normal around the fourth week. Although leukocytosis is common, leukopenia may be seen in some persons during the first 3 days of the illness. Atypical lymphocytes are common, constituting more than 20% of the total lymphocyte count. Heterophil antibodies usually appear during the second or third week and decline after the acute illness has subsided. They may, however, be detectable for up to 9 months after onset of the disease.

Most persons with infectious mononucleosis recover without incident. The acute phase of the illness usually lasts for 2 to 3 weeks, after which recovery occurs rapidly. Some degree of debility and lethargy may persist for 2 to 3 months.

Diagnosis and Treatment

Diagnosis is based on the clinical features of fever, pharyngitis, and lymphadenopathy, coupled with the presence of atypical lymphocytes and heterophil antibodies. EBV-specific antibody studies may facilitate diagnosis in heterophil-negative cases. Treatment usually is symptomatic and supportive. It includes bed rest and analgesics such as aspirin to relieve the fever, headache, and sore throat. In cases of severe pharyngotonsillitis, corticosteroids are given to reduce inflammation.

In summary, infectious mononucleosis is a self-limited lymphoproliferative disorder caused by the B lymphocytotropic EBV, a member of herpesvirus family. The highest incidence of infectious mononucleosis is found in adolescents and young adults and is seen more frequently in the upper socioeconomic classes of developed countries The disease is characterized by fever, generalized lymphadenopathy, sore throat (i.e., pharyngitis), and the appearance in the blood of atypical lymphocytes and several antibodies, including the well-known heterophil antibodies that are used in the diagnosis of infectious mononucleosis.

Neoplastic Disorders of Hematopoietic and Lymphoid Origin

After you have completed this section of the chapter, you should be able to meet the following objectives:

- Use the predominant white blood cell type and classification of acute or chronic to describe the four general types of leukemia
- State the warning signs of acute leukemia

- Explain the manifestations of leukemia in terms of altered cell differentiation
- Describe the following complications of acute leukemia and its treatment: leukostasis, tumor lysis syndrome, hyperuricemia, and blast crisis
- State the difference between syngeneic, allogeneic, and autologous bone marrow transplantation

The leukemias are malignant neoplasms of cells originally derived from the hematopoietic stem cell. They are characterized by diffuse replacement of bone marrow with unregulated proliferating immature neoplastic cells. In most cases, the leukemic cells spill out into the blood, where they are seen in large numbers. The term *leukemia* (*i.e.,* white blood) was first used by Virchow to describe a reversal of the usual ratio of red blood cells to white blood cells. Leukemia is thought to arise after the malignant transformation of a single hematopoietic cell line. The leukemic cells proliferate mainly in the bone marrow, circulate in the blood, and infiltrate the spleen, lymph nodes, and other tissues.

Leukemia strikes about 28,000 persons in the United States each year. In 1996, approximately 27,600 new cases were diagnosed, and about 21,000 persons died of this disease.[11] More children are stricken with leukemia than with any other form of cancer, and it is the leading cause of death in children between the ages of 3 and 14 years. Although leukemia commonly is thought of as a childhood disease, it strikes more adults than children: 27,600 adults per year compared with 2500 children.

Advances in molecular biology have contributed greatly to an understanding of leukemic cell types, including the early stages of cell differentiation and gene function. This information has greatly influenced the diagnosis, treatment, and prognosis of patients with leukemia.

Classification

The leukemias commonly are classified according to their predominant cell type (*i.e.,* lymphocytic or myelocytic) and whether the condition is acute or chronic. A rudimentary classification system divides leukemia into four types: acute lymphocytic (lymphoblastic) leukemia (ALL), chronic lymphocytic leukemia (CLL), acute myelocytic (myeloblastic) leukemia (AML), and chronic myelocytic leukemia (CML). The lymphocytic leukemias involve immature lymphocytes and their progenitors that originate in the bone marrow but infiltrate the spleen, lymph nodes, CNS, and other tissues. The myelocytic leukemias, which involve the pluripotent myeloid stem cells in bone marrow, interfere with the maturation of all blood cells, including the granulocytes, erythrocytes, and thrombocytes.

ALL is the most common leukemia in childhood, with a peak incidence between the ages of 2 and 4 years. Approximately 2000 children are diagnosed with ALL in the United States yearly, whereas roughly 500 children are diagnosed with AML.[12] CLL affects older persons; fewer than 10% of those who develop the disease are younger than 50 years old. AML is seen most often between the ages of 13 and 39 years and CML between the ages of 30 and 50 years.

Causes

The causes of leukemia are unknown. The incidence of leukemia among persons who have been exposed to high levels of radiation is unusually high. The number of cases of leukemia reported in the most heavily exposed survivors of the atomic blasts at Hiroshima and Nagasaki during the 20-year period from 1950 to 1970 was nearly 30 times the expected rate.[13] An increased incidence of leukemia also is associated with exposure to benzene and the use of antitumor drugs and chloramphenicol. Leukemia may occur as a second cancer after aggressive chemotherapy for other cancers, such as Hodgkin's disease,[14] gastrointestinal cancers,[15] ovarian cancer,[16] and ALL.[17,18] AML is the most common type of secondary cancer.

A significant number of cases of leukemia have been reported in identical twins. An identical twin of a person with acute leukemia has a 25% chance of developing the disease, whereas a fraternal twin has little excess risk. Leukemia is relatively frequently associated with congenital chromosomal abnormalities such as Down syndrome, Klinefelter's syndrome, and Turner's syndrome.

Advances in cytogenetic studies have made it increasingly evident that many forms of leukemia are associated with nonrandom chromosomal changes (usually translocations). For example, the Philadelphia chromosome (*i.e.,* translocation from chromosome 22 to chromosome 9)[19] is present in about 90% of persons with CML.[20] In many cases, these chromosomal aberrations, which are present at diagnosis, disappear with treatment and remission and then reappear with relapse. The underlying cause of these chromosomal changes is unknown. It is possible, however, to try to correlate the chromosomes that are affected with the genes involved. This may lead to increased understanding of the pathogenesis of leukemia and to the discovery of new methods of diagnosis and treatment.

Clinical Manifestations

A leukemic cell is an immature and mobile type of white blood cell. As explained in Chapter 5, differentiation of a cell line determines its structure, function, and life span. Because leukemic cells are immature and poorly differentiated, they are capable of an increased rate of proliferation and have a prolonged life span. They cannot perform the functions of mature leukocytes and are therefore ineffective as phagocytes. Because they proliferate rapidly, leukemic cells interfere with the maturation of normal bone marrow cells, including the erythroblasts (red blood cells) and the megakaryoblasts (platelets). The mobile cells can travel throughout the circulatory system, cross the blood-brain barrier, and infiltrate many body organs.

Acute Leukemias

Acute leukemia is a cancer of the hematopoietic stem cells. It usually has a sudden and stormy onset of signs and symptoms related to depressed bone marrow function (Table 9-2). Most patients present for medical evaluation within 3 months of the onset of symptoms. They may have mild pancytopenia (*i.e.*, anemia, thrombocytopenia, and neutropenia), a normal leukocyte count and absence of blast cells, or leukocytosis and circulating blast cells. Generalized lymphadenopathy, splenomegaly, and hepatomegaly caused by infiltration of leukemic cells occur in all acute leukemias but are more common in ALL. The patients may also complain of malaise, lethargy, weight loss, fever, night sweats, bone or joint pain, and genitourinary manifestations such as cystitis. They may exhibit hematuria, renal failure, hyperuricemia, uric acid nephropathy, and testicular involvement.[21]

According to the American Cancer Society, the warning signs and symptoms of acute leukemia are fatigue, pallor, weight loss, repeated infections, easy bruising, nosebleeds and other types of hemorrhage.[23] These features may appear suddenly in children. Both ALL and AML are characterized by fatigue resulting from anemia; bleeding because of a decreased platelet count; and bone marrow involvement, including subperiosteal infiltration, marrow expansion, and bone resorption, which causes bone tenderness and pain. Infection results from neutropenia, with the risk of infection becoming high as the neutrophil count falls below 500/μl.

A definitive diagnosis of acute leukemia is based on blood and bone marrow studies; it requires the demonstration of leukemic cells in the peripheral blood, bone marrow, or extramedullary tissue. Laboratory findings reveal the presence of immature (blasts) white blood cells in the circulation and bone marrow, where they may constitute 60% to 100% of the cells.[22] As these cells proliferate and begin to crowd the bone marrow, the development of other cell lineages in the marrow is suppressed. Consequently, there is a loss of mature myeloid cells, such as erythrocytes, granulocytes, and platelets. Anemia is almost always present, and the platelet count is decreased.

Signs and symptoms of CNS involvement occur in ALL and AML and include headache, nausea, vomiting, cranial nerve palsies, papilledema, and occasionally seizures and coma. The latter two are more common in children than in adults and in ALL than in AML. *Leukostasis*, a condition in which the circulating blast count is markedly elevated (usually >100,000μl), leading to impaired circulation, presents as headache, confusion, and dyspnea. Once identified, this condition requires immediate and effective treatment, including leukapheresis (*i.e.*, removal of white blood cells) and chemotherapy.

Hyperuricemia occurs as the result of increased proliferation or increased purine breakdown secondary to leukemic cell death that results from chemotherapy. It may increase before and during treatment. Prophylactic therapy with allopurinol is routinely administered to prevent renal complications secondary to uric acid

TABLE 9-2

Clinical Manifestations of Leukemia and Their Pathologic Basis*

Clinical Manifestations	Pathologic Basis
Bone marrow depression	
Malaise, easy fatigability	Anemia
Fever	Infection or increased metabolism by neoplastic cells
Bleeding	Decreased thrombocytes
Petechiae	
Ecchymosis	
Gingival bleeding	
Epistaxis	
Bone pain and tenderness upon palpation	Subperiosteal bone infiltration, bone marrow expansion, and bone resorption
Headache, nausea, vomiting, papilledema, cranial nerve palsies, seizures, coma	Leukemic infiltration of central nervous system
Abdominal discomfort	Generalized lymphadenopathy, hepatomegaly, splenomegaly due to leukemic cell infiltration
Increased vulnerability to infections	Immaturity of the white cells and ineffective immune function
Hematologic abnormalities	Physical and metabolic encroachment of leukemia cells on red blood cell and thrombocyte precursors
Anemia	
Thrombocytopenia	
Hyperuricemia and other metabolic disorders	Abnormal proliferation and metabolism of leukemic cells

*Manifestations vary with the type of leukemia.

crystallization in the urine. Chemotherapy and selective irradiation (*e.g.*, CNS irradiation) are used in the treatment of acute leukemia. Chemotherapy includes induction therapy designed to elicit a remission, intensification therapy after a remission is achieved to further reduce the leukemic cell population, and maintenance therapy to maintain remission. Remission is defined as eradication of leukemic cells as detectable by conventional technology. Massive necrosis of malignant cells can occur during the initial phase of treatment. This phenomenon, known as *tumor lysis syndrome*, can lead to life-threatening metabolic disorders, including hyperkalemia, hyperphosphatemia, hyperuricemia, hypomagnesemia, hypocalcemia, and acidosis, with the potential for causing acute renal failure. Prophylactic aggressive hydration with alkaline solutions and administration of allopurinol to reduce uric acid levels is given to counteract these effects.[24]

Bone marrow transplantation (BMT) from an identical twin (*i.e.*, syngeneic transplantation) or an HLA-matched sibling or unrelated donor (*i.e.*, allogeneic transplantation) has proved effective in treating ALL and AML. BMT is usually considered after the patient has achieved remission from the induction therapy. The BMT procedure involves first treating the recipient of the transplant with lethally high doses of chemotherapy alone or with irradiation (the conditioning regimen) to eliminate all the leukemic cells, followed by infusion of the bone marrow from the donor. Potential complications that can result from the conditioning regimen include gastrointestinal side effects such as nausea, vomiting, diarrhea, mucositis, and anorexia; hemorrhagic cystitis from high-dose cyclophosphamide, syndrome of inappropriate antidiuretic hormone from cyclophosphamide, tumor lysis syndrome, veno-occlusive disease, diffuse lung damage, and irreversible cardiac damage[25]

A complication unique to allogeneic transplantation is graft-versus-host disease (see Chapter 12), in which the donor's immune system engrafts in the recipient and proceeds to recognize the recipient's tissues as foreign subsequently mounting an immune response. Autologous (self) transplantation has also been used in the treatment of acute leukemia. In this approach, the leukemic patient's own bone marrow is collected during remission, cryopreserved, and then reinfused after treatment to destroy all the leukemic cells. One of the problems with autologous bone marrow transplantation is the probable contamination of the bone marrow with leukemic cells. Various chemotherapeutic and immunologic agents have been used to eradicate residual tumor cells. One method under investigation involves purging the marrow with monoclonal antibodies that specifically bind and destroy the leukemic cells.

Acute Lymphocytic Leukemia

ALL primarily strikes children and young adults, accounting for 80% of childhood acute leukemias. The peak incidence occurs at about age 4. ALL can be classified according to the origin of the lymphocytes: early B-cell precursor, pre-B cell, mature B cell, early T-cell precursor, and mature T cell.[26] Most ALLs are of B-cell origin, mainly of the early B-precursor type.

ALL treatment usually consists of three phases, remission induction therapy, consolidation therapy, and maintenance therapy, in which combination chemotherapy is administered. Because systemic chemotherapeutic agents cannot cross the blood-brain barrier and eradicate leukemic cells that have entered the CNS, cranial irradiation combined with intrathecal chemotherapy often is used as a prophylactic measure to prevent CNS recurrence. Concern about the potential adverse effects of intracranial therapy, however, has prompted reappraisal of the treatment strategies. CNS irradiation usually is reserved for children with initial CNS leukemia or who are at high risk for CNS relapse.[23] The long-term effects of treatment on childhood cancer survivors is discussed in Chapter 5. Although CNS involvement is a major problem in children, the incidence in adults at the time of diagnosis is less than 10%.

ALL is one of the outstanding examples of a once-fatal disease that is now treatable and potentially curable with combination chemotherapy. Current chemotherapy regimens cure approximately 70% of children with ALL.[22] The prognosis for adults is more variable.

Acute Myelocytic Leukemia

AML, also called acute nonlymphocytic leukemia, is chiefly an adult disease with more than 50% of cases occurring in patients older than 60 years. However, it is also seen in children and young adults. Complete remission rates for younger patients are higher than 70%, with 30% experiencing a prolonged disease-free survival. However, survival rates for the elderly seldom exceed 50% to 55%.[27]

Of all the leukemias, AML is most strongly linked with toxins and underlying congenital and hematologic disorders. It is the type of leukemia associated with Down syndrome and is the most frequent second cancer seen in persons who have been treated for other types of cancer.[24]

The AMLs are an extremely heterogeneous group of disorders. Some arise from the pluripotent stem cells in which myeloblasts predominate, and others arise from the monocyte-granulocyte precursor, which is the cell of origin for myelomonocytic leukemia. Based on the line of differentiation and the maturity of the cells, AMLs have been divided into seven subtypes in the widely used French-American-British classification system (Table 9-3). In addition to the common manifestations of acute leukemia (*e.g.*, fatigue, weight loss, fever, easy bruising), certain presentations are distinctive for the subtypes. Infiltration of malignant cells in the skin, gums, and other soft tissue is particularly common in the monocytic form (M5) of leukemia, whereas disseminated intravascular coagulation poses a serious complication of promyelocytic leukemia (M3).

AML is treated with intensive chemotherapy to effect aplasia of the bone marrow. During this period, supportive transfusion and antibiotic therapy often are needed. If remission is achieved, some type of continu-

TABLE 9-3
FAB Classification for AML

Class	Type of Leukemia	Percentage of AML
M1	AML without differentiation*	20
M2	AML with differentiation	29–30
M3	Promyelocytic leukemia	5–7
M4	Acute myelomonocytic leukemia	22–30
M5	Acute monocytic leukemia	10–19
M6	Acute erythroleukemia	1–5
M7	Acute megakaryoblastic leukemia	2–5

FAB, French-American-British; AML, acute myelocytic leukemia. Developed from information in Kumar V.K., Cotran R.S., Robbins S.L. [1992]. *Basic pathology* (5th ed., pp. 365–372), Philadelphia: W.B. Saunders; Champlin R., Gold D.W. [1991]. The leukemias. In Wilson J.D., Braunwald E., Isselbacher K.J. (Eds.). *Harrison's principles of internal medicine* (12th ed.). New York: McGraw-Hill.

ing chemotherapy is used. In some cases, bone marrow transplantation may be performed. Chemotherapy induces complete remission in 70% of persons with AML, about one fourth of whom achieve long-term, disease-free survival or cure.

Chronic Leukemias

Chronic leukemias have a more insidious onset than acute leukemias and may be discovered during a routine medical examination by a blood count. CLL is a disorder of older adults. CML is predominantly a disorder of adults, but it can affect children as well.

Chronic Lymphocytic Leukemia

Mainly a disease of older persons, CLL typically follows a slow, chronic course. For these persons, reassurance that they can live a normal life for many years is important. Complications such as autoimmune thrombocytopenia and hemolytic anemia may be managed with corticosteroid treatment, or a splenectomy may be necessary. CLL is a disorder characterized by the proliferation and accumulation of relatively mature lymphocytes that are immunologically incompetent. The malignant cell lineage is predominantly the B lymphocyte in the United States and the T lymphocyte in Asia. Individuals initially experience fatigue and reduced exercise tolerance, enlargement of superficial lymph nodes, or splenomegaly. The onset of CLL is insidious with approximately 25% of the cases diagnosed on a routine examination when enlarge lymph nodes are discovered. As the disease progresses, lymph nodes gradually increase in size and new nodes are involved, sometimes in unusual areas such as the scalp, orbit, pharynx, pleura, the gastrointestinal tract, liver, prostate, and gonads. Severe fatigue, recurrent or persistent infections, pallor, edema, thrombophlebitis, and pain are also experienced. As the malignant cell population increases, the proportion of normal marrow precursors is reduced until only lymphocytes remain in the marrow.[21] The treatment of CLL is variable. Most early cases require no specific treatment. Indications for chemotherapy include progressive fatigue, troublesome lymphadenopathy, anemia, and thrombocytopenia.

Hairy cell leukemia, a rare leukemia of B-lymphocyte origin, is characterized by the presence of leukemic cells that have fine, hairlike cytoplasmic projections. It occurs mainly in older men. The most common physical finding is splenomegaly, which commonly is massive and may be the only presenting sign. Pancytopenia occurs from failure of the bone marrow and splenic sequestration of cells is seen in more than 50% of cases. The course of the disease is chronic, and the median survival has been about 6 years. In the past, the treatment of choice was splenectomy, which has produced beneficial results in approximately two thirds of the patients. This procedure raises the blood count and relieves symptoms in many persons. Interferon-α (IFN-α) has produced responses in 67% to 90% of cases and has led to the disappearance of the disease for some time. Two experimental drugs, deoxycoformycin and 2-chlorodeoxyadenosine, have proved promising.[10]

Chronic Myelocytic Leukemia

A myeloproliferative disorder, CML involves expansion of all bone marrow elements and accounts for 15% of all leukemias. The bone marrow cells from which CML is derived express a chromosomal translocation in which a proto-oncogene is translocated from chromosome 9 onto chromosome 22.[28] This chromosome is called the Philadelphia chromosome. CML is divided into three stages: chronic or stable, accelerated, and acute or blast crisis. Early in the course, the clinical features are mild and nonspecific. CML usually progresses to a more aggressive phase within 30 to 40 months, at which time the patients experience leukocytosis, weakness, splenomegaly, and weight loss.

The finding of abnormal blood counts on routine testing frequently leads to the diagnosis of CML. The most characteristic laboratory finding at presentation is leukocytosis with immature cell types in the peripheral blood. Anemia and, eventually, thrombocytopenia develop. Anemia causes weakness, easy fatigability, and exertional dyspnea. Splenomegaly is present in 50% of cases at the time of diagnosis; hepatomegaly is less common, and lymphadenopathy is relatively uncommon. Splenomegaly often causes a feeling of abdominal fullness and discomfort. Bleeding and easy bruising may arise from dysfunctional platelets.

Within an average of 3 to 4 years, most cases undergo transformation to the blast phase, which is heralded by the accelerated phase. During the accelerated phase, constitutional symptoms such as low-grade fever, night sweats, and weight loss develop because of rapid proliferation and hypermetabolism of the leukemic cells. Erratic fluctuations in white blood cell and platelet counts may accompany the accelerated phase. The blast crisis represents evolution to acute leukemia and is characterized by an increasing number of myeloid precursors, especially blast cells. Constitutional symptoms become more pronounced during this period, and splenomegaly may increase significantly. Isolated infiltrates of leukemic cells can involve the skin, lymph nodes, bones, and CNS. With very high blast counts (>100,000/μl), symptoms of leukostasis may occur. The prognosis for patients who are in the blast crisis phase is poor, with survival rates averaging 2 to 4 months.

The treatment of chronic leukemia varies with the type of leukemic cell, the stage of the disease, other health problems, and the person's age. Often, the treatment is palliative. The median survival is 3 to 4 years, with fewer than 30% of persons living 5 years after diagnosis. Standard treatment for CML in the chronic phase has consisted of single-agent chemotherapy, producing remissions in 70% to 80% of patients. However, more than 90% of these patients continue to express Philadelphia chromosome–positive cells. During the blast crisis phase, combination therapy frequently used to treat AML is administered, although response rates are low (20% to 30%) and remissions vary from 2 to 12 months. Allogeneic BMT provides the only cure for CML, yielding a 5-year survival for 50% to 60% of patients. IFN-α has been evaluated in the treatment of the chronic phase of CML and has been found to produce complete responses in 50% to 75% of patients, with 20% to 40% exhibiting eradication of the Philadelphia chromosome.[28]

In summary, leukemias are malignant neoplasms of the hematopoietic stem cells with diffuse replacement of bone marrow. Leukemias are classified according to cell type (*i.e.*, lymphocytic or myelocytic) and whether the disease is acute or chronic. The lymphocytic leukemias, most common in children, involve the lymphoid precursors that originate in bone marrow but infiltrate the spleen, lymph nodes, CNS, and other tissues. The myelocytic leukemias, which are seen more often in adults, involve the pluripotent myeloid stem cells in the bone marrow and interfere with the maturation of all blood cells, including granulocytes, erythrocytes, and thrombocytes. The warning signs and symptoms of acute leukemia are fatigue, paleness, weight loss, repeated infections, easy bruising, and nosebleeds and other hemorrhages. In children, these symptoms may appear suddenly.

Malignant Lymphomas

After you have completed this section of the chapter, you should be able to meet the following objectives:

- Compare the lymphoproliferative disorders associated with Hodgkin's disease and non-Hodgkin's lymphoma
- Contrast and compare the signs and symptoms of Hodgkin's disease and non-Hodgkin's lymphoma

The lymphomas, Hodgkin's disease and non-Hodgkin's lymphoma, represent malignant neoplasms of cells derived from lymphoid tissue (*i.e.*, lymphocytes and histiocytes) and their precursors or derivatives.[10] The seventh most common cancer in the United States, the lymphomas are among the most studied human tumors and among the most curable.

Hodgkin's Disease

Hodgkin's disease is a malignant neoplasm of the lymphatic structures. An English physician, Thomas Hodgkin, first described the disease in 1832. It is estimated that approximately 7500 new cases of Hodgkin's disease would be diagnosed in 1996 with 1510 deaths.[11] Distribution of the disease is bimodal; the incidence rises sharply after age 10, peaks in the early 20s, and then declines until age 50. After age 50, the incidence again increases steadily with age. The younger adult group consists equally of men and women, but after 50, the incidence is higher among men.[29] In 60% to 90% of persons with localized Hodgkin's disease, the possibility exists of a definitive cure, defined as normal life expectancy for the patient's age for 10 or more years after treatment.

The cause of Hodgkin's disease is unknown. There is a long-standing suspicion that the disease may begin as an inflammatory reaction to an infectious agent, possibly a virus. This belief is supported by epidemiologic data that include the clustering of the disease among family members and among students who have attended the same school. A suspected etiologic agent is the EBV, because a significant percentage of biopsy specimens have exhibited EBV DNA. Contradictory findings to the proposed viral hypothesis include an absence of occurrence in marital partners. There also seems to be an association between the presence of the disease and a deficient immune state.[29] As with other forms of cancer, it is likely that no single agent is responsible for the development of Hodgkin's disease.

Manifestations

Hodgkin's disease is characterized by painless and progressive enlargement of a single node or group of nodes. It is believed to originate within one area of the lymphatic system, and if unchecked, it spreads throughout the lymphatic network. The initial lymph node involvement typically is above the level of the diaphragm, and the cervical chain or supraclavicular nodes most commonly are affected. An exception is in elderly persons, in whom the subdiaphragmatic lymph nodes may be the first to be involved. Involvement of the retroperitoneal lymph nodes, liver, spleen, and bone marrow occurs after the disease becomes generalized.

The malignant proliferating cells may invade almost any area of the body and may produce a wide variety of signs and symptoms. A common symptom is the development of a progressive, painless, rubbery, lymph node enlargement that is predominantly found in the neck area in 60% to 80% of patients. Approximately 40% of patients exhibit the "B" symptoms, which include low-grade fever, night sweats, and unexplained weight loss.[29] Other symptoms such as fatigue, pruritus, and anemia are indicative of disease spread. In the advanced stages of Hodgkin's disease, the liver, lungs, digestive tract, and occasionally, CNS may be affected. As the disease progresses, the rapid proliferation of abnormal lymphocytes leads to an immunologic defect, particularly in cell-mediated responses, rendering the person more susceptible to bacterial, viral, fungal, and protozoal infections. Neutrophilic leukocytosis and mild normocytic normochromic anemia are common. Eosinophilia may also occur. Leukopenia usually is a late manifestation. Hypergammaglobulinemia is common during the early stages of the disease, and hypogammaglobulinemia may develop in advanced disease.

Diagnosis and Treatment

A definitive diagnosis of Hodgkin's disease requires that the Reed-Sternberg cell be present in a biopsy specimen of lymph node tissue. Although the question of neoplastic lineage remains unclear, evidence suggests that the Reed-Sternberg cell, a distinctive giant tumor cell, is derived from the macrophage-monocyte line. This cell may also be found in other disorders, such as infectious mononucleosis.

Computed tomographic scans of the abdomen commonly are used in screening for involvement of abdominal and pelvic lymph nodes. Radiologic visualization of the abdominal and pelvic lymph structures can be achieved through the use of bipedal lymphangiography. In this diagnostic test, radiopaque dye is injected into the lymphatic channels of the lower leg, enabling visualization of the iliac and paraaortic nodes. Nuclear studies, such as a gallium scan in which the tumor takes up the radionuclide or a staging laparotomy to detect abdominal nodes and inspect the liver, also may be done.

The staging of Hodgkin's disease is of great clinical importance, because the choice of treatment and the prognosis are ultimately related to the distribution of the disease. Staging is determined by the number of lymph nodes that are involved, whether the lymph nodes are on one or both sides of the diaphragm, and whether there is disseminated disease involving the bone marrow and liver. A modification of the frequently used Ann Arbor Classification of Hodgkin's Disease includes extent of disease, location, bulk, and number of anatomic locations of involvement. Patients are designated stage A if they lack constitution symptoms and stage B if they experience significant weight loss, fever, and night sweats.

Irradiation and chemotherapy are used in treating the disease. Most patients with localized disease are treated with radiation therapy. As the accuracy of staging techniques, delivery of radiation, and developments of curative combination chemotherapy regimens have improved, the survival of patients with Hodgkin's disease has also improved. Nonetheless, long-term survivors of Hodgkin's disease are at increased risk of dying from cardiac disease caused primarily from mediastinal radiation, infections resulting from immunosuppressive chemotherapy and intensive irradiation, and secondary malignancies caused by the use of alkylating chemotherapy agents used in the chemotherapy protocols. These risks have prompted the development of clinical trials to evaluate the reduction of aggressive therapy with the intent of decreasing the risk of long-term complications. Recommendations from these early studies include performing staging laparotomies in patients with early-stage disease with the aim of potentially reducing the use of chemotherapy and reducing the extent of radiation therapy and the amount of chemotherapy.[30]

Non-Hodgkin's Lymphomas

The non-Hodgkin's lymphomas are a heterogeneic group of neoplastic disorders of the lymphoid tissue, usually the lymph nodes. Unlike Hodgkin's disease, which is initially localized to a single group of lymph nodes, the non-Hodgkin's lymphomas typically are multicentric in origin and spread early to various tissues throughout the body, especially the liver, spleen, and bone marrow. Non-Hodgkin's lymphomas occur three times more frequently than Hodgkin's disease. In 1996, approximately 52,700 new cases were diagnosed in the United States and about 23,300 deaths resulted from these disorders.[11]

A viral cause is suspected in at least some of the lymphomas. Cell cultures and immunologic studies of one type of lymphoma, Burkitt's lymphoma, which is found in some parts of Africa, have implicated EBV without proving a causal association. Serologic studies have also demonstrated an association between the HTLV-I retrovirus and T-cell leukemia or lymphoma. Non-Hodgkin's lymphomas are also seen with increased frequency in persons with acquired immunodeficiency syndrome, in those who have received chronic immunosuppressive therapy after kidney or liver transplantation, and in individuals with acquired or congenital immunodeficiencies.

As tumors of the immune system, non-Hodgkin's lymphomas may originate from B cells (70% to 80%), T cells, or histiocytes (*i.e.*, macrophage-monocytes). Histiocytic forms of lymphoma are rare, accounting for less than 1% of cases. Non-Hodgkin's lymphomas commonly are divided into three groups, depending on the grade of the tumor: low-grade lymphomas, which are predominantly B-cell tumors; intermediate-grade lymphomas, which include B-cell and some T-cell lymphomas; and high-grade lymphomas, which are largely immunoblastic (B-cell), lymphoblastic (T-cell), Burkitt's, and non-Burkitt's lymphomas.

Manifestations

The signs and symptoms of non-Hodgkin's lymphomas are similar to those of Hodgkin's disease. The most frequently occurring clinical manifestation in Hodgkin's and non-Hodgkin's lymphoma is painless, superficial lymphadenopathy. Other differences include a noncontiguous nodal spread of the disease in non-Hodgkin's and contiguous spread in Hodgkin's disease; more common extranodal disease in non-Hodgkin's with more frequent involvement of the gastrointestinal tract, testes, and bone marrow while uncommon in Hodgkin's disease; more frequent mediastinal disease in Hodgkin's disease (50%) but a lower occurrence in non-Hodgkin's lymphoma (20%); bone marrow and liver involvement that are more common in non-Hodgkin's but uncommon in Hodgkin's; and disease often localized and B symptoms that are more common in Hodgkin's disease than non-Hodgkin's lymphomas.

Leukemic transformation with high peripheral lymphocytic counts occurs in about 13% of persons with non-Hodgkin's lymphomas. Patient have increased susceptibility to bacterial, viral, and fungal infections associated with hypogammaglobulinemia, and poor humoral antibody response, rather than impaired cellular immunity, is seen with Hodgkin's disease.

Diagnosis and Treatment

As with Hodgkin's disease, a lymph node biopsy is used to confirm the diagnosis. Bone marrow biopsy, blood studies, abdominal computed tomographic scans, and nuclear medicine studies often are used to determine the stage of the disease.

For early-stage disease, radiation therapy is used as a single treatment. However, because most persons present with late-stage disease, combination chemotherapy, combined adjuvant radiation therapy, or both are recommended. Combination regimens frequently include aggressive multiple chemotherapy agents that result in a variety of distressing symptoms such as nausea, vomiting, infection, and alopecia. For rapidly progressive intermediate or high-grade lymphoma, CNS prophylaxis is achieved with high doses of chemotherapeutic agents that can cross the blood-brain barrier such as methotrexate, intrathecal chemotherapy (administered by spinal tap), or cranial irradiation. Bone marrow and peripheral stem cell transplantation are being investigated as a potentially curative treatment modality in patients with highly resistant disease. These treatments have been found to produce increases in disease-free survival with complete remission rates of 60%.[31]

> The lymphomas, Hodgkin's disease and non-Hodgkin's lymphomas, represent malignant neoplasms of cells native to lymphoid tissue (i.e., lymphocytes and histiocytes) and their precursors or derivatives. They are among the most studied human tumors and among the most curable. Hodgkin's disease is characterized by painless and progressive enlargement of a single node or group of nodes. It is believed to originate within one area of the lymphatic system and, if unchecked, spreads throughout the lymphatic network. Non-Hodgkin's lymphomas are a group of neoplastic disorders of the lymphoid tissue, usually the lymph nodes. Unlike Hodgkin's disease, which is initially localized to a single group of lymph nodes, most non-Hodgkin's lymphomas are multicentric in origin and spread early to various tissues throughout the body, especially the liver, spleen, and bone marrow.

Multiple Myeloma

After you have completed this section of the chapter, you should be able to meet the following objectives:

- Describe the lymphoproliferative disorder that occurs with multiple myeloma
- Explain the origin of the Bence Jones protein that appears in the urine of a patient with multiple myeloma

Multiple myeloma is a plasma cell cancer of the osseous tissue and accounts for 10% to 15% of all hematologic malignancies. In the course of its dissemination, it also may involve nonosseous sites. It is characterized by the uncontrolled proliferation of an abnormal clone of plasma cells, which secrete primarily immunoglobulin G or immunoglobulin A. In 1996, approximately 14,400 new cases were diagnosed and more than 10,400 deaths from this disease occurred in the United States.[11] Fewer than 2% of cases occur before the age of 40, with the 68 years the median age at time of onset for men and 70 years for women. The cause of multiple myeloma is unknown, but several risk factors have been associated with the disease. Occupational exposure to wood, metal, rubber, textile, and petroleum; exposure to high- and low-dose ionizing radiation; recurrent infections; and drug allergies have all been associated with its pathogenesis.[32]

In multiple myeloma, there is an atypical proliferation of one of the immunoglobulins called the M protein, a monoclonal antibody. Although there is an abundance of immunoglobulin, it is not effective in maintaining humoral immunity.[32] Myeloma cells secrete osteoclast-activating factors (OAF) that stimulate the proliferation and activation of osteoclasts and leads to bone destruction and resorption. This increased bone resorption predisposes the individual to pathologic fractures and hypercalcemia.[33] Paraproteins secreted by the plasma cells may cause a hyperviscosity of body fluids and may break down into amyloid, a proteinaceous substance deposited between cells, causing heart failure and neuropathy. In some forms of multiple myeloma, the plasma cells produce only *Bence Jones proteins*, abnormal proteins that consist of the light chains of the immunoglobulin molecule. Because of their low molecular weight, Bence Jones proteins are partially excreted in the urine. Many of these abnormal proteins are directly toxic to renal tubular structures, which may lead to tubular destruction and, eventually, to renal failure. The malignant plasma cells can also form tumors (*i.e.*, plasmacytomas) that have a tendency to cause spinal cord compression.

Bone pain is one of the first symptoms to occur and one of the most common, occurring in 75% to 80% of all individuals diagnosed with multiple myeloma. Bone destruction also impairs the production of erythrocytes and leukocytes and predisposes the patient to anemia and recurrent infections. Many patients experience weight loss and weakness. Renal insufficiency occurs in 50% of patients.[32] Neurologic manifestations caused by neuropathy or spinal cord compression may also be present.

Although numerous treatment options have been attempted for multiple myeloma in the last 3 decades, the results have been disappointing. With standard chemotherapy, the median survival may reach 2 to 3 years. Multiple myeloma is a radiosensitive disease, but most radiation therapy is used primarily for palliation, specifically to treat lytic bone lesions, compression fractures, and decrease pain. IFN-α has produced response rates of 15% when used alone and 68% when used with chemotherapy. Some investigators discourage the use of IFN-α, because it has been found in vitro to stimulate myeloma cells by inducing the autocrine production of interleukin-6. Syngeneic, allogeneic, or autologous BMT has produced complete remission rates of 50% to 60%, but 5-year survival rates are predicted to be approximately 40% to 50%. Peripheral stem cell transplantation has been used as well, but there exists an unsubstantiated concern of possible contamination with peripheral myeloma cells.[32]

In summary, multiple myeloma results in the uncontrolled proliferation of immunoglobulin secreting plasma cells, usually a single clone of immunoglobulin G– or immunoglobulin A–producing cells, that results in increased bone resorption, leading to pathologic bone lesions.

REFERENCES

1. Lydyard P., Grossi C. (1996). The development of the immune system. In Roitt I.M., Brostoff J., Male D.K. (Eds.). *Immunology* (4th ed., pp. 10.2–10.14), St. Louis: Mosby.
2. Bell A. (1992). Hematopoiesis: Morphology of human blood and marrow cells. In Harmening D.M. (Ed.). *Clinical hematology and fundamentals of hemostasis* (pp. 21–41). Philadelphia: F.A. Davis.
3. Malarkey L.M., McNorrow M.E. (Eds.). (1996). Hematologic function. In *Nurse's manual of laboratory tests and diagnostic procedures* (pp. 392–444). Philadelphia: W.B. Saunders.
4. Montiel M. (1992). Bone marrow. In Harmening D.M. (Ed.). *Clinical hematology and fundamentals of hemostasis* (pp. 42–53). Philadelphia: F.A. Davis.
5. Abbas A. K., Lichtman A.H., Pober J.S. (Eds.). (1994). Cytokines. In *Cellular and molecular immunology* (2nd ed., pp. 240–260). Philadelphia: W.B. Saunders.
6. Strauss R.G. (1992). Cell biology and disorders of neutrophils. In Harmening D.M. (Ed.). *Clinical hematology and fundamentals of hemostasis* (pp. 241–257). Philadelphia: F.A. Davis.
7. Koenig J.M., Christensen R.D. (1989). Incidence, neutrophil kinetics, and natural history of neonatal neutropenia associated with maternal hypertension. *New England Journal of Medicine* 321, 775–562.
8. Workman M.L., Ellerhorst-Ryan J., Hargrave-Koertge V. (1993). (Eds.). Infections in the immunocompromised host. In *Nursing care of the immunocompromised patient* (pp. 229–262). Philadelphia: W.B. Saunders.
9. Schooley R.T. (1994). Epstein-Barr virus infections, including infectious mononucleosis. In Isselbacher K.J., Braunwald E., Wilson J.D., Martin J.B., Fauci A.S., Kasper D.L. (Eds.). *Harrison's principles of internal medicine* (2nd ed., pp. 790–793). New York: McGraw-Hill.
10. Cotran R.S., Kumar V., Robbins S.L. (Eds.). (1994). Diseases of white cells, lymph nodes, and spleen. In *Pathologic basis of disease* (5th Ed., pp. 629–672). Philadelphia: W.B. Saunders.
11. Parker S.L., Tong T., Bolden S., et al. (1996). Cancer Statistics, 1996. *CA. Cancer Journal for Clinicians* 46 (1), 5–27.
12. Pui C.H. (1995). Childhood leukemias. *New England Journal of Medicine, 332* (24), 1618–1630.
13. Jablon S., Kato H. (1972). Studies of the mortality of A-bomb survivors. *Radiation Research* 50, 658.
14. Pederson-Bjergaard J., Larsen S.O. (1982). Incidence of acute nonlymphocytic leukemia, preleukemia and acute myeloproliferative syndrome up to 10 years after treatment for Hodgkin's disease. *New England Journal of Medicine* 307, 964.
15. Boise J.D., Greene M.H., Killen I.Y., et al. (1983). Leukemia and preleukemia after adjuvant treatment of gastrointestinal cancer with semustine. *New England Journal of Medicine* 309, 107.
16. Collman C.A., Dahlberg S. (1990). Treatment-related leukemia. *New England Journal of Medicine* 322, 52–53.
17. Pui C., Behm F.G., Raimondi S. (1989). Secondary acute myeloid leukemia in children treated for acute lymphoid leukemia. *New England Journal of Medicine* 321, 136–142.
18. Negalia J.P., Meadows A.T., Robison L.L. (1991). Secondary neoplasms after acute lymphoblastic leukemia in children. *New England Journal of Medicine* 325, 1330–1336.
19. Golde D.W., Gulati S.C. (1994). The myeloproliferative diseases. In Isselbacher K.J., Braunwald E., Wilson J.D., Martin J.B., Fauci A.S., Kasper D.L. (Eds.). *Harrison's principles of internal medicine* (13th ed., pp. 1758–1760). New York: McGraw-Hill.
20. Kurzrock R., Gulterman J.U., Talpaz M. (1988). The molecular genetics of Philadelphia chromosome-positive leukemia. *New England Journal of Medicine* 319, 990–998.
21. Callaghan M.E. (1996). Leukemia. In McCorkle R., Grant M., Frank-Stromborg M., Baird S.B. (Eds.). *Cancer nursing: A comprehensive textbook.* (2nd ed., pp. 752–771). Philadelphia: W.B. Saunders.
22. American Cancer Society. (1987). *Cancer facts and figures 1987*. Atlanta: American Cancer Society.
23. Pui C., Rivera G.K. (1991). Childhood leukemia. In Hollieb A.L., Fink D.J., Murphy G. (Eds.). *American Cancer Society textbook of clinical oncology* (pp. 433–452). Atlanta: American Cancer Society.
24. Mitus A.J., Rosenthal D.S. (1991). Adult leukemias. In Hollieb A.L., Fink D.J., Murphy G. (Eds.). *American Cancer Society textbook of clinical oncology* (pp. 410–432). Atlanta: American Cancer Society.
25. Ford R., McDonald J., Mitchell-Supplee K.J., Jagels B.A. (1996). Marrow transplant and peripheral blood stem cell transplantation. In McCorkle R., Grant M., Frank-Stromborg M., Baird S.B. (Eds.). *Cancer nursing: A comprehensive textbook* (2nd ed., pp. 504–530). Philadelphia: W.B. Saunders.
26. Devine S.M., Larson R.A. (1994). Acute leukemia in adults: Development in diagnosis and treatment. *Cancer* 44 (6), 326–352.
27. Stasi R., Venditti A., Del Poeta G., et al. (1996). Intensive treatment of patients age 60 years and older with de novo acute myeloid leukemia. *Cancer* 77 (12), 2476–2488.
28. Wujick D. (1996). Update on the diagnosis of and therapy for acute promyelocytic leukemia and chronic myelogenous leukemia. *Oncology Nursing Forum* 23 (3), 478–487.
29. Carson C. (1996). Hodgkin's disease and non-Hodgkin's lymphomas. In McCorkle R., Grant M., Frank-Stromborg M., Baird S.B. (Eds.). *Cancer nursing: A comprehensive textbook* (2nd ed., pp. 729–751). Philadelphia: W.B. Saunders.

30. Mauch P.M., Kalish L.A., Marcus C.K., et al. (1995). Long-term survival in Hodgkin's disease: Relative impact of mortality, second tumors, infection, and cardiovascular disease. *The Cancer Journal* 1 (1), 33–42.
31. Engelking C., Hubbard S.M. (1996). Current issues and controversies in the management of non-Hodgkin's lymphoma, monograph #2: For the oncology nurse (pp. 1–39). New York: Triclinical Communications.
32. Sheridan C.A. (1996). Multiple Myeloma. *Seminars in Oncology Nursing* 12 (1), 59–69.
33. Collins-Hattery A.M. (1996). Multiple myeloma. In McCorkle R., Grant M., Frank-Stromborg M., Baird S.B. (Eds.). *Cancer nursing: A comprehensive textbook* (2nd ed., pp. 840–849). Philadelphia: W.B. Saunders Company.

ADDITIONAL READINGS

Aschan J., Ringden O., Andstrom E., et al. (1994). Individualized prophylaxis against graft-versus-host disease in leukemic marrow transplant recipients. *Bone Marrow Transplantation* 14, 79–87.

Buchsel P.C., Kapustay P.M. (1995). Peripheral stem cell transplantation. *Oncology Nursing* 2 (2), 1–14.

Cozad J. (1996). Infectious mononucleosis [review]. Nurse Practitioner, 21 (3), 14–28.

Deeg H.J. (1994). Prophylaxis and treatment of acute graft-versus-host disease: Current state, implications of new immunopharmacologic compounds and future strategies to prevent and treat acute GVHD in high-risk patients. *Bone Marrow Transplantation* 14 (Suppl. 4), S56–S60.

Ferrara J.L.M. (1994). Paradigm shift for graft-versus-host disease. *Bone Marrow Transplantation* 14, 183–184.

Hays K. (1990). Physiology of normal bone marrow. *Seminars in Oncology Nursing* 6 (1), 3–8.

Tabbara I.A. (1996). Allogenic bone marrow transplantation [review]. *Southern Medical Journal* 89 (9), 857–868.

Thomas E.D. (1994). Bone marrow transplantation—past, present, future. *Scandinavian Journal of Immunology* 39 (4), 339–345.

Immunity and Inflammation

The quest to understand the mechanism of disease and ways to prevent it permeates humankind's history. Many civilizations contributed to the storehouse of knowledge. Among the early accomplishments of the Chinese are a number of practices they developed to prevent disease, one of which took the form of inoculation.

The deadly smallpox had been one of the world's most dreaded diseases. During the Middle Ages, epidemics were frequent; they swept across Asia and other parts of the world, leaving widespread death in their wake. In the 1400s, the Chinese created a technique to protect themselves during an epidemic. They collected the crusts of smallpox sores and allowed them to dry. The dried material was ground into a powder and inhaled. The procedure was found to be hazardous, but it remains one of the first attempts at vaccination.

UNIT III

CHAPTER 10

Mechanisms of Infectious Disease

W. Michael Dunne, Jr.

All living creatures share two basic purposes in life—survival and reproduction. This tenet applies equally to humans and to members of the microbial world, including bacteria, viruses, fungi, and protozoa. To satisfy these goals, organisms must extract from the environment nutrients essential for growth and proliferation; for countless organisms, that environment is the human body. Normally, the contact between humans and microorganisms is incidental and, in certain situations, may actually benefit both organisms. Under extraordinary circumstances, however, the invasion of the human body by microorganisms can produce harmful and potentially lethal consequences. These consequences are collectively called *infectious diseases.*

Terminology

After you have completed this section of the chapter, you should be able to meet the following objectives:

- Define the terms host, infectious disease, colonization, microflora, virulence, pathogen, and saprophyte
- Describe the concept of host-microorganism interaction using the concepts of commensalism, mutualism, and parasitic relationships

All scientific disciplines evolve with a distinct vocabulary, and the study of infectious diseases is no exception. The most appropriate way to approach this subject is with a brief discussion of the terminology used to characterize interactions between humans and microbes.

Any organism capable of supporting the nutritional and physical growth requirements of another is called a *host*. Throughout this chapter, the term *host* most often refers to humans supporting the growth of microorganisms. The term *infection* describes the presence and multiplication of a living organism on or within the host. Occasionally, the terms infection and *colonization* are used interchangeably.

One common misconception should be dispelled: not all contacts between microorganisms and humans are injurious. The internal and external exposed surfaces of the human body are normally and harmlessly inhabited by a multitude of bacteria, collectively referred to as the *normal microflora* (Table 10–1). Although the colonizing bacteria acquire nutritional needs and shelter, the host is not adversely affected by the relationship. An

TABLE 10-1

Location and Variety of Nonpathogenic Normal Human Microflora

Area	Sites	Bacteria	
		Gram-positive	Gram-negative
Upper respiratory tract	Mouth, nose	+++	+++
	Nasopharynx	(Aerobes and	Aerobes and
	Throat	anaerobes)	anaerobes)
Lower respiratory tract	Larynx	0	0
	Trachea	0	0
	Lungs	0	0
External surfaces	Skin	++++	+
	Outer ear	(Aerobes and	(Transient)
	Eyes	Anaerobes)	0
Upper gastro-intestinal tract	Stomach	+	+
	Duodenum	(Transient)	(Transient)
	Esophagus	0	0
	Jejunum	0	0
Lower gastrointestinal tract	Ileum	+++	++++
	Colon	(Predominantly anaerobes)	(Predominantly anaerobes)
External genitourinary tract	Vagina	++	++
	Anterior urethra	0	0
Internal genitourinary tract	Cervix, ovaries	0	0
	Fallopian tubes	0	0
	Uterus, prostate	0	0
	Bladder, kidney	0	0
	Testes, epididymis	0	0
Body fluids	Blood, urine	0	0
	Spinal fluid	0	0
	Synovial fluid	0	0
	Peritoneal fluid	0	0

Key: 0 = none; + = rare; + + = few; + + + = moderate; + + + + = many.

interaction such as this is called *commensalism*. The term *mutualism* is applied to an infection in which the microorganism and the host derive benefits from the interaction. For example, certain inhabitants of the human intestinal tract extract nutrients from the host and secrete essential vitamin byproducts of metabolism (*e.g.*, vitamin K), which are absorbed and used by the host. A *parasitic relationship* is one in which only the infecting organism benefits from the relationship. If the host sustains injury or pathologic changes in response to a parasitic infection, the process is called an *infectious disease*.

The severity of an infectious disease can range from mild to life threatening, depending on many variables, including the health of the host at the time of infection and the *virulence* (*i.e.*, disease-producing potential) of the microorganism. A select group of microorganisms called *pathogens* are so virulent that they are rarely found in the absence of disease. Fortunately, there are few human pathogens in the microbial world. Most microorganisms are harmless *saprophytes*, which are free-living organisms obtaining their growth from dead or decaying organic material from the environment. All microorganisms, even saprophytes and members of the normal flora, can be *opportunistic pathogens*, capable of producing an infectious disease when the health and immunity of the host have been severely weakened by illness, famine, or medical therapy.

In summary, throughout life, humans are continuously and harmlessly colonized by a multitude of microscopic organisms. This relationship is kept in check by the intact defense mechanisms of the host (*e.g.*, mucosal and cutaneous barriers, normal immune function) and the innocuous nature of most environmental microorganisms. Those factors that weaken the resistance of the host or increase the virulence of colonizing microorganisms can disturb the equilibrium of the relationship and cause disease. The degree to which the balance is shifted in favor of the microorganism determines the severity of illness.

Agents of Infectious Disease

After you have completed this section of the chapter, you should be able to meet the following objectives:

Mycobacteria	Parasites	Mycoplasmas	Fungi	Chlamydia/ Rickettsia	Spirochetes
+	+	+	+	0	+
0	(Protozoans)	0	(Yeast)	0	0
0	0	0	0	0	0
0	0	0	0	0	0
0	0	0	0	0	0
+	0	0	+	0	0
0	0	0	(Yeast)	0	0
0	0	0	0	0	0
+	0	0	0	0	0
(Transient)					
0	0	0	0	0	0
0					
+	+	0	+	0	+
0	(Protozoans)	0	(Yeast)		0
0	0	+	+	0	0
0	0	0	(Yeast)	0	0
0	0	0	0	0	0
0	0	0	0	0	0
0	0	0	0	0	0
0	0	0	0	0	0
0	0	0	0	0	0
0	0	0	0	0	0
0	0	0	0	0	0
0	0	0	0	0	0
0	0	0	0	0	0

- Describe the structural characteristics and mechanisms of reproduction for viruses, bacteria, rickettsiae, and chlamydiae, fungi, and parasites
- Use the concepts of incidence, portal of entry, source of infection, symptomatology, disease course, site of infection, agent, and host characteristics to explain the mechanisms of infectious diseases

The agents of infectious disease include viruses, bacteria, rickettsiae, and chlamydiae, fungi, and parasites.

Viruses

Viruses are the smallest obligate intracellular pathogens. They are incapable of replication outside of a living cell. They have no organized cellular structures but instead consist of a protein coat (*i.e.*, capsid) surrounding a nucleic acid core (*i.e.*, genome) of RNA or DNA—never both (Fig. 10–1). Some viruses are enclosed within a lipoprotein envelope derived from the cytoplasmic membrane of the parasitized host cell. Certain viruses are continuously shed from the infected cell surface enveloped in buds pinched from the cytoplasmic membrane. Enveloped viruses include members of the herpesvirus group and paramyxoviruses such as influenza.

Viruses must penetrate a susceptible living cell and use the biosynthetic machinery of the cell to produce viral progeny. The process of viral replication is shown in Figure 10–2. Not all viral agents cause lysis and death of the host cell during the course of replication. Still other viruses enter the host cell and insert their genome into the host cell chromosome, where the genome remains in a latent, nonreplicating state for long periods without causing disease. Under the appropriate stimulation, the virus undergoes active replication and produces symptoms of disease months to years later. Members of the herpesvirus group and adenovirus are the best examples of latent viruses. Herpesviruses include the viral agents of chickenpox and zoster (*i.e.*, shingles), genital herpes, cytomegalovirus infections, infectious mononucleosis, and fever blisters. In each of these, the resumption of the latent viral replication may produce symptoms of primary disease (*e.g.*, genital herpes) or cause an entirely different symptomatology (*e.g.*, shingles instead of chickenpox).

Within the past 15 years, members of the retrovirus group have received considerable attention after

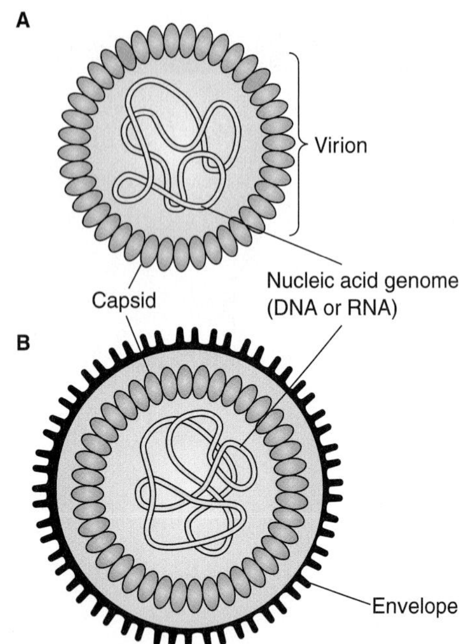

Figure 10-1
(**A**) The basic structure of a virus includes a protein coat surrounding an inner core of nucleic acid (DNA or RNA). (**B**) Some viruses may also be enclosed in a lipoprotein outer envelope.

identification of the human immunodeficiency viruses (HIV) as the causative agent of acquired immunodeficiency syndrome (AIDS). The retroviruses have a unique mechanism of replication. After entry into the host cell, the viral RNA genome is first translated into DNA by a viral enzyme called reverse transcriptase. The viral DNA copy is integrated into the host chromosome and exists in a latent state similar to the herpesviruses. Reactivation and replication require a reversal of the entire process. Some retroviruses lyse the host cell during the process of replication. In the case of HIV, the infected cells regulate the immunologic defense system of the host and their lysis leads to a permanent suppression of the immune response.

In addition to causing infectious diseases, certain viruses also have the ability to transform normal host cells into malignant cells during the replication cycle. This group of viruses is referred to as *oncogenic* and includes certain retroviruses and DNA viruses such as the herpesviruses, adenoviruses, papovaviruses.

The viruses of humans and animals have been categorized somewhat arbitrarily according to various characteristics, including the type of viral genome (*i.e.*, single-stranded or double-stranded DNA or RNA), the mechanism of replication (*e.g.*, retroviruses), the mode of transmission (*e.g.*, anthropod-borne viruses, enteroviruses), and the type of disease produced (*e.g.*, hepatitis A, B, C, D, and E viruses), just to name a few.

Bacteria

Bacteria are autonomously replicating unicellular organisms known as *prokaryotes* because they lack an organized nucleus. Compared with nucleated eukaryotic cells (see Chapter 1), the structure of the bacterial cell is small and relatively primitive (Fig. 10–3). Bacteria approximate the size of the eukaryotic mitochondria (about 1 μm in diameter) and may be the evolutionary ancestors of mitochondria.

Bacteria contain no organized intracellular organelles, and the genome consists of only a single chromosome of DNA. Many bacteria transiently harbor smaller extrachromosomal pieces of circular DNA called plasmids. Occasionally, plasmids contain genetic information that increases the virulence of the organism. Similar to eukaryotic cells, but unlike viruses, bacteria contain DNA and RNA.

The prokaryotic cell is organized into an internal compartment called the *cytoplasm*, which contains the reproductive and metabolic machinery of the cell (Fig. 10–4). The cytoplasm is surrounded by a flexible lipid membrane, called the cytoplasmic membrane, which is enclosed within a rigid cell wall. The structure and synthesis of the cell wall determine whether the microscopic shape of the bacterium is spherical (*cocci*), helical

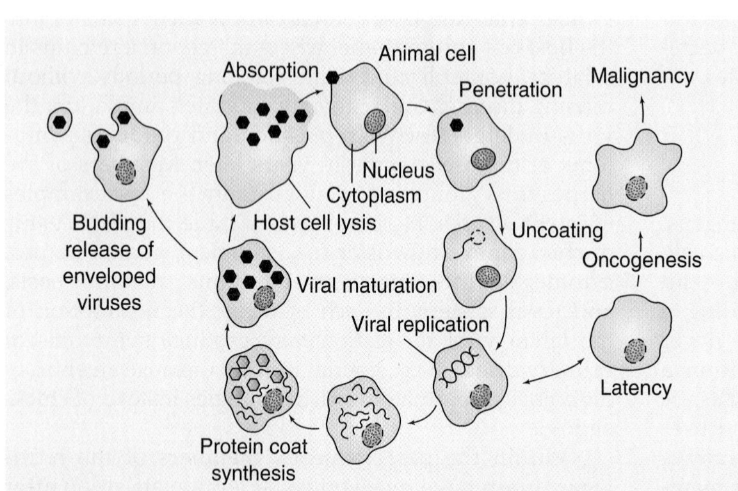

Figure 10-2
Schematic representation of the many possible consequences of viral infection of host cells, including cell lysis (poliovirus), continuous release of budding viral particles, or latency (herpesviruses) and oncogenesis (papovaviruses).

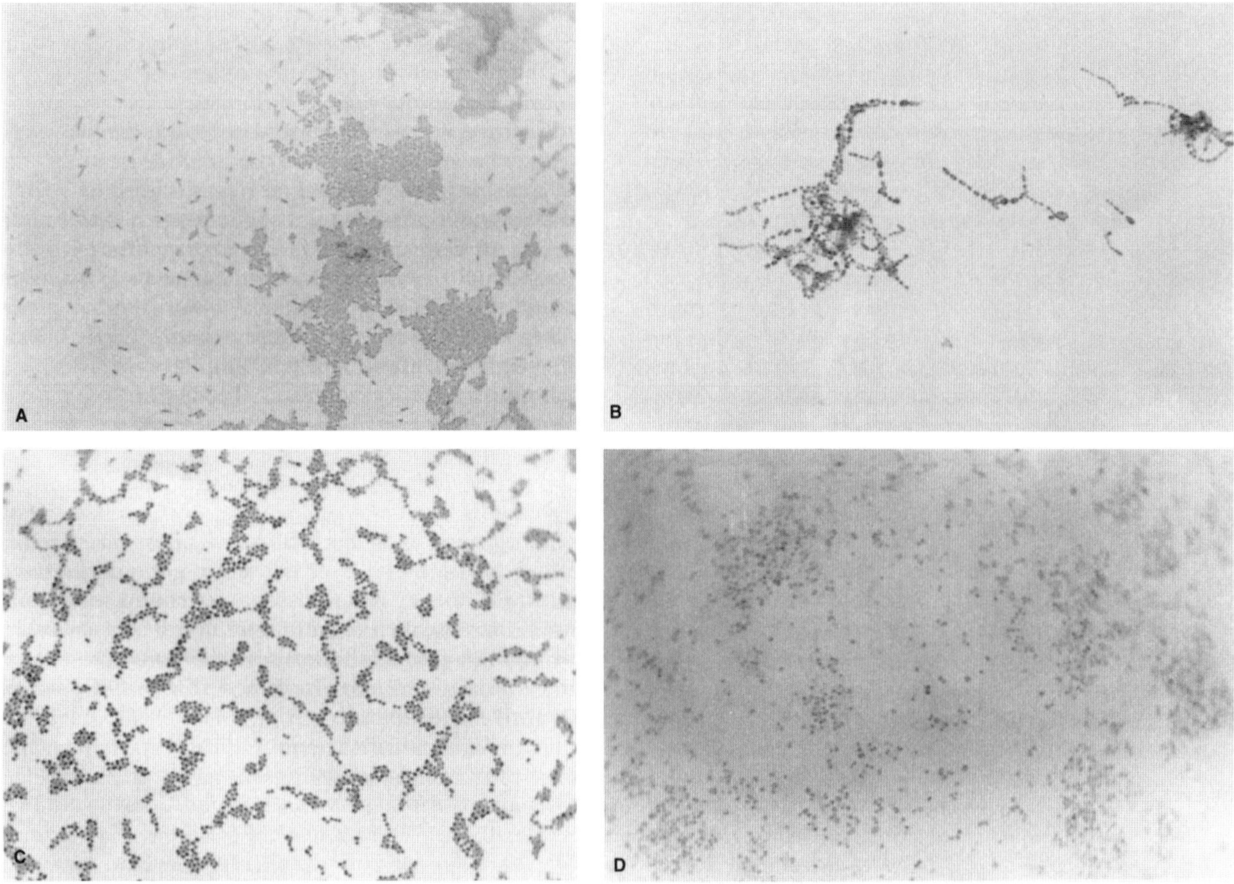

Figure 10-3
A sampling of the microscopic morphology of bacteria demonstrating the variability of size and shape including bacilli (**A**), streptococci (**B**), staphylococci (**C**), and diplococci (**D**).

(*spirilla*), or elongate (*bacilli*). Most bacteria produce a cell wall composed of a distinctive polymer known as *peptidoglycan*. This polymer is only produced by prokaryotes and is therefore an ideal target for antibacterial therapy. Several bacteria synthesize an extracellular capsule composed of protein or carbohydrate. The capsule protects the organism from environmental hazards such as the immunologic defenses of the host.

Certain bacteria are motile as the result of external whiplike appendages called *flagella*. The rotary action of the flagella transports the organism through a liquid environment like a propeller. Bacteria can also produce hairlike structures projecting from the cell surface called *pili* or *fimbriae*, which enable the organism to adhere to surfaces such as mucous membranes or other bacteria.

Most prokaryotes reproduce asexually by simple cellular division. The number of planes in which an organism divides can influence the microscopic morphology. For instance, when the cocci divide in chains, they are called *streptococci*; in pairs, *diplococci*; and in clusters, *staphylococci*. The growth rate of bacteria varies significantly among different species and depends greatly on physical growth conditions and the availability of nutrients. In the laboratory, a single bacterium placed in a suitable growth environment such as an agar plate reproduces to the extent that it forms a visible colony composed of millions of bacteria within a few hours.

The physical appearance of the colony can be distinctive for each type of bacteria. Some bacteria produce highly resistant *spores* when faced with an unfavorable environment. The spores exist in a quiescent state almost indefinitely until suitable growth conditions are encountered. The spores germinate, and the organism resumes normal metabolism and replication.

Bacteria are extremely adaptable life forms. They inhabit almost every environmental extreme on earth, including humans. However, each individual bacterial species has a well-defined set of growth parameters, including nutrition, temperature, light, humidity, and atmosphere. Bacteria with extremely strict growth requirements are called *fastidious*. For example, *Neisseria gonorrhoeae*, the bacterium that causes gonorrhea, cannot live for extended periods outside the human body. Some bacteria require oxygen for growth and metabolism and are called *aerobes;* others cannot survive in an oxygen-containing environment and are called *anaerobes*. An organism capable of adapting its metabolism to aerobic or anaerobic conditions is called *facultatively anaerobic*.

In the laboratory, bacteria are generally classified according to the microscopic appearance and staining

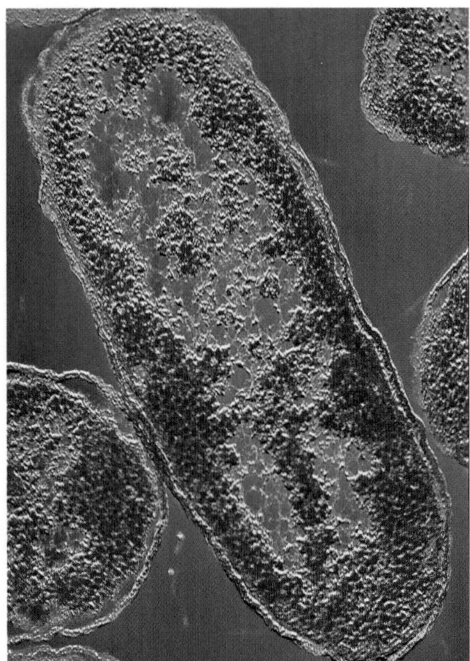

Figure 10-4
False-color transmission electron micrograph of the rod-shaped, gram-negative bacterium *Escherichia coli*, showing the simple procaryotic cell structure including the cytoplasm, the cytoplasmic membrane, and the rigid cell wall. (© Science Source/Photo Researchers)

properties of the cell. Gram's stain, originally developed in 1884 by the Danish bacteriologist Christian Gram, is still the most widely used staining procedure. Bacteria are designated as *gram-positive* organisms if they are stained purple by a primary basic dye (usually crystal violet); those that are not stained by the crystal violet but are counterstained a red color by a second dye (safranin) are called *gram-negative* organisms. Staining characteristics and microscopic morphology are used in combination to describe bacteria. For example, *Streptococcus pyogenes*, the agent of scarlet fever and rheumatic fever, is a gram-positive streptococcal organism that is spherical, grows in chains, and stains purple by Gram's stain. *Legionella pneumophila*, the bacterium responsible for legionnaire's disease, is a gram-negative rod.

For purposes of identification and classification, each member of the bacterial kingdom is categorized into a small group of biochemically and genetically related organisms called the *genus* and further subdivided into distinct individuals within the genus called *species*. The genus and species assignment of the organism is reflected in its name (*e.g.*, *Staphylococcus* [genus] *aureus* [species]).

Spirochetes

The spirochetes are an eccentric category of bacteria that are mentioned separately because of their unusual cellular morphology and mechanism of motility. Technically, the spirochetes are gram-negative rods but are distinctive in that the cell' shape is helical and the length of the organism is many times its width. A series of filaments are wound about the cell wall and extend the entire length of the cell. These filaments propel the organism through an aqueous environment in a corkscrew motion.

Spirochetes are anaerobic or facultatively anaerobic organisms and contain three genera: *Leptospira*, *Borrelia*, and *Treponema*. Each genus has saprophytic and pathogenic strains. The pathogenic leptospires infect a wide variety of wild and domestic animals. Infected animals shed the organisms into the environment through the urinary tract. Transmission to humans occurs by contact with infected animals or urine-contaminated surroundings. Leptospires gain access to the host directly through mucous membranes or breaks in the skin and can produce a severe and potentially fatal illness called Weil's syndrome. In contrast, the borreliae are transmitted from infected animals to humans through the bite of an arthropod vector such as lice or ticks. Included among the genus *Borrelia* are the agents of relapsing fever (*B. recurrentis*) and Lyme disease (*B. burgdorferi*). Pathogenic *Treponema* species require no intermediates and are spread from person to person by direct contact. The most important member of the genus is *Treponema pallidum*, the cause of syphilis.

Mycoplasmas

The mycoplasmas are unicellular prokaryotes capable of independent replication. These organisms are less than one third the size of bacteria and contain a small DNA genome approximately one-half the size of the bacterial chromosome. The cell is composed of cytoplasm surrounded by a membrane, but unlike bacteria, the mycoplasmas do not produce a rigid peptidoglycan cell wall. As a consequence, the microscopic appearance of the cell is highly variable, ranging from coccoid forms to filaments, and the mycoplasmas are resistant to cell wall–inhibiting antibiotics (*e.g.*, penicillins, cephalosporins).

The mycoplasmas of humans are divided into three genera: *Mycoplasma*, *Ureaplasma*, and *Acholeplasma*. The first two of these require cholesterol from the environment to produce the cell membrane; the *Acholeplasma* do not. In the human host, mycoplasmas are commensals. However, a number of species are capable of producing serious diseases, including pneumonia (*Mycoplasma pneumoniae*), genital infections (*Mycoplasma hominis* and *Ureaplasma urealyticum*), and maternally transmitted respiratory infections to low-birth-weight infants (*U. urealyticum*).

Rickettsiae, Chlamydiae, Ehrichieae, and *Coxiella*

This interesting group of organisms combine the characteristics of viral and bacterial agents to produce disease in humans. All are obligate intracellular pathogens like the viruses but produce a rigid peptidoglycan cell wall, reproduce asexually by cellular division, and contain RNA and DNA similar to the bacteria.

The rickettsiae depend on the host cell for essential vitamins and nutrients, but the chlamydiae appear to scavenge intermediates of energy metabolism such as adenosine triphosphate (ATP). The rickettsiae infect but do not produce disease in the cells of certain arthropods such as fleas, ticks, and lice. The organisms are accidentally transmitted to humans through the bite of the arthropod (*i.e.,* vector) and produce a number of potentially lethal diseases, including Rocky Mountain spotted fever and epidemic typhus.

The chlamydiae are slightly smaller than the rickettsiae but are structurally similar. Unlike the rickettsiae, chlamydiae are transmitted directly between susceptible vertebrates without an intermediate arthropod host. Transmission and replication of chlamydiae occur through a defined life cycle. The infectious form, called an *elementary body*, attaches to and enters the host cell where it transforms into a larger *reticulate body*. The latter undergoes active replication into multiple elementary bodies, which are shed into the extracellular environment to initiate another infectious cycle. Chlamydial diseases of humans include sexually transmitted genital infections (see Chapter 52); ocular infections and pneumonia of newborns (*Chlamydia trachomatis*); upper and lower respiratory tract infections in children, adolescents, and young adults (*Chlamydia pneumoniae*); and respiratory disease acquired from infected birds (*Chlamydia psittaci*).

The ehrlichieae are also obligate intracellular organisms that resemble the rickettsiae in structure and produce and variety of veterinarian and human diseases some of which have a tick vector. These organisms target host mononuclear and polymorphonuclear white blood cells for infection and, similar to the chlamydiae, multiply within the cytoplasm of infected within vacuoles called *morulae*. Unlike the chlamydiae, however, the ehrlichieae do not have a defined life cycle and are independent of the host cell for energy production. In the far East, *E. sennetsu* produces a disease in humans called sennetsu fever that resembles infectious mononucleosis. In the United States, the most frequent manifestation of *Ehrlichia* infection is human monocytic ehrlichiosis—a disease cause by *E. chaffeensis* that is easily confused with Rocky mountain spotted fever.

The genus *Coxiella* contains only one species, *C. burnetii*. Like its rickettsial counterparts, it too is a gram-negative intracellular organism that infects a variety of animals, including cattle, sheep, and goats. In humans, *Coxiella* infection produces a disease called *Q fever*, characterized by a nonspecific febrile illness often accompanied by headache, chills, arthralgias, and mild pneumonia. The organism produces a highly resistant spore stage that is transmitted to humans when animal tissue is aerosolized (*e.g.,* during meat processing) or by ingestion of contaminated milk.

Fungi

The fungi are free-living, eukaryotic saprophytes found in every habitat on earth. Some are members of the normal human microflora. Fortunately, few fungi are capable of causing diseases in humans, and most of these are incidental self-limited infections of skin and subcutaneous tissue. Serious fungal infections are rare and usually initiated through puncture wounds or inhalation. Despite their normally harmless nature, fungi can cause serious life-threatening opportunistic diseases when host defense capabilities have been disabled.

The fungi can be separated into two groups, yeasts and molds, based on rudimentary differences in their morphology (Fig. 10–5). The yeasts are single-celled organisms, approximately the size of a red blood cell, that reproduce by a budding process. The buds separate from the parent cell and mature into identical daughter cells. Molds produce long, hollow, branching filaments called *hyphae*. Some molds produce cross walls, which segregate the hyphae into compartments, and others do not. A limited number of fungi are capable of growing as yeasts at one temperature and as molds at another. These organisms are called *dimorphic fungi* and include a number of human pathogens such as the agents of blastomycosis, histoplasmosis, and coccidioidomycosis (*i.e.,* San Joaquin fever).

The visual appearance of a fungal colony tends to reflect its cellular composition. Colonies of yeast are generally smooth with a waxy or creamy texture. Molds tend to produce cottony or powdery colonies composed of mats of hyphae collectively called a *mycelium*. The mycelium can penetrate the growth surface or project above the colony like the roots and branches of a tree. Yeasts and molds produce a rigid cell wall layer that is chemically unrelated to the peptidoglycan of bacteria and is therefore not susceptible to the effects of penicillinlike antibiotics.

Most fungi are capable of sexual or asexual reproduction. The former process involves the fusion of zygotes with the production of a recombinant zygospore. Asexual reproduction involves the formation of highly resistant spores called *conidia* or *sporangiospores*, which are borne by specialized structures that arise from the hyphae. Molds are identified in the laboratory by the characteristic microscopic appearance of the asexual fruiting structures and spores.

Just like the bacterial pathogens of humans, fungi can only produce disease in the human host if they can grow at the temperature of the infected body site. For example, a number of fungal pathogens called the *dermatophytes* are incapable of growing at core body temperature (37°C) and the infection is limited to the cooler cutaneous surfaces. Diseases caused by these organisms (*e.g.,* ringworm, athlete's foot, jock itch) are collectively called superficial mycoses. Systemic mycoses are serious fungal infections of deep tissues and, by definition, are caused by organisms capable of growth at 37°C. Yeasts such as *Candida albicans* are commensals of the skin, mucous membranes, and gastrointestinal tract and are capable of growth at a wider range of temperatures. Intact immune mechanisms and competition for nutrients provided by the bacterial flora normally keep colonizing fungi in check. Alterations in either of these components by disease states or antibiotic therapy can upset the balance, permitting fungal overgrowth and setting the stage for opportunistic infections.

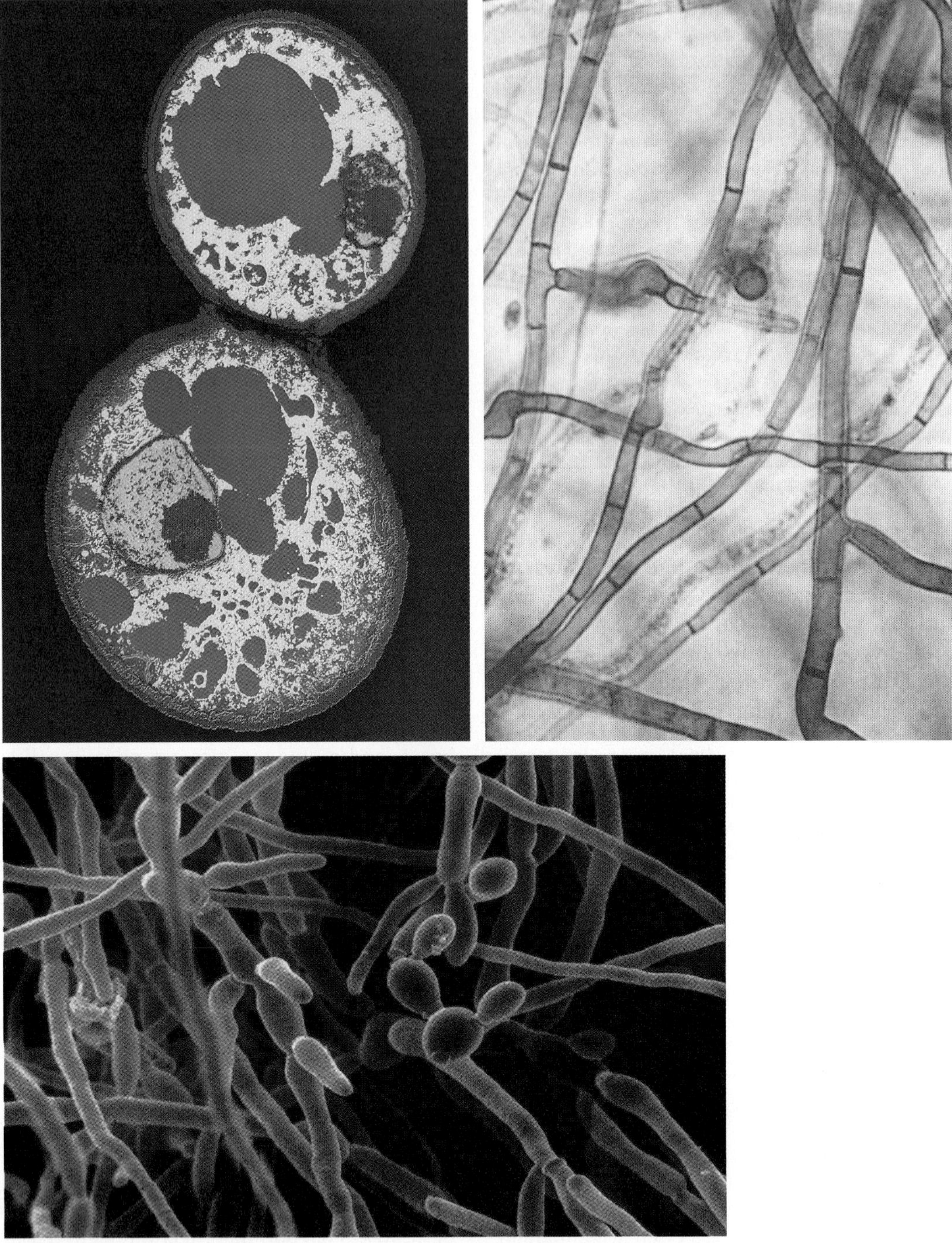

Figure 10-5
The microscopic morphology of fungal pathogens in humans. The yeasts are single-celled organisms that reproduce by the budding process (**upper left**). The molds (**right**) produce long branched or unbranched filaments called hyphae. *Candida albicans* (**lower left**) is a budding yeast that produces pseudohyphae both in culture and in tissues and exudates. (Upper left and lower left © Science Source/Photo Researchers)

Parasites

In a strict sense, any organism that derives benefits from its biologic relationship with another organism is a parasite. In the study of microbiology, the term *parasite* has evolved to designate members of the animal kingdom that infect and cause disease in other animals and includes protozoa, helminths, and arthropods.

The protozoa are unicellular animals with a complete complement of eukaryotic cellular machinery, including a well-defined nucleus and organelles. Reproduction may be sexual or asexual, and life cycles may be simple or complicated with several maturation stages requiring more than one host for completion. Most are saprophytes, but a few have adapted to the accommodations of the human environment and produce a variety of diseases, including malaria, amebic dysentery, and giardiasis. Protozoan infections can be passed directly from host to host (*e.g.*, sexual contact), indirectly through contaminated water or food, or by way of an arthropod vector. Direct or indirect transmission results from the ingestion of highly resistant cysts or spores that are shed in the feces of an infected host. When the cysts reach the intestine, they mature into vegetative forms called trophozoites, which are capable of asexual reproduction or cyst formation. Most trophozoites are motile by means of flagella, cilia, or ameboid motion.

The helminths are a collection of wormlike parasites, which include the roundworms (*i.e.*, nematodes), tapeworms (*i.e.*, cestodes), and flukes (*i.e.*, trematodes). The helminths reproduce sexually within the definitive host, and some require an intermediate host for the development and maturation of offspring. Humans can serve as the definitive or intermediate host and, in certain diseases such as trichinosis, as both. Transmission of helminth diseases occurs primarily through the ingestion of fertilized eggs (ova) or the penetration of infectious larval stages through the skin—directly or with the aid of an arthropod vector. Helminth infections can involve many organ systems and sites, including the liver and lung, urinary and intestinal tracts, circulatory and central nervous systems, and muscle. Although most helminth diseases have been eradicated from the United States, they are still a major health concern of developing nations.

The parasitic arthropods of humans and animals include the vectors of infectious diseases (e.g., ticks, mosquitoes, biting flies) and the ectoparasites. The ectoparasites infest external body surfaces and cause localized tissue damage or inflammation secondary to the bite or burrowing action of the arthropod. The most prominent human ectoparasites are mites (*i.e.*, scabies), chiggers, lice (*i.e.*, head, body, and pubic), and fleas. Transmission of ectoparasites occurs directly by contact with immature or mature forms of the arthropod or its eggs found on the infested host or the host's clothing, bedding, or grooming articles (*e.g.*, combs, brushes). Many of the ectoparasites are vectors of other infectious diseases, including endemic typhus and bubonic plague (*i.e.*, fleas) and epidemic typhus (*i.e.*, lice). A summary of the salient characteristics of human microbial pathogens is presented in Table 10–2.

In summary, this section of the chapter underscores the extreme diversity of prokaryotic and eukaryotic microorganisms capable of causing infectious diseases in humans. With the advent of immunosuppressive medical therapy and immunosuppressive diseases such as AIDS, the number and type of potential microbic pathogens, the so-called opportunistic pathogens, have increased dramatically. However, most infectious illnesses in humans continue to be caused by only a small fraction of the organisms that comprise the microscopic world.

Mechanisms of Infection

After you have completed this section of the chapter, you should be able to meet the following objectives:

- Differentiate between incidence and prevalence and among endemic, epidemic, and panepidemic
- Describe the stages of an infectious disease after the point at which the potential pathogen enters the body
- List the systemic manifestations of infectious disease
- Describe mechanisms and significance of antimicrobial and antiviral drug resistance
- Explain the actions of intravenous immunoglobulin and cytokines in treatment of infectious illnesses

TABLE 10-2 Comparison of Characteristics of Human Microbial Pathogens

Organism	Defined Nucleus	Genomic Material	Size*	Intracellular Extracellular	Motility
Virus	No	DNA or RNA	0.02–0.3	I	−
Bacteria	No	DNA	0.5–15	I/E	±
Mycoplasmas	No	DNA	0.2–0.3	E	−
Spirochetes	No	DNA	6–15	E	+
Rickettsias	No	DNA	0.2–2	I	−
Chlamydia	No	DNA	0.3–1	I	−
Yeasts	Yes	DNA	2–60	I/E	−
Molds	Yes	DNA	2–15 (hyphal width)	E	−
Protozoans	Yes	DNA	1–60	I/E	+
Helminths	Yes	DNA	2 mm–>1 m	E	+

*Micrometers unless indicated.

Epidemiology of Infectious Diseases

Epidemiology, in the context of this chapter, is the study of factors, events, and circumstances that influence the transmission of infectious diseases among humans. The ultimate goal of the epidemiologist is to devise strategies that interrupt or eliminate the spread of an infectious agent. To accomplish this, infectious diseases must be classified according to incidence, portal of entry, source, symptoms, disease course, site of infection, and virulence factors so that potential outbreaks may be predicted and averted or appropriately treated. Each of these categories is discussed in detail with the exception of agents and host, which have already been reviewed.

Epidemiology is a science of rates. The expected frequency of any infectious disease must be calculated so that gradual or abrupt changes in frequency can be observed. The term *incidence* is used to describe the number of new cases of an infectious disease that occur within a defined population (*e.g.*, per 100,000 persons) over an established period of time (*e.g.*, monthly, quarterly, yearly). Disease *prevalence* indicates the number of active cases at any given time. A disease is considered *endemic* in a particular geographic region if the incidence and prevalence are expected and relatively stable. An *epidemic* describes an abrupt and unexpected increase in the incidence of disease over endemic rates. A *pandemic* refers to the spread of disease beyond continental boundaries. The advent of rapid worldwide travel increased the likelihood of pandemic transmission of pathogenic microorganisms.

Portal of Entry

The portal of entry refers to the process by which a pathogen enters the body, gains access to susceptible tissues, and causes disease. Among the potential modes of transmission are penetration, direct contact, ingestion, and inhalation.

Penetration

Any disruption in the integrity of the body's surface barrier (*e.g.*, skin, mucous membranes) is a potential site for invasion of microorganisms. The break may be the result of an accidental injury (*e.g.*, abrasions, burns, penetrating wounds), medical procedures such as surgery or catheterization, a primary infectious process that produces surface lesions such as chickenpox or impetigo, or direct inoculation from intravenous drug use or from animal or arthropod bites. The latter mode of transmission can be extremely dangerous, because large numbers of organisms can be introduced directly into vital sites, bypassing the host's primary immune defense systems.

Direct Contact

Some pathogens are transmitted directly from infected tissue or secretions to exposed, intact mucous membranes without a prerequisite for damaged mucosal barriers. This is especially true of certain sexually transmitted diseases (STDs) such as gonorrhea, syphilis, chlamydia, and herpes, for which exposure of uninfected membranes to pathogens occurs during intimate contact.

The transmission of STDs is not limited to sexual contact. *Vertical transmission* of these agents (i.e., from mother to child) can occur across the placenta or during birth when the mucous membranes of the child come in contact with infected vaginal secretions of the mother. When an infectious disease is transmitted from mother to child during gestation or birth, it is classified as a *congenital infection*. The most frequently observed congenital infections include the parasite *Toxoplasma gondii*, rubella, cytomegalovirus, herpes simplex viruses, and syphilis (the so-called *TORCH* infections), varicella-zoster (*i.e.*, chickenpox) parvovirus B19, and HIV. Of these, cytomegalovirus is by far the most common cause of congenital infection in the United States, affecting nearly 1% of all newborns. However, more than 6000 HIV-infected women give birth each year in the U.S., and the numbers are likely far greater in developing nations. With a 13% to 30% chance of vertical transmission, HIV is rapidly gaining in stature as a congenitally transmitted infection.

The severity of congenital defects associated with these infections depends greatly on the gestational age of the fetus when transmission occurs, but most of these agents can cause profound mental retardation and neurosensory deficits, including blindness and hearing loss. HIV rarely produces overt signs and symptoms in the infected newborn, and it sometimes takes years for the effects of the illness to manifest.

Ingestion

The entry of pathogenic microorganisms or their toxic products through the oral cavity and gastrointestinal tract represents one of the more efficient means of disease transmission in humans. Many bacterial, viral, and parasitic infections, including cholera, typhoid fever, dysentery (amoebic and bacillary), food poisoning, traveler's diarrhea, and hepatitis A, are initiated through the ingestion of contaminated food and water. This mechanism of transmission necessitates that an infectious agent survives the low pH and enzyme activity of gastric secretions and the peristaltic action of the intestines in numbers sufficient to establish infection (*i.e.*, infectious dose). Ingested pathogens also must compete successfully with the normal bacterial flora of the bowel for nutritional needs. Persons with reduced gastric acidity (*i.e.*, achlorhydria) due to disease or medication are more susceptible to infection by this route because the number of ingested microorganisms surviving the gastric environment is greater. Ingestion has also been postulated as a means of transmission of HIV infection from mother to child through breast-feeding.

Inhalation

The respiratory tract of healthy persons is equipped with a multitiered defense system to prevent potential pathogens from entering the lungs. The surface of the respiratory tree is lined with a layer of mucus that is continuously swept up and away from the lungs and toward the mouth by the beating motion of ciliated epithelial cells. Humidification of inspired air increases the size of aerosolized particles, which are effectively filtered by the mucous membranes of the upper respiratory tract. Coughing also aids in the removal of particulate matter from the lower respiratory tract. Respiratory secretions contain antibodies and enzymes capable of inactivating infectious agents. Particulate matter and microorganisms that ultimately reach the lung are cleared by phagocytic cells.

Despite this impressive array of protective mechanisms, a number of pathogens can invade the human body through the respiratory tract, including agents of bacterial pneumonia (*Streptococcus pneumoniae, Legionella pneumophila*), meningitis and sepsis (*N. meningitidis* and *Haemophilus influenzae*), tuberculosis, and the viruses responsible for measles, mumps, chickenpox, influenza, and the common cold. Defective pulmonary function or mucociliary clearance caused by noninfectious processes such as cystic fibrosis, emphysema, or smoking can increase the risk of inhalation-acquired diseases.

The portal of entry does not dictate the site of infection. Ingested pathogens may penetrate the intestinal mucosa, disseminate through the circulatory system, and cause diseases in other organs such as the lung or liver. Whatever the mechanisms of entry, the transmission of infectious agents is directly related to the number of infectious agents absorbed by the host.

Source

The source of an infectious disease refers to the location, host, object, or substance from which the infectious agent was acquired: essentially the who, what, where, and when of disease transmission. The source may be endogenous (*i.e.*, acquired from the host's own microbial flora as would be the case in an opportunistic infection) or exogenous (*i.e.*, acquired from sources in the external environment such as the water, food, soil, or air). The infectious agent can originate from another human being, as from mother to child during gestation (*i.e.*, congenital infections) or birth (*i.e.*, perinatal infections). Zoonoses are a category of infectious diseases passed from other animal species to humans. Examples of zoonoses include cat-scratch disease, rabies, and visceral or cutaneous larval migrans. The spread of infectious diseases, including Lyme disease, malaria, yellow fever, and trypanosomiasis, through biting arthropod vectors has already been mentioned.

Source can denote a place. For instance, infections that develop in patients while they are hospitalized are called *nosocomial*, and those that are acquired outside of health care facilities are called *community acquired*. The source may also pertain to the body substance that is the most likely vehicle for transmission, such as feces, blood, body fluids, respiratory secretions, and urine. Infections can be transmitted from person to person through shared inanimate objects (fomites) contaminated with infected body fluids. An example of this mechanism of transmission would include the spread of the HIV and hepatitis B virus through the use of shared syringes by intravenous drug users. Infection can also be spread through a complex combination of source, portal of entry, and vector. The well-publicized 1993 outbreak of hantavirus pulmonary syndrome in the southwestern United States is a prime example. This viral illness was transmitted to humans by inhalation of dust contaminated with saliva, feces, and urine of infected rodents.

Symptomatology

The term *symptomatology* refers to the collection of signs and symptoms expressed by the host during the disease course. This is also known as the *clinical picture* or disease presentation and can be characteristic of any given infectious agent. In terms of pathophysiology, symptoms are the outward expression of the struggle between invading organisms and the retaliatory inflammatory and immune responses of the host (see Chapter 11). The symptoms of an infectious disease may be specific and reflect the site of infection (*e.g.*, diarrhea, rash, convulsions, hemorrhage, pneumonia). Conversely, symptoms such as fever, myalgia, headache, and lethargy are relatively nonspecific and can be shared by a number of diverse infectious diseases. The symptoms of a diseased host can be obvious, as in the cases of chickenpox or measles. Other covert symptoms, such as hepatitis or an increased white blood cell count, may require laboratory testing to detect. Accurate recognition and documentation of symptomatology can aid in the diagnosis of an infectious disease.

Disease Course

The course of any infectious disease can be divided into several distinguishable stages after the point of time in which the potential pathogen enters the host. These stages are the incubation period, the prodromal stage, the acute stage, the convalescent stage, and the resolution stage (Fig. 10–6). The stages are based on the progression and intensity of the host's symptoms over time. The duration of each phase and the pattern of the overall illness can be specific for different pathogens, thereby aiding in the diagnosis of an infectious disease.

The *incubation period* is the phase during which the pathogen begins active replication without producing recognizable symptoms in the host. The incubation period may be short, as in the case of salmonellosis (6 to 24 hours) or prolonged such as that of hepatitis B (50 to 180 days) or HIV (months to years). The duration of the incubation period can be influenced by additional factors, including the general health of the host, the portal of entry, and the infectious dose of the pathogen.

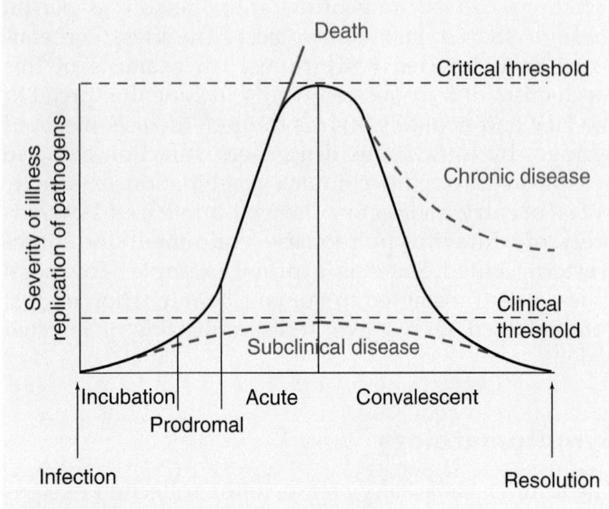

Figure 10-6
The stages of a primary infectious disease as they appear in relation to the severity of symptoms and the numbers of infectious agents. The clinical threshold corresponds with the initial expression of recognizable symptoms whereas the critical threshold represents the peak of disease intensity.

The hallmark of the *prodromal stage* is the initial appearance of symptoms in the host, although the clinical presentation during this time may be only a vague sense of malaise. The host may experience mild fever, myalgia, headache, and fatigue. These are constitutional changes shared by a great number of disease processes. The duration of the prodromal stage can vary considerably from host to host.

The *acute stage* is the period during which the host experiences the maximum impact of the infectious process corresponding to rapid proliferation and dissemination of the pathogen. During this phase, toxic byproducts of microbial metabolism, cell lysis, and the immune response mounted by the host combine to produce tissue damage and inflammation. The symptoms of the host are pronounced and more specific than the prodromal stage, usually typifying the pathogen and sites of involvement.

The *convalescent period* is characterized by the containment of infection, progressive elimination of the pathogen, repair of damaged tissue, and resolution of associated symptoms. Similar to the incubation period, the time required for complete convalescence may be days, weeks, or months, depending on the type of pathogen and the voracity of the host's immune response. The *resolution* is the total elimination of a pathogen from the body without residual signs or symptoms of disease.

Several notable exceptions of the classic presentations of an infectious process have been recognized. *Chronic* infectious diseases have a markedly protracted and sometimes irregular course. The host may experience symptoms of the infectious process continuously or sporadically for months or years without a convalescent phase. In contrast, *subclinical* or *subacute* illness progresses from infection to resolution without clinically apparent symptoms. A disease is called *insidious* if the prodromal phase is protracted; a *fulminant* illness is characterized by abrupt onset of symptoms with little or no prodrome. Fatal infections are variants of the typical disease course.

Site of Infection

Inflammation of an anatomic location is usually designated by adding the suffix *-itis* to the name of the involved tissue (*e.g.*, bronchitis, infection of the bronchi and bronchioles; encephalitis, brain infection; carditis, infection of the heart). These are general terms, however, and they apply equally to inflammation from infectious and noninfectious causes. The suffix *-emia* is used to designate the presence of a substance in the blood; the terms *bacteremia, viremia,* and *fungemia* describe the presence of these infectious agents in the bloodstream. The term *sepsis*, or *septicemia*, refers to the presence of microbial toxins in the blood.

The site of an infectious disease is determined ultimately by the type of pathogen, the portal of entry, and competence of the host's immunologic defense system. Many pathogenic microorganisms are restricted in their capacity to invade the human body. *M. pneumoniae*, influenza viruses, and *L. pneumophila* rarely cause disease outside the respiratory tract; infections caused by *N. gonorrhoeae* are generally confined to the genitourinary tract; and shigellosis and giardiasis seldom extend beyond the gastrointestinal tract. These are considered localized infectious diseases. The bacterium *Helicobacter pylori* is an extreme example of a site-specific pathogen. *H. pylori* is considered a probable agent of gastric ulcers and has not been implicated in disease processes elsewhere in the human body. Bacteria such as *H. influenzae* type b, a prominent pathogen of young children; *Salmonella typhi*, the cause of typhoid fever; and *B. burgdorferi*, the agent of Lyme disease, tend to disseminate from the primary site of infection to involve other locations and organ systems. These are examples of systemic pathogens. Most systemic infections disseminate throughout the body by way of the circulatory system.

An abscess is a localized pocket of infection composed of devitalized tissue, microorganisms, and the host's phagocytic white blood cells—in essence, a stalemate in the infectious process. The spread of the pathogen has been contained by the host, but white cell function within the toxic environment of the abscess is hampered, and the elimination of microorganisms is retarded. Abscesses usually must be surgically drained to effect a complete cure. Similarly, infections of biomedical implants such as catheters, artificial heart valves, and prosthetic bone implants are seldom cured by the host's immune response and antimicrobial therapy. The infecting organism colonizes the surface of the implant producing a dense matrix of cells, host proteins, and capsular material, called a *biofilm*, necessitating the removal of the device.

Virulence Factors

Virulence factors are substances or products generated by infectious agents that enhance their ability to cause disease. Although the number and type of microbial products that fit this description are numerous, they can generally be grouped into four categories: toxins, adhesion factors, evasive factors, and invasive factors (Table 10–3).

Toxins

Toxins are substances that alter or destroy the normal function of the host or host's cells. Toxin production is a trait chiefly monopolized by bacterial pathogens, although certain fungal and protozoan pathogens also elaborate substances toxic to humans. Bacterial toxins have a diverse spectrum of activity and exert their effects on a wide variety of host target cells. For classification purposes, however, the bacterial toxins can be divided into two main types: *exotoxins* and *endotoxins*.

Exotoxins are proteins released from the bacterial cell during growth. Bacterial exotoxins enzymatically inactivate or modify key cellular constituents leading to cell death or dysfunction. Diphtheria toxin, for example, inhibits cellular protein synthesis; botulism toxin decreases the release of neurotransmitter from cholinergic neurons, causing flaccid paralysis; tetanus toxin decreases the release of neurotransmitter from inhibitory neurons, producing spastic paralysis; and cholera toxin induces fluid secretion into the lumen of the intestine, causing diarrhea. Other examples of exotoxin-induced diseases include pertussis (whooping cough), anthrax, traveler's diarrhea, toxic shock syndrome, and a host of foodborne illnesses (*i.e.*, food poisoning).

Bacterial exotoxins that produce vomiting and diarrhea are sometimes referred to as *enterotoxins*. There has been a resurgent interest in streptococcal pyrogenic exotoxin A (SPEA), an exotoxin produced by certain strains of group A, beta-hemolytic streptococci (*Streptococcus pyogenes*) that causes a life-threatening toxic shock–like syndrome similar to the disease associated with tampon use produced by *Staphylococcus aureus*. The streptococcal form of intoxication is sometimes called *Henson's disease*, because it was this infection that caused the death of the famous puppeteer Jim Henson. Other exotoxins that have gained notoriety include the Shiga-like toxins produced by *Escherichia coli* O157:H7. The ingestion of undercooked hamburger meat contaminated with organism produces hemorrhagic colitis and a sometimes fatal illness called hemolytic-uremic syndrome (HUS), characterized by vascular endothelial damage, acute renal failure, and thrombocytopenia. HUS occurs primarily in infants and young children who have not developed antibodies to the Shiga-like toxins.

Endotoxins do not contain protein, are not actively released from the bacterium during growth, and have no enzymatic activity. Rather, endotoxins are complex molecules composed of lipid and polysaccharides found in the cell wall of gram-negative bacteria. Studies of different endotoxins have indicated that the lipid portion of the endotoxin confers the toxic properties to the molecule. Endotoxins are potent activators of a number of regulatory systems in humans. A small amount of endotoxin in the circulatory system (*i.e.*, endotoxemia) can induce clotting, bleeding, inflammation, hypotension, and fever. The sum of the physiologic reactions to endotoxins is sometimes called *endotoxic shock*.

Adhesion Factors

No interaction between microorganisms and humans can progress to infection or disease if the pathogen is unable to attach to and colonize the host. The process of microbial attachment may be site specific (*e.g.*, mucous membranes, skin surfaces), cell specific (*e.g.*, T lymphocytes, respiratory epithelium), or nonspecific (*e.g.*, moist areas, charged surfaces). In any of these cases, adhesion requires a positive interaction between the surfaces of host cells and the infectious agent.

The site to which microorganisms adhere is called a *receptor*, and the reciprocal molecule or substance that binds to the receptor is called a *ligand* or *adhesin*. Receptors may be proteins, carbohydrates, lipids, or complex

TABLE 10-3 **Examples of Virulence Factors Produced by Pathogenic Microorganisms**

Factor	Category	Organism	Effect on Host
Cholera toxin	Exotoxin	*Vibrio cholerae* (bacterium)	Secretory diarrhea
Diphtheria toxin	Exotoxin	*Corynebacterium diphtheriae* (bacterium)	Inhibits protein synthesis
Lipopolysaccharide	Endotoxin	Many gram-negative bacteria	Fever, hypotension, shock
Toxic shock toxin	Enterotoxin	*Staphylococcus aureus* (bacterium)	Rash, diarrhea, vomiting, hepatitis
Hemagglutinin	Adherence	Influenzae virus	Establishment of infection
Pili	Adherence	*Neisseria gonorrhoeae* (bacterium)	Establishment of infection
Leukocidin	Evasive	*Staphylococcus aureus*	Kills phagocytes
IgA protease	Evasive	Haemophilus influenzae (bacterium)	Inactives antibody
Capsule	Evasive	*Cryptococcus neoformans* (yeast)	Prevents phagocytosis
Collagenase	Invasive	*Pseudomonas aeruginosa* (bacterium)	Penetration of tissue
Protease	Invasive	*Aspergillus* (mold)	Penetration of tissue
Phospholipase	Invasive	*Clostridium perfringens* (bacterium)	Penetration of tissue

molecules composed of all three. Similarly, ligands may be simple or complex molecules and, in some cases, highly specific structures. Ligands that bind to specific carbohydrates are called *lectins*. Certain bacteria produce hairlike structures protruding from the cell surface called *pili* or *fimbriae*, which anchor the organism to receptors on host cell membranes to establish an infection. Many viral agents, including influenza, mumps, measles, and adenovirus produce filamentous appendages or spikes called *hemagglutinins*, which recognize carbohydrate receptors on the surfaces of specific cells in the upper respiratory tract of the host.

After initial attachment, a number of bacterial agents become embedded in a gelatinous matrix of polysaccharides called a slime or mucous layer. The slime layer serves two purposes: it anchors the agent firmly to host tissue surfaces, and it protects the agent from the immunologic defenses of the host.

Evasive Factors

A number of factors produced by microorganisms enhance virulence by evading various components of the host's immune system. Extracellular polysaccharides (*e.g.*, capsules, slime, mucous layers) discourage engulfment and killing of pathogens by the phagocytic white blood cells (*i.e.*, neutrophils and macrophages) of the host. Encapsulated organisms such as *Streptococcus agalactiae*, *Streptococcus pneumoniae*, *N. meningitidis*, and (before the vaccine) *H. influenza* are a cause of significant morbidity and mortality in neonates and children who lack protective anticapsular antibodies. Certain bacterial, fungal, and parasitic pathogens avoid phagocytosis by excreting leukocidins—toxins that deplete the host of neutrophils and macrophages by causing specific and lethal damage to the cytoplasmic membrane of white blood cells. Other pathogens, such as the bacterial agents of listeriosis and legionnaires' disease are adapted to survive and reproduce within phagocytic white blood cells after ingestion, avoiding or neutralizing the usually lethal products contained within the lysosomes of the cell.

Other unique strategies employed by pathogenic microbes to evade immunologic surveillance have evolved solely to avoid recognition by host antibodies. Strains of *S. aureus* produce a surface protein (protein A) that immobilizes immunoglobulin G, holding the antigen-binding region harmlessly away from the organisms. This pathogen also secretes a unique enzyme called coagulase. Coagulase converts soluble human coagulation factors into a solid clot, which envelops and protects the organism from phagocytic host cells and antibody. *H. influenzae* and *N. gonorrhoeae* secrete enzymes that cleave and inactivate secretory immunoglobulin A, neutralizing the primary defense of the respiratory and genital tracts at the site of infection.

Borrelia species, including the agents of Lyme disease and relapsing fever, alter surface antigens during the disease course to avoid immunologic detection. It appears that the ingenuity to devise strategic defense systems and stealth technologies is not limited to humans. Viruses such as HIV impair the function of immunoregulatory cells. Although this property increases the virulence of these agents, it is not considered a virulence factor in the true sense of the definition.

Invasive Factors

Invasive factors are products produced by infectious agents that facilitate the penetration of anatomic barriers and host tissue. Most invasive factors are enzymes capable of destroying cellular membranes (*e.g.*, phospholipases), connective tissue (*e.g.*, elastases, collagenases), intercellular matrices (*e.g.*, hyaluronidase), and structural protein complexes (*e.g.*, proteases). It is the combined effects of invasive factors, toxins, and antimicrobial and inflammatory substances released by host cells to counter infection that mediate the tissue damage and pathophysiology of infectious diseases.

Diagnosis of Infectious Diseases

After you have completed this section of the chapter, you should be able to meet the following objectives:

- State the two criteria used in the diagnosis of an infectious disease
- Explain the differences in culture, serology, and antigen or metabolite detection methods for diagnosis of infectious disease

The diagnosis of an infectious disease requires two criteria: the recovery of a probable pathogen or evidence of its presence from the infected sites of a diseased host and accurate documentation of clinical signs and symptoms (*i.e.*, symptomatology) compatible with an infectious process. In the laboratory, the diagnosis of an infectious agent is accomplished using three basic techniques: culture, serology, or the detection of characteristic antigens, genomic sequences, or metabolites produced by the pathogen.

Culture refers to the propagation of a microorganism outside of the body, usually on or in artificial growth media such as agar plates or broth (Fig. 10–7). The specimen from the diseased host is inoculated into broth or on to the surface of an agar plate, and the culture is placed in a controlled environment (*e.g.*, incubator) until the growth of microorganisms becomes detectable. In the case of a bacterial pathogen, identification is based on microscopic appearance and Gram's stain reaction, shape, texture, and color (*i.e.*, morphology) of the colonies and by a panel of reactions that "fingerprint" salient biochemical characteristics of the organism. Certain bacteria such as *Mycobacterium leprae*, the agent of leprosy, and *T. pallidum*, the syphilis spirochete, do not grow on artificial media and require additional methods of identification. Fungi and mycoplasmas are cultured in much the same way as bacteria but with more reliance on microscopic and colonial morphology for identification.

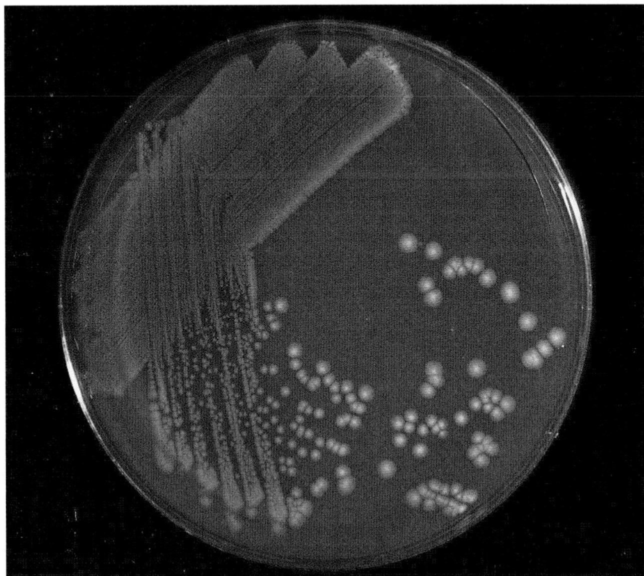

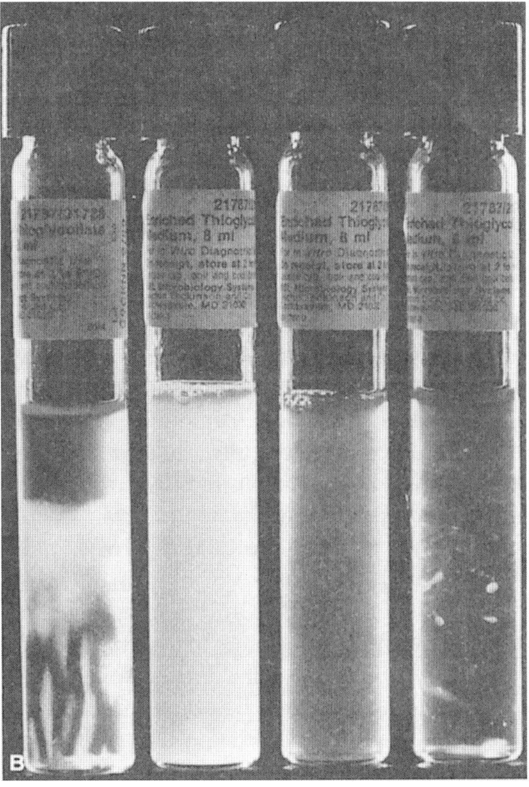

Figure 10-7
Variability of the macroscopic appearance of bacterial cultured on solid, agar-containing medium (**left**) and liquid broth medium (**right**). On solid surfaces, bacteria form distinct colonies as demonstrated by the β-hemolytic streptococcus (*Streptococcus pyogenes*) on sheep blood agar (**left**). Bacteria cultured in broth form a variety of growth patterns, ranging from particulate to homogenous, turbid suspensions. Anaerobic bacteria cultured in liquid medium tend to grow best at the bottom of the tube, where the concentration of molecular oxygen is lowest. (Left © Science Source/Photo Researchers)

Chlamydiae, rickettsiae, and all human viruses are obligate intracellular pathogens. As a result, the propagation of these agents in the laboratory requires the inoculation of eukaryotic cells grown in culture (*i.e.,* cell cultures). A cell culture consists of a flask containing a single layer, or monolayer, of eukaryotic cells covering the bottom and overlaid with broth containing essential nutrients and growth factors. When a virus infects and replicates within cultured eukaryotic cells, it produces pathologic changes in the appearance of the cell called cytopathic effect (CPE) (Fig. 10–8). The CPE can be detected microscopically, and the pattern and extent of cellular destruction is often characteristic of a particular virus.

Although culture media have been developed for the growth of certain human protozoa and helminths in the laboratory, the diagnosis of parasitic infectious diseases has traditionally relied on microscopic, or in the case of worms, visible identification of organisms, cysts, or ova directly from infected patient specimens.

Serology, the study of serum, is an indirect means of identifying infectious agents by measuring serum antibodies in the diseased host. A tentative diagnosis can be made if the antibody level, also called *antibody titer,* against a specific pathogen rises during the acute phase of the disease and falls during convalescence. Serologic identification of an infectious agent is not as accurate as culture, but it may be a useful adjunct, especially for the diagnosis of diseases caused by pathogens that cannot be cultured (*e.g.,* hepatitis B virus). The measurement of antibody titers has another advantage in that specific antibody types such as IgM and IgG are produced by the host during different phases of an infectious process; IgM-specific antibodies generally rise and fall during the acute phase, whereas the synthesis of the IgG class of antibodies increases during the acute phase and remains elevated until or beyond resolution. Measurements of class-specific antibodies are also useful in the diagnosis of congenital infections. IgM antibodies do not cross the placenta, but certain IgG antibodies are transferred passively from mother to child during the final trimester of gestation. Consequently, an elevation of pathogen-specific IgM antibodies found in the serum of a neonate must have originated from the child and therefore indicates congenital infection. A similarly increased IgG titer in the neonate does not differentiate congenital from maternal infection.

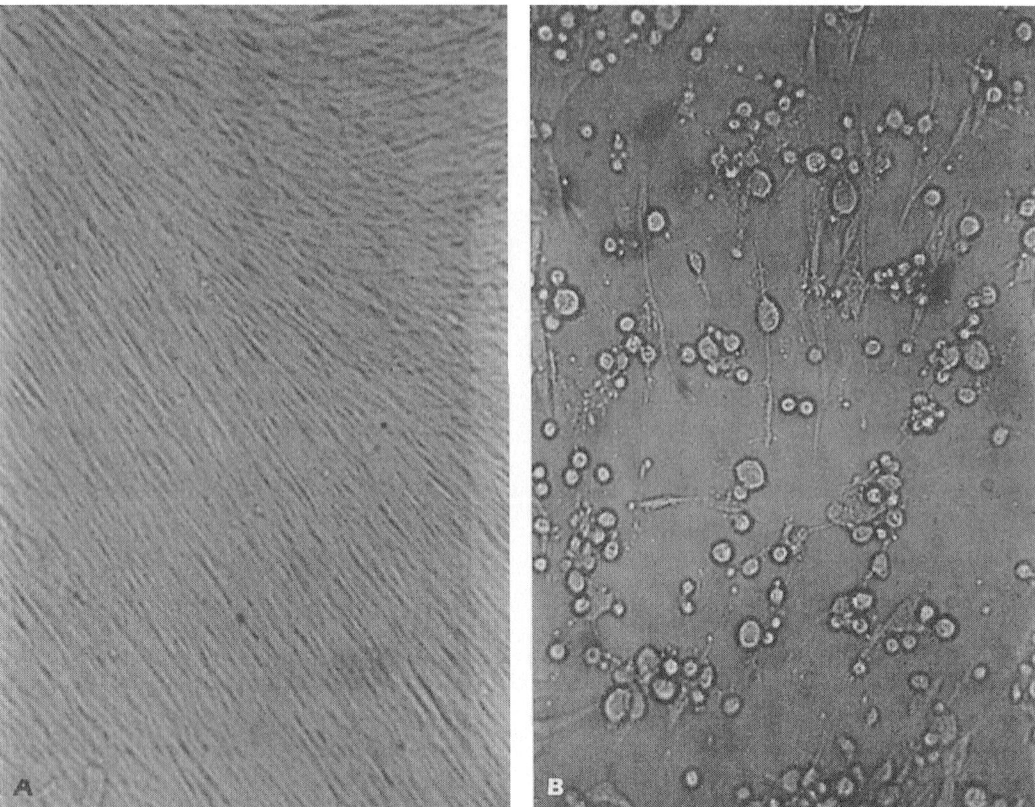

Figure 10-8
The microscopic appearance of a monolayer of uninfected human fibroblasts grown in cell culture (**A**) and the same cells after infection with herpes simplex virus (**B**), demonstrating the cytopathic effect caused by viral replication and concomitant cell lysis.

The technology of *direct antigen detection* has evolved rapidly over the past decade and in the process has revolutionized the diagnosis of infectious diseases. Antigen detection incorporates features of culture and serology but reduces by a fraction the time required for diagnosis. In principle, this method relies on purified antibodies to detect antigens of infectious agents in specimens obtained from the diseased host. The source of antibodies used for antigen detection can be animals immunized against a particular pathogen or *hybridomas.* Hybridomas are created by fusing normal antibody-producing spleen cells from an immunized animal with malignant myeloma cells, which synthesize large quantities of antibody. The result is a cell that produces an antibody called a *monoclonal antibody,* which is highly specific for a single antigen and a single pathogen. Regardless of the source, the antibodies are labeled with a substance that allows microscopic or overt detection when bound to the pathogen or its products. Generally, the three types of labels used for this purpose are fluorescent dyes, enzymes, and particles such as latex beads. Fluorescent antibodies allow visualization of an infectious agent with the aid of a fluorescent microscope. Depending on the type of fluorescent dye used, the organism may appear a bright green or orange color against a black background, making detection extremely easy. Enzyme-labeled antibodies function in a similar manner. The enzyme is capable of converting a colorless compound into a colored substance, thereby permitting detection of antibody bound to an infectious agent without the use of a fluorescent microscope. Particles coated with antibodies clump together, or agglutinate, when the appropriate antigen is present in a specimen. Particle agglutination is especially useful when examining infected body fluids such as urine, serum, or spinal fluid.

The identification of infectious agents through the detection of sequences of DNA or RNA unique to a single agent has undergone rapid development and use during the past few years. Several techniques have been devised to accomplish this goal, each having different degrees of sensitivity regarding the number of organisms that need to be present in a specimen for detection. The first of these methods is called *DNA probe hybridization.* Small fragments of DNA are cut from the genome of a specific pathogen and labeled with compounds (*e.g.,* radioisotopes, photo-emitting chemicals) that allow detection. The labeled DNA "probes" are added to specimens from an infected host. If the pathogen is present, the probe attaches to the complementary strand of DNA on the genome of the infectious agent, permitting rapid diagnosis. The use of labeled probes has allowed visualization of particular agents within and around individual cells in histologic sections of tissue.

The second and most sensitive method of DNA detection to be developed is called the *polymerase chain reaction* (PCR) (Fig. 10–9). This method incorporates two unique reagents: a specific pair of oligonucleotides (usually more than 25 nucleotides long) called primers and a heat-stable DNA polymerase. To perform the assay, the primers are added to the specimen containing the suspect pathogen, and the sample is heated to melt all the DNA in the specimen and then allowed to cool. The primers locate and bind only to the complementary target DNA of the pathogen in question. The heat-stable polymerase begins to replicate the DNA from the point at which the primers attached, similar to two trains approaching one another on separate but converging tracks. After the initial cycle, DNA polymerization ceases at the point where the primers were located, producing a strand of DNA with a distinct size, depending on the distance separating the two primers. The specimen is heated again, and the process starts anew. After many cycles of heating, cooling, and polymerization, a large number of uniformly sized DNA fragments are produced only if the specific pathogen (or its DNA) is present in the specimen. The polymerized DNA fragments are separated by electrophoresis and visualized with a dye or identification by hybridization by a specific probe.

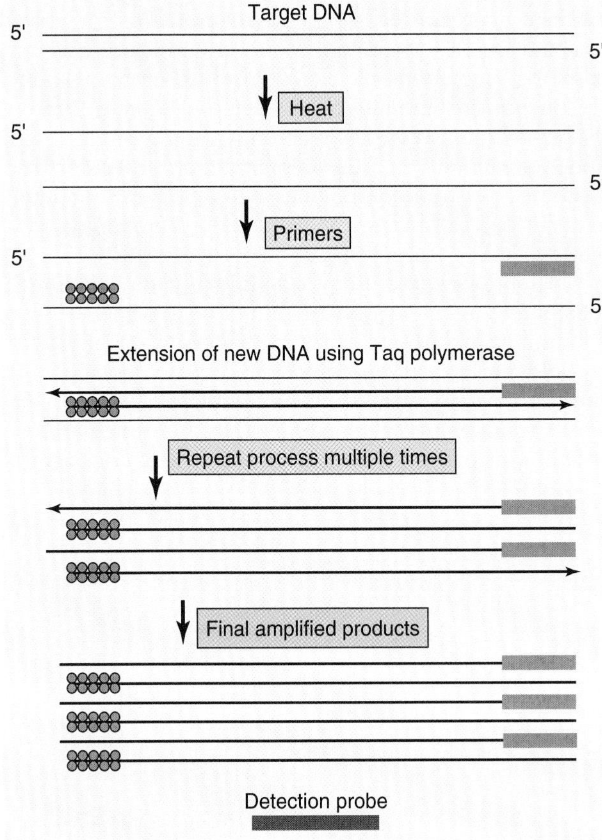

Figure 10-9
The polymerase chain reaction is depicted. The target DNA is first melted using heat (generally around 94°C) to separate the strands of DNA. Primers that recognize specific sequences within the target DNA are allowed to bind as the reaction cools. Using a unique, thermostable DNA polymerase called Taq and an abundance of deoxynucleoside triphosphates, new DNA strands are amplified from the point of the primer attachment. The process is repeated many times (called cycles) until millions of copies of DNA are produced, all of which have the same length defined by the distance (in base pairs) between the primer binding sites. These copies are then detected by electrophoresis and staining or through the use of labeled DNA probes that similar to the primers, recognize a specific sequence located within the amplified section of DNA.

PCR is an extremely useful and powerful tool. In some circumstances, this method can detect as little as one virus or bacterium in a single specimen. This method also allows laboratorians to diagnose infections caused by microorganisms that are impossible or difficult to grow in culture.

Many variations of *gene amplification* techniques related to PCR are being developed with the promise of increased sensitivity and automated methods that would bring this technology out of research laboratories and into routine diagnostic laboratories. One of the newer applications of gene amplification technology is the quantitation of HIV and hepatitis C virus DNA in serum of plasma of the infected patient. If the therapy is effective, viral replication is suppressed and the viral load in the peripheral blood is low. Conversely, if mutations in the viral genome lead to resistant strains or if the antiviral therapy is ineffective, viral replication and the patient's viral load rises, indicating a need to change the therapeutic approach.

Therapy for Infectious Diseases

After you have completed this section of the chapter, you should be able to meet the following objectives:

- Cite three general intervention methods that can be used in treatment of infectious illnesses
- State four basic mechanisms by which antibiotics exert their action
- Differentiate bactericidal from bacteriostatic

The goal of treatment for an infectious disease is complete removal of the pathogen from the host and the restoration of normal physiologic function to damaged tissues. Most infectious diseases of humans are self-limiting (*i.e.*, they require little or no medical therapy for a complete cure). When an infectious process gains the upper hand and therapeutic intervention is essential, the choice of treatment may be medicinal through the use of antimicrobial agents; immunologic with antibody preparations, vaccines, or substances that stimulate and improve the host's immune function, or surgical by removing infected tissues. The decision of which therapeutic modality or combination of therapies is based on the extent, urgency, and location of the disease process, the pathogen, and the availability of effective antimicrobial agents.

Antimicrobial Agents

The use of chemicals, potions, and elixirs in the treatment of infectious diseases dates back to the earliest records of human medicine. More than 2000 years ago, Greek and Chinese physicians recognized that certain substances were useful for preventing or curing wound infections. Although the biologic activity of these compounds was not understood, some may have inadvertently contained byproducts of molds that resemble modern antibiotics. From that time until the late 1800s, when the relation between infection and microorganisms was finally accepted, the evolution of antiinfective therapy was less than explosive. It was not until the advent of World War II, after the introduction of sulfonamides and penicillin, that the development of antimicrobial compounds matured into a science of great consequence. Today, the comprehensive list of effective antiinfective agents is burgeoning. Most antimicrobial compounds can be categorized roughly according to mechanism of antiinfective activity, chemical structure, and target pathogen (*e.g.*, antibacterial, antiviral, antifungal, or antiparasitic agents).

Antibacterial Agents

Antibacterial agents are generally called antibiotics. Most antibiotics are actually produced by other microorganisms—primarily bacteria and fungi—as byproducts of metabolism and usually are only effective against other prokaryotic organisms. An antibiotic is considered *bactericidal* if it causes irreversible and lethal damage to the bacterial pathogen and *bacteriostatic* if its inhibitory effects on bacterial growth are reversed when the agent is eliminated. Antibiotics can be classified into families of compounds with related chemical structure and activity (Table 10–4).

Not all antibiotics are effective against all pathogenic bacteria. Some agents are only effective against gram-negative bacteria, and others are specific for gram-positive organisms. The so-called broad-spectrum antibiotics, such as the newest class of cephalosporins, are active against a wide variety of gram-positive and gram-negative bacteria. Members of the *Mycobacterium* genus, including *Mycobacterium tuberculosis*, are extremely resistant to the effects of the major classes of antibiotics and require an entirely different spectrum of agents for therapy. The four basic mechanisms of the antibiotics are inhibition of bacterial peptidoglycan synthesis (*e.g.*, penicillins, cephalosporins, glycopeptides); inhibition of bacterial protein synthesis (*e.g.*, aminoglycosides, macrolides, tetracyclines, chloramphenicol, and rifampin); interruption of nucleic acid synthesis (*e.g.*, fluoroquinolones, nalidixic acid); and interference with normal metabolism (*e.g.*, sulfonamides, trimethoprim).

Despite lack of antibiotic activity against eukaryotic cells, many agents cause unwanted or toxic side effects in humans, including allergic responses (*e.g.*, penicillins, cephalosporins, sulfonamides, glycopeptides), hearing and kidney impairment (*e.g.*, aminoglycosides), and liver or bone marrow toxicity (*e.g.*, chloramphenicol). Of greater concern is the increasing prevalence of bacteria

TABLE 10-4

Classification and Activity of Antibacterial Agents (Antibiotics)

Family	Example	Target Site	Side Effects
Penicillins	Ampicillin	Cell wall	Allergic reactions
Cephalosporins	Cephalexin	Cell wall	Allergic reactions
Monobactams	Aztreonma	Cell wall	Rash
Aminoglycosides	Tobramycin	Ribosomes (protein synthesis)	Hearing loss Nephrotoxicity
Tetracyclines	Doxycycline	Ribosomes (protein synthesis)	Gastrointestinal irritation Allergic reactions Teeth and bone dysplasia
Macrolides	Clindamycin	Ribosomes (protein synthesis)	Colitis Allergic reactions
Sulfonamides	Sulfadiazine	Folic acid synthesis	Allergic reactions Anemia Gastrointestinal irritation
Glycopeptides	Vancomycin	Ribosomes (protein synthesis)	Allergic reactions Hearing loss Nephrotoxicity
Quinolones	Ciprofloxacin	DNA synthesis	Gastrointestinal irritation
Miscellaneous	Chloramphenicol	Ribosomes (protein synthesis)	Anemia Hepatotoxicity
	Rifampin	Ribosomes (protein synthesis)	Allergic reactions
	Trimethoprim	Folic acid synthesis	Same as sulfonamides

resistant to the effects of antibiotics. The ways in which bacteria acquire resistance to antibiotics are becoming as numerous as the number of antibiotics. Bacterial resistance mechanisms include the production of enzymes that inactivate antibiotics such as β-lactamases, genetic mutations that alter antibiotic binding sites, alternative metabolic pathways that bypass antibiotic activity, and changes in the filtration qualities of the bacterial cell wall that prevent access of antibiotics to the target site within the organism. It is the continuous search for a better mousetrap that makes antiinfective therapy such a fascinating aspect of infectious diseases.

Antiviral Agents

Until recently, few effective antiviral agents were available for treating human infections. The reason for this is host toxicity; viral replication requires the use of eukaryotic host cell enzymes, and the drugs that effectively interrupt viral replication are likely to interfere with host cell reproduction as well. However, in response to the AIDS epidemic, there has been massive, albeit delayed, development of antiretroviral agents. Almost all antiviral compounds are synthetic, and with few exceptions, the primary target of antiviral compounds is viral RNA or DNA synthesis. Agents such as acyclovir, ganciclovir, vidarabine, and ribavirin mimic the nucleoside building blocks of RNA and DNA. During active viral replication, the nucleoside analogues inhibit the viral DNA polymerase, preventing duplication of the viral genome and spread of infectious viral progeny to other susceptible host cells. Similar to the specificity of antibiotics, antiviral agents may be active against RNA viruses only, DNA viruses only, or occasionally both. Other nucleoside analogues such as zidovudine, lamivudine, didanosine, stavudine, and zalcitabine were developed specifically for the treatment of AIDS by targeting the HIV-specific enzyme, reverse transcriptase, for inhibition. This key enzyme is essential for viral replication and has no counterpart in the infected eukaryotic host cells.

Another class of antiviral agents, developed solely for the treatment of HIV infections are called protease inhibitors and include indinavir, ritonavir, and saquinavir. These drugs inhibit an HIV-specific enzyme that is necessary for late maturation events in the virus life cycle.

Experimental approaches to antiviral therapy include compounds that inhibit viral attachment to susceptible host cells and drugs that prevent uncoating of the viral genome once inside the host cell and agents, such as foscarnet, that directly inhibit viral DNA polymerase. Although the treatment of viral infections with antimicrobial agents is a relatively recent endeavor, reports of viral mutations resulting in resistant strains have become increasingly more common. This is an especially troubling in the case of HIV, in which resistance to relatively new antiviral agents, including nuceoloside analogues and protease inhibitors, has already been described, prompting the need for combination or alternating therapy with multiple antiretroviral agents.

Antifungal Agents

The target site of the two most important families of antifungal agents is the cytoplasmic membranes of yeasts or molds. Fungal membranes differ from human cell membranes in that they contain the sterol ergosterol instead of cholesterol. The polyene family of antifungal compounds (*e.g.*, amphotericin B, nystatin) preferentially bind to ergosterol and form holes in the cytoplasmic membrane, causing leakage of the fungal cell contents and, eventually, lysis of the cell. The imidazole class of drugs (*e.g.*, fluconazole, itraconazole, ketoconazole) inhibit the synthesis of ergosterol, thereby damaging the integrity of the fungal cytoplasmic membrane. Both types of drugs bind to a certain extent to the cholesterol component of host cell membranes and elicit a variety of toxic side effects in treated patients. The nucleoside analogue 5-fluorocytosine (5-FC) disrupts fungal RNA and DNA synthesis but without the toxicity associated with the polyene and imidazole drugs. Unfortunately, 5-FC demonstrates little or no antifungal activity against molds or dimorphic fungi and is primarily reserved for infections caused by yeasts.

A novel class of antifungal compounds called *pneumocandins* have received considerable attention, because they inhibit the synthesis of β-1,3-glucan, a major cell wall polysaccharide that is found in fungi, including *C. albicans*, *Aspergillus*, and *Pneumocystis carinii*.

Antiparasitic Agents

Because of the extreme diversity of human parasites and their growth cycles, a review of antiparasitic therapies and agents would be highly impractical and lengthy. Similar to other infectious disease caused by eukaryotic microorganisms, treatment of parasitic illnesses is based on exploiting essential components of the parasite's metabolism or cellular anatomy that are not shared by the host. Any relatedness between the target site of the parasite and the cells of the host increases the likelihood of toxic reactions in the host.

Continued development of improved antiparasitic agents suffers greatly from economic considerations. Parasitic diseases of humans are primarily the scourge of poor, developing nations of the world. As a result, financial incentives to produce more effective therapies are nonexistent. Resistance among human parasites to standard, effective therapy is also a major concern. In Africa, Asia, and South America, the incidence of chloroquine-resistant malaria (*Plasmodium falciparum*) is on the rise. Resistant strains require more complicated, expensive, and potentially toxic therapy with a combination of agents.

Immunotherapy

An exciting approach to the treatment of infectious diseases is immunotherapy. This strategy involves supplementing or stimulating the host's immune response so that the spread of a pathogen is limited or reversed.

Several products are available for this purpose, including intravenous immune globulin (IVIG) and cytokines. IVIG is a pooled preparation of antibodies obtained from normal, healthy immune human donors that is infused as an intravenous solution. In theory, pathogen-specific antibodies present in the infusion facilitate neutralization, phagocytosis, and clearance of infectious agents above and beyond the capabilities of the diseased host. Hyperimmune immunoglobulin preparations, which are also commercially available, contain high titers of antibodies against specific pathogens, including hepatitis B virus, cytomegalovirus, rabies, and varicella-zoster virus.

Cytokines are substances produced by human white blood cells that, in small quantities, stimulate white cell replication, phagocytosis, antibody production, and the induction of fever, inflammation, and tissue repair—all of which counteract infectious agents and hasten recovery. With the advent of genetic engineering and cloning, many cytokines, including interferons and interleukins, have been produced in the laboratory and are being evaluated experimentally as antiinfective agents. As we learn more about the action of cytokines, we are beginning to appreciate that some of the adverse reactions associated with infectious processes result from our own inflammatory response. Interventional therapies designed to inactivate certain cytokines (e.g., tumor necrosis factor) have proven to be helpful in animal models of infection. It is not unlikely that therapies based on the regulation of the inflammatory response will become widely used in human medicine over the next few years.

One of the most efficient but often overlooked means of preventing infectious diseases is immunization. Proper and timely adherence to recommended vaccination schedules in children and boosters in adults effectively reduces the senseless spread of vaccine-preventable illnesses such as measles, mumps, pertussis, and rubella, which still occur in the United States with alarming frequency.

Surgical Intervention

Before the discovery of antimicrobial agents, surgical removal of infected tissues, organs, or limbs was occasionally the only option available to prevent the demise of the infected host. Today, medicinal therapy with antibiotics and other antiinfective agents is an effective solution for most infectious diseases. However, surgical intervention is still an important option for cases in which the pathogen is resistant to available treatments; containment of rapidly progressing infectious process is the only means of saving the patient (*e.g.*, gas gangrene); or access to an infected site by antimicrobial agents is limited and surgical drainage (*e.g.*, abscesses), cleaning of the site (debridement), or removal of organs or necrotic tissue (*e.g.*, appendectomy) can hasten the recovery process. In certain situations, surgery may be the only means of effecting a complete cure, as in the case of endocarditis (*i.e.*, infected heart valves), in which the diseased valve must be replaced with a mechanical or biologic valve to restore normal function.

In summary, the ultimate outcome of any interaction between microorganisms and the human host is decided by a complex and ever-changing set of variables that take into account the overall health and physiologic function of the host and the virulence and infectious dose of the microbe. In many instances, disease is an inevitable consequence, but with continued advancement of science and technology, the vast number of cases can be eliminated or rapidly cured with appropriate therapy. It is the intent of those who study infectious diseases to understand thoroughly the pathogen, the disease course, the mechanisms of transmission, and the host response to infection. This knowledge will lead to development of improved diagnostic techniques, revolutionary approaches to antiinfective therapy, and eradication or control of microscopic agents that cause frightening devastation and loss of life throughout the world.

BIBLIOGRAPHY

Blaser M.J. (1992). *Helicobacter pylori*: Its role in disease. *Clinical Infectious Diseases* 15, 386–391.

Brenner D.J., O'Connor S.P., Winkler H.H., Steigerwalt A.G. (1993) Proposals to unify the genera *Bartonella* and *Rochalimaea,* with descriptions of *Bartonella quintana* comb. nov., *Bartonella vinsonii* comb. nov., *Bartonella henselae* comb. nov., and *Bartonella elizabethae* comb. nov., and to remove the family *Bartonellaceae* from the order *Rickettsiales. International Journal of Systematic Bacteriology* 43, 777–786.

Bush K., Jacoby G.A., Medeiros A.A. (1995). A functional classification scheme for β-lactamases and its correlation with molecular structure. *Antimicrobial Agents and Chemotherapy* 39, 1211–1233.

Butler J.C., Peters C.J. (1994). Hantaviruses and hantavirus pulmonary syndrome. *Clinical Infectious Diseases* 19, 387–395.

Carpenter C.C.J., Fischl M.A., Hammer S.M., et al. (1996). Antiviral therapy for HIV infection in 1996. *Journal American Medical Association* 276, 146–54.

Christensen G.D. (1993). The "sticky" problem of *Staphylococcus epidermis* sepsis. *Hospital Practice* 28, 27–38.

Dumler J.S., Bakken J.S. (1995). Ehrlichial diseases in humans: Emerging tick-borne infections. *Clinical Infectious Diseases* 20, 1102–1110.

Eisenstein B.I. (1990) The polymerase chain reaction. *New England Journal of Medicine* 322, 178–83.

Gold H.S., Moellering R.C., Jr. (1996). Drug resistance: Antimicrobial-drug resistance. *New England Journal of Medicine* 335 (19), 1445–1453.

Jacobsen H., Hanggi M., Ott M., et al. (1996). In vivo resistance to a human immunodeficiency virus type 1 proteinase inhibitor: Mutations, kinetics, and frequencies. *Journal Infectious Diseases* 173, 1379–87.

Krogfelt K.A. (1991). Bacterial adhesion: Genetics, biogenetics, and role in pathogenesis of fimbrial adhesions of *Escherichia coli*. *Review of Infectious Disease* 13, 721–735.

Lennette E.H., Balows A., Hausler W.J., Jr., et al. (Eds.). (1985). *Manual of clinical microbiology*. Washington, DC: American Society for Microbiology.

Livermore D.M. (1995). β-Lactamases in laboratory and clinical resistance. *Clinical Microbiology Review* 8, 557–84.

Moore S.S. (1996). Pattern and predictability of emerging infections. *Hospital Practice* 31, 85–108.

Petri W.A. (1988). Tick-borne diseases. *American Family Practice* 37 (6), 95.

Richman D.D. (1996). New strategies to combat HIV drug resistance. *Hospital Practice* Aug 15, 47–58.

Rosenthal N. (1994). Tools of the trade–recombinant DNA. *New England Journal of Medicine* 331 (5), 315–317.

Walker D.H. (1996). Human ehrlichiosis: More trouble than ticks. *Hospital Practice* Apr 15, 47–57.

White N.J. (1996). Current concepts: The treatment of malaria. *New England Journal of Medicine* 335 (11), 800–806.

Zanetti G., Glauser M.P., Baumgartner J.D. (1991). Use of immunoglobulins in prevention and treatment of infection in critically ill patients: Review and critique. *Review of Infectious Diseases* 13, 985–992.

CHAPTER 11

Immunity and Inflammation

Cynthia Sommers

The human body constantly defends itself against bacteria, viruses, and foreign substances it encounters. It also must detect and respond to abnormal cells and molecules that periodically develop in the body so that diseases such as cancers do not occur. These external and internal threats are efficiently handled by two cooperative defense systems. One system is our nonspecific or general defenses that can protect us from any pathogen and does not distinguish one type of pathogen from another (Table 11–1). The second defense system, the immune system, responds specifically to each type of foreign invader or molecule.

Nonspecific or innate resistance results from two lines of general defenses. Microorganisms encounter the first line of resistance on exposure to the epithelial layers that line our skin and mucous membranes. The second line of nonspecific defenses involves chemical signals, antimicrobial proteins, and phagocytic cells associated with the inflammatory response. These two lines of nonspecific defense mechanisms are important for the control of microbial growth. They also aid in proper signaling of the second defense system–specific immunity.

The major focus of this chapter is to present an overview of the immune cells, molecules, and tissues and to describe the normal mechanisms used to protect the body against foreign invaders.

Immune System

After you have completed this section of the chapter, you should be able to meet the following objectives:

- State the properties associated with specific immunity
- Define and describe the characteristics of an antigen
- Characterize the significance and function of the major histocompatibility complex molecules
- Describe the functions of the macrophage
- Contrast and compare the development and function of the T and B lymphocytes from stem cell to a regulator or effector immune cell
- Describe the function and characteristics of natural killer cells

TABLE 11-1 Immune Defenses

First Line of Defense	Second Line of Defense	Third Line of Defense
Intact skin Mucous membranes and their secretions	Phagocytic white blood cells Inflammation and fever Antimicrobial substances Natural killer cells	Specialized lymphocytes Antibodies

- State the function of the five classes of immunoglobulins
- Differentiate between the central and peripheral lymphoid structures
- Describe the properties of cytokines and how they influence an immune responses
- Compare passive and active immunity
- Characterize the role of the complement system in the immune response

The immune system consists of the immune cells and the central and peripheral lymphoid structures. It produces an enormous variety of white blood cells and molecules that can recognize and remove the large variety of intruders it encounters. Several different types of immune cells and the molecules they produce interact to form a dynamic network that protects the body from foreign invaders, while also recognizing and sparing host cells identified as self.

Fundamental to the appropriate functioning of this defense system is the ability to regulate the recognition, amplification, and response of the immune cells to the antigen. The immune system must recognize and differentiate one foreign pathogen from another, while simultaneously distinguishing these foreign molecules from normal cells and proteins in the body. This phenomenal ability to differentiate nonself or dangerous agents from self or nonharmful agents is unique to this system. Immune cells and molecules must also be quickly produced but not made in excess. An evolutionary adaptation that is unique to the immune system is a memory response–the ability to recall and produce an increased immune response on subsequent exposure to the same foreign agents. After a person has had the mumps, the immune system remembers the experience and protects the person against having the disease again. Although the immune response is normally protective, it can also produce undesirable effect such as when the response is excessive or when it recognizes self tissue as foreign. Regulation of the immune response is important because of the tremendous energy requirements needed to produce new immune cells and the molecules they produce and because inappropriate or excessive responses can lead to permanent tissue damage.

Antigen

Before discussing the cells and responses inherent in immunity, it is important to understand the substances that elicit the host to produce a response. *Antigens* are substances foreign to the host that stimulate an immune response. These foreign molecules are recognized by receptors on immune cells and by binding proteins generated in response to the stimulus. The term *immunogen* is synonymous with antigen. Antigens include molecules of bacteria, fungi, viruses, protozoans, and parasitic worms. Antigens are also present on foreign material such as pollen, poison ivy plant resin, insect venom, and transplanted organs. Most antigens are macromolecules such as proteins and polysaccharides. Rarely, lipids and nucleic acids serve as antigens. Molecules differ in their ability to stimulate an immune response. Chemically complex foreign molecules tend to be good stimulators of immunity.

Antigens, which are generally very large and complex, are degraded to expose smaller chemical units that can be recognized by lymphocytes. These discrete, immunologically active sites on antigens are called *antigenic determinants* or *epitopes* (Fig. 11–1). It is the unique molecular shape of an epitope that is recognized by a

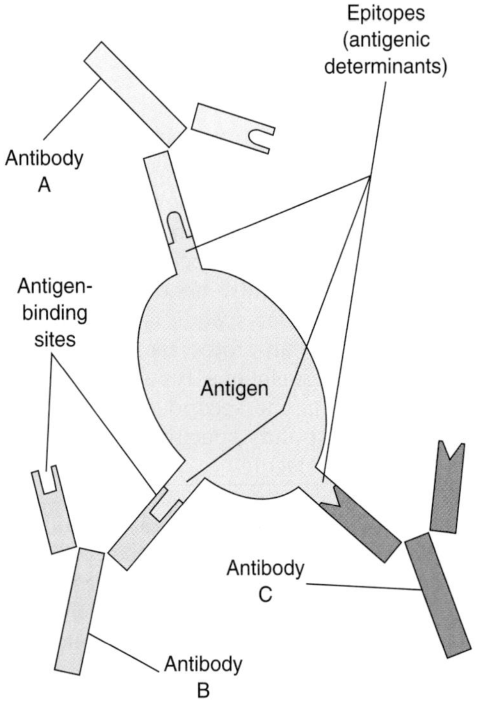

FIGURE 11–1 Multiple epitopes (A,B,C) on a complex antigen being recognized by different antibodies.

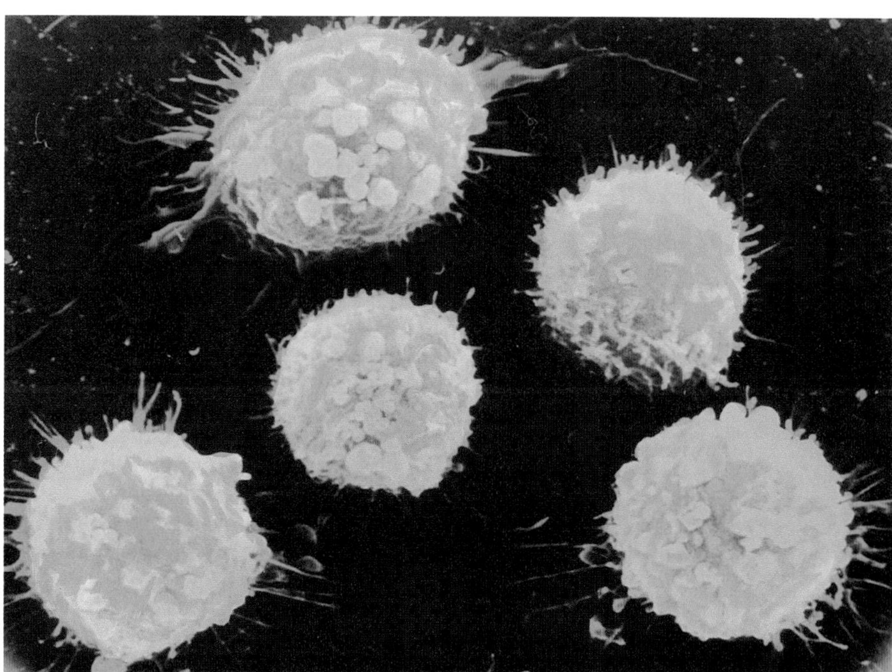

FIGURE 11–2
A scanning micrograph of two lymphocytes. (© CNRI/Science Photo Library, Science Source/Photo Researchers)

specific receptor molecule found on the surface of the lymphocyte. A single antigen such as a viral protein may contain several antigenic determinants; each can stimulate a distinct clone of lymphocytes to respond. Different parts of the virus may have different antigens. Hundreds of antigenic determinants are found on complex structures such as the bacterial cell wall.

Smaller substances (molecular masses less than 10,000 daltons) are usually unable to stimulate an adequate immune response by themselves. When these low-molecular-weight compounds, known as *haptens*, combine with larger protein molecules, they act as antigens. The larger proteins act as carrier molecules to form antigenic *hapten-carrier complexes*. Some allergic responses can be generated by hapten-carrier complexes. For example, penicillin (molecular mass of approximately 350 daltons) is incapable of causing an immune response by itself. However, penicillin can chemically combine with body proteins in some individuals to form larger complexes that can then generate an immune response to the penicillin epitope. An allergic response can be generated by hapten-carrier complexes.

Immune Cells

The primary cells of the immune system are white blood cells, called *lymphocytes* (Fig. 11–2). Other accessory cells, such as macrophages and dendritic cells, aid in the processing of antigen and activation of lymphocytes. There are two types of immune cells: regulatory cells and effector cells. The regulatory cells assist in orchestrating the immune response. For example, helper T lymphocytes activate other immune cells. The final stages of the immune response are aided by effector cells such as cytotoxic T lymphocytes that ensure efficient removal of the foreign invader.

Lymphocytes represent 25% to 35% of blood leukocytes and 99% of the cells in the lymph. Like other blood cells, lymphocytes are generated from stem cells in the bone marrow (Fig. 11–3). These undifferentiated cells locate into the central lymphoid tissues, where they mature into distinct types of lymphocytes. One class of lymphocyte, the *B lymphocyte* (B cell) matures in the bone marrow and is essential for humoral or antibody-mediated immunity. The other class of lymphocyte, the *T lymphocytes* (T cell), completes its maturation in the thymus and functions to produce cell-mediated immunity, as well as aiding in antibody production. About 60% to 70% of blood lymphocytes are T cells, and 10% to 20% are B cells. The various types of lymphocytes are distinguished by their function and response to antigen, cell membrane molecules and receptors, types of secreted proteins, and tissue location. High concentrations of mature T and B lymphocytes are found in the lymph nodes, spleen, and mucosal tissues where they can respond to antigen.

The B-cell antigen receptor consists of membrane-bound immunoglobulin proteins that can bind a specific antigen. The T-cell receptor recognizes the antigen in association with a self-recognition protein, called a major histocompatibility complex molecule.

The immune system enlists specialized antigen-presenting cells (APCs), such as the macrophage, to ensure the appropriate processing and presentation of antigen. On recognition of antigen and after additional stimulation by various secreted signaling molecules called *cytokines*, the B and T lymphocytes divide several times to form populations or clones of cells that continue to differentiate into effector cells and memory cells. Effector cells help in causing destruction and removal of

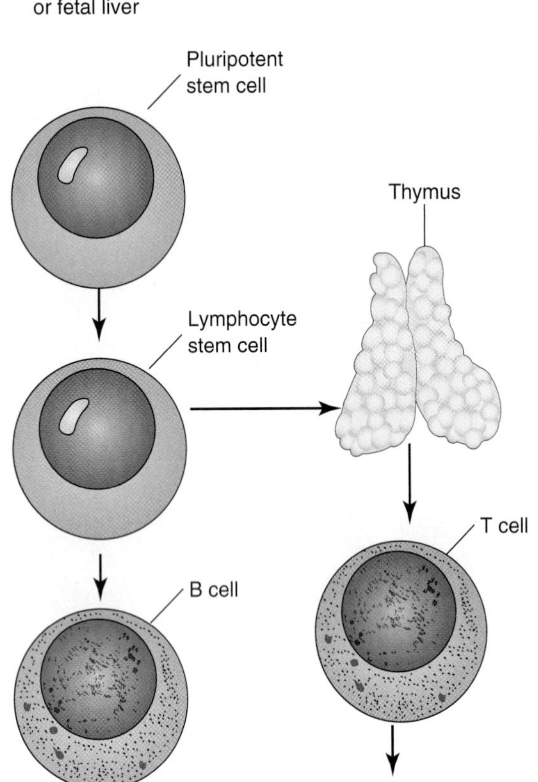

FIGURE 11–3
Pathway for T and B cell differentiation.

the antigen. Several types of effector cells and molecules defend the body in an immune response (Fig. 11–4). In humoral or antibody-mediated immunity, activated B cells produce effector cells called *plasma cells,* which secrete protein molecules called *antibodies* or *immunoglobulins.* Antibodies bind and aggregate foreign cells and molecules to aid their efficient removal. Phagocytic cells can more efficiently bind, engulf, and digest antigen-antibody aggregates or *immune complexes* than they can antigen alone.

Mature T and B cells display surface molecules called *clusters of differentiation* (CD). These molecules serve to define functionally distinct T-cell subsets such as $CD4^+$ and $CD8^+$ cells. The many cell surface *CD molecules* detected on immune cells have allowed scientists to identify cells and learn the process of activation and maturation of cells. For example, the human immunodeficiency virus (HIV) that causes acquired immunodeficiency syndrome (AIDS) infects and destroys the helper T cell. In cell-mediated immunity, regulatory $CD4^+$ *helper T cells* enhance the response of other T and B cells, and effector *cytotoxic T cells* ($CD8^+$) kill tumor cells and virus-infected cells (see Fig. 11–4).

T and B lymphocytes possess all of the key properties associated with the specific immune response—*specificity, diversity, memory,* and *self-nonself recognition.* These cells can exactly recognize and remove a particular microorganism or foreign molecule. Each lymphocyte targets a specific antigen and differentiates that invader from other molecules that may be similar. The approximately 10^{12} lymphocytes in the body have tremendous diversity. They can respond to the millions of different kinds of microorganisms encountered daily. This diversity occurs because an enormous variety of lymphocyte populations have been programmed during development, each to respond to a particular antigen. After the lymphocytes are stimulated by their antigen, they acquire a memory response. The memory T and B lymphocytes that are generated remain in the body for a long time and can respond more rapidly on repeat exposure than naive cells (see Fig. 11–4). Because of this heightened state of immune reactivity, the immune system can usually respond to commonly encountered microorganism so efficiently that we are unaware of the response.

Major Histocompatibility Complex Molecules

An essential feature of specific immunity is the ability to discriminate between the body's own molecules and foreign antigens. Failure to distinguish self from nonself can lead to conditions such as autoimmune disease where the immune system destroys the body's own cells. Key molecules essential for distinguishing self from nonself are the cell surface glycoproteins called *major histocompatibility complex (MHC).* These molecules, which are coded by closely linked genes on chromosome 6, were first identified because of their role in organ and tissue transplantation.

The MHC cell membrane molecules involved in self recognition and cell-to-cell communication fall into two classes: MHC I and MHC II molecules (Fig. 11–5). *MHC I* molecules are cell surface glycoproteins that interact with antigen receptors on $CD8^+$ T lymphocytes and are found on the cell membranes of nearly all nucleated cells in the body. *MHC II* molecules, which are found primarily on macrophages and other APCs involved in an immune response, communicate with antigen receptors on $CD4^+$ T lymphocytes. A third group of genes located on the same chromosome as the MHC I and MHC II genes encode other proteins involved in the immune response. Complement and cytokines important for signaling an immune response are examples of MHC III proteins. These are structurally and functionally unrelated to MHC I or II molecules. Each individual has a unique collection of MHC proteins. Because of the number of MHC genes and the possibility of several alleles for each gene, it is almost impossible for any two individuals to be identical, except if they are identical twins. MHC molecules serve as the self components that the immune system uses to distinguish self from nonself. They also function as antigen-binding molecules. In contrast to the receptors on lymphocytes that bind a unique antigen molecule, each MHC protein binds a broad spectrum of antigens. Antigens bound to MHC molecules are then presented to

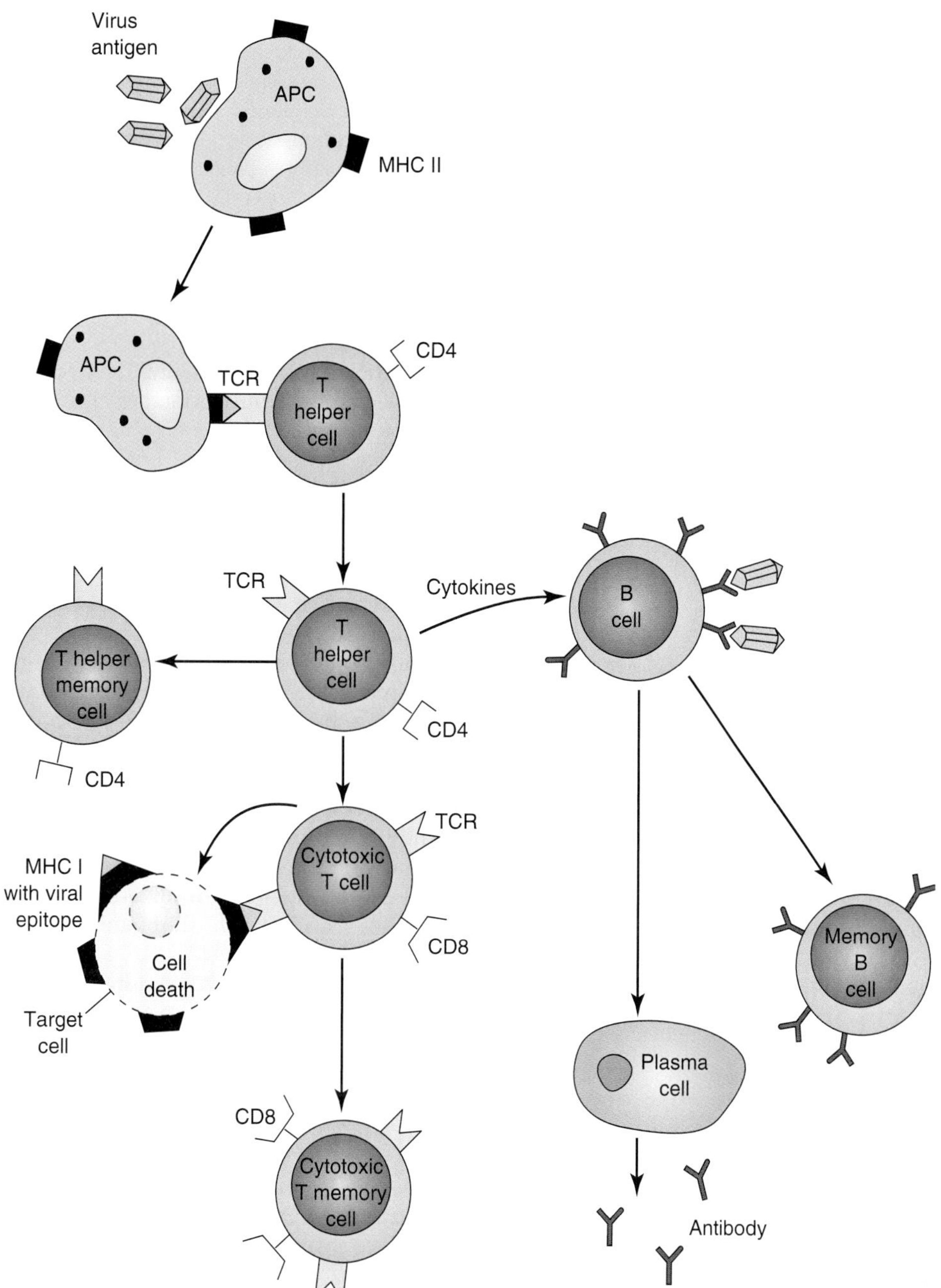

FIGURE 11–4
Pathway for immune cell participation in an immune response.

T lymphocytes, which become activated on recognition of the antigen associated with the MHC molecule.

Human MHC proteins are called human leukocyte antigens (HLA) because they were first detected on white blood cells. Because these molecules play a role in transplant rejection and are detected by immunologic tests, they are commonly called antigens. The human MHC I proteins are designated HLA-A, HLA-B, and HLA-C, and the MHC II proteins are identified as HLA-DR, HLA-DP, and HLA-DQ (Table 11–2). Additional, less well defined MHC class I and II genes have also been described. Each of these gene loci in a population can be occupied by multiple alleles or alternate genes. For example, there are more than 24 possible genes for the A locus and 50 genes for the B locus. Each of the gene products or antigens is designated by a number, such as HLA-A1 or HLA-B27.

Because the MHC I and II genes are closely linked, the combination of HLA genes is usually inherited as a unit, called a *haplotype*. Each person inherits a chromosome from each parent and therefore has two HLA haplotypes. The identification or typing of HLA molecules is impor-

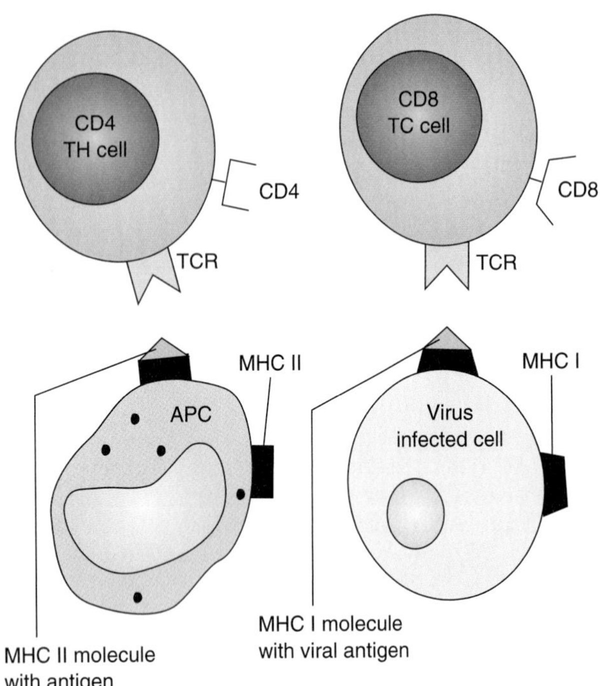

FIGURE 11–5
Interaction of a CD4 helper T (TH) cell with class II MHC molecule on an antigen presenting (APC) cell and CD8 cytotoxic (TC) T cell with class I MHC molecule on a virus infected cell.

tant in tissue or organ transplants, forensics, and paternity evaluations. In organ or tissue transplantation, the closer the matching of HLA types, the greater is the probability of identical antigens and the less is the chance of rejection.

Monocytes and Macrophages

Monocytes and tissue macrophages are a part of the *mononuclear phagocyte system* included in the reticuloendothelial system. All of the cells of the mononuclear phagocytic system arise from common precursors in the bone marrow that produces the blood monocytes. The monocytes migrate to the various tissues where they mature into macrophages. The tissue macrophages are scattered in connective tissue or clustered in organs such as the lung (*i.e.*, alveolar macrophages), liver (*i.e.*, Kupffer's cells), spleen, lymph nodes, peritoneum, central nervous system (*i.e.*, microglial cells), and other areas. Langerhans' cells are macrophages that are located in the skin. These skin macrophages are involved in cell-mediated immune reactions of the skin such as delayed allergic contact hypersensitivity (see Chapter 12).

Macrophages serve several important functions in an immune response. Macrophages are activated by the presence of antigen to engulf and digest foreign particles (Fig. 11–6). The ingestion process can be aided by the presence of antibody. The phagocytic destruction of microorganisms helps to contain infectious agents until specific immunity can be marshaled. Early in the host response, the macrophage functions as an accessory cell to insure amplification of the inflammatory response and initiation of specific immunity. Macrophages also secrete *cytokines* (*e.g.*, tumor necrosis factor [TNF], interleukin-1 [IL-1]) that produce fever and prime T and B lymphocytes that have encountered antigen. Activated macrophages act as APCs that breakdown complex antigens into peptide fragments that can associate with MHC II proteins. Macrophages can then present these complexes to the helper T cell so that nonself-self recognition and activation of the immune response can occur. The macrophages can serve as phagocytic effector cells in humoral and cell-mediated immune responses. They can remove antigen-antibody aggregates, or under the influence of T-cell cytokines, they can destroy virus-infected cells or tumor cells.

B Lymphocytes

The B lymphocytes are responsible for humoral immunity. Humoral immunity provides for elimination of bacterial invaders, neutralization of bacterial toxins, prevention of viral infection, and immediate allergic responses (see Chapter 12).

B lymphocytes can be identified by the presence of surface immunoglobulin that functions as the antigen receptor, class II MHC proteins, complement receptors, and specific CD molecules. During the maturation of B cells, which occurs in the bone marrow, stem cells first change into immature precursor (pre-B) cells. A rearrangement of genes produces a unique receptor and type of effector antibody (e.g., IgG or IgA). This stage of maturation is programmed into the B cells and does not require antigen; it is an antigen-independent process. The mature B cell leaves the bone marrow, enters the circulation, and migrates to the various peripheral lymphoid tissues where it is stimulated to respond to a specific antigen.

TABLE 11-2
Properties of MHC Class I and MHC Class II Molecules

Properties	MHC Class I	MHC Class II
HLA antigens	HLA-A, HLA-B, HLA-C	HLA-DR, HLA-DP, HLA-DQ
Distribution	Virtually all nucleated cells	Restricted to immune cells, antigen-presenting cells, B cells, and macrophages
Functions	Present processed antigen to cytotoxic CD8$^+$ T cells; restricts cytolysis to virus-infected cells, tumor cells, transplanted cells	Present processed antigenic fragments to CD4$^+$ T cells; necessary for effective interaction among immune cells

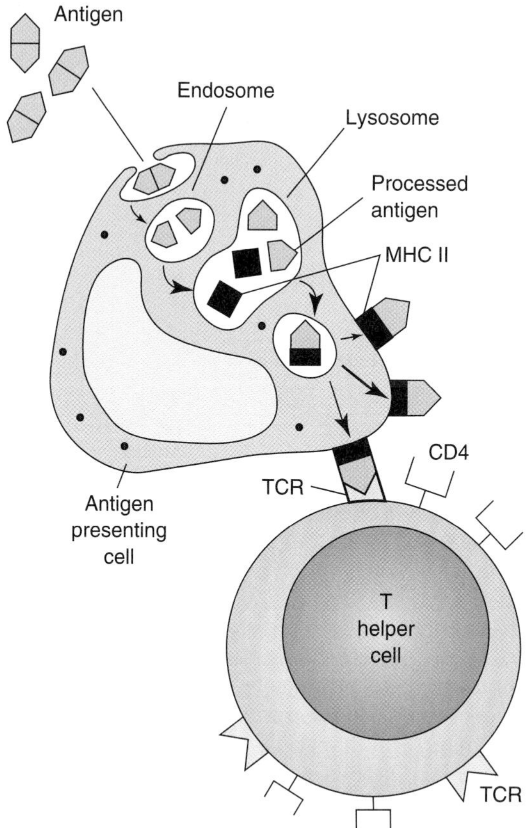

FIGURE 11–6
Presentation of antigen to T helper cell by an antigen presenting cell (APC).

The commitment of a B-cell line to a specific antigen is evident by the expression of the surface immunoglobulin antigen receptor molecule. B cells that encounter antigen complementary to their surface immunoglobulin receptor and receive T-cell help undergo a series of changes that transform the B cell into an antibody secreting plasma cells or into memory B cells (Fig. 11–7). B lymphocytes can also function as APCs by ingesting the surface-bound antigen, processing it into small peptides, and recycling the peptide now complexed to the MHC class II molecules to its surface. The antigen peptide–MHC II complex is recognized by helper T cells, which are then stimulated to secrete various cytokines. These cytokines cause multiplication and maturation of antigen-activated B and T cells. The activated B cell divides and undergoes terminal maturation into a plasma cell, which can produce thousands of antibody molecules per second. The antibodies are released into the blood and lymph where they bind and remove their unique antigen. Longer-lived memory B cells also are generated and distributed into the peripheral tissues in preparation for subsequent antigen exposure.

Immunoglobulins

Antibodies form a class of proteins called immunoglobulins. The immunoglobulins (Ig) have been divided into five classes: IgG, IgA, IgM, IgD, and IgE (Table 11–3). Immunoglobulins have a characteristic four-polypeptide structure consisting of at least two identical antigen binding sites (Fig. 11–8). Each immunoglobulin is composed of two identical light (L) chains and two identical heavy (H) chains to form a Y-shaped molecule. The two forklike ends of the immunoglobulin molecule bind antigen and are called *Fab* (*i.e.*, antigen binding) *fragments*, and the tail of the molecule, which is called the *Fc fragment*, directs the biologic properties that are characteristic of a particular class of immunoglobulins. The amino acid sequence of the heavy and light chains shows constant (C) regions and variable (V) regions. The constant regions have sequences of amino acids that vary little among the antibodies of a particular class of immunoglobulin. The constant regions allow separation of immunoglobulins into classes (*e.g.*, IgM, IgG) and provide the different immunoglobulin types with distinct functions. The wide variation in the amino acid sequence of the variable regions seen from antibody to antibody allows this region to serve as the antigen binding site. It is in this region that a unique amino acid sequence determines a distinctive three-dimensional pocket where several weak chemical bonds complementary to the antigen allow recognition and binding to occur. Each B-cell clone produces antibody with one specific antigen-binding variable region or domain. During the course of the immune response, class switching (*e.g.*, from IgM to IgG) can occur, causing the B-cell clone to produce any of the following antibody types.

IgG (gamma-globulin) is the most abundant of the circulating immunoglobulins. It is present in body fluids and readily enters the tissues. IgG is the only immunoglobulin that crosses the placenta and can transfer immunity from the mother to the fetus. This class of immunoglobulin protects against bacteria, toxins, and viruses in body fluids and activates the complement system. There are four subsets of IgG (*i.e.*, IgG1, IgG2, IgG3, and IgG4) that have some restrictions in their response to certain types of antigens. For example, IgG2 appears to be specific for bacteria that are encapsulated with a polysaccharide covering such as *Streptococcus pneumoniae*, *Haemophilus influenzae*, and *Neisseria meningitides*.

IgA, a secretory immunoglobulin, is found in saliva, tears, colostrum (*i.e.*, first milk of a nursing mother), and in bronchial, gastrointestinal, prostatic, and vaginal secretions. This dimeric secretory immunoglobulin is considered a primary defense against local infections in mucosal tissues. IgA prevents the attachment of viruses and bacteria to epithelial cells.

IgM is a macromolecule that forms a polymer of five basic immunoglobulin units. It is too large to cross the placenta and does not transfer maternal immunity. It is the first circulating immunoglobulin to appear in response to an antigen and is the first antibody type made by a newborn. This is diagnostically useful, because the presence of IgM usually suggests a current infection by a specific pathogen. The identification of newborn IgM rather than maternally transferred IgG to a specific pathogen is indicative of an *in utero* or newborn infection.

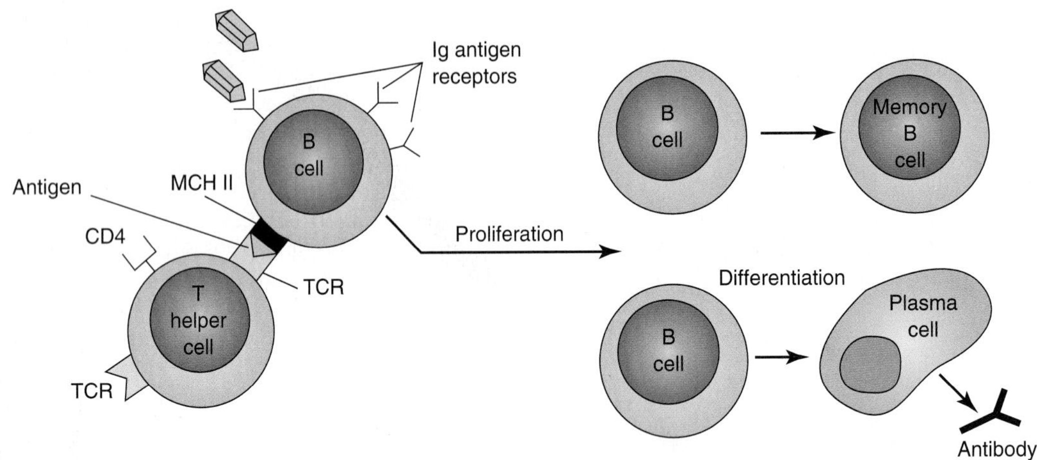

FIGURE 11–7
Pathway for B cell differentiation.

IgD is mostly found on the cell membranes of B lymphocytes. It serves as an antigen receptor needed for initiating the differentiation of B cells.

IgE is involved in combating parasitic infections, inflammation, allergy, and some hypersensitivity reactions. It binds to mast cells and basophils. The binding of antigen to the bound IgE triggers the release from these cells of histamine and other mediators of inflammation and allergic reactions.

T Lymphocytes

T lymphocytes function in the activation of other T cells and B cells, in the control of viral infections, in the rejection of foreign tissue grafts, and in delayed hypersensitivity reactions (see Chapter 12). Collectively, these immune responses are called cell-mediated or cellular immunity. Besides the ability to respond to cell-associated antigens, the T cell is integral to immunity because it regulates and amplifies the response of B and T lymphocytes.

T lymphocytes arise from bone marrow stem cells, but unlike B cells, pre-T cells migrate to the thymus for their maturation. There the immature T lymphocytes undergo rearrangement of the genes needed for expression of a unique T-cell antigen receptor similar to that of the B cell. The *T-cell receptor* (TCR) is composed of two polypeptides that fold to form a groove that recognizes processed antigen peptide-MHC complexes. The TCR is associated with other surface molecules known as the *CD3 complex* that participate in antigen recognition. Maturation of subpopulations of T cells (*i.e.,* $CD4^+$ and $CD8^+$) also occurs in the thymus. Mature T cells migrate to the peripheral lymphoid tissues and, on encountering antigen, multiply and differentiate into memory T cells and various effector T cells.

Helper T Cells. The $CD4^+$ helper T cell (T_H) serves as a master switch for the immune system. Activation of helper T cells depends on the recognition of antigen in association with MHC class II molecules. Activated helper T cells secrete cytokines that influence the function of nearly all other cells of the immune system. These cytokines attract and activate B cells, cytotoxic T cells, natural killer cells, macrophages, and other immune cells. Distinct subpopulations of helper T cells (*i.e.,* T_H1 and T_H2) have been identified and shown to produce different types of cytokines. The pattern of cytokine production determines whether an antibody or cell-mediated immune response develops. This differential expressions of cytokines can influence expressions of some diseases (i.e., lepromatous and tuberculoid leprosy).

Cytotoxic T Cells. Activated $CD8^+$ T cells become cytotoxic T cells (T_C cells or CTLs) after recognition of antigen–MHC I complexes on target cell surfaces (Fig. 11–9). The recognition of antigen–MHC I complexes on infected target cells ensures that neighboring uninfected host cells, which express MHC I molecules alone, are not indiscriminately destroyed. The $CD8^+$ T cells destroy target cells by releasing cytolytic enzymes, toxic cytokines, and pore-forming molecules (*i.e.,* perforins). The perforin proteins produce pores in the target cell membrane, allowing entry of toxic molecules and loss of cell constituents. The $CD8^+$ T cells are especially important in controlling viruses and intracellular bacteria, because antibody is inefficient at attacking these internally replicating microorganisms.

Cell-mediated immunity involves $CD4^+$ and $CD8^+$ T lymphocytes. Activated helper T cells release various cytokines that recruit and activate other lymphocytes and inflammatory cells. Cytokines can induce positive migration or chemotaxis of several types of inflammatory cells, including macrophages, granulocytes, and basophils. Activation of macrophages enhances their phagocytic, metabolic, and enzymatic potential, resulting in more efficient destruction of infected cells. This type of

TABLE 11-3

Classes and Characteristics of Immunoglobulins

Figure	Class	Percentage of Total	Characteristics
	IgG	75.0	Displays antiviral, antitoxin, and antibacterial properties; only Ig that crosses the placenta; responsible for protection of newborn; activates complement and binds to macrophages
J	IgA	15.0	Predominant Ig in body secretions, such as saliva, nasal and respiratory secretions, and breast milk; protects mucous membranes
	IgM	10.0	Forms the natural antibodies such as those for ABO blood antigens; prominant in early immune responses; activates complement
–C	IgD	0.2	Found on B lymphocytes; needed for maturation of B cells
–C	IgE	0.004	Binds to mast cells and basophils; involved in parasitic infections, allergic and hypersensitivity reactions

defense is important against intracellular pathogens such as *Mycobacteria* and *Listeria monocytogenes*.

A similar sequence of T-cell and macrophage activation, but with sometimes excessive inflammation, can be elicited in delayed hypersensitivity reactions. Contact dermatitis due to a poison ivy reaction or dye sensitivity are examples of delayed hypersensitivity caused by hapten-carrier complexes of cell-mediated immune reactions.

Natural Killer Cells

Natural killer (NK) cells are lymphocytes that are functionally, genotypically, and phenotypically distinct from T cells, B cells, and monocyte-macrophages. The NK cell is a nonspecific effector cell that can kill tumor cells and virus-infected cells. This cell is programmed to automatically kill foreign cells, in contrast to the $CD8^+$ T cells, which need to be activated to become cytotoxic. Programmed killing is inhibited by contact of NK cell membrane molecules with MHC self molecules on normal host cells.

NK cells appear as large granular lymphocytes with an indented nuclei and abundant, pale cytoplasm containing red granules. These cells characteristically express CD16 and CD56 cell surface molecules but lack the typical T-cell markers (*i.e.*, TCR-CD3, CD4/8). The mechanism of NK cytotoxicity is similar to T-cell cytotoxicity in that it depends on production of pore-form-

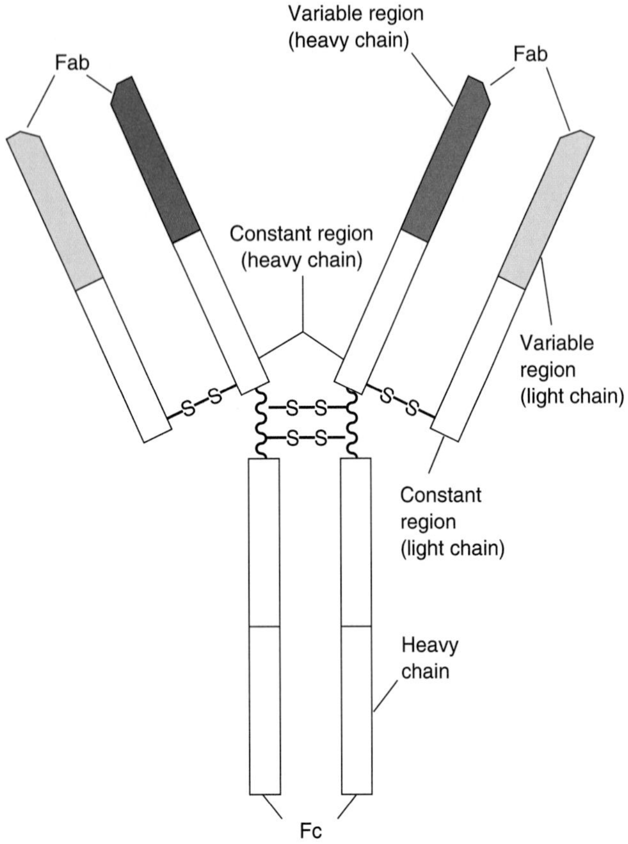

FIGURE 11–8
Schematic model of an IgG molecule showing the constant and variable regions of the light and dark chains.

ing proteins (*i.e.,* NK perforins), enzymes, and toxic cytokines. NK cell activity can be enhanced in vitro on exposure to interleukin-2 (IL-2), a phenomenon called *lymphokine-activated killer* (LAK) activity. NK cells also participate in antibody-dependent cellular cytotoxicity (ADCC), a mechanism by which a cytotoxic effector cell can kill an antibody-coated target cell. The role of NK cells is probably one of immune surveillance for cancerous or virally infected cells.

Lymphoid Organs

The cells of the immune system are present in large numbers in the central and peripheral lymphoid organs. These organs and tissues are widely distributed in the body and provide different, but often overlapping functions (Fig. 11–10). The central lymphoid organs, the bone marrow and the thymus, provide the environment for immune cell production and maturation. The peripheral lymphoid organs function to trap and process antigen and promote its interaction with mature immune cells. These structures consist of lymph nodes, spleen, tonsils, appendix, Peyer's patches in the intestine, and mucosa-associated lymphoid tissues in the respiratory, gastrointestinal, and reproductive systems. The lymphoid organs are connected by networks of lymph channels, blood vessels, and capillaries. The immune cells continuously circulate through the various tissues and organs to seek out and destroy foreign material.

Thymus

The thymus is an elongated, bilobed structure that is located in the neck region above the heart. Each lobe is surrounded by a connective tissue capsule layer and is divided into lobules. Each lobule is composed of two compartments: an outer area or *cortex,* which is densely packed with *thymocytes* or immature T cells, and an inner area or *medulla* that contains few lymphocytes but more dendritic cells, macrophages and the distinctive morphologic structure of the thymus, the Hassall's corpuscles (Fig. 11–11).

The thymus is a fully developed organ at birth, weighing approximately 15 to 20 g. At puberty, when the immune cells are well established in peripheral lymphoid tissues, the thymus begins regressing and is replaced by adipose tissue. Nevertheless, some thymus tissue persists into old age. The function of the thymus is central to the development of the immune system. Precursor T (pre-T) cells enter the thymus as functionally and phenotypically immature T cells. They progressively differentiate into mature T cells as they transverse the organ from the cortical to medullary

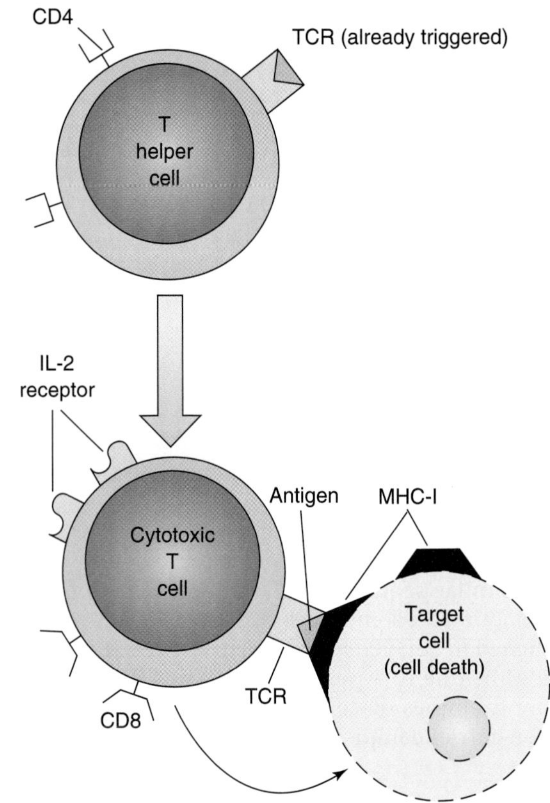

FIGURE 11–9
Helper T cell activation of cytotoxic T cell and destruction of target cell with antigen -MHC I complex by the cytotoxic T cell.

areas. Rapid cell multiplication and maturation occurs in the cortex under the influence of thymic hormones (*e.g.*, thymulin, thymopoietin). Cortical thymocytes undergo TCR gene rearrangement and TCR and CD4+/CD8+ surface expression. More than 95% of the thymocytes die in the cortex and never leave the thymus, probably because of production of inappropriate receptors or cell components. Only those T cells able to recognize foreign antigen and not react to self (*i.e.*, MHC or self antigens) are allowed to mature. This process is called *thymic selection.* The thymus must be extremely thorough in eliminating self-reactive cells to ensure that autoimmune reactivity and disease do not result. Mature immunocompetent T cells leave the thymus in 2 to 3 days and enter the peripheral lymphoid tissues through the bloodstream.

Impairment of the thymus function has been associated with immunologic deficiency disorders. If the thymus is removed from certain animals at birth or it is congenitally absent, as it is in certain human conditions, the result is a decrease of lymphocytes in the blood and a marked depletion or absence of T lymphocytes in the circulation and peripheral lymphoid tissues.

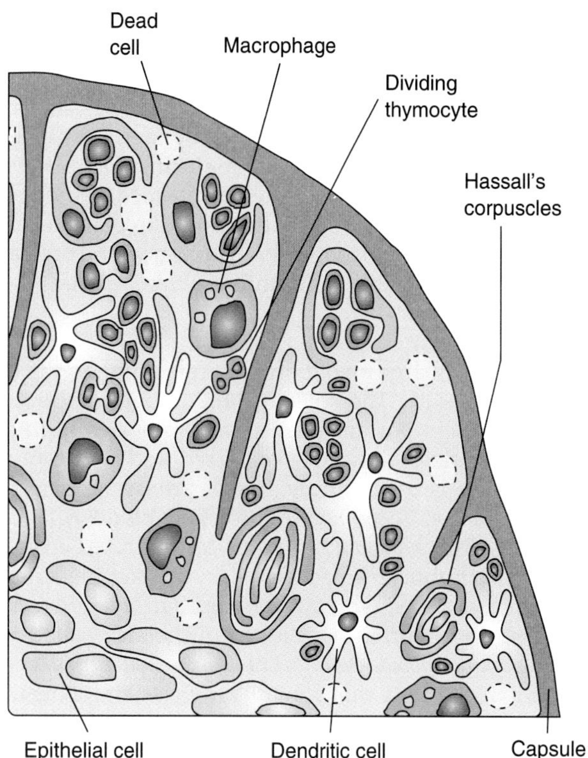

FIGURE 11–11
Structural features of the thymus gland. The thymus gland is divided into lobules containing an outer cortex densely packed with dividing thymocytes or premature T cells and an inner medulla that contains macrophages, dendritic cells, and Hassall's corpuscles.

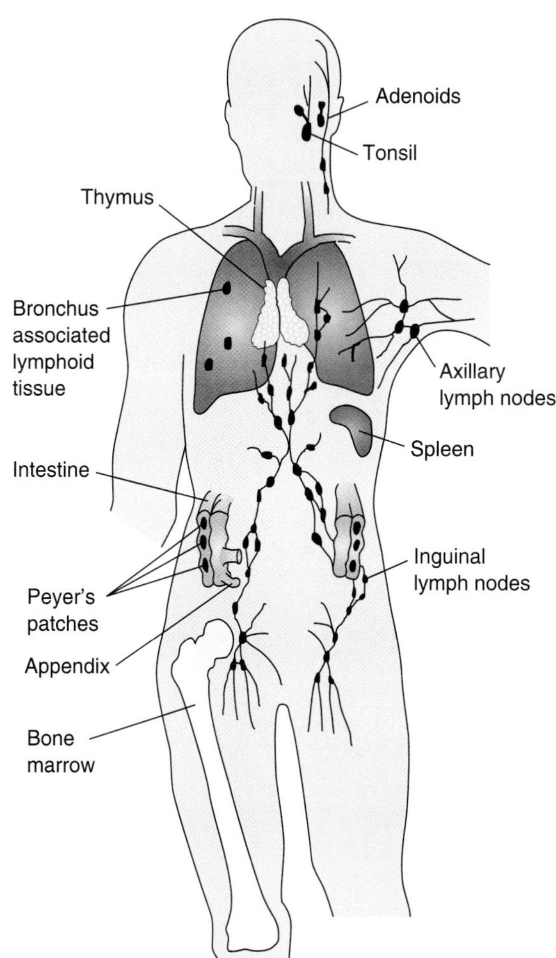

FIGURE 11–10
Central and peripheral lymphoid organs and tissues.

Lymph Nodes

Lymph nodes are small aggregates of lymphoid tissue located along lymphatic channels throughout the body. Each lymph node processes lymph from a discrete, adjacent anatomic site. Many lymph nodes are in the axillae, groin, and along the great vessels of the neck, thorax, and abdomen. Lymph nodes have two functions: removal of foreign material from lymph before it enters the bloodstream and serving as centers for proliferation of immune cells. These tissues are located along the lymph ducts, which lead from the tissues to the thoracic duct.

A lymph node is a bean-shaped tissue surrounded by a connective tissue capsule. Lymph enters the node through afferent channels that penetrate the capsule, and it leaves through the efferent lymph vessels located in the deep indentation of the hilus. Lymphocytes and macrophages flow slowly through the node and allow trapping and interaction of antigen and immune cells. The reticular meshwork serves as a surface on which macrophages attach and phagocytose antigens. Dendritic cells, which also permeate the lymph node, aid antigen presentation.

A lymph node can be divided into an outer cortex, a paracortex, and inner medulla (Fig 11–12). The T lymphocytes are more abundant in the paracortex area of the node, and the B lymphocytes are more abundant in the follicles and germinal centers located in the outer cortex. The T lymphocytes proliferate on antigenic stimulation and migrate to the follicles, where they interact with B lymphocytes. These activated follicles become germinal centers, containing macrophages, follicular dendritic cells, and dividing and maturing T and B cells. Activated B cells then migrate to the medullary area, where they complete their maturation into plasma cells. These cells stay localized in the lymph node but release large quantities of antibodies into the circulation.

Spleen

The spleen is a large, ovoid organ located high in the left abdominal cavity. The spleen filters antigens from the blood and is important in response to systemic infections. The spleen is composed of red and white pulp. The *red pulp* is well supplied with arteries and is the area where senescent and injured red blood cells are destroyed. The *white pulp* contains concentrated areas of B and T lymphocytes permeated by macrophages and dendritic cells. The lymphocytes (primarily T cells) that surround the central arterioles form the area called the *periarterial lymphoid sheath*. The diffuse *marginal zone*, which is B cell rich, that contains follicles and germinal centers separates the white pulp from the red pulp. A similar sequence of activation occurs in the spleen as is seen in the lymph nodes.

Other Secondary Lymphoid Tissues

Other secondary lymphoid tissues include the mucosa-associated lymphoid tissues (MALT). They are located around membranes lining the respiratory, digestive, and urogenital tract. In some tissues, the lymphocytes are organized in loose clusters, but in other tissues such as the tonsils, Peyer's patches in the intestine, and the appendix, organized structures are evident. These tissues contain all the necessary cell components (*i.e.*, T cells, B cells, and macrophages) for an immune response. Because of the continuous stimulation of the lymphocytes in these tissues by microorganisms constantly entering the body, large numbers of plasma cells are evident. Immunity at the mucosal layers help to minimize damage of vulnerable internal organs caused by systemic infections.

Cytokines and the Immune Response

Cytokines are small (usually with molecular weights <20,000), secreted hormone-like polypeptides produced during all phases of an immune response. Cytokines act

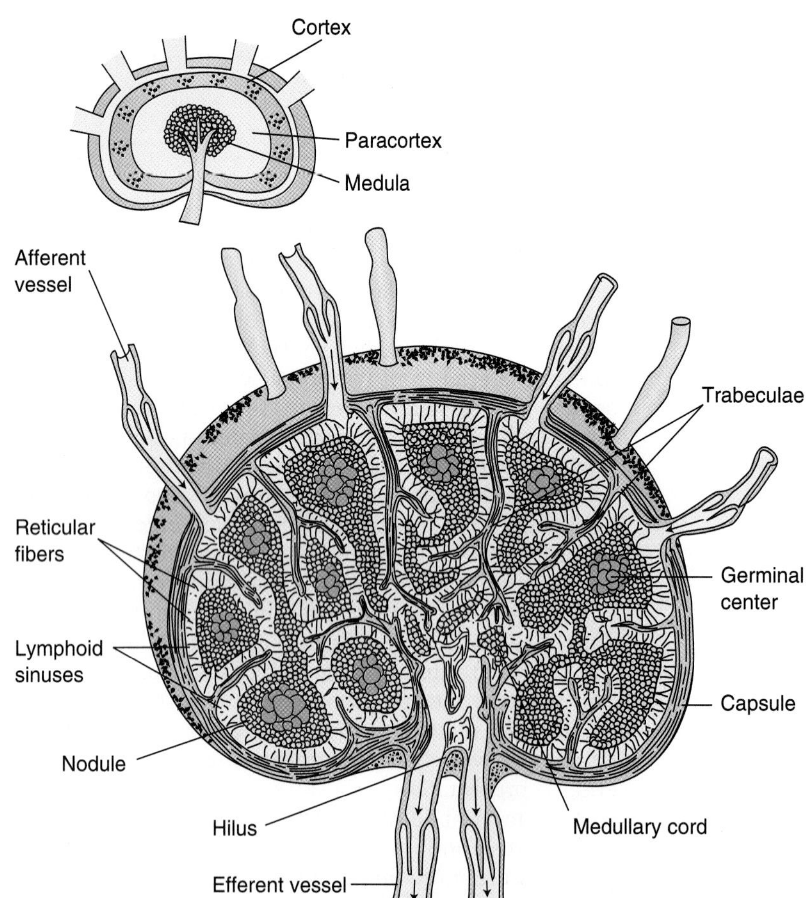

FIGURE 11–12 Structural features of a lymph node. Bacteria that gain entry to the body are filtered out of the lymph as it flows through the node.

predominantly on immune cells and are induced regulators of the immune response. These proteins function as intercellular signals that regulate local and, at times, systemic inflammatory responses. Cytokines modulate reactions of the host to foreign antigens or injurious agents by regulating the movement, proliferation, and differentiation of leukocytes and other cells (Table 11–4). Cytokines are synthesized by many cells types but are made primarily by activated T lymphocytes and macrophages.

Cytokines can be named for the general cell type that produces them (*e.g.,* lymphokines, monokines). More specifically, they are named by an international nomenclature (*i.e.,* interleukins 1 through 17) or for the biologic property that was first ascribed to them. For example, interferons were named because they interfered with virus multiplication. Cytokines commonly affect more than one cell type and have more than one biologic effect. It is now known that interferon-gamma (IFN-γ) inhibits virus replication and is a potent activator of macrophages and NK cells. Specific cytokines have biologic activities that overlap. Maximization of the immune response and protection against detrimental mutations in a single cytokine are possible benefits of redundancy in cytokines and their overlapping actions.

The production of cytokines often occurs in a cascade in which one cytokine affects the production of subsequent cytokines or cytokine receptors. Some cytokines have been shown to inhibit the biologic effects of earlier cytokines. This pattern of expression and feedback ensures appropriate control of cytokine synthesis. Excessive cytokine production can lead to serious symptoms including those associated with septic shock, food poisoning, and some types of cancer.

Cytokines generate their responses by binding to specific receptors on their target cells. Many cytokine receptors share a common structural motif and a similar family of cytoplasmic signaling proteins that direct the activation of genes for cell responses. The biologic responses associated with cytokines are partially regulated by the cells expressing their receptor and by when the receptors are produced. Most cytokines are released at cell-to-cell interfaces, where they bind to receptors on nearby cells. The short half-life of cytokines ensures that excessive immune responses and general systemic activation does not occur.

The biologic properties of cytokines fall into several major groups. One group of cytokines (*e.g.,* IL-1, TNF) mediate inflammation by producing fever and the acute-phase response and by attracting and activating phagocytes (*e.g.,* IL-8, IFN-γ). Other cytokines are maturation factors for hematopoiesis of white or red blood cells (*e.g.,* IL-3, granulocyte-macrophage colony-stimulating factor [GM-CSF], granulocyte colony-stimulating factor [G-CSF]). Recombinant CSF molecules are being used to increase the success rates of bone marrow transplants. Most of the interleukin cytokines function as cell communication molecules among T cells, B cells, macrophages, and other immune cells. The availability of recombinant cytokines offers the possibility of several clinical therapies where stimulation or inhibition of the immune response is desirable. IL-2 therapy for several malignancies has lead to some clinical success.

Interleukin-1

The major function of IL-1 is as a mediator of the inflammatory response. However, IL-1 also serves as a second signal in the activation of $CD4^+$ T cells and the growth and differentiation of B cells. The major source of IL-1 is the macrophage, although it is also produced by keratinocytes, Langerhans' cells, normal B cells, cultured T cells, fibroblasts, neutrophils, and smooth muscle cells.

Interleukin-2

The presence of IL-2, formerly known as T-cell growth factor, is necessary for the proliferation and function of helper T, cytotoxic T, B, and NK cells. IL-2 interacts with T lymphocytes by binding to specific membrane receptors that are present on activated T cells but not on resting T cells. The expression of IL-2 receptors can be triggered by the binding of a specific antigen to the cell surface. Sustained T-cell proliferation relies on the presence of IL-2 and IL-2 receptors; if either is missing, cell proliferation ceases, and the cell dies. Severe combined immunodeficiency diseases have been associated with mutations in IL-2 and the IL-2 receptor. This cytokine ensures maximum amplification of immune responses if antigen is present. Cyclosporine, a drug used to prevent rejection of heart, kidney, and liver transplants, functions primarily by inhibiting the synthesis of IL-2.

Interferons

The interferons are a family of cytokines that protect neighboring cells from invasion by intracellular parasites, including viruses, rickettsiae, malarial parasites, and other organisms. Bacterial toxins, complex polysaccharides, and several other chemical substances can induce interferon production. Not all the substances that induce interferon are antigenic.

There are at least three types of interferon (IFN): IFN-α, produced by leukocytes; IFN-β, produced by fibroblasts; and IFN-γ, produced by T cells. Secreted IFN interacts with receptors on neighboring cells to stimulate the translation of an antiviral protein that affects viral synthesis. The actions of IFN are not pathogen specific; they are effective against different types of viruses and intracellular parasites. They are, however, species specific. Animal IFNs do not provide protection in humans. IFN produced during immune reactions is primarily IFN-γ. The function of IFN-γ is comparable to that of interleukins and includes the activation of macrophages, generation of cytotoxic lymphocytes, and enhancement of NK cell activity.

Tumor Necrosis Factor

Like IL-1, TNF is a cytokine with multiple immunologic and inflammatory effects. It was first described as an activity in serum that induced hemorrhagic necrosis in

TABLE 11-4

Characteristic Biologic Properties of Human Cytokines

Cytokine	Biologic Activity
Interluekin-1 (alpha and beta)	Activates resting T cells; is cofactor for hematopoietic growth factor; induces fever, sleep, ACTH release, neutropenia, and other systemic acute-phase responses; stimulates synthesis of cytokines, collagen, and collegenases; activates endothelial and macrophagic cells; mediates inflammation, catabolic process, and nonspecific resistance to infection
Interleukin-2	Growth factor for activated T cells; induces synthesis of other cytokines; activates cytotoxic lymphocytes
Interleukin-3	Support growth of pluripotent (multilineage) bone-marrow stem cells; is growth factor for mast cells
Interleukin-4	Growth factor for activated B cells, resting T cells, and mast cells; induces MHC class I antigen expression on B cells; enhances cytotoxic T cells; activates macrophages
Interluekin-5	B cell differentiating and growth factor; promotes differentiation of eosinophils; promotes antibody production (IgA)
Interleukin-6	Acts as cofactor for immunoglobulin production by B cells; stimulates hepatocytes to produce acute phase proteins
Interleukin-7	Stimulates pre-B cells and thymocytes; stimulates myeloid precursors and megokaryocytes
Interleukin-8	Chemoattracts neutrophils and T lymphocytes; regulates lymphocyte homing and neutrophil infiltration
Interleukin-10	Suppresses cytokine production by T helper cells; inhibits antigen presentation
Interleukin-12	Enhances activation of cytotoxic T, NK, and macrophages; acts opposite to IL-10
Interferon-gamma	Induces MHC class I, class II, and other surface antigens on a variety of cells; activates macrophages and endothelial cells; augments or inhibits other cytokine activities; augments NK cell activity; exerts antiviral activity
Interferon (alpha and beta)	Exerts antiviral activity; induces class I antigen expression; augments NK cell activity; has fever-inducing and antiproliferative properties
Tumor necrosis factor (alpha and beta)	Direct cytotoxin for some tumor cells; induces fever, sleep, and other acute-phase responses; stimulates the synthesis of other cytokines, collagen, and collagenases; activates endothelial and macrophagic cells; mediates inflammation, catabolic processes, and septic shock
Colony-stimulating factor (CSF)	
Granulocyte-macrophage CSF	Promotes neutrophilic, eosinophic, and macrophage bone marrow colonies; actives mature granulocytes
Granulocyte CSF	Promotes neutrophilic colonies
Macrophage CSF	Promotes macrophagic colonies
T-cell growth factor-beta	Chemotactic for fibroblasts; inhibits proliferation of endothelial cells; epithelial cells, and T and B lymphocytes; suppresses NK cell activity

certain tumors and later independently discovered as *cachectin*, a circulating mediator of wasting during parasitic disease. TNF is produced by activated macrophages and other activated cells, such as T cells and NK cells. Besides functioning as a major chemical mediator in the inflammatory response and indirectly effecting the fever response, TNF may function as a costimulator of T cells. This cytokine is an especially potent stimulator of IL-1, IL-6, and IL-8. In the setting of bacterial sepsis, high serum levels of TNF may mediate endotoxic shock. TNF is primarily responsible for the tissue wasting seen in cases of chronic inflammation.

Hematopoietic Colony-Stimulating Factors

CSFs are cytokines that stimulate bone marrow pluripotent stem and progenitor or precursor cells to produce large numbers of platelets, erythrocytes, neutrophils, monocytes, eosinophils, and basophils. The CSFs were named according to the type of target cell on which they act (see Table 11–4). GM-CSF acts on the granulocyte-monocyte progenitor cells to produce monocytes and neutrophils; G-CSF more specifically induces neutrophils proliferation; and M-CSF specifically directs the mononuclear phagocyte progenitor. Other cytokines, including IL-1, IL-2, IL-3, IL-4, IL-5, IL-6, IL-7, and IL-11, may influence hematopoiesis, directly or indirectly, during the immune response.

Immunity and the Immune Response

Immunity is a normal adaptive response designed to protect the body against potentially harmful foreign substances, infections, and other sources of nonself antigens. Immunity can be innate or acquired. *Innate (non-*

specific) immunity is the natural resistance with which a person is born. General factors such heredity, age, health, species, race, and sex can influence innate immunity. For example, humans get mumps but dogs do not because they lack on their cells virus-specific binding sites needed for infection. Natural or innate resistance also depends on several internal and external barriers and responses that are grouped as anatomic, physiologic, phagocytic, and inflammatory.

Acquired immunity is the protection that a person gains through exposure to antigens or through transfer of protective antibodies against an antigen. The process of acquiring the ability to respond to an antigen after administration by injection (or oral route as in the polio vaccine) is known as immunization. The *immune response* describes the interaction between an antigen (*i.e.*, immunogen) and an antibody (*i.e.*, immunoglobulin) or reactive T lymphocyte.

Active immunity is acquired through immunization or actually having a disease. It is called active because it depends on a response by the person's immune system. Active immunity, although long lasting once established, does require a few days to weeks on first exposure before the immune response is sufficiently developed to contribute to the destruction of the pathogen. However, the immune system is usually able to react within hours to subsequent exposure to the same agent because of the presence of memory B and T lymphocytes.

Passive immunity is immunity transferred from another source. An infant receives passive immunity from its mother in utero and from antibodies that it receives from its mother's breast milk. Passive immunity also can be transferred through injection of antiserum, which contains the antibodies for a specific disease, or through pooled gamma-globulin or immune serum, which contains antibodies for many infectious agents. Passive immunity only produces short-term protection that lasts for weeks or months.

Humoral Immunity

Humoral immunity depends on maturation of B lymphocytes into plasma cells, which produce antibodies. The combination of antigen with antibody can result in several effector responses such as precipitation of antigen-antibody complexes, agglutination or clumping of cells, neutralization of bacterial toxins and viruses, lysis and destruction of pathogens or cells, adherence of antigen to immune cells, facilitation of phagocytosis, and complement activation. For example, antibodies can neutralize a virus by binding the sites on the virus that it uses to bind to the host cell, negating its ability to infect the cell.

Two types of responses occur in the development of humoral immunity: a primary or secondary response (Fig. 11–13). A *primary* immune response occurs when the antigen is first introduced into the body. During this primary response, there is a latent or lag period before the antibody can be detected in the serum. This latent period involves the processing of antigen by the APCs and recognition by helper T cells. The antigen receptors on helper T cells match the antigenic peptide in association with class II MHC molecules on the APCs. The activated helper T cell produces cytokines to further stimulate the immune system. In humoral immunity, activated helper T cells trigger B cells to proliferate and differentiate into a clone of plasma cells that produce antibody. Detectable antibody continues to rise for a few weeks. Recovery from many infectious diseases occurs at the time during the primary response when the antibody concentration is reaching its peak. The *secondary or memory response* occurs on second or subsequent exposures to the antigen. During the secondary response, the rise in antibody occurs sooner and reaches a higher level because of the available memory cells.

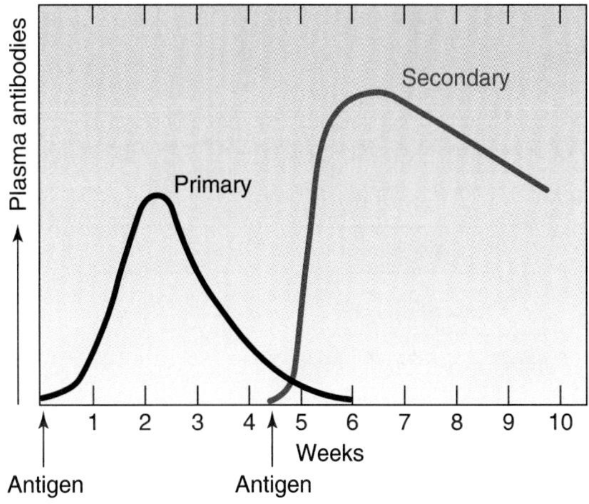

FIGURE 11–13
Primary and secondary phases of the humoral immune response to the same antigen.

During the primary response, B cells are activated to proliferate and differentiate into antibody-secreting plasma cells. A fraction of activated B cells do not differentiate in plasma cells. Such B cells form a pool of memory cells. During the secondary response, the memory cells recognize the antigen and stimulate production of plasma cells, which produce the specific antibody. The booster immunization given for some diseases, such as tetanus, makes use of the secondary response. For a person who has been previously immunized, administration of a booster shot causes an almost immediate rise in antibody to a level sufficient to prevent development of the disease.

Cell-Mediated Immunity

Cell-mediated immunity provides protection against viruses and cancer cells. In cell-mediated immunity, the action of the T lymphocytes and the macrophages predominate. The most aggressive phagocyte, the macrophage, becomes activated only after exposure to T-cell cytokines. As in humoral immunity, the initial stages of cell-mediated immunity are directed by an APC displaying the antigen peptide–MHC II complex to the helper T cell. Helper T cells become activated

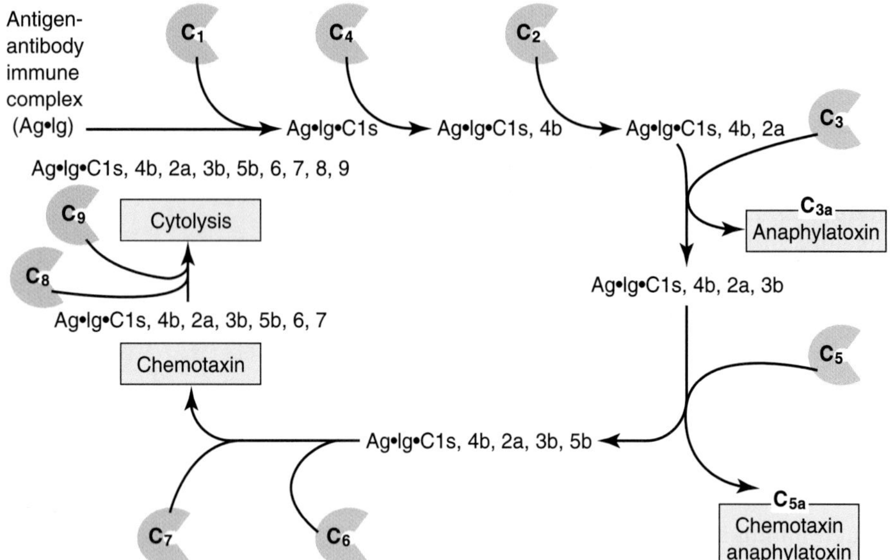

FIGURE 11–14
Classic complement pathway and major biologic activities (in blocks).

after recognition by the TCR of the antigen–MHC complex on the APC and by priming with interleukin-1, which is secreted by the macrophage. The activated helper T cell then synthesizes interleukin-2 and the IL-2 receptor. These molecules drive the multiplication of clones of helper T cells, which amplify the response. Further differentiation of the helper T cells leads to production of additional cytokines (*e.g.*, IFN-γ, TNF-β, IL-12), which enhances the activity of cytotoxic T cells and effector macrophages. A cell-mediated immune response usually occurs through the cytotoxic activity of T_C cells and the enhanced engulfment and killing by macrophages.

Complement System

The complement system is a primary mediator of the humoral immune response that enables the body to produce inflammation and help the localization of an infective agent. The complement system, like the blood coagulation system, consists of a group of proteins that is normally present in the circulation as functionally inactive precursors (Fig. 11–14). These proteins make up 10% to 15% of the plasma-protein fraction. For a complement reaction to occur, the complement components must be activated in the proper sequence. Uncontrolled activation of the complement system is prevented by inhibitor proteins and the instability of the activated complement proteins at each step of the process. There are two parallel but independent mechanisms for activation of the complement system: the classic and alternate pathways.

The classic complement pathway is activated when complement-fixing antibody binds to antigens on a cell surface or in soluble aggregates (Fig. 11–15). Only immune responses involving immunoglobulins IgG and IgM activate complement. The immune complex triggers a series of enzyme reactions that act in a cascade fashion. Modified or split complement proteins released during activation function in the next step of the pathway or are released into the tissue fluid to produce biologic effects important in inflammation. Several structurally modulated complement proteins bind to form pores in the membrane of foreign cells in a manner similar to the perforin proteins. Table 11–5 lists immune responses that occur as the result of complement fixation.

The alternate (properdin) pathway is activated by complex polysaccharides or enzymes. This system sub-

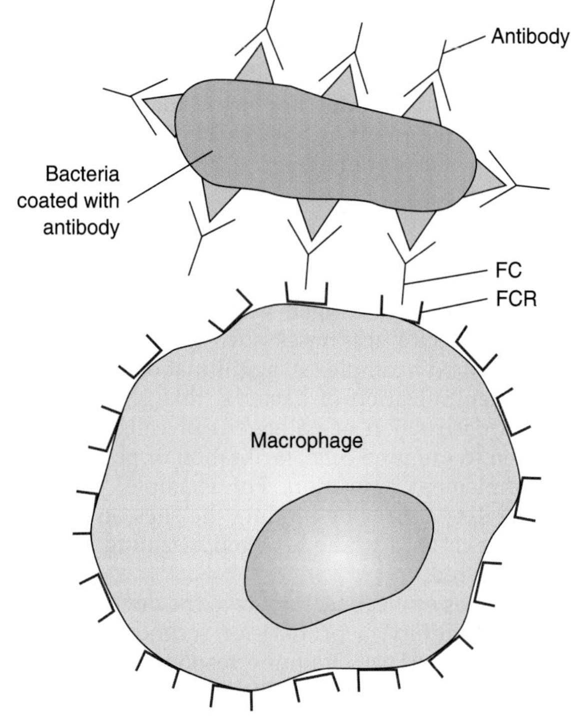

FIGURE 11–15
Complement-mediated interaction between macrophage and bacterium.

TABLE 11-5
Complement-Mediated Immune Responses

Response	Effects
Cytolysis	Destruction of cell membranes of body cells or pathogens
Adherence of immune cells	Adhesion of antigen-antibody complexes to surfaces of cells or tissues such as phagocytes that line blood vessels and various other cells
Chemotaxis	Chemical attraction of phagocytic cells to foreign agents
Anaphylaxis	Degranulation of mast cells with release of histamine and other inflammatory mediators
Opsonization	Targeting of the antigen so it can be easily engulfed and digested by macrophages and other phagocytic cells

stitutes other molecules for the proteins used in the first two steps of the classic complement pathway but requires the presence of C3b and subsequent complement proteins. The biologic effects produced are similar to the classic complement pathway. After activation of the complement system, interactions occur that range from lysis of a spectrum of different kinds of cells to direct mediation of the inflammatory process. First, complement has been shown to mediate the lytic destruction of many kinds of cells, including red blood cells, platelets, bacteria, and lymphocytes. Both complement pathways may induce cytolysis. Second, a major biologic function of complement activation is opsonization—the coating of antigen-antibody complexes such that aggregates are engulfed and cleared more efficiently by macrophages. Third, chemotactic complement products can trigger an influx of leukocytes. These white blood cells remain fixed in the area of complement activation through attachment to specific sites on C3b and C4b molecules. Fourth, production of anaphylatoxin (C3a and C5a) can lead to contraction of smooth muscle, increased vascular permeability, and edema.

Regulation of the Immune Response

Self-regulation is an essential property of the immune system. An inadequate immune response may lead to immunodeficiency, but an inappropriate or excessive response may lead to conditions varying from allergic reactions to autoimmune diseases. This regulation is not well understood and involves all aspects of the immune response—the antigen, antibody, cytokines, regulatory T cells, and the neuroendocrine system.

With each exposure to antigen, the immune system must determine the branch of the immune system to be activated, the extent of the immune response, and its duration. After exposure to an antigen, the immune response to that antigen develops after a brief lag, reaches a peak, and then recedes. The reason that normal immune responses are self-limited is because the response eliminates the antigen and the products of the response, such as cytokines and antibodies, have a short half-life and are only secreted for brief periods after antigen recognition. Effector cells such as plasma cells and cytotoxic T cells have short half-lives. There is also evidence of helper T-cell feedback inhibition of the immune response.

Another facet of immune self-regulation is inhibition of immune responses by tolerance. The term *tolerance* is used to define the ability of the immune system to be nonreactive to self antigens while allowing immunity to foreign agents. Tolerance to self antigens protects an individual from harmful autoimmune reactions. Exposure of an individual to foreign antigens may lead to tolerance and the inability to respond to potential pathogens that cause infection. Tolerance exists not only to self tissues, but also to maternal-fetal tissues. Special regulation of the immune system is also evident in defined privileged sites such as the brain, testes, ovaries, and eyes. Immune damage in these areas could result in serious consequences to the individual and the human species.

In summary, immunity is the resistance to a disease that is provided by the immune system. It can be acquired actively through immunization or having a disease or acquired passively by receiving antibodies or immune cells from another source. Antigens have antigenic determinant sites or epitopes, which the immune system recognizes with specific receptors that distinguish them as nonself and as unique antigens. Immune mechanisms can be classified into two types: specific and nonspecific. Specific immunity involves humoral and cellular mechanisms where the immune cells differentiate self from nonself and can recognize and respond to a unique antigen. The humoral immune response involves antibodies produced by activated B lymphocytes. Cell-mediated immunity depends on T-cell responses to cellular antigens. Nonspecific immune mechanisms can distinguish between self and nonself but cannot differentiate among antigens. They include the complement system, cytokines, and the phagocytic functions of the neutrophils and macrophages. The cytokines, produced largely by T cells, function as intercellular signals that regulate immune and inflammatory responses.

Developmental Aspects of the Immune System

After you have completed this section of the chapter, you should be able to meet the following objectives:

- Explain the transfer of passive immunity from mother to fetus and from mother to infant during breast-feeding
- Characterize the development of active immunity in the infant and small child
- Describe changes in the immune response that occur with aging

Embryologically, the immune system develops in several stages, beginning at 5 to 6 weeks as the fetal liver becomes active in hematopoiesis. Development of the primary lymphoid organs (*i.e.,* thymus and bone marrow) begins during the middle of the first trimester and proceeds rapidly. Secondary lymphoid organs (*i.e.,* spleen, lymph nodes, and tonsils) develop soon after. These secondary lymphoid organs are rather small but well developed at birth and mature rapidly during the postnatal period. The thymus is largest relative to body size and is normally about two thirds its mature weight, which it achieves during the first year of life.

Transfer of Immunity From Mother to Infant

Protection of a newborn to antigens occurs through transfer of maternal antibodies. Maternal IgG antibodies cross the placenta during fetal development and remain functional in the newborn for the first months of life. IgG is the only class of immunoglobulins to cross the placenta. Maternal IgG disappears during the first 6 to 8 months of life while infant synthesis of immunoglobulins increases. Maternally transmitted IgGs are effective against most gram-positive organisms and against most viruses. The neonate is, however, quite susceptible to infections with gram-negative organisms, because he or she has not received maternal antibodies to these organisms. The largest amount of IgG crosses the placenta during the last weeks of pregnancy and is stored in fetal tissues, and infants born prematurely may be deficient. Because of transfer of IgG antibodies to the fetus, a baby born to a mother infected with HIV will have a positive HIV antibody test result, although he or she may not be infected with the virus.

Cord blood does not normally contain IgM or IgA. If present, these antibodies are of fetal origin and represent exposure to intrauterine infection. The infant begins producing IgM antibodies soon after birth, in response to immense antigenic stimulation of his or her new environment. Premature infants appear to be able to produce IgM as well as term infants. At about 6 days of age the IgM rises sharply and this rise continues until about 1 year of age when the adult level is achieved.

Serum IgA is normally first detected at about 13 days after birth. The level increases during early childhood until adult levels are reached between the sixth and seventh year. In addition to placentally transferred antibodies, IgA is transferred by breast-feeding in colostrum or mother's milk. These antibodies provide local immunity for the intestinal system and have been shown to decrease diarrheal infections in underdeveloped countries. These evolutionary adaptations of the immune system have increased the survival of our species and optimized the development of other important organs in the early months of life.

Immune Response in the Elderly

Aging is characterized by a declining ability to adapt to environmental stresses. One of the factors thought to contribute to this problem is a decline in immune responsiveness. This includes changes in cell-mediated and antibody-mediated immune responses. Elderly persons tend to be more susceptible to infections, they have more evidence of autoimmune and immune complex disorders than younger persons, and they have a higher incidence of cancer. Experimental evidence suggests that vaccination is less successful in inducing immunization in older persons than younger adults. However, the effect of altered immune function on the health of elderly persons is clouded by the fact that age-related changes or disease may affect the immune response.

The alterations in immune function that occur with advanced age are not fully understood. There is a decrease in the size of the thymus gland, which is thought to affect T-cell function. The size of the gland begins to decline shortly after sexual maturity, and by age 50, it has usually diminished to 15% or less of its maximum size. There are conflicting reports regarding age-related changes in the peripheral lymphocytes. Some researchers have reported a decrease in the absolute number of lymphocytes, and others have found little if any change. The most common finding is a slight decrease in the proportion of T cells to other lymphocytes and decrease in CD4 and CD8 cells.

More evident are altered responses of the immune cells to antigen stimulations; increasing proportions of lymphocytes become unresponsive while the remainder continue to function relatively normally. T and B cells show deficiencies in activation. In the T-cell types, the $CD4^+$ subset is most severely affected. Evidence indicates that aged T cells have decreased synthesis of cytokines that drive the proliferation of lymphocytes and diminished expression of the receptors that interact with those cytokines. For example, it has been shown that IL-2 synthesis decreases markedly with aging. Although B-cell function is compromised with age, the range of antibodies that can be recognized is not diminished. If anything, the repertoire is increased to the extent that B cells begin to recognize some self-antigens as foreign antigens. This may be the basis for the increased incidence of autoimmune disease in the elderly.

In summary, a newborn is protected against antigens in early life by passive transfer of maternal antibodies through the placenta (IgG) and colostrum (IgA) through breast-feeding. Some changes are seen with aging, including an increase in autoimmune diseases. The impact of alterations in immune function that occur with aging is not fully understood.

The Inflammatory Response

After you have completed this section of the chapter, you should be able to meet the following objectives:

- State the purpose of inflammation
- State the five cardinal signs of acute inflammation and describe the physiologic mechanisms involved in production of these signs

- Compare the hemodynamic and cellular phases of the inflammatory response
- Contrast acute and chronic inflammation
- List four types of inflammatory mediators and state their function
- Name and describe the five types of inflammatory exudates
- Define the characteristics of an acute-phase response

Inflammation is the reaction of vascularized tissue to local injury. Although the effects of inflammation are often viewed as undesirable because they are unpleasant and cause discomfort, the process is essentially a beneficial one that allows a person to live with the effects of everyday stress. Without the inflammatory response, wounds would not heal, and minor infections would become overwhelming. However, inflammation also produces undesirable effects. The crippling effects of rheumatoid arthritis, for example, result from inflammation.

The causes of inflammation are many and varied. Inflammation commonly results because of an immune response to infectious microorganisms. Other causes of inflammation are trauma, surgery, caustic chemicals, extremes of heat and cold, and ischemic damage to body tissues.

Although the inflammatory response can be initiated by a variety of injurious agents and the extent can vary, the sequence of events that follow is remarkably similar. The body, however, uses only those responses that are needed to minimize tissue damage. A small area of local swelling and redness may be sufficient to prevent injury from a mosquito bite, whereas more serious conditions, such as appendicitis, may incite fever, leukocytosis, and body fluid and protein influx.

Inflammatory conditions are named by adding the suffix *-itis* to the affected organ or system. For example, appendicitis refers to inflammation of the appendix, pericarditis to inflammation of the pericardium and neuritis to inflammation of a nerve. More descriptive expressions of the inflammatory process might indicate whether the process was acute or chronic and what type of exudate was formed (*e.g.*, acute fibrinous pericarditis).

Acute Inflammation

The classic description of acute inflammation has been handed down through the ages. In the first century A.D., the Roman physician Celsus described the local reaction of injury in terms known as the cardinal signs of inflammation. These signs are *rubor* (redness), *tumor* (swelling), *calor* (heat), and *dolor* (pain). In the second century, A.D., the Greek physician Galen added a fifth cardinal sign, *functio laesa,* or loss of function. An acute inflammatory response is characterized by a rapid onset and the resolution of the tissue changes and damage in a short time period. Changes occur locally at the site of injury as well as systemically. A general alarm and recruitment system sent throughout the body is known as the *acute-phase response*. A rapid increase and decrease in several plasma proteins is characteristic of the acute-phase component of inflammation.

The manifestation of acute inflammation can be divided into two categories, vascular and cellular blood responses. At the biochemical level, many of the responses that occur during acute inflammation are associated with the release of chemical mediators. The hemodynamic and white blood cell responses contribute to the *inflammatory exudates,* the extravascular influx of fluid containing high concentrations of proteins, salts, cells, and cellular debris.

Vascular Response

The vascular, or hemodynamic changes that occur with inflammation begin almost immediately after injury and are initiated by a momentary constriction of small vessels in the area. This vasoconstriction is followed immediately by vasodilation of the arterioles and venules that supply the area. As a result, the area become congested, causing the redness(erythema) and warmth associated with acute inflammation. Accompanying this hyperemic response is an increase in capillary permeability, which allows fluid to escape into the tissue and cause swelling (*i.e.*, edema). Pain and impaired function follow as a result of tissue swelling and release of chemical mediators.

These responses benefit the host by controlling the effects of the injurious agent. The movement of the fluid out of the capillaries and into the tissue spaces dilutes the toxic and irritating agent. As fluid moves out of the capillaries, stagnation of flow and clotting of blood in the small capillaries occurs at the site of injury. This aids in localizing the spread of infectious microorganisms.

Depending on the severity of injury, the hemodynamic changes that occur with inflammation follow one of three patterns of responses. The first is an immediate transient response, which occurs with minor injury. The second is an immediate sustained response, which occurs with more serious injury and continues for several days and damages the vessels in the area. The third type of response is a delayed hemodynamic response; the increase in capillary permeability occurs after 4 to 24 hours after injury. A delayed response often accompanies radiation types of injuries, such as a sunburn.

Cellular Responses

The cellular stage of acute inflammation is marked by movement of white blood cells (leukocytes) into the area of injury. The phagocytic cells that respond early are primarily neutrophils and possibly other granulocytes. As the process continues, monocytes exit the blood and mature into macrophages in the tissue environment. These longer-lived phagocytes help to destroy the agent, aid signaling of specific immunity, and serve to resolve the inflammatory process. The cellular response of the phagocytes includes the margination or pavementing of white blood cells to capillary walls, emigration of the white blood cells, chemotaxis or positive migration of the cells to the site of injury, and phagocytosis.

Granulocytes. Granulocytes are identifiable because of their characteristic cytoplasmic granules. These white blood cells have distinctive multilobar nuclei. The granulocytes are divided into three types (*i.e.*, neutrophils, eosinophils, and basophils) according to the staining properties of the granules (see Chapter 6).

The *neutrophil* is the primary phagocyte that arrives early at the site of inflammation, usually within 90 minutes of injury. Their cytoplasmic granules contain enzymes and other antibacterial substances that are used in destroying and degrading the engulfed particles. Because these white blood cells have nuclei that are divided into three to five lobes, they are often called *polymorphonuclear* (PMNs) or *segmented neutrophils* (segs). The neutrophil count in the blood often increases greatly during the inflammatory process. After being released from the bone marrow, circulating neutrophils have a life span of only about 10 hours and therefore must be constantly replaced if their numbers are to be adequate. This requires an increase in circulating white blood cells, a condition called *leukocytosis*. With excessive demand for phagocytes, immature forms of neutrophils are released from the bone marrow. These immature cells are often called *bands* because of the horseshoe shape of their nuclei. The phrase a *shift to the left* in a white blood cell differential count refers to the increase in immature neutrophils seen in severe infections.

The characteristic reddish staining cytoplasmic granules of the *eosinophils* identifies these granulocytes. These leukocytes increase in the blood during allergic reactions and parasitic infections. For large parasitic worms that cannot be phagocytized, eosinophils are activated to release their granule armament. They also regulate inflammation and allergic reactions by controlling specific chemical mediator release during these processes. The dark purple staining granules of the *basophils* contain histamine and other bioactive mediators of inflammation. The basophils are involved in producing symptoms in inflammation and allergic reactions. They may also play a role in parasitic infections. The mast cell, which is found in the tissues, is very similar in many of its properties to the basophil.

Mononuclear Phagocytes. The monocytes are the largest of the blood white blood cells and constitute 3% to 8% of the total blood leukocytes. The circulating life span of the monocyte is three to four times longer than that of the granulocytes and these cells survive for a longer time in the tissues. The monocytes, which migrate in increased number into the tissues on response to inflammatory stimuli, mature into *macrophages*. Within 5 hours, mononuclear cells arrive at the inflammatory site, and by 48 hours, monocytes and macrophages are the predominant cell types. The macrophages engulf larger and greater quantities of foreign material than the neutrophils. They also migrate to the local lymph nodes to prime specific immunity. These leukocytes play an important role in chronic inflammation where they can surround and wall off foreign material that cannot be digested.

Margination and Emigration of Leukocytes. During the early stages of the inflammatory response, fluid leaves the capillaries, causing blood viscosity to increase. The release of chemical mediators (*i.e.*, histamine, leukotrienes, and kinins) and cytokines affect the endothelial cells of the capillaries and cause the leukocytes to increase their expression of adhesion molecules. The leukocytes begin to *marginate*, or move to and along the periphery of the blood vessels. The cobblestone appearance of the vessel lining due to margination of leukocytes has led to the term *pavementing*. After adherence of the phagocyte to the endothelial cells, emigration occurs.

Emigration is a mechanism by which the leukocyte extend pseudopodia, pass through the capillary walls by ameboid movement, and migrate into the tissue spaces (Fig. 11–16). The movement of white blood cells through the capillary walls occurs by a process called *diapedesis*. Along with the emigration of leukocytes, there may also be an escape of red cells.

Chemotaxis. The leukocytes wander through the tissue guided by secreted cytokines (chemokines; interleukin-8), bacterial and cellular debris, and complement fragments (C3a, C5a). This process by which leukocytes are caused to migrate in response to a chemical signal is called chemotaxis. The positive movement up the concentration gradient of chemical mediators to the site of injury increases the probability of a sufficiently localized cellular response.

Phagocytosis. In the next stage of the cellular response, the neutrophils and macrophages engulf and degrade the bacteria and cellular debris in a process called *phagocytosis* (see Fig. 11–16). Phagocytosis involves four distinct steps: chemotaxis, adherence plus opsonization, engulfment, and intracellular killing. Neutrophil and macrophage chemotaxis can be stimulated by many factors, including complement, chemotactic factors produced by leukocytes, and even bacteria. Contact between the bacteria or antigen with the phagocyte cell membrane is essential for trapping the agent and triggering the final steps of phagocytosis. If the antigen is coated with antibody or complement, its adherence is increased because of binding to Fc or complement receptors These receptors recognize the constant part (Fc fragment) of the antibody molecule or the products of processed complement (C3b molecule). This process of enhanced binding of an antigen due to antibody or complement is called *opsonization*. Engulfment follows the recognition of the agent as foreign. Cytoplasmic extensions (pseudopods) surround and enclose the particle in a membrane-enclosed phagocytic vesicle or phagosome. In the cell cytoplasm, the phagosome merges with a lysosome containing antibacterial molecules and enzymes that can digest the microbe.

Intracellular killing of pathogens is accomplished through several mechanisms, including enzymes, defensins, and toxic oxygen and nitrogen products produced by oxygen-dependent metabolic pathways. The metabolic burst pathways that generate toxic oxygen and

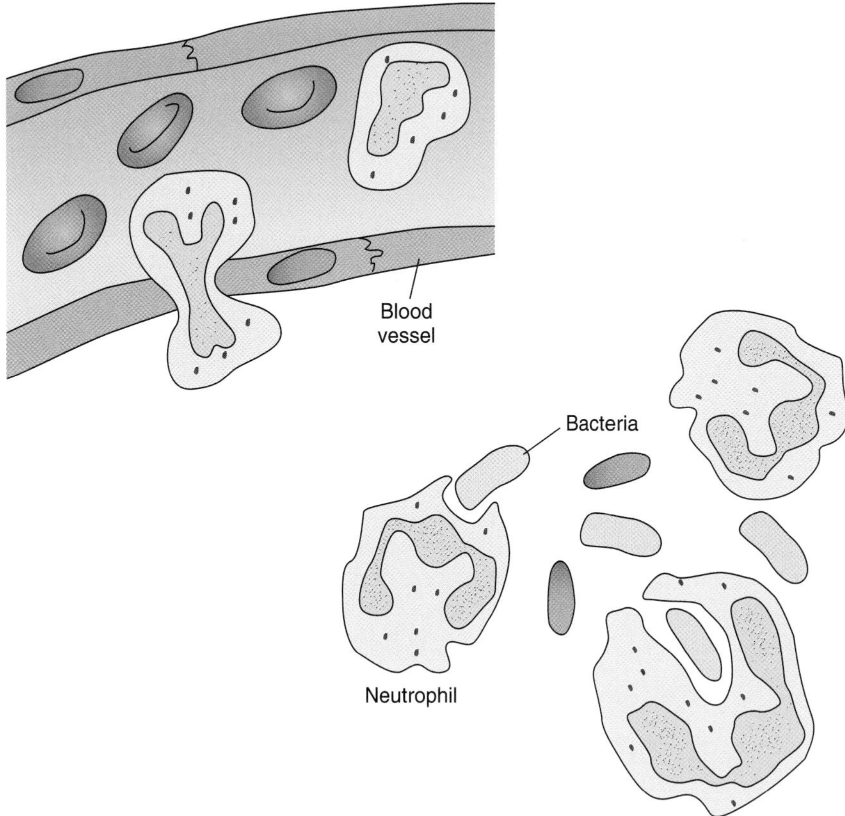

FIGURE 11–16
Neutrophil emigration and phagocytosis.

nitrogen products (*i.e.,* nitric oxide, peroxyonitrites, hydrogen peroxide, and hypochlorous acid) require oxygen and metabolic enzymes such as myeloperoxidase, NADPH-oxidase and nitric oxide synthetase. Individuals born with genetic defects in some of these enzymes have immunodeficiency conditions that make them susceptible to repeated bacterial infection.

Acute-Phase Response

Along with the cellular responses, a constellation of systemic effects called the *acute-phase response* occurs. The acute-phase response, which usually begins within hours or days of the onset of inflammation or infections includes changes in the concentrations of plasma proteins, increased erythrocyte sedimentation rate (ESR), fever, increase in the number of leukocytes, skeletal muscle catabolism, and negative nitrogen balance. These responses are generated after the release of the cytokines, interleukin-1 (IL-1), TNF-α, and interleukin-6. These cytokines effect the thermoregulatory center in the hypothalamus to produce fever, the most obvious sign of the acute-phase response. IL-1 and other cytokines induce an increase in the number and immaturity of circulating neutrophils by stimulating their production in the bone marrow. Lethargy, a common feature of the acute-phase response, results from the effects of IL-1 and TNF-α on the central nervous system.

During the acute-phase response, the liver dramatically increases the synthesis of acute-phase proteins such as fibrinogen and C-reactive protein that serve several different nonspecific host defense functions. The change in the types of plasma proteins contribute to the increased sedimentation rate of erythrocytes (see Chapter 6). The metabolic changes that include skeletal muscle catabolism provide amino acids that can be used in the immune response and for tissue repair. The total systemic process coordinates various activities in the body to enable an optimum host response.

Inflammatory Mediators

Although inflammation is precipitated by injury, its signs and symptoms are produced by chemical mediators. Mediators can be classified by function: those with vasoactive and smooth muscle constricting properties such as histamine, prostaglandins, leukotrienes, and platelet-activating factor (PAF); chemotactic factors such as complement fragments (C5a) and cytokines (IL-8); plasma proteases that can activate complement and components of the clotting system; reactive molecules and cytokines liberated from leukocytes, which when released into the extracellular environment can cause damage to the surrounding tissue. Table 11–6 describes some chemical mediators and their major impact on inflammation.

Histamine. Histamine is widely distributed throughout the body. It is found in high concentration in platelets, basophils, and mast cells. Histamine causes dilation and increased permeability of capillaries. It is one of the first mediator of an inflammatory response. Antihistamine drugs suppress this immediate, transient response.

TABLE 11-6

Signs of Inflammation and Corresponding Chemical Mediator

Inflammatory Response	Chemical Mediator
Swelling, redness, and tissue warmth (vasodilation and increased capillary permeability)	Histamine, prostaglandins, leukotrienes, bradykinin, platelet-activating factor
Tissue damage	Lysosomal enzymes and products released from neutrophils, macrophages, and other inflammatory cells.
Chemotaxis	Complement fragments
Pain	Prostaglandins
	Bradykinin
Fever	Interleukin-1 and interleukin-6
Leukocytosis	Tissue necrosis factor and interleukin-8

Plasma Proteases. The plasma proteases consist of the kinins, activated complement proteins, and clotting factors. One kinin, bradykinin, causes increased capillary permeability and pain. The clotting system (see Chapter 7) contributes to the vascular phase of inflammation, mainly through fibrinopeptides that are formed during the final steps of the clotting process.

Prostaglandins. The prostaglandins are ubiquitous lipid-soluble molecules derived from arachidonic acid, a fatty acid liberated from cell membrane phospholipids. Several prostaglandins are synthesize from arachidonic acid through the cyclooxygenase metabolic pathway. Prostaglandins contribute to vasodilation, capillary permeability and the pain and fever that accompany inflammation. The stable prostaglandins (PGE_1 and PGE_2) induce inflammation and potentiate the effects of histamine and other inflammatory mediators. The prostaglandin, thromboxane A_2, promotes platelet aggregation and vasoconstriction. Drugs such as aspirin and indomethacin inhibit prostaglandin synthesis. The glucocorticoid hormones or drugs are known to curtail the availability of arachidonic acid needed for prostaglandin synthesis.

Leukotrienes. The leukotrienes are chemical mediators first discovered in leukocytes and chemically have a triene structure. Like the prostaglandins, the leukotrienes are formed from arachidonic acid through the lipoxygenase pathway. One leukotriene causes slow and sustained constriction of the bronchioles and is an important inflammatory mediator in bronchial asthma and immediate hypersensitivity reactions (see Chapters 12 and 24). The leukotrienes have also been reported to affect the permeability of the postcapillary venules, the adhesion properties of endothelial cells, and the chemotaxis and extravascularization of neutrophils, eosinophils, and monocytes.

Platelet-Activating Factor. Generated from a complex lipid stored in cell membranes, platelet activating factor affects a variety of cell types and induces platelet aggregation. It activates neutrophils and is a potent eosinophil chemoattractant. When injected into the skin, PAF causes a wheal-and-flare reaction and leukocyte infiltrate characteristic of immediate hypersensitivity reactions. When inhaled, PAF cause bronchospasm, eosinophil infiltration, and nonspecific bronchial hyperreactivity.

Inflammatory Exudates

Characteristically, the acute inflammatory response involves production of exudates. These exudates can vary in terms of fluid, plasma protein, and cell content. Acute inflammation can produce serous, fibrinous, membranous, purulent and hemorrhagic exudates. Inflammatory exudates are often composed of a combination of these types. Serous exudates are watery exudates low in protein content and result from plasma entering the inflammatory site. Fibrinous exudates contain large amounts of fibrinogen and form a thick and sticky meshwork, much like the fibers of a blood clot. Membranous or pseudo membranous exudates develop on mucous membrane surfaces and are composed of necrotic cells enmeshed in a fibrinopurulent exudate. A purulent or suppurative exudate contains pus, which is composed of degraded white blood cells, proteins and tissue debris. An abscess or cellulitis are examples of purulent exudates. Hemorrhagic exudates occur where severe tissue injury causes damage to blood vessels or when there is significant leakage of red cells from the capillaries.

Chronic Inflammation

Acute infections are usually self-limiting and are rapidly controlled by the host defenses. In contrast, chronic inflammation is self-perpetuating and may last for weeks, months, or even years. It may develop during a recurrent or progressive acute inflammatory process or from low-grade, smoldering responses that fail to evoke an acute response. Characteristic of chronic inflammation is an infiltration by mononuclear cells (macrophages and lymphocytes) instead of the influx of neutrophils commonly seen in acute inflammation. Chronic inflammation also involves the proliferation of fibroblasts instead of exudates. As a result, the risk of scaring and deformity developing is usually considered greater than in acute inflammation. Agents that evoke chronic inflammation are typically low-grade persistent irritants that are unable to penetrate deeply or spread rapidly. Among the causes of chronic inflammation are foreign bodies such as talc, silica, asbestos, and surgical suture materials. Many viruses provoke chronic inflammatory responses, as do certain bacteria, fungi, and larger parasites of moderate to low virulence. Examples are the tubercle bacillus, the treponema of syphilis, and the actinomyces. The presence of injured tissue such as that surrounding a healing fracture also may incite chronic inflammation. Immunologic mechanisms are thought to play an important role in chronic inflammation. The two patterns of chronic inflammation are a nonspecific chronic inflammation and granulomatous inflammation.

Nonspecific chronic inflammation involves a diffuse accumulation of macrophages and lymphocytes at the site of injury. Macrophages accumulate at the site because of infiltration from the tissue because of chemotaxis and prolonged survival and immobilization of these cells within the inflammatory areas. These mechanisms lead to fibroblast proliferation, with subsequent scar formation that in many cases replaces the normal connective tissue or the functional parenchymal tissues of the involved structures. For example, scar tissue resulting from chronic inflammation of the bowel causes narrowing of the bowel lumen.

A granulomatous lesion results from chronic inflammation. A granuloma is typically a small, 1- to 2-mm lesion in which there is a massing of macrophages surrounded by lymphocytes. These modified macrophages resemble epithelial cells and are sometimes called *epithelioid cells*. Like other macrophages, these epithelioid cells are derived originally from blood monocytes. Granulomatous inflammation is associated with foreign bodies such as splinters, sutures, silica, and asbestos and with microorganisms that cause tuberculosis, syphilis, sarcoidosis, deep fungal infections, and brucellosis. These types of agents have one thing in common: they are poorly digested and are usually not easily controlled by other inflammatory mechanisms. The epithelioid cells in granulomatous inflammation may clump in a mass (granuloma) or coalesce, forming a large multinucleated giant cell that attempts to surround the foreign agent. A dense membrane of connective tissue eventually encapsulates the lesion and isolates it.

A tubercle is a granulomatous inflammatory response to *Mycobacterium tuberculosis*. Peculiar to the tuberculosis granuloma is the presence of a caseous (cheesy) necrotic center.

In summary, inflammation describes a local response to tissue injury and can present as an acute or chronic condition. Acute inflammation is the local response of tissue to a nonspecific form of injury. The classic signs of inflammation are redness, swelling, local heat, pain, and loss of function. The inflammatory response is orchestrated by chemical mediators such as histamine, prostaglandins, platelet activating factor, complement fragments, and reactive molecules that are liberated by leukocytes. Acute inflammation involves a hemodynamic phase during which blood flow and capillary permeability are increased and a cellular phase during which phagocytic white blood cells called granulocytes move into the area to engulf and degrade the inciting agent. Cytokines also influence the cellular responses. Acute inflammation involves the production of exudates containing serous fluid (serous exudate), red blood cells (hemorrhagic exudate), fibrinogen (fibrinous exudate) products of mucous membrane, and fibrinogen breakdown products (membranous exudate) and tissue debris and white blood cell breakdown products (purulent exudate).

In contrast to acute inflammation, which is self-limiting, chronic inflammation is more prolonged and is usually caused by persistent irritants, most of which are insoluble and resistant to phagocytosis and other inflammatory mechanisms. Chronic inflammation involves the presence of mononuclear cells (lymphocytes and macrophages) rather than granulocytes. Exudates are formed in acute inflammation compared with the proliferation of fibroblasts that cause scaring and deformity in chronic inflammation.

BIBLIOGRAPHY

Ahmed R., Gray D. (1996). Immunological memory and protective immunity: Understanding their relation. *Science* 272, 54–60.

Baumann H., Gauldie J. (1994). The acute phase response. *Immunology Today* 15, 74–80.

Caligaris-Cappio F., Ferrarini M. (1996). B cells and their fate in health and disease. *Immunology Today* 17, 206–208.

Cotran R.S., Kumar V., Robbins S.L.. (1994). *Pathologic basis of disease* (5th ed., pp. 51–92, 171–178). Philadelphia: W.B. Saunders.

Fearon D., Locksley R.M. (1996). The instructive role of Innate Immunity in the acquired immune response. *Science* 272, 50–54.

Galli S.J. (1993). New concepts about the mast cells. *New England Journal of Medicine* 328, 257–265.

Gallin J.I., Goldstein I.M., Snyderman R., ed. *Inflammation: Basic principles and clinical correlates* (2nd ed.). New York: Raven Press, 1992.

Janeway C.A., Jr., Travers P. (1996). *Immunobiology: The immune system in health and disease* (3rd ed.). New York: Garland Publishing.

Kuby J. (1997). *Immunology* (3rd ed.). San Francisco: W.H. Freeman.

Miller R.A. (1996). The aging immune system: Primer and prospectus. *Science* 273, 70–73.

Moretta L. (1996). Receptors for HLA class-I molecules in human natural killer cells. *Annual Review of Immunology* 14, 619–648.

Roitt I., Brostoff J., Male D. (1996). *Immunology* (4th ed.). St. Louis: Mosby.

Sell S., Berkower I., Max E. (1996). *Immunology, immunopathology and immunity* (5th ed.). East Norwalk, CT: Appleton & Lange.

Stites D., Terr A., Parslow T.G. (Eds). (1994). *Basic and clinical immunology* (8th ed.). East Norwalk, CT: Appleton & Lange.

CHAPTER 12

Alterations in the Immune Response

Carol Mattson Porth and W. Michael Dunne, Jr.

The human immune network is a multifaceted defense system that has evolved to protect against invading microorganisms, prevent the proliferation of cancer cells, and mediate the healing of damaged tissue. Under normal conditions, the immune response deters or prevents disease. Occasionally, however, the inadequate, inappropriate, or misdirected activation of the immune system can produce debilitating or life-threatening illnesses, typified by immunodeficiency states, allergic or hypersensitivity reactions, transplantation pathophysiology, and autoimmune disorders. The variety of immunologic disorders that directly or indirectly lead to pathologic conditions in humans are discussed in this chapter.

Immunodeficiency Disease

After you have finished this section of the chapter, you should be able to do the following:

- List the most important categories of immunodeficiency disease

CHART **12-1**
Immunodeficiency States

Humoral (B-Cell) Immunodeficiency

Primary
- Transient hypogammaglobulinemia of infancy
- X-linked hypogammaglobulinemia
- Common variable immunodeficiency
- Selective deficiency of IgG, IgA, IgM

Secondary
- Increased loss of immunoglobulins (nephrotic syndrome)*

Cellular (T-Cell) Immunodeficiency

Primary
- Congenital thymic aplasia (DiGeorge's syndrome)
- Abnormal T-cell production (Nezelof's syndrome)

Secondary
- Malignant disease (Hodgkin's disease and others)
- Transient suppression of T-cell production and function due to an acute viral infection such as measles
- AIDS
- Purine nucleoside phosphorylase (PNP) or adenosine deaminase (ADA) deficiency

Combined B-Cell and T-Cell immunodeficiency

Primary
- Severe combined immunodeficiency (autosomal or sex-linked recessive)
- Wiskott-Aldrich syndrome (immunodeficiency, thrombocytopenia, and eczema)
- Ataxia and telangiectasia

Secondary
- Irradiation
- Immune suppressant and cytotoxic drugs
- Aging

Complement Disorders

Primary
- Angioneurotic edema (complement 1 inactivator deficiency)
- Selective deficiency in a complement component

Secondary
- Acquired disorders that involve complement utilization

Phagocytic Dysfunction

Primary
- Chronic granulomatous disease
- Glucose-6-phosphate dehydrogenase deficiency
- Job's syndrome
- Chédiak-Higashi syndrome
- CD11/CD18 deficiency

Secondary
- Drug induced (corticosteroid and immunosuppressive therapy)
- Diabetes mellitus

*Examples are not inclusive

- State the difference between primary and secondary immunodeficiency states
- Compare and contrast immunodeficiency disorders caused by B-cell and T-cell disorders
- State the function of the complement system and relate to the manifestations of hereditary angioneurotic edema
- State the proposed mechanisms of dysfunction and manifestations in primary disorders of phagocytosis

Immunodeficiency can be defined as an abnormality in one or more branches of the immune system that renders a person susceptible to diseases normally prevented by an intact immune system. Four major categories of immune mechanisms defend the body against infectious or neoplastic disease: humoral or antibody-mediated immunity (*i.e.*, B lymphocytes); cell-mediated immunity (*i.e.*, T lymphocytes and lymphokines); the complement system; and phagocytosis (*i.e.*, neutrophils and macrophages). Although not usually included in a discussion of the immune system, disorders that breech the integrity of natural barriers such as skin, mucous membranes, and secretory antimicrobial enzymes (*e.g.*, lysozyme in tears, the hydrolytic enzymes in saliva) can also produce a state of immunodeficiency.

Abnormalities of the immune system can be classified as primary (*i.e.*, congenital or inherited) or secondary if the immunodeficiency is acquired later in life. Secondary immunodeficiency can be the result of infection (*e.g.*, acquired immunodeficiency syndrome [AIDS]), neoplastic disease (*e.g.*, lymphoma), or immunosuppressive therapy (*e.g.*, cyclosporine). Regardless of the cause, primary and secondary deficiencies can produce the same spectrum of disease. The severity and symptomatology of the various immunodeficiencies depend on the disorder and extent of immune system involvement. The various categories of immunodeficiency are summarized in Chart 12–1. AIDS is discussed in Chapter 13.

Humoral (B-Cell) Immunodeficiencies

Humoral immunodeficiency can range from a transient decrease in immunoglobulin levels during early infancy to inherited disorders that interrupt the production of one or all of the immunoglobulins. During the first few months of life, infants are protected from infection by IgG class antibodies that have been transferred from the maternal circulation during fetal life. IgA, IgM, IgD, and IgE do not normally cross the placenta. The presence of elevated levels of IgA or IgM in the infant cord blood suggests premature antibody production in response to an intrauterine infection. An infant's level of maternal IgG gradually declines over a period of about 6 months. Concomitant with the loss of maternal antibody, the infant's immature humoral immune system begins to function, and between the ages of 1 and 2 years, the child's antibody production reaches adult levels.

Antibody production depends on the differentiation of B stem cells within the bone marrow to mature, immunoglobulin-producing plasma cells. This maturation cycle initially involves the production of surface IgM, migration from the marrow to the peripheral lymphoid tissue, and switching to the specialized production of IgG, IgA, IgD, IgE, or IgM antibodies after antigenic stimulation (Fig. 12–1).

Transient Hypogammaglobulinemia of Infancy

Any abnormality that blocks or prevents the maturation of B stem cells can produce a state of immunodeficiency. For example, certain infants may experience a delay in the maturation process of B cells that leads to a prolonged deficiency in IgG levels (IgM and IgA levels are normal) beyond 6 months of age. The total number and antigenic response of circulating B cells is normal, but the chemical communication between B and T cells that leads to clonal proliferation of antibody-producing plasma cells seems to be reduced. This condition is referred to as *transient hypogammaglobulinemia of infancy*. The result of this condition is usually limited to repeated bouts of upper respiratory and middle ear infections, and this condition usually resolves by the time the child is 2 to 4 years of age.

Primary B-Cell Immunodeficiency

At the opposite end of the spectrum of B-cell immunodeficiencies is a serious X-linked recessive genetic disorder called *Bruton's agammaglobulinemia* that only affects males.[1] As the name implies, children with this disorder have essentially undetectable levels of all serum immunoglobulins. They are susceptible to meningitis and recurrent otitis media and to sinus and pulmonary infections with encapsulated organisms such as *Streptococcus pneumoniae, Haemophilus influenzae* type b, or *Neisseria meningitidis*.[2] Many children with this disorder have severe tooth decay. The central defect in this syndrome is a block in differentiation of pre-B cells, creating an absence of mature circulating B cells and plasma cells. T lymphocytes, however, are normal in number and function. Symptoms of the disorder usually coincide with the loss of maternal antibodies. A clue to the presence of the disorder is failure of an infection to respond completely and promptly to antibiotic therapy. Diagnosis is based on demonstration of low or absent serum immunoglobulins. Therapy is based on monthly administration of intravenous immunoglobulin and prompt antimicrobial therapy for suspected infections. The prognosis of this condition depends on the prompt recognition and treatment of infections. Chronic pulmonary disease is an ever-present danger.

Another disorder of B-cell maturation, which is similar to Bruton's hypogammaglobulinemia, is a condition called *common variable immunodeficiency* or *late-onset hypogammaglobulinemia*. In this syndrome, the terminal differentiation of mature B cells to plasma cells is blocked. The result is markedly reduced serum immunoglobulin levels, normal numbers of circulating B lymphocytes, and a complete absence of germinal centers and plasma cells in lymph nodes and the spleen. The symptomatology is similar to that of Bruton's hypogammaglobulinemia (*i.e.*, recurrent otitis media and sinus and pulmonary infections with encapsulated organisms), but the onset of symptoms occurs much later, usually between the ages of 15 and 35 years, and distribution of disease between males and females is equal. Persons with late-onset hypogammaglobulinemia also have an increased tendency to develop chronic lung disease, autoimmune disorders, hepatitis, gastric carcinoma, and chronic diarrhea with associated intestinal malabsorption. Approximately one

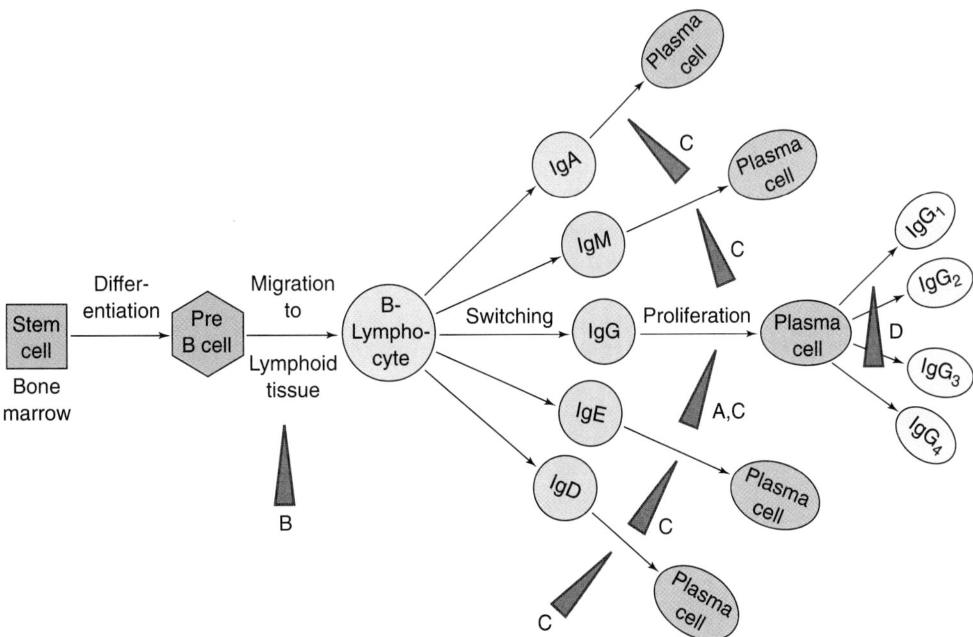

FIGURE 12–1
Stem cells to mature immunoglobulin-secreting plasma cells. *Arrows* indicate the stage of the maturation process that is interrupted in (**A**) transient hypoglobulinemia, (**B**) Bruton's hypogammaglobulinema, (**C**) common variable immunodeficiency, and (**D**) IgG subclass deficiency.

half of persons with the disorder have evidence of abnormal T-cell immunity, suggesting that this syndrome is a complex immunodeficiency.Treatment methods for late-onset hypogammaglobulinemia are similar to those used for Bruton's hypogammaglobulinemia.

Selective IgA deficiency is the most common type of immunoglobulin deficiency, affecting 1 in 400 to 1 in 1000 persons.[1] The syndrome is characterized by moderate to marked reduction in levels of serum and secretory IgA. It is likely that the cause of this deficiency is a block in the pathway that promotes terminal differentiation of mature B cells to IgA secreting plasma cells. Approximately two thirds of persons with selective IgA deficiency have no overt symptoms, presumably because IgG and IgM levels are normal and compensate for the defect. At least 50% of affected children overcome the deficiency by the age of 14 years. Persons with markedly reduced levels of IgA often experience repeated upper respiratory and gastrointestinal infections and have increased incidence of allergies such as asthma, of autoimmune disorders, and of malignancies. They also can develop antibodies against IgA, which can lead to an anaphylactic response when given blood components containing IgA.[1] There is no treatment available for selective IgA deficiency unless there is a concomitant reduction in IgG levels. Administration of IgA is of little benefit because it has a short half-life and is not secreted across the mucosa. There is also the risk associated with IgA antibodies.

An *IgG subclass deficiency* is another type of selective immunoglobulin deficiency. Children who are prone to multiple upper respiratory and middle ear infections throughout the year are sometimes afflicted with an IgG subclass deficiency. This deficiency alters their ability to produce antibodies against polysaccharide antigens. As discussed in Chapter 11, IgG immunoglobulins can be divided into four subclasses (IgG1 through IgG4) based on structure and function. Most circulating IgG belongs to IgG1 (70%) and IgG2 (20%) subclasses. In general, antibod˘es directed against protein antigens belong to IgG1 and IgG3 subclasses, and antibodies directed against carbohydrate and polysaccharide antigens are primarily IgG2 subclass. As a result, persons who are deficient in IgG2 subclass antibodies can be at greater risk for developing sinusitis, otitis media, and pneumonia caused by polysaccharide-encapsulated microorganisms such as *S. pneumoniae, H. influenzae* type b, and *N. meningitidis.* Children with mild forms of the deficiency can be treated with prophylactic antibiotics to prevent repeated infections. Intravenous immune globulin (IVIG) can be given to children with severe manifestations of this deficiency. The use of polysaccharide vaccines conjugated to protein carriers can provide protection against some of these infections because protein conjugated to protein carriers stimulates an IgG1 response.

Secondary B-Cell Immunodeficiencies

Secondary deficiencies in humoral immunity can develop as a consequence of selective loss of immunoglobulins through the gastrointestinal or genitourinary tracts. Such is the case in persons with nephrotic syndrome who, because of abnormal glomerular filtration, lose serum IgA and IgG in their urine (see Chapter 28). Because of its larger molecular size, IgM is not filtered into the urine, and serum levels remain normal.

Cellular (T-Cell) Immunodeficiency

Unlike the B-cell lineage in which a well-defined series of differentiation steps ultimately leads to the production of immunoglobulins, mature T lymphocytes are composed of distinct subpopulations whose immunologic assignments are diverse. T cells can be functionally divided into helper, suppressor, and cytotoxic subtypes and a population of T cells that promote delayed hypersensitivity reactions. Collectively, T lymphocytes protect against fungal, protozoan, viral, and intracellular bacterial infections; control malignant cell proliferation; and are responsible for coordinating the overall immune response.

Primary T-Cell Immunodeficiency

There are few primary forms of T-cell immunodeficiency, probably because defects in this branch of the immune response are usually lethal mutations. One such abnormality, called *DiGeorge's syndrome,* stems from an embryonic developmental defect. The defect is thought to occur before the 12th week of gestation, at the time when the thymus gland, parathyroid gland, and parts of the head, neck, and heart are developing. Formerly thought to be caused by a variety of factors including extrinsic teratogens, this defect has been traced to gene on chromosome 22 (22q11).[1] Babies born with this defect have partial or complete failure to develop the thymus and parathyroid glands and have congenital defects of the head, neck, and heart.

The extent of immune and parathyroid abnormalities is highly variable, as are the other defects. Occasionally, a child has no heart defect. In some babies, the thymus is not absent but is in an abnormal location and is extremely small. These babies can have partial DiGeorge's syndrome, in which hypertrophy of the thymus occurs with development of normal immune function. The facial disorders can include hypertelorism (*i.e.,* increased distance between the eyes), micrognathia (*i.e.,* fish mouth), low-set posterior angulated ears, split uvula, and high-arched palate (Fig. 12–2). Urinary tract abnormalities are also common. The most frequent presenting sign is hypocalcemia and tetany that develops in the first 24 hours of life. It is caused by the absence of the parathyroid gland and is resistant to standard therapy.

Children who survive the immediate neonatal period may develop recurrent or chronic infections because of impaired T-cell immunity. Children may also have an absence of immunoglobulin production, caused by a lack of helper T-cell function. For children who do require treatment, thymus transplantation can be performed to reconstitute T-cell immunity. Bone marrow transplantation has also been successfully used to restore normal

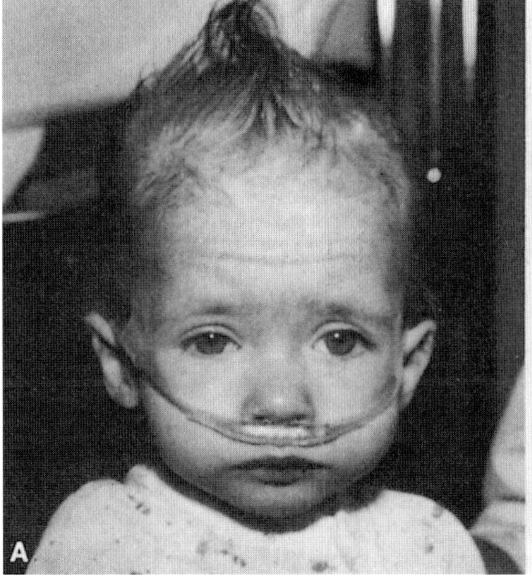

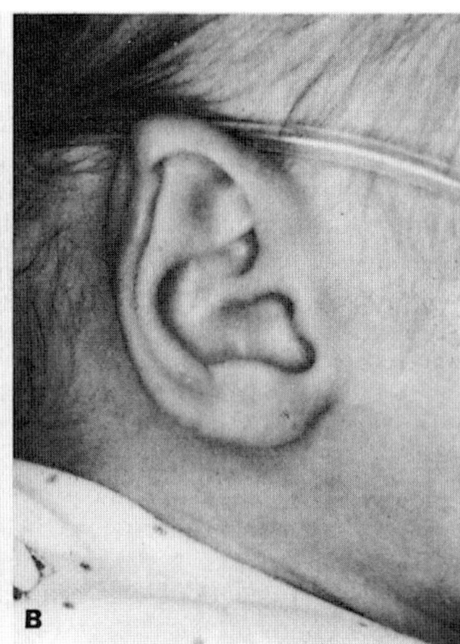

FIGURE 12–2
(**A**) Facial abnormalities in a child with DiGeorge's syndrome, as illustrated by hypertelorism, defective low-set ears, hypoplastic mandible, and bowing upward of the upper lip and (**B**) by a closeup of the ears showing a notched pinna and deficient helix formation.

T-cell populations. If blood transfusions are needed, as during corrective heart surgery, special processing is required to prevent graft-versus-host disease.

A related disorder, called *Nezelof's syndrome,* is caused by a defect in thymus gland development with T-cell deficiency but without associated parathyroid dysfunction and other congenital deformities. This syndrome occurs in males and females. The cause of the disorder is unknown. Children with the disorder experience recurrent or chronic pulmonary infections, failure to thrive, oral or cutaneous candidiasis, chronic diarrhea, gram-negative infections, and severe varicella (chickenpox) in infancy. It is the primary immunodeficiency disease in children most often confused with AIDS.[3]

Secondary T-Cell Immunodeficiency

Secondary deficiencies of T-cell function are more common than primary deficiencies and have been described in conjunction with acute viral infections (*e.g.,* measles virus, cytomegalovirus) and with certain malignancies such as Hodgkin's disease and other lymphomas. In the case of viruses, direct infection of specific T lymphocyte subpopulations (e.g., helper cells) by lymphotropic viruses such as the human immunodeficiency virus (HIV) and human herpesvirus type 6 can lead to loss of cellular function and selective subtype depletion with a concomitant loss of immunologic responsibility associated with that subtype. Persons with neoplastic disorders can have impaired T-cell function based on unregulated multiplication or dysfunction of one particular subclone of T cells. The outward expression of this may be an increased susceptibility to infections caused by normally harmless pathogens (called *opportunistic infections*) or failure to generate delayed-type hypersensitivity reactions (called *anergy*).

Persons with anergy have a diminished or absent reaction to a battery of skin-test antigens, including *Candida* antigen and the tuberculin test, even when infected with *Mycobacterium tuberculosis.* In persons with anergy, a negative skin test result for tuberculosis can mean a true lack of exposure to tuberculosis or indicate the person's inability to mount an appropriate T-cell response. One of the methods of testing for anergy is the use of a control skin test with an antigen that most persons have been exposed to. The antigens most commonly used for this purpose are *Candida,* mumps, and tetanus. Most adults have had previous exposure to these antigens and should display a positive result if they have normal T-cell function. Usually, two control tests are done along with the tuberculin test. If the person has a positive reaction to one or both of the control tests, a negative tuberculin test result usually means that the person is not infected *M. tuberculosis*. The limitations of the control test depends on previous exposure to the allergen.

A particularly severe secondary T-cell disorder stems from an inherited (autosomal recessive) deficiency in the enzyme *purine nucleoside phosphorylase* (PNP). Reduced levels of PNP lead to the accumulation of toxic intermediates of purine metabolism within T lymphocytes, causing cell death or loss of cell function. The B-cell immune response is usually normal.[4] A related but distinct genetic defect leads to abnormally low levels of a lymphocytic cell enzyme called *adenosine deaminase* (ADA). Similar to PNP deficiency, the ADA defect leads to accumulation of toxic metabolites within T lymphocytes and causes cell death. This condition can be treated using enzyme replacement therapy.

Combined T-Cell and B-Cell Immunodeficiencies

Disorders of the immune response that have elements of B- and T-cell dysfunction fall under the broad classification of combined immunodeficiency syndrome (CIDS) and include a spectrum of inherited (autosomal recessive and X-linked) conditions. A single mutation in any one of the many genes that influence the lymphocyte development or response including lymphocyte receptors, cytokines, or major histocompatibility antigens could lead to combined immunodeficiency. Regardless of the affected gene, the net result is a disruption in the normal communication system of B and T lymphocytes and deregulation of the immune response. The spectrum of disease resulting from CIDS ranges from mild to severe to ultimately fatal forms.

The most severe form T- and B-cell deficiency is often referred to as *severe combined immunodeficiency syndrome* (SCIDS). Children with SCIDS have a disease course that resembles AIDS, with failure to thrive, chronic diarrhea, and opportunistic infections that usually lead to death by the age of 2 years. Treatment consists of measures to prevent and control infections. Specific antibiotic treatment depends on the type of microorganism that is present. Intramuscular or intravenous gamma globulin may also be used. Immunizations with live attenuated viruses such as the poliovirus should be avoided. SCIDS has been successfully treated with bone marrow transplantation.

About 50% of persons with the autosomal recessive form of SCID have an associated deficiency in the enzyme ADA. Absence of this enzyme leads to accumulation of toxic metabolites that kill dividing and resting T cells. Enzyme replacement therapy is used in the management of persons with this form of SCIDS.[4,5] Gene therapy has been used to insert the missing gene into stem cells from cord blood of neonates who were diagnosed prenatally with the disease.[5] The gene-treated stem cells, which are then infused into infant, home to the bone marrow, where they begin producing ADA-containing T cells. Only a few children have been treated with gene therapy, and it is probably too early to know what the long-term effects of the treatment will be.

Ataxia-telangiectasia syndrome is also an inherited (autosomal recessive) disorder, which is thought to result from a mutation in a single gene located at chromosome 11q22.23. As the name implies, this syndrome is heralded by worsening cerebellar ataxia (*i.e.*, poor muscle coordination) and the appearance of telangiectasias (*i.e.*, lesions consisting of dilated capillaries and arterioles) on skin and conjunctival surfaces (Fig. 12–3). The ataxia usually goes unnoticed until the toddler begins to walk; the telangiectasias develop thereafter, especially on skin surfaces exposed to the sun. The ataxia progresses slowly and relentlessly to severe disability. Intellectual development is normal at first but seems to stop at the 10-year level in many of these children. Children with this syndrome have associated deficiencies in cellular and humoral components of the immune response, including reduced levels of IgA, IgE, and IgG2, absolute lymphopenia, and a decrease in the ratio of $CD4^+$ helper T cells to $CD8^+$ suppressor T cells. About 70% have an IgA deficiency, and about half also have an IgG subclass deficiency. They are susceptible to recurrent upper and lower respiratory tract infections (particularly those caused by encapsulated bacteria) and have an increased risk for the development of malignancies. Death from malignant lymphoma is common.

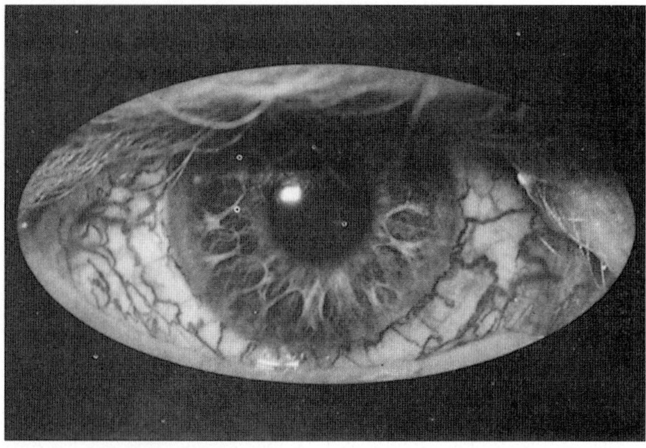

FIGURE 12–3
Striking telangiectasis on the bulbar conjunctiva of a 22-year-old patient with ataxia-telangectasia. These dilated vessels typically appear between the ages of 2 and 5.

Wiskott-Aldrich syndrome is an X-linked recessive disorder that becomes symptomatic during the first year of life. Infants with this syndrome are plagued by eczema, recurrent infections, and low platelet counts. Bleeding episodes or symptoms due to infection usually begin within the first 6 months of life. Abnormalities of humoral immunity include decreased serum levels of IgM, and markedly elevated serum IgA and IgE concentrations. T-cell dysfunction is initially mild but progressively deteriorates, and patients become increasingly susceptible to develop malignancies of the mononuclear phagocytic system including Hodgkin's lymphoma and leukemia. Children with Wiskott-Aldrich syndrome typically are unable to produce antibody to polysaccharide antigens and therefore are susceptible to infections caused by encapsulated microorganisms. They are also prone to septicemia and meningitis with these organisms. Varicella infection can be lethal to children with this condition. Bone marrow transplantation has been successful in children with Wiskott-Aldrich syndrome. Splenectomy may be used to control the thrombocytopenia in situations in which bone marrow transplantation cannot be done.

Disorders of the Complement System

The complement system is an integral part of the normal immune response (see Chapter 11). The activation of the complement network, through the classic (*i.e.*, antigen-antibody complexes) or alternative (*i.e.*, binding of activated C3 to surfaces) pathways, promotes chemotaxis, opsonization, and phagocytosis of invasive pathogens, bacteriolysis, and anaphylactic reactions. It seems reasonable to predict that alterations in normal levels of complement or the absence of a particular complement component could create a state of immunodeficiency. As with B- and T-cell deficiencies, complement disorders can be classified as primary if the deficiency is inherited or secondary if the condition develops due to another disease process.

Primary Disorders of the Complement System

Most primary disorders of the complement system are transmitted as autosomal recessive traits and can involve one or more complement components. A C2 deficiency causes a susceptibility to multiple and potentially life-threatening infections caused by encapsulated bacteria, especially *S. pneumoniae*. Persons with C2 deficiency are also at risk to develop autoimmune disorders that resemble lupus erythematosus. Similarly, persons with *C3 deficiency* are predisposed to develop serious and recurrent infections caused by encapsulated bacteria and *Staphylococcus aureus* because of their inability to opsonize and lyse bacteria. Unlike persons with C2 and C3 deficiencies, persons with deficiencies in factors C1 (C1q, r, and s) and C4 are not necessarily at increased risk for recurrent infections because the alternative pathway can be activated normally through C3. However, many of them develop autoimmune diseases. Although persons with deficiencies in the terminal components of complement (C5 through C9) are susceptible to repeated episodes of meningitis and sepsis caused by *N. meningitides* or systemic gonococcal disease, they are less likely to develop autoimmune disorders than persons with other complement deficiencies.[6]

Hereditary angioneurotic edema is a particularly interesting form of complement deficiency.[7] Persons with this disorder do not produce a functional C1 inhibitor. Activation of the classic complement pathway is uncontrolled, leading to increased breakdown of C4 and C2 with concomitant release of C-kinin, a vasodilator. This causes episodic attacks of localized edema involving the face, neck, joints, abdomen, and sites of trauma. Swelling of the subcutaneous tissues, especially of the face, can be disfiguring and swelling of the gastric mucosa causes nausea, vomiting, and diarrhea. If the trachea or larynx is involved, the episode can prove fatal. The attacks associated with this inherited disease usually begin before the age of 2 and become progressively worse with age. Symptoms can last from 1 to 4 days, and most persons with the disorder have more than one attack a month. A vapor-heated C1 inhibitor concentrate has been developed. This concentrate can be used to prevent and treat an acute attack of hereditary angioedema.[8,9]

Secondary Disorders of the Complement System

Secondary complement deficiencies can also occur in persons with functionally normal complement systems due to rapid activation and turnover of complement components (as is seen in immune complex disease) or reduced synthesis of components as would be the case in chronic cirrhosis of the liver or malnutrition.

Disorders of Phagocytosis

The phagocytic system is composed primarily of polymorphonuclear leukocytes (*i.e.*, neutrophils and eosinophils) and mononuclear phagocytes (*i.e.*, circulating monocytes and tissue and fixed [spleen] macrophages). The primary purpose of phagocytic cells is to migrate to the site of infection (*i.e.*, chemotaxis), aggregate around the affected tissue (*i.e.*, adherence), envelope invading microorganisms or foreign substances (*i.e.*, phagocytosis), and generate microbactericidal substances (*e.g.*, enzymes or byproducts of metabolism) to kill the ingested pathogens. A defect in any of these functions or a reduction in the absolute number of available cells can essentially disrupt the phagocytic system. As with other alterations in immune function, defects in phagocytosis can be a primary or secondary disorder.

Primary Disorders of the Phagocytosis

The best known disorders of phagocytosis are the *chronic granulomatous diseases* (CGD). The CGD are a group of inherited disorders (X-linked or autosomal recessive) that greatly reduce or inactivate the ability of phagocytic cells to produce the so-called "respiratory burst" which results in the generation of toxic derivatives of oxygen (superoxide anion and hydrogen peroxide). These oxygen species participate in creating an intracellular environment that kills ingested microorganisms. Recurrent infections, along with granulomatous lesions in persons with CGD is thought to be due to persistence of viable microorganisms within impaired phagocytic cells. Other aspects of phagocyte function, such as engulfment of microorganisms, are normal.

Children with CGD are subject to chronic and acute infections of the skin, liver, lung, and other soft tissues.[10] Organisms responsible for the infections include *S. aureus, S. epidermis, Serratia marcescens, Pseudomonas, Escherichia coli, Candida*, and *Aspergillus*.[11] These infections usually begin during the first 2 years of life. The disorder is diagnosed by examining the ability of a person's phagocytes to reduce a yellow dye (*i.e.*, nitroblue tetrazolium) to a blue compound during active respiration. Treatment of the disorder is generally limited to the use of prophylactic antibiotics or white blood cell infusions. Other disorders of phagocyte metabolism include myeloperoxidase deficiency, glucose-6-phosphate dehydrogenase deficiency, and glutathione peroxidase deficiency. Each of these metabolic disorders promotes an increased rate of infection in affected persons but usually not with the frequency or severity seen in CGD.

Job's syndrome is a multisystem disorder that is inherited as an autosomal dominant trait. It is characterized by unregulated IgE synthesis, delayed or diminished polymorphonuclear neutrophil chemotaxis, recurrent infections of the skin and respiratory tract, and chronic eczema. The manifestations of the disorder become apparent early in infancy with the development of chronic mucocutaneous candidiasis and "cold" cutaneous abscesses (*i.e.*, without the usual symptoms of warmth, redness, and pain).

Similar to CGD, the most common pathogen is *S. aureus*, but children with the disorder are also susceptible to a multitude of bacterial and fungal infections. In addition to elevated IgE levels and poor chemotactic response, children with Job's syndrome frequently have coarse facial features, red hair, retarded growth, broad nasal bridge, eosinophilia, and osteoporosis.

By contrast, *Chédiak-Higashi syndrome* is an autosomal recessive disorder in which the central defect in phagocytic function is thought to be caused by abnormal cell membrane fluidity, poor cytoskeletal coordination, and poor fusion of neutrophilic granules with phagocytosed microorganisms. The end result is poor mobility of the phagocytes and delayed killing of ingested bacteria. As with other disorders of phagocytosis, children with Chédiak-Higashi syndrome are subject to repeated cutaneous and respiratory tract infections, usually caused by beta-hemolytic streptococci (*e.g., S. pyogenes*) and *S. aureus*. Other characteristics of the syndrome include partial albinism and bleeding disorders. Giant granules in the cytoplasm of neutrophils are pathognomonic of the condition.

An unusual but interesting disorder of phagocytic function is based on the absence or deficiency of glycoproteins that are normally present on the cell membrane of neutrophils and monocytes called the *CD11/CD18 complex*. These glycoproteins are essential for almost all of the surveillance functions performed by phagocytes, including adhesion, chemotaxis, phagocytosis, and the stimulation of oxidative metabolism that follows phagocytosis. The first indication of this deficiency in an infant is delayed umbilical separation followed by severe, recurrent infections caused by a wide variety of gram-positive and gram-negative bacteria. Children with complete lack of CD11/CD18 glycoproteins rarely survive beyond the first year of life, but those with a deficiency in CD11/CD18 production have a longer life span. Therapy for this deficiency includes prophylactic antibiotic therapy and bone marrow transplantation. In the future, this condition may be amenable to gene replacement therapy.

Secondary Disorders of Phagocytosis

Secondary deficiencies of the phagocytic system can be caused by a number of circumstances, such as opsonins, which are factors such as antibody and complement that coat the surface of a foreign substance and enhance phagocytosis, and chemotactic factors, such as antibody and complement that coat the surface of microorganisms and promote increased migration of phagocytes to the site of infection and stimulate phagocytosis. Deficiencies of either of these opsonins reduce the overall effectiveness of phagocytes. Drugs that impair or prevent inflammation and T-cell function such as corticosteroids or cyclosporin A also alter phagocytic response through modulation of cytokines.

Persons with diabetes mellitus also demonstrate poor phagocytic function, primarily from altered chemotaxis. The reason for this dysfunction is not understood, but it is unrelated to the age or the severity of the metabolic disorder. Apparently, this is a separate genetic disorder that is coinherited at a higher frequency among persons with diabetes and among family members.

Persons with HIV infection and AIDS represent another form of acquired or secondary deficiency of phagocytic function. However, in this case, the deficiency is due to direct infection and destruction of helper T cells and monocytes-macrophages by the virus (see Chapter 13).

In summary, an immunodeficiency is defined as an absolute or partial loss of the normal immune response, which places a person in a state of compromise and increases the risk of developing infections or malignant complications. Immunodeficiency states can affect one or more of the four main components of the immune response: antibody or humoral (B-cell) immunity; cellular or T-cell immunity; the complement system; and the phagocytic system. The variety of defects known to involve the immune response can be classified as primary (i.e., endogenous or inherited) or secondary (i.e., caused by exogenous factors such as drugs or infection). The extent to which any or all of these components are compromised dictates the severity of the immunodeficiency.

Allergic and Hypersensitivity Disorders

On completion of this section of the chapter, you should be able to do the following:

- Compare the causes of immediate and delayed-type immune responses
- Describe the immune mechanisms involved in a type I, type II, type III, and type IV hypersensitivity reaction
- State the difference between an atopic and nonatopic hypersensitivity response
- Describe the pathogenesis of allergic rhinitis, food allergy, serum sickness, Arthus reaction, contact dermatitis, and hypersensitivity pneumonitis
- Characterize the differences in latex allergy caused by a type I, IgE-mediated hypersensitivity response and that caused by a type IV, cell-mediated response

Allergic or hypersensitivity disorders are caused by immune responses to environmental antigens that produce inflammation and cause tissue injury. When used to describe an allergic response, these antigens are usually referred to as *allergens*. Allergens are any foreign substance capable of inducing and immune response. Many different chemicals of natural and chemical origin are known allergens. Complex natural organic chemical, especially proteins are more likely to cause and immediate hypersensitivity response; whereas, simple organic compounds, inorganic chemicals, and metals more commonly cause delayed hypersensitivity reactions. Exposure to the allergen can be through inhalation, ingestion, injection, or skin contact. Sensitization of a specific individual to a specific allergen is the result of a particular interplay between the chemical or physical properties of the allergen, the mode and quantity of exposure, and the unique genetic makeup of the person.

The manifestations of allergic responses reflect the effect of an immunologically induced inflammatory response in the organ or tissue involved. These manifestations generally are independent of the agent involved. For example, the symptoms of hay fever are the same whether the allergy is caused by ragweed pollen or mold spores. The diversity of allergic responses derives from the different immunologic effector pathways that are involved (*e.g.*, hay fever versus allergic dermatitis).

Historically, allergic disorders have been categorized as two basic types: immediate and delayed-type hypersensitivity. The criteria for this classification involve the time between exposure to the inducing antigen or allergen, and the appearance of symptoms. Immediate hypersensitivity are terms used to described antibody-mediated allergy and delayed-type hypersensitivity to T-lymphocyte–mediated responses.

Allergic reactions can be divided into four categories: type I, IgE-mediated disorder; type II, antibody-mediated (cytotoxic) disorders; type III, complement-mediated immune disorders; and type IV, T-cell–mediated hypersensitivity reactions.

Type I, IgE-Mediated Disorders

Type I reactions are immediate-type hypersensitivity reactions that are triggered by binding of an allergen to a specific IgE that is found on the surface of a mast cell or basophil. In addition to their role in allergic responses, the IgE are involved in acquired immunity to parasitic infections. Serum IgE levels may be elevated in response to the presence of either a parasitic infection or an allergy.

The mast cells, which are tissue cells, and basophils, which are blood cells, are derived from hematopoietic (blood) precursor cells. Mast cells are normally distributed throughout connective tissue, especially in areas beneath the skin and mucous membranes of the respiratory, gastrointestinal, and genitourinary tracts, and adjacent to blood and lymph vessels.[12] This location places mast cells near surfaces that are exposed to environmental antigens and parasites. Mast cells in different parts of the body and even in a single site can have significant differences in mediator content and sensitivity to agents that produce mast cell degranulation. For example skin mast cells differ from lung mast cells in being more sensitive to morphine, substance P, and other neuropeptides and in the ideal temperature at which degranulation occurs (30° in skin versus 37° in the lungs).[12]

Mast cells and basophils have granules that contain potent mediators of allergic reactions. These mediators are preformed within the cell or activated through enzymatic processing. During the sensitization or priming stage, the allergen-specific IgE antibodies attach to receptors on the surface of these mast cells and basophils. With subsequent exposure, the sensitizing allergen binds to the cell-associated IgE and triggers a series of events that ultimately leads to degranulation of the sensitized mast cells or basophils causing release of their allergy-producing mediators (Fig. 12–4).

The most notable mediators of allergic reactions include histamine, complement, acetylcholine, slow-reacting substances of anaphylaxis, kinins, and eosinophil chemotactic factor (see Chapter 11). *Histamine* is a potent vasodilator that increases the permeability of capillaries and venules and causes smooth muscle contraction and bronchial constriction. *Complement*, when activated, leads to further release of histamine, stimulates the inflammatory response, and promotes leukocyte chemotaxis with secondary release of cytokines. *Acetylcholine* produces bronchial smooth muscle contraction and dilation of small blood vessels. The *slow-reacting substances of anaphylaxis* include leukotrienes and prostaglandins. They produce responses similar to histamine and acetylcholine, although their effects are delayed and prolonged by comparison. The *kinins*, which are a group of potent inflammatory peptides, require activation through enzymatic modification. Once activated, these peptide mediators produce vasodilatation, smooth muscle contraction, leukocyte chemotaxis, and increased vascular permeability. *Eosinophil chemotactic factor* includes peptides released from mast cells and basophils after binding of surface IgE to allergen. These peptides prompt chemotaxis of eosinophils and leukocytes to the site of allergen contact, contributing to the inflammatory response.

Types of Disorders

There are two types of IgE-mediated allergic reactions—atopic and nonatopic disorders. The immunologic pathogenesis of the two disorders is same, but predisposing factors and manifestations are different. The atopic diseases are characterized by a hereditary predisposition and production of a local reaction to IgE antibodies produced in response to common environmental agents. The nonatopic disorders lack the genetic component and organ specificity of the atopic disorders The nonatopic disorders include anaphylactic reactions (Chapter 20), urticaria or hives (Chapter 15), and angioedema.

Atopic Disorders

The term *atopic* refers to a genetically determined hypersensitivity to common environmental allergens mediated by an IgE–mast cell reaction. Persons with atopic disorders are commonly allergic to more than one, and often many, environmental allergens. The disorder tends to run in families and affects about 1 of 10 persons in the United States. The most common atopic disorders are allergic rhinitis and allergic asthma. Atopic dermatitis is less common and food allergy even less common. The discussion in this section focuses on allergic rhinitis and food allergy. Allergic asthma is discussed in Chapter 24 and atopic dermatitis in Chapter 15. Latex allergy is a newly emerging disorder that can result from IgE-mediated or T-cell–mediated hypersensitivity response. It discussed separately at the end of this section.

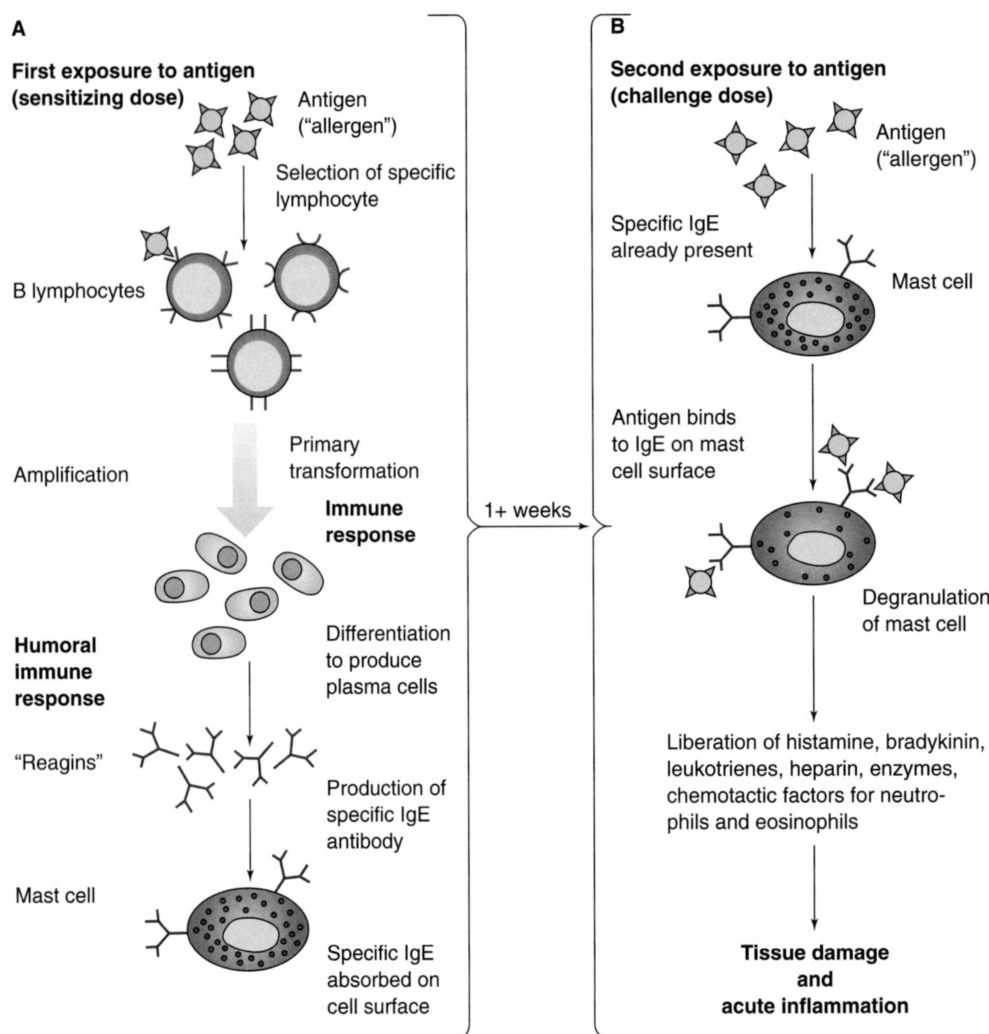

FIGURE 12–4
Type I, IgE-Mediated hypersensitivity reaction. (Chandrasoma P., Taylor C. R. [1995]. *Concise pathology* [2nd ed.]. Norwalk, CT: Appleton and Lange. p. 104)

The cause of atopic disorders is complex and involves a genetic component and environmental allergen exposure. Persons afflicted with atopic allergic conditions tend to have high serum levels of IgE and increased numbers of basophils and mast cells. Although the IgE-triggered response is likely a key factor in the pathophysiology of atopic allergic disorders, it is not the only factor and may not be responsible for conditions such as atopic dermatitis and certain forms of asthma. Many stimuli can induce conditions that are indistinguishable from atopic disorders yet bypass the immune response. It is possible that persons with atopic disorders are exquisitely responsive to the chemical mediators of allergic reactions rather than having hyperactive IgE immunity.

Allergic Rhinitis. Allergic rhinitis (*i.e.,* allergic rhinoconjunctivitis) is characterized by symptoms of sneezing, itching, and watery discharge from the eyes and nose. Severe attacks may be accompanied by systemic malaise, fatigue, and muscle soreness from sneezing. Fever is absent. Sinus obstruction may cause headache. Typical allergens include pollens from ragweed, grasses, trees, and weeds; fungal spores; house dust mites; animal dander; and feathers. Allergic rhinitis can be divided into perennial and seasonal allergic rhinitis depending on the chronology of symptoms. Persons with the perennial type of allergic rhinitis experience symptoms throughout the year, but those with seasonal allergic rhinitis (*i.e.,* hay fever) are plagued with intense symptoms in conjunction with periods high allergen (*e.g.,* pollens, fungal spores) exposure. Symptoms that become worse at night suggest a household allergen, and symptoms that disappear on weekends suggest occupational exposure.

Diagnosis depends on a careful history and physical examination, microscopic identification of nasal eosinophilia, and skin testing to identify the offending allergens.

Treatment is symptomatic in most cases and includes the use of oral antihistamines and decongestants. Nasal corticosteroids are often effective when used appropriately. Intranasal cromolyn, a drug that prevents mast cell degranulation, may be useful, especially when administered before expected contact with an offending allergen. When possible, avoidance of the offending allergen is recommended. A program of desensitization may be used when symptoms are particularly bothersome. Desensitization involves frequent (usually weekly) injections of the offending antigens. The antigens, which are given in increasing doses, stimulate production of high levels of IgG, which acts as a blocking antibody by combining with the antigen before it can combine with the cell-bound IgE antibodies.

Food Allergies. Virtually any food can produce atopic or nonatopic allergies. Sea foods (*i.e.*, crustaceans and mollusks) are important causes of nonatopic anaphylactic reactions. Legumes, cow's milk, and egg white allergies are common. The allergenicity of a food may be changed by heating or cooking. A person may be allergic to drinking milk but may not have symptoms when milk is included in cooked foods.

Food allergies can occur at any age but, similar to atopic dermatitis and rhinitis, they tend to manifest during childhood. The allergic response is thought to occur after contact between specific food allergens and sensitizing IgE found in the intestinal mucosa causing local and systemic release of histamine and other mediators of the allergic response. In this disorder, allergens are usually food proteins and partially digested food products. Carbohydrates, lipids, or food additives, such as preservatives, colorings, or flavorings, are also potential allergens. Closely related food groups can contain common cross-reacting allergens. For example, some persons are allergic to all legumes (i.e., beans, peas, and peanuts).

Diagnosis of food allergies is usually based on careful food history and provocative diet testing. Provocative testing involves careful elimination of a suspected allergen from the diet for a period of time to see if the symptoms disappear and reintroducing the food to see the symptoms reappear. Only one food should be tested at a time. Treatment focuses on avoidance of the food or foods that are responsible for the allergy.

Type II, Antibody-Mediated Disorders

Type II (cytotoxic) hypersensitivity reactions are the end result of direct interaction between IgG and IgM class antibodies and tissue or cell surface antigens, with subsequent activation of complement or antibody-dependent cell-mediated cytotoxicity (Fig. 12–5). Examples of type II reactions include mismatched blood transfusion reactions, hemolytic disease of the newborn due to ABO or Rh incompatibility, and certain drug reactions. In the latter, the binding of certain drugs to the surface of red or white blood cells elicits an antibody and complement response that lyses the drug-coated cell. Lytic drug reactions can produce transient anemia, leukopenia, or thrombocytopenia, which are corrected by the removal of the offending drug.

Type III, Immune Complex Allergic Disorders

Immune complex allergic disorders are mediated by the formation of insoluble antigen-antibody complexes that activate complement (Fig. 12–6). Activation of complement by the immune complex generates chemotactic and vasoactive mediators that cause tissue damage by a variety of mechanisms including alterations in blood flow and vascular permeability, and the destructive action of inflammatory cells. Immune complexes formed in the circulation produce damage when they come in contact with the vessel wall or become trapped in filtering structures such as the glomerulus. Immune complexes are eventually deposited within blood vessels; because immune complexes can activate complement, localized tissue damage can occur wherever these complexes are deposited. Type III reactions are responsible for the vasculitis seen in certain autoimmune diseases such as systemic lupus erythematosus (SLE) or the kidney damage seen with acute glomerulonephritis. Unlike type II reactions in which the damage is caused by direct and specific binding of antibody to tissue, the harmful effects of type III reactions are indirect (*i.e.*, secondary to the inflammatory response induced by activated complement). Immune complex disorders can present with local manifestations as in the Arthus reaction, which produces local manifestations, or serum sickness, which is a systemic disorder.

Arthus Reaction

The *Arthus reaction* is a term used by pathologists and immunologists to describe localized tissue necrosis (usually in the skin) caused by immune complexes. In the laboratory, an Arthus reaction can be produced by injecting an antigen preparation into the skin of an immune animal with high levels of circulating antibody. Within 4 to 10 hours, a red, raised lesion appears on the skin at the site of the injection. An ulcer often forms in the center of the lesion. Unlike type I immune reactions, the Arthus reaction is not caused by IgE. It is thought that the injected antigen diffuses into local blood vessels, where it comes in contact with specific antibody (IgG) to incite a localized vasculitis (*i.e.*, inflammation of a blood vessel). Tissue sections of Arthus lesions show deposited immunoglobulin, complement, and fibrinolytic products within blood vessels. If the blood vessel bursts, hemorrhage into surrounding tissue occurs. If the blood vessel is occluded, the oxygen supply to surrounding tissue is interrupted (*i.e.*, an ischemic event), causing cell death and tissue necrosis.

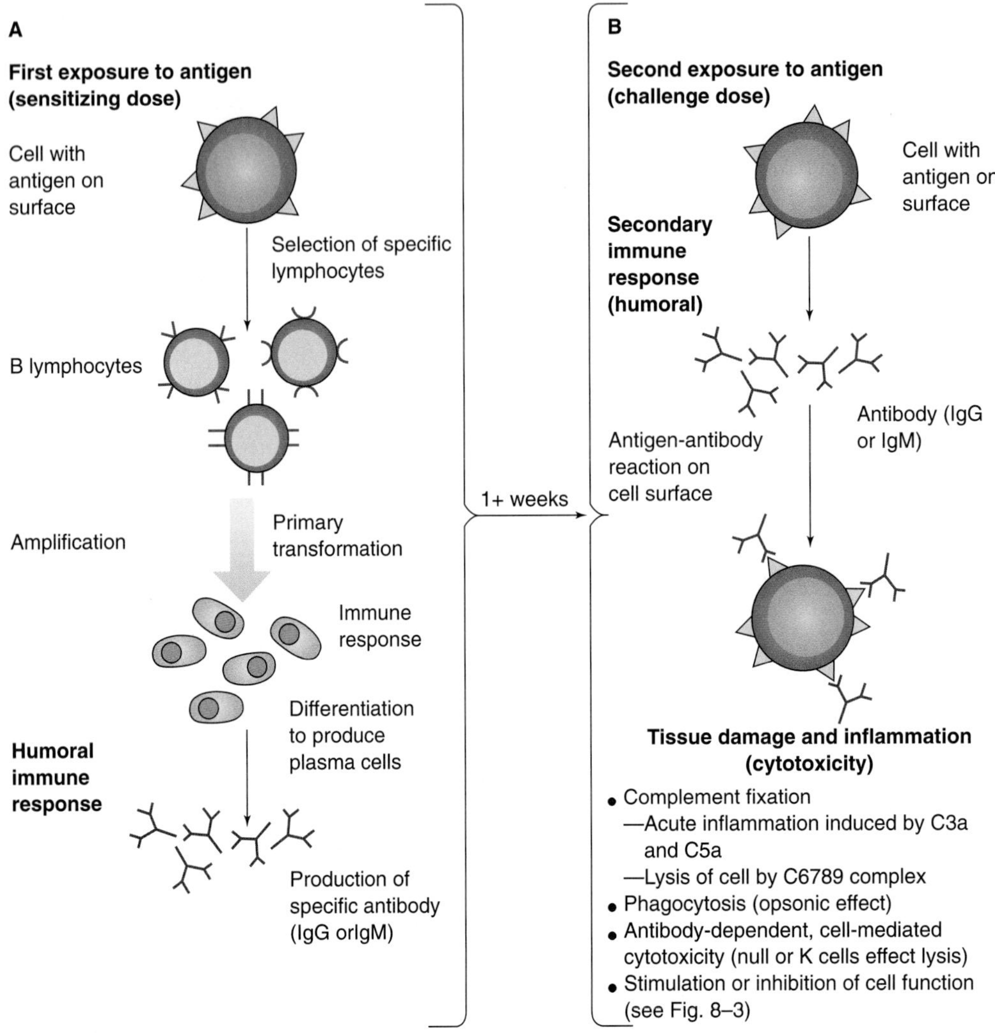

FIGURE 12–5
Type II, cytotoxic hypersensitivity reaction. (Chandrasoma P., Taylor C.R. [1995]. *Concise pathology*. [2nd ed.]. Norwalk, CT: Appleton & Lange. p. 105)

Serum Sickness

The term *serum sickness* was originally coined to describe a syndrome consisting of rash, lymphadenopathy, arthralgias, and occasionally neurologic disorders that appeared 7 or more days after injections of horse antisera. Although this therapy is rarely used today, the name remains. The most common contemporary causes of this allergic disorder include antibiotics (especially penicillin), various foods, drugs, and insect venoms. Serum sickness is triggered by the deposition of insoluble antigen-antibody (IgM and IgG) complexes within blood vessels, joints, heart, and kidney tissue. The deposited complexes activate complement, increase vascular permeability, and recruit phagocytic cells, all of which can promote focal tissue damage and edema. The signs and symptoms include urticaria, patchy or generalized rash, extensive edema (usually of the face, neck, and joints), and fever. In most cases, the damage is temporary, and symptoms resolve within a few days. However, a prolonged and continuous exposure to the sensitizing antigen can lead to irreversible damage. In previously sensitized persons, severe and even fatal forms of serum sickness may occur immediately or within several days after the sensitizing drug or serum is administered.

Treatment of serum sickness is generally directed toward removal of the sensitizing antigen and symptomatic relief. This may include aspirin for joint pain and antihistamines for pruritus. Epinephrine or systemic corticosteroids may be used for severe reactions.

Type IV, Cell-Mediated Hypersensitivity Disorders

Unlike other hypersensitivity reactions, type IV, delayed hypersensitivity is mediated by cells, not antibodies. Type IV hypersensitivity reactions usually occur 24 to 72 hours after exposure of a sensitized individual to the offending antigen. It is mediated by T lymphocytes that are directly cytotoxic ($CD8^+$ T cells) or secrete lymphokines ($CD4^+$ T cells) that cause tissue changes (Fig. 12–7). The reac-

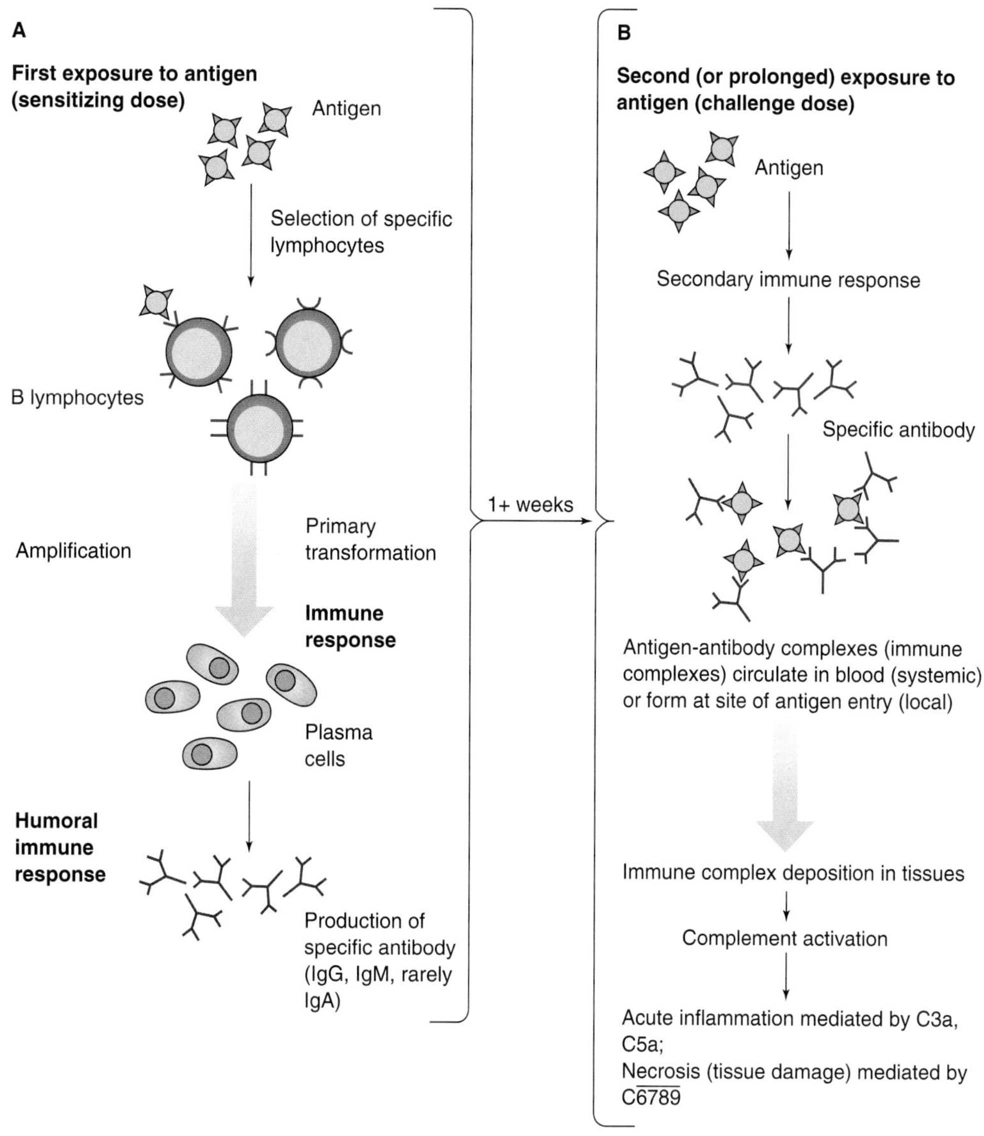

FIGURE 12–6
Type III, immune complex-mediated, hypersensitivity reaction. (Chandrasoma P., Taylor C. R. [1995]. *Concise pathology* [2nd ed.]. Norwalk, C.T: Appleton and Lange. p. 107)

tion is initiated by antigen specific CD4+ helper T cells, which release numerous immunoregulatory and proinflammatory cytokines into the surrounding tissue. These substances attract antigen-specific and nonspecific T or B lymphocytes and monocytes, neutrophils, eosinophils, and basophils. Some of the cytokines promote differentiation and activation of macrophages that function as phagocytic and antigen-presenting cells. Activation of the coagulation cascade leads to formation and deposition of fibrin.

The best known type of delayed hypersensitivity response is the reaction to the tuberculin test, in which inactivated tuberculin or purified protein derivative is injected under the skin. In a previously sensitized person, redness and and induration of the area develops with 8 to 12 hours, reaching a peak in 24 to 72 hours. A positive tuberculin test indicates that a person has had sufficient exposure to the the *M. tuberculosis* organism to incite a hypersensitivity reaction, it does not mean that he or she has tuberculosis.

Certain types of antigens induce cell-mediated immunity with an especially pronounced macrophage response. This type of delayed hypersensitivity commonly develops in response to particulate antigens that are large, insoluble, and difficult to eliminate. The accumulated macrophages are often transformed into epithelioid cells. A microscopic aggregation of epithelioid cells, which are usually surrounded by a layer of lymphocytes, is called a granuloma. Inflammation that is characterized by this type of type IV hypersensitivity is called granulomatous inflammation (see Chapter 11).

Direct T-cell–mediated cytotoxicity, which causes necrosis of antigen-bearing cells, is believed to be important in eradication of virus-infected cells, autoimmune

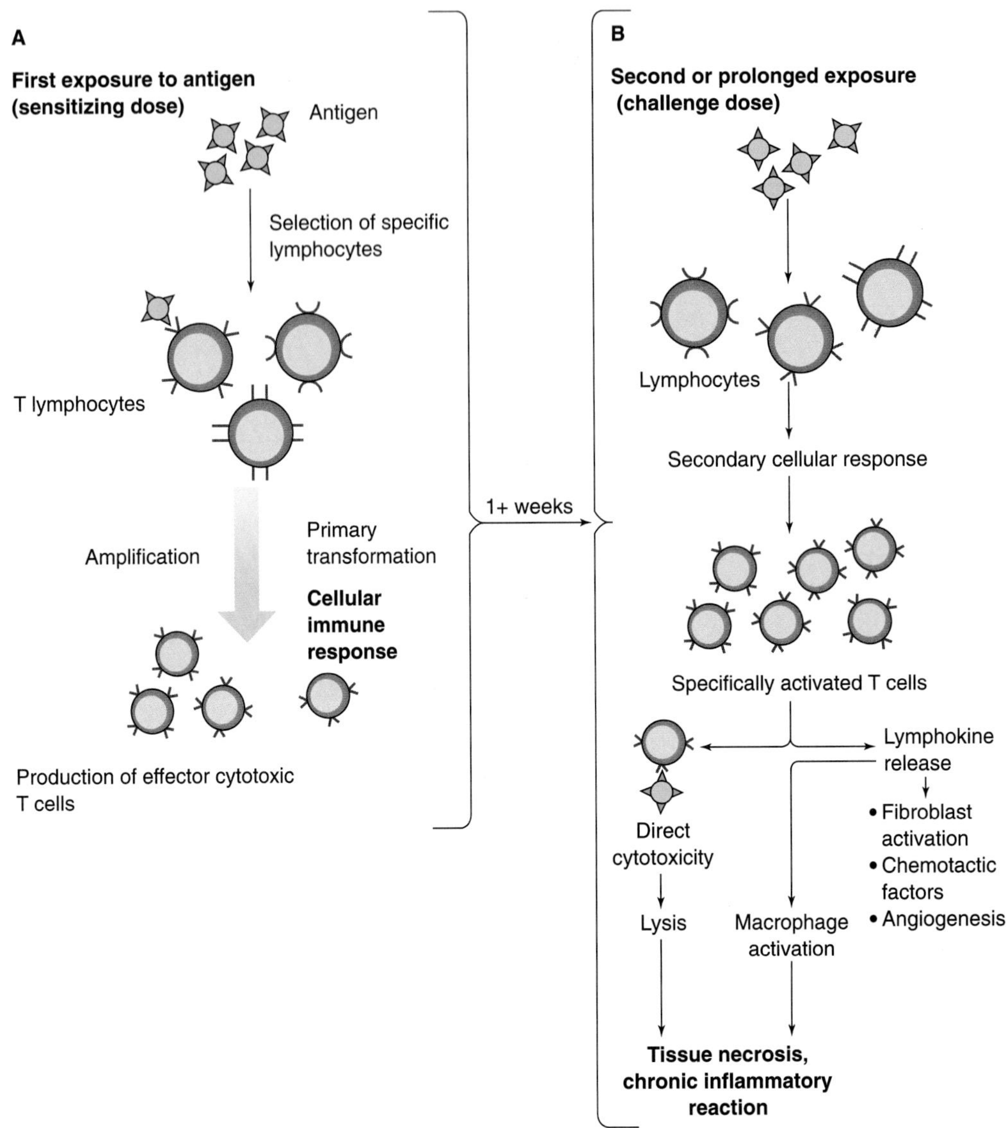

FIGURE 12–7
Type IV, cell-mediated, delayed-type hypersensitivity reaction. (Chandrasoma P., Taylor C. R. [1995]. *Concise pathology* [2nd ed.]. Norwalk, C.T: Appleton and Lange. p. 108)

diseases such as Hashimoto's thyroiditis, and host-versus-graft or graft-versus-host transplant rejection. Allergic contact dermatitis and hypersensitivity pneumonitis are presented as examples of cell-mediated hypersensitivity reactions.

Allergic Contact Dermatitis. Allergic contact dermatitis denotes an inflammatory response confined to the skin that is initiated by reexposure to an allergen to which a person has previously become sensitized (*e.g.*, cosmetics, hair dyes, metals, topical drugs). Contact dermatitis usually consists of erythematous macules, papules, and vesicles (*i.e.*, blisters). The affected area often becomes swollen and warm, with exudation, crusting, and development of a secondary infection. The location of the lesions often provides a clue about the nature of the antigen causing the disorder. The most common form of this condition is the dermatitis that follows an intimate encounter with poison ivy or oak antigens, although many other substances can trigger a reaction.

The mechanism of events that lead to prior sensitization to an antigen is not completely understood. It is likely that sensitization follows transdermal transport of an antigen, with subsequent presentation to T lymphocytes. Subpopulations of sensitized lymphocytes are distributed throughout the body so that subsequent cutaneous exposure to the offending antigen promotes a localized reaction regardless of the initial site of contact. The severity of the reaction associated with contact dermatitis ranges from mild to intense, depending on the person and the allergen. Because this condition follows the mechanism of a delayed hypersensitivity response, the reaction does not become apparent for at least 12 hours and usually more than 24 hours after exposure.

Depending on the antigen and the duration of exposure, the reaction may last from days to weeks and is typified by erythematous, vesicular, or papular lesions associated with intense pruritus and weeping.

Diagnosis of contact dermatitis is made by observing the distribution of lesions on the skin surface and associating a particular pattern with exposure to possible allergens. If a particular allergen is suspected, a patch test can be used to confirm the suspicion. For this, the suspected allergen is applied to a gauze or patch that is taped to a hair-free surface for 48 hours. The patch is removed, and the surface is inspected daily for a response. Treatment is generally limited to the removal of the irritant, and topical application (*e.g.*, ointments, corticosteroid creams) to relieve symptomatic skin lesions and to prevent secondary bacterial infections. Severe reactions may require systemic corticosteroid therapy.

Hypersensitivity Pneumonitis. Hypersensitivity pneumonitis or allergic alveolitis is associated with exposure to inhaled organic dusts or related occupational antigens. The disorder is thought to involve a susceptible host and activation of pulmonary T cells, followed by the release of cytokine mediators of inflammation.[13] The inflammatory response that ensues (generally several hours after exposure) produces labored breathing, dry cough, chills and fever, headache, and malaise. The symptoms usually subside within hours after the sensitizing antigens are removed. A primary example of hypersensitivity pneumonitis is "farmers lung," a condition resulting from exposure to moldy hay. Other sensitizing antigens include tree bark, sawdust, animal danders, and *Actinomycetes* bacteria that are occasionally found in humidifiers, hot tubs, and swimming pools. Exposure to small amounts of antigen for a long period may lead to chronic lung disease with minimal reversibility. This can happen to persons exposed to avian or animal antigens or a contaminated home air humidifier.[13]

The most important element in the diagnosis of hypersensitivity pneumonitis is to obtain a good history (occupational and otherwise) of exposure to possible antigens. Skin tests, when available, and serum tests for precipitating antibody can be done. Occasionally, direct observation of the person's work and other environments may help to establish a diagnosis. Treatment consists of identifying and avoiding the offending antigens. Severe forms of the disorder may be treated with systemic corticosteroid therapy.

Latex Allergy

With the advent of HIV and other blood-borne diseases, the use of natural latex gloves has spiraled. Between 1988 and 1992, an estimated 11.8 billion examining gloves and 1.8 billion surgical gloves were used in the United States.[14] Accompanying the increased use of latex gloves has come reports of latex allergy among health care workers. Patients exposed to use of latex gloves or other products have also become sensitized to latex. It has been estimated that 7% to 10% of health care workers regularly exposed to latex and 28% to 67% of children with spina bifida have a positive skin test result for latex proteins, indicating increased blood levels of IgE antibody.[14–16] Life-threatening anaphylactic reactions and deaths have been reported from exposure to natural latex rubber during medical and surgical procedures.

Natural rubber latex is derived from the milky sap of the *Heva brasiliensis* plant or rubber tree.[16] Various accelerants, curing agents, antioxidants, and stabilizers are added to the liquid latex during the manufacturing process. Allergic reactions to latex products can be triggered by the latex proteins or by the additives used in the manufacturing process. The cornstarch glove powder has an important role in the allergic response. Latex proteins are readily absorbed by glove powder and become airborne.

Latex allergy can involve a type I, IgE-mediated, hypersensitivity reaction or a type IV, T-cell–mediated, response. The most common type of allergic reaction to latex gloves is a contact dermatitis caused by a type IV, delayed-hypersensitivity reaction to rubber additives. The type I, IgE-mediated, hypersensitivity reactions that occur in response to the latex proteins are less common but far more serious. The distinction between the type I and type IV reactions to latex products is not always clear. Afflicted individuals may experience both types of reactions. Persons with latex allergy commonly show cross sensitivity to avocado, kiwi, and chestnut, probably because latex proteins are similar to proteins in these products.

Allergic contact dermatitis is a delayed hypersensitivity that develops 48 to 96 hours after direct contact with latex additives. It usually affects the dorsum of the hands and is characterized by a vesicular rash. When latex contact is continued, the area becomes crusted and thickened in appearance. Type I, Ig-E mediated latex allergy may manifest as urticaria, rhinoconjunctivitis, asthma, or anaphylaxis.

Exposure to latex may occur by cutaneous, mucous membrane, inhalation, internal tissue, or intravascular routes. Most severe reactions have resulted from latex proteins coming in contact with the mucus membranes of the mouth, vagina, urethra, or rectum. Children with spina bifida who undergo frequent examinations and treatments involving the mucosal surface of the bladder or rectum are at particular risk for development of latex allergy. A large number of latex products are used in dentistry and oral mucosal contact is common during dental procedures. Anaphylactic reactions have been caused by exposure of the internal organs to the surgeon's gloves during surgery. Indirect contact also occurs when aerosolized latex proteins disperse on the clothes of health care workers and on the drapes and sponges used during surgery.

Diagnosis of latex allergy is often based on careful history and evidence of skin reactions due to latex exposure. Because many of the reported reactions to latex gloves have been the result of a nonimmunologic dermatitis, it is important to differentiate between nonallergic and allergy types of dermatitis. Latex skin-prick testing can be done, but it should be done in an allergy center familiar with the test and with equipment available to treat possible anaphylactic reactions. Serum tests for latex-specific IgE antibodies can also be done.

Treatment of latex allergy consists of avoiding latex exposure. Use of powder-free gloves can reduce the amount of airborne latex particles. Health care workers with severe and life-threatening allergy may be forced to change employment. Patients at high risk for latex allergy (*e.g.*, children with spina bifida, health care workers with atopy) should be offered clinical testing for latex allergy before undergoing procedures that expose them to natural rubber latex. All surgical or other procedures on persons with latex allergy should be done in a latex-free environment.

In summary, hypersensitivity and allergic disorders are responses to environmental, food, or drug antigens that would not affect most of the population. There are four basic categories of hypersensitivity responses: type I responses, which are mediated by the IgE-class immunoglobulins and include anaphylactic shock, hay fever, angioedema, and bronchial asthma; type II cytotoxic reactions, which are characterized by hemolytic transfusion reactions and caused by immunoglobulin (IgG and IgM) activation of complement; type III reactions, which result from the formation of insoluble antigen-antibody complexes that become deposited within blood vessels or in the kidney and cause localized tissue injury; and type IV cell-mediated responses in which sensitized T lymphocytes promote an inflammatory response when presented with the sensitizing antigen.

Transplantation Immunopathology

On completion of this section of the chapter, you should be able to do the following:

- Discuss the rationale for matching of human leukocyte antigen and major histocompatibility complex types in organ transplantation
- Compare the immune mechanisms involved in host-versus-graft and graft-versus-host transplant rejection

Not long ago, transplantation of solid organs (*e.g.*, liver, kidney, heart) and bone marrow was considered experimental and reserved for persons for whom alternative methods of therapy were exhausted and survival was unlikely. However, with a greater understanding of humoral and cellular immune regulation, the development of immunosuppressive drugs such as cyclosporine, and an appreciation of the role of the major histocompatibility complex (MHC) antigens, transplantation has become nearly routine, and the subsequent success rate has been greatly enhanced.

Regardless of the type of transplant, the cell surface antigens that determine whether transplanted tissue is recognized as foreign or native are the MHC, also called human leukocyte antigen (HLA) in humans (see Chapter 11). Transplanted tissue can be categorized as *allogenic* if the donor and recipient are related or unrelated but share similar HLA types, *syngeneic* if the donor and recipient are identical twins, and *autologous* if donor and recipient are the same person. Donors of solid organ transplants can be living or dead (cadaver) and related or nonrelated (heterologous). When cells bearing foreign MHC antigens are transplanted, the recipient's immune system attempts to eliminate the donor cells, a process referred to as *host-versus-graft disease* (HVGD). Conversely, the cellular immunity of the transplanted tissue can attack unrelated recipient tissue causing a *graft-versus-host disease* (GVHD). The likelihood of rejection varies indirectly with the degree of HLA or MCH relatedness between donor and recipient. The two-year graft survival rate for kidney transplants is 85% for cadaveric graft recipients treated with immunosuppressant drugs and 90% for related-donor transplantation patients.[11]

Host-Versus-Graft Disease

In HVGD, the immune cells of the transplant recipient attack the donor cells of the transplanted organ. HVGD is usually limited to allogenic organ transplants, although even HLA-identical siblings may differ in some minor HLA loci, which can evoke slow rejection. Rejection due to HVGD is a complex process that involves cell-mediated and circulating antibodies. The activation of $CD8^+$ cytotoxic T cells and $CD4^+$ helper T cells is triggered in response to the donor's HLA antigens. Activation of $CD4^+$ helper cells leads to proliferation of B-cell–mediated antibody production and delayed-type hypersensitivity reaction. The initial target of the recipient antibodies is graft vasculature. The antibodies can produce injury to the transplanted organ by complement-mediated cytotoxicity, generation of antigen-antibody complexes, or antibody-mediated cytolysis.[17]

There are three basic patterns of transplant rejections: hyperacute, acute, and chronic. A *hyperacute* reaction occurs almost immediately after transplantation; in kidney transplants, it can often be seen at the time of surgery. As soon as blood flow from the recipient to the donor organ begins, it develops a cyanotic, mottled appearance. Sometimes, the reaction takes hours to days to develop. The hyperacute response is produced by existing recipient antibodies to graft antigens that initiate an Arthus-type reaction in the blood vessels of the graft. These antibodies have usually developed in response to previous blood transfusions, pregnancies in which the mother develops antibodies to fetal antigens, or infections with bacteria or viruses possessing antigens that mimic MHC antigens.

Acute rejection generally occurs within the first few months after transplantation. In the patient with an organ transplant, acute rejection is evidenced by signs of organ failure. Acute rejection often involves humoral and cell-mediated immune responses. Acute rejection may involve subacute vasculitis characterized by lesions that often lead to arterial narrowing or obliteration.[17]

Chronic host-versus-graft rejection occurs over a prolonged period. It manifests with dense intimal fibrosis of blood vessels of the transplanted organ. In renal transplantation, it is characterized by a gradual rise in serum creatinine over a period of 4 to 6 months. The actual mechanism of this type of response is unclear but may include release of cytokines such as interleukin-1 and platelet-derived growth factor.[11]

Graft-Versus-Host Disease

Three basic requirements are necessary for GVHD to develop: the transplant must have a functional cellular immune component; the recipient tissue must bear antigens foreign to the donor tissue; and the recipient immunity must be compromised to the point that it cannot destroy the transplanted cells.[18] The primary agents of GVDH are T cells, and the antigens they recognize and attack are HLA. The greater the difference in tissue antigens between the donor and recipient, the greater is the likelihood of GVHD. If the recipient has a normally functioning immune system, it quickly eradicates HLA-mismatched transplants, making immunosuppression a necessity. Without appropriate therapy, most allogeneic (and even syngeneic or autologous) bone marrow transplant recipients develop some form of GVHD.

If GVHD occurs, the primary targets of the acute illness are the skin, liver, intestine, and cells of the immune system. *Acute GVHD* is characterized by a pruritic, maculopapular rash, which begins on the palms and soles and frequently extends over the entire body, with subsequent desquamation. The epithelial layer is the primary site of injury. When the intestine is involved, symptoms include nausea, bloody diarrhea, and abdominal pain. GVHD of the liver can lead to bleeding disorders and coma. GVHD is considered chronic if symptoms persist or begin 100 days or more after transplantation. *Chronic GVHD* is characterized by abnormal humoral and cellular immunity, severe skin disorders, and liver disease.

The pathogenesis of acute GVHD is initiated in three stages: recognition and presentation by donor T cells of foreign recipient antigens, activation of T cells through cytokines, and multiplication of activated T cells. The actual tissue pathology observed with GVHD is produced directly by the action of cytotoxic T cells or indirectly through the release of inflammatory mediators such as tissue necrosis factor-alpha, interleukins, and complement. Conversely, chronic GVHD has all the markings of an autoimmune disorder in which activated T cells recognize minor MHC antigens common to all persons and that are therefore not foreign.

A third type of GVHD has been recognized that follows the transplantation of genetically identical tissue (*i.e.*, syngeneic or autologous). This variety of GVHC stems from the pretreatment conditioning regimen (*e.g.*, total body irradiation) or treatment with cytotoxic drugs. The conditioning therapy disrupts the normal immune surveillance system and allows "rogue" autoreactive T cells to proliferate and attack native tissue. Syngeneic GVHD is usually self-limited and not severe.

GVHD can be prevented by blocking any of the three steps of pathogenesis. For example, donor T cells can be selectively removed from the transplanted tissue or destroyed using various treatments such as monoclonal antibodies with attached toxins, equivalent to heat-seeking missiles. Alternatively, immunosuppressive or antiinflammatory drugs such as cyclosporine or glucocorticoids can be used to block T-cell activation and the action of cytokines.

In summary, organ and bone marrow transplantation has been enhanced by a greater understanding of humoral and cellular immune regulation, the development of immunosuppressive drugs such as cyclosporine, and an appreciation of the role of the MHC antigens. The likelihood of rejection varies indirectly with the degree of HLA (or MHC) relatedness between donor and recipient. A rejection can involve an attempt by the recipient's immune system to eliminate the donor cells (HVGD) or an attack by the cellular immunity of the transplanted tissue on the unrelated recipient tissue (GVHD).

Autoimmune Disease

After you have finished this section of the chapter, you should be able to do the following:

- Relate the mechanisms of self-tolerance to the possible explanations for development of autoimmune disease
- Compare the effector mechanisms involved in allergy with those involved in autoimmune disease
- Name four or more diseases attributed to autoimmunity
- Describe three or more postulated mechanisms underlying autoimmune disease
- State the criteria for establishing an autoimmune basis for a disease

To function properly, the immune system must be able to differentiate foreign antigens from self antigens. Normally, there is a high degree of immunologic tolerance to self antigens, which prevents the immune system from destroying the host. Autoimmune disorders result from the breakdown in the integrity of immune tolerance such that a humoral or cellular immune response can be mounted against host tissue or antigens leading to localized or systemic injury.

The autoimmune responses that give rise to disease are limited to the same effector responses that operate in immunity and allergy. These include anaphylaxis, cytotoxic, antigen-antibody complex, and cell-mediated mechanisms. Although a single effector mechanism may appear to be the cause of the disease, many diseases are mediated by several mechanisms.

Autoimmune diseases can affect almost any cell or tissue in the body. There are known or suspected hematologic, rheumatologic, neurologic, and endocrine disorders associated with autoimmunity. Some autoimmune disorders, such as Hashimoto's thyroiditis, are tissue specific; others, such as SLE, affect multiple organs and systems. Chart 12–2 lists some of the probable autoimmune diseases. Many of these disorders are discussed elsewhere in this book.

Normal Versus Disease-Associated Autoimmunity

The ability of the immune system to differentiate foreign from self antigens is the responsibility of HLA.[19] HLA is encoded by MHC genes (see Chapter 11). To elicit a T-cell response, the antigen must first be processed and presented on the surface of a phagocytic cell, such as a macrophage that also displays MHC antigen. This dual recognition requirement acts like a security system and affects all T-cell subpopulations: cytotoxic T cells, which damage target cells directly, and the helper and suppressor T cells, which augment or restrict B- or T-cell function, respectively. Helper and suppressor T cells are the positive and negative feedback circuits of the immune system. Without these controls, an immune response would never accelerate to an effective level or it would continue unabated causing undue destruction of the host.

CHART **12–2**
*Probable Autoimmune Disease**

Systemic
Mixed connective-tissue disease*
Polymyositis-dermatomyositis
Rheumatoid arthritis
Scleroderma
Sjögren's syndrome
Systemic lupus erythematosus

Blood
Autoimmune hemolytic anemia
Autoimmune neutropenia and lymphopenia
Idiopathic thrombocytopenic purpura

Other Organs
Acute idiopathic polyneuritis
Atrophic gastritis and pernicious anemia
Autoimmune adrenalitis
Goodpasture's syndrome
Hashimoto's thyroiditis
Insulin-dependent diabetes mellitus
Myasthenia gravis
Premature gonadal (ovarian) failure
Primary biliary cirrhosis
Sympathetic ophthalmia
Temporal arteritis
Thyrotoxicosis (Graves' disease)
Ulcerative colitis

*Examples are not inclusive.

Genetic Predisposition

Genetic factors can increase the incidence and severity of autoimmune diseases,[20] as shown by the familial clustering of several autoimmune diseases and the observation that certain inherited HLA types occur more frequently in persons with a variety of immunologic and lymphoproliferative disorders. For example, 90% of persons with ankylosing spondylitis carry the HLA-B27 antigen, but only 7% of a control group without the disease have the antigen. Other HLA-associated diseases are Reiter's syndrome and HLA-B27, rheumatoid arthritis and HLA-DR4, and SLE and HLA-DR3. The molecular basis for these associations is unknown. In the case of SLE, as many as six potentially abnormal gene loci may be involved in providing a veritable matrix of disease patterns. Because not all persons with genetic predisposition develop autoimmunity, it appears that other factors such as a "trigger event" interact to precipitate the altered immune state. The event or events that trigger the development of an autoimmune response are unknown. It has been suggested that the "trigger" may be a virus or other microorganism, a chemical substance, or a self antigen from a body tissue that has been hidden from the immune system during development.

Self-Tolerance

Self-tolerance is the absence of an immune response directed against a person's own antigens. Because of the need for MHC recognition, a T-cell response directed against self antigens is rare. B cells sometimes recognize self antigens complexed with smaller molecules or haptens as foreign and, without the control afforded by suppressor T cells, can ultimately mount an immune response. With a normally functioning cellular immune system, an abnormal B-cell response is held in check. Among the mechanisms that serve to maintain self-tolerance are clonal deletion, clonal anergy, and peripheral suppression. Defects in any of these mechanisms could result the development of an immune response to self antigens.

Clonal deletion refers to the elimination of self-reactive T and B lymphocytes during their maturation. Self-reactive T cells are eliminated in the thymus. T cells develop from bone marrow–derived progenitor cells that undergo maturation in the thymus. T cells that display the host's MHC antigens and T cell receptors for a nonself antigen are allowed to mature within the thymus (*i.e.*, positive selection) and those that have a high affinity for host cells are sorted out and destroyed (*i.e.*, negative selection). Self-reactive B cells are eliminated in the bone marrow in a similar manner.

Another mechanism of self-tolerance is clonal anergy. Clonal anergy refers to the functional inactivation of lymphocytes induced through an encounter with antigens under certain conditions. Activation of CD4+ T cells requires two signals: recognition of the antigen in association with MHC class II molecule on the surface of the antigen-presenting cell. When both parts of this signal are not adequately presented, the T cell becomes anergic. For example, T cells reactive to an organ-specific antigen may not be deleted in the thymus. When that happens, the self-reactive T cell clone may develop anergy when interacting with organ cells that do not express the MHC class II molecule. Clonal anergy affects B cells as well. It is probably the major mechanism for B-cell tolerance to self-reactive antigens. It seems likely that some self-reactive T cells escape clonal deletion and clonal anergy. It is thought that there are peripheral mechanisms that suppress self-reactive T cells. One such mechanism is the suppressor T cell. These cells are believed to be a distinct subset of CD8+ T cells. The mechanism by which these T cells exert their suppressor function is unclear. These cells may secrete cytokines that suppress the activity of self-reactive immune cells.

Mechanisms of Autoimmune Disease

There are multiple explanations for the formation of autoantibodies or failure to recognize host antigens as self. Among the possible mechanisms responsible for development of autoimmune disease are aberrations in antigen, receptor, T-cell, and MHC interactions; disorders of immune regulatory or surveillance function; cross-reactivity or molecular mimicry; and superantigens. Estrogens also may play a role in the immune response and development of autoimmune disease. For example, a number of autoimmune disorders such as lupus erythematosus are seen more commonly in women. Evidence suggest that estrogens stimulate and androgens suppress the immune response.[21] Because of the complexity of the immune system, it seems unlikely that autoimmune disorders arise from a single defect.

Aberrations in Antigen, T-Cell Receptor, and Major Histocompatibility Complex Interactions

The immune system recognizes antigen in the context of T-cell receptor and MCH interactions. An autoimmune response could develop due to an aberration in any of these three stages of the immune response–antigen structure, T-cell receptor function, or MHC antigen presentation. Because B-cell immunity requires support of helper T cells, the development of autoantibodies also depends on these interactions. Cytokines that function as mediators in the immune response may also be involved. For example, estrogen stimulates a DNA sequence that promotes the production of interferon-gamma, which is thought to assist in the induction of an autoimmune response.[22]

Antigen Structure. There are many ways in which chemical or microbial antigens can be modified to evoke an altered immune response, leading to an autoimmune disorder. Autoantigenic drugs and viruses can be complexed to a carrier that is recognized by nontolerant helper T cells as foreign. Virus-encoded antigens expressed on the cell surface could act as carriers for self antigens. In this case, the self antigen would appear as a hapten for which an immune response could be induced.

Partial degradation of self antigens may also occur. For example, partially degraded collagen or enzymatically altered thyroglobulin or gamma globulin may be sufficiently foreign to promote an autoimmune response.

T-Cell Receptor and Major Histocompatibility Complex Interactions. Activation of antigen-specific CD4+ T cells requires two signals: recognition of the antigen in association with class II MHC molecules on the surface of the antigen-presenting cells (APCs) and set of costimulatory signals provided by the APCs. One of the functions of the costimulatory signals provided by the APCs is to initiate clonal anergy to self-reactive T cells. The costimulatory signal requires a special binding ligand that is present on the APC and the T cell. The possibility for development of autoimmune disorders arises when self-reactive antigens are presented to the T-cell receptors by the MHC molecules of the APC. The costimulatory signal may also be defective, preventing the development of anergy in self-reactive T cells.

One of the more interesting aspects of the T-cell receptor and MHC interaction is research designed to develop mechanisms for interrupting the process as a means of treating autoimmune disease. For example, monoclonal antibodies that would target the T-cell receptor are being investigated, as is the development of strategies to block the binding part of the responsible MHC molecule.[23]

Disorders of Immune Regulatory or Surveillance Function

Because T cells regulate the immune response, an increasing ratio of helper T to suppressor T cells may lead to the development of autoimmune disorders. An example of this can be seen in persons with multiple sclerosis, in whom fluctuations in suppressor T-cell numbers parallel the intensity of the disease process.

Molecular Mimicry

It is possible that certain autoimmune disorders are caused by *molecular mimicry,* in which a foreign antigen so closely resembles a self antigen that antibodies produced against the former react with the latter.[24] A humoral or cellular response can be mounted against antigenically altered or injured tissue creating an immune process. In rheumatic fever and acute glomerulonephritis, for example, a protein in the cell wall of group A hemolytic streptococci has considerable homology with antigens in heart and kidney tissue, respectively. After infection, antibodies directed against the microorganism cause a classic case of mistaken identity, which leads to inflammation of the heart or kidney. Certain drugs, when bound to host proteins or glycoproteins, form a complex to which a humoral response is directed with substantial cross-reactivity to the original self protein. The antihypertensive agent methyldopa can bind to surface antigens on red cells to induce an antibody-mediated hemolytic anemia.

Not everyone exposed to group A hemolytic streptococci develops an autoimmune reaction. The reason that only certain persons are targeted for autoimmune reactions to a particular self-mimicry molecule may be determined by differences in HLA types. The HLA type determines exactly which fragments of a pathogen are displayed on the cell surface for presentation to T cells. One individual's HLA may bind self-mimicry molecules for presentation to T cells and another HLA type may not.

Superantigens

Superantigens are a family of related substances, including staphylococcal and streptococcal exotoxins that can short circuit the normal sequence of events, leading to activation of helper T cells. Superantigens do not require processing and presentation by macrophages to induce a T-cell response. Instead, they are able to interact with a T-cell receptor outside the normal antigen binding site. Normally, only a small percentage of the T-cell population (<0.01%) is stimulated by the presence of processed antigens on the surface of macrophages, compared with superantigens that can interact with 5% to 30% of T cells. Superantigens directly link the MHC II complex molecules of APCs such as macrophages to T-cell receptors, causing a massive release of T-cell inflammatory cytokines, primarily interleukin-2 and tumor necrosis factor, and an uncontrolled proliferation of T cells. At least one disease in adults, toxic shock syndrome, is mediated by superantigens. Kawasaki's disease in children (Chapter 19) probably has a similar cause. Superantigens may also participate in other autoimmune diseases such as rheumatoid arthritis.[25]

Diagnosis and Treatment of Autoimmune Disease

Suggested criteria for determining that a disorder is an autoimmune disorder are evidence of an autoimmune reaction, determination that the immunologic findings are not secondary to another condition, and the lack of other identified causes for the disorder. In the future, it is likely that autoimmune disorders will be diagnosed by directly identifying the genes responsible for the condition, as is the case for cystic fibrosis. The current diagnosis of autoimmune disease is based primarily on clinical findings and serologic testing.

The basis for most serologic assays is the demonstration of antibodies directed against tissue antigens or cellular components. For example, a child with chronic or acute history of fever, arthritis, and a macular rash along with high levels of antinuclear antibody has a probable diagnosis of lupus erythematosus. The detection of autoantibodies in the laboratory is usually accomplished by one of three methods: indirect fluorescent antibody assays (IFA), enzyme-linked immunosorbent assay (ELISA), or particle agglutination of some kind. The rationale behind each of these methods is similar: the patient's serum is diluted and allowed to react with an antigen-coated surface (*i.e.*, whole, fixed cells for the detection of antinuclear antibodies). In the case of IFA and ELISA, a second "labeled" antibody is added, which binds to the patient's antibody and forms a visible reaction. Particle agglutination assays are much simpler. The binding of the patient's antibody to antigen-coated particles causes a visible agglutination reaction. For most serologic assays, the patient's serum is serially diluted until it no longer produces a visible reaction (e.g., 1:100 dilution). This is called a positive titer. Healthy persons sometimes have low titers of antibody against cellular and tissue antigens, but the titers are usually far less than patients with autoimmune disease.

Treatment of autoimmune disease is based on tissue or organ involvement, the effector mechanism involved, and the magnitude and chronicity of the effector processes. Ideally, treatment should focus on the mechanism underlying the autoimmune disorder. Research into the development of vaccines to target critical pathways in the emergence of autoimmune responses is ongoing.

Intravenous IgG has been effectively used in treatment of some autoimmune disorders such as platelet depletion in immune thrombocytopenia. The mechanisms responsible for its effectiveness are not precisely known, but the effect is thought to occur because the exogenous antibodies bind to macrophages, which are prevented from attacking host cells coated with autoantibodies.[26]

In summary, autoimmune diseases represent a disruption in self-tolerance that results in damage to body tissues by the immune system. Autoimmune diseases can affect almost any cell or tissue of the body. Autoimmune responses that give rise to disease are limited to the same effector responses that operate in immunity and allergy. These include immediate-type hypersensitivity, cytotoxic, antigen-antibody complex, and cell-mediated mechanisms. Although a single effector mechanism may appear to be the cause of the disease, many diseases are mediated by several mechanisms. Normally, self-tolerance is maintained through clonal deletion, clonal anergy, and peripheral suppression. Defects in any of these mechanisms could impair self-tolerance and predispose to development of autoimmune disease.

The ability of the immune system to differentiate foreign from self antigens is the responsibility of HLA encoded by MHC genes. Antigen is presented to receptors of T cells in combination with MHC molecules. Among the possible mechanisms responsible for development of autoimmune disease are aberrations in antigen, T-cell, and MHC interactions; disorders of immune regulatory or surveillance function; cross-reactivity or molecular mimicry; and superantigens.

Suggested criteria for determining that a disorder results from an autoimmune disorder are evidence of an autoimmune reaction, determination that the immunologic findings are not secondary to another condition, and the lack of other identified causes for the disorder.

REFERENCES

1. Shyur S., Hill H.R. (1996). Recent advances in the genetics of primary immunodeficiency syndromes. *The Journal of Pediatrics* 129 (1), 8–24.
2. Ledermman H.M. (1994). Disorders of humoral immunity. In Oski F.A. (Ed.). *Principles and practices of pediatrics* (3rd ed., pp. 184–191). Philadelphia: J.B. Lippincott.
3. Buckley R. (1996). Combined B- and T-cell diseases. In Behrman R.E., Kliegman R.M., Arvin A.M. (Eds.). *Nelson textbook of pediatrics* (15th ed., pp. 571–577). Philadelphia: W.B. Saunders.
4. Hong R. (1994). Combined immunodeficiency diseases. In Oski F.A. (Ed.). *Principles and practices of pediatrics* (3rd ed., pp. 198–205). Philadelphia: JB Lippincott.
5. Blaese R.M. (1995). Steps toward gene therapy. *Hospital Practice* 30(11), 33–40.
6. Johnston R.B. (1996). The complement system. In Behrman R.E., Kliegman R.M., Arvin A.M. (Eds.). *Nelson textbook of pediatrics* (15th ed., pp. 577–583). Philadelphia: W.B Saunders.
7. Cotten H.R. (1987). Hereditary antioneurotic edema, 1887–1987. *New England Journal of Medicine* 317, 43–45.
8. Cicardi M., Agostoni A. (1996). Hereditary angioedema. *New England Journal of Medicine* 334 (25), 1666–1667.
9. Waytes A.T., Rosen F.S., Frank M.M. (1996). Treatment of hereditary angioedema with a vapor-heated C1 inhibitor concentrate. *New England Journal of Medicine* 334 (25), 1630–1634.
10. Baebner R.L. (1996). Chronic granulomatous disease. In Behrman R.E., Kliegman R.M., Arvin A.M. (Eds.). *Nelson textbook of pediatrics* (15th ed., pp. 596–598). Philadelphia: W.B. Saunders.
11. Stites D.P., Terr A.I., Parslow T.G. (1994). *Basic and clinical immunology* (8th ed., pp. 8, 266–78, 279–285, 286–302, 303–308, 317–326, 363–370, 380–386, 747–753).). Norwalk: Appleton & Lange.
12. Galli S.J. (1993). New concepts about the mast cell. *New England Journal of Medicine* 328 (4), 257–265.
13. Salvaggio J.E. (1995). The identification of hypersensitivity pneumonitis. *Hospital Practice* 30(5), 57–66.
14. Sussman G.L. (1995). Allergy to latex rubber. *Annals of Internal Medicine* 122 (1), 43–46.
15. Sussman G.L., Beezhold D.H. (1996). Safe use of natural rubber latex. *Allergy and Asthma Proceedings* 17 (2), 101–102.
16. Steelman V.M. (1995). Latex allergy precautions. *Nursing Clinics of North America* 30 (3), 475–493.
17. Cotran R.S., Kumar V., Robbins S.L. (1994). *Robbins' pathologic basis of disease* (5th ed., pp.171–240). Philadelphia: W.B. Saunders.
18. Ferrara J.L.M., Deeg H.J. (1991). Graft-versus-host disease. *New England Journal of Medicine* 324, 667–674.
19. Theofilopoulos A.N. (1995). The basis of autoimmunity: Part I: Mechanisms of aberrant self-recognition. *Immunology Today* 16 (2), 90–97.
20. Theofilopoulos A.N. (1995). The basis of autoimmunity: Part II: Genetic predisposition. *Immunology Today* 16 (3), 150–158.
21. Cutolo M., Sulli A., Seriolo S., Accardo S., Masi A.T. (1995). Estrogens, the immune response and autoimmunity. *Clinical and Experimental Rheumatology* 13, 217–226.
22. Steinman L. (1993). Autoimmune disease. *Scientific American* 269(3), 106–14.
23. Fathman C.G. (1995). Ternary complex therapy for autoimmune disease. *Hospital Practice* 30(8), 57–65.
24. Barnett L.A., Fujinami R.S. (1992). Molecular mimicry: A mechanism for autoimmune injury. *FASEB J* 6, 840–844.
25. Kotzin B.L. (1994). Superantigens and their role in disease. *Hospital Practice* 29(11), 59–70.
26. Schenkein D.E. (1992). Intravenous IgG for treatment of autoimmune disease. *Hospital Practice* 27(10A), 29–51.

ADDITIONAL READINGS

Buckley R.H., Schiff R.L. (1991). The use of intravenous immune globulin in immunodeficiency diseases [review]. *New England Journal of Medicine* 325, 109–117.

Clark R.A. (1990). Genetic variations in chronic granulomatous disease. *Hospital Practice* 25(5A), 51–72.

D'Andrea A.D. (1994). Cytokine receptors in congenital hematopoietic disease. *New England Journal of Medicine* 330 (12), 839–846.

Dalton T.A., Bennett J.C. (1992). Autoimmune disease and the major histocompatibility complex: Therapeutic implications. *American Journal of Medicine* 92, 183–188.

Hassner A., Adelman D.C. (1991). Biologic response modifiers in primary immunodeficiency disorders. *Annals of Internal Medicine* 115 (4), 294–307.

Hollingsworth H.M. (1996). Allergic rhinoconjunctivitis. *Hospital Practice* 31(6), 61–63.

Johnson H.M., Russell J.K., Pontzer C.H. (1992). Superantigens in human disease. *Scientific American* 266, 92–101.

Leonard W.J. (1996). The molecular basis of X-linked severe combined immunodeficiency: Defective cytokine receptor signaling. *Annual Review of Medicine* 47, 229–239.

Pedinoff A.J. (1996). Approaches to treatment of seasonal allergic rhinitis. *Southern Medical Journal* 89 (12), 1130–1139.

Reiser H., Stadecker M.J. (1996). Costimulatory B7 molecules in the pathogenesis of infectious and autoimmune diseases. *New England Journal of Medicine* 335 (18), 1369–1377.

Schwartz R.H. (1993). T cell anergy. *Scientific American* 267(8), 62–71.

Simon R.A. (1996). Adverse reactions to food and drug additives. *Immunology and Allergic Clinics of North America* 16 (1), 137–171.

Subramaniam A. (1995). The chemistry of natural rubber latex. *Immunology and Allergic Clinics of North America* 15 (1), 1–19. [The entire issue is devoted to latex allergy.]

Tabbara I.A. (1996). Allogenic bone marrow transplantation. *Southern Medical Journal* 89 (9), 857–867.

Yunginger J.W. (1992). Lethal food allergy in children. *New England Journal of Medicine.* 327 (6), 321–322.

Wilkin T.J. (1990). Receptor autoimmunity in endocrine disorders. *New England Journal of Medicine* 323 (19), 1318–1324.

CHAPTER 13

Acquired Immunodeficiency Syndrome

Susan E. Dietz

At the beginning of the AIDS epidemic, many Americans had little sympathy for people with AIDS. The feeling was that somehow people from certain groups deserved their illness. Let us put those feelings behind us. We are fighting a disease, not people. Those who are already afflicted are sick people and need our care as do all sick patients. The country must face this epidemic as a unified society. We must prevent the spread of AIDS while at the same time preserving humanity and intimacy.[1]

C. EVERETT KOOP, MD, ScD
Surgeon General (1981–1989)
U.S. Public Health Service

Acquired immunodeficiency syndrome (AIDS) is caused by a retrovirus that selectively attacks and destroys the immune system. The Centers for Disease Control and Prevention (CDC) estimates that 650,000 to 900,000 persons in the United States were living with human immunodeficiency virus (HIV) infection in 1992.[2] The prevalence of HIV infection and AIDS in the United States has been highest in the East and West Coast regions and lowest in the northern Midwest and Mountain states. Prevalence is greater in urban than in rural areas. Cases of HIV infection and AIDS have been concentrated among men between the ages of 20 and 39, although women and children are increasingly affected. More than 500,000 cases of AIDS had been diagnosed in the United States through December 1995.[3] The total number of deaths increased from 31 deaths before 1981 to more than 315,000 through December 1995.[3] At least 15,000 new HIV infections are diagnosed each year in the United States.[3] Some populations, such as African Americans and Hispanics, are disproportionately affected by this epidemic.[3]

During the 1980s, AIDS emerged as a leading cause of death in the United States. In 1994, HIV infection was the most common cause of death among persons between the ages of 25 and 44 years.[4] In the same year, HIV was the eighth leading cause of death overall, accounting for 2% of all deaths.[4] In 1994, the death rate from HIV infection per 100,000 population among persons between the ages of 25 and 44 years was almost four times as high for black men (177.9) as for white men (47.2) and nine times as high for black women (51.2) as for white women (5.7).[4] In 1994, HIV infection or AIDS was the fourth leading cause of years of potential life lost before the age of 65 years (compared with sixth in 1990).[4] These trends reflect the youthfulness of those who have died of AIDS and the increasing number of deaths.

The AIDS Epidemic and Transmission of HIV Infection

On completion of this section of the chapter, you should be able to do the following:

- Briefly trace the history of the AIDS epidemic

- State the virus responsible for AIDS and explain how it differs from most other viruses
- Describe the mechanisms of HIV transmission and relate them to the need for public awareness and concern regarding the spread of AIDS

The AIDS Epidemic

The first recognized cases of AIDS occurred in the summer of 1981, when pneumonia caused by *Pneumocystis carinii*, a previously rare fungus, and Kaposi's sarcoma, a previously rare malignancy, were reported in otherwise healthy persons.[5] Both of these conditions previously occurred only in severely immunocompromised persons. The condition became known in 1982 as the *acquired immunodeficiency syndrome*, although its causes and modes of transmission were not immediately obvious.[5] An understanding of the virology of AIDS progressed with amazing efficiency; within 3 years after the first cases were recognized, the virus causing AIDS was identified.[5] The virus was initially known by various names, including human T-cell lymphotropic virus type 3 (HTLV-III), lymphadenopathy-associated virus (LAV), and AIDS-associated retrovirus (ARV).[6] The internationally accepted term since 1986 has been human immunodeficiency virus (HIV).[7] HIV selectively attacks CD4+ T lymphocytes, the immune cells responsible for orchestrating and coordinating the immune response to infection. As a consequence, persons with HIV infection are susceptible to severe infections with ordinarily harmless organisms.

Before the virus was discovered, however, much was learned about how it could be transmitted. First described among homosexual men in June 1981, AIDS was recognized among injecting drug users the following year and among persons with hemophilia, infants born to infected mothers, and as early as 1983, among heterosexual sex partners of persons with AIDS.[8] Studies of these diverse groups led to the conclusion that AIDS is an infectious disease spread by blood, sexual contact, and perinatally from mother to child. The cumulative world total of AIDS cases was 11,965 at the end of 1984.[9]

Because HIV or AIDS occurs throughout the world and affects an exceptionally high proportion of the population, it is often referred to as a pandemic. As of June 30, 1996, 1,393,649 cases of AIDS were reported officially to the Joint United Nations Programme on AIDS.[10] Because of underrecognition, underreporting, and reporting delays, a more realistic estimate may be that over 7 million persons (including 1.6 million children) worldwide have developed AIDS since it was first recognized.[10] Because reporting of cases is not uniform throughout the world, many countries may not be accurately represented in these figures.

The absence of a cure and preventive vaccine has led to broad and increasing public concern. Estimated inpatient hospital costs for a person with AIDS average $24,000, and outpatient costs average $8000, for a total of $32,000 per year (in 1990 dollars).[10] Medical care costs for a person with HIV infection (not diagnosed with AIDS) are estimated at $5150 per year (in 1990 dollars).[10]

HIV infection can be detected by a blood test for antibody to the virus. Nearly 100% of infected persons have antibody to the virus. AIDS is a state of severe immunodeficiency that develops in persons after they have been infected with HIV for several years. Cohort studies show that 51% of persons will develop AIDS within 10 years after seroconverting (*i.e.*, developing antibodies as a result of acquiring infection with HIV).[11]

The virus responsible for most HIV infection worldwide is called HIV type 1. A second type of HIV, human immunodeficiency virus type 2 (HIV-2) is endemic in many countries in West Africa but generally much rarer in other parts of the world.[12] HIV-2 appears to be transmitted in the same manner as HIV-1. HIV-2 can also cause immunodeficiency evidenced by a reduction in the number of CD4+ T lymphocytes and the development of AIDS. The spectrum of disease for HIV-2 is similar to that of HIV-1. However, HIV-2 spreads more slowly and causes disease more slowly than HIV-1. Through 1991, 17 cases of HIV-2 were reported in the United States as compared with the estimated 40,000 new cases of HIV-1 infection each year.[12] Because of the relatively rare occurrence of HIV-2 in the United States, there is little reason to believe it will have a major impact on morbidity and mortality over the short term.[12] Long-term consequences will depend on its spread in the population.

Transmission of HIV Infection

HIV is transmitted from one person to another through sexual contact, by blood contact, or perinatally. HIV is not transmitted through casual contact. Several studies involving more than 1000 uninfected, nonsexual household contacts with persons with HIV infection (including siblings, parents, and children) have shown no evidence of transmission.[13] HIV is not spread by mosquitoes or other insect vectors.[7] When infected blood, semen, or vaginal secretions from one person are deposited onto a mucous membrane or into the bloodstream of another person, transmission can occur.

Blood, semen, and vaginal or cervical secretions contain sufficient concentrations of HIV to transmit the infection.[7] Contact with semen occurs during vaginal and anal sexual intercourse, oral sex (*i.e.*, fellatio), and donor insemination. Exposure to vaginal or cervical secretions occurs during vaginal intercourse and oral sex (*i.e.*, cunnilingus). In most cities in the United States, sexual transmission of HIV is primarily related to vaginal or anal intercourse. In the United States, 58% of AIDS cases are among men who have sex with men, and 6% of AIDS cases are related to infection through heterosexual contact.[4] In the developing world, heterosexual transmission is the major route of HIV infection.[7]

The use of injection needles, syringes, and other drug-injection paraphernalia contaminated with blood containing HIV is a direct route for transmission of HIV. Of the reported cases of AIDS in the United States, 32% occurred among persons who use injecting drugs, including 25% among persons in whom injecting drug use was the only risk factor.[3] HIV-infected injecting drug users can pass the virus to their needle-sharing and sex partners and, in the case of pregnant women, to their offspring.[7] Although alcohol, cocaine, and other noninjecting drugs do not directly transmit infection, their use alters perception of risk and reduces inhibitions about engaging in behaviors that pose a high risk of transmitting HIV infection. Transfusions of whole blood, plasma, platelets, or blood cells before 1985 resulted in the transmission of HIV.[7] However, these routes of transmission now account for only a small and declining percentage of AIDS in the United States (*i.e.*, 1% in adults and 5% in children).[3] All blood donations in the United States have been screened for HIV since mid-1985. There may continue to be cases of AIDS identified as being transmitted by transfusions for some time because of the long incubation period for AIDS.

The clotting factor used by persons with hemophilia is derived from the pooled plasma of many donors. Before HIV testing of plasma donors was implemented in 1985, the virus was transmitted to persons with hemophilia through infusions of clotting factor concentrates.[7] Although the clotting factor is heat-treated to kill HIV, 70% to 80% of persons with hemophilia born before 1985 may have already been infected. Other blood products, such as gamma globulin or hepatitis B immune globulin, have not been implicated in the transmission of HIV.[7]

HIV may be transmitted from infected women to their offspring by three routes: *in utero* through the maternal-placental circulation, by inoculation during labor and delivery, and through breast-feeding after birth.[14] Transmission probably occurs during labor and delivery or shortly thereafter. Several prospective studies have reported perinatal transmission rates ranging from 13% to 40%, depending on factors such as the stage of infection in the mother.[15]

AIDS among health care workers in the United States results primarily from infection that occurs outside the work setting. Small numbers of health care workers have been infected with HIV through occupational exposure.[3] The CDC recommends that Universal Blood and Body Fluid Precautions be used in encounters with all patients in the health care setting (Chart 13–1).[16] Because health care workers may be caring for persons whose HIV status is unknown, adherence to the precautions with all patients is the most prudent way to prevent occupational exposure.[17] Studies show that the occupational risk of acquiring HIV in the health care setting is low. Occupational risk of infection for health care workers is most often associated with percutaneous inoculation (*i.e.*, needlestick) of blood from a patient with HIV.[18] The average risk for HIV infection from percutaneous exposure to HIV-infected blood is 0.3%.[18]

Evidence from CDC investigations suggests that the risk of transmission from infected health care workers to patients during invasive procedures is small. When recommended infection-control procedures are followed, the risk of transmitting hepatitis B virus (HBV) from an infected health care worker to a patient is small, and the risk of transmitting HIV is likely to be even smaller. Although rare, the likelihood of patient exposure to an infected health care worker's blood may vary, depending on the procedure and on the skill and physical health of the infected worker (Chart 13–2).[19]

CHART 13-1

General Principles of Universal Precautions*

1. Take care to prevent injuries when using needles, scalpels, and other sharp instruments or devices. Do not recap used needles by hand, and do not bend, break, or otherwise manipulate used needles by hand. Place used disposable syringes and needles, scalpel blades, and other sharp items in puncture-resistant containers located as close to the treatment area as possible.
2. Use protective barriers (*i.e.*, gloves, gowns, masks, and protective eyewear) to prevent exposure to blood, body fluids containing visible blood, and other fluids to which universal precautions apply. The type of protective barrier should be appropriate for the procedure being performed and the type of exposure anticipated.
3. Immediately and thoroughly wash hands and other skin surfaces that are contaminated with blood, body fluids containing visible blood, or other body fluids to which universal precautions apply.

*This list is abbreviated.

(Centers for Disease Control. [1988]. Update: Universal precautions for prevention of transmission of human immunodeficiency virus, hepatitis B virus, and other blood-borne pathogens in health-care settings. *Morbidity and Mortality Weekly Report, 37,* 377)

Evidence increasingly shows that persons with another sexually transmitted disease (STD) are at increased risk for HIV infection. Research supports the hypothesis that the risk of HIV transmission is increased in the presence of genital ulcerative STDs (*i.e.*, syphilis, herpes simplex virus [HSV], and chancroid) and nonulcerative STDs (*i.e.*, gonorrhea, chlamydia, and trichomoniasis). Available data also suggest that HIV increases the duration and recurrence of lesions, treatment failures, and atypical presentation of genital ulcerative diseases. This "epidemiologic synergy" may be responsible for the explosive increase in HIV infection among some populations.[20]

The HIV-infected person is infectious even when no symptoms are present. The point at which antibodies to the virus can first be detected in the blood of an infected person—when the person converts from being negative for HIV antibody in the blood to positive for the presence of antibodies—is called *seroconversion*. Seroconversion typically occurs within 1 to 3 months after exposure to HIV but can take up to 6 months or, in rare cases, even longer.[20] An HIV-infected person can transmit the virus to others even before seroconversion. The time after infection and before seroconversion is known as the "window

CHART 13-2

Recommendations for Preventing The Transmission of HIV and HBV to Patients During Exposure-Prone Invasive Procedures

To minimize the risk of HIV or HBV transmission, the following measures are recommended:

- All health-care workers (HCWs) should adhere to universal precautions, including the appropriate use of handwashing, protective barriers, and care in the use and disposal of needles and other sharp instruments. HCWs who have exudative lesions or weeping dermatitis should refrain from all direct patient care and from handling patient-care equipment and devices used in performing invasive procedures until the condition resolves. HCWs should also comply with current guidelines for disinfection and sterilization of reusable devices used in invasive procedures.
- Currently available data provide no basis for recommendations to restrict the practice of HCWs infected with HIV or HBV who perform invasive procedures not identified as exposure-prone, provided the infected HCWs practice recommended surgical or dental technique and comply with universal precautions and current recommendations for sterilization or disinfection.
- Exposure-prone procedures should be identified by medical, surgical, or dental organizations and institutions at which the procedures are performed.
- HCWs who perform exposure-prone procedures should know their HIV antibody status. HCWs who perform exposure-prone procedures and who do not have serologic evidence of immunity to HBV from vaccination or from previous infection should know their HBsAg status and, if that is positive, should also know their HBeAg status.
- HCWs who are infected with HIV or HBV and who are HBeAg positive should not perform exposure-prone procedures unless they have sought counsel from an expert review panel and been advised under what circumstances, if any, they may continue to perform these procedures.* Such circumstances include notifying prospective patients of the HCWs seropositivity before they undergo exposure-prone invasive procedures.
- Mandatory testing of HCWs for HIV antibody, HBsAg is not recommended. The current assessment of the risk that infected HCWs will transmit HIV or HBV to patients during exposure-prone procedures does not support the diversion of resources that would be required to implement mandatory testing programs. Compliance by HCWs with recommendations can be increased through education, training, and appropriate confidentiality safeguards.

*The review panel should include experts who represent a balanced perspective. Such experts might include all of the following: the HCW's personal physicians, an infectious disease specialist with expertise in the epidemiology of HIV and HBV transmission, a health professional with expertise in the procedures performed by the HCW, and state or local public health officials. If the HCW's practice is institutionally based, the expert review panel might also include a member of the infection-control committee, preferably a hospital epidemiologist. HCWs who perform exposure-prone procedures outside the hospital or institutional setting should seek advice from appropriate state and local public health officials regarding the review process.

(Centers for Disease Control. [1991]. Recommendations for preventing transmission of human immunodeficiency virus and hepatitis B virus to patients during exposure-prone invasive procedures. *Morbidity and Mortality Weekly Report 40,* 1–9)

period."[20] Rarely, infection can occur from transfused blood that was screened for HIV antibody and found negative, because the donor was recently infected and still in the window period. Consequently, the U.S. Food and Drug Administration (FDA) requires blood collection centers to screen potential donors through interviews designed to identify behaviors known to present risk for HIV infection.

In summary, AIDS is an infectious disease of the immune system caused by the HIV. First described in June 1981, the disease is prevalent worldwide and is one of the leading causes of death among young adults in the United States. The severity of the clinical disease and the absence of a cure or preventive vaccine have increased public awareness and concern. HIV is transmitted from one person to another through sexual contact, through blood exchange, or perinatally. Transmission occurs when the infected blood, semen, or vaginal secretions of one person are deposited onto a mucous membrane or into the bloodstream of another person. The primary routes of transmission are through sexual intercourse and the use of contaminated injection equipment. Although blood transmission may occur with blood transfusion or occupational exposure in a health care setting, only a small percentage of HIV transmission is attributable to blood transfusion or occupational infection. HIV infection is not transmitted through casual contact or by insect vectors. There is growing evidence of an association between HIV infection and other STDs. Infected persons can transmit the virus to others before their own infections can be detected by antibody tests.

Pathophysiology of AIDS

On completion of this section of the chapter, you should be able to do the following:

- Describe diagnosis of AIDS using the CDC AIDS case definition
- Describe the alterations in immune function that occur in persons with AIDS

- Relate the altered immune function in persons with HIV infection and AIDS to the development of opportunistic infections, tuberculosis, and Kaposi's sarcoma
- Explain the possible significance of a positive antibody test for HIV infection
- Differentiate between the EIA (ELISA) and Western blot antibody detection tests for HIV infection
- List the four stages of HIV Infection and describe the symptoms, psychosocial issues, and management concerns for each stage

Since the first description of AIDS, considerable strides have been made in understanding the pathophysiology of the disease. The virus and its mechanism of action, HIV antibody screening tests, and some treatment methods were discovered within a few years after the recognition of the first cases. Further progress on understanding the pathophysiology of AIDS and development of more powerful treatments continues to be made.

HIV belongs to a class of viruses called retroviruses, which carry their genetic information in RNA rather than DNA. HIV infects a limited number of cell types in the body, including a subset of lymphocytes called CD4+ T cells (also known as helper cells or T4 lymphocytes)[7] and macrophages.[21] The CD4+ T cells are necessary for normal immune function (see Chapter 11). Among other functions, the CD4+ T cell recognizes foreign antigens and infected cells and helps activate the antibody-producing B lymphocytes. The CD4+ T cells also orchestrate cell-mediated immunity, in which cytotoxic CD8+ T cells and natural killer (NK) cells directly destroy virus-infected cells and foreign antigens. Phagocytic monocytes and macrophages are also influenced to fight infection by CD4+ T cells.

The CD4 protein molecule on the surface of CD4+ cells enables HIV to establish infection. A surface protein on the viral envelope of HIV, gp120, binds to the CD4 molecule on the surface of the lymphocyte (Fig. 13–1). Although T lymphocytes seem to have the highest number of CD4 molecules, the molecule is also present on other cells, such as monocytes and macrophages.[22] After attaching to the CD4 molecule, the virus enters the lymphocyte and sheds its protein coat. Viral RNA is transcribed into DNA using a unique enzyme called reverse transcriptase. A second strand is produced to form a DNA duplex, called proviral DNA, the DNA that is integrated into the host cell DNA.[22]

In some cells, the infection enters a latent phase that serves as a reservoir from which the virus can continue to be released for several years.[22] In other cells, the virus replicates, killing the cell and releasing copies of HIV into the bloodstream. These viral particles, or virions, invade other CD4+ T cells, allowing the infection to progress. Everyday, millions of infected CD4+ T cells are destroyed, releasing billions of viral particles into the bloodstream, but each day nearly all the CD4+ T cells are replaced and nearly all the viral particles are destroyed. Over years, however, the CD4+ T-cell count gradually decreases through this process, and the number of viruses detected in the blood of persons infected with HIV increases.[22]

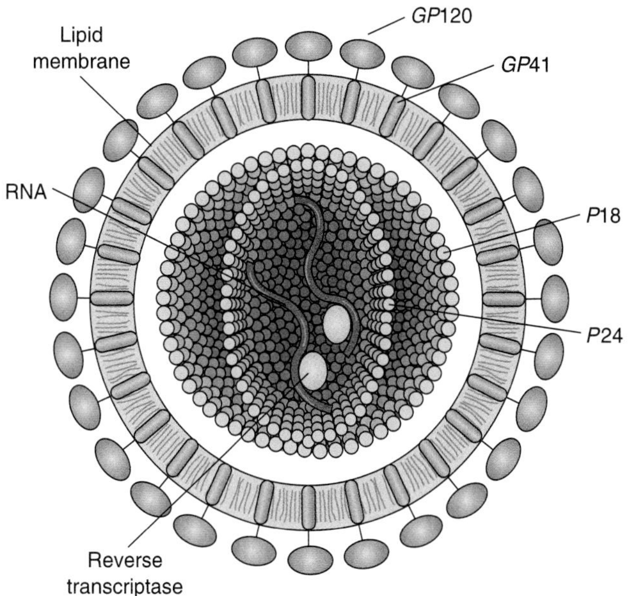

FIGURE 13–1
The human immunodeficiency virus (HIV).

Until the CD4+ T-cell count falls to a very low level, infected persons remain asymptomatic, although there is active viral replication[23] and serologic tests can identify antibodies to HIV proteins. These antibodies are usually detectable as early as 1 to 3 months after infection.[21] These antibodies unfortunately do not convey protection against the virus.[21] Although symptoms are not evident, the infection proceeds on a microbiologic level, including the invasion and selective destruction of CD4+ T cells. The continual decline of CD4+ T cells, which are pivotal cells in the immune response, strips the person with AIDS of protection against common organisms and cancerous cells.[22]

Diagnosis

The most accurate and inexpensive method for identifying HIV is the HIV antibody test. The first commercial assays for HIV were introduced in 1985 to screen donated blood. Since then, use of antibody detection tests has been expanded to include evaluating persons at increased risk for HIV infection and as a component of the case definition of AIDS. The HIV antibody test procedure consists of screening with an enzyme immunoassay (EIA), also known as enzyme-linked immunosorbent assay (ELISA), followed by a confirmatory test, the Western blot assay, which is performed if the EIA is positive.[24] Because this procedure usually takes several days, rapid on-site assay tests show promise of improving the delivery of services and increasing the number of persons who learn their serostatus.[25] In light of the psychosocial issues related to HIV and AIDS, sensitivity and confidentiality must be maintained whenever testing is implemented. Counseling before and after testing to allay fears, to provide accurate information, to ensure appropriate follow-up testing, and to provide referral to needed medical and psychosocial services is essential.

The EIA detects antibodies produced in response to HIV infection and is based on the light absorbance of antigen-antibody complexes in sample wells compared with control wells.[21] The test kit contains beads or microtiter wells coated with HIV antigens. When a serum sample is added, HIV antibodies in the serum bind to the antigen-coated surface. A second antibody linked to an enzyme is added to combine with the antigen-antibody complexes. These steps are separated by washings and incubations before a substrate for the enzyme is added. Color development, indicating the amount of bound HIV antibody, is measured with a spectrophotometer. The test is considered reactive if the measured light absorbance is greater than a cutoff value established from known positive and negative controls.[21] Samples that are repeatedly reactive are tested by a supplemental test such as the Western blot.[24]

The Western blot assay allows identification of antibodies to specific viral antigens. For the test, HIV antigens prepared from a virus culture are separated by electrophoresis and transferred (blotted) to nitrocellulose paper, which is subsequently cut into strips.[21] The serum sample is added to a strip, allowing specific HIV antibodies to bind with specific viral antigen bands. The reaction is carried out similarly to the EIA. This technique permits the identification of antibodies to specific HIV proteins and glycoproteins.[21] When certain combinations of the antibody bands are identified, the test result is considered positive. The Western blot test is more specific than the EIA, and in the rare case with a false-positive EIA test result, the Western blot test can identify the person as uninfected.

Serologic tests for detecting HIV antibodies are sensitive and specific. When serum test results are strongly reactive or borderline by EIA and positive by Western blot, the person is considered to be infected with HIV.[24] Both tests are important because, in some situations, misinformation can be generated by EIA testing alone. The EIA test has a high predictive value when used in groups with a high prevalence of infection (*e.g.*, sexually active homosexual men).[26] However, when the EIA test is used in groups of low prevalence of infection (*e.g.*, blood donors), most of the positive results turn out to be false-positive results.[26] The Western blot test is therefore essential to determine which persons with positive EIA tests are truly infected.

An estimated 34 million HIV antibody tests are performed in the United States each year.[27] New technology has led to the development of consumer-controlled (e.g., home test kits available without a prescription) HIV testing. The kits approved by the FDA allow persons to collect their own blood sample through a finger-stick process, mail the specimen to a laboratory for the EIA and confirmatory tests, and receive results by telephone.[27] Wherever the test is performed, it is important to understand that testing is not an end in itself but a pathway to prevention, treatment, and care.

Polymerase chain reaction (PCR) is a specialized technique for detecting HIV DNA, although availability of the test is limited.[28] Because the amount of viral DNA in the HIV-infected cell is small compared with the amount of human DNA, direct detection of viral genetic material is difficult.[28] PCR is a method for amplifying the viral DNA up to 1 million times or more to increase the probability of detection.[28] PCR detects the presence of the virus rather than the antibody to the virus, which the EIA and Western blot tests detect. PCR is useful in diagnosing HIV infection in infants born to infected mothers, because these infants have their mothers' HIV antibody whether the children are infected or not.[28]

Effective January 1, 1993, the CDC implemented a new classification system for HIV infection and a new AIDS case definition for adolescents and adults emphasizing the clinical importance of the $CD4^+$ T-cell count in the categorization of HIV-related clinical conditions.[29] The new classification system defines three categories that correspond to $CD4^+$ T-cell counts per microliter (μL) of blood:

Category 1: $\geq$500 cells/μL

Category 2: 200 to 499 cells/μL

Category 3: <200 cells/μL[29]

There are also three clinical categories. Clinical category A includes persons who are asymptomatic or have persistent generalized lymphadenopathy or symptoms of primary retroviral syndrome (*i.e.*, acute seroconversion illness).[29] Clinical category B includes persons with symptoms of immune deficiency not serious enough to be included in Category C.[29] Category C includes conditions listed in the AIDS surveillance case definition shown in Chart 13–3.[29] Each HIV-infected person has a $CD4^+$ T-cell category and a clinical category. The combination of these two categorizations, $CD4^+$ T-lymphocyte categories 1, 2, and 3 and clinical categories A, B, and C, can guide clinical and therapeutic actions in the management of HIV infection. According to the 1993 case definition, persons in category 3 or category C are considered to have AIDS (see Chart 13–3).

Clinical Course of the Disease

The typical course of disease for persons infected with HIV consists of four stages: primary or initial infection; clinical latency; clinically apparent disease with constitutional symptoms; and development of AIDS indicator diseases.[23]

Many persons, when they are initially infected with HIV, have an acute mononucleosis-like syndrome known as acute retroviral syndrome.[30] This acute phase may include fever, myalgias, malaise, sore throat, nausea, lethargy, retro-orbital pain, photophobia, lymphadenopathy, maculopapular rash, and headache.[31] During this time, there is a burst of viral replication, which can temporarily lower the $CD4^+$ T-cell count. After several

CHART 13-3

Conditions Included in the 1993 AIDS Surveillance Case Definition

Candidiasis of bronchi, trachea, or lungs
Candidiasis, esophageal
Cervical cancer, invasive*
Coccidioidomycosis, disseminated or extrapulmonary
Cryptococcosis, extrapulmonary
Cryptosporidiosis, chronic intestinal (>1 month's duration)
Cytomegalovirus disease (other than liver, spleen, or nodes)
Cytomegalovirus retinitis (with loss of vision)
Encephalopathy, HIV-related
Herpes simplex: chronic ulcer(s) (>1 month's duration) or bronchitis, pneumonitis, or esophagitis
Histoplasmosis, disseminated or extrapulmonary
Isosporiasis, chronic intestinal (>1 month's duration)
Kaposi's sarcoma
Lymphoma, Burkitt's (or equivalent term)
Lymphoma, immunoblastic (or equivalent term)
Lymphoma, primary, of brain
Mycobacterium avium complex or *M kansasii,* disseminated or extrapulmonary
Mycobacterium tuberculosis, any site (pulmonary* or extrapulmonary)
Mycobacterium, other species or unidentified species, disseminated or extrapulmonary
Pneumocystis carinii pneumonia
Pneumonia, recurrent*
Progressive multifocal leukoencephalopathy
Salmonella septicemia, recurrent
Toxoplasmosis of brain
Wasting syndrome due to HIV

*Added to the 1993 expansion of the AIDS surveillance case definition
(Centers for Disease Control and Pervention. [1992]. 1993 Revised classification system for HIV infection and expanded surveillance case definition for AIDS among adolescents and adults. *Morbidity and Mortality Weekly Report* 41 [RR-17], 19)

weeks, the immune system acts to control viral replication and reduces it to a lower level, where it remains for several more years.

The acute phase may be followed by a latent period of as many as 10 years before many other symptoms occur.[23] During this time, the $CD4^+$ T-lymphocyte count falls gradually from the normal range (800 to 1000 cells/μL) to 200 cells/μL or lower. Some persons with HIV infection develop lymphadenopathy during this phase. *Persistent generalized lymphadenopathy* is usually defined as lymph nodes that are chronically swollen for more than 3 months in at least two locations, not including the groin. The lymph nodes may be sore or visible externally.[23]

When the immune system reaches a point of being severely compromised, an opportunistic infection or malignancy may occur. Opportunistic infections involve common organisms that normally do not produce infection unless there is impaired immune function. The most common is *Pneumocystis carinii* pneumonia (PCP). The most common opportunistic malignancies are Kaposi's sarcoma and lymphoma. Although a person with AIDS may live for many years after the first serious illness, because of immune system failure, these opportunistic illnesses become progressively more severe and difficult to treat. The complications of AIDS include opportunistic diseases of the respiratory, gastrointestinal, and nervous systems and the wasting syndrome.[23]

Respiratory Manifestations

PCP is the most common respiratory opportunistic disease in persons with AIDS.[32] PCP is caused by a fungus that is common in soil, houses, and many other places in the environment. In persons with healthy immune systems, the fungus does not cause infection or disease. In persons with AIDS, *P. carinii* can multiply quickly in the lungs and cause pneumonia.[32] These symptoms may be acute or gradually progressive. Persons may complain of fever, chest pain, sputum production, or shortness of breath. Physical examination may demonstrate only fever and tachypnea; rales may be absent and breath sounds may be normal. The chest x-ray film may show interstitial infiltrates, but a normal chest film does not exclude PCP.[32] The specific diagnosis can be made in some persons by examination of induced sputum, but most require bronchoscopy and bronchoalveolar lavage or lung biopsy.[32]

Other organisms that cause pulmonary infections in persons with AIDS include *Mycobacterium tuberculosis,* cytomegalovirus (CMV), *Mycobacterium avium* complex (MAC), *Toxoplasma gondii,* and *Cryptococcus neoformans.*[24] Pneumonia may also occur because of more common pulmonary pathogens, including *Streptococcus pneumoniae, Haemophilus influenzae,* and *Legionella pneumophila.* Some persons may be infected with multiple organisms.[32] Kaposi's sarcoma can also occur in the lungs.

Mycobacterium tuberculosis

From 1985 to 1991, there was a 16% increase in the number of cases of tuberculosis reported annually in the United States—a marked change from the average annual decline of 6% during the preceding 30 years.[33] A number of factors contributed to this increase; the most profound is the epidemic of HIV infection. Persons infected with *M. tuberculosis* (i.e., those with positive tuberculin skin tests) are more likely to develop tuberculosis if they are infected with HIV.[33] Equally important, HIV-infected persons exposed to tuberculosis are likely to have rapidly progressive primary disease instead of a subclinical tuberculosis infection.[33] The clinical presentation of tuberculosis in persons with advanced HIV infection differs from that in persons with normal cellular immunity. With advanced HIV infection, tuberculosis often presents diffuse pulmonary infiltrates or thoracic lymphadenopathy and extrapulmonary involvement in the central nervous system (CNS).[33]

During the last 3 decades, most persons with tuberculosis have responded well to therapy. However, from

1988 to 1991, there were at least six outbreaks of tuberculosis that were resistant to multiple drugs.[33] The transmission of drug-resistant disease has occurred between patients, from patients to health care workers or prison guards, and from patients to family members.[33] About 90% of the cases of drug-resistant tuberculosis have occurred in HIV-infected persons.[33] Mortality rates from disease of this type among HIV-infected persons range from 70% to 90%, with a median of 4 to 16 weeks from diagnosis to death.[33]

Gastrointestinal Manifestations

Esophageal candidiasis is another common opportunistic infection occurring among persons with AIDS.[32] Other opportunistic organisms causing esophagitis include CMV and herpes simplex virus.[32] Persons experiencing these infections usually complain of painful swallowing or retrosternal pain. Endoscopy, with esophageal brushings or biopsy, is required for definitive diagnosis.[32]

Diarrhea or gastroenteritis also occurs commonly in persons with AIDS. Symptoms may be the result of protozoal infection by *Cryptosporidium parvum*.[32] This watery diarrhea may produce large volumes of stool per day and last for months. Such severe symptoms can lead to weakness and death from fluid loss. Other organisms causing gastroenteritis and diarrhea may be *Isospora belli*, MAC, and microsporidia. These organisms are identified by examining the stool specimen with special stains. Unfortunately, there is no effective treatment for diarrhea due to cryptosporidia, microsporidia, or most viruses.

Nervous System Manifestations

Neurologic complications of HIV infections occur frequently and may affect the peripheral or CNS. These complications arise from the direct effects of the retrovirus on the CNS and from opportunistic infections.[34] Neurologic symptoms may occur in HIV-infected persons who are otherwise asymptomatic.[34]

Toxoplasmosis is a common opportunistic infection affecting the CNS in persons with AIDS. The organism, *T. gondii* , is a parasite. The typical presentation includes fever, altered mental status, seizures, or motor deficits.[32] Computed tomography (CT scans) or magnetic resonance imaging (MRI) generally show lesions, but in some cases, brain biopsy is necessary for definitive diagnosis. Primary CNS lymphoma may also occur in persons with AIDS.[34] The clinical course of these lymphomas often includes rapid progression and death, despite treatment.[34]

Progressive multifocal leukoencephalopathy is a subacute demyelinating disease of the CNS.[35] Multiple lesions in the white matter of the brain or brain stem cause dementia, blindness, paralysis, and in most cases, death within 1 year.[35]

C. neoformans is a fungus that typically causes fever, cough, dyspnea, pleuritic chest pain, and meningitis.[35] Disseminated infection may be found in the bone marrow, kidneys, liver, spleen, lymph nodes, heart, skin, and other organs.[35] Cryptococcal meningitis is diagnosed by laboratory testing of the cerebrospinal fluid.

A common neurologic syndrome attributed directly to HIV is called *AIDS dementia complex*.[34] This neurologic syndrome may occur in as many as 15% of persons with AIDS.[34] Marked by subtle cognitive or behavioral dysfunction occurring over weeks to months, persons may initially develop memory loss, difficulty in concentrating, euphoria, social withdrawal, or lethargy.[34] These early signs are easily confused with depression or drug abuse and may be ignored until they eventually progress to severe dementia with motor disturbances, ataxia, tremor, spasticity, and paraplegia.[34] A characteristic pattern of cerebral atrophy with prominent sulci and ventricles is shown on CT and MRI.[34] Examination of the cerebrospinal fluid typically shows a mild pleocytosis with an elevated protein or lowered glucose concentration.[34] AIDS dementia complex may initially occur without any other signs or symptoms of AIDS.[34]

Cancers and Malignancies

Kaposi's sarcoma is a malignancy of endothelial cells that line small blood vessels. An opportunistic cancer, Kaposi's sarcoma occurs in immunosuppressed persons (*e.g.*, transplantation patients, persons with AIDS). Before 1981, most cases of Kaposi's sarcoma were found in North America among elderly men of Mediterranean or Eastern European Jewish descent and in Africa among young black adults and children.

There is a great diversity in the clinical manifestations of Kaposi's sarcoma.[32] The disease usually begins as one or more macules, papules, or violet skin lesions that enlarge and become darker. They may enlarge to form raised plaques or tumors. These irregularly shaped tumors can be from one eighth of an inch to silver dollar size. Tumor nodules are frequently located on the trunk, neck, and head, especially the tip of the nose. They are usually painless in the early stages, but discomfort may develop as the tumor ages. Invasion of internal organs, including the lungs, gastrointestinal tract, and lymphatic system, occurs commonly. The tumors may obstruct organ function or rupture and cause internal bleeding. The progression of Kaposi's sarcoma may be slow or rapid. Biopsy of suspicious lesions is needed to make a definitive diagnosis. Chemotherapy and radiation therapy are effective for palliative treatment of the tumors.[32] Treatment of the malignancy alone is unlikely to improve survival, because most patients die of opportunistic infections rather than tumor effects.[32]

Epidemiologic studies indicate that women with HIV infection experience a higher incidence of cervical dysplasia than non-HIV–infected women.[36] These lesions, usually a slowly developing precursor to cervical carcinoma, progress rapidly in women with HIV infection.[36] They are thought to result from infection with human papillomavirus (HPV). In addition to the rapid progression from mild dysplasia to carcinoma in situ, women with HIV infection may be less responsive to standard treatments and have a poorer prognosis than uninfected women.[36] Occurrence of cervical dysplasia is detected by Papanicolaou (Pap) smear and cervical colposcopy.

Wasting Syndrome

HIV wasting syndrome is one of the criteria for AIDS in the case definition.[24] The syndrome is common in persons with HIV infection or AIDS. In Africa, AIDS has become known as "slim disease" because of this condition, which is characterized by profound involuntary weight loss (>10% of baseline body weight), severe diarrhea, and chronic weakness with fever.[24] This diagnosis is made when no other opportunistic infections or neoplasms can be identified as causing these symptoms.[24]

Early Management

After HIV infection is confirmed, laboratory and other test results are combined with the results of the physical examination to determine the stage of the disease. Therapeutic intervention is based on the stage of the infection and the appearance of specific opportunistic diseases and conditions. A careful physical examination and evaluation of recent complaints and symptoms are components of the initial staging process. Early recognition of HIV is becoming more common and medical intervention in the early stages may delay life-threatening symptoms and slow the spread of disease. Because of frequent advances in the management of HIV infection, primary care givers must be prepared to update their knowledge of diagnosis, testing, evaluation, and medical intervention. The United States Public Health Service issued Early HIV Infection Clinical Practice Guidelines in 1994 to assist clinicians in caring for persons with HIV disease[37] and the Guidelines for the Prevention of Opportunistic Infections in HIV-Infected Persons in 1995.[38]

Treatment

There is no cure for AIDS. An increasing number of therapeutics, however, are being approved by the FDA for treatment of HIV infection. Opportunistic diseases are treated individually with standard and experimental protocols such as antibiotics, antifungals, and anticancer therapies.[39] Although still under investigation, there is currently no vaccine to prevent HIV infection.

Many drugs aimed at stopping the replication of HIV in cells are under investigation. Actions of these drugs vary from interfering with the time the HIV attaches to the host cell to the phase when new virions are released. Most of the currently available drugs are inhibitors of reverse transcriptase or of protease.[39] Nucleoside analogues, a class of reverse transcriptase inhibitors, have been shown to prevent the spread of HIV to new cells.[39] Although these drugs can prevent the spread of infectious virus to new cells, they do not interfere with the replication of the virus after infection has been established inside the host cell.[39] Protease inhibitors target events later in the replication cycle and have shown dramatic success in treating HIV infection.[39] For example, noninfectious particles are formed inside the host cell when HIV protease, an essential element for producing virions, is blocked with a protease inhibitor drug.[39]

Combining multiple drugs as a therapeutic approach has also been shown to reduce problems of drug failure, viral resistance, and drug toxicity.[39] The synergistic effects of the different drugs allows smaller dosages, and the variety of mechanisms act on different cells and stages of the replication cycle.[39] In general, antiviral therapies are prescribed to improve the overall survival time of persons with HIV infection and to slow the progression to AIDS. Other drugs have been approved and are commonly used for the prevention and treatment of opportunistic infections and conditions, including *P. carinii* pneumonia, toxoplasmosis, Kaposi's sarcoma, cryptococcal meningitis, and cytomegalovirus retinitis.[35]

Theoretically, other infections may increase HIV-related disease progression through activation of the immune system.[40] Persons with HIV should be advised to avoid infections as much as possible and seek evaluation promptly when they occur. Immunization is important, because persons infected with HIV are at risk of developing many infectious diseases. Some of these diseases can be avoided by vaccination while the immune system's responsiveness is relatively intact. Pneumococcal vaccine should be given once, as soon as possible after HIV infection is diagnosed, and influenza vaccine should be given yearly. Bacille Calmette-Guérin (BCG), oral typhoid vaccine, or live-virus vaccines should not be given to persons with HIV infection or AIDS.[41] Persons with asymptomatic HIV infection should be vaccinated against measles, mumps, and rubella.[41] Persons with HIV infection should be encouraged to avoid excessive use of alcohol, other drugs, and smoking. A balanced diet, moderate exercise, and stress management are all positive factors in maintaining a healthy lifestyle, although none have been shown to prolong life or change the prognosis of HIV infection. After a diagnosis of AIDS has been made, the survival rate is approximately 50% at 1 year and 15% at 5 years.[42]

Psychosocial Issues

The psychologic effects of HIV infection or AIDS may be just as significant as the physical effects. The dramatic impact of this catastrophic illness is compounded by complex reactions on the part of the person with HIV or AIDS, his or her partner, friends and family, members of the health care team, and the community. These reactions may be influenced by inadequate information, fear of contagion, shame, prejudices, and condemnation of risk behaviors.[43] In addition to the fear and grief associated with death, the person with HIV or AIDS may also experience guilt, anger, and uncertainty.[43] Questioning and self-examination are common as the person attempts to cope with the disease.[43] Preexisting psychiatric conditions may include alcohol and drug abuse. Appropriate treatment should be made available when alcohol or other drug dependence is evident.

The person with HIV infection or AIDS may feel helpless, hopeless, stigmatized, and out of control.[44] HIV or AIDS affects all spheres of life. Isolated from peers and with a threatened sense of identity, the person may be anxious, depressed, and miserable.[44] Acknowledging a diagnosis of AIDS may be the first indication to family and colleagues of otherwise hidden lifestyles (*i.e.*, homosexuality or drug use). This increases the strain on relationships with important support persons.

Diagnosis and treatment of cognitive and affective disorders are essential parts of ongoing care for the HIV-infected person.[44] The emotional stress, feelings of isolation, and sadness experienced by the person with HIV or AIDS can be overwhelming. Most persons, however, manage to learn to cope and live with their HIV infection. Persons with the disease must have as much information and control over activities as possible. They should be encouraged to direct their energies in a positive manner and continue with their social and group activities as long as such activities are helpful. Appropriate social support systems (*e.g.*, AIDS service organizations, community groups, religious organizations) should be called on to assist whenever possible. When they learn they can live with HIV infection, often for several years, many persons develop a positive outlook based on living their lives to the fullest.

To deal with these complex issues, the health care team must recognize and accept their fears, prejudices, and emotions concerning those with HIV or AIDS. Personal feelings must not prevent caregivers from acknowledging the intrinsic human worth of all persons and their right to be treated with dignity and respect. Members of the health care team should have adequate support for their own emotional needs generated from working with persons with AIDS. Grief, anxiety, and concern over stigmatization are normal feelings and should be acknowledged and dealt with through peer support or professional counseling to reduce burnout and emotional strain of members of the health care provider team.

In summary, HIV, a retrovirus, infects the body's CD4+ T cells and macrophages. HIV genetic material becomes integrated into the host cell DNA. Manifestations of infection, such as acute mononucleosis like symptoms, may occur shortly after infection or appear after a latent phase that may last many years. The end of the latent period is marked by the onset of severe opportunistic infections and cancers. The complications of these infections, manifested throughout the respiratory, gastrointestinal, and nervous systems, include pneumonia, esophagitis, diarrhea, gastroenteritis, tumor, wasting syndrome, altered mental status, seizures, and motor deficits. HIV is diagnosed by the enzyme immunoassay and the Western blot assay–antibody detection tests that are sensitive, specific, and reliable. The emotional stress, feelings of isolation, and sadness experienced by the person with HIV or AIDS can be overwhelming, but most persons adjust to living with HIV infection. Diagnosis and treatment of cognitive and affective disorders are an essential part of ongoing care for the HIV-infected person. Appropriate treatment should be made available when alcohol or other drug dependence is noticed.

Prevention of HIV Infection

On completion of this section of the chapter, you should be able to do the following:

- Discuss the CDC recommendations for preventing the transmission of HIV and HBV to patients during exposure-prone invasive procedures
- Describe the universal precautions for HIV infection

Preventive Strategies

Because there is no cure for HIV or AIDS, adopting risk-free or low-risk behavior is the best protection against the disease. Abstinence or long-term, mutually monogamous sexual relationships between two uninfected partners are ways to avoid HIV infection and other sexually transmitted diseases. Correct and consistent use of latex condoms can provide protection from the disease by not allowing contact with semen or vaginal secretions during intercourse.[45] "Natural" or "lambskin" condoms do not provide the same protection from HIV as latex because of the larger pores in the material.[45] Only water-based lubricants should be used with condoms; petroleum (oil-based) products weaken the structure of the latex.[45]

The use of injecting drugs provides another opportunity for HIV transmission. Avoiding recreational drug use and particularly avoiding the practice of using syringes that may have been used by another person are important to AIDS prevention. Medical and public health authorities recommend that persons who inject drugs use a new sterile syringe for each injection, or if this is not possible, clean their syringes thoroughly with full-strength household bleach.

Substances that alter inhibitions can lead to risky sexual behavior. For example, smoking cocaine (*i.e.*, "crack") heightens the perception of sexual arousal, and this can influence the user to practice unsafe sexual behavior.[46] The addictive nature of many recreational drugs can lead to an increase in the frequency of unsafe sexual behavior and the number of partners as the user engages in sex exchanged for money or drugs.[46] Persons concerned about their risk should be encouraged to get information and counseling about their infection status.

Public health programs in the United States have been profoundly affected by the HIV epidemic. Although standard methods for disease intervention and statistical analysis are applied to HIV, public health programs have become more responsive to community concerns, confidentiality, and long-term follow-up of clients as a direct result of the HIV epidemic. Testing for HIV antibodies and counseling have become widely available in the

United States. Whenever HIV testing is performed, counseling should be offered. HIV prevention counseling should be culturally competent, sensitive to issues of sexual identity, developmentally appropriate, and linguistically relevant.[47]

The essential elements of any HIV prevention counseling interaction include a personalized risk assessment and prevention plan.[48] Education and behavioral intervention continue to be the mainstay of HIV prevention programs. Individual risk assessment and education regarding HIV transmission and possible prevention techniques or skills are delivered to persons in clinical settings and to those at high risk of infection in community settings. Community-wide education is provided in schools, in the workplace, and in the media. Training for professionals can have an impact on HIV spread and is an important element of prevention. The constant addition of new information on HIV makes prevention ever changing and challenging.

Universal Precautions

Universal precautions are intended to prevent parenteral, mucous membrane, and nonintact skin exposures of health care workers to blood-borne pathogens. These procedures are referred to as "universal" because they are intended for use with all patients. The precautions apply to all body fluids that may contain HIV (*i.e.*, blood, semen, vaginal or cervical secretions, and other bodily fluids if they are visibly contaminated with blood).[16] Blood is the single most important source of HIV pathogens in the occupational setting, although universal precautions also apply to semen and vaginal or cervical secretions. Because the associated risk of transmission is unknown, universal precautions should also be used with tissues and fluids that ordinarily would be handled with aseptic technique, such as cerebrospinal, pleural, peritoneal, pericardial, and amniotic fluids.[16]

Universal precautions do not apply to the following fluids, unless they contain visible blood, because the risk of transmission is extremely low or nonexistent: feces, nasal secretions, sputum, sweat, tears, urine, saliva, and vomitus. Epidemiologic studies have not shown HIV to be transmitted by any of these fluids in health care or community settings.[16]

General infection control practices include the use of gloves for digital examinations of mucous membranes and endotracheal suctioning and handwashing after all contact with patients or their body fluids. The general principles of universal precautions are listed in Chart 13–1. The U.S. Occupational Safety and Health Administration (OSHA) has enacted regulations that mandate hospitals and other health care employers to provide personal protective equipment to employees who may come in contact with blood or other potentially infectious materials.[49] Personal protective equipment includes gloves, gowns, laboratory coats, face shields or masks, eye protection, mouth pieces, resuscitation bags, and pocket masks or other ventilation devices.[49]

Study results indicate that HIV is sensitive to chemical disinfectants. Commonly used germicides at the manufacturer recommended concentrations inactivate HIV within 2 to 10 minutes. Sodium hypochlorite (*i.e.*, household bleach) in a water dilution from 1:10 to 1:100 and 70% alcohol (*e.g.*, ethyl, isopropyl) inactivated the virus within 1 minute of contact.[50]

In summary, risk-free or low-risk behavior is the best protection against HIV infection, because there is no cure for AIDS. Abstinence or long-term mutually monogamous sexual relationships between two uninfected partners, use of condoms, avoiding drug use and the use of nonsterile syringes, and the practice of universal precautions by health care workers are essential to stopping the spread of HIV.

HIV Infection in Infants and Children

On completion of this section of the chapter, you should be able to do the following:

- Discuss the vertical transmission of HIV from mother to child and recommended prevention measures
- Cite problems with diagnosis of HIV infection in the infant
- Compare the progress of HIV infection in infants and children with HIV infection in adults

Although early in the epidemic children with AIDS might have become infected through receiving blood products or blood transfusions, almost all of the current transmission of HIV infection to children in the United States occurs perinatally. Infected women may transmit the virus to their offspring *in utero*, during labor and delivery, or through breast milk. Diagnosis of HIV infection in children born to HIV-infected mothers is complicated by the presence of maternal HIV antibody, which crosses the placenta to the fetus.[51] Consequently, all infants born to HIV-infected women are HIV-antibody positive at birth, although only 15% to 30% are actually infected.[51] In uninfected infants, this antibody usually persists until the child is 9 to 18 months of age.[51]

Although a positive antibody test alone does not diagnose HIV infection in the newborn, the test does identify a perinatally exposed infant who requires careful follow-up and management. Clinical evaluation and repeated testing are the primary means of diagnosis in these infants. Children born to mothers with HIV infection are considered uninfected with HIV if they become HIV-antibody negative after 6 months of age, have no other laboratory evidence of HIV infection, and have not met the surveillance case definition criteria for AIDS in children.[51] Infected infants usually appear well for the first few months of life, although immune abnormalities can sometimes be detected. A number of children have remained well or with mild symptoms for more than 5 years.[14]

Although transmission of HIV to a fetus can take place as early as the 8th week of gestation, research data suggest that at least one half of perinatally transmitted infections occur during or shortly after the birth process.[15] The risk of transmission is increased if the mother has a low CD4+ T-cell counts, high level of HIV in the blood, or advanced HIV disease and if there is increased exposure of the fetus to maternal blood, premature rupture of membranes, premature delivery, or the mother breast-feeds the baby.[15]

Among children with AIDS reported to CDC in 1995, 27% had PCP, 19% had lymphoid interstitial pneumonitis, 15% had recurrent serious bacterial infections, and 16% had *Candida* esophagitis. Wasting syndrome was reported in 18%, and HIV encephalopathy was reported in 17% of the children.[3] Clinical presentation and age at diagnosis are related to survival of children with AIDS. Overall, 57% of the children reported to CDC in 1988 and 1989 were alive 12 months after diagnosis. A major cause of early mortality for HIV-infected children is PCP.[14] The 1-year survival rate was only 30% for children younger than 12 months of age with PCP, compared with 55% for children younger than 12 months with other conditions.[14] One-year survival rates for older children were 48% for those with PCP and 72% for those with other conditions.[14]

Infants clearly progress faster than adults in developing immunodeficiency and related illnesses.[14] Modeling of the incubation period for infants suggests that 3 years is the median age at which AIDS is diagnosed.[14] In adults, the median incubation period is about 10 years. Few adults develop AIDS in the first 3 years after infection.[14] The relative immaturity of the immune system of infants may account for the more rapid progression, as may many other factors such as route of infection and dose of virus.[14] Infants born to infected mothers are significantly more likely to develop AIDS in the first year of life than infants infected by blood transfusions.[14]

Perinatal transmission can be lowered by two thirds by treating the mother during the end of her pregnancy and the baby when it is born with the antiviral medication zidovudine.[52] The United States Public Health Service and the American Academy of Pediatrics therefore recommend that HIV counseling and testing should be offered to all pregnant women and women of childbearing age in the United States.[15] The recommendations also stress that women who test positive for HIV antibodies should be informed of the perinatal prevention benefits of zidovudine therapy and offered this treatment.[15] Additional benefits of voluntary testing for mothers and newborns include reduced morbidity because of intensive treatment and supportive health care, the opportunity for early antiviral therapy, and information regarding the risk of transmission from breast milk.[53]

In summary, Infected women may transmit the virus to their offspring *in utero,* during labor and delivery, or through breast milk. Diagnosis of HIV infection in children born to HIV-infected mothers is complicated by the presence of maternal HIV antibody, which crosses the placenta to the fetus. This antibody usually disappears within 9 and 18 months in uninfected children. Perinatal transmission can be lowered by treating the mother during the end of her pregnancy and the baby when it is born with the antiviral medication zidovudine.

REFERENCES

1. Koop C.E. (1986). *The Surgeon General's report on acquired immune deficiency syndrome* (p. 6). Washington, DC: U.S. Department of Health and Human Services.
2. Karon J.M., Rosenberg P.S., McQuillan G., et al. (1996). Prevalence of HIV infection in the United States, 1984 to 1992. *Journal of the American Medical Association* 276, 126–131.
3. Centers for Disease Control and Prevention. (1995). HIV/AIDS surveillance report. *Morbidity and Mortality Weekly Report* 7, 1–39.
4. Centers for Disease Control and Prevention. (1996). Update: Mortality attributable to HIV infection among persons aged 25–44 years—United States. *Morbidity and Mortality Weekly Report* 45, 121–125.
5. Curran J.W., Morgan W.M., Hardy A.M., et al. (1985). The epidemiology of AIDS: Current status and future prospects. *Science* 229, 1352.
6. Montagnier L., Alizon M. (1986). The human immune deficiency virus (HIV): An update. In Gluckman J.C., Vilmer E. (Eds.). *Proceedings of the Second International Conference on AIDS* (p. 13). Paris: Elsevier.
7. Friedland G.H., Klein R.S. (1987). Transmission of the human immunodeficiency virus. *New England Journal of Medicine* 317, 1125.
8. Centers for Disease Control. (1982). Update on acquired immune deficiency syndrome (AIDS)—United Stated. *Morbidity and Mortality Weekly Report* 31 (37), 507–514.
9. Joint United Nations Programme on AIDS. (1996). *The HIV/AIDS situation in mid-1996: Global and regional highlights.* Geneva, Switzerland: UNAIDS.
10. Hellinger F.J. (1991). Forecasting the medical care costs of the HIV epidemic: 1991–1994. *Inquiry* 28, 213–225.
11. Rutherford G.W., Lifson A.R., Hessol N.A., et al. (1990). Course of HIV-1 infection in a cohort of homosexual and bisexual men: An 11-year follow-up study. *British Medical Journal* 301, 1183–1188.
12. O'Brien T.R., George J.R., Holmberg S.D. (1992). Human immunodeficiency virus type-2 infection in the United States—epidemiology, diagnosis, and public health implications. *Journal of the American Medical Association* 267, 2775–2779.
13. Gershon R.R.M., Vlahov D., Nelson K.E. (1990). The risk of transmission of HIV-1 through non-percutaneous, nonsexual modes—a review. *AIDS* 4, 645–650.
14. Oxtoby M.J. (1990). Perinatally acquired human immunodeficiency virus infection. *Pediatric Infectious Disease Journal* 9, 609–619.
15. Centers for Disease Control and Prevention. (1995). U.S. Public Health Service recommendations for human immunodeficiency virus counseling and voluntary testing for pregnant women. *Morbidity and Mortality Weekly Report* 44(RR-7), 1–15.

16. Centers for Disease Control. (1988). Update: Universal precautions for prevention of transmission of human immunodeficiency virus, hepatitis B virus, and other blood-borne pathogens in health-care settings. *Morbidity and Mortality Weekly Report* 37, 377.
17. Centers for Disease Control and Prevention. (1996). Update: Provisional public health service recommendations for chemoprophylaxis after occupational exposure to HIV. *Morbidity and Mortality Weekly Report* 45, 468–469.
18. Centers for Disease Control. (1991). Recommendations for preventing transmission of human immunodeficiency virus and hepatitis B virus to patients during exposure-prone invasive procedures. *Morbidity and Mortality Weekly Report* 40, 1–9.
19. Wasserheit J.N. (1992). Epidemiological synergy–interrelationships between human immunodeficiency virus infection and other sexually transmitted diseases. *Sexually Transmitted Diseases* 19(2), 61–77.
20. Horsburgh C.R., Jason J., Longini I.M., et al. (1989). Duration of human immunodeficiency virus infection before detection of antibody. *Lancet* 16, 637–639.
21. Levy J.A. (1988). The human immunodeficiency virus (HIV) and its pathogenic properties. In Schinaz R.F., Nahmias A.J. (Eds.). *AIDS in children, adolescents and heterosexual adults* (pp. 117–125). New York: Elsevier.
22. Fauci A.S. (1988). The human immunodeficiency virus: Infectivity and mechanisms of pathogenesis. *Science* 239, 617–622.
23. Pantaleo G., Graziosi C., Fauci A.S. (1993). The immunopathogenesis of human immunodeficiency virus infection. *New England Journal of Medicine* 328, 327–335.
24. Centers for Disease Control. (1987). Revision of the CDC surveillance case definition for acquired immunodeficiency syndrome. *Morbidity and Mortality Weekly Report* 36, 3S.
25. Kassler W.J., Alwano-Edyegu M.G., Marum E., et al. (1996). The performance of rapid on-site HIV assay in Uganda: Results of a field trial. *XI International Conference on AIDS*, Vancouver, British Columbia, Canada.
26. Francis D.P., Chin J. (1987). The prevention of acquired immunodeficiency syndrome in the United States. *Journal of the American Medical Association* 257, 1357.
27. Branson B.M. (1966). Home testing for HIV—It's coming. Are you ready? *International AIDS Society Newsletter* March 4.
28. Rogers M.F., Ou C.Y., Kilbourne B., Schochetman G. (1991). Advances and problems in the diagnosis of human immunodeficiency virus infection in infants. *Pediatric Infectious Disease Journal* 10, 523–531.
29. Centers for Disease Control and Prevention. (1992). 1993 Revised classification system for HIV infection and expanded surveillance case definition for AIDS among adolescents and adults. *Morbidity and Mortality Weekly Report* 41 (RR-17), 1–23.
30. Ho D.D., Sarngadharan M.G., Resnick L., et al. (1985). Primary human T-lymphotropic virus type III infection. *Annals of Internal Medicine* 103, 880.
31. Tindall B., Cooper D.A. (1991). Primary HIV infection: Host responses and intervention strategies. *AIDS* 5, 1–14.
32. Sherertz R.A. (1985). Acquired immune deficiency syndrome. *Medical Clinics of North America* 69, 637.
33. Snider D.E., Roper W.L. (1992). The new tuberculosis. *New England Journal of Medicine* 326, 703–705.
34. Price R.W., Brew B., Sidtis J., et al. (1988). The brain in AIDS: Central nervous system HIV-1 infection and AIDS dementia complex. *Science* 239, 586.
35. Flaskerud J.H., Ungvarski P.J. (1995). *HIV/AIDS: A guide to nursing care* (3rd ed.). Philadelphia: W.B. Saunders.
36. Centers for Disease Control. (1990). Risk of Cervical disease in HIV infected women. *Morbidity and Mortality Weekly Report* 39, 846–849.
37. Agency for Health Care Policy and Research. (1990). Clinical practice guideline No. 7: *Evaluation and management of early HIV infection.* AHCPR Publication No. 94–0572. Bethesda, MD: U.S. Department of Health and Human Services.
38. Centers for Disease Control and Prevention. (1995). USPHS/IDSA guidelines for prevention of opportunistic infections in persons infected with human immunodeficiency virus: A summary. *Morbidity and Mortality Weekly Report* 44(RR-8), 1–34.
39. Hirsch M.S., D'Aquila R.T. (1993). Therapy for human immunodeficiency virus infection. *New England Journal of Medicine* 328, 1686–1695.
40. Quinn T.C., Piot P., McCormick J.B., et al. (1987). Serologic and immunologic studies in patients with AIDS in North America and Africa. The potential role of infectious agents as cofactors in human immunodeficiency virus infection. *Journal of the American Medical Association* 257, 2617.
41. Centers for Disease Control. (1991). Update on adult immunization–recommendations of the Immunization Practices Advisory Committee (ACIP). *Morbidity and Mortality Weekly Report* 40, 13.
42. Rothenberg R., Woelfel M., Stoneburner R., et al. (1987). Survival with the acquired immunodeficiency syndrome. *New England Journal of Medicine* 317, 1297.
43. Lippman S.W., James W.A., Frierson R.L. (1993). AIDS and the family: Implications for counselling. *AIDS Care* 5, 71–78
44. O'Brien A.M., Oerlemans-Bunn M., Blachfield J.C. (1987). Nursing the AIDS patient at home. *AIDS Patient Care* 1, 21.
45. Centers for Disease Control. (1988). Condoms for the prevention of sexually transmitted diseases. *Morbidity and Mortality Weekly Report* 37, 133–137.
46. Edlin B.R., Irwin K.L., Faruque S., et al. and the Multicenter Crack Cocaine and HIV Infection Study Team. (1994). Intersecting epidemics—Crack cocaine use and HIV infection among inner-city young adults. *New England Journal of Medicine* 331, 1422–1427.
47. Valdiserri R.O., Moore M., Gerber A.R., et al. (1993). A study of clients returning for counseling after HIV testing: Implications for improving rates of return. *Public Health Reports* 108, 12–18.
48. Centers for Disease Control and Prevention. (1993). Recommendations for HIV testing services for inpatients and outpatients in acute-care hospital settings and technical guidance on HIV counseling. *Morbidity and Mortality Weekly Report* 42 (RR-2), 1–5 and 11–16.
49. Department of Labor, Occupational Safety and Health Administration. (1991). *Occupational exposure to bloodborne pathogens: Final rule* (29 CFR 1910.1030) (pp. 64004–64182). Washington, DC: Federal Register December 6, 1991.
50. Resnick L., Veren K., Salhuddin S.K., et al. (1986). Stability and inactivation of HTLV-III/LAV under clinical and laboratory environments. *Journal of the American Medical Association* 255, 1887.
51. Centers for Disease Control and Prevention. (1994). 1994 Revised classification system for human immunodeficiency virus infection in children less than 13 years of age. *Morbidity and Mortality Weekly Report* 43 (RR-12), 1–10.
52. Connor E.M., Sperling R.S., Gleber R., et al. (1994). Reduction of maternal-infant transmission of human immunodeficiency virus type 1 with zidovudine treatment. *New England Journal of Medicine* 331, 1173 1180.

53. American Academy of Pediatrics. (1992). Perinatal human immunodeficiency virus (HIV) testing. *Pediatrics* 89, 791–793.

ADDITIONAL READINGS

Agency for Health Care Policy and Research (AHCPR), Public Health Service, USDHHS. (1994). *Evaluation and management of early HIV infection. Clinical Practice Guideline. No. 7.* AHCPR publication No. 94–0572. Rockville, MD: U.S. Department of Health and Human Services.

American Medical Association. (1996). *A Physician Guide to HIV Prevention.* Chicago: American Medical Association.

Burroughs M.H., Edelson P.J. (1991). Medical care of the HIV-infected child. *Pediatric Clinics of North America* 38, 45–67.

Caldwell M.B., Rogers M.F. (1991). Epidemiology of pediatric HIV infection. *Pediatric Clinics of North America* 38, 1–16.

Centers for Disease Control. (1992). Recommendations for prophylaxis against *Pneumocystis carinii* pneumonia for adults and adolescents infected with human immunodeficiency virus. *Morbidity and Mortality Weekly Report* 41 (RR-4), 1–11.

Darrow W.W. (1991). AIDS: Socioepidemiologic responses to an epidemic. In Ulack R., Skinner W.F. (Eds.). *AIDS and the social sciences: Common threads* (pp. 82–99). Lexington: The University Press of Kentucky.

Farizo K.M., Buehler J.W., Chamberland M.E., et al. (1992). Spectrum of disease in persons with human immunodeficiency virus infection in the United States. *Journal of the American Medical Association* 267, 1798–1805.

Flaskerud J.H., Ungvarski P.J. (1995). *HIV/AIDS: A guide to nursing care* (3rd ed.). Philadelphia: W.B. Saunders.

Goldschmid R.H., Moy A. (1996). Antiretroviral drug treatment for HIV / AIDS. *American Family Physician* 54, 574–580.

Graham N., Zeger S.L., Park L.P., et al. (1992). The effects on survival of early treatment of human immunodeficiency virus infection. *New England Journal of Medicine* 326, 1037–1042.

Hinman A.R. (1991). Strategies to prevent HIV infection in the United States. *American Journal of Public Health* 81, 1557–1559.

Hoyt M.J., Staats A. (1991). Wasting and malnutrition in patients with HIV / AIDS. *Journal of the Association of Nurses in AIDS Care* 2, 16–26.

Kassler W.J., Wu A.W. (1992). Addressing HIV infection in office practice. *Primary Care* 19, 19–33.

Phillips T.J., Dover J.S. (1992). Human immunodeficiency virus infection. *New England Journal of Medicine* 326, 172–178.

Prober C.G., Gershon A.A. (1991). Medical management of newborns and infants born to human immunodeficiency virus seropositive mothers. *Pediatric Infectious Disease Journal* 10, 684–695.

Wei X., Ghosh SK., Taylor ME., Johnson VA., et al. (1995). Viral dynamics in human immunodeficiency virus type 1 infection. *Nature* 373 (6510), 117–122.

UNIT IV

Integumentary Function

Dermatoglyphics, or the study of the ridges on the skin of the fingertips and palms of the hand, has intrigued cultures throughout the ages. These ridges, which are unique to each individual, develop early in fetal life. In the days before written signatures, the fingerprint was often used as a personal seal on land sales, loans, and other transactions. Some of the first evidence of the use of fingerprints comes from China, where the practice of imprinting fingers extends over centuries. In the 16th century, when the sale of children was common among the Chinese, whole palm and sole prints were often included on the deed of sale.

Although elements of symbolism, magic, and superstition abound with deciphering of palm creases and fingertip ridges in areas such as fortune-telling, scientific interest was delayed until the late 18th and early 19th centuries. In 1823, J.E. Purkinje (1787–1869) developed the first classification of patterns for fingerprint ridges, providing the basis for the use of fingerprints as a means of personal identification. This was followed by an 1880 publication of Henry Faulds (1843–1930), who suggested that fingerprints left at the crime scene could serve as positive identification of offenders when apprehended.

CHAPTER 14

Control of Integumentary Function

Gladys Simandl

The skin is primarily an organ of protection. It is the largest organ of the body and forms the major barrier between the internal organs and the external environment. The skin accounts for roughly 16% of the body's weight. As the body's first line of defense, the skin is continuously subjected to potentially harmful environmental agents, including solid matter, liquids, gases, sunlight, and microorganisms. Although the skin may become bruised, lacerated, burned, or infected, it has remarkable properties that allow for a continuous cycle of healing, shedding, and cell regeneration.

In its protective role, the skin has a constant flora of microorganisms. Relatively harmless strains protect the skin surface from other, more virulent organisms. A thin layer of lipid film covers the skin that contains fatty acids that are bactericidal, protecting against entry of harmful microorganisms. The skin also serves as an immunologic barrier. The Langerhans' cells detect foreign antigens, playing an important part in allergic skin conditions and skin graft rejections. As a chemical barrier, the skin controls substances entering or leaving the body.

The skin serves several other important functions. The skin is richly innervated with pain, temperature, and touch receptors. Skin receptors relay the numerous qualities of touch, such as pressure, sharpness, dullness, and pleasure to the central nervous system (CNS) for localization and fine discrimination. The skin is important in regulating body temperature (see Chapter 56). The skin also plays an essential role in vitamin D_3 synthesis, which controls calcium and phosphate metabolism.

The skin may demonstrate outwardly what occurs in the body systemically. A number of systemic diseases are manifested by skin disorders (*e.g.*, systemic lupus erythematosus, several forms of cancer, Kaposi's sarcoma associated with acquired immunodeficiency syndrome [AIDS]). This means that, although skin eruptions frequently represent primary disease of the skin, they may also be a manifestation of systemic disease.

The skin also has an elusive quality of reflecting emotional states, regardless of disease. It is through the skin that warmth and human affection are given and received. The skin conveys notions of health, beauty, integrity, and love. Human beings emphasize the body and, in particular, the skin to the degree that even slight imperfections may evoke a wide variety of human responses. As more is learned about the skin through scientific investigations, the importance of considering mind-body connections when working with persons who have skin disorders is becoming increasingly apparent.

Structure of the Skin

After you have completed this chapter, you should be able to do the following:

- List and describe the functions of skin
- Describe the changes in a keratinocyte from its inception in the basal lamina to its arrival on the outer surface of the skin
- List the four specialized cells of the epidermis and describe what is known about their functions
- Describe the structure and function of the dermis and subcutaneous layers of skin

- Describe the following skin appendages and their functions: sebaceous gland, eccrine gland, apocrine gland, nails, and hair
- Characterize the skin in terms of sensory and immune function

Because there are great variations in skin structure on different parts of the body, normal skin is difficult to describe. Variations are found in the properties of the skin, such as the thickness of skin layers, the distribution of sweat glands, and the number and size of hair follicles. For example, the skin is thicker on the palms of the hands and soles of the feet (0.8 mm) than elsewhere on the body (0.07 to 0.12 mm). Hair follicles are densely distributed on the scalp, axillae, and genital areas, but it is sparse on the inner arms and abdomen. The apocrine sweat glands are confined to the axillae and the anogenital area.

Nevertheless, certain structural properties are common to all skin in all areas of the body. The skin is composed of two layers: the epidermis (outer layer) and the dermis (inner layer). A basal lamina (formerly called the basement membrane) divides the two layers. The subcutaneous tissue, a layer of loose connective and fatty tissues, binds the dermis to the underlying tissues of the body (Fig. 14–1).

Epidermis

The functions of the skin depend on the properties of its outermost layer, the epidermis. The epidermis covers the body, and it is specialized to form the various skin appendages: hair, nails, and glandular structures. The keratinocytes of the epidermis produce a fibrous protein called *keratin*, which is essential to the protective function of skin. In addition to the keratinocytes, the epidermis has three other types of cells that arise from its basal layer: melanocytes that produce a pigment called melanin, which protects against ultraviolet radiation; Merkel's cells that provide sensory information, and Langerhans' cells

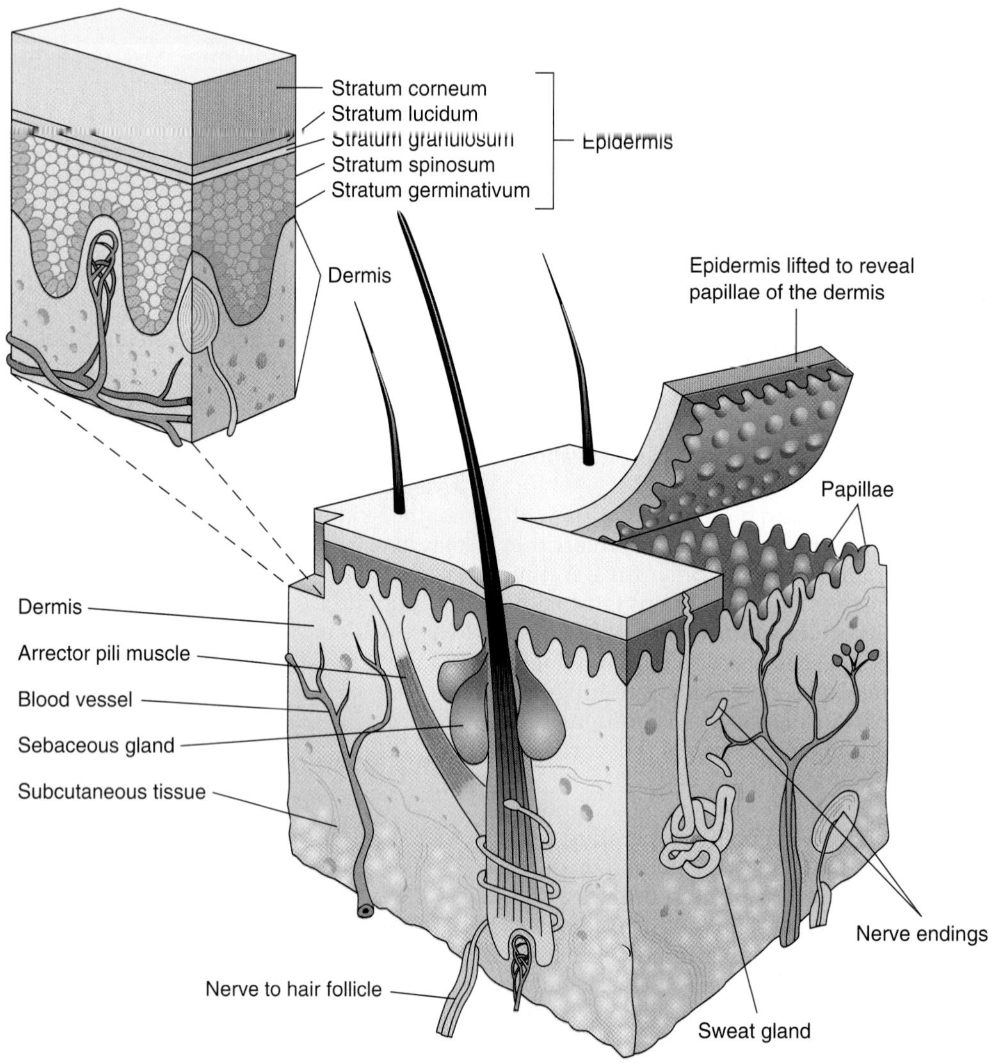

FIGURE 14–1
Three-dimensional view of the skin.

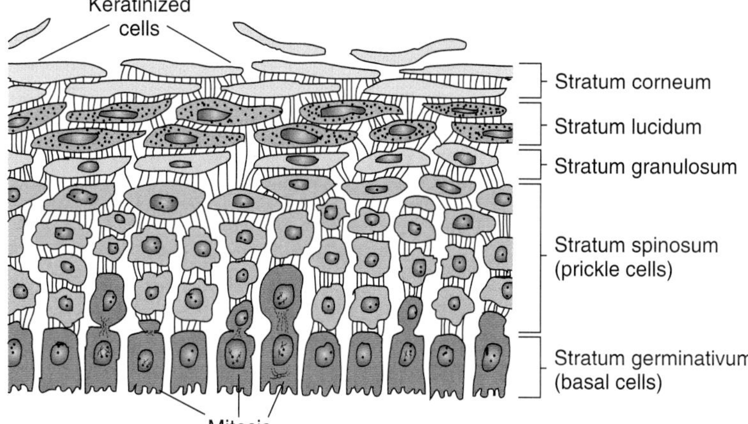

FIGURE 14–2 Epidermal cells. The basal cells undergo mitosis, producing keratinocytes that change their size and shape as they move upward, replacing cells that are lost during normal cell shedding.

that link the epidermis to the immune system. The epidermis contains openings for two types of glands, sweat glands, which produce watery secretions, and sebaceous glands, which produce an oily secretion called *sebum*.

Keratinocyte

The keratinocyte is the major cell of the epidermis. The epidermis is composed of stratified squamous keratinized epithelium, which when viewed under the microscope is seen to consist of five distinct layers, or strata, that represent a progressive differentiation or maturation of the keratinocytes: the stratum germinativum, or basal layer; the stratum spinosum; the stratum granulosum; the stratum lucidum; and the stratum corneum.

The deepest layer, the stratum germinativum or stratum basale, consists of a single layer of basal cells that are attached to the basal lamina. The basal cells, which are columnar, undergo mitosis to produce new keratinocytes that move toward the skin surface to replace cells lost during normal skin shedding. Unlike the other layers of the epidermis, the basal cells do not migrate toward the skin surface, but remain stationary in the stratum germinativum.

The next layer, the stratum spinosum, is formed as the progeny of the basal cell layer move outward toward the skin surface. This layer is two to four layers thick, and its cells become differentiated as they migrate outward. The cells of this layer are commonly referred to as prickle cells, because they develop a spiny appearance as their cell borders interact.

The stratum granulosum is only a few cells thick; it consists of granular cells that are the most differentiated cells of the living skin. The cells in this layer are unique in that two opposing functions are occurring simultaneously. While some cells are losing cytoplasm and DNA structures, others continue to synthesize keratin.

The stratum lucidum, which lies just superficial to the stratum granulosum, is thin and transparent. It consists of transitional cells that retain some of the functions of living skin cells from the layers below and resemble the cells of the stratum corneum. This layer can be seen on the palms of the hands and soles of the feet.

The top or surface layer, the stratum corneum, consists of dead, keratinized cells. This layer contains the most cell layers and the largest cells of any zone of the epidermis. It ranges from 15 layers thick in areas such as the face to 25 layers or more on the arm. Specialized areas, such as the palms of the hands or soles of the feet, have 100 or more layers.

The keratinocyte that originates in the basal layer changes morphologically as it is pushed toward the outer layer of the epidermis. For example, in the basal layer, the keratinocyte is round. As it is pushed into the stratum spinosum, the keratinocyte becomes multisided. It becomes flatter in the granular layer and is flattened and elongated in the stratum corneum (Fig. 14–2). The migration time of a keratinocyte from basal layer to the stratum corneum is 20 to 30 days. Keratinocytes also change cytoplasmic structure and composition as they are pushed outward. This transformation from viable cells to the dead cells of the stratum corneum is called *keratinization*.

The movement of the cells to the surface of the skin can best be described as random or nonsynchronized. Keratinocytes pass other keratinocytes, melanocytes, and Langerhans' cells as they migrate in a seemingly random fashion. However, the cells are connected with minute points of attachment called *desmosomes*. Desmosomes keep the cells from detaching and provide some structure to the skin while it is in perpetual motion. The basal layer provides the underlying structure and stability for the epidermis.

Melanocytes

Melanocytes are pigment-synthesizing cells that are located at or in the basal layer. They function to produce pigment granules called *melanin*, the black or brown substance that gives skin its color. The ability to synthesize melanin depends on the ability of the melanocytes to produce an enzyme called *tyrosinase*, which converts the amino acid tyrosine to a precursor of melanin. A genetic lack of this enzyme results in a clinical condition called *albinism*. Persons with this disorder lack pigmentation in the skin, hair, and iris of the eye. Tyrosinase is synthesized in the rough endoplasmic reticulum of the melanocytes and then routed to membranous vesicles in the Golgi complex called *melanosomes*. Melanin is subsequently synthesized in the melanosomes. Melano-

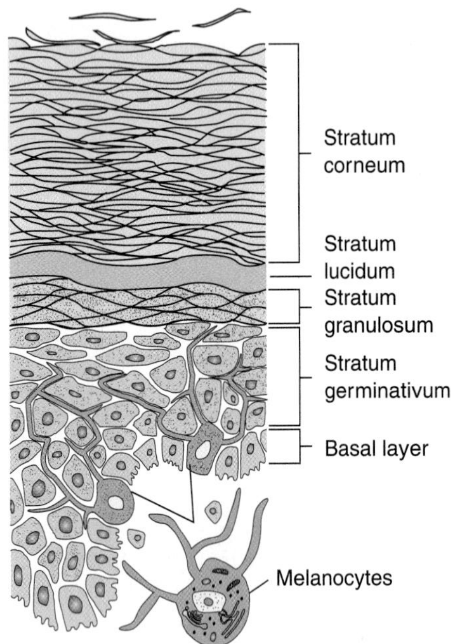

FIGURE 14–3
Melanocytes. The melanocytes, which are located in the basal layer of the skin, produce melanin pigment granules that give skin its color. The melanocytes have threadlike cytoplasmic-filled extensions that are used in passing the pigment granules to the keratinocytes.

cytes have long cytoplasm-filled extensions that extend between the keratinocytes. Although the melanocytes remain in the basal layer, the melanosomes are transferred to the keratinocytes through these dendritic processes. The dendrite tip containing the melanosome is engulfed by a nearby keratinocyte, and the melanin transferred (Fig. 14–3). Each melanocyte is capable of supplying several keratinocytes with melanin.

Exposure to the sun's ultraviolet rays increases the production of melanin, causing tanning to occur. The primary function of melanin is to protect the skin from harmful ultraviolet sun rays, which are implicated in skin cancers. Melanin protects by absorbing and scattering the radiation. The amount of melanin in the keratinocytes determines a person's skin color. Black-skinned and white-skinned people have the same amount of melanocytes. However, in the skin of African Americans, more melanosomes are produced. The greater number of melanosomes produced and transferred to the keratinocyte is responsible for the darker pigmentation in African Americans; African Americans do not have more melanocytes than whites, but the production of pigment is increased. All people have relatively few or no melanocytes in the epidermis of the palms of the hands or soles of the feet. In light-skinned people, the number of melanocytes decreases with age; the skin becomes lighter and is more susceptible to skin cancer.

Merkel's Cells

Merkel's cells consist of free nerve endings attached to modified epidermal cells. Their origin remains unknown, and they are the least densely populated cell of the epidermis. Merkel's cells are found over the entire body, but are most plentiful on the skin of the fingers, toes, lips, oral cavity, and outermost sheath of hair follicles (*i.e.*, the touch areas). It is believed that Merkel's cells function as mechanoreceptors, or touch receptors. Other encapsulated nerve endings (*e.g.*, Pacinian corpuscles, Meissner's corpuscles, Ruffini corpuscles, Krause end bulbs) are present in the dermis.

Langerhans' Cells

Langerhans' cells are located in the suprabasal layers of the epidermis among the keratinocytes. They are few compared with the keratinocytes. They are derived from precursor cells originating in the bone marrow and continuously repopulate the epidermis. Like melanocytes, they have a dendritic shape and a clear cytoplasm. *Birbeck granules* that often resemble tennis racquets are their most distinguishing characteristic microscopically.

Langerhans' cells are the immunologic cells responsible for recognizing foreign antigens harmful to the body (Fig. 14–4). As such, the Langerhans' cells play an important role in defending the body against foreign antigens. Langerhans' cells bind antigen to their surface, process it, and bearing the processed antigen, they migrate from the epidermis into lymphatic vessels and then into regional lymph nodes where they become known as *dendritic cells*. During their migration in the lymph channels, the Langerhans' cells become potent antigen-presenting cells (see Chapter 11). Langerhans' cells are innervated by sympathetic nerve fibers, which may explain why the skin's immune system is altered under stress. An example of this is the exacerbations of acne seen in persons under stress. Keratinocytes also are involved the immunologic functions of the skin. Langerhans' cells are antigen-presenting cells, and the keratinocytes produce a number of cytokines that stimulate maturation of skin-localizing T cells.

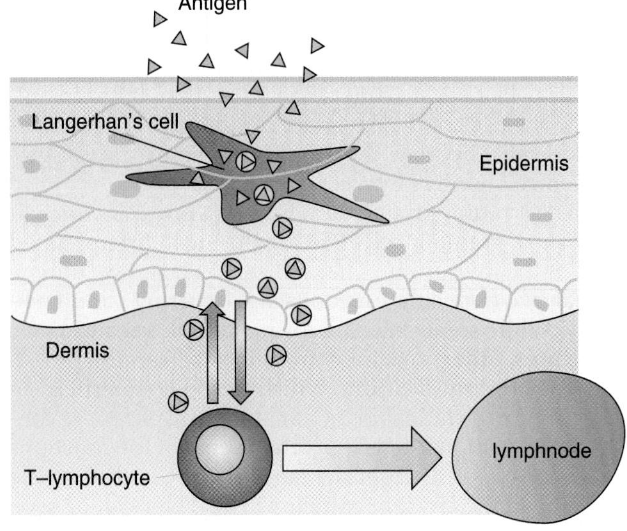

FIGURE 14–4
Langerhans' cells.

Basal Lamina

The basal lamina is a layer of intercellular matrix that connects the epidermis to the dermis, with both structures contributing to its formation. Characteristics of the basal lamina have become increasingly defined over the years. The basal lamina contains collagen fibers and glycoproteins and consists of four distinct layers, all contributing to the adhesion and elasticity of the skin. The collagen fibers provide the skin with tensile strength, anchorage, and elasticity. Compared with white skin, black skin has fewer elastic fibers throughout this layer, which may account for the decreased wrinkling associated with sun exposure and aging among black people. The glycoproteins are believed to be associated with cohesion.

The function of the basal lamina as a barrier remains debatable, because many substances are able to penetrate it. Lymphocytes, neutrophils, and Langerhans' cells easily penetrate it, but the basal lamina has been found to bar larger molecules.

Fibroblasts synthesize the intercellular matrix. They also secrete enzymes needed to break down and thereby remodel the matrix.

Dermis

The dermis is the connective tissue layer that separates the epidermis from the subcutaneous fat layer. It supports the epidermis and serves as its primary source of nutrition. The two layers of the dermis, the papillary dermis and the reticular dermis, are composed of cells, fibers, ground substances, nerves, and blood vessels. The pilar (hair) structures and glandular structures are embedded in this layer and continue through the epidermis. In general, the black dermis is more compact than the white dermis, thereby lessening wrinkling in darker-skinned people.

Papillary Dermis

The *papillary dermis* (pars papillaris) is a thin, superficial layer that lies adjacent to the epidermis. It consists of collagen fibers and ground substance. This layer is densely covered with conical projections called *dermal papillae* (see Fig. 14–1). The basal cells of the epidermis project into the papillary dermis, forming *rete ridges*. Microscopically, the junction between the epidermis and the dermis appears like undulating ridges and valleys. It is believed that the dense structure of the dermal papillae serves to minimize the separation of the dermis and the epidermis. Dermal papillae contain capillary venules, which serve to nourish the epidermal layers of the skin. This layer of the dermis is well vascularized. Lymph vessels and nerve tissue are also found in this layer.

Reticular Dermis

The *reticular dermis* (pars reticularis) is the thicker area of the dermis and forms the bulk of the dermal layer. This is the layer from which the tough leather hides of animals are made. The reticular dermis is characterized by a complex meshwork of three-dimensional collagen bundles interconnected with large elastic fibers and ground substance, a viscid gel that is rich in mucopolysaccharides. The collagen fibers are oriented parallel to the body's surface in any given area. Collagen bundles may be organized lengthwise, as on the abdomen, or in round clusters, as in the heel. The direction of surgical incisions is often determined by this organizational pattern.

Immune Cells

Immune cells found in the dermis include macrophages, T cells, mast cells, and fibroblasts. Dermal macrophages and venular epithelial cells may present antigen to T cells in the dermis. Most of these T cells are previously activated or memory T cells. T-cell responses to macrophage or endothelium-associated antigens in the dermis are probably more important in generating an immune response to antigen challenge in previously immunized persons than in initiating a response to a new antigen. The major type of T-cell–mediated immune response in the skin is delayed-type hypersensitivity (see Chapter 12).

Mast cells, which have a prominent role in IgE-mediated immediate hypersensitivity, are also present in the dermis. These cells are strategically located at body interfaces such as the skin and mucous membranes and are thought to interact with antigens that come in contact with the skin.

Blood Vessels

The arterial vessels that nourish the skin form two plexuses (*i.e.*, collection of blood vessels), one located between the dermis and the subcutaneous tissue and the other between the papillary and reticular layers of the dermis. The pink color of the skin results primarily from blood seen in the vessels of this plexus. Capillary flow that arises from vessels in this plexus also extends up and nourishes the overlaying epidermis by diffusion. Blood leaves the skin by way of small veins that accompany the subcutaneous arteries. The lymphatic system of the skin, which aids in combating certain skin infections, is also limited to the dermis.

The skin is richly supplied with arteriovenous anastomoses in which blood flows directly between an artery and a vein, bypassing the capillary circulation. These anastomoses are important in terms of temperature regulation. They can open up, letting blood flow through the skin vessels when there is a need to dissipate body heat, and close off, conserving body heat if the environmental temperature is cold.

Innervation

The innervation of the skin is complex. The skin, with its accessory structures, serves as an organ for receiving sensory information from the environment. Accordingly, the dermis is well supplied with sensory nerves. It contains nerves that supply the blood vessels, sweat glands, and arrector pili muscles.

The receptors for touch, pressure, heat, cold, and pain are widely distributed in the dermis. The papillary layer of the dermis is supplied with free nerve endings that serve as nociceptors (*i.e.,* pain) and thermoreceptors. The dermis also contains encapsulated pressure-sensitive receptors that detect pressure and touch. The largest of these are the *pacinian corpuscles,* which are widely distributed in the dermis and subcutaneous tissue. The afferent nerve endings of the pacinian corpuscle are surrounded by concentric layers of modified Schwann cells such that they resemble an onion when sectioned. Flat, encapsulated nerve endings found on the palmer surfaces of fingers and palmar surfaces and planter surfaces of the feet are called *Meissner's corpuscles.* These are highly sensitive mechanoreceptors for touch. The deep dermis is supplied with small spindle-shaped mechanoreceptors called *Ruffini corpuscles.* They register tension in the supporting collagen fibers. A few regions of the skin are supplied by *Krause end bulbs,* nerve endings contained in an ill-defined capsule. Although their function is uncertain, they are thought to function as mechanoreceptors.

Because of the variations in function among the different types of nerve endings, it is generally agreed that sensory modalities are not associated with a particular type of receptor. For example, the sensations of pain, touch, and pressure probably result from multiple stimuli. The final sensation may be the result of central summation in the CNS, which mediates patterned responses.

Most of the skin's blood vessels are under sympathetic nervous system control. The sweat glands are innervated by cholinergic fibers but controlled by the sympathetic nervous system. Likewise, the sympathetic nervous system controls the arrector pili (pilomotor) muscles that cause elevation of hairs on the skin. Contraction of these muscles tends to cause the skin to dimple, producing "goose bumps."

Subcutaneous Tissue

The subcutaneous tissue layer consists primarily of fat and connective tissues that lend support to the vascular and neural structures supplying the outer layers of the skin. There is controversy about whether the subcutaneous tissue should be considered an actual layer of the skin. Because the eccrine glands and deep hair follicles extend to this layer and several skin diseases involve the subcutaneous tissue, the subcutaneous tissue may be considered part of the skin.

Skin Appendages

The skin houses a variety of appendages, including hair, nails, and sebaceous and sweat glands. The distribution and the functions of the appendages vary.

Sweat Glands

There are two types of sweat glands: eccrine and apocrine. *Eccrine sweat glands* are simple tubular structures that originate in the dermis and open directly to the skin surface. They are numerous (several million), vary in density, and are located over the entire body surface. Their purpose is to transport sweat to the outer skin surface to regulate body temperature. *Apocrine sweat glands* are fewer in number than eccrine sweat glands. They are larger and located deep in the dermal layer. They open through a hair follicle, even though a hair may not be present, and are found primarily in the axillae and groin. The major difference between these glands and the eccrine glands is that apocrine glands secrete an oily substance. In animals, apocrine secretions give rise to distinctive odors that enable animals to recognize the presence of others. In humans, apocrine secretions are sterile until mixed with the bacteria on the skin surface; then they produce what is commonly known as body odor.

Sebaceous Glands

The sebaceous glands are located over the entire skin surface except for the palms, soles, and sides of the feet. They are part of the pilosebaceous unit. They secrete a mixture of lipids, including triglycerides, cholesterol, and wax. This mixture is called *sebum;* it lubricates hair and skin. Sebum is not the same as the surface lipid film. Sebum prevents undue evaporation of moisture from the stratum corneum during cold weather and helps to conserve body heat. Sebum production is under the control of genetic and hormonal influences. Sebaceous glands are relatively small and inactive until an individual approaches adolescence. The glands then enlarge, stimulated by the rise in sex hormones. Gland size directly influences the amount of sebum produced, and the level of androgens influences gland size. The sebaceous glands are the structures that become inflamed in acne (see Chapter 15).

Hair

Hair is a structure that originates from hair follicles in the dermis. Most hair follicles are associated with sebaceous glands, and these structures combine to form the *pilosebaceous unit.* The entire hair structure consists of the hair follicle, sebaceous gland, hair muscle (arrector pili), and in some instances, the apocrine gland (Fig. 14–5). Hair is a keratinized structure that is pushed upward from the hair follicle. Growth of the hair is centered in the bulb (*i.e.,* base) of the hair follicle, and the hair undergoes changes as it is pushed outward. Hair has been found to go through cyclic phases identified as anagen (*i.e.,* the growth phase), catagen (the atrophy phase), and telogen (*i.e.,* the resting phase). A vascular network at the site of the follicular bulb nourishes and maintains the hair follicle. Melanocytes are found in the bulb and are responsible for the color of the hair. The arrector pili muscle, located under the sebaceous gland, provides a thermoregulation function by contracting to cause "goose bumps," thereby reducing the skin surface area that is available for the dissipation of body heat.

Nails

The nails are hardened keratinized plates that protect the fingers (fingernails) and toes (toenails) and enhance dexterity. The nails grow out from curved transverse groove

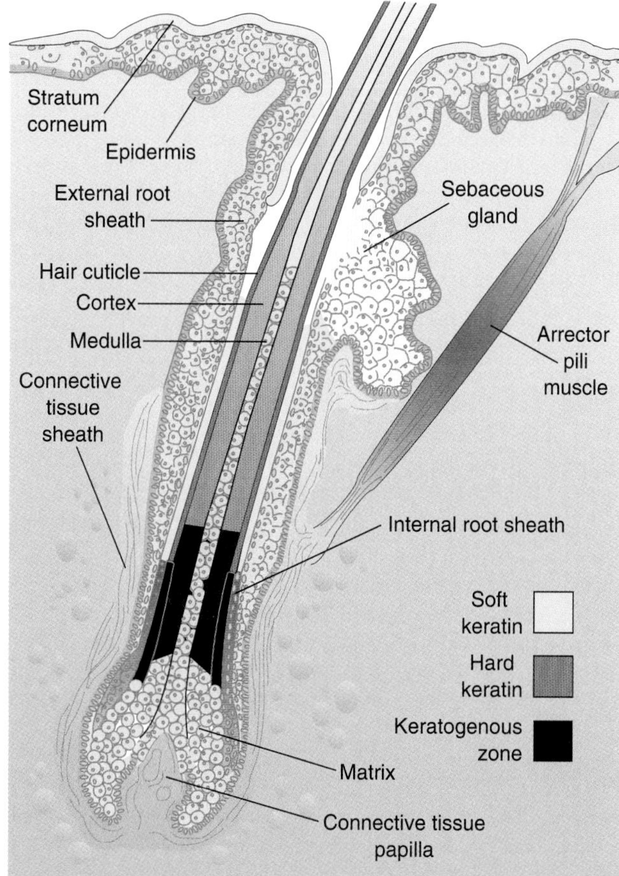

FIGURE 14–5
Parts of a hair follicle.

called the nail groove. The floor of this groove, called *nail matrix* is the germinal region of the nail plate (Fig. 14–6). The underlying epidermis, attached to the nail plate, is called the *nail bed*. Like hair, nails are the end product of dead matrix cells that are pushed outward from the nail matrix. Unlike hair, nails grow continuously rather than cyclically, unless permanently damaged or diseased. The epithelium of the fold of skin that surrounds the nail consists of the usual layers of skin. The stratum corneum forms the *eponychium* or cuticle. The nearly transparent nail plate provides a useful window for viewing the amount of oxygen in the blood, allowing a view of the color of the blood in the dermal vessels.

In summary, the skin is primarily an organ of protection. It is the largest organ of the body and forms the major barrier between the internal organs and the external environment. The skin is richly innervated with pain, temperature, and touch receptors; it synthesizes vitamin D and plays an essential role in fluid and electrolyte balance. It contributes to glucose metabolism through its glycogen stores. The skin is composed of two layers, the epidermis and the dermis, separated by a basal lamina. A layer of subcutaneous tissue binds the dermis to the underlying organs and tissues of the body. The epidermis, the outermost layer of the skin, contains five layers, or strata. The major cells of the epidermis are the keratinocytes, melanocytes, Langerhans' cells, and Merkel's cells. The stratum germinativum, or basal layer, is the source of the cells in all five layers of the epidermis. The keratinocytes, which are the major cells of the epidermis, are transformed from viable keratinocytes to dead keratin as they move from the innermost layer of the epidermis (*i.e.*, stratum germinativum) to the outermost layer (*i.e.*, stratum corneum). The melanocytes are pigment-synthesizing cells that give skin its color. The dermis provides the epidermis with support and nutrition and is the source of blood vessels, nerves, and skin appendages (*i.e.*, hair follicles, sebaceous glands, nails, and sweat glands). Sensory receptors for touch, pressure, heat, cold, and pain are widely distributed in the dermis. The skin serves as a first line of defense against microorganisms and other harmful agents. The epidermis contains Langerhans' cells, which process foreign antigens for presentation to T cells, and the dermis contains macrophages, T cells, mast cells, and fibroblasts.

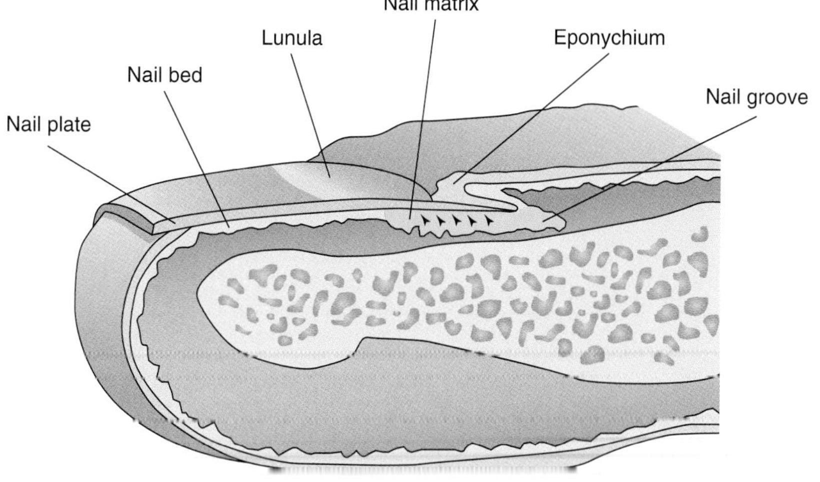

FIGURE 14–6
Parts of a fingernail. *Arrowheads* indicate the direction of displacement of nail cells in the germinal region of the nail plate.

BIBLIOGRAPHY

Cormack D.H. (1993). *Essential histology* (pp. 255–268). Philadelphia: J.B. Lippincott.

Fawcett D.W. (1994). *A textbook of histology* (12th ed., p. 525). New York: Chapman & Hall.

Montagna W., Prota G., Kenney J.A. (1993). *Black skin: Structure and function* (pp. 22–54). San Diego: Academic Press.

Moschella S.L., Hurley H.J. (1992). *Dermatology* (3rd ed.). Philadelphia: W.B. Saunders.

Rogers A.W. (1992). *Textbook of anatomy*. New York: Churchill Livingstone.

Rotstein H. (1993). *Principles and practice of dermatology* (3rd ed.). Boston: Butterworth-Heinemann.

Sternberg S.S. (1992). *Histology for pathologists*. New York: Raven Press.

CHAPTER 15

Alterations in Skin Function and Integrity

Gladys Simandl

The skin is a unique organ in that numerous signs of disease or injury are immediately observable. As an interface between the external and internal environment, skin disorders represent the culmination of environmental forces and internal functioning of the body. Sunlight, arthropods and insects, infectious agents, chemicals, and physical agents may all play a role in the pathogenesis of skin disorders. In many cases, the skin relays signs of other organic dysfunction.

Manifestations of Skin Disorders

After you have completed this section of the chapter, you should be able to meet the following objectives:

- Describe the following skin rashes and lesions: macule, patch, papule, plaque, nodule, tumor, wheal, vesicle, bulla, pustule

- Cite two physiologic explanations for pruritus
- State common alterations found in black skin
- Describe common pigmentary disorders of the skin

No two skin disorders look exactly alike, nor are they necessarily caused by the same agents. The appearance of many skin disorders are influenced by the discomfort, such as itching, that they produce or by self-treatment of the disorder. Skin color may also influence the appearance of skin disorders. Nevertheless, most skin disorders have some unique characteristics. Recognition of these characteristics contribute to accurate diagnosis and treatment. This section of the chapter covers lesions and rashes, dry skin, pruritus, skin disorders due to mechanical forces, variations in black skin, and pigmentary skin disorders.

Lesions and Rashes

Rashes are temporary eruptions of the skin, such as those associated with childhood diseases, heat, diapers, or drug-induced reactions. The term *lesion* refers to a traumatic or pathologic loss of normal tissue continuity, structure, or function. The components of a rash sometimes are referred to as lesions. Rashes and lesions may range in size from a fraction of a millimeter (e.g., the pinpoint spots of petechiae) to many centimeters (e.g., decubitus ulcer, pressure sore). They may be blanched (white), reddened (erythematous), hemorrhagic or purpuric (containing blood), or pigmented. Repeated rubbing and scratching can lead to lichenification (i.e., thickened and rough skin characterized by prominent skin markings due to repeated scratching or rubbing) or excoriation (i.e., lesion caused by breakage of the epidermis, causing a raw, linear area, often self-induced). Skin lesions may occur as primary lesions arising in previously normal skin, or they may develop as secondary lesions resulting from other disease conditions. Figure 15–1 illustrates various types of skin lesions.

Pruritus

Pruritus, or itching, is a symptom common to many skin disorders. Pruritus often accompanies skin disorders. Itching may also be symptomatic of other organ disorders, such as diabetes mellitus or biliary disease, when no skin anomaly exists.

Itch is mediated by cutaneous receptors. Itch and pain are carried by small, unmyelinated afferent C fibers found in the dermis of the skin, mucous membranes, and cornea. The C fibers enter the dorsal horn of the spinal cord, synapse, cross the midline to the opposite side of the cord, and ascend in the spinothalamic tract to the thalamus. From there, the impulse travels to the sensory cortex. A variety of mediators stimulate the C fiber endings and induce itching. Substances such as histamine, bradykinin, substance P, and bile salts act locally to stimulate the itch receptors. Warmth can also act locally to trigger the itch phenomenon. Prostaglandins are modulators of the itch response, lowering the threshold for other mediators. Morphine promotes itch while relieving pain by acting on central opioid receptors.

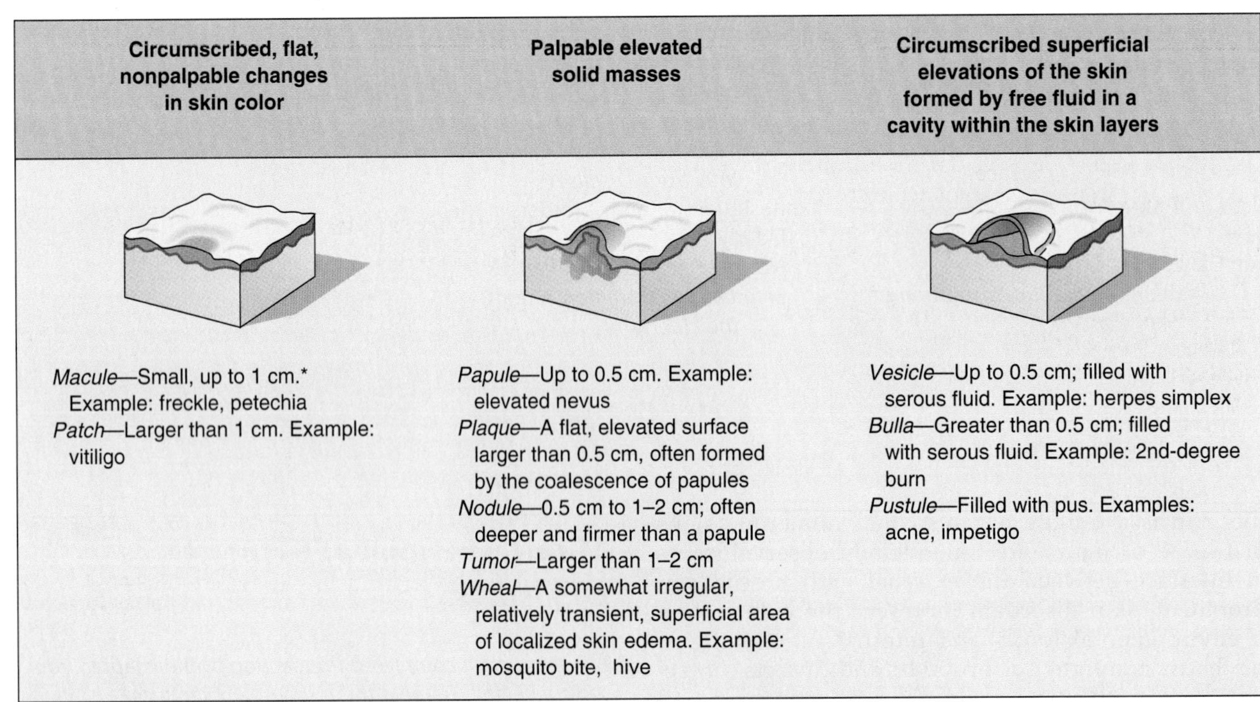

Circumscribed, flat, nonpalpable changes in skin color
Palpable elevated solid masses
Circumscribed superficial elevations of the skin formed by free fluid in a cavity within the skin layers
Macule—Small, up to 1 cm.* Example: freckle, petechia
Patch—Larger than 1 cm. Example: vitiligo
Papule—Up to 0.5 cm. Example: elevated nevus
Plaque—A flat, elevated surface larger than 0.5 cm, often formed by the coalescence of papules
Nodule—0.5 cm to 1–2 cm; often deeper and firmer than a papule
Tumor—Larger than 1–2 cm
Wheal—A somewhat irregular, relatively transient, superficial area of localized skin edema. Example: mosquito bite, hive
Vesicle—Up to 0.5 cm; filled with serous fluid. Example: herpes simplex
Bulla—Greater than 0.5 cm; filled with serous fluid. Example: 2nd-degree burn
Pustule—Filled with pus. Examples: acne, impetigo

Figure 15–1
Primary lesions may arise form previously normal skin. Authorities vary somewhat in their definitions of skin lesions by size. Dimensions given should be considered approximate.

The well-known response to an itch is scratching, which can cause skin excoriations. Because excoriated skin is more susceptible to infectious processes, measures should be taken to reduce pruritus and prevent scratching. Persons with pruritus should be instructed to keep fingernails trimmed and use the entire hand to rub over large body surfaces.[1]

Because vasodilatation increases itching, a common method of reducing pruritus is cold applications. Other treatment measures for self-limited or seasonal cases of pruritus include moisturizing lotions, bath oils, and the use of humidifiers. Application of topical corticosteroids may be helpful in some situations, such as for allergy-mediated urticaria. Administration of systemic antihistamines, opiate antagonists, and corticosteroids may be indicated for persons with severe pruritus. Some chronic forms of itching, such as chronic urticaria, are uncomfortable and psychologically debilitating. The selective use of antidepressant medications may help these persons.

Dry Skin

Dry skin (i.e., xerosis) may be a natural occurrence, as in the drying of skin associated with aging, or it may be symptomatic of underlying skin or systemic disorders. Most cases of dry skin are caused by dehydration of the stratum corneum. Any number of symptoms may accompany dry skin, such as pruritus or pain.

Treatment should be directed toward alleviation of the dry skin condition with lubricants that maintain skin hydration by serving as a barrier to evaporative water loss. Lubricants can be emollients, humectants, or occlusives. *Emollients* are lotions that contain fatty acids that generally do not leave a residue on the skin. The fatty acids replace the oils lost on the skin surface. Emollients are generally short lived and need to be reapplied frequently. *Humectants* are the additives in lotions, such as urea, that draw out water from the deeper layers and hold it on the skin surface. *Occlusives* are thick creams that contain petroleum or some other moisture-proof material; they prevent water loss. Occlusives are the most effective, but because of their greasiness and lack of cosmetic appeal, some persons do not wish to use them. Use of room humidifiers and keeping the room temperature as low as possible to prevent sweating and water loss from the skin may also be helpful.

Skin Injury From Mechanical Processes

Mechanical processes consist of rubbing, pressure, and frictional forces applied to the skin. Repeated rubbing of skin may result in necrosis of the stratum spinosum and can cause blisters, calluses, or corns.

A *blister* is a vesicle or fluid-filled papule. Blisters of mechanical origin form from the friction caused by repeated rubbing on a single area of the skin. Blisters also develop from first-degree and second-degree partial-thickness burns. Histologically, there is degeneration of epidermal cells and a disruption of intercellular junctions that causes the layers of the skin to separate. As a result, fluid accumulates, and a noticeable bleb forms on the skin surface. Blisters are best protected by adding layers of padding (*e.g.*, adhesive bandages, gauze) to prevent further blister formation. Breaking the skin of a blister to remove the fluid is inadvisable because of the risk of secondary infections.

Prolonged repeated rubbing or pressure can produce a *callus*, or area of increased skin production (*i.e.*, hyperkeratosis). Increased cohesion between cells results in hyperkeratosis and decreased skin shedding. A callus may be filed down but is likely to recur if the pressure continues.

Corns are small, well-circumscribed, conical keratinous thickenings of the skin. They usually appear on the toes from rubbing or ill-fitting shoes. The actual corn is a small, encapsulated body of hardened keratinous material. Pain often accompanies corns. Corns may be surgically removed, but they recur if the causative agent is not removed.

Alterations in Black Skin

Several skin disorders common to African Americans are not commonly found in European Americans. Similarly, some skin disorders such as skin cancers affect light-skinned persons more commonly than dark-skinned persons. Because of these differences, serious

TABLE 15-1

Common Normal Variations in Black Skin

Variation	Appearance
Futcher (Voigt's) line	Demarcation between darkly pigmented and lightly pigmented skin in upper arm; follows spinal nerve distribution; common in black and Japanese populations
Midline hypopigmentation	Line or band of hypopigmentation over the sternum, dark or faint, lessens with age; common in Latin American and black populations
Nail pigmentation	Linear dark bands down nails or diffuse nail pigmentation, brown, blue or blue-black
Oral pigmentation	Blue to blue-gray pigmentation of oral mucosa; gingivae also affected
Palmar changes	Hyperpigmented creases, small hyperkeratotic papules, and tiny pits in creases
Plantar changes	Hyperpigmented macules, can be multiple with patchy distribution, irregular borders, and variance in color

(Developed from information in Rosen T., Martin S. [1981]. *Atlas of black dermatology*. Boston: Little Brown)

skin disorders may be overlooked, and common occurrences in black skin may be mistaken for anomalies.

Because of the darker pigmentation in black skin, skin pallor, cyanosis, and erythema are more difficult to observe in African Americans. Normal variations in skin structure and skin tones make evaluation of black skin difficult (Table 15–1). Verbal histories must therefore be relied on to assess skin changes. The verbal history should include clients' descriptions of their normal skin tone. Observing for two major signs, hypopigmentation and hyperpigmentation, is also important. *Hypopigmentation* refers to a loss of pigmentation; *hyperpigmentation* refers to excessive melanin production. Loss of color and excess of color are important signs often accompanying black skin disorders. The appearances of skin disorders listed in Table 15–2 are common to the African American who represents a blend of African Negro, European Caucasian, and Native American.

Pigmentary Skin Disorders

Pigmentary skin disorders involve the melanocytes. In some cases, there is an absence of melanin production, as in vitiligo or albinism. In other cases, there is an increase in melanin or some other pigment, as in mongolian spots or melasma. In either case, the emotional impact can be devastating. Because pigmentary changes can result in social ostracism, it is also important to treat the emotional and social components of these skin disorders.

Vitiligo

Vitiligo is a pigmentary problem of concern to darkly pigmented persons of all races. It also affects whites, but not as often, and the effects are usually not as socially problematic. The lesion is a macular depigmentation with definite borders on the face, axillae, neck, or extremities (Fig. 15–2). The borders are smooth. The patches vary in size from small macules to ones involving large skin surfaces. The large macular type is more common. Depigmented areas appear white, pale colored, or sometimes grayish blue. These areas burn easily in sunlight, and they enlarge over time. The depigmented areas contain no melanocytes.

Vitiligo appears at any age, but the peak incidence is in the second and third decades. Women have a higher incidence. It has been on the rise in India, Pakistan, and Far Eastern countries. Although the cause is unknown, autoimmune factors have been implicated. The condition accompanies other autoimmune diseases, such as diabetes mellitus and pernicious anemia. Vitiligo may also be a cutaneous expression of a systemic disorder, especially thyroid disease. Although there is a familial tendency, vitiligo may be precipitated by emotional stress or physical trauma, such as sunburn.

Although treatment regimens for vitiligo are many, none is curative. Suntan lotions, skin stains, and cosmetics are used for camouflage. Topical corticosteroids have been used, and the combination of psoralen and ultraviolet A radiation treatment has been successful in patients who have involvement of 40% or more of the skin surface. If extensive skin surfaces are involved, the treatment may

TABLE 15–2
Appearance of Common Disorders of Black Skin

Disorder	Appearance
Hot-comb alopecia	Well-defined patches of scalp alopecia on crown; extends down; decreased number of follicular orifices, hair loss irreversible; due to use of hot comb with petroleum, more common with Afro hairstyles
Infantile acropustulosis	Crops of vesicopustules for 7 to 10 days, followed by a 2- to 3-week remission before recurrence; pruritus; affects palms and soles of feet in children 2 to 10 months of age; resolves by 3 years of age
Keloids	Firm, smooth, shiny hairless elevated scars, sometimes hyperpigmented; often with symptomatic pruritus, tenderness, or pain; extremely common even with simple wounds on ears, neck, jaw, cheeks, upper chest, shoulders, and back
Mongolian spot	Very common; ill-defined light blue to slate gray macule in lumbosacral area; usually disappears but may persist through adulthood
Atopic dermatitis	Follicular lesion development that progresses to a lichenification stage; hyperpigmented lichenifications are interspersed with excoriated pink patches; common in blacks
Pityriasis rosea	Lesions are salmon-pink, dull-red, or dark-brown; profuse fine scales, not commonly seen in white skin; postinflammatory pigmentary changes are more common in blacks
Psoriasis	Does not commonly occur in blacks; distribution is similar, but the plaques are bright red, violet, or blue-black; pigment changes may persist after treatment
Tinea versicolor	Common in blacks, increased incidence in tropical climates; hypopigmented or extremely hyperpigmented patches, gray to dark brown; occurs more often on the face in blacks than in whites
Lichen planus	Papules are deep purple from pigmentary leakage; oral lesions are uncommon; hypertrophic lesions are more common in blacks than in whites

(Developed from information in Rosen T., Martin S. [1981] *Atlas of black dermatology.* Boston: Little, Brown)

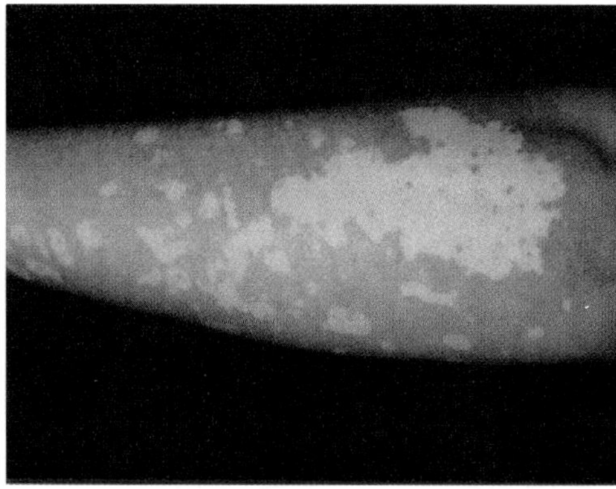

Figure 15–2
Vitiligo of the forearm of a black person. (Neutrogena Skin Care Institute)

be reversed and the pigmented areas are bleached to match the remainder of the skin color.

Albinism

Albinism is a congenital disorder in which there are a normal number of melanocytes, but they lack tyrosinase, the enzyme needed for synthesis of melanin. The most common type is oculocutaneous albinism, which is recessively inherited. It affects the skin, hair, and eyes. Individuals have pale or pink skin, white or yellow hair, and light-colored or sometimes pink eyes. Persons with albinism have ocular problems, such as extreme sensitivity to light, refractive errors, and nystagmus. They are also at great risk for developing skin cancers and must protect themselves from solar radiation.

Melasma

Melasma is a common disorder characterized by darkened macules on the face. It occurs in men but is more common in women, particularly during pregnancy or while using oral contraceptives. It may or may not resolve after giving birth or discontinuing hormonal birth control. Melasma is exacerbated by sun exposure. It is most common in brown-skinned people from Asia, India, and South America.

In summary, skin lesions, rashes, pruritus, and dry skin are the most common manifestations of skin disorders. Rashes are temporary skin eruptions. Lesions result from traumatic or pathologic loss of the normal continuity, structure, or function of the skin. Lesions may be vascular in origin; they may occur as primary lesions in previously normal skin; or they may develop as secondary lesions resulting from primary lesions. Pruritus and dry skin are symptoms common to many skin disorders. Scratching because of pruritus can lead to excoriation, infection, and other complications. Mechanical processes may also lead to skin alterations. The manifestations of several skin disorders vary among light-skinned and dark-skinned persons. Providers must understand numerous variations when describing and assessing skin.

Primary Disorders of the Skin

After you have completed this section of the chapter, you should be able to meet the following objectives:

- Relate the behavior of fungi to the production of superficial skin lesions associated with tinea or ringworm
- State the cause and describe the appearance of impetigo and ecthyma
- Compare the viral causes, manifestations, and treatment of verrucae, herpes simplex, and herpes zoster lesions
- Compare acne vulgaris, acne conglobata, and rosacea in terms of appearance and location of lesions
- Describe the pathogenesis of acne vulgaris and relate to measures used in treating the disorder
- Differentiate allergic and contact dermatitis and atopic and nummular eczema
- Describe the differences and similarities between erythema multiforme minor, Stevens-Johnson syndrome, and toxic epidermal necrolysis
- Define the term papulosquamous and use the term to describe the lesions associated with psoriasis, pityriasis rosea, and lichen planus
- Relate the life cycle of the *Sarcoptes scabiei* to the skin lesions seen in scabies
- Use knowledge of the life cycles of *Pediculus humanus corporis* and *Pediculus humanus capitis* to explain the lesions associated with body and head lice
- Explain the mechanism whereby ticks transmit disease to humans and name the organism transmitted in Rocky Mountain spotted fever and Lyme disease

Primary skin disorders are those originating in the skin. They include infectious processes, acne and rosacea, papulosquamous dermatoses, allergic disorders and drug reactions, and arthropod infestations. Although most of these disorders are not life threatening, they can affect the quality of life.

Infectious Processes

The skin is subject to invasion by a number of microorganisms, including fungi, bacteria, and viruses. Normally, the skin flora, sebum, immune responses, and other protective mechanisms guard the skin against infection. Depending on the virulence of the infecting agent and the competence of the host's resistance, infections may result.

Superficial Fungal Infections

A fungus is a free-living saprophytic plantlike organism (see Chapter 10). Certain strains of fungi are considered normal flora. Fungal (mycotic) infections of the skin are classified as superficial or deep types. The superficial infections are called *dermatophytoses;* they are commonly known as *tinea* or *ringworm.* Deep fungal infections involve the epidermis, dermis, and subcutis. Infections that are typically superficial may exhibit deep involvement in immunosuppressed individuals.

Fungi causing superficial skin infections live on the dead, keratinized cells of the epidermis. They emit an enzyme that enables them to digest keratin, which results in superficial skin scaling, nail disintegration, and hair structure breakage. An exception to this is the invading fungus of tinea versicolor, which does not produce a keratolytic enzyme. Deeper reactions involving vesicles, erythema, and infiltration are thought to be caused by inflammation resulting from exotoxins liberated by the fungus. Fungi are also capable of producing an allergic or immune response. Superficial fungal infections affect various parts of the body, with the lesions varying according to site and fungal species. Tinea can affect the body (*i.e.,* tinea corporis), face and neck (*i.e.,* tinea faciei), scalp (*i.e.,* tinea capitis), hands (*i.e.,* tinea manus), feet (*i.e.,* tinea pedis), or nails (*i.e.,* tinea unguium).

Individual species of three genera have been identified as the invading fungi in most forms of tinea: *Microsporum* (*M. audouinii, M. canis, M. gypseum*), *Epidermophyton* (*E. floccosum*), and *Trichophyton* (*T. schoenleinii, T. violaceum, T. tonsurans*). Only *Microsporum* and *Trichosporon* invade the hair. Anthropophilic species (*M. audouinii, M. tonsurans, T. violaceum*) are parasitic on humans and are spread by other infected humans. Zoophilic species (*M. canis and M. mentagrophytes*) cause parasitic infections in animals, but can be spread by other infected humans.

Diagnosis of superficial fungal infections is primarily done by microscopic examination of skin scrapings. Hyphae are threadlike filaments that grow from spores and are visible microscopically. Mycelia are macroscopic aggregations of hyphae. The fungal spores, the reproducing bodies of fungi, are rarely seen on skin scrapings. Potassium hydroxide preparations are used to prepare slides of skin scrapings. The potassium hydroxide disintegrates human tissue and leaves behind the hyphae for examination. With another method of diagnosis, a Wood's light (ultraviolet light) is directed onto the affected area. Under the light, many fungi fluoresce a green to yellow-green color (Fig. 15–3).

Griseofulvin is the prototype oral prescription antifungal agent. It is used for severe or recalcitrant cases. Synthetic antifungal agents, called *azole compounds* and *allylamines*, such as ketoconazole and fluconazole, have been used effectively in the treatment of tinea corporis and other fungal infections. These agents have replaced tolnaftate or undecylenic acid based ointments. Although griseofulvin is a fungistatic agent (*i.e.,* stops fungal growth), the synthetic agents are considered to be fungicidal (*i.e.,* kills the fungus) and therefore more effective. Terbinafine, a newer allylamine derivative, has been effective in severe cases; it resolves skin problems in a shorter amount of time (2 weeks rather than 4).[2] Some of the synthetic agents, however, have more serious side effects, such as hepatic toxicity. Topical preparations of some synthetic fungicides (*e.g.,* ketoconazole, miconazole, clotrimazole) are available and produce less severe side effects. Topical corticosteroids may be used in conjunction with antifungal agents to relieve itching and erythema secondary to inflammation.

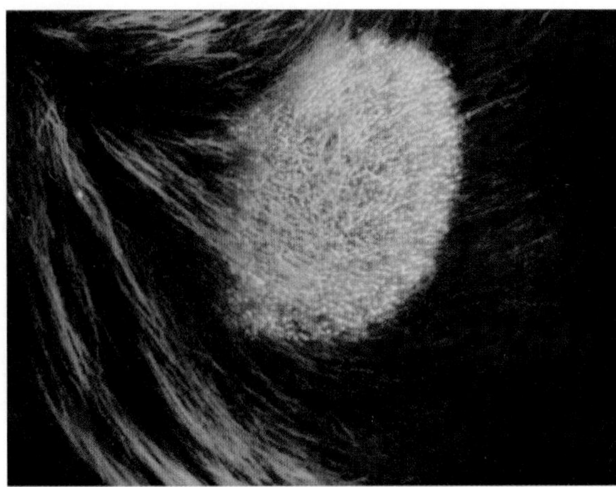

Figure 15–3
Tinea hairs fluorescing under Wood's light.

Tinea of the Body or Face. Tinea corporis (*i.e.,* ringworm of the body) can be caused by any of the fungi, but it is usually caused by *M. canis* or *M. audouinii;* less frequently, it is caused by *T. rubrum* or *T. mentagrophytes.* The lesions vary, depending on the fungal agent, but the most common types of lesions are round, oval, or circular patches (Fig. 15–4). Patches have central clearings with raised red borders consisting of vesicles, papules, or pustules. The lesion begins as a red papule and enlarges with central healing. The borders are sharply defined, but lesions may coalesce. Pruritus, a mild burning sensation, and erythema frequently accompany the skin lesion.

Tinea corporis affects all ages. However, children seem most prone to infection. Transmission is most commonly from kittens, puppies, and other children who

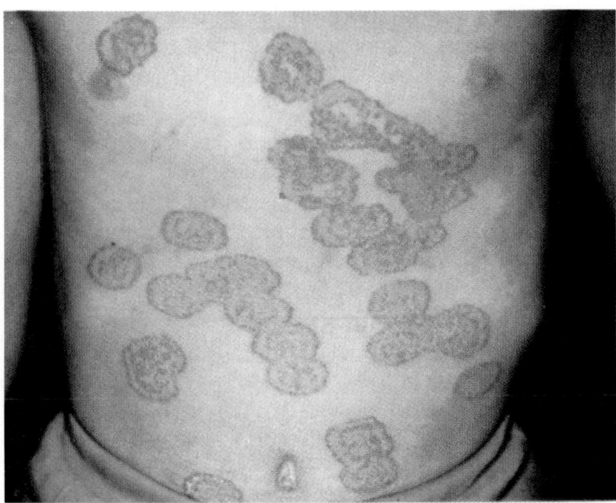

Figure 15–4
Tinea of the body caused by *Microsporum canis.*

have infections. Less common forms are from foot and groin infections.

Tinea faciale, or ringworm of the face, is an infection caused by *T. mentagrophytes* or *T. rubrum*. Tinea faciale may mimic the annular, erythematous, scaling, pruritic lesions characteristic of tinea corporis. It may also appear as flat erythematous patches. In either case, misdiagnosis is not uncommon.

Topical antifungal agents are usually effective in treating tinea corporis and tinea faciale. Oral antifungal agents may be used in resistant cases.

Tinea of the Scalp. There are two common types of tinea capitis or ringworm of the scalp: primary (*i.e.*, noninflammatory) and secondary (*i.e.*, inflammatory). Primary lesions characteristically manifest as grayish, round, hairless patches or as balding spots on the head. The lesions vary in size and are most commonly seen on the back of the head (Fig. 15–5). Mild erythema, crust, or scale may be present. The individual is usually asymptomatic, although pruritus may exist. The primary form of tinea capitis is caused by *M. audouinii* and *M. canis* transferred from kittens, puppies, and other humans. Epidemics have occurred from *T. tonsurans* and *M. audouinii*, representing human-to-human transmission, with *T. tonsurans* being the most common infectious agent.[3,4]

Children between 3 and 8 years of age are primarily affected. Tinea capitis seldom occurs in adults. This has been partially attributed to the higher content of fatty acids in the sebum after puberty.

The inflammatory type of tinea capitis is caused by virulent strains of *T. mentagrophytes*, *T. verrucosum*, and *M. gypseum*. The onset is rapid, and lesions are usually localized to one area. The initial lesion consists of a pustular scaly round patch with broken hairs. A secondary bacterial infection is common and may lead to a painful, circumscribed, boggy, and indurated lesion called a *kerion*. The highest incidence is among children and farmers who work with infected animals.

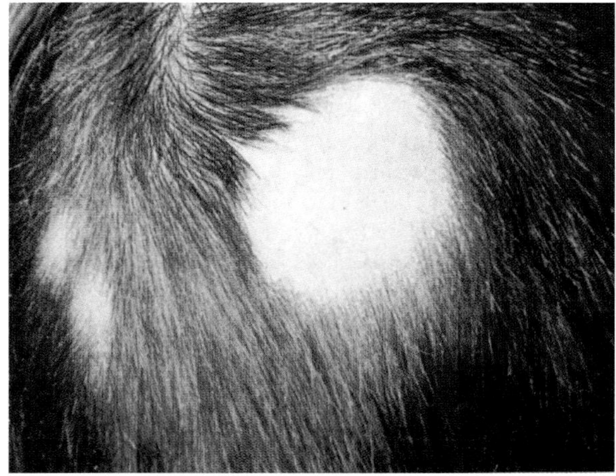

Figure 15–5
Tinea of the scalp caused by *Microsporum audouini*.

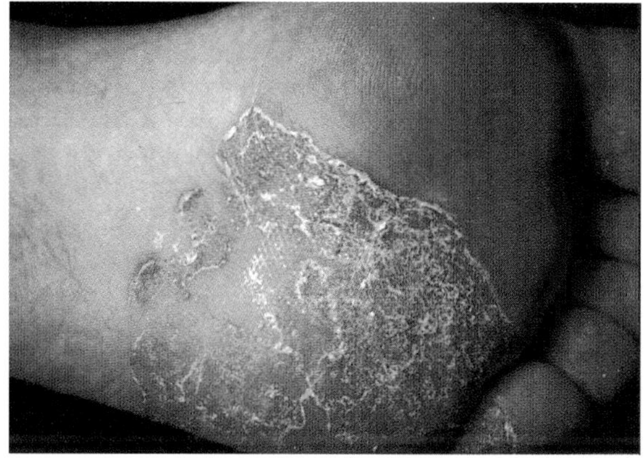

Figure 15–6
Chronic tinea of sole of the foot caused by *Trichophyton rubrum*. (Schering Corp.)

The treatment for both forms of tinea capitis is griseofulvin, an oral antifungal agent. The synthetic antifungals have been effective modalities as well. Topical ointments are sometimes indicated in addition to oral medications. Because of the lower fatty acid content in sebum of children, several antifungal agents have been prepared with fatty acid bases. These antifungal agents have revolutionized treatment, replacing the old remedies in which children were often subjected to head shavings and the use of harsh shampoos and salves. Wet packs, medicated shampoos, and antibiotics may be prescribed for the secondary types of infection.

Tinea of the Foot. Tinea of the foot (*i.e.*, tinea pedis, athlete's foot, or ringworm of the feet) is a common skin disorder primarily affecting the spaces between the toes, the soles of the feet, or the sides of the feet (Fig. 15–6). It is caused by *T. mentagrophytes* and *T. rubrum*. The lesions vary from a mild scaling lesion to a painful, exudative, erosive, inflamed lesion with fissuring. Lesions are often accompanied by pruritus, pain, and foul odor.

Some persons are prone to chronic tinea pedis. Mild forms are more common during dry environmental conditions. Exacerbations of the mild form occur as a result of hot weather, sweating, and exercise or when the feet are exposed to moisture or occlusive shoes. Tinea pedis may occur alone or in combination with other infections such as tinea corporis or tinea cruris. Patches may occur on the hands, a condition known as the intradermal (dermatophytid) reaction.

Simple forms of tinea pedis are treated with topical applications of antifungals. Complex cases are treated with oral griseofulvin, ketoconazole, or terbinafine; the latter is the most effective.[2] Other treatment and preventive modalities include scrupulous cleaning and drying of affected areas; use of clean, dry socks; and at least daily sock changes. When bathed, the feet should be dried after other parts of the body to prevent spread of the disease.

Tinea of the Hand. Tinea of the hand (*i.e.*, tinea manus or ringworm of the hands), is rarely a primary infection. The primary infection is usually tinea pedis, with tinea manus occurring as a secondary infection. Tinea manus usually occurs only on one hand, but other infectious processes, such as contact dermatitis and psoriasis, affect both hands.

The same fungal agents responsible for tinea pedis, *T. rubrum* and *T. mentagrophytes*, cause tinea manus. The characteristic lesion is a blister on the palm or finger surrounded by erythema (Fig. 15–7). Chronic lesions are scaly and dry. Cracking and fissuring may occur. The lesions may spread to the plantar surfaces of the hand. If chronic, tinea manus may lead to tinea of the fingernails.

The treatment of choice is oral griseofulvin therapy for approximately 3 months. Synthetic antifungal (*i.e.*, ketoconazole and terbinafine) drugs have also been effective.

Tinea of the Nail. Tinea of the nail (*i.e.*, tinea unguium or onychomycosis) is a chronic fungal infection of the nails of the hands or feet. Tinea of the toenails is common; tinea of the fingernails is less common. Toenail infection is common in persons prone to chronic infections of tinea pedis. Often, the infection in the toenails becomes a ready source for future infections of the foot. It may begin from a crushing injury to a toenail or from the spread of tinea pedis.

Tinea unguium usually is caused by *T. rubrum* or *T. mentagrophytes*. The infection usually begins at the tip of the nail, where the fungus digests the nail keratin. Initially, the nail appears opaque, white, or silvery (Fig. 15–8). The nail then turns yellow or brown. This condition remains unchanged for years and may involve only one or two nails and produce no discomfort. Gradually, the nail thickens and becomes frail as the infection spreads and includes the nail plate. The nail cracks and thickens. The nail plate separates from the nail bed, and permanent discoloration and distortion result. It may spread to other nails.

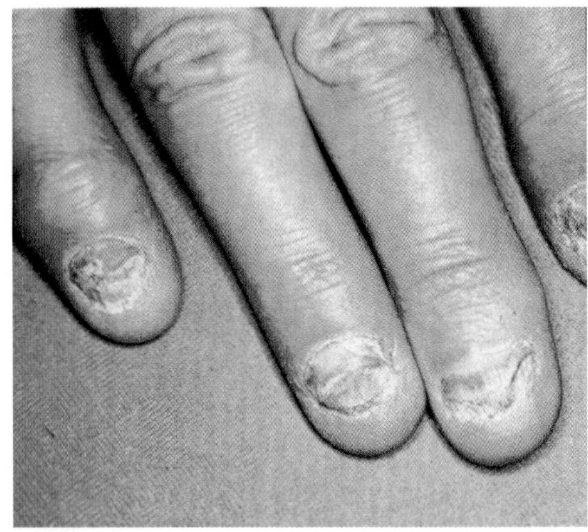

Figure 15–8
Tinea of the fingernail caused by *Trichophyton rubrum.* (Duke Laboratories, Inc.)

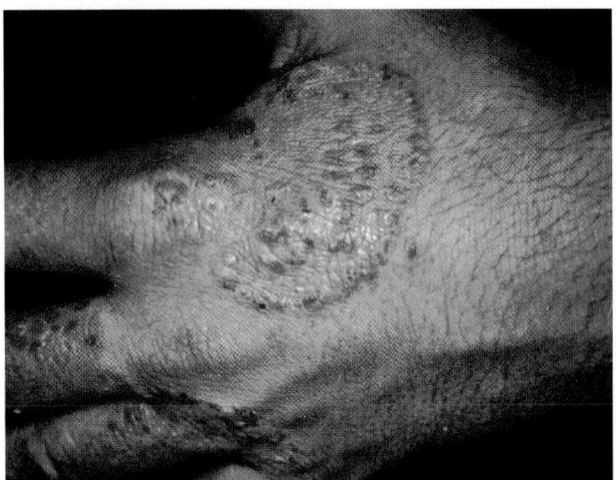

Figure 15–7
Tinea of the dorsum of the hand caused by *Trichophyton mentagrophytes.* (Duke Laboratories, Inc.)

The prognosis for fungal infections of the toenail is poor. The recurrence rate even after treatment is high. Oral griseofulvin for as long as 1 year in conjunction with topical antifungals is the treatment choice. Oral synthetic antifungal agents, especially terbinafine, have been effective. Patients should be monitored closely for the side effects of the drugs. Some authorities recommend removal of the infected toenails, with or without antifungal therapy. Fingernail infections are more easily treated. Successful therapy seems to depend on the persistence of the therapist and the patient.

Tinea Versicolor. Tinea versicolor is a fungal infection involving the upper chest, the back, and sometimes the arms. The causative agent is *Malassezia furfur*. The infection occurs primarily in young adults in tropic and temperate regions, but cases have been reported in the northern states.

The characteristic lesion is a yellow, pink, or brown sheet of scaling skin. The name *versicolor* is derived from the multicolored variations of the lesion. The patches are depigmented and do not tan when exposed to ultraviolet light. The skin has an overall appearance of being "dirty." These cosmetic defects often bring the patient to the physician in the summer months. It is believed that the fungus filters the ultraviolet light, preventing tanning. In darker-skinned persons, the depigmented areas are more apparent.

Selenium sulfide, found in several shampoo preparations, has been an effective fungistatic treatment measure. Boiling or steam-pressing clothes may help in the prevention of recurrence. Miconazole or ketoconazole creams or shampoos, because of their fungicidal properties, have become the drugs of choice. The infection may recur after drug therapy.

Tinea Incognito. Tinea incognito is a form of dermatophyte infection that developed with the widespread use topical corticosteroids. It is often seen in cases where tinea infections are misdiagnosed as eczema and treated with corticosteroids. Because the corticosteroids suppress the inflammation, scaling and erythema may not be present. There has also been an increased incidence of tinea incognito in persons with acquired immunodeficiency syndrome (AIDS). Patients with the disorder often present with thickened plaques with lichenification, papules, pustules, and nodules. Telangiectasias, atrophy, and striae may be present. Tinea incognito is most often seen on the groin, on the hand, or on the dorsal aspect of the hand.

Treatment measures include the discontinuing of topical corticosteroids while using low-dose oral corticosteroids to prevent the flare-up associated with stopping potent topical steroids. Topical or oral antifungal agents may be used, depending on the severity of the infection. Persons who must remain on potent topical corticosteroids are difficult to treat.

Dermatophytid Reaction. A secondary skin eruption may occur in persons allergic to the fungus responsible for the dermatophytes. This dermatophytid or intradermal reaction may occur during an acute episode of a fungal infection. The most common reaction occurs on the hands in response to tinea pedis. The lesions are vesicles with erythema extending over the palms and fingers of the hand and sometimes to other areas. Less commonly, a more generalized reaction occurs in which papules or vesicles erupt on the trunk or extremities. These eruptions may resemble tinea corporis. Lesions may become excoriated and infected with bacteria. Treatment is directed at the primary site of infection. The intradermal reaction resolves in most cases without intervention if the primary site is cleared.

Candidal Infections. Candidiasis (i.e., moniliasis) is a fungal infection caused by *Candida albicans*. This yeastlike fungus is a normal inhabitant of the gastrointestinal tract, mouth, and vagina (see Chapter 52). The skin problems result from the release of irritating toxins on the skin surface. Some persons are predisposed to candidal infections by conditions such as diabetes mellitus, antibiotic therapy, pregnancy, use of birth control pills, poor nutrition, and immunosuppressive diseases. Oral candidiasis may be the first sign of infection with human immunodeficiency virus (HIV).

C. albicans thrives in warm, moist intertriginous areas of the body. The rash is red with well-defined borders. Patches erode the epidermis, and there is scaling. Mild to severe itching and burning often accompany the infection. Severe forms of infection may involve pustules or vesiculopustules. A candidial infection can be differentiated from a tinea infection by the presence of satellite lesions. These satellite lesions are maculopapular and are found outside the clearly demarcated borders of the candidal infection. Satellite lesions are often diagnostic of diaper rash complicated by *Candida*. The appearance of candidal infections varies according to the site. Table 15–3 summarizes site characteristics.

Treatment measures vary according to the location. Preventive measures, such as wearing rubber gloves, are encouraged for persons with infections of the hands. Intertriginous areas are often separated with clean cotton cloth and allowed to air dry as a means of decreasing the macerating effects of heat and moisture. Nystatin (Mycostatin), an antibiotic available in tablets, powder, or vaginal suppositories, is effective for control of infection. Oral synthetic agents, such as ketoconazole and fluconazole, have also been effective.

Bacterial Infections

Bacteria are considered normal flora of the skin. Most bacteria are not pathogenic, but when pathogenic bacteria invade the skin, superficial or systemic infections may develop. Bacterial infections are classified as primary (*i.e.*, superficial) or secondary (*i.e.*, deep). Impetigo is an example of a primary bacterial infection; infected ulcers are an example of a secondary bacterial infection.

Samples from infected sites are usually cultured for diagnosis. In addition to antibiotic therapy, the

TABLE 15–3
Candidal Infections: Locations and Appearance of Lesions

Location	Appearance
Breasts, groin, axillae, anus, umbilicus, toe or fingerwebs	Red lesions with well-defined borders and presence of satellite lesions; lesions may be dry or moist
Vagina	Red, oozing lesions with sharply defined borders and inflamed vagina; cervix may be covered with moist, white plaque, cheesy, foul-smelling discharge; presence of pruritus and burning
Glans penis (balanitis)	Red lesions with sharply defined borders; penis may be covered with white plaque; presence of pruritus and burning
Mouth (thrush)	Creamy white flakes on a red, inflamed mucous membrane; papillae on tongue may be enlarged
Nails	Red, painful swelling around nail bed; common in persons who often have their hands in water

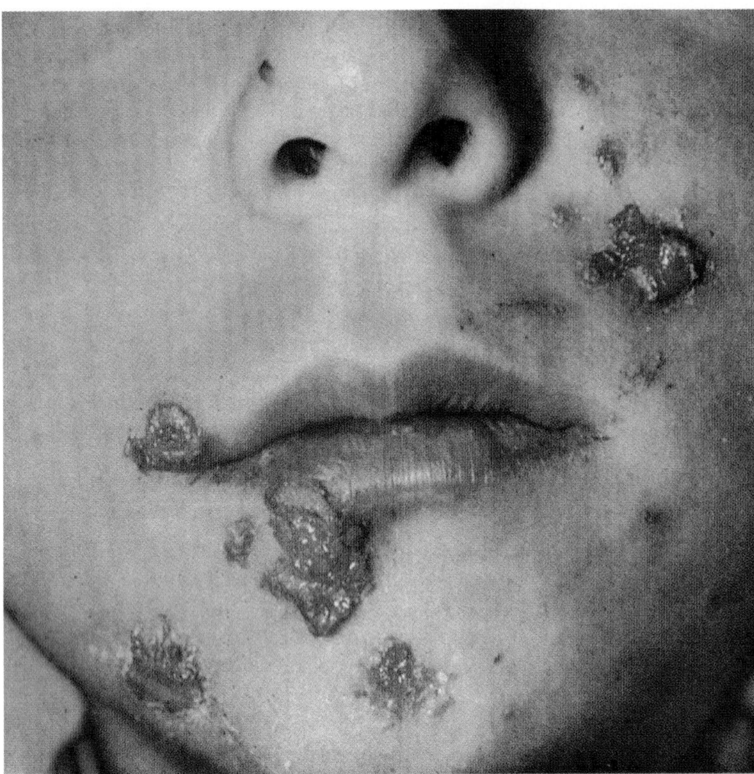

Figure 15–9
Impetigo of the face. (Abner Kurten, *Folia Dermatologica.* No. 2. Geigy Pharmaceuticals.)

treatment of bacterial infections often includes hygiene education, general isolation procedures, and dietary management.

Impetigo. Impetigo is a common superficial bacterial infection caused by *staphylococci* or *group A β-hemolytic streptococci* (GABHS). Historically, there has been a shift from a higher incidence of GABHS-type impetigo to *Staphylococcus aureus* as the predominant causal agent. Impetigo is common among young infants and children, although older children and adults occasionally contract the disease. It is highly communicable in the younger population.

Impetigo initially appears as a small vesicle or pustule or as a large bulla. The primary lesion ruptures, leaving a denuded area that discharges a honey-colored serous liquid. The liquid hardens on the skin surface and dries as a honey-colored crust with a stuck-on appearance (Fig. 15–9). New vesicles erupt within hours. Pruritus often accompanies the lesions, and the skin excoriations that result from scratching multiply the infection sites. A possible complication of untreated GABHS impetigo is poststreptococcal glomerulonephritis (see Chapter 28). Lesions are most often found on the face, but they can occur anywhere on the body. Topical mupirocin (Bactroban) has proved clinically effective with few side effects for cases of impetigo. Many practitioners treat with systemic antibiotics, such as dicloxacillin or erythromycin, depending on the extent of skin involvement.

A less common form of *S. aureus* infection, called *Ritter's disease,* manifests with a diffuse scarlet fever–like rash, followed by skin separation and sloughing (Fig. 15–10). the patient may have fever. It is also called *staphylococcal scalded-skin syndrome,* because the skin looks scalded. It usually affects children younger than 5 years of age, but immunosuppressed adults are also

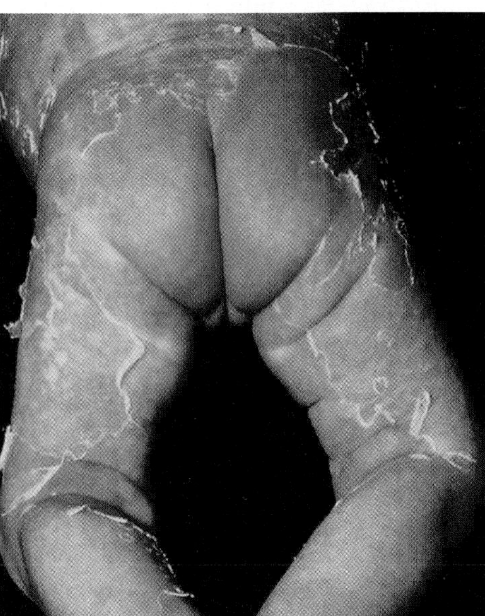

Figure 15–10
Staphylococcal scalded-skin syndrome. (Fitzpatrick T.B., Johnson R.A., Polono M.K., Suurmond D., Wolff K. [1992]. *Color atlas and synopsis of clinical dermatology* [2nd ed., p. 297]. New York: McGraw-Hill)

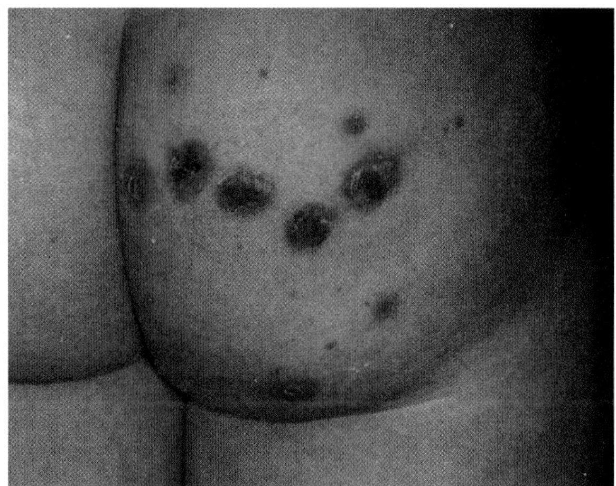

Figure 15–11
Ecthyma on the buttocks of a 13-year-old boy. (Glaxo-Wellcome Co.)

at risk. Ritter's disease is considered a deeper skin infection because the superficial layers of the epidermis are separated and shed. Systemic antibiotics, either oral or parenteral, are used to treat the disorder.

Ecthyma is an ulcerative form of impetigo, usually secondary to minor trauma. It is caused by GABHS, *S. aureus*, or *Pseudomonas*. It frequently occurs on the buttocks and thighs of children (Fig. 15–11). The lesions are similar to those of impetigo. A vesicle or pustule ruptures, leaving a skin erosion or ulcer that weeps and dries to a crusted patch, often resulting in scar formation. With extensive ecthyma, there is a low-grade fever and extension of the infection to other organs. Treatment usually involves systemic antibiotics, such as dicloxacillin or erythromycin.

Viral Infections

Viruses are intracellular pathogens. They have no organized cell structure but consist of a DNA or RNA core surrounded by a protein coat. Viruses rely completely on live cells for reproduction. The viruses seen in skin lesion disorders tend to be DNA-containing viruses. Viruses invade the keratinocyte, begin to reproduce, and cause cellular proliferation or cellular death. The rapid increase in viral skin diseases has been attributed to the use of corticosteroid drugs, which have immunosuppressive qualities, and the use of antibiotics, which alter the bacterial flora of the skin. As the number of bacterial infections has decreased, there has been a proportional rise in viral skin diseases.

Verrucae. Verrucae, or warts, are common, benign papillomas caused by DNA-containing papovaviruses. Although warts vary in gross appearance depending on their location, they all have a similar histologic appearance (Table 15–4). The wart is not a mass of uniform tumor cells but, like other skin diseases, is an exaggeration of the normal skin composition. There is an irregular thickening of the stratum spinosum and greatly increased thickening of the stratum corneum.

Human papillomavirus (HPV) is the subgroup of the papovaviruses that causes human warts. There are more than 60 types of HPVs found on the skin and mucous membranes of humans. Many are genital warts that are sexually transmitted; some types of HPV may increase the risk of cervical cancer (see Chapter 51). The remainder account for warts that commonly appear on the hands and feet (Fig. 15–12). The nongenital warts, types 1, 2, 3, and 4, are generally not precancerous. They are known as plantar warts, common warts, and flat warts. Wart transmission occurs usually through skin contact.

Warts resolve spontaneously when immunity to the virus develops. The immune response may be delayed for years. After 5 years, most warts that are left untreated have disappeared. In earlier years, treatment measures were directed at eradicating all wart tissue, primarily by excision. Because this frequently left scars, treatment was directed at irritation of the wart with liquid nitrogen or acid chemicals. Cryotherapy and salicylic acid paint or plasters have been effective. Various types of laser therapy also have been successful in wart eradication. Given the resolution rate of most warts, self-hypnosis

TABLE 15-4
Types and Characteristics of Verrucae (Warts)

Type	Location	Appearance
Verruca vulgaris (common warts)	Anywhere on the skin, usually on the hands	Ragged dome-shape with growth above the skin surface
Verruca filiformis	Eyelids, face, neck	Long fingerlike projections
Verruca plana (flat wart)	Forehead, dorsum of hand	Small flat tumors, may be barely visible
Verruca plantaris (plantar wart)	Sole of foot	Flat to slightly raised growth extending deep into skin; painful; bleeding occurs with superficial trimming; coalesced plantar warts are referred to as mosaic warts
Condyloma acuminata	Mucous membrane of the penis, female genitalia, perianal areas, and rectum	Large moist projections with rough surfaces; usually pink or purple in color

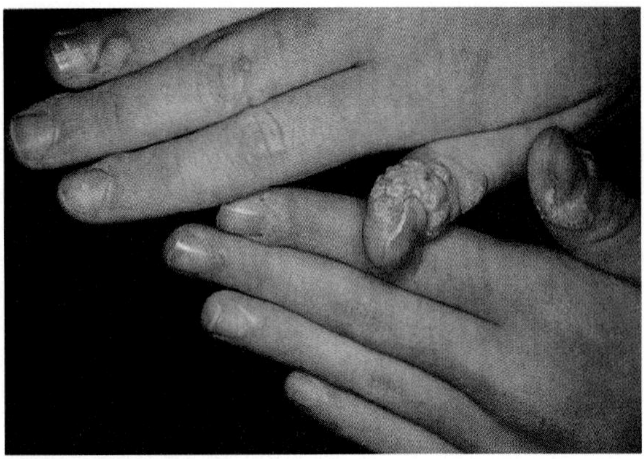

Figure 15–12
Common and periungal warts. (Reed and Carnick Pharmaceuticals)

with imagery has also been successful in their mitigation and elimination.[5]

Herpes Simplex. Herpes simplex virus (HSV) infections of the skin and mucous membrane are common (i.e., cold sore or fever blister). Two types of herpesviruses infect humans: type I and type II. HSV-I and HSV-II can cause genital herpes, but most commonly the latter form is involved. HSV-I may be transmitted to other parts of the body through the occupational hazards that exist in athletics and some professions, such as dentistry and medicine. HSV-I and HSV-II may also be transmitted by kissing or oral sex. It is likely that many adults were exposed to HSV-I during childhood and therefore have antibodies to that virus. However, most adults are unlikely to have been exposed to HSV-II before becoming sexually active. This explains why so few adults develop cold sores due to HSV-I. However, there is a high risk of getting HSV-II when exposed for the first time as an adult (see Chapter 52.)

Herpesvirus lesions usually begin with a burning or tingling sensation. Vesicles and erythema follow and progress to pustules, ulcers, and crusts before healing (Fig. 15–13). The lesion is most common on the lips, face, and mouth. Pain is common, and healing takes place within 10 to 14 days.

HSV infections are of two types: primary and secondary. The primary infection usually consists of a high fever, sore throat, painful vesicles, and ulcers of the tongue, palate, gingiva, buccal mucosa, and lips. The primary infection results in the development of antibodies to the virus so that recurrences (*i.e.*, secondary infections) are more localized and less severe. After an initial infection, the herpesvirus persists in the trigeminal and other ganglia in the latent state. Recurrent lesions are common in a small percentage of persons. Precipitating factors may be stress, sunlight exposure, menses, or injury. Individuals who are immunocompromised may have severe attacks.

There is no cure for herpes simplex; most treatment measures are palliative. Topical application of lidocaine, an anesthetic agent, or diphenhydramine, an antihistamine, along with aspirin helps to relieve pain. Cold compresses help in the acute stages. The most effective treatment has been the antiviral drug acyclovir. Acyclovir is an antimetabolite that inhibits herpesvirus replication. It is given orally or intravenously and is the prototype of all the antiviral drugs. Severe forms have been treated with idoxuridine, an antiviral agent, which prevents certain aspects of DNA synthesis and thereby inhibits viral reproduction without causing cell injury.

Herpes Zoster. Herpes zoster (*i.e.*, shingles) is an acute localized inflammatory disease of a dermatome segment of the skin. It is caused by the same herpesvirus, varicella-zoster, that causes chickenpox. It is believed to be the result of reactivation of a latent varicella-zoster virus that was dormant in the sensory dorsal ganglia since a childhood infection. During an episode of shingles, the reactivated virus travels from the ganglia to the skin of the corresponding dermatome.

The clinical picture of herpes zoster is the eruption of vesicles with erythematous bases that are restricted to skin areas supplied by sensory neurons of a single or associated group of dorsal root ganglia (Fig. 15–14). Eruptions are generally unilateral in the thoracic region, trunk, and face. In immunosuppressed persons, the lesions may extend beyond the dermatome. New crops of vesicles erupt for 3 to 5 days along the nerve pathway. The lesions are deeper and more confluent than those of chickenpox (Fig. 15–15). The vesicles dry, form crusts, and eventually fall off. The lesions usually clear in 2 to 3 weeks. Severe pain and paresthesia are common. In the elderly, herpes zoster is a particularly serious condition that may be long-lasting and eventually lead to death. Pain reports from elderly persons indicate an increased severity and lengthy episodes of up to 1 year. The reason may be greater involvement of small nerve fibers from the loss of large nerve fibers associated with aging. Postherpetic neuralgia is the most important complica-

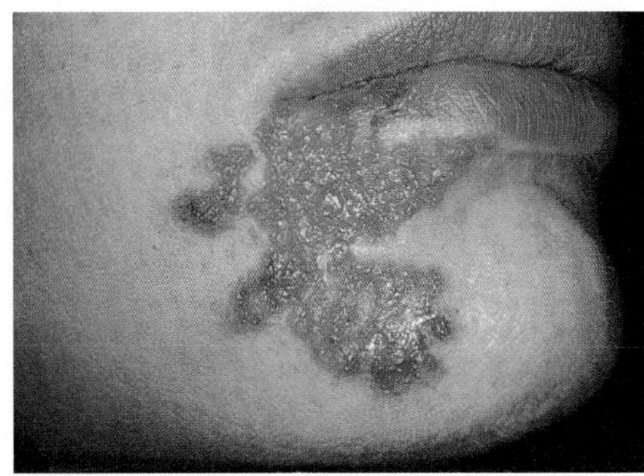

Figure 15–13
Recurrent herpes simplex of the face. (Dermick Laboratories, Inc.)

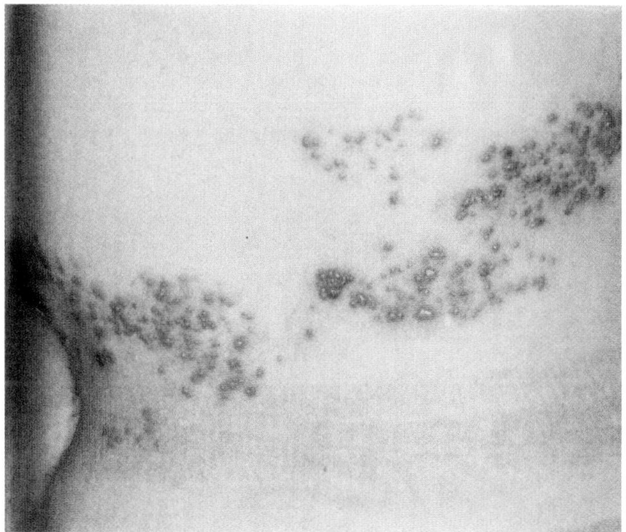

Figure 15–14
Herpes zoster in a common presentation, with involvement of a single dermatome. (Habif T.P. [1996]. *Clinical dermatology* [3rd ed., p. 351]. St Louis: CV Mosby)

tion occurring in persons older than 50. Eye involvement can result in permanent blindness and occurs in a large percentage of cases involving the ophthalmic division of the trigeminal nerve. The occurrence of herpes zoster in any person warrants careful assessment, because development of herpes zoster may be the first sign of the immunosuppression associated with AIDS.

The treatment of choice for herpes zoster is early oral or intravenous doses of acyclovir. Valacyclovir and famciclovir, newer and more potent antivirals, have demonstrated increased rash healing. When given in the acute vesicular stage, the antiviral drugs have decreased the amount of lesion development and pain.[6] However, many persons present in the prevesicular stage, making diagnosing more difficult. Persons also present after the vesicles have erupted, when the antivirals are much less useful. Narcotic analgesics have been used to decrease pain. Nerve blocks also have been used in the early management of herpetic pain. Systemic corticosteroids have been effective in some cases, but their use remains controversial. Local treatment measures include Burow's solution compresses, aqueous alcohol lotions, calamine lotion, and starch shake lotions. Treatment of pain associated with herpetic neuralgia is discussed further in Chapter 40.

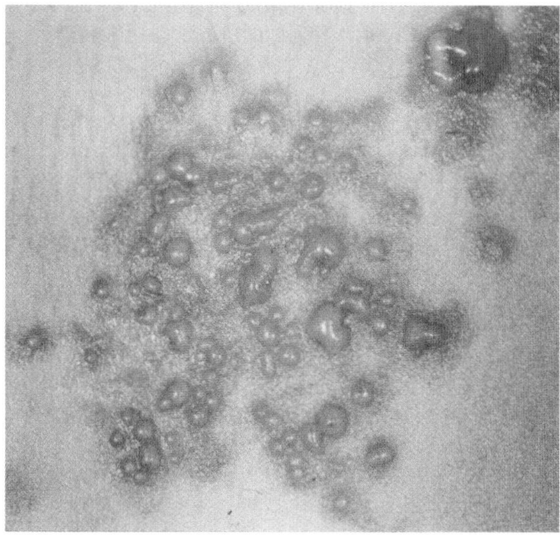

Figure 15–15
Herpes zoster is characterized by various sizes of vesicles. Vesicles of herpes simplex are uniform in size. (Habif T.P. [1996]. *Clinical dermatology* [3rd ed., p. 353]. St Louis: CV Mosby)

Acne and Rosacea

Acne is commonly referred to as a disorder of the pilosebaceous unit (*i.e.,* hair and sebaceous gland). The hair follicle is a tubular invagination of the epidermis in which hair is produced. Cornified epidermal cells from the surface skin layer line the upper portion of the follicle (see Fig. 14–5). The sebaceous glands empty into the hair follicle, and the pilosebaceous unit opens to the skin surface by means of a widely dilated opening called a *pore.* The sebaceous glands are largest on the face, scalp, and scrotum but are present in all areas of the skin except for the soles of the feet and palms of the hands. The cells of the sebaceous gland are derived from the epidermal keratin cell and have a structure similar to epidermal cells, except that they accumulate lipid droplets. The sebaceous glands produce a complex lipid mixture called *sebum,* from the Latin word meaning tallow or grease. Sebum consists of a mixture of free fatty acids, triglycerides, diglycerides, monoglycerides, sterol esters, wax esters, and squalene. Sebum production occurs as a holocrine process in which the sebaceous gland cells that produce the sebum are completely broken down and their lipid contents are emptied through the sebaceous duct into the hair follicle.

The flow of sebum is continuous, and a disturbance in flow is one of the major causes of acne. The amount of sebum produced depends on two factors: the size of the sebaceous gland and the rate of cellular growth. Sebaceous cell proliferation and sebum production are uniquely responsive to direct hormonal stimulation by androgen. In men, testicular androgens are the main stimulus for sebaceous activity; in women, adrenal and ovarian androgens maintain sebaceous activity.

Acne lesions consist of comedones (*i.e.,* whiteheads and blackheads), papules, pustules, and in severe cases, cysts. Blackheads are plugs of material that accumulate in sebaceous glands that open to the skin surface. The color of blackheads results from melanin that has moved into the sebaceous glands from adjoining epidermal cells. Whiteheads are pale, slightly elevated papules with no visible orifice. Papules are raised areas less than 5 mm in diameter. Pustules have a central core of purulent material. Nodules are larger than 5 mm in diameter and may become suppurative or hemorrhagic. Suppurative nodules are often referred to as cysts because of their resemblance to inflamed epidermal cysts. Acne lesions are divided into noninflammatory and inflammatory lesions. Noninflammatory acne consists primarily of comedones, and inflammatory acne consists of papules, pustules, and nodules or cysts. The inflammatory lesions are believed to develop from the escape of sebum into the dermis and the irritating effects of the fatty acids that are contained in the sebum.

There are numerous forms of acne with various etiologic agents and influences. Two types of acne occur during different stages of the life cycle: acne vulgaris, which is the most common form among adolescents and young adults, and acne conglobata, which develops later in life.

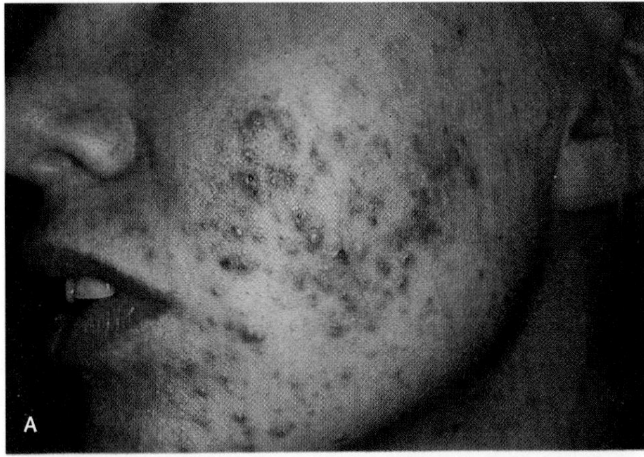

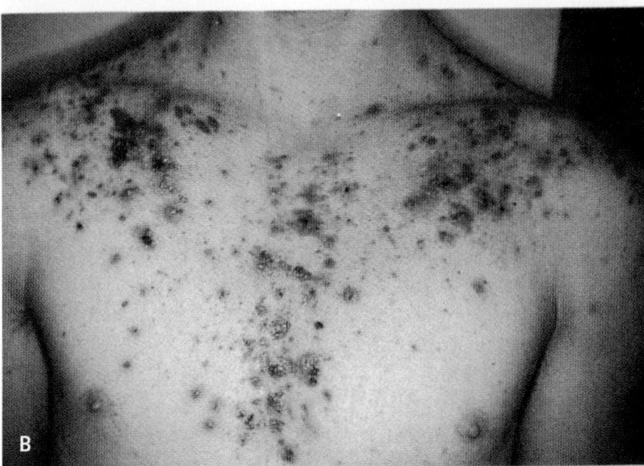

Figure 15–16
(A) Acne of the face and **(B)** acne of the chest.

Acne Vulgaris

The prevalence of acne vulgaris during adolescence is approximately 100%, because almost all teenagers experience at least a few comedones. The difference is the severity of the condition, rather than incidence.[7] In women, acne may begin earlier and persist until 30 years of age; however, the overall incidence and severity is greater in men.

Acne vulgaris lesions form primarily on the face and neck and, to a lesser extent, on the back, chest, and shoulders (Fig. 15–16). The lesions are thought to result from increased production of sebum by the sebaceous glands and plugging of the pilosebaceous ducts. The presence of *Propionibacterium acnes* contributes to the development of acne. The *P. acnes* organism contains lipases. These enzymes can result in breakdown of the free fatty acids that produce inflammation. The *P. acnes* organism depends on the presence of sebum for its survival.

The cause of acne vulgaris remains unknown. Several contributing factors have been examined including the influence of androgens on sebaceous cell activity, increased proliferation of the keratinizing epidermal cells that form the sebaceous cells, increased sebum production in relation to the severity of the disease, decreased amounts of linoleic acid in the sebum, and presence of *P. acnes*. There is a genetic predisposition to acquiring acne, and stress is thought to play an important part in the longer prevalence of the condition among women. The exact link between stress and acne is unknown, but it is believed that stress increases the secretion of androgen.[7]

Over the years, several factors have been studied empirically and rejected as causal or contributing agents: acne as an infectious process, makeup, diets high in fatty content, and certain foods, such as chocolate. However, many therapists continue to advise general hygienic and preventive measures as a child nears puberty. These include washing the face gently with soap and water; avoiding touching the face with the hands; shampooing hair and scalp regularly; keeping hair away from the face; avoiding the use of creams and moisturizers; and using water-based, rather than oil-based, makeup. Exposure to sunlight may be helpful, but is a debatable therapy. A balanced diet is recommended. Stressful or fatigue-producing activities should be minimized.

Mild forms of acne respond well to stringent hygiene measures in addition to the topical application of acne creams, ointments, and lotions. A mainstay of acne therapy is avoiding any mechanical trauma, such as squeezing, rubbing, or picking comedones. Even resting the chin, forehead, or cheek on a hand can exacerbate the condition. Hats, sweatbands, and shirt collars have contributed to acne. Numerous commercial products are available that contain drying and antibiotic agents. Oil-based preparations should be avoided, because they may contribute to the problem. Many acne creams and lotions contain keratolytic agents such as sulfur, salicylic acid, phenol, and resorcinol. These agents act chemically to break down keratin and loosen comedones and exert a peeling effect on the skin. With the advent of more effective products, these preparations are seldom prescribed anymore. Some of these preparations may contribute to the acne problem by forming comedones, and more effective topical agents are available.

Treatment of moderate to severe acne is based on four objectives supported by current knowledge of the condition: correction of the defect in epidermal cell proliferation, lessening of sebaceous gland activity, reduction of the *P. acnes* population, and reduction of the inflammatory process. Many of the treatment modalities may be used alone or in combination with other treatments. An important treatment measure is sensitivity to the client's emotional needs.

Benzoyl peroxide, which has been in existence since the early 1900s, is an antibacterial agent especially effective in reducing the *P. acnes* population. Bacterial proteins are oxidized by the oxygen free radicals released from metabolism of benzoyl peroxide on the skin. Because of its mechanism of action, bacterial resistance does not develop to benzoyl peroxide. The irritant effect of the drug also causes vasodilation and increased blood flow, which may hasten resolution of the inflammatory lesions.

Tretinoin (Retin-A), an acid derivative of vitamin A, is a strong topical agent that has been tremendously effective. It works indirectly by reducing sebum production and helps remove comedones by increasing mitotic activity at the base of the follicle. Comedones are pushed out from below. It further interferes with comedone formation by preventing the follicle from sticking together, lessening the chance of an impacted pore. It also aids in blood flow, thereby helping to clear papules and pustules. Because tretinoin is applied topically, it remains chiefly on the epidermis, with minimal absorption into the circulation.

Topically applied antibiotics are also effective in treating mild to moderate acne. Topical tetracycline, erythromycin, and clindamycin are used most commonly. They do not affect existing lesions but prevent future lesions by decreasing *P. acnes* colonization and the subsequent formation of sebaceous fatty acid metabolites that act as inflammatory stimuli. Treatment failure can result from development of antibiotic resistance. Oral low-dose tetracycline has been used effectively for many years. Tetracycline has no effect on sebum production, but it decreases bacterial growth and the amount of free fatty acids produced. Tetracycline requires a sufficient treatment period to establish effective blood levels. Side effects are minimal, which is why the drug has remained so useful. However, it does have teratogenic effects on skeletal and tooth development and should not be given to pregnant women, lactating women, and children. Erythromycin, another antibiotic, also has been effective in acne treatment. Of the antimicrobial drugs, dapsone has been effective in severe cystic acnes. However, side effects are many. The drug should be used with caution and close monitoring.

Estrogens reduce the size and the secretion of the sebaceous gland, but because of the high dosages required, they are contraindicated in men. In women, estrogen therapy or birth control pills may be administered. Side effects are those associated with any estrogen therapy, such as nausea, weight gain, spotting, breast tenderness, amenorrhea, thromboembolic disorders, and a possible increased risk of breast cancer.

Corticosteroid therapy has been limited primarily to severe, resistant cases. The therapy results in remarkable healing, but acne usually returns after the therapy has been terminated. Isotretinoin (Accutane), an orally administered synthetic retinoid or acid form of vitamin A, has revolutionized the treatment of recalcitrant cases of acne and cystic acnes. In carefully planned dosages, oral isotretinoin has cleared major cases of acne and initiated long-term remissions of the disease. It is administered for 3- to 4-month treatment periods. Although the exact mode of action is unknown, it decreases sebaceous gland activity, prevents new comedones from forming, reduces the *P. acnes* count by sebum reduction, and has an anti-inflammatory effect. Because of its many side effects, it is used only in persons with severe acne. Side effects are dryness of the mouth and other mucous membranes, conjunctivitis, musculoskeletal system abnormalities, and elevated liver and serum lipid levels. Isotretinoin is also a major teratogen that causes brain, heart, and ear malformations. Women taking isotretinoin are strongly advised not to become pregnant; some health care providers require written contracts from women to this end.

Other treatment measures for acne include surgery, ultraviolet irradiation, cryotherapy, and intralesional glucocorticosteroid injection. Acne surgery involves the aspiration of comedones with small-bore needles or devices designed to extract comedone contents. Scarring is a common sequela if done improperly. The use of ultraviolet irradiation, which involves exposure to hot or cold quartz lights for specified periods, remains controversial. It continues to be used in treatment of some forms of acne. Cryotherapy (*i.e.*, freezing with carbon dioxide slushes, liquid nitrogen, dry ice, or acetone) has been effective in promoting healing of lesions by removing the outer layers of skin. Intralesional injection of corticosteroids using a syringe or needleless injector is limited to severe nodulocystic forms of acne. It has been effective in promoting cyst healing, but usually has to be repeated frequently.

Acne Conglobata

Acne conglobata occurs later in life and is a chronic form of acne. Comedones, papules, pustules, nodules, abscesses, cysts, and scars occur on the back, buttocks, and chest. Lesions occur to a lesser extent on the abdomen, shoulders, neck, face, upper arms, and thighs. The comedones have multiple openings. Their discharge is odoriferous, serous, and purulent or mucoid. Healing leaves deep keloidal lesions. Afflicted persons have anemia with increased white blood cell counts, sedimentation rates, and neutrophil counts. The treatment is difficult and stringent. It often includes debridement, systemic corticosteroid therapy, oral retinoids, and systemic antibiotics.

Other Forms of Acne

There are numerous other forms of acne. The symptoms vary depending on the source or age of onset. Treatment measures for these acnes depend on the precipitating agent and the extent of the lesions. Many of the previously discussed treatment measures have been used with various degrees of success.

Acne fulminans is manifested by a sudden eruption of large, inflamed lesions on the back and chest that ulcerate, heal, and scar. The lesions are extremely painful, and the person often limps in a bent-over position. Teenage boys, often with a mild form of acne, are most affected by this type. *Steatocystoma multiplex* consists of an eruption of many cystic lesions of various sizes on the trunk of men and women of young adult age. *Neonatal acne* occurs on newborn infants, mostly males. Typically, it is found on the nose and cheeks; it usually clears without treatment. *Drug acnes* occur as an untoward reaction to certain pharmacologic agents, most commonly steroids, iodides (in cough mixtures), and bromides (in sedatives). Acne that results from the exposure to occupational compounds or chemicals is called *occupational acne*. Many of the precipitating agents are the same as those that cause allergic responses; cutting oils are the most offensive.

Acne cosmetica is believed to be caused by women's use of cosmetic, cleaning, and self-adornment products. The exact causes are unknown because of the variety of cosmetic agents used by women. Even after cosmetic use has been discontinued, this acne usually persists and is difficult to heal. *Acne detergicans* is believed to be caused by compulsive washing of the face with soaps, and *acne mechanica* develops from repeated trauma to the skin. A common form of acne mechanica is seen on football players from the rubbing of their helmets. *Pomade acne* follows the hairline and is most commonly seen on African-American males. *Acne excoriée des jeunes filles* is a mild form of acne seen in adolescent girls. The lesions spread from scratching and picking that are believed to be of emotional origin.

Rosacea

Rosacea, formerly called acne rosacea, is a chronic inflammatory process that occurs in middle-aged and older adults. It is easily confused with acne and may coexist with it. In the early stage of development, there are repeated episodes of blushing, eventually becoming a permanent dark red erythema on the nose and cheeks that sometimes extends to the forehead and chin (Fig. 15–17). This stage often occurs before the age of 20. As the person ages, the erythema persists, and telangiectasia with or without acneiform components (*e.g.*, comedones, pustules, nodules) develops. After years of affliction, acne rosacea may develop into an irregular, bullous hyperplasia (thickening) of the nose, known as *rhinophyma*. The sebaceous follicles and openings enlarge, and the skin color changes to a purple red. The cause remains unknown. It is more common in fair-skinned persons and has been called "the curse of the Celts." An early characteristic and diagnostic sign is persons who "flush and blush." It is more common in women; rhinophyma is more common in men.

Alcoholic intake has been rejected as a causative agent. However, persons with rosacea are heat sensitive. They are instructed to avoid vascular-stimulating agents such as heat, cold, sunlight, hot liquids, highly seasoned foods, and alcohol. Treatment measures are similar to those used for acne vulgaris. Rhinophyma can be treated surgically.

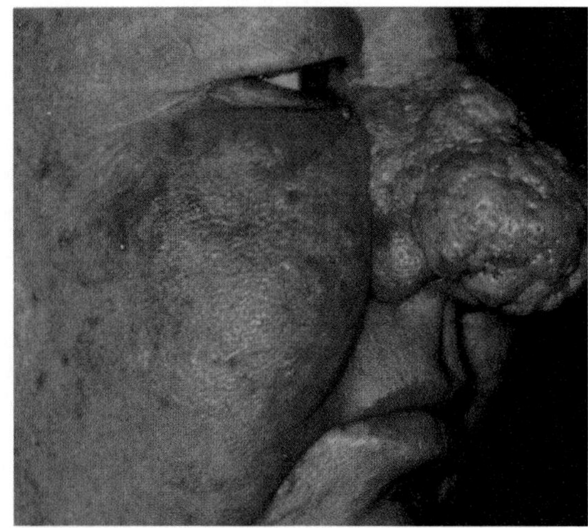

Figure 15–17
Chronic rosacea with rhinophyma. (Hoechst Marion Rouseel Pharmaceuticals, Inc.)

Eczematous Dermatoses

Eczema is an inflammatory skin response to any injurious agent. It is characterized by epidermal edema with separation of epidermal cells. Eczematous dermatoses may be related to hypersensitivity reactions and include irritant contact dermatitis, allergy contact dermatitis, atopic eczema, and nummular eczema.

Contact or Irritant Dermatitis

Contact dermatitis is a common inflammation of the skin. There are two types of contact dermatitis: *allergic contact dermatitis* and *irritant contact dermatitis*. Allergic contact dermatitis is the cell-mediated allergic response brought about by sensitization to an allergen. It is a type IV sensitivity reaction (see Chapter 12). This type depends on hapten migration into the skin to produce an immune reaction. More than 2000 allergens have been identified as capable of producing the inflammatory skin response. Some are listed in Table 15–5. Crude forms of many naturally occurring substances are less allergenic than alloys and synthetic products. Additives such as dyes and perfumes account for the major sources of known allergens. An example is the increased incidence of contact dermatitis from synthetic latex products, specifically the use of rubber gloves and condoms because of the HIV epidemic. Additional examples are poison ivy, chemicals, and metal alloys found in jewelry.

The lesions of allergic contact dermatitis range from a mild erythema with edema to vesicles or large bullae (Fig. 15–18). Secondary lesions from bacterial infection may occur. Lesions can occur almost anywhere on the body. The typical poison ivy lesion consists of vesicles or bullae

TABLE 15-5 Sources of Contact Dermatitis Allergens

Sources	Possible Allergens
Clothing	Raw material such as wool, polyester, cotton, dyes and sizers in new fabrics and clothing; detergents used to wash clothing
Cosmetics	Dyes, perfumes, oil (*e.g.*, lanolin, coconut oil, olive oil, palm oil)
Cleaning products (e.g., soaps, detergents)	Fats, alkali, perfumes, dyes, formaldehyde, hydrochloric acid, sodium carbonate, ammonium hydroxide, and germicidal agents
Occupational exposure	Metals, metal salts, and alloys (nickel); resin, natural and synthetic; tung oil, linseed oil, turpentine; usually the allergens are from the processing of rubber rather than crude rubber (acids, alkalis, solvents, soaps, dust, heat) and are more common from rubber products (gloves, footwear, condoms)
Plants and woods	Ragweed; lichens; poison ivy, oak, and sumac; pine (more from resin and turpentine); caterpillars; and growth on trees and plants
Soap ingredients	
Fats	Coconut oil, olive oil, palm oil, rosin, and fish or whale oil
Alkali	Sodium hydroxide, potassium hydroxide, sodium carbonate, trisodium phosphate, sodium tripolyphosphate, pyrophosphate, sodium silicate
Perfumes	Seed oil, oil of bergamot, bitter almond oil, eucalyptus oil, geranium oil, lavender oil, peppermint oil, rosemary oil, musk
Coloring agents	D&C yellow No. 11, eosin, rhodamine, fuchsin, ultramarine green

in a linear pattern. The vesicles and bullae break and weep, leaving an excoriated area. Irritant contact dermatitis occurs in persons who are in contact with a sufficient amount of the irritant to cause a reaction. It can occur from mechanical means such as rubbing (*e.g.*, wool, fiberglass), chemical irritants (*e.g.*, household cleaning products), or environmental irritants (*e.g.*, plants, urine). An example is the skin burn that may occur from contact with cement products. Irritant contact dermatitis ranges from acute to chronic cases. Skin reactions range from mild erythema and scaling to acute necrotic burns. Several factors contribute to the condition besides the initial irritant: friction, trauma, humidity, and age.

In allergic contact dermatitis and irritant contact dermatitis, the location of the lesions are of great benefit in diagnosing the causative agent. Treatment measures for both are aimed at removing the source of the irritant or allergen. This may mean that the person needs to modify his or her behavior or even change employment to avoid the irritant or allergen. Modification measures may include wearing protective clothing such as goggles or impenetrable gloves. Another modification measure may be alerting persons who have irritant contact dermatitis and work in heavy industrial areas to avoid strong hand cleansers and remove grease and grime with an inert oil (*e.g.*, salad oil, mineral oil) before washing with soap and water.

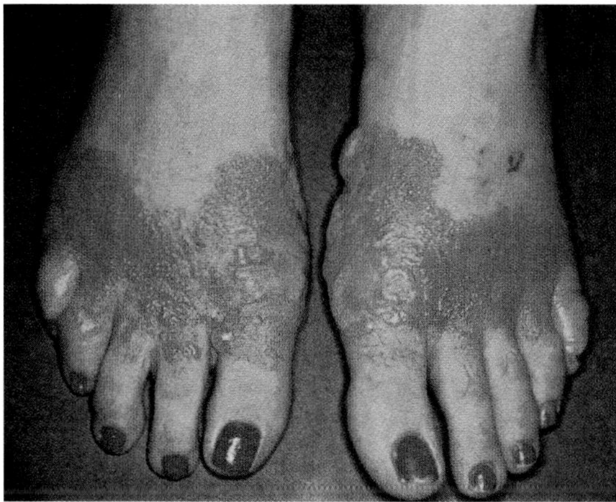

Figure 15–18 Contact dermatitis from shoe material. (Glaxo Wellcome Co.)

Minor cases are treated by washing the affected areas to remove further contamination by the irritant or allergen, applying antipruritic creams or lotions, and bandaging the exposed areas. Topical corticosteroids may be helpful in these cases. Systemic treatment regimens differ according to the type of irritant or allergen and the severity of the reaction. More extreme cases are treated with wet dressings, systemic corticosteroids, and oral antihistamines.

Atopic Eczema and Nummular Eczema

Atopic eczema (*i.e.*, atopic dermatitis) is a common skin disorder that occurs in two clinical forms, infantile and adult. It is associated with a type I hypersensitivity reaction (see Chapter 12). There is usually a family history of asthma, hay fever, or atopic dermatitis. The infantile form is characterized by vesicle formation, oozing, and crusting with excoriations. It usually begins in the cheeks and may progress to involve the scalp, arms, trunk, and legs (Fig. 15–19). The skin of the cheeks may be paler, with extra creases under the eyes (*i.e.*, Denny Morgan folds). There is marked follicle involvement in persons with black skin. Lesions may be hypopigmented or

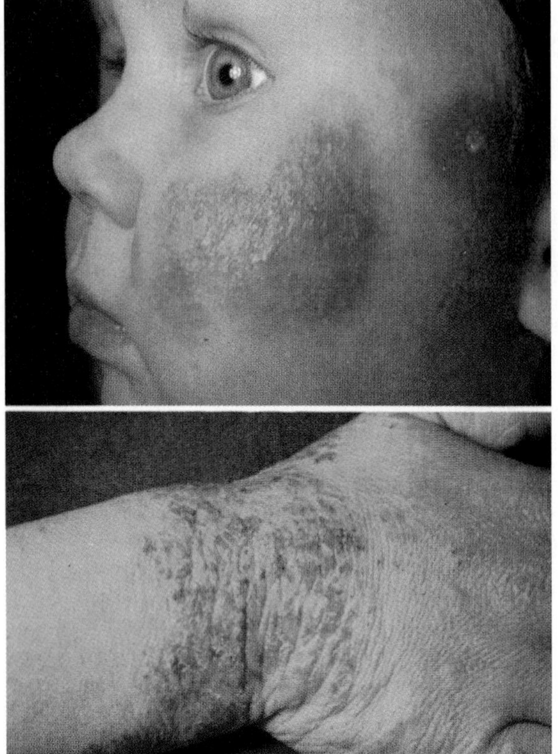

Figure 15–19
Atopic eczema on an infant's face and wrist. (Dome Chemicals.)

hyperpigmented or both on a black-skinned person. The infantile form usually becomes milder as the child ages, often disappearing by the age of 15. Adolescents and adults generally have dry, leathery, and hyperpigmented or hypopigmented lesions located in the antecubital and popliteal areas. These may spread to the neck, hands, feet, eyelids, and behind the ears. Itching may be severe with both forms. Secondary infections are common.

Treatment measures for atopic eczema are designed for the chronic nature of the disease. Avoiding exposure to environmental irritants and foods that cause exacerbation of the symptoms is recommended. Wool and lanolin (*i.e.,* wool fat) often aggravate the condition. Dryness of the skin often causes the condition to become worse. For this reason, bathing and the use of soap and water should be reduced. Avoidance of temperature changes and stress helps to minimize abnormal and cutaneous vascular and sweat responses. Acute weeping lesions are treated with soothing lotions, soaps, baths, or wet dressings. Subacute or subsiding lesions may be treated with lotions containing mild antipruritic agents. Chronic dry lesions are treated with ointments and creams containing lubricating, keratolytic, or antipruritic agents. Topical or systemic corticosteroid therapy may be indicated for severe cases.

The lesions of nummular eczema are coin-shaped (nummular), papulovesicular patches mainly involving the arms and legs (Fig. 15–20). Lichenification and secondary bacterial infections are common. The exact cause of *nummular eczema* is unknown. There is usually a history of asthma, hay fever, or atopic dermatitis. The disease is chronic and most often occurs in elderly men. Ingestion of iodides and bromides usually aggravates the condition. The treatment is palliative. Frequent bathing and foods rich in iodides and bromides should be avoided. Topical corticosteroids and antibiotics are prescribed as necessary.

Urticaria

Urticaria, also called hives, is characterized by edematous plaques called *wheals* accompanied by intense itching. The wheals typically appear as raised pink or red areas surrounded by a paler halo. They blanch with pressure and vary in size from a few millimeters to centimeters. Thicker lesions that result from massive transudation of fluid into the dermis or subcutaneous tissue are referred to angioedema. Although angioedema lesions can occur on any skin surface, they typically involve the larynx, causing hoarseness or sore throat, or mucosal surface of the gastrointestinal tract, causing abdominal pain.

Histamine is the most common mediator of urticaria. Histamine causes hyperpermeability of microvessels of the skin and surrounding tissue, allowing fluid to leak into the tissues and causing edema and wheal formation.[8,9] Histamine is contained in the granules of mast cells. A variety of immunologic, nonimmunologic, physical, and chemical stimuli can cause mast cell degranulation with release of histamine into the surrounding tissues and circulation.

Urticaria can be acute or chronic. If daily or almost daily episodes of urticaria persist for longer that 6 weeks, the condition is considered chronic. The most common causes of acute urticaria are foods or drinks, medications, or exposure to pollens or chemicals. Food is the most common cause of acute urticaria in children. Although nonsteroidal antiinflammatory drugs, including aspirin, do not normally cause urticaria, they may exacerbate preexisting disease.

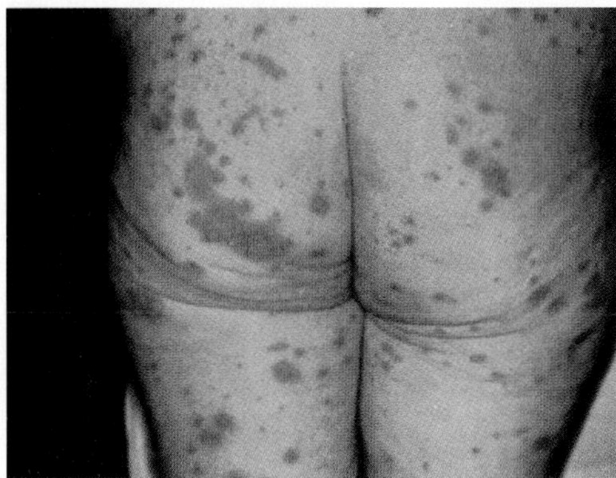

Figure 15–20
Nummular eczema of the buttocks. (Johnson and Johnson.)

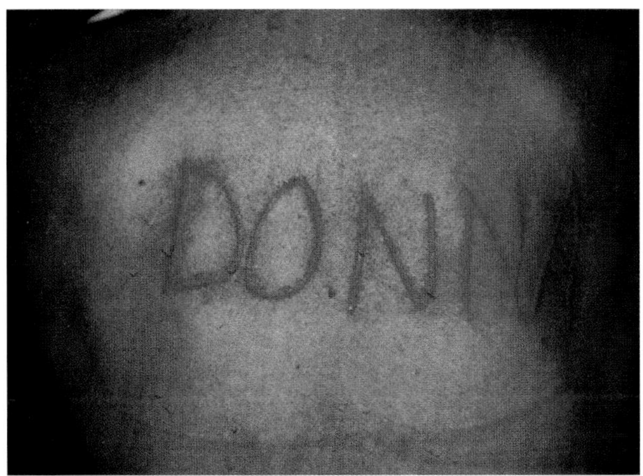

Figure 15–21
Dermographism on a patient's back. Dermik Laboratories, Inc.

Chronic urticaria affects primarily adults and is twice as common in women as in men. Usually, its cause cannot be determined despite extensive laboratory tests. There is increasing evidence that some forms of chronic urticaria are associated with histamine-releasing autoantibodies. In rare cases, urticaria is a manifestation of underlying disease. Conditions that have been implicated are certain types of cancers, collagen diseases, hepatitis, and thyroid abnormalities. There is a significant association between chronic urticaria and autoimmune thyroid disease (*e.g.,* Hashimoto's thyroiditis, Graves' disease, toxic multinodular thyroiditis). A hereditary deficiency of complement (*i.e.,* C1 esterase inhibitor) can also cause urticaria and angioedema.

Physical urticarias constitute another form of chronic urticaria.[9] Physical urticarias are intermittent, usually last less than 2 hours, are produced by appropriate stimulus, have a distinctive appearance and locations, and are seen most frequently in young adults. In dermographism (*i.e.,* skin writing), which is one form of physical urticaria, wheals and flares occur in response to simple rubbing of the skin (Fig. 15–21). The wheals that follow the pattern of the scratch or rubbing appear within 5 to 10 minutes and dissolve completely with 15 to 20 minutes. Other types of physical urticaria are cholinergic (*i.e.,* exercise-induced), cold, delayed pressure, solar (*i.e.,* sunlight), aquagenic (*i.e.,* water), vibratory, and external (localized heat-induced). Table 15–6 summarizes the features of common types of physical urticaria. Appropriate challenge tests (*e.g.,* application of an ice cube to the skin to initiate development of cold urticaria) can be used to differentiate physical urticaria from chronic urticaria due to other causes.

Most types of urticaria are treated with antihistamines: drugs that block histamine type 1 (H_1) and, less frequently H_1 in combination with histamine type 2 (H_2). They control urticaria by inhibiting vasodilation and escape of fluid into the surrounding tissues. Severe urticaria and angioedema are treated with epinephrine. Oral corticosteroids may be used in treatment of refractory urticaria. Tricyclic antidepressant drugs, particularly those with antihistamine actions, may also be used. Starch or colloid-type (e.g., Aveno) baths may be used as a comfort measure.

Drug-Induced Skin Eruptions

Without exception, any drug can cause a localized or generalized skin eruption. Topical drugs usually are responsible for a localized contact dermatitis type of rash, and systemic drugs cause generalized skin lesions. Most drug eruptions are morbilliform (*i.e.,* measlelike) or exanthematous. They usually disappear in a few days. Some progress to more severe skin eruptions, necessitating prompt medical attention. Table 15–7 describes the characteristics of selected drug-induced skin eruptions. Drug-induced skin reactions mimic almost all other skin lesions described in this chapter.

The diagnosis of a drug sensitivity depends almost entirely on accurate reporting by the person, because the lesions from drug sensitization differ greatly. Treatment is aimed at eliminating the offending drug. Mild skin eruptions are treated symptomatically, but severe drug eruptions often require systemic corticosteroid therapy and antihistamines.

Three types of bullous skin manifestations that result from drug reactions end in epidermal skin detachment:

TABLE **15-6**

Clinical Features of Physical Urticaria

Type	Clinical Features
Dermographism	Itchy linear wheals with surrounding bright red flair; last no longer than 15 to 30 minutes
Cholinergic urticaria	Small wheals with surrounding bright red flare and intense pruritus develop in response to a rise in core temperature, as with exercise, external heat, emotion, or eating spicy foods; last no longer than 1 to 2 hours
Cold urticaria	Itchy, pale or red swelling at site of contact with cold surfaces, air, or water; lasts no longer than 30 to 60 minutes
Pressure urticaria	Large, painful, or itchy swelling at site of pressure (*e.g.,* waist, palms, hands); appears 1 to 4 hours after pressure application and lasts 24 hours or more
Solar urticaria	Itchy, pale or red swelling at site of exposure to ultraviolet light

TABLE 15-7

Types of Rashes Associated With Drug-Induced Skin Eruptions

Drugs	Type of Rash
Barbiturates, arsenic, sulfonamides, quinine	Resembles measles
Barbiturates, arsenic, codeine, morphine	Resembles scarlet fever
Bismuth, gold, barbiturates	Resembles pityriasis rosea
Quinine, procaine, antihistamines	Eczematous
Isoniazid, para-aminosalicylic acid combinations	Resembles nummular eczema
Penicillin, salicylates, opium	Urticaria
Bromides, iodides, testosterone, corticotropin	Pustular (acne)
Sulfonamides, penicillin, phenylbutazone	Vesicular, bullous
Quinacrine, arsenic, gold	Lichen planus
Contraceptive drugs, quinacrine	Pigment changes
Arsenic, mercury	Keratosis and epitheliomas

erythema multiforme minor, Stevens-Johnson syndrome (*i.e.*, erythema multiforme major), and *toxic epidermal necrolysis*. The latter two are rare occurrences, but they can be life threatening. Both are usually caused by sensitivity to drugs, mostly sulfonamides and anticonvulsants. *Erythema multiforme minor* may be drug induced, but more frequently it occurs after infections, especially with herpes simplex. It is self-limiting, with a small amount of skin detachment at the lesion sites.

The lesions of *erythema multiforme minor* and *Stevens-Johnson syndrome* are similar. The primary lesion of both is a round, erythematous papule, resembling an insect bite. Within hours to days, these lesions change into several different patterns. The individual lesions may enlarge and coalesce, producing small plaques, or they may change to concentric zones of color appearing as "target" or "iris" lesions (Fig. 15–22). The outermost rings of the target lesions are usually erythematous; the central portion is usually opaque white, yellow, or gray

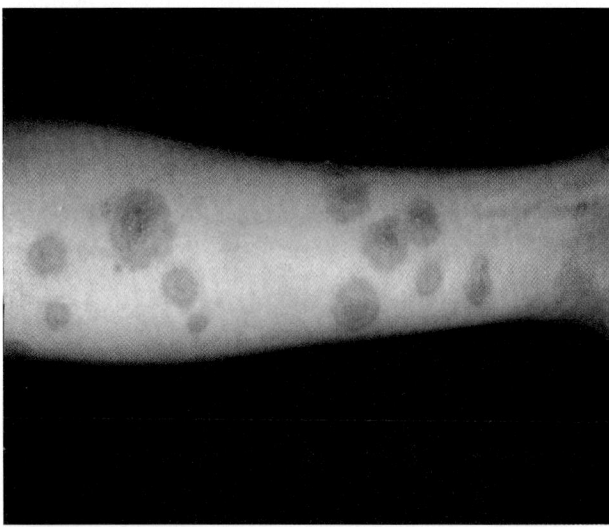

Figure 15–22
Erthyema-muliforme–like eruption on the patient's arm. Notice the dusky, target-like appearance. (Dermick Laboratories, Inc.)

(dusky). In the center, small blisters on the dusky purpuric macules may form, giving them the characteristic target-like appearance. Although there is wide distribution of lesions over the body surface area, there is a propensity for the face and trunk. With Stevens-Johnson syndrome, there is more skin detachment.

Toxic epidermal necrolysis is the most serious and life-threatening drug reaction. The person experiences a prodromal period of malaise, low-grade fever, and sore throat. Within a few days, widespread erythema and large flaccid bullae appear, followed by the loss of the epidermis. This leaves a denuded and painful dermis. The skin surrounding large denuded areas may have the typical target-like lesions seen with Stevens-Johnson syndrome. The skin separates easily from the dermis with lateral pressure; this is called *Nikolsky's sign*. The epithelium of mucosal surfaces, especially the mouth and eyes, may be involved.

These three types of bullous skin eruptions are seemingly quite similar. The diagnostic boundary for erythema multiforme minor is that it usually occurs after herpes simplex infection and is self-limiting. Precise diagnostic boundaries between Stevens-Johnson syndrome and toxic epidermal necrolysis have not been established. However, it is generally agreed that cases involving less than 10% of the body surface area are called Stevens-Johnson syndrome, and detachment of more than 30% of the epidermis is labeled toxic epidermal necrolysis.[10,11] The mortality rate for Stevens-Johnson syndrome is less than 5%, and that for toxic epidermal necrolysis is 30% or greater.[11]

The skin detachment of these drug reactions is different from the desquamation (*i.e.*, peeling) discussed with other skin disorders. For example, with scarlet fever, peeling of the stratum corneum, the dead keratinized layer, occurs. In the bullous disorders discussed here, full-thickness detachment (*i.e.*, peeling of the entire epidermis down to the dermis) occurs. This leaves the person vulnerable to multiple associated problems, such as loss of body fluid, nutritional deficits, thermal control, and electrolyte imbalance.

Treatment of erythema multiforme minor and minor cases of Stevens-Johnson syndrome include relief of symptoms using compresses, antipruritic drugs, and topical anesthetics. Corticosteroid therapy may be indicated in more moderate cases, although its use is controversial. For major cases of Stevens-Johnson syndrome or toxic epidermal necrolysis, hospitalization is required for fluid replacement, antibiotics, respiratory care, analgesics, and moist dressings. When large areas of skin are detached, the care is similar to thermal burn patients.

Papulosquamous Dermatoses

Papulosquamous dermatoses are a group of skin disorders that are characterized by scaly papules and plaques. Among the major papulosquamous diseases discussed in this section are psoriasis, pityriasis rosea, and lichen planus.

Psoriasis

Psoriasis is a common, papulosquamous disease characterized by white, scaling patches of various sizes. Psoriasis occurs worldwide, although the incidence is lower in warmer, sunnier climates. In the United States, it affects 1% to 2% of the population.[12] The average age of onset is in the third decade. Approximately one third of the patients have a genetic history, indicating an hereditary factor. Childhood onset of the disease is more associated with a familial history than psoriasis occurring in adults older than 30.[12] The disease, which can persist throughout life and exacerbate at unpredictable times, is classified as a chronic ailment. A few cases, however, have been known to clear and not recur.

The cause of psoriasis is uncertain. There is strong evidence of a T-lymphocyte–mediated dermal immune response to an unidentified antigen.[13,14] It is thought that the activated T lymphocytes (mainly CD4-positive helper T cells) produce chemical messengers called *cytokines,* which stimulate keratinocyte proliferation. The accompanying inflammatory changes are caused by infiltration of neutrophils and monocytes (see Chapter 11). Skin trauma (*i.e.,* prepsoriasis) is a common precipitating factor in those predisposed to the disease. This reaction of the skin to the original trauma, which can be of any type, is called the *Koebner reaction.* There appears to be an association between psoriasis and arthritis. Psoriatic arthritis occurs in 5% to 7% of persons with psoriasis (see Chapter 47).

Psoriasis is characterized by increased migration of keratinocytes from the basal layer of the epidermis. Histologically, the migration time of the keratinocyte from the basal cell layer of the stratum corneum decreases from the normal 14 days to approximately 4 to 7 days. Cell turnover and metabolism increases, a process called *hyperkeratosis.* There is thinning of the suprapapillary plate, with elongation and edema of the dermal papillae. Capillary blood flow increases to support the metabolic demands. Capillary beds show permanent damage even when the disease is in remission or has resolved. There is absence of the granular layer of the epidermis, and neutrophils are found in the stratum corneum.

A chronic stationary form of psoriasis, called *psoriasis vulgaris,* is the most common form. The lesions may occur anywhere on the skin, but most often involve the elbows, knees, and scalp (Fig. 15–23). The primary lesions are papules that vary in shape. The papules form into plaques with thick and silvery scales. A differential diagnostic finding is that the plaques bleed from minute points when removed, which is known as *Auspitz sign.*

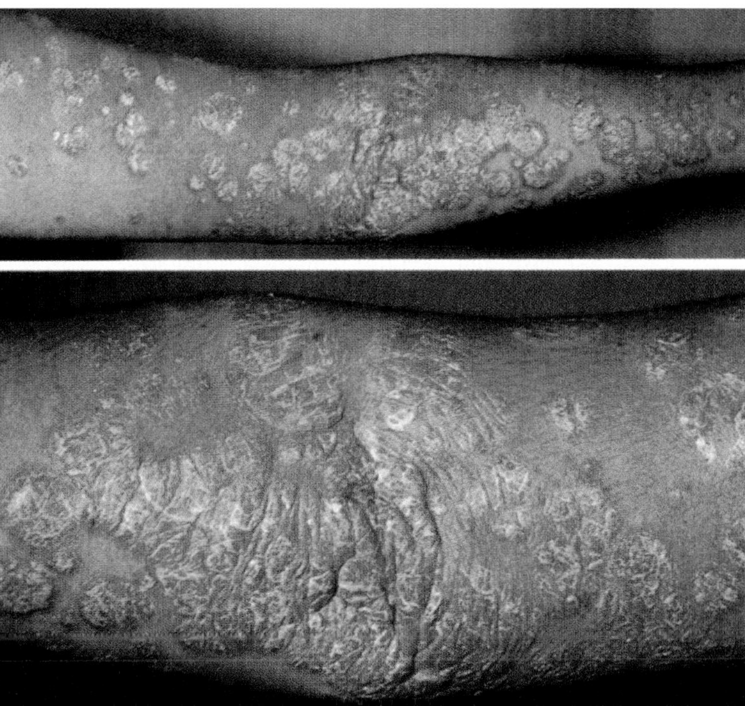

Figure 15–23
Psoriasis on the elbows of a 17-year-old girl. (Roche Laboratories)

Secondary lesions are uncommon, but there may be excoriation, thickening, or oozing. In African Americans, the plaques may turn purple.

Other forms of psoriasis exist. One form is called *guttate psoriasis,* which occurs in children and young adults. Its lesions are small and usually limited to the upper trunk and extremities. This form is generally brought on by a streptococcal infection. Sometimes this form resolves after several weeks, or it may progress into the chronic form. Generalized *pustular psoriasis* is a distinct form of the disease that is distinguished by a fever that lasts for several days after eruptions of small pustules. The pustules occur over the trunk and extremities and may include nail beds, palms of the hands, and soles of the feet. *Erythrodermic psoriasis* affects all body surfaces, including the hands, feet, nails, trunk, and extremities. It is characterized by a process in which the lesions scale and become confluent, leaving much of the body surface a bright red, with continued skin shedding. This form is rare. *Psoriasis annularis* is another rare form of the disease. As its name implies, the lesions have an annular shape.

Treatment. The goal of treatment is to suppress the signs and symptoms of the disease. There is no cure. Treatment measures are divided into topical and systemic approaches. Generally, topical agents are used first in any treatment regimen and when less than 20% of the body surface is involved.[13,14]

Topical agents include emollients, keratolytic agents, coal tar, anthralin, corticosteroids, and calcipotriene. Emollients hydrate and soften the psoriatic plaques. Petroleum based products are more effective than water based, but they are less acceptable cosmetically to persons with psoriasis. Keratolytic agents are peeling agents. Salicylic acid is the most widely used. It softens and removes plaques. It has been used alone or in conjunction with other topical agents. Coal or wood tar (*i.e.,* crude tar or wood extract) is one of the oldest yet effective forms of treatment. The skin is covered with a film of coal tar for up to several weeks. The exact mechanism of action of the tar products is unknown, but the side effects of the treatment are few. Newer preparations of coal tar lotions and shampoos make them more aesthetically pleasing to persons with psoriasis, but the odor remains a problem. Anthralin has remained a topical treatment of choice. Applied topically, it has been effective in resolving lesions in approximately 2 weeks. A treatment variation, called the Ingram method, involves coal tar applications, ultraviolet B (UVB) radiation, followed by anthralin paste application. A major disadvantage to anthralin is that it stains the skin and clothes brown or purple.

Topical corticosteroids are widely used and relatively effective. They are more acceptable to persons with psoriasis because they do not stain and are relatively easy to use. Their effectiveness is increased when used under occlusive dressings, but the side effects increase.

Calcipotriene, a topical vitamin D derivative, is a newer drug and has been shown to be effective and safe for short-term and long-term treatment of psoriasis. It inhibits epidermal cell proliferation and enhances cell differentiation. Calcipotrol treatment does not seem to affect calcium or bone metabolism.

Systemic treatments include phototherapy, photochemotherapy, methotrexate, retinoids, corticosteroids, and cyclosporine. The positive effects of sunlight have long been established. Climatotherapy (*i.e.,* warm climate and saltwater baths for 4 to 6 weeks) and heliotherapy (*i.e.,* sunbathing in a suitable climate) have been effective treatment measures for those who can afford to travel.

Photochemotherapy involves using a light-activated form of the drug methoxsalen. Methoxsalen, a psoralen, exerts its actions when exposed to ultraviolet A (UVA) radiation in the 320- to 400-nm wavelength range. The combination treatment regimen of psoralen (P) and UVA is known by the acronym PUVA. Methoxsalen is given orally before UVA exposure. Activated by the UVA energy, methoxsalen inhibits DNA synthesis preventing cell mitosis, decreasing the hyperkeratosis that occurs with psoriasis. Unfortunately, this regimen increases the risk of subsequently developing melanoma.

Retinoids are derivatives of vitamin A. Etretinate has been effective, and isotretinoin (used for acne) is less effective in treating psoriasis. Etretinate suppresses inflammation and DNA synthesis in the epidermis. The drug may be used as short-term adjunctive therapy in combination with PUVA and UVB treatment.

Systemic corticosteroids have been effective in treating severe or pustular psoriasis. However, they cause severe side effects, including Cushing's syndrome. Intralesional injection of the corticosteroid drug, triamcinolone, has proven effective in resistant lesions. Methotrexate, which is used for cancer treatment, is an antimetabolite that inhibits DNA synthesis and prevents cell mitosis. Methotrexate is given orally and has been effective in treating psoriasis when other approaches fail. The drug has many side effects, including nausea, malaise, leukopenia, thrombocytopenia, and liver function abnormalities. Cyclosporine is a potent immunosuppressive drug used to prevent rejection in organ transplantation. It suppresses inflammation and the proliferation of T cells in persons with psoriasis. Its use is limited to severe psoriasis because of serious toxic and side effects, including nephrotoxicity, hypertension, and increased risk of cancers. Intralesional cyclosporine has also been effective.

Pityriasis Rosea

Pityriasis rosea is a rash of unknown origin that primarily affects young adults. The incidence is highest in winter. It may be viral, and the picornavirus is under investigation. Cases occur in clusters and among persons who are in close contact with each other, indicating an infectious spread. However, there are no data to support communicability. It may be an immune response to any number of agents.

The characteristic lesion is an oval macule or papule with surrounding erythema (Fig. 15–24). The lesion spreads with central clearing, much like tinea corporis.

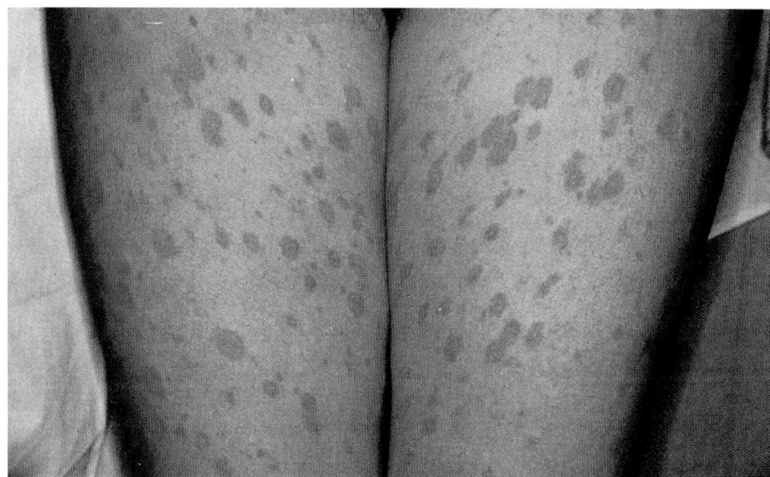

Figure 15–24
Pityriasis rosea of the thighs. (Syntex Laboratories.)

This initial lesion is a solitary lesion called the *herald patch* and is usually on the trunk or neck. As the lesion enlarges and begins to fade away (2 to 10 days), successive crops of lesions appear on the trunk and neck. The lesions on the back have a characteristic "Christmas tree" pattern. The extremities, face, and scalp may be involved. Mild to severe pruritus may occur.

The disease is self-limited and usually disappears within 6 to 8 weeks. Treatment measures are palliative and include topical steroids, antihistamines, and colloid baths. Systemic corticosteroids may be indicated in severe cases.

Lichen Planus

The term *lichen* is of Greek origin and means *tree moss*. The term is applied to skin disorders characterized by small (2 to 10 mm), flat-topped papules with irregular, angulated borders (Fig. 15–25). Lichen planus is a relatively common chronic, pruritic disease. It involves inflammation and papular eruption of the skin and mucous membranes. Idiopathic lichen planus is associated with a variety of drugs and chemicals in susceptible persons. Lichen planus may involve a cell-mediated immune response that occurs in the basal cells. There is basal cell degeneration with reduced cell mitosis. There are variations in the pattern of lesions (e.g., annular, linear) and differences in the sites (e.g., mucous membranes, genitalia, nails, scalp). The characteristic lesion is a purple, polygonal papule covered with a shiny, white, lacelike pattern. These lesions appear on the wrist, ankles, and trunk of the body. Most persons who have skin lesions also have oral

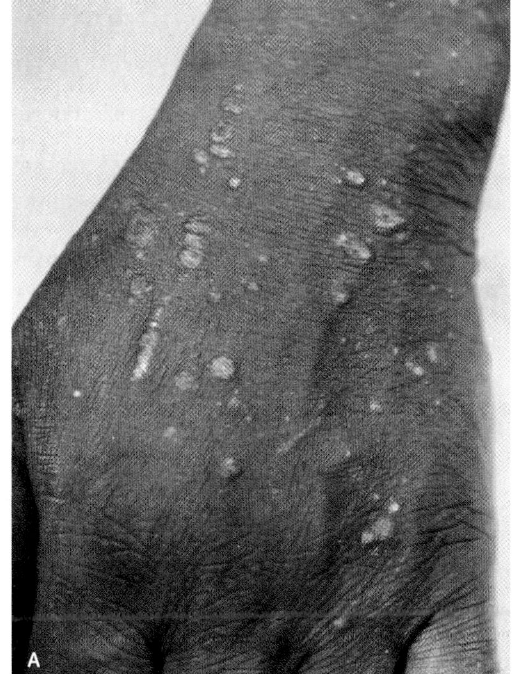

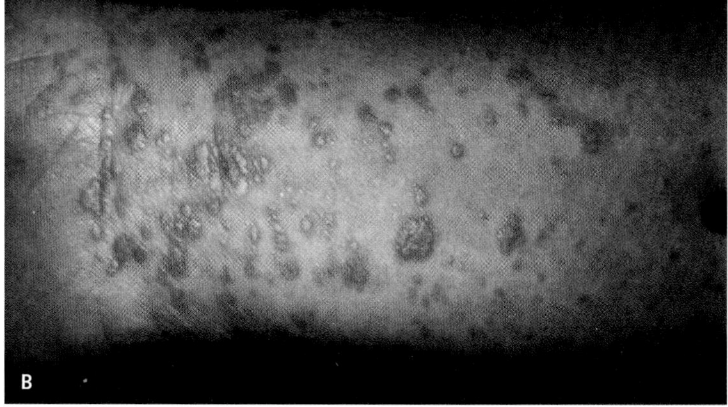

Figure 15–25
(A) Lichen planus of the dorsum of the hand and wrist. Notice the violacenous color of the papules and the linear Koebner phenomenon. **(B)** Lichen planus. (E.R. Squibb, Johnson & Johnson)

lesions. These appear as milky white lacework on the buccal mucosa or tongue.

For most persons, lichen planus is a self-limited disease. Treatment measures include discontinuation of all medications, followed by treatment with topical corticosteroids and occlusive dressings. Systemic corticosteroids may be indicated in severe cases. Intralesional injections of triamcinolone acetonide suspension, a corticosteroid preparation, has produced some cures. Antipruritic agents are helpful in reducing itch.

Lichen Simplex Chronicus

Lichen simplex chronicus is a localized lichenoid dermatitis. It is characterized by the occurrence of patches of itchy, reddened, thickened, and scaly, dry skin (Fig. 15–26). Persons with the condition may have a single or, less frequently, multiple lesions. The lesions are seen most commonly at the nape of the neck, wrist, ankles, or anal area. The condition usually begins as a small pruritic patch, which culminates in a cycle of itching, scratching, more itching and scratching, and development of a chronic dermatosis. Excoriations and lichenification with thickening of the skin develops because of the chronic itching and scratching. Treatment consists of measures to decrease scratching of the area. A moderate-potency corticosteroid is often prescribed to decrease the itching and subsequent inflammatory process.

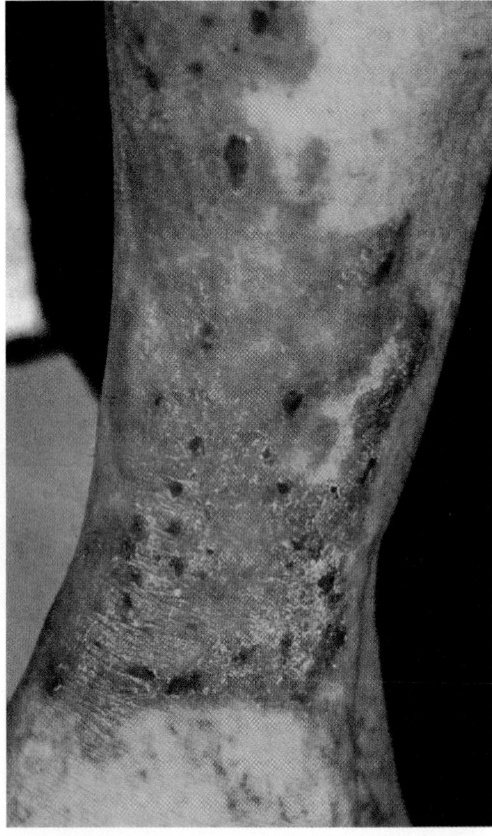

Figure 15–26
Localized lichen simplex chronicus of the leg. (Duke Laboratories, Inc.)

Arthropod Infestations

The skin is susceptible to a variety of disorders as a result of an invasion or infestation by bugs, ticks, or parasites. The type of rash or sometimes singular lesion depends on the causative agent.

Scabies

Scabies is caused by a mite, *Sarcoptes scabiei*, that burrows into the epidermis. After a female mite is impregnated, she burrows into the skin and lays two to three eggs each day for 4 or 5 weeks. The eggs hatch after 3 to 4 days, and the larvae migrate to the skin surface. At this point, they burrow into the skin only for food or protection. The larvae molt and become nymphs; they molt once more to become adults. After the new adult females are impregnated, the cycle is repeated.

The characteristic lesion is a small burrow, approximately 2 mm long, that may be red to reddish brown. Small vesicles may cover the burrows. The areas most commonly affected are the interdigital web of the finger, flexor surface of the wrist, inner surface of the elbow, axilla, female nipple, penis, belt line, and gluteal crease. Pruritus is common and may result from the burrows, the fecal material of the mite, or both. Excoriations may develop from scratching. Secondary bacterial infections and severe skin lesions may occur if the condition is untreated.

Scabies is transmitted by person-to-person contact, including sexual contact. It is also transmitted by contact with mite-infested sheets in hospitals and nursing homes, because the mite can live up to 2 days on sheets or clothing. Scabies affects all people in all socioeconomic classes, although African Americans seem more resistant. Usually more prevalent in times of war and famine, it reached pandemic proportions in the 1970s, perhaps as a result of poverty, sexual promiscuity, and worldwide travel. Outbreaks continue to occur, but they are mostly sporadic and localized to nursing homes and families.

Diagnosis is done by skin scrapings. A positive diagnosis relies on the presence of mites, ova, or feces. The treatment is simple and curative. After bathing, Permethrin, lindane, Malathion, or other effective mite-killing agents are applied over the entire skin surface for 12 hours. Repeat applications may be recommended in certain cases, but one treatment is usually sufficient. Care must be taken to ensure that close contacts are treated. Clothes and towels are disinfected with hot water and detergent or they can be isolated for 4 weeks. If symptoms persist after treatment, the patient should be advised not to retreat the condition without consulting a health care provider. A red-brown nodule, thought to be an allergic response from the mite parts left on the skin, may form after treatment.

Pediculosis

Pediculosis is the term for infestation with lice (genus *Pediculus*). Lice are gray, gray-brown, or red-brown, oval, wingless insects that live off the blood of humans and animals. Lice are host specific; lice that live on animals do not transfer to humans and vice versa. Lice are also host dependent; they cannot live apart from the host beyond a few hours. As with scabies, the incidence of pediculosis increased in the 1970s to pandemic levels, probably because of increases in poverty, sexual experiences, and worldwide travel.

Three types of lice affect humans: *Pediculus humanus corporis* (body lice), *Phthirus pubis* (pubic lice), and *Pediculus humanus capitis* (head lice). Although these three types differ biologically, they have similar life cycles. The life cycle of a louse consists of an unhatched egg or "nit," three molt stages, an adult reproductive stage, and death. Before adulthood, lice live off the host and are incapable of reproduction. After fertilization, the egg is laid by the female louse along a hair shaft. These nits appear pearl gray to brown. Depending on the site, a female louse can lay between 150 and 300 nits in her life. The life span of a feeding louse is 30 to 50 days. Lice are equipped with stylets that pierce the skin. Their saliva contains an anticoagulant that prevents host blood from clotting while the louse is feeding. A louse takes up to 1 ml of blood during a feeding.

Pediculosis Corporis. Pediculosis corporis is infestation with *Pediculus humanus corporis*, or body lice. The lice are chiefly transferred through contact with an infested person, clothing, or bedding. The lice live in fibers of clothes, coming out only to feed. Unlike the pubic louse and the head louse, the body louse can survive 10 to 14 days without the host.

The typical lesion is a macule at the site of the bite. Papules and wheals may develop. The infestation is pruritic and evokes scratching that brings about a characteristic linear excoriation. Eczematous patches are frequently found. Secondary lesions may become scaly and hyperpigmented and leave scars. Areas typically affected are the shoulders, trunk, and buttocks. The presence of nits in the seams of clothes confirms a diagnosis of body lice.

Treatment measures consist of eradicating the louse and nits on the body and on clothing. Dry-cleaning clothes, washing them in hot water, or steam pressing are recommended methods. Special attention is given to the seams. Merely storing clothing in plastic bags for 2 weeks also rids clothes of lice. Many physicians prefer not to treat the body unless nits are in evidence on hair shafts. If treatment is indicated, lindane shampoo or topical preparations containing Malathion or other pediculicides are recommended. Care must be taken to ensure that close contacts are treated.

Pediculosis Pubis. Pediculosis pubis, the infestation known as crabs or pubic lice, is a nuisance disease that is uncomfortable and embarrassing. The disease is spread by intimate contact with someone harboring *Phthirus pubis*. Lice and nits are located in the pubic area of males and females. Occasionally, they may be found in sites of secondary sex characteristics, such as the beard in males or the axilla in males and females. Symptoms include intense itching and irritation of the skin. Diagnosis is made on the basis of symptoms and microscopic examination. The treatment is the same as for head lice.

Pediculosis Capitis. Pediculosis capitis, or infestation with head lice, primarily affects white-skinned persons; it is relatively unknown in darker-skinned persons. The incidence is higher among female children, although hair length has not been indicated as a contributing factor. Infestations of head lice are usually confined to the nape of the neck and behind the ears. Less frequently, head lice are found on the beard, pubic areas, eyebrows, and body hairs. Head lice are transmitted by human-to-human contact and by sharing combs and brushes. A positive diagnosis depends on the presence of firmly attached nits on hair shafts. Crawling adults are occasionally seen. Pruritus and scratching of the head are the primary indicators that head lice may be present. The scalp may appear red and excoriated from scratching. In severe cases, the hair becomes matted together in a crusty, foul-smelling "cap." An occasional morbilliform rash, which may be misdiagnosed as rubella, may occur with lymphadenopathy.

Head lice are treated with Permethrin, lindane, or Malathion shampoos or rinses. Retreatment may be needed to eliminate the hatching nits. Dead nits may be removed with a fine-toothed comb. Newer, over-the-counter nit removal hair rinses have also been effective.

Ticks

Ticks are insects that live in woods and underbrush. They attach to human and animal hosts and burrow into the epidermis, where they feed on blood. The tick bite is not problematic; the dangers stem from the infectious bacteria or viruses that they carry to human hosts. There are many tickborne illnesses, including Central European encephalitis, Q fever, babesiasis, and relapsing fever. Common tickborne diseases in the United States include Rocky Mountain spotted fever and Lyme disease.

Rocky Mountain Spotted Fever. *Rocky Mountain spotted fever* is caused by a tick that carries *Rickettsia rickettsii*. Rocky Mountain spotted fever used to be localized but now occurs throughout the United States, mostly from April to September. The initial tick bite appears as a papule or macule, with or without a central punctum. The tick burrows in and enlarges as it feeds. The tick must be attached to the human host for 4 to 6 hours before the rickettsiae are activated by the blood. Rickettsiae are found in the tick feces and body parts. They enter the bloodstream and multiply in the body tissues. Within 4 to 8 days, the patient experiences fever, headache, muscle aches, nausea, and vomiting. A rash that starts on the wrist or ankle follows. The characteristic rash is macular or maculopapular and spreads to the rest of the body. Other symptoms include generalized edema, conjunctivitis, petechial lesions, photophobia, lethargy, confusion, and cranial nerve deficits.

Treatment requires hospitalization and antibiotic therapy. The most important measure is to prevent tick bites by using insect repellents while engaged in activities in the woods. After a tick has attached itself, it is important to remove all the body parts to limit the possibility of infection. Ticks may be removed by slowly pulling them out with a tweezers, dousing them with mineral oil or alcohol before removal, or applying a hot match to the end of the tick. The heat method is the least effective because the tick may regurgitate into the open wound. Alternately, a thread may be used for persons who are out in the woods. The thread is looped, pulled over the tick at its smallest part at the skin surface, and both ends of the thread are then tightened to lift up the skin. The tension on the thread is held for 4 to 5 minutes, allowing the tick to slowly back out.[15] It is important to not handle the tick with bare hands, because infectious material may enter the through breaks in the skin.

Lyme Disease. *Lyme disease* is the most common tick-borne disease in the United States, characterized by a distinctive skin lesion, erythema chronicum migrans (ECM). It is a red macule or papule that expands in an annular fashion with a central clearing at the bite site. The average time from bite to appearance of the ECM is 9 days (range of 1 to 28 days).

The disease is caused by a spirochete, *Borrelia burgdorferi*, and occurs in three stages that may overlap. In the first or acute stage, there is the appearance of the ECM, often accompanied by malaise, fatigue, fever, headache, and lymphadenopathy. In the second or intermediate stage, there may be cardiac and neurologic manifestations in addition to the recurrence of the ECM weeks to months later. The third or chronic stage is characterized by arthritis that develops weeks to years later in about 60% of cases. Occasionally, chronic neurologic problems develop.

Lyme disease was first reported in Europe in the early 1900s and in 1976 in the United States. It was named after the town in Connecticut where the disease was discovered by a mother who reported eight cases of juvenile arthritis. Differences exist in the symptoms between Europe and the United States. For example, arthritis symptoms occur more frequently in the United States. Acrodermatitis chronica atrophicans (i.e., atrophy or sclerosis of the dermis resulting in "cigarette paper skin" through which blood vessels and muscles are easily seen) occurs more frequently in Europe with a similar tick bite. Incidence rates are highest in three geographic areas in the United States: coastal northeastern states (*i.e.*, Massachusetts to Maryland), Midwest states (*i.e.*, Minnesota and Wisconsin), and western states (*i.e.*, California, Utah, Nevada, Oregon, and Washington).

Preventive measures include using tick repellents, wearing clothing that covers the body, and regularly checking for ticks and promptly removing attached ticks. Transmission of the disease occurs only if the tick has fed for several hours on the host. Lyme disease can be reliably diagnosed by the presence of the ECM, but diagnosis without the rash is difficult. Serologic tests are the only practical method for diagnosing Lyme disease, but they lack specificity and can yield false-positive tests. Interlaboratory variation in test results also remains a problem. It is hoped that detection of bacterial DNA by the polymerase chain reaction method may become a useful method for establishing the diagnosis (see Chapter 10).

Tetracycline is effective against the spirochete, and penicillin is moderately so. Antibiotics such as doxycycline, amoxicillin, cefuroxime axetil, and erythromycin can be used if initiated during the first stage. Ceftriaxone is recommended for treatment of disseminated disease. Long-term courses of therapy are indicated in later forms of the disease. Corticosteroids and other antiinflammatory drugs may be used to provide relief from musculoskeletal manifestations.

In summary, primary disorders of the skin include infectious processes, inflammatory conditions, immune disorders, allergic reactions, and arthropod infestations. Superficial fungal infections are called dermatophytoses and are commonly known as tinea or ringworm. Impetigo, which is caused by staphylococci or β-hemolytic streptococci, is the most common superficial bacterial infection. Viruses are responsible for verrucae (warts), herpes simplex I lesions (cold sores or fever blisters), and herpes zoster (shingles). Noninfectious inflammatory skin conditions such as acne, lichen planus, psoriasis, and pityriasis rosea are of unknown origin. They are usually localized to the skin and are rarely associated with specific internal disease. Allergic skin responses involve the body's immune system and are caused by hypersensitivity reactions to allergens, environmental agents, drugs, and other substances. The skin is sensitive to a number of disorders resulting from invasion or infestation by bugs, ticks, or parasites. The tick bite is not problematic; the dangers stem from the infectious bacteria or viruses that they carry to human hosts.

Nevi and Skin Cancers

After you have completed this section of the chapter, you should be able to meet the following objectives:

- Cite changes in a nevus (mole) that are suggestive of cancerous transformation
- Describe the three types of ultraviolet radiation and relate them to sunburn, aging skin changes, and the development of skin cancer
- List three drugs that produce photosensitivity
- State the properties of an effective sun screen
- Compare the appearance and outcome of basal cell carcinoma, squamous cell carcinoma, and malignant melanoma

Nevi

Nevi, or moles, are common congenital or acquired tumors of the skin that are benign. Almost all adults have nevi, some in greater numbers than others. Nevi can be pigmented or nonpigmented, flat or elevated, and hairy or nonhairy.

Nevocellular nevi are pigmented nevi that are derived from cells in the neural crest. They contain modified melanocytes and come in various shapes. Nevocellular nevi are tan to deep brown, uniformly pigmented, small papules with well-defined and rounded borders. Blue nevi are bluish black. *Junctional nevi* are aggregates of well-defined cells located within the lower epidermal layer that lies adjacent to the dermis (Fig. 15–27).

Histologically, most nevi begin as junctional nevi. Eventually, nevus cells begin to grow into the dermis. *Compound nevi* contain epidermal and dermal components. *Dermal nevi* are located within the dermis. Nevi or moles are important because of their capacity to transform to malignant melanomas. The relation between preexisting benign nevi and malignant melanoma is unclear. Although the average person has about 20 moles, only 4 of 100,000 persons develop malignant melanoma. Two types of pigmented nevi are associated with malignant transformation. These are the congenital melanocytic nevus and the dysplastic nevus, which are discussed later. Because of the possibility of malignant transformation, any mole that undergoes a change warrants immediate medical attention. The changes to observe and report are size, thickness, color, itching, or bleeding.

Skin Cancer

There has been an alarming increase of skin cancers over the past 2 decades. The American Cancer Society reported that there were an estimated 500,000 new cases of skin cancer in 1994. New melanomas accounted for 32,000 of them; the remainder were basal or squamous cell carcinomas.[16]

Ultraviolet radiation and harsh weather exposure are related to the increase in malignant skin lesions in white-skinned persons. The decrease in the ozone layer is another factor. Persons have more leisure time and spend increasing amounts of time in the sun with uncovered skin. The type of person prone to skin cancers is a white, fair-skinned person who burns easily and usually has a history of sunburns during childhood. The incidence among persons who tan easily and do not burn is lower. For darker-skinned persons, the incidence is low: 3.4 per 100,000 African Americans compared with 232.6 per 100,000 whites.[17]

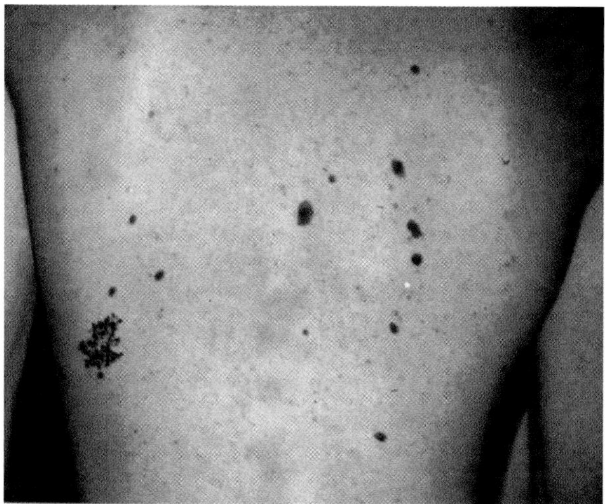

Figure 15–27
Junctional nevi of the back of a 16-year-old patient. (Owen Laboratories, Inc.)

Ultraviolet Radiation Promotion of Skin Cancer

The skin is the protective shield against harmful ultraviolet rays from the sun. The increased production of melanin as a result of exposure to ultraviolet radiation is believed to be the body's protective response. However, melanin alone cannot prevent skin cancer. Skin cancers have been increasing at an alarming rate over the past 20 years, and most forms are directly related to sun exposure. Other skin alterations, such as senile lentigines, have been linked to ultraviolet radiation exposure. Exposure to the sun and harsh weather has also been linked to early wrinkling and aging of the skin. Efforts are now aimed at understanding the skin's response to ultraviolet radiation exposure and informing the public about the dangers of the sun.

The earth's sunlight is measured in wavelengths. Wavelengths range from about 290 nm in the ultraviolet region up to about 2500 nm in the infrared region. Ultraviolet radiation accounts for roughly 5% of solar radiation, but the amount of radiation human beings are exposed to has increased because of artificial sources, such as tanning salons and occupational exposure. Ultraviolet radiation is divided into three types: UVC, UVB, and UVA. UVC rays are 100 to 280 nm long. They are short and do not pass through the earth's atmosphere. However, they are produced artificially and are damaging to the eyes. UVB rays are 280 to 315 nm. These are the rays primarily responsible for nearly all skin effects after exposure to sunlight. They are more commonly referred to as "sunburn rays." UVA rays are 315 to 400 nm. These rays, which can pass through window glass, are more commonly referred to as "sun tanning rays." Generally, it takes about 1000 times more UVA to match the untoward effects of UVB. Nonetheless, UVA contributes to many skin alterations. Artificial sources of UVA, such as tanning salons, may produce the same effects as UVB.[18,19]

The wavelength of sunlight in an area is determined by the ozone layer. Ozone absorbs wavelengths shorter than 320 nm; the shortest wavelength of sunlight reaching the earth is about 290 nm. The diminishing ozone layer is believed to be a critical factor in increased ultraviolet light exposure and the concomitant increased incidence of cancerous skin lesions over the past 2 decades.[18] Smoke and fog may play a part in reducing the intensity of ultraviolet radiation.

With ultraviolet radiation exposure, human cells release vasoactive and injurious chemicals, resulting in vasodilation and sunburn. Melanin in the stratum corneum absorbs ultraviolet radiation. The skin responds to ultraviolet radiation exposure by increasing its melanin content as a means of preventing destruction of the lower skin layers. The immune system in the skin, especially the Langerhans' cells are also involved. The number of cells are decreased and their activity is lessened by ultraviolet radiation exposure.[20]

Sunburn. Sunburn is caused by excessive exposure of the epidermal and dermal layers of the skin to ultraviolet radiation exposure, resulting in an erythematous inflammatory reaction. Sunburn ranges from mild to severe. A mild sunburn consists of various degrees of redness after exposure to the sun. Inflammation, vesicle eruption, weakness, chills, fever, malaise, and pain accompany more severe forms of sunburn. Scaling and peeling follow any overexposure to sunlight. Black skin also burns and may appear grayish or gray-black.

Severe sunburns are treated with boric acid soaks and topical creams to limit pain and maintain skin moisture. Extensive second-degree and third-degree burns require hospitalization and specialized burn care techniques, as described under thermal burns.

Drug-Induced Photosensitivity. Some drugs are classified as photosensitive drugs because they produce an exaggerated response to ultraviolet light when the drug is taken in combination with sun exposure. Examples are sulfonamides, thiazide diuretics, tetracycline, sulfonylurea hypoglycemia agents, phenothiazine, and antipsychotic drugs. Photosensitivity is sometimes a desired effect when treating skin conditions that respond well to ultraviolet radiation exposure. An example is psoriasis. However, an increased incidence of cancerous lesions has been found in persons who have been treated therapeutically with photosensitive agents. Their use requires caution and careful surveillance.

Sunscreens and Other Protective Measures. The Food and Drug Administration requires a rating on all commercial suntan preparations based on their ability to obstruct ultraviolet radiation absorption. The ratings are generally on a scale of 1 to 35; higher ratings block more sunlight. Total sun-blocking agents with ratings of 35 and higher are available. *Para*-aminobenzoic acid (PABA) is a common blocking ingredient in many suntan creams, but it blocks mostly the UVB rays. Some suntan lotions protect against UVA. These products contain oxybenzone, dioxybenzone, or avobenzone. Sunless suntan creams, such as dihydroxyacetone, produce a tan without exposure to the sun. Unlike earlier forms of sunless tanning creams, they produce a more natural-looking tan.

Suntan creams should be used diligently and according to the person's tendency to burn rather than tan. It is recommended that suntan creams be applied 30 minutes before sun exposure and reapplied every 2 hours. Early morning and late afternoon sun exposures are less harmful because the ultraviolet rays are longer. Because many skin cancers are correlated with childhood sunburns, children younger than 18 should use sunscreens with a blocking agent of at least 15. However, sun screens may encourage a false sense of security. Prolonged sun exposure as a result of using sun screens may still increase the chance of getting skin cancers.[21] Other preventive measures include a knowledge about sunlight and how to protect the skin. Shade does not necessarily protect persons from the sun's rays, because UV rays are reflected from many surfaces. Sand is a good reflector of sunlight. A person can become sunburned even while sitting under an umbrella on a sandy beach. Water absorbs ultraviolet radiation rather than reflecting it. However, ultraviolet radiation penetrates the upper few inches of clear water. This, combined with the scattered reflection of water, can increase the exposure to ultraviolet radiation. Shielding the skin with clothing and hats or head coverings also decreases ultraviolet radiation exposure.

Basal Cell Carcinoma

Basal cell carcinoma is the most common form of skin cancer (Fig. 15–28). Like other skin cancers, basal cell carcinoma has increased in occurrence over the past two decades. Fair-skinned persons with a history of significant long-term sun exposure are more susceptible. Black- and brown-skinned persons are occasionally affected.

Basal cell carcinoma is usually a nonmetastasizing tumor that extends widely and deeply if left untreated. These tumors are most frequently seen on the head and neck. They also occur less frequently on other skin surfaces that were not exposed to the sun. However, basal cell carcinoma usually occurs in persons who were exposed to great amounts of sunlight. The incidence is twice as high among men than women and greatest in the 55- to 75-year-old age group.[22]

Although there are several histologic types of basal cell carcinoma, nodular ulcerative and superficial basal cell carcinomas are the most frequently occurring types. *Nodular ulcerative basal cell carcinoma* is the most common type. It is a nodulocystic structure that begins as a small, flesh-colored or pink, smooth, translucent nodule that enlarges over time. Telangiectatic vessels are frequently

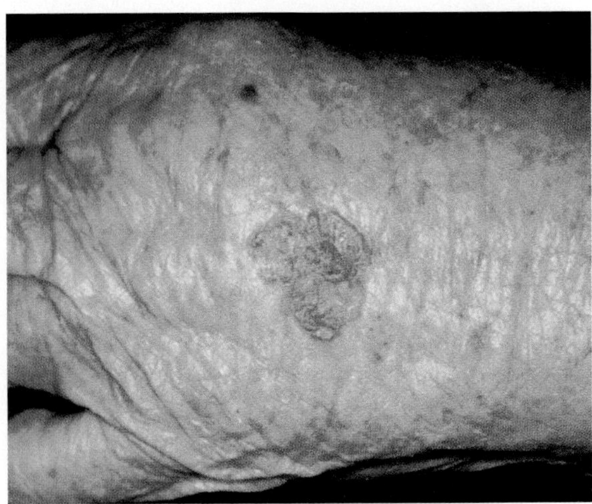

Figure 15–28
Basal cell carcinoma and wrinkling of the hand. (Syntex Laboratories, Inc.)

seen beneath the surface. Over the years, a central depression forms that progresses to an ulcer surrounded by the original shiny, waxy border.

The second most common form is *superficial basal cell carcinoma,* which is most often seen on the chest or back. It begins as a flat, nonpalpable, erythematous plaque. The red, scaly areas slowly enlarge, with nodular borders and telangiectatic bases. This type of skin cancer is difficult to diagnose because it mimics other dermatologic problems.

All suspected basal cell carcinomas are biopsied for diagnosis. The treatment depends on the site and extent of the lesion. The most important treatment goal is complete elimination of the lesion. Also important is the maintenance of function and optimal cosmetic effect. Curettage with electrodesiccation, surgical excision, irradiation, and chemosurgery are effective in removing all cancerous cells. Patients should be checked at regular intervals for recurrences.

Squamous Cell Carcinoma

Squamous cell carcinomas are malignant tumors of the outer epidermis. The increase in the incidence of squamous cell carcinomas is consistent with increased ultraviolet radiation exposure. Squamous cell carcinoma metastasis is more common than metastasis of basal cell carcinoma. There are two types of squamous cell carcinoma: intraepidermal and invasive. *Intraepidermal squamous cell carcinoma* remains confined to the epidermis for a long time. However, at some unpredictable time, it may penetrate the basement membrane to the dermis and metastasize to the regional lymph nodes. It then converts to *invasive squamous cell carcinoma.* The invasive type can develop from intraepidermal carcinoma or from a premalignant lesion (*e.g.,* actinic keratoses). It may be slow or fast growing with metastasis.

Squamous cell carcinoma is a scaly, keratotic, slightly elevated lesion with an irregular border, usually with a shallow chronic ulcer (Fig. 15–29). Later lesions grow outward, show large ulcerations, and have persistent crusts and raised, erythematous borders. These lesions occur on sun-exposed areas of the skin, particularly the nose, forehead, helixes of the ears, lower lip, and back of the hands.

The mechanisms of squamous cell carcinoma development are unclear. Sunlight is implicated as a causative factor. Most squamous cell cancers occur in sun-exposed areas of the skin, and persons who spend much time outdoors, have lighter skin, and live in lower latitudes are more affected. Other suspected causes include exposure to arsenic (*i.e.,* Bowen's disease), gamma radiation, tars, and oils.

Treatment measures are aimed at the removal of all cancerous tissue using methods such as electrosurgery, excision surgery, chemosurgery, or radiation therapy. After treatment, the person is observed for the remainder of his or her life for signs of recurrence. The recurrence rate is roughly 50%, with a 70% metastatic rate.[23]

Malignant Melanoma

Malignant melanoma is a malignant tumor of the melanocytes. It is a rapidly progressing, metastatic form of cancer. There has been a dramatic increase in the incidence of malignant melanoma over the past 2 decades, with the incidence almost tripling over the past 4 decades. There has been a 5% to 6% annual increase, and it is anticipated that 1 of every 75 Americans will have melanoma by the year 2000.[24] The thinning of the ozone layer in the earth's stratosphere has been an important factor in this incidence rate. Society's emphasis on sun tanning is also implicated. Public health screening measures, early diagnosis, increased knowledge of precursor lesions, and greater public knowledge of the disease may account for increased reporting and rising rates. These factors have contributed to earlier intervention and increased survival rates of persons who have malignant melanoma.

The incidence is highest in white, professional, indoor workers of middle to high social class. Severe, blistering sunburns in early childhood and intermittent intense sun exposures (trips to sunny climates) contribute to increased susceptibility to melanoma in young and middle-aged adults. The rate of incidence is increased for persons who immigrate to sunny locations. Incidence rates are higher for persons who burn easily and tan minimally. The use of suntanning salons has also been implicated in the development of malignant melanoma. Roughly 90% of malignant

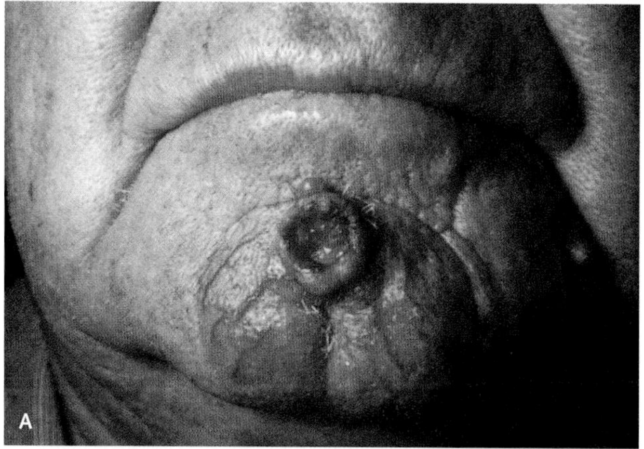

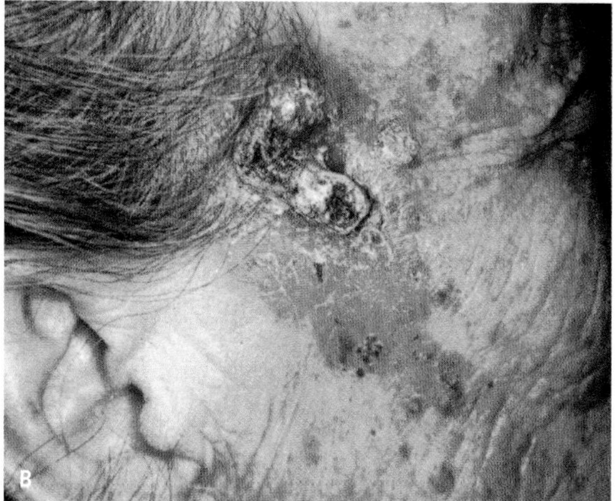

Figure 15–29
(A) Squamous cell carcinoma of the chin. **(B)** Squamous cell carcinoma and keratosis of aged skin. (Syntex Laboratories, Inc., Westwood Pharmaceuticals)

melanomas in whites occur on sun-exposed skin. However, in African Americans and Asians, roughly 67% occur on non–sun-exposed areas, such as mucous membranes and subungual, palmar, and plantar surfaces.[17]

Malignant melanomas differ in size and shape. Their exact cause—specifically how and when a nevus converts to a melanoma—remains unknown. Most seem to arise from preexisting benign nevi or as new, molelike growths (Fig. 15–30). Usually, they are slightly raised and black or brown. Borders are irregular, and surfaces are uneven. Periodically, melanomas ulcerate and bleed. There may be surrounding erythema, inflammation, and tenderness. Dark melanomas are often mottled with red, blue, and white shades. These three colors represent three concurrent processes: melanoma growth (blue), inflammation and the body's attempt to localize and destroy the tumor (red), and scar tissue formation (white). Malignant melanomas can appear anywhere on the body. Although they are frequently found on sun-exposed areas, sun exposure alone does not account for their development. In men, they are frequently found on the trunk, head, neck, and arms; in women, they are also found on the legs.

Four types of melanomas have been identified: superficial spreading, lentigo maligna, nodular, and

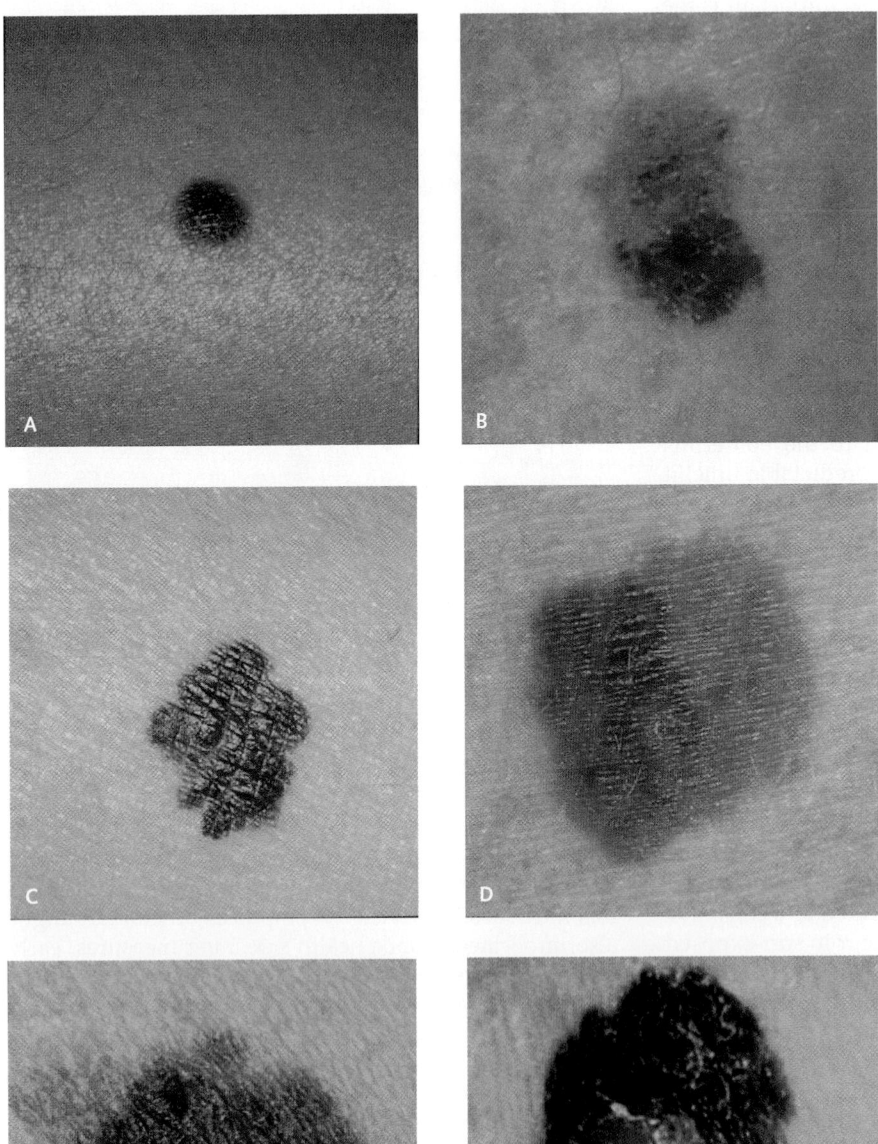

Figure 15–30 **(A)** Normal mole with even, round contour and sharply defined borders. **(B)** Changes in appearance of a mole: *asymmetry.* **(C)** Changes in appearance of a mole: *border irregularity*. **(D)** Changes in appearance of a mole: *color and uneven pigmentation*. **(E)** Changes in the appearance of a mole: *diameter greater than 6 mm.* **(F)** Changes in the surface of a mole: *scaliness, oozing, and bleeding.* (American Cancer Society. [1995]. *What you should know about melanoma.* Dallas: American Cancer Society)

acral-lentiginous.[25] *Superficial spreading melanoma* is characterized by a raised-edged nevus with lateral growth. It has a disorderly appearance in color and outline. This lesion tends to have biphasic growth, horizontally and vertically. It typically ulcerates and bleeds with growth. This type of lesion accounts for 70% of all melanomas and is most prevalent in persons who sunburn easily and have intermittent sun exposure. *Lentigo maligna melanoma* accounts for 4% to 10% of all melanomas. It is a slow-growing, flat nevus and occurs primarily on sun-exposed areas of elderly persons. This type is most closely associated with cumulative exposure to the sun. *Nodular melanoma* is raised and initially grows vertically, is a uniform blue-black color, and is sharply delineated. These lesions tend to look like blood blisters. *Acral-lentiginous melanoma* occurs primarily in black- and brown-skinned persons on the palms of the hands, soles of the feet, nail beds, and mucous membranes. It has the appearance of lentigo maligna.

Three precursor lesions have been identified in the development of melanoma: lentigo maligna, congenital melanocytic nevi, and dysplastic nevi. Recognition of these precursors is important to the early diagnosis and treatment of melanoma. *Lentigo maligna* is a flat lesion that looks like an irregular freckle. The tan-brown to black lesion has irregular pigmentation and borders. It spreads and may look like a stain. Lentigo malignas frequently occur in elderly persons on sun-exposed areas. *Congenital melanocytic nevi* are large, brown to black hyperpigmented nevi that are present at birth. Generally, they are found on the hands, shoulders, buttocks, entire arm, or trunk of the body. Some involve large areas of the body in garmentlike fashion. These nevi darken with age. Hairs that are present in the lesion become coarser. Malignant changes often occur at an early age, usually by age 10. *Dysplastic nevi* are flat to slightly raised lesions consisting of neural crest derived cells (*i.e.*, nevocellular nevi) and often have a diameter greater than 1 cm. A person may have hundreds of these lesions; they occur on sun-exposed and covered areas of the body. They vary in shade from brown and red to flesh tones and have irregular borders. There is some familial tendency to develop dysplastic nevi.

The prognosis of malignant melanoma is varied. It depends on a host of factors, including lesion thickness, stage of the disease process, anatomic site, age, and the type of lesion. Ten-year survival rates have increased steadily over the past 30 years, but the mortality rate continues to increase. This inconsistency may reflect the rapidly rising incidence of melanoma.

Stage I patients have no evidence of tumor growth in regional lymph nodes. The disease process is limited to the localized lesion area. The 10-year survival rate for these patients after surgical intervention is 81%. *Stage II* melanomas have metastasized to the regional lymph nodes. The 10-year survival rate reported for these persons is 47%. *Stage III* malignant melanoma involves metastasis to distant organs in the body. The prognosis is poor, with survival ranging up to 16 months.[26]

Early detection is critical with melanoma. An *ABCD rule* has been developed to aid in early diagnosis and timely treatment of malignant melanoma. The acronym stands for *a*symmetry, *b*order irregularity, *c*olor variegation, and *d*iameter greater than 0.6 cm (*i.e.*, pencil eraser size). Patients should be taught to watch for these changes in existing nevi or the development of new nevi, as well as other alterations such as bleeding or itching. All persons should use sun-blocking agents when exposed to the sun, but it is imperative with those whose skin burns easily. Regular self-examination of the total skin surface with good lighting in front of a mirror is recommended. Any change in nevi should be brought to the attention of a health care provider.

Treatment measures depend on the severity. Deep and wide excisions with skin grafts are used. Current cancer treatment, such as immunotherapy, chemotherapy or radiation therapy, is indicated when the disease becomes systemic.

In summary, nevi are moles that are usually benign. Because they may undergo cancerous transformation, any mole that undergoes a change warrants immediate medical attention. There has been an alarming increase of skin cancers over the skin over the past 2 decades. Repeated exposure to the ultraviolet rays of the sun has been implicated as the principal cause of skin cancer. Neoplasms of the skin include basal cell carcinoma, squamous cell carcinoma, and malignant melanoma. Squamous cell carcinoma and basal cell carcinoma are of epidermal origin. Basal cell carcinomas are the most common form of skin cancer. They are slow-growing tumors that rarely metastasize. Squamous cell carcinoma is also common, especially in older persons, and usually arises on sun-exposed areas of the body. The two types of squamous cell carcinoma are intraepidermal and invasive. Intraepidermal squamous cell carcinoma remains confined to the epidermis for a long time. Invasive squamous cell carcinoma can develop from intraepidermal carcinoma or from a premalignant lesion (e.g., actinic keratoses). Malignant melanoma is a malignant tumor of melanocyte origin. It is a rapidly progressing, metastatic form of cancer. Clinically, malignant melanoma of the skin is usually asymptomatic. The most important clinical sign is the change in color of pigmented skin lesion such as a mole. As the result of increased public awareness, most melanomas can be cured surgically.

Burns

After you have completed this section of the chapter, you should be able to meet the following objectives:

- Compare the tissue involvement for first-degree, second-degree partial-thickness, second-degree full-thickness, and third-degree burns
- State how the rule of nine is used in determining the body surface area involved in a burn
- Cite the determinants for grading burn severity using the American Burn Association classification of burns

- Describe the systemic complications of burns
- Describe major considerations in treatment of burn injury

Most burns occur accidentally in the home or workplace. Severe burn patients are surviving at a higher rate in the 1990s than they did previously. The number of deaths has decreased proportionately since the 1970s. Approximately 60,000 to 80,000 persons with burns are admitted to the hospital annually.[27] Of those admitted, 5500 die.[28] The remainder of those with serious burns require extensive medical burn treatment, which has improved greatly over the years.

Inhalation injury remains the major problem contributing to mortality from burns. Sepsis and pneumonia are other important contributing factors to mortality. Burns are caused by a number of sources. Flame burns occur because of exposure to direct fire. Scald burns result from hot liquids spilled or poured on the skin surface. In a child, a scald burn may be indicative of child abuse. Chemical burns occur from industrial agents used in occupational sites. Electrical burns occur from contact with live electrical wires in fields or in the home. Electrical burns are usually more extensive because of internal tissue injury and the entrance and exit wounds. Lightening, electromagnetic radiation, and ionizing radiation can also cause skin burns.

Classification

The four classifications for the depth of burn injuries are: first-degree, second-degree partial-thickness, second-degree full-thickness, and third-degree burns. The depth of a burn is largely influenced by the length of time exposed to the heat source and the temperature of the heating agent.

First-degree burns (*i.e.*, superficial partial-thickness burns) involve only the outer layers of the epidermis. They are red or pink, dry, and painful. There is usually no blister formation. A mild sunburn is an example. The skin maintains its ability to function as a water vapor and bacterial barrier, and heals in 3 to 10 days. First-degree burns usually require only palliative treatment, such as pain relief measures and adequate fluid intake. Extensive first-degree burns on infants, the elderly, and persons who receive radiation therapy for cancer may need more care.

Second-degree partial-thickness burns involve the epidermis and various degrees of the dermis. They are painful, moist, red, and blistered. Underneath the blisters is weeping, bright pink or red skin that is sensitive to temperature changes, air exposure, and touch. The blisters prevent the loss of body water and superficial dermal cells. Excluding excision of large burn areas, it is important to maintain intact blisters after injury because they serve as a good bandage and may promote wound healing.[29] These burns heal in about 1 to 2 weeks.

The *second-degree full-thickness burn* involves the entire epidermis and dermis. Structures that originate in the subcutaneous layer, such as hair follicles and sweat glands, remain intact. These burns can be very painful because the pain sensors remain intact. Tactile sensors may be absent or greatly diminished in the areas of deepest destruction. These burns appear as mottled pink, red, or waxy white areas with blisters and edema. The blisters resemble flat, dry tissue paper, rather than the bullous blisters seen with superficial partial-thickness injury. After healing, in about 1 month, these burns maintain their softness and elasticity, but there may be the loss of some sensation. Scar formation is usual. These burns heal with supportive medical care aimed at preventing further tissue damage, providing adequate hydration, and ensuring that the granular bed is adequate to support reepithelialization.

Third-degree full-thickness burns extend into the subcutaneous tissue and may involve muscle and bone. Thrombosed vessels can be seen under the burned skin, indicating that the underlying vasculature is involved. Third-degree burns vary in color from waxy white or yellow to tan, brown, deep red, or black. These burns are hard, dry, and leathery. Edema is extensive in the burn area and surrounding tissues. There is no pain because the nerve sensors have been destroyed. However, there is no such thing as a "pure" third-degree burn. Third-degree burns are almost always surrounded by second-degree burns, which are surrounded by an area of first-degree burns. The injury sometimes has an almost target-like appearance because of the various degrees of burn. Full-thickness burns wider than 1.5 inches usually require skin grafts because all the regenerative (*i.e.*, dermal) elements have been destroyed. Smaller injuries usually heal from the margins inward toward the center, the dermal elements regenerating from the healthier margins. However, regeneration may take many weeks and leave a permanent scar, even in smaller burns.

In addition to the depth of the wound, the extent of the burn is also important. Extent is measured by estimating the amount of total body surface area (TBSA) involved. Several tools exist for estimating the TBSA. For example, the *Rule of Nines* counts anatomic body parts as multiples of 9%, with the perineum being 1%. The Lund and Browder chart includes a body diagram table that estimates the TBSA by age and anatomic part.[30] Children are more accurately assessed using this method because it takes into account the difference in relative size of body parts.

These estimates are then converted to the American Burn Association Classification of Extent of Injury (Table 15–8). Together, the depth and the extent of the burn indicate the severity of the burn and the need for treatment. Other factors, such as age, location, other injuries, and preexisting conditions, are taken into consideration for a full assessment of burn injury. These factors can increase the severity of the burn and the length of treatment. A first-degree burn is reclassified as a more severe burn if other factors exist, such as burns to the hands, face, and feet; inhalation injury; electrical burns; other trauma; or existence of psychosocial problems. Genital burns almost always require hospitalization, because

TABLE 15-8

American Burn Association Grading of Burn Severity

Burn Type	Minor	Moderate	Major
Partial thickness	<15% TBSA, adult <10% TBSA, child	15–25% TBSA, adult 10–20% TBSA, child	>25% TBSA, Adult >20% TBSA, child
Full thickness	<2% TBSA, adult	2–10% TBSA, adult	≥10% TBSA

TBSA, total body surface area

(American Burn Association [1976]. *American Burn Association Committee on Specific Optimal Criteria for Hospital Resources for Care of Patients with Burn Injury.* San Antonio: American Burn Association)

edema may cause difficulty voiding and the location complicates maintenance of a bacteria free environment.

Systemic Complications

Burn victims often are confronted with hemodynamic instability, impaired respiratory function, hypermetabolic response, major organ dysfunction, and sepsis. The magnitude of the response is proportional to the extent of injury, usually reaching a plateau when about 60% of the body is burned. The treatment challenge is for immediate resuscitation efforts and for more long-term maintenance of physiologic function. Pain and emotional problems are additional problems faced by persons with burns.

Hemodynamic Instability

Hemodynamic instability begins almost immediately with injury to capillaries in the burned area and surrounding tissue. Because of a loss of vascular volume, major burn victims often present in the emergency room in a form of hypovolemic shock (Chapter 20) known as *burn shock.* The patient has a decrease in cardiac output, increased peripheral vascular resistance, and impaired perfusion of vital organs. Burn shock is proportional to the extent and depth of injury. Fluid is lost from the vascular, interstitial, and cellular compartments. Sodium is lost from the vascular and interstitial fluid compartments, and potassium is lost from the intracellular compartment.

The major hemodynamic derangement results from a rapid shift of plasma from the vascular system into interstitial fluid compartment, resulting in edema. The loss of plasma fluid and proteins decreases vascular colloidal osmotic pressure and results in additional edema formation in the burned and nonburned areas. Because plasma fluid rather than whole blood is lost from the vascular compartment, there is an increase in hematocrit and concentration of other blood components. Consequently, damaged red cells within the capillaries may sludge, leading to thrombosis and further impairment of blood flow to vital organs. Because of the increased concentration of coagulation factors, burn victims are at increased risk of developing disseminated intravascular coagulation (see Chapter 7). In persons with hemodynamic instability, adequate fluid resuscitation is essential to survival. The amounts of fluid needed are great. The type and amount of fluid are calculated according to the extent of the burn and the age and weight of the person, balanced with the increased fluid expended through burn sites. In persons receiving adequate fluid resuscitation, cardiac output usually returns to normal in about 24 hours.

Respiratory Dysfunction

Smoke inhalation and postburn lung dysfunction are frequent problems in burn victims. Victims are often trapped in a burning structure and inhale significant amounts of smoke, carbon monoxide, and other toxic fumes. Water-soluble gases, such as ammonia, sulfur dioxide, and chlorine, that are found in smoke from burning plastics and rubber react with mucous membranes to form strong acids and alkalis that induce ulceration of the mucous membrane, bronchospasm, and edema. Lipid-soluble gases such nitrous oxide and hydrogen chloride are transported to the lower airways, where they produce their damage. These substances damage cell membranes and impair the function of the mucociliary blanket. There may also be thermal injury to the respiratory passages.

Symptoms of inhalation injury include hoarseness, drooling, an inability to handle secretions, rales and rhonchi, strider, hacking cough, and labored and shallow breathing. Serial blood gases show a fall in PO_2. Signs of mucosal injury and airway obstruction often are delayed for 24 to 48 hours after a burn. It is necessary to continually monitor the patient for early signs of respiratory distress. Humidified oxygen is administered to prevent drying and sloughing of the mucosa. Intubation and ventilatory support may be needed. Other pulmonary conditions, such as pneumonia, pulmonary embolism, or pneumothorax, may occur secondarily to the burn.

Hypermetabolic Response

The stress of burn injury increases the metabolism and nutritional requirements. Secretion of stress hormones such as catecholamines and cortisol is increased in an effort to maintain homeostasis. Heat production is increased in an effort to balance heat losses from the burned area. Hypermetabolism characterized by increased oxygen consumption and increased glucose use, and protein and fat wasting are characteristic responses to burn trauma and infection. The metabolic rate of persons with burns covering 40% of total surface area are often twice normal.[31] The hypermetabolic state peaks at about 7 to 17 days after the burn, and tissue breakdown diminishes as the wounds heal. Persons with 40% total surface area burns have been shown to lose 25% of their preadmission weight by 3 weeks after the injury. Nutritional support is essential to recovery from burn injury. Enteral and parenteral hyperalimentation is used to deliver sufficient nutrients to prevent tissue breakdown and postburn weight loss.

Organ Dysfunction

Burn shock results in impaired perfusion of vital organs. The patient may have impaired function of kidneys, gastrointestinal tract, and nervous system. Although the initial insult is often one of hypovolemic shock and impaired organ perfusion, sepsis may contribute to impaired organ function after the initial resuscitation period.

Renal insufficiency can occur in burn patients as a result of the hypovolemic state, damage to the kidneys at the time of the burn, or from drugs that are administered. Immediately after the burn, a person goes into a short period of relative anuria, followed by a phase of hypermetabolism characterized by increased urine output and nitrogen loss. The effects of burn injury on the gastrointestinal tract include gastric dilation and decreased peristalsis. These effects are compounded by immobility and narcotic analgesics. Burn victims are observed carefully for vomiting and fecal impaction. A complication called *Curling's ulcer* is relatively common in burn victims and is thought to be the result of stress and gastric ischemia. Enteral feeding tubes are inserted almost immediately. Tube feeding is intended to mitigate ulcer formation, maintain the integrity of the intestinal mucosa, and provide sufficient calories and protein for the hypermetabolic state. Burn patients are encouraged to begin eating as soon as possible to maintain gastrointestinal integrity.

Neurologic changes can occur from periods of hypoxia. Neurologic damage may result from head injuries, drug or alcohol abuse, carbon monoxide poisoning, fluid volume deficits, and hypovolemia. With an electrical burn, the brain or spine can be directly injured. The responses to physiologic damage may include confusion, memory loss, insomnia, lethargy, and combativeness.

Musculoskeletal effects include fractures that occur at the time of the accident, deep burns extending to the muscles and bone, hypertrophic scarring, and contractures. The hypermetabolic state increases tissue catabolism and severe protein and fat wasting.

Sepsis and Immune Function

A significant complication of the acute phase of burn injury is sepsis. It may arise from the burn wound, pneumonia, urinary tract infection or infection elsewhere in the body, or the use of invasive procedures or monitoring devices. Immunologically, the skin is the body's first line of defense. When the skin is no longer intact, the body is open to bacterial infection. Destruction of the skin also prevents the delivery of cellular components of the immune system to the site of injury. There is also loss of normal protective skin flora and a shift to colonization by more pathogenic flora.

Suppression of the immune system after burn trauma contributes to the development of sepsis. B-cell and T-cell immunity are involved (Chapter 11). The cause of immunosuppression is unclear, but undoubtedly, multiple factors are involved. It has been suggested that immunosuppression factors are produced by tissues away from the site of injury (*e.g.,* liver, gastrointestinal tract, endocrine system) and by the burned tissue itself. The capillary leak that occurs in the immediate postburn period removes immune cells and immunoglobulins from the circulation. Stress also contributes to immunosuppression through the hypothalamic-pituitary-adrenal axis (see Chapter 53). Persons with prior immunodeficiency, those with chronic debilitating conditions, and known alcoholics are particularly at risk. The very young and the elderly are also at risk for immunosuppression.

Pain

Burn injuries are extremely painful, and pain management must be a major priority in the care of these patients. The degree of pain in the resuscitative and acute phases of care is influenced by the depth and extent of the burn injury. During this stage, pain medications are usually given intravenously because of injury to the skin and because of impaired blood flow to the subcutaneous and intramuscular tissues.

Emotional Trauma

Burns are emotionally devastating because of the impact of disfigurement, pain, and lengthy recovery. These are persons who at one moment were well and extensively burned the next. Burn patients are faced with enormous physiologic, psychologic, and social challenges. Any number of human responses are expected and normal for the person experiencing a major burn. Patients may exhibit responses such as anger, denial, and refusal to cooperate. The patient and family usually need psychologic support in addition to all the physiologic forms of life support.

Treatment

Regardless of the type of burn, the first step in any burn situation is stopping the causal agent to prevent further tissue damage. Copious amounts of water over the burned area are extremely helpful. Immediate submersion is more important than removal of clothing, which may delay cooling the involved areas. Cold (ice) applications are not recommended, because ice can further limit blood flow to an area, turning a partial-thickness into a full-thickness burn.

Depending on the depth and extent of the burn, medical treatment is necessary. Emergency care consists of resuscitation and stabilization with intravenous fluids while maintaining cardiac and respiratory function. Once hospitalized, the treatment regimen includes fluid replacement, maintenance of nutritional demands, antibiotic therapy, maintenance of cardiac and respiratory functions, pain alleviation, and emotional support.

After hemodynamic stability and pulmonary stability have been established, treatment is directed toward initial care of the wound. The wound is cleaned, debrided, and covered with a topical antimicrobial agent. Because of alterations in immune function, protective isolation measures may be instituted.

Eschar (*i.e.*, burned tissue) is excised as soon as possible, because the skin regenerates faster with less chance of microbial infection. Early excision and dressing limits fluid loss, thereby decreasing the hypermetabolic response and improving the cosmetic results.[32] Antimicrobial agents, such as silver sulfadiazine, mafenide acetate, or silver nitrate, are applied to burned areas, which are dressed with various gauzes. Systemic antibiotics are seldom useful at the burn sites because of the loss of the functional components of the skin. The dressings are changed according to the specific practice of the health care provider.

Burns that encircle the entire surface of the body or a body part (*e.g.*, arms, legs, torso) act like tourniquets and can cause major tissue damage to the muscles, tendons, and vasculature under the area of the leathery eschar skin. These burns are called *circumferential burns*. The eschar is incised longitudinally (*i.e.*, escharotomy), and sometimes a fasciotomy (*i.e.*, surgical incision through the fascia of the muscle) is performed. The timing of these incisions is important. Incision is done after the patient's circulatory condition stabilizes to some degree, thereby limiting some of the massive fluid loss. However, the incisions must occur before the eschar formation can cause hypoxia and necrosis of the tissues and organs under it. This is extremely important when torso burns occur, because the pressure placed on a chest can cause an inability to breathe and decreased blood return to the heart.

Skin grafts are surgically implanted as soon as possible, often at the same time the burns are debrided, to promote new skin growth, limit fluid loss, and act as a dressing. Skin grafts can be permanent or temporary and split-thickness or full-thickness. *Permanent skin grafts* are used over newly excised tissue. *Temporary skin grafts* are used to cover a burned area until the tissue underneath it has healed.

A *split-thickness skin graft* is one that includes the epidermis and part of the dermis. The thickness of these grafts depends on the donor site and the need of the burn patient. A split-thickness skin graft can be sent through a skin mesher that cuts tiny slits into the skin, allowing it to expand up to nine times its size. These grafts are used frequently because they can cover large surface areas and there is less autorejection. *Full-thickness skin grafts* include the entire thickness of the dermal layer. They are used primarily for reconstructive surgery or for deep, small areas. The donor site of a full-thickness skin graft requires a split-thickness skin graft to help it heal.

Various sources of skin grafts exist: *homograft* (*i.e.*, skin obtained from another human being, alive or recently dead), *heterograft* (*i.e.*, skin obtained from another species, such as pigs), and *autograft* (*i.e.*, skin obtained from the person's own body). The best choice is autografting when there is enough uninterrupted skin on the person's body. *Synthetic skin grafts* are evolving as the research in this area continues.

Rehabilitation

Because the normal body response to disuse is flexion, the contractures that occur with a burn are disfiguring and cause loss of limb or appendage use. Contractures are unnecessary. Treatment measures include splinting (*i.e.*, anatomically positioning and wrapping appendages) and physical therapy to prevent contractures and maintain muscle tone. Firm splint devices and elastic Jobst stockings, sometimes of the full body, are often used.

Psychologic and emotional resources are also provided to burn patients and their families. Rehabilitation can take long periods, considering the numerous hospitalizations, skin grafting procedures, and plastic surgeries. Burn centers across the country specialize in total care for patients and have many of the additional supportive services needed for burn patients.

In summary, burns cause damage to skin structures, ranging from first-degree burns, which damage to the epidermis, to third-degree full-thickness burns, which extend into the subcutaneous tissue and may involve muscle and bone. The extent of injury is determined by the thickness of the burn and the total body surface area involved. In addition to skin involvement, burn injury can cause hemodynamic instability with hypovolemic shock, inhalation injury with respiratory involvement, a hypermetabolic state, organ dysfunction, immune suppression and sepsis, pain, and emotional trauma. Treatment methods vary with the severity of injury and include immediate resuscitation and maintenance of physiologic function, wound cleaning and debridement, application of antimicrobial agents and dressings, and skin grafting. Efforts are directed toward preventing or limiting disfigurement and disability.

Age-Related Skin Manifestations

After you have completed this section of the chapter, you should be able to meet the following objectives:

- Differentiate of a strawberry hemangioma from a port-wine stain hemangioma in terms of appearance and outcome

- Describe the distinguishing features of rashes associated with the common infectious childhood diseases: roseola infantum, rubeola, rubella, chickenpox, and scarlet fever
- Characterize the physiologic changes of aging skin
- Describe the appearance of skin tags, keratoses, lentigines, and vascular lesions that are commonly seen in the elderly

Many skin problems occur more commonly in certain age groups. Because of aging changes, infants, children, and elderly persons tend to have different skin problems.

Skin Manifestations Infancy and Childhood

Skin Disorders of Infancy

Infancy connotes the image of perfect, unblemished skin. For the most part, this is true. However, several congenital skin lesions, such as mongolian spots, hemangiomas, and nevi, are associated with the early neonatal period. Table 15–9 summarizes common skin problems of the infant and small child.

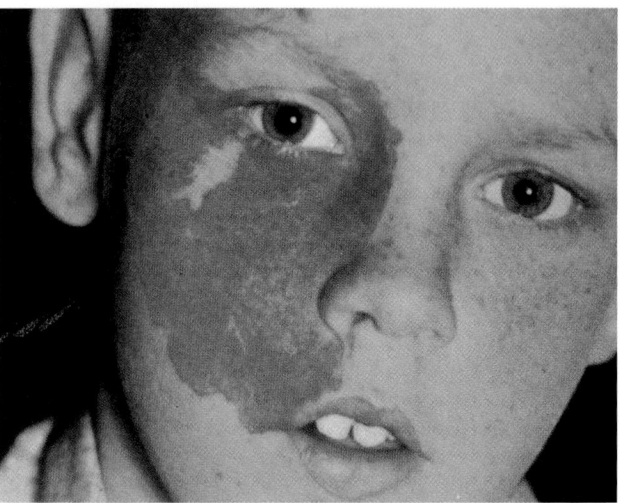

Figure 15–31
Port-wine stain on the face of a boy. (Ortho Dermatology Corp.)

Mongolian Spots and Hemangiomas. Mongolian spots are caused by selective pigmentation. They usually occur on the buttocks or sacral area and are commonly seen in the yellow and black races.

Hemangiomas are vascular disorders of the skin. Two types of hemangiomas are commonly seen in infants and small children: bright red, raised strawberry hemangiomas and flat, reddish purple port-wine stain hemangiomas. The strawberry hemangiomas begin as small, red lesions that are noticed shortly after birth. They may remain as small superficial lesions or extend to involve the subcutaneous tissue. Strawberry hemangiomas usually disappear before 5 to 7 years of age without leaving an appreciable scar. Port-wine stain hemangiomas are rare, usually occur on the face, and are noticeable (Fig. 15–31). They do not disappear with age. Cover-up cosmetics are used in an attempt to conceal their disfiguring effects. Laser surgery has been used effectively in the treatment of port-wine stain hemangiomas.

The term *nevus* is used to denote any common congenital or acquired skin tumor. They are commonly referred to as moles. Most are benign. Nevi vary in shape, color, and size.

Because of its newness, infant skin is sensitive to irritation, injury, and extremes of temperature. The contents of soiled diapers, if not changed frequently, can lead to contact dermatitis and bacterial infections. Prolonged exposure to a warm humid environment can lead to prickly heat, and too-frequent bathing can cause dryness and lead to skin problems. Baby lotions are helpful in maintaining skin moisture, and baby powder

TABLE 15-9
Common Skin Lesions of Infants and Small Children

Lesion	Appearance
Congenital Dermatoses	
Hemangiomas	
Strawberry	Bright-red raised and rounded lesions; may enlarge with growth of infant and then a regress; usually disappear by 5 to 7 years of age
Port-wine stain	Flat reddish-purple disfiguring lesion; usually found on the face; does not disappear with age
Mongolian spot	Light blue, gray-green to slate gray macule; commonly located in the lumbosacral area; usually disappears with age
Nevi (moles)	Vary in size, shape, and location; usually brown-black, flat or raised macules or papules; borders are usually well defined and rounded
Irritative and Inflammatory Dermatoses	
Cradle cap	Yellowish, greasy, and crusted collection of vernix and shedding skin on scalp
Prickly heat	Tiny vesicles usually located on the neck, back, chest, trunk, abdomen, and folds of skin; pruritus is common
Diaper rash	Erythematous macular rash; blister formation, excoriation, and infection may develop

acts as a drying agent. Both are useful aids when used selectively and according to the nature of the skin problem (*i.e.*, excessive moisture or dryness). Unnecessary bathing should be avoided, and clothing appropriate to the environment should be worn.

Diaper Rash. The appearance of diaper rash ranges from simple (*i.e.*, widely distributed macules on the buttocks and anogenital areas) to severe (*i.e.*, beefy, red, excoriated skin surfaces in the diaper area). It results from a combination of ammonia and other breakdown products of urine. The treatment includes frequent diaper changes with careful cleaning of the irritated area to remove the waste products. This is particularly important in hot weather. Exposing the irritated area to air is helpful. Use of plastic pants should be discouraged. Diapers washed in gentle detergent and thoroughly rinsed to remove all traces of waste products help to reduce the risk of diaper rash. Although disposable diapers may help in some cases, their plastic backing may further augment the problem unless they are changed frequently. For intractable, severe cases, the child should be seen by a health care provider for treatment of any secondary infections. Secondary candidal (*i.e.*, yeast) infections are common (Fig. 15–32).

Prickly Heat. Prickly heat (i.e., heat rash) results from constant maceration of the skin because of prolonged exposure to a warm, humid environment. Maceration leads to midepidermal obstruction and rupture of the sweat glands. Although commonly seen during infancy, prickly heat may occur at any age. The treatment includes the removal of excessive clothing, cooling the skin with warm water baths, drying the skin with powders, and avoiding hot, humid environments.

Cradle Cap. Cradle cap is a greasy crust or scale formation on the scalp. It is usually attributed to infrequent and inadequate washing of the scalp. Cradle cap is treated by mild shampooing and gentle combing to remove the scales. Sometimes oil can be left on the head for 3 minutes, softening the scales before scrubbing. Selenium sulfate may be helpful in difficult cases. Caretakers should be advised about the need to rub the scalp firmly to remove the buildup of keratinized cells.

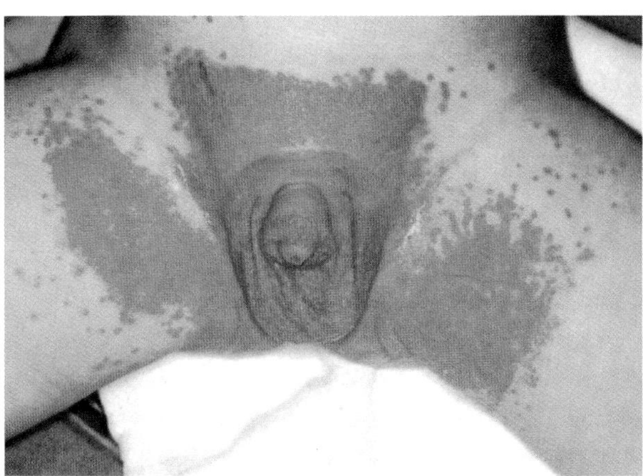

Figure 15–32
Candida intertrigo after a course of oral antibiotics in a 1-year-old child. (Owen Laboratories, Inc.)

Skin Manifestations of Common Infectious Diseases

Infectious childhood diseases that produce rashes include roseola infantum, rubella, rubeola, varicella, and scarlet fever. Although these diseases are seen less frequently because of successful immunization programs (*i.e.*, rubella and rubeola) and use of antibiotics (*i.e.*, scarlet fever), they still occur.

Roseola Infantum. Roseola infantum (*i.e.*, exanthem subitum) is a contagious viral disease of infants and small children, most frequently between 6 and 18 months of age. It is caused by human herpesvirus-6 and produces a characteristic maculopapular rash covering the trunk and spreading to the appendages. The rash is preceded by an abrupt onset of high fever (≤105°F), inflamed tympanic membranes, and coldlike symptoms usually lasting 3 to 4 days. These symptoms improve at about the same time the rash appears. Unlike rubella, no cervical or postauricular lymph node adenopathy occurs. Roseola infantum is frequently mistaken for rubella. Rubella can usually be excluded by the age of the child and the absence of lymph node adenopathy. Generally, children younger than 6 to 9 months do not develop rubella, because they retain some maternal antibodies. Blood antibody titers may be taken to determine the actual diagnosis. In most cases, there are no long-term effects from this disease.

Treatment for roseola infantum is palliative. There is no vaccine for prevention. Antipyretic drugs such as acetaminophen and cooling baths are used to reduce the fever. Rest and fluids are recommended for recuperation and body rehydration. Pruritus may accompany the other symptoms, but this is rare.

Rubella. Rubella (i.e., 3-day measles or German measles) is a childhood disease caused by the rubella virus (a togavirus). It is characterized by a diffuse, punctate, macular rash that begins on the trunk and spreads to the arms and legs (Fig. 15–33). Mild febrile states occur; generally, the fever is less than 100°F. Postauricular, suboccipital, and cervical lymph node adenopathy is common. Coldlike symptoms usually accompany the disease in the form of cough, congestion, and coryza.

Rubella usually has no long-lasting sequelae; however, the transmission of the disease to pregnant women early in the gestation period may result in congenital rubella syndrome. Among the clinical signs of congenital rubella syndrome are cataracts, microcephaly, mental retardation, deafness, patent ductus arteriosus, glaucoma, purpura, and bone defects. Most states have laws requiring immunization to prevent transmission of rubella. Immunization is accomplished by live-virus injection. A single injection after 12 to 15 months of age has

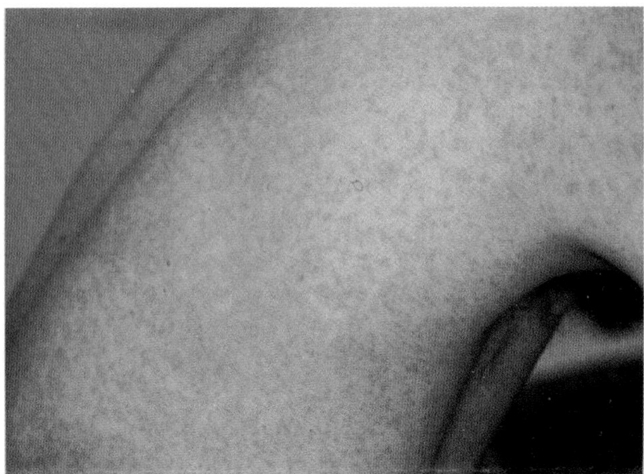

Figure 15–33
Rubella (*i.e.*, German or 3-day measles) rash of the trunk. (Fitzpatrick T.B., Johnson R.A., Polono M.K., Suurmond D., Wolff K. [1992]. *Color atlas and synopsis of clinical dermatology* [2nd ed., p. 289]. New York: McGraw-Hill)

produced a 98% to 99% immunity response in immunized children and is considered adequate in the prevention of rubella.[33] Many areas, however, require a second preschool or later dose of rubella vaccine to increase the immunity response of the vaccine and prevent congenital rubella. Cases of rubella in unimmunized children are rare when the level of immunization in the general population remains high. Treatment is symptomatic and supportive.

Rubeola. *Measles* (*i.e.*, rubeola, hard measles, 7-day measles) is an acute, highly communicable viral disease caused by morbillivirus. The characteristic rash is macular and blotchy; sometimes, the macules become confluent (Fig. 15–34). The rubeola rash usually begins on the face and spreads to the appendages. There are several accompanying symptoms: a fever of 100°F or greater, Koplik's spots (*i.e.*, small, irregular red spots with a bluish white speck in the center) on the buccal mucosa, and mild to severe photosensitivity. The patient commonly has coldlike symptoms, general malaise, and myalgia. In severe cases, the macule may hemorrhage into the skin tissue or onto the outer body surface. This form is called hemorrhagic measles. The course of measles is more severe in infants, adults, and malnourished children. There may be severe complications, including otitis media, pneumonia, and encephalitis. Antibody titers are determined for a conclusive diagnosis of rubeola.

The treatment for measles is symptomatic. Children are isolated in a darkened room, antipyretic medications are given to reduce the fever, and rest and relaxation are encouraged. If marked dehydration exists or the symptoms are severe, a health care provider should be consulted.

Measles is a disease preventable by vaccine and immunization is required by law in the United States. Immunization is accomplished by injection of a live-virus vaccine. A single injection after 12 months of age is sufficient to produce initial immunity. A second injection should be given on entry to elementary school, although it can be given in middle school. There has been a notable increase in the number of measles cases in the United States and other countries over the past few years. Measles outbreaks occur among unimmunized and underimmunized children.

Varicella. Chickenpox (*i.e.*, varicella) is a common communicable childhood disease. It is caused by the herpes zoster virus, which is also the agent in shingles (*i.e.*, herpes zoster). The characteristic skin lesion occurs in three stages: macule, vesicle, and granular scab. The macular stage is characterized by development within hours of macules over the trunk of the body, spreading to the limbs, buccal mucosa, scalp, axillae, upper respiratory tract, and conjunctiva (Fig. 15–35). During the second stage, the macules vesiculate (*i.e.*, filled with water or blister) and may become depressed or umbilicated (*i.e.*, raised blisters with depressed centers). The vesicles break open and a scab forms during the third stage. Crops of lesions occur successively, so that all three forms of the lesion are usually visible by the third day of the illness.

Mild to extreme pruritus accompanies these lesions, which can lead to scratching and subsequent development of secondary bacterial infections. Chickenpox is also accompanied by coldlike symptoms, including cough, coryza (*i.e.*, nasal discharge), and sometimes photosensitivity. Mild febrile states usually occur, typically beginning 24 hours before lesion outbreak. Side effects,

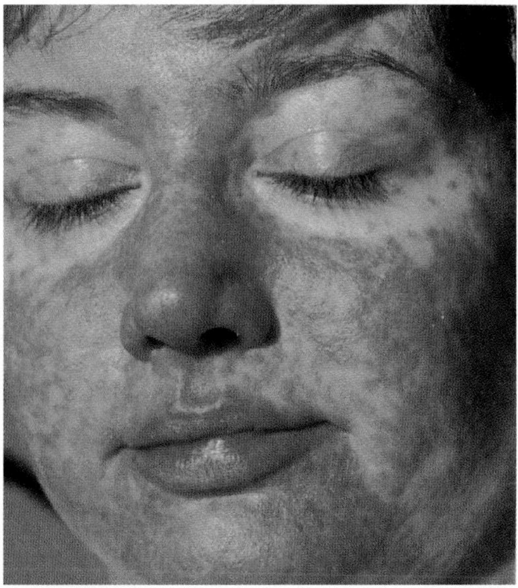

Figure 15–34
Rubeola rash on the face of a young woman. (Fitzpatrick T.B., Johnson R.A., Polono M.K., Suurmond D., Wolff K. [1992]. *Color atlas and synopsis of clinical dermatology* [2nd ed., p. 291]. New York: McGraw-Hill)

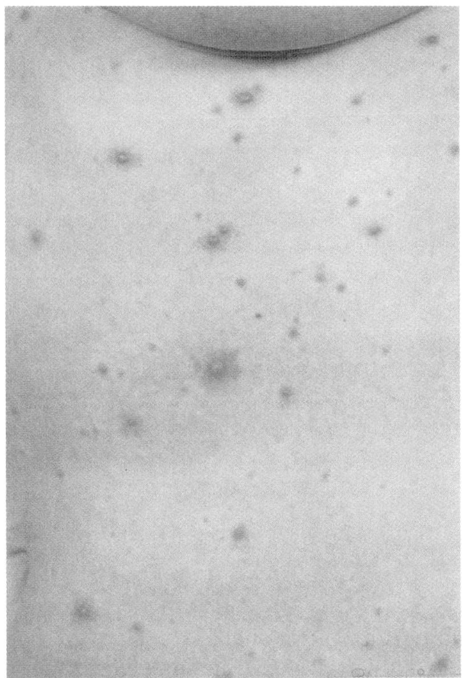

Figure 15–35
Varicella (*i.e.*, chickenpox), with characteristic erythematous papules and vesicles. (Fitzpatrick T.B., Johnson R.A., Polono M.K., Suurmond D., Wolff K. [1992]. *Color atlas and synopsis of clinical dermatology* [2nd ed., p. 289]. New York: McGraw-Hill)

such as pneumonia, septic complications, and encephalitis, are rare.

Live attenuated varicella vaccine has been demonstrated to be highly effective in the prevention of chickenpox in healthy children (70% to 90%) and children who have leukemia (100%).[34,35] The vaccine is available in the United States, but in most states immunization is not required by law.

Acyclovir has been effective in reducing the number of lesions and length of illness with healthy children when given within the first 24 hours of disease onset.[36] However, because the disease is relatively benign in children, treatment measures remain primarily palliative. Antipyretic drugs such as acetaminophen are given to reduce fever; they may also relieve local discomfort. Pruritus is relieved with lukewarm baths and applications of topical antipruritics such as Caladryl lotion. Home remedies, such as baking soda or colloidal oatmeal baths, also relieve itching. A health care provider should be notified in cases of severe pruritus. Oral administration of diphenhydramine (Benadryl) or other antihistamines may be prescribed. Rest and fluids are important in recuperation and rehydration. Varicella may be more complicated. For example, it may be complicated with Reye's syndrome when children have been treated with aspirin. Varicella in adults may be more severe, with a prolonged recovery rate and greater chances of developing varicella pneumonitis or encephalitis. Immunocompromised persons may experience a chronic, painful type. These persons should seek professional help. Acyclovir or other antivirals may be helpful along with other, more potent, symptomatic care.

Scarlet Fever. Scarlet fever (*i.e.*, scarlatina) is a systemic reaction to the toxins produced by group A β-hemolytic streptococci. The circulating toxin is responsible for the rash and systemic symptoms. Scarlet fever frequently is associated with streptococcal sore throat (*i.e.*, strep throat). Scarlet fever was a feared disease in the 19th and early 20th century, when it was more virulent and before the advent of penicillin. Scarlet fever is characterized by a pink punctate skin rash on the neck, chest, axillae, groin, and thighs. When palpated, the rash feels like fine sandpaper. The patient has flushing of the face with circumoral pallor. Other symptoms include high fever, nausea, vomiting, strawberry tongue (*i.e.*, white-coated tongue through which enlarged and red lingual papillae project), raspberry tongue (*i.e.*, bright red), and skin desquamation. Complications of scarlet fever include otitis media, peritonsillar abscess, rheumatic fever, acute glomerulonephritis, and cholera. Penicillin is the drug of choice for treatment.

Skin Manifestations and Disorders in the Elderly

Elderly persons experience a variety of age-related skin disorders and exacerbations of earlier skin problems. Aging skin is believed to involve a complex process of actinic (*i.e.*, solar) damage, normal aging, and hormonal influences.[37] Actinic changes primarily involve increased occurrence of lesions on sun-exposed surfaces of the body.

Normal Age-Related Changes

Normal aging consists of changes that occur on areas of the body that have not been exposed to sun. They include thinning of the dermis and the epidermis, diminution in subcutaneous tissue, lessening and thickening of blood vessels, and a decrease in the number of melanocytes, Langerhans' cells, and Merkel's cells. The keratinocytes shrink, but the number of dead keratinized cells at the surface increase. This results in less padding and thinner skin, with color and elasticity changes. The skin also loses its resistance to environmental and mechanical trauma. Tissue repair takes longer.

With aging, there is also less hair and nail growth, with permanent hair pigment loss. Hormonally, there is less sebaceous gland activity, although the glands in the facial skin may increase in size. Hair growth reduction may also be hormonally influenced.[2] Although the reason is poorly understood, the skin in most elderly persons becomes dry, rough, and scaly. Dryness becomes worse during the winter, when the need for home heating lowers the humidity. Treatment includes increasing humidification of the air; bathing less frequently, using warm rather than hot water; using mild soap; and applying moisturizers while the skin is still moist.

Skin Lesions Common Among the Elderly

The most common skin lesions in the elderly are skin tags, keratoses, lentigines, and vascular lesions. Most are actinic manifestations; they occur as a result of exposure to sun and weather over the years.

Skin Tags. *Skin tags* are soft, brown or flesh-colored papules. They occur on any skin surface, but most frequently the neck, axilla, and intertriginous areas. They range in size from a pinhead to the size of a pea. Skin tags have the normal texture of the skin. They are benign and can be removed with scissors or electrodesiccation for cosmetic purposes.

Keratoses. A *keratosis* is a horny growth or an abnormal growth of the keratinocytes. A *seborrheic keratosis* (*i.e.,* seborrheic wart) is a benign, sharply circumscribed, wartlike lesion that has a stuck-on appearance (Fig. 15–36). They vary in size up to several centimeters. They are usually round or oval. They are usually pigmented tan, brown, or black, although less pigmented ones may appear yellow or pink. Keratoses can be found on the face or trunk, as a solitary lesion or sometimes by the hundreds. Seborrheic keratoses are benign, but they must be watched for changes in color, texture, or size, which may indicate malignant transformation to a melanoma.

Actinic keratoses are the most common premalignant skin lesions that develop on sun-exposed areas. The lesions are usually less than 1 cm in diameter and appear as dry, brown scaly areas, often with a reddish tinge. Actinic keratoses are often multiple and more easily felt than seen (Fig. 15–37). They are often indistinguishable from squamous cell carcinoma without biopsy. A hyperkeratotic form also exists that is more prominent and palpable. Often, there is a weathered appearance of the surrounding skin. Slight changes, such as enlargement or ulceration, may indicate malignant transformation. Most actinic keratoses are treated with 5-fluorouracil cream, which erodes the lesions. Roughly 20% of actinic keratoses convert to squamous cell carcinomas.

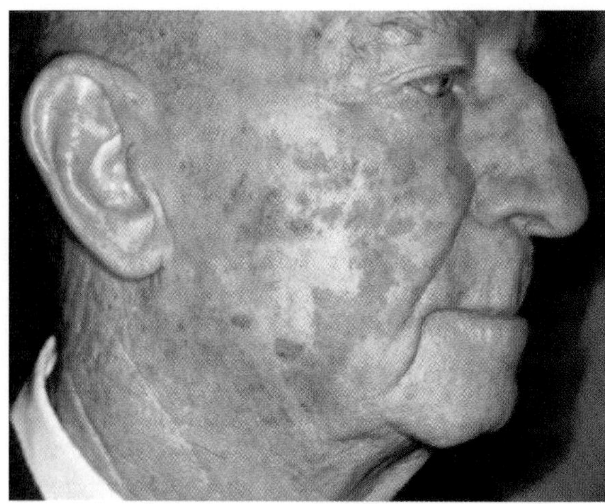

Figure 15–37
Multiple actinic keratoses of the face of an 80-year-old man. (Dermick Laboratories, Inc.)

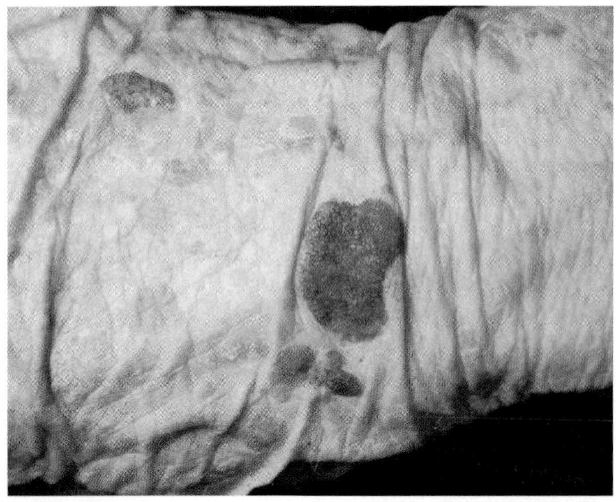

Figure 15–36
Large seborrheic keratoses on the hand of an 84-year-old woman.

Lentigines. A *lentigo* is a well-bordered brown to black macule, usually less than 1 cm in diameter. *Solar lentigines* are tan to brown, benign spots on sun-exposed areas (Fig. 15–38). They are commonly referred to as liver spots. Creams and lotions containing hydroquinone (*e.g.,* Eldoquin, Solaquin) may be used to temporarily bleach the spots. These agents inhibit the synthesis of new pigment without destroying existing pigment. Higher concentrations are available by prescription. Successful treatment depends on avoiding sun exposure and consistent use of sunscreens. Liquid nitrogen applications have been successful in eradicating senile lentigines.

Lentigo maligna (*i.e.,* Hutchinson's freckle) is a slowly progressive (≤20 years) preneoplastic disorder of melanocytes. It occurs on sun-exposed areas, particularly the face. The lesion is a pigmented macule with a well-defined border and grows to 5 cm or sometimes larger. Over the years, it grows and may become slightly raised and wartlike. If untreated, a true malignant melanoma often develops. Surgery, curettage, and cryotherapy have been effective at removing the lentigines. Careful monitoring for conversion to melanoma is important.

Vascular Lesions. *Vascular lesions* are vascular tumors with chronically dilated blood vessels. Small blood vessels lie within the middle to upper dermis. *Senile angiomas* (*i.e.,* cherry angiomas) are smooth, cherry red or purple, dome-shaped papules. They are usually found on the trunk. *Telangiectases* are single dilated blood vessels, capillaries, or terminal arteries that appear on areas exposed to sun or harsh weather, such as the cheeks and the nose. The lesions can become large and disfiguring.

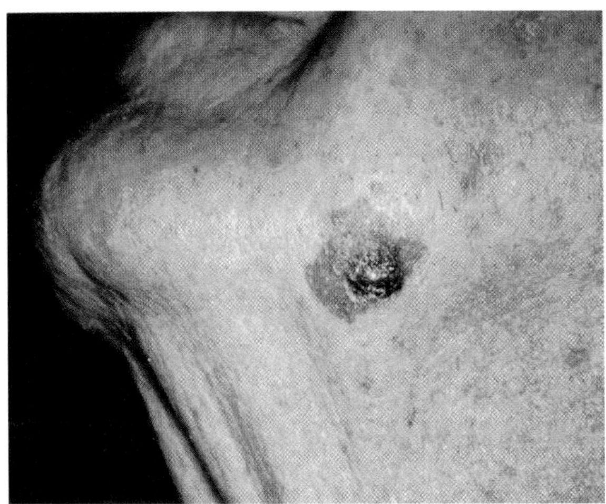

Figure 15–38
Lentigo on the cheek. (Syntex Laboratories, Inc.)

Pulsed dye lasers have been effective in removing them. *Venous lakes* are small, dark blue, slightly raised papules that have a lake-like appearance. They occur on exposed body parts, particularly the backs of the hands, ears, and lips. They are smooth and compressible. Venous lakes can be removed by electrosurgery, laser therapy, or surgical excision if a person desires.

In summary, some skin problems occur in specific age groups. Common in infants are diaper rash, prickly heat, and cradle cap. Infectious childhood diseases that are characterized by rashes include roseola infantum, rubella (i.e., German measles), rubeola (i.e., 7-day measles), varicella (i.e., chickenpox), and scarlet fever (i.e., scarlatina). Vaccines are available to protect against rubella, rubeola, and varicella. Changes in skin that occur with aging involve a complex process of actinic damage, normal aging, and hormonal influences. With aging, there is thinning of the dermis and the epidermis; diminution in subcutaneous tissue; lessening and thickening of blood vessels; and a slowing of hair and nail growth. Dry skin is common among the elderly, becoming worse during the winter months. Among the skin lesions seen in the elderly are skin tags, keratoses, lentigines, and vascular skin lesions.

REFERENCES

1. Greco P.J., Ende J. (1992). An office-based approach to the patient with pruritus. *Hospital Practice* 27, 121.
2. Evans E.G.V., Dodman B., Williamson D.M., Brown G.J., Bowen R.G. (1993). Comparison of terbinafine and clotrimazole in treating tinea pedis. *British Medical Journal* 307, 645–647.
3. Honig P.J., Caputo G.L., Leyden J.J., McGinley K., Selbst S.M., McGravey A.R. (1994). Treatment of kerions. *Journal of Pediatric Dermatology* 11, 69–71.
4. Benenson A.S. (Ed.). (1995). *Control of communicable diseases manual* (16th ed., p. 134). Washington, DC: American Public Health Association.
5. Spanes N.P., Williams V., Gwynn M.I. (1990). Effects of hypnotic, placebo, and salicylic acid treatments on wart regression. *Psychosomatic Medicine* 52, 109.
6. Tyring S.K. (1996). Early treatment of herpes zoster. *Hospital Practice* 31, 137–144.
7. Plewig G., Klingman A.M. (1993). *Acne and rosacea* (2nd ed., pp. 3, 341). New York: Springer-Verlag.
8. Scott C.B., Moloney M.F. (1996). Physical urticaria. *The Nurse Practitioner* 21 (11), 42–59.
9. Greaves M.W. (1995). Chronic urticaria. *New England Journal of Medicine* 332 (26), 1767–1772.
10. Bastuji-Garin S., Rzany B., Stern R.S., Shear N.H., Naldi L., Roujeau J.C. (1993) Clinical classification of cases of toxic epidermal necrolysis, Stevens-Johnson syndrome, and erythema multiforme. *Archives of Dermatology* 129, 92–96.
11. Roujeau J.C., Stern R.S. (1994). Severe adverse cutaneous reactions to drugs. *New England Journal of Medicine* 331, 1272–1284.
12. Camisa C. (1994). Psoriasis (pp. 3, 30–31, 55). Boston: Blackwell.
13. Phillips T.J. (1996). Current treatment options in psoriasis. *Hospital Practice* 31, 155–166.
14. Greaves M.W., Weinstein G.D. (1995). Treatment of psoriasis. *New England Journal of Medicine* 332, 581–588.
15. Habif T.P. (1996). *Clinical Dermatology* (3rd ed., p. 474). St. Louis: Mosby.
16. Boring C.C., Squires T.S., Tong T., Montgomery S. (1994). Cancer statistics. *Cancer* 44, 7–26.
17. Halder R.M., Bridgeman-Shah S. (1995). Skin cancer in African Americans. *Cancer* 75, 667–673.
18. Diffey B.L. (1992). Human exposure to ultraviolet radiation. In Marks R, Plewig G. (Eds.). *The environmental threat to the skin* (pp 3–9). London: Martin Dunitz.
19. Armstrong R.B. (1992). Photobiology of ultraviolet radiation. In Abel E.A. (Ed.). *Photochemotherapy in dermatology* (pp. 17–31). New York: Igaku-Shoin.
20. Jeevan A., Kripke M.L. (1995). Ozone depletion and the immune system. *Lancet* 342, 1159–1160.
21. Garland C.F., Garland F.C., Gorham E.D. (1993). Rising trends in melanoma: A hypothesis concerning sunscreen effectiveness. *Annals of Epidemiology* 3, 103–110.
22. Preston D.S., Stern R.S. (1992). Nonmelanoma cancers of the skin. *New England Journal of Medicine* 327, 1649–1662.
23. Frankel D.H. (1992). Squamous cell carcinoma of the skin. *Hospital Practice* 27, 99–106.
24. Marks R. (1995). An overview of skin cancers: Incidence and causation. *Cancer* 75, 607–612.
25. NIH Consensus Conference. (1992). Diagnosis and treatment of early melanoma. *Journal of the American Medical Association* 268, 1314.
26. Rigel D.S., Sober A.J., Friedman R.J. (1991). Prognostic factors influencing survival in persons with cutaneous melanoma (pp. 198–206). In Friedman R.J., Rigel D.S., Kopf A.W., Harris M.N., Baker D. (Eds.). *Cancer of the skin*. Philadelphia: W.B. Saunders.
27. Nguyen T.T., Gilpin D.A., Meyer N.A., Herndon D.N. (1996). Current treatment of severely burned patients. *Annals of Surgery* 223, 14–25.
28. Brigham P.A., McLoughlin E. (1996). Burn incidence and medical care use in the United States: Estimates, trends, and data sources. *Journal of Burn Care Rehabilitation* 17, 95–107.

29. Wilson Y., Goberdhan N., Dawson R.A., Smith J., Freelander E., MacNeil S. (1994). Investigation of the presence and role of calmodulin and other mitogens in human burn blister fluid. *Journal of Burn Care and Rehabilitation* 15, 303–314.
30. Hudak C.M., Gallo B.M. (1994). *Critical care nursing* (6th ed., pp. 978–1005). Philadelphia; J.B. Lippincott.
31. Lund C.C., Browder N.C. (1944). Estimation of areas of burns. *Journal of Surgical Gynecological Obstetrics* 79:352–358.
32. Caldwell F.T., Wallace B.H., Cone J.B. (1996). Sequential excision and grafting of the burn injuries of 1507 patients treated between 1967 and 1986: End results and the determinants of death. *Journal of Burn Care and Rehabilitation* 17, 137–146.
33. Benenson A.S. (Ed.). (1995). *Control of communicable diseases manual* (16th ed., p. 89). Washington, DC: American Public Health Association.
34. Hardy I., Gershon A.A., Steinberg S.P., et al. (1991). Varicella Vaccine Collaborative Study Group: The incidence of zoster after immunization with live attenuated varicella vaccine: A study in children with leukemia. *New England Journal of Medicine* 325, 1545–1550.
35. Dunkle L.M., Arvin A.M., Whitley R.J., et al. (1991). A controlled trial of acyclovir for chickenpox in normal children. *New England Journal of Medicine* 325, 1539–1554.
36. Benenson A.S. (Ed.). (1995). *Control of communicable diseases manual* (16th ed., p. 407). Washington, DC: American Public Health Association.
37. Bolognia J.L. (1995). Aging skin. *American Journal of Medicine* 98, 99S–103S.

ADDITIONAL READINGS

Abel E.A. (Ed.). (1992). *Photochemotherapy in dermatology*. New York: Igaku-Shoin.

Arnold M.L., Odam R.B., James W.D. (Eds.). (1990). *Andrew's diseases of the skin: Clinical dermatology* (8th ed.). Philadelphia: W.B. Saunders.

Balch C.M., Houghton A.N., Milton G.W., Sober A.J., Soong S. (Eds.). (1992). *Cutaneous melanoma* (2nd ed.). Philadelphia: W.B. Saunders.

Baran R., Dawber R.P.R. (Eds.). (1994). *Diseases of the nails and their management* (2nd ed.). Oxford: Blackwell.

Bennett J.E., Hay R.J., Peterson P.K. (Eds.). (1992). *New strategies in fungal disease: Proceedings of an international symposium*. Edinburgh: Churchill Livingstone.

Brunnel P.A. (1991). Chickenpox—Examining our options. *New England Journal of Medicine* 325, 1577–1579.

Epstein J.H. (1990). Phototherapy and photochemistry. *New England Journal of Medicine* 322, 1149–1151.

Fine J. (1995). Management of acquired bullous skin diseases. *New England Journal of Medicine* 333, 1475–1484.

Fitzpatrick T.B., Johnson R.A., Polano M.K., Suurmond D., Wolff K. (1992). *Color atlas and synopsis of clinical dermatology: Common and serious diseases* (2nd ed.). New York: McGraw-Hill.

Friedman R.J., Rigel D.S., Kopf A.W., Harris M.N., Baker D. (1991). *Cancer of the skin*. Philadelphia: W.B. Saunders.

Hashimoto K., Mehregan A.H. (1990). *Tumors of the epidermis*. Boston: Butterworths.

Holleb A.I., Fink D.J., Murphy G.P. (Eds.). (1991). *Clinical oncology* (7th ed.). New York: American Cancer Society.

Koh H.K. (1991). Cutaneous melanoma. *New England Journal of Medicine* 325, 171–182.

Lowe N.J. (1991). Systemic treatment of severe psoriasis. *New England Journal of Medicine* 324, 33–34.

Malloy B.M., Perez-Wood R.C. (1991). Neonatal skin care: Prevention of skin breakdown. *Pediatric Nursing* 17 (1), 41–48.

Marks R. (1993). *Eczema*. Cardiff, UK: Martin Dunitz.

Marks R. (1993). *Roxburgh's common skin diseases* (16th ed.). New York: Chapman & Hall.

Marks R., Plewig G. (1992). *The environmental threat to the skin*. London: Martin Dunitz.

Marzulli F.N., Maibach H.I. (Eds.). (1991). *Dermatotoxicology*. New York: Hemisphere.

Phillips R.J., Dover J.S. (1992). Recent advances in dermatology. *New England Journal of Medicine* 326, 167–178.

Sauer G.C., Hall J.C. (1996). *Manual of skin diseases* (7th ed.). Philadelphia: Lippincott-Raven Publishers.

Sober A.J., Fitzpatrick T.B. (Eds.). (1993). *The year book of dermatology*. St. Louis: Mosby.

Trofino R.B. (1991). *Nursing care of the burn-injured patient*. Philadelphia: Davis.

Van der Valk P.G., Maibach H.I. (1996). *The irritant contact dermatitis syndrome*. New York: CRC Press.

Circulatory Function

Of all body systems, the heart and circulation presented the most difficult puzzle to solve. From the fifth century B.C.*, theories about blood and its movement were linked to the concept of the four elements (fire, earth, air, and water) and the* pneuma*, or life force. According to the Greek physician Galen (130–200), the starting point of the circulatory system was the gut, where food was made into "chyle" and then carried to the liver where it was converted into blood. From the liver, which was believed to be the center of the circulation, a small amount of blood was sent to the heart and lungs where heat from the heart and pneuma from the air were added, producing an ultimate concoction of "vital spirits" that was carried in the arteries to all parts of the body.*

It was not until the work of the English physician William Harvey (1578–1657) that answers to the mysteries of the circulation began to emerge. It was he who first proposed that blood traveled in a circuitous route through the body, being pumped by the active phase of the heart's contraction, not relaxation as had been previously believed. In his studies, Harvey showed that a cut artery in an animal spurts during the heart's contraction. He also demonstrated that the atria of the heart had the same relationship to the veins as the veins do to the arteries and that blood from the heart was circulated through the lungs where it was oxygenated. As strange as it may seem today, these concepts were so revolutionary to Harvey's contemporaries that the world's basic understanding of how the body functions was thrown into turmoil.

UNIT V

CHAPTER 16

Control of the Circulation

The circulatory system, which consists of the heart and blood vessels, has one main function—transport. The circulatory system delivers oxygen and nutrients needed for metabolic processes to the tissues, carries waste products from cellular metabolism to the kidneys and other excretory organs for elimination, and circulates electrolytes and hormones needed to regulate body function. Temperature regulation relies on the circulatory system for transport of core heat to the periphery, where it can be dissipated into the external environment. The circulatory system also plays a vital role in the transport of various immune substances that contribute to the body's defense mechanisms. Amazingly, the blood flow to each tissue of the body is controlled in relation to tissue need. The purpose of this chapter is to discuss the organization of the circulatory system, the function of the heart as a pump, blood vessels and the systemic circulation, neural control of circulatory function, and the microcirculation and lymphatic system.

Organization of the Circulatory System

After you have completed this section of the chapter, you should be able to meet the following objectives:

- Compare the functions and distribution of blood flow and blood pressure in the systemic and pulmonary circulations
- State the relation between blood volume and blood pressure in the circulatory system

Pulmonary and Systemic Circulations

The circulatory system can be divided into two parts: the *pulmonary circulation*, which moves blood through the lungs and links the gas exchange function of the respiratory system, and the *systemic circulation*, which supplies all of the other tissues of the body (Fig. 16–1). The blood that is in the heart and pulmonary circulation is sometimes referred to as the *central circulation* and that outside the central circulation as the *peripheral circulation*.

Both the pulmonary and systemic circulations have a pump, an arterial system, capillaries, and a venous system. Arteries and arterioles function as a distribution system to move blood to the tissues. Capillaries serve as an exchange system where transfer of gases, nutrients, and wastes takes place. Venules and veins serve as collection and storage vessels that return blood to the heart. The pulmonary circulation consists of the right heart, the pulmonary artery, the pulmonary capillaries, and the pulmonary veins. The large pulmonary vessels are unique in that the pulmonary artery is the only artery that carries venous blood and the pulmonary veins, the only veins that carry arterial blood.

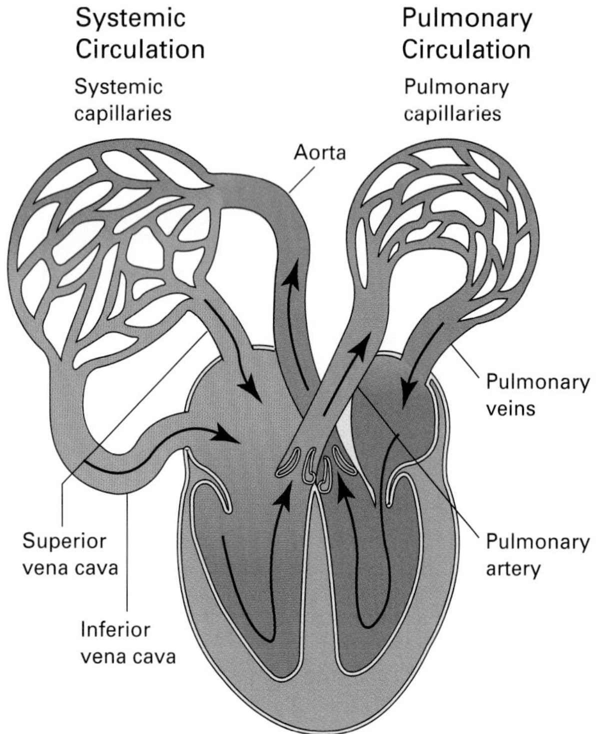

Figure 16–1
Systemic and pulmonary circulations. The right side of the heart pumps blood to the lungs, and the left side of the heart pumps blood to the systemic circulation.

The systemic circulation consists of the left heart, the aorta and its branches, the capillaries that supply the brain and peripheral tissues, and the systemic venous system and the vena cava. The veins from the lower portion of the body converge into the inferior vena cava and those from the head and upper extremities converge into the superior vena cava. The inferior vena cava and superior vena cava empty into the right heart.

Although the pulmonary and systemic systems function similarly, they have some important differences. The pulmonary circulation is the smaller of the two, and it functions with a much lower pressure. Because the pulmonary circulation is located in the chest and in close proximity to the heart, it functions as a low-pressure system with a mean arterial pressure of about 12 mm Hg. The low pressure of the pulmonary circulation allows blood to move through the lungs more slowly, which is important for gas exchange. Because the systemic circulation must transport blood to distant parts of the body, often against the effects of gravity, it functions as a high-pressure system, with a mean arterial pressure of 90 to 100 mm Hg.

The circulatory system is a closed system in which the heart consists of two pumps in series: one to propel blood through the lungs (*i.e.*, pulmonary circulation) and the other to propel blood to all other tissues of the body (*i.e.*, systemic circulation). Unidirectional flow through the heart is ensured by the heart valves. Both sides of the heart are further divided into two chambers, an atrium and a ventricle. The atria function as collection chambers for blood returning to the heart and as auxiliary pumps that assist in filling the ventricles. The ventricles are the main pumping chambers of the heart. The right ventricle pumps blood through the pulmonary artery to the lungs and the left ventricle pumps blood through the aorta into the systemic circulation. The ventricular chambers of the right and left heart have inlet and outlet valves that act reciprocally (*i.e.*, one set of valves is open while the other is closed) to control the direction of blood flow through the cardiac chambers.

The effective function of the circulatory system requires that the outputs of both sides of the heart pump the same amount of blood over time. If the output of the left heart were to fall below that of the right heart, blood would accumulate in the pulmonary circulation. Likewise, if the right heart were to pump less effectively than the left heart, blood would accumulate in the systemic circulation. The left and right heart seldom eject exactly the same amount of blood with each beat. This is because blood return to the heart is affected by activities of daily living such as taking a deep breath or moving from the seated to standing position. These beat-by-beat variations in cardiac output are accommodated by the storage capabilities of the venous system that allow for temporary changes in volume. Fluid accumulation only occurs when the storage capacity of the venous system has been exceeded.

Volume and Pressure Distribution

Blood flow in the circulatory system depends on a blood volume that is sufficient to fill the blood vessels and a pressure that provides the force to move blood forward. The total blood volume is a function of age and body weight, ranging from 85 to 90 ml/kg in the neonate to 70 to 75 ml/kg in the adult. As shown in Figure 16–2, about 4% of the blood at any given time is in the left heart, 16% is in the arteries and arterioles, 4% is in the capillaries, 64% is in the venules and veins, and 4% is in the right heart. The arteries and arterioles, which have thick elastic walls and function as a distribution system, have the highest pressure. The capillaries are small, thin-walled vessels that link the arterial and venous sides of the circulation. Because of their small size and large surface area, the capillaries contain the smallest amount of blood. The venules and veins, which contain largest amount of blood, are thin-walled distensible vessels that function as a reservoir to collect blood from the capillaries and return it to the right heart.

Blood moves from the arterial to the venous side of the circulation along a pressure difference, moving from an area of higher pressure to one of lower pressure. As shown in Figure 16–2, the pressure distribution in the different parts of the circulation is almost an inverse of the volume distribution. The pressure in the arterial side of the circulation, which contains only about one sixth of the blood volume, is much greater than the pressure on the venous side of the circulation, which contains about two thirds of the blood. This pressure and volume distribution is due in a large part to the structure and relative elasticity of the arteries and veins. It is the pressure difference between the arterial and venous sides of the circulation (about 84 mm Hg) that provides the driving force for flow of blood in the systemic circulation. The pulmonary circulation has similar arterial-venous pressure differences, albeit of a lesser magnitude, that facilitate blood flow.

Because the pulmonary and systemic circulations are connected and function as a closed system, blood can be shifted from one circulation to the other. In the pulmonary circulation, the blood volume (about 450 ml in the adult) can vary from as low as 50% of normal to as high as 200% of normal. Increases in intrathoracic pressure, which impede venous return to the right heart, can produce a transient shift from the central to the systemic circulation of as much as 250 ml of blood. Body position also affects the distribution of blood volume. In the recumbent position, about 25% to 30% of the total blood volume is in the central circulation. On standing, this blood is rapidly displaced to the lower part of the body because of the forces of gravity. Because the volume of the systemic circulation is about seven times that of the pulmonary circulation, a shift of blood from one system to the other has a much greater effect in the pulmonary than in the systemic circulation.

In summary, the circulatory system functions as a transport system that circulates nutrients and other materials to the tissues and removes waste products. The circulatory system can be divided into two parts: the systemic and the pulmonary circulation. The heart pumps blood throughout the system, and

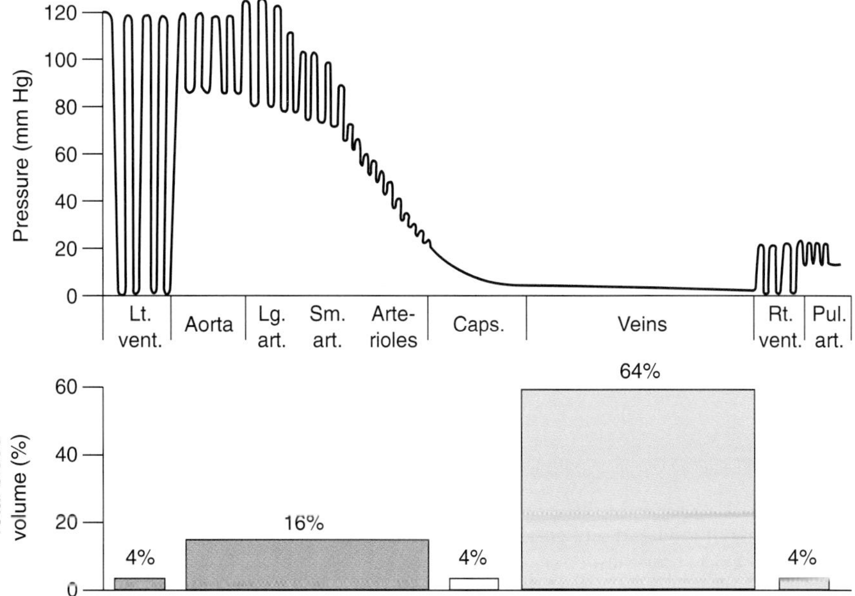

Figure 16–2
Pressure and volume distribution in the systemic circulation. The graphs show the inverse relation between internal pressure and volume in different portions of the circulatory system. (Smith J.J., Kampine J.P. [1984]. *Circulatory physiology: The essentials* [2nd ed.]. Baltimore: Williams & Wilkins)

the blood vessels serve as tubes through which blood flows. The arterial system carries fluids from the heart to the tissues, and the veins carry them back to the heart. The cardiovascular system is a closed system with a right and left heart connected in series. The systemic circulation, which is served by the left heart, supplies all the tissues except the lungs, which are served by the right heart and the pulmonary circulation. Blood moves throughout the circulation along a pressure gradient, moving from the high-pressure arterial system to the low-pressure venous system. In the circulatory system, pressure is inversely related to volume. The pressure on the arterial side of the circulation, which contains only about one sixth of the blood volume, is much greater than the pressure on the venous side of the circulation, which contains about two thirds of the blood.

The Heart as a Pump

After you have completed this section of the chapter, you should be able to meet the following objectives:

- Describe the structural components and function of the pericardium, myocardium, endocardium, and the heart valves and fibrous skeleton
- Draw a figure of the cardiac cycle, incorporating volume, pressure, phonocardiogram, and electrocardiographic changes that occur during atrial and ventricular systole and diastole
- Define the terms *preload* and *afterload*
- State the formula for calculating the cardiac output and explain the effects that venous return, cardiac contractility, and heart rate have on cardiac output
- Describe the cardiac reserve and relate it to the Frank-Starling mechanism

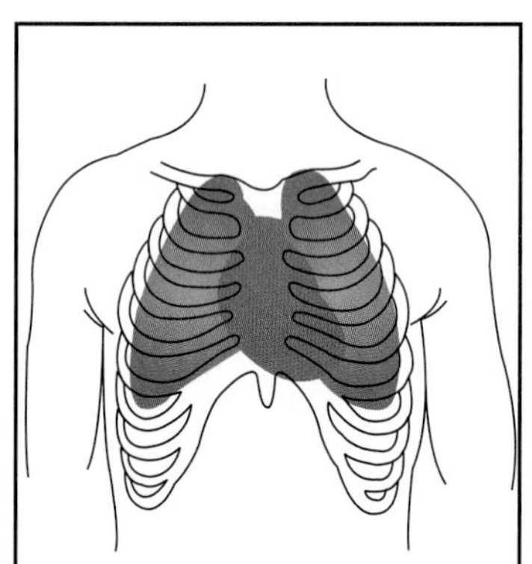

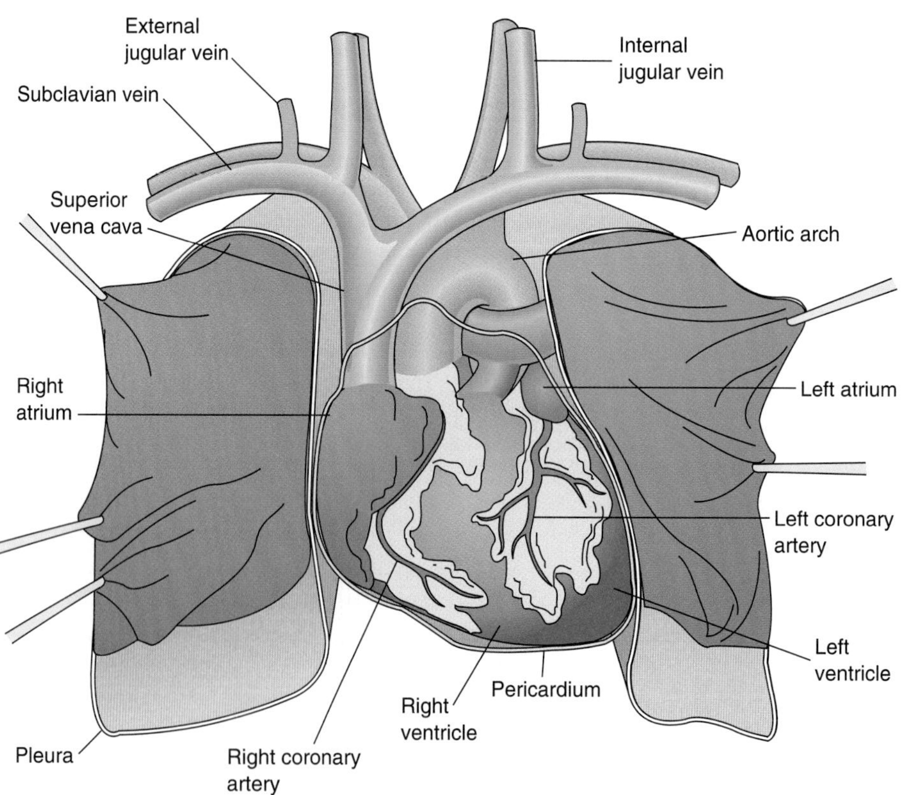

Figure 16–3
Anterior view of the heart and great vessels and their relationship to lungs and skeletal structures of the chest cage (upper left box).

The heart is a four-chambered muscular pump about the size of a man's fist that beats an average of 70 times each minute, 24 hours each day, 365 days each year for a lifetime. In 1 day, this pump moves more than 1800 gallons of blood throughout the body, and the work performed by the heart over a lifetime would lift 30 tons to a height of 30,000 ft.

Functional Anatomy of the Heart

The heart is located between the lungs in the mediastinal space of the intrathoracic cavity within a loose-fitting sac called the *pericardium.* It is suspended by the great vessels, with its broader side (*i.e.,* base) facing upward and its tip (*i.e.,* apex) pointing downward, forward, and to the left. The heart is positioned obliquely, so that the right side of the heart is almost fully in front of the left side of the heart, with only a small portion of the lateral left ventricle on the frontal plane of the heart (Fig. 16–3). When the hand is placed on the thorax, the main impact of the heart's contraction is felt against the chest wall at a point between the fifth and sixth ribs, a little below the nipple and about 3 inches to the left of the midline. This is called the *point of maximum impulse* (*PMI*).

The wall of the heart is composed of an outer epicardium, which lines the pleural cavity; the myocardium or muscle layer; and the smooth endocardium, which lines the chambers of the heart. A fibrous skeleton supports the valvular structures of the heart. The intraatrial and intraventricular septum divide the heart into a right and a left pump, each composed of two muscular chambers: a thin-walled atrium, which serves as a reservoir for blood coming into the heart, and a thick-walled ventricle, which pumps blood out of the heart. The increased thickness of the left ventricular wall results from the additional work this ventricle is required to perform.

Pericardium

The pericardium forms a fibrous covering around the heart, holding it in a fixed position in the thorax. It provides physical protection and a barrier to infection. The pericardium consists of a tough outer fibrous layer and a thin inner serous layer. The outer fibrous layer is attached to the great vessels that enter and leave the heart, the sternum, and the diaphragm. The fibrous pericardium is highly resistive to distention; it prevents acute dilatation of the heart chambers and exerts a restraining effect on the left ventricle. The inner serous layer consists of a visceral layer and a parietal layer. The visceral layer, also known as the *epicardium,* covers the entire heart and great vessels and then folds over to form the parietal layer that lines the fibrous pericardium (Fig. 16–4). Between the visceral and parietal layers is the pericardial cavity, a potential space that contains 30 to 50 ml of serous fluid. This fluid acts as a lubricant to minimize friction as the heart contracts and relaxes.

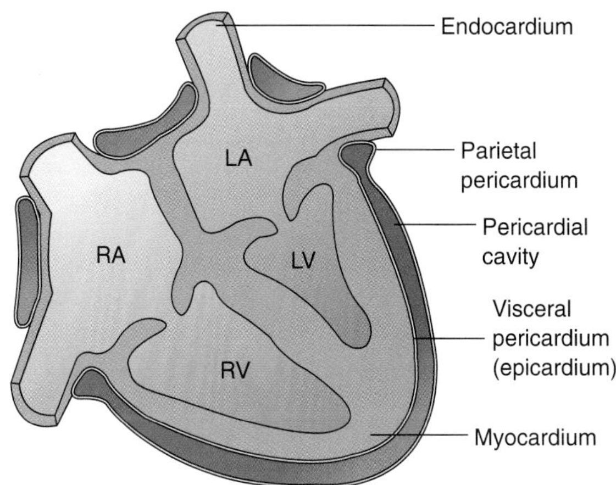

Figure 16–4
Layers of the heart, showing the visceral pericardium, the pericardial cavity, and the parietal pericardium. RA, right atrium; LA, left atrium; RV, right ventricle; LV, left ventricle.

Myocardium

The myocardium, or muscular portion of the heart, forms the wall of the atria and ventricles. Cardiac muscle cells, like skeletal muscle, are striated and composed of sarcomeres that contain actin and myosin filaments (see Fig. 1–25). They are smaller and more compact than skeletal muscle cells and contain many large mitochondria, reflecting their continuous energy needs. The extracellular matrix of cardiac muscle is filled with a loose connective tissue, called the *endomysium,* containing numerous capillaries that support the function of the contracting muscle cells.

Cardiac muscle contracts much like skeletal muscle, except the contractions are involuntary and the duration of contraction is much longer. Unlike the orderly longitudinal arrangement of skeletal muscle fibers, cardiac muscle cells are arranged as an interconnecting latticework, with their fibers dividing, then recombining, and dividing again (Fig. 16–5). The cell membranes of the interconnecting fibers are joined by darkly staining structures called *intercalated disks.* The intercalated disks, which are unique to cardiac muscle, consist of adhering and "communicating" gap junctions that serve as low-resistance pathways for the passage of ions and electrical impulses from one cardiac cell to another (Fig. 16–6). The myocardium therefore behaves as a single unit, or *syncytium,* rather than as a group of isolated units, as does skeletal muscle. When one myocardial cell becomes excited, the impulse travels rapidly so the heart can beat as a unit.

As in skeletal muscle, cardiac muscle contraction involves actin and myosin filaments, which interact and slide along one another during muscle contraction. Compared with skeletal muscle cells, cardiac muscle cells have less well defined sarcoplasmic reticulum for storing calcium and have a shorter distance from the cell membrane to the myofibrils. Be-

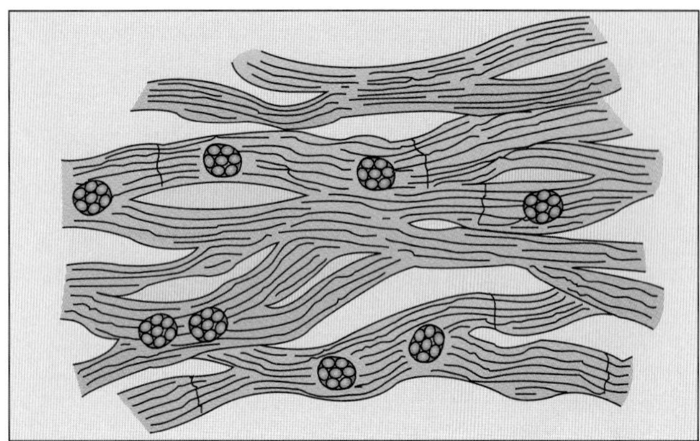

Figure 16–5
Cardiac muscle fibers, showing the branching structure and intercalated disks.

cause less calcium can be stored in the muscle cells, cardiac muscle relies more heavily than skeletal muscle on an influx of extracellular calcium ions for contraction. Extracellular calcium, which enters through channels in the cell membrane and T-tubules of the muscle cell, triggers the release of intracellular calcium from the sarcoplasmic reticulum, and it participates in muscle contraction. Muscle relaxation results from cessation of calcium release, its removal from the actin-myosin sites, and its energy-dependent reuptake from the cytoplasm into the sarcoplasmic reticulum and other storage sites.

Endocardium

The endocardium is a thin, three-layered membrane that lines the heart. The innermost layer consists of smooth endothelial cells supported by a thin layer of connective tissue. The endothelial lining of the endocardium is continuous with the lining of the blood vessels that enter and leave the heart. The middle layer consists of dense connective tissue with elastic fibers. The outer layer, composed of irregularly arranged connective tissue cells, contains blood vessels and branches of the conduction system and is continuous with the myocardium.

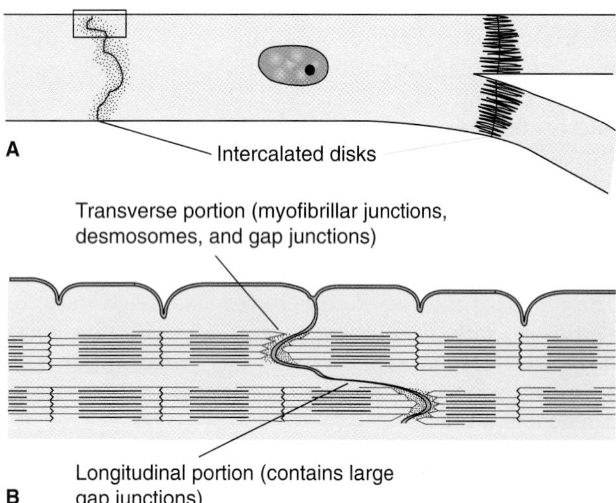

Figure 16–6
(**A**) Cardiac muscle with an intercalated disk at each end. (**B**) Area indicated in **A**, showing where cell junctions lie in the intercalated disks.

Heart Valves and Fibrous Skeleton

For the heart to function effectively, blood must move through its chambers. This directional flow is provided by the heart's two atrioventricular (*i.e.*, tricuspid and mitral) valves and two semilunar (*i.e.*, pulmonic and aortic) valves (Fig. 16–7). An important structural feature of the heart is its fibrous skeleton, which consists of four interconnecting valve rings and surrounding connective tissue. It separates the atria and ventricles and forms a rigid support for attachment of the valves and insertion of the cardiac muscle (Fig. 16–8). The tops of the valve rings are attached to the muscle tissue of the atria, pulmonary trunks, aorta, and valve rings. The bottoms are attached to the ventricular walls.

The atrioventricular (AV) valves control the flow of blood between the atria and the ventricles. The thin edges of the AV valves form cusps, two on the left side of the heart (*i.e.*, bicuspid valve) and three on the right side (*i.e.*, tricuspid valve). The bicuspid valve is also known as the mitral valve. The AV valves are supported

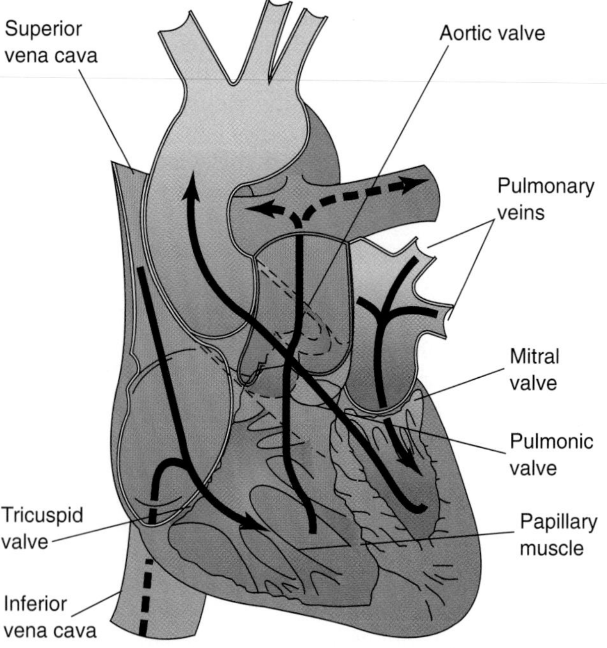

Figure 16–7
Valvular structures of the heart. The atrioventricular valves are in an open position, and the semilunar valves are closed. There are no valves to control the flow of blood at the inflow channels (*i.e.*, vena cava and pulmonary veins) to the heart.

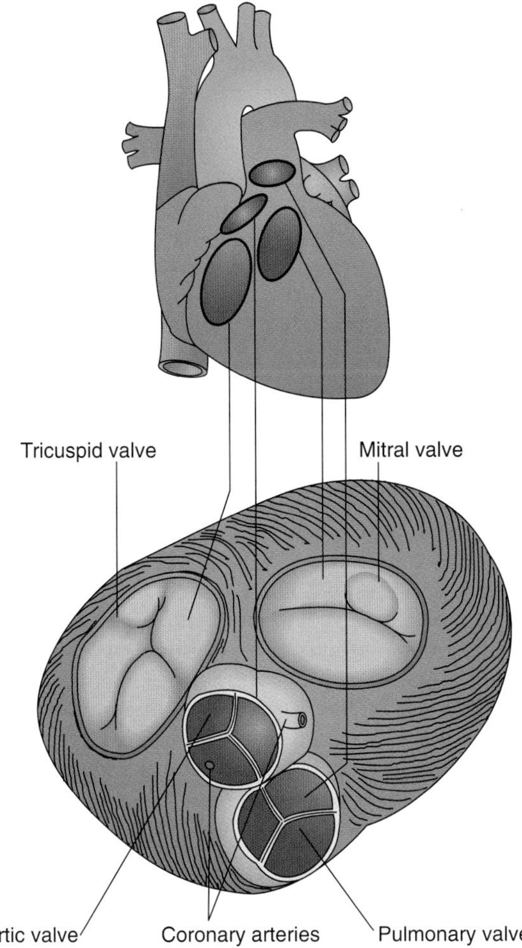

Figure 16–8
Fibrous skeleton of the heart, which forms the four interconnecting valve rings and support for attachment of the valves and insertion of cardiac muscle.

by the papillary muscles, which project from the wall of the ventricles, and the chordae tendineae, which attach to the valve. Contraction of the papillary muscles at the onset of systole ensures closure by producing tension on the leaflets of the AV valves before the full force of ventricular contraction pushes against them. The chordae tendineae are cordlike structures that support the AV valves and prevent them from everting into the atria during systole.

The semilunar valves control the movement of blood out of the ventricles. The aortic valve controls the flow of blood into the aorta; the pulmonic valve, also known as the pulmonary valve, controls blood flow into the pulmonary artery. The aortic and pulmonic valves often are referred to as the semilunar valves because their flaps are shaped like half-moons. The pulmonic and the aortic valve have three little teacup-shaped leaflets. These cuplike structures collect the retrograde, or backward, flow of blood that occurs toward the end of systole, enhancing

Heart Sounds

Closure of the heart valves produces vibrations of the surrounding heart tissues and blood that can be detected as the audible "lub-dup" sounds heard with a stethoscope during cardiac auscultation. There are four heart sounds (see Fig. 16–10). The first and second sounds are heard in all healthy individuals. The third and fourth heart sounds usually are not heard and may or may not indicate pathology.

The first and second heart sounds represent closure of the atrioventricular and semilunar valves, respectively. The first heart sound (lub), which has a lower pitch and lasts longer (about 0.14 second) than the second sound, marks the onset of systole and the closure of the atrioventricular valves. The second heart sound (dup) occurs with the closure of the semilunar valves; it is shorter (0.10 second) and has a higher pitch than the first heart sound. The second heart sound is a composite sound resulting from the closure of both the aortic and the pulmonic valve. The aortic valve normally closes slightly before the pulmonic valve, causing a separation of the two components of the second heart sound. During expiration, aortic valve closure precedes pulmonic valve closure by 0.02 to 0.04 second. During inspiration, this difference is increased to 0.04 to 0.06 second, because during inspiration, there is an increase in venous return to the right heart, and it takes longer for the right ventricle to empty and the pulmonic valve to close. At the same time, less blood is returning to the left ventricle, causing the aortic valve to close slightly earlier. An audible widening of the second heart sound that occurs with inspiration is a normal finding. It often is referred to as a physiologic splitting and can be heard only in the left second intercostal space.

The third heart sound is low pitched and occurs during rapid filling of the ventricles early in diastole, about 0.12 second after the second heart sound. It usually is heard only in young persons or in patients with heart failure. The fourth heart sound is produced by atrial contraction during the last third of diastole; it is audible only in conditions in which resistance to ventricular filling occurs during late diastole. The heart sounds and their relation to the cardiac cycle are shown in Figure 16–10.

Heart murmurs are caused by abnormal vibrations produced by turbulent blood flow. In the heart, turbulence occurs when the velocity of blood flow is increased, the valve diameter is decreased, or the viscosity of the blood is decreased. For example, very high velocities of flow may be reached when blood is ejected through a narrowed, or stenotic, heart valve. Severe anemia may reduce blood viscosity to the point at which turbulence occurs. Auscultation to detect murmurs or abnormalities of the heart sounds is a valuable diagnostic procedure. Although auscultation of the heart does not involve the use of expensive equipment, it does require a trained ear and a thorough understanding of the physiologic events associated with valvular function and the cardiac cycle.

closure. For the development of a perfect seal along the free edges of the semilunar valves, each valve cusp must have a triangular shape, which is facilitated by a nodular thickening at the apex of each leaflet (Fig. 16–9). The openings for the coronary arteries are located in the aorta just above the aortic valve. There are no valves at the atrial sites (*i.e.*, venae cavae and pulmonary veins) where blood enters the heart. This means that excess blood is pushed back into the veins when the atria become distended. For example, the jugular veins typically become prominent in severe right-sided heart failure when they normally should be flat or collapsed. Likewise, the pulmonary venous system becomes congested when outflow from the left atrium is impeded.

Cardiac Cycle

The term *cardiac cycle* is used to describe the rhythmic pumping action of the heart. The cardiac cycle can be divided into two parts: *systole*, the period during which the ventricles are contracting, and *diastole*, the period during which the ventricles are relaxed and filling with blood. Simultaneous changes occur in left atrial pressure, left ventricular pressure, aortic pressure, ventricular volume, the electrocardiogram (ECG), and heart sounds during the cardiac cycle (Fig. 16–10).

During diastole, the ventricles increase their volume to about 120 ml (*i.e.*, the *end-diastolic volume*), and at the end of systole, about 50 ml of blood (*i.e.*, the *end-systolic volume*) remains in the ventricles (Fig. 16–11). The difference between the end-diastolic and end-systolic volumes (about 70 ml) is called the *stroke volume*. The stroke volume divided by the end-diastolic volume, which is called the *ejection fraction*, represents the fraction of the diastolic volume that is ejected from the heart during systole.

The electrical activity, recorded on the ECG, precedes the mechanical events of the cardiac cycle. The small rounded P wave of the ECG represents depolarization of the sinoatrial node (*i.e.*, pacemaker of the heart), the atrial conduction tissue, and the atrial muscle mass. The QRS complex registers the depolarization of the ventricular conduction system and the ventricular muscle mass. The T wave on the ECG occurs during the last half of systole and represents repolarization of the ventricles. The cardiac conduction system and the ECG is discussed further in Chapter 21.

Ventricular Systole and Diastole

Ventricular systole can be divided into three periods: the isovolumetric contraction period, the ejection period, and the period of isovolumetric relaxation. The isovolumetric contraction period, which begins with the closure of the AV valves and occurrence of the first heart sound, heralds the onset of systole. Immediately after closure of the AV valves, there is an additional 0.02 to 0.03 second during which the semilunar outlet (pulmonic and aortic) valves remain closed. This period, during which the volume remains the same but the ventricles are contracting, is called the *isovolumetric contraction period*. The ventricular pressures rise abruptly during the isovolumetric period because no blood is leaving the heart; the ventricles continue to contract until left ventricular pressure is slightly higher than aortic pressure, and right ventricular pressure is higher than pulmonary artery pressure. At this point, the semilunar valves open, signaling the onset of the *ejection period*. About 60% of the stroke volume is ejected during the first quarter of systole, and the remaining 40% is ejected during the next two quarters of systole. Little blood is ejected from the heart during the last quarter of systole, although the ventricle remains contracted. At the end of systole, the ventri-

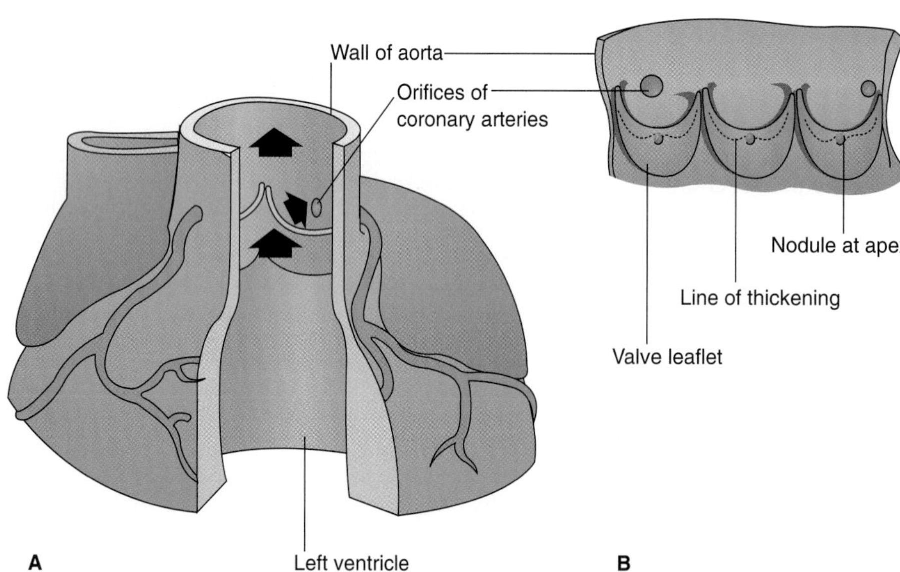

Figure 16–9 Diagram of the aortic valve. (**A**) Its position at the base of the ascending aorta is indicated. (**B**) The appearance of its three leaflets when the aorta is cut open and spread out, flat.

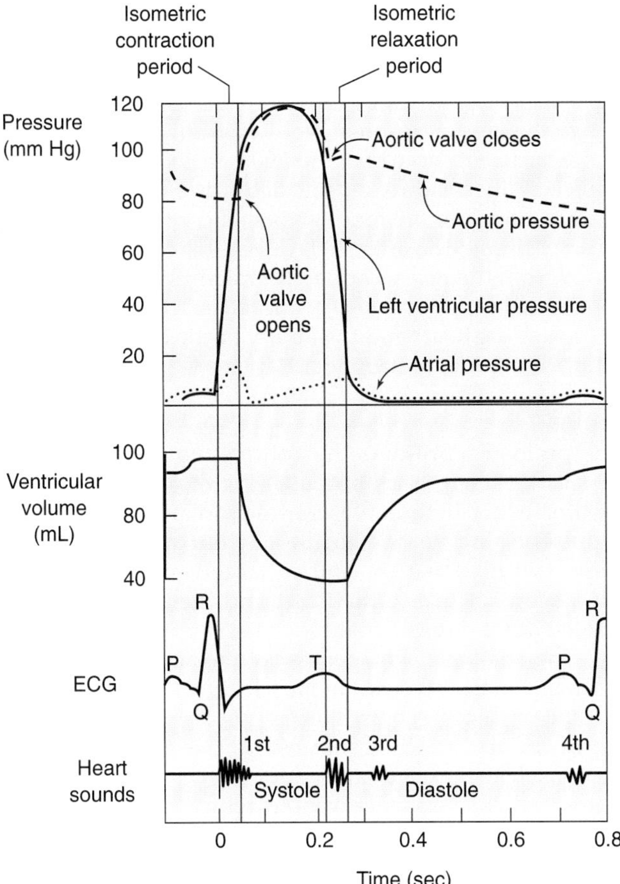

Figure 16–10
Events in the cardiac cycle, showing changes in aortic pressure, left ventricular pressure, atrial pressure, left ventricular volume, the electrocardiogram (ECG), and heart sounds.

cles relax, causing a precipitous fall in intraventricular pressures. As this occurs, blood from the large arteries flows back toward the ventricles, causing the aortic and pulmonic valves to snap shut—an event that is marked by the second heart sound.

The aortic pressure reflects changes in the ejection of blood from the left ventricle. There is a rise in pressure and stretching of the elastic fibers in the aorta as blood is ejected into the aorta at the onset of the ejection period. The aortic pressure continues to rise and then begins to fall during the last quarter of systole as blood flows out of the aorta into the peripheral vessels. At the end of ejection, the left ventricle begins to relax and its pressure falls below that in the aorta, at which point the aortic valve closes giving rise to the second heart sound. The incisura, or notch, in the aortic pressure tracing represents closure of the aortic valve. Recoil of the elastic fibers in the aorta that were stretched during systole maintain arterial blood pressure during the diastolic phase of the cardiac cycle.

Ventricular diastole is marked by filling of the ventricles. After closure of the semilunar valves, the ventricles continue to relax for another 0.03 to 0.06 second (*i.e.*, the *isovolumetric relaxation period*); during this time, ventricular volume remains the same but the ventricular pressure drops until it becomes less than atrial pressure. As this happens, the AV valves open, and the blood that has been accumulating in the atria during systole flows into the ventricles. Most of ventricular filling occurs during the first third of diastole, which is called the *rapid filling period*. During the middle third of diastole, inflow into the ventricles is almost at a standstill. The last third of diastole is marked by atrial contraction, which gives an additional thrust to ventricular filling. When audible, the third heart sound is heard during the rapid filling period of diastole as blood flows into a distended or noncompliant ventricle. A fourth heart sound can occur during the last third of diastole as the atria contract.

Atrial Filling and Contraction

Atrial contraction occurs during the last third of diastole. It is preceded by the P wave on the ECG. There are three main atrial pressure waves that occur during the cardiac cycle. The *a* wave is caused by atrial contraction. The *c* wave occurs as the ventricles begin to contract, and their increased pressure causes the AV valves to bulge into the atria. The *v* wave results from a slow buildup of blood in the atria toward the end of systole

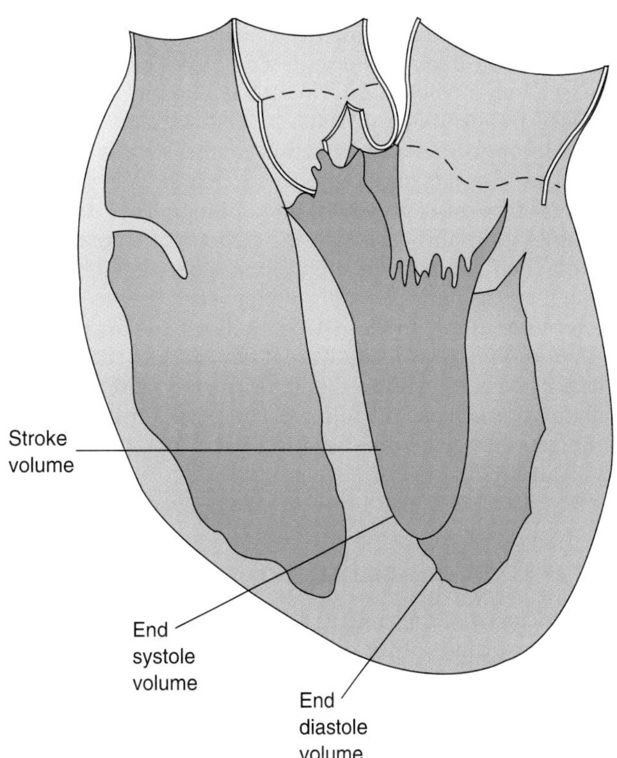

Figure 16–11
The ejection fraction, which represents the difference between the end-diastolic and end-systolic volumes.

when the AV valves are still closed. The right atrial pressure waves are transmitted to the internal jugular veins as pulsations. These pulsations can be observed visually and may be used to assess cardiac function. For example, exaggerated *a* waves occur when the volume of the right atrium is increased because of impaired emptying into the right ventricle.

Because there are no valves between the junctions of the central veins (*i.e.*, venae cava and pulmonary veins) and the atria, atrial filling occurs during both systole and diastole. During normal quiet breathing, right atrial pressure usually varies between −2 mm Hg and +2 mm Hg. It is this low atrial pressure that maintains the movement of blood from the systemic circulation into the right atrium and from the pulmonary veins into the left atrium. Right atrial pressure is regulated by a balance between the ability of the heart to move blood out of the right heart and through the left heart into the systemic circulation and the tendency of blood to flow from the peripheral circulation into the right atrium.

The difference between the venous and atrial pressure is called the *atrial filling pressure*. When the heart pumps strongly, right atrial pressure is decreased and atrial filling is enhanced. Right atrial pressure is also affected by changes in intrathoracic pressure. It is decreased during inspiration when intrathoracic pressure becomes more negative, and it is increased during coughing or forced expiration when intrathoracic pressure becomes more positive. Venous return reflects the amount of blood in the systemic circulation that is available for return to the right heart and the force that moves blood back to the right side of the heart. It is increased when the blood volume is expanded and decreased in hypovolemic shock.

Although the main function of the atria is to store blood as it enters the heart, these chambers also act as pumps that aid in ventricular filling. This function becomes more important during periods of increased activity when the diastolic filling time is decreased because of an increase in heart rate or when heart disease impairs ventricular filling. In these two situations, the cardiac output would fall drastically were it not for the action of the atria. It has been estimated that atrial contraction can contribute as much as 30% to cardiac reserve during periods of increased need, while having little or no effect on cardiac output during rest.

Regulation of Cardiac Performance

The efficiency of the heart as a pump often is measured in terms of cardiac output or the amount of blood the heart pumps each minute. The cardiac output (CO) is the product of the stroke volume (SV) and the heart rate (HR) and can be expressed by the equation: $CO = SV \times HR$. The CO varies with body size and the metabolic needs of the tissues. It increases with physical activity and decreases during rest and sleep. The average cardiac output in normal adults ranges from 3.5 to 8.0 L/minute. In the highly trained athlete, this value can increase to levels as high as 32 L/ minute during maximum exercise.

The *cardiac reserve* refers to the maximum percentage of increase in cardiac output that can be achieved above the normal resting level. The normal young adult has a cardiac reserve of about 300% to 400%. The heart's ability to increase its output according to body needs mainly depends on four factors: the preload, or ventricular filling; the afterload, or resistance to ejection of blood from the heart; cardiac contractility; and the heart rate. Cardiac performance is influenced by the work demands of the heart and the ability of the coronary circulation to meet its metabolic needs (see Chapter 19).

Preload

The preload represents the volume work of the heart. It is called the *preload* because it is the work imposed on the heart before the contraction begins. Preload represents the amount of blood that the heart must pump with each beat and is largely determined by the venous return to the heart and the accompanying stretch of the muscle fibers.

The anatomic arrangement of the actin and myosin filaments in the myocardial muscle fibers is such that the tension or force of contraction is greatest when the muscle fibers are stretched just before the heart begins to contract. The maximum force of contraction and cardiac output is achieved when venous return produces an increase in left ventricular end-diastolic filling (*i.e.*, preload) such that the muscle fibers are stretched about two and one-half times their normal resting length (Fig. 16–12). When the muscle fibers are stretched to this degree, there is optimal overlap of the actin and myosin filaments and number of crossbridge attachments needed for maximal contraction.

The increased force of contraction that accompanies an increase in ventricular end-diastolic volume is referred to as the *Frank-Starling mechanism* or *Starling's law of the heart*. The Frank-Starling mechanism allows the heart to adjust its pumping ability to accommodate various levels of venous return. Cardiac output is less when decreased filling causes excessive overlap of the actin and myosin filaments or when the filaments are pulled too far apart because of excessive filling.

Afterload

The afterload is the pressure or tension work of the heart. It is the pressure that the heart must generate to move blood into the aorta. It is called the afterload because it is the work presented to the heart after the contraction has commenced. The systemic arterial blood pressure is the main source of afterload work on the left heart and the pulmonary arterial pressure the main source of afterload work for right heart. The afterload work of the left ventricle is also increased with narrowing (*i.e.*, stenosis) of the aortic valve. For example, in the late stages of aortic stenosis, the left ventricle may need to generate systolic pressures up to 300 mm Hg to move blood through the diseased valve.

Cardiac Contractility

Cardiac contractility refers to the ability of the heart to change its force of contraction without changing its resting (*i.e.*, diastolic) length. The contractile state of the myocardial muscle is determined by biochemical and biophysical properties that govern the actin and myosin interactions within the myocardial cells. It is strongly influenced by the number of calcium ions that are available to participate in the contractile process.

An *inotropic* influence is one that modifies the contractile state of the myocardium independent of the Frank-Starling mechanism (see Fig. 16–12, *curve B*). For instance, sympathetic stimulation produces a positive inotropic effect by increasing the calcium that is available for interaction between the actin and myosin filaments. Hypoxia exerts a negative inotropic effect by interfering with the generation of adenosine triphosphate (ATP), which is needed for muscle contraction.

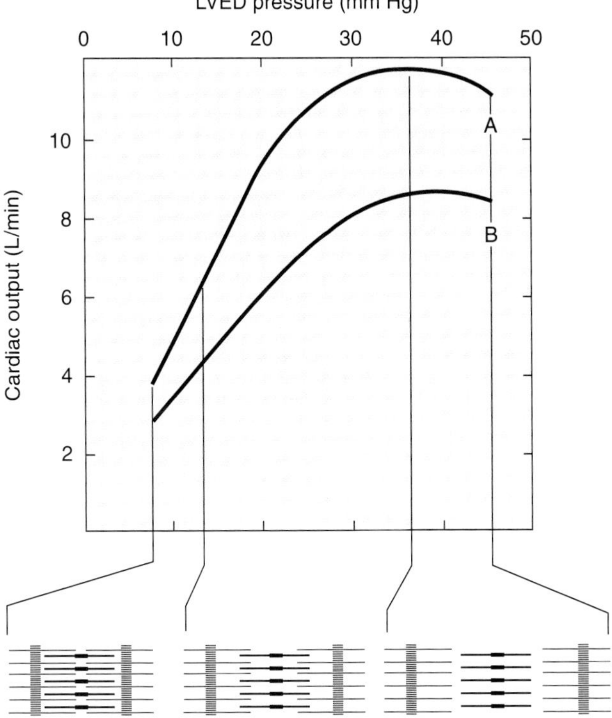

Figure 16–12
(**Top**) Starling ventricular function curve. An increase in left ventricular end-diastolic (LVED) pressure produces an increase in cardiac output (*curve B*) by means of the Frank-Starling mechanism. The maximum force of contraction and increased stroke volume are achieved when diastolic filling causes the muscle fibers to be stretched about two and one half times their resting length. In *curve A*, an increase in cardiac contractility produces an increase in cardiac output without a change in LVED volume and pressure. (**Bottom**) Stretching of the actin and myosin filaments at the different LVED filling pressures.

Heart Rate

The heart rate determines the frequency with which blood is ejected from the heart. As the heart rate increases, the time spent in diastole is reduced, and there is less time for the filling of the ventricles before the onset of systole. At a heart rate of 75 beats per minute, one cardiac cycle lasts 0.8 second, of which about 0.3 second is spent in systole and about 0.5 second in diastole. As the heart rate increases, the time spent in systole remains about the same, whereas that spent in diastole decreases. This leads to a decrease in stroke volume; at high heart rates, it may cause a decrease in cardiac output. One of the dangers of ventricular tachycardia is a reduction in cardiac output because the heart does not have time to fill adequately.

The *double product*, which is calculated by multiplying the heart rate by the mean arterial blood pressure, is used clinically to estimate cardiac oxygen consumption or cardiac work. The blood pressure represents systole and the time that the heart is contracting to eject blood into the aorta. The heart rate gives the number of times per minute that the pressure must be generated.

In summary, the heart is a four-chambered muscular pump that lies in the pericardial sac within the mediastinal space of the intrathoracic cavity. The wall of the heart is composed of an outer epicardium, which lines the pericardial cavity; a fibrous skeleton; the myocardium, or muscle layer; and the smooth endocardium, which lines the chambers of the heart. The four heart valves control the direction of blood flow.

The cardiac cycle describes the pumping action of the heart. It is divided into two parts: systole, during which the ventricles contract and blood is ejected from the heart, and diastole, during which the ventricles are relaxed and blood is filling the heart. The stroke volume (about 70 ml) represents the difference between the end-diastolic volume (about 120 ml) and the end-systolic volume (about 50 ml). The electrical activity of the heart, as represented on the ECG, precedes the mechanical events of the cardiac cycle. The heart sounds signal the closing of the heart valves during the cardiac cycle. Atrial contraction occurs during the last third of diastole. Although the main function of the atria is to store blood as it enters the heart, the atrial contraction acts to increase cardiac output during periods of increased activity when the filling time is reduced or in disease conditions in which ventricular filling is impaired.

The heart's ability to increase its output according to body needs depends on the preload, or filling of the ventricles (i.e., end-diastolic volume); the afterload, or resistance to ejection of blood from the heart; cardiac contractility, which is determined by the interaction of the actin and myosin filaments of cardiac muscle fibers; and the heart rate, which determines the frequency with which blood is ejected from the heart. The maximum force of cardiac contraction occurs when an increase in preload stretches muscle fibers of the heart to about two and one-half times their resting length (i.e., Frank-Starling mechanism).

Blood Vessels and the Systemic Circulation

After you have completed this section of the chapter, you should be able to meet the following objectives:

- Compare the structure and function of arteries, arterioles, veins, and capillaries
- Describe the structure and function of vascular smooth muscle
- Use the term *compliance* to describe the characteristics of arterial and venous blood vessels
- Define the term *hemodynamics* and describe the effects of blood pressure; vessel radius, length, and cross sectional area; and blood viscosity on the characteristics of blood flow
- Use Laplace's law to explain the effect of radius size on the pressure and wall tension in a vessel
- Use the equation, blood pressure = cardiac output × peripheral vascular resistance, to explain the regulation of arterial blood pressure
- Describe mechanisms involved in short-term and long-term regulation of blood pressure
- Define autoregulation and characterize mechanisms responsible for short-term and long-term regulation of blood flow

The vascular system functions in the delivery of oxygen and nutrients and removal of wastes from the tissues. It consists of arteries and arterioles, the capillaries, and the venules and veins. Although blood vessels are often compared with a system of plumbing pipes, this analogy only serves as a starting point. Blood vessels are dynamic structures that constrict and relax to adjust blood pressure and flow to meet the varying needs of the many different tissue types and organ systems. Structures such as the heart, brain, liver, and kidneys require a large and continuous flow to carry out their vital functions. In other tissues such as the skin and skeletal muscle the need for blood flow varies with the level of function. For example, there is need for increased blood flow to the skin during fever, and there is a need for increased skeletal blood flow during exercise.

Blood Vessels

All blood vessels, except the capillaries, have walls composed of three layers, or coats, called *tunicae* (Fig. 16–13). The *tunica externa,* or *tunica adventitia,* is the outermost covering of the vessel. This layer is composed of fibrous and connective tissues that support the vessel. The *tunica media,* or *middle layer,* is largely a smooth muscle layer that constricts to regulate and control the diameter of the vessel. The *tunica intima,* or *inner layer,* has an elastic layer that joins the media and a thin layer of endothelial cells that lie adjacent to the blood. The endothelial layer provides a smooth and slippery inner surface for the vessel. This smooth inner lining, as long as it remains intact, prevents platelet adherence and blood clotting. The layers of the different types of blood vessels vary with vessel function. The walls of the arterioles, which control blood pressure, have large amounts of smooth muscle. Veins are thin-walled, distensible, and collapsible vessels. Capillaries are single-cell–thick vessels designed for the exchange of gases, nutrients, and waste materials.

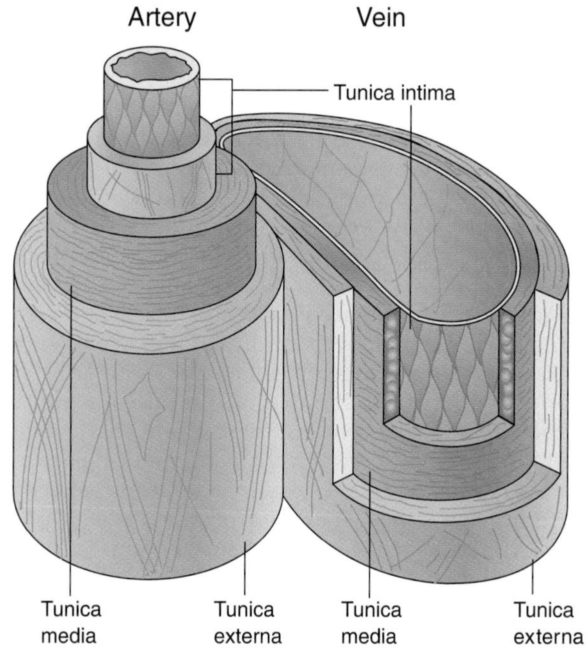

Figure 16–13
Medium-sized artery and vein, showing the relative thickness of the three layers.

Arteries and Arterioles

The arterial system consists of the large and medium-sized arteries and the arterioles. Arteries are thick-walled vessels with large amounts of elastic fibers. The elasticity of these vessels allows them to stretch during cardiac systole, when the heart contracts and blood enters the circulation, and to recoil during diastole, when the heart relaxes. The arterioles, which are predominantly smooth muscle, serve as resistance vessels for the circulatory system. They act as control valves through which blood is released as it moves into the capillaries. Sympathetic vasoconstrictor tone enables these vessels to constrict or to relax as needed to maintain blood pressure.

Capillaries

Capillaries are microscopic, single-cell–thick vessels that connect the arterial and venous segments of the circulation. In each person, there are about 10 billion capillaries, with a total surface area of 500 to 700 m^2. The capillary wall is composed of a single layer of endothelial cells surrounded by a basement membrane (Fig. 16–14).

Intracellular junctions join the capillary endothelial cells; these are called the *capillary pores.* Lipid-soluble materials diffuse directly through the capillary cell membrane. Water and water-soluble materials leave and enter the capillary through the capillary pores. The size of the capillary pores varies with capillary function. In the brain, the endothelial cells are joined by tight junctions that form the blood-brain barrier. This prevents substances that would alter neural excitability from leaving the capillary. In organs that process blood contents, such as the liver, capillaries have large pores so that substances can pass easily through the capillary wall. In the kidneys, the glomerular capillaries have small openings called *fenestrations,* which pass directly through the middle of the endothelial cells. Fenestrated capillary walls are consistent with the filtration function of the glomerulus.

Veins and Venules

The veins and venules are thin-walled, distensible, and collapsible vessels. The venules collect blood from the capillaries, and the veins transport blood back to the heart. The veins are capable of enlarging and storing large quantities of blood, which can be made available to the circulation as needed. Even though the veins are thin-walled, they are muscular. This allows them to contract or expand to accommodate varying amounts of blood. Veins are innervated by the sympathetic nervous system. When blood is lost from the circulation, the veins constrict as a means of maintaining intravascular volume.

The venous system is a low-pressure system, and when a person is in the upright position, blood flow in the venous system must oppose the effects of gravity. Valves in the veins of extremities prevent retrograde flow (Fig. 16–15), and with the help of skeletal muscles that surround and intermittently compress the veins in a milking manner, blood is moved forward to the heart. Their pressure ranges from about 10 mm Hg at the end of the venules to about 0 mm Hg at the entrance of the vena cavae into the heart. There are no valves in the abdominal or thoracic veins, and blood flow in these veins is heavily influenced by the pressure in the abdominal and thoracic cavities, respectively.

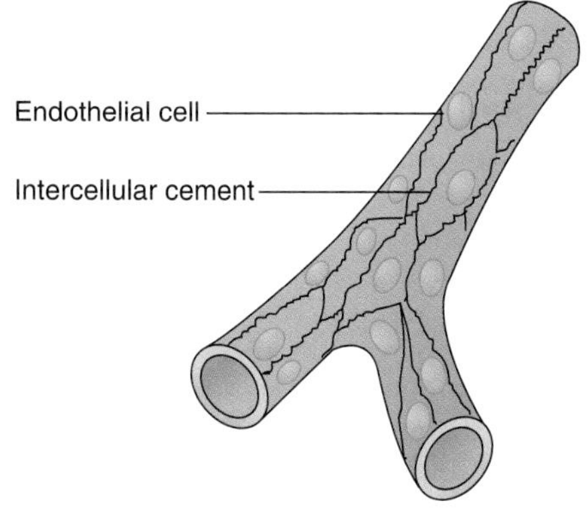

Figure 16–14
Endothelial cells and intercellular cement in a section of capillary.

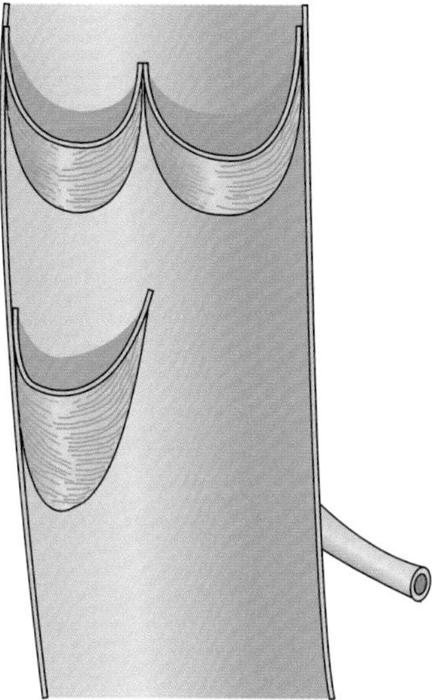

Figure 16–15
Portion of a femoral vein opened, to show valves. The direction of blood flow is upward.

Vascular Smooth Muscle

Smooth muscle contracts slowly and generates high forces for long periods with low energy requirements; it uses only 1/10 to 1/300 the energy of skeletal muscle. These characteristics are important in structures, such as blood vessels, that must maintain their tone day in and day out.

Although vascular smooth muscle contains actin and myosin filaments, these contractile filaments are not arranged in striations as they are in skeletal and cardiac muscle. The smooth muscle fibers are instead linked together in a strong cablelike system that generates a circular pull as it contracts. Smooth muscle also lacks the regulatory protein, troponin, which initiates crossbridge formation in skeletal and cardiac muscle (see Chapter 1). Instead smooth muscle has a regulatory protein called *calmodulin* that binds calcium. The calcium-calmodulin complex activates myosin kinase, a phosphorylating enzyme that initiates crossbridge formation (Fig. 16–16).

Compared with skeletal and cardiac muscle, smooth muscle has less well developed sarcoplasmic reticulum for storing intracellular calcium, and it has very few fast sodium channels. Depolarization of smooth muscle instead relies largely on extracellular calcium, which enters through calcium channels in the muscle membrane.

Smooth muscle has voltage-gated calcium channels that respond to changes in membrane potential and receptor-activated calcium channels. Receptor-activated channels respond to chemical messengers such as norepinephrine that can act in an excitatory manner that causes the channels to remain closed. Sympathetic nervous system control of vascular smooth muscle tone occurs by way of receptor-activated chan-

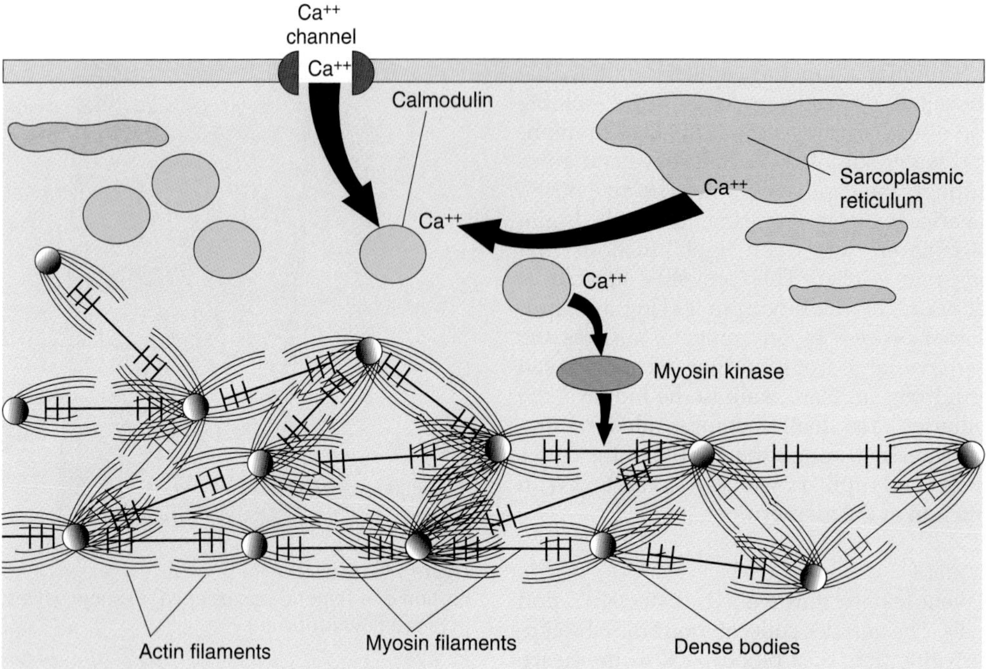

Figure 16–16
Mechanism of vascular smooth muscle contraction. Calmodulin binds calcium that enters through calcium channels in the cell membrane or is released from the sarcoplasmic reticulum. The calcium-calmodulin complex, in turn, activates myosin kinase, a phosphorylating enzyme, which initiates cross-bridge formation. Smooth muscle, which lacks the striations of cardiac and skeletal muscle, relies on the dense bodies to form a cable-like structure that produces a circular pull as the muscle contracts.

nels. In general, α-adrenergic receptors are excitatory and produce vasoconstriction, and β-adrenergic receptors are inhibitory and produce vasodilation. Calcium-channel blocking drugs cause vasodilation by blocking calcium entry through the calcium channels.

Smooth muscle contraction and relaxation also occurs in response to local tissue factors such as lack of oxygen, increased hydrogen ion concentrations, and excess carbon dioxide. Nitric oxide, formerly known as the endothelial relaxing factor, acts locally to produce smooth muscle relaxation and regulate blood flow. These factors are discussed more fully under local control of blood flow.

Principles of Blood Flow

The term *hemodynamics* (*hemo* means blood, and *dynamic* refers to the relation between motion and forces) describes the physical principles governing pressure, flow, and resistance as they relate to the cardiovascular system. The hemodynamics of the circulatory system are complex. The heart is an intermittent pump, and as a result, blood flow in the arterial circulation is pulsatile. The blood vessels are branched, distensible tubes of various dimensions. The blood is a suspension of blood cells, platelets, lipid globules, and plasma proteins. Despite this complexity, the function of the circulatory system can be explained by the principles of basic fluid mechanics that apply to nonbiologic systems, such as household plumbing systems.

Pressure, Flow, and Resistance

The most important factors governing the function of the circulatory system are *volume, pressure, resistance,* and *flow*. Optimal function requires a volume that is sufficient to fill the vascular compartment and a pressure that is sufficient to ensure blood flow to all body tissues.

Blood flow is determined by two factors: a pressure difference between the two ends of a vessel or group of vessels and the resistance that blood must overcome as it moves through the vessel or vessels (Fig. 16–17). The relation between pressure, resistance, and flow is expressed by the equation, $F = P/R$, in which F is the blood flow, P is the difference in pressure between the two ends of the system, and R is the resistance to flow through the system.

The total resistance that the blood encounters as it flows through the systemic circulation is referred to as the *systemic vascular resistance* (SVR) or *total peripheral resistance*. The systemic vascular resistance cannot be measured directly. Instead, it is estimated by rearranging the variables in the previous equation ($SVR = P/CO$) and using the pressure difference between the left and right sides of the circulation as a measure of resistance and cardiac output as a measure of flow. This equation considers

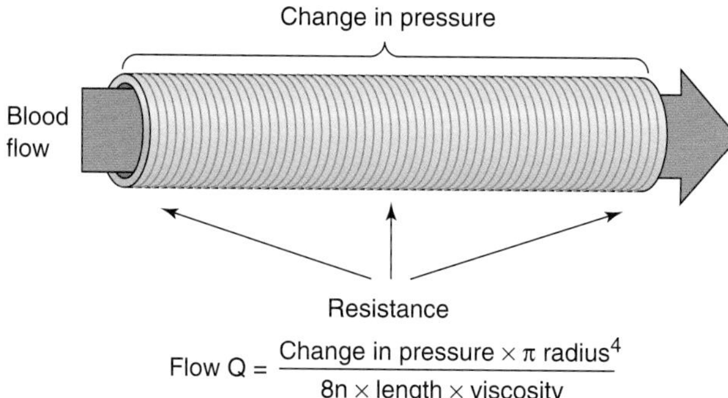

Figure 16–17
Factors affect blood flow (Poiseuille's law). Increasing the pressure difference between the two ends of the vessel increases flow. Flow diminishes as resistance increases. Resistance is directly proportional to blood viscosity and the length of the vessel and inversely proportional to the fourth power of the radius.

the entire systemic circulation as a single tube that begins in the aorta and ends in the right atrium. The pressure difference between these two points is the mean arterial pressure (about 100 mm Hg) minus the right atrial pressure (about 0 mm Hg). The flow or cardiac output is about 100 ml/second at rest. The SVR is 100/100 or 1 peripheral resistance unit (PRU). The total resistance in the pulmonary circulation is only about 0.12 PRU. In this case, the blood flow is the same as in the systemic circulation, but the pressure difference between the pulmonary artery and left atrium (16 − 4 mm Hg) is much less.

A helpful equation for understanding factors that affect blood flow ($F = \Delta P \times \pi \times r^4 / 8n \times L \times \text{viscosity}$) was derived by the French Physician Poiseuille more than a century ago (see Fig. 16–17). According to this equation, the two most important determinants of flow in the circulatory system are change in pressure (ΔP) and the vessel radius^4 (r^4). The length (L) of vessels does not usually change and 8n are constants that do not change. Because flow is directly related to the fourth power of the radius, small changes in vessel radius can cause large changes in flow to an organ or tissue. For example, the rate of flow is 16 times greater in a vessel with a radius of 2 mm than in a vessel with a radius of 1 mm. The reader is asked to consider the consequences of a 25%, 50%, and 75% narrowing of a coronary artery in terms of blood flow to the myocardium.

According to Poiseuille's equation, blood flow is inversely related to a third factor, the viscosity of the blood. Viscosity is the resistance to flow caused by the friction of molecules in a fluid. The viscosity of a fluid is largely related to its thickness. The more particles that are present in a solution, the greater the frictional forces that develop between the molecules. Unlike water that flows through plumbing pipes, blood is a nonhomogeneous liquid. It contains blood cells, platelets, fat globules, and plasma proteins that increase its viscosity. The red blood cells, which constitute 40% to 45% of the formed elements of the blood, largely determine the viscosity of the blood. When measured in relation to water, the relative viscosity of plasma is 1.5, and at a normal hematocrit of 42 to 45, that of whole blood is 3.0. Under special conditions, temperature may affect viscosity. There is a 2% rise in viscosity for each 1°C decrease in body temperature, a fact that helps explain the sluggish blood flow that is seen in persons with hypothermia.

Cross-sectional Area and Velocity of Flow

Velocity is a distance measurement; it refers to the speed or linear movement with time (centimeters per second) with which blood flows through a vessel. *Flow* is a volume measurement (milliliters per second); it is determined by the cross-sectional area of a vessel and the velocity of flow (Fig. 16–18). When the flow through a given segment of the circulatory system is constant—as it must be for continuous flow—the velocity is inversely proportional to the cross-sectional area of the vessel (i.e., the smaller the cross-sectional area, the greater the velocity of flow). This phenomenon can be compared with cars moving from a two-lane to a single-lane section of a highway. To keep traffic moving at its original pace, cars would have to double their speed in the single-lane section of the highway. So it is with flow in the circulatory system.

The linear velocity of blood flow in the circulatory system varies widely from 30 to 35 cm/second in the aorta to 0.2 to 0.3 mm/second in the capillaries. This is because even though each individual capillary is very small, the total cross-sectional area of all the systemic capillaries greatly exceeds the cross-sectional area of other parts of the circulation. As a result of this large surface area, the slower movement of blood allows ample time for exchange of nutrients, gases, and metabolites between the tissues and the blood.

Laminar and Turbulent Flow

Blood flow normally is laminar with the blood components arranged in layers so that the plasma is adjacent

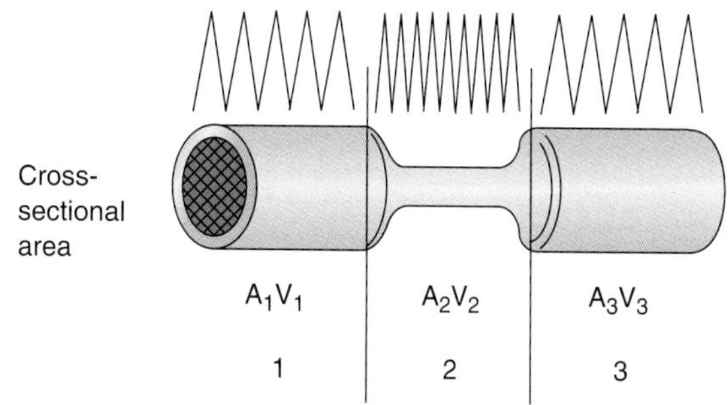

Figure 16–18
Effect of cross-sectional area (A) on velocity (V) of flow. In section 1, velocity is low because of an increase in cross-sectional area. In section 2, velocity is increased because of a decrease in cross-sectional area. In section 3, velocity is again reduced because of an increase in cross-sectional area.

to the smooth, slippery endothelial surface of the blood vessel and the blood cells, including the platelets, are in the center or axis of the bloodstream (Fig. 16–19). This arrangement reduces friction by allowing the blood layers to slide smoothly over one another, with the axial layer having the most rapid rate of flow.

Under certain conditions, blood flow switches from laminar to turbulent flow (see Fig. 16–19). Turbulent flow is flow in which blood moves crosswise and lengthwise along a vessel in a manner similar to the eddy currents seen in a rapidly flowing river at a point of obstruction . Turbulent flow is influenced by a number of conditions, including high velocity of flow, large vessel diameter, and low blood viscosity. The tendency for turbulence to occur increases in direct proportion to the velocity of flow. Imagine the chaos as cars from a two- or three-lane highway converge on a single-lane section of the highway. The same type of thing happens in blood vessels that have been narrowed by disease processes, such as atherosclerosis. Low blood viscosity allows the blood to move faster and accounts for the transient occurrence of heart murmurs in some persons who are severely anemic. Turbulent flow predisposes to clot formation as platelets and other coagulation factors come in contact with the endothelial lining of the vessel.

Turbulent flow often can be heard through a stethoscope. An audible murmur in a blood vessel experiencing turbulent flow is referred to as a *bruit*.

Wall Tension, Radius, and Pressure

In a blood vessel, wall tension is the force in the vessel wall that opposes the distending pressure inside the vessel. The relation between wall tension, pressure, and the radius of a vessel or sphere was described more than 200 years ago by the French astronomer and mathematician Pierre de Laplace. This relation, which has come to be known as *Laplace's law*, can be expressed by the equation,

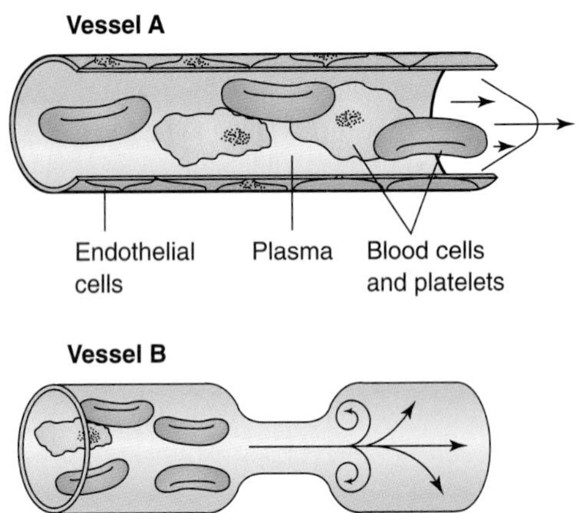

Figure 16–19
Laminar and turbulent flow in blood vessels. Vessel A shows streamlined or laminar flow in which the plasma layer is adjacent to the vessel endothelial layer and blood cells are in the center of the bloodstream. Vessel B shows turbulent flow in which the axial location of the platelets and other blood cells is disturbed.

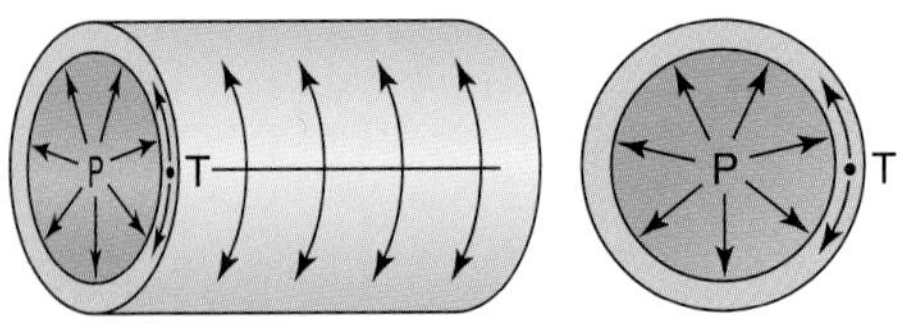

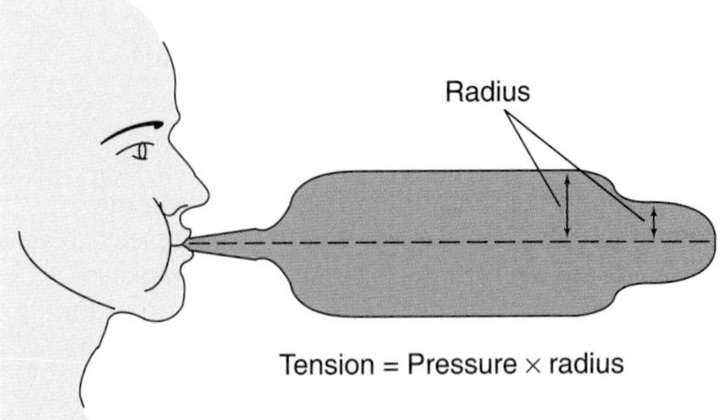

Figure 16–20
(**A**) Pressure and tension in a cylindric blood vessel. The tension (T) tends to open an imaginary slit along the length of the blood vessel. Laplace's law relates pressure, radius, and tension as described in the text. (**B**) Effect of the radius of a cylinder on tension. In a balloon, the tension in the wall is proportional to the radius because the pressure is the same everywhere inside the balloon. The tension is lower in the portion of the balloon with the smaller radius. (Rhoades R.A., Tanner G.A. [1996]. *Medical physiology* [p.627]. Boston: Little, Brown).

$P = T/r$, in which T is wall tension, P is the intraluminal pressure, and r is vessel radius. Using Laplace's law, wall tension can also be expressed as the product of vessel pressure times its radius (Fig. 16–20). In this case, the internal pressure expands the vessel until it is exactly balanced by wall tension. The larger the radius, the greater is the tension needed to balance a particular pressure. This correlation can be compared with a partially inflated long balloon, in which the tension in the more inflated part of the balloon with the larger radius is greater than in the less inflated section with the smaller radius, because the pressure is the same throughout the balloon. These same principles apply to the increased radius of an arterial aneurysm, which is characterized by an outpouching of a segment of the arterial wall. Because of the increased wall tension, an aneurysm tends to progress and may eventually rupture (see Chapter 17).

Laplace's law was later expanded to include wall thickness ($T = P \times r/\text{wall thickness}$). Wall tension is inversely related to wall thickness such that, the thicker the vessel wall, the lower the tension and vice versa. In hypertension, arterial vessel walls hypertrophy and become thicker, thereby minimizing wall stress.

Laplace's law ($P = T/r$) can also be applied to the pressure required to maintain the patency of small blood vessels. Providing that the thickness of a vessel wall and its tension remain constant, it takes more pressure to overcome wall tension and keep a vessel open as its radius decreases in size. The *critical closing pressure* refers to the point at which vessels collapse so that blood can no longer flow through them. In circulatory shock, for example, there is a decrease in blood volume and vessel radii, along with a drop in blood pressure. As a result, many of the small vessels collapse as blood pressure drops to the point where it can no longer overcome the wall tension. The collapse of peripheral veins often makes it difficult to insert venous lines that are needed for fluid and blood replacement.

Distention and Compliance

Compliance refers to the total quantity of blood that can be stored in a given portion of the circulation for each millimeter rise in pressure. *Compliance* (C) is defined by the equation, $C = V/P$, in which V is the change in volume and P is the change in distending pressure. The distending pressure is the difference between the pressure inside the vessel minus the pressure outside the vessel. This is called the *transmural pressure*. The more compliant a vessel, the greater is the change in volume for any transmural pressure.

Compliance reflects the distensibility of the blood vessel (*i.e.*, increase in volume/increase in pressure × original volume). The distensibility of the arteries allows them to accommodate the pulsatile output of the heart. The most distensible of all vessels are the veins that can increase their volume with only slight changes in pressure, allowing them to function as reservoir for storing large quantities of blood that can be returned to the circulation when it is needed. The compliance of a vein is about 24 times that of its corresponding artery, because it is eight times as distensible and has a volume three times as great.

Arterial Blood Pressure

The arterial blood pressure, often referred to as the *blood pressure*, results from the intermittent ejection of blood from the left ventricle into the aorta. It rises during systole as the left ventricle contracts and falls as the heart relaxes during diastole. Under ordinary conditions, there are moment-by-moment variations in blood pressure related to activities of daily living such as moving from the lying to standing position, exercise, and emotional stress. Normally, blood pressure is regulated at levels sufficient to ensure adequate tissue perfusion. Blood pressure regulation requires the use of short-term and long-term mechanisms.

Blood enters the arterial circulation during ventricular systole. The intermittent pumping action of the ventricles produces a *pressure pulse* that serves as the driving force for the circulation (Fig. 16–21). In the systemic circulation, the pressure pulse has its origin in the rapid ejection of blood from the left ventricle into the aorta at the onset of systole. This creates an impulse or pressure wave that is transmitted from molecule to molecule along the length of the vessel. In the aorta, this pressure wave is transmitted at a velocity of 4 to 6 m/second, which is about 20 times faster than the flow of blood.

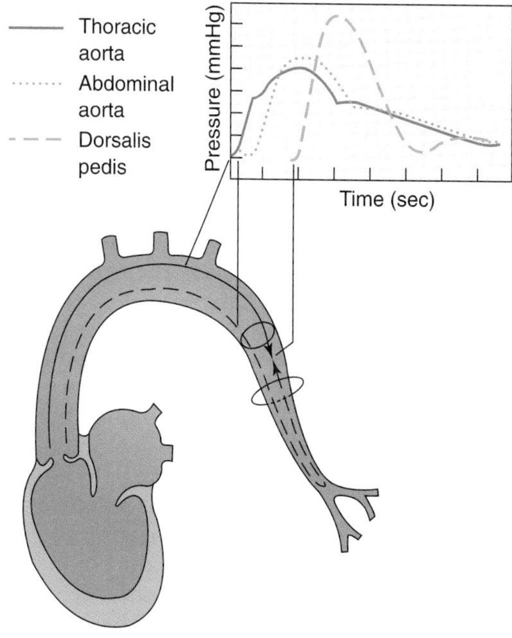

Figure 16–21
Amplification of the arterial pressure wave as it moves forward in the peripheral arteries. This amplification occurs as a forward-moving pressure wave merges with a backward-moving reflected pressure wave. **(Inset)** The amplitude of the pressure pulse increases in the thoracic aorta, abdominal aorta, and dorsalis pedis.

These pressure waves are similar to those created by splashing water in a basin or tub. When taking a pulse, it is the pressure pulses that are felt, and it is the pressure pulses that produce the Korotkoff sounds heard during blood pressure measurement. The tip or maximum deflection of the pressure pulse coincides with the systolic blood pressure, and the minimum point of deflection coincides with the diastolic pressure.

As the pressure wave moves out through the aorta into the arteries, it changes as it collides with reflected waves from the periphery. Just as the waves created by splashing water in a tub increase in amplitude as they hit the edge of the tub and reverse their direction of movement, the pressure pulse increases as it moves to the peripheral arteries. This is why the systolic pressure is higher in the medium-sized arteries than in the aorta even though the diastolic pressure is lower. With peripheral arterial disease, resistance to transmission of the pressure wave increases and a delay occurs in the transmission of the reflected wave, so that the pulse decreases rather than increases in amplitude.

After its initial amplification, the pressure pulse becomes smaller and smaller as it moves through the smaller arteries and arterioles, until it disappears almost entirely in the capillaries. This damping of the pressure pulse is caused by the resistance and distensibility characteristics of these vessels. The increased resistance of these small vessels impedes the transmission of the pressure waves. The distensibility of these vessels is great enough, however, that any small change in flow does not cause a pressure change. Although the pressure pulses usually are not transmitted to the capillaries, there are situations in which this does occur. For example, injury to a finger or other area of the body often results in a throbbing sensation. In this case, extreme dilatation of the small vessels in the injured area produces a reduction in the dampening of the pressure pulse. Capillary pulsations also occur in conditions that cause exaggeration of aortic pressure pulses, such as aortic regurgitation or patent ductus arteriosus (see Chapter 19).

Two major factors affect the pressure pulse in the arterial system and thereby affect the arterial blood pressure. These two factors are the cardiac output and the resistance that the blood encounters as it moves through the peripheral circulation. The cardiac output is determined by the stroke volume and heart rate (*i.e.*, stroke volume × heart rate). The peripheral vascular resistance reflects the resistance of the arterial vessels, mainly the arterioles. Blood pressure (BP) can be viewed as the product of the cardiac output (CO) and the total peripheral resistance (TPR) and can be represented by the equation, $BP = CO \times TPR$.

In healthy adults, the pressure at the height of the pressure pulse, called the *systolic pressure*, normally is about 120 mm Hg, and the lowest pressure, called the *diastolic pressure*, is about 80 mm Hg. The difference between the systolic and diastolic pressure (about 40 mm Hg) is called the *pulse pressure*. It reflects the magnitude or height of the pressure pulse. The *mean arterial pressure* (about 90 to 100 mm Hg) represents the average pressure in the arterial system during ventricular contraction and relaxation.

Short-Term Regulation

Neural and hormonal mechanisms function in the short-term regulation of blood pressure. The short-term adjustments occurring over seconds, minutes, or hours are intended to correct temporary imbalances that occur during the performance of everyday activities such as physical exercise and changes in body position. These mechanisms are also responsible for maintenance of blood pressure at survival levels during life-threatening situations.

Neural Mechanisms. The neural control of blood pressure is mediated by the autonomic nervous system through control mechanisms that include intrinsic circulatory reflexes, extrinsic reflexes, and higher neural control centers. The intrinsic reflexes, including the baroreflex and chemoreceptor-mediated reflex, are located within the circulatory system and are essential for rapid and short-term regulation of blood pressure (discussed under neural control of circulatory function). The extrinsic reflexes are found outside the circulation. They include blood pressure responses associated with factors such as pain, cold, and isometric handgrip exercise. The neural pathways for these reactions are largely unknown, and their responses are less consistent than those of the intrinsic reflexes. Among higher center responses are the central nervous system (CNS) ischemic response and those caused by changes in mood and emotion.

Humoral Mechanisms. A number of hormones and humoral mechanisms contribute to blood pressure regulation, including the renin-angiotensin-aldosterone mechanism and vasopressin. The *renin-angiotensin-aldosterone system* plays a central role in blood pressure regulation. Renin is an enzyme that is synthesized, stored, and released from the juxtaglomerular cells of the kidneys in response to a fall in blood pressure, sympathetic stimulation, or decreased extracellular sodium concentration. Most of the renin that is released leaves the kidney and enters the bloodstream, where it acts enzymatically to convert a circulating plasma protein called *angiotensinogen* to *angiotensin I* (Fig. 16–22). Angiotensin I travels to the small blood vessels of the lung, where it is converted to *angiotensin II* by the *angiotensin-converting enzyme* that is present in the endothelium of the lung vessels. Although angiotensin II has a half-life of several minutes, renin persists in the circulation for 30 minutes to 1 hour and continues to cause production of angiotensin II during this time.

Angiotensin II functions in short-term and long-term regulation of blood pressure. It is a strong vasoconstrictor, particularly of arterioles and to a lesser extent of veins. The vasoconstrictor effect raises peripheral vascular resistance (and blood pressure) and functions in the short-term regulation of blood pressure. For example, the renin-angiotensin system, which is activated during blood loss, produces an increase in systemic vascular resistance even before the blood pressure starts to fall. A second major function of angiotensin II, stimulation of aldosterone from the adrenal gland, contributes to the long-term regulation of blood pressure by increasing salt and water retention by the kidney. It also acts directly on the kidney to decrease the elimination of salt and water. Angiotensin II plays a significant role in maintaining blood volume in persons on a low-sodium diet.

Vasopressin, or antidiuretic hormone, is released from the posterior pituitary gland in response to decreases in blood volume and blood pressure, an increase osmolality of body fluids, and other stimuli. The antidiuretic actions of vasopressin are discussed in Chapter 26. Vasopressin has a direct vasoconstrictor effect on blood vessels, particularly those of the splanchnic circulation. However, long-term increases in vasopressin cannot maintain volume expansion or hypertension, and it does not enhance hypertension produced by sodium-retaining hormones or other vasoconstricting substances. It has been suggested that vasopressin plays a permissive role in hypertension through its fluid-retaining properties or as a neurotransmitter that serves to modify autonomic nervous system (ANS) function.

Long-Term Regulation

Neural and hormonal regulation of blood pressure are short-term mechanisms that act rapidly to restore blood pressure. They are, however, ineffective in the long-term

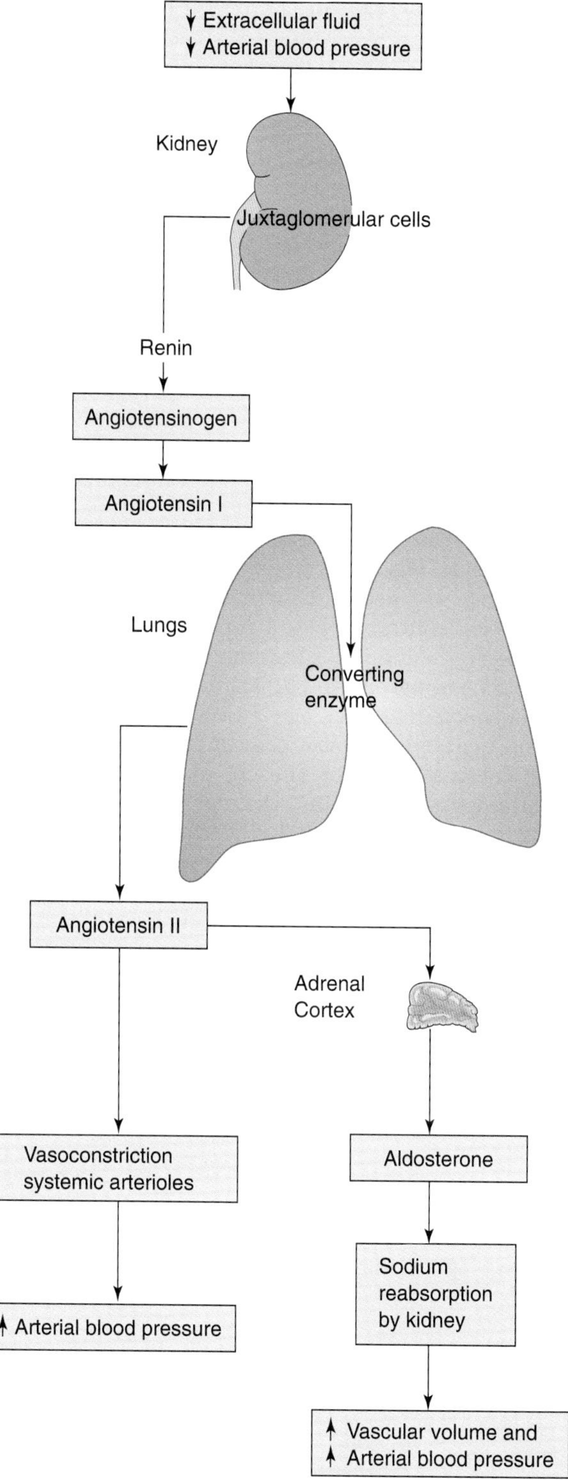

Figure 16–22
Control of blood pressure by the renin-angiotensin-aldosterone system. Renin combines with the plasma protein angiotensinogen to form angiotensin I; angiotensin-converting enzyme in the lung converts angiotensin I to angiotensin II; and angiotensin II produces vasoconstriction and increases salt and water retention through direct action on the kidney and through increased aldosterone secretion by the adrenal cortex.

regulation of blood pressure. Instead, responsibility for the long-term regulation of blood pressure appears to be vested in the kidneys and in the extracellular fluid volume.

Renal–Body Fluid System. According to Arthur Guyton, a noted physiologist, the long-term regulation of blood pressure is vested in the renal–body fluid system which regulates extracellular fluid volume. Accordingly, when the body contains too much extracellular fluid, the arterial pressure increases; when too little fluid is present, blood pressure decreases. For example, an increase in arterial pressure greatly increases the rate at which water (*i.e.*, pressure diuresis) and sodium (*i.e.*, pressure natriuresis) are excreted by the kidney.

Figure 16–23 illustrates the control of blood pressure by the renal–body fluid system. This graph consists of two intersecting curves: the renal output curve and the straight line that represents the net salt and water intake or level at which the blood pressure is regulated. The only point on the graph at which the intake and output are balanced is at the equilibrium point, which in this case is 100 mm Hg.

As an example of how the renal–body fluid mechanism works, first assume that the blood pressure rises to 150 mm Hg; when this happens, the renal output of water and salt increases and blood pressure returns to the equilibrium point. However, if the blood pressure were to decrease to 70 mm Hg, the kidneys would decrease their output of water and salt, causing the blood pressure to rise. The kidneys continue to increase or decrease their elimination of water and salt until the blood pressure has returned to the equilibrium point.

The only way to change the long-term regulation of blood pressure using the concept of the renal–body fluid control system is to change the level of the water and salt line or the pressure range of the renal output curve. For example, a defect in pressure diuresis or natriuresis can shift the curve to the right so that blood pressure is maintained at a higher level. Likewise, a shift in the water and salt intake line raises the equilibrium point to a higher level of pressure.

Increased Fluid Volume. Increased extracellular volume elevates blood pressure through an increase in cardiac output. There are two different ways in which cardiac output increases blood pressure: one is through a direct effect on blood pressure, and the second is an indirect effect resulting from local autoregulation of blood flow. When excess blood flows through a tissue, local blood vessels constrict and return the flow to normal. When cardiac output is increased, all of the tissues of the body are exposed to increased blood flow and autoregulation constricts blood vessels throughout the body; this increases the systemic vascular resistance, producing an increase in blood pressure. Normally, an increase in blood pressure should produce pressure diuresis with an increased output of salt and water by the kidney, returning the pressure to normal. In hypertension, renal control mechanisms are

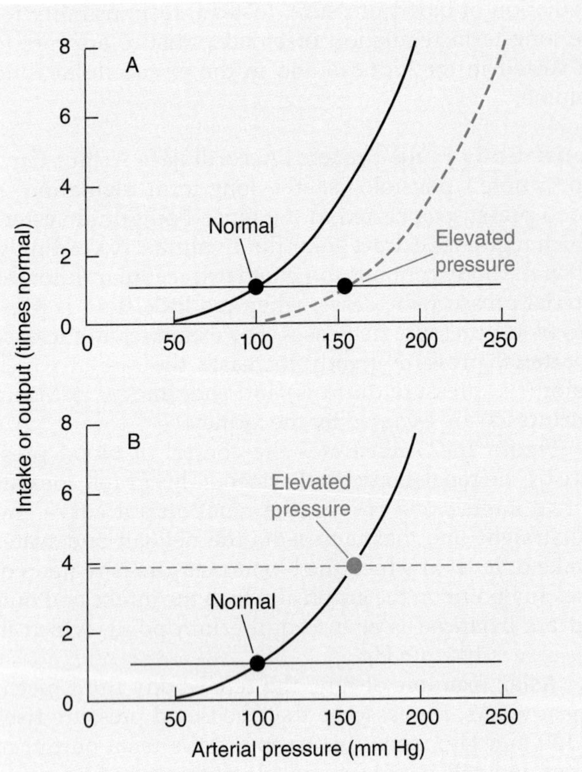

Figure 16–23
Two ways in which the arterial pressure can be increased: (**A**) by shifting the renal output curve in the right-hand direction toward a higher pressure level and (**B**) by increasing the intake level of salt and water. (Guyton A.C., Hall JE. [1996] *Textbook of medical physiology* [9th ed., p. 223]. Philadelphia: W.B. Saunders)

altered such that the renal output curve is shifted to the right and blood pressure is maintained at a higher level.

Local Control of Blood Flow

Tissue blood flow is regulated on a minute-to-minute basis in relation to tissue needs and on a longer-term basis through the development of collateral circulation. Neural mechanisms regulate the cardiac output and blood pressure needed to support these local mechanisms.

Short-Term Autoregulation

Local control of blood flow is governed largely by the nutritional needs of the tissue. For example, blood flow to organs such as the heart, brain, and kidneys remains relatively constant, although blood pressure may vary over a range of 60 to 180 mm Hg (Fig. 16–24). The ability of the tissues to regulate their own blood flow over a wide range of pressures is called *autoregulation*. Autoregulation of blood flow is maintained by blood vessel distention or by local tissue factors, such as lack of oxygen or accumulation of tissue metabolites (i.e., potassium, lactic acid, or adenosine, which is a breakdown product of ATP). It involves the selective opening and closing of capillary channels. Local control is particularly important in tissues such as skeletal muscle, which has varying blood flow requirements according to the level of activity.

An increase in local blood flow is called *hyperemia*. The ability of tissues to increase blood flow in situations of increased activity, such as exercise, is called *functional hyperemia*. When the blood supply to an area has been occluded and then restored, local blood flow through the tissues increases within seconds to restore the metabolic equilibrium of the tissues. This increased flow is called *reactive hyperemia*. The transient redness seen on an arm after leaning on a hard surface is an example of reactive hyperemia. Local control mechanisms rely on a continuous flow from the main arteries; therefore, hyperemia cannot occur when the arteries that supply the capillary beds are narrowed. For example, if a major coronary artery becomes occluded, the opening of channels supplied by that vessel cannot restore blood flow.

Tissue Factors Contributing to Local Control of Blood Flow. Vasodilator substances, formed in tissues in response to a need for increased blood flow, also aid in the local control of blood flow. The most important of these are histamine, serotonin (*i.e.*, 5-hydroxytryptamine), the kinins, and the prostaglandins.

Histamine increases blood flow. Most blood vessels contain histamine in mast cells and nonmast cell stores; when these tissues are injured, histamine is released. In certain tissues, such as skeletal muscle, the activity of the mast cells is mediated by the sympathetic nervous system; when sympathetic control is withdrawn, the mast cells release histamine. Vasodilation then results from increased histamine and the withdrawal of vasoconstrictor activity.

Serotonin is liberated from aggregating platelets during the clotting process; it causes vasoconstriction and plays a major role in control of bleeding. Serotonin is

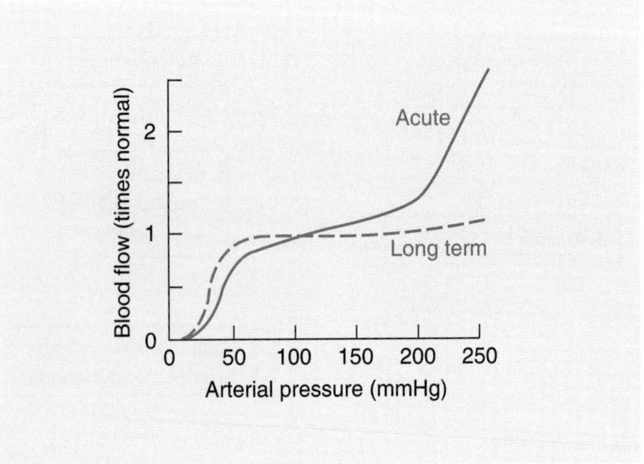

Figure 16–24
Effect on blood flow through a muscle of increasing arterial pressure. The *solid curve* shows the effect if pressure is raised over a few minutes. The *dashed curve* shows the effect if the arterial pressure is raised slowly over many weeks. (Guyton A.C., Hall J.E. [1996]. *Textbook of medical physiology* [9th ed., p. 203]. Philadelphia: W.B. Saunders)

found in brain and lung tissues, and there is some speculation that it may be involved in the vascular spasm associated with some allergic pulmonary reactions and migraine headaches.

The *kinins* (i.e., kallidins and bradykinin) are liberated from the globulin kininogen, which is present in body fluids. The kinins cause relaxation of arteriole smooth muscle, increase capillary permeability, and constrict the venules. In exocrine glands, the formation of kinins contributes to the vasodilation needed for glandular secretion.

Prostaglandins are synthesized from constituents (*i.e.*, the long-chain fatty acid arachidonic acid) of the cell membrane. Tissue injury incites the release of arachidonic acid from the cell membrane, which initiates prostaglandin synthesis. There are several prostaglandins (*e.g.*, E_2, F_2, D_2), which are subgrouped according to their solubility; some produce vasoconstriction and some produce vasodilation. As a rule of thumb, those in the E group are vasodilators, and those in the F group are vasoconstrictors. The adrenal glucocorticoid hormones produce an antiinflammatory response by blocking the release of arachidonic acid, preventing prostaglandin synthesis.

Endothelial Control of Vasodilation and Vasoconstriction. The endothelium, which lies between the blood and the vascular smooth muscle, serves as a physical barrier for vasoactive substances that circulate in the blood. Once thought to be nothing more than a single layer of cells that line blood vessels, it is now known that the endothelium plays an active role in controlling vascular function. In capillaries, which are composed of a single layer of endothelial cells, the endothelium is active in transporting cell nutrients and wastes. In addition to its function in capillary transport, the endothelium removes vasoactive agents such as norepinephrine from the blood, and it produces enzymes that convert precursor molecules to active products (*e.g.*, angiotensin I to angiotensin II in lung vessels).

One of the important functions of the normal endothelium is to synthesize and release factors that control vessel dilation. Of particular importance was the discovery, first reported in the early 1980s, that the intact endothelium was able to produce a factor that caused relaxation of vascular smooth muscle. This factor was originally named *endothelium-derived relaxing factor* and is now known to be nitric oxide. Many other cells types produce nitric oxide by means of similar enzymes. In these tissues, nitric oxide affords other functions, including modulation of nerve activity in the nervous system.

The normal endothelium maintains a continuous release of nitric oxide, which is formed from L-arginine through the action of the enzyme nitric oxide synthase (Fig. 16–25). The production of nitric oxide can be stimulated by a variety of endothelial agonists, including acetylcholine, bradykinin, histamine, and thrombin. Shear stress resulting from an increase in blood flow or blood pressure also stimulates nitric oxide production and vessel relaxation. Nitric oxide also inhibits platelet aggregation and secretion of platelet contents, many of which cause vasoconstriction. The fact that nitric oxide is released into the vessel lumen (to inactivate platelets) and away from the lumen (to relax smooth muscle) suggests that it protects against both thrombosis and vasoconstriction.

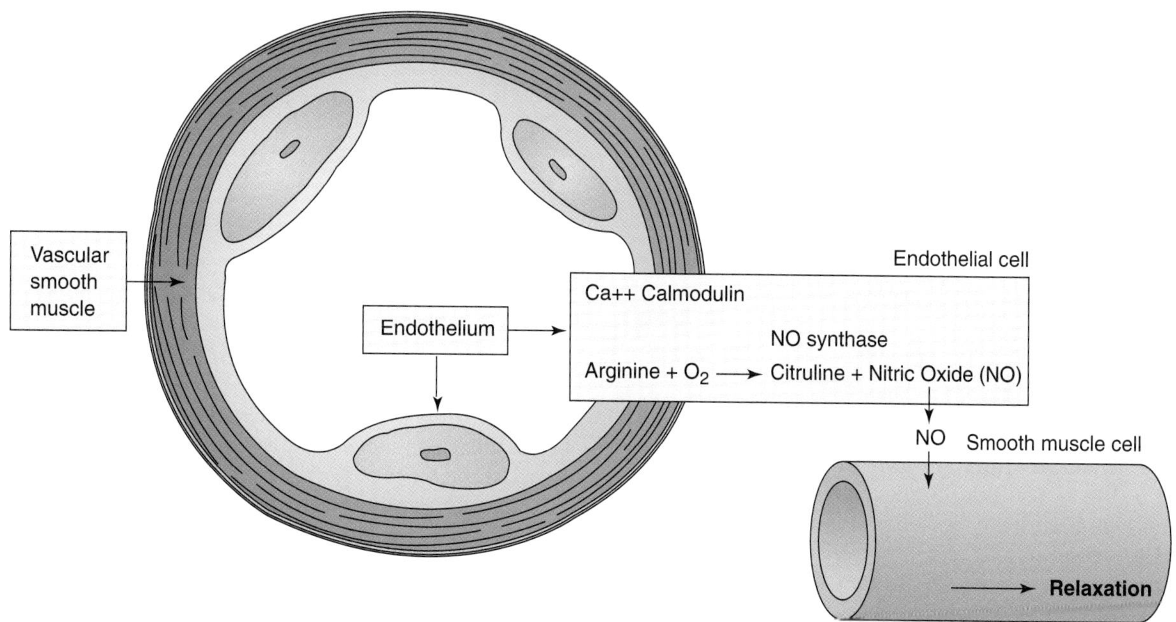

Figure 16–25
Function of nitric oxide in smooth muscle relaxation.

In addition to nitric oxide, the endothelium also produces other vasodilating substances such as the prostaglandin, prostacyclin, which produces vasodilation and inhibits platelet aggregation. It has been suggested that the tendency to vasoconstriction that characterizes atherosclerotic vessels may be related to impaired vasodilator function due to disruption of the vessel endothelial layer.

The endothelium also produces a number of vasoconstrictor substances, including angiotensin II, vasoconstrictor prostaglandins, and a family of peptides called *endothelins*. There are at least three endothelins. Endothelin-1 made by human endothelial cells, is the most potent endogenous vasoconstrictor known. Receptors for endothelins also have been identified.

Long-Term Regulation

Collateral circulation is a mechanism for the long-term regulation of local blood flow. In the heart and other vital structures, anastomotic channels exist between some of the smaller arteries. These channels permit perfusion of an area by more than one artery. When one artery becomes occluded, these anastomotic channels increase in size, allowing blood from a patent artery to perfuse the area supplied by the occluded vessel. For example, persons with extensive obstruction of a coronary blood vessel may rely on collateral circulation to meet the oxygen needs of the myocardial tissue normally supplied by that vessel. As with other long-term compensatory mechanisms, the recruitment of collateral circulation is most efficient when obstruction to flow is gradual rather than sudden.

In summary, the walls of all blood vessels, except the capillaries, are composed of three layers: the tunica externa, tunica media, and tunica intima. The layers of the vessel vary with its function. Arteries are thick-walled vessels with large amounts of elastic fibers. The walls of the arterioles, which control blood pressure, have large amounts of smooth muscle. Veins are thin-walled, distensible, and collapsible vessels. Venous flow is designed to return blood to the heart. It is a low-pressure system and relies on venous valves and the action of muscle pumps to offset the effects of gravity. Capillaries are single-cell–thick vessels designed for the exchange of gases, nutrients, and waste materials.

Blood flow is controlled by many of the same mechanisms that control fluid flow in nonbiologic systems. It is influenced by vessel length, pressure differences, vessel radius, blood viscosity, cross-sectional area, and wall tension. The rate of flow is directly related to the pressure difference between the two ends of the vessel and the vessel radius and inversely related to vessel length and blood viscosity. The cross-sectional area of a vessel influences the velocity of flow; as the cross-sectional area decreases, the velocity is increased, and vice versa. Laminar blood flow is flow in which there is layering of blood components in the center of the bloodstream. This reduces frictional forces and prevents clotting factors from coming in contact with the vessel wall. In contrast to laminar flow, turbulent flow is disordered flow, in which the blood moves crosswise and lengthwise in blood vessels. The relation between wall tension, transmural pressure, and radius is described by Laplace's law, which states that wall tension becomes greater as the radius increases. Wall tension is also affected by wall thickness; it increases as the wall becomes thinner and decreases as the wall becomes thicker.

Blood pressure is determined by the cardiac output and systemic vascular resistance. Normally, blood pressure is regulated at levels sufficient to ensure adequate tissue perfusion. Blood pressure regulation requires the use of short-term and long-term mechanisms. Short-term regulation of blood pressure involves neural and hormonal mechanisms; it occurs over minutes and hours and is intended to correct temporary imbalances in blood pressure, such as those caused by postural changes, exercise, or hemorrhage. Long-term mechanisms control the daily, weekly, and monthly regulation of blood pressure and involve a change in the excretion of salt and water by the kidneys (i.e., the renal–body fluid pressure control system).

The mechanisms that control blood flow are designed to ensure adequate delivery of blood to the capillaries in the microcirculation, where the exchange of cellular nutrients and wastes occurs. Local control is governed largely by the needs of the tissues and is regulated by local tissue factors such as lack of oxygen and the accumulation of metabolites. Hyperemia is a local increase in blood flow that occurs after a temporary occlusion of blood flow. It is a compensatory mechanism that decreases the oxygen debt of the deprived tissues. Collateral circulation is a mechanism for long-term regulation of local blood flow that involves the development of collateral vessels.

Neural Control of Circulatory Function

After you have completed this section of the chapter, you should be able to meet the following objectives:

- Describe the distribution of sympathetic and parasympathetic nervous system in innervation of the circulatory system and their effects on heart rate and cardiac contractility
- List the types of sympathetic and parasympathetic receptors and characterize their neurotransmitters in terms of circulatory function
- Describe the role of the central nervous system in terms of regulating circulatory function
- Explain the role of the autonomic nervous system in the circulatory response to postural stress, increased intrathoracic pressure, and face immersion

The neural control of the circulatory system occurs primarily through the sympathetic and parasympathetic divisions of the ANS. The ANS contributes to control of cardiovascular function control through cardiac (*i.e.*, heart rate and cardiac contractility) and vascular (*i.e.*, peripheral vascular resistance) function.

The neural control centers for the integration and modulation of cardiac function and blood pressure are located bilaterally in the medulla oblongata. The medullary cardiovascular neurons are grouped into three distinct pools that lead to sympathetic innervation of the heart and blood vessels and parasympathetic innervation of the heart. The first two, which control sympathetic-mediated acceleration of heart rate and blood vessel tone, are called the *vasomotor center*. The third, which controls parasympathetic-mediated slowing of heart rate, is called the *cardioinhibitory center*. These brain stem centers receive information from many areas of the nervous system, including the hypothalamus. The arterial baroreceptors and chemoreceptors provide the medullary cardiovascular center with continuous information regarding the function of the circulatory system.

Baroreceptors

Baroreceptors are pressure-sensitive receptors located in the walls of blood vessels and the heart. The carotid and aortic baroreceptors are located in strategic positions between the heart and the brain (Fig. 16–26). The baroreceptors respond to a change in the stretch of the vessel wall by sending impulses to cardiovascular centers in the brain stem to effect appropriate changes in heart rate and vascular smooth muscle tone. For example, the fall in blood pressure that occurs on moving from the lying to the standing position produces a decrease in the stretch of the aortic and carotid baroreceptors with a resultant increase in heart rate and peripheral vascular resistance due to vasoconstriction. The rapidity with which the baroreflex response occurs is such that an increase in heart rate can usually be observed within several heart beats, and the adjustment of blood pressure is usually complete within 1 to 2 minutes. This rapid response is needed to prevent the occurrence of orthostatic hypotension with dizziness and even fainting (see Chapter 18).

The carotid and aortic baroreceptors are often referred to as the high-pressure baroreceptors because they are located in the high-pressure arterial side of the circulation. There are also low-pressure baroreceptors, which are located in the right atria and pulmonary artery (*i.e.*, the low-pressure side of the circulation). As with other neural receptors, the baroreceptors adapt to prolonged changes in blood pressure and are probably of limited importance in the long-term regulation of blood pressure.

Chemoreceptors

The chemoreceptors are sensitive to changes in the oxygen, carbon dioxide, and hydrogen ion content of the blood. The arterial chemoreceptors are located in the carotid bodies, which lie in the bifurcation of the two common carotids, and in the aortic bodies of the aorta (see Fig. 16–26). Because of their location, these chemoreceptors are always in close contact with the arterial blood. Although the main function of the chemoreceptors is to regulate ventilation, they also communicate with the vasomotor center and can induce widespread vasoconstriction. Whenever the arterial pressure drops below a critical level, the chemoreceptors are stimulated because of diminished oxygen supply and a buildup of carbon dioxide and hydrogen ions. Persons with chronic lung disease may develop systemic and pulmonary hypertension due to hypoxemia (see Chapter 24).

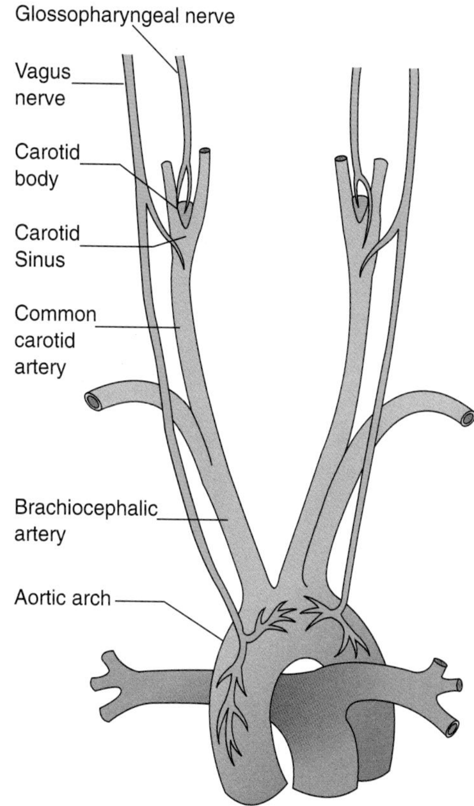

Figure 16–26
Location and innervation of the aortic arch and carotid sinus baroreceptors and the carotid body chemoreceptors.

Autonomic Regulation of Cardiac Function

The heart is innervated by the parasympathetic and sympathetic nervous systems. Parasympathetic innervation of the heart is achieved by means of the vagus nerve. The parasympathetic outflow to the heart originates from the vagal nucleus in the medulla. The axons of these neurons pass to the heart in the cardiac branches of the vagus nerve. The effect of vagal stimulation on heart function is largely limited to heart rate, with increased vagal activity producing a slowing of the pulse. Sympathetic outflow to the heart and blood vessels arises from neurons located in the reticular formation of the brain stem. The axons of these neurons descend in the intermediolateral columns of the spinal cord; they exit from the upper thoracic segments of the spinal cord and synapse in the paravertebral ganglia with the postganglionic neurons that innervate the heart. Cardiac sympathetic fibers are widely distributed to the sinoatrial and AV nodes and the myocardium. Increased sympathetic activity produces an increase in the heart rate and the velocity and force of cardiac contraction.

Autonomic Regulation of Vascular Function

The sympathetic nervous system serves as the final common pathway for controlling the smooth muscle tone of the blood vessels. Most of the sympathetic preganglionic fibers that control vessel function originate in the vasomotor center of the brain stem and travel in the intermediolateral column of the spinal cord and exit with the ventral nerves; they then synapse with postganglionic fibers in the paravertebral ganglia. The sympathetic neurons that supply the blood vessels maintain them in a state of tonic activity, so that even under resting conditions, the blood vessels are partially constricted. Vessel constriction and relaxation are accomplished by altering this basal input. Increasing sympathetic activity causes constriction of some vessels, such as those of the skin, the gastrointestinal tract, and the kidneys. Some blood vessels are supplied by vasoconstrictor and vasodilator fibers. Skeletal muscle, for example, is innervated by both types of fibers; activation of sympathetic vasodilator fibers provides the muscles with increased blood flow during exercise. Although the parasympathetic nervous system contributes to the regulation of heart function, it has little or no control over blood vessels.

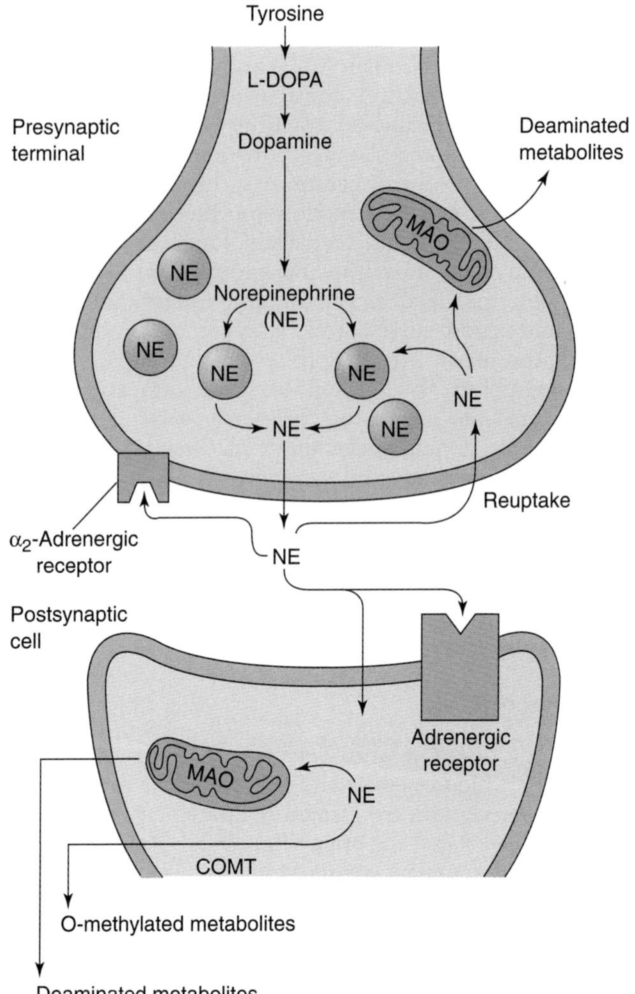

Figure 16–27
Mechanisms of norepinephrine synthesis, release, metabolism, and reuptake. Presynaptic α_2-adrenergic receptors act in the feedback regulation of norepinephrine synthesis and release. Norepinephrine is both removed from the synapse by the uptake process and degraded by monoamine oxidase (MAO) and catechol-O-methyltransferase (COMT).

Autonomic Neurotransmitters

The actions of the ANS are mediated by chemical neurotransmitters. Acetylcholine is the postganglionic neurotransmitter for parasympathetic neurons and norepinephrine is the main neurotransmitter for postganglionic sympathetic neurons. Sympathetic neurons also respond to epinephrine, which is released into the bloodstream by the adrenal medulla. The neurotransmitter dopamine can also act as a neuromediator for some sympathetic neurons. The sympathetic neurotransmitters are called *catecholamines.*

The catecholamines are synthesized in the axoplasm of sympathetic nerve terminal endings from the amino acid tyrosine (Fig. 16–27). In the process of catecholamine synthesis, tyrosine is hydroxylated (*i.e.,* has a hydroxyl group added) to form DOPA. DOPA is decarboxylated (*i.e.,* has a carboxyl group removed) to form dopamine, and dopamine is hydroxylated to form norepinephrine. In the adrenal gland, an additional step occurs during which norepinephrine is methylated (*i.e.,* a methyl group is added) to form epinephrine. Epinephrine is also called *adrenaline,* and sympathetic neurons are also called *adrenergic* neurons.

Each of the steps in neurotransmitter synthesis requires a different enzyme, and the type of neurotransmitter that is produced depends on the type of enzymes that are available in a nerve terminal. For example, the postganglionic sympathetic neurons that supply blood vessels synthesize norepinephrine, whereas postganglionic neurons in the adrenal medulla produce epinephrine or norepinephrine. Epinephrine accounts for about 80% of the catecholamines released from the adrenal gland. The synthesis of epinephrine by the adrenal medulla is influenced by the glucocorticoid secretion from the adrenal cortex. These hormones are transported by way of an intraadrenal vascular network from the adrenal cortex to the adrenal medulla, where they cause the sympathetic neurons to increase their production of epinephrine by way of increased enzyme activity. Thus, any stress situation sufficient to evoke increased levels of glucocorticoids also increases epinephrine levels.

As the catecholamines are synthesized, they are stored in vesicles. The final step of norepinephrine synthesis occurs in these vesicles. During an action potential, the neurotransmitter molecules are released from the storage vesicles. The storage vesicles not only provide a means for concentrated storage of the catecholamines, but they also protect them from the cytoplasmic enzymes that are capable of degrading the neurotransmitter. In addition to neuronal synthesis, there is a second major mechanism for replenishment of norepinephrine in sympathetic nerve terminals. This mechanism consists of the active recapture or reuptake of the released neurotransmitter into the nerve terminal. From 50% to 80% of the norepinephrine that is released during an action potential is removed from the synaptic area by an active reuptake process. This process terminates the action of the neurotransmitter and allows it to be reused by the neuron. The remainder of the released catecholamines diffuse into the surrounding tissue fluids or are degraded by two special enzymes: catechol-O-methyltransferase (COMT), which is diffusely present in all tissues, and monoamine oxidase (MAO), which is found in the nerve endings themselves.

Some drugs, such as the tricyclic antidepressants, are thought to increase the level of catecholamines at the site of nerve endings in the brain by blocking the reuptake process. Others, such as the MAO inhibitors, decrease the enzymatic degradation of the neurotransmitters and thereby increase their levels.

Autonomic Receptors

The neuromediators exert their effect through membrane proteins called *receptors*. The neuromediators and receptors interact in a lock and key fashion, which ensures specificity of action. Receptors that interact with acetylcholine are called *cholinergic* receptors, and those that interact with the sympathetic neuromediators are called *adrenergic* receptors. There are two types of adrenergic receptors: alpha (α) and beta (β) receptors. In vascular smooth muscle, stimulation of α receptors produces vasoconstriction; stimulation of β receptors causes vasodilatation. The α receptors have been further subdivided into α_1 and α_2 receptors. The α_1 receptors are found primarily at postsynaptic effector sites such as vascular smooth muscle. The α_2 receptors are abundant in the CNS and act at presynaptic sites to produce feedback inhibition of sympathetic outflow. The β_1 receptors are found primarily in the heart, and β_2 receptors are found in the bronchioles and in other sites that have β-mediated functions. In many tissues, the response that occurs is determined by the presence of a particular receptor type, which can vary from tissue to tissue. For example, in vascular smooth muscle that has α_1 receptors, sympathetic stimulation produces vasoconstriction; similar stimulation produces vasodilatation in other vessels that have β_2 receptors.

The role of the ANS in control of blood pressure is only beginning to be understood. For example, central α_2-adrenergic receptors are known to inhibit sympathetic outflow from the brain. Several antihypertensive medications exert their effect at this level. The α- and β-adrenergic receptors respond to endogenous catecholamines or exogenous pharmacologic agents (*e.g.*, drugs). Drugs that can selectively activate or block specific types of adrenergic receptors have been developed to treat high blood pressure.

Central Nervous System Responses

It is not surprising that the CNS, which plays an essential role in regulating vasomotor tone and blood pressure, would have a mechanism for controlling the blood flow to the cardiovascular centers that control circulatory function. When the blood flow to the brain has been sufficiently interrupted to cause ischemia of the vasomotor center, these vasomotor neurons become strongly excited, causing massive vasoconstriction as a means of raising the blood pressure to levels as high as the heart can pump against. This response is called the CNS ischemic response, and it can raise the blood pressure to levels as high as 270 mm Hg for as long as 10 minutes. The CNS ischemic response is a last-ditch stand to preserve the blood flow to vital brain centers; it does not become activated until blood pressure has fallen to at least 60 mm Hg, and it is most effective in the range of 15 to 20 mm Hg. If the cerebral circulation is not reestablished within 3 to 10 minutes, the neurons of the vasomotor center cease to function, so that the tonic impulses to the blood vessels stop and the blood pressure falls precipitously.

The *Cushing reflex* is a special type of CNS reflex resulting from an increase in intracranial pressure. When the intracranial pressure rises to levels that equal intraarterial pressure, blood vessels to the vasomotor center become compressed, initiating the CNS ischemic response. The purpose of this reflex is to produce a rise in arterial pressure to levels above intracranial pressure so that the blood flow to the vasomotor center can be reestablished. Should the intracranial pressure rise to the point that the blood supply to the vasomotor center becomes inadequate, vasoconstrictor tone is lost, and the blood pressure begins to fall. The elevation in blood pressure associated with the Cushing reflex is usually of short duration and should be considered a protective homeostatic mechanism. The brain and other cerebral structures are located within the rigid confines of the skull, with no room for expansion, and any increase in intracranial pressure tends to compress the blood vessels that supply the brain.

Autonomic Response to Circulatory Stresses

The response of the cardiovascular system to the stresses of everyday living is mediated largely through the autonomic nervous system. These stresses include postural stress, Valsalva's maneuver, and face immersion.

Postural Stress

During movement from the supine to the standing position, about 20% of the blood in the heart and lungs is displaced into the legs. The venous filling of the heart is decreased, the stroke volume falls, and blood pressure decreases. As the blood pressure drops, the baroreceptors are stimulated and produce a reflex-mediated increase in heart rate and peripheral vascular resistance. These responses prevent the blood pressure from falling excessively when the standing position is assumed. With prolonged standing, an increase in plasma volume and the action of the skeletal muscle pumps aid in the return of blood to the heart. Decreased tolerance of the upright position causes orthostatic hypotension, which is discussed in Chapter 18.

Valsalva's Maneuver

Valsalva's maneuver, which involves forced expiration against a closed glottis, incites a sequence of rapid changes in preload and afterload stresses along with autonomically mediated changes in the heart rate and systemic vascular resistance. Valsalva's maneuver is a normal accompaniment of many everyday activities. It is used in coughing, lifting, pushing, vomiting, and straining at stool. The pushing that occurs during the final stages of childbirth makes extensive use of the maneuver.

The rise in intrathoracic pressure (often to levels of 40 mm Hg or greater) during the strain of Valsalva's maneuver causes a decrease in venous return to the heart, with a resultant decrease in stroke volume output from the heart, a decrease in systolic and pulse pressures, and a baroreflex-mediated increase in the heart rate and systemic vascular resistance. After the release of the strain, venous return is suddenly reestablished; stroke volume and arterial blood pressure undergo marked but transient elevations. The sudden rise in arterial pressure that occurs at a time when reflex vasoconstriction is still present causes a vagal slowing of the heart rate that normally lasts for several beats. Valsalva's maneuver may be used as a method of testing circulatory reflexes, because the increase in heart rate and total peripheral resistance that occur during Valsalva's strain and the bradycardia that follows its release are mediated through the baroreceptors and the autonomic nervous system.

Face Immersion

The diving reflex (i.e., face immersion) is a potent protective mechanism against asphyxia in birds and submerged vertebrates; it allows for gross redistribution of the circulation to ensure the oxygenation of the brain and heart. The diving response has three main features: apnea, an intense vagal slowing of heart rate, and a powerful peripheral vasoconstriction. Except for the coronary and cerebral blood vessels, there is massive vasoconstriction to the extent that the circulation becomes in effect a heart-brain circuit. Because of the severe vasoconstriction, arterial pressure remains relatively unchanged.

In humans, application of cold water to the face produces a similar reduction in the heart rate and in the skin and muscle blood flow. The slowing of the heart rate is greater with ice water than with cool water and greater with cool water than with cool air. Immersion of the face in ice water may be used clinically to terminate supraventricular paroxysmal tachycardia. Because the reflex is potent in the neonate, it may protect against asphyxia during the birth process. It has also been credited with increasing the chance of survival of children who have accidentally fallen into cold water and remained submerged for longer periods than are normally associated with survival.

In summary, the neural control centers for the regulation of cardiac function and blood pressure are located in the reticular formation of the lower pons and medulla of the brain stem, where the integration and modulation of ANS responses occur. These brain stem centers receive information from many areas of the nervous system, including the hypothalamus. The heart is innervated by the parasympathetic and sympathetic nervous systems. The parasympathetic nervous system functions in regulating heart rate through the vagus nerve, with increased vagal activity producing a slowing of heart rate. The sympathetic nervous system has an excitatory influence on heart rate and contractility, and it serves as the final common pathway for controlling the smooth muscle tone of the blood vessels.

Autonomic control of the circulatory system occurs through neurotransmitters that exert their effect through membrane receptors. There are two types of adrenergic receptors: alpha (α) and beta (β) receptors. In vascular smooth muscle, stimulation of α receptors produces vasoconstriction; stimulation of β receptors causes vasodilatation. Alpha receptors have been further subdivided into $\alpha 1$ and $\alpha 2$ receptors. The $\alpha 1$ receptors are found primarily at postsynaptic effector sites such as vascular smooth muscle.

The response of the cardiovascular system to the stresses of everyday living such as postural stress, Valsalva's maneuver, and face immersion is mediated largely through the autonomic nervous system. Many of these stresses can be used to evaluate the function of the autonomic nervous system.

The Microcirculation and Lymphatic System

After you have completed this section of the chapter, you should be able to meet the following objectives:

- Describe the structure and function of the microcirculation
- Relate the effects of the capillary pressure, interstitial fluid pressure, capillary colloidal osmotic pressure, and

interstitial colloidal osmotic pressure to the exchange of fluids at the capillary level
- Describe the structures of the lymphatic system and relate them to the role of the lymphatics in controlling interstitial fluid volume
- Define the term *edema*

The capillaries, venules, and metarterioles of the circulatory system are collectively referred to as the *microcirculation*. It is here that exchange of gases, nutrients, and metabolites move between the tissues and the circulating blood.

The Microcirculation

Blood enters the microcirculation through an arteriole, passes through the capillaries, and leaves by way of a small venule. The metarterioles serve as thoroughfare channels that link arterioles and capillaries (Fig. 16–28). Small cuffs of smooth muscle, the precapillary sphincters, are positioned at the arterial end of the capillary. The smooth muscle tone of the arterioles, venules, and precapillary sphincters serves to control blood flow through the capillary bed. Dependent on venous pressure, blood flows through the capillary channels when the precapillary sphincters are open.

Blood flow through capillary channels, designed for exchange of nutrients and metabolites, is called *nutrient flow*. In some parts of the microcirculation, blood flow bypasses the capillary bed, moving through a connection called an *arteriovenous shunt*, which directly connects an arteriole and a venule. This type of blood flow is called *nonnutrient flow* because it does not allow for nutrient exchange. Nonnutrient channels are common in the skin and are important in terms of heat exchange and temperature regulation.

The lymphatic system represents an accessory system that removes excess fluid, including osmotically active proteins, and large particles from the interstitial spaces and returns it to the circulation. Because of their size, these proteins and large particles cannot be reabsorbed into the venous capillaries. The removal of proteins from the interstitial spaces is an essential function, without which death would occur in about 24 hours.

Capillary-Interstitial Fluid Exchange

About one sixth of the body consists of spaces between body cells called the *interstitium*. The interstitium is supported by collagen and elastin fibers and filled with proteoglycan (sugar-protein) molecules that combine with water to form a tissue gel (see Chapter 1). The tissue gel acts like a sponge to entrap the interstitial fluid and provide for even distribution to all the cells, even those that are most distant from the capillary. Although most of the fluid is entrapped in the tissue gel, small "trickles" of free fluid develop between the proteoglycan molecules. Normally, only small amounts of free fluid is present. In a condition called *edema* where excess fluid is present in the interstitial spaces, the amount of *free* fluid can expand tremendously.

Four forces determine the movement of fluid between capillaries and the interstitial spaces: the intracapillary pressure, the interstitial fluid pressure, the plasma colloidal osmotic pressure, and the interstitial colloidal osmotic pressure. The intracapillary and tissue pressures can be viewed as pushing pressures that force fluid out of the capillary or interstitial space and the osmotic pressures as pulling pressures that draw fluid into the capillary or interstitium. The intracapillary pressure causes fluids to move through the capillary pores into the interstitial spaces and the capillary colloidal osmotic pressure pulls the fluids back into the capillary. Also important to this exchange mechanism is the lymphatic system, which returns osmotically active proteins and excess interstitial fluids to the circulatory system.

Normally, the movement of fluid between the capillary bed and the interstitial spaces is continuous. A state of equilibrium exists as long as equal amounts of fluid enter and leave the interstitial spaces (Fig. 16–29). The approximate average forces at the arterial and venous ends of a capillary in the systemic circulation that causes fluid movement across the capillary membrane are shown in Figure 16–30. In the diagram, the capillary pressure is 28 mm Hg. The capillary pressure, along with a negative interstitial pressure (3 mm Hg) and an interstitial fluid colloidal osmotic pressure (8 mm Hg), contributes to the outward movement of fluid. Plasma proteins and other nondiffusible particles that remain in the capillary exert an osmotic pressure (28 mm Hg) that pulls fluids back into the venous end of the capillary. This yields a total outward pushing pressure of about 39 mm Hg and an inward pulling pressure of 28 mm Hg at the arterial end of the capil-

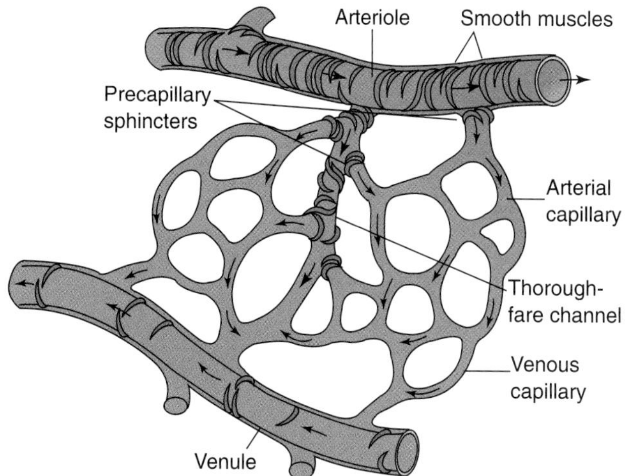

Figure 16–28
Capillary bed. Precapillary sphincters control the flow of blood through the capillary network. Thoroughfare channels (*i.e.*, arteriovenous shunts) allow blood to move directly from the arteriole into the venule without moving through nutrient channels of the capillary.

lary. On the venous end, the outward pushing pressures drop to 21 mm Hg, and the inward pulling forces remain at 28 mm Hg. A slight imbalance in forces (*i.e.,* 11 mm Hg outward forces and 7 mm Hg inward forces) causes slightly more filtration of fluid into interstitial spaces than is pulled back into the capillary; it is this fluid that is returned to the circulation by the lymphatic system.

Capillary Filtration Pressure

The intracapillary pressure, also called the *capillary filtration pressure,* is the force that pushes water through the capillary pores into the interstitial spaces. Capillary filtration pressure reflects the arterial pressure, the venous pressure, and the hydrostatic effects of gravity. Because arterial pressure decreases as blood moves away from the heart, the pressure at the arterial end of the capillary is normally higher than the pressure at its venous end. This pressure difference, or gradient, contributes to the outward movement of fluid from the capillary. Venous pressure can also be transmitted back to the capillary, thereby increasing intracapillary pressure and the outward movement of fluid. For example, venous thrombosis can obstruct venous flow, producing an increase in venous and capillary pressures. Capillary pressure also reflects changes in capillary volume. For example, intracapillary pressure can be expected to increase when the tone of the precapillary sphincters and the arterioles that supply the capillary bed is decreased. The swelling that occurs with inflammation develops because of a histamine-induced dilatation of the precapillary sphincters and arterioles that supply the affected area.

The pressure due to gravity is called the *hydrostatic pressure.* In a person in the standing position, the weight of the blood in the vascular column causes an increase of 1 mm Hg in pressure for every 13.6 mm of distance below the level of the heart. The hydrostatic pressure in the veins of an adult male can reach a level of 90 mm Hg. This pressure is then transmitted to the capillary bed. Gravity has no effect on blood pressure in a person in the recumbent position, because the blood vessels are then at the level of the heart. Because of the passive nature of pressure in the capillary bed, the terms *capillary pressure* and *hydrostatic pressure* are often used interchangeably.

Interstitial Fluid Pressure

The *interstitial fluid pressure* reflects the pressure exerted on the interstitial fluids. It can be positive or negative. In organs, such as the kidneys, which are encased in a tough fibrous capsule, the interstitial fluid pressure is positive, thereby opposing filtration of fluid out of the capillaries. Atmospheric pressure is usually negative in relation to capillary pressure. In the skin that is exposed to atmospheric pressure, the interstitial pressure is usually several millimeters of mercury less than capillary pressures. A negative interstitial fluid pressure increases the outward forces that pull fluid out of the capillary into the interstitium.

Capillary Colloidal Osmotic Pressure

The capillary colloidal osmotic pressure reflects the osmotic effect of the plasma proteins in drawing fluid into the capillary. Osmosis represents the movement of water across a semipermeable membrane along its concentration gradient moving from the side of the membrane

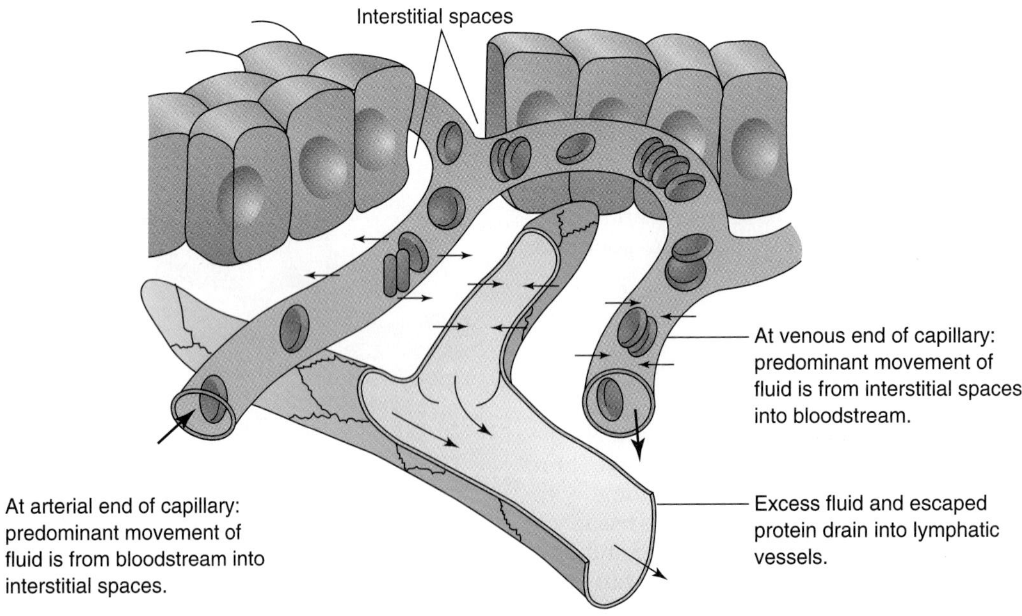
Interstitial spaces
At venous end of capillary: predominant movement of fluid is from interstitial spaces into bloodstream.
Excess fluid and escaped protein drain into lymphatic vessels.
At arterial end of capillary: predominant movement of fluid is from bloodstream into interstitial spaces.

Figure 16–29
Exchanges through capillary membranes in the formation and removal of interstitial fluid.

Outward Forces	
Capillary pressure	28 mm Hg
Negative interstitial pressure	3 mm Hg
Interstitial colloidal osmotic pressure	8 mm Hg
Total forces	39 mm Hg
Inward forces	
Plasma colloidal osmotic pressure	28 mm Hg
Total forces	28 mmHg
Summation of Forces	
Outward	39 mm Hg
Inward	28 mm Hg
Net outward force	11 mm Hg

Inward Forces	
Plasma colloidal osmotic pressure	28 mm Hg
Total forces	28 mm Hg
Outward forces	
Capillary pressure	10 mm Hg
Negative interstitial pressure	3 mm Hg
Interstitial colloidal osmotic pressure	8 mm Hg
	21 mm Hg
Summation of Forces	
Inward	28 mm Hg
Outward	21 mm Hg
Net inward force	7 mm Hg

Figure 16–30
Inward and outward forces in the capillary.

that has the greatest number of particles to the one that has the least number. A colloid solution is one in which there are evenly dispersed particles, much as cream particles become dispersed when milk is homogenized. The term *colloidal osmotic pressure* is used to differentiate the osmotic effects of the particles in a colloidal solution from those of the dissolved crystalloids such as sodium. The pressure units (mm Hg) used for measuring osmotic pressure represent the mechanical pressure or force that would be needed to oppose the osmotic movement of water.

The plasma proteins are large molecules that disperse in the blood and occasionally escape into the tissue spaces. Because the capillary membrane is almost impermeable to the plasma proteins, these particles exert a force that draws fluid into the capillary and offsets the pushing force of the capillary filtration pressure. The plasma contains a mixture of plasma proteins, including albumin, the globulins, and fibrinogen. Albumin, which is the smallest and most abundant of the plasma proteins, accounts for about 70% of the total osmotic pressure. It is the number, not the size, of the particles in solution that controls the osmotic pressure. One gram of albumin (molecular weight of 69,000) contains almost six times as many molecules as 1 gram of fibrinogen (molecular weight of 400,000). (Normal values for the plasma proteins are albumin, 4.5 g/dl; globulins, 2.5 g/dl; and fibrinogen, 0.3 g/dl.)

Tissue Colloidal Osmotic Pressure

Although the size of the capillary pores prevents most plasma proteins from leaving the capillary, small amounts do leak into the interstitial spaces to exert an osmotic force that favors movement of capillary fluid into the interstitium. This amount is often increased in conditions such inflammation that increase capillary permeability. The lymph system is responsible for removing proteins from the interstitium; in the absence of a functioning lymphatic system, tissue colloidal osmotic pressure increase, causing fluid to accumulate. Normally, a few white blood cells, plasma proteins, and other large molecules enter the interstitial spaces; these cells and molecules, which are too large to reenter the capillary, rely on the loosely structured wall of the lymphatic vessels for return to the vascular compartment.

The Lymphatic System

The lymphatic system, commonly called the *lymphatics*, serves almost all body tissues, except cartilage, bone, epithelial tissue, and tissues of the central nervous system. Most of these tissues, however, have prelymphatic channels that eventually flow into areas supplied by the lymphatics. Lymph is derived from interstitial fluids that flow through the lymph channels. It contains plasma proteins and other osmotically active particles that rely on the lymphatics for movement back into the circulatory system. When lymph flow is obstructed, a condition called *lymphedema* occurs. Involvement of lymph structures by malignant tumors and removal of lymph nodes at the time of cancer surgery are common causes of lymphedema. The lymphatic system is also the main route for absorption of nutrients, particularly fats, from the gastrointestinal tract. The lymph system also filters the fluid at the lymph nodes and removes foreign particles such as bacteria.

The lymphatic system is made up of vessels similar to those of the circulatory system. These vessels commonly travel along with an arteriole or venule or with its companion artery and vein. The terminal lymphatic vessels are made up of a single layer of connective tissue with an endothelial lining and resemble blood capillaries. The lymphatic vessels lack tight junctions and are loosely anchored to the surrounding tissues by fine filaments (Fig. 16–31). The loose junctions permit the entry of large particles, and the filaments hold the vessels open under conditions of edema, when the pressure of the surrounding tissues would otherwise cause them to collapse. The lymph capillaries drain into larger lymph vessels that ultimately empty into the right and left thoracic ducts (Fig. 16–32). The thoracic ducts empty into the circulation at the junctions of the subclavian and internal jugular veins.

Although not as distinct as in the circulatory system, the larger lymph vessels show evidence of having intimal, medial, and adventitial layers similar to blood vessels. The intima of these channels contain elastic tissue and an endothelial layer, and the larger collecting lymph channels contain smooth muscle in their medial layer. Contraction of this smooth muscle assists in propelling lymph fluid toward the thorax. External compression of the lymph channels by pulsating blood vessels in the vicinity and active and passive movements of body parts also aid in forward propulsion of lymph fluid. The rate of flow through the lymphatic system by way of all of the various lymph channels, about 120 ml per hour, is determined by the interstitial fluid pressure and the activity of lymph pumps.

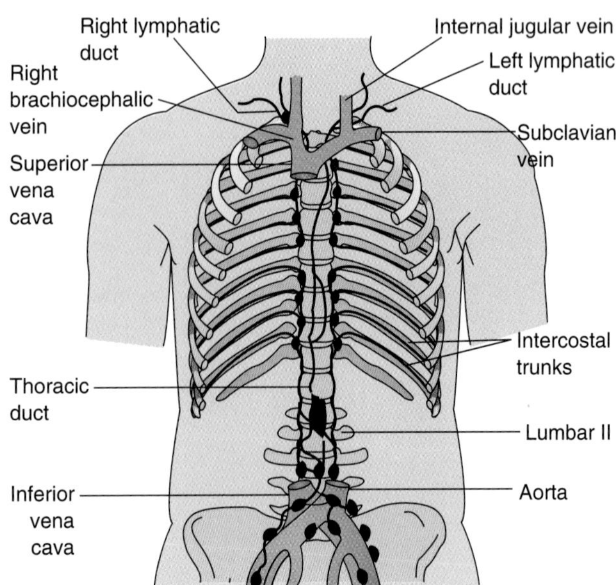

Figure 16–32
The diagram shows the course of the thoracic duct and right lymphatic duct. Deep lymphatic vessels and nodes are also shown.

Edema

Edema refers to excess interstitial fluid in the tissues (see Chapter 26). Edema can result from any of the factors that control movement of water between the vascular compartment and the tissue spaces. It can occur because of an disproportionate increase in capillary pressure, decreased colloidal osmotic pressure, capillary permeability, or impaired lymph flow. Edema is not a disease but rather the manifestation of altered physiologic function and can occur in healthy and sick individuals. In hot weather, the superficial blood vessels dilate, and sodium and water retention increases, which causes swelling of the hands and feet. Edema of the ankles and feet becomes more pronounced during prolonged periods of standing, when the forces of gravity are superimposed on the heat-induced vasodilatation and increased extracellular fluid volume.

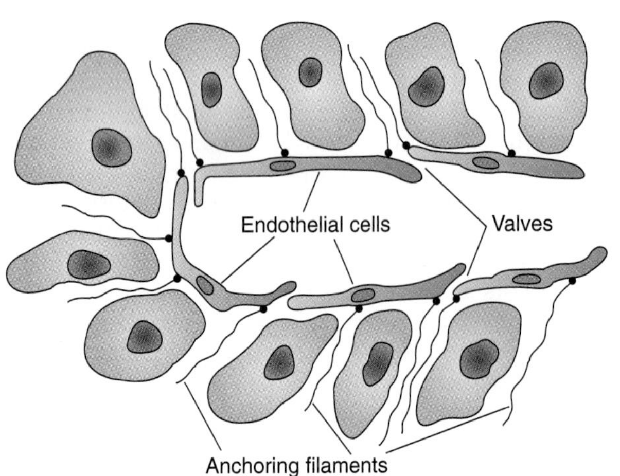

Figure 16–31
Special structure of the lymphatic capillaries that permits passage of substances of high molecular weight back into the lymph. (Guyton A.C., Hall J.E. [1996]. *Textbook of medical physiology* [9th ed., p. 194]. Philadelphia: W.B. Saunders)

In summary, exchange of fluids between the vascular compartment and the interstitial spaces occurs at the capillary level. The capillary filtration pressure pushes fluids out of the capillaries, and the colloidal osmotic pressure exerted by the plasma proteins pulls fluids back into the capillaries. Albumin, which is the smallest and most abundant of the plasma proteins, provides the major osmotic force for return of fluid to the vascular compartment. Normally, slightly more fluid leaves the capillary bed than can be reabsorbed. This excess fluid is returned to the circulation by way of the lymphatic channels.

BIBLIOGRAPHY

Berne R.M., Levy M.N. (1993). *Physiology* (3rd ed., pp. 361–478). St. Louis: C.V. Mosby.

Guyton A.C., Hall J.E. (1996). *Medical physiology* (9th ed., pp. 107–294). Philadelphia: W.B. Saunders.

Katz A.M. (1992). *Physiology of the heart*. New York, Raven Press.

Shepard J.T., Vanhoutte P.M. (1979). *The human cardiovascular system*. New York: Raven Press.

Johansen K. (1982). Aneurysms. *Scientific American* 247 (1), 110.

Porth C.J.M., Bamrah V.S., Tristani F.E., et al. (1984). The Valsalva: Mechanisms and clinical implications. *Heart and Lung* 13 (5), 507.

McCormack D.H. (1987). *Ham's histology* (9th ed., p. 448). Philadelphia: J.B. Lippincott.

Rhoades R.S., Tanner G.A. (1996). *Medical physiology* (pp. 207–301). Boston, Little, Brown.

Smith J.J., Kampine J.P. (1989). *Circulatory physiology* (3rd ed.). Baltimore: Williams & Wilkins.

Vanhoutte P.M. (1987). Endothelium and the control of vascular tissue. *News in Physiological Sciences* 2 (2), 21.

CHAPTER 17

Alterations in Blood Flow in the Systemic Circulation

Blood flow in the arterial and the venous system depends on a system of patent blood vessels and adequate perfusion pressure. A disturbance in blood flow in the arterial or venous systems disrupts the delivery of oxygen and nutrients, removal of waste products, and the return of blood to the heart. Unlike disorders of the respiratory system or central circulation that cause hypoxia and impair oxygenation of tissues throughout the body, the effects of blood vessel disease is usually limited to local tissues supplied by a particular vessel or group of vessels. With arterial disorders, there is decreased blood flow to the tissues along with impaired delivery of oxygen and nutrients. Venous disorders interfere with the outflow of blood from the capillaries, removal of tissue wastes, and return of blood to the heart. Arterial and venous disorders can lead to tissue injury and death.

Disturbances in flow can result from pathologic changes within the vessel wall (*i.e.,* atherosclerosis and vasculitis), acute vessel obstruction due to thrombus or embolus, vasospastic constriction (*i.e.,* Raynaud's phenomenon), abnormal vessel dilation (*i.e.,* arterial aneuryoms or varicose veins), or compression of blood vessels by extravascular forces (*i.e.,* tumors, edema, or firm surfaces such as those associated with pressure ulcers).

This chapter is organized into three sections: disorders of the arterial circulation, disorders of the venous circulation, and disorders of blood vessel compression.

Disorders of the Arterial Circulation

After you have completed this section of the chapter, you should be able to meet the following objectives:

- List the five types of lipoproteins and state their function in terms of lipid transport and development of atherosclerosis.
- Describe the role of low-density lipoprotein receptors in removal of cholesterol from the blood
- Cite the criteria for diagnosis of hypercholesteremia
- List the vessels most commonly affected by atherosclerosis and describe the vessel changes that occur

- Describe possible mechanisms involved in the development of atherosclerosis
- List risk factors in atherosclerosis
- State the signs and symptoms of acute arterial occlusion
- Describe the pathology associated with the vasculitides relate to four disease conditions associated with vasculitis
- Compare the mechanisms and manifestations of ischemia associated with atherosclerotic peripheral vascular disease, Raynaud's phenomenon, and thromboangiitis obliterans (*i.e.*, Buerger's disease)
- Distinguish among berry aneurysms, aortic aneurysms, and dissecting aneurysms
- Compare the pathology and manifestation of thoracic or abdominal and dissecting aneurysm

The arterial system distributes blood to all the various tissues in the body. There are three types of arteries: large elastic arteries, including the aorta and its distal branches; medium-sized arteries, such as the coronaries and renal arteries; and small arteries and arterioles that pass through the tissues. The large arteries function mainly in transport of blood. The medium-sized arteries are composed predominately of circular and spirally arranged smooth muscle cells. Distribution of blood flow to the various organs and tissues of the body is controlled by contraction and relaxation of the smooth muscle of these vessels. The small arteries and arterioles regulate capillary blood flow. Each of these different types of arteries tend to be affected by different disease processes.

Pathology of the arterial system affects body function through impaired blood flow. The effect that impaired blood flow has on the body depends on the structures involved and the extent of altered flow. The term *ischemia* (*i.e.*, holding back of blood) denotes a reduction in arterial flow to a level that is insufficient to meet the oxygen demands of the tissues. *Infarction* refers an area of ischemic necrosis within an organ, produced by occlusion of its arterial blood supply or its venous drainage. The discussion in this section focuses on cholesterol and hyperlipidemia, atherosclerosis, vasculitis, arterial disease of the extremities, and arterial aneurysms. Atherosclerosis and vasculitis produce their effects through altered blood flow caused by damage to blood vessels.

Cholesterol and Hyperlipidemia

Elevated levels of blood cholesterol are implicated in the development of atherosclerosis. An estimated 38.3 million Americans (20.5%) have high cholesterol levels that could contribute to a heart attack, stroke, or other cardiovascular event associated with atherosclerosis.[1] A review of the normal process of cholesterol transport and metabolism is included to assist the reader in understanding of the pathogenesis of atherosclerosis.

Lipoproteins

Cholesterol is a waxy, fatlike substance that is essential to the growth and viability of body cells. It is an important component of cell membranes and is used in the synthesis of steroid hormones (e.g., estrogens, testosterone, cortisol). Although most cholesterol is found in cells, about 7% circulates in the blood serum.[2] It is the serum cholesterol that contributes to the formation of atherosclerotic plaques in arteries throughout the body.

Because cholesterol and triglycerides are insoluble in plasma, they are encapsulated by special fat-carrying proteins called *lipoproteins* for transport in the blood. There are five classes of lipoproteins: chylomicrons, very-low-density lipoprotein (VLDL), intermediate-density lipoprotein (IDL), low-density lipoprotein (LDL), and high-density lipoprotein (HDL). The naming of these lipoproteins is based on the results of ultracentrifugation, by which the lipoproteins are separated according to their density. Triglycerides have a lower density than cholesterol. Accordingly, VLDL carries large amounts of triglycerides compared with LDL, which is the main carrier of cholesterol.

Each type of lipoprotein consists of a large molecular complex of lipids and proteins called *apoproteins*.[3,5] The major lipid constituents are cholesterol esters, triglycerides, nonesterified cholesterol, and phospholipids. The insoluble cholesterol esters and triglycerides are located in the hydrophobic core of the lipoprotein macromolecule, surrounded by the soluble phospholipids, nonesterified cholesterol, and apoproteins (Fig. 17–1). Nonesterified cholesterol and phospholipids provide a negative charge that allows the lipoprotein to be soluble in plasma.

There are four major classes of apoproteins: A (*i.e.*, A-I, A-II, A-III, and A-IV), B (*e.g.*, B-48, B-100), C (*i.e.*, CI, CII, and CIII), and E.[3,4] The apoproteins control the interactions and ultimate metabolic fate of the lipoproteins. Some of the apoproteins activate the lipolytic enzymes that facilitate the removal of lipids from the lipoproteins; others serve as a reactive site that cellular receptors can recognize and use in endocytosis and the metabolism of the lipoproteins. The major apoprotein in

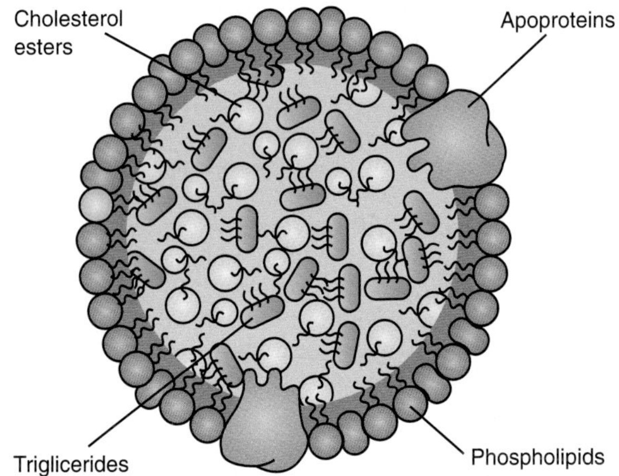

Figure 17-1
General structure of a lipoprotein. The cholesterol esters and triglycerides are located in the hydrophobic core of the macromolecule, surrounded by phospholipids and aproproteins

LDL is B-100. Research findings suggest that genetic defects in apoproteins may be involved in hyperlipidemia and accelerated atherosclerosis.[2]

There are two sites of lipoprotein synthesis: the small intestine and the liver. The chylomicrons, which are the largest lipoprotein molecules, are synthesized in the wall of the small intestine and carry large amounts of triglycerides. They are involved in the transport of dietary (exogenous) triglycerides and cholesterol that have been absorbed from the gastrointestinal tract. Chylomicrons travel to the capillaries of adipose and skeletal muscle tissue, where they transfer their triglycerides to fat and muscle cells. The remaining cholesterol-containing chylomicron remnant particles are taken up by the liver and their cholesterol used in the synthesis of VLDL or excreted in the bile.

The liver synthesizes and releases VLDL and HDL. The VLDLs contain large amounts of triglycerides and lesser amounts of cholesterol esters. They provide the primary pathway for transport of the endogenous triglycerides produced in the liver, as opposed to those obtained from the diet. Like chylomicrons, VLDLs carry their triglycerides to tissue capillaries of fat and muscle cells, where they are removed. The resulting IDL fragments are reduced in triglyceride content and enriched in cholesterol. They are taken to the liver and recycled to form VLDL or converted to LDL in the vascular compartment. IDLs are the main source of LDL. The exogenous and endogenous pathways for triglyceride and cholesterol transport are shown in Figure 17–2.

LDL, sometimes called the "bad cholesterol," is the main carrier of cholesterol. LDL is removed from the circulation by receptor-dependent and non–receptor-dependent mechanisms. Receptor-mediated removal involves binding of LDL to cell surface receptors, followed by endocytosis, a phagocytic process in which LDL is engulfed and moved into the cell in the form of a membrane-covered endocytic vesicle. Within the cell, the endocytic vesicles fuse with lysosomes, and the LDL molecule is enzymatically degraded, causing free cholesterol to be released into the cytoplasm.

About 70% of LDL is removed by way of the receptor-dependent pathway in the liver. Other nonhepatic tissues (*i.e.,* adrenal glands, smooth muscle cells, endothelial

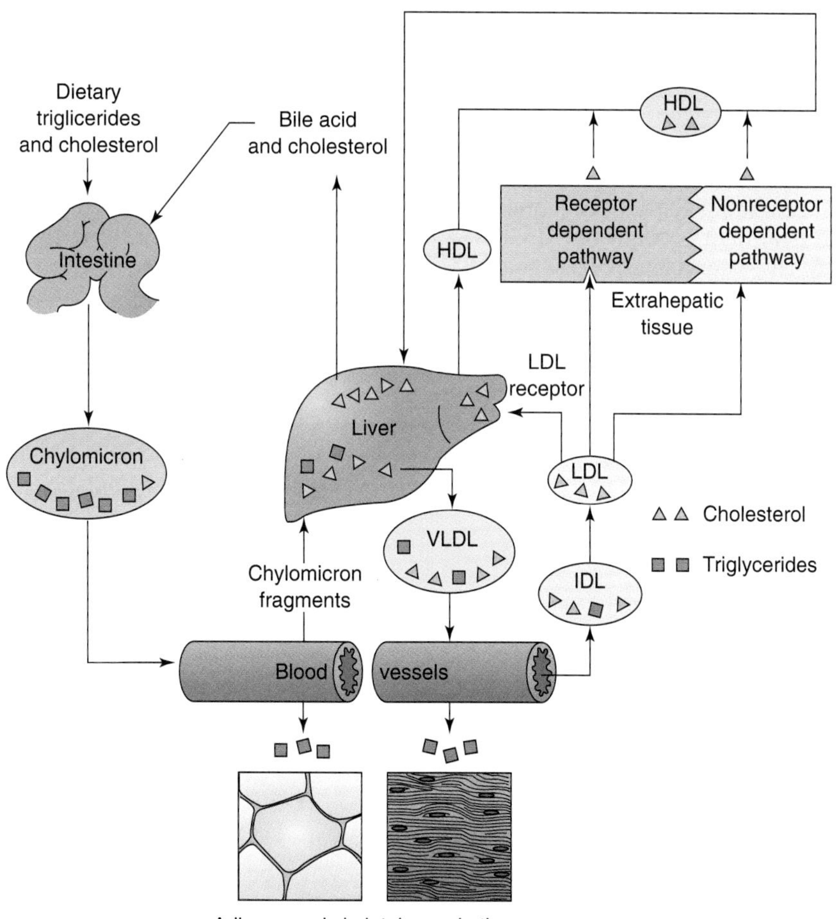

Figure 17-2
Schematic representation of the exogenous and endogenous pathways for triglyceride and cholesterol transport.

cells, and lymphoid cells) also use the receptor-dependent pathway to obtain cholesterol needed for membrane and hormone synthesis. These tissues can control their cholesterol intake by adding or removing LDL receptors. The remaining LDL is removed by nonreceptor-dependent mechanisms, including ingestion by phagocytic monocytes. Macrophage uptake of LDL within the arterial wall can result in the accumulation of insoluble cholesterol ester, the formation of foam cells, and the development of atherosclerosis. When there is a decrease in LDL receptors or when LDL levels exceed receptor availability, the amount of LDL that must be removed by the non–receptor-dependent mechanisms is increased.

HDL is synthesized in the liver and often is referred to as the "good cholesterol." HDL participates in the reverse transport of cholesterol. Epidemiologic studies show an inverse relation between HDL levels and the development of atherosclerosis. It is thought that HDL, which is low in cholesterol and rich in surface phospholipids, facilitates the clearance of cholesterol from atheromatous plaques and transports it to the liver where it may be excreted rather than reused in the formation of VLDL. HDL is also believed to inhibit cellular uptake of LDL. It has been observed that regular exercise and moderate alcohol consumption increase HDL levels. Smoking and diabetes, which are in themselves risk factors for atherosclerosis, are associated with decreased levels of HDL.

Hypercholesteremia

According to the guidelines developed by the National Cholesterol Education Program's Expert Panel on Detection, Evaluation, and Treatment of High Blood Cholesterol in Adults, a blood cholesterol level of less than 200 mg/dl is considered desirable; levels between 200 and 239 mg/dl are borderline-high; and levels equal to or greater than 240 mg/dl are high. HDL levels of less than 35 mg/dl are considered a risk factor.[5]

Serum cholesterol levels may be elevated as a result of an increase in any of the lipoproteins—the chylomicrons, VLDL, IDL, LDL, or HDL. The commonly used classification system for hyperlipidemia is based on the type of lipoprotein involved (Table 17–1). Three factors—nutrition, genetics, and metabolic diseases—can raise blood lipid levels. Most cases of elevated levels of cholesterol are probably multifactorial. Some persons may have increased sensitivity to dietary cholesterol; others have a lack of LDL receptors; and still others have an altered synthesis of the apoproteins, including oversynthesis of apoprotein B-100, the major apoprotein in LDL.

Hypercholesteremia can be classified as primary or secondary hypercholesterolemia. Primary hypercholesteremia describes elevated cholesterol levels that develop independent of other health problems or life style behaviors. Secondary hypercholesterolemia is associated with other health problems and behaviors.

Many types of *primary hypercholesterolemia* have a genetic basis. There may be a defective synthesis of the apoproteins, a lack of receptors, defective receptors, or defects in the handling of cholesterol within the cell that are genetically determined. For example, the LDL receptor is deficient or defective in the genetic disorder known as *familial hypercholesterolemia* (type IIA). This autosomal dominant type of hyperlipoproteinemia results from a mutation in the gene specifying the receptor for LDL. Because most of the circulating cholesterol is removed by receptor-dependent mechanisms, blood cholesterol levels are markedly elevated in persons with this disorder. The disorder is probably one of the most common of all mendelian disorders; the frequency of heterozygotes is 1 in 500 persons in the general population.[2] Heterozygotes have a twofold to threefold eleva-

TABLE 17–1

Classification of Hyperlipidproteinemias and Their Genetic Basis

Type	Familiar Name	Lipoprotein abnormality	Known underlying genetic defects
1	Exogenous dietary hypertriglyceridemia	Elevated chylomicrons and triglycerides	Mutation in lipoprotein lipase gene
2a	Familial hypercholesterolemia	Elevated LDL-cholesterol	Mutation in LDL receptor gene or in apoprotein B gene
2b	Combined hyperlipidemia	Elevated LDL, VLDL, and triglycerides	Mutation in LDL receptor gene or apoprotein B gene
3	Remnant hyperlipidemia	Increased remnants (chylomicrons), IDL triglycerides, and cholesterol	Mutation in apolipoprotein E gene
4	Endogenous hypertriglyceridemia	Elevated VLDL and triglycerides	Unknown
5	Mixed hypertriglyceridemia	Elevated VLDL, chylomicrons, cholesterol, triglycerides greatly elevated	Mutation in apolipoprotein CII gene

(Data developed from Cotran R.S., Kumar V., Robbins S.L. [1994] *Robbins pathologic basis of disease* [5th ed., pp. 481–82], Philadelphia: W.B. Saunders, and Gotto A.M. [1988]. Lipoprotein metabolism and etiology of hyperlipidemia. *Hospital Practice,* 23 (Suppl 1), 4)

tion of plasma cholesterol levels; in homozygotes, the elevation may be fivefold or greater. Although heterozygotes commonly have an elevated cholesterol level from birth, they do not develop symptoms until adult life, when they develop xanthomas (*i.e.*, cholesterol deposits) along the tendons and atherosclerosis. Myocardial infarction before age 40 is common. Homozygotes are much more severely affected; they develop cutaneous xanthomas in childhood and may develop myocardial infarction by age 20.[2]

Causes of *secondary hyperlipoproteinemia* include obesity with high-caloric intake and diabetes mellitus. High-calorie diets increase the production of VLDL, with triglyceride elevation and high conversion of VLDL to LDL. Excess ingestion of cholesterol may reduce the formation of LDL receptors and thereby decrease LDL removal. Diets that are high in triglycerides and saturated fats increase cholesterol synthesis and suppress LDL receptor activity. In diabetes mellitus, metabolic derangements cause an elevation of lipoproteins.

Measures to Control Blood Cholesterol Levels. The Expert Panel on Detection, Evaluation, and Treatment of High Blood Cholesterol in Adults recommends that all adults 20 years of age and older have their blood cholesterol level measured at least once every 5 years.[5] HDL levels should be measured at the same time. These measurements may be made in the nonfasting state. It is particularly important that persons at high risk, such as those with a strong family history of coronary heart disease, be tested. This recommendation applies to children and adult family members. In persons with cholesterol levels above 240 mg/dl, repeat measurements of serum cholesterol along with lipoprotein analysis may be indicated. LDL cholesterol can be estimated using this approach. A subsequent recommendation by the American College of Physicians recommends that the ages for initial cholesterol screening be raised from 20 to 35 years for men and to 45 years for women unless there is evidence of a familial lipoprotein disorder or at least other characteristics that increase the risk of coronary heart disease.[6]

Management of Hyperlipidemia. The management of hypercholesterolemia focuses on dietary and lifestyle modifications; when these are unsuccessful, pharmacologic treatment may be necessary. The second report of the Expert Panel on Detection, and Treatment of High Blood Cholesterol in Adults (Adult Treatment Panel II) continues to identify reduction in LDL as the primary target for cholesterol-lowering therapy.[7] The Panel recommended increased emphasis on absolute risk of coronary heart disease as a guide to type and intensity of therapy; more attention to increasing HDL levels; and increased emphasis on physical activity and weight loss as components in the dietary treatment of high blood cholesterol.

Three elements affect dietary cholesterol and its lipoprotein fractions: excess caloric intake, saturated fats, and cholesterol. Excess calories consistently lower HDL and less consistently elevate LDL. Saturated fats in the diet can strongly influence cholesterol levels. Each 1% of saturated fat relative to caloric intake increases the cholesterol level an average of 2.8 mg/dl.[8] Depending on individual differences, it raises the VLDL and the LDL. Dietary cholesterol tends to increase LDL cholesterol. On average, each 100 mg/dl of ingested cholesterol raises the serum cholesterol 8 to 10 mg/dl.[8]

Lipid-lowering drugs ultimately work by affecting cholesterol production, increasing intravascular breakdown, or removing cholesterol from the bloodstream. Drugs that act directly to decrease cholesterol levels also have the beneficial effect of further lowering cholesterol levels by stimulating the production of additional LDL receptors. Unless lipid levels are severely elevated, it is recommended that a minimum of six months intensive diet therapy be undertaken before considering drug therapy.[7]

Four types of medications are available for treating hypercholesterolemia: bile acid–binding resins, niacin and its congeners, HMG-CoA reductase inhibitors, and fibric acid agents. Estrogen replacement therapy may be used as a possible alternative or adjunct to drug therapy in postmenopausal women. The *bile acid–binding resins*, cholestyramine and colestipol, bind and sequester cholesterol-containing bile acids in the intestine and prevent the reabsorption of cholesterol by way of the chylomicrons. *Nicotinic acid*, a niacin congener, blocks the synthesis and release of VLDL by the liver, thereby lowering not only VLDL levels but IDL and LDL levels as well. *Inhibitors of HMG-CoA reductase* (i.e., statins), a key enzyme in the cholesterol biosynthetic pathway, can reduce or block the hepatic synthesis of cholesterol. The *fibric acid derivatives*, clofibrate and gemfibrozil, decrease the synthesis of VLDL from chylomicron fragments and enhance the intravascular lipolysis of VLDL and IDL. Because many of these drugs have significant adverse effects, they usually are used only in persons with significant hyperlipidemia that cannot be controlled by other means, such as diet.

Atherosclerosis

Atherosclerosis is a type of arteriosclerosis or hardening of the arteries. The term *atherosclerosis*, which comes from the Greek word *atheros* (meaning gruel or paste) and *sclerosis* (meaning hardness), is characterized by the formation of fibrofatty lesions in the intimal lining of the large and medium-sized arteries such as the aorta and its branches, the coronary arteries, and the large vessels that supply the brain. Of these, the coronaries are the most commonly affected arteries.

Although there has been a gradual decline in deaths from atherosclerosis over the past several decades, coronary heart disease remains the leading cause of death among men and women in the United States.[1] The reported decline in death rate probably reflects new and improved methods of medical treatment and improved health care practices resulting from an increased public awareness of the factors that predispose to the development of this disorder.

Atherosclerosis begins as an insidious process, and clinical manifestations of the disease typically do not become evident for 20 to 40 years or longer. Fibrous plaques commonly begin to appear in the arteries of Americans in their twenties. Necropsy findings from 300 American soldiers (average age of 22) killed during the Korean war indicated that 77% had gross evidence of atherosclerosis.[9]

Risk Factors

The cause or causes of atherosclerosis have not been determined with certainty. Epidemiologic studies have, however, identified predisposing risk factors, which are listed in Chart 17–1.[9] In terms of health care behaviors, some of these risk factors can be affected by a change in health behavior and others cannot.

The major risk factor for atherosclerosis is hypercholesteremia. Nonlipid risk factors such as increasing age, family history of premature coronary heart disease, and male sex cannot be changed. The tendency to develop atherosclerosis appears to run in families. Persons who come from families with a strong history of heart disease or stroke due to atherosclerosis are at greater risk for developing atherosclerosis than those with a negative family history. Several genetically determined alterations in lipoprotein and cholesterol metabolism have been identified, and it seems likely that others will be identified in the future. The incidence of atherosclerosis increases with age. Men (after age 45) are at greater risk for developing coronary heart disease than are women; even though the death rate of women increases after menopause (after age 55 without estrogen replacement therapy), it never reaches that of men.

The major risk factors that can be affected by a change in health care behaviors include cigarette smoking, hypertension, high blood cholesterol levels, and diabetes mellitus. Cigarette smoking is closely linked with coronary heart disease and sudden death. One hypothesis is that components of cigarette smoke may be toxic, causing oxidative insult and damage to the endothelial lining of blood vessels.[10] Endothelial dysfunction may be worsened by cigarette smoke, which is why cessation of smoking by high-risk individuals is often followed within a few years by reduced risk of ischemic heart disease.

High blood pressure and high blood cholesterol levels often can be controlled with a change in health care behaviors and medications. There is evidence that elevated serum cholesterol not only contributes to development of atherosclerotic lesions that block arteries, but also interferes with vessel relaxation.[10,11] Observational research indicates that a linear relation exists between serum cholesterol levels and coronary heart disease; a 10% decrease in serum cholesterol is associated with a 20% decrease in coronary heart disease.[12]

The association between coronary heart disease and contributing or "soft" factors is not as convincing as for the established risk factors. These "soft" risk factors commonly are linked with the established and other contributing risk factors. For example, obesity and physical inactivity often are observed in the same person. Both conditions are reported to bring about elevations in blood lipid levels. Likewise, major risk factors such as cigarette smoking are closely associated with stress and personality patterns. Diabetes mellitus (type 2) typically develops in middle-aged persons and those who are overweight. Diabetes elevates blood lipid levels and otherwise increases the risk of atherosclerosis (see Chapter 36). Controlling other risk factors is particularly important in those with diabetes.

CHART 17-1
Risk Factors in Coronary Heart Disease Other Than Low-Density Lipoproteins

Positive Risk Factors

Age
- Men: ≥45 years
- Women: ≥55 years or premature menopause without estrogen replacement therapy

Family history of premature coronary heart disease (definite myocardial infarction or sudden death before 55 years of age in father or other male first-degree relative, or before 65 years of age in mother or other female first-degree relative)

Current cigarette smoking

Hypertension (≥140/90 mm Hg* or on antihypertensive medication)

Low HDL cholesterol (≤35 mg/dL*)

Diabetes mellitus

Negative Risk Factor

High HDL cholesterol (≥60 mg/dL)

HDL, high-density lipoprotein.
*Confirmed by measurements on several occasions.
(Modified from National Cholesterol Program. [1994]. Second report of the Expert Panel on Detection, Evaluation, and Treatment of High Blood Pressure in Adults (Adult Treatment Panel II). *Circulation* 89 (3), 1350)

Mechanisms of Development

Fatty streaks are thin, flat yellow streaks in the intima (Fig. 17–3). They consist of macrophages and smooth muscle cells that have become distended with lipid to form foam cells. Fatty streaks appear in the aortas of some children younger than 1 year and all children by 10 years.[2] This occurs regardless of geographic setting, sex, or race. Fatty streaks in the coronary arteries begin to appear in adolescence. There is controversy about whether fatty streaks are precursors of atherosclerotic lesions.

Atherosclerotic lesions are characterized by the accumulation of intracellular and extracellular lipids, proliferation of vascular smooth muscle cells, and for-

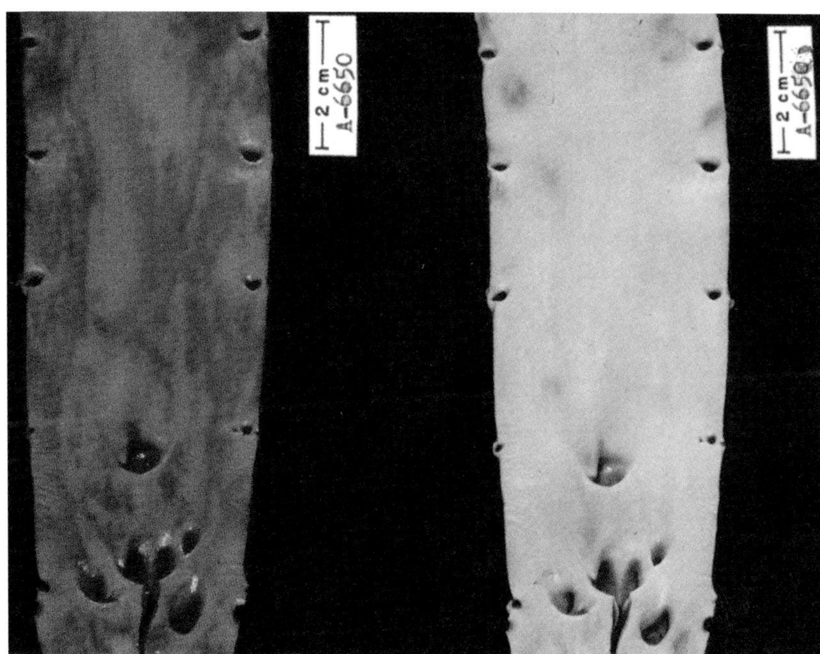

Figure 17-3
Fatty streak of atherosclerosis. The aorta of the young man shows numerous fatty streaks on the luminal surface when stained with Sudan red. The unstained specimen is shown on the right.

mation of scar tissue and connective tissue proteins. The lesions begin as a gray to pearly white elevated thickening of the vessel intima with a core of extracellular lipid (mainly cholesterol, which usually is complexed to proteins) covered by a fibrous cap of connective tissue and smooth muscle. More advanced lesions contain hemorrhage, ulceration, and scar tissue deposits. As the lesions increase in size, they encroach on the lumen of the artery and eventually may occlude the vessel or predispose to thrombus formation, causing a reduction of blood flow (Fig. 17–4). Because blood flow is related to the fourth power of the radius, reduction in blood flow becomes more severe as the disease progresses.

Although the risk factors associated with atherosclerosis have been identified through epidemiologic studies, many unanswered questions remain regarding the mechanisms by which these risk factors contribute to the development of atherosclerosis. There is increasing evidence suggesting that atherosclerosis is at least partially the result of endothelial injury, lipid (*i.e.*, LDL and cholesterol) infiltration, recruitment of inflammatory cells (*i.e.*, predominantly monocytes and T lymphocytes), and smooth muscle proliferation. The vascular endothelial layer, which consists of a single layer of cells with cell-to-cell attachments, normally serves as a selective barrier that protects the subendothelial layers by interacting with blood cells and other blood components.

One hypothesis of plaque formation is that injury to the endothelial vessel layer is the initiating factor in the development of atherosclerosis. Endothelial injury allows monocytes, platelets, cholesterol, and other blood components to come in contact with and stimulate abnormal proliferation of smooth muscle cells and connective tissue within the vessel wall (Fig. 17–5). A number of factors are regarded as possible injurious agents, including products associated with smoking, immune mechanisms, and mechanical stress such as that associated with hypertension. If the injury is a single event, the damage usually is reversible. However, if the factors that led to vessel damage persists, there is less time for healing to occur, and the lesion may become chronic.

Evidence also suggests that locally modified LDLs may act as cofactors that are necessary for growth and proliferation of vascular smooth muscle cells.[2] Interactions between the endothelial layer of the vessel wall and white blood cells, particularly the monocytes (blood macrophages), normally occur throughout life; these

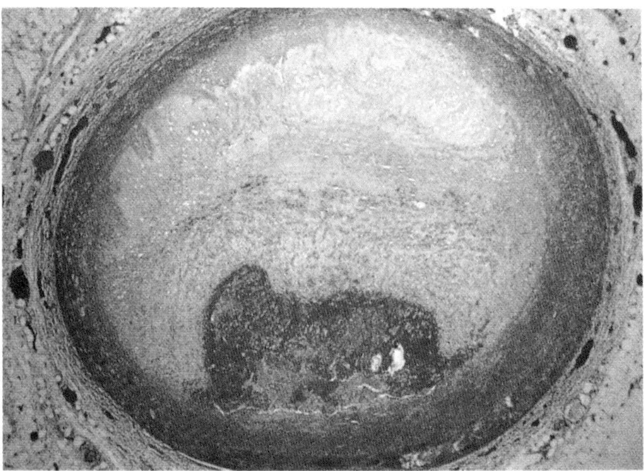

Figure 17-4
Atherosclerotic coronary occlusion. A coronary artery of a patient who died from an acute myocardial infarction shows severe atherosclerosis and a recent thrombus in the narrowed lumen.

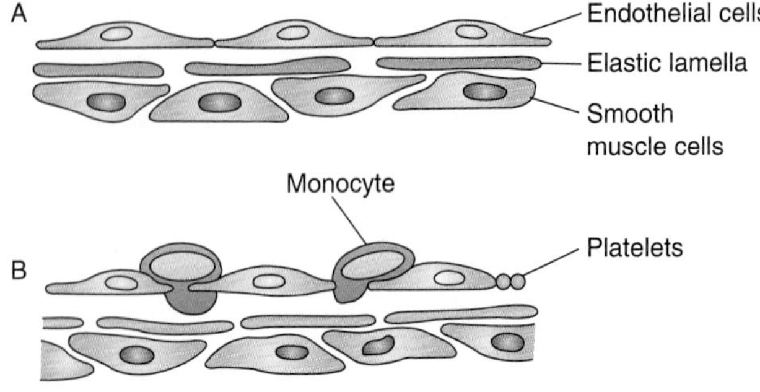

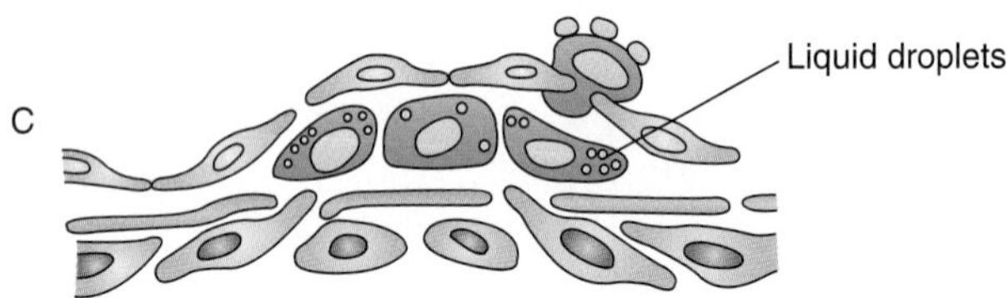

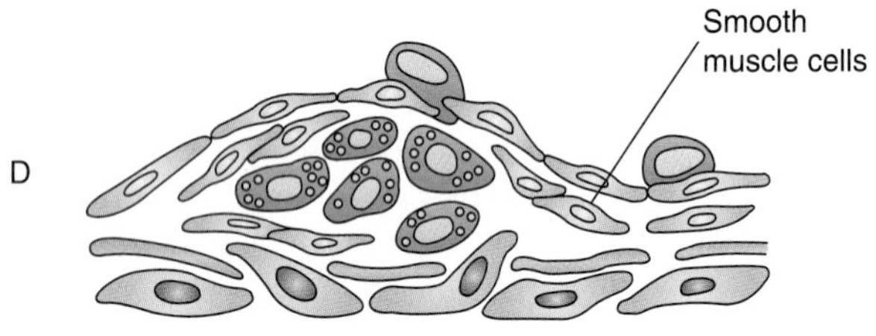

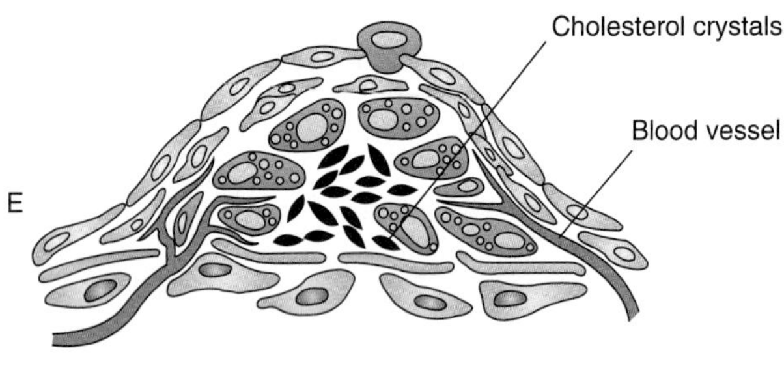

Figure 17-5
Process in the response to injury hypothesis. (**A**) Normal. (**B**) Endothelial injury with adhesion if monocytes and platelets (latter to denuded endothelium). (**C**) Migration of monocytes (from lumen) and smooth muscle cells (from media) into intima. (**D**) Smooth muscle cell proliferation in the intima. (**E**) Well-developed plaque. (From Cotram RS, Vumar V, Robbins S. [1994]. *Robbins' pathologic basis of disease* [5th ed.]. Philadelphia: WB Saunders.)

interactions increase when blood cholesterol levels are elevated. One of the earliest responses to elevated cholesterol levels is the attachment of monocytes to the endothelium.[2] The monocytes have been observed to move through the cell-to-cell attachments of the endothelial layer into the subendothelial spaces, where they ingest lipid and in the process become foam cells (Fig. 17–6). Foam cells, which are present in all stages of atherosclerotic plaque formation, are thought to promote growth factors that modulate the proliferation of smooth muscle cells and deposition of extracellular matrix in the lesions.

Clinical Manifestations

The clinical manifestations of atherosclerosis depend on the vessels involved and the extent of vessel obstruction. Atherosclerotic lesions produce their effects through narrowing of the vessel and production of ischemia; sudden vessel obstruction due to plaque hemorrhage or rupture; thrombosis and formation of emboli resulting from damage to the vessel endothelium; and aneurysm formation due to weakening of the vessel wall.[2] In larger vessels such as the aorta, the important complications are those of thrombus formation and weakening of the vessel wall. In medium-sized arteries such as the coronaries and cerebral arteries, ischemia and infarction due to vessel occlusion is more common. Although atherosclerosis can affect any organ or tissue, the arteries supplying the heart, brain, kidneys, lower extremities, and small intestine are most frequently involved.

Vasculitis

The vasculitides are group of vascular disorders that cause inflammatory injury and necrosis of the blood vessel wall (*i.e.*, vasculitis). The vasculitides, which are a common pathway for tissue and organ involvement in many different disease conditions, involve the endothelial cells and smooth muscle cells of the arterial wall.[13,14] Because they may also affect veins and capillaries, the terms *vasculitis, angiitis,* and *arteritis* are often used interchangeably. Vasculitis may result from direct injury to the vessel, infectious agents, immune processes, or secondary to other disease states such as systemic lupus erythematosus (Fig. 17–7). Physical agents such as cold (*i.e.*, frostbite), irradiation (*i.e.*, sunburn), mechanical injury, and toxins may secondarily cause vessel damage, often leading to necrosis of the vessels.

The vasculitides are commonly classified based on clinical findings, pathology, and prognosis. One classification system divides the conditions into four groups (see Table 17–2).[13] Group I vasculitides produce necrotizing damage to small and medium-sized muscular arteries of major organ systems. Group II vasculitides involve hypersensitivity reactions that produce a venulitis. They commonly involve the skin and are often a complication of an underlying disease (*i.e.*, vasculitis associated with neoplasms or connective tissue disease) and exposure to environmental agents (*i.e.*, serum sickness and urticarial vasculitis; see Chapter 12). Group III vasculitides involve large elastic arteries; they are called giant cell arterides because they involve infiltration of the vessel wall with giant cells and mononuclear cells. Group IV consists of miscellaneous vasculitides; it includes conditions such as Kawasaki syndrome (see Chapter 19) and thromboangiitis obliterans (discussed with arterial diseases of the

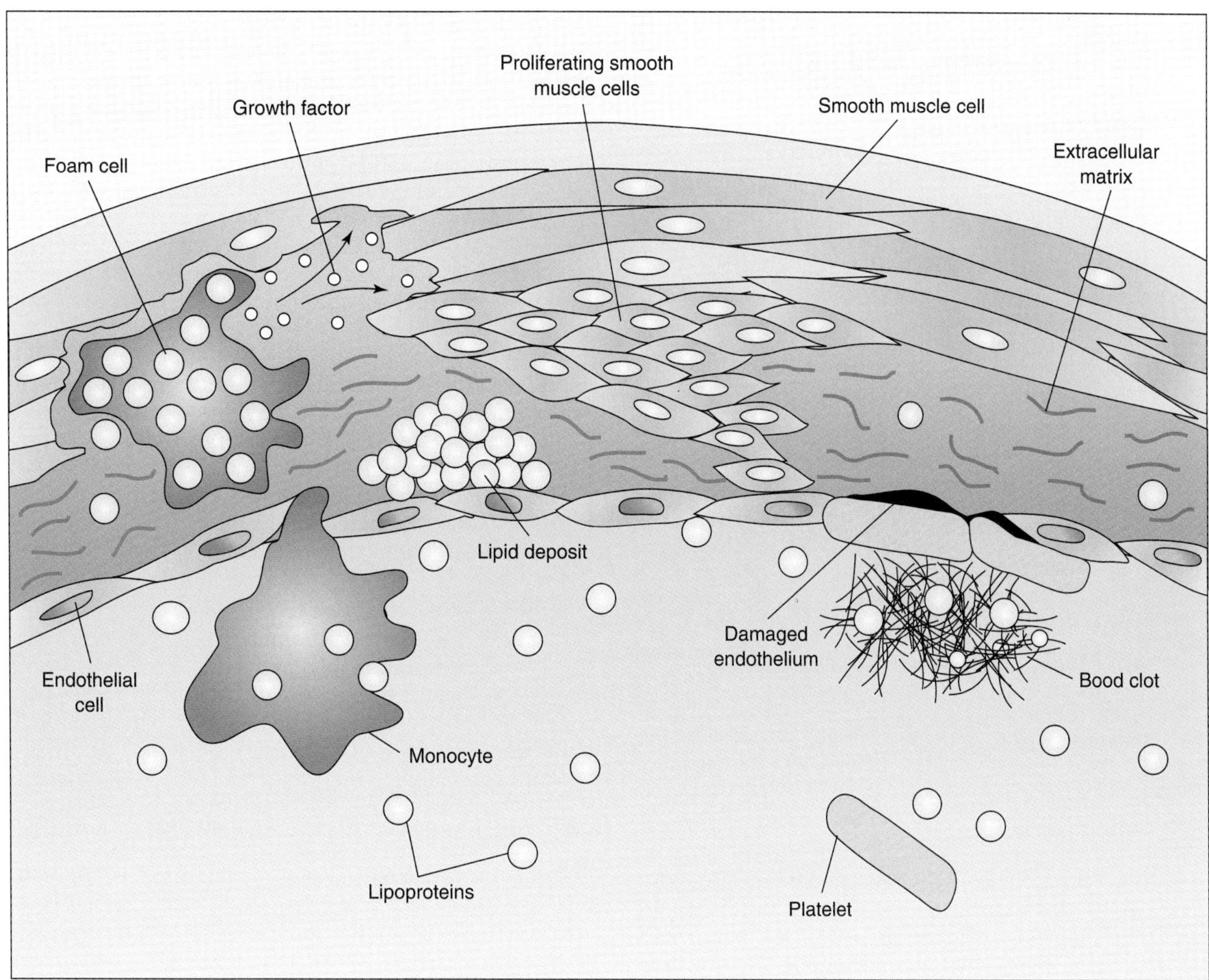

Figure 17-6
Role of excess lipoprotein and monocyte in the pathogenesis of atherosclerosis. Elevated levels of cholesterol-carrying lipoproteins cause monocytes to attach to and move through cell-to-cell attachmnents in the endothelium. Monocytes that consume excess lipoproteins become foam cells, which release growth factors that encourage proliferation of smooth muscle cells and extracellular matrix, leading to atherosclerotic plaque formation, endothelial injury, and blood clot formation.

extremities). Two examples of vasculitides are included in this section: polyarteritis nodosa and giant cell temporal arteritis.

Polyarteritis Nodosa

Polyarteritis nodosa, so named because of the numerous nodules found along the course of muscular arteries, is a primary multisystem inflammatory disease of small and medium-sized blood vessels, especially those of the kidney, liver, intestine, peripheral nerve, skin, and muscle. The disease is seen more commonly in men than women.

The cause of the polyarteritis nodosa remains unknown. It can occur in drug abusers and may be associated with use of certain drugs such as allopurinol and the sulfonamides. There is an association between polyarteritis nodosa and hepatitis B infection, with 10% to 40% of persons with disease having antibodies to hepatitis in their serum. Other associations include serous otitis media, hairy cell leukemia, and hyposensitization therapy for allergies. Persons with connective tissue diseases such as systemic lupus erythematosus, rheumatoid arthritis, and primary Sjögren's syndrome may develop manifestations similar to those of primary polyarteritis nodosa.

Manifestations. The onset of polyarteritis nodosa is usually abrupt with complaints of anorexia, weight loss, fever, and fatigue often accompanied by signs of organ involvement. The kidney is the most frequently affected organ, and hypertension is a common manifestation of the disorder. Gastrointestinal involvement may manifest

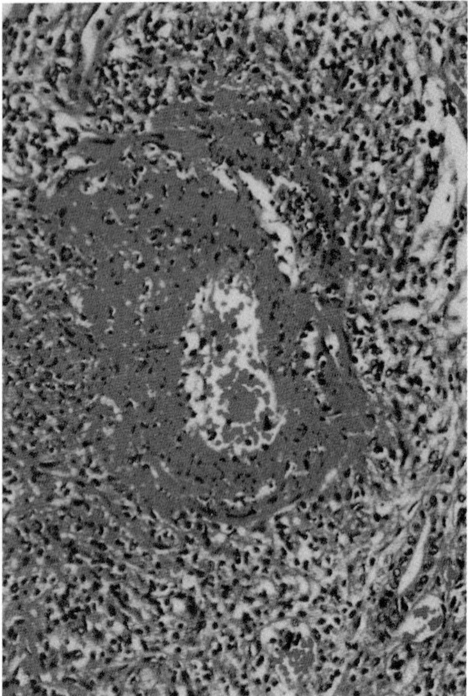

Figure 17-7
Polyarteritis nodosa. The intense inflammatory cell infiltrate in the arterial wall and surrounding connective tissue is associated with fibrinoid necrosis and disruption of the vessel wall.

as abdominal pain, nausea, vomiting, or diarrhea. Myalgia, arthralgia, and arthritis are common as are peripheral neuropathies such as parasthesias, pain, and weakness. Central nervous system complications include thrombotic and hemorrhagic stroke. Cardiac manifestations result from involvement of the coronary arteries. Skin lesions may also occur and are highly variable. They include reddish blue mottled areas of discoloration of the skin of the extremities called *livedo reticularis*, purpura (*i.e.*, black and blue discoloration from bleeding into the skin), urticaria (*i.e.*, hives), and ulcers.

Diagnosis and Treatment. Laboratory findings, although variable, include an elevated erythrocyte sedimentation rate, leukocytosis, anemia, and signs of organ involvement such as hematuria and abnormal liver function tests. The diagnosis is confirmed through biopsy specimens demonstrating necrotizing vasculitis of the small and large arteries. Treatment involves use of high-dose corticosteroid therapy and often cytotoxic immunosuppressant agents (*e.g.*, azathioprine, cyclophosphamide). Before the availability of corticosteroids and immunosuppressive agents, the disease was commonly fatal. With the use of these agents, the 5-year survival rate is more than 80%.[14] After the disease is under control, treatment is usually continued for at least 1 year and then gradually tapered. Intravenous immunoglobulin is being used with increasing frequency and with very promising results.

Giant Cell Temporal Arteritis

Temporal arteritis (*i.e.*, giant cell arteritis) is a focal inflammatory condition of medium and large size arteries. It predominantly affects branches of arteries originating from the aortic arch, including the superficial temporal, vertebral, ophthalmic, and posterior ciliary arteries. The disorder progresses to involve the entire artery wall with focal necrosis and granulomatous inflammation involving multinucleated giant cells. It is more common in elderly persons, with a 2:1 female to male ratio. The cause is unknown, although an autoimmune origin has been suggested.

Manifestations. The disorder is often insidious in onset and may be heralded by the sudden onset of headache, tenderness over the artery, swelling and redness of the overlying skin, and blurred vision or diplopia, and facial pain. Almost one half of affected persons have systemic involvement in the form of polymyalgia rheumatica (see Chapter 47).

Diagnosis and Treatment. Diagnosis is based on the clinical manifestations, a characteristically elevated erythrocyte sedimentation rate, and temporal artery biopsy. Treatment includes use of corticosteroids. Before persons with the disorder were treated with corticosteroids, blindness developed in almost 80% of cases.[14]

Arterial Disease of the Extremities

Disorders of the circulation in the extremities are often referred to as *peripheral vascular disorders*. In many respects, the disorders that affect arteries in the extremities is the same as those affecting the coronary and cerebral arteries in that they produce ischemia, pain, impaired function, and in some cases infarction and tissue necrosis. Not only are the effects similar, but the pathologic conditions that impair circulation in the extremities are identical. This section focuses on acute arterial occlusion of the extremities, atherosclerotic occlusive disease, thromboangiitis obliterans, and Raynaud's disease and phenomenon.

Acute Arterial Occlusion

Acute arterial occlusion is a sudden event that interrupts arterial flow to the affected tissues or organ. Most acute arterial occlusions are the result of an embolus or a thrombus. Rarely, the tips of catheters that have been inserted into a vessel can break off and become emboli. Although much less common than emboli and thrombus, trauma or arterial spasm caused by arterial cannulation can be another cause of acute arterial occlusion.

An *embolus* is a freely moving particle such a blood clot that breaks loose and travels in the larger vessels of the circulation until lodging in a smaller vessel and occluding blood flow. Most emboli arise in the heart and are caused by conditions that cause blood clots to develop on the wall of a heart chamber or valve surface. Emboli are usually a complication of heart disease:

TABLE 17-2

Examples of Vasculitides Classified by Group and Characteristics

Group	Examples	Characteristics
Group I—systemic necrotizing vasculitides	Polyartertis nodosa Rheumatoid vaculitis	Affects medium-sized vessels of major organ systems; usually associated with an underlying disease or environmental agent
	Allergic angiitis and granulmatosis (Churg-Straus syndrome)	Churg-Strauss syndrome involves eosinophil-rich and granulomatous inflammation that affects the respiratory tract and is associated with asthma and allergic rhinitis.
Group II—hypersensitivity vasculitides	Serum sickness Vasculits associated with infectious diseases (*e.g.*, bacterial endocarditis) Hepatitis B Vasulitis associated with neoplasms Vasculitis associated with connective tissue disease Urticarial vasculitis	Produces a venulitis with endothelial swelling, red blood cell extravasation, and fibrinoid necrosis Predominance of skin involvement with sporodic damage to major organ systems Thought to be mediated by immunologic mechanisms
Group III—giant cell arteriitis	Temporal arteritis	Affects large elastic arteries; infiltration of vessel wall with giant cells and mononuclear cells, producing periarteritis with dramatic ischemic consequences Temporal arteriitis affects extracranial branches of the carotid artery and often affects the temporal artery.
	Takayasu's arteriitis	Takayasu's arteriitis affects the aorta and its branches.
Group IV—miscellaneous	Thromboangiitis obliterans	
	Kawasaki syndrome	Kawasaki syndrome is an arteritis involving large, medium-sized, and small arteries (frequently the coronaries) and is associated with mucocutaneous lymph node syndrome, usually in young children.

(Developed from Pariser K.M., Wolff S.M. [1992]. The clinical spectrum of vasculitis. In Loscalzo J., Creager M.A., Dzau V.J. [Eds.]. *Vascular medicine: A textbook of vascular biology and disease* [pp. 1012–1013]. Boston: Little, Brown, and Cotran R.S., Kumar V., Robbins S.L. [1994]. *Pathologic basis of disease* [4th ed., pp. 489–499]. Philadelphia, W.B. Saunders)

ischemic heart disease with or without infarction, atrial fibrillation, or rheumatic heart disease. Prosthetic heart valves can be another source of emboli. Other types of emboli are fat emboli that originate from bone marrow of fractured bones, air emboli from the lung, and amniotic fluid emboli that develop during childbirth.

A *thrombus* is a blood clot that forms on the wall of a vessel and continues to grow until reaching a size that obstructs blood flow. Atherosclerosis, which causes narrowing of and disruption of the intimal lining of affected vessels, is a frequent cause of thrombotic occlusion.

Manifestations. The signs and symptoms of acute arterial occlusion depend on the artery involved and the adequacy of the collateral circulation. Emboli tend to lodge in bifurcations of the major arteries, including the aorta and iliac, femoral, and popliteal arteries. Occlusion in an extremity causes sudden onset of acute pain with numbness, tingling, weakness, pallor, and coldness. There often is a sharp line of demarcation between the oxygenated tissue above the line of obstruction and that below the line of obstruction. Pulses are absent below the level of the occlusion. These changes are rapidly followed by cyanosis, mottling, and loss of sensory, reflex, and motor function. Tissue dies unless blood flow is restored.

Diagnosis and Treatment. Diagnosis of acute arterial occlusion is based on signs of impaired blood flow. It uses visual assessment, palpation of pulses, and methods to assess blood flow. Treatment of acute arterial occlusion is aimed at restoring blood flow. Thrombolytic therapy (*i.e.*, streptokinase or tissue plasminogen activator) may be used in an attempt to dissolve the clot. Anticoagulant therapy (*i.e.*, heparin) usually is given to prevent extension of the embolus. Application of heat and cold should be avoided, and the extremity should be protected from injury resulting from hard surfaces and overlying bedclothes. An embolectomy—surgical removal of the embolus—may be indicated.

Atherosclerotic Occlusive Disease

Atherosclerosis is an important cause of peripheral vascular disease and is seen most commonly in the vessels of the lower extremities. The condition is sometimes referred to as *arteriosclerosis obliterans*. The superficial femoral and popliteal arteries are the most commonly affected vessels. When lesions develop in the lower leg and foot, the tibial, common peroneal, or pedal vessels are the arteries most commonly affected. The disease is seen most commonly in men in their sixties and seventies.[15] The risk factors for this disorder are similar to those for atherosclerosis. Cigarette smoking contributes to the progress of the atherosclerosis of the lower extremities and to the development of symptoms of ischemia. Persons with diabetes mellitus develop more extensive and more rapidly progressive vascular disease than do nondiabetic individuals.

Manifestations. As with atherosclerosis in other locations, the signs and symptoms of vessel occlusion are gradual. Usually, there is at least a 50% narrowing of the vessel before symptoms of ischemia arise. The primary symptom of chronic obstructive arterial disease is intermittent claudication or pain with walking. Typically, persons with the disorder complain of calf pain, because the gastrocnemius muscle has the highest oxygen consumption of any muscle group in the leg during walking. Some persons may complain of a vague aching feeling or numbness, rather than pain. Other activities such as swimming, bicycling, and climbing stairs use other muscle groups and may not incite the same degree of discomfort as walking. Other signs of ischemia include atrophic changes and thinning of the skin and subcutaneous tissues of the lower leg and diminution in the size of the leg muscles. The foot often is cool, and the popliteal and pedal pulses are weak or absent. Limb color blanches with elevation of the leg because of the effects of gravity on perfusion pressure and becomes deep red when the leg is in the dependent position because of an autoregulatory increase in blood flow and a gravitational increase in perfusion pressure.

When blood flow is reduced to the extent that it no longer meets the minimal needs of resting muscle and nerves, ischemic pain at rest, ulceration, and gangrene develop. As tissue necrosis develops there is typically severe pain in the region of skin breakdown, which is worse at night with limb elevation and is improved with standing.[15].

Diagnosis and Treatment. Diagnostic methods include inspection of the limbs for signs of chronic low-grade ischemia such a subcutaneous atrophy, brittle toenails, hair loss, pallor, coolness, or dependent rubor. Palpation of the femoral, popliteal, posterior tibial, and dorsalis pedis pulses allows for an estimation of the level and degree of obstruction. The ratio of ankle to arm (*i.e.*, tibial and brachial arteries) systolic blood pressure is used detect significant obstruction, with a ratio of less than 0.9 indicating occlusion. Normally, systolic pressure in the ankle exceeds that in the brachial artery, because systolic pressure and pulse pressure tend to increase as the pressure wave moves away from the heart (see Chapter 16). Blood pressures may be taken at various levels on the leg to determine the level of obstruction. A Doppler ultrasound stethoscope may be used for detecting pulses and measuring blood pressure. Ultrasound imaging, radionuclide imaging, and contrast angiography may also be used as diagnostic methods.

The tissues of extremities affected by atherosclerosis are easily injured and slow to heal. Treatment includes measures directed at protection of the affected tissues and preservation of functional capacity. Walking (slowly) to the point of claudication usually is encouraged, because it increases collateral circulation.

Assessment of Arterial Flow In the Extremities

The methods for assessing arterial blood flow and detecting arterial disease include monitoring of capillary refill time and peripheral pulses. Angiography, Doppler ultrasonic flow studies, and magnetic resonance imaging (MRI) may be used for a more definitive diagnosis.

Capillary refill time is an indicator of the efficiency of the microcirculation. It is measured by depressing the nail bed of a finger or toe until the underlying skin blanches. The refill time is normal if the capillary vessels refill within 3 seconds after pressure is released.[25] The volume of the peripheral pulses and capillary refill time are useful indirect methods for assessing peripheral perfusion. Peripheral pulses can be palpated over vessels in the head, neck (*i.e.*, carotid), and extremities. In situations associated with potential vessel spasm or thrombosis, it may be necessary to check only for the presence of pulses. In many situations, however, the pulse volume (weak and thready to strong and bounding) provides useful information about vascular volume and the condition of the arterial circulation. Arterial auscultation is used to listen to the flow of blood with a stethoscope. The term *bruit* is used to describe an audible murmur heard over a peripheral artery. It is caused by turbulent blood flow and is suggestive of obstructive arterial disease.

Doppler ultrasound flow studies use reflected ultrasound waves, which are transmitted back to the skin surface from a blood vessel to determine the direction and velocity of blood flow. Doppler studies can be used to establish the patency of a given blood vessel. They are useful in studying blood flow in the carotid arteries, abdominal vessels, fetal blood vessels, and peripheral blood vessels.

MRI is a noninvasive technique that can be used to study blood flow. The method uses a magnetic filed to align the charges on blood components as they move through blood vessels. The aligned charges emit measurable radiofrequency signals, which can be detected electronically and recorded.

Surgery (*i.e.,* femoropopliteal bypass grafting using a section of saphenous vein) may be indicated in severe cases. In persons with diabetes, the peroneal arteries between the knees and ankles are commonly involved, making revascularization difficult.[15] Thromboendarterectomy with removal of the occluding core of atherosclerotic tissue may be done if the section of diseased vessel is short. Percutaneous transluminal angioplasty, in which a balloon catheter is inserted into the area of stenosis and the balloon inflated to increase vessel diameter, is another form of treatment.

Thromboangiitis Obliterans

Thromboangiitis obliterans (e.g., Buerger's disease) is an inflammatory (*i.e.,* vasculitis) arterial disorder that causes thrombus formation. The disorder affects the medium-sized arteries, usually the plantar and digital vessels in the foot and lower leg. Arteries in the arm and hand may also be affected. Although primarily an arterial disorder, the inflammatory process often extends to involve adjacent veins and nerves. It usually is a disease of men between the ages of 25 and 40 who are heavy cigarette smokers, but it can occur in women. The pathogenesis of Buerger's disease remains speculative, although cigarette smoking and in some instances tobacco chewing seem to be involved. It has been suggested that the tobacco may trigger an immune response in susceptible persons or it may unmask a clotting defect, either of which could incite an inflammatory reaction of the vessel wall.[16]

Manifestations. Pain is the predominant symptom of the disorder. It is usually related to distal arterial ischemia. During the early stages of the disease, there is intermittent claudication in the arch of the foot and the digits. In severe cases, pain is present even when the person is at rest. The impaired circulation increases sensitivity to cold. The peripheral pulses are diminished or absent, and there are changes in the color of the extremity. In moderately advanced cases, the extremity becomes cyanotic when the person assumes a dependent position, and the digits may turn reddish blue even when in a nondependent position. With lack of blood flow, the skin assumes a thin, shiny look and hair growth and skin nutrition suffer. Chronic ischemia causes thick, malformed nails. If the disease continues to progress, tissues eventually ulcerate and gangrenous changes arise that may necessitate amputation.

Diagnosis and Treatment. Diagnostic methods are similar to those for atherosclerotic disease of the lower extremities. As part of the treatment program for thromboangiitis obliterans, it is mandatory that the person stop smoking cigarettes or using tobacco. Other treatment measures are of secondary importance and focus on methods for producing vasodilation and preventing tissue injury. Sympathectomy may be done to alleviate the vasospastic manifestations of the disease.

Raynaud's Disease and Phenomenon

Raynaud's disease or phenomenon is a functional disorder caused by intense vasospasm of the arteries and arterioles in the fingers and, less often, the toes. The disorder is divided into two types: the primary type, called *Raynaud's disease,* occurs without demonstrable cause, and the secondary type, called *Raynaud's phenomenon,* is associated with other disease states or known causes of vasospasm.[17,18]

Vasospasm implies an excessive vasoconstrictor response to stimuli that normally produce only moderate vasoconstriction. In contrast to other regional circulations that are supplied by vasodilator and vasoconstrictor fibers, the cutaneous vessels of the fingers and toes are innervated only by sympathetic vasoconstrictor fibers. In these vessels, vasodilation occurs by withdrawal of sympathetic stimulation. Cooling of specific body parts such as the head, neck, and trunk produces a sympathetic-mediated reduction in digital blood flow, as does emotional stress.

Raynaud's disease is seen in otherwise healthy young women, and it often is precipitated by exposure to cold or by strong emotions and is usually limited to the fingers. It also follows a more benign course than Raynaud's phenomenon, seldom causing tissue necrosis. The cause of vasospasm in primary Raynaud's disease is unknown. Hyperreactivity of the sympathetic nervous system has been suggested as a contributing cause.[19] Raynaud's phenomenon is associated with previous vessel injury, such as frostbite, occupational trauma associated with the use of heavy vibrating tools, collagen diseases, neurologic disorders, and chronic arterial occlusive disorders. Another occupation-related cause is the exposure to alternating hot and cold temperatures such as that experienced by butchers and food preparers.[20] Raynaud's phenomenon often is the first symptom of collagen diseases. It occurs in 80% to 90% of persons with scleroderma and in 10% to 35% of persons with systemic lupus erythematosus.[18]

Manifestations. In Raynaud's disease and Raynaud's phenomenon, ischemia due to vasospasm causes changes in skin color that progress from pallor to cyanosis, a sensation of cold, and changes in sensory perception, such as numbness and tingling. The color changes usually are first noticed in the tips of the fingers, later moving into one or more of the distal phalanges. After the ischemic episode, there is a period of hyperemia with intense redness, throbbing, and paresthesias. The period of hyperemia is followed by a return to normal color. Although all of the fingers are usually affected symmetrically, the involvement may affect only one or two digits. In some cases, only a portion of the digit is affected.

In severe, progressive cases usually associated with Raynaud's phenomenon, trophic changes may develop. The nails may become brittle, and the skin over the tips of the affected fingers may thicken. Nutritional impairment of these structures may give rise to arthritis. Ulceration and superficial gangrene of the fingers, although infrequent, may occur.

Diagnosis and Treatment. The initial diagnosis is based on history of vasospastic attacks supported by other evidence of the disorder. Immersion of the hand in cold water may be used to initiate an attack as an aid to diagnosis. Raynaud's disease is differentiated from Raynaud's phenomenon by excluding secondary disorders known to cause vasospasm.

Treatment measures are directed toward eliminating factors that cause vasospasm and protecting the digits from trauma during an ischemic episode. Abstinence from smoking and protection from cold are priorities. The entire body must be protected from cold, not just the extremities. Avoidance of emotional stress is another important factor in controlling the disorder, because anxiety and stress may precipitate a vascular spasm in predisposed persons. Biofeedback training may be helpful in persons with Raynaud's disease but does not seem to be as effective for those with Raynaud's phenomenon. Vasoconstrictor medications, such as the decongestants contained in allergy and cold preparations, should be avoided. Treatment with vasodilator drugs may be indicated, particularly if episodes are frequent, because frequency encourages the potential for development of thrombosis and gangrene. The calcium-channel blocking drugs (*e.g.*, diltiazem, nifedipine, and nicardipine) decrease the severity and frequency of attacks. Prazosin, an α-adrenergic receptor–blocking drug, may also be used. Surgical interruption of sympathetic nerve pathways (sympathectomy) may be used for persons with severe symptoms.

Aneurysms

An aneurysm is an abnormal localized dilatation of a blood vessel. Aneurysms can occur in arteries and veins, but they are most common in the aorta. There are two types of aneurysms: true aneurysms and false aneurysms. A *true aneurysm* is one in which the aneurysm is bounded by a complete vessel wall. The blood in a true aneurysm remains within the vascular compartment. A *false* or *pseudo aneurysm* represents a localized rupture or tear in the inner wall of the artery with formation of an extravascular hematoma that causes vessel enlargement. Unlike true aneurysms, false aneurysms are bounded only by the outer layers of the vessel wall or supporting tissues.

Aneurysms can assume several forms and may be classified according to their cause, location, and anatomic features (Fig. 17–8). A *berry aneurysm* consists of a

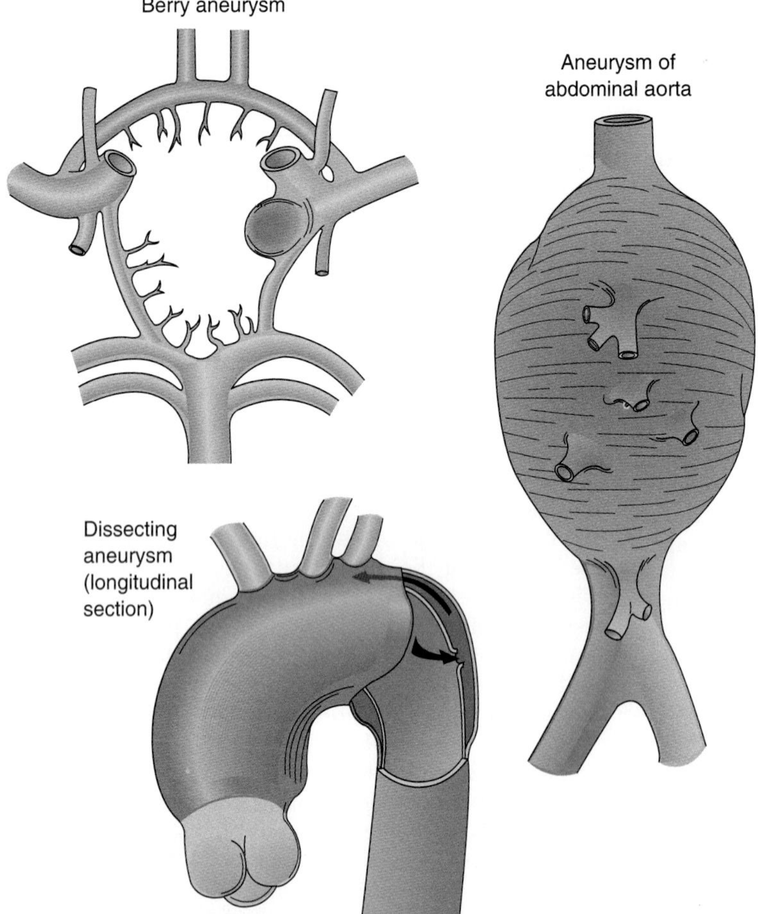

Figure 17-8
Three forms of aneurysms—berry aneurysm in the circle of WIllis, fusiform-type aneurysm of the abdominal aorta, and a dissecting aortic aneurysm.

small, spherical dilatation of the vessel and seldom is larger than 1.5 cm in diameter.[2] This type of aneurysm usually is found in the circle of Willis in the cerebral circulation. A *fusiform aneurysm* involves the entire circumference of the vessel and is characterized by a gradual and progressive dilatation of the vessel. These aneurysms, which vary in diameter (up to 20 cm) and length, may involve the entire ascending and transverse portions of the thoracic aorta or may extend over large segments of the abdominal aorta. A *saccular aneurysm* extends over part of the circumference of the vessel and appears saclike. They can vary from 5 to 20 cm in diameter and are often partially or completely filled by thrombi.[2] A *dissecting aneurysm*, is a false aneurysm resulting from a tear in the intimal layer of the vessel that allows blood to enter the vessel wall, dissecting its layers to create a blood-filled cavity.

The weakness that leads to aneurysm formation may be caused by several factors, including congenital defects, trauma, infections, and atherosclerosis. Once initiated, the aneurysm grows larger as the tension in the vessel increases. This is because the tension in the wall of a vessel is equal to the pressure multiplied by the radius (*i.e.*, tension = pressure × radius; see Chapter 16). In this case, the pressure in the segment of the vessel affected by the aneurysm does not change but remains the same as that of adjacent portions of the vessel. As an aneurysm increases in diameter, the tension in the wall of the vessel increases in direct proportion to its increased size. If untreated, the aneurysm may rupture because of the increased tension. Even an unruptured aneurysm can cause damage by exerting pressure on adjacent structures and interrupting blood flow.

Aortic Aneurysms

Aortic aneurysms may involve any part of the aorta: the ascending aorta, aortic arch, descending aorta, thoracoabdominal, or abdominal aorta. Multiple aneurysms may be present. The two most common causes of aortic aneurysms are atherosclerosis and degeneration of the vessel media. Aortic aneurysms are more common after age 50 and affect men more often than women.

Manifestations. The signs and symptoms of aortic aneurysms depend on the size and location. An aneurysm may also be asymptomatic, with the first evidence of its presence being associated with vessel rupture. With aneurysms of the thoracic aorta, substernal, back, and neck pain may occur. There may also be dyspnea, stridor, or a brassy cough caused by pressure on the trachea. Hoarseness may result from pressure on the recurrent laryngeal nerve, and there may be difficulty swallowing because of pressure on the esophagus.[21] The aneurysm may also compress the superior vena cava, causing distention of neck veins and edema of the face and neck.

Abdominal aortic aneurysms are most commonly located below the level of the renal artery and involve the bifurcation of the aorta and proximal end of the common iliac arteries. Most abdominal aneurysms are asymptomatic. Because an aneurysm is of arterial origin, a pulsating mass may provide the first evidence of the disorder. Typically, aneurysms larger than 4 cm are palpable. The mass may be discovered during a routine physical examination or the affected person may complain of its presence. Calcification, which frequently exists on the wall of the aneurysm, may be detected during abdominal radiologic examination. Pain may be present and varies from mild midabdominal or lumbar discomfort to severe abdominal and back pain. As the aneurysm expands, it may compress the lumbar nerve roots, causing lower back pain that radiates to the posterior aspects of the legs. The aneurysm may extend to and impinge on the renal, iliac, mesenteric arteries, or vertebral arteries that supply the spinal cord. An abdominal aneurysm may also cause erosion of vertebrae. Stasis of blood favors thrombus formation along the wall of the vessel, and peripheral emboli may develop, causing symptomatic arterial insufficiency.

With thoracic and abdominal aneurysms, the most dreaded complication is rupture. The likelihood of rupture correlates with increasing aneurysm size.

Diagnosis and Treatment. Diagnostic methods include use of ultrasound imaging, computed tomographic (CT) scans, and magnetic resonance imaging (MRI). Surgical repair, in which the involved section of the aorta is replaced with a synthetic graft of woven Dacron, frequently is the treatment of choice.

Dissecting Aneurysms

A dissecting aneurysm is an acute life-threatening condition. It involves hemorrhage into the vessel wall with longitudinal tearing (*i.e.*, dissection) of the vessel wall to form a blood-filled channel. Unlike atherosclerotic aneurysms, dissecting aneurysms often occur without evidence of previous vessel dilatation. They can originate anywhere along the length of the aorta. The most common site in the ascending aorta is within a few centimeters of the aortic valve.[22] The second most common site is the thoracic aorta just distal to the origin of the subclavian artery.

Dissecting aneurysms are caused by conditions that weaken or cause degenerative changes in the elastic and smooth muscle of the layers of the aorta. They are most common in the 40- to 60-year-old age group and more prevalent in men than in women.[2] There are two risk factors that predispose to a dissecting aneurysm: hypertension and degeneration of the medial layer of the vessel wall. There is a history of hypertension in 94% of cases.[2] Dissecting aneurysms are also associated with connective tissue diseases, such as Marfan's syndrome. Aortic dissection may also occur during pregnancy because of histochemical changes in the aorta that occur during this time. Other factors that predispose to aortic dissection are congenital defects of the aortic valve (*i.e.*, bicuspid or unicuspid valve structures) and aortic coarctation. Aortic dissection is a potential complication of cardiac surgery or catheterization. Surgically related dissection may occur at the points where the aorta has been incised or cross-clamped; it has also been reported at the site where the saphenous vein was sutured to the aorta during coronary artery bypass surgery.

There are several systems for classifying dissecting aortic aneurysms. The Stanford system uses two classifications: type A and type B. Those in the ascending aorta regardless of the site of the primary tear are designated type A (IA and IIA) and those not involving the ascending aorta are designated type B (Fig. 17–9). Dissections usually extend distally from the intimal tear. When the ascending aorta is involved, expansion of the wall of the aorta may impair closure of the aortic valve. There is also risk of aortic rupture with blood moving into the pericardium and compressing the heart. Although the length of dissection varies, it is possible for the abdominal aorta to be involved with progression into the renal, iliac, or femoral arteries. Partial or complete occlusion of the arteries that arise from the aortic arch or the intercostal or lumbar arteries may lead to stroke, ischemic peripheral neuropathy, or impaired blood flow to the spinal cord.

Manifestations. A major symptom of a dissecting aneurysm is the abrupt presence of excruciating pain, described as tearing or ripping. The location of the pain may point to the site of dissection.[20] Pain associated with dissection of the ascending aorta frequently is located in the anterior chest, and pain associated with dissection of the descending aorta often is located in the back. In the early stages, blood pressure typically is moderately or markedly elevated. Later, the blood pressure and the pulse rate become unobtainable in one or both arms as the dissection disrupts arterial flow to the arms. Syncope, hemiplegia, or paralysis of the lower extremities may occur because of occlusion of blood vessels that supply the brain or spinal cord. Heart failure may develop when the aortic valve is involved.

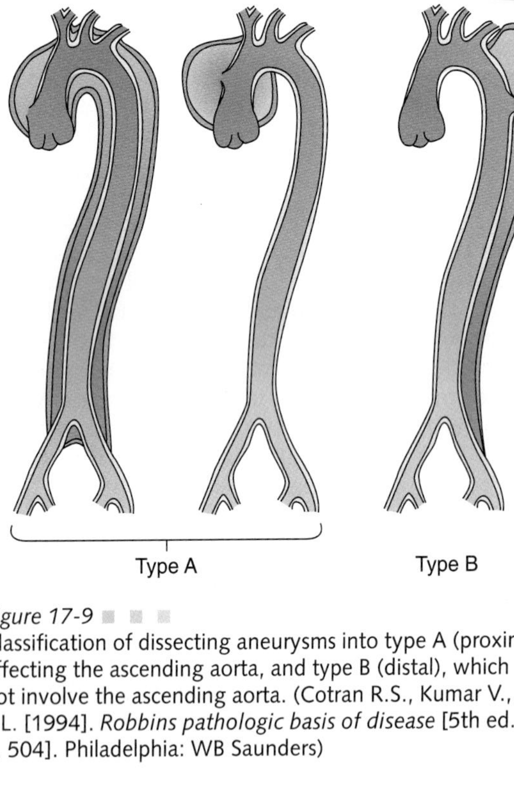

Type A

Type B

Figure 17-9
Classification of dissecting aneurysms into type A (proximal), affecting the ascending aorta, and type B (distal), which does not involve the ascending aorta. (Cotran R.S., Kumar V., Robbins S.L. [1994]. *Robbins pathologic basis of disease* [5th ed., p. 504]. Philadelphia: WB Saunders)

Diagnosis and Treatment. Diagnosis of aortic dissection is based on history and physical examination. Aortic angiography, transesophageal echocardiography, CT scans, and MRI studies aid in the diagnosis.

The treatment of dissecting aortic aneurysm may be medical or surgical. Aortic dissection is a life-threatening emergency situation; persons with a probable diagnosis are stabilized medically even before the diagnosis is confirmed. Two important factors that participate in propagating the dissection are high blood pressure and the steepness of the pulse wave. Without intervention, these forces continue to cause extension of the dissection. Medical treatment therefore focuses on control of hypertension and the use of drugs that lessen the force of systolic blood ejection from the heart. Two commonly used drugs are intravenous sodium nitroprusside and a β-adrenergic blocking drug, given in combination. Surgical treatment consists of resection of the involved segment of the aorta and replacement with a prosthetic graft. Mortality caused by dissecting aneurysm is high. If untreated, the mortality rate exceeds 50% within the first 48 hours, and 80% die within 6 weeks.[23]

In summary, the arterial system distributes blood to all the various tissues of the body, and pathology of the arterial system exerts its effects through ischemia or impaired blood flow. There are two types of arterial disorders: diseases such as atherosclerosis, vasculitis, and peripheral arterial diseases that obstruct blood flow and disorders such as aneurysms that weaken the vessel wall.

Atherosclerosis, a leading cause of death in the United States, affects large and medium-sized arteries, such as the coronary and cerebral arteries. It has an insidious onset, and its lesions usually are far advanced before symptoms appear. Although the mechanisms of atherosclerosis are uncertain, risk factors associated with its development have been identified. These include factors such as heredity, sex, and age, which cannot be controlled; factors such as smoking, high blood pressure, high serum cholesterol levels, and diabetes, which can be controlled; and other contributing factors such as obesity, lack of exercise, and stress. Cholesterol relies on lipoproteins (LDLs and HDLs) for transport in the blood. The LDLs, which are atherogenic, carry cholesterol to the peripheral tissues. The HDLs, which are protective, remove cholesterol from the tissues and carry it back to the liver for disposal. LDL receptors play a major role in removing cholesterol from the blood; persons with reduced numbers of receptors are at particularly high risk for development of atherosclerosis. The vasculitides are group of vascular disorders characterized by vasculitis or inflammation and necrosis of the blood vessels in various tissues and organs of the body. It can be caused by injury to the vessel, infectious agents, immune processes, or secondary to other disease states such as systemic lupus erythematosus.

Occlusive disorders interrupt arterial flow of blood and interferes with the delivery of oxygen and nutrients to the tissues. Occlusion of flow can result from a thrombus, emboli, vessel compression, vasospasm, or structural changes within the vessel. Peripheral arterial diseases affect blood vessels outside the heart and thorax. They include Raynaud's phenomenon, caused by vessel spasm; thromboangiitis obliterans (Buerger's disease), characterized by an inflammatory process that involves medium-sized arteries. Aneurysms are localized areas of vessel dilation caused by weakness of the arterial wall. A berry aneurysm, most often found in the circle of Willis in the brain circulation, consists of a small spherical vessel dilation. Fusiform and saccular aneurysms, most often found in the thoracic and abdominal aorta, are characterized by gradual and progressive enlargement of the aorta. They can involve part of the vessel circumference (saccular) or extend to involve the entire circumference of the vessel (fusiform). A dissecting aneurysm is an acute life-threatening condition. It involves hemorrhage into the vessel wall with longitudinal tearing (dissection) of the vessel wall to form a blood-filled channel. The most serious effect of aneurysms is rupture.

Disorders of the Venous Circulation

After you have completed this section of the chapter, you should be able to meet the following objectives:

- Describe venous return of blood from the lower extremities, including the function of the muscle pumps and the effects of gravity and relate to the development of varicose veins
- Differentiate primary from secondary varicose veins
- Characterize the pathology of venous insufficiency and relate to the development of stasis dermatitis and venous ulcers
- Cite risk factors associated with venous thrombosis and describe the manifestation of the disorder and its treatment

Veins are low-pressure, thin-walled vessels that rely on the ancillary action of skeletal muscle pumps and changes in abdominal and intrathoracic pressure to return blood to the heart. Unlike the arterial system, the venous system is equipped with valves that prevent retrograde flow of blood. Although its structure enables the venous system to serve as a storage area for blood, it also renders the system susceptible to problems related to stasis and venous insufficiency. This section focuses on three common problems of the venous system: varicose veins, venous insufficiency, and venous thrombosis. Varicosities of the anal and perianal veins (hemorrhoids) are discussed in Chapter 32 and esophageal varices in Chapter 33.

Venous Circulation of the Lower Extremities

The venous system in the legs consists of two components: the superficial veins (*i.e.*, saphenous vein and its tributaries) and the deep venous channels (Fig. 17–10). Perforating or communicating veins connect these two systems. Blood from the skin and subcutaneous tissues in the leg collects in the superficial veins and is then transported across the communicating veins into the deeper venous channels for return to the heart. Venous valves prevent the retrograde flow of blood and play an important role in the function of the venous system. Although these valves are irregularly located along the length of the veins, they are almost always found at junctions where the communicating veins merge with the larger deep veins and where two veins meet. The number of venous valves differs somewhat from one person to another, as does the structural competence, factors that may help to explain the familial predisposition to development of varicose veins.

The action of the leg muscles assist in moving venous blood from the lower extremities back to the heart. When a person walks, the action of the leg muscles serves to increase flow in the deep venous channels and return venous blood to the heart (Fig. 17–11). The function of the so-called *muscle pump*, located in the gastrocnemius and soleus muscles of the lower extremities, can be compared with pumping action of the heart.[24] During muscle contraction, which is similar to systole, valves in the communicating channels close to prevent backward flow of blood into the superficial system, as blood in the deep veins is moved forward by the action of the contracting muscles. During relaxation, which is similar to diastole, the communicating valves open allowing blood from the superficial veins to move into the deep veins.

Varicose Veins

Varicose, or dilated, tortuous veins of the lower extremities are common and often lead to secondary problems of venous insufficiency. Varicose veins are described as being primary or secondary. Primary varicose veins originate in the superficial saphenous veins, and secondary varicose veins result from impaired flow in the deep venous channels. About 80% to 90% of venous blood from the lower extremities is transported through the deep channels. The development of secondary varicose veins becomes inevitable when flow in these deep channels is impaired or blocked. The most common cause of secondary varicose veins is deep vein thrombosis. Other causes include congenital or acquired arteriovenous fistulas, congenital venous malformations, and pressure on the abdominal veins caused by pregnancy or a tumor.

It has been estimated that 10% to 20% of persons develop primary varicose veins in the lower extremities. The condition is more common after age 50 and in obese

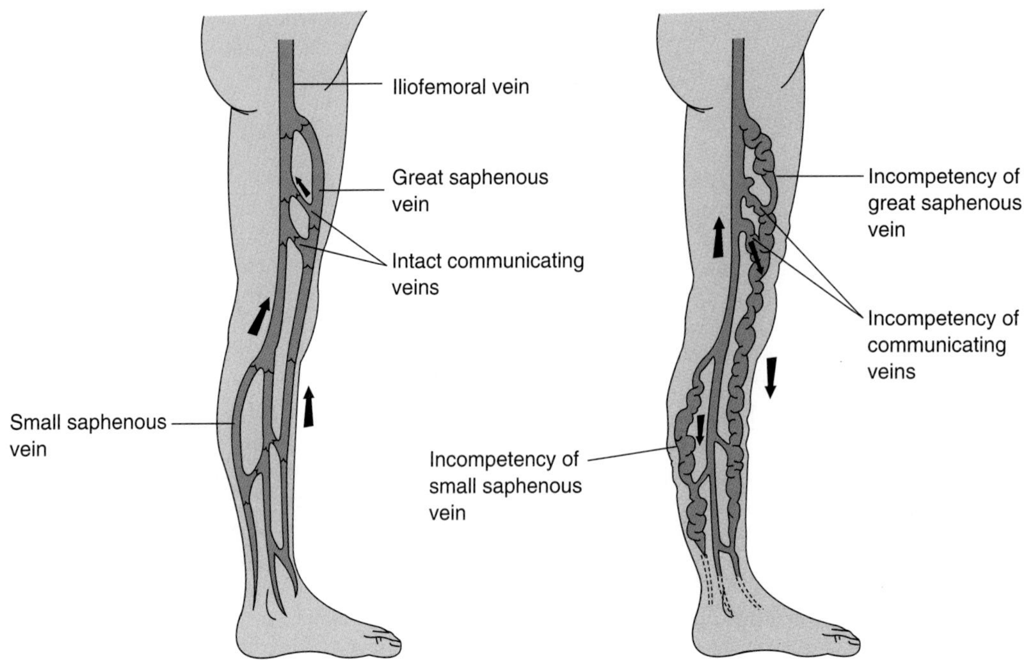

Figure 17-10
Superficial and deep venous channels of the leg. (**A**) Normal venous structures and flow patterns. (**B**) Varicosities in the superficial venous system are the result of incompetent valves in the communicating veins. The *arrows* in both views indicate the direction of blood flow. (Modified from Abramson D.I. [1974]. *Vascular disorders of the extremities* [2nd ed.]. New York: Harper & Row)

persons, and it occurs more often in women than men, probably because of venous stasis caused by pregnancy.[2] More than 50% of persons with primary varicose veins have a family history of the disorder, suggesting that heredity may play a role.

Mechanisms of Development

Prolonged standing and increased intraabdominal pressure are important contributing factors in the development of primary varicose veins. Prolonged standing increases venous pressure and causes dilatation and stretching of the vessel wall. One of the most important factors in the elevation of venous pressure is the hydrostatic effect associated with the standing position. When a person is in the erect position, the full weight of the venous columns of blood is transmitted to the leg veins. The effects of gravity are compounded in persons who stand for long periods without using their leg muscles to assist in pumping blood back to the heart.

Because there are no valves in the inferior vena cava or common iliac veins, blood in the abdominal veins must be supported by the valves located in the external iliac or femoral veins. When intraabdominal pressure increases, as it does during pregnancy, or when the valves in these two veins are absent or defective, the stress on the saphenofemoral junction is increased. The high incidence of varicose veins in women who have been pregnant also suggests a hormonal effect on venous smooth muscle contributing to venous dilatation and valvular incompetence. Lifting also increases intraabdominal pressure and decreases flow of blood through the abdominal veins. Occupations that require repeated heavy lifting, also predispose to development of varicose veins.

Prolonged exposure to increased pressure causes the venous valves to become incompetent so they no longer close properly. When this happens, the reflux of blood causes further venous enlargement, pulling the valve leaflet apart and causing more valvular incompetence in sections of adjacent distal veins. Another consideration in the development of varicose veins is the fact that the superficial veins have only subcutaneous fat and superficial fascia for support, but the deep venous channels are supported by muscle, bone, and connective tissue. Obesity reduces the support provided by the superficial fascia and tissues, increasing risk of developing varicose veins.

Manifestations. The signs and symptoms associated with primary varicose veins vary. Most women with superficial varicose veins complain of their unsightly appearance. In many cases, aching in the lower extremities and edema, especially after long periods of standing, may occur. The edema usually subsides at night when the legs are elevated. When the communicating veins are incompetent, symptoms are more common.

Diagnosis and Treatment

The diagnosis of varicose veins can often be made after physical inspection. Several procedures are used to assess the extent of venous involvement associated with varicose veins. In one of these, the Trendelenburg's test, a tourniquet is applied to the affected leg while it is elevated and the veins are empty. The person then assumes the standing position, and the tourniquet is removed. If the superficial veins are involved, the veins distend quickly. To assess the deep channels, the tourniquet is applied while the person is standing and the veins are filled. The person then lies down and the affected leg is elevated. Emptying of the superficial veins indicates that the deep channels are patent. The Doppler ultrasonic flow probe may also be used to assess the flow in the large vessels. Angiographic studies using a radiopaque contrast medium are also used to assess venous function.

After the venous channels have been repeatedly stretched and the valves rendered incompetent, little can be done to restore normal venous tone and function. Ideally, measures should be taken to prevent the development and progression of varicose veins. These measures center on avoiding activities such as continued standing that produce prolonged elevation of venous pressure. Treatment measures for varicose veins focus on improving venous flow and preventing tissue injury. When correctly fitted, elastic support stockings or leggings compress the superficial veins and prevent distention. The most precise control is afforded by prescription stockings, measured to fit properly. These stocking should be applied before the standing position is assumed at a time when the leg veins are empty.

Sclerotherapy, which is often used in treatment of small residual varicosities, involves the injection of a sclerosing agent into the collapsed superficial veins to produce fibrosis of the vessel lumen. Surgical treatment consists of removing the varicosities and the incompetent perforating veins, but it is limited to persons with patent deep venous channels.

Chronic Venous Insufficiency

The term *venous insufficiency* refers to the physiologic consequences of deep vein thrombosis, valvular incompetence, or a combination of both conditions. The most common cause is deep vein thrombosis, which causes deformity of the valve leaflets, rendering them incapable of closure. In the presence of valvular incompetence, effective unidirectional flow of blood and emptying of the deep veins cannot occur. The muscle pumps are also ineffective, often driving blood in retrograde directions. Secondary failure of the communicating and superficial veins, subject the subcutaneous tissues to high pressures.

With venous insufficiency, there are signs and symptoms associated with impaired blood flow. In contrast to the ischemia caused by arterial insufficiency, venous insufficiency leads to tissue congestion, edema, and eventual impairment of tissue nutrition. The edema is exacerbated by long periods of standing. Necrosis of subcutaneous fat deposits occur, followed by skin atrophy. Brown pigmentation of the skin caused by hemosiderin

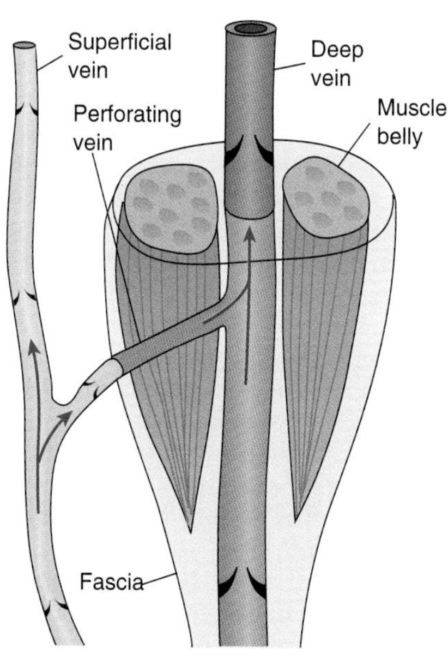

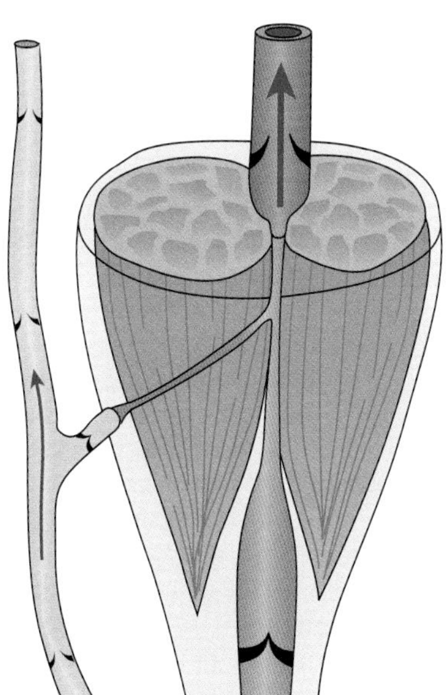

Figure 17-11
The skeletal muscle pumps and their function in promoting blood flow in the deep and superficial calf vessels of the leg. The majority of perforating veins lie below the knee. When the calf muscle is relaxed (**A**), blood moves from the superficial to the deep veins. Muscle contraction (**B**) propels blood in the deep veins toward the heart, and closure of the venous valves prevents backflow. (Margolis D.J. [1992]. Management of venous ulcerations. *Hospital Practice* 27[5], 37. © 1992, The McGraw-Hill Companies).

deposits resulting from the breakdown of red blood cells is common. Secondary lymphatic insufficiency occurs, with progressive sclerosis of the lymph channels in the face of increased demand for clearance of interstitial fluid.

In its advanced form, impairment of tissue nutrition causes *stasis dermatitis* and the development of *stasis* or *venous ulcers*. Stasis dermatitis is characterized by the presence of thin, shiny, bluish brown, irregularly pigmented desquamative skin that lacks the support of the underlying subcutaneous tissues. Minor injury leads to relatively painless ulcerations that are difficult to heal. The lower part of the leg is particularly prone to develop stasis dermatitis and venous ulcers. Most lesions are located medially over the ankle and lower leg, with the highest frequency just above the medial malleolus. Persons with long-standing venous insufficiency may develop stiffening of the ankle joint and loss of muscle mass and strength.

Venous Thrombosis

The term venous thrombosis, sometimes called *thrombophlebitis*, describes the presence of thrombus within a vein and the accompanying inflammatory response in the vessel wall. Thrombi can develop in the superficial or the deep veins. Deep vein thrombosis (DVT) most commonly occurs in the lower extremities. DVT of the lower extremity is a serious disorder, complicated by pulmonary embolism (see Chapter 24), recurrent episodes of deep venous thrombosis, and development of chronic venous insufficiency. Most postoperative thrombi arise in the soleal sinuses or the large veins draining the gastrocnemius muscles.[25] Isolated calf thrombi are often asymptomatic. If left untreated, they may extend to the larger, more proximal veins, with an increased risk of pulmonary emboli.

In 1846, Virchow described the triad that has come to be associated with venous thrombosis: stasis of blood, increased blood coagulability, and vessel wall injury.[26] Risk factors for venous thrombosis are summarized in Chart 17–2.

Stasis of blood occurs with immobility of an extremity or the entire body. Bed rest and immobilization are associated with decreased blood flow and venous pooling in the lower extremities and with increased risk of DVT. Persons who are immobilized by a hip fracture, joint replacement, or spinal cord injury are particularly vulnerable to DVT. The risk of DVT is increased in situations of impaired cardiac function. This may account for the relatively high incidence in persons with acute myocardial infarction and congestive heart failure. Elderly persons are more susceptible than younger persons, probably because disorders that produce venous stasis occur more frequently in older persons. Long airplane travel poses a particular threat in persons predisposed to DVT because of prolonged sitting and increased blood viscosity due to dehydration.[27]

CHART 17-2
*Risk Factors Associated With Venous Thrombosis**

Venous Stasis

Bed rest
Immobility
Spinal cord injury
Acute myocardial infarction
Congestive heart failure
Shock
Venous obstruction

Hyperreactivity of Blood Coagulation

Stress and trauma
Pregnancy
Childbirth
Oral contraceptive use
Dehydration
Cancer

Vascular Trauma

Indwelling venous catheters
Surgery
Massive trauma or infection
Fractured hip
Orthopedic surgery

*Many of these disorders involve more than one mechanism.

Hypercoagulability is a homeostatic mechanism designed to increase clot formation, and conditions that increase the concentration or activation of clotting factors predispose to DVT. Thrombosis can also be caused by deficiencies in certain plasma proteins that normally inhibit thrombus formation, such as antithrombin III, protein C, and protein S.[25] The postpartum state is associated with increased levels of fibrinogen, prothrombin, and other coagulation factors. The use of oral contraceptives appears to increase coagulability and predispose to venous thrombosis, a risk that is further increased in women who smoke. Certain cancers are associated with increased clotting tendencies, and although the reason for this is largely unknown, substances that promote blood coagulation may be released from the tissues because of the cancerous growth. When body fluid is lost because of injury or disease, the resulting hemoconcentration causes clotting factors to become more concentrated.

Vessel injury can result from a trauma situation or from surgical intervention. It may also occur secondary to infection or inflammation of the vessel wall. Persons undergoing hip surgery and total hip replacement are at particular risk because of trauma to the femoral and iliac veins, and in the case of hip replacement, thermal damage from heat generated by the polymerization of the acrylic cement that is used in the procedure.[25] Venous catheters are another source of vascular injury.

Manifestations

Many persons with venous thrombosis are asymptomatic, probably because the vein is not totally occluded or because of collateral circulation. When present, the most common signs and symptoms of venous thrombosis are those related to the inflammatory process: pain, swelling, and deep muscle tenderness. Fever, general malaise, and an elevated white blood cell count and sedimentation rate are accompanying indications of inflammation. There may be tenderness and pain along the vein. Swelling may vary from minimal to maximal. As many as 50% of persons with DVT are asymptomatic.

The site of thrombus formation determines the location of the physical findings. The most common site is in the venous sinuses in the soleus muscle and posterior tibial and peroneal veins (Fig. 17–12). Swelling in these cases involves the foot and ankle, although it may be slight or absent. Calf pain and tenderness are common. Femoral vein thrombosis with calf thrombosis produces pain and tenderness in the distal thigh and popliteal area. Thrombi in ileofemoral veins produce the most profound manifestations with swelling, pain, and tenderness of the entire extremity. With DVT in the calf veins, active dorsiflexion produces calf pain (*Homans' sign*). Another assessment measure, the *Bancroft sign* involves compression of the anterior calf muscles against the interosseous membrane. When tenderness is reported, the test result is positive.

Diagnosis and Treatment

The risk of pulmonary embolism emphasizes the need for early detection and treatment of DVT. Several tests are useful for this purpose: ascending venography, impedance plethysmography, and ultrasonography (*e.g.*, real-time, B-mode, duplex).

Whenever possible, venous thrombosis should be prevented in preference to being treated. Early ambulation after childbirth and surgery is one measure that decreases the risk of thrombus formation. Exercising the legs and wearing support stockings improve venous flow. A further precautionary measure is to avoid assuming body positions that favor venous pooling. Antiembolism stockings of the proper fit and length should be used routinely in persons at risk for DVT. Another strategy used for immobile persons at risk for developing DVT is a sequential pneumatic compression device. It consist of a plastic sleeve that encircle the legs and provides alternating periods of compression on the lower extremity. When properly used, these devices enhance venous emptying to augment flow and reduce stasis. Prophylactic anticoagulation is often used in persons who are at high risk for development of venous thrombi.

The objectives of treatment of venous thrombosis are to prevent formation of additional thrombi, prevent extension and embolization of existing thrombi, and minimize venous valve damage. A 15- to 20-degree elevation of the legs prevents stasis. It is important that the entire

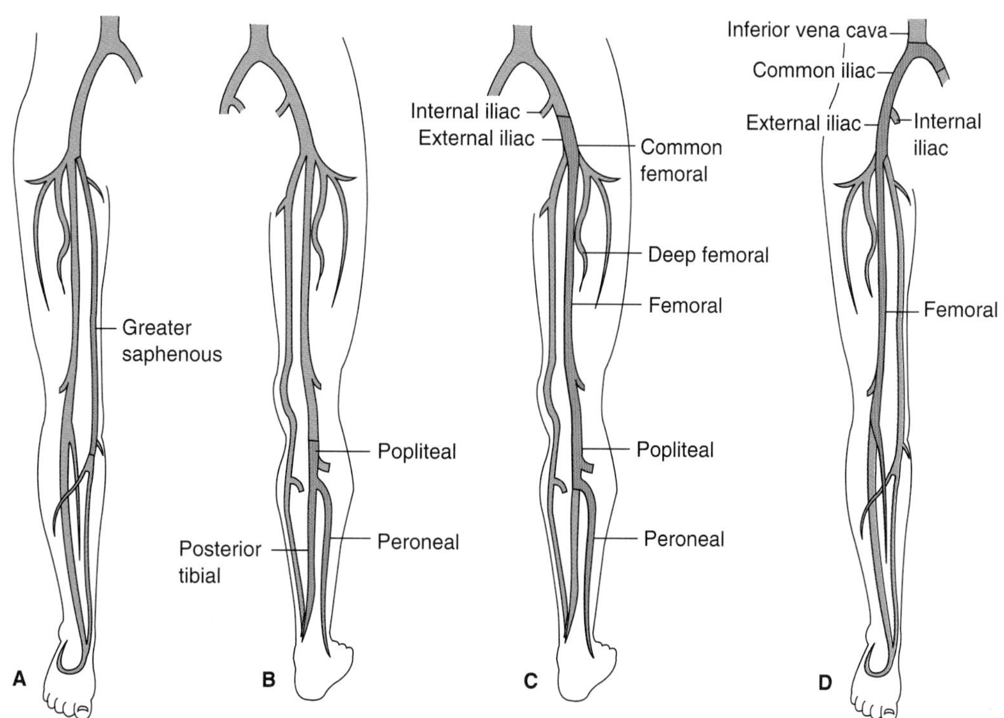

Figure 17-12

Common sites of venous thrombosis. (**A**) Superficial thrombophlebitis. (**B**) Most common form of deep thrombophlebitis. (**C** and **D**) Deep thrombophlebitis from the calf to iliac veins. (Haller J.A. Jr. [1967]. *Deep thrombophlebitis: Pathophysiology and treatment.* Philadelphia: W.B. Saunders)

lower extremity or extremities be carefully extended to avoid acute flexion of the knee or hip. Heat often is applied to the leg to relieve venospasm and to aid in the resolution of the inflammatory process. Bed rest usually is maintained until local tenderness and swelling have subsided. Gradual ambulation with elastic support is then permitted. Standing and sitting increase venous pressure and are to be avoided. Elastic support is needed for 3 to 6 months to permit recanalization and collateralization and to prevent venous insufficiency.

Anticoagulation therapy (*i.e.*, heparin and warfarin) is used to treat and to prevent venous thrombosis. Treatment typically is initiated with continuous infusion or subcutaneous injections of heparin. Subcutaneous injections of low-molecular-weight heparin may be given on an outpatient basis. This is usually followed by prophylactic therapy with oral anticoagulant therapy to prevent further thrombus formation. The mechanisms of action of the anticoagulant drugs are discussed in Chapter 7. Thrombolytic therapy (*i.e.*, streptokinase, urokinase, or tissue plasminogen activator) may be used in an attempt to dissolve the clot.

Surgical removal of the thrombus may be undertaken in selected cases. Surgery interruption of the vena cava may be done in persons at high risk of developing pulmonary emboli. This procedure involves ligating the vena cava with a suture or clamp or in creating a filterlike insertion to prevent large clots from moving through the vessel. Percutaneous insertion (through the skin) of intracaval devices has largely replaced direct surgical procedures.

In summary, the storage function of the venous system renders it susceptible to venous insufficiency, stasis, and thrombus formation. Varicose veins occur with prolonged distention and stretching of the superficial veins owing to venous insufficiency. Varicosities can arise because of defects in the superficial veins (i.e., primary varicose veins) or because of impaired blood flow in the deep venous channels (i.e., secondary varicose veins). Venous insufficiency reflects chronic venous stasis resulting from valvular incompetence. It is associated with stasis dermatitis and stasis or venous ulcers. Venous thrombosis describes the presence of thrombus within a vein and the accompanying inflammatory response in the vessel wall. It is associated with vessel injury, stasis of venous flow, and hypercoagulability states. Thrombi can develop in the superficial or the deep veins (i.e., DVT). Thrombus formation in deep veins is a precursor to venous insufficiency and embolus formation.

Disorders of Blood Flow Due to Extravascular Forces

After you have completed this section of the chapter, you should be able to meet the following objectives:

- State five possible causes of compartment syndrome
- Explain why pulses and capillary refill time are not good assessment measures for compartment syndrome
- Cite two causes of pressure ulcers
- Explain how shearing forces contribute to ischemic skin damage
- List four measures that contribute to the prevention of pressure ulcers

Blood flow occurs along a pressure gradient, moving from the arterial to the venous side of the circulation. For blood to move through the vessels of the systemic circulation, arterial pressure must be greater than venous pressure, and the arterial and venous pressures must be greater that the external pressure of the surrounding tissues. Injury or infections that cause tissue swelling can compromise blood flow, particularly in parts of the body where the skin or other supporting tissues cannot expand to accommodate the increased volume. In other situations, external pressure may compress the tissues and the blood vessels. Two conditions that compromise blood flow because of increased external pressure are compartment syndrome and pressure ulcers.

Compartment Syndrome

The muscles and nerves of an extremity are enclosed in a tough and inelastic fascial envelope called a *muscle compartment* (Fig. 17–13). Compartment syndrome describes a condition of increased pressure within a limited anatomic space, usually a muscle compartment, that impairs circulation and produces ischemic tissue injury.[28] If the pressure in the compartment is sufficiently high, tissue circulation is compromised, causing death of nerve and muscle cells. Permanent loss of func-

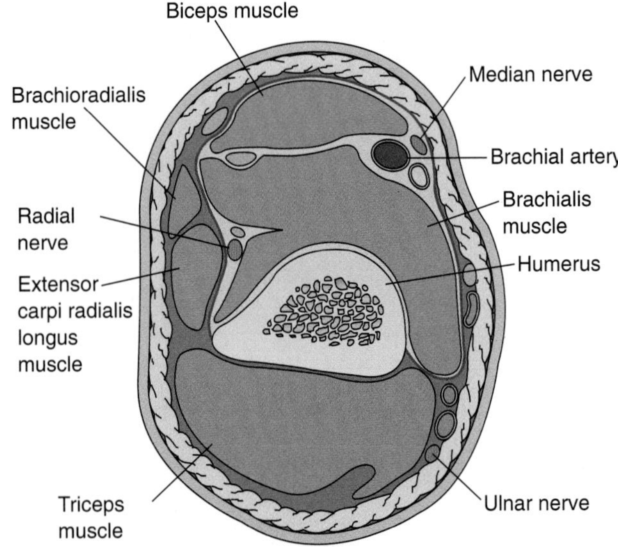

Figure 17-13
Distal anterior arm muscle compartment, showing the location of fascia, muscles, nerves, and blood vessels.

tion and limb contracture may occur. The amount of pressure required to produce a compartmental syndrome depends on many factors, including the duration of the pressure elevation, the metabolic rate of the tissues, vascular tone, and local blood pressure. Less tissue pressure is required to stop circulation when hypotension or vasoconstriction is present. Intracompartmental pressures of 30 to 40 mm Hg (normal is about 6 mm Hg) are considered sufficient to impair capillary blood flow.[29] Nerve dysfunction (*i.e.*, paresthesia and hypoesthesia) develops within 30 minutes of ischemia; muscle dysfunction, within 2 to 4 hours; and irreversible loss of function (*e.g.*, contractures, sensory aberrations, muscle weakness) begins after 12 to 24 hours of total ischemia.[30] Prompt diagnosis and decompression are essential to reinstate capillary pressure and prevent permanent disability.

Causes

Compartment syndrome can result from a decrease in compartment size or an increase in the volume of its contents (Chart 17–3). The most common causes are crushing injuries, fractures, contusions, snake bites, postischemic swelling after arterial injury or thrombosis, severe exercise, limb compression due to drug or alcohol overdose, and venous occlusion.

Decreased Compartment Size. Among the causes of decreased compartment size are constrictive dressings and casts, closure of fascial defects, and thermal injuries or frostbite. Splitting a cast or releasing the dressing usually is sufficient to relieve most of the pressure. The appearance of a muscle hernia or fascial defect may be the result of increased compartmental pressure. This commonly is seen in persons with chronic exercise-related compartment syndrome. Surgical closure of the hernia decreases compartmental size and may result in an acute compartment syndrome. In persons with circumferential third-degree burns, the inelastic and constricting eschar produces a decrease in the size of the underlying compartments. Burns are also associated with the formation of massive edema and an increase in compartment volume. The combination of the two problems may lead to necrosis of the underlying neuromuscular tissues. Frostbite produces neuromuscular injury for similar reasons.

Increased Compartment Volume. Increased compartment volume can be caused by postischemic swelling, trauma, vascular injury and bleeding, infiltration of intravenous infusions, and venous obstruction. One of the most important causes of compartment syndrome is bleeding and edema caused by fractures and osteotomies (see Chapter 45). Contusions and soft tissue injury are also common causes of compartment syndrome. Bleeding can occur as a complication of arterial punctures, particularly in persons with bleeding disorders or those who are receiving anticoagulant drugs. Infiltration of intravenous fluids can also restrict compartment size and cause compartment ischemia and postischemic swelling. Increased compartment volume may follow ischemic events, such as arterial occlusion, that are of sufficient duration to produce capillary damage, causing increased capillary permeability and edema. During unattended coma caused by drug overdose or carbon monoxide poisoning, high compartment pressures are produced when an extremity is compressed by the weight of the overlying head or torso. Exercise may produce acute or chronic elevations in compartment pressure.

Diagnosis and Treatment

It is important that a person at risk for development of compartment syndrome be identified and that proper assessment methods be instituted. Assessment should include pain assessment, examination of sensory (*i.e.*, light touch and two-point discrimination) and motor function (*i.e.*, movement and muscle strength), test of passive stretch, and palpation of the muscle compartments.

The most important symptom of compartment syndrome is unrelenting pain, usually described as a deep, throbbing sensation, that is greater than that expected for the primary problem, such as fracture or contusion. Pain with passive stretch is a common finding. Tenseness and tenderness of the involved compartment are specific symptoms of compartment syndrome. The skin over the compartment may become taut, shiny, warm, and red. Paresthesias progressing to anesthesia occur secondary to nerve involvement. Muscle weakness results from muscle ischemia. Although peripheral pulses and capillary refill time are parts of a complete assessment, they frequently are normal in the presence of compartment syndrome because the major arteries are located outside the muscle compartments. Although edema may make it difficult to palpate the pulse, the increased compartment pressure seldom is sufficient to occlude flow in a major artery. Doppler methods usually confirm the existence of a pulse. Direct measurements of tissue pressure can be obtained using a needle or wick catheter inserted into the muscle compartment. This method is particularly useful in persons who are unresponsive and in those with nerve deficits. Compartment

CHART **17-3**
Causes of Compartment Syndrome

Decreased Compartment Size

Constrictive dressings and casts
Infiltration of intravenous fluids
Thermal injury and frostbite
Surgical closure of fascial defects

Increased Compartment Volume

Fractures and orthopedic surgery
Trauma and bleeding
Postischemic injury
Severe exercise
Prolonged immobilization with limb compression (*e.g.*, drug overdose)
Thermal injury and frostbite
Intravenous infiltration

decompression is recommended when pressures rise to 30 mm Hg.

Treatment consists of reducing compartmental pressures. This entails cast splitting or removal of restrictive dressings. These procedures are often sufficient to relieve most of the underlying pressure and symptoms. Limb elevation is not recommended when compartment syndrome is suspected. Although elevation is widely used to promote venous drainage of an injured extremity, it may be detrimental in compartment syndrome. Because venous pressure must exceed tissue pressure, elevation of an extremity cannot augment venous drainage after intracompartment pressures are elevated. When an extremity is elevated, its arterial pressure falls because of the effects of gravity. Blood flow to an extremity can be arrested because of diminution of arterial pressure in the elevated extremity.

When compartment syndrome cannot be relieved by the measures described, a fasciotomy may become necessary. During this procedure, the fascia is incised longitudinally and separated so that the compartment volume can expand and blood flow can be reestablished. Because of potential problems with wound infection and closure, this procedure is performed as a last resort.

Pressure Ulcers

Pressure ulcers are ischemic lesions of the skin and underlying structures caused by external pressure that impairs the flow of blood and lymph. Pressure ulcers often are referred to as decubitus ulcers or bedsores. The word *decubitus* comes from the Latin term meaning lying down. A pressure ulcer, however, may result from pressure exerted in the seated or the lying position. Pressure ulcers are most likely to develop over a bony prominence, but they may occur on any part of the body that is subjected to external pressure, friction, or shearing forces.

The reported incidence and prevalence of pressure ulcers in hospital settings has ranged from 2.7% to 29.5% [31–33] and in skilled care and nursing home settings, from 2.4% to 23%.[33,34] Several subpopulations are at particular risk, including persons with quadriplegia, elderly persons with restricted activity and hip fractures, and persons in the critical care setting.

Mechanisms of Development

Two factors contribute to the development of pressure ulcers external pressure that compress blood vessels and the friction and shearing forces that tear and injure vessels.

External Pressure. External pressure that exceeds capillary pressure (about 25 mm Hg) interrupts the blood flow in the capillary beds. When this pressure is greater than the pressure in the arterioles, it also interrupts the flow in these vessels. When the pressure between a bony prominence and a support surface exceeds the normal capillary filling pressure of about 32 mm Hg, capillary flow is essentially obstructed.[35] If this pressure is applied constantly for 2 hours, oxygen deprivation coupled with an accumulation of metabolic end products leads to irreversible tissue damage. The same amount of pressure causes more damage when it is distributed over a small area than when it is distributed over a larger area. If a person weighing 70 kg with a total surface area of 1.8 m^2 were in the supine position, with pressure evenly distributed, the pressure at any given point would be 5.7 mm Hg.[36] About 7 lb of pressure per square inch of tissue surface is sufficient to obstruct blood flow.

Whether a person is sitting or lying down, the weight of the body is borne by tissues covering the bony prominences. Ninety-six percent of pressure ulcers are located on the lower part of the body, most often over the sacrum, the coccygeal areas, the ischial tuberosities, and the greater trochanter.[37] Pressure over a bony area is transmitted from the surface to the underlying dense bone; all the underlying tissue is compressed, with the greatest pressure at the surface of the bone and dissipating in a conelike manner toward the surface of the skin (Fig. 17–14).

Extensive underlying tissue damage can be present when a small superficial skin lesion is first noticed. The skin lesion often is just the "tip of the iceberg." Altering the distribution of pressure from one skin area to another prevents tissue injury. Persons unconsciously shift their weight to redistribute pressure on the skin

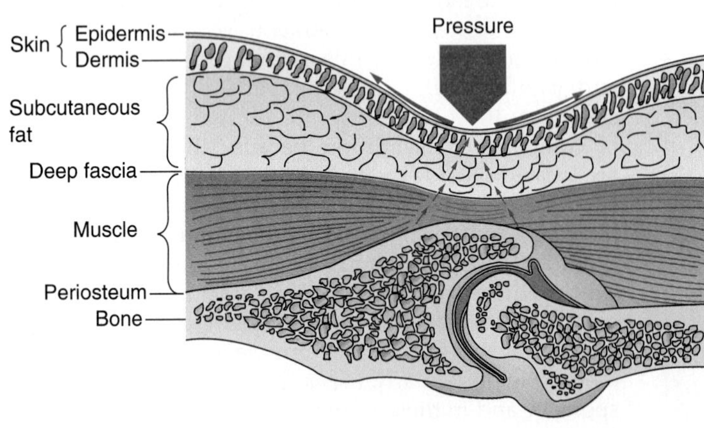

Figure 17-14
Pressure over a bony prominence compresses all intervening soft tissue, with a resulting wide, three-dimensional pressure gradient that causes various degrees of ischemia and damage. (Shea J.D. [1975]. Pressure sores: Classification and management. *Clinical Orthopaedics and Related Research* 112, 90)

and underlying tissues. During the night, for example, they turn in their sleep, preventing ischemic injury of tissues that overlie the bony prominences that support the weight of the body; the same is true for sitting for any length of time. The movements needed to shift the body weight are made unconsciously, and only when movement is restricted do they become aware of discomfort. Pressure ulcers most commonly occur with conditions in which normal sensation and movement to effect redistribution of body weight are impaired, such as spinal cord injury.

Friction and Shearing Forces. Shearing forces are caused by the sliding of one tissue layer over another with stretching and angulation of blood vessels, causing injury and thrombosis. Injury caused by shearing forces commonly occurs when the head of the bed is elevated, causing the torso to slide down toward the foot of the bed. When this happens, friction and perspiration cause the skin and superficial fascia to remain fixed against the bed linens while the deep fascia and skeleton slide downward. The same thing can happen when a person sitting up in a chair slides downward.

Another source of shearing forces is pulling rather than lifting a person up in bed. In this case, the skin remains fixed to the sheet while the fascia and muscles are pulled upward.

Prevention

The prevention of pressure ulcers is preferable to treatment. In 1992, a special panel of the Agency for Health Care Policy and Research, the Panel for the Prediction and Prevention of Pressure Ulcers in Adults, released the Clinical Practice Guidelines for Pressure Ulcers in Adults.[38] The recommendations developed by the panel target four overall goals: identifying at-risk persons who need prevention and the specific factors placing them at risk; maintaining and improving tissue tolerance to pressure to prevent injury; protecting against the adverse effects of external mechanical forces (*i.e.*, pressure, friction, and shear); and reducing the incidence of pressure ulcers through educational programs.[38]

Risk Factor Assessment. Risk factors identified as contributing to the development of pressure ulcers were those related to sensory perception (*i.e.*, ability to respond meaningfully to pressure-related discomfort), level of skin moisture, urine and fecal continence, nutrition and hydration status, mobility, circulatory status, and presence of shear and friction forces.

Numerous risk assessment tools exist; however, only the Braden Scale and the Norton Scale have been extensively tested. The Norton Scale ranks risk according to physical condition, mental condition, activity, mobility, and incontinence,[39] and the Braden Scale ranks sensory perception, moisture, activity, nutrition, and friction and shear.[40] Identifying persons who are at risk for development of pressure ulcers allows health care facilities to focus prevention measures on this group to reduce the incidence of pressure ulcers.

Skin Care and Early Treatment. Methods for preventing pressure ulcers include frequent position change, meticulous skin care, and frequent and careful observation to detect early signs of skin breakdown. All persons at risk for pressure ulcers should have systematic skin inspection done at least once each day, with particular attention to bony prominences.[38] The bed linens should be kept clean, dry, and wrinkle free. The skin should be cleaned at the time of urine and fecal soiling with a mild cleaning agent that minimizes irritation and skin dryness. When soiling of the skin cannot be controlled, it is recommended that absorbent underpads or briefs be used to present a quick-drying surface for the skin. Topical agents that act as moisture barriers can also be used.

Adequate hydration of the stratum corneum appears to protect the skin against mechanical insult.[38] The skin should be kept clean and protected from environmental factors that cause drying. The level of skin hydration decreases with decreasing ambient air temperature, particularly when the relative humidity of the ambient air is low.[38] Dry skin should be treated with moisturizers. The prevention of dehydration also improves the circulation. It also decreases the concentration of urine, thereby minimizing skin irritation in persons who are incontinent, and it reduces urinary problems that contribute to incontinence. Maintenance of adequate nutrition is important. Anemia and malnutrition contribute to tissue breakdown and delay healing after tissue injury has occurred.

The panel also recommended that the age-old practice of massaging over the bony prominences be avoided. Research suggests that using massage to stimulate blood and lymph flow may decrease skin blood flow and increase the risk of deep tissue injury.

Protection Against Mechanical Forces. Frequent change of position prevents tissue injury owing to pressure. Persons who are in bed and at risk for development of pressure ulcers should be repositioned at least every 2 hours if this is consistent with the overall treatment goals. It is recommended that persons who are in a chair or wheelchair be repositioned every hour or put back to bed. Persons who are able to shift their weight should be advised to do so every 15 minutes.

Special pads and mattresses that distribute weight more evenly may be used. Silicone-filled pads, egg-crate cushions, turning frames, flotation pads, and other devices minimize contact pressure. Adequate exposure of the skin to air is necessary to avoid the buildup of heat and perspiration. Care should be taken to maintain the person at a position of 30 to 40 degrees to minimize slipping and shearing forces from sliding against the sheets. It is also important that the person be lifted and not dragged across the sheet. A lifting sheet works well for this purpose. Elevation of the ankles and heels off the sheets with foam pads can reduce skin breakdown in these areas of the body. The use of air cushions (*i.e.*, donuts) is not recommended. Casts, braces, and splints can exert extreme pressure on underlying tissues, and persons with these devices require special attention to avoid skin breakdown.

Staging and Treatment

Pressure ulcers can be staged according to the following four categories recommended by the Panel for Prediction and Prevention of Pressure Sores in Adults[38] and the National Pressure Ulcer Advisory Panel[41]:

> Stage I: nonblanchable erythema of intact skin; the heralding of skin ulceration. Reactive hyperemia normally can be expected to be present for one half to three fourths as long as the pressure occluded blood flow to the area; it should not be confused with a stage I pressure ulcer.
>
> Stage II: partial-thickness skin loss involving epidermis or dermis, or both. The ulcer is superficial and presents clinically as an abrasion, a blister, or a shallow crater.
>
> Stage III: full-thickness skin loss involving damage and necrosis of subcutaneous tissue that may extend down to but not through underlying fascia. The ulcer manifests as a deep crater with or without undermining of adjacent tissue.
>
> Stage IV: full-thickness skin loss with extensive destruction, skin necrosis, or damage to muscle, bone, or supporting structures (e.g., tendon or joint capsule). Undermining and sinus tracts may also be associated with stage IV pressure ulcers.

These staging criteria have limitations. Identification of stage I pressure ulcers may be difficult in persons with darkly pigmented skin, and when eschar is present, accurate staging of the pressure may be difficult until the eschar has sloughed or the wound has been debrided.

After skin breakdown has occurred, special treatment measures are needed to prevent further ischemic damage, reduce bacterial contamination and infection, and promote healing. A major advance in the treatment of pressure ulcers has occurred in the area of wound dressings that offer moist wound healing. Dry dressings favor the formation of a dry crust over the wound, through which granulation tissue and advancing epithelium must burrow as it heals the area. Moist dressings, on the other hand, encourages formation of granulation and epithelization.[42]

Treatment methods are selected based on the stage of the ulcer.[35] Stage I ulcers usually are treated with frequent turning and measures to remove pressure. Stage II or III ulcers with little exudate are treated with petroleum gauze, semipermeable, or occlusive dressings to maintain a moist healing environment. Transparent semipermeable dressings (*e.g.*, Op-Cit, Tegaderm) allow wound visibility and seal in the body's own defenses against invasion—leukocytes, plasma, fibrin, and growth factors. Stage III ulcers usually require debridement (*i.e.*, removal of necrotic tissue and eschar). This can be done surgically, with wet-to-dry dressings, through the use of proteolytic enzymes (*e.g.*, fibrinolysin-desoxyribonuclease [Elase], streptokinase-stretodornase [Varidase]), or autolytic debridement, which involves the use of synthetic dressings to cover the wound and allow for devitalized tissues to self-digest from enzymes normally present in wound fluids.[43] Stage IV wounds often require packing to obliterate dead space and are covered with nonadherent dressings. Care is taken to avoid overpacking the wound, because it may produce pressure and cause additional tissue damage. Dressings are usually changed every 8 to 12 hours, depending on severity, degree of infection, and amount of exudate. Stage IV ulcers may require surgical interventions, such as skin grafts or myocutaneous flaps.

In summary, blood flow in the circulatory system is brought about by pressure differences between the arterial and venous systems and a transmural pressure (i.e., internal minus external) that holds the vessel open. Under certain conditions, such as compartment syndrome and pressure ulcers, increases in external pressures can exceed intravascular pressure and interrupt blood flow. Compartment syndrome is a condition of increased pressure within a muscle compartment that compromises blood flow and affords the potential for death of nerve and muscle tissue. It can result from a decrease in compartment size (e.g., constrictive dressings, closure of fascial defects, thermal injury, frostbite) or an increase in compartment volume (e.g., postischemic swelling, fractures, contusion and soft tissue trauma, bleeding caused by vascular injury, venous congestion).

Pressure ulcers are caused by ischemia of the skin and underlying tissues. They result from external pressure, which disrupts blood flow, or shearing forces, which cause stretching and injury to blood vessels. Pressure ulcers are divided into four stages, according to the depth of tissue involvement. The prevention of pressure ulcers is preferable to treatment. The goals of prevention should include identifying at-risk persons who need prevention and the specific factors placing them at risk; maintaining and improving tissue tolerance to pressure to prevent injury; protecting against the adverse effects of external mechanical forces (i.e., pressure, friction, and shear), and reducing the incidence of pressure ulcers through educational programs.

REFERENCES

1. American Heart Association. *1997 Heart Facts*. (1997). Dallas: American Heart Association.
2. Cotran R.S., Kumar V., Robbins S.L. (1994). *Pathologic basis of disease* (5th ed., pp. 135–137, 467–507). Philadelphia: W.B. Saunders.
3. Gotto A.M. (1988). Lipoprotein metabolism and the etiology of hyperlipidemia. *Hospital Practice* 23 (Suppl 1), 4.
4. Gwynne J.T. (1988). Lipoprotein structure and metabolism. *Consultant* 28 (6), 6.
5. Expert Panel on Detection, Evaluation, and Treatment of High Blood Cholesterol in Adults. (1993). Report of the National Cholesterol Education Program (NCEP) Expert

Panel on detection, evaluation, and treatment of high blood cholesterol in adults. *JAMA* 269 (23), 3015–3023.
6. American College of Physicians. (1996). Guidelines for using serum cholesterol, high-density lipoprotein, cholesterol, and triglyceride levels as screening test for preventing coronary heart disease in adults. *Annals of Internal Medicine* 124, 515–517.
7. Expert Panel on Detection, Evaluation, and Treatment of High Blood Cholesterol in Adults (Adult Treatment Panel II). (1994). *Circulation* 89:1329–1445.
8. Goldberg R.B. (1988). Dietary modification of cholesterol levels. *Consultant* 28 (Suppl 6), 35.
9. Enos W.F., Beyer J.C., Holmes R.F. (1955). Pathogenesis of coronary artery disease in American soldiers killed in Korea. *Journal of the American Medical Association* 158, 912.
10. Glasser S.P., Selwyn A.P., Ganz P. (1996). Atherosclerosis: Risk factors and the vascular endothelium. *American Heart Journal* 31 (2), 379–384.
11. Levine G.N., Keaney J.F., Vita J.A.(1995). Cholesterol reduction in cardiovascular disease. *New England Journal of Medicine* 332 (8), 512–521.
12. Gaziano J.M., Hebert P.R., Hennekens C.H. (1996). Cholesterol reduction: Weighing the benefits and risks. *Annals of Internal Medicine* 124 (10), 914–918.
13. Pariser K.M., Wolff S.M. (1992) The clinical spectrum of vasculitis. In Loscalzo J., Creager M.A., Dzau V.J. (Eds.). *Vascular medicine: A textbook of vascular biology and diseases* (p. 1011). Boston: Little, Brown.
14. Clark J.A. (1995). Unraveling the mystery: Clues to systemic vasculitic disorders. *AACN Clinical Issues* 6 (4), 645–656.
15. Halperin J.L., Creager M.A. (1992). Arterial obstructive diseases of the extremities. In Loscalzo J., Creager M.A., Dzau V.J. (Eds.). *Vascular medicine: A textbook of vascular biology and diseases* (pp. 835–859). Boston: Little, Brown.
16. Colburn M.D., Moore W.S. (1993). Buerger's disease. *Heart Disease and Stroke* 2(5), 424–432.
17. Bacharach J.M., Olin J.W. (1994). Raynaud's phenomenon. *Heart Disease and Stroke* 3(5), 255–259.
18. Creager M.A., Halperin J.L., Coffman J.D. (1992) Vasospastic disorders and vasculitis. In Loscalzo J., Creager M.A., Dzau V.J. (Eds.). *Vascular medicine: A textbook of vascular biology and diseases* (pp. 975–995). Boston: Little, Brown.
19. Wigley F.M. (1991). The differential diagnosis of Raynaud's phenomenon. *Hospital Practice* 26 (7A), 63–84.
20. Lennihan R., Porter J.M., Summer D.S., et al. (1988). Raynaud's phenomenon: A wrap-up. *Patient Care* 22 (3), 94.
21. Creager M.A., Halperin J.L., Whittemore A.D. (1992). Aneurysm disease of the aorta and its branches. In Loscalzo J., Creager M.A., Dzau V.J. (Eds.). *Vascular medicine: A textbook of vascular biology and diseases* (pp. 903–923). Boston: Little, Brown.
22. DeSanchis R.W., Doroghazi R.M., Austen W.G., et al. (1987). Aortic dissection. *New England Journal of Medicine* 317, 1060.
23. House-Fancher M.A. (1996). Aortic dissection: Pathophysiology, diagnosis, and acute care management. *AACN Clinical Issues* 6 (4), 602–614.
24. Donaldson M.C. (1992). Chronic venous disorders. In Loscalzo J., Creager M.A., Dzau V.J. (Eds.). *Vascular medicine: A textbook of vascular biology and diseases* (pp. 1075–1094). Boston: Little, Brown.
25. Weinmann E.E., Salzman E.W. (1994). Deep-vein thrombosis. *New England Journal of Medicine* 331 (24), 1630–1641.
26. Virchow R. (1846). Weinere untersuchungen uber dic verstropfung der lungenrarterie und ihre folgen. *Beitrage zur Experimentelle Pathologie und Physiologie* 2, 21.
27. Hirsch J., Williams W.J. (1995). Deep vein thrombosis: Recovery or recurrence? *Hospital Practice* 30(3), 71–79.
28. Slye D.A. (1991). Orthopedic complications: Compartment syndrome, fat embolism, and venous thrombosis. *Nursing Clinics of North America* 26 (1), 113–124.
29. Matsen F. (1975). Compartment syndrome: A unified concept. *Clinical Orthopaedics and Related Research* 113, 8–13.
30. Ashton H. (1962). Critical closing pressure in human peripheral vascular beds. *Clinical Science* 22, 79.
31. Clark M., Kadhom H.M. (1988). The nursing prevention of pressure sores in hospital and community patients. *Journal of Advanced Nursing* 13, 365–373.
32. Meehan M. (1990). Multisite pressure sore prevalence survey. *Decubitus* 3, 14–17.
33. Langema D.K., Olson B., Hunter S., et al. (1989). Incidence and prediction of pressure ulcers in five patient care settings, extended care, home health, and hospice in one locale. *Decubitus* 2 (2), 42.
34. Young L. (1989). Pressure ulcer prevalence and associated patient characteristics in one long-term facility. *Decubitus* 2 (2), 52.
35. Patterson J.A., Bennett R.G. (1995). Prevention and treatment of pressure sores. *Journal of the American Geriatric Society* 43, 919–927.
36. Beland I., Passos J.Y. (1981). *Clinical nursing* (4th ed., p. 1112). New York: Macmillan.
37. Reuler J.B., Cooney T.G. (1981). The pressure sore: Pathophysiology and principles of management. *Annals of Internal Medicine* 94, 661.
38. Panel for the Prediction and Prevention of Pressure Ulcers in Adults. (1992). *Pressure ulcers in adults: Prediction and prevention (clinical practice guidelines*. DHHS, AHCPR Publication No. 92–0047. Washington, DC: U.S. Government Printing Office.
39. Braden B.J. (1989). Clinical utility of the Braden scale for predicting pressure ulcer risk. *Decubitus* 2 (3), 44–46, 50–51.
40. Norton D. (1989). Calculating the risk: Reflections on the Norton Scale. *Decubitus* 2 (3), 24–31.
41. National Pressure Ulcer Advisory Panel. (1989). Pressure ulcers, incidence, economics, and risk assessment. Consensus Development Conference Statement. *Decubitus* 2 (2), 24–28.
42. Findlay D. (1996). Practical management of pressure ulcers. (1996). *American Family Physician* 54 (5), 1519–1528.
43. Patterson J.A., Bennett R.G. (1995). Prevention and treatment of pressure sores. *Journal of the American Geriatric Society* 43, 919–927.

ADDITIONAL READINGS

Cohn L.H. (1994). Aortic aneurysm: New aspects of diagnosis and treatment. *Hospital Practice* 29(3), 47–56.

Coffman J.D. (1992). Venous thrombosis and the diagnosis of pulmonary embolism. *Hospital Practice* 27(4A), 99–112.

Eftychiou V. (1996). Clinical diagnosis and management of the patient with deep venous thromboembolism and acute pulmonary edema. *Nurse Practitioner* 21 (3), 50–69.

Garber A.M., Browner W.S., Hulley S.B. (1996). Cholesterol screening in asymptomatic adults, revisited. *Annals of Internal Medicine* 124 (5), 518–531.

Gotto A.M. (1994). Cholesterol levels in young adults: Screen or intervene? *Hospital Practice* 29(3), 109–116.

Gourdin F.W. (1993). Etiology of venous ulceration. *Southern Medical Journal* 86 (10), 1142–1145.

Grundy S.M., Mazzaferri E.L. (1996). Addressing the spectrum of hypercholesteremia. *Hospital Practice* 31(6), 43–60.

Hutchinson M.R., Ireland M.L. (1994). Common compartment syndromes in athletes. *Sports Medicine* 17 (3), 200–208.

Hyers T.M. (1996). Integrated management of venous thromboembolism. *Southern Medical Journal* 89 (1), 20–26.

O'Brien K.D., Chait A. (1994). The role of the artery wall atherogenesis. *Medical Clinics of North America* 78 (1), 41–67.

Robinson J.G., Hunninghake D.G. (1995). Practical management of hyperlipidemia. *Contemporary Internal Medicine* 7 (2), 15–27.

Rocchini A.P. (1994). Diagnosis and management of lipid disorders in children. *Heart Disease and Stroke* 3(5), 247–254.

Writing Group PEPI Trial. (1995). Effects of estrogen and estrogen/progestin regimens on heart disease risk factors in postmenopausal women. *JAMA* 273 (3), 199–208

CHAPTER 18

Alterations in Blood Pressure: Hypertension and Orthostatic Hypotension

The arterial blood pressure is the driving force for blood flow in the circulatory system. Although blood pressure varies from moment to moment, it is perhaps the most controlled variable in the circulatory system. The importance of measuring blood pressure and treating high blood pressure has been recognized for more than 50 years. A speaker at the 1938 meeting of the Chicago Society of Internal Medicine stated[1]

> . . . while it [measurement of blood pressure] does not carry an immediate purport in cases of acute illness as do the temperature and pulse; yet for long-term evaluation of health of the average person it is far more significant. No other commonly used test gives such quick and reasonably exact information regarding life expectancy.

The discussion in this chapter focuses on determinants of blood pressure and conditions of altered arterial pressure hypertension and orthostatic hypotension.

Arterial Blood Pressure

After you have completed this section of the chapter, you should be able to meet the following objectives:

- Define the terms *arterial blood pressure, systolic blood pressure, diastolic blood pressure, pulse pressure,* and *mean arterial blood pressure*
- Explain how cardiac output and peripheral vascular resistance interact in determining systolic and diastolic blood pressure.

Blood flow in the circulatory system depends on a series of patent vessels and a pressure that moves blood throughout the system. It is the arterial blood pressure that distributes blood to all of the tissues of the body. The arterial blood pressure depends on the pumping action of the heart as it propels blood into the arterial system, the elastic properties of the blood vessels and their ability to accept various amounts of blood as it is ejected from the heart, and the resistance blood vessels that control the runoff of blood into the microcirculation.

Determinants of Blood Pressure

The arterial pressure reflects the intermittent ejection of blood from the left ventricle into the aorta. It rises during systole as the left ventricle contracts, and falls as the heart relaxes during diastole, giving rise to a *pressure pulse* (see Chapter 16). The contour of the arterial pressure tracing shown in Figure 18–1 is typical of the pressure changes that occur in the large arteries of the systemic circulation. There is a rapid rise in the pulse contour during left ventricular contraction, followed by a slower rise to peak pressure. About 70% of the blood that leaves the left ventricle is ejected during the first one third of systole (*i.e.*, the *rapid ejection period*); this accounts for the rapid rise in the pulse contour. The end of systole is marked by a brief downward deflection and formation of the *dicrotic notch*, which occurs when ventricular pressure falls below that in the aorta. The sudden closure of the aortic valve and the rebound energy it produces cause a brief rise in pressure immediately after the notch. As the ventricles relax and blood flows into the peripheral vessels during diastole, the arterial pressure falls rapidly at first and then declines slowly as the driving force decreases.

In healthy adults, the pressure at the height of the pressure pulse, called the *systolic pressure*, normally is about 120 mm Hg, and the lowest pressure, called the *diastolic pressure*, is about 80 mm Hg. The difference between the systolic and diastolic pressure (about 40 mm Hg) is called the *pulse pressure*. It reflects the magnitude or height of the pressure pulse. The *mean arterial pressure* represents the average pressure in the arterial system during ventricular contraction and relaxation (about 90 to 100 mm Hg) and is depicted by the darker area under the pressure tracing in Figure 18–1.

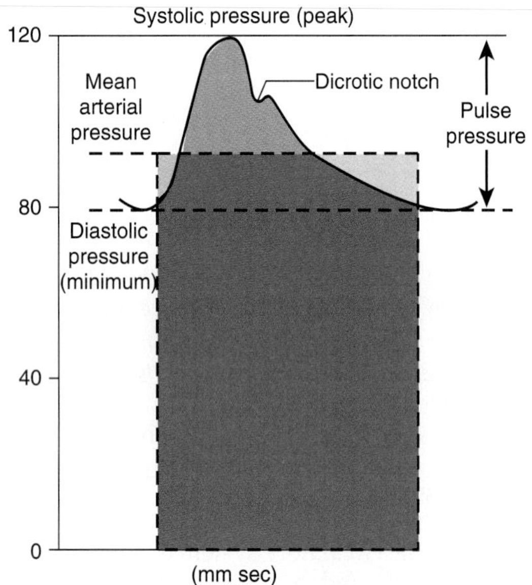

Figure 18–1
Intraarterial pressure tracing made from the brachial artery. Pulse pressure is the difference between systolic and diastolic pressures. The *darker area* represents the mean arterial pressure, which can be calculated by using the formula of mean arterial pressure =diastolic pressure +pulse pressure/3.

In hypertension and disease conditions that affect blood pressure, changes in blood pressure are often described in terms of systolic, diastolic, pulse pressure, and mean arterial pressures. Each of these pressures contribute individually and collectively to blood flow in the various tissue beds of the body. The levels to which these pressures rise and fall is influenced by the stroke volume, the rapidity with which blood is ejected from the heart, the elastic properties of the aorta, and the total peripheral resistance.

Mean Arterial Pressure

The mean arterial blood pressure represents the average blood pressure in the systemic circulation. The mean arterial pressure (MABP) is determined by the cardiac output (CO) or amount of blood that the heart pumps each minute (*i.e.*, stroke volume × heart rate) and the total resistance that the blood encounters as it is being pumped through the peripheral circulation, called the total peripheral resistance (TPR). The mean arterial pressure can represented by the equation, $MABP = CO \times TPR$.

Mean arterial pressure can be estimated by adding one third of the pulse pressure to the diastolic pressure (*i.e.*, diastolic blood pressure + pulse pressure/3). Hemodynamic monitoring equipment in intensive and coronary care units measures or computes mean arterial pressure automatically. Because it is a good indicator of tissue perfusion, the mean arterial pressure is often monitored, along with systolic and diastolic blood pressures, in critically ill patients.

Systolic Blood Pressure

The systolic blood pressure reflects the intermittent ejection of blood into the aorta (Fig. 18–2). As blood is ejected into the aorta, it stretches the vessel wall and produces a rise in aortic pressure. The extent to which the systolic pressure rises or falls with each cardiac cycle is determined by the amount of blood ejected into the aorta with each heart beat (*i.e.*, stroke volume) and the velocity of ejection and by the elastic properties of the aorta. Systolic pressure increases when there is a rapid ejection of a large stroke volume or when the stroke volume is ejected into a rigid aorta. Only about one third of the ejected blood leaves the aorta during ventricular systole, and the elastic walls of the aorta normally stretch to accommodate the varying amounts of blood that are ejected into the aorta; this prevents the pressure from rising excessively during systole and maintains pressure during diastole. In some elderly persons, the elastic fibers of the aorta lose some of their resiliency, and the aorta becomes more rigid. When this occurs, the aorta is less able to stretch and buffer the pressure that is generated as blood is ejected into the aorta, resulting in an elevated systolic pressure.

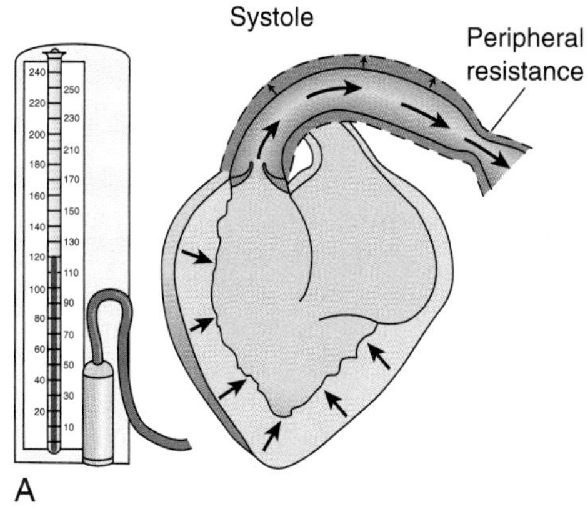

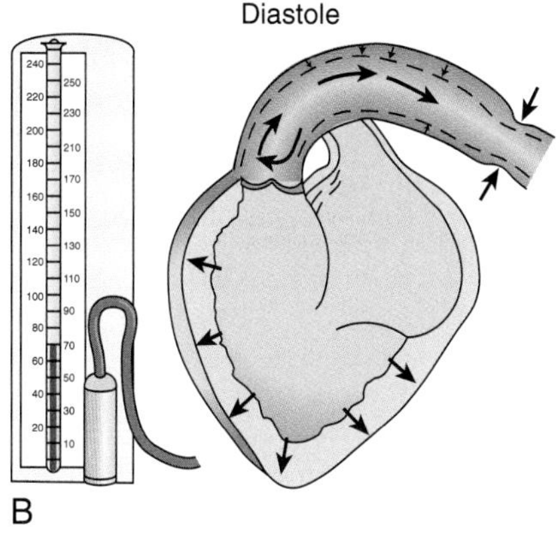

Figure 18–2
Diagram of the left side of the heart. (**A**) Systolic blood pressure represents the ejection of blood into the aorta during ventricular systole; it reflects the stroke volume, the distensibility of the aorta, and the velocity with which blood is ejected from the heart. (**B**) Diastolic blood pressure represents the pressure in the arterial system during diastole; it is largely determined by the peripheral vascular resistance.

Diastolic Blood Pressure

The diastolic blood pressure is maintained by the energy that has been stored in the elastic walls of the aorta during systole (see Fig. 18–2). The level at which the diastolic pressure is maintained depends on the condition of the aorta and large arteries and their ability to stretch and store energy, the competency of the aortic valve, and the resistance of the arterioles that control outflow of blood into the microcirculation. When there is an increase in peripheral vascular resistance, as with sympathetic stimulation, diastolic blood pressure rises. The arteries are located between the outlet of the aorta and the arterioles, which control the total peripheral vascular resistance and runoff of blood from the arterial circulation. With arteriosclerosis, the smaller arteries may become rigid and unable to accept the runoff of blood from the aorta without producing an increase in diastolic pressure. Closure of the aortic valve at the onset of diastole is essential to the maintenance of the diastolic pressure. When there is incomplete closure of the aortic valve, as in aortic regurgitation (Chapter 19), the diastolic pressure drops as blood flows backward into the left ventricle rather than moving forward into the arterial system.

Pulse Pressure

The pulse pressure reflects the pulsatile nature of arterial blood flow and is an important component of blood pressure. During the rapid ejection period of ventricular systole, the volume of blood that is ejected into the aorta exceeds the amount that exits the arterial system. The pulse pressure reflects this difference. The pulse pressure rises when additional amounts of blood are ejected into the arterial circulation, and it falls when the resistance to outflow is decreased. In hypovolemic shock, the pulse pressure declines because of a decrease in stroke volume and systolic pressure. This occurs despite an increase in peripheral vascular resistance, which maintains the diastolic pressure.

Blood Pressure Measurement

Arterial blood pressure measurements are usually obtained by the indirect method using a sphygmomanometer and the auscultatory method. In the measurement of blood pressure, a cuff that contains a rubber bladder is placed around the upper arm. The bladder of the cuff

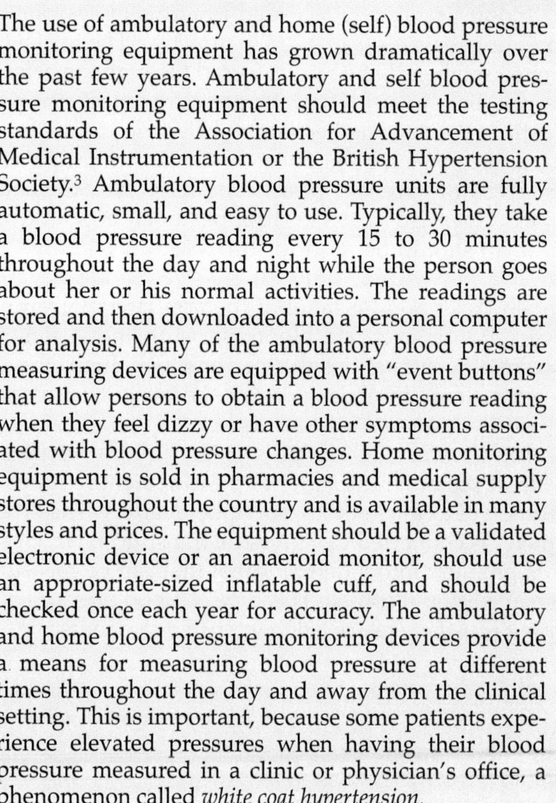

Ambulatory and Home Blood Pressure Monitoring

The use of ambulatory and home (self) blood pressure monitoring equipment has grown dramatically over the past few years. Ambulatory and self blood pressure monitoring equipment should meet the testing standards of the Association for Advancement of Medical Instrumentation or the British Hypertension Society.[3] Ambulatory blood pressure units are fully automatic, small, and easy to use. Typically, they take a blood pressure reading every 15 to 30 minutes throughout the day and night while the person goes about her or his normal activities. The readings are stored and then downloaded into a personal computer for analysis. Many of the ambulatory blood pressure measuring devices are equipped with "event buttons" that allow persons to obtain a blood pressure reading when they feel dizzy or have other symptoms associated with blood pressure changes. Home monitoring equipment is sold in pharmacies and medical supply stores throughout the country and is available in many styles and prices. The equipment should be a validated electronic device or an anaeroid monitor, should use an appropriate-sized inflatable cuff, and should be checked once each year for accuracy. The ambulatory and home blood pressure monitoring devices provide a means for measuring blood pressure at different times throughout the day and away from the clinical setting. This is important, because some patients experience elevated pressures when having their blood pressure measured in a clinic or physician's office, a phenomenon called *white coat hypertension*.

CHART **18-1**
Korotkoff Sounds

Phase I	Period marked by the first tapping sounds, which gradually increase in intensity
Phase II	Period during which a murmur or swishing sound is heard
Phase III	Period during which sounds are crisper and greater in intensity
Phase IV	Period marked by distinct, abrupt muffling or by a soft blowing sound
Phase V	Point at which sounds disappear

is inflated to a point at which its pressure exceeds that of the artery, occluding the blood flow. The cuff is then slowly deflated until the pressure in the vessel again exceeds the pressure in the cuff. A small amount of blood is then forced through the partially obstructed artery, and by placing a stethoscope over the brachial artery distal to the cuff, the examiner can audibly monitor the tapping sounds that are produced. The auscultatory sounds, or tapping sounds, heard during blood pressure measurement are often referred to as Korotkoff sounds, after the Russian physician who first described them (Chart 18–1). Automated or semiautomated methods of blood pressure measurement use a microphone, pulse sensor, or Doppler equipment for detecting the equivalent of the Korotkoff sounds.

Blood pressure is recorded in terms of systolic and diastolic pressures (*e.g.*, 120/70 mm Hg). The initial tapping sound heard as blood is forced through the artery is the systolic pressure. Diastolic pressure reflects the point at which the sounds become muffled or are no longer heard; it represents the point at which arterial pressure is sufficient to prevent vessel compression by the cuff. It is recommended that the disappearance of sound (*i.e.*, phase V) should be used for the diastolic reading.[2] The use of a cuff with an appropriate-size bladder (*i.e.*, one that encircles 80% or more of the arm circumference) is necessary for accurate blood pressure measurements. Too small a cuff can result in erroneously high pressure measurements in obese persons, because it takes more pressure to compress the artery.

Intraarterial methods provide for direct measurement of blood pressure. Intraarterial measurement requires the insertion of a catheter into a peripheral artery. The arterial catheter is connected to a pressure transducer, which converts pressure into a digital signal that can be measured, displayed, and recorded. This type of blood pressure monitoring is usually restricted to intensive care units.

In summary, the alternating contraction and relaxation of the heart produce a pressure pulse that moves the blood through the circulatory system. The elastic walls of the aorta stretch during systole and relax during diastole to maintain the diastolic pressure. The pressure pulse is responsible for the Korotkoff sounds heard when blood pressure is measured using a blood pressure cuff, and it is this impulse that is felt when the pulse is taken. Systolic pressure denotes the highest point of the pulse pressure, and diastolic denotes the lowest point. The pulse pressure is the difference between these two pressures. The mean arterial pressure reflects the average pressure throughout the cardiac cycle. It can be estimated by adding one third of the pulse pressure to the diastolic pressure.

Physical (i.e., blood volume and the elastic properties of the blood vessels) and physiologic factors (i.e., cardiac output and peripheral vascular resistance) influence mean arterial blood pressure. Mean arterial blood pressure is determined by the cardiac output and total peripheral vascular resistance (MABP = CO × TPR). Systolic pressure is determined primarily by the characteristics of the stroke volume, whereas diastolic pressure is determined largely by the conditions of the arteries and arterioles and their abilities to accept the runoff of blood from the aorta. The pulse pressure reflects the pulsatile nature of the arterial blood flow and is an important component of blood pressure.

Hypertension

After you have completed this section of the chapter, you should be able to meet the following objectives:

- Cite the definition of *hypertension* put forth by the Joint National Committee on Detection, Evaluation, and Treatment of Hypertension
- Differentiate among essential, systolic, secondary, and malignant forms of hypertension
- Describe the possible influence of genetics, age, race, obesity, sodium and other cation (*i.e.*, potassium, calcium, and magnesium) intake, alcohol consumption, and stress on development of essential hypertension
- Cite the risks of hypertension in terms of target organ damage
- Describe behavior modification strategies used in treatment of hypertension
- List the different categories of drugs used to treat hypertension and state their action in control of high blood pressure
- Explain the changes in blood pressure that accompany normal pregnancy and describe the four types of hypertension that can occur during pregnancy
- Cite the criteria for the diagnosis of high blood pressure in children
- Define *systolic hypertension* and relate the circulatory changes that occur with aging and that predispose to the development of systolic hypertension
- Describe possible problems related to blood pressure measurement in the elderly

Hypertension, or high blood pressure, is probably the most common of all cardiovascular disorders. The prevalence of hypertension increases with age, and the rate among African Americans is higher than among white Americans. It occurs in all geographic areas of the country and affects persons from low-, middle-, and upper-income groups. It has been estimated that in the United States as many as 50 million adults have high blood pressure.[2]

In 1972, the National Institutes of Health founded the National High Blood Pressure Education Program. The purpose of the program was to increase awareness among health professionals and the public about the importance of detecting and treating hypertension. When the program began, only 51% of persons with hypertension (blood pressure >160/95) were aware that they had elevated blood pressure, and only 36% were being treated with medications for their hypertension. This data can be compared with information collected between 1988 and 1991, in which 84% of persons with hypertension were aware that they had an elevated blood pressure and 73% of these were being treated with medications. During this same period, the mortality rate from coronary heart disease decreased about 50% and that from stroke fell by 57%. Despite these trends, hypertension remains one of the most frequently encountered chronic health problems and continues as one of the most significant risk factors for morbidity and mortality from coronary heart disease, congestive heart failure, chronic renal failure, and stroke.[2]

Hypertension is commonly divided into the categories of primary and secondary hypertension. In primary hypertension, often called essential hypertension, the chronic elevation in blood pressure occurs without evidence of other disease. In secondary hypertension, the elevation of blood pressure results from some other disorder, such as kidney disease. Malignant hypertension, as the name implies, is an accelerated form of hypertension.

Essential Hypertension

The fifth (1993) report of the Joint National Committee (JNC-V) on Detection, Evaluation, and Treatment of High Blood Pressure of the National Institutes of Health recommended criteria for the diagnosis of high blood pressure in individuals 18 years of age and older.[2] According to recommendations contained in the JNC-V report, the diagnosis of hypertension is made if the systolic blood pressure is 140 mm Hg or higher and diastolic blood pressure is 90 mm Hg or higher when at least two blood pressure measurements are averaged on two or more subsequent visits, unless the systolic pressure is 210 mm Hg or higher or diastolic pressure is 120 mm Hg or higher. The 1993 report of the JNC includes a category of high normal blood pressure (*i.e.*, systolic pressure of 130 to 139 mm Hg and diastolic pressure of 85 to 89 mm Hg) and categorizes high blood pressure into four stages based on systolic and diastolic blood pressures (Table 18–1). A consistently elevated systolic pressure of 160 mm Hg or higher with a diastolic pressure of less than 90 mm Hg is classified as isolated systolic hypertension.

The report emphasizes that obtaining one elevated blood pressure reading should not constitute the diagnosis of hypertension. Blood pressure measurements should be taken when the person is relaxed and has rested for at least 5 minutes and has not smoked or ingested caffeine within 30 minutes. Because blood pressure in many individuals is highly variable, blood pressure should be measured on different occasions over a period of several months for a diagnosis of hypertension is made unless the pressure is extremely elevated or associated with symptoms (see Table 18–1). At least two measurements should be made at each visit in the same arm while the person is seated. The diastolic pressure is recorded at the disappearance of sound, or phase V of the Korotkoff sounds.[2]

Mechanisms of Blood Pressure Elevation

Several factors, including hemodynamic, neural, humoral, and renal mechanisms, are thought to interact in producing long-term elevations in blood pressure. As with other disease conditions, it is improbable that there

TABLE 18–1

Classification and Follow-up of Blood Pressure Measurements for Adults Age 18 and Older

Category*	Systolic Blood Pressure (mm Hg)	Diastolic Blood Pressure (mm Hg)	Follow-up Recommended
Normal	<130	<85	Recheck in 2 years
High Normal	130–139	85–89	Recheck in 1 year†
Hypertension			
Stage 1 (mild)	140–159	90–99	Confirm within 2 months
Stage 2 (moderate)	160–179	100–109	Evaluate or refer within 1 month
Stage 3 (severe)	180–209	110–119	Evaluate or refer within 1 week
Stage 4 (very severe)	≥210	≥120	Evaluate or refer immediately

*Based on the average of two or more readings taken at each of two or more visits after an initial screening of those not taking antihypertensive drugs and not acutely ill. When systolic and diastolic pressure fall into different categories, the higher category should be selected to classify the individual's blood pressure status. For instance, 160/92 should be classified as stage 2, and 180/120 should be classified as stage 4. Isolated systolic hypertension (ISH) is defined as SBP >140 mm Hg and DBP <90 mm Hg and staged appropriately (*e.g.*, 170/85 mm Hg is defined as stage 2 ISH).
†Consider offering counseling in lifestyle modifications.
(Adapted from the National Heart, Lung, and Blood Institute. [1993]. The fifth report of the National Committee on Detection, Evaluation, and Treatment of High Blood Pressure (pp. 4, 6). Bethesda: National Institutes of Health)

is a single cause responsible for the development of essential hypertension or that the condition is a single disease. Because arterial blood pressure is the product of cardiac output and total peripheral resistance, all forms of hypertension involve hemodynamic mechanisms—an increase in cardiac output or total peripheral vascular resistance or a combination of the two. Other factors such as sympathetic nervous system activity, kidney function in terms of salt and water retention, the electrolyte composition of the intracellular and extracellular fluids, cell membrane transport mechanisms, and humoral influences such as the renin-angiotensin-aldosterone mechanism play an active or permissive role in regulating the hemodynamic mechanisms that control blood pressure. Blood pressure regulation is discussed in Chapter 16.

Considerable evidence suggests that the kidney is directly or indirectly involved in most and perhaps all forms of hypertension.[4,5] Normally, the kidney maintains blood pressure within a very narrow range by conserving or eliminating sodium and water. The relation between arterial pressure and the elimination of sodium and water has been called *pressure natriuesis*. When blood pressure rises, the kidney normally responds by increasing its excretion of salt and water. Evidence suggests that persons who develop hypertension require a higher arterial pressure to regulate the elimination of salt and water by the kidney. This does not mean that the abnormality leading to hypertension is internal to the kidney. For example, excess sympathetic nerve activity or the release of vasoconstrictor substances that alter the transmission of pressure to the kidney could initiate hypertension. Similarly, changes in neural and humoral control of kidney function could shift the pressure natriuresis relation to higher pressures and initiate hypertension. The role of the kidney in the development of essential hypertension is further supported by the fact that many hypertension medications produce their blood pressure–lowering effects by increasing salt and water excretion.

Contributing Factors

Although the cause or causes of essential hypertension are largely unknown, several factors have been implicated as contributing to its development. These risk factors include family history of hypertension, race, and age-related increases in blood pressure. Other lifestyle factors can contribute to the development of hypertension by interacting with the risk factors. These lifestyle factors include high sodium intake, excessive calorie intake and obesity, physical inactivity, excessive alcohol consumption, and low intake of potassium. Oral contraceptive drugs also may increase blood pressure in predisposed women. Although stress can raise blood pressure acutely, there is less evidence linking it to chronic elevations in blood pressure. It has also been suggested that a diet that is low in calcium and magnesium may contribute to long-term elevations in blood pressure; however, there is no convincing evidence to justify increased intake of either of these minerals for the purpose of preventing or treating hypertension. Although dietary fats and cholesterol are independent risk factors for coronary heart disease, there is no evidence that they raise blood pressure. Although not identified as a primary risk factor in hypertension, smoking is an independent risk factor in coronary heart disease and should be avoided.

Family History. The inclusion of heredity as a contributing factor in the development of hypertension is supported by the fact that hypertension is seen most frequently among persons with a family history of hypertension. Persons with two or more first-degree relatives with hypertension before age 55 have a 3.8 times greater risk of developing hypertension before age 50 than persons without a family history.[6] The inherited predisposition does not seem to rely on other risk factors, but when they are present, the risk is apparently additive. The pattern of heredity is unclear; it is unknown whether a single gene or multiple genes are involved. Whatever the explanation, the high incidence of hypertension among close family members seems significant enough to be presented as a case for recommending that persons from these high-risk families be encouraged to participate in hypertensive screening programs.

Age-Related Changes in Blood Pressure. Maturation and growth are known to cause predictable increases in blood pressure. For example, in the newborn, arterial blood pressure is normally only about 50 mm Hg systolic and 40 mm Hg diastolic. Sequentially, blood pressure increases with physical growth from a value of 78 mm Hg systolic at 10 days of age to 120 mm Hg at the end of adolescence. Blood pressure usually continues to undergo a slow rate of increase during the adult years.

The relation between the aging process and hypertension is commonly accepted. The author can recall a number of older persons describing the normal range of blood pressure as being "100 plus your age." Although it is known that this is not true, it is possible that the cardiovascular and autonomic nervous system changes that occur as part of the normal aging process do contribute to the increased blood pressures observed in older persons. Individuals tend to age differently, and this factor undoubtedly accounts for some of the great variations in blood pressure among elderly persons. Isolated systolic hypertension is discussed in a later section.

Race. Hypertension is not only more prevalent in African Americans than whites, it is also more severe. The National Health and Nutrition Examination Survey II (1988 to 1991) reported that diastolic blood pressures were significantly greater for African Americans than for white men and women 35 years of age and older and that systolic pressures of African-American women at every age were greater than those of white women.[7,8] Hypertension tends to occur earlier in African Americans than in whites, and it is often not treated early enough or aggressively enough. Blacks also tend to experience greater cardiovascular and renal damage at any level of pressure.[9]

The reasons for the increased incidence of hypertension among African Americans is unknown. Studies have shown that many African-American persons with hypertension have lower renin levels than white persons with hypertension.[10] They also do not respond to increased salt intake by increasing their renal excretion of sodium at normal levels of arterial blood pressure. Instead, sodium elimination requires a higher level of blood pressure. These changes in sodium excretion have been linked to what has been called a *salt-thrifty gene.* It has been suggested that the genetic trait may have developed as an evolutionary adaptation to the severe demands for sodium conservation in the western African environment and the slavery environment of the Western hemisphere. In both environments, survival under conditions of heavy exertion in a warm climate along with salt and water deprivation depended on the body's ability to conserve sodium.[11]

Evidence suggests that blacks, when provided equal access to diagnosis and treatment, can achieve overall reductions in blood pressure and experience fewer cardiovascular complications similar to whites. Barriers that limit access to the health care system include inadequate financial support, inconveniently located health care facilities, long waiting times, and inaccessibility to culturally relevant health education about hypertension. With the high prevalence of salt sensitivity, obesity, and smoking among blacks, health education and lifestyle modifications are particularly important. Because of their increased salt sensitivity and low-renin profile, African Americans are reported to respond better to drugs, such as diuretics and calcium-channel–blocking drugs that do not exert their primary actions through renin mechanisms.[2]

Unfortunately, there is little information regarding hypertension in other racial groups, including Native Americans, Asians and Pacific Islanders, and Hispanics.

High Salt Intake. Increased salt intake has long been suspected as an etiologic factor in the development of hypertension. The relation between body levels of sodium and hypertension is based, at least partially, on the finding of a decreased incidence of hypertension among primitive, unacculturated people from widely different parts of the world. For example, among the Yanomamo Indians of northern Brazil, who excrete only about 1 mEq of sodium per day, the average blood pressure in men 40 to 49 years of age was 107/67 mm Hg and 98/62 mm Hg in women of the same age.[12] From childhood through adult life, acculturated societies consume 10 to 20 g of salt daily. Drinking water may be another source of increased sodium intake; some cities have considerable sodium in the water supply.

Just how increased salt intake contributes to the development of hypertension is still unclear. It may be that salt causes an elevation in blood volume, increases the sensitivity of cardiovascular or renal mechanisms to adrenergic influences, or exerts its effects through some other mechanism such as the renin-angiotensin-aldosterone mechanism. There is little evidence that restriction of salt intake reduces blood pressure in normotensive persons,[13] nor is there evidence that salt restriction reduces blood pressure in all cases of hypertension. The impact of long-term, nationwide restriction of sodium consumption in the normotensive population is unknown; it could, for example, create problems in persons who respond poorly to volume-depleting stresses in the absence of readily available salt in their diet. Identification of persons at risk who would specifically benefit from salt reduction would facilitate hypertension management.

Obesity. Excessive weight is commonly associated with hypertension. In a large, nationwide screening program of more than 1 million persons, it was found that the frequency of hypertension among those who were overweight and between 20 and 39 years of age was double that of persons of normal weight and triple that of underweight persons.[14] It has been suggested that fat distribution might be a more critical indicator of hypertension risk than actual overweight. The waist-to-hip ratio is commonly used to differentiate central or upper body obesity (*i.e.,* fat cell deposits in the abdomen) from peripheral or lower body obesity with fat cell deposits in the buttocks and legs (see Chapter 54). Studies have found an association between hypertension and increased waist-to-hip ratio (*i.e.,* central obesity) even when body mass index and skinfold thickness are taken into account.[15,16] Abdominal or visceral fat seems to be more insulin resistant than fat deposited over the buttocks and legs.

Hyperinsulinemia. Insulin resistance and an accompanying compensatory hyperinsulinemia have been suggested as possible etiologic links to the development of hypertension and associated metabolic disturbances such as hyperlipidemia and obesity.[17] Although insulin resistance is common in obesity and type 2 (non–insulin-dependent) diabetes mellitus, it has also been observed in nonobese persons and those without type 2 diabetes. In persons with obesity and type 2 diabetes and in those with hypertension, the defect appears to be in the ability of insulin to stimulate the uptake and disposal of glucose by skeletal muscle.[18]

At least four mechanisms have been proposed for the effects of hyperinsulinemia on blood pressure: activation of the sympathetic nervous system and its effects on cardiac output, peripheral vascular resistance, and renal sodium retention; insulin-stimulated changes in growth of vascular smooth muscle that results in an increase in peripheral vascular resistance; the effect of insulin on salt and water retention by the kidney; and changes in sodium and calcium transport across the cell membrane of vascular smooth muscle, thereby sensitizing blood vessels to vasopressor stimuli.[19]

It has been suggested that the insulin-mediated increase in sympathetic activity is directed at increasing the metabolic rate as a means of burning the calories that cannot be stored because of insulin resistance. Unfortunately, the increase in sympathetic activity also contributes to the development of hypertension by stimulating the heart, the blood vessels, and the kidney.

Hyperinsulinemia also is associated with high plasma triglyceride levels and low concentrations of high-density lipoproteins.

Insulin resistance may be a genetic or acquired trait. For example, it has been shown that insulin-mediated glucose disposal declines by 30% to 40% in persons who are 40% over ideal weight. Nonpharmacologic interventions, such as caloric restriction, weight loss, and exercise, tend to decrease insulin resistance, sympathetic nervous system activity, and blood pressure.[18]

Excess Alcohol Consumption. Regular alcohol drinking plays a role in the development of hypertension. The effect is seen with different types of alcoholic drinks, in men and women, and in a variety of ethnic groups.[20,21] One of the first reports of a link between alcohol consumption and hypertension came from the Oakland-San Francisco Kaiser-Permanente Medical Care Program study of 84,000 persons that correlated known drinking patterns and blood pressure levels.[22] This study revealed that the regular consumption of three or more drinks per day increased the risk of hypertension. Systolic pressures were more markedly affected than diastolic pressures. Blood pressure may improve or return to normal when alcohol consumption is decreased or eliminated. The mechanism whereby alcohol exerts its effect on blood pressure is unclear. It has been suggested that lifestyle factors such as obesity and lack of exercise may be accompanying factors.

Intake of Potassium, Calcium, and Magnesium. It appears that the ratio of sodium to potassium in the diet, rather than increased sodium intake alone, influences blood pressure.[23–25] In terms of food intake, a diet high in sodium is generally low in potassium; conversely, a diet high in potassium is generally low in sodium. One of the major benefits of increased potassium intake is increased elimination of sodium. Other effects include a dampening of vasoconstrictor responses that are induced by norepinephrine and other vasoactive agents. A high-potassium diet does not appear to alter blood pressure in normotensive persons, nor is there evidence to suggest a significant effect from use of potassium supplements in hypertensive persons with normal potassium levels. The use of potassium supplements is expensive and possibly hazardous for some persons. Instead, it is recommended that high-potassium, low-sodium foods be substituted for high-sodium, low-potassium foods in the diet.

The associations of high blood pressure, calcium, and magnesium levels have been investigated.[26] Although there have been reports of high blood pressure in persons with low calcium intake or lowering of blood pressure with increased calcium intake, the link between low calcium intake and hypertension is inconclusive.[27] Magnesium, which has been described as "nature's physiologic calcium blocker," is credited with blocking calcium entry into vascular smooth muscle cells, thereby decreasing vascular reactivity.[28] As with calcium, the benefits of supplementing magnesium intake in persons with hypertension are controversial.

Stress. Physical and emotional stress undoubtedly contribute to transient alterations in blood pressure. Studies in which arterial blood pressure was continually monitored on a 24-hour basis as persons performed their normal activities showed marked fluctuations in pressure associated with normal life stresses—increasing during periods of physical discomfort and family crisis and declining during rest and sleep.[29,30] As with other risk factors, the role of stress-related episodes of transient hypertension in producing the chronically elevated pressures seen in essential hypertension is still speculative. It may be that vascular smooth muscle hypertrophies with increased activity in a manner similar to that of skeletal muscle or that the central integrative pathways in the brain become adapted to the frequent stress-related input.

Psychologic techniques involving biofeedback, relaxation, and transcendental meditation have emerged as possible methods for controlling blood pressure. It is still too early to tell whether these techniques offer information about the role of stress in the production of hypertension or will prove useful in its treatment.

Oral Contraceptive Drugs. Oral contraceptives cause a mild increase in blood pressure in many women and overt hypertension in about 5%.[31] Why this occurs is largely unknown, although it has been suggested that estrogen and progesterone are responsible for the effect. Various contraceptive drugs contain different amounts and combinations of estrogen and progestational agents, and these differences may contribute to the occurrence of hypertension in some women but not others. Fortunately, the hypertension associated with oral contraceptives usually disappears after the drug has been discontinued, although it may take as long as 6 months for this to happen. However, in some women the blood pressure may not return to normal; they may be at risk for developing hypertension. The risk of hypertension-associated cardiovascular complications is found primarily in women older than 35 years of age and in those who smoke.[2]

Signs and Symptoms

Essential hypertension is typically asymptomatic, and diagnosis is often made by chance during screening procedures or when a person seeks medical care for other purposes. Although headache is often considered to be an early symptom of hypertension, it affects only a small number of hypertensives at the time of diagnosis. When present, the headache associated with hypertension is believed to result from intense vasodilatation. It occurs most frequently on awakening and is usually felt in the back of the head or neck.

A common early symptom of target-organ damage in long-term hypertension is nocturia, which indicates that the kidneys are losing their ability to concentrate urine. Other signs and symptoms commonly attributed to hypertension are probably related to the long-term effects of blood pressure elevation on other organ systems in the body, such as the eyes, heart, and blood vessels.

Aside from elevated blood pressure measurements, few diagnostic tests are useful in detecting and diagnosing essential hypertension. The increased availability of hypertensive screening clinics provides one of the best means for early detection. Laboratory tests, x-ray films, and other diagnostic tests are usually done to exclude secondary hypertension and determine the presence or extent of target-organ disease.

Target-Organ Damage

The complications associated with hypertension are associated with the presence of atherosclerosis that frequently accompanies or is the result of sustained levels of high blood pressure or from the direct effects of hypertension on the heart and blood vessels. The 1993 JNC-V report uses the term *target-organ disease* to describe the cardiac, cerebrovascular, peripheral vascular, renal, and retinal complications associated with hypertension.[2] The excess morbidity and mortality related to hypertension is progressive over the whole range of systolic and diastolic pressures. Target-organ damage varies markedly among persons with similar levels of hypertension.

Hypertension is a major risk factor for atherosclerosis; it predisposes the patient to all major atherosclerotic cardiovascular disorders, including heart failure, stroke, coronary artery disease, and peripheral artery disease. The risk of coronary artery disease and stroke depend to a great extent on other risk factors such as obesity, smoking, and elevated cholesterol levels. If all else is favorable, the risk of a coronary event in persons with mild hypertension is no greater than the average population of the same age. However, if a cluster of risk factors exists, the risk is greatly increased.[32] The same is true for stroke. The risk of stroke occurring in persons with hypertension occurs over an eightfold range, depending on the number of associated risk factors. Cerebrovascular complications are more closely related to systolic than diastolic hypertension. The incidence of these complications is greatly reduced by antihypertensive therapy.

Hypertension increases the workload of the left ventricle by increasing the pressure against which the heart must pump as it ejects blood into the systemic circulation. As the workload of the heart increases, the left ventricular wall hypertrophies to compensate for the increased pressure work. The prevalence of left ventricular hypertrophy increases with age and is highest in persons with blood pressures over 160/95 mm Hg. It was observed in 12% to 20% of persons with mild hypertension and in 50% of asymptomatic persons with mild to moderate hypertension.[33] Despite its adaptive advantage, left ventricular hypertrophy is a major risk factor for ischemic heart disease, cardiac dysrhythmias, sudden death, and congestive heart failure. Hypertensive left ventricular hypertrophy regresses with therapy. Regression is most closely related to systolic pressure reduction and does not appear to reflect the particular type of medication used.

Hypertension can also lead to nephrosclerosis, a common cause of renal insufficiency (see Chapter 29). Hypertensive kidney disease is more common in blacks than whites. Hypertension also plays an important role in accelerating the course of other types of kidney disease, particularly diabetic nephropathy.

Treatment

The main objective for treatment of essential hypertension is to achieve and maintain arterial blood pressure below 140/90 mm Hg, with the goal of preventing morbidity and mortality. For persons with secondary hypertension, efforts are made to correct or control the disease condition causing the hypertension. Antihypertensive medications and other measures supplement the treatment for the underlying disease. The JNC-V report on Detection, Evaluation, and Treatment of High Blood Pressure contains a treatment algorithm for hypertension that includes lifestyle modification and, when necessary, guidelines for use of pharmacologic agents to achieve and maintain systolic pressure below 140 mm Hg and diastolic pressure below 90 mm Hg (Fig. 18–3).[2]

Lifestyle Modification. Lifestyle modification, previously referred to as nonpharmacologic therapy, includes weight reduction, reduction of sodium intake, regular physical activity, modification of alcohol intake, and smoking cessation. Other lifestyle modification strategies, such as increased intake of potassium, calcium, and magnesium or the use of relaxation and biofeedback, were not included in the JNC-V report because of a lack of convincing data to justify recommendation.[2] For persons with stage 1 hypertension, an attempt to control blood pressure with weight loss and other lifestyle modifications should be tried for at least 3 to 6 months before initiating pharmacologic treatment.

Recognizing obesity as a major risk factor in essential hypertension, the committee recommended that all obese hypertensive adults be encouraged to participate in weight reduction programs with the goal of achieving a body weight within 15% of their desirable weight.

A high-salt diet may play a critical role in maintaining blood pressure elevation, and it may limit the effectiveness of some antihypertensive drugs. The report recommends that persons with hypertension limit their salt intake to 70 to 100 mEq per day (*i.e.*, 1.5 to 2.5 g sodium or 4 to 6 g of salt). Because many prepared foods are high in sodium, merely refraining from use of the salt shaker is usually not sufficient. Instead, it was recommended that persons consult package labels for the sodium content of canned foods, frozen foods, soft drinks, and other foods and beverages to reduce sodium intake adequately.

A sedentary lifestyle has been cited as a risk factor in cardiovascular disease. A regular program of physical exercise (*e.g.*, walking, biking, swimming) is protective, especially for those at increased risk for cardiovascular disease because of hypertension. Exercise may have further indirect benefits, such as weight loss or motivation for changing other risk factors. Persons with hypertension should be evaluated before beginning an exercise program of appropriate types of exercise. Weight lifting

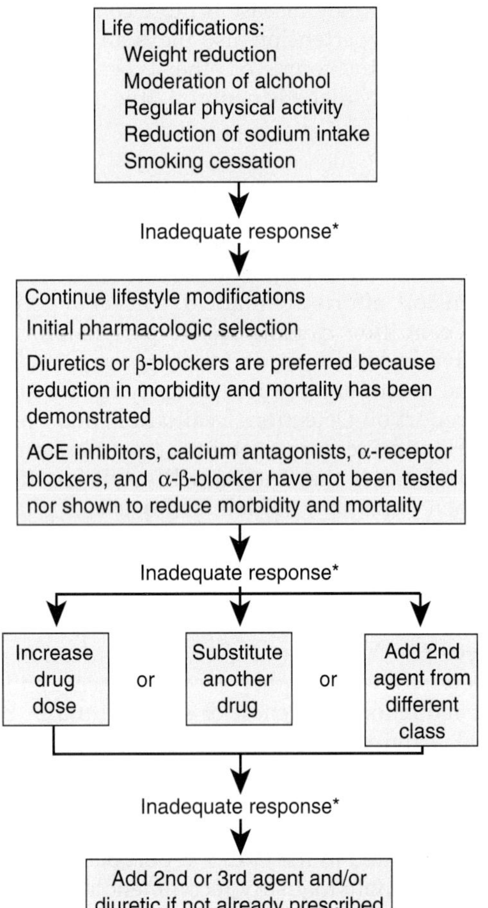

Figure 18–3
Treatment algorithm. *Asterisks* indicate that response means the patient achieved goal blood pressure or is making considerable progress toward this goal. ACE, angiotensin-converting enzyme. (National Heart, Lung, and Blood Institute. [1993]. *The fifth report of the National Committee on Detection, Evaluation, and Treatment of High Blood Pressure.* [p. 16]. Bethesda, MD: NIH Publication No. 93–1088)

and other forms of isometric exercise can raise blood pressure acutely and should be done with caution.

Because of alcohol's association with high blood pressure, the JNC-V report recommended restriction of alcohol consumption to no more than 1 oz per day (equal to 2 oz of 100-proof whiskey, approximately 8 oz of wine, or 24 oz of beer). Significant hypertension may develop during withdrawal from heavy alcohol consumption, but the pressor effects of alcohol withdrawal usually subside within a few days after alcohol consumption is reduced.

Although nicotine has not been associated with long-term elevations in blood pressure as in essential hypertension, it has been shown to increase the risk of heart disease. The fact that smoking and hypertension are major cardiovascular risk factors should be reason enough to encourage the hypertensive smoker to quit. Studies have also reported an interaction between smoking and the antihypertensive drug propranolol, in which smokers required larger doses of the drug to achieve similar reductions in blood pressure compared with nonsmokers.

There is conflicting evidence about the direct effects of dietary fats on blood pressure. As with smoking, however, the interactive effects of saturated fats and high blood pressure as cardiovascular risk factors would seem to warrant dietary modification to reduce the intake of foods high in cholesterol and saturated fats.

Pharmacologic Treatment. The decision to initiate pharmacologic treatment is based on the severity of the hypertension, the presence of target-organ disease, and the existence of other conditions and risk factors. Drug selection is based on the stage of hypertension. Among the drugs used in the treatment of hypertension are diuretics, adrenergic inhibitors, vasodilators, angiotensin-converting enzyme inhibitors, and calcium-channel–blocking drugs. Only diuretics and β-adrenergic–blocking drugs have been shown to reduce mortality and morbidity related to coronary heart disease in major clinical trials. However, clinical trials require considerable time to complete, and these are two of the older drugs used in hypertension treatment. Clinical trials with newer drugs are in progress. A brief discussion of the physiologic action of the commonly used antihypertensive drugs is provided.

Diuretics, such as the thiazides, loop diuretics, and the aldosterone antagonist (potassium-sparing) diuretics, lower blood pressure initially by decreasing vascular volume (by suppressing renal reabsorption of sodium and increasing salt and water excretion) and cardiac output (see Chapter 25). With continued therapy, a reduction in total peripheral resistance becomes the major mechanism of blood pressure reduction.

β-Adrenergic–blocking drugs are effective in hypertension because they decrease heart rate and cardiac output. The β-blockers also decrease renin release. There are two types of β-adrenergic receptors: β_1 and β_2. The β_1-blocking drugs are cardioselective, exerting their effects on the heart, whereas the β_2-adrenergic receptor–blocking drugs affect bronchodilation, relaxation of skeletal blood vessels, and other beta-mediated functions. Both cardioselective (β_1) and nonselective (β_1 and β_2) adrenergic-blocking drugs are used in the treatment of hypertension.

The *angiotensin-converting enzyme (ACE) inhibitors* act by decreasing angiotensin II levels and reducing its effect on vasoconstriction, aldosterone levels, intrarenal blood flow, and the glomerular filtration rate. They also inhibit bradykinin degradation and stimulate prostaglandin synthesis, and sometimes reduce sympathetic nervous system activity. These latter effects may explain why they work in some persons with low renin hypertension. These drugs are increasingly used as the initial medication in mild to moderate hypertension. Because of their effect on the renin-angiotensin system, these drugs are contraindicated in persons with renal artery stenosis in which the renin-angiotensin mechanism functions as a compensatory mechanism to maintain adequate renal perfusion. Because they inhibit aldosterone, these agents can also increase serum potassium levels and cause hyperkalemia.

A newcomer to the field of antihypertensive medications is the *angiotensin II receptor–blocking drugs*. These drugs have the advantage of not producing cough, which was a frequent side effect of ACE inhibitors.

The *calcium-channel receptor–blocking drugs* inhibit the movement of calcium into cardiac and vascular smooth muscle. Each of the different agents in this group acts in a slightly different way. They probably reduce blood pressure by several mechanisms, including a reduction of smooth muscle tone in the venous and arterial systems. Some calcium blockers have a direct myocardial effect that reduces the cardiac output through a decrease in cardiac contractility and a fall in heart rate. Other calcium-blocking drugs influence venous tone and reduce the cardiac output through a decrease in venous return. Still others influence arterial vascular smooth muscle by inhibiting calcium transport across the cell membrane channels or inhibiting the vascular response to norepinephrine or angiotensin.

The *centrally acting adrenergic inhibitors* block sympathetic outflow from the central nervous system. These agents are actually α-adrenergic (α_2) agonists that act in negative-feedback manner to decrease sympathetic outflow from presynaptic sympathetic neurons in the central nervous system. The α_2-adrenergic inhibitors are effective as single therapy for some persons, but they are often used as second- or third-line agents because of the high incidence of side effects. One of the agents, clonidine, is available as a transdermal patch that is replaced weekly.

The *α_1-receptor antagonists* block postsynaptic α_1-receptors and reduce the effect of the sympathetic nervous system on the vascular smooth muscle tone of the blood vessels that regulate the total peripheral vascular resistance. These drugs produce a pronounced fall in blood pressure after the first dose; therefore, treatment is initiated with a smaller dose given at bedtime. Postdosing palpitations, headache, and nervousness may continue with chronic treatment.

Vasodilator drugs promote a decrease in total peripheral vascular resistance by directly producing relaxation of vascular smooth muscle, particularly of the arterioles. These drugs often produce initial stimulation of the sympathetic nervous system and tachycardia and salt and water retention as a result of the decreased filling of the vascular compartment.

Treatment Strategies. The pharmacologic treatment of stage 1 and 2 hypertension is usually initiated when blood pressure remains elevated after a 3 to 6 months of vigorous encouragement of lifestyle modification. Drug therapy is usually initiated with a single drug, usually a diuretic or a β blocker. The alternative drugs—calcium antagonists, ACE inhibitors, α_1-receptor blockers and α-β blockers—are considered to be equally effective and may be used.

If the response to the initial drug is not adequate after 1 to 3 months, one of three approaches is used: the dose can be increased if the initial dose was below the maximum recommended; an agent from another class can be added; or the initial drug can be discontinued and another drug substituted. Combining antihypertensive drugs with different modes of action often allows smaller doses of drugs to be used to achieve blood pressure control, minimizing the possibility of dose-dependent side effects from any one drug. In treating stage 3 or 4 hypertension, it is often necessary to add a second or third drug after a short interval if the treatment goal is not achieved.

Factors considered when hypertensive drugs are prescribed are the person's lifestyle (*i.e.*, someone with a busy schedule may have problems with medications that must be taken three times each day); demographics (*e.g.*, some drugs are more effective in elderly or African-American persons); motivation for adhering to the drug regimen (*e.g.*, some drugs can produce undesirable and even life-threatening consequences if discontinued abruptly); other disease conditions and therapies; and potential for side effects (*e.g.*, some drugs may impair sexual functioning or mental acuity; others have not been proved safe for women of childbearing age). Another factor to be considered is the cost of the drug in relation to financial resources. There is a wide variation in the prices of antihypertensive medications that should be considered when medications are prescribed. This is particularly important for low-income persons with moderate to severe hypertension, because keeping costs at an affordable level may be the key to compliance.

For persons with mild hypertension who have satisfactorily controlled their blood pressure through treatment for at least 1 year, reduction of medication using a reverse stepwise approach may be used, particularly if there has been successful adherence to nonpharmacologic methods of treatment.

Secondary Hypertension

Only 5% to 10% of hypertensive cases are classified as secondary hypertension (*i.e.*, hypertension due to another disease condition). Unlike essential hypertension, many of the conditions causing secondary hypertension can be corrected or cured by surgery or specific medical treatment. Secondary hypertension tends to be seen in persons before age 30 and after age 50.[34] Renal artery stenosis and coarctation of the aorta are more common in younger persons. Cocaine and cocaine-like substances can cause significant hypertension. In older persons, the sudden onset of secondary hypertension is often associated with atherosclerotic disease of the renal blood vessels.

Among the most common causes of secondary hypertension are kidney disease (i.e., renovascular hypertension), adrenal cortical disorders, pheochromocytoma, and coarctation of the aorta. To avoid duplication in descriptions, the mechanisms associated with elevations of blood pressure in these disorders are discussed briefly, and a more detailed discussion of specific disease disorders is reserved for other sections of this book.

Renal Hypertension

With the dominant role that the kidney assumes in blood pressure regulation, it is not surprising that the largest single cause of secondary hypertension is renal disease. Most acute kidney disorders result in decreased urine formation, retention of salt and water, and hypertension. This includes acute glomerulonephritis, acute renal failure, and acute urinary tract obstruction. Hypertension is also common among persons with chronic pyelonephritis, polycystic kidney disease, diabetic nephropathy, and end-stage renal disease, regardless of cause. Renovascular hypertension refers to hypertension caused by reduced renal blood flow and activation of the renin-angiotensin-aldosterone mechanism. It is the most common cause of secondary hypertension and is sometimes a reversible cause of renal failure. In about two thirds of cases, the hypertension results from ischemia due to renal artery stenosis.[34,35]

The reduced renal blood flow that occurs with renovascular disease causes the affected kidneys to release excessive amounts of renin, increasing circulating levels of angiotensin II. Angiotensin II increases blood pressure by producing arteriolar vasoconstriction to increase peripheral vascular resistance, and it increases aldosterone levels to increase sodium retention by the kidney. One or both of the kidneys may be affected. When the renal artery of only one kidney is involved, the unaffected kidney is subjected to the detrimental effects of the elevated blood pressure so that the affected kidney can maintain its function.

Among the causes of renal artery stenosis are fibromuscular dysplasia and atherosclerosis. In contrast to renal artery disease due to atherosclerosis, which most commonly occurs in older persons, fibromuscular renal artery disease is more common in women and tends to occur in younger age groups, often persons in their twenties. Genetic factors may be involved, and the incidence tends to increase with risk factors such as smoking and hyperlipidemia. Renal artery stenosis should be suspected when hypertension develops in a previously normotensive person older than 50 (i.e., atherosclerotic form) or younger than 30 (i.e., fibromuscular hyperplasia) or when accelerated hypertension occurs in a person with previously controlled hypertension. An abdominal bruit may be present. Because renal blood flow depends on the increased blood pressure generated by the renin-angiotensin system, administration of ACE inhibitors can cause a rapid decline in renal function. Persons with atherosclerotic renal artery stenosis often have evidence of atherosclerotic lesions in the coronary, cerebral, or peripheral arteries.

Diagnosis of renovascular disease often involves the use of angiographic studies. The captopril renal scintigram (scan) is a noninvasive test that is often used to screen for the disorder. This test is based on the assumption that captopril, an ACE inhibitor, can decrease renal blood flow, thereby decreasing the uptake radionuclide by the affected kidney. Three-dimensional phase control magnetic resonance imaging may also be used.

The goal of treatment is to control the blood pressure and stabilize renal function. Angioplasty or revascularization has been shown to be an effective long-term treatment for the disorder. Drug therapy may be used to control blood pressure and prevent renal insufficiency. β-Adrenergic–blocking drugs inhibit renin release and are used for this purpose. Renovascular hypertension also responds to ACE inhibitors, but these agents must be used with caution because of their ability to decrease renal function.

Disorders of Adrenocorticosteroid Hormones

Increased levels of adrenocorticosteroid hormones can also give rise to hypertension. Primary hyperaldosteronism (*i.e.*, excess production of aldosterone by the adrenal cortex) and excess levels of glucocorticoids (i.e., Cushing's disease or syndrome) tend to raise the blood pressure (see Chapter 35). These hormones facilitate salt and water retention by the kidney; the hypertension that accompanies excessive levels of either hormone is probably related to this factor. For patients with primary hyperaldosteronism, a salt-restricted diet often produces a reduction in blood pressure. Because aldosterone acts on the distal renal tubule to increase sodium absorption in exchange for potassium elimination in the urine, persons with hyperaldosteronism usually have decreased potassium levels. Potassium-sparing diuretics, such as spironolactone, which is an aldosterone antagonist, are often used in the medical management of persons with the disorder.

Licorice is an extract from the *Glycyrrhiza glabra* that has been used in medicine since ancient times. European licorice (not licorice flavoring) is associated with sodium retention, edema, hypertension, and hypokalemia. It produces a syndrome similar to primary hyperaldosteronism. Licorice is an effective analogue of the 11β-steroid dehydrogenase enzyme that modulates access to the aldosterone receptor in the kidney.[36]

Pheochromocytoma

A pheochromocytoma is a tumor of chromaffin tissue, which contains sympathetic nerve cells that stain with chromium salts. The tumor is most commonly located in the adrenal medulla but can arise in other sites such as sympathetic ganglia, where there is chromaffin tissue.[37] Although only 0.1% to 0.5% of persons with hypertension have an underlying pheochromocytoma, the disorder can cause serious hypertensive crises. Eight percent to 10% of the tumors are malignant.

Like adrenal medullary cells, the tumor cells of a pheochromocytoma produce and secrete the catecholamines epinephrine and norepinephrine. The hypertension that develops results from the massive release of these catecholamines. Their release may be paroxysmal rather than continuous, causing periodic episodes of headache, excessive sweating, and palpations. Headache is the most common symptom and can be quite severe. Nervousness, tremor, pallor of the face, weakness, fatigue, and weight loss occur less frequently. Marked variability in blood pressure between episodes is typical. About 50% of persons with pheochromocytoma have paroxysmal episodes of hypertension, sometimes to dangerously high levels. The other 50% have sustained hypertension, and some may even be normotensive.[37,38]

Several tests are available to differentiate hypertension due to pheochromocytoma from other forms of hypertension. The most commonly used diagnostic measure is the determination of urinary catecholamines and their metabolites, including vanillylmandelic acid. Although measurement of plasma catecholamines may also be used, other conditions can cause catecholamines to be elevated. After the presence of a pheochromocytoma has been established, the tumor needs to be located. Computed tomographic (CT) scans may be used for this purpose. Metaiodobenzylguanidine (MIBG) scintigraphic imaging may be done. MIBG resembles the norepinephrine structure and enters adrenergic tissues by the same mechanism. Surgical removal of operable tumors is curative.[37]

Coarctation of the Aorta

Coarctation represents a narrowing of the aorta. In the adult form of coarctation, the narrowing most commonly occurs just distal to the origin subclavian arteries (see Chapter 19).[39] Because of the narrowing, blood flow to the lower parts of the body and kidneys is reduced. In the infantile form of coarctation, the narrowing occurs proximal to the ductus arteriosus, in which case heart failure and other problems may occur. Many affected babies die within their first year of life.

In the adult form of coarctation, an increase in cardiac output may result from renal compensatory mechanisms. The ejection of a large stroke volume into a narrowed aorta with limited ability to accept the runoff results in an increase in systolic blood pressure and blood flow to the upper part of the body. Blood pressure in the lower extremities may be normal, although it is frequently low. It has been suggested that the increase in cardiac output and maintenance of the pressure to the lower part of the body is achieved through the renin-angiotensin-aldosterone mechanism in response to a decrease in renal blood flow. Pulse pressure in the legs is almost always narrowed, and the femoral pulses are weak. Because the aortic capacity is diminished, there is usually a marked increase in pressure (measured in the arms) during exercise, when the stroke volume and heart rate are exaggerated. For this reason, blood pressures in both arms and one leg should be determined; a 20 mm Hg or higher pressure in the arms than in the legs suggests coarctation of the aorta. Involvement of the left subclavian artery or an anomalous origin of the right subclavian may produce decreased or absent left or right brachial pulses, respectively. Palpation of both brachial pulses and measurement of blood pressure in both arms are important.

Treatment consists of surgical repair or balloon angioplasty. Although balloon angioplasty is a relatively recent form of treatment, it has been used in children and adults with good results. However, there are few data on long-term follow-up.

Malignant Hypertension

A small number of persons with secondary hypertension develop an accelerated and potentially fatal form of the disease—malignant hypertension. This is usually a disease of younger persons, particularly young African-American men, women with toxemia of pregnancy, and persons with renal and collagen diseases.

Malignant hypertension is characterized by sudden marked elevations in blood pressure, with diastolic values above 120 mm Hg, renal disorders, vascular changes, and retinopathy. There may be intense arterial spasm of the cerebral arteries with hypertensive encephalopathy. Cerebral vasoconstriction is probably an exaggerated homeostatic response designed to protect the brain from excesses of blood pressure and flow. The regulatory mechanisms are often insufficient to protect the capillaries, and cerebral edema frequently develops. As it advances, papilledema (*i.e.*, swelling of the optic nerve at its point of entrance into the eye) ensues, giving evidence of the effects of pressure on the optic nerve and retinal vessels. The patient may have headache, restlessness, confusion, stupor, motor and sensory deficits, and visual disturbances. In severe cases, convulsions and coma follow.

Prolonged and severe exposure to exaggerated levels of blood pressure in malignant hypertension injures the walls of the arterioles, and intravascular coagulation and fragmentation of red blood cells may occur. The renal blood vessels are particularly vulnerable to hypertensive damage. Renal damage due to vascular changes is probably the most important prognostic determinant in malignant hypertension. Elevated levels of blood urea nitrogen and serum creatinine, metabolic acidosis, hypocalcemia, and proteinuria provide evidence of renal impairment.

The complications associated with a hypertensive crisis demand immediate and rigorous medical treatment. With proper therapy, the death rate from this cause can be markedly reduced, as can additional episodes. Two drugs, diazoxide and sodium nitroprusside, are used to treat hypertensive emergencies, although others also may be required to bring the blood pressure down to a safe level. Diazoxide, which causes arteriolar dilatation, and sodium nitroprusside, a vasodilator that also affects the venous system, are administered intravenously.

High Blood Pressure in Pregnancy

About 10% of all pregnancies are accompanied by hypertension. The National High Blood Pressure Education Program's Working Group Report on High Blood Pressure in Pregnancy recommends four diagnostic categories for hypertension that occurs during pregnancy: chronic hypertension, preeclampsia-eclampsia, chronic hypertension with superimposed preeclampsia-eclampsia, and transient hypertension.[40] The report emphasizes a need to differentiate hypertension that precedes pregnancy from that developing during pregnancy. The criteria for diagnosing hypertension in pregnancy are systolic pressure increases of 30 mm Hg or greater and diastolic pressure increases of 15 mm Hg or greater compared with the average values before 20 weeks' gestation. When previous blood pressures are not known, values of 140/90 mm Hg or above are considered abnormal.

Chronic Hypertension

Chronic hypertension is considered as hypertension that is unrelated to the pregnancy. It is defined as a history of high blood pressure before pregnancy, identification of hypertension before 20 weeks of pregnancy, and hypertension that persists after pregnancy. In women with chronic hypertension, blood pressure often decreases in early pregnancy and increases during the last trimester (3 months) of pregnancy, resembling preeclampsia. Consequently, women with undiagnosed chronic hypertension who do not present for medical care until the later months of pregnancy may be incorrectly diagnosed as having preeclampsia. Women with chronic hypertension are at increased risk for developing preeclampsia. *Transient hypertension* is a condition of high blood pressure that occurs during the last trimester or early postdelivery period but resolves to normotensive levels within 10 days after delivery.

Preeclampsia and Eclampsia

Preeclampsia, sometimes called *pregnancy-induced hypertension,* is characterized by the triad of hypertension of pregnancy as previously defined, proteinuria (≥300 mg/L in 24 hours), and edema (weight gain of >2 kg/wk) developing after the 20th week of pregnancy. Preeclampsia occurs primarily during first pregnancies and during subsequent pregnancies in women with chronic hypertension, multiple fetuses, diabetes mellitus, or coexisting renal disease. It is associated with a condition called a *hydatidiform mole* (*i.e.*, abnormal pregnancy caused by a pathologic ovum, resulting in a mass of cysts). Of interest is the reversal of the diurnal pattern of blood pressure in preeclamptic hypertension; it is often highest during the night.[41]

Pregnancy-induced hypertension is thought to involve a decrease in placental blood flow leading to the release of toxic mediators that alter the function of endothelial cells in blood vessels throughout the body, including those of the kidney, brain, liver, and heart.[37,42,43] The endothelial changes result in signs and symptoms of preeclampsia and, in more severe cases, of intravascular clotting and hypoperfusion of vital organs. The complications of pregnancy-induced hypertension are life threatening to both the mother and the fetus. These include convulsions and sometimes coma (*i.e.*, eclampsia). The *HELLP syndrome* is an acronym for *h*emolysis, *e*levated *l*iver function tests, and *l*ow *p*latelet counts used to describe a severe complication of preeclampsia and eclampsia.

Defining the causes of pregnancy-induced hypertension is difficult because of the normal circulatory changes that occur during pregnancy. Blood pressure normally decreases during the first trimester, reaches its lowest point during the second trimester, and gradually rises during the third trimester. The fact that there is a 40% to 60% increase in cardiac output during early pregnancy means the fall in blood pressure that occurs during the first part of pregnancy must result from a decrease in peripheral vascular resistance. Because the cardiac output remains high throughout pregnancy, the gradual rise in blood pressure that begins during the second trimester probably represents a return of the peripheral vascular resistance to normal. Pregnancy is normally accompanied by increased levels of renin, angiotensin I and II, estrogen, progesterone, prolactin, and aldosterone, all of which may alter vascular reactivity. Women who develop preeclampsia are thought to be particularly sensitive to the vasoconstrictor responses of the renin-angiotensin-aldosterone system. They are also particularly responsive to other vasoconstrictors, including the catecholamines and vasopressin. It has been proposed that some of the sensitivity may be caused by a prostacylin-thromboxane imbalance. Thromboxane is a prostaglandin with vasoconstrictor properties, and prostacylin is a prostaglandin with vasodilator properties.

Diagnosis and Treatment

Early prenatal care is important in the detection of high blood pressure during pregnancy. It is recommended that all pregnant women, including those with hypertension, refrain from alcohol and tobacco use. Salt restriction is usually not recommended during pregnancy, because pregnant women with hypertension tend to have lower plasma volumes than normotensive pregnant women and because the severity of hypertension may reflect the degree of volume contraction. There has been interest in the use of low-dose aspirin for its effects on prostacylin-thromboxane balance in high-risk women; although its effects have been disappointing,[44] there is continued interest in its use for selected cases.

In women with preeclampsia, delivery of the fetus is curative. The timing of delivery becomes a difficult decision in preterm pregnancies, because the welfare of both the mother and the infant must be taken into account. Bed rest is a traditional therapy. Antihypertensive medications, when required, must be carefully chosen because of their potential effects on uteroplacental blood flow and on the fetus. For example, the ACE inhibitors can cause injury and even death of the fetus when given during the second and third trimesters of pregnancy.

High Blood Pressure in Children

Blood pressure is known to rise from infancy to late adolescence. The average systolic blood pressure at 1 day of age is approximately 70 mm Hg and increases to about 85 mm Hg at 1 month of age.[45] During the preschool years, blood pressure begins to follow a pattern that tends to be maintained as the children grow older. This pattern continues into adolescence and adulthood, suggesting the roots of essential hypertension are established early in life. A familial influence on blood pressure can often be identified early in life. Children of parents with high blood pressure tend to have higher blood pressures than children with normotensive parents.

In 1977, the Task Force on Hypertension in Children published its first recommendations on blood pressure measurement and control in children. This report was updated in 1987 and again in 1996. In its update of the 1987 Task Force Report on High Blood Pressure in Children and Adolescents, the 1996 Task Force included height as a variable in determination of blood pressure.[45] They recommended continued classification of blood pressure into three ranges: normal (*i.e.*, systolic and diastolic pressures below the 90th percentile for age, height, and sex); high normal (*i.e.*, systolic or diastolic blood pressures between the 90th and 95th percentile for age, height, and sex); and high blood pressures or hypertension (*i.e.*, average systolic and diastolic blood pressures equal to or greater than the 95th percentile for age, height, and sex on at least three occasions).

High blood pressure in children has been further defined as significant hypertension (*i.e.*, blood pressure between the 95th and 99th percentile for age and sex) and severe hypertension (*i.e.*, blood pressure above the 99th percentile for age and sex). Table 18–2 presents percentile of blood pressure for boys and girls ages 3 to 16 years of age according to height. The Task Force recommended that children 3 years of age through adolescence should have their blood pressure taken once each year. They recommended that phase V Korotkoff sounds should be used for determining diastolic pressure for children of all ages. As with adults, blood pressure should be obtained using the proper-sized cuff and a well-functioning manometer. Repeated measurements over time, rather than a single, isolated determination, are required to establish consistent and significant observations. Accurate blood pressure measurements are often difficult to obtain in infants and children who are restless; errors are easily generated in Korotkoff sounds if heavy pressure is exerted on the stethoscope. The Task Force recommended the use of auscultatory methods of blood pressure measurement in children, rather than automated methods. Automated methods are acceptable in infants, in the intensive care unit, and children in whom auscultation is difficult.

Secondary hypertension is most common in infants and children. In later childhood and adolescence, essential hypertension is more common. Approximately 75% to 80% of secondary hypertension is caused by kidney abnormalities.[46] Coarctation of the aorta is another cause of hypertension in children and adolescents. Endocrine causes of hypertension such as pheochromocytoma and adrenal cortical disorders are rare. Hypertension in infants is most commonly associated with high umbilical catheterization and renal artery obstruction due to thrombosis.[47] Most cases of essential hypertension is associated with obesity or a family history of hypertension.[48]

A number of drugs of abuse, therapeutic agents, and toxins may also increase blood pressure. Alcohol should be considered as a risk factor in adolescents. Oral contraceptives are a common cause of hypertension in adolescent females. The nephrotoxicity of the drug cylclosporine, an immunosuppressant used in transplant therapy, may cause hypertension in children after bone marrow, heart, kidney, or liver transplantation. The

TABLE 18–2

95th Percentile Blood Pressure in Boys and Girls 1 to 16 Years of Age, According to Height*

Blood Pressure	Age (yrs)	Height Percentile for Boys				Height Percentile for Girls			
		5th	*25th*	*75th*	*95th*	*5th*	*25th*	*75th*	*95th*
Systolic									
	1	98	101	104	106	101	103	105	107
	3	104	107	111	113	104	105	108	110
	6	109	112	115	117	108	110	112	114
	10	114	117	121	123	116	117	120	122
	13	121	124	128	130	121	123	126	128
	16	129	132	136	138	125	127	130	132
Diastolic									
	1	55	56	58	59	57	57	59	60
	3	63	64	66	67	65	65	67	68
	6	72	73	75	76	71	72	73	75
	10	77	79	80	82	77	77	79	80
	13	79	81	83	84	80	81	82	84
	16	83	84	86	87	83	83	85	86

*The height percentiles were determined with standard growth curves
(Data adapted from Update on the 1987 Task Force Report on High Blood Pressure in Children and Adolescents: A Working Group Report From the National High Blood Pressure Education Program. (1996). *Pediatrics* 98(4), 653–654.)

coadministration of glucocorticosteroid drugs appears to increase the incidence of hypertension.

Children with high blood pressure, significant high blood pressure, or severe high blood pressure should be referred for medical evaluation and treatment as indicated. Treatment includes nonpharmacologic methods and, if necessary, pharmacologic therapy. The Task Force suggested use of the stepped-care approach for drug treatment of children who require antihypertensive medications.

High Blood Pressure in the Elderly

The prevalence of hypertension in the elderly population (65 to 74 years) of the United States ranges from 53% for whites to 55% for Mexican Americans and 72% for African Americans.[49] The most common type of hypertension in the elderly is isolated systolic hypertension in which systolic pressure is elevated while diastolic pressure remains within normal range. The JNC guidelines (see Table 18–1) have been recommended for in defining systolic hypertension.[50] According to this definition, systolic hypertension is defined as a systolic pressure greater than 140 mm Hg and a diastolic pressure of 90 mm Hg or less. This definition is controversial, and the former definition, a systolic pressure of at least 160 mm Hg and a diastolic pressure of less than 90 mm Hg, continues to be used by some experts.[51]

Aging processes that contribute to an increase blood pressure are a stiffening of the large arteries, particularly the aorta; decreased baroreceptor sensitivity; increased peripheral vascular resistance; and decreased renal blood flow. The increased arterial stiffness offsets the increase in diastolic pressure that normally should accompany an increase in peripheral vascular resistance. The disproportionate rise in systolic pressure observed in some elderly persons is explained in terms of the increased rigidity of the aorta and peripheral arteries that accompanies the aging process. These changes are largely caused by a loss of elastin fibers in the wall of the aorta and larger blood vessels. Normally, the elastic properties of the aorta allow it to stretch during systole as a means of buffering the rise in pressure that occurs as blood is ejected from the heart. During diastole, the recoil of the elastin fibers transmit the stored pressure to the peripheral arterioles as a means of maintaining the diastolic blood pressure. As the aorta loses its elasticity and becomes more rigid as a result of the aging process, the pressure generated during ventricular systole is transmitted to the peripheral arteries practically unchanged.

Isolated systolic hypertension is recognized as an important risk factor for cardiovascular morbidity and mortality in older persons. Stroke is two to three times more common in elderly hypertensives than in age-matched normotensive subjects.[52] Treatment of hypertension in the elderly has beneficial effects in terms of reducing the incidence of cardiovascular events such as stroke. The Systolic Hypertension in the Elderly Program (SHEP) showed a a reduction of 36% in stroke and a 27% reduction in myocardial infarction in persons who were treated for hypertension compared with those who were not.[53]

Diagnosis

The recommendations for measurement of blood pressure in the elderly are similar to those for the rest of the population. Blood pressure variability is particularly prevalent among older persons, and it is therefore especially important to obtain six to nine measurements (*i.e.*, two or three readings on two or three occasions) to establish a diagnosis of hypertension. The effects of food, position, and other environmental factors are also exaggerated in older persons. Special care is also warranted when the blood pressure is being taken, because blood pressure measurement methods can produce pressures that are too low (*i.e.*, auscultatory gap) or falsely elevated (*i.e.*, pseudohypertension). In some elderly persons with hypertension, a silent interval, called the auscultatory gap, may occur between the end of the first and beginning of the third phases of the Korotkoff sounds, providing the potential for underestimating the systolic pressure, sometimes by as high as 50 mm Hg.[54] Because the gap occurs only with auscultation, it is recommended that a preliminary determination of systolic blood pressure be made by palpation and the cuff be inflated above this value for auscultatory measurement of blood pressure. It is also recommended that the cuff be deflated slowly to avoid missing the first Korotkoff sounds.

In some older persons, the indirect measurement of blood pressure using a blood pressure cuff and the Korotkoff sounds has been shown to give falsely elevated readings compared with the direct intraarterial method. This is because excessive cuff pressure is needed to compress the sclerotic arteries of some older persons. A simple procedure called *Osler's maneuver* has been reported to differentiate persons with true hypertension from those whose blood pressure is spuriously elevated because of excessive sclerosis of the large arteries.[55] This procedure involves inflating the blood pressure cuff above systolic pressure and carefully palpating the radial or brachial artery. Whenever either of these arteries remains clearly palpable (despite being pulseless), the peson is said to be Osler positive; when the artery is collapsed and not palpable, the person is said to be Osler negative.

Although sitting has been the standard position for blood pressure measurement, it is recommended that blood pressure also be taken in the supine and standing positions in the elderly. There is often a transient fall in blood pressure on standing, after which baroreflex-mediated increases in heart rate and total peripheral resistance (*i.e.*, vascular constriction) usually return blood pressure to normal values. Because these reflexes are often less responsive in the elderly and may be impaired by hypertensive medications, it has been recommended that blood pressure be measured in the supine position and at 2 to 5 minutes after assumption of the standing position. This should be done during pretreatment examinations and during follow-up examinations after treatment has been instituted. This approach can detect the complication of postural hypotension, which can occur with some medications.

Treatment

The treatment of hypertension in the elderly is similar to that for younger age groups. However, blood pressure should be reduced slowly and cautiously. When possible, appropriate lifestyle modification measures should be tried first. Antihypertensive medications should be prescribed carefully, because the older person may have impaired baroreflex sensitivity and renal function. Usually, medications are initiated at smaller doses, and doses are increased more gradually. Care givers must be alert to the hazards of adverse drug interactions in older persons, who may be on multiple medications, including over-the-counter preparations.

In summary, hypertension is probably one of the most common cardiovascular disorders. It may occur as a primary disorder (i.e., essential hypertension) or as a symptom of some other disease (i.e., secondary hypertension). Secondary forms of hypertension include renal disorders that increase salt and water retention, adrenal cortical disorders such as hyperaldosteronism and Cushing's disease that increase salt and water retention, pheochromocytomas that increases catecholamine levels, and coarctation of the aorta, which produces a compensatory increase in blood pressure.

The incidence of essential hypertension increases with age, is seen more frequently among African Americans, and is linked to a family history of high blood pressure, obesity, and increased salt intake. Uncontrolled hypertension increases the risk of heart disease, renal complications, retinopathy, and stroke. Because hypertension occurs as a silent disorder, screening programs provide an effective means of early detection. The importance of screening lies in the fact that hypertension can usually be controlled and its complications can be prevented or minimized with appropriate treatment measures. Treatment of essential hypertension focuses on nonpharmacologic methods such as weight reduction, reduction of sodium intake, regular physical activity, modification of alcohol intake, and smoking cessation. The decision to initiate pharmacologic treatment is based on the severity of the hypertension, the presence of target-organ disease, and the existence of other conditions and risk factors. Among the drugs used in the treatment of hypertension are diuretics, adrenergic inhibitors, vasodilators, ACE inhibitors, and calcium-channel–blocking drugs.

Hypertension that occurs during pregnancy can be divided into four categories: chronic hypertension, preeclampsia-eclampsia, chronic hypertension with superimposed preeclampsia-eclampsia, and transient hypertension. Preeclampsia-eclampsia is hypertension that develops after 20 weeks' gestation and is accompanied by proteinuria and edema. This form of hypertension, which is thought to result from impaired placental perfusion along with the release of toxic vasoactive substances that alter blood vessel tone and blood clotting mechanisms, poses a particular threat to the mother and the fetus.

Blood pressure is known to rise from infancy to late adolescence. During childhood, blood pressure is influenced by growth and maturation; therefore, blood pressure norms have been established using age and height, race, and sex-specific percentiles to identify children for further follow-up and treatment. Although hypertension occurs infrequently in children, it is recommended that children 3 years of age through adolescence should have their blood pressure taken once each year.

The most common type of hypertension in the elderly is isolated systolic hypertension (systolic pressure >140 mm Hg and diastolic pressure >90 mm Hg). Its pathogenesis is related to the loss of elastin fibers in the aorta and the inability of the aorta to stretch during systole. Untreated systolic hypertension is recognized as an important risk factor for stroke and other cardiovascular morbidity and mortality in older persons. Indirect blood pressure measurement can be falsely elevated because of sclerotic blood vessels that require excessive cuff pressures or blood pressure may be underestimated because of an auscultatory gap.

Orthostatic Hypotension

After you have completed this section of the chapter, you should be able to meet the following objectives:

- Define the term *orthostatic hypotension*
- Explain how fluid deficit, medications, aging, disorders of the autonomic nervous system, and bed rest contribute to the development of orthostatic hypotension

Orthostatic or postural hypotension is an abnormal drop in blood pressure on assumption of the standing position. In the absence of normal circulatory reflexes or blood volume, blood pools in the lower part of the body when the standing position is assumed, cardiac output falls, and blood flow to the brain is inadequate. Dizziness, syncope (*i.e.*, fainting), or both may occur.

Mechanisms

After the assumption of the upright posture from the supine position, approximately 500 to 700 ml of blood are momentarily shifted to the lower part of the body, with an accompanying fall in central blood volume and arterial pressure.[56] Normally, this fall in blood pressure is transient, lasting through several cardiac cycles, because the baroreceptors located in the thorax and carotid sinus area sense the decreased pressure and initiate reflex constriction of the veins and arterioles and an increase in heart rate, which brings blood pressure back to normal. Within a few minutes of standing, blood levels of antidiuretic hormone and sympathetic neuromediators increase as a secondary means of ensuring maintenance of normal blood pressure in the standing position. Muscle movement in the lower extremities also aids venous return to the heart by pumping blood out of the legs.

In persons with healthy blood vessels and normal autonomic function, cerebral blood flow is usually not reduced in the upright position unless arterial pressure falls below 70 mm Hg. The strategic location of the arterial baroreceptors between the heart and brain is designed to ensure that the arterial pressure is maintained within a range sufficient to prevent a reduction in cerebral blood flow.

Classification

Although there is no firm agreement on the definition of orthostatic hypotension, many authorities consider a drop in systolic of 20 mm Hg or more or a drop in diastolic blood pressure of 10 mm Hg or more as diagnostic of the condition.[57] Some authorities regard the presence of orthostatic symptoms (*e.g.*, dizziness, syncope) as being more relevant than the numerical fall in blood pressure.[58] Kochar developed a functional classification of orthostatic hypotension that uses the drop in blood pressure and orthostatic symptoms (Chart 18–2).[59]

Causes

A wide variety of conditions, acute and chronic, are associated with orthostatic hypotension. These include reduced blood volume, drug-induced hypotension, altered vascular responses associated with aging, bed rest, and autonomic nervous system dysfunction.

CHART **18-2**
Functional Classification of Orthostatic Hypotension

Class 1 Asymptomatic postural hypotension (fall in either systolic or diastolic BP ≥20 mmHg)
Class 2 Lightheadedness (dizziness, giddiness) associated with postural hypotension but no history of syncope
Class 3 History of syncope (fainting) accompanied with postural hypotension
Class 4 Incapacitated because of severe dizziness or frequent syncope due to documented postural hypotension

(Kochar M. S. [1990]. Orthostatic hypotension. In Smith J.J. [Ed.]. *Circulatory response to the upright posture* [p. 171]. Boca Raton, FL: CRC Press)

Reduced Blood Volume

Orthostatic hypotension is often an early sign of reduced blood volume or fluid deficit. When blood volume is decreased, the vascular compartment is only partially filled; although cardiac output may be adequate when a person is in the recumbent position, it often decreases to the point of causing weakness and fainting when the person assumes the standing position. Common causes of orthostatic hypotension related to hypovolemia are excessive use of diuretics, excessive diaphoresis, loss of gastrointestinal fluids through vomiting and diarrhea, and loss of fluid volume associated with prolonged bed rest.

Drug-Induced Hypotension

Antihypertensive drugs and psychotropic drugs are the most common cause of chronic orthostatic hypotension. In most cases, the orthostatic hypotension is well tolerated. If postural hypotension is of class 2 or more, it is recommended that the dosage of the drug be reduced or a different drug be used.[59] Table 18–3 lists some drugs that have the potential for causing orthostatic hypotension.

Aging

Weakness and dizziness on standing are common complaints of elderly persons. The Cardiovascular Health Study reports a 16.2% prevalence of asymptomatic orthostatic hypotension among persons 65 years of age and older.[60] Orthostatic hypotension was associated with systolic hypertension, major electrocardiographic abnormalities, and carotid artery stenosis.[60] Because cerebral blood flow primarily depends on systolic pressure, patients with impaired cerebral circulation may experience symptoms of weakness, ataxia, dizziness, and syncope when their arterial pressure falls even slightly. This may happen in older persons who are immobilized for brief periods or whose blood volume is decreased owing to inadequate fluid intake or overzealous use of diuretics.

Postprandial blood pressure often decreases in elderly persons.[61] The greatest postprandial changes occur after a high carbohydrate meal.[62] Although the mechanism responsible for these changes is not fully understood, it is thought to result from glucose-mediated impairment of baroreflex sensitivity and increased splanchnic blood flow mediated by insulin and vasoactive gastrointestinal hormones.

Bed Rest

Prolonged bed rest promotes a reduction in plasma volume, a decrease in venous tone, failure of peripheral vasoconstriction, and weakness of the skeletal muscles that support the veins and assist in returning blood to the heart (see Chapter 55). Physical deconditioning follows even short periods of bed rest. After 3 to 4 days, the blood volume is decreased. Loss of vascular and skeletal muscle tone is less predictable but probably becomes maximal after about 2 weeks of bed rest. Orthostatic intolerance is a recognized problem of space flight—a

TABLE 18-3
Drugs Known to Cause Orthostatic Hypotension

Drug Groups*	Specific Drugs	Mechanism of Action
Antihypertensive drugs	Pentolinium (Ansolysen) Trimetaphan (Arfonad)	Blocks transmission of sympathetic impulses at the autonomic ganglia
	Guanethidine (Ismelin)	Blocks sympathetic impulses at the postganglionic sites
	Methyldopa (Aldomet) Clonidin (Catapres)	Decreases sympathetic outflow from the CNS
	Hydralazine (Apresoline) Prazosin (Minipres) Minoxidil (Loniten)	Direct vasodilator action
Antiparkinsonian drugs	Levodopa preparation Amantadine (Symmetrel)	Vasodilatation due to β-adrenergic stimulation or α blockade of the peripheral vascular system
Antipsychotic drugs	Chlorpromazine (Thorazine) Thiethylperazine (Torecan) Thioridazine (Mellaril)	Loss of reflex vasoconstriction due to blocking of α receptors; these drugs also impair sympathetic outflow from the brain
Calcium-channel blockers	Diltiazem (Cardizem) Nifedipine (Procardia) Verapamil (Calan, Isoptin)	Direct vasodilator action
Tricyclic and related antidepressant drugs	Amitriptyline (Elavil, Endep, Amitid, Amtril, others) Amoxapine (Asendin) Desipramine (Norepramine, Pertofrane) Doxepin (Adapin, Sinequan) Imipramine (Tofranil, Imavate, others) Nortriptyline (Aventyl, Pamelor) Maprotiline (Ludiomil) Traxodone (Desyrel)	Blocks norepinephrine uptake in central adrenergic neurons, with a resultant increase in stimulation of central α-adrenergic receptors, causing a decrease in peripheral sympathetic nervous system activity
Vasodilator drugs	Nitrates (nitroglycerin and long-acting nitrates)	Direct vasodilator action

*This list is not intended to be inclusive; it encompasses some of the widely prescribed drugs.

potential risk after reentry into the earth's gravitational field.

Disorders of Autonomic Nervous System Function

The sympathetic nervous system plays an essential role in adjustment to the upright position. Sympathetic stimulation increases heart rate and cardiac contractility and causes constriction of peripheral veins and arterioles. Orthostatic hypotension caused by altered autonomic function is common in peripheral neuropathies associated with diabetes mellitus, after injury or disease of the spinal cord, or as the result of a cerebral vascular accident in which sympathetic outflow from the brain stem is disrupted.

Idiopathic Orthostatic Hypotension

Idiopathic orthostatic hypotension is unrelated to drug therapy or pathologic conditions. It may be of two types: idiopathic orthostatic hypotension not accompanied by other signs of neurologic deficits or idiopathic hypotension accompanied by multiple neurologic deficits (*i.e.*, Shy-Drager syndrome). The Shy-Drager syndrome usually develops in middle to late life as orthostatic hypotension associated along with uncoordinated movements, urinary incontinence, constipation, and other signs of neurologic deficits referable to the corticospinal, extrapyramidal, corticobulbar, and cerebellar systems.

Diagnosis and Treatment

Orthostatic hypotension can be assessed with the blood pressure cuff. A reading should be made when the patient is supine, immediately after assumption of the seated or upright position, and at 2- to 3-minute intervals for 5 minutes. Because it takes about 5 to 10 minutes for the blood pressure to stabilize after lying down, it is recommended that the patient be supine for this period before standing.[63] It is strongly recommended that a second person be available when blood pressure is measured in the standing position to prevent injury should the patient become faint. A tilt table can also be used for this purpose. With a tilt table, the recumbent patient can be moved to a head-up position without voluntary movement when the table is tilted.

Persons with a drop in blood pressure to orthostatic levels should be evaluated to determine the cause and seriousness of the condition. A history should be done to elicit information about symptoms, particularly dizziness and history of syncope and falls; medical conditions, particularly those such as diabetes mellitus that predispose to orthostatic hypotension; use of prescription and over-the-counter drugs; and symptoms of autonomic nervous system dysfunction, such as impotence or bladder dysfunction. A physical examination should document blood pressure in both arms and the heart rate while in the supine, sitting, and standing positions and should note the occurrence of symptoms.

Treatment of orthostatic hypotension is usually directed toward alleviating the cause or, if this is not possible, toward helping the person learn ways to cope with the disorder and prevent falls and injuries. Correcting the fluid deficit and trying a different antihypertensive medication are examples of measures designed to correct the cause. Measures designed to help persons prevent symptomatic orthostatic drops in blood pressure include gradual ambulation (*i.e.*, sitting on the edge of the bed for several minutes and moving the legs to initiate skeletal muscle pump function before standing) to allow the circulatory system to adjust; avoidance of situations that encourage excessive vasodilatation (*e.g.*, drinking alcohol, exercising vigorously in a warm environment); and avoidance of excess diuresis (*e.g.*, use of diuretics), diaphoresis, or loss of body fluids. Tight-fitting elastic support hose or an abdominal support garment may help prevent pooling of blood in the lower extremities and abdomen.

In summary, orthostatic hypotension refers to an abnormal fall in systolic and diastolic blood pressures that occurs on assumption of the upright position. An important consideration in orthostatic hypotension is the occurrence of dizziness and syncope. Among the factors that contribute to its occurrence are decreased fluid volume, medications, aging, defective function of the autonomic nervous system, and the effects of immobility. Diagnosis of orthostatic hypotension includes blood pressure measurement in the supine and upright positions, a history of symptomatology, medication use, and disease conditions that contribute to a postural drop in blood pressure. Treatment includes correcting the reversible causes and assisting the person to compensate for the disorder and prevent falls and injuries.

REFERENCES

1. Robinson S.C., Brucer M. (1939). Range of normal blood pressure: A statistical study of 11,383 persons. *Archives of Internal Medicine* 64 (3), 409.
2. National Heart, Lung, and Blood Institute. (1993). The fifth report of the Joint National Committee on Detection, Evaluation, and Treatment of High Blood Pressure. NIH Publication No. 93–1088. Bethesda: National Institutes of Health.
3. Pickering T., American Society for Blood Pressure Ad Hoc Panel. (1995). Recommendations for use of home (self) and ambulatory blood pressure monitoring. *American Journal of Hypertension* 9, 1–11.
4. Cowley A.W., Roman R.J. (1996). The role of the kidney in hypertension. *Journal of the American Medical Association* 275(20), 1581–1589.
5. Hall J.E., Guyton A.C., Brands M.W. (1996). Pressure-volume regulation in hypertension. *Kidney International* 49 (Suppl. 55), S35–S41.
6. Williams R.R., Hunt S.C., Hassstedt S.J., et. al. (1991). Are there interactions and relations between genetic and environmental factors predisposing to high blood pressure? *Hypertension* 18 (Suppl. I), S29–S37.
7. Burt V.L., Whelton P., Rocella E.J., et al. (1995). Prevalence of hypertension in the US population: Results from the Third National Health and Nutrition Examination Survey, 1988–91. *Hypertension* 25, 305–313.
8. Gillum R.F. (1996). Epidemiology of hypertension in African American Women. *American Heart Journal* 131, 385–395.
9. Kaplan N.M. (1994). Ethnic aspects of hypertension. *Lancet* 344, 450–452.
10. Blaustein M.P., Grim C.E. (1991). The pathogenesis of hypertension: Black-white differences. *Cardiovascular Clinics* 21 (3), 97–114.
11. Wilson T.W., Grim C.E. (1991). Biohistory of slavery and blood pressure differences in blacks today: A hypothesis. *Hypertension* 17 (Suppl. I), I122–I128.
12. Oliver W.J., Cohen E.L., Neel J.V. (1975). Blood pressure, sodium intake, and sodium related hormones in the Yanomamo Indians, a "no-salt" culture. *Circulation* 52 (1), 146.
13. Midgley J.P., Mathew A.G., Greenwood C.M.T., et al. (1996). Effect of reduced dietary sodium on blood pressure. *Journal of the American Medical Association* 275 (20), 1590–1597.
14. Stamler R., Stamler J., Riedlinger W.R. (1978). Weight and blood pressure. *Journal of the American Medical Association* 240, 1607.
15. Cassano P.A., Segal M.R., Vokonas P.S., Weiss S.T. (1990). Body fat distribution, blood pressure, and hypertension: A prospective study of men in the normative aging study. *Annals of Epidemiology* 1, 33–48.
16. Peiris A.N., Sothmann M.S., Hoffmann R.G., et al. (1989). Obesity, fat distribution, and cardiovascular risk. *Annals of Internal Medicine* 110, 867–872.
17. Ward K.D., Sparrow D., Landsberg L. (1996). Influence of insulin, sympathetic nervous system activity, and obesity on blood pressure: The Normative Aging Study. *Journal of Hypertension* 14, 301–306.
18. Reaven G.M., Lithell H., Landsberg L. (1996). Hypertension and associated metabolic abnormalities—The role of insulin resistance and the sympathoadrenal system. *New England Journal of Medicine* 334 (6), 374–381.
19. Williams B. (1994). Insulin resistance: The shape of things to come. *Lancet* 344, 521–524.
20. Beilin L.J., Puddy I.B., Burke V. (1996). Alcohol and hypertension–Kill or cure. *Journal of Human Hypertension* 10 (Suppl. 2), S1–S5.
21. Marmot M.G., Elliott P., Shipley M.J., Dyer A.R., Ueshima U., Beevers D.G., et.al. (1994). Alcohol and blood pressure: The INTERSALT study. *British Medical Journal* 308, 1263–1267.
22. Klatsky A.L., Freidman G.D., Siegelaub A.B. (1977). Alcohol consumption and blood pressure. *New England Journal of Medicine* 296 (21), 1194.
23. Fregly M.J. (1983). Estimates of sodium and potassium intake. *Annals of Internal Medicine* 98 (Part 2), 792.
24. Lanford G.H. (1983). Dietary potassium and hypertension: Epidemiologic data. *Annals of Internal Medicine* 98 (Part 2), 770.
25. Kaplan N.M. (1994). *Clinical Hypertension* (6th ed., pp. 175–180). Baltimore, Williams & Wilkins.

26. McCarron D.A. (1983). Calcium and magnesium in human hypertension. *Annals of Internal Medicine* 98 (Part 2), 800.
27. Allender P.S., Cutler J.A., Follman D., et al. (1996). Dietary calcium and blood pressure: A meta-analysis of randomized clinical trials. *Annals of Internal Medicine* 124 (9), 825–831.
28. Iseri L.T., French J.H. (1984). Magnesium: Nature's physiologic calcium blocker. *American Heart Journal* 108 (1), 188.
29. Bevan A.T., Hanour A.J., Stott F.H. (1969). Direct arterial pressure recording in unrestricted man. *Clinical Science and Molecular Medicine* 36, 329.
30. Pickering T., Harshfield G.A., Kleinert H.D., et al. (1982). Blood pressure during normal daily activities, sleep, and exercise. *Journal of the American Medical Association* 247 (7), 992.
31. Kaplan N.M. (1995). The treatment of hypertension in women. *Archives of Internal Medicine* 155, 563–567.
32. Kannel W.B. (1996). Blood pressure as a cardiovascular risk factor. *Journal of the American Medical Association* 275 (24), 1571–1576.
33. Frohlich E.D., Chobanian A.B., Devereux R.G., et al. (1992). The heart in hypertension. *New England Journal of Medicine* 327 (24), 998–1008.
34. Ram C.V. (1994). Secondary hypertension: Workup and Correction. *Hospital Practice* 4, 137–155.
35. Aristizabal D., Frohlich E.D. (1992). Hypertension due to renal arterial disease. *Heart Disease and Stroke* 1(4), 227–234.
36. Gomez-Sanchez C.E., Gomez-Sanchez E.P., Yamakita N. (1995). Endocrine causes of hypertension. *Seminars in Nephrology* 15 (2), 106–115.
37. Zamorski M.A., Green L.A. (1996). Preeclampsia and hypertensive disorders of pregnancy. *American Family Physician* 53 (5), 1595–1604.
38. Venkata C., Ram S., Fierro-Carrion G.A. (1995). Pheochromocytoma. *Seminars in Nephrology* 15 (2), 126–137.
39. Roa P.S. (1995). Coarctation of the aorta. *Seminars in Nephrology* 15 (2), 87–105.
40. National High Blood Pressure Education Program Working Group. (1990). Report on high blood pressure in pregnancy. *American Journal of Obstetrics and Gynecology* 63 (5, Part I), 1689–1712.
41. Olofsson P. (1995). Characteristics of a reversed circadian blood pressure rhythm in pregnant women with hypertension. *Journal of Human Hypertension* 9, 565–570.
42. Duda J. (1996). Preeclampsia. *Western Journal of Medicine* 164, 315–320.
43. Lindheimer M.D., Katz A.I. (1985). Hypertension in pregnancy. *New England Journal of Medicine* 313 (11), 675.
44. CLASP (Collaborative Low-Dose Aspirin Study in Pregnancy) Collaborative Group: CLASP. (1994). A randomized trial of low-dose aspirin for the prevention and treatment of pre-eclampsia among 9364 pregnant women. *Lancet* 343, 619–629.
45. Sinaiko A.R. (1996). Hypertension in children [review]. *New England Journal of Medicine* 335 (26), 1968–1973.
46. National Heart, Lung and Blood Institute. (1996). Update of the 1987 Task Force Report of the Second Task Force on High Blood Pressure in Children and Adolescents: A Working Group report from the National High Blood Pressure Education Program. *Pediatrics* 88 (4), 649–658.
47. Pruitt A.W. System Hypertension. In Behrman R.E., Kliegman R.M., Arvin A.M. (1996). *Nelson Textbook of Pediatrics* (15th ed., pp. 1368–1374). Philadelphia: W.B. Saunders.
48. Gobble M.M. Hypertension in Infancy. (1993). *Pediatric Clinics North America* 40 (1), 105–121.
49. Loggie J.M.H. (1994). Hypertension in Children. *Heart Disease and Stroke* May / June, 147–154.
50. National High Blood Pressure Education Program Working Group. (1994). National High Blood Pressure Education Working Group report on hypertension in the elderly. *Hypertension* 23, 275–285.
51. Kaplan N.M. (1995). Hypertension in the elderly. *Annual Review of Medicine* 45:27–38.
52. Kannel J.P., Levy D. (1993). Isolated systolic hypertension in the elderly. *Hospital Practice* (9), 57–74.
53. SHEP Cooperative Research Group. (1991). Prevention of stroke by antihypertensive drug treatment in older persons with isolated systolic hypertension. *Journal of the American Medical Association* 265:3255–3264.
54. Messerli F.H., Ventura H.O., Amodeo C. (1985). Osler's maneuver and pseudohypertension. New England Journal of Medicine 312 (24), 1548.
55. Nicharas AP., Laragh JH. (1980). Hypertension in the elderly: Diagnosis and treatment. *Modern Concepts in Cardiovascular Disease* 69, 49.
56. Smith J.J. Porth C.J.M. (1990). Age and the response to orthostatic stress. In Smith J.J. (Ed.). *Circulatory response to the upright posture* (pp. 121–138). Boca Raton, FL: CRC Press.
57. Lipsitz L.A. (1989). Orthostatic hypotension in the elderly. *New England Journal of Medicine* 321, 952–957.
58. Hollister A.S. (1992). Orthostatic hypotension: Causes, evaluation, and management. *Western Journal of Medicine* 157, 652–657.
58. Kochar M.S. (1990). Orthostatic hypotension. In J.J. Smith (Ed.). *Circulatory response to the upright posture* (pp. 170–179). Boca Raton, FL: CRC Press.
59. Rutan G.H., Hermanson B., Bild D.E., Kittner S.J., LaBaw F., Tell G.S. (1992). Orthostatic hypotension in older adults: The Cardiovascular Study. *Hypertension* 19, 508–519.
60. Jansen R.W.M.M., Lipsitz L.A. (1995). Postprandial hypotension: Epidemiology, pathophysiology, and clinical management. *Annals of Internal Medicine* 122 (4), 286–295.
61. Lipsitz L.A., Lyquist R.P., Wei J.Y., et al. (1983). Postprandial reduction in blood pressure in the elderly. *New England Journal of Medicine* 309, 81–86.
62. Potter J.F., Heseltine D., Matthews J., et al. (1989). Effects of meal composition on the postprandial blood pressure, catecholamine and insulin changes in elderly subjects. *Clinical Science* 77, 226.
63. Porth C.J.M. (1996). Unpublished data from Orthostatic Hypotension in the Elderly Study.

ADDITIONAL READINGS

Anastos K., Charney P., Charon R.A., et al. (1991). Hypertension in women: What is really known. *Annals of Internal Medicine* 115, 287–293.

Applegate W.B. (1991). Systolic hypertension in older people. *Advances in Internal Medicine* 37, 37–54.

Brunner H.R. (1990). The renin–angiotensin system in hypertension: An update. *Hospital Practice* 25 (8A), 71–81.

Cunha U.V. (1987). Management of orthostatic hypotension in the elderly. *Geriatrics* 42 (9), 61.

Cunningham F.G., Lindheimer M.D. (1992). Hypertension in pregnancy. *New England Journal of Medicine* 326, 927–932.

Daniels S.R. (1992). Primary hypertension in childhood and adolescence. *Pediatric Annals* 21, 226–234.

Fletcher A.E., Bulpitt C.J. (1992). How far should blood pressure be lowered? *New England Journal of Medicine* 326, 251–253.

Francis C.K. (1991). Hypertension, cardiac disease and compliance in minority patients. *American Journal of Medicine* 91 (Suppl. A), 29S–36S.

Frohlich E.D., Chobanian A.V., Devereux R.B., et al. (1992). The heart in hypertension. *New England Journal of Medicine* 327, 998–1008.

Gistrap L.C., Gant N.F. (1990). Pathophysiology of preeclampsia. *Seminars in Perinatology* 14, 147–151.

Hoeldtke R.D., Carabello B. (1987). Hemodynamic changes during food ingestion in a patient with postprandial hypotension. *Journal of the American Geriatric Society* 35, 354.

Hollister A.S. (1992). Orthostatic hypotension: Causes, evaluation, and management. *Western Journal of Medicine* 157, 652–657.

Kaplan N.M. (1992). Treatment of hypertensive emergencies and urgencies. *Heart Disease and Stroke* 1, 373–378.

Laragh J.H. (1992). The modern evaluation and treatment of hypertension: The causal role of the kidneys. *Journal of Urology* 147, 1469–1477.

Lipsitz L.A. (1989). Hypertension in the elderly. *Hospital Practice* 24, 119–142.

Mann S.J. (1992). Detection of renovascular hypertension—State of the art: 1992. *Annals of Internal Medicine* 117, 845–853.

Memmer M.K. (1988). Acute orthostatic hypotension. *Heart and Lung* 17, 134.

Psaty B.M., Furberg C.D., Kuller L.H., et al. (1992). Isolated systolic hypertension and subclinical cardiovascular disease in the elderly. *Journal of the American Medical Association* 268, 1287–1291.

Rousseau P.C. (1988). Postural hypotension in the elderly. *Hospital Practice* 23, 74.

Schneider R.E., Messerli F.H. (1987). Obesity hypertension. *Medical Clinics of North America* 71, 991.

Shea S., Misra D., Ehrlich M.H., et al. (1992). Predisposing factors for severe, uncontrolled hypertension in an inner city minority population. *New England Journal of Medicine* 327, 776–781.

Smith J.J., Porth C.J.M. (1990). Age and the response to orthostatic stress. In Smith J.J. (Ed.). *Circulatory response to the upright posture* (pp. 121–138). Boca Raton, FL: CRC Press.

Walczak M. (1991). Prevalence of orthostatic hypotension. *Journal of Gerontological Nursing* 17 (11), 26–29.

CHAPTER 19

Alterations in Cardiac Function

More than 57 million persons in the United States have some form of cardiovascular disease. About 42% of all deaths (954,720 in 1994) result from cardiovascular disease.[1] Heart attack is the nation's number one killer; it is responsible for more than one fifth of all deaths and is the predominant cause of early disability in the American labor force. Each year, about 32,000 children are born with congenital heart defects, and 1,380,000 children and adults are affected with rheumatic fever. In 1997, it was estimated that heart and blood vessel disease cost the nation an average of $259.1 billion. In an attempt to focus on common heart problems that affect persons in all age groups, this chapter is organized into six sections: disorders of the pericardium, coronary heart disease, disorders of the myocardium, infectious and immunologic disorders, valvular heart disease, and heart disease in infants and children.

Disorders of the Pericardium

After you have completed this section of the chapter, you should be able to meet the following objectives:

- Describe the function of the pericardium and relate to the manifestations of acute pericarditis, pericardial effusion, constrictive pericarditis and cardiac tamponade
- Describe the physiology of pericardial effusion
- Compare the manifestations of acute pericarditis with those of chronic pericarditis with effusion and constrictive pericarditis
- Relate the cardiac compression that occurs with cardiac tamponade to the clinical manifestations of the disorder, including pulsus paradoxus

The pericardium isolates the heart from other thoracic structures, maintains its position in the thorax, and prevents it from overfilling. The two layers of the pericardium are separated by a thin layer of serous fluid, which prevents frictional forces from developing as the inner visceral layer, or epicardium, comes in contact with the outer parietal layer of the fibrous pericardium. The mechanisms that control the movement of fluid between the capillaries and the pericardial space are the same as those that control fluid movement between the capillaries and the interstitial spaces of other body tissues (see Chapter 26). The pericardial sac normally contains 30 to 50 ml of clear, straw-colored fluid. Although 1 L or more of fluid may accumulate, volumes of more than 500 ml are uncommon. Conditions that produce edema in other structures of the body, such as kidney disease and heart failure, may also produce an accumulation of fluid in the pericardial sac. This is called *pericardial effusion*.

The pericardium is subject to many of the same pathologic processes (*e.g.*, inflammation, neoplastic disease, congenital disorders) that affect other structures of the body. Pericardial disorders usually are associated with or result from another disease within the heart or in the surrounding structures (Chart 19–1). The discussion in this section focuses on the pathologic processes associated with acute inflammation of the pericardium (*i.e.*, pericarditis), pericardial effusion, and constrictive pericarditis.

CHART 19-1 Classification of Disorders of the Pericardium

Inflammation

Acute inflammatory pericarditis

1. Infectious
   Viral (echo, coxsackie and others)
   Bacterial (*e.g.*, tuberculosis, staphylococcus, streptococcus)
   Fungal
2. Immune and collagen disorders
   Rheumatic fever
   Rheumatoid arthritis
   Systemic lupus erythematosus
3. Metabolic disorders
   Uremia and dialysis
   Myxedema
4. Ischemia and tissue injury
   Myocardial infarction
   Cardiac surgery
   Chest trauma
5. Physical and chemical agents
   Radiation therapy
   Untoward reactions to drugs, such as hydralazine, procainamide, and anticoagulants

Chronic inflammatory pericarditis
   Can be associated with most of the agents causing an acute inflammatory response

Neoplastic Disease

1. Primary
2. Secondary (*e.g.*, carcinoma of the lung or breast, lymphoma)

Congenital Disorders

1. Complete or partial absence of the pericardium
2. Congenital pericardial cysts

Types of Pericardial Disorders

Acute Pericarditis

Acute pericarditis represents an acute inflammatory process and is usually characterized by chest pain, pericardial friction rub, and serial electrocardiographic (ECG) abnormalities.[2–4] It can result from a number of diverse causes. In many cases, the condition is self-limited, resolving in 2 to 6 weeks, but in other cases, pericarditis from the same cause may persist and produce recurrent subacute or chronic disease.

Acute pericarditis can be classified according to cause (*e.g.*, infections, trauma, rheumatic fever) or the nature of the exudate (*e.g.*, serous, fibrinous, purulent, hemorrhagic). Like other inflammatory conditions, acute pericarditis often is associated with increased capillary permeability. The capillaries that supply the serous pericardium become permeable, allowing plasma proteins, including fibrinogen, to leave the capillaries and enter the pericardial space. This results in an exudate that varies in type and amount according to the causative agent. Acute pericarditis frequently is associated with a fibrinous (fibrin-containing) exudate, which heals by resolution or progresses to deposition of scar tissue and formation of adhesions between the layers of the serous pericardium. Inflammation may also involve the superficial myocardium and the adjacent pleura and sternum.

Viral infections, especially infections with coxsackievirus, echoviruses, influenza, Epstein-Barr, varicella, hepatitis, mumps, and the human immunodeficiency virus (HIV), are the most common cause of acute pericarditis and are probably responsible for many cases classified as idiopathic pericarditis. Acute viral pericarditis is seen more frequently in men than in women and often is preceded by a prodromal phase during which fever, malaise, and other flulike symptoms are present. In some cases, a well-defined infection elsewhere in the body, such as a upper respiratory tract infection, precedes the onset of pericarditis and is the primary site of infection. Although the acute symptoms usually subside in several weeks, easy fatigability often continues for several months.

Other causes of acute pericarditis are rheumatic fever, the postpericardiotomy syndrome, posttraumatic pericarditis, metabolic disorders (*e.g.*, uremia, myxedema), and pericarditis associated with connective tissue diseases (*e.g.*, systemic lupus erythematosus, rheumatoid arthritis). With the increased use of open heart surgery in the treatment of various heart disorders, the postpericardiotomy syndrome has become a commonly recognized form of pericarditis. Pericarditis with effusion is a common complication in persons with renal failure, in those with untreated uremia, and in those being treated with hemodialysis. Irradiation may initiate a subacute pericarditis, with an onset usually within the first year of therapy. It is most commonly associated with high doses of radiation delivered to areas near the heart.

The manifestations of acute pericarditis include a triad of chest pain, pericardial friction rub, and ECG changes. Acute pericarditis may also cause dyspnea. This symptom is related in part to having to breathe shallowly to avoid pain from the rubbing of inflamed pericardial and adjacent pleural surfaces. The clinical findings and other manifestations may vary according to the causative agent. Leukocytosis and an elevation in the erythrocyte sedimentation rate are common.

Nearly all persons with acute pericarditis have chest pain. The pain usually is abrupt in onset, occurs in the precordial area, and is described as sharp. It may radiate to the neck, back, abdomen, or side. It typically is worse with deep breathing, coughing, swallowing, and positional changes because of changes in venous return and cardiac filling. Many persons seek relief by sitting up and leaning forward. Only a small portion of the pericardium, the outer layer of the lower parietal pericardium below the fifth and sixth intercostal spaces, is sensitive to pain. This means that pericardial pain probably results from inflammation of the surrounding structures, particularly the pleura. Pain is more common when a considerable amount of fluid is in the pericardial sac, probably because of the increased stretching of the lower parietal pericardium.

A pericardial friction rub, which is heard when a stethoscope is placed on the chest, results from the rubbing and friction between the inflamed pericardial surfaces. The sound associated with a friction rub has been described as leathery or close to the ear. It is heard best when the patient is leaning forward in the seated position and the diaphragm of the stethoscope is placed firmly along the left sternal border over the xiphoid process or near the lower border of the sternum.

Four stages of ECG changes occur during acute pericarditis. In stage 1, there is an acute elevation of the ST segment; in stage 2, the ST segment becomes isoelectric; in stage 3, the T wave becomes inverted; and in stage 4, the ECG pattern returns to normal.[3–5] The ST segment changes begin within hours to days after the onset of acute pericarditis. Serial electrocardiograms are useful in differentiating acute pericarditis from myocardial infarction.

Pericardial Effusion

Pericardial effusion refers to the presence of fluid in the pericardial cavity. Its major threat is compression of the heart chambers. The amount of fluid, the rapidity with which it accumulates, and the elasticity of the pericardium determine the effect the effusion has on cardiac function. Small pericardial effusions may produce no symptoms or abnormal clinical findings. Even a large effusion that develops slowly may cause few or no symptoms, providing the pericardium is able to stretch and avoid compressing the heart. However, a sudden accumulation of 200 ml may raise intracardiac pressure to levels that seriously limit the venous return to the heart. Symptoms of cardiac compression may also occur with relatively small accumulations of fluid when the pericardium has become thickened by scar tissue or neoplastic infiltrations.

Cardiac Tamponade. Cardiac tamponade is cardiac compression caused by excess fluid or blood in the pericardial sac. It can occur as the result of trauma, cancer, uremia, cardiac rupture due to myocardial infarction or diagnostic procedures, or dissecting aneurysm. The seriousness of the condition results from the restriction in ventricular filling, with a subsequent critical reduction in stroke volume, and the severity depends on the amount of fluid present and the rate at which it accumulates. A rapid accumulation of fluid results in an increase in central venous pressure, a decrease in venous return to the heart, distention of the jugular veins, a decrease in cardiac output despite an increase in heart rate, a decrease in systolic blood pressure, and signs of circulatory shock.

Pulsus paradoxus refers to an exaggeration of the normal inspiratory decrease in systolic blood pressure and is a clinical indicator of cardiac tamponade.[6] The decreased intrathoracic pressure that occurs during inspiration normally accelerates venous flow, increasing right atrial and ventricular filling. This causes the interventricular septum to bulge to the left, producing internal compression of the left ventricle. In cardiac tamponade, the left ventricle is compressed from within by movement of the interventricular septum and from without by fluid in the pericardium (Fig. 19–1). With pulsus paradoxus, left ventricular output can decrease within a beat of the beginning of inspiration.

Pulsus paradoxus can be determined by palpation or cuff sphygmomanometry. In this condition, the arterial pulse, as palpated at the carotid or femoral artery, is reduced or absent during inspiration. Palpation provides

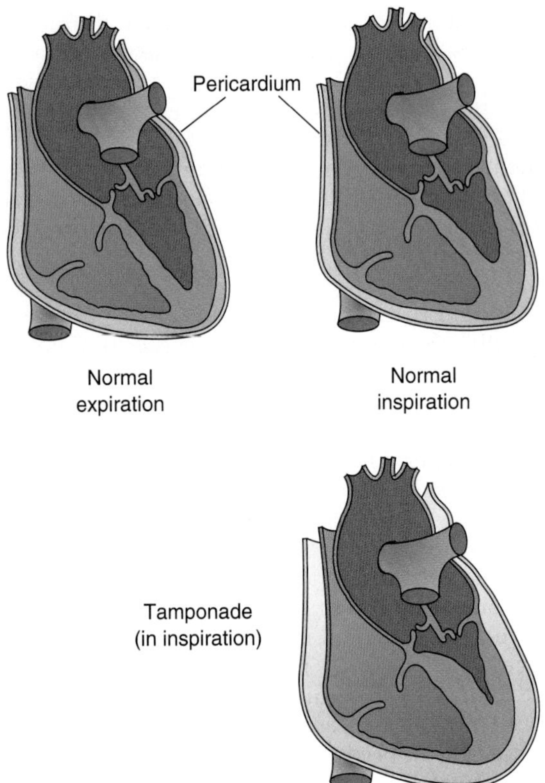

Figure 19–1
Effects of respiration and cardiac tamponade on ventricular filling and cardiac output. During inspiration venous flow into the right heart increases, causing the interventricular septum to bulge into the left ventricle. This produces a decrease in left ventricular volume, with a subsequent decrease in stroke volume output. In cardiac tamponade, the fluid in the pericardial sac produces further compression of the left ventricle, causing an exaggeration of the normal inspiratory decrease in stroke volume and systolic blood pressure.

only a gross estimate of the degree of paradoxus. Pulsus paradoxus is more sensitively estimated when the blood pressure cuff is inflated to a value above the systolic pressure and then deflated slowly at a rate of 2 mm Hg per second until the first Korotkoff sound is detected with expiration. After notation of this pressure, the cuff is deflated until the Korotkoff sounds can be heard throughout the respiratory cycle. A difference greater than 10 mm Hg between inspiration and expiration is indicative of pulsus paradoxus. In cardiac tamponade, this implies a large reduction in ventricular volume.

Chronic Pericarditis With Effusion. Chronic pericarditis with effusion is characterized by an increase in inflammatory exudate that continues beyond the anticipated period. In some cases, the exudate persists for several years. In most cases of chronic pericarditis, no specific pathogen can be identified. The process commonly is associated with other forms of heart disease, such as rheumatic fever, congenital heart lesions, or hypertensive heart disease. Systemic diseases, such as lupus erythematosus, rheumatoid arthritis, scleroderma, and myxedema, are also causes of chronic pericarditis, as are metabolic disturbances associated with acute and chronic renal failure. Unlike those of acute pericarditis, the signs and symptoms of chronic pericarditis often are minimal; often the disease is detected for the first time on routine chest x-ray films. As the condition progresses, the fluid may accumulate and compress the adjacent cardiac structures and impair cardiac filling.

Constrictive Pericarditis

In constrictive pericarditis, fibrous scar tissue develops between the visceral and parietal layers of the serous pericardium. In time, the scar tissue contracts and interferes with diastolic filling of the heart, at which point cardiac output and cardiac reserve become fixed. Ascites is a prominent early finding and may be accompanied by pedal edema, dyspnea on exertion, and fatigue. The jugular veins are also distended. *Kussmaul's sign* is an inspiratory distention of the jugular veins caused by the inability of the right atrium, encased in its rigid pericardium, to accommodate the increase in venous return that occurs with inspiration.

Diagnosis and Treatment

Various diagnostic tests are used to confirm the presence of pericardial disease. These measures include auscultation, chest radiology, electrocardiography, echocardiography, radiation-scanning procedures, computed tomography, and magnetic resonance imaging. The echocardiogram is the most definitive of these studies. Aspiration and laboratory analysis of the pericardial fluid may be used to identify the causative agent.

Treatment depends on the cause. When infection is present, antibiotics specific for the causative agent usually are prescribed. Antiinflammatory drugs such as aspirin and nonsteroidal antiinflammatory agents may be given to minimize the inflammatory response and the accompanying undesirable effects. Pericardiocentesis, the removal of fluid from the pericardial sac, may be a lifesaving measure in severe cardiac tamponade. Surgical treatment may be required for traumatic lesions of the heart or for constrictive pericarditis in which cardiac filling is severely impaired.

In summary, the pericardium is a two-layered membranous sac that isolates the heart from other thoracic structures, maintains its position in the thorax, and prevents it from overfilling. The mechanisms that control the movement of fluid between the capillaries and the space that separates the two layers of the pericardium are the same as those that control fluid movement between the capillaries and the interstitial spaces of other body tissues.

Disorders of the pericardium include acute pericarditis, pericardial effusion, cardiac tamponade, and constrictive pericarditis. The major threat of pericardial disease is compression of the heart chambers.

Acute pericarditis is characterized by chest pain, ECG changes, and a friction rub. Among its causes are infections, uremia, rheumatic fever, connective tissue diseases, and myocardial infarction. Pericardial effusion refers to the presence of an exudate in the pericardial cavity, and the condition can be acute or chronic. It can increase intracardiac pressure, compress the heart, and interfere with venous return to the heart. The amount of exudate, the rapidity with which it accumulates, and the elasticity of the pericardium determine the effect the effusion has on cardiac function. Cardiac tamponade is a life-threatening cardiac compression resulting from excess fluid in the pericardial sac. In constrictive pericarditis, scar tissue develops between the visceral and parietal layers of the serous pericardium. In time, the scar tissue contracts and interferes with cardiac filling.

Coronary Heart Disease

After you have completed this section of the chapter, you should be able to meet the following objectives:

- Describe blood flow in the coronary circulation and relate it to the metabolic needs of the heart
- Describe the use of the electrocardiogram, stress testing, nuclear imaging, and cardiac catheterization in assessment of the coronary circulation
- State the physiologic cause of myocardial ischemia
- Distinguish among classic angina, variant angina, unstable angina, silent myocardial ischemia, and myocardial infarction in terms of pathophysiology and symptomatology
- Compare the treatment goals for angina and silent myocardial ischemia with those for myocardial infarction
- Compare the procedures used in percutaneous transluminal coronary angioplasty and coronary bypass surgery
- Explain the mechanisms, criteria for use, and benefits of thrombolytic therapy in patients with myocardial infarction
- Cite the benefits of an exercise program in patients with coronary heart disease

The term *coronary heart disease* (CHD), also called *coronary artery disease*, describes heart disease caused by impaired coronary blood flow. Disease of the coronary vessels can cause angina, myocardial infarction, cardiac dysrhythmias, conduction defects, heart failure, and sudden death. Almost half of all cardiovascular deaths result from CHD. In 1994, CHD caused 487,490 deaths; 13,670,000 persons have a history of angina, heart attack, or both.[1] In most cases, CHD is caused by atherosclerosis (see Chapter 17). In 1993, 51.1% of CHD deaths were men and 48.9 % women.[1] CHD often is a silent disorder; most men and women older than 50 have moderately advanced coronary atherosclerosis, although most have no symptoms of heart disease.

CHD can affect one or all of the major epicardial coronary arteries and their branches (*i.e.*, one-, two-, or three-vessel disease) and can be diffuse or localized to one area of a single vessel. At least 75% of the vessel lumen is usually occluded before there is a significant reduction in blood flow. The effects of CHD range from ischemia to infarction and death of myocardial tissue. Although atherosclerosis reduces blood flow by producing a fixed narrowing of the coronary arteries, acute myocardial ischemia and infarction are usually precipitated by disruption of an atherosclerotic plaque with hemorrhage, fissuring, and ulceration.

Coronary Circulation

There are two main coronary arteries, the left and the right, which arise from the coronary sinus just above the aortic valve (Fig. 19–2). The left coronary artery extends for about 3.5 cm as the *left main coronary artery* and then divides into the anterior descending and circumflex branches. The *left anterior descending artery* passes down through the groove between the two ventricles, giving off *diagonal branches,* which supply the left ventricle, and *perforating branches*, which supply the anterior portion of the interventricular septum and the anterior papillary muscle of the left ventricle. The *circumflex* branch of the left coronary artery passes to the left and moves posteriorly in the groove that separates the left atrium and ventricle, giving off branches that supply the left lateral wall of the left ventricle. The *right coronary artery* lies in the right atrioventricular groove, and its branches supply the right ventricle. The right coronary artery usually moves to the back of the heart where it forms the *posterior descending artery*, which supplies the posterior portion of the heart (the interventricular septum, atrioventricular node, and posterior papillary muscle). The sinoatrial node usually is supplied by the right coronary artery. In 10% to 20% of persons, the left circumflex rather than the right coronary artery moves posteriorly to form the posterior descending artery.

Because the openings for the coronary arteries originate in the root of the aorta just outside the aortic valve, the primary factor responsible for perfusion of the coronary arteries is the aortic pressure. Changes in aortic pressure produce parallel changes in coronary blood flow.

In addition to providing the aortic pressure that moves blood through the coronary vessels, the contracting heart muscle influences its own blood supply by compressing the intramyocardial and subendocardial blood vessels. The large epicardial coronary arteries lie on the surface of the heart, with the smaller intramyocardial branching off and penetrating the myocardium before merging with a network or plexus of subendocardial vessels. During systole, contraction of the cardiac muscle compresses the intramyocardial vessels that feed the subendocardial plexus and the increased pressure in the ventricle causes further compression of the

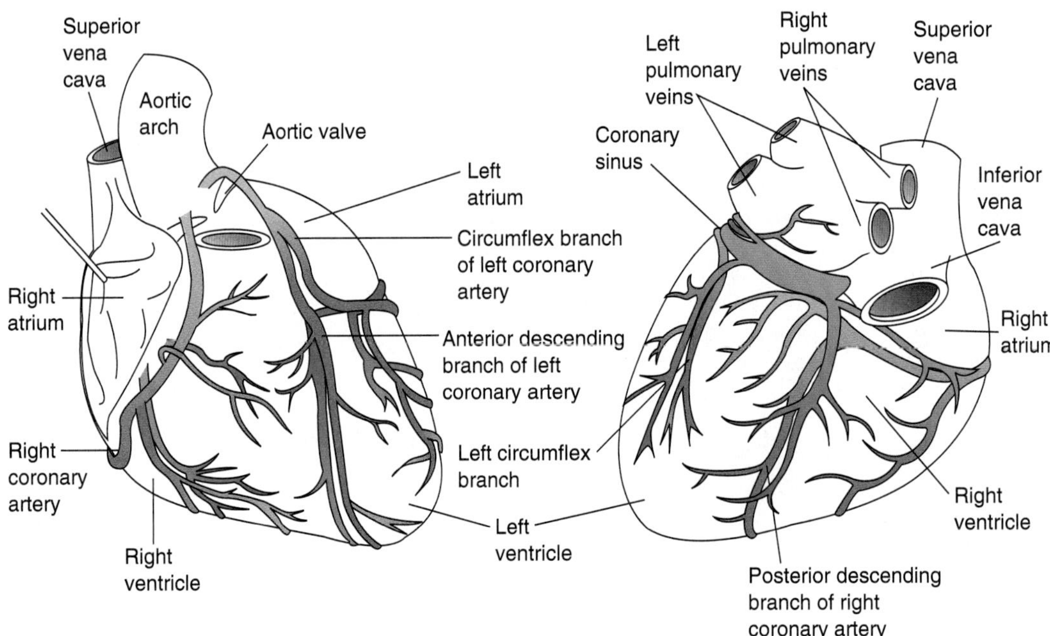

Figure 19–2
Coronary arteries and some of the coronary sinus veins.

subendocardial vessels (Fig. 19–3). As a result, blood flow through the subendocardial vessels is less during systole than in the outer coronary vessels. To compensate, the subendocardial vessels are far more extensive than the outermost arteries, allowing a disproportionate increase in subendocardial flow during diastole. Because subendocardial blood flow mainly occurs during diastole, there is risk of myocardial ischemia and infarction when diastolic pressure is low and when there is an elevation in diastolic intraventricular pressure sufficient to compress the vessels in the subendocardial plexus.[7] Intramyocardial blood flow is also affected by heart rate because at rapid heart rates, the time spent in diastole is greatly reduced.

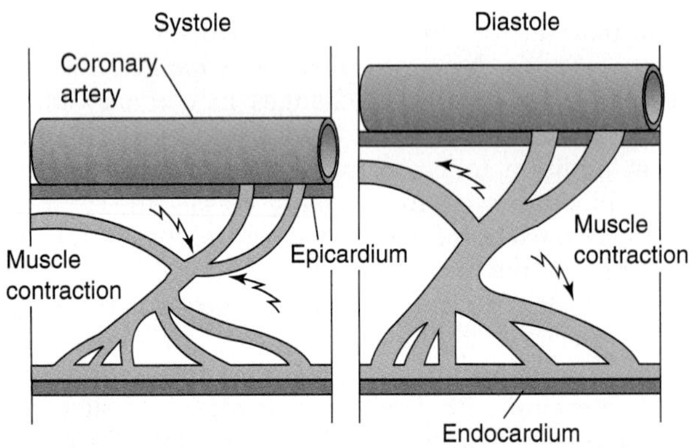

Figure 19–3
The compressing effect of the contracting myocardium on intramyocardial blood vessels and subendocardial blood flow during systole and diastole.

Metabolic influences

Heart muscle relies primarily on fatty acids and aerobic metabolism to meet its energy needs. Although the heart can engage in aerobic metabolism, this process relies on the continuous delivery of glucose and results in the formation of large amounts of lactic acid. Blood flow is usually regulated by the need of the cardiac muscle for oxygen. Even under normal resting conditions, the heart extracts and uses 60% to 80% of oxygen in blood flowing through the coronary arteries, compared with the 25% to 30% extracted by skeletal muscle. Because there is little oxygen reserve in the blood, the coronary arteries must increase their flow to meet the metabolic needs of the myocardium during periods of increased activity. The normal resting blood flow through the coronary arteries averages about 225 ml per minute.[7] During strenuous exercise, coronary flow may increase fourfold to fivefold to meet the energy requirements of the heart.

One of the major determinants of coronary blood flow is the metabolic activity of the heart. Although the link between cardiac metabolic rate and coronary blood flow remains unsettled, it appears to result from the release of metabolic mediators that are generated as a result of a decrease in the ratio of oxygen supply to oxygen demand.[8] Numerous agents, referred to as *metabolites,* have been suggested as mediators of vasodilation that accompanies increased cardiac work. These substances include lactic acid, potassium ions, and adenosine that is released from working myocardial cells.

Endothelial Control of Coronary Vascular Tone

The endothelial cells that line blood vessels, including the coronaries, normally present a barrier between the blood and the arterial wall, and they have antithrombogenic properties that inhibit platelet aggregation and clot formation. The endothelial cells also produce vasodilating and vasoconstricting factors. It has been suggested that endothelial dysfunction may contribute to the conditions that lead to plaque instability and fissuring.[9]

The endothelium synthesizes a powerful vasodilator called *endothelium-derived relaxing factor* (EDRF), one form of which is nitric oxide. EDRF communicates directly with vascular smooth muscle, causing relaxation. Only a few vasodilators, including nitroglycerin that is used in the treatment of angina, are thought to act directly on vascular smooth muscle, independent of EDRF, to produce vasodilation. It has been proposed that EDRF contributes to the regulation of blood flow by producing relaxation of vascular smooth muscle and preventing platelet aggregation and release of platelet factors that promote thrombus formation. Some of the reported stimuli for release of EDRF are acetylcholine, thrombin, histamine, norepinephrine, vessel distention, or shear stress associated with blood flow. Atherosclerosis tends to replace EDRF-producing endothelial cells. Responses to endothelium-dependent stimuli that normally dilate healthy coronary arteries have been found to be impaired in persons with atherosclerosis.[9] It has been suggested that the tendency for vasospasm that occurs in atherosclerotic vessels may impair EDRF function.

The endothelium is also the source of vasoconstricting factors; the best known are the endothelins. Although there are several endothelins, endothelin-1 (ET-1), seems to be important in producing vasoconstriction. The formation of ET-1 is stimulated by thrombin, epinephrine, and vasopressin. Plasma levels of ET-1 are elevated in atherosclerosis, acute myocardial infarction, congestive heart failure, and hypertension. ET-1 is also reportedly produced by activated macrophages in atherosclerotic lesions of persons with acute ischemic coronary disease and plaque rupture.[9]

Collateral Circulation

Although there are no connections between the large coronary arteries, there are anastomotic channels that join the small arteries (Fig. 19–4). With gradual occlusion of the larger vessels, the smaller collateral vessels increase in size and provide alternative channels for blood flow.[10] One of the reasons CHD does not produce symptoms until it is far advanced is that the collateral channels develop at the same time the atherosclerotic changes are occurring.

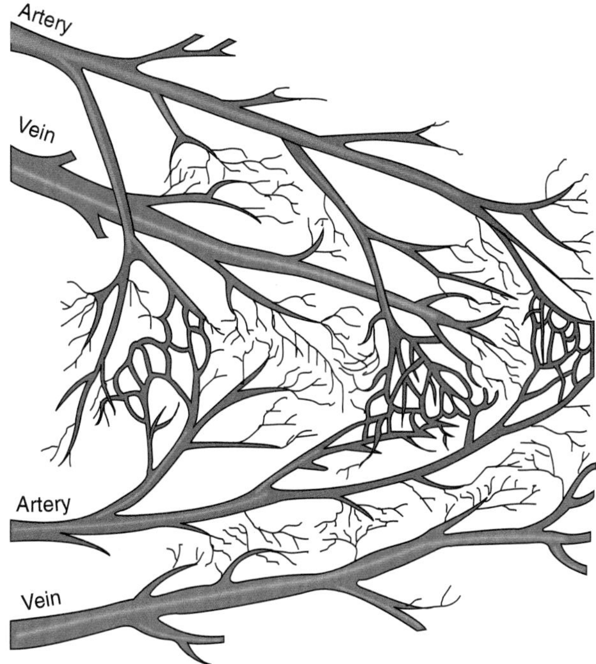

Figure 19–4
Anastomoses of the smaller coronary arterial vessels. (Guyton A.C., Hall J.E. [1996]. *Textbook of medical physiology* [9th ed., p.260]. Philadelphia: W.B. Saunders)

Evaluation of the Coronary Circulation

Among the methods used in evaluating coronary blood flow and myocardial perfusion are electrocardiography, exercise and pharmacologic stress testing, nuclear imaging, and cardiac catheterization.

Electrocardiography. Electrocardiography is the most frequently used method for detecting myocardial ischemia due to CHD (see Chapter 21). The usual criteria for diagnosis of ischemia is a horizontal depression or downsloping of the ST segment of at least 1 mm (0.1 mV) at 80 msec beyond the junction of the QRS and ST segment (*i.e.,* J point) or inversion, flattening, or peaking of the T wave.[11] The ECG pattern is also used to determine dysrhythmias that manifest as a result of myocardial ischemia due to CHD, and it can provide evidence of old myocardial infarction. A newer method called signal-averaged for high-resolution electrocardiography accentuates the QRS complex so that low-amplitude afterpotentials that correlate with high risk of ventricular dysrhythmias and sudden death can be detected.

Continuous ambulatory ECG monitoring can be done using a Holter monitor (see Chapter 21). Ambulatory ECG monitoring is often done to detect transient ST segment and T wave changes that occur and are not accompanied by symptoms (*i.e.,* silent ischemia).

Stress Testing. Exercise stress testing is a means of observing cardiac function under stress. Two types of tests are commonly used: the motorized treadmill and the bicycle ergometer. Of these two, the treadmill is the most popular, probably because it uses walking, an activity that is familiar to most persons. The treadmill test also requires higher levels of myocardial performance than other forms of exercise. Bicycle exercise does not require as high a level of myocardial oxygen demand as treadmill walking, and the person can become fatigued before myocardial ischemia is reached. Blood pressure is monitored during exercise testing and the ECG pattern recorded for the purpose of determining heart rate and detecting myocardial ischemic changes. Chest pain, severe shortness of breath, dysrhythmias,

ST-segment changes on the ECG, or a decrease in blood pressure suggests CHD, and if one or more of these signs or symptoms are present, the test is usually terminated.

Under some conditions pharmacologic agents are used to stress the heart. There are two basic types of pharmacologic stress tests. One uses drugs such as the synthetic catecholamine dobutamine to mimic the effects of exercise. The second type uses vasodilator drugs, such as dipyridamole and adenosine, that produce profuse vasodilation, increasing heart rate and stroke volume, thereby increasing myocardial oxygen demand.

Nuclear Imaging. Nuclear cardiology techniques involve the use of radionuclides (*i.e.*, radioactive substances) and essentially are noninvasive. Three types of nuclear cardiology tests commonly are used: myocardial perfusion imaging, infarct imaging, and radionuclide angiocardiography. With all three types of tests, a scintillation (gamma) camera is used to record the radiation emitted from the radionuclide. A computer processing system, which is linked to the scintillation camera, is an essential part of all nuclear imaging systems.

Myocardial perfusion imaging is used to visualize the regional distribution of blood flow. Myocardial perfusion imaging uses thallium-201 or one of the newer technetium-based agents that are extracted from the blood and taken up by functioning myocardial cells. Thallium-201, an analogue of potassium, is distributed to the myocardium in proportion to the magnitude of blood flow. After injection, an external detection device describes the distribution of the radioactive material. An ischemic area appears as a "cold spot" that lacks radioactive uptake. The most important application of this technique has been its use during stress testing for evaluation of ischemic heart disease.

Acute infarct imaging uses a radionuclide such as technetium pyrophosphate that is taken up by the cells in the infarcted zone. With this method, the radionuclide becomes concentrated in the damaged myocardium, allowing its visualization as a "hot spot," or positive area, of increased uptake of the radionuclide.

Radionuclide angiocardiography provides actual visualization of the ventricular structures during systole and diastole and provides a means for evaluating ventricular function during rest and exercise stress testing. A radioisotope such as technetium-labeled albumin, which does not leave the capillaries but remains in the blood and is not bound to the myocardium, is used for this type of imaging. This type of nuclear imaging can be used to determine right and left ventricular volumes, ejection fractions, regional wall motion, and cardiac contractility. This method is also useful in the diagnosis of intracardiac shunts.

Cardiac Catheterization. Cardiac catheterization involves the passage of flexible catheters into the great vessels and chambers of the heart. In right heart catheterization, the catheters are inserted into a peripheral vein (usually the basilic or femoral) and then advanced into the right heart. The left heart catheter is inserted retrograde through a peripheral artery (usually the brachial or femoral) into the aorta and left heart. The cardiac catheterization laboratory, where the procedure is done, is equipped for viewing and recording fluoroscopic images of the heart and vessels in the chest and for measuring pressures within the heart and great vessels. It also has equipment for cardiac output studies and for obtaining samples of blood for blood gas analysis. Angiographic studies are made by injecting a contrast medium into the heart, so that an outline of the moving structures can be visualized and filmed. Coronary arteriography involves the injection of a contrast medium into the coronary arteries; this permits visualization of lesions within these vessels.

Ischemic Heart Disease

The term *ischemia* means to suppress or withhold blood flow. Myocardial ischemia occurs when the ability of the coronary arteries to supply blood is inadequate to meet the metabolic demands of the heart. Limitations in coronary blood flow may be caused by atherosclerotic lesions, vasospasm, thrombosis, or a combination of the three conditions. More than 90% of persons with myocardial ischemia have advanced coronary atherosclerosis.[2] Metabolic demands of the heart are increased with everyday activities such as mental stress, exercise, and exposure to cold. In certain disease states, such as thyrotoxicosis, the metabolic demands may be so excessive that blood supply is inadequate despite normal coronary arteries. In other situations, such as aortic stenosis, the coronary arteries may not be diseased, but the perfusion pressure may be insufficient to provide adequate blood flow. Symptomatic myocardial ischemia (*i.e.*, angina pectoris) and silent, or painless, myocardial ischemia are important functional indicators of active CHD and increased risk of myocardial infarction or sudden death.

Angina

The term *angina* is derived from a Latin word meaning to choke. Angina pectoris is a symptomatic paroxysmal chest pain or pressure sensation associated with transient myocardial ischemia. The pain typically is described as constricting, squeezing, or suffocating. It usually is steady, increasing in intensity only at the onset and end of the attack. The pain of angina commonly is located in the precordial or substernal area of the chest; it is similar to myocardial infarction in that it may radiate to the left shoulder, jaw, arm, or other areas of the chest (Fig. 19–5). In some persons, the arm or shoulder pain may be confused with arthritis; in others, epigastric pain is confused with indigestion. The duration of angina is brief—seldom does it last for more than 5 minutes.

There are three types of angina: classic angina, variant angina, and unstable angina. The Canadian Cardiovascular Society Classification (CCSC) system can be

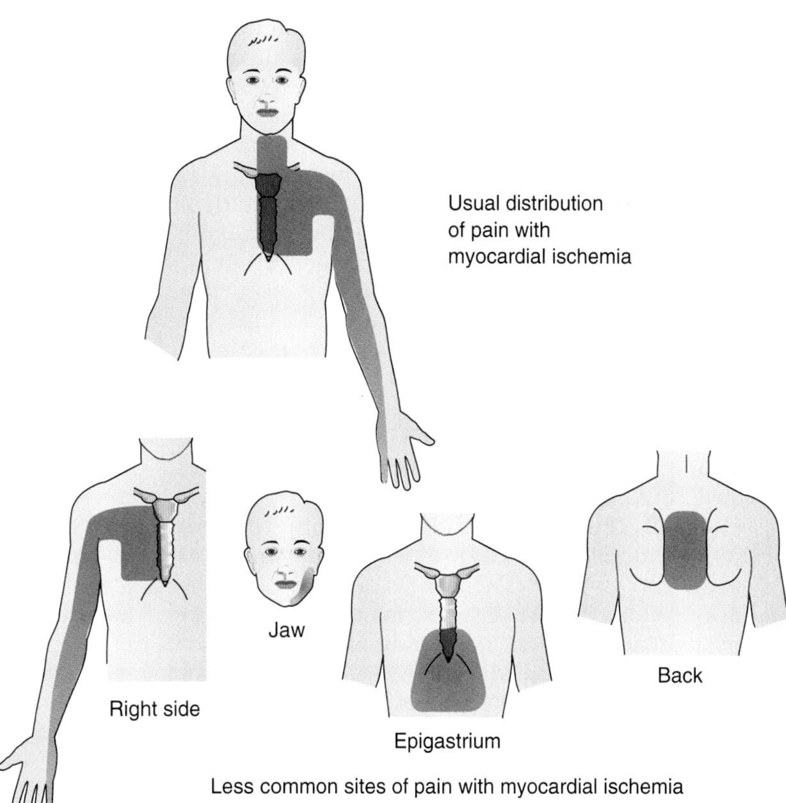

Figure 19–5
Pain patterns with myocardial ischemia. The usual distribution is referral to all or part of the sternal region, the left side of the chest, the neck, and down the ulnar side of the left forearm and hand. With severe ischemic pain, the right chest and right arm are often involved as well, although isolated involvement of these areas is rare. Other sites sometimes involved, either alone or together with pain in other sites, are the jaw, epigastrium, and back.

used to grade the severity of anginal pain and discomfort (Table 19–1).[12]

Classic Angina. Classic angina, sometimes called exertional angina, is associated with atherosclerotic disease that produces fixed obstruction of the coronary arteries. It occurs when the metabolic needs of the myocardium exceed the ability of the occluded coronary arteries to deliver adequate blood flow. Pain usually is precipitated by situations that increase the work demands of the heart, such as physical exertion, exposure to cold, and emotional stress. Despite the fact that most persons with angina have atherosclerotic heart disease, angina does not develop in a considerable number of persons with advanced coronary atherosclerosis. This is probably because of their sedentary lifestyle, the development of adequate collateral circulation, or the inability of these persons to perceive pain. In many instances, myocardial infarction occurs without a history of angina.

Variant Angina. The syndrome of variant or Prinzmetal's angina was first described by Prinzmetal and associates in 1959.[13] Subsequent evidence indicated that variant angina is caused by spasms of the coronary arteries; the condition is also called *vasospastic angina.*[14] In most instances, the spasms occur in the presence of

TABLE 19–1

Canadian Cardiovascular Society Classification for Angina

Class	Description of Stage
Class I	Ordinary physical activity, such as walking or climbing stairs, does not cause angina. Angina occurs with strenuous, rapid, or prolonged exertion at work or recreation.
Class II	Slight limitation of ordinary activity. Angina occurs on walking or climbing stairs rapidly, walking uphill, walking or stair climbing after meals, or in cold, in wind, under emotional stress, or only during the few hours after awakening. Walking more than two blocks on the level and climbing more than one flight of ordinary stairs at a normal pace and in normal conditions can elicit angina.
Class III	Marked limitations of ordinary physical activity. Angina occurs on walking one to two blocks on the level and climbing one flight of stairs in normal conditions and at a normal pace.
Class IV	Inability to carry on any physical activity without discomfort—anginal symptoms may be present at rest.

(Campeau L. [1976]. Grading of angina pectoris [letter]. *Circulation* 54, 522–523. Copyright 1976, American Heart Association, Inc. Used with permission.)

coronary artery stenosis; however, variant angina has occurred in the absence of visible disease. Unlike the classic form of angina, which occurs with exertion or stress, variant angina usually occurs during rest or with minimal exercise and frequently occurs nocturnally. It may be associated with the rapid eye movement stage of sleep. It commonly follows a cyclic or regular pattern of occurrence (*e.g.*, it happens at the same time each day). The mechanism of coronary vasospasm is uncertain. It has been suggested that it may result from hyperactive sympathetic nervous system responses, from a defect in the handling of calcium in vascular smooth muscle, or from a reduced production of prostaglandin I_2, which promotes vasodilation.

Dysrhythmias often occur when the pain is severe, and most persons are aware of their presence during an attack. ECG changes are significant if recorded during an attack. These abnormalities include ST segment elevation or depression, T wave peaking, inversion of U waves, and rhythm disturbances. The ECG abnormalities may be recorded by continuous ECG monitoring or ambulatory Holter monitoring and are reversed by nitroglycerin. Ergonovine, a nonspecific vasoconstrictor, may be administered during cardiac catheterization to evoke an anginal attack and demonstrate the presence and location of coronary vasospasm.

Treatment of variant angina involves avoidance of precipitating vasospastic stimuli such as exposure to cold, smoking, and emotional stress. Because of their vasodilating effects, nitroglycerin and the calcium-channel blocking drugs are used in treating variant angina.

Unstable Angina. Unstable angina is considered to be a clinical syndrome of myocardial ischemia that falls between stable angina and myocardial infarction. Unlike classic angina, which is caused by a fixed obstruction, or variant angina, which results from vasospasm, unstable angina results from atherosclerotic plaque disruption. Because of its propensity to lead to infarction, it is sometimes referred to as *preinfarction angina.*

The Agency for Health Care Policy and Research Clinical Practice Guidelines defines unstable angina as having three presentations: symptoms at rest (usually prolonged [>20 minutes]); new-onset (<2 months) exertional angina as evidenced by an increase in severity of at least one CCSC class to at least CCSC class III; or recent (<2 months) acceleration of angina to at least CCSC class III.[12] Most cases of unstable angina are caused by significant CHD. Classic angina and variant angina may manifest as unstable angina. Cocaine has been implicated as a risk factor for unstable angina. Cocaine is thought to induce myocardial ischemia through increased myocardial oxygen demand, decreased oxygen supply from coronary artery spasm or thrombosis, or direct myocardial toxicity.[12]

Unstable angina is thought to be triggered by a subtle or minor injury to a coronary atherosclerotic plaque. Although plaque disruption may occur with or without thrombosis, it increases the degree of coronary artery obstruction. When the plaque injury is mild, intermittent thrombotic occlusions may occur and cause episodes of anginal pain at rest. Vasoconstricting factors (*i.e.*, thromboxane, serotonin, and platelet-derived growth factor) are released from platelets that aggregate at the site of injury. These platelet factors contribute, even at rest, to episodes of reduced coronary blood flow and silent or symptomatic myocardial ischemia. Thrombus formation can progress until the coronary artery becomes occluded, leading to myocardial infarction.

Diagnosis of unstable angina is usually based on pain history, ECG evidence of ischemia, and other signs of impaired myocardial function such as acute congestive heart failure. The risk of sudden death or ischemic complications with unstable angina are greater than with stable angina but lower than with myocardial infarction. The risk of death or ischemic complications is greater when the symptoms first appears and gradually declines to approach those of stable angina within about 2 months.[12] Because of the risk, initial evaluation is usually done in a health care facility capable of providing ECG monitoring and advanced life support. Persons who are deemed to be at high risk for sudden cardiac death or myocardial infarction are admitted to an intensive care unit for observation and treatment.

Silent Myocardial Ischemia

Silent myocardial ischemia occurs in the absence of anginal pain. The factors that cause silent myocardial ischemia appear to be the same as those responsible for angina—impaired blood flow from the effects of coronary atherosclerosis or vasospasm. Silent myocardial ischemia affects three populations: persons who are asymptomatic without other evidence of CHD, persons who have had a myocardial infarct and continue to have episodes of silent ischemia, and persons with angina who also have episodes of silent ischemia.[15] The reason for the painless episodes of ischemia is unclear. The episodes may be shorter and involve less myocardial tissue than those producing pain. Another explanation is that persons with silent angina have defects in pain threshold, pain transmission, or autonomic neuropathy with sensory denervation. There is evidence of an increased incidence of silent myocardial ischemia in persons with diabetes mellitus, probably the result of autonomic neuropathy, which is a common complication of diabetes.[16] Exercise stress tests or Holter monitoring is usually used to confirm the diagnosis of silent myocardial ischemia.

Treatment

Measures for the treatment of myocardial ischemia usually are directed toward reducing the work demands of the heart or vessel constriction when coronary spasm or thrombosis is present. Treatment measures include nonpharmacologic and pharmacologic methods directed at reducing the preload and afterload work of the heart and measures such as percutaneous transluminal coronary angioplasty (PTCA) and coronary artery bypass surgery, which are used to improve blood flow to the myocardium. Treatment methods for persons with unstable angina who are at high risk for myocardial infarction or cardiac complications are similar to those for myocardial infarction.

Nonpharmacologic Methods. Nonpharmacologic treatment methods include the selective pacing of physical activities, smoking cessation in persons who smoke, stress reduction, avoidance of cold or other stresses that produce vasoconstriction, and weight reduction if obesity is present. Immediate cessation of activity often is sufficient to abort an anginal attack. Sitting down or standing quietly may be preferable to lying down, because these positions decrease preload by producing pooling of blood in the lower extremities. Sudden exposure to cold increases vasoconstriction and afterload stress; persons with myocardial ischemia are cautioned against rapidly drinking large amounts of cold liquids (>240 ml) and breathing extremely cold air. Anxiety often precipitates angina and silent myocardial ischemia, because it causes an increase in heart rate and blood pressure.

Pharmacologic Methods. Pharmacologic methods include the selective use of a combination of nitroglycerin and long-acting nitrates, β-adrenergic–blocking drugs, calcium-channel–blocking drugs, and antiplatelet drugs.

Nitroglycerin (glycerol trinitrate) and long-acting nitrates such as isosorbide dinitrate and pentaerythritol tetranitrate are used to relieve anginal pain and silent myocardial ischemia. They are vasodilating drugs that relax venous and arterial vessels. Venous dilatation decreases venous return to the heart (*i.e.*, preload), thereby reducing ventricular volume and compression of the subendocardial vessels, and returns the end-diastolic length of the ventricular muscle fibers to a more favorable position on the Starling curve. They also decrease the tension in the wall of the ventricle so that less pressure is needed to pump blood, and they reduce the amount of blood that needs to be pumped. Relaxation of the arteries reduces the pressure against which the heart must pump (*i.e.*, afterload). In addition to their vasodilator effects, the nitrates are thought to have an inhibitory effect on platelet activation and aggregation that may contribute to their beneficial effects in persons with CHD.

Nitroglycerin is absorbed into the portal circulation and destroyed by the liver when it is taken orally; therefore, it is administered by methods such as sublingual pills or sprays or with topical ointments or patches that bypass the portal circulation. Sublingual absorption is rapid, and pain relief usually begins in 30 seconds. Topical ointments have a duration of action of 4 to 6 hours. The adhesive patches have a longer duration of action (24 hours). Two long-acting oral nitrate preparations are available: isosorbide dinitrate and isosorbide-5-mononitrate. These medications are given two to three times each day. Administration of any of the nitrates leads to drug tolerance, a condition in which the drug is no longer effective in relieving angina. The only effective method preventing the development of tolerance is to use an intermittent dosing that provides for an 8- to 10-hour drug-free period. This can be accomplished by measures such as removing nitroglycerin patches at night or using an asymmetric dosing regimen (*e.g.*, 8 AM and 3 PM) for administration of the long-acting nitrates.

The *β-adrenergic–blocking drugs* act as antagonists that block β-receptor–mediated functions of the sympathetic nervous system. There are two types of β receptors: β_1 and β_2. The β_1 receptors are found in the heart, and β_2 receptors are found in other parts of the body. Blockade of β_1 receptors in the heart reduces the heart rate, cardiac contractility, and myocardial oxygen consumption. The β_2 receptors are located primarily in vascular and bronchial smooth muscle. Blocking of these receptors produces vasoconstriction and bronchoconstriction. In angina, the primary benefits of β-adrenergic–blocking drugs are derived from their effects on β_1 receptors in the heart that decrease cardiac work and myocardial oxygen consumption.

The *calcium-channel–blocking drugs* sometimes are called calcium antagonists. Free intracellular calcium serves to link many membrane-initiated events with cellular responses, such as action potential generation and muscle contraction. Vascular smooth muscle lacks the sarcoplasmic reticulum and other structures necessary for intracellular storage of calcium; instead, it relies on the influx of calcium from the extracellular fluid into the cell to initiate and sustain contraction. In cardiac muscle, the slow inward calcium current contributes to the plateau of the action potential and to cardiac contractility. The slow calcium current is particularly important in the pacemaker activity of the sinoatrial node and the conduction properties of the atrioventricular (AV) node. The therapeutic effect of the calcium antagonists results from coronary and peripheral artery dilatation and decreased myocardial metabolism associated with the decrease in myocardial contractility.

Aspirin is often used as an *antiplatelet drug*. It is used to prevent platelet aggregation and myocardial infarction. Platelet aggregation is initiated by the prostaglandin, thromboxane A_2. The actions of aspirin (*i.e.*, acetylsalicylic acid) are related to the presence of the acetyl group, which irreversibly acetylates the critical platelet enzyme, cyclooxygenase, which is required for thromboxane A_2 synthesis. Because the action is irreversible, the effect of aspirin on platelet function lasts for the lifetime of the platelet—about 8 to 10 days. The recommended doses of aspirin range from 75 to 325 mg per day. Higher doses of aspirin do not increase its efficacy but do increase gastric irritation. Dipyridamole and ticlopidine are other antiplatelet agents that may be used for treatment of ischemic heart disease.[17] Dipyridamole affects platelet aggregation by increasing platelet cyclic adenosine monophosphate. Ticlopidine inhibits platelet aggregation through adenosine phosphate, but the exact mechanism is unknown. Ticlopidine can cause rash and diarrhea. Although rare, it can cause severe neutropenia; frequent blood counts may be needed.

Revascularization Procedures. Revascularization procedures, including PTCA, coronary stent implantation, and coronary artery bypass surgery, may be done to relieve coronary artery obstruction caused by atherosclerotic lesions.

Coronary Angioplasty. Coronary angioplasty (*i.e.*, PTCA) is used to reduce atherosclerotic plaque obstruction. Although angioplasty usually produces immediate relief of anginal symptoms, its use is associated with death or nonfatal myocardial infarction in about 5% of persons and with restenosis requiring repeated angioplasty or bypass surgery in about 30% of persons undergoing the procedure.[18] Implantation of coronary stents reduces the occurrence of restenosis. Measures to reduce thrombosis during angioplasty also decrease the risk of death and myocardial infarction.

PTCA involves balloon dilatation of a stenotic coronary vessel. The procedure is done under local anesthesia in the cardiac catheterization laboratory and is similar to cardiac catheterization for coronary angiography. With PTCA, a double-lumen balloon dilatation catheter is introduced percutaneously into the femoral or brachial artery and then advanced under fluoroscopic view to the coronary ostium. It is then directed into the affected coronary artery and advanced until the balloon segment is within the stenotic area of the vessel. When in place, the balloon is inflated for 15 seconds to 2 or 3 minutes using a pressure-controlled pump.[19] The mechanism of dilation is compression and rupture of the atherosclerotic plaque and stretching of the plaque free vessel wall (Fig. 19–6). PTCA can also be used to dilate coronary artery bypass grafts. Acute complications of PTCA include thrombosis and vessel dissection; longer-term complications involve restenosis of the dilated vessel. Refinements in the balloon catheters have resulted in decreased risk of vessel perforation and ischemic complications.

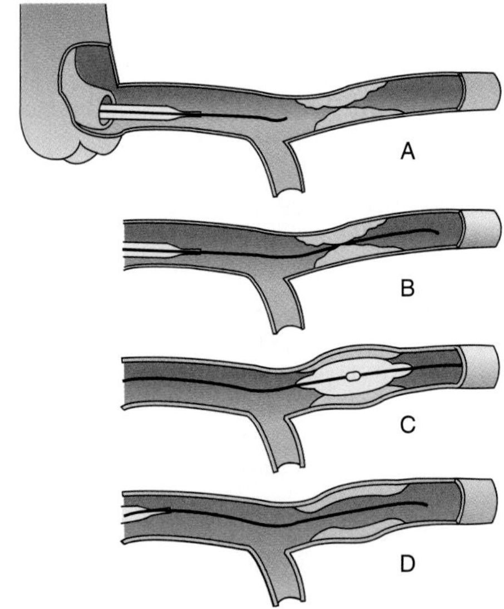

Figure 19–6
(**A**) PTCA dilation catheter and guidewire exiting the guiding catheter. (**B**) Guidewire advanced across the stenosis. (**C**) Dilation catheter advanced across the stenosis and inflated. (**D**) Dilation catheter pulled back to assess luminal diameter. (Reprinted with permission of Advanced Cardiovascular Systems [ACS], Inc., Santa Clara, CA.)

Coronary stents are fenestrated, stainless-steel tubes that can be inserted into a coronary artery and then expanded to prevent vessel restenosis (Fig. 19–7). Stents are also used to prevent abrupt vessel closure caused by vessel dissection that occurs as a complication of PTCA. Stenting is used in high-risk situations that are not likely to managed successfully by PTCA alone. Persons undergoing stent procedures are treated with antiplatelet and anticoagulant drugs to prevent thrombosis, which is a major risk after the procedure.

Research has focused on antithrombin therapies to prevent thrombosis and complications associated with PTCA. One such development is a monoclonal antibody, called *Abciximab*, which blocks the platelet glycoprotein IIb/IIIa receptor that binds fibrinogen.[18]

Atherectomy (*i.e.*, cutting of the atherosclerotic plaque with a high-speed circular blade from within the vessel) is being tested as a mechanical technique to remove atherosclerotic tissue during angioplasty. Laser angioplasty devices are also being tested.[18]

Coronary Artery Bypass Grafting. The surgical treatment of CHD—*coronary artery bypass grafting* (CABG)—remains popular for patients who have significant CHD uncontrolled by angioplasty or pharmacologic therapy. In this surgical procedure, revascularization of the myocardium is effected by placing a saphenous vein graft between the aorta and the affected coronary artery distal to the site of occlusion or by using the internal mammary artery as a means of revascularizing the left anterior descending artery or its branches. Figure 19–8 shows the placement of a saphenous vein graft and a mammary artery graft. One to five distal anastomoses are commonly done. Although it cannot be documented that this surgery significantly alters the progress of the disease, it does relieve pain, and patients may have more productive lives.

Myocardial Infarction

Acute myocardial infarction (AMI), also known as a heart attack, refers to the ischemic death of myocardial tissue associated with atherosclerotic disease of the coronary arteries. Heart attack is the largest killer of

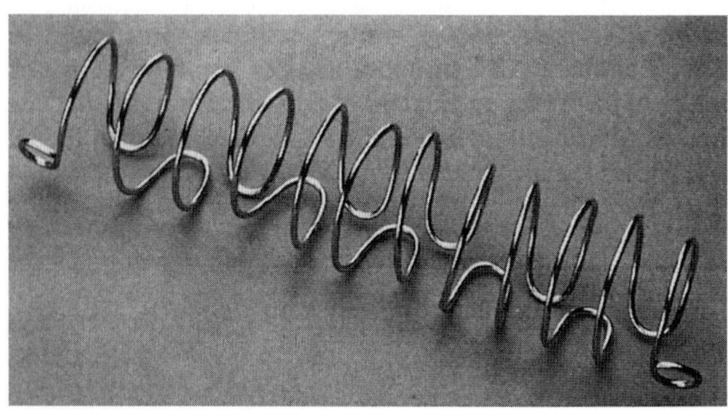

Figure 19–7
The Gianturco-Roubin Flex-Stent. (Courtesy of Cook, Inc., Bloomington, IN)

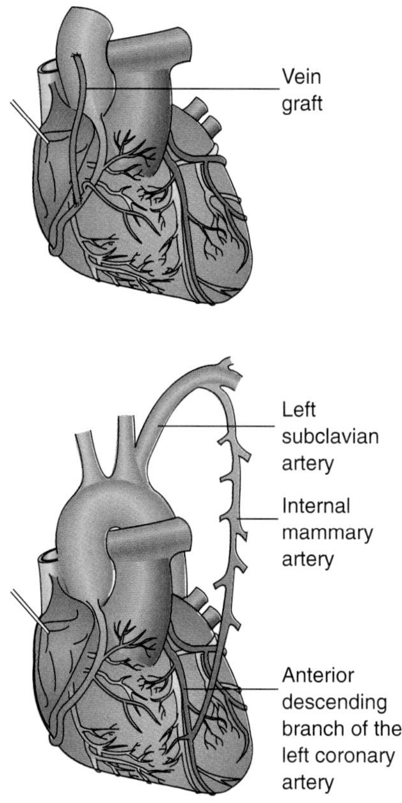

Figure 19–8
Coronary artery revascularization. **(Top)** Saphenous vein bypass graft. The vein segment is sutured to the ascending aorta and the right coronary artery at a point distal to the occluding lesion. **(Bottom)** Mammary artery bypass. The mammary artery is anastomosed to the anterior descending left coronary artery, bypassing the obstructing lesion.

American men and women[1]: 1.5 million Americans have new or recurrent heart attacks each year, and one third of those die within the first hour, usually as the result of cardiac arrest resulting from ventricular fibrillation.

Myocardial infarction occurs three times more frequently during the early morning hours (between 6:00 AM to 12:00 NOON) than during evening hours, suggesting that physiologic factors in early morning, including surges in coronary artery tone and blood pressure, may promote atherosclerotic plaque disruption and subsequent platelet deposition. It has been suggested that cortisol levels, which are elevated above basal levels in the morning, may enhance the sensitivity of the coronary vessels to the vasoconstricting actions of the catecholamines, which have a prominent surge after arising in the morning.[20]

Pathology

AMI usually results from rupture or fissuring of an atherosclerotic plaque (Fig. 19–9). Although fixed atherosclerotic lesions of the epicardial coronary arteries may progress to complete occlusion, they do not usually precipitate AMI, probably because of the development of collateral circulation. As atherosclerotic lesions develop, they become lipid laden and vulnerable to rupture or fissuring with release of substances that cause platelet activation and thrombin generation; it is the resultant thrombus that interrupts blood flow and leads to myocardial infarction.[21] Although AMI most often results from atherosclerotic plaque disruption, some persons may experience AMI because of prolonged severe vasospasm, as in Prinzmetal's variant angina.

A myocardial infarct may involve the endocardium, myocardium, epicardium, or a combination of these. AMI can be divided into two major types: transmural and subendocardial infarcts. Transmural infarcts involve the full thickness of the ventricular wall and most commonly occur when there is obstruction of a single artery. Subendocardial infarcts involve the inner one third to one half of the ventricular wall and occur more frequently in the presence of severely narrowed but still patent arteries. Most infarcts are transmural, involving the free wall of the left ventricle and the interventricular septum (Fig. 19–10). The area of infarction is determined by the coronary artery that is affected and by its distribution of blood flow. About 30% to 40% of infarcts affect the right coronary artery, 40% to 50% affect the left anterior descending artery, and the remaining 15% to 20% affect the left circumflex artery.[2]

Although gross tissue changes are not apparent for hours after onset of an AMI, the ischemic area ceases to function within a matter of minutes, and irreversible damage to cells occurs in about 40 minutes. The principal biochemical consequence of AMI is the onset of anaerobic metabolism with inadequate production of energy to sustain normal myocardial function. As a result, a striking loss of contractile function occurs within 60 seconds of AMI onset. Changes in cell structure (*i.e.*, glycogen

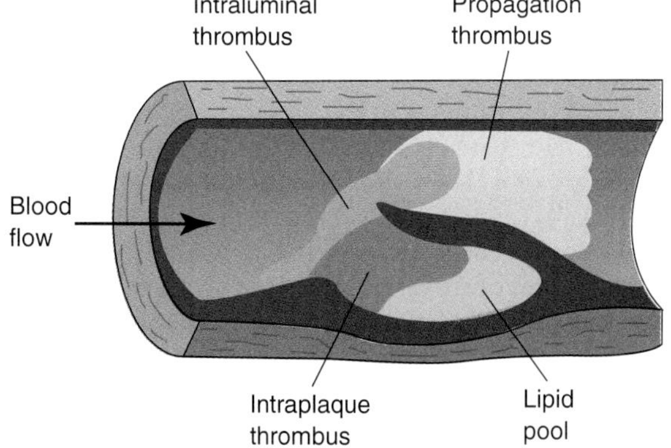

Figure 19–9
Representation of a longitudinal reconstruction of a coronary artery showing the histological components of an occluding thrombus. Much of the thrombus at the site of occlusion is contained within the plaque and compresses the lumen from outside. Intraluminal thrombus develops adjacent to a plaque fissure and then propagates downstream. A plug of lipid has extruded into the lumen. (Redrawn from Davies M.J. [1990]. A macro and micro view of coronary vascular insult in ischemic heart disease. *Circulation 82*[Suppl. II]:38. Copyright 1990 American Heart Association)

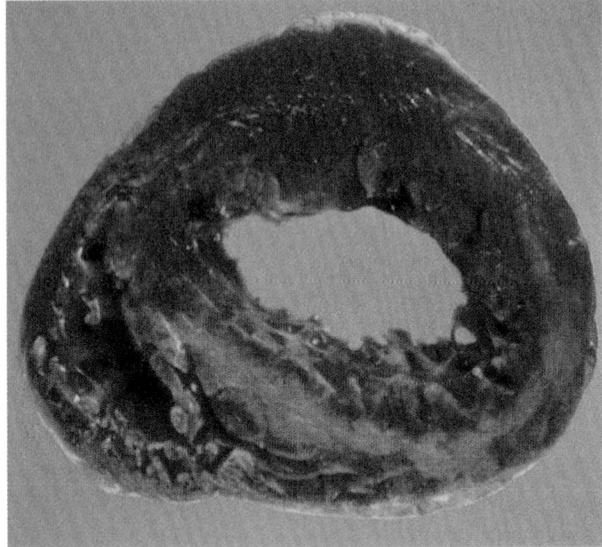

Figure 19–10
Acute myocardial infarct. A cross-section of the ventricles of a man who died a few days after the onset of severe chest pain shows a transmural infarct in the posterior and septal regions of the left ventricle. The necrotic myocardium is soft, yellowish, and sharply demarcated.

depletion and mitochondrial swelling) develop within several minutes. These early changes are reversible if blood flow is restored. Myocardial ischemia also contributes to cardiac dysrhythmias and sudden death, usually as the result of ventricular fibrillation. Many resuscitated survivors of "sudden death" do not develop AMI, indicating that the event resulted from ischemia caused by acute plaque change with minimal thrombus formation.

Irreversible myocardial cell death occurs after 20 to 40 minutes of severe ischemia. Microvascular injury occurs in about 1 hour and follows irreversible cell injury. If blood flow can be restored within this 20- to 40-minute timeframe, loss of cell viability does not occur or is minimal. The progression of ischemic necrosis usually begins in the subendocardial area of the heart and extends through the myocardium to involve progressively more of the transmural thickness of the ischemic zone. The extent of the infarct depends on the location, rapidity of development, severity of coronary vessel occlusion and vasospasm, amount of heart tissue supplied by the vessel, duration of the occlusion, metabolic needs of the affected tissue, extent of collateral circulation, and other factors such as heart rate, blood pressure, and cardiac rhythm.[2]

After a myocardial infarction, there usually are three zones of tissue damage: a zone of myocardial tissue that becomes necrotic because of an absolute lack of blood flow; a surrounding zone of injured cells, some of which will recover; and an outer zone in which cells are ischemic and can be salvaged if blood flow can be reestablished (Fig. 19–11). The boundaries of these zones may change with time after the infarction and with the success of treatment measures to reestablish flow.

The term *reperfusion* refers to reestablishment of blood flow through use of thrombolytic therapy. Early reperfusion (within 15 to 20 minutes) after onset of ischemia can prevent necrosis. Reperfusion after a longer interval can salvage some of the myocardial cells that would have died owing to longer periods of ischemia. It may also prevent microvascular injury that occurs over a longer period. Although much of the viable myocardium existing at the time of reflow ultimately recovers, critical abnormalities in biochemical function may persist, causing impaired ventricular function. The recovering area of the heart is often referred to as a *stunned myocardium*. Because myocardial function is lost before cell death occurs, a stunned myocardium may not be capable of sustaining life, and persons with large areas of dysfunctional myocardium may require life support until the stunned regions regain their function.[2]

Myocardial cells that undergone necrosis are gradually replaced with scar tissue (Table 19–2). An acute inflammatory response develops in the area of necrosis about 2 to 3 days after infarction. Thereafter, macrophages begin removing the necrotic tissue; the damaged area is gradually replaced with an ingrowth of highly vascularized granulation tissue, which gradually becomes less vascular and more fibrous.[2] At about 4 to 7 days, the center of infarcted area is soft and yellow; if rupture of the ventricle, interventricular septum, or valve structures occurs, it usually happens at this time. Replacement of the necrotic myocardial tissue is usually complete by the seventh week. Areas of the myocardium that have been replaced with scar tissue lack the ability to contract and initiate or conduct action potentials.

Manifestations

The manifestations of myocardial infarction can be categorized into four groups: pain and autonomic responses associated with the ischemic event; weakness and signs related to impaired myocardial function; dysrhythmias and ECG changes associated with changes in electrical

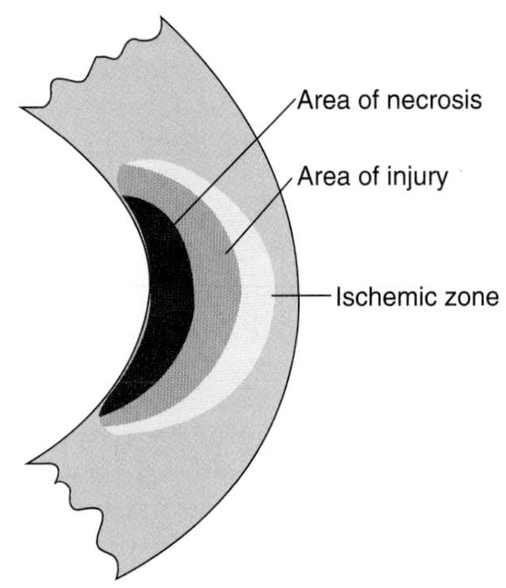

Figure 19–11
Areas of tissue damage after myocardial infarction.

TABLE 19-2
Tissues Changes after Myocardial Infarction

Time After Onset	Type of injury and Gross Tissue Changes
0–0.5 hours	Reversible injury
1–2 hours	Onset of irreversible injury
4–12 hours	Beginning of coagulation necrosis
18–24 hours	Continued coagulation necrosis; gross pallor of infarcted tissue
2–3 days	Total coagulation necrosis; continued gross pallor of infarcted area and sometimes hyperemia due to onset of acute inflammatory process.
3–7 days	Infarcted area becomes soft with a yellow-brown center and hyperemic edges
10 days	Maximally soft and yellow with vascularized edges; fibroblastic activity at edges denotes beginning of scar tissue generation
7th week	Scar tissue replacement complete

(Developed from information in Cotran R.S., Kumar V., Robbins S.L. [1994]. *Robbins pathologic basis of disease* [5th ed., pp. 532–534]. Philadelphia: W.B. Saunders.

conduction secondary to ischemia and death of myocardial cells; and symptoms of inflammation and elevated serum enzyme levels indicative of tissue death.

The onset of myocardial infarction usually is abrupt, with pain as the significant symptom. The pain typically is severe and crushing, often described as being constricting, suffocating, or like "someone sitting on my chest." The pain usually is substernal, radiating to the left arm, neck, or jaw, although it may be experienced in other areas of the chest. Unlike that of angina, the pain associated with myocardial infarction is more prolonged and not relieved by rest or nitroglycerin, and narcotics frequently are required.

Gastrointestinal complaints are common. There may be a sensation of epigastric distress; nausea and vomiting may occur. These symptoms are thought to be related to the severity of the pain and vagal stimulation. The epigastric distress may be mistaken for indigestion, and the patient may seek relief with antacids or other home remedies, which only delays getting medical attention. Complaints of fatigue and weakness, especially of the arms and legs, are common. Pain and sympathetic stimulation combine to give rise to tachycardia, anxiety, restlessness, and feelings of impending doom. The skin often is pale, cool, and moist. The impaired myocardial function may lead to hypotension and shock.

ECG changes may not be present immediately after the onset of symptoms, except as dysrhythmias. Premature ventricular contractions are common dysrhythmias after myocardial infarction. The occurrence of other dysrhythmias and conduction defects depends on the areas of the heart and conduction pathways that are included in the necrotic myocardium.

In the infarcted area, cell death causes inflammation and the release of intracellular proteins and enzymes into the extracellular fluid. The white blood cell count usually begins to rise. Fever and leukocytosis usually develop within about 24 hours and continue for 3 to 7 days. The erythrocyte sedimentation rate begins to rise during the first day or two after infarction, reaches a peak on the fourth or fifth day, and may remain elevated for several weeks.

Diagnosis

The diagnosis of myocardial infarction is based on the history of prolonged chest pain and other signs of distress, ECG changes characteristic of ischemia, and a rise in plasma markers indicative of myocardial injury.

Electrocardiographic Changes. During the period of impaired blood flow, injured and ischemic cells revert to anaerobic metabolism, with a resultant increase in lactic acid production, much of which is released into the local extracellular fluid. The necrotic cells become electrically inactive, and their membranes become disrupted, such that their intracellular contents, including potassium, are released into the surrounding extracellular fluid. This causes local areas of hyperkalemia, which can affect the membrane potentials of functioning myocardial cells. As a result of membrane injury and local changes in extracellular potassium and pH levels, some parts of the infarcted myocardium are unable to conduct or generate impulses, other areas are more difficult to excite, and still others are overly excitable. These different levels of membrane excitability in the necrotic, injured, and ischemic zones of the infarcted area set the stage for development of dysrhythmias and conduction defects after myocardial infarction. Each of these zones in the infarcted area conducts impulses differently. These changes in impulse conduction can be detected on the electrocardiogram and are the basis for determining whether an infarct has occurred and the area of the heart in which it is located.

Typical ECG changes associated with death of myocardial tissue include prolongation of the Q wave, elevation of the ST segment, and inversion of the T wave. (The ECG changes are variable and complex, and interested readers and those intending to work in the coronary care unit are referred to specialty texts.)

Molecular Markers. The diagnosis of myocardial infarction can be confirmed by increased levels of molecular markers that are released into the blood as a result of myocardial cell death. These markers include myoglobin, intracellular enzymes, and cardiac muscle troponins that are part of the actin-myosin unit. As indicated in Figure 19–12, concentrations of these proteins and enzymes become elevated at different times after infarction and provide useful diagnostic information.[21] The level of myoglobin, an oxygen-carrying protein normally in cardiac and skeletal muscle, becomes elevated within 1 hour after myocardial cell death, with peak levels reached within 4 to 8 hours.

Enzymes released from the damaged myocardial cells include creatine kinase (CK, formerly called creatinine phosphokinase) and lactate dehydrogenase (LDH). CK exceeds normal range within 4 to 8 hours and declines to normal within 2 to 3 days. There are three isoenzymes of CK, with the MB isoenzyme (CK-MB) being highly specific for injury to myocardial tissue. LDH exceeds the normal range by 24 to 48 hours, reaches a peak in 3 to 6 days, and returns to normal within 8 to 14 hours.

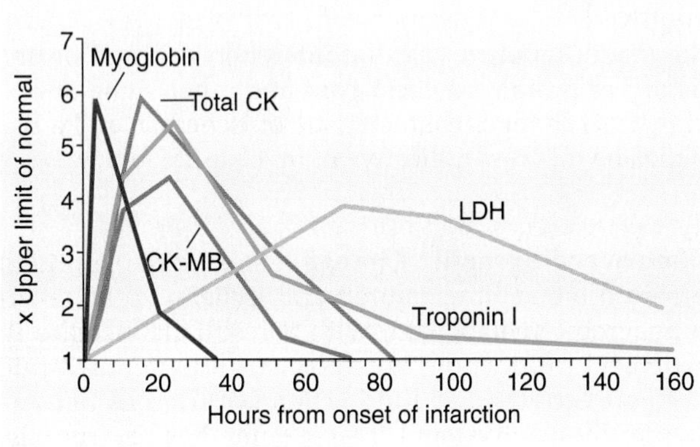

Figure 19–12
Time course of elevations of serum markers after AMI. This figure summarizes the relative timing, rate of rise, peak values, and duration of elevation above the upper limit of normal for multiple serum markers following AMI. Although traditionally total CK, CK-MB, and lactic dehydrogenase (LDH [with isoenzymes]) are measured, the relatively slow rate of rise above normal for CK and the potential confusion with noncardiac sources of enzyme release for both total CK and LDH have inspired the search for additional serum markers. The smaller myoglobin molecule is released quickly from infarcted myocardium but is not cardiac specific. Therefore, elevations of myoglobin that may be detected quite early after the onset of infarction require confirmation with a more cardiac-specific marker such as CK-MB or troponin I. Troponin I (and troponin T; not shown) rises more slowly than myoglobin and may be useful for diagnosis of infarction even up to 3 to 4 days after the event. Assays for cardiac-specific troponin I and troponin T using monoclonal antibodies are now available. (From Antman E.M. [1994]. General hospital management. In: Julian D.G., & Braunwald E. (eds.): *Management of acute myocardial infarction.* London: W.B. Saunders Ltd., p. 63)

The troponin complex consists of three subunits (*i.e.*, troponin C, troponin I, and troponin T) that regulate calcium-mediated contractile process in striated muscle. These subunits are released during myocardial infarction. Cardiac muscle forms of both troponin T and troponin I are used in diagnosis of myocardial infarction. It has been suggested that the cardiac troponin assay is more capable of detecting episodes of myocardial infarction in which cell damage is below that detected by CK-MB levels.[21]

Treatment

The methods used in treatment of AMI are directed at rapid recanalization of the occluded coronary artery, adequate pain relief, managing life-threatening complications, and rehabilitation to maximize physical and psychologic well-being during and after recovery. Controlled clinical trials have demonstrated that intravenously administered thrombolytic agents recanalize coronary arteries, reduce the size of the infarct, preserve left ventricular function, and reduce mortality.

The American College of Cardiology and American Heart Association (ACC/AHA) Task Force guidelines for management of AMI recommend that the initial emergency department management of myocardial infarction include administration of oxygen by nasal prongs; sublingual nitroglycerin (unless systolic blood pressure is less than 90 mm Hg or the heart rate is less than 50 or more than 100 beats/min); adequate analgesia; and aspirin (160 to 325 mg).[22] ECG monitoring should be instituted, and a 12-lead electrocardiogram should be performed. Persons with ECG evidence of infarction should receive immediate reperfusion therapy with thrombolytic agents or PTCA.[22]

The administration of oxygen augments the oxygen content of inspired air and increases the oxygen saturation of hemoglobin. Arterial oxygen levels may fall precipitously after myocardial infarction, and oxygen administration helps to maintain the oxygen content of the blood perfusing the coronary circulation. The severe pain of myocardial infarction gives rise to anxiety and recruitment of autonomic nervous system responses, both of which increase the work demands of the heart. Morphine and meperidine (Demerol) often are given intravenously for pain relief because they have a rapid onset of action and the intravenous route does not elevate enzyme levels. The intravenous route bypasses the variable rate of absorption of subcutaneous or intramuscular sites, which often are underperfused because of a decrease in cardiac output that occurs after infarction. Morphine has vasodilator properties and often is used as the narcotic of choice in treatment of AMI.[22] Sublingual nitroglycerin is given because of its vasodilating effect and ability to relieve coronary pain. Vasodilating drugs commonly decrease venous return (*i.e.*, reduce preload) and arterial blood pressure (*i.e.*, reduce afterload) and thereby reduce oxygen consumption.

Aspirin inhibits platelet aggregation, and it is thought that it may promote reperfusion and reduce the likelihood of rethrombosis.[23] It has been suggested that because of its antiplatelet effects, aspirin may also help to stabilize arterial patency after thrombolytic therapy.

Intravenous nitroglycerin may be given to limit infarction size and is most effective if given within 4 hours of symptom onset. Because sympathetic activity increases the metabolic activity of the myocardium and, consequently, myocardial oxygen consumption, β-adrenergic–blocking drugs may be used to reduce sympathetic stimulation of the heart after myocardial infarction. These drugs decrease myocardial contractility and cardiac workload; alter resting myocardial membrane potentials and decrease dysrhythmia frequency; and may also redistribute coronary artery blood flow and improve myocardial blood supply.

Thrombolytic Agents. Thrombolytic drugs are used to dissolve blood and platelet clots; they react with plasminogen to create plasmin, which lyses fibrin clots and digests clotting factors V and VIII, prothrombin, and fibrinogen. Several thrombolytic agents are approved by the Food and Drug Administration, including non–fibrin-selective agents such as streptokinase, anisoylated plasminogen-streptokinase activator complex (APSAC), and urokinase and fibrin-selective agents such as recombinant tissue plasminogen activator (rtPA) and prourokinase. Studies that have compared the three thrombolytic agents—streptokinase, APSAC, and rtPA—found no significant differences between them in relation to mortality, morbidity, and left ventricular function.

Thrombolytic therapy can reduce mortality and limit infarct size. The best results occur if treatment is initiated within 1 to 2 hours.[21] The magnitude of benefit declines after this period, but it is possible that some benefit can be achieved for up to 12 hours after the onset of pain. The person must be a low-risk candidate for complications caused by bleeding.

Percutaneous Transluminal Coronary Angioplasty. Coronary revascularization includes the use of PTCA, and if needed, CABG surgery may be used when the administration of a thrombolytic agent is contraindicated or ineffective. PTCA can be used as a primary coronary angioplasty to achieve refusion without prior administration of thrombolytic agents; an immediate adjunctive therapy applied as soon as possible after administration of a thrombolytic agent; a "salvage" or "rescue" procedure performed in persons for whom thrombolytic therapy has failed; or a deferred adjunctive coronary angioplasty which is done within the first 7 days after AMI to prevent recurrent ischemia.[24] When used as the primary treatment for AMI, PTCA must be done within a few hours after the onset of infarction for maximal effectiveness.

Coronary Artery Bypass Grafting Surgery. Although thrombolytic therapy and PTCA are the therapies of choice for AMI, emergency CABG surgery is the next therapy of choice if the first two fail. The operation is used to improve circulation to the myocardium, as described earlier in the chapter. The procedure should be done within 4 to 6 hours of symptom onset.[21]

Complications

The stages of recovery from AMI are closely related to the size of the infarct and the changes that have taken place within the infarcted area. Fibrous scar tissue lacks the contractile, elastic, and conductive properties of normal myocardial cells; the residual effects and the complications are determined essentially by the extent and location of the injury. Among the complications of AMI are sudden death, heart failure and cardiogenic shock, pericarditis and Dressler's syndrome, thromboemboli, rupture of the heart, and ventricular aneurysms.

Sudden death from CHD is death that occurs within 1 hour of symptom onset. It usually is attributed to fatal dysrhythmias, which may occur without evidence of infarction. About 30% to 50% of persons with AMI die of ventricular fibrillation within the first few hours after symptoms begin. Early hospitalization after onset of symptoms greatly improves chances of averting sudden death, because appropriate resuscitation facilities are immediately available when the fatal ventricular dysrhythmia occurs.

Depending on its severity, myocardial infarction has the potential for compromising the pumping action of the heart. Heart failure and cardiogenic shock (Chapter 20) are dreaded complications of AMI.

Pericarditis may complicate the course of AMI. It usually appears on the second or third day after infarction. The person experiences a new type of pain that is sharp and stabbing and is aggravated with deep inspiration and positional changes. A pericardial friction rub may or may not be heard in all persons who have postinfarction pericarditis, and it often is transitory, usually resolving uneventfully. Dressler's syndrome describes the signs and symptoms associated with pericarditis, pleurisy, and pneumonitis: fever, chest pain, dyspnea, and abnormal laboratory test results (*i.e.*, elevated white blood cell count and sedimentation rate) and ECG findings. The symptoms may arise between 1 day and several weeks after infarction and are thought to represent a hypersensitivity response to tissue necrosis. Antiinflammatory agents or corticosteroid drugs may be used to reduce the inflammatory response.

Thromboemboli are a potential complication, arising as venous thrombi or occasionally as clots from the wall of the ventricle. Immobility and impaired cardiac function contribute to stasis of blood in the venous system. Elastic stockings, along with active and passive leg exercises, usually are included in the postinfarction treatment plan as a means of preventing thrombus formation. If a clot is detected on the wall of the ventricle (usually by echocardiography), treatment with anticoagulants is indicated.

The acute postmyocardial infarction period can be complicated by rupture of the myocardium, the interventricular septum, or a papillary muscle. Myocardial rupture, occurring on the fourth to seventh day when the injured ventricular tissue is soft and weak, often is fatal. Necrosis of the septal wall or papillary muscle may also lead to the rupture of either of these structures, with worsening of ventricular performance. Surgical repair usually is indicated, but whenever possible, it is delayed until the heart has had time to recover from the initial infarction. Vasodilator therapy and the aortic balloon counterpulsation pump may provide supportive assistance during this period.

An *aneurysm* is an outpouching of the ventricular wall. Scar tissue does not have the characteristics of normal myocardial tissue; when a large section of ventricular muscle is replaced by scar tissue, an aneurysm may develop (Fig. 19–13). This section of the myocardium does not contract with the rest of the ventricle during systole. Instead, it diminishes the pumping efficiency of the heart and increases the work of the left ventricle, predisposing the patient to heart failure. Ischemia in the surrounding area predisposes the patient to development of dysrhythmias, and stasis of blood within the aneurysm can lead to thrombus formation. Surgical resection often is corrective.

Cardiac Rehabilitation Programs

Rehabilitation programs for persons with myocardial infarction incorporate rest, exercise, and risk factor modification. Protecting the oxygen supply of the heart and decreasing the myocardial oxygen consumption as much as possible are concerns during the early treatment of myocardial infarction. Most persons with myocardial infarction are maintained on bed rest for at least 12 hours.[22] This 12-hour period is followed by a gradual increase in activity, depending on the severity of the infarction and on complications. Modifying the diet to include foods that are low in salt and cholesterol and easy to digest is another treatment measure used to decrease cardiac work. Stool softeners may be prescribed to prevent constipation and avoid straining with defecation.

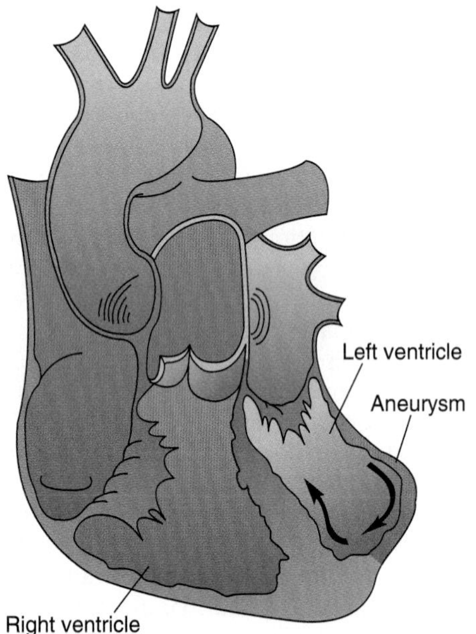

Figure 19–13
Paradoxical movement of a ventricular aneurysm during systole.

An exercise program is an integral part of a cardiac rehabilitation program. It includes activities such as walking, swimming, and bicycling. These exercises involve changes in muscle length and rhythmic contractions of muscle groups. Most exercise programs are individually designed to meet each person's physical and psychologic needs. The goal of the exercise program is to increase the maximal oxygen consumption by the muscle tissues, so that these persons are able to perform more work at a lower heart rate and blood pressure. In addition to exercise, cardiac risk factor modification incorporates strategies for smoking cessation, weight loss, stress reduction, and control of hypertension and diabetes.

In summary, CHD usually is caused by atherosclerosis. It frequently is a silent disorder, and symptoms do not occur until the disease is far advanced. Myocardial ischemia occurs when there is a disparity between the metabolic needs of the myocardium and the amount of blood that the coronary arteries can deliver, and it may manifest as angina. There are three types of angina. Classic angina is associated with atherosclerosis of the coronary arteries, in which pain is precipitated by increased work demands on the heart and relieved by rest; variant angina results from spasms of the coronary arteries. Unstable angina is an accelerated form of angina in which the pain occurs more frequently, is more severe, and lasts longer. Silent myocardial ischemia occurs without symptoms. Diagnostic methods for CHD include ECG methods, exercise testing, nuclear imaging studies, and angiographic studies in the cardiac catheterization laboratory. Treatment includes nonpharmacologic methods such as pacing of activities and avoidance of activities that cause angina. Pharmacologic methods include the use of nitrates, β blockers, and calcium-channel–blocking drugs. Revascularization procedures include percutaneous transluminal coronary angioplasty along with the use of coronary artery stents and CABG.

Myocardial infarction refers to the ischemic death of myocardial tissue associated with obstructed blood flow in the coronary arteries owing to atherosclerosis or thrombosis. The infarct can involve the endocardium, myocardium, epicardium, or a combination of all three layers and the pericardium. Diagnostic methods include the use of electrocardiograph monitoring, serum markers such as CK-MB, myoglobin, and cardiac troponin I and T. Treatment goals focus on reestablishment of myocardial blood flow through rapid recanalization of the occluded coronary artery, prevention of clot extension, alleviation of pain, measures such as administration of oxygen to increase the oxygen saturation of hemoglobin, and the use of vasodilators to reduce the work demands of the heart.

Thrombolytic agents, PTCA, or CABG are measures used to recanalize or bypass the occluded artery. Aspirin is given for its effects on platelet aggregation. The complications of myocardial infarction include potentially fatal dysrhythmias, heart failure, cardiogenic shock, pericarditis, thromboemboli, rupture of cardiac structures, and ventricular aneurysms.

Myocardial Disease

After you have completed this section of the chapter, you should be able to meet the following objectives:

- Define and cite causes of myocarditis
- Characterize the pathogenesis of viral myocarditis
- Describe the possible outcomes of viral myocarditis
- Define the term *cardiomyopathy* and compare the heart changes that occur with dilated, hypertrophic, constrictive cardiomyopathies, and arrhythmogenic right ventricular cardiomyopathy

Myocardial diseases are those originating in the myocardium, but not from cardiovascular disease, and include myocarditis and cardiomyopathies. Both conditions are causes of sudden death and heart failure. Of the more than 3 million persons in the United States who suffer from heart failure, about 25% result from idiopathic dilated cardiomyopathy.[25]

Myocarditis

The term *myocarditis* is used to describe an inflammation of the heart muscle and conduction system without evidence of myocardial infarction.[26] Myocarditis can occur as a primary disease or as a secondary disorder, as in rheumatic fever. Viral myocarditis accounts for about 80% of cases and is the one that most often manifests as a primary infection.[26] Myocarditis is a frequent pathologic cardiac finding in persons with acquired immunodeficiency disease (AIDS) because of the AIDS virus and other infectious agents. Bacterial myocarditis is uncommon compared with viral forms of the disease; the most common forms are associated with rheumatic fever and diphtheria toxins. Other causes of myocarditis are radiation therapy, hypersensitivity reactions, and exposure to chemical or physical agents that induce acute myocardial necrosis and secondary inflammatory changes.

Myocardial injury from myocarditis is thought to result from necrosis caused by direct invasion of the offending organism, toxic effects of exogenous or endotoxins produced by a systemic pathogen, or destruction of cardiac tissue by immunologic mechanisms initiated by the infectious agent. The immunologic response may be directed at foreign antigens of the infectious agent that share molecular characteristics with those of the host cardiac myocytes (*i.e.*, molecular mimicry; see Chapter 12), providing a continuous stimulus for the immune response even after the infectious agent has been cleared from the body.

Infectious myocarditis is most often caused by enteroviruses, principally coxsackie B viruses. Two phases of coxsackie B virus infection are damaging to the heart. During the initial 10 days to 2 weeks of infection, the virus replicates in the myocardium, destroying heart cells. During the second phase, the inflammatory response continues even though viral replication has become quiescent. During this time, sustained myocardial injury may continue owing to immune responses. The inflammation may resolve within 2 weeks, or it may become chronic.[26] Depending on the severity of the process, left ventricular function may be sufficiently impaired to cause congestive heart failure during the acute course of the disease or later. Depending on the extent of inflammation and destruction of myocardial cells, some persons may develop idiopathic dilated cardiomyopathy.

Manifestations

Manifestations of myocarditis vary from an absence of symptoms to profound heart failure or sudden death. When viral myocarditis occurs in children or young adults, it often is symptomatic. It affects twice as many males as females.[2] Acute symptomatic myocarditis typically manifests as malaise, dyspnea, low-grade fever, and tachycardia that is more pronounced than would be expected with the level of fever that is present. The patient commonly has a history of an upper respiratory tract or gastrointestinal tract infection, followed by a latent period of several days.

Clinical manifestations include a flulike syndrome, fever, fatigue, palpitations, chest pain, leukocytosis, and elevated erythrocyte sedimentation rate. There is a rise in the CK level, with or without an elevated MB fraction. Cardiac auscultation may reveal an S_3 ventricular gallop rhythm and a transient pericardial or pleurocardial rub. In about one half of the cases, myocarditis is transient, and symptoms subside within 1 to 2 months. In other cases, fulminant heart failure and life-threatening dysrhythmias develop, causing sudden death. Still others progress to subacute and chronic disease.[27]

Diagnosis and Treatment

The diagnosis of myocarditis can be suggested by clinical manifestations. The ECG changes of acute myocarditis include ECG conduction disturbances such as ventricular dysrhythmias, AV junctional block, ST-segment elevation, T-wave inversion, and transient Q waves. Confirmation of active myocarditis requires endomyocardial biopsy.[26]

Treatment measures focus on symptom management and prevention of myocardial damage. Bed rest is necessary, and activity restriction must be maintained until fever and cardiac symptoms subside to decrease the myocardial workload. Activity is gradually increased but kept at a sedentary level for 6 months to 1 year. The restriction includes the avoidance of swimming, jogging, weight lifting, and carrying heavy objects. According to the American College of Cardiology, athletes should not be allowed to return to competitive sports for at least 6 months and then only if the ECG and ventricular function test results have returned to normal values.[28]

The use of corticosteroids and immunosuppressant drugs such as azathioprine and cyclosporine remain controversial. The National Institutes of Health–sponsored multicentered Myocarditis Treatment Trial was established to evaluate the effectiveness of immunosuppression in the treatment of acute myocarditis. The results of this trial are being analyzed.[26] Although treatment of myocarditis is successful in many persons, some develop congestive heart failure and can expect only a limited lifespan. For these persons, heart transplantation becomes an alternative.

Cardiomyopathies

The cardiomyopathies are a group of disorders that affect the heart muscle. They can develop as primary or secondary disorders. The primary cardiomyopathies, which are discussed in this chapter, are heart muscle diseases of unknown origin. Secondary cardiomyopathies are conditions in which the cardiac abnormality results from another cardiovascular disease, such as myocardial infarction. In the United States, an estimated 1% of cardiac deaths can be attributed to primary cardiomyopathies. The onset of the primary cardiomyopathies often is silent, and symptoms do not occur until the disease is well advanced. The diagnosis is suspected when a young, previously healthy, normotensive person develops cardiomegaly and heart failure.

In 1989, the International Society and Federation of Cardiology and the World Health Organization categorized the primary cardiomyopathies into three groups: dilated, hypertrophic, and restrictive (Fig. 19–14).[29] This classification was enlarged in 1996 to include arrhythmogenic right ventricular cardiomyopathy.[30] Peripartum cardiomyopathy is a disorder of pregnancy.

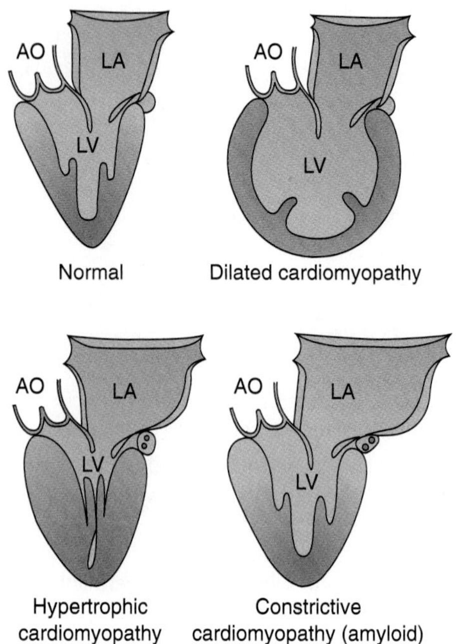

Figure 19–14
The various types of cardiomyopathies compared with the normal heart. (Roberts W.C., & Ferrans V.J. [1975]. Pathologic anatomy of the cardiomyopathies. *Human Pathology, 6*, 289)

Dilated Cardiomyopathies

Dilated cardiomyopathies are characterized by enlargement of the heart chambers (often all four) and the impaired pumping function of the ventricles. Dilated cardiomyopathy may be idiopathic (*i.e.*, of unknown origin), familial or genetic, viral, immunologic, metabolic, alcoholic, or from toxic disorders, or they may be associated with an underlying heart disease such as CHD. Many cases of idiopathic cardiomyopathy may have a genetic or inherited basis. One study found that 20% of affected persons have first-degree relatives with myocardial dysfunction.[31] Among the proposed patterns of genetic transmission are autosomal dominant, autosomal recessive, and X-linked inheritance patterns.

The most common initial manifestation of dilated cardiomyopathy is heart failure. There is a profound reduction in the left ventricular ejection fraction (*i.e.*, ratio of stroke volume to end-diastolic volume) to 40% or less, compared with a normal value of about 67%. Microscopic study reveals evidence of scarring and atrophy of myocardial cells. The ventricular wall usually is thickened, and mural thrombi are common, most often found in the left ventricle but also seen in the right ventricle or either atrium.

After symptoms have developed, the course of the disorder is distinguished by a propensity for development of heart failure, embolism, and ventricular dysrhythmias and has a poor prognosis. Fifty percent of persons with dilated cardiomyopathy are alive 5 years after initial diagnosis, and 25% are alive 10 years after diagnosis.[1] The most striking symptoms of dilated cardiomyopathy are right- and left-sided heart failure, dyspnea on exertion, paroxysmal nocturnal dyspnea, orthopnea, weakness, fatigue, ascites, and peripheral edema. On physical examination, an enlarged apical beat with the presence of a third and fourth heart sound and a murmur associated with regurgitation of one or both AV valves frequently are found. The systolic pressure is normal or low, and the peripheral pulses often are of low amplitude. Pulsus alternans, in which the pulse regularly alternates between weaker and stronger volume, may be present. Basilar rales frequently are detected. Sinus tachycardia, atrial fibrillation, and complex ventricular dysrhythmias leading to sudden cardiac death are common.

The treatment of dilated cardiomyopathy is directed toward relieving the symptoms of heart failure and reducing the workload of the heart (see Chapter 20). Digoxin, diuretics, and afterload-reducing drugs are used to improve myocardial contractility and decrease left ventricular filling pressures. Avoiding myocardial depressants, including alcohol, and pacing rest with asymptomatic levels of exercise or activity are imperative. Proper electrolyte balance and internal cardioverter defibrillators are effective in controlling recurrent ventricular dysrhythmias associated with dilated cardiomyopathy. In persons with severe heart failure that is refractory to treatment, cardiac transplantation may be considered.

Hypertrophic Cardiomyopathies

Hypertrophic cardiomyopathy is characterized by left, right, or left and right ventricular hypertrophy. Although the hypertrophy may be symmetric, the involvement of the ventricular septum often is disproportionate, producing obstruction of the left ventricular outflow channel and dilated atria. It is characterized by a small left ventricular volume with hypertrophy of ventricular muscle mass. Synonyms for this disorder include *idiopathic hypertrophic subaortic stenosis* and *asymmetric septal hypertrophy.*

Symptomatic hypertrophic cardiomyopathy commonly is a disease of young adulthood. The cause of the disorder is unknown, although it often is of familial origin, with the disorder being inherited as an autosomal dominant trait. Molecular studies of the genetic alterations responsible for hypertrophic cardiomyopathy suggest that the disease is caused by mutation in one of four genes encoding the proteins of the cardiac sarcomeres (*i.e.,* muscle fibers): the β-myosin heavy-chain, cardiac troponin T, α-tropomyosin, and myosin-binding protein C genes.[32]

A distinctive microscopic finding in hypertrophic cardiomyopathy is myofibril disarray. Instead of the normal parallel arrangement of myofibrils, the myofibrils branch off at random angles, sometimes at right angles to an adjacent fiber with which they connect. Small bundles of fibers may course haphazardly through normally arranged muscle fibers.[2] These disordered fibers may produce abnormal movements of the ventricles, with uncoordinated contraction and impaired relaxation.[33] Arrhythmias and premature sudden death are common with this disorder. Study results have shown that 36% of young athletes who die suddenly have probable or definite hypertrophic myocardiopathy.[1]

The manifestations of hypertrophic cardiomyopathy are variable; for reasons that are unclear, some persons with the disorder remain stable for many years and gradually develop more symptoms as the disease progresses, but others experience sudden cardiac death as first evidence of the disease.[32] Atrial fibrillation is a common precursor to sudden death in those who die of dysrhythmias. Dyspnea is the most common symptom associated with a gradual elevation in left ventricular diastolic pressure resulting from impaired ventricular filling and increased wall stiffness caused by ventricular hypertrophy. Because of the obstruction to outflow from the left ventricle, increasingly greater levels of ventricular pressure are needed to eject blood into the aorta, limiting cardiac output. Chest pain, fatigue, and syncope are common and worsen during exertion.[33]

The treatment of hypertrophic cardiomyopathy includes medical and surgical management. The goal of medical management is to relieve the symptoms by lessening the pressure difference between the left ventricle and the aorta, thereby improving cardiac output. Drugs that block the β-adrenergic receptors may be used in persons with chest pain, dysrhythmias, or dyspnea. These drugs reduce the heart rate and myocardial contractility by allowing more time for ventricular filling and reducing ventricular stiffness. The calcium-channel–blocking drug verapamil has proved useful in relieving the symptoms of dyspnea, chest pain, and syncope.[34] Increased calcium uptake and increased intracellular calcium content are associated with an increased contractile state, a characteristic finding in patients with hypertrophic cardiomyopathy. Disopyramide and amiodarone are effective in controlling the supraventricular and complex ventricular tachydysrhythmias associated with hypertrophic cardiomyopathies. Both drugs may also reduce the subaortic gradient because of their negative inotropic effects.[34]

Surgical treatment may be used if severe symptoms persist despite medical treatment. It involves incision of the septum (*i.e.,* myotomy) with or without the removal of part of the tissue (*i.e.,* myectomy). It is accompanied by all the risks of open heart surgery.

Restrictive Cardiomyopathies

Of the three categories of cardiomyopathies, the restrictive type is the least common in Western countries. With this form of cardiomyopathy, ventricular filling is restricted because of excessive rigidity of the ventricular walls, although the contractile properties of the heart remain relatively normal. The condition is endemic in parts of Africa, India, South and Central America, and Asia.[35] Outside the tropics, the most common causes of restrictive cardiomyopathy are endocardial infiltrations such as amyloidosis. Amyloid infiltrations of the heart are common in the elderly. The idiopathic form of the disorder may have a familial origin.

Symptoms of restrictive cardiomyopathy include dyspnea, paroxysmal nocturnal dyspnea, orthopnea, peripheral edema, ascites, fatigue, and weakness. The manifestations of restrictive cardiomyopathy resemble those of constrictive pericarditis. In the advanced form of the disease, all the signs of heart failure are present except cardiomegaly.

Arrhythmogenic Right Ventricular Cardiomyopathy

In arrhythmogenic right ventricular cardiomyopathy, right ventricular myocardium is replaced with a fibrofatty deposit. This condition frequently has a familial predisposition, with an autosomal dominant inheritance pattern. Sudden death due to arrhythmias is common, particularly in the young.[30]

Peripartum Cardiomyopathy

Although it is rare, dilated cardiomyopathy can develop during the peripartum period. Most cases of peripartum cardiomyopathy have their onset within 5 weeks after giving birth, but a few women begin to develop symptoms during the last month of pregnancy.[36] The incidence of peripartum cardiomyopathy is significantly higher in black women older than 30, in women with a third or subsequent pregnancy, in women having twins, or in those with toxemia.[36] In the United States, the incidence of peripartum cardiomyopathy is 1 case in 1300 to 4000 normal pregnancies.[37]

The cause of peripartum cardiomyopathy is uncertain. A viral cause or exposure of the maternal immune system to myometrial, placental, or fetal antigens has been proposed. The signs and symptoms of the disorder resemble those of previously described dilated cardiomyopathy. Treatment methods are also similar to those used in dilated cardiomyopathy.

There are two possible outcomes of peripartum cardiomyopathy. In about one half of cases, the heart returns to normal within 6 months, and the chances for long-term survival are good. In these women, heart failure returns only during subsequent pregnancies. In the other one half of cases, cardiomegaly persists, and the prognosis is poor and death is probable if another pregnancy occurs. In women with cardiomyopathy from documented viral myocarditis, the likelihood of recurrence is low.

In summary, myocarditis is an acute inflammation of the myocardium, most often of viral origin. Myocardial injury from myocarditis is thought to result from necrosis due to direct invasion of the offending organism, toxic effects of exogenous or endotoxins produced by a systemic pathogen, and destruction of cardiac tissue by immunologic mechanisms initiated by the infectious agent. Although the disease usually is benign and self-limited, it can result in sudden death or chronic heart failure, for which heart transplant may be considered.

The cardiomyopathies represent disorders of the heart muscle. Cardiomyopathies may manifest as primary or secondary disorders. Secondary cardiomyopathies are conditions in which damage to the cardiac muscle results from another disease process, such as myocardial infarction. There are four main types of primary cardiomyopathies: dilated, or congestive, cardiomyopathy, in which fibrosis and atrophy of myocardial cells with dilatation of all four heart chambers occur; hypertrophic cardiomyopathy, characterized by a disproportionate involvement of the ventricular septum, causing obstruction of the left ventricular outflow channel and a disarray in the organization of myocardial fibers and ventricular hypertrophy; restrictive cardiomyopathy, in which there is excessive rigidity of the ventricular wall; and arrhythmogenic right ventricular cardiomyopathy. Peripartum cardiomyopathy occurs during pregnancy.

The cause of the primary cardiomyopathies is largely unknown. The disease is suspected when a young, previously healthy person develops cardiomegaly and heart failure.

Infectious and Immunologic Disorders

After you have completed this section of the chapter, you should be able to meet the following objectives:

- Distinguish between the role of infectious organisms and the immune system in rheumatic fever, infective endocarditis, and Kawasaki's disease
- Compare the effects of rheumatic fever, bacterial endocarditis, and Kawasaki's disease on cardiac structures and their function
- Describe the relation between the infective vegetations associated with infective endocarditis and the extracardiac manifestations of the disease
- Explain measures that can be used to prevent infective endocarditis

Infective Endocarditis

Infective endocarditis is a condition involving microbial invasion of the endocardial surface of the heart. The disorder is characterized by the development of easily fragmented vegetative lesions laden with the infective agent.[2] The disease commonly affects persons with preexisting heart defects; the vegetative lesions attach to these defects. Heart valves are most commonly involved, but the lesions may affect a septal defect or the endocardial surface of the heart wall. In the preantibiotic era, infective endocarditis was almost always a fatal disease.

Factors that determine the clinical presentation and outcome of infective endocarditis are the nature of the infecting organism and the presence of preexisting heart defects. Because endocarditis in intravenous drug users and infections acquired during heart surgery have special features, the source of infections is also important.[38]

Predisposing Factors

Two predisposing factors contribute to the development of infective endocarditis: a damaged endocardial surface and a portal of entry by which the organism gains access to the bloodstream. The presence of valvular disease, prosthetic heart valves, or congenital heart defects provides an environment conducive to bacterial growth. In persons with preexisting valvular or endocardial defects, simple gum massage or an innocuous oral lesion may afford the pathogenic bacteria access to the bloodstream. Transient bacteremia may emerge in the course of seemingly minor health problems, such as an upper respiratory tract infection, a skin lesion, or a dental procedure.

The risk of infective endocarditis is increased among intravenous drug users to an incidence of 2% to 3% per year, which is several-fold greater than that for persons with rheumatic heart disease and prosthetic heart valves. The mode of infection is a contaminated drug solution or a needle contaminated with skin flora. Intravenous drug abuse is the most common source of right-sided (tricuspid) lesions.[39] Although staphylococcal infections are common, intravenous drug users may be infected with unusual organisms, such as gram-negative bacilli, yeasts, and fungi.

In hospitalized patients, infective endocarditis may arise as a complication of infected intravascular or urinary tract catheters. Infective endocarditis may also complicate prosthetic heart valve replacement. It can develop as an early infection that follows surgery or as a later infection that results from the long-term presence of the prosthesis. Infections of prosthetic valves account for 10% to 20% of cases of infectious endocarditis.

Depending on the duration of the disease, presenting manifestations, and complications, cases of infective endocarditis can be classified as acute, subacute, or chronic types.[40] *Acute infective endocarditis* is thought to primarily affect persons with normal hearts and are usually caused by *Staphylococcus aureus, Streptococcus pneumoniae, Streptococcus pyogenes*, and *Neisseria. S. aureus* in particular produces a rapidly progressive and destructive form of the disease. Subacute endocarditis is most frequently seen in patients with damaged hearts and is usually caused by less virulent organisms such as *Streptococcus viridans*, enterococci, and varieties of other gram-negative and gram-positive bacilli, yeasts, and fungi. Certain low-virulence organisms such as *Legionella* and *Brucella* may produce a chronic form of the disease.[40]

Pathophysiology

The pathophysiology of infective endocarditis involves the formation of intracardiac vegetative lesions that have local and distant systemic effects. The vegetative lesion that is characteristic of infective endocarditis consists of a collection of infectious organisms and cellular debris enmeshed in the fibrin strands of clotted blood. The infectious loci continuously release bacteria into the bloodstream and are a source of persistent bacteremia. These lesions may be singular or multiple, may grow to be as large as several centimeters, and usually are found loosely attached to the free edges of the valve surface (Fig. 19–15). As the lesions grow, they cause valve destruction, leading to valvular regurgitation, ring abscesses with heart block, and valve perforation. The loose organization of these lesions permits the organisms and fragments of the lesions to form emboli and travel in the bloodstream. The fragments may lodge in small blood vessels, causing small hemorrhages, abscesses, and infarction of tissue. The bacteremia can also initiate immune responses thought to be responsible for the skin manifestations, arthritis, glomerulonephritis, and other immune disorders associated with the condition.

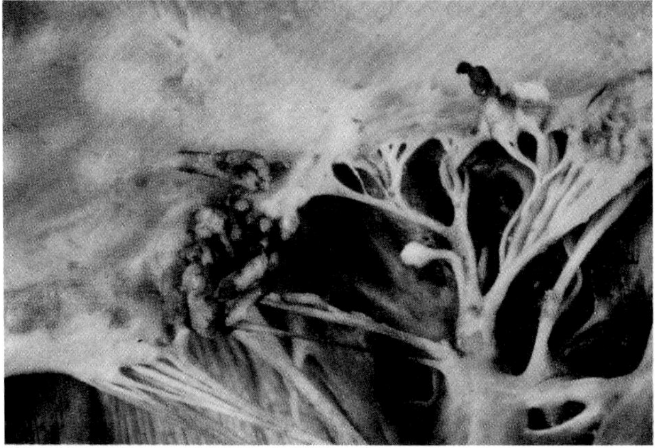

Figure 19–15
Bacterial endocarditis. The mitral valve shows destructive vegetations, which have eroded through the free margin of the valve leaflet.

Manifestations

The signs and symptoms of infective endocarditis include fever and signs of systemic infection, change in the character of an existing heart murmur, and evidence of embolic distribution of the vegetative lesions. In the acute form, the fever usually is spiking and accompanied by chills. In the subacute form, the fever usually is low grade, of gradual onset, and frequently accompanied by other systemic signs of inflammation, such as anorexia, malaise, and lethargy. Small petechial hemorrhages frequently result when emboli lodge in the small vessels of the skin, nail beds, and mucous membranes. Splinter hemorrhages (*i.e.*, dark red lines) under the nails of the fingers and toes are common. Cough, dyspnea, arthralgia or arthritis, diarrhea, and abdominal or flank pain may occur as the result of systemic emboli.

The clinical course of infective endocarditis is determined by the extent of heart damage, the type of organism involved, site of infection (*i.e.*, right or left side of the heart), and whether embolization from the site of infection occurs. Destruction of infected heart valves is common with certain forms of organisms, such as *S. aureus*. Peripheral embolization can lead to metastatic infections and abscess formation; these are particularly serious when they affect organs such as the brain and kidneys. Right-sided endocarditis, which usually involves the tricuspid valve, leads to septic emboli traveling to the lung, causing infarction and lung abscesses.

Diagnosis and Treatment

The blood culture is the most definitive diagnostic procedure and is essential to guide treatment. At least six cultures should be obtained to increase the probability of obtaining a positive culture. The optimal time to obtain cultures is during a chill, just before a temperature rise. Positive cultures are usually obtainable for infections caused by gram-positive cocci, but cultures may fail to grow gram-negative organisms or fungi. The echocardiogram is useful in detecting underlying valvular pathology.

The Duke University criteria can be used in making a definitive diagnosis of infective endocarditis. A diagnosis of infective endocarditis using the Duke criteria requires the presence of two major criteria, one major and three minor criteria, or five minor criteria.[39] The two major criteria are persistently positive blood cultures (at least two positive cultures separated by 12 hours or at least three cultures at least 1 hour apart or 70% of blood cultures are positive if at least four are drawn) and evidence of endocardial involvement as demonstrated by a positive echocardiogram or new valvular regurgitation. The six minor criteria are: a predisposing heart condition; fever; vascular phenomenon such as emboli, mycotic aneurysm, or intracranial hemorrhage; immunologic phenomenon such as glomerulonephritis or rheumatoid factor; positive blood cultures not meeting the major criteria; and positive echocardiogram not meeting the major criteria.

Treatment of infective endocarditis focuses on identifying and eliminating the causative microorganism, minimizing the residual cardiac effects, and treating the pathology induced by the emboli. Antibiotic therapy is used to eradicate the pathogen. Blood cultures are used to identify the causative organism and determine the most appropriate antibiotic regimen. Surgery may be indicated for moderate to severe heart failure, progressive renal failure, significant emboli, dysrhythmias, or left-sided endocarditis. Infected prosthetic valves may need to be replaced.

Of great importance is the prevention of infective endocarditis in persons with known risk factors. Prevention can be largely accomplished through prophylactic administration of an antibiotic before dental and other procedures that may cause bacteremia.[41]

Rheumatic Heart Disease

Rheumatic fever is an acute, recurrent inflammatory disease that follows a throat infection with group A β-hemolytic streptococci. The most serious aspect of rheumatic fever is chronic valvular heart disease that produces permanent cardiac dysfunction and sometimes causes fatal heart failure years later. In the United States and other industrialized countries, the incidence of rheumatic fever and prevalence of rheumatic heart disease has markedly declined in recent years. In 1994, 5540 persons in the United States died of rheumatic fever or rheumatic heart disease, compared with 22,000 deaths in 1950.[1] These figures include persons who died from complications of rheumatic heart disease contracted at an earlier date. This decline has been attributed to the introduction of antimicrobial agents for improved treatment of streptococcal pharyngitis, increased access to medical care, and improved economic standards, along with better and less crowded housing. Unfortunately, rheumatic fever and rheumatic heart disease continues to be a major health problem in many underdeveloped countries of the world where inadequate health care, poor nutrition, and crowded living conditions still prevail.

Rheumatic fever is primarily a disease of school-aged children. The incidence of acute rheumatic fever peaks between ages 5 and 15.[2] The disease usually follows an inciting streptococcal throat infection by 1 to 4 weeks. Rheumatic fever and its cardiac complications can be prevented by antibiotic treatment of the initial streptococcal throat infection.

The pathogenesis of the disease is unclear, and why only 3% of persons with uncomplicated streptococcal infections develop rheumatic fever remains to be answered. The time frame for development of symptoms in relation to the sore throat and the presence of antibodies to the *Streptococcus* organism strongly suggest an immunologic origin. Like other immunologic phenomena, rheumatic fever requires an initial sensitizing exposure to the offending streptococcal agent, and the risk of recurrence is high after each subsequent exposure.

Manifestations

Rheumatic fever can manifest as an acute, recurrent, or chronic disorder. The acute stage of rheumatic fever includes a history of an initiating streptococcal infection and subsequent involvement of the mesenchymal connective tissue of the heart, blood vessels, joints, and subcutaneous tissues. Common to all is a lesion called the *Aschoff body*.[2] The Aschoff body is a localized area of tissue necrosis surrounded by immune cells. The recurrent phase usually involves extension of the cardiac effects of the disease. The chronic phase of rheumatic fever is characterized by permanent deformity of the heart valves and is a common cause of mitral valve stenosis. Chronic rheumatic heart disease usually does not appear until at least 10 years after the initial attack, sometimes decades later.

Most children with rheumatic fever have a history of sore throat, headache, fever, abdominal pain, nausea, vomiting, swollen glands (usually at the angle of the jaw), and other signs and symptoms of streptococcal infection. Other clinical features associated with an acute episode of rheumatic fever are related to the acute inflammatory process and the structures involved in the disease process. There are five major manifestations of rheumatic fever: carditis, polyarthritis, chorea, erythema marginatum, and subcutaneous nodules. Minor manifestations can include arthralgia, fever, laboratory test results indicating elevated levels of acute-phase reactants, and a prolonged RR interval on the electrocardiogram.

Carditis. Rheumatic fever can affect the pericardium, myocardium, or endocardium, and all of these layers of the heart usually are involved. Rheumatic pericarditis causes the production of a fibrinous or serofibrinous exudate. For the most part, the myocarditis is reversible and produces minimal changes in cardiac function. The involvement of the endocardium and valvular structures produces the permanent and disabling effects of the disease. Although any of the four valves can be involved, the mitral and aortic valves most often are affected. During the acute inflammatory stage of the disease, the valvular structures become red and swollen; small vegetative lesions develop on the valve leaflets. The acute inflammatory changes gradually proceed to development of fibrous scar tissue, which tends to contract and cause deformity of the valve leaflets and shortening of the chordae tendineae. In some cases, the edges or commissures of the valve leaflets fuse together as healing occurs.

The manifestations of rheumatic carditis include a heart murmur in a child without a previous history of rheumatic fever, change in the character of a murmur in a person with a previous history of the disease, cardiomegaly or enlargement of the heart, friction rub or other signs of pericarditis, and congestive heart failure in a child without discernible cause.[42]

Polyarthritis. Although not a cause of permanent disability, polyarthritis is the most common finding in rheumatic fever. The inflammatory process affects the synovial membrane of the joint, causing swelling, heat, redness, pain, tenderness, and limited motion. The arthritis is almost always migratory, affecting one joint and then moving to another. The joints most frequently affected are the larger ones, particularly the knees, ankles, elbows, and wrists. In untreated cases, the arthritis lasts about 4 weeks. A striking feature of rheumatic arthritis is the dramatic response (usually within 48 hours) to salicylates.[43]

Chorea. Chorea (*i.e.*, Sydenham's chorea), sometimes called St. Vitus' dance, is the major central nervous system manifestation. It most frequently is seen in girls. There typically is an insidious onset of irritability and other behavior problems. The child often is fidgety, cries easily, begins to walk clumsily, and drops things. The choreic movements are spontaneous, rapid, purposeless, jerking movements that interfere with voluntary activities. Facial grimaces are common, and even speech may be affected. The chorea is self-limited, usually running its course within a matter of weeks or months.

Erythema Marginatum. Erythema marginatum lesions are maplike macular areas most commonly seen on the trunk or inner aspects of the upper arm and thigh. Skin lesions are present only in about 10% of patients who have rheumatic fever; they are transitory and disappear during the course of the disease.

Subcutaneous Nodules. The subcutaneous nodules are 1 to 4 cm in diameter. They are hard, painless, and freely movable and usually overlie the extensor muscles of the wrist, elbow, ankle, and knee joints. Subcutaneous nodules are rare, but when present, they most often occur in persons with carditis.

Minor Manifestations. The minor manifestations provide evidence of an acute inflammatory process and cardiac manifestations. Elevated levels of acute-phase reactants are not specific for rheumatic fever but provide evidence of an acute inflammatory response. The erythrocyte sedimentation rate, C-reactive protein, and white blood cell count commonly are used; unless corticosteroids or salicylates have been used, the results of these tests are almost always elevated in persons who present with polyarthritis, carditis, or chorea. These tests are also used to determine when the acute phase of the illness has subsided. A prolonged PR interval on the electrocardiogram is a nonspecific finding. It does not correlate with the ultimate development of chronic rheumatic heart disease.

Diagnosis and Treatment

The diagnosis of rheumatic fever is based on the Jones criteria, which were initially proposed in 1955 and revised in 1984 and 1992 by a committee of the American Heart Association.[42] The criteria were developed because no single laboratory test, sign, or symptom is pathognomonic of the disease, although several combinations of them are diagnostic. The signs and symptoms of rheumatic fever are grouped into major and minor categories. The presence of two major signs (*i.e.*, carditis, polyarthritis, chorea, erythema marginatum, and subcutaneous nodules) or one major and two minor signs (*i.e.*, arthralgia, fever, elevated levels of acute-phase reactants, and prolonged PR interval) accompanied by evidence of a preceding group A streptococcal infection indicates a high probability of rheumatic fever.

Evidence of a streptococcal infection is established through the use of throat cultures, antigen tests, and antibodies to products liberated by the streptococci. Throat cultures taken at the time of the acute infection usually are positive for group A streptococcal infection. It takes several days to obtain the results of a throat culture. The development of rapid tests for direct detection of group A streptococcal antigens have provided at least a partial solution for this problem. These tests use latex agglutination or an enzyme immunoassay and can be completed in a few minutes. Both types of tests are highly specific for group A streptococcal infection but are limited in terms of their sensitivity (*e.g.*, the person may have a negative test result but have a streptococcal infection), and a negative antigen test result should be confirmed with a throat culture when a streptococcal infection is suspected. Group A streptococci elaborate a large number of extracellular products, including streptolysin O and deoxyribonuclease (DNase) B. The antibodies to these products are measured for retrospective confirmation of recent streptococcal infections in persons thought to have acute rheumatic fever.[43]

Treatment is designed to control the acute inflammatory process and to prevent cardiac complications and recurrence of the disease. During the acute phase, prevention of residual cardiac effects is of primary concern; antibiotics, antiinflammatory drugs, and selective restriction of physical activities are prescribed. Recurrences of rheumatic fever are high, particularly in children and in patients who have had carditis during their initial episode. Penicillin (or another antibiotic in penicillin-sensitive patients) is used prophylactically for at least 5 years to prevent recurrence. Penicillin is also the antibiotic of choice for treating the acute illness. Salicylates and corticosteroids are also widely used.

Secondary prevention and compliance with a plan for prophylactic administration of penicillin require that the patient and the family understand the rationale for such measures and the measures themselves. Patients also need to be instructed to report possible streptococcal infections to their physicians. They should be instructed to inform their dentists about the disease so that they can be adequately protected during dental procedures that may traumatize the oral mucosa.

Kawasaki's Disease

Kawasaki's disease, also known as mucocutaneous lymph node syndrome, is an acute febrile disease of young children. First described in Japan in 1967 by Dr. Tomisaku Kawasaki, the disease affects the skin, brain, eyes, joints, liver, lymph nodes, and heart.[44–46] The disease can produce aneurysmal disease of the coronary arteries and is the most common cause of acquired heart disease in young children. More than 3000 children with Kawasaki's disease are diagnosed annually in the United States, and 0.5% to 1.0% of those die of complications of coronary artery involvement. Although first reported in Japanese children, the disease affects children of many races, occurs worldwide, and is increasing in frequency.

The disease is characterized by a vasculitis (*i.e.*, inflammation of the blood vessels) that begins in the small vessels (*i.e.*, arterioles, venules, and capillaries) and progresses to involve some of the larger arteries, such as the coronaries. The cause of Kawasaki's disease is unknown, but it is thought to be of immunologic origin. Immunologic abnormalities that include increased activation of helper T cells and increased levels of immune mediators and antibodies that destroy endothelial cells have been detected during the acute phase of the disease. It has been hypothesized that some unknown antigen triggers the immune response; it is speculated to be a common infectious agent, probably a virus, that triggers the response in a genetically predisposed child.

Manifestations

The course of the disease is triphasic and includes an *acute febrile phase* that lasts about 7 to 14 days; a *subacute phase* that follows the acute phase and lasts until days 10 through 24; and a *convalescent phase* that follows the subacute stage and continues until the signs of the acute-phase inflammatory response have subsided and the signs of the illness have disappeared.

The acute phase begins with an abrupt onset of fever, followed by conjunctivitis, rash, involvement of the oral mucosa, redness and swelling of the hands and feet, and enlarged cervical lymph nodes. The fever typically is high, reaching 40°C (104°F) or more; has an erratic spiking pattern; is unresponsive to antibiotics; and persists for 5 or more days. The conjunctivitis, which is bilateral, begins shortly after the onset of fever, persists throughout the febrile course of the disease, and may last as long as 3 to 5 weeks. There is no exudate, discharge, or conjunctival ulceration, differentiating it from many other types of conjunctivitis. The rash usually is deeply erythematous and may take several forms, the most common of which is a nonpruritic urticarial rash with large erythematous plaques or a measles-type rash. Although the rash usually is generalized, it may be accentuated centrally or peripherally. Some children develop a perianal rash with a diaper-like distribution. Oropharyngeal manifestations include fissuring of the lips, diffuse erythema of the oropharynx, and hypertrophic papillae of the tongue, creating a strawberry appearance. The hands and feet become swollen, painful, and have reddened palms and soles. The rash, oropharyngeal manifestations, and changes in hands and feet appear within 1 to 3 days of fever onset and usually disappear as the fever subsides. Lymph node involvement is the least constant feature of the disease. It is cervical and unilateral, with a single, firm, enlarged lymph node mass that is usually larger than 1.5 cm in diameter.

The subacute phase begins with the defervescence of fever and lasts until all signs of the disease have disappeared. During the subacute phase, desquamation (*i.e.*, peeling) of the skin of the fingers and toe tips begins and progresses to involve the entire surface of the palms and soles. Patchy peeling of skin areas other than the hands and feet may occur in some children.

The convalescent stage persists from the complete resolution of symptoms until all signs of inflammation have disappeared. This usually takes about 8 weeks.

In addition to the major manifestations that occur during the acute stage of the illness, there are several associated, less specific characteristics of the disease, including arthritis, urethritis and pyuria, gastrointestinal manifestations (*e.g.*, diarrhea, abdominal pain), hepatitis, and hydrops of the gallbladder. Arthritis or arthralgia occurs in about 30% of children with the disease, characterized by symmetric joint swelling that involves large and small joints. Central nervous system involvement occurs in almost all children and is characterized by pronounced irritability and lability of mood.

Cardiac involvement is the most important manifestation of Kawasaki's disease. Between 10% and 40% of children develop coronary vasculitis within the first 2 weeks of the illness, manifested by dilatation and aneurysm formation in the coronary arteries, as seen on two-dimensional echocardiography. The manifestations of coronary artery involvement include signs and symptoms of myocardial ischemia or, rarely, overt myocardial infarction or rupture of the aneurysm. Pericarditis, myocarditis, endocarditis, heart failure, and dysrhythmias may also develop.

Diagnosis and Treatment

As with rheumatic fever, the diagnosis of Kawasaki's disease is based on clinical findings, because no specific laboratory test for the disease exists.[47] In 1987, the Centers for Disease Control and Prevention published diagnostic criteria that are used in establishing a diagnosis of Kawasaki's disease.[48] The diagnosis is confirmed by the presence of a fever that lasts 5 or more days without another more reasonable explanation and by at least four of the following acute-stage manifestations of the disease: bilateral conjunctivitis; oropharyngeal manifestations (*e.g.*, injected or fissured lips, injected pharynx, strawberry tongue); extremity changes (*e.g.*, redness of the palms or soles, edema of the hands or feet, generalized peeling of the skin of the hands or feet, usually beginning around the nails); rash; and cervical lymphadenopathy. Chest radiographs, ECG tests, and two-dimensional echocardiography are used to detect coronary artery involvement and follow its progress. Coronary angiography may be used to determine the extent of coronary artery involvement.

Intravenous gamma globulin and aspirin are considered the best therapy for prevention of coronary artery abnormalities in children with Kawasaki's disease. During the acute phase of the illness, aspirin usually is given in larger doses and for its antiinflammatory and antipyretic effects. After the fever is controlled, the aspirin dose is lowered, and the drug is given for its anti–platelet-aggregating effects.

Recommendations for cardiac follow-up evaluation (*i.e.*, stress testing and sometimes coronary angiography) are based on the level of coronary artery changes. Anticoagulant therapy may be recommended for children with multiple or large coronary aneurysms. Some restrictions in activities such as competitive sports may be advised for children with significant coronary artery abnormalities.[47]

In summary, infective endocarditis involves the invasion of the endocardium by pathogens that produce vegetative lesions on the endocardial surface. The loose organization of these lesions permits the organisms and fragments of the lesions to be disseminated throughout the systemic circulation. The condition can be caused by several organisms. Two predisposing factors contribute to the development of infective endocarditis: a damaged endocardium and a portal of entry through which the organisms gain access to the bloodstream.

Rheumatic fever, which is associated with an antecedent group A streptococcal infection, is an important cause of heart disease. Its most serious and disabling effects result from involvement of the heart valves. Because there is no single laboratory test, sign, or symptom that is pathognomonic of acute rheumatic fever, the Jones criteria are used to establish the diagnosis during the acute stage of the disease.

Kawasaki's disease is an acute febrile disease of young children that affects the skin, brain, eyes, joints, liver, lymph nodes, and heart. The disease can produce aneurysmal disease of the coronary arteries and is the most common cause of acquired heart disease in young children.

Valvular Heart Disease

After you have completed this section of the chapter, you should be able to meet the following objectives:

- State the function of the heart valves and relate alterations in hemodynamic function of the heart that occurs with valvular disease
- Compare the effects of stenotic and regurgitant mitral and aortic valvular heart disease on cardiovascular function
- Compare the methods of and diagnostic information obtained from cardiac auscultation, phonocardiography, and echocardiography as they relate to valvular heart disease

The function of the heart valves is to promote directional flow of blood through the chambers of the heart. Dysfunction of the heart valves can result from a number of disorders, including congenital defects, trauma, ischemic damage, degenerative changes, and inflammation. In 1993, 15,200 persons in the United States died of valvular heart disease.[1] Although any of the four heart valves can become diseased, the most commonly affected are the mitral and aortic valves. Disorders of the pulmonary and tricuspid valves are uncommon, probably because of the low pressure in the right side of the heart.

Hemodynamic Derangements

The heart valves are composed of leaflets that are covered on both sides by endocardium and have a middle supporting core of dense fibrous connective tissue containing collagen and elastic fibers. Capillaries and smooth muscle are present at the base of the leaflet but do not extend up into the valve. The leaflets of the heart valves may be injured or become the site of an inflammatory process that can deform their line of closure. Healing of the leaflets is often associated with increased collagen content and scarring, causing the leaflets to shorten and become stiffer. The edges of the valve leaflets can heal together so that the valve does not open or close properly.

Two types of mechanical disruptions occur with valvular heart disease: narrowing of the valve opening so it does not open properly and distortion of the valve so it does not close properly (Fig. 19–16). *Stenosis* refers to a narrowing of the valve orifice and failure of the valve leaflets to open normally. The reduction in orifice areas produces an energy loss as laminar flow is converted to less efficient turbulent flow. This increases the work of the chamber emptying through the narrowed valve—the left atria in the case of mitral stenosis and the

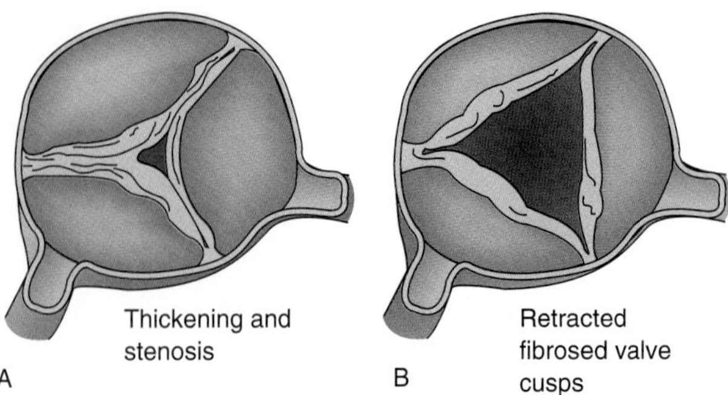

Figure 19–16
Disease of the aortic valve as viewed from the aorta. (**A**) Stenosis of the valve opening. (**B**) An incompetent or regurgitant valve that is unable to close completely.

left ventricle in aortic stenosis. Blood flow through a normal valve can increase five to seven times the resting value; consequently, valvular stenosis must be severe before it causes life-threatening problems. Symptoms usually are first noticed during situations of increased flow, such as exercise. An *incompetent* or *regurgitant* valve permits blood flow to continue while the valve is closed—flowing into the left ventricle during diastole when the aortic valve is affected and into the left atrium during systole when the mitral valve is diseased. Valvular disorders may cause stenosis (Fig. 19–17) and regurgitation.

The effect that valvular heart disease has on cardiac function is related to alterations in blood flow across the valve and to the resultant increase in work demands on the heart that the disorder generates. Many valvular heart defects are characterized by heart murmurs resulting from turbulence that occurs when blood flows through a diseased valve. Disorders in valve flow and heart chamber size for mitral and aortic value disorders are illustrated in Figure 19–18.

Mitral Valve Disorders

The mitral valve controls the directional flow of blood between the left atrium and the left ventricle. The edges or cusps of the AV valves are thinner than those of the semilunar valves; they are anchored to the papillary muscles by the chordae tendineae. During much of systole, the mitral valve is subjected to the high pressure generated by the left ventricle as it pumps blood into the systemic circulation, and the chordae tendineae prevent the eversion of the valve leaflets into the left atrium.

Mitral Valve Stenosis

Mitral valve stenosis most commonly is the result of rheumatic fever. Less frequently, the defect is congenital and manifests during infancy or early childhood.[49] Mitral valve stenosis is characterized by fibrous replacement of valvular tissue, along with stiffness and fusion of valve commissures (see Fig. 19–17). Involvement of the chordae tendineae causes shortening, which pulls the valvular structures more deeply into the ventricles. As the resistance to flow through the valve increases, the left atrial pressure rises, and dilatation of this heart chamber eventually occurs. The increased left atrial pressure is transmitted to the pulmonary venous system, causing pulmonary congestion. The rate of flow across the valve depends on the size of the valve orifice, the driving pressure (*i.e.*, atrial minus ventricular pressure), and the time available for flow during diastole. As the condition progresses, symptoms of decreased cardiac output occur during extreme exertion or other situations that cause tachycardia and thereby reduce diastolic filling time. In the late stages of the disease, pulmonary vascular resistance increases with the development of pulmonary hypertension; this increases the arterial pressure against which the right side of the heart must pump and eventually leads to failure of this side of the heart.

The signs and symptoms of mitral valve stenosis depend on the severity of the obstruction and are related to elevation in left atrial pressure and pulmonary congestion, decreased cardiac output owing to impaired left ventricular filling, and left atrial enlargement with development of atrial arrhythmias and mural thrombi. The symptoms are those of pulmonary congestion, including nocturnal paroxysmal dyspnea and orthopnea. Premature atrial beats, paroxysmal atrial tachycardia, and atrial fibrillation may occur as a result of distention of the left atrium. Together, the fibrillation and distention predispose to mural thrombus formation, from which systemic emboli may form. Palpitations, chest pain, weakness, and fatigue are common complaints.

The murmur of mitral valve stenosis is heard during diastole when blood is flowing through the constricted valve orifice; it is characteristically a low-pitched rumbling murmur, best heard at the apex of the heart. The first heart sound often is accentuated and somewhat delayed because of the increased left atrial pressure; an

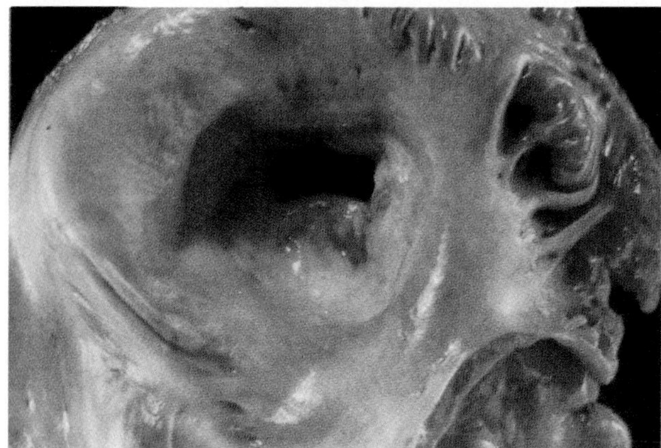

Figure 19–17
Chronic rheumatic valvulitis. A view of the mitral valve from the left atrium shows rigid, thickened, and fused leaflets with a narrow orifice, creating the characteristic "fish mouth" appearance of the rheumatic mitral stenosis.

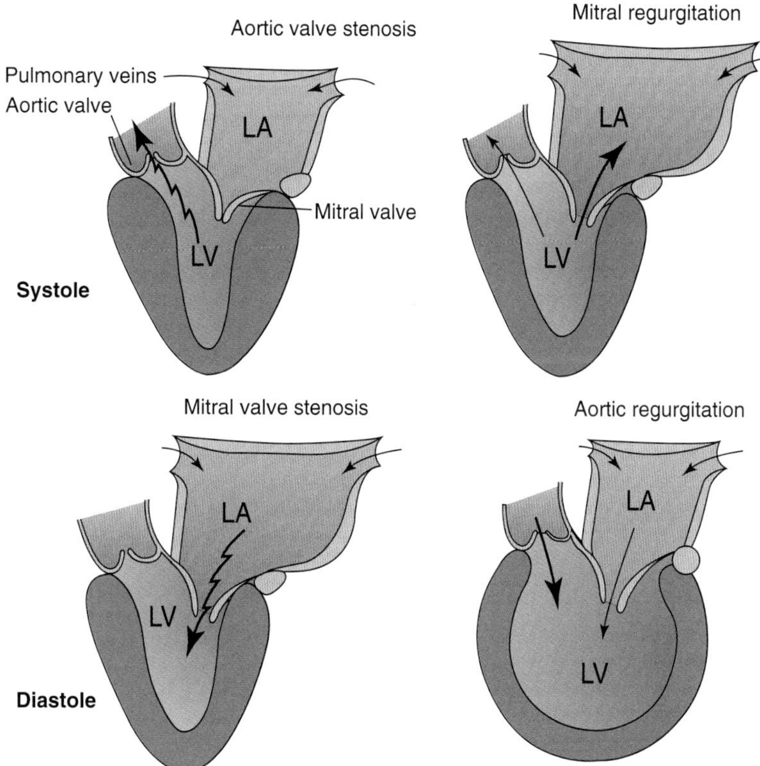

Figure 19–18
Alterations in hemodynamic function that accompany aortic valve stenosis, mitral valve regurgitation, mitral valve stenosis, and mitral valve regurgitation. *Thin arrows* indicate direction of normal flow, and *thick arrows* the direction of abnormal flow.

opening snap may precede the diastolic murmur as a result of the elevation in left atrial pressure.

Mitral Valve Regurgitation

Mitral valve regurgitation can result from many processes. Rheumatic heart disease is associated with a rigid and thickened valve that does not open or close completely. In addition to rheumatic disease, mitral regurgitation can result from rupture of the chordae tendineae or papillary muscles, papillary muscle dysfunction, or stretching of the valve structures due to dilatation of the left ventricle or valve orifice. Mitral valve prolapse is a common cause of mitral valve prolapse. Acute mitral valve regurgitation may occur abruptly, such as with papillary muscle dysfunction after myocardial infarction, valve perforation in infective endocarditis, or ruptured chordae tendineae in mitral valve prolapse.

With mitral valve insufficiency, blood from the left ventricle moves back into the left atrium during systole and is returned to the left ventricle during diastole. In acute regurgitation, left atrial pressure rises rapidly, leading to pulmonary edema if severe. With chronic mitral regurgitation, the left atrium enlarges gradually. Mitral regurgitation, like mitral stenosis, predisposes to atrial fibrillation. The degree of left ventricular enlargement reflects the severity of regurgitation. As the disorder progresses, left ventricular function becomes impaired, and the left atrial pressure increases, with the subsequent development of pulmonary hypertension. The increased volume work associated with mitral regurgitation is relatively well tolerated, and many persons with the disorder remain asymptomatic for 10 to 20 years despite severe regurgitation. A characteristic feature of mitral valve regurgitation is an enlarged left ventricle, a hyperdynamic left ventricular impulse, and a pansystolic (throughout systole) murmur.

Mitral Valve Prolapse

Sometimes referred to as the floppy mitral valve syndrome, mitral valve prolapse occurs in 2.5% of males and 7.6% of females in the general population.[50] The disorder is seen three times more frequently in women than in men and may have a familial basis. Although the cause of the disorder is unknown, it has been associated with Marfan's syndrome, osteogenesis imperfecta, and other connective tissue disorders and with cardiac, hematologic, neuroendocrine, metabolic, and psychologic disorders.

Pathologic findings in persons with mitral valve prolapse include a myxedematous (mucinous) degeneration of the spongiosum, which lies between the collagen and elastic tissue covering the atrial aspect of the valve and the thick layer of connective tissue that provides the main support for the valve, causing a redundancy of valve tissue and ballooning of the valve leaflets into the left atrium during systole when the ventricular pressure is high. Certain forms of mitral valve prolapse may arise from disorders of the myocardium that result in abnormal movement of the ventricular wall or papillary muscle; this places undue stress on the mitral valve.

The most commonly encountered symptoms in the clinical setting are chest pain, weakness, dyspnea, fatigue, anxiety, palpitations, and lightheadedness. Unlike angina, the chest pain often is prolonged, ill defined, and not associated with exercise or exertion. The pain has been attributed to ischemia resulting from traction of the prolapsing valve leaflets. The anxiety, palpitations, and dysrhythmias sometimes experienced by these patients may result from abnormal function of the autonomic nervous system that accompanies the disorder. Rare cases of sudden death have been reported for persons with mitral valve prolapse, mainly those with a family history of similar occurrences. The disorder is characterized by a spectrum of auscultatory findings, ranging from a silent form to one or more midsystolic clicks followed by a late systolic murmur.[50] Various abnormal ECG changes can occur. Dysrhythmias may be brought out by exercise stress testing or 24-hour ECG monitoring. Echocardiographic studies have become a method for the diagnosis of mitral valve prolapse, and the availability of this technique has undoubtedly contributed to increased recognition of the problem, particularly in its asymptomatic form.

The treatment of mitral valve prolapse focuses on the relief of symptoms and the prevention of complications. The β-adrenergic blocking drugs have proved useful in treating the autonomic manifestations, chest discomfort, and dysrhythmias that occur in the symptomatic form of the disease. Infective endocarditis is an uncommon complication in patients with a murmur; antibiotic prophylaxis usually is recommended before dental treatments or surgery.

Aortic Valve Disorders

The aortic valve is located between the aorta and left ventricle. The aortic valve has three cusps and is sometimes referred to as the aortic semilunar valve because its leaflets are crescent shaped. The aortic valve has no chordae tendineae. Although their structures are similar, the cusps of the aortic valve are thicker than those of the mitral valve. The middle layer of the aortic valve is thickened near the middle, where the three leaflets meet, ensuring a tight seal. Between the thickened tissue and their free margins, the leaflets are more thin and flimsy.

An important aspect of the aortic valve is the location of the orifice for the two main coronary arteries, which are located behind the valve and at right angles to the direction of blood flow. It is the lateral pressure in the aorta that propels blood into the coronary arteries (Fig. 19–19). During the ejection phase of the cardiac cycle, the lateral pressure is diminished by conversion of potential energy to kinetic energy as blood moves forward into the aorta. This process is grossly exaggerated in aortic stenosis because of the high flow velocities.

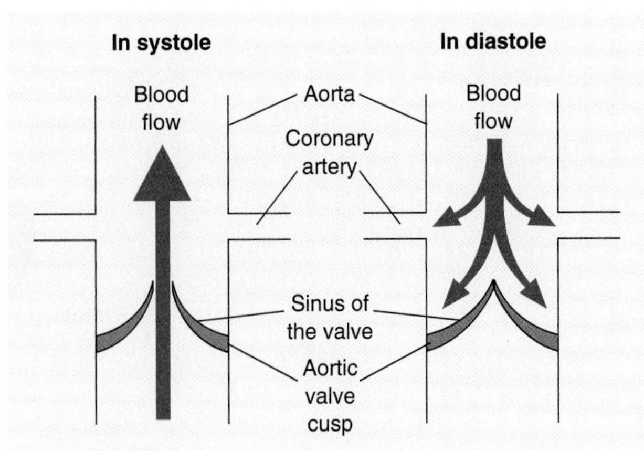

Figure 19–19
Location of the orifices for the coronary arteries and the direction of blood flow during systole and diastole.

Aortic Valve Stenosis

Because aortic stenosis causes resistance to ejection of blood into the aorta, the work demands on the left ventricle are increased, and the volume of blood ejected into the systemic circulation is decreased. The most common causes of aortic stenosis are rheumatic fever and congenital valve malformations. Congenital malformations may result in unicuspid, bicuspid, or misshaped valve leaflets. In elderly persons, stenosis may be related to degenerative atherosclerotic changes of the valve leaflets.

Obstruction to aortic outflow causes a decrease in stroke volume, along with a reduction in systolic blood pressure and pulse pressure. Because of the narrowed opening, it takes longer for the heart to eject blood; the heart rate often is slow, the pulse is of low amplitude, and there is a systolic ejection murmur.

The onset of signs and symptoms of aortic stenosis largely depends on the person's activity level. In persons who lead sedentary lives, the disease may be far advanced before symptoms are noticed. Exertional dyspnea is a common presenting symptom. It is characterized by vertigo and syncope when the stroke volume falls to levels insufficient for cerebral needs. The combination of increased work demands on the hypertrophied left ventricle and decreased perfusion of the coronary vessels may cause angina. Persons with aortic stenosis tend to be asymptomatic for many years despite severe obstruction.[49]

Aortic Valve Regurgitation

An incompetent aortic valve allows blood to return to the left ventricle during diastole. This defect may result from conditions that cause scarring of the valve leaflets or from enlargement of the valve orifice to the extent that the valve leaflets no longer meet. Rheumatic fever ranks first on the list of causes of aortic regurgitation. Failure of a prosthetic valve is another cause of aortic regurgitation. Acute aortic regurgitation is most commonly caused by infective endocarditis, trauma, or aortic dissection.

Chronic aortic regurgitation is characterized by a widening of the pulse pressure—the systolic pressure is high and the diastolic pressure low. Widening of the pulse pressure has two underlying mechanisms. First, there is an increase in the stroke volume (and systolic blood pressure) as the left ventricle ejects blood entering from the lungs and the blood that has leaked back across the aortic valve into the ventricle during diastole. Second, because the aortic valve fails to close completely, diastolic pressure cannot be maintained. Dilation of the left ventricle increases left ventricular systolic tension required to develop any level of systolic pressure; this leads to volume overload hypertrophy.[49]

Signs and symptoms of chronic aortic regurgitation include exertional dyspnea, orthopnea, and paroxysmal nocturnal dyspnea. In aortic regurgitation, failure of aortic valve closure during diastole causes an abnormal drop in diastolic pressure; because coronary blood flow is greatest during diastole, this decreases the pressure needed to perfuse the coronary arteries. Although angina is rare, it may occur when the heart rate and diastolic pressure fall to low levels. Systolic pressure is elevated, and diastolic pressure is abnormally low. Korotkoff sounds may persist to zero, even though intraarterial pressure rarely falls below 30 mm Hg.[49] The large stroke volume, wide pulse pressure, and rapid runoff of blood from the aorta that occur in aortic regurgitation also produce characteristic changes in the peripheral pulses: prominent carotid pulsations in the neck, throbbing peripheral pulses, and a left ventricular impulse that causes the chest to move with each beat. Persons often complain of an uncomfortable awareness of heart beat, particularly when lying down. The hyperkinetic pulse of more severe aortic stenosis, called a *water-hammer pulse,* is characterized by distention and quick collapse of the artery. In persons with severe aortic stenosis, the head may bob with each heart beat (*i.e.,* de Musset's sign). The turbulence of the flow across the aortic valve during diastole produces a high-pitched or blowing type of murmur.

Persons with chronic aortic regurgitation often remain asymptomatic for a long time. This contrasts with acute aortic regurgitation, in which there is no time for the left ventricle to undergo adaptation. As a result, there is severe elevation in left ventricular end-diastolic pressure, which is transmitted to the left atrium and pulmonary veins, culminating in pulmonary edema. A fall in cardiac output leads to sympathetic stimulation and a resultant increase in heart rate and peripheral vascular resistance that cause the regurgitation to worsen.

Diagnosis and Treatment

Valvular defects usually are detected through cardiac auscultation. Diagnosis is aided by cardiac auscultation (*i.e.,* heart sounds), phonocardiography, echocardiography, and cardiac catheterization. A permanent recording of the heart sounds can be made through the use of a *phonocardiogram.* This is obtained by placing a high-fidelity microphone on the chest wall over the heart while a recording is made. An ECG tracing usually is made simultaneously for timing purposes.

Echocardiography uses ultrasonography to record an image of heart structures. An ultrasound signal has a frequency greater than 20,000 Hz (cycles per second) and is inaudible to the human ear. Echocardiography uses ultrasound signals in the range of 2 million to 5 million Hz. The ultrasound signal is reflected (*i.e.,* echoes) whenever tissue resistance to the transmission of the sound beam changes. It is possible to create an image of the internal structures of the heart because the chest wall, blood, and different heart structures all reflect ultrasound differently.

The echocardiogram is useful for determining ventricular dimensions and valve movements, obtaining data on the movement of the left ventricular wall and septum, estimating diastolic and systolic volumes, and viewing the motion of individual segments of the left ventricular wall during systole and diastole. It can also be used for studying valvular disease and detecting pericardial effusion.

The treatment of valvular defects consists of medical management of heart failure and associated problems and surgical intervention to repair or replace the defective valve. Mitral commissurotomy is the surgical enlargement of a stenotic valve. It may be performed as an open or a closed procedure. The open procedure requires extracorporeal circulation (*i.e.,* cardiopulmonary bypass) but has the advantage of affording the surgeon direct visualization of the operative site. Valvular replacement, with a prosthetic device or a homograft, usually is reserved for severe disease because the ideal substitute valve has not yet been invented. Percutaneous balloon valvuloplasty involves the opening of a stenotic valve by guiding an inflated balloon through the valve orifice. The procedure is done in the cardiac catheterization laboratory and involves the insertion of a balloon catheter into the heart by way of a peripheral blood vessel.

In summary, dysfunction of the heart valves can result from a number of disorders, including congenital defects, trauma, ischemic heart disease, degenerative changes, and inflammation. Rheumatic endocarditis is a common cause. Valvular heart disease produces its effects through disturbances of blood flow. A stenotic valvular defect is one that causes a decrease in blood flow through a valve, resulting in impaired emptying and increased work demands on the heart chamber that empties blood across the diseased valve. A regurgitant valvular defect permits the blood flow to continue when the valve is closed. Valvular heart disorders produce blood flow turbulence and often are detected through cardiac auscultation.

Heart Disease in Infants and Children

After you have completed this section of the chapter, you should be able to meet the following objectives:

- Trace the flow of blood in the fetal circulation, and state the function of the foramen ovale and ductus arteriosus

- State the changes in circulatory function that occur at birth
- Compare the effects of left-to-right and right-to-left shunts on the pulmonary circulation and production of cyanosis
- Describe the anatomic defects and altered patterns of blood flow in children with atrial septal defects, ventricular septal defects, endocardial cushion defects, pulmonary stenosis, tetralogy of Fallot, patent ductus arteriosus, transposition of the great vessels, and coarctation of the aorta

This section of the chapter provides an overview of congenital heart defects, including the embryonic development of the heart, fetal and postnatal circulation, hemodynamic manifestations of congenital heart defects, and a description of the more common defects.

About 32,000 babies are born each year with a congenital heart defect.[1] About 25% of these have a severe defect that would cause death within the first year if not corrected. Premature infants have a higher incidence of congenital heart defects, most commonly patent ductus arteriosus and atrial septal defects. Depending on the type of defect, children with congenital heart disease experience various signs and symptoms associated with altered heart action, heart failure, pulmonary vascular disorders, and difficulty in supplying the peripheral tissues with oxygen and other nutrients.

Embryonic Development of the Heart

The heart is the first functioning organ in the embryo; its first pulsatile movements begin during the third week after conception. This early development of the heart is essential to the rapidly growing embryo as a means of circulating nutrients and removing waste products. Most of the development of the heart and blood vessels occurs between the third and eighth weeks of embryonic life.

The developing heart begins as two endothelial tubes that fuse into a single tubular structure.[51,52] The early heart structures develop as the tubular heart elongates and forms alternate dilations and constrictions. A single atrium and ventricle along with the bulbus cordis develop first. This is followed by formation of the truncus arteriosus and the sinus venosus, a large venous sinus that receives blood from the embryo and developing placenta (Fig. 19–20). The early pulsatile movements of the heart begin in the sinus venosus and move blood out of the heart by way of the bulbus cordis, truncus arteriosus, and aortic arches.

A differential growth rate in the early cardiac structures, along with fixation of the heart at the venous and arterial ends, causes the tubular heart to bend over on itself. As the heart bends, the atrium and the sinus venosus come to lie behind the bulbus cordis, truncus arteriosus, and ventricle. This looping of the primitive heart results in the heart's alignment in the left side of the chest with the atrium located behind the ventricle. Malrotation during formation of the ventricular loop can cause various malpositions, such as dextroposition of the heart.

The embryonic heart undergoes further development as partitioning of the chambers occurs. Partitioning of the AV channel, atrium, and ventricle begins in the fourth week and essentially is complete by the fifth week. The separation of the heart begins as tissue bundles, called the *endocardial cushions,* form in the midportion of the dorsal and ventral walls of the heart in the region of the AV canal and begin to grow inward. Until the separation begins, a single AV channel exists between the atria and the ventricles. As the endocardial cushions enlarge, they meet and fuse to form separate right and left AV channels (Fig. 19–21). The mitral and tricuspid valves develop in these channels. The endocardial cushions also contribute to formation of parts of the atrial and ventricular septum. Defects in endocardial cushion formation can result in atrial and ventricular septal defects, complete AV canal defect, and anomalies of the mitral and tricuspid valves.

Compartmentalization of the ventricles begins with the growth of the intraventricular septum from the floor

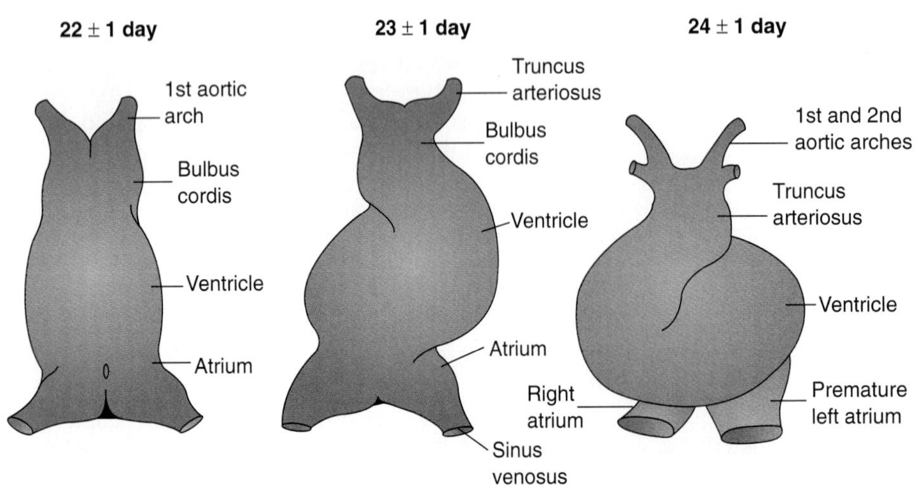

Figure 19–20 Ventral view of the developing heart (20–25 days). (Adapted from Moore K.L. [1977]. *The developing human* [2nd ed.]. Philadelphia: W.B. Saunders)

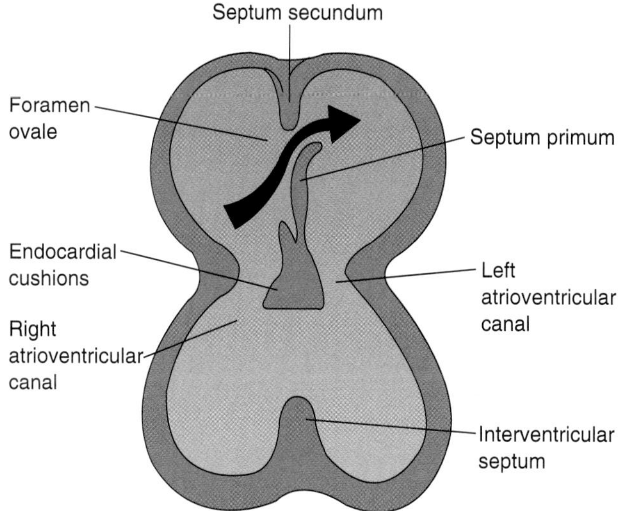

Figure 19–21
Development of the endocardial cushions, right and left atrioventricular canals, interventricular septum, and septum primum and septum secundum of the foramen ovale. Note that blood from the right atrium flows through the foramen ovale to the left atrium.

of the ventricle moving upward toward the endocardial cushions. Fusion of the endocardial cushions with the intraventricular septum usually is completed by the end of the seventh week.

Partitioning of the atrial septum is more complex and occurs in two stages, beginning with the formation of a thin, crescent-shaped membrane called the *septum primum* that emerges from the anterosuperior portion of the heart and grows toward the endocardial cushions, leaving an opening called the *foramen primum* between its lower edge and the endocardial cushions. A second membrane, called *septum secundum,* also begins to grow from the upper wall of the atrium on the right side of the septum primum. As this membrane grows toward the endocardial cushions, it gradually overlaps an opening in the upper part of the septum primum, forming an oval opening with a flap-type valve called the *foramen ovale* (see Fig. 19–21). The upper part of the septum primum gradually disappears; the remaining part becomes the valve of the foramen ovale. The foramen ovale forms a communicating channel between the two upper chambers of the heart. This opening, which closes shortly after birth, allows blood from the umbilical vein to pass directly into the left heart, bypassing the lungs. An ostium secundum defect, which is one type of atrial septal defect, is thought to arise from excessive absorption of the septum primum.

To complete the transformation into a four-chambered heart, provision must be made for separating the blood pumped from the right side of the heart, which is to be diverted into the pulmonary circulation, from the blood pumped from the left side of the heart, which is to be pumped to the systemic circulation. This separation of blood flow is accomplished by developmental changes in the outlet channels of the tubular heart, the bulbus cordis, and the truncus arteriosus, which undergo spiral twisting and vertical partitioning (Fig. 19–22). As these vessels spiral and divide, the location of the aorta becomes posterior and to the right of the pulmonary artery. Impaired spiraling during this stage of development can lead to defects such as transposition of the great vessels.

In the process of forming a separate pulmonary trunk and aorta, a vessel called the *ductus arteriosus* develops. This vessel, which connects the pulmonary artery and the aorta, allows blood entering the pulmonary

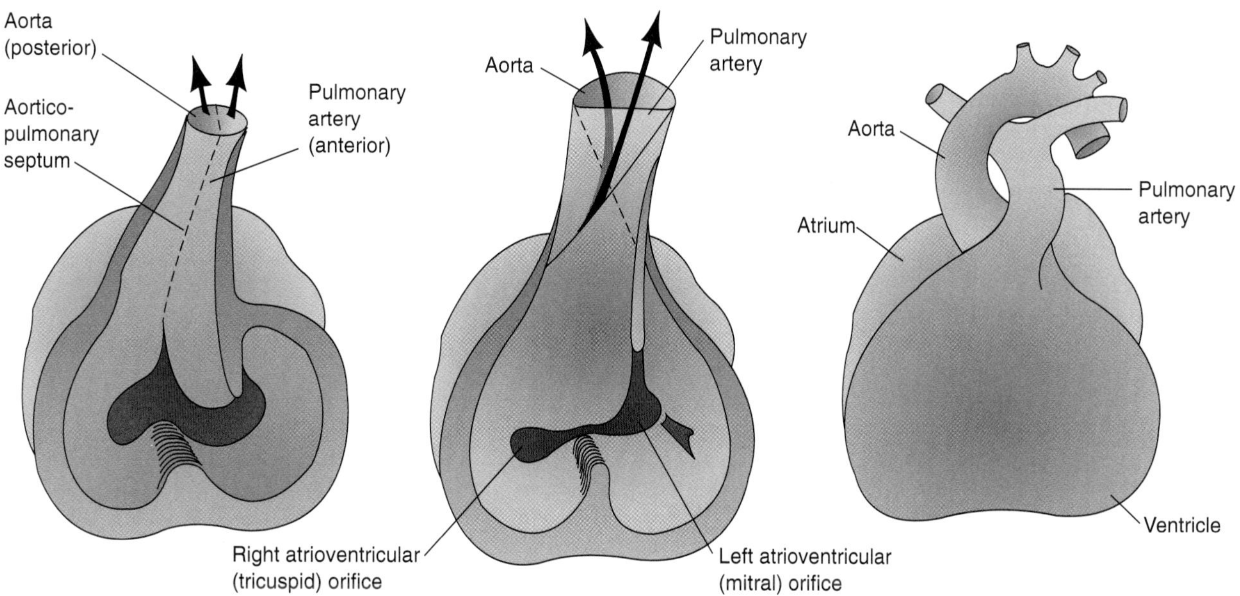

Figure 19–22
Separation and twisting of the truncus arteriosus to form the pulmonary artery and aorta.

trunk to be shunted into the aorta as a means of bypassing the lungs. Like the foramen ovale, the ductus arteriosus usually closes shortly after birth.

Fetal and Perinatal Circulation

The fetal circulation is different anatomically and physiologically from the postnatal circulation. Before birth, oxygenation of blood occurs by way of the placenta, and after birth, it occurs by way of the lungs. The fetus is maintained in a low-oxygen state (PO_2 to 30 mm Hg) and 60% to 70% saturation.[53,54] To compensate, fetal cardiac output is higher than at any other time (400 to 500 ml/ kg/min).

In the fetus, blood enters the circulation by way of the umbilical vein and returns to the placenta by way of the two umbilical arteries (Fig. 19–23). A vessel called the *ductus venosum* allows blood from the umbilical vein to bypass the hepatic circulation and pass directly into the inferior vena cava. From the inferior vena cava, blood flows into the right atrium and then is directed through the foramen ovale into the left atrium. Blood then passes into the left ventricle and is ejected into the ascending aorta to perfuse the head and upper extremities. In this way, the best-oxygenated blood from the placenta is used to perfuse the brain. At the same time, venous blood from the head and upper extremities returns to the right side of the heart by way of the superior vena cava, moves into the right ventricle, and is ejected into the pulmonary artery. The pulmonary vascular resistance is very high because the lungs are fluid filled and the resultant alveolar hypoxia contributes to intense vasoconstriction. Because of the high pulmonary vascular resistance, the blood that is ejected into the pulmonary artery is diverted through the ductus arteriosus into the descending aorta. This blood perfuses the lower extremities and is returned to the placenta by way of the umbilical arteries.

At birth, the infant takes its first breath and switches from placental to pulmonary oxygenation of the blood. The most dramatic alterations in the circulation after birth are the elimination of the low-resistance placental vascular bed and the marked pulmonary vasodilation that is produced by initiation of ventilation. The pressure in the pulmonary circulation and the right side of the heart fall as fetal lung fluid is replaced by air and as lung expansion decreases the pressure transmitted to the pulmonary blood vessels. With lung inflation, the alveolar oxygen tension increases, causing reversal of the hypoxemic-induced pulmonary vasoconstriction of the fetal circulation. Cord clamping and removal of the low-resistance placental circulation produce an increase in systemic vascular resistance and a resultant increase in left ventricular pressure. The resultant fall in right atrial pressure and rise in left atrial pressure produce closure of the foramen ovale. Reversal of the fetal hypoxemic state also produces constriction of ductal smooth muscle, contributing to closure of the ductus arteriosus. The foramen ovale and the ductus arteriosus normally close within the first day of life, effectively separating the pulmonary and systemic circulations.

After the initial precipitous fall in pulmonary vascular resistance, a more gradual decrease in pulmonary

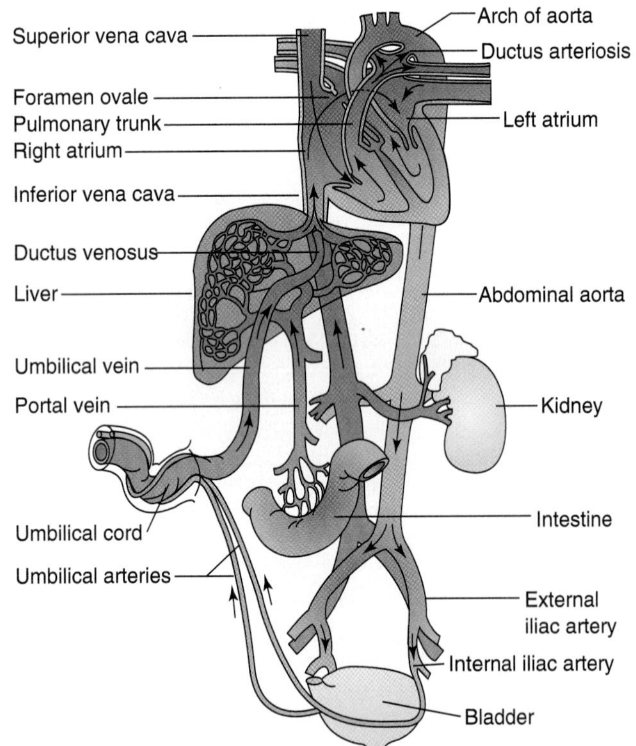

Figure 19–23
Fetal circulation.

vascular resistance is related to regression of the medial smooth muscle layer in the pulmonary arteries. During the first 2 to 9 weeks of life, gradual thinning of the medial smooth muscle layer of pulmonary arteries results in further decreases in pulmonary vascular resistance.[54] By the time a healthy, term infant is several weeks old, the pulmonary vascular resistance has fallen to adult levels.

Several factors, including prematurity, alveolar hypoxia, lung disease, and congenital heart defects, may affect postnatal pulmonary vascular development.[54] If a baby is born prematurely, the smooth muscle layers of the pulmonary vasculature may develop incompletely or regress in a shorter period. Much of the development of the smooth muscle layer in the pulmonary arterioles occurs during the latter part of gestation; as a result, infants who are born prematurely have less medial smooth muscle. These infants follow the same pattern of smooth muscle regression, but because less muscle exists, the muscle layer may regress in a shorter period. The pulmonary vascular smooth muscle in premature infants may also be less responsive to hypoxia. For these reasons, a premature infant may demonstrate a larger fall in pulmonary vascular resistance and a resultant shunting of blood from the aorta through the ductus arteriosus to the pulmonary artery within hours of birth.

Hypoxia during the first days of life may delay or prevent the normal fall in pulmonary vascular resistance. During this period, the pulmonary arteries remain reactive and can constrict in response to hypoxia, acidosis, hyperinflation of the alveoli, and hypothermia. Alveolar hypoxia is one of the most potent stimuli of pulmonary vasoconstriction and of pulmonary hypertension in the neonate.

Congenital Heart Defects

The major development of the fetal heart occurs between the fourth and seventh weeks of gestation, and during this time, most congenital heart defects arise. The development of the heart may be altered by environmental, genetic, and chromosomal influences.

Most congenital heart defects are thought to be multifactorial in origin, resulting from an interaction between a genetic predisposition to develop a heart defect and environmental influences. Infants born to parents with congenital heart defects or with siblings who have congenital heart defects are at higher risk. Some heart defects, such as coarctation of the aorta, atrial septal defect of the secundum type, and pulmonary valve stenosis, and certain ventricular septal defects have a stronger familial predisposition than others.

Chromosomal defects are thought to account for about 5% of congenital heart defects. Characteristic of these influences is the increased number of cardiac lesions observed in children born with Down syndrome (*i.e.*, trisomy of chromosome 21). Another 2% to 4% of cases result from adverse maternal conditions and teratogenic influences, including maternal diabetes, congenital rubella, maternal alcohol ingestion, and treatment with anticonvulsant drugs.

Acyanotic and Cyanotic Disorders

Congenital heart defects produce their effects through abnormal shunting of blood and through alterations in pulmonary blood flow. They commonly are classified as congenital heart disease with cyanosis or congenital heart disease with little or no cyanosis.[55,56] Left-to-right shunts are commonly categorized as acyanotic disorders and right-to-left shunt with obstruction as cyanotic disorders. Of the congenital defects discussed in this chapter, patent ductus arteriosus, atrial and ventricular septal defects, endocardial cushion defects, pulmonary valve stenosis, and coarctation of the aorta are considered defects with little or no cyanosis; tetralogy of Fallot and transposition of the great vessels are considered defects with cyanosis.

Shunting of blood refers to the diverting of blood flow from one system to the other—from the arterial to the venous system (*i.e.*, left-to-right shunt) or from the venous to the arterial system (*i.e.*, right-to-left shunt). The shunting of blood in congenital heart defects is determined by the presence of an *abnormal opening* between the right and left circulations and the degree of resistance to flow through the opening.

A right-to-left shunt results in unoxygenated blood moving from the right side of the heart into the left side of the heart and then being ejected into the systemic circulation. Cyanosis develops when sufficient unoxygenated blood mixes with oxygenated blood in the left side of the heart. In left-to-right shunt, blood intended for ejection into the systemic circulation is recirculated through the right side of the heart and back through the lungs; this increased volume distends the right side of the heart and pulmonary circulation and increases the workload placed on the right ventricle. A child with a septal defect that causes left-to-right shunting usually has an enlarged right side of the heart and pulmonary blood vessels.

The vascular resistance of the systemic and pulmonary circulations may influence the direction of shunting. Because of the high pulmonary vascular resistance in the neonate, atrial and septal defects usually do not produce significant shunt or symptoms during the first weeks of life. As the pulmonary vascular smooth muscle regresses in the neonate, the resistance in the pulmonary circulation normally falls below that of the systemic circulation; in uncomplicated atrial or ventricular septal defects, blood shunts from the left side of the heart to the right. In more complicated ventricular septal defects, increased resistance to outflow may affect the pattern of shunting. For example, defects that increase resistance to aortic outflow (*e.g.*, aortic valve stenosis, coarctation of the aorta) increase left-to-right shunting, and defects that obstruct pulmonary outflow (*e.g.*, pulmonary valve stenosis, increased pulmonary vascular resistance) increase right-to-left shunting. Crying may increase right-to-left shunting in infants with septal defects by increasing pulmonary vascular resistance. This may be one of the reasons some infants with congenital heart defects become cyanotic during crying.

Changes in Pulmonary Vascular Resistance and Blood Flow

In contrast to the arterioles in the systemic circulation, the mature pulmonary arterioles are thin-walled vessels, and they can accommodate various levels of stroke volume from the right heart. Many of the complications of congenital heart disorders result from their effect on the pulmonary circulation, which may be exposed to an increase or a decrease in blood flow.

In a term infant who has a congenital heart defect that produces markedly increased pulmonary blood flow (*e.g.*, ventricular septal defect), the increased flow stimulates pulmonary vasoconstriction and prevents normal thinning of pulmonary vascular smooth muscle. These conditions delay or reduce the normal drop in pulmonary vascular resistance. As a result, symptoms related to increased pulmonary blood flow often are not apparent until the infant is 4 to 12 weeks old.

Congenital heart defects that persistently increase pulmonary blood flow or pulmonary vascular resistance have the potential of causing pulmonary hypertension and producing pathologic changes in the pulmonary vasculature. When shunting of systemic blood flow into the pulmonary circulation threatens permanent injury to the pulmonary vessels, a surgical procedure may be done in an attempt to reduce the flow by increasing resistance to outflow from the right ventricle. This procedure, called *pulmonary banding*, consists of placing a constrictive band around the main pulmonary artery. The banding technique is used as a temporary measure to alleviate the symptoms and protect the pulmonary vessels in anticipation of later surgical repair of the defect. This procedure requires thoracotomy (*i.e.*, opening the chest cavity) but does not necessitate cardiopulmonary bypass (*i.e.*, use of the heart-lung machine).

Some congenital heart defects, such as pulmonary valve stenosis, decrease pulmonary blood flow, producing inadequate oxygenation of blood. The affected child may experience fatigue, exertional dyspnea, impaired growth, and even syncope.

Manifestations and Treatment

Congenital heart defects manifest with numerous signs and symptoms. Some defects, such as patent ductus arteriosus and small ventricular septal defects, close spontaneously, and in other, less severe defects, there are no signs and symptoms. The disorder typically is discovered during a routine health examination. Pulmonary congestion, cardiac failure, and decreased peripheral perfusion are the chief concerns in children with more severe defects. Such defects often cause problems shortly after birth or early in infancy. The child may exhibit cyanosis, respiratory difficulty, and fatigability and is likely to have difficulty with feeding and failure to thrive. A generalized cyanosis that persists longer than 3 hours after birth suggests congenital heart disease.

One technique for evaluating the infant consists of administering 100% oxygen for 10 minutes. If the infant "pinks up," the cyanosis probably was caused by respiratory problems. Because infant cyanosis may appear as a duskiness, it is important to assess the color of the mucous membranes, fingernails, toenails, tongue, and lips. Pulmonary congestion in the infant causes an increase in respiratory rate, orthopnea, grunting, wheezing, coughing, and rales. The baby whose peripheral perfusion is markedly decreased may appear to be in a shocklike state.

The manifestations and treatment of heart failure in the infant and young child are similar to those in the adult, but the infant's small size and limited physical reserve make the manifestations more serious and treatment more difficult. The treatment plan usually includes supportive therapy designed to help the infant compensate for the limitations in cardiac reserve and to prevent complications. Surgical intervention often is required for severe defects; it may be done in the early weeks of life or, conditions permitting, delayed until the child is older. A discussion of congestive heart failure in children is presented in Chapter 20.

Most children with structural congenital heart disease and those who have had corrective surgery are at risk for development of infectious endocarditis. These children should receive prophylactic antibiotic therapy during periods of increased risk of bacteremia.

Types of Defects

Congenital heart defects, whose frequencies are summarized in Table 19–3, can affect almost any of the cardiac

TABLE 19–3

Relative Frequency of Congenital Heart Lesions*

Lesions	Percentage of all Lesions
Ventricular septal defect	25–30
Atrial septal defect (secundum)	6–8
Patent ductus arteriosus	6–8
Coarctation of the aorta	5–7
Tetralogy of Fallot	5–7
Pulmonic valve stenosis	5–7
Aortic valve stenosis	4–7
Transposition of the great vessels	3–5
Hypoplastic left ventricle	1–3
Hypoplastic right ventricle	1–3
Truncus arteriosus	1–2
Total anomalous pulmonary venous return	1–2
Tricuspid atresia	1–2
Single ventricle	1–2
Double-outlet right ventricle	1–2
Others	5–10

*Excluding patent ductus arteriosus in preterm neonate, bicuspid aortic valve, peripheral pulmonary stenosis, and mitral valve prolapse. (From Behrman, R.E. [Ed.]. [1996]. *Nelson's textbook of pediatrics* [15th ed., p. 1286]. Philadelphia: W.B. Saunders)

structures or central blood vessels. Defects include communication between heart chambers, interrupted development of the heart chambers or valve structures, malposition of heart chambers and great vessels, and altered closure of fetal communication channels. The particular defect reflects the embryo's stage of development at the time it occurred. Some congenital heart disorders, such as tetralogy of Fallot, involve several defects. The development of the heart is simultaneous and sequential; a heart defect may reflect the multiple developmental events that were occurring simultaneously or sequentially.

Patent Ductus Arteriosus. Patent ductus arteriosus results from persistence of the fetal ductus beyond the prenatal period. In fetal life, the ductus arteriosus is the vital link by which blood from the right side of the heart bypasses the lungs and enters the systemic circulation (Fig. 19–24G). After birth, this passage is no longer needed, and it usually closes during the first 24 to 72 hours. The physiologic stimulus and mechanisms associated with permanent closure of the ductus are not entirely known, but the fact that infant hypoxia predisposes to a delayed closure suggests that the increase in arterial oxygen levels that occur immediately after birth play a role. Additional factors that contribute to closure are a fall in endogenous levels of prostaglandins and adenosine levels and the release of vasoactive substances. After constriction, the lumen of the ductus becomes permanently sealed with fibrous tissue within 2 to 3 weeks. Ductal closure may be delayed or prevented in very premature infants, probably as a result of a combination of factors, including decreased medial muscle in the ductus wall, decreased constrictive response to oxygen, and increased circulating levels of vasodilating prostaglandins. Hemodynamically significant patent ductus arteriosus is observed in about one half of infants with birth weights less than 1000 g.[54] Ductal closure may also be delayed in infants with congenital heart defects that produce a decrease in oxygen tension.

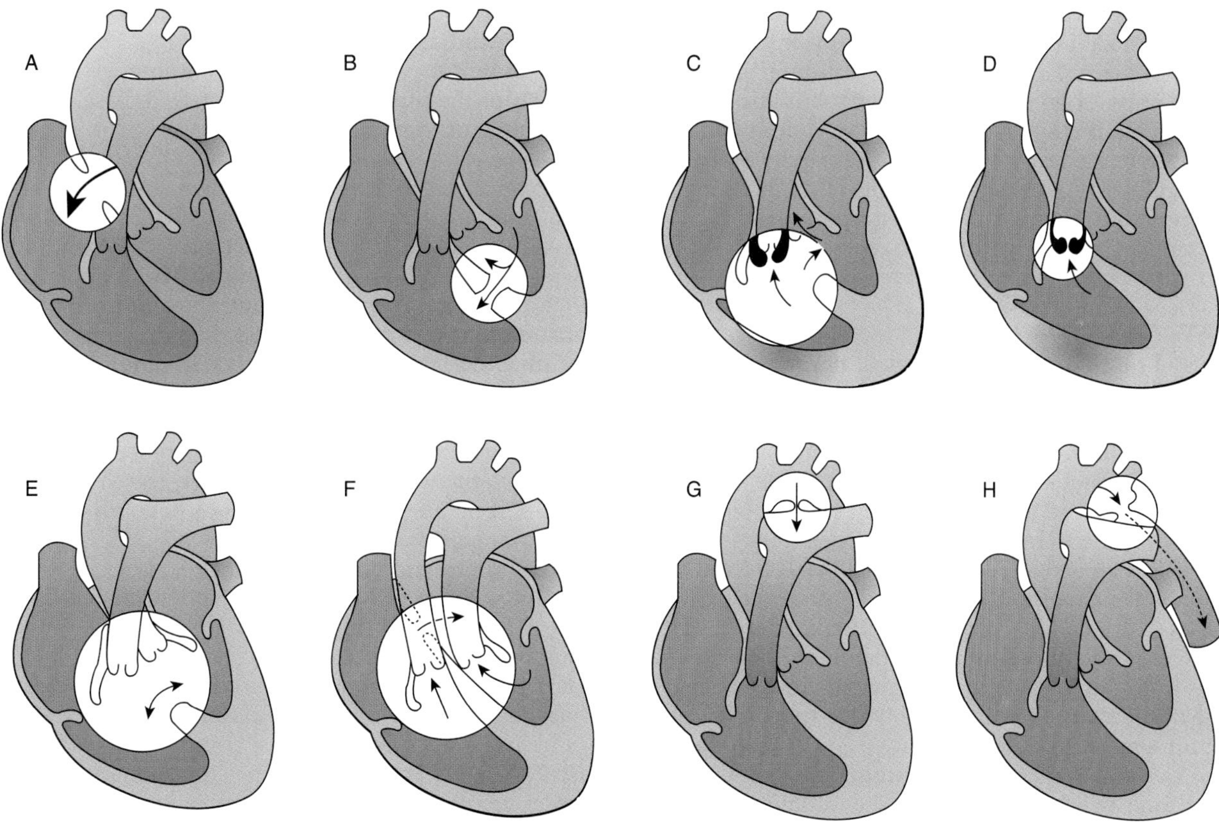

Figure 19–24
Congenital heart defects. (**A**) Atrial septal defect. Blood is shunted from left to right. (**B**) Ventricular septal defect. Blood is usually shunted from left to right. (**C**) Tetralogy of Fallot. This involves a ventricular septal defect, dextroposition of the aorta, right ventricular outflow obstruction, and right ventricular hypertrophy. Blood is shunted from right to left. (**D**) Pulmonary stenosis, with decreased pulmonary blood flow and right ventricular hypertrophy. (**E**) Endocardial cushion defects. Blood flows between the chambers of the heart. (**F**) Transposition of the great vessels. The pulmonary artery is attached to the left side of the heart and the aorta to the right side. (**G**) Patent ductus arteriosus. The high-pressure blood of the aorta is shunted back to the pulmonary artery. (**H**) Postductal coarctation of the aorta.

As is true of other heart and circulatory defects, patency of the ductus arteriosus may vary; the size of the opening may be small, medium, or large. After the infant's pulmonary vascular resistance falls, the patent ductus arteriosus provides for a continuous runoff of aortic blood into the pulmonary artery, causing a decrease in aortic diastolic and mean arterial pressure and a widening of the pulse pressure. With a large patent ductus, the runoff is continuous, resulting in increased pulmonary blood flow, pulmonary congestion, and increased resistance against which the right side of the heart must pump. Increased pulmonary venous return and increased work demands may lead to left ventricular failure.

Administration of indomethacin, an inhibitor of prostaglandin synthesis, is used as a treatment to induce closure of a patent ductus arteriosus. If this method of treatment fails, surgical ligation may be needed. Transcatheter closure in the cardiac catheterization laboratory using a Teflon plug, occlusive umbrella, or intravascular coil can be used in selected cases.[55] A visually assisted thoracoscopic surgical technique allows closure to be accomplished without thoracotomy.

The function of the ductus arteriosus in providing a right-to-left shunt in prenatal life has prompted the surgical creation of an aortic-pulmonary shunt as a means of improving pulmonary blood flow in children with severe pulmonary outflow disorders. Research has focused on the role of type E prostaglandins in maintaining the patency of the ductus. By injecting prostaglandin E into the umbilical vein of infants who require a ductal shunt, closure has been delayed or prevented.

Atrial Septal Defects. In atrial septal defects, a hole in the atrial septum persists as a result of improper septal formation (Fig. 19–24*A*). Two common types of atrial septal defects are those that involve the ostium primum and ostium secundum (most common). The defect occurs more frequently in females than males. It may be single or multiple and varies from a small, asymptomatic opening to a large, symptomatic opening.

Most atrial septal defects are small, and the defect is discovered inadvertently during a routine physical examination. In the case of an isolated septal defect that is large enough to allow shunting, the flow of blood usually is from the left side to the right side of the heart because of the more compliant right ventricle and because the pulmonary vascular resistance is lower than the systemic vascular resistance. This produces right ventricular volume overload and increased pulmonary blood flow. The increased volume of blood that must be ejected from the right heart also prolongs closure of the pulmonary valve and produces a separation (*i.e.*, fixed splitting) of the aortic and pulmonary components of the second heart sound. Most children with atrial septal defects are asymptomatic. Adolescents and young adults may develop atrial fibrillation or atrial flutter and palpations because of atrial dilation.

Because spontaneous closure occurs in some children, surgical treatment usually is delayed until the child is of school age. Transcatheter closure in the cardiac catheterization laboratory has proved effective. This procedure uses a double-umbrella catheter, with an umbrella placed on each side of the defect.[54] It often is used in children who have complex congenital heart defects that require multistage surgical procedures. This approach can eliminate one surgical procedure. Surgical closure may be necessary when the defect does not close spontaneously or transcatheter closure is not deemed appropriate.

Ventricular Septal Defects. A ventricular septal defect is an opening in the ventricular septum that results from a imperfect separation of the ventricles during early fetal development (Fig. 19–24*B*). Ventricular septal defects are the most common form of congenital heart defect; they may be the only cardiac defect, or they may be one of multiple cardiac anomalies. In 20% of all persons with congenital heart disease, a ventricular defect is the only abnormality.

The ventricular septum originates from two sources: the interventricular groove of the folded tubular heart that gives rise to the muscular part of the septum and the endocardial cushions that extend to form the membranous portion of the septum. The upper membranous portion of the septum is the last area to close, and it is here that most defects occur.

Depending on the size of the opening, the signs and symptoms of a ventricular septal defect may range from an asymptomatic murmur to congestive heart failure. If the defect is small, it allows a small shunt and small increases in pulmonary blood flow. These defects produce few symptoms, and about one third close spontaneously.[54] With medium-sized defects, a larger shunt occurs, producing a larger increase in pulmonary blood flow (*i.e.*, twice as much blood may pass through the pulmonary circulation as through the systemic circulation). The increased pulmonary flow most often occurs under relatively low pressure. Most of the children with such defects are asymptomatic and have a low risk of developing pulmonary vascular disease.

Children with large defects have a large amount of pulmonary blood flow. Because the defect is nonrestrictive, the pressure in the left and right sides of the heart is equalized, and blood is shunted from the left side of the heart into the pulmonary artery under high pressures that are sufficient to produce pulmonary hypertension. In these children, left-to-right shunting through the ventricular defect is lessened when pulmonary and systemic circulations offer equal resistance to flow. The child's symptoms improve during this time.[54] As the child's pulmonary vascular resistance increases further, a right-to-left shunt develops, and the child demonstrates cyanosis. This reversal of the direction of shunt flow is called *Eisenmenger's syndrome*.

Most infants with a ventricular septal defect are asymptomatic during early infancy, because the higher pulmonary vascular resistance prevents shunting from occurring. After an infant's pulmonary vascular resistance falls and a shunt develops, a characteristic systolic murmur develops. The infant with a large, uncomplicated ventricular septal defect usually is asymptomatic until pulmonary vascular resistance begins to fall at about 4 to 12 weeks. After a large shunt develops, the mother reports that the infant breathes rapidly, feeds poorly, and is diaphoretic (*i.e.*, signs of congestive heart failure). Right-to-left shunting produces cyanosis.

The treatment of a ventricular septal defect depends on the size of the defect and accompanying hemodynamic derangements. Children with small or medium-sized defects are followed closely in the hope that the defect will close spontaneously. Prophylactic antibiotic therapy is given during periods of increased risk for bacteremia. Cardiac catheterization may be performed in children with medium-sized or large defects who become symptomatic to document the location of the lesion, identify any associated heart defects, and determine the pulmonary vascular resistance. Congestive heart failure is treated medically. Surgical intervention is required for infants who do not respond to medical management. When possible, surgical closure of the defect is performed. Pulmonary artery banding may be done in cases of complex congenital defects with the risk of pulmonary vascular involvement, in children with defects that are not amenable to medical or surgical treatment, or when the ventricular defect is only one of several defects present. The pulmonary band is removed when the ventricular defect is closed during open heart surgery at a later time.

Endocardial Cushion Defects. The endocardial cushions form the AV canals, the upper part of the ventricular septum, and the lower part of the atrial septum. Endocardial cushion defects are responsible for about 5% of all congenital heart defects. As many as 50% of children with Down syndrome have endocardial cushion defects.

Because endocardial cushions contribute to multiple aspects of heart development, several variations with this type of defect are possible. The terms most commonly used to categorize endocardial cushion defects are partial and complete AV canal defects.[54] In partial AV canal defects, the two AV valve rings are complete and separate. The most common type of partial AV canal defect is an ostium primum defect, with a cleft in the mitral valve. In complete canal defect, there is a common AV valve orifice along with defects in the atrial and the ventricular septal tissue. Many variations of these two forms of endocardial cushion defect are possible (Fig. 19–24*E*). *Ebstein's anomaly* is a defect in endocardial cushion development characterized by displacement of tricuspid valvular tissue into the ventricle. The displaced tricuspid leaflets are attached directly to the right ventricular endocardial surface or to shortened or malformed chordae tendineae.

The direction and magnitude of a shunt in a child with endocardial cushion defects are determined by the combination of defects and the child's pulmonary and systemic vascular resistance. The hemodynamic effects of an isolated ostium primum defect are those of the previously described atrial septal defect. These children are largely asymptomatic during childhood. If a ventricular septal defect is present, pulmonary blood flow is increased after pulmonary vascular resistance falls. Many children with ventricular septal defects have effort intolerance, easy fatigability, and recurrent infections, particularly when the shunt is large. The larger the defect, the greater is the shunt, and the higher is the pressure in the pulmonary vascular system.

With complete AV canal defects, congestive heart failure and intercurrent pulmonary infections appear early in infancy. There is left-to-right shunting and transatrial and transventricular mixing of blood. Pulmonary hypertension and increased pulmonary vascular resistance are common. Cyanosis develops with progressive shunting.

The treatment for endocardial cushion defects is determined by the severity of the defect. With an ostium primum defect, surgical repair usually is planned on an elective basis before the child enters school. Palliative or corrective surgery is required in infants with complete AV canal defects who develop congestive heart failure and do not respond to medical treatment. Total surgical repair of complete AV canal defects can be accomplished with low operative risk.

Pulmonary Stenosis. Pulmonary stenosis may occur as an isolated valvular lesion or in conjunction with more complex defects, such as tetralogy of Fallot. In isolated valvular defects, the pulmonary cusps may be absent or malformed, or they may remain fused at their commissural edges; all three abnormalities often coexist.

Pulmonary valvular defects usually cause some impairment of pulmonary blood flow and increase the work load imposed on the right side of the heart (Fig. 19–24*D*). Most children with pulmonic valve stenosis have mild to moderate stenosis that does not increase in severity. These children are largely asymptomatic. Severe defects are manifested by marked impairment of pulmonary blood flow that begins during infancy and is likely to become more severe as the child grows. About one third of children younger than 2 years develop cyanosis.[54] The ductus arteriosus may provide the vital accessory route for perfusing the lungs in infants with severe stenosis. When pulmonary stenosis is extreme, increased pressures in the right side of the heart may delay closure of the foramen ovale.

Treatment measures designed to maintain the patency of the ductus arteriosus may be used as a palliative measure to maintain or increase pulmonary blood flow in infants with severe pulmonary stenosis. Pulmonary valvotomy often is the treatment of choice. Transcatheter balloon valvuloplasty may be used in some infants with moderate degrees of obstruction. Introduction of an expandable intravascular stent may be used to prevent restenosis.[55]

Tetralogy of Fallot. As the name implies, tetralogy of Fallot consists of four associated congenital heart defects: ventricular septal defects that involve the membranous septum and the anterior portion of the muscular septum; dextroposition or shifting to the right of the aorta, so that it overrides the right ventricle and is in communication with the septal defect; obstruction or narrowing of the pulmonary outflow channel, including pulmonic valve stenosis, a decrease in the size of the pulmonary trunk, or both; and hypertrophy of the right ventricle because of the increased work required to pump blood through the obstructed pulmonary channels (Fig. 19–24C).

Most children with tetralogy of Fallot display some degree of cyanosis—hence the term *blue babies*. The cyanosis develops as the result of decreased pulmonary blood flow and because the right-to-left shunt causes mixing of unoxygenated blood with the oxygenated blood, which is ejected into the peripheral circulation. Hypercyanotic spells may occur during the first months of life. These spells typically occur in the morning during crying, feeding, or defecating. These activities increase the infant's oxygen requirements. Crying and defecating may further increase pulmonary vascular resistance, thereby increasing right-to-left shunting and decreasing pulmonary blood flow. With the hypercyanotic spell, the infant becomes acutely cyanotic, hyperpneic, irritable, and diaphoretic. Later in the spell, the infant becomes limp and may lose consciousness. Placing the infant in the knee-chest position increases systemic vascular resistance, which increases pulmonary blood flow and decreases right-to-left shunting. During a hypercyanotic spell, toddlers and older children may spontaneously assume the squatting position, which functions like the knee-chest position to relieve the spell.[54]

Because of the hypoxemia that occurs in these children, palliative surgery designed to increase pulmonary blood flow often is needed during early infancy, with corrective surgery being done at a later age. Palliative surgery involves the creation of a surgical shunt to increase pulmonary blood flow. The most popular procedures use the subclavian artery or prosthetic material to create a shunt between the aorta and pulmonary artery.

Transposition of the Great Vessels. In complete transposition of the great vessels, the aorta originates in the right ventricle, and the pulmonary artery originates in the left ventricle (Fig. 19–24*F*). The defect is more common in infants whose mothers have diabetes and in male infants. In infants born with this defect, survival depends on communication between the right and left sides of the heart in the form of a patent ductus arteriosus or septal defect. Prostaglandin E_1 may be administered in an effort to maintain the patency of the ductus arteriosus. Balloon atrial septostomy may be done to increase the blood flow between the two sides of the heart. In this procedure, a balloon-tipped catheter is inserted into the heart through the vena cava and then passed through the foramen ovale into the left atrium. The balloon is then inflated and brought back through the foramen ovale, enlarging the opening as it goes.

Corrective surgery is essential for long-term survival.[55] An arterial switch procedure (*i.e.*, Jatene operation) may be done. This procedure, which corrects the relation of the systemic and pulmonary blood flows, is preferably performed in the first 2 to 3 weeks of life, before postnatal reduction in pulmonary vascular resistance. An atrial switch procedure (*i.e.*, Mustard or Senning operation) is performed on older children. Both of these procedures reverse the blood flow at the atrial level by the surgical formation of intraatrial baffles.

Coarctation of the Aorta. Coarctation of the aorta is a localized narrowing of the aorta, proximal (preductal or coarctation of infancy) or distal (postductal) to the ductus (Fig. 19–24*H*). About 98% of coarctations are postductal. The anomaly occurs twice as often in males as in females. Coarctation of the aorta may be a feature of Turner's syndrome (see Chapter 4).

The classic sign of coarctation of the aorta is a disparity in pulsations and blood pressures in the arms and legs. The femoral, popliteal, and dorsalis pedis pulsations are weak or delayed compared with the bounding pulses of the arms and carotid vessels. The systolic blood pressure in the legs obtained by the cuff method normally is 10 to 20 mm Hg higher than in the arms.[55] In coarctation, the pressure is lower and may be difficult to obtain. The differential in blood pressure is common in children older than age 1, about 90% of whom have hypertension in the upper extremities greater than the 95th percentile for age (see Chapter 18).

Children with significant coarctation should be treated surgically; the optimal age for surgery is 2 to 4 years. If untreated, most persons with coarctation of the aorta die between 20 and 40 years of age. The common serious complications are related to the hypertensive state.

In *preductal* or *infantile coarctation,* the ductus remains open and shunts blood from the pulmonary artery through the ductus arteriosus into the aorta. It frequently is seen with other cardiac anomalies and carries a high mortality rate. Because of the position of the defect, blood flow throughout the systemic circulation is reduced, and the affected infant develops heart failure at an early age because of the increased work load imposed on the left ventricle. Medical and surgical methods are used to treat these infants.

In summary, the embryonic development of the heart occurs during weeks 3 through 8 after conception. During this time, development of the atrial and ventricular septa divides the embryonic tubular heart into a right side and a left side. The endocardial cushions develop to form separate right and left AV canals, and the separation and spiraling of the bulbus cordis and truncus arteriosus separate the blood flow for the pulmonary and systemic circulations. At birth, the fetus takes its first breath and switches from placental to pulmonary oxygenation of blood. The foramen ovale and ductus arteriosus close, separating the pulmonary and systemic circulations. There is an almost immediate increase in systemic vascular resistance and left heart pressures and a decrease in pulmonary vascular resistance and right heart pressures. The smooth muscle layer in the pulmonary blood vessels undergoes gradual thinning during the first weeks of life, producing a further decrease in pulmonary vascular resistance.

Congenital heart defects affect about 8 of every 1000 neonates and arise during the period of fetal heart development. The defect reflects the stage of development at the time the causative event occurred. Several factors contribute to the development of congenital heart defects, including genetic and chromosomal influences, viruses, and environmental agents such as drugs and radiation. The cause of the defect often is unknown. The defect may produce no effects, or it may markedly affect cardiac function. Congenital heart defects commonly produce shunting of blood from the right to the left side of the heart or from the left to the right side of the heart. Left-to-right shunts typically increase the volume of the right side of the heart and pulmonary circulation, and right-to-left shunts transfer unoxygenated blood from the right side of the heart to the left side, diluting the oxygen content of blood that is being ejected into the systemic circulation and causing cyanosis. The direction and degree of shunt depend on the size of the defect that connects the two sides of the heart and the difference in resistance between the two sides of the circulation. Congenital heart defects commonly are classified as defects that produce cyanosis and those that produce little or no cyanosis. Depending on the severity of the defect, congenital heart defects may be treated medically or surgically. Medical and surgical treatment often is indicated in children with severe defects.

REFERENCES

1. American Heart Association. (1997). *1997 Heart and stroke facts.* Dallas: American Heart Association.
2. Cotran R.S., Kumar V., Robbins S.L. (1994). *Pathologic basis of disease* (5th ed., pp. 528, 566–656). Philadelphia: W.B. Saunders.
3. Lorell B.H. (1997). Pericardial diseases. In Braunwald E. (Ed.). *Heart disease* (5th ed., pp. 1478–1515). Philadelphia: W.B. Saunders.
4. Fowler N.O. (1992). Pericardial disease. *Heart Disease and Stroke* 1 (2), 85–94.
5. Spodick D. (1989). Pericarditis, pericardial effusion, cardiac tamponade, and constriction. *Critical Care Clinics* 5, 455.
6. Sulzbach L.M. (1989). Measurement of pulsus paradoxus. *Focus on Critical Care* 16, 142.
7. Guyton A. (1996). *Medical physiology* (9th ed., pp. 238–239, 256–263). Philadelphia: W. B. Saunders.
8. Berne R.M., Levy L.M. (1992). *Cardiovascular physiology* (6th ed., pp. 266, 156–157). St. Louis: Mosby Year Book.
9. Ganz P., Braunwald E. (1997). Coronary blood flow and myocardial ischemia. In Braunwald E. (Ed.). *Heart disease* (5th ed., pp. 1164–1168). Philadelphia: W.B. Saunders.
10. Gregg D.E., Patterson R.E. (1980). Functional importance of coronary collaterals. *New England Journal of Medicine* 303 (24), 1404.
11. Crawford M.H. (1995). Unstable angina. In Crawford M.H. (Ed.). *Diagnosis and Treatment in Cardiology* (pp. 41–49). Norwalk CT: Appleton & Lange.
12. Unstable Angina Guideline Panel. (1994). *Unstable Angina: Diagnosis and Management.* AHCPR Publication No. 94–0602. Rockville, MD: U.S. Department of Health and Social Services.
13. Prinzmetal M., Kennamer, R., Merliss R., et al. (1959). A variant form of angina pectoris. *American Journal of Medicine* 27, 375–388.
14. Pepine C.J., El-Tamimi H., Lambert C.R. (1992). Prinzmetal's angina (variant angina). *Heart Disease and Stroke* 1, 281–286.
15. Cohn P.F. (1994). Silent myocardial ischemia: To treat or not to treat. *Hospital Practice* 29 (6), 107–116.
16. Chiariello M., Indolfi C. (1996). Silent myocardial ischemia in patients with diabetes mellitus. *Circulation* 93, 2089– 2091.
17. Clem J.R. (1995). Pharmacotherapy of ischemic heart disease. *AACN Clinical Issues* 6 (3), 404–417.
18. Bittl J.A. (1997). Advances in coronary angioplasty. *New England Journal of Medicine* 337 (17), 1290–1302.
19. Lincoff A.M., Topol E.J. (1997). Interventional catheterization techniques. In Braunwald E. (Ed.). *Heart disease* (5th ed., pp. 1366–1383). Philadelphia: W.B. Saunders.
20. Johnstone M.T., Mittleman M., Tofler G., Muller J.E. (1996). The pathophysiology of the onset of morning cardiovascular events. *American Journal of Hypertension* 9, 22S–28S.
21. Antman E.M., Braunwald E. (1997). Acute myocardial infarction. In Braunwald E. (Ed.). *Heart disease* (5th ed., pp. 1184–1288). Philadelphia: W.B. Saunders.
22. Ryan T.J., Anderson J.L., Antman E.M., et al. (1996). ACC/AHA guidelines for the management of patients with acute myocardial infarction: A report of the American College of Cardiology/American Heart Association Task Force on Practice Guidelines (Committee on Management of Acute Myocardial Infarction). *Journal of American College of Cardiology* 28, 1328–1428.
23. Eisenberg M.J., Topol E.J. (1996). Prehospital administration of aspirin in patients with unstable angina and acute myocardial infarction. *Archives of Internal Medicine* 156, 1506–1510.
24. Coombs V.J., Brinker J.A. (1995). Primary angioplasty in the acute myocardial infarction setting. *AACN Clinical Issues* 6 (3), 387–397.
25. Brown C.A., O'Connell J.B. (1995). Myocarditis and idiopathic dilated cardiomyopathy. *American Journal of Medicine* 99, 309–314.
26. Olinde K.D., O'Connell J.B. (1994). Inflammatory heart disease: Pathogenesis, clinical manifestations, and treatment of myocarditis. *Annual Review of Medicine* 45, 481–490.
27. Stevenson L.W. (1996). Diseases of the myocardium. In Bennett J.C., Plum F. *Cecil textbook of medicine* (20th ed., pp. 327–336). Philadelphia, W.B. Saunders.
28. Maron B.J., Gaffney F.A., Jeresaty R.M., McKenna W.J., Miller W.W. (1985). Task force III: Hypertrophic cardiomyopathy, other myopericardial diseases and mitral valve prolapse. *Journal American College of Cardiology* 6, 1215–1217.
29. Committee Members. (1982). Report of WHO/ISF Task force on the Definition and Classification of Cardiomyopathies. *British Heart Journal* 44, 672–673.
30. Richardson P., Rapporteur W., McKenna W., et al. (1996). Report of the 1995 World Health Organization/International Society and Federation of Cardiology Task Force on Definition and Classification of Cardiomyopathies. *Circulation* 93, 841–842.

31. Dec G.W., Fuster V. (1994). Idiopathic dilated cardiomyopathy. *New England Journal of Medicine* 331 (23), 1564–1575.
32. Spirito P., Seidman C.E., McKenna W.J., Maron B.J. (1997). The management of hypertrophic cardiomyopathy. *New England Journal of Medicine* 336 (11), 775–783.
33. Courtney-Jenkins A. (1987). The patient with hypertrophic cardiomyopathy. *Journal of Cardiovascular Nursing* 2, 33.
34. Maron B.J., Bonow R.D., Cannon R.D., et al. (1987). Hypertrophic cardiomyopathy. Part 2: Interrelations of clinical manifestations, pathophysiology, and therapy. *New England Journal of Medicine* 316, 844–852.
35. Kushwaha S.S., Fallon J.T., Fuster V. (1997). Restrictive cardiomyopathy. *New England Journal of Medicine* 336 (4), 267–274.
36. Cragin P. (1988). Peripartum cardiomyopathy. *Focus on Critical Care* 15, 39.
37. McMullan M.R., Moore C.K., O'Connell J.B. (1993). Diagnosis and management of peripartum cardiomyopathy. *Hospital Practice* 28 (11), 89–104.
38. Massie B.M., Amidon T.A. (1997). Cardiovascular disease. In Tierney L.M., McPhee S.J., Papadakis M.A. (Eds.). *Current medical diagnosis and treatment* (36th ed., pp. 341–344). Norwalk, CT: Appleton & Lange.
39. Durek D.T., Lukas A.S., Bright D.R. (1994). New criteria for diagnosis of infective endocarditis. *American Journal of Medicine* 96, 200.
40. Bansal R.C. (1995). Infective endocarditis. *Medical Clinics of North America* 79 (5), 1205–1239.
41. Durback D.T. (1995). Prevention of infective endocarditis. *New England Journal of Medicine* 332 (1), 38–44.
42. Ad Hoc Committee to Revise Jones Criteria (modified) of the Council on Rheumatic Fever and Congenital Heart Disease of the American Heart Association. (1984). Jones criteria (revised) for guidance in the diagnosis of rheumatic fever. *Circulation* 69, 203A–208A.
43. Committee on Rheumatic Fever, Endocarditis, and Kawasaki Disease of the Council on Cardiovascular Disease in the Young of the American Heart Association. (1993). Guidelines for the diagnosis of rheumatic fever. *Journal of the American Medical Association* 268, 2069–2073.
44. Shulman S.T., DeInocencio J., Hirsch R. (1995). Kawasaki disease. *Pediatric Clinics of North America* 42 (5), 1205–1222.
45. Barron K.S., Murphy D.J. (1989). Kawasaki syndrome: Still a fascinating enigma. *Hospital Practice* 24 (10A), 51–60.
46. Rowley A.H., Gonzalez-Crussi F., Schulman F. (1988). Kawasaki syndrome: A review article. *Review of Infectious Diseases* 10, 1–15.
47. Schulman S.T. (Ed.). (1989). Management of Kawasaki syndrome: A consensus statement prepared by North American participants of The Third International Kawasaki Disease Symposium, Tokyo, Japan, December, 1988. *Pediatric Infectious Disease Journal* 8, 663–665.
48. Rauch A.M. (1987). Kawasaki's syndrome: Review of new epidemiologic and laboratory evidence. *Pediatric Infectious Disease Journal* 6, 1016–1021.
49. Braunwald E. (Ed.). (1997). *Heart disease* (5th ed, pp. 1007–1076). Philadelphia: W.B. Saunders.
50. Levy D., Savage D. (1987). Prevalence and clinical features of mitral valve prolapse. *American Heart Journal* 113, 1281.
51. Moore K.L. (1988). *The developing human* (4th ed., pp. 286–308). Philadelphia: W.B. Saunders.
52. Hazinski M.F. (1983). Congenital heart disease in the neonate: Epidemiology, cardiac development, and fetal circulation. *Neonatal Network* 1 (2), 29–43.
53. Heyman M.A., Rudolph A.M. (1972). Effects of congenital heart disease on fetal and neonatal circulations. *Progress in Cardiovascular Diseases* 14 (2), 115–143.
54. Hazinski M.F. (1992). *Nursing care of the critically ill child* (2nd ed., pp. 12–131, 271–361). St. Louis: Mosby–Year Book.
55. Behrman R.E. (Ed.). (1996). *Nelson textbook of pediatrics* (15th ed., pp. 1286–1335). Philadelphia: W.B. Saunders.
56. Nouri S. (1997). Congenital heart defects: Cyanotic and acyanotic. *Pediatric Annals* 26 (2), 92–98.

ADDITIONAL READINGS

Alyn I.B., Baker L.K. (1992). Cardiovascular anatomy and physiology of the fetus, neonate, infant, child, and adolescent. *Journal of Cardiovascular Nursing* 6 (3), 1–11.

Ardinger R.H. (1997). Genetic counseling in congenital heart disease. *Pediatric Annals* 26 (2), 99–104.

Bayer A.S. (1993) Infective endocarditis. *Clinical Infectious Diseases* 17, 313–322.

Creel C.A. (1994). Silent myocardial ischemia and nursing implications. *Heart and Lung* 23 (3), 218–227.

Davies M.J. (1995). Stability and instability: Two faces of coronary atherosclerosis. *Circulation* 94, 2013–2020.

Effat M.A. (1995). Pathophysiology of ischemic heart disease: An Overview. *AACN Clinical Issues* 6 (3), 369–374.

Fishbein M.C., Siegel R.J. (1996). How big are coronary atherosclerotic plaques that rupture. *Circulation* 94, 2662–2666.

Friedman W.F. (1997). Congenital heart disease in infancy and childhood. In Braunwald E. (Ed.). *Heart disease* (5th ed., pp. 877–962). Philadelphia, WB Saunders.

Gessner I.H. (1997). What makes a heart murmur innocent? *Pediatric Annals* 26 (2), 82–104.

Hartz R.S. (1996). Minimally invasive heart surgery. *Circulation* 94, 2669–2670.

Hollander J.E. (1995). The management of cocaine-associated myocardial ischemia. *New England Journal of Medicine* 333 (19), 1267–1272.

Hoffman J.I.E. (1990). Congenital heart disease. *Pediatric Clinics of North America* 37 (1), 25–44.

Kelly D.P., Strauss A.W. (1994). Inherited cardiomyopathies. *New England Journal of Medicine* 330 (13), 913–919.

Lange L.G., Schreiner G.F. (1994). Immune mechanisms of cardiac disease. *New England Journal of Medicine* 330 (16), 1129–1134.

Marian A.J., Roberts R. (1995). Molecular genetics of hypertrophic cardiomyopathy. *Annual Review of Medicine* 46, 213–223.

McNulty C.M. (1992). Active viral myocarditis: Application of current knowledge to clinical practice. *Heart Disease and Stroke* 1, 135–140.

Molavi A. (1992). Endocarditis: Recognition, management, and prophylaxis. *Cardiovascular Clinics* 23, 139.

Pinsky W.W., Arciniegas E. (1990). Tetralogy of Fallot. *Pediatric Clinics of North America* 37 (1), 179–192.

Ruygrok P.N, Serrys P.W. (1996). Intracoronary stenting. *Circulation* 94, 882–890.

Schwartz M.L., Cox G., Lin A.E., et al. (1996). Clinical approach to genetic cardiomyopathy in children. *Circulation* 94, 2021–2038.

Shiffman R.N. ( ). Guidelines and revision: 30 years of the Jones criteria for diagnosis of rheumatic fever. *Archives Pediatric and Adolescent Medicine* 149, 727–732.

Zales V.R., Wright K.L. (1997). Endocarditis, pericarditis, and myocarditis. *Pediatric Annals* 26 (2), 116–121.

CHAPTER 20

Heart Failure and Circulatory Shock

Nancie Urban and Carol M. Porth

Adequate perfusion of body tissues depends on the pumping ability of the heart, a vascular system that transports blood to the cells and back to the heart, sufficient blood to fill the circulatory system, and tissues that are able to extract and use oxygen and nutrients from the blood. Impaired pumping ability of the heart and circulatory shock are separate conditions that reflect failure of the circulatory system. Both conditions exhibit common compensatory mechanisms even though they differ in terms of pathogenesis and causes.

Heart Failure

After you have completed this section of the chapter, you should be able to meet the following objectives:

- Explain the effect of cardiac reserve on symptom development in heart failure
- Define the terms *preload*, *afterload*, and *cardiac contractility*
- Explain how increased sympathetic activity, fluid retention, the Frank-Starling mechanism, and myocardial hypertrophy act as compensatory mechanisms in heart failure
- Differentiate high-output versus low-output heart failure, systolic versus diastolic heart failure, and right-sided versus left-sided heart failure
- Describe the physiologic mechanisms underlying the manifestations of congestive heart failure
- Describe the methods used in diagnosis and assessment of cardiac function in persons with heart failure
- Describe the actions of diuretics, inotropic agents, and vasodilators on the physiologic manifestations of heart failure
- Compare the indications for use of assistive devices, heart transplant, and cardiomyoplasty in treatment of heart failure

- Relate the effect of left ventricular failure to the development of and manifestations of pulmonary edema
- Describe the pathophysiology of cardiogenic shock

The term *heart failure* denotes the failure of the heart as a pump. Although morbidity and mortality from other cardiovascular diseases has decreased over the past several decades, the incidence of heart failure is increasing at an alarming rate. This change undoubtedly reflects treatment improvements and survival from other forms of cardiac illness. It has been estimated that more than 2 million Americans have heart failure, with approximately 400,000 new cases diagnosed each year. Despite advances in treatment, the mortality rate for even mild to moderate heart failure exceeds 50%.[1] In its more advanced form, heart failure may progress to pulmonary edema and cardiogenic shock, which are immediate life-threatening forms of heart failure. Aggressive management of acute and chronic heart failure is critical to prevent its shock state. After cardiogenic shock ensues, mortality rates rise to 85% or more.[2]

This section of the chapter is divided into four parts: physiology of heart failure, congestive heart failure, acute pulmonary edema, and cardiogenic shock.

Physiology of Heart Failure

The heart has the amazing capacity to adjust its activity to meet the varying needs of the body. During sleep, its output declines, and during exercise, it increases markedly. The ability to increase cardiac output during increased activity is called the *cardiac reserve*. For example, competitive swimmers and long-distance runners have large cardiac reserves. During exercise the cardiac output of these athletes rapidly increases to as much as five to six times their resting level. In sharp contrast with healthy athletes, persons with heart failure often use their cardiac reserve at rest. For them, just climbing a flight of stairs may cause shortness of breath, because they have exceeded their cardiac reserve.

The physiology of heart failure involves an interplay between two factors: the inability of the failing heart to maintain sufficient cardiac output to support body functions and the recruitment of compensatory mechanisms designed to maintain the cardiac reserve.

Cardiac Output

The cardiac output is the amount of blood that the heart pumps each minute. It reflects how often the heart beats each minute (*i.e.*, heart rate) and how much blood the heart pumps with each beat (*i.e.*, stroke volume) and can be expressed as the product of the heart rate and stroke volume: cardiac output = heart rate × stroke volume. Heart rate is regulated by balancing sympathetic, or adrenergic, activity, which accelerates heart rate, with parasympathetic, or vagal, activity, which slows it down. Stroke volume is a function of preload, afterload, and cardiac contractility.

Preload and Afterload. The work that the heart performs consists mainly of ejecting blood that has returned to the ventricles during diastole into the pulmonary or systemic circulations. As with skeletal muscle, the work of cardiac muscle is determined by what are called loading conditions—the stretch imposed by the load and the force that the muscle must generate to move the load. The terms preload and afterload are often used to describe the workload of the heart. *Preload* reflects the loading condition of the heart at the end of diastole. It is the force stretching the resting heart muscle just before contraction and is mainly determined by the venous return to the heart. As the ventricles fill during diastole, the tension rises much like that which occurs when a balloon is filled with water.

For any given cardiac cycle, the maximum volume of blood filling the ventricle is present at the end of the diastolic filling period. Referred to as the *end-diastolic volume*, this volume causes the tension and the pressure within the ventricles to rise. End-diastolic pressure can be measured clinically, providing an estimate of preload status. Within limits, as preload increases, the stroke volume increases in accord with the Frank-Starling mechanism. In heart failure, the ventricles may become overstretched because of excessive filling. When this happens, intraventricular pressure rises, and stroke volume may decrease. Preload may be excessively elevated in conditions such as myocardial infarction in which the ventricles become distended due to impaired pumping ability; in valvular heart disease such as aortic regurgitation, in which a portion of the ejected systole volume moves back into the ventricle and is added to the diastolic volume; and renal failure, in which an increase in blood volume produces an increase in venous return.

Afterload represents the force that the contracting heart must generate to eject blood from the filled heart. The main components of afterload are ventricular wall tension and the systemic (peripheral) vascular resistance. The greater the systemic vascular resistance, the higher are the wall tension and resulting intraventricular pressure that must be generated to open the semilunar (aortic and pulmonic) valves. As a result, excessive afterload may impair ventricular ejection if the ventricles cannot generate sufficient pressure. Aortic stenosis and severe hypertension may excessively elevate left ventricular afterload and contribute to the development of heart failure.

Cardiac Contractility. *Cardiac contractility* refers to the mechanical performance of the heart—the ability of the contractile elements of the heart muscle (*i.e.*, actin and myosin filaments) to interact and shorten against a load. The ejection of blood from the heart during systole depends on cardiac contractility. Contractility increases cardiac output independent of preload filling and muscle stretch.

An *inotropic influence* is one that increases cardiac contractility. Sympathetic stimulation increases the strength of cardiac contraction (*i.e.*, positive inotropic action), and hypoxia and ischemia decrease contractility (*i.e.*, negative inotropic effect). The drug digitalis, which is classified as an inotropic agent, increases cardiac contractility such that the heart is able to eject more blood at any level of preload filling. A decrease of cardiac contractility can result from loss of functional muscle tissue due to myocardial infarction or from conditions such as cardiomyopathy that diffusely affect the myocardium.

Compensatory Mechanisms

In heart failure, the cardiac reserve is largely maintained through compensatory mechanisms, the most important of which are the Frank-Starling mechanism; activation of neurohumoral mechanisms, particularly the release of norepinephrine from sympathetic nerve terminals and recruitment of the renin angiotensin system; and myocardial remodeling and hypertrophy.[3] The healthy and the failing heart may use the same compensatory mechanisms. In the failing heart, early decreases in cardiac function may go unnoticed because these compensatory mechanisms maintain the cardiac output. This state is called *compensated heart failure*. Unfortunately, these mechanisms were not intended for long-term use. In severe and prolonged *decompensated heart failure* the compensatory mechanisms are no longer effective, and the compensatory mechanisms may themselves worsen the failure. Figure 20–1 diagrams the mechanisms of compensated and decompensated heart failure.

Frank-Starling Mechanism. The Frank-Starling mechanism increases stroke volume by means of an increase in ventricular end-diastolic volume (*i.e.*, preload). With increased diastolic filling, there is increased stretching of the myocardial fibers, more optimal approximation of the actin and myosin filaments, and a resultant increase in the force of the next contraction (see Chapter 16). In the normally functioning heart, the Frank-Starling mechanism serves to match the outputs of the two ventricles. Figure 20–2 illustrates the cardiac reserve in relation to the end-diastolic volume and stroke volume output of the normal and failing heart.

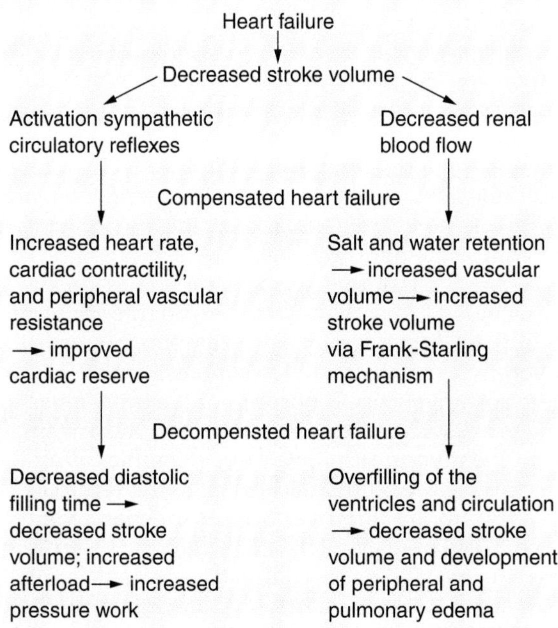

Figure 20–1
Sequence of events in compensated and decompensated heart failure.

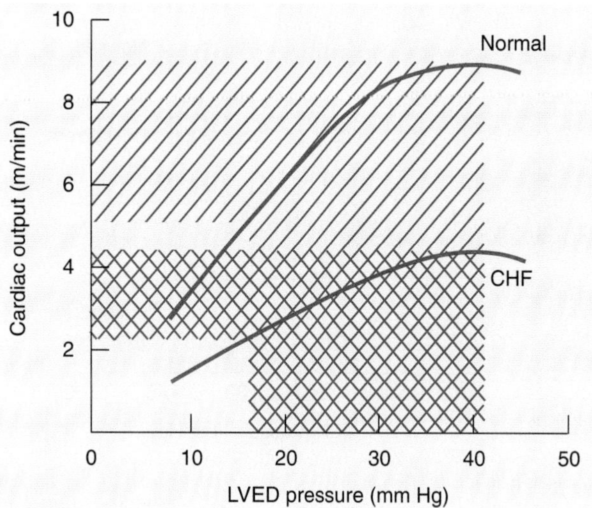

Figure 20–2
The cardiac reserve as represented on the Frank-Starling curve in the normal and failing heart. The lighter colored area represents the cardiac reserve in a person with normal cardiac function, and the darker crosshatched portion represents the cardiac reserve in a person with heart failure.

In heart failure, the Frank-Starling mechanism also helps to support the cardiac output. Cardiac output may be normal at rest in persons with heart failure because of increased ventricular end-diastolic volume and the Frank-Starling mechanism. However, this mechanism becomes ineffective when the heart becomes overfilled and the muscle fibers are overstretched. With deterioration of myocardial function, the ventricular function curve depicted in Figure 20–2 flattens, and when an increase in cardiac output is needed, as occurs with increased physical activity, there is a lesser increase in cardiac output and a greater rise in left ventricular end-diastolic volume and pressure. The maximal increase in cardiac output that can be achieved may severely limit activity, while at the same time producing an elevation in pulmonary capillary pressure and development of dyspnea and pulmonary congestion (Fig. 20-3). At the point where the heart becomes overfilled to the extent that actin and myosin filaments cannot produce an effective contraction, further increases in ventricular filling may produce a fall in cardiac output.

An important determinant of myocardial energy consumption is ventricular wall tension. Overfilling of the ventricle produces a decrease in wall thickness and an increase in wall tension. Because increased wall tension increases myocardial oxygen requirements, it can produce ischemia and further impairment of cardiac function. The use of diuretics in persons with heart failure helps to reduce vascular volume and ventricular filling, thereby unloading the heart and reducing ventricular wall tension.

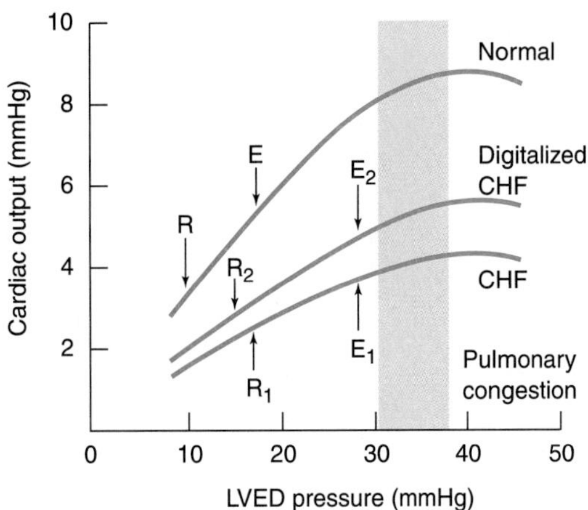

Figure 20–3
Frank-Starling curves. R, resting; E, exercise; LVED, left ventricular end-diastolic; CHF, congestive heart failure. (Iseri L.T., Benvenuti D.J. [1983]. Pathogenesis and management of congestive heart failure—revisited. *American Heart Journal* 105 (2), 346)

Increased Sympathetic Nervous System Activity. Stimulation of the sympathetic nervous system plays an important role in the compensatory response to decreased cardiac output and to the pathogenesis of heart failure.[4] Both cardiac sympathetic tone and catecholamine levels are elevated during the late stages of most forms of heart failure. By direct stimulation of heart rate and cardiac contractility and by regulation of vascular tone, the sympathetic nervous system helps to maintain perfusion of the various organs, particularly the heart and brain. In persons with more severe heart failure, blood from the skin, kidneys, and gastrointestinal tract is diverted to the more critical cerebral and coronary circulations.

The negative aspects of these adaptations include an increase in vascular resistance and the afterload against which the heart must pump. There is also evidence that prolonged sympathetic stimulation may exhaust myocardial stores of norepinephrine and may lead to destruction of sympathetic nerve endings. Moreover, these effects are distributed unevenly across the myocardium and may have deleterious effects on cardiac structure and function over time. For example, they may adversely affect the balance between oxygen supply and demand in persons in whom this ratio is precariously balanced. The catecholamines may also contribute to the high rate of sudden death by promoting dysrhythmias.[4]

In addition to its effect on the heart, excessive sympathetic stimulation produced by heart failure also affects other organ systems. Because of vasoconstrictor effects, it can decrease blood flow to skin, muscle, kidney and abdominal organs. This not only decreases tissue perfusion, but also contributes to an increase in peripheral vascular resistance and afterload stress of the heart.[5]

Renin-Angiotensin Mechanism. One of the most important effects of a lowered cardiac output in heart failure is a reduction in renal blood flow and glomerular filtration rate, which leads to salt and water retention. Normally, the kidneys receive about 25% of the cardiac output, but this may be decreased to as low as 8% to 10% in persons with heart failure. With decreased renal blood flow, there is a progressive increase in renin secretion by the kidneys along with parallel increases in circulating levels of angiotensin II. The increased concentration of angiotensin II contributes to a generalized and excessive vasoconstriction and provides a powerful stimulus for aldosterone production by the adrenal cortex (see Chapter 16). Aldosterone increases tubular reabsorption of sodium with an accompanying increase in water retention. Because aldosterone is metabolized in the liver, its levels are further increased when heart failure causes liver congestion. Angiotensin II also increases levels of antidiuretic hormone (ADH), which serves as a vasoconstrictor and inhibitor of water excretion (see Chapter 26).

Angiotensin II is also thought to contribute to the myocardial hypertrophy that occurs in heart failure, possibly acting as a growth factor.[6] Angiotensin-converting enzyme (ACE) inhibitor drugs, which block the conversion of angiotensin I to angiotensin II, have become common therapy for heart failure.[7]

Atrial Natriuretic Peptide. A hormone called the *atrial natriuretic peptide* (ANP), or *atriopeptin*, affects fluid balance in heart failure.[8,9] ANP is a peptide hormone released from atrial cells in the heart in response to increased atrial stretch and pressure. The hormone produces rapid and transient natriuresis, diuresis, and moderate loss of potassium in the urine. Increased ANP levels have been found in adults with congestive heart failure, but the role of ANP in compensating for alterations in cardiac function that occur with heart failure is still unclear.

Myocardial Hypertrophy. Myocardial hypertrophy is a long-term compensatory mechanism. Cardiac muscle, like skeletal muscle, responds to an increase in work demands by undergoing hypertrophy. Hypertrophy increases the number of contractile elements (*i.e.*, actin and myosin) in myocardial cells as a means of increasing their contractile performance.

Heart diseases that increase resistance to the ejection of blood from the ventricles provide the greatest stimulus for hypertrophy. For example, the wall of the left ventricle may increase to six times its normal size in severe aortic stenosis. If portions of the heart muscle are damaged and replaced with scar tissue, the undamaged part of the myocardium often hypertrophies as a means of improving the pumping capacity of the ventricle. Cardiac hypertrophy improves cardiac function by increasing ventricular wall thickness, which normalizes wall stress so that the heart contracts more efficiently. Research suggests that hypertrophy alters the way that the muscle contracts and handles the calcium needed for actin-myosin interactions; it contracts more slowly and energetically.[6]

Although hypertrophy increases the systolic function of the heart, it can also eventually lead to diastolic dysfunction and myocardial ischemia. Some forms of hypertrophy may lead to abnormal remodeling of the ventricular wall with reduction in chamber size and reduced diastolic filling and increased wall tension. For example, untreated hypertension causes hypertrophy that may preserve systolic function for a time but also create diastolic dysfunction that worsens the failure syndrome.[10] This can have its greatest effect during conditions that increase heart rate, further limiting diastolic filling and coronary blood flow.[11] The hypertrophied heart also has impaired coronary vascular reserve and susceptibility to ischemia. When the oxygen requirements of the increased muscle mass exceed the ability of the coronary vessels to bring blood to the area, myocardial hypertrophy is no longer beneficial and may result in ischemia with decreased contractility. Abnormal growth of nonmyocardial tissue (*e.g.*, fibrous tissue) may produce stiffness of the ventricle and further impair ventricular function.

Congestive Heart Failure

Heart failure occurs when the pumping ability of the heart becomes impaired. Congestive heart failure is heart failure that is accompanied by congestion of body tissues. After an initial compensatory period, the clinical manifestations of heart failure become complicated with pulmonary congestion or systemic venous congestion.

Heart failure may be caused by a variety of conditions, including acute myocardial infarction, hypertension, or degenerative conditions of the heart muscle known collectively as cardiomyopathies. Heart failure may also occur because of excessive work demands on the heart such as occurs with hypermetabolic states or with volume overload such as occurs with renal failure. Either of these states may exceed the work capacity of even a healthy heart. In persons with asymptomatic heart disease, heart failure may be precipitated by an unrelated illness or stress. Table 20–1 lists major causes of heart failure.

Heart failure may be described as high-output or low-output failure, systolic or diastolic failure, and right-sided or left-sided failure.

High-Output Versus Low-Output Failure

An uncommon type of heart failure that is caused by an excessive need for cardiac output is often referred to as *high-output failure*. With high-output failure, the function of the heart may be supranormal but inadequate owing to excessive metabolic needs. Causes of high-output failure include severe anemia, thyrotoxicosis, conditions that cause arteriovenous shunting, and Paget's disease. High-output failure tends to be specifically treatable.

Low-output failure is caused by disorders that impair the pumping ability of the heart, such as ischemic heart disease and cardiomyopathy. As a result, treatment options tend to be more limited and focus primarily on symptom management, with attempts to slow the natural progress of the etiologic disease state.

Systolic Versus Diastolic Failure

Until recently, congestive heart failure was viewed mainly in terms of backward and forward failure. *Backward failure* represented failure of one the ventricles to effectively empty the heart during diastole such that blood backs up in the venous system, causing congestion. *Forward failure* was characterized by impaired forward movement of blood into the arterial system emerging from the heart. Forward failure has been associated with high-output failure in which the heart was unable to

TABLE 20–1

Causes of Heart Failure

Impaired Cardiac Function	Excess Work Demands
Myocardial Disease	**Increased Pressure Work**
Cardiomyopathies	Systemic hypertension
Myocarditis	Pulmonary hypertension
Coronary insufficiency	Coarctation of the aorta
Myocardial Infarction	
Valvular Heart Disease	**Increased Volume Work**
Stenotic valvular disease	Arteriovenous shunt
Regurgitant valvular disease	Excessive administration of intravenous fluids
Congenital Heart Defects	**Increased Perfusion Work**
	Thyrotoxicosis
	Anemia
Constrictive Pericarditis	

maintain sufficient forward flow because of excessive demand.

A later classification separates the pathophysiology of congestive failure into two new categories—systolic dysfunction and diastolic dysfunction. With *systolic dysfunction*, there is impaired ejection of blood from the heart during systole; with *diastolic dysfunction*, there is impaired filling of the heart during diastole (Fig. 20–4). Many persons with heart disease fall into an intermediate category, with elements of systolic and diastolic dysfunction.[3,12,13]

Systolic Dysfunction. Systolic dysfunction involves a decrease in cardiac contractility and ejection fraction. It commonly results from conditions that impair the contractile performance of the heart (*e.g.*, ischemic heart disease and cardiomyopathy) or from hemodynamic conditions that produce a volume overload (*e.g.*, valvular insufficiency and anemia) or a pressure overload (*e.g.*, hypertension and valvular stenosis).

A normal ventricle ejects about 50% to 65% of the blood in the ventricle at the end of diastole when it contracts. This is called the *ejection fraction*. In systolic heart failure, the ejection fraction declines progressively with increasing degrees of myocardial dysfunction. In very severe forms of heart failure, the ejection fraction may drop to a single-digit percentage. With a decrease in ejection fraction, there is a resultant increase in diastolic volume, ventricular dilation, and ventricular wall tension and a rise in ventricular end-diastolic pressure. The symptoms of persons with systolic dysfunction mainly result from reductions in ejection fraction and cardiac output.

Diastolic Dysfunction. Diastolic dysfunction, which reportedly accounts for 25% to 40% of all cases of congestive heart failure, is characterized by smaller ventricular chamber size, ventricular hypertrophy, and poor ventricular compliance (*i.e.*, ability to stretch during filling).[10,12] Because of impaired filling, congestive symptoms tend to predominate in diastolic dysfunction. Among the conditions that cause diastolic dysfunction are those that restrict diastolic filling (*e.g.*, mitral stenosis), those that increase ventricular wall thickness and reduce chamber size (*e.g.*, myocardial hypertrophy due to lung disease and hypertrophic cardiomyopathy), and those that delay diastolic relaxation (*e.g.*, aging, ischemic heart disease). Aging is often accompanied by a delay in relaxation of the heart during diastole; diastolic filling begins while the ventricle is still stiff and resistant to stretching to accept an increase in volume.[14] A similar delay occurs with myocardial ischemia, resulting from a lack of energy to break the rigor bonds that form between the actin and myosin filaments of the contracting cardiac muscle and to remove the calcium that activates muscle contraction.[15] Because tachycardia produces a decrease in diastolic filling time, persons with diastolic dysfunction often become symptomatic during activities and situations that increase heart rate.

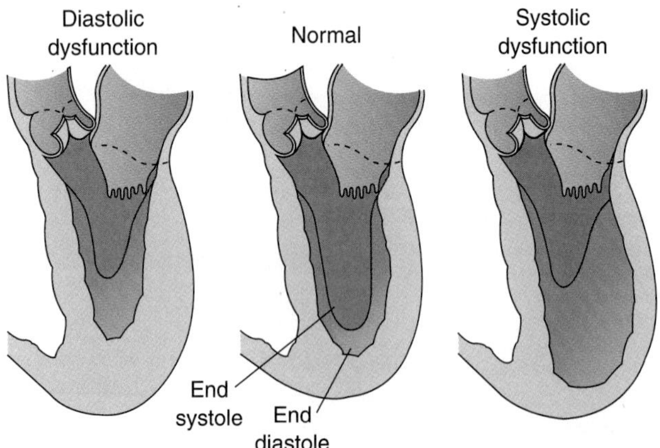

Figure 20–4
Congestive heart failure due to systolic and diastolic dysfunction. The ejection fraction represents the difference between end-diastolic function and end-systolic volume. (**Middle**) Normal systolic and diastolic function with normal ejection fraction; (**left**) diastolic dysfunction with decreased ejection fraction due to decreased diastolic filling; (**right**) systolic dysfunction with decreased ejection fraction due to impaired systolic function.

Right-Sided Versus Left-Sided Heart Failure

Heart failure also can be classified according to the side of the heart (right or left) that is affected. An important feature of the circulatory system is that the right and left ventricles act as two pumps that are connected in series. To function effectively, the right and left ventricles must maintain an equal output. Although the initial event that leads to heart failure may be primarily right sided or left sided in origin, long-term heart failure usually involves both sides. It is often easier, however, to understand the physiologic mechanisms associated with heart failure when right- and left-sided failure are considered separately.

Right-Sided Heart Failure. The right heart pumps deoxygenated blood from the systemic circulation into the pulmonary circulation. Consequently, when the right heart fails, there is accumulation or damming back of blood in the systemic venous system. This causes an increase in right atrial, right ventricular end-diastolic, and systemic venous pressures.

The clinical result is manifested in development of edema in the peripheral tissues and congestion of the abdominal organs (Fig. 20–5). Because of the effects of gravity, the edema is most pronounced in the dependent parts of the body—in the lower extremities when the person is in the upright position and in the area over the sacrum when the person is supine. The accumulation of edema fluid is evidenced by a gain in weight (*i.e.*, 1 pint of accumulated fluid results in a 1-lb weight gain). Daily measurement of weight can be used as a means of assessing fluid accumulation in a patient with chronic congestive heart failure. As a rule, a weight gain of more than 2 lb in 24 hours or 5 lb in 1 week is considered a sign of worsening failure.

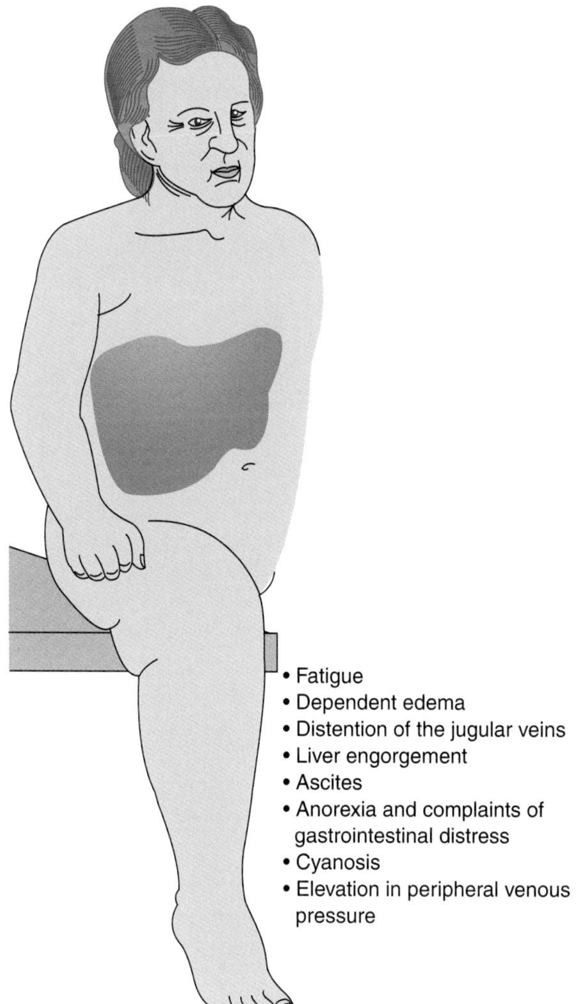

• Fatigue
• Dependent edema
• Distention of the jugular veins
• Liver engorgement
• Ascites
• Anorexia and complaints of gastrointestinal distress
• Cyanosis
• Elevation in peripheral venous pressure

Figure 20–5
Manifestations of right-sided heart failure.

Right-sided heart failure causes congestion of the viscera. As venous distention progresses, blood backs up in the hepatic veins that drain into the inferior vena cava, and the liver becomes engorged. This may cause hepatomegaly and right upper quadrant pain. In severe and prolonged right-sided failure, liver function is impaired and hepatic cells may die. Congestion of the portal circulation may also lead to engorgement of the spleen and development of ascites. Congestion of the gastrointestinal tract may interfere with digestion and absorption of nutrients, causing anorexia and abdominal discomfort. The jugular veins, which are above the level of the heart, are normally collapsed in the standing position or when sitting with the head at higher than a 30-degree angle. In severe right-sided failure, the external jugular veins become distended and can be visualized when the person is sitting up or standing.

The causes of right-sided heart failure include conditions that restrict blood flow into the lungs. Stenosis or regurgitation of the tricuspid or pulmonic valves, right ventricular infarction, cardiomyopathy, and persistent left-sided failure are common causes. Acute or chronic pulmonary disease, such as severe pneumonia, pulmonary embolus, or pulmonary hypertension, can cause right heart failure, referred to as *cor pulmonale.* The combination of atrial fibrillation and pulmonary changes seen with aging have been associated with tricuspid regurgitation and right heart failure in the elderly.[16]

Left-Sided Heart Failure. The left side of the heart pumps blood from the low-pressure pulmonary circulation into the high-pressure arterial side of the systemic circulation. With impairment of left heart function, there is a decrease in cardiac output; an increase in left atrial and left ventricular end-diastolic pressures; and congestion in the pulmonary circulation. When the pulmonary capillary pressure (normally about 10 mm Hg) exceeds the capillary osmotic pressure (normally about 25 mm Hg), there is a shift of intravascular fluid into the interstitium of the lung and development of pulmonary edema (Fig. 20–6). An episode of pulmonary edema often occurs at night, after the person has been reclining for some time and the gravitational forces have been removed from the circulatory system. It is then that the edema fluid that had been sequestered in the lower extremities during the day is returned to the vascular compartment and redistributed to the pulmonary circulation. The manifestations of left-sided heart failure are illustrated in Figure 20–7.

The most common causes of left-sided heart failure are acute myocardial infarction and cardiomyopathy. Left-sided heart failure and pulmonary congestion can develop very rapidly in persons with acute myocardial infarction. Even when the infarcted area is small, there may be a surrounding area of ischemic tissue. This may result in a large area of nonpumping ventricle and rapid onset pulmonary edema. Mechanical defects associated with myocardial infarction such as papillary muscle dysfunction or rupture (which produces mild to severe mitral valve regurgitation) or left ventricular aneurysm development may contribute to pulmonary edema (see Chapter 19). Stenosis or regurgitation of the aortic or mitral valves also creates the level of left-sided backflow that results in pulmonary congestion. Pulmonary edema may also develop during rapid infusion of intravenous fluids or blood transfusions in an elderly person or in a person with limited cardiac reserve.

Manifestations of Congestive Heart Failure

The manifestations of congestive heart failure depend on the extent of right-sided and left-sided failure. The signs and symptoms include edema, nocturia, shortness of breath, fatigue and limited exercise tolerance, signs of increased sympathetic activity, cyanosis, ascites, and cachexia. The severity and progression of symptoms depend on the extent and type of cardiac dysfunction that is present. Some persons with heart failure appear comfortable at rest. Others become dyspneic during conversation or with minor activity.

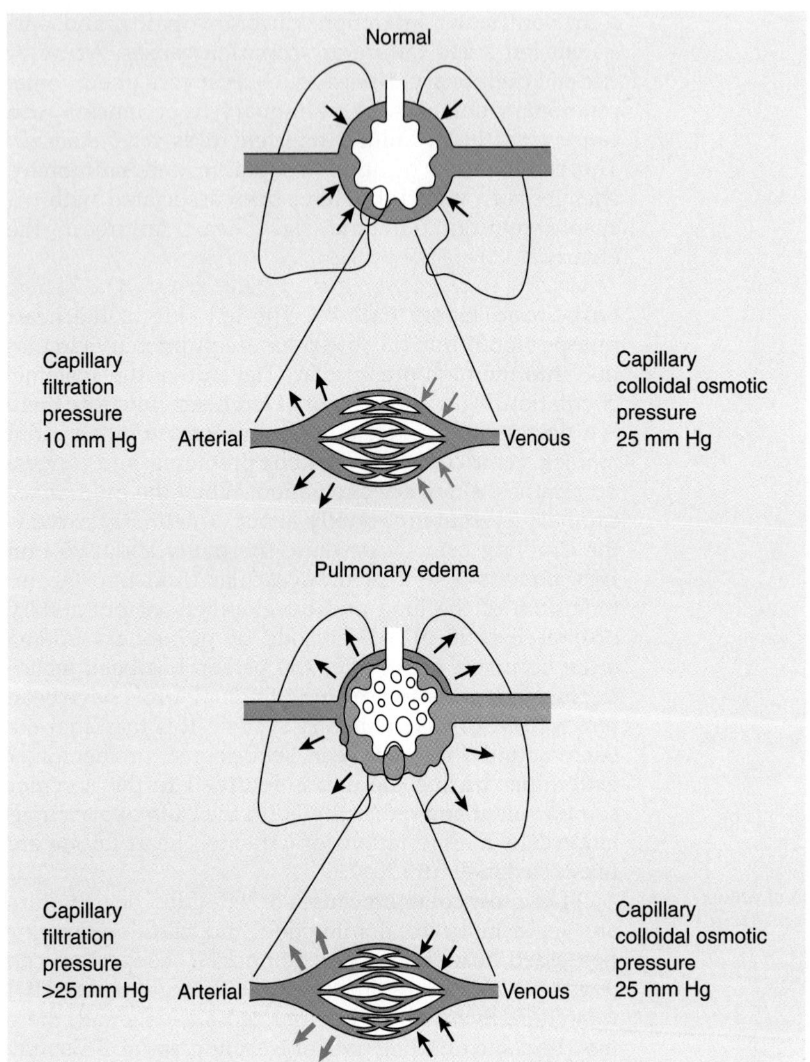

Figure 20–6
Mechanism of respiratory symptoms in left-sided heart failure. *Black arrows* indicate major force, and *red arrows* indicate a minor force.

Although a major compensatory mechanism in heart failure, the sympathetic nervous system is responsible for a number of physical signs and symptoms of heart failure. Peripheral vasoconstriction is manifested by pallor and coldness of the extremities and cyanosis of the nail beds and digits. Patients may also exhibit diaphoresis and tachycardia. Vasoconstriction may impede the loss of body heat and result in low-grade fever.

Fluid Retention and Edema. Many of the manifestations of congestive heart failure result from the increased capillary pressures that develop in the peripheral circulation in right-sided heart failure and in the pulmonary circulation in left-sided heart failure. The increased capillary pressure reflects an overfilling of the vascular system because of increased salt and water retention and venous congestion resulting from the impaired pumping ability of the heart.[17]

Nocturia is a nightly increase in urine output that occurs relatively early in the course of congestive heart failure. It results from the return to the circulation of edema fluids from the dependent parts of the body when the person assumes the supine position for the night. As a result, the cardiac output, renal blood flow, glomerular filtration, and urine output increase. Oliguria is a late sign related to a severely reduced cardiac output and resultant renal failure.

Respiratory Manifestations. Shortness of breath due to congestion of the pulmonary circulation is one of the major manifestations of left-sided heart failure. Perceived shortness of breath (*i.e.*, breathlessness) is called *dyspnea*. Dyspnea related to an increase in activity is called *exertional dyspnea*. *Orthopnea* is shortness of breath that occurs when a person is supine. The gravitational forces that cause fluid to become sequestered in the lower legs and feet when the person is standing or sitting

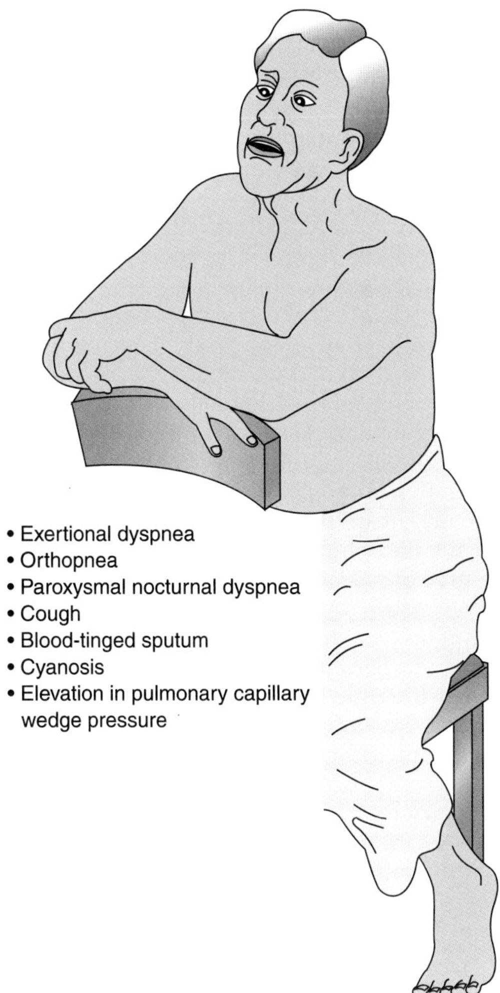

• Exertional dyspnea
• Orthopnea
• Paroxysmal nocturnal dyspnea
• Cough
• Blood-tinged sputum
• Cyanosis
• Elevation in pulmonary capillary wedge pressure

Figure 20–7
Manifestations of left-sided heart failure.

are removed when a person with congestive heart failure assumes the supine position; fluid from the legs and dependent parts of the body is mobilized and redistributed to an already distended pulmonary circulation. *Paroxysmal nocturnal dyspnea* is a sudden attack of dyspnea that occurs during sleep. It disrupts sleep, and the person awakens with a feeling of extreme suffocation that resolves when he or she sits up. Initially, the experience may be interpreted as awakening from a bad dream.

A subtle and often overlooked symptom of heart failure is a chronic dry, nonproductive cough, which becomes worse when the person is lying down. Bronchospasm due to congestion of the bronchial mucosa may cause wheezing and difficulty in breathing. This condition is sometimes referred to as *cardiac asthma*.

Cheyne-Stokes respiration, also known as periodic breathing, is characterized by a slow waxing and waning of respiration. The person breathes deeply for a period when the PCO_2 is high and then slightly or not all when the PCO_2 falls. In persons with left-sided heart failure, the condition is thought to be caused by a prolongation of the heart-to-brain circulation, particularly in persons with hypertension and associated cerebral vascular disease.

Fatigue and Weakness. Fatigue and limb weakness often accompany diminished output from the left ventricle. Cardiac fatigue is different from general fatigue in that it is not present in the morning but appears and progresses as activity increases during the day. In acute or severe left-sided failure, cardiac output may fall to levels that are insufficient for providing the brain with adequate oxygen, and there are indications of mental confusion and disturbed behavior. Confusion, impairment of memory, anxiety, restlessness, and insomnia are common in elderly persons with advanced heart failure, particularly in those with cerebral atherosclerosis. Unfortunately, these very symptoms may confuse the diagnosis of heart failure in the elderly, because this population may manifest these changes because of the myriad other causes associated with aging.

Cachexia and Malnutrition. Cardiac cachexia is a condition of malnutrition and tissue wasting that occurs in persons with end-stage heart failure. A number of factors probably contribute to its development, including the fatigue and depression that interfere with food intake, congestion of the liver and gastrointestinal structures that impair digestion and absorption and produce feelings of fullness, and the circulating toxins and mediators released from poorly perfused tissues that impair appetite and contribute to tissue wasting.

Cyanosis. Cyanosis is the bluish discoloration of the skin and mucous membranes caused by excess desaturated hemoglobin in the blood; it is often a late sign of heart failure. Cyanosis may be central, caused by arterial desaturation resulting from impaired pulmonary gas exchange, or peripheral, caused by venous desaturation resulting from extensive extraction of oxygen at the capillary level. *Central cyanosis* is caused by conditions that impair oxygenation of the arterial blood, such as pulmonary edema, left heart failure, or right-to-left shunting. *Peripheral cyanosis* is caused by conditions such as low output failure that cause delivery of poorly oxygenated blood to the peripheral tissues or by conditions such as peripheral vasoconstriction that cause excessive removal of oxygen from the blood. Central cyanosis is best monitored in the lips and mucous membranes, because these areas are not subject to conditions such as cold that cause peripheral cyanosis. Persons with right-sided or left-sided heart failure may develop cyanosis especially around the lips and in the peripheral parts of the extremities.

Diagnostic Methods

Diagnostic methods in heart failure are directed toward establishing the cause of the disorder and determining the extent of the dysfunction. Because heart failure represents the failure of the heart as a pump and can occur in the course of a number of heart diseases or other systemic disorders, the diagnosis of heart failure is often based on signs and symptoms related to the failing heart itself, such as shortness of breath and fatigue. The functional classification of the New York Heart Association is one guide to classifying the extent of dysfunction (Table 20–2).[18]

Electrocardiographic findings may indicate atrial or ventricular hypertrophy, underlying disorders of cardiac rhythm, or conduction abnormalities such as right or left bundle branch block. Chest radiographs provide information about the size and shape of the heart and pulmonary vasculature. The cardiac silhouette can be used to detect cardiac hypertrophy and dilatation. X-ray films can indicate the relative severity of the failure by revealing if pulmonary edema is predominantly vascular, interstitial, or advanced to the alveolar and bronchial stages. Echocardiographic studies are used to reveal the size and function of cardiac valvular structures and the size and motion of both ventricles. It can also indicate pericardial effusion and determine the ventricular ejection fraction. Radionuclide angiography and cardiac catheterization are other diagnostic tests used to describe the underlying causes of heart failure such as heart defects and cardiomyopathy. Because other health problems contribute to heart failure, diagnostic methods are used to detect conditions such as anemia, thyroid dysfunction, or kidney disease.

Invasive hemodynamic monitoring is often used in the management of acute, life-threatening episodes of heart failure. These monitoring methods include central venous pressure (CVP), pulmonary capillary wedge pressure (PCWP), thermodilution cardiac output measurements, and intraarterial measurements of blood pressure.

CVP reflects the amount of blood returning to the heart. Measurements of central venous pressure are best obtained by means of a catheter inserted into the right atrium through a peripheral vein or by means of the right atrial port (opening) in a pulmonary artery catheter. This pressure is decreased in hypovolemia and increased in right heart failure. The changes that occur in CVP over time are usually more significant than the absolute numeric values obtained during a single reading.

PCWP is obtained by means of a flow-directed, balloon-tipped pulmonary artery (Swan-Ganz) catheter. This catheter is introduced through a peripheral or central vein and then advanced into the right atrium. The balloon is then inflated with air enabling the catheter to float through the right ventricle into the pulmonary artery until it becomes wedged in a small pulmonary vessel (Fig. 20–8). After the catheter is in place, the balloon is inflated *only* when the PCWP is being measured. Continuous inflation of the balloon with its accompanying occlusion of a small pulmonary artery would cause necrosis of pulmonary tissue. With the balloon inflated, the catheter monitors pulmonary capillary pressures in direct communication with pressures from the left heart. The pulmonary capillary pressures provide a means of assessing the pumping ability of the left heart.

One type of pulmonary artery catheter is equipped with a thermistor probe to obtain *thermodilution measurements of cardiac output*. A known amount of solution of a known temperature (iced or room temperature) is injected into the right atrium through an opening in the catheter, and the temperature of the blood is measured downstream in the pulmonary artery by means of a thermistor probe located at the end of that catheter. A microcomputer calculates the cardiac output from the time-temperature curve resulting from the rate of change of the temperature of the blood that flows past the thermistor. Catheters with oximeters built into their tips that permit continuous monitoring of oxygen saturation (SvO_2) are also available, as are catheters that provide continuous output data.

Intraarterial blood pressure monitoring provides a means for continuous monitoring of blood pressure. It is used in persons with acute heart failure when aggressive intravenous drug therapy or mechanical assist devices are required. Measurements are obtained through the use of a small catheter inserted into a peripheral artery, usually the radial artery. The catheter is connected to a

TABLE 20–2

New York Heart Association Functional Classification of Patients With Heart Disease

Classification	Characteristics
Class I	Patients with cardiac disease but without the resulting limitations in physical activity. Ordinary activity does not cause undue fatigue, palpitation, dyspnea, or anginal pain.
Class II	Patients with heart disease resulting in slight limitations of physical activity. They are comfortable at rest. Ordinary physical activity results in fatigue, palpitation, dyspnea, or anginal pain.
Class III	Patients with cardiac disease resulting in marked limitation of physical activity. They are comfortable at rest. Less than ordinary physical activity causes fatigue, palpitation, dyspnea, or anginal pain.
Class IV	Patients with cardiac disease resulting in inability to carry on any physical activity without discomfort. The symptoms of cardiac insufficiency or of the anginal syndrome may be present even at rest. If any physical activity is undertaken, discomfort increases.

(Criteria Committee of the New York Heart Association. [1964]. *Diseases of the heart and blood vessels: Nomenclature and criteria for diagnosis* [6th ed., pp. 112–113]. Boston: Little, Brown)

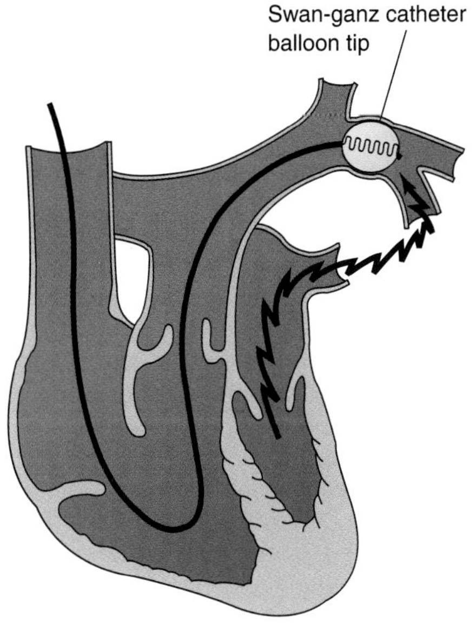

Figure 20–8
Swan-Ganz balloon-tipped catheter positioned in a pulmonary capillary. The pulmonary capillary wedge pressure, which reflects the left ventricular diastolic pressure, is measured with the balloon inflated.

pressure transducer, and beat-by-beat measurements of blood pressure are recorded. The monitoring system displays the contour of the pressure waveform and a digital reading of the systolic, diastolic, and mean arterial pressures along with heart rate and rhythm. Contemporary monitors can also provide continuous digital display of respiratory rate and core temperature from the thermistor located at the end of the pulmonary artery catheter.

Treatment Methods

The goals of treatment for chronic heart failure are directed toward relieving the symptoms and improving the quality of life, with a long-term goal of slowing, halting, or reversing the cardiac dysfunction.[19] Treatment measures include correction of reversible causes such as anemia or thyrotoxicosis, surgical repair of a ventricular defect or an improperly functioning valve, pharmacologic and nonpharmacologic control of afterload stresses such as hypertension, modification of activities and lifestyle to a level consistent with the functional limitations of a reduced cardiac reserve, and the use of medications to improve cardiac function and limit excessive compensatory mechanisms. Restriction of salt intake and diuretic therapy facilitate the excretion of edema fluid. Counseling, health teaching, and other assistive measures such as follow-up or ongoing surveillance programs help persons with heart failure to manage their treatment regimen and cope with activity limitations and other manifestations of the disorder.

In severe heart failure, restriction of activity, including bed rest if necessary, often facilitates temporary recompensation of cardiac function. However, there is no convincing evidence that continued bed rest is of benefit or that it changes the course of the disease for persons who are able to maintain some degree of activity.

Pharmacologic Treatment. A number of medications are used in the treatment of heart failure, including inotropic agents, diuretics, and vasodilators.[19–21] The choice of pharmacologic agents is determined by problems caused by the disorder (*i.e.*, systolic or diastolic dysfunction) and those brought about by activation of compensatory mechanisms (*e.g.*, excess fluid retention, inappropriate activation of sympathetic mechanisms).

Diuretics are among the most frequently prescribed medications for heart failure. They promote the excretion of edema fluid and help to sustain cardiac output and tissue perfusion by reducing preload and allowing the heart to operate at a more optimal part of the Frank-Starling curve. Thiazide and loop diuretics are used. In emergency situations, such as acute pulmonary edema, loop diuretics such as furosemide or bumetanide can be administered intravenously. When given intravenously, these drugs act quickly to reduce venous return through vasodilation so that right ventricular output and pulmonary vascular pressures are decreased. This response to intravenous drug administration is extrarenal and precedes the onset of diuresis.

Inotropic agents increase cardiac contractility regardless of end-diastolic volume and pressure (*i.e.*, preload). They include digitalis preparations, β-adrenergic agonists such as dopamine and dobutamine, and the newer nondigitalis, noncatecholamine inotropic agents. *Digitalis* has been a recognized treatment for congestive heart failure for the past 200 years. The various forms of digitalis are called *cardiac glycosides*. They improve cardiac function by increasing the force and strength of ventricular contraction. By decreasing sinoatrial node activity and decreasing conduction through the atrioventricular node, they also slow the heart rate and increase diastolic filling time. Although not a diuretic, digitalis promotes urine output by improving cardiac output and renal blood flow. The digitalis drugs act by binding to sodium-potassium ATPase on the cell membrane and inhibiting the sodium-potassium pump. When intracellular sodium is increased because of inhibition of the sodium-potassium pump by digitalis, the exchange of intracellular calcium for extracellular sodium is inhibited; as a result, more calcium is available to activate the myocardial actin-myosin contractile apparatus.

The margin between therapeutic and toxic doses of digitalis is very narrow. Toxic signs and symptoms may range from mild gastrointestinal disturbance to more serious and life-threatening cardiac dysrhythmias. Unfortunately, these indicators of toxicity may be attributed to other causes. For example, confusion is a common sign of digitalis toxicity in the elderly. Low potassium, high calcium, and low magnesium blood levels predispose to digitalis toxicity, an important consideration in patients who are on digitalis because many of them are also taking diuretics, which promote potassium and magnesium losses. The elderly are at particular risk for developing digitalis toxicity because a decrease in renal function that occurs with aging interferes with elimination of the drug. Several drugs are known to affect digitalis levels, and this should be taken into consideration in persons who are on the drug. Laboratory methods allow monitoring of serum digitalis levels.

A relatively new group of inotropic agents, the nondigitalis, noncatecholamine phosphodiesterase inhibitors (*e.g.*, amrinone, milrinone, enoximone, piroximone), increase cardiac contractility without inhibiting the sodium-potassium membrane pump or activating adrenergic receptors. These drugs inhibit the breakdown of cAMP, with a subsequent increase in calcium influx similar to that caused by the β-adrenergic agonists. Amrinone and milrinone also have a vasodilator effect, which may contribute to their usefulness in treating congestive heart failure. However, the value of these drugs for long-term use is still uncertain owing to the high incidence of adverse reactions such as dysrhythmias.[11]

Vasodilator drugs produce relaxation of vascular smooth muscle. These drugs induce venous pooling of blood, relax the pulmonary arterial and venous vessels, and reduce the peripheral vascular resistance. With pooling of blood in the peripheral veins, less blood returns to the right heart for delivery to the pulmonary circulation. Up to 2 L of fluid can be displaced by the tremendous capacity of the venous beds in the gut and lower extremities. Relaxation of the pulmonary vessels diminishes the pressure in the pulmonary capillaries and allows fluid to be reabsorbed from the interstitium of the lung and from the alveoli. With a decrease in peripheral vascular resistance, there is less pressure against which the left heart must pump, and the work of the left ventricle is decreased.

The vasodilators currently in use are the nitrates, hydralazine, prazosin, and the angiotensin converting enzyme (ACE) inhibitors. The *nitrates* produce relaxation of arteriolar and venous smooth muscle. Sodium nitroprusside is a form of nitroglycerin given by continuous intravenous infusion in situations of acute heart failure. Oral and topical forms of nitroglycerin are used in the long-term management of ischemic heart disease. *Hydralazine* is a potent arteriolar dilator; it markedly reduces afterload and increases cardiac output. The combination of nitrates and oral hydralazine has proved effective in the management of persons with mild to moderate heart failure symptoms. *Prazosin*, an oral α-adrenergic blocking drug that relaxes arterial smooth muscle, is being used selectively in the treatment of heart failure. However, its long-term benefits are unknown.

ACE inhibitors, which prevent the conversion of angiotensin I to angiotensin II, have been effectively used in the treatment of heart failure. In heart failure, renin activity is frequently elevated because of decreased renal blood flow. The net result is an increase in angiotensin II, which causes vasoconstriction and increased aldosterone production with a subsequent increase in salt and water retention by the kidney. Both mechanisms increase the workload of the heart. There is also evidence that the ACE inhibitors may decrease the progression of ineffective hypertrophy in persons with heart failure.[6] Some studies have shown that the ACE inhibitors can relieve symptoms and increase survival in persons with symptomatic congestive heart failure.[22,23] The newer angiotensin II receptor blockers have the advantage of not causing a cough, which is a troublesome side effect of the ACE inhibitors for many persons.

Mechanical Support. In addition to pharmacologic methods, several types of mechanical support have been developed as a temporary measure to treat persons with acute myocardial pump failure. Mechanical support is typically reserved for end-stage heart failure, used as a bridge to heart transplantation or for stabilizing the effects of cardiogenic shock.

Continuous hemofiltration is an external process for removing, filtering, and returning blood volume using a compact device and peripheral vascular access. When used early in the management of moderate to severe heart failure, hemofiltration can increase mean arterial pressure, reduce preload and afterload, reverse cardiac dysfunction, help restore renal function, and eliminate cardiopulmonary toxic metabolites from the plasma, all of which improve survival.[24]

An *intraaortic balloon pump* is a more invasive device that pumps in synchrony with the heart (Fig. 20–9). It consists of a 10-inch-long balloon that is inserted through a catheter into the descending aorta. The balloon is positioned so that the distal tip lies about 1 inch from the aortic arch. The balloon is filled with helium and is timed to inflate during ventricular diastole and

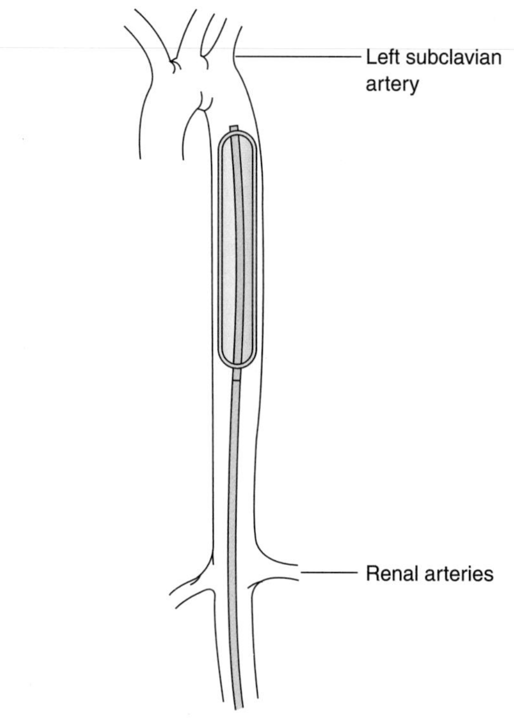

Figure 20–9
Aortic balloon pump.

deflate just before ventricular systole. Diastolic inflation creates a pressure wave in the ascending aorta that increases coronary artery flow and a less intense wave in the lower aorta that enhances organ perfusion. The sudden balloon deflation at the onset of systole lowers the resistance to ejection of blood from the left ventricle, thereby increasing the heart's pumping efficiency and decreasing myocardial oxygen consumption.

Ventricular assist devices (VADs) are mechanical pumps that are used to support ventricular function.[25] They are used to decrease the workload of the myocardium while maintaining cardiac output and systemic arterial pressure. This decreases the workload on the ventricle and allows it to rest and recover. Most VADs require an invasive open-chest procedure for implantation. They may be used in patients who fail or have difficulty being weaned from cardiopulmonary bypass after cardiac surgery; those who develop cardiogenic shock after myocardial infarction; those with end-stage cardiomyopathy; and those who are awaiting cardiac transplantation. Earlier and more aggressive use of VADs as a bridge to transplantation has been shown to increase survival.[26] VADs can be used to support the function of the left ventricle, right ventricle, or both ventricles.

A newer VAD-like device, called the *hemopump*, has been developed. An advantage of the hemopump is that it consists of a single catheter that can be inserted from the femoral artery, passed through the aorta, and positioned inside the left ventricle. The device draws oxygenated blood from the ventricle using a rapidly rotating pump device (much like a jet turbine) and propels it into the aorta. Although the nonpulsative flow and risk of blood cell trauma increase with use of this device, 40% survival rates have been reported in persons with profound heart failure.[27]

Heart Transplantation. Heart transplantation, once a scientific curiosity, has become an established method of treatment for a growing number of persons with end-stage heart disease. Many of the successes of heart transplantation can be credited to improved methods of immunosuppressive therapy, which optimize survival and rehabilitation. The number of successful heart transplantations has been steadily climbing, with over 2000 procedures performed per year and an average survival rate of 80% or better, depending on the transplantation center.[28] Despite the overall success of heart transplantation, donor availability and complications from infection, rejection, and immunosuppression drug therapy remain problems.

Surgery is performed by placing the recipient on cardiopulmonary bypass and excising the diseased heart. An orthotopic cardiac approach is typically used to attach the donor heart (Fig. 20–10). Pacing wires are loosely attached to the right ventricle to assist with temporary pacing of the heartbeat in the event of bradycardia during the immediate postoperative phase. The heterotopic approach to heart transplantation is the surgical "piggy-backing" of a donor heart beside the recipient's own heart. The transplanted heart functions like a ventricular assist device. This procedure results in two beating hearts within a single chest cavity.[29] Immediate postoperative care is directed toward maintaining hemodynamic stability, observing for bradyrhythmias and postoperative hemorrhage, and monitoring for transient renal failure. Subsequent postoperative management focuses on recognition and prevention of infection or rejection of the donor heart and monitoring of immunosuppressive therapy.

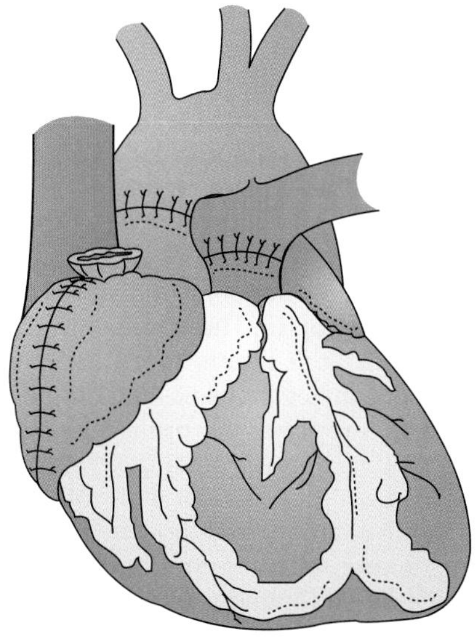

Figure 20–10
Orthotopic heart transplantation and sites of donor heart attachment.

Cardiomyoplasty. An alternative to heart transplantation that is growing in success and acceptance is a procedure called *cardiomyoplasty*.[30] This procedure involves fashioning one of the patient's latissimus dorsi back muscles into a wrap that embraces the heart. Because the muscle is native tissue, rejection is not a problem. Because the proximal end of the muscle remains intact, perfusion is optimal with enhanced potential for healing and performance. A pacemaker, which is placed between the heart and the back muscle, stimulates the muscle to contract. After several weeks of rest and healing, the skeletal muscle is gradually stimulated by the pacemaker to condition it in a necessary transformation into a more fatigue-resistant type of muscle tissue. Although more work is needed to identify the optimal way to wrap the muscle and condition it for maximum ventricular assist, cardiomyoplasty provides an alternative to transplantation for some persons, particularly when a donor heart is not available.

Acute Pulmonary Edema

Acute pulmonary edema is a life-threatening condition. In severe pulmonary edema, capillary fluid moves into the alveoli. The accumulated fluid in the alveoli and respiratory airways causes lung stiffness, makes lung expansion more difficult, and impairs the gas exchange function of the lung. With the decreased ability of the lungs to oxygenate the blood, the hemoglobin leaves the pulmonary circulation without being fully oxygenated. Cyanosis and shortness of breath result.

Manifestations

A person with acute pulmonary edema is usually seen sitting and gasping for air. The apprehension is obvious. The pulse is rapid, the skin is moist and cool, and the lips and nail beds are cyanotic. As the lung edema worsens and oxygen supply to the brain falls off, confusion and stupor appear. Dyspnea and air hunger are accompanied by a cough productive of frothy (resembling beaten egg whites) and often blood-tinged sputum—the effect of air mixing with serum albumin and red blood cells that have moved into the alveoli. The movement of air through the alveolar fluid produces fine crepitant sounds called *crackles,* which can be heard through a stethoscope placed on the chest. As fluid moves into the larger airways, the breathing becomes louder. The crackles heard earlier become louder and more coarse. In the terminal stage the breathing pattern is called the *death rattle.* Patients with severe pulmonary edema literally drown in their own secretions.

Treatment

Treatment of acute pulmonary edema is directed toward reducing the fluid volume in the pulmonary circulation. This can be accomplished by reducing the amount of blood that the right heart delivers to the lungs or by improving the work performance of the left heart. Several measures can decrease the blood volume in the pulmonary circulation; the seriousness of the pulmonary edema determines which are used. One of the simplest measures to relieve orthopnea is assumption of the seated position. For many persons, sitting up or standing is almost instinctive and may be sufficient to relieve the symptoms associated with mild accumulation of fluid.

Measures to improve left heart performance focus on decreasing the preload by reducing the filling pressure of the left ventricle and on reducing the afterload against which the left heart must pump. This can be accomplished through the use of vasodilator drugs, treatment of arrhythmias that impair cardiac function, and improvement of the contractile properties of the left ventricle with digitalis. Rapid digitalization can be accomplished with intravenous administration of the drug.

Oxygen therapy increases the oxygen content of the blood and helps relieve anxiety. Positive-pressure breathing increases the intraalveolar pressure, opposes the capillary filtration pressure in the pulmonary capillaries, and is sometimes used as a temporary measure to decrease the amount of fluid moving into the alveoli. Positive-pressure breathing can be administered through a specially designed continuous positive airway pressure (CPAP) mask. In the most severe cases, however, endotracheal intubation and mechanical ventilation may be necessary. Although its mechanisms of action are unclear, morphine sulfate is usually the drug of choice in acute pulmonary edema. Morphine relieves anxiety and depresses the pulmonary reflexes that cause spasm of the pulmonary vessels. It also increases venous pooling by vasodilation. Aminophylline is another drug, administered intravenously, that may be useful. It reduces bronchospasm, increases the glomerular filtration rate, and promotes urinary excretion of sodium and water.

Cardiogenic Shock

Cardiogenic shock implies failure of the heart to pump blood adequately. Cardiogenic shock can occur with relative speed because of the damage to the heart that occurs during myocardial infarction; ineffective pumping caused by cardiac dysrhythmias; mechanical defects that may occur as a complication of myocardial infarction, such as ventricular septal defect; ventricular aneurysm; acute disruption of valvular function; or problems associated with open heart surgery. Cardiogenic shock may also ensue as an end-stage condition of coronary artery disease or cardiomyopathy.

The most common cause of cardiogenic shock is myocardial infarction. It develops in 15% to 20% of persons admitted to hospitals with a diagnosis of myocardial infarction, and its severity and progression appear to be related to the amount of myocardium involved.[31] Most patients who die of cardiogenic shock have lost at least 40% of the contracting muscle of the left ventricle because of a recent infarct or a combination of recent and old infarcts.[32] Cardiogenic shock can follow other types of shock associated with inadequate coronary blood flow, or it can develop because substances released from ischemic tissues impair cardiac function. One such substance, myocardial depressant factor, is released into the circulation during severe shock. Myocardial depressant factor produces reversible (although often severe) myocardial depression, ventricular dilation, decreased left ventricular ejection fraction, and left ventricular diastolic pressure.[33] It is a key factor in the high mortality associated with septic shock and the syndrome of multiple organ failure.

In all cases of cardiogenic shock, there is failure to eject blood from the heart, hypotension, and inadequate cardiac output. Increased systemic vascular resistance often contributes to the deterioration of cardiac function by increasing afterload or the resistance to ventricular systole. The filling pressure, or preload of the heart, is also increased as blood returning to the heart is added to blood that was previously returned but not pumped forward, resulting in an increase in end-systolic ventricular volume. Increased resistance to ventricular systole (*i.e.,* afterload) combined with the decreased myocardial contractility causes the increased end-systolic ventricular volume and increased preload, which further complicate cardiac status.

Manifestations

The signs and symptoms of cardiogenic shock are consistent with those of heart failure. The lips, nail beds, and skin are cyanotic because of stagnation of blood flow and increased extraction of oxygen from the hemoglobin as it passes through the capillary bed. The CVP and PCWP rise as a result of volume overload caused by the pumping failure of the heart.

Treatment

Treatment of cardiogenic shock requires a precarious balance between improving cardiac output, reducing the workload and oxygen needs of the myocardium, and preserving coronary perfusion. Fluid volume must be regulated within a level that maintains the filling pressure (*i.e.*, venous return) of the heart and maximum use of the Frank-Starling mechanism without causing pulmonary congestion.

Catecholamines increase cardiac contractility but must be used with caution, because they also produce vasoconstriction and increase cardiac workload by increasing the afterload. The intra-aortic balloon pump provides a means of increasing aortic diastolic pressure and enhances coronary and peripheral blood flow without increasing systolic pressure and the afterload, against which the left ventricle must pump.[32] When greater support is needed, a VAD for the left ventricle or both ventricles may be needed. The use of extracorporeal membrane oxygenation (ECMO), once considered only effective in infants and small children, has been used with limited success in adults.[34]

When cardiogenic shock is caused by myocardial infarction, several aggressive interventions can be successfully used. The rapid and aggressive administration of tissue plasminogen activator (tPA) to dissolve intracoronary thrombi has been shown to significantly improve aortic pressure and survival.[35,36] The tPA was found to be more effective than streptokinase, another thrombolytic agent. Another promising alternative includes emergent direct percutaneous transluminal angioplasty (see Chapter 19). Compared with emergent coronary bypass surgery, thrombolytic therapy and percutaneous transluminal angioplasty are dispelling old beliefs that acutely infarcting myocardium could not withstand the rigors of these procedures.[37]

In summary, heart failure occurs when the heart fails to pump sufficient blood to meet the metabolic needs of body tissues. The physiology of heart failure reflects an interplay between a decrease in cardiac output that accompanies impaired function of the failing heart and the compensatory mechanisms designed to preserve the cardiac reserve. Four compensatory mechanisms contribute to the cardiac reserve: increased activity of the sympathetic nervous system, salt and water retention, the Frank-Starling mechanism, and myocardial hypertrophy. In the failing heart, early decreases in cardiac function may go unnoticed because these compensatory mechanisms maintain the cardiac output. This is called compensated heart failure. Unfortunately, the mechanisms were not intended for long-term use, and in severe and prolonged decompensated heart failure, the compensatory mechanisms are no longer effective, and the mechanisms themselves further impair cardiac function. In congestive heart failure, there is a decrease in cardiac output along with fluid accumulation in body tissues.

Heart failure may be described as high-output or low-output failure, systolic or diastolic failure, and right-sided or left-sided failure. With high-output failure the function of the heart may be supranormal but inadequate because of excessive metabolic needs, and low-output failure is caused by disorders that impair the pumping ability of the heart. With systolic dysfunction there is impaired ejection of blood from the heart during systole; with diastolic dysfunction there is impaired filling of the heart during diastole. Right-sided failure is characterized by congestion in the peripheral circulation, and left-sided failure by congestion in the pulmonary circulation.

The manifestations of heart failure include edema, nocturia, fatigue and impaired exercise tolerance, cyanosis, signs of increased sympathetic nervous system activity, and impaired gastrointestinal function and malnutrition. In right-sided failure there is dependent edema of the lower parts of the body, engorgement of the liver, and ascites. In left-sided failure, shortness of breath and chronic nonproductive cough are common.

The diagnostic methods in heart failure are directed toward establishing the cause of the disorder and determining the extent of the dysfunction. Treatment is directed toward correcting the cause whenever possible, improving cardiac function, maintaining the fluid volume within a compensatory level, and developing an activity pattern consistent with individual limitations in cardiac reserve. Among the medications used in the treatment of heart failure are inotropic agents, diuretics, and vasodilator drugs. Heart transplantation is becoming an established method of treatment for some persons with end-stage heart disease. The intra-aortic balloon pump or ventricular assist devices may be used as temporary support measures for severe heart failure.

Acute pulmonary edema is a life-threatening condition. The accumulation of fluid in the interstitium of the lung and alveoli interferes with lung expansion and gas exchange. It is characterized by extreme breathlessness, rales, frothy sputum, cyanosis, and signs of hypoxemia. Measures to improve left heart performance focus on decreasing the preload by reducing the filling pressure of the left ventricle and reducing the afterload against which the left heart must pump. In cardiogenic shock, there is a failure to eject blood from the heart, hypotension, inadequate cardiac output, and impaired perfusion of peripheral tissues. Treatment of cardiogenic shock requires a precarious balance between improving cardiac output, reducing the work load and oxygen needs of the myocardium, and preserving coronary perfusion.

Circulatory Failure (Shock)

After you have completed this section of the chapter, you should be able to meet the following objectives:

- State a clinical definition of *shock*
- Describe the compensatory mechanisms that are activated in circulatory shock
- List the chief characteristics of hypovolemic shock, cardiogenic shock, obstructive shock, and distributive shock
- List and describe the four stages of hypovolemic shock
- Compare the pathophysiology of neurogenic shock, anaphylactic shock, and septic shock
- Characterize changes in thirst, skin blood flow, pulse rate, urine output, and sensorium that are indicative of shock
- Describe the complications of shock as they relate to the lung, kidney, gastrointestinal tract, and blood clotting
- State the rationale for treatment measures to correct and reverse shock
- Define *multiple organ dysfunction syndrome* and cite its significance in shock

The functions of the circulatory system are to perfuse body tissues and to supply them with oxygen. Vascular failure, often referred to as *circulatory shock,* can be described as a failure of the circulatory system, with decreased peripheral perfusion and inadequate oxygenation of vital organs and cells of the body. It is not a specific disease but can occur in the course of many life-threatening, traumatic, or disease states. Although circulatory shock produces hypotension, it should not be equated with a drop in blood pressure. Hypotension often is a late sign and indicates a failure of compensatory mechanisms.

Physiology of Shock

Adequate perfusion of body tissues depends on the pumping ability of the heart, a vascular system that transports blood to the cells and back to the heart, sufficient blood to fill the vascular system, and tissues that are able to use and extract oxygen and nutrients from the blood. As with heart failure, vascular failure produces compensatory physiologic responses that eventually decompensate into various shock states if not properly treated in a timely manner.

In severe and prolonged shock, the vascular system fails. When this occurs, there is relaxation of the arterioles and venules, a fall in arterial pressure, and venous pooling of blood. At the capillary level, hypoxia and the products of cell deterioration cause increased capillary permeability, stagnation of blood flow, the formation of small blood clots, and shifting of intravascular volume into the interstitium, a condition called *third spacing*.

Flow in the Microcirculation

The delivery of oxygen and nutrients to body cells and the removal of metabolic waste products depend on adequate blood flow throughout the capillaries of the microcirculation. There are two types of capillary flow: *nutrient flow* and *nonnutrient flow.* Nutrient flow describes flow in the true capillary pathways that supply cells with oxygen and nutrients. In nonnutrient flow, blood is shunted directly from the arterial to the venous side of the circulation without passing through the true capillary pathways. Nonnutrient flow provides warmth, but not oxygen and nutrients, to the tissues. In distributive shock, nonnutrient flow is increased, and the skin is warm and flushed. Nutrient and nonnutrient flow are decreased in hypovolemic shock, and the skin is cool and clammy.

Compensatory Mechanisms

Without compensatory mechanisms to maintain cardiac output and blood pressure, the loss of vascular volume would result in a rapid progression from the initial to the progressive and irreversible stages of shock.

The most immediate of the compensatory mechanisms are the sympathetic-mediated responses designed to maintain cardiac output and blood pressure. Within seconds after the onset of hemorrhage or the loss of blood volume, signs of sympathetic and adrenal medullary activity appear: tachycardia, increased cardiac contractility, and widespread vasoconstriction. The sympathetic vasoconstrictor response affects the arterioles and the veins. Arteriolar constriction helps to maintain blood pressure by increasing the systemic vascular resistance, and venous constriction mobilizes blood that has been stored in the capacitance side of the circulation as a means of increasing venous return to the heart. There is considerable capacity for blood storage in the large veins of the abdomen and liver. About 350 ml of blood that can be mobilized in shock is stored in the liver. Sympathetic stimulation does not cause constriction of the cerebral and coronary vessels, and blood flow through the heart and brain is maintained at essentially normal levels as long as the mean arterial pressure remains above 70 mm Hg.[38]

During the early stages of hypovolemic shock, vasoconstriction causes a reduction in the size of the vascular compartment and an increase in systemic vascular resistance. This response usually is all that is needed when the injury is slight, and blood loss is arrested at this point. As hypovolemic shock progresses, there are further increases in heart rate and cardiac contractility, and vasoconstriction becomes more intense. There is vasoconstriction of the blood vessels that supply the skin, skeletal muscles, kidneys, and abdominal organs, with a resultant decrease in blood flow. When acidosis becomes evident, the arterial chemoreceptors are activated and add an additional vasoconstrictor effect.

Compensatory mechanisms designed to restore blood volume include absorption of fluid from the interstitial spaces, conservation of salt and water by the kidneys, and thirst. Extracellular fluid is distributed between the interstitial spaces and the vascular compartment (see Chapter 26). When there is a loss of vascular volume, capillary pressures decrease, and water is drawn into the vascular compartment from the interstitial spaces. The maintenance of vascular volume is further enhanced by renal mechanisms that conserve fluid. The previously described decrease in renal blood flow, which results from sympathetic vasoconstriction, lowers the glomerular filtration rate and activates the renin-angiotensin mechanism (see Chapter 18), which increases the release of aldosterone by the adrenal cortex, producing a further increase in sodium reabsorption by the kidney tubules. The decrease in blood volume also stimulates centers in the hypothalamus that regulate ADH release and thirst. A decrease in blood volume of 10% is sufficient to stimulate ADH release and thirst.[39] ADH, also known as *vasopressin,* constricts the peripheral arteries and veins and greatly increases water retention by the kidneys.

The compensatory mechanisms that the body recruits in hypovolemic and other forms of circulatory shock were not intended for long-term use. When injury is severe or its effects prolonged, the compensatory mechanisms begin to exert their own detrimental effects. The intense vasoconstriction causes a decrease in tissue perfusion, impaired cellular metabolism, release of vasoactive inflammatory mediators such as histamine, liberation of lactic acid, and cell death. After circulatory function has been reestablished, whether the shock will be irreversible or the patient will survive is determined largely at the cellular level.

Cellular Changes

At the cellular level, oxygen and nutrients supply the energy needed to maintain cellular function. Within the cell, oxygen and fuel substrates are converted to adenosine triphosphate (ATP), the cell's energy source. The cell uses ATP for a number of purposes, including operation of the sodium-potassium membrane pump that moves sodium out of the cell and potassium back into the cell.

The cell uses two pathways to convert nutrients to energy (see Chapter 1). The first is the *anaerobic* (nonoxygen) *glycolytic* pathway, which is located in the cytoplasm. Glycolysis converts glucose to ATP and pyruvate. The second pathway is the *aerobic* (oxygen-dependent) pathway, called the *citric acid cycle* or *Krebs' cycle,* which is located in the mitochondria. When oxygen is available, pyruvate from the glycolytic pathway moves into the mitochondria and enters the citric acid cycle, where it is transformed into ATP and the metabolic byproducts carbon dioxide and water. Fatty acids and proteins can also be metabolized in the mitochondrial pathway. When oxygen is lacking, pyruvate does not enter the citric acid cycle; instead, it is converted to lactic acid. In severe shock, cellular metabolic processes are essentially anaerobic, which means that excess amounts of lactic acid accumulate in the cellular and the extracellular compartment.

The anaerobic pathway, while allowing energy production to continue in the absence of oxygen, is relatively inefficient and produces significantly less ATP than does the aerobic pathway. Without sufficient energy production, normal cell function cannot be maintained, and the activity of the sodium-potassium membrane pump is impaired. As a result, sodium chloride accumulates within cells and potassium is lost from cells. The cells then swell, and their membranes become more permeable. Mitochondrial activity becomes severely depressed and lysosomal membranes rupture, resulting in the release of enzymes that cause further intracellular destruction. This is followed by cell death and the release of intracellular contents into the extracellular spaces. Intracellular enzymes (*e.g.,* myocardial depressant factor from pancreatic enzymes) and inflammatory mediators (*e.g.,* histamine, serotonin, tissue necrosis factor) are released.[33] These and many other substances like them produce adverse changes in the microcirculation that reduce the chance of recovery.

Circulatory Shock

Circulatory shock is the result of actual or relative loss of intravascular volume. Actual or direct volume losses, referred to as hypovolemia, are seen in cases of hemorrhage, burns, or extreme diuresis, when whole blood is lost through redistribution to the interstitial tissues (*i.e.,*

CHART **20-1**
Classification of Circulatory Shock

Hypovolemic
Loss of whole blood
Loss of plasma
Loss of extracellular fluid

Obstructive
Inability of the heart to fill properly (cardiac tamponade)
Obstruction to outflow from the heart (pulmonary embolus, cardiac myxoma, pneumothorax, or dissecting aneurysm)

Distributive
Loss of sympathetic vasomotor tone
Presence of vasodilating substances in the blood (anaphylactic, septic, or toxic shock syndrome)
Shunting of vascular fluid to the interstitial space (third spacing)
Arteriovenous shunting
Failure of body cells to use oxygen

third spacing) or when volume cannot circulate because of vascular obstruction. In either case, perfusion and oxygenation at the cellular level is decreased producing generalized organ failure. Aside from cardiogenic shock, which directly results from failure of the heart as a pump, circulatory shock can be classified as hypovolemic, obstructive, or distributive. These three main types of shock are summarized in Chart 20–1. Figure 20–11 compares normal circulation with the circulatory changes in each shock classification.

Hypovolemic Shock

Hypovolemic shock is characterized by diminished blood volume such that there is inadequate filling of the vascular compartment (see Fig. 20–11). It occurs when there is an acute loss of 15% to 20% of the circulating blood volume. The decrease may be caused by an external loss of whole blood (*e.g.*, hemorrhage), plasma (*e.g.*, severe burns), or extracellular fluid (*e.g.*, gastrointestinal fluids lost in vomiting or diarrhea). Hypovolemic shock can also result from an internal hemorrhage or from third-space losses, when extracellular fluid is shifted from the vascular compartment to the interstitial space or compartment.

Hypovolemic shock has been the most widely studied and usually serves as a prototype in discussions of the manifestations of shock. Figure 20–12 shows the effect of removing blood from the circulatory system during about 30 minutes.[38] About 10% can be removed without changing the cardiac output or arterial pressure. The average blood donor loses a pint of blood without suffering adverse effects. As increasing amounts of blood (10% to 25%) are removed, the cardiac output falls while the arterial pressure is maintained. This is because of sympathetic-mediated increases in heart rate and vasoconstriction. Because blood pressure is the product of cardiac output and systemic vascular resistance ($BP = CO \times SVR$), an increase in systemic vascular resistance maintains blood pressure in the presence of decreased blood volume and cardiac output for a short period. Cardiac output and tissue perfusion decrease before signs of hypotension occur. Cardiac output and arterial pressure fall to zero when about 35% to 45% of the total blood volume has been removed.[38]

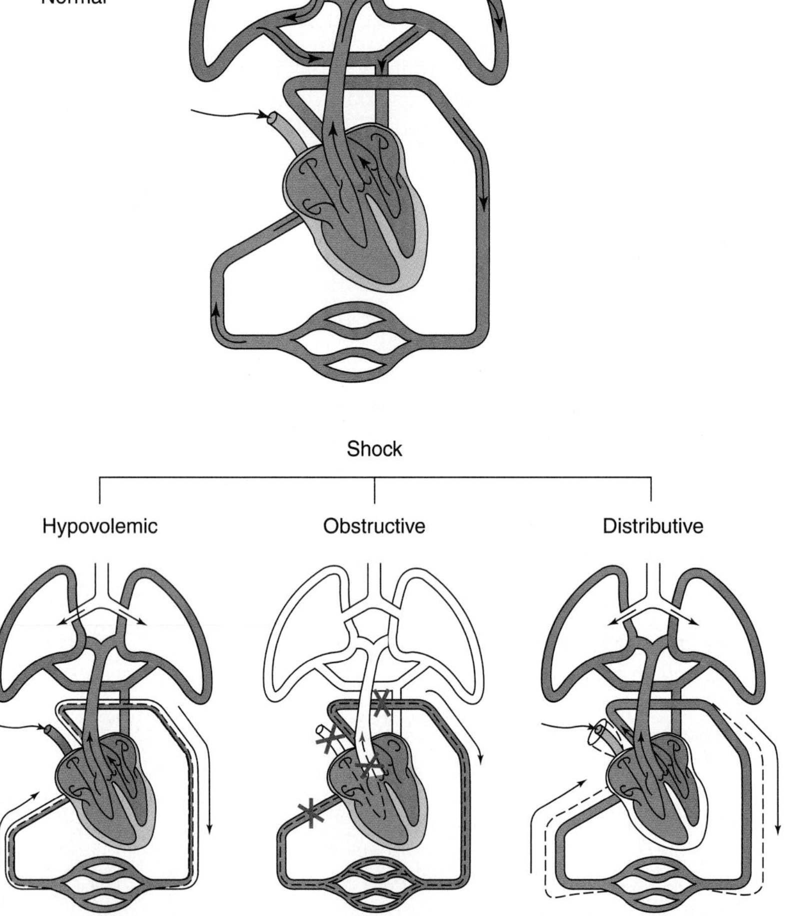

Figure 20–11 Types of shock.

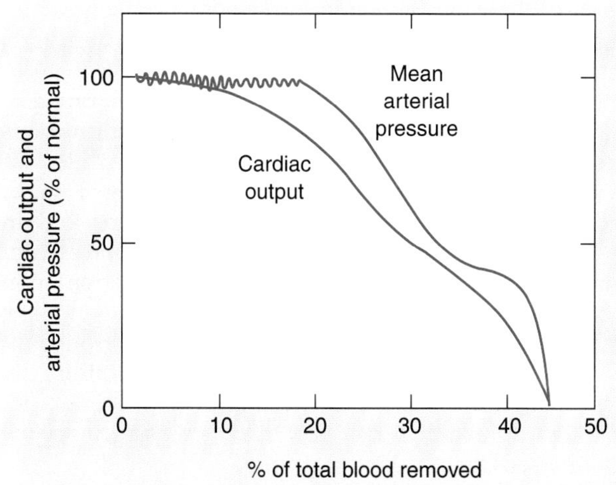

Figure 20–12
Effect of hemorrhage on cardiac output and arterial pressure. (Guyton A.C. [1986]. *Textbook of medical physiology* [7th ed.]. Philadelphia: W.B. Saunders)

The progression of hypovolemic shock can be divided into four stages. During the *initial stage*, the circulatory blood volume is decreased but not enough to cause serious effects. The second stage is the *compensatory stage*; although the circulating blood volume is reduced, compensatory mechanisms are able to maintain blood pressure and tissue perfusion at a level sufficient to prevent cell damage. The third stage is the *progressive stage* or *stage of decompensated shock*. At this point, unfavorable signs begin to appear: the blood pressure begins to fall, blood flow to the heart and brain is impaired, capillary permeability is increased, fluid begins to leave the capillary, blood flow becomes sluggish, and the body cells and their enzyme systems are damaged. The fourth and final stage is the *irreversible stage*. In irreversible shock, even though the blood volume may be restored and vital signs stabilized, death ensues eventually. Although the factors that determine recovery from severe shock have not been clearly identified, it appears that they are related to blood flow at the level of the microcirculation. The severity and clinical findings associated with hypovolemic shock are summarized in Table 20–3.

Obstructive Shock

The term *obstructive shock* is used to describe circulatory shock that results from mechanical obstruction of the flow of blood through the central circulation (great veins, heart, or lungs; see Fig. 20–11). Obstructive shock may be caused by a number of conditions, including dissecting aortic aneurysm, cardiac tamponade, pneumothorax, atrial myxoma, or evisceration of abdominal contents into the thoracic cavity because of a ruptured hemidiaphragm. The most frequent cause of obstructive shock is pulmonary embolism.

The primary physiologic results of obstructive shock are elevated right heart pressure and impaired venous

TABLE 20–3
Correlation of Clinical Findings and the Magnitude of Volume Deficit in Hemorrhagic Shock

Severity of Shock	Clinical Findings	Percentage of Reduction in Blood Volume (mL)
None	None; normal blood donation	Up to 10 (500 mL)*
Mild	Minimal tachycardia Slight decrease in blood pressure Mild evidence of peripheral vasoconstriction with cool hands and feet	15–25 (750–1250)
Moderate	Tachycardia, 100–120 bpm Decrease in pulse pressure Systolic pressure, 90–100 mm Hg Restlessness Increased sweating Pallor Oliguria	25–35 (1250–1750)
Severe	Tachycardia over 120 bpm Blood pressure below 60 mm Hg systolic and frequently unobtainable by cuff Mental stupor Extreme pallor, cold extremities Anuria	Up to 50 (2500)

*Based on blood volume of 7% in a 70-kg male of medium build.
(Adapted from Weil M., Shubin H. [1967]. *Diagnosis and treatment of shock*. [p. 118]. Baltimore: Williams & Wilkins)

return to the heart. The signs of right heart failure are seen, including elevation of CVP and jugular venous distention. Treatment modalities focus on correcting the cause of the disorder, frequently with surgical interventions such as pulmonary embolectomy, pericardiocentesis (*i.e.*, removal of fluid from the pericardial sac) for cardiac tamponade, or the insertion of a chest tube for correction of a tension pneumothorax or hemothorax. In select cases of pulmonary embolus, thrombolytic drugs may be used to dissolve the clots causing the obstruction.

Distributive Shock

Distributive shock is characterized by loss of blood vessel tone, enlargement of the vascular compartment, and displacement of the vascular volume away from the heart and central circulation. With distributive shock, the capacity of the vascular compartment expands to the extent that a normal volume of blood does not fill the circulatory system (see Fig. 20–11). Loss of vessel tone has two main causes: a decrease in the sympathetic control of vasomotor tone and the presence of vasodilator substances in the blood. Venous return is decreased in distributive shock, which leads to a diminished cardiac output but not a decrease in total blood volume; this type of shock is also referred to as *normovolemic shock*. There are three shock states that share the basic circulatory pattern of distributive shock: neurogenic shock, anaphylactic shock, and septic shock.

Neurogenic Shock. *Neurogenic shock* describes shock caused by decreased sympathetic control of blood vessel tone caused by a defect in the vasomotor center in the brain stem or the sympathetic outflow to the blood vessels. Output from the vasomotor center can be interrupted by brain injury, the depressant action of drugs, general anesthesia, hypoxia, or lack of glucose (*e.g.*, insulin reaction). Fainting due to emotional causes is a transient form of neurogenic shock. Spinal anesthesia or spinal cord injury above the midthoracic region can interrupt the transmission of outflow from the vasomotor center. The term *spinal shock* is used to describe the neurogenic shock that occurs in persons with spinal cord injury. Many general anesthetic agents can cause a neurogenic shocklike reaction, especially during induction, because of interference with sympathetic nervous system function. In contrast to hypovolemic shock, the heart rate in neurogenic shock often is slower than normal, and the skin is dry and warm. This type of distributive shock is rare and usually transitory.

Anaphylactic Shock. Anaphylactic shock is characterized by massive vasodilation, pooling of blood in the peripheral blood vessels, and increased capillary permeability.[40] This type of shock, which is a manifestation of systemic anaphylaxis, is caused by an immunologically mediated reaction in which vasodilator substances such as histamine are released into the blood (see Chapter 12). These substances cause dilatation of arterioles and venules along with a marked increase in capillary permeability. The vascular response in anaphylactic shock is accompanied by bronchospasm, contraction of gastrointestinal and uterine smooth muscle, and urticaria or angioedema.

Among the most frequent causes of anaphylactic shock are reactions to drugs, such as penicillin; foods, such as nuts and shellfish; and animal sera, such as tetanus antitoxin. The most common cause is stings from insects of the order Hymenoptera (*i.e.*, bees, wasps, and fire ants). Latex allergy has caused serious life-threatening anaphylaxis in a growing segment of the population. Health care workers and others who are exposed to latex are developing latex sensitivities that range from mild urticaria, contact dermatitis, and mild respiratory distress to anaphylactic shock.[41] Children with spina bifida are also at extreme risk for this increasingly serious allergy (see Chapter 12).

The onset of anaphylaxis depends on the sensitivity of the person and the rate and quantity of antigen exposure. Anaphylactic shock often develops suddenly; death can occur within a matter of minutes unless appropriate medical intervention is promptly instituted. Signs and symptoms associated with impending anaphylactic shock include abdominal cramps, apprehension, burning and warm sensation of the skin, itching, urticaria (*i.e.*, hives), coughing, choking, wheezing, chest tightness, and difficulty in breathing. After blood begins to pool peripherally, there is a precipitous drop in blood pressure and the pulse becomes so weak that it is difficult to detect. Life-threatening airway obstruction may ensue as a result of laryngeal edema or bronchial spasm.

The prevention of anaphylactic shock is preferable to treatment. After a person has been sensitized to an antigen, the risk of a fatal outcome always exists. All patients should be carefully questioned about earlier drug reactions and should be told what medications they are to receive before the medications are administered. Persons with known hypersensitivities should carry some form of medical identification to alert medical personnel if they become unconscious or unable to relate this information. Persons with allergies should also be informed about what procedures to follow in case they are inadvertently exposed to the antigen that causes the anaphylactic reaction (*e.g.*, bee sting). In some situations, it may be medically necessary to administer agents known to cause anaphylaxis. Protocols that have been developed to prevent or decrease the severity of the reaction involve pharmacologic pretreatment to block or blunt the reaction.

Because it is not always possible to prevent anaphylactic shock, all health care personnel should be aware of the characteristic signs and symptoms so that appropriate care can be instituted promptly. Treatment includes prompt discontinuance of the inciting agent and measures to decrease absorption; close monitoring of cardiovascular and respiratory function; and maintenance of adequate respiratory gas exchange, cardiac output, and tissue perfusion. Epinephrine constricts the blood vessels and relaxes the smooth muscle in the bronchioles; it usually is the first drug to be given to a patient believed to be experiencing an anaphylactic reaction. Other treatment measures include the administration of oxygen, antihistaminic drugs, and corticosteroids. Resuscitation measures may be required. It may be helpful to institute measures to decrease absorption when the antigenic agent has been injected into the tissues. This can be accomplished by the application of ice, which constricts the blood vessels. Measures to reduce absorption should not replace other treatment measures, but they may be particularly helpful in situations in which medical treatment is not immediately available. For example, application of ice may delay the absorption of the antigen from a bee sting so that there is time to secure medical attention.

Septic Shock. *Septic shock* is associated with severe infection and the systemic response to infection. It most frequently is associated with gram-negative bacteremia, although it can be caused by gram-positive bacilli and other microorganisms such as fungi, which carry even a greater risk of mortality.[42] Unlike other types of shock, septic shock commonly is associated with pathologic complications, such as pulmonary insufficiency (*i.e.*, shock lung), disseminated intravascular coagulation (DIC), and multiple organ dysfunction syndrome.

Septic shock has become the most common type of distributive shock. It has a mortality rate of about 50%. The rise in incidence of septic shock has been attributed to advances in health care and technology and to an increase in the population of immunocompromised persons. The presence of intravenous and urinary catheters are potential sources of infection and sepsis. Especially susceptible are high-risk neonates and young infants with immature immune systems and the elderly who have debilitating chronic illnesses and poor nutritional status.[43] Septic shock has been described within the context of the systemic inflammatory response. Although usually associated with infection, the systemic inflammatory response can be initiated by noninfectious disorders such as acute trauma and pancreatitis. To enable recognition, description, and classification of persons with sepsis, the American College of Chest Physicians and the Society of Critical Care Medicine published consensus terminology to describe and define the clinical manifestations and progression of sepsis (Chart 20–2).[44]

Septic shock typically manifests with fever, vasodilation, and warm, flushed skin. Mild hyperventilation, respiratory alkalosis, and abrupt alterations in personality and inappropriate behavior due to reduction in cerebral blood flow may be the earliest signs and symptoms of septic shock. These manifestations, which are thought to be a primary response to the bacteremia, commonly precede the usual signs and symptoms of sepsis by several hours or days. Unlike other forms of shock (*i.e.*, cardiogenic, hypovolemic, and obstructive) that are characterized by a compensatory increase in systemic vascular resistance, septic shock often presents with hypovolemia due to arterial and venous dilatation and leakage of plasma into the interstitial spaces.[45]

Aggressive treatment of the hypovolemia in septic shock leads to an decrease in systemic vascular resistance and increased cardiac output and tachycardia. In the past, this hyperdynamic pattern of response was thought to be present early in shock and was called *warm shock*. A second pattern of *cold shock* that was accompanied by a low cardiac output and cold extremities was thought to indicate the late stages of septic shock and a poor prognosis. With the development of refined resuscitation methods and better hemodynamic monitoring systems, about 90% of patients in septic shock demonstrate a hyperdynamic response with high cardiac output and low systemic vascular resistance.[45] However, despite the fact that cardiac output is normal or increased, cardiac function is depressed, the heart becomes dilated, and the ejection fraction decreases.

CHART 20–2
Definitions of Sepsis and Septic Shock

Infection: Microbial phenomenon characterized by an inflammatory response to the presence of microorganisms and the invasion of normally sterile host tissue by these organisms.

Bacteremia: The presence of viable bacteria in the blood.

Systemic Inflammatory Response Syndrome: The systemic inflammatory response to a variety of severe clinical insults. The response is manifested by two or more of the following conditions:
- Temperature >38°C or <36°C
- Heart rate >90 beats/min
- Respiratory rate >20 breaths/min or Pa_{CO_2} <32 torr (<4.3 kPa)
- WBC >12,000 cells/mm^3, <4000 cells/mm^3, or 10% immature (band) forms

Sepsis: The systemic response to infection. This systemic response is manifested by two or more of the above conditions (temperature, heart rate, respiratory rate, and WBC) as a result of infection:

Severe Sepsis: Sepsis associated with organ dysfunction, hypoperfusion, or hypotension. Hypoperfusion and perfusion abnormalities may include, but are not limited to lactic acidosis, oliguria, or an acute alteration in mental status.

Septic Shock: Sepsis with hypotension, despite adequate fluid resuscitation, along with the presence of perfusion abnormalities that may include but are not limited to lactic acidosis, oliguria, or an acute alteration in mental status. Patients who are on inotropic or vasopressor agents may not be hypotensive at the time that perfusion abnormalities are measured.

Hypotension: A systolic BP of <90 mm Hg or a reduction of >40 mm Hg from baseline in the absence of other causes of hypotension.

Multiple Organ Dysfunction Syndrome: Presence of altered organ function in an acutely ill patient such that homeostasis cannot be maintained without intervention.

(American College of Chest Physicians/Society of Critical Care Medicine Consensus Conference. [1992]. Definitions for sepsis and organ failure and guidelines for use of innovative therapies in sepsis. *Critical Care Medicine* 20 [6], 866)

The mechanisms of septic shock are thought to be related to mediators of the inflammatory response. One possibility is that toxins from the sepsis-producing organisms incite an immune reaction, which leads to decreased vascular tone and increased permeability. The resulting vasodilatation and third spacing of extracellular fluids combine to magnify the hypotensive effects of septic shock to decrease oxygen delivery to the cells and increase the mortality. Another theory is that cytokines (see Chapter 11) are involved, including elevated levels of tumor necrosis factor-α (TNF-α) that incite neutrophil activation, capillary leak syndrome, and development of DIC.[46] Another hypothesis is that cellular metabolism is abnormal in persons with septic shock, as evidenced by increased blood lactate concentrations, metabolic acidosis, increased glycolysis, and decreased extraction of oxygen from the circulating blood. Considerable research has been generated regarding the relationship between mortality from septic shock and oxygen delivery or the ability of cells to use oxygen effectively. Many cases of septic shock demonstrate high mixed venous oxygen saturation, indicating a cellular inability to use delivered oxygen. Because of this, oxygen delivery for these persons may need to exceed normal levels to preserve cellular oxygenation.[47]

The treatment of septic shock focuses on the causative agent and support of the circulation. The administration of antibiotics specific to the infectious agent is essential. The cardiovascular status of the patient must be supported to maintain oxygen delivery to the cells. Swift and aggressive fluid administration is needed to compensate for third spacing, and equally aggressive use of vasopressors, such as epinephrine, norepinephrine bitartrate, and phenylephrine, is needed to counteract the vasodilation caused by endotoxins.[19] Studies support the early and aggressive use of positive inotropic drugs, such as dobutamine, to increase cardiac contractility and maintain oxygen delivery.[48] Of particular interest has been the development of human monoclonal antibodies to the endotoxins produced by the gram-negative sepsis. Supplemental immune globulins have been used to treat sepsis but without great success unless used early or prophylactically in persons at risk for septic shock such as high-risk cardiac surgery patients.[49]

Toxic Shock. *Toxic shock* is a unique manifestation of a septic shock pattern and is typically a life-threatening event. First described in the 1980s, it is characterized by extreme hypotension, high fever, headache, dizziness, myalgia, confusion, rash, conjunctivitis, sore throat, vomiting, and watery diarrhea.[50] Desquamation (*i.e.*, peeling) of the skin on the hands and feet frequently occurs during convalescence.

Although some cases of toxic shock syndrome have been reported in men and children, by far the greatest number of cases occur in menstruating women. Tampon use is considered a primary risk factor for toxic shock. The most common organism associated with toxic shock is *Staphylococcus aureus*. The onset of menstrual toxic shock syndrome occurs 1 to 11 days (median, 2 days) after vaginal bleeding begins. Nonmenstrual toxic shock syndrome has been associated with surgical infections, nonsurgical infections of the skin or the subcutaneous or osseous tissues, and childbirth or abortion.

Manifestations of Shock

The signs and symptoms of hypovolemic shock are closely related to low peripheral blood flow and excessive sympathetic stimulation. For purposes of discussion, the manifestations of hypovolemic shock have been divided into the following categories: thirst, skin and body temperature changes, arterial and venous pressure, pulse rate, urine output, and changes in sensorium.

Thirst. An early symptom in hypovolemic shock, thirst is easily overlooked in situations in which concealed bleeding occurs. Explanations regarding the causes of thirst are many, although the underlying cause is probably related to decreased blood volume and increased serum osmolality (see Chapter 26). Many patients with trauma have a decreased renal blood flow because of an intense sympathetic nervous system stimulation, along with an increase in ADH levels, which causes water retention. Water should be given cautiously, because water intoxication can occur in a patient who continues to drink water in the face of altered renal function.

Skin and Body Temperature. In hypovolemic shock, sympathetic stimulation leads to intense vasoconstriction of the skin vessels and activation of the sweat glands. As a result, the skin is cool and moist. When shock is caused by hemorrhage, the loss of red blood cells leaves the skin and mucous membranes looking pale. The decrease in body temperature that is often observed in shock reflects a decrease in the body's metabolic rate.

Pulses and Pressures. An increase in heart rate often is an early sign of shock. Like vasoconstriction, the tachycardia of early shock is a sign of sympathetic nervous system response to injury. Tachycardia may also reflect emotional aspects surrounding injury or the pain associated with trauma. Blood volume and vessel tone are reflected in the quality of the pulse. A weak and thready pulse indicates vasoconstriction and a reduction in filling of the vascular compartment. Decreased intravascular volume results in decreased venous return to the heart and a fall in CVP.

Considerable controversy exists over the value of blood pressure measurements in the diagnosis and management of shock. This is because compensatory mechanisms tend to preserve blood pressure until shock is relatively far advanced. Furthermore, an adequate arterial pressure does not ensure adequate perfusion and oxygenation of vital organs at the cellular level. This does not imply that blood pressure should not be measured in patients at risk for developing shock, but it does indicate the need for other assessment measures by which shock may be detected at an earlier stage.

In shock, blood pressure commonly is measured intraarterially, because the sphygmomanometer may not always provide an accurate measurement. Systolic pressures measured by cuff methods typically are lower than those measured intraarterially, because in shock, increased vascular resistance in the upper extremities alters the hemodynamic events that produce the Korotkoff sounds. The first tapping sounds detectable with the stethoscope may be heard at a pressure that is considerably lower than that measured from the artery. The *Doppler method,* in which blood pressure is measured noninvasively by ultrasound, may provide a more accurate estimate of Korotkoff sounds when they are no longer audible through the stethoscope. In some instances, this method may be used as an alternative to continuous intraarterial monitoring.

Urine Output. Urine output decreases very quickly in hypovolemic and other forms of shock. Compensatory mechanisms decrease renal blood flow as a means of diverting blood flow to the heart and brain. Oliguria of 20 ml/hour or less indicates severe shock and inadequate renal perfusion. Continuous measurement of urine output is essential for assessing the circulatory status of the patient in shock.

Sensorium. Restlessness and apprehension are common behaviors in early shock. As the shock progresses and blood flow to the brain decreases, restlessness is replaced by apathy and stupor. If shock is unchecked, the apathy progresses to coma. Coma caused by blood loss alone and not related to head injury or other factors is an unfavorable sign.

Treatment Measures

The treatment of circulatory shock is directed toward correcting or controlling the underlying cause and improving tissue perfusion. In hypovolemic shock, the goal of treatment is to restore vascular volume. This can be accomplished through intravenous administration of fluids and blood. Plasma expanders, including *dextrans and colloidal albumin solutions,* have a high molecular weight, do not necessitate blood typing, and remain in the circulation for longer periods than the crystalloids, such as glucose and saline. The dextrans must be used with caution, because they may induce serious or fatal reactions, including anaphylaxis. Fluids and blood are best administered based on volume indicators such as CVP and PCWP. This is particularly important in pediatric patients, whose fluid balance allows less variation from normal before compromise to tissue perfusion results[46] and who may respond better to hypertonic saline instead of other crystalloid or colloid solutions.[51]

Caution must be used in fluid resuscitation to prevent "reperfusion injury," which is caused by excess generation of free radicals when oxygen is reintroduced after prolonged hypotension (see Chapter 2).[52] To prevent such injury, several techniques are being tested, such as infusing moderately hypothermic solutions (28°C to 32°C).[53] Other techniques include using hemoglobin-based blood substitutes, as opposed to the perfluorocarbons used in earlier studies. Bovine hemoglobin is much like human hemoglobin in that it has a low affinity for oxygen and readily releases oxygen to the cells.[54] There are also attempts at producing recombinant human hemoglobin for use in plasma preparations.[55]

Circulatory Assistance. In hypovolemic shock, a pneumatic antishock garment (PASG) may be used. The PASG, which encases the legs and abdomen and can be inflated separately or wholly, compresses the blood vessels of the legs or abdomen and increases venous return to the heart. This *autotransfusion* effect is potentially lifesaving when used by emergency personnel in the field to manage hemorrhagic shock or traumatic shock. However, no benefit has been shown from the PASG in terms of hospital stay or mortality.[55] The PASG has been associated with the incidence of compartment syndrome (see Chapter 17) when used on trauma patients without lower leg injury.[56] Compartment syndrome frequently results in muscle necrosis, loss of limb function, potential limb loss, and occasionally death. The PASG is contraindicated in cardiogenic shock, because the increased venous return further overloads the failing heart. The use of PASG must be carefully considered and used judiciously in select situations. Ironically, the simple act of passively elevating the legs has been verified as an effective intervention to increase preload and significantly improve cardiovascular performance.[57]

Vasoactive Drugs. Vasoactive drugs are agents capable of constricting or dilating blood vessels. Considerable controversy exists about the advantages or disadvantages related to the use of these drugs.

There are two types of receptors for the sympathetic nervous system: alpha and beta. The β receptors are further subdivided into β_1 and β_2. In the cardiorespiratory system, stimulation of the α receptors causes vasoconstriction; stimulation of β_1 receptors causes an increase in heart rate and the force of myocardial contraction; and stimulation of β_2 receptors produces vasodilation of the skeletal muscle beds and relaxation of the bronchioles.

Dopamine is often prescribed to treat shock, because it induces a more favorable array of α- and β-receptor actions than many of the other adrenergic drugs. Dopamine is thought to increase blood flow to the kidneys, liver, and other abdominal organs while maintaining vasoconstriction of less vital structures, such as the skin and skeletal muscles, when given in low doses (<20 μg/kg/ minute). In severe shock, higher doses may be needed to maintain blood pressure. After dopamine administration exceeds this low-dose range, it has vasoconstrictive effects on blood flow to the kidneys and abdominal organs that is similar to that of epinephrine.

The vasodilators nitroprusside (Nipride) and nitroglycerin are used to treat cardiogenic shock. Nitroprusside causes arterial and venous dilatation, producing a decrease in venous return to the heart, with a reduction in arterial resistance against which the left heart must pump. Nitroglycerin focuses its effects on the venous vascular beds until, at high doses, it begins to dilate the arterial beds as well. The arterial pressure is maintained by an increased ventricular stroke volume ejected against a lowered systemic vascular resistance; this allows blood to be redistributed from the pulmonary vascular bed to the systemic circulation.

Complications of Shock

Wiggers, a noted circulatory physiologist, stated, "Shock not only stops the machine, but it wrecks the machinery."[58] Many body systems are wrecked by severe shock. Five major complications of severe shock are shock lung, acute renal failure, gastrointestinal ulceration, DIC, and multiple organ dysfunction syndrome. The complications of shock are serious and often fatal.

Shock Lung

Shock lung, or adult respiratory distress syndrome (ARDS), is a potentially lethal form of respiratory failure that can follow severe shock (see Chapter 24). The term *shock lung* was introduced during the Vietnam war to describe the progressive pulmonary failure seen in soldiers who suffered major trauma. The symptoms usually do not develop until 24 to 48 hours after the initial trauma; in some instances, they occur later. ARDS is thought to result from increased permeability of the pulmonary capillaries to water and plasma proteins.[59] Protein-rich fluids leak into the alveolar and interstitial spaces, impairing gas exchange and making the lung stiffer and more difficult to inflate. Some patients develop a hyaline membrane syndrome similar to that seen in respiratory distress syndrome in the neonate. The respiratory rate and effort of breathing increase. Arterial blood gas analysis establishes the presence of profound hypoxemia with hypercapnia, resulting from impaired matching of ventilation and perfusion and from the greatly reduced diffusion of blood gases across the thickened alveolar membranes.

The exact cause of ARDS is unknown. It has been suggested that the problem results from one or more factors:

- A decrease in lung perfusion and ischemia of the type II alveolar cells, which produce surfactant
- Oxygen toxicity
- Pulmonary venoconstriction and pulmonary edema related to sympathetic stimulations and hypoxemia
- Fluid overload with stretching and disruption of the pulmonary capillaries
- Damage to the lungs by endotoxins and substances released as the result of sepsis
- Activation of neutrophils that contribute to the formation of free oxygen radicals that not only destroy surfactant but the cells that produce surfactant
- Embolization of the microcirculation of the lung with resulting infarctions
- Prolonged hypotension

It is possible that multiple mechanisms operate to cause a similar pattern of injury or to trigger a common response (*e.g.*, intravascular clotting), which produces the pulmonary damage.

Interventions for shock lung have typically focused on supporting ventilation mechanically to optimize gas exchange. Despite high levels of oxygen and mechanical alterations in intrapulmonary pressure using pressure support and positive end-expiratory pressure (PEEP), most persons with ARDS remain hypoxic with deadly results.

New interventions have focused on more aggressive treatment of the underlying cause, such as rapid infusion of high doses of the thrombolytic drug streptokinase for the treatment of obstructive shock due to massive pulmonary emboli.[60] Some improvement in mortality has been shown with the use of inhaled nitric oxide in stabilizing the pulmonary vasculature in ARDS associated with anaphylactic and septic shock.[61–63]

Acute Renal Failure

The renal tubules are particularly vulnerable to ischemia, and *acute renal failure* is one important late cause of death in severe shock. Sepsis and trauma account for most cases of acute renal failure. The endotoxins implicated in septic shock are powerful vasoconstrictors that are capable of activating the sympathetic nervous system and causing intravascular clotting. They have been shown to trigger all the separate physiologic mechanisms that contribute to the onset of acute renal failure. The degree of renal damage is related to the severity and duration of shock. The normal kidney is able to tolerate severe ischemia for 15 to 20 minutes. The renal lesion most frequently seen after severe shock is *acute tubular necrosis.* Acute tubular necrosis usually is reversible, although return to normal renal function may require weeks or months (see Chapter 29). Continuous monitoring of urine output during shock provides a means of assessing renal blood flow. Frequent monitoring of serum creatinine and blood urea nitrogen levels also provides valuable information regarding renal status.

Gastrointestinal Complications

The gastrointestinal tract is particularly vulnerable to ischemia because of the changes in distribution of blood flow to its mucosal surface. In shock, there is widespread constriction of blood vessels that supply the gastrointestinal tract, causing a redistribution of blood flow that severely diminishes mucosal perfusion. There is growing evidence that the splanchnic and mesenteric vascular beds experience disproportionately greater vasoconstriction in response to circulating catecholamines and angiotensin II than do other vascular beds.[62] Superficial mucosal lesions of the stomach and duodenum can develop within hours of severe trauma, sepsis, or burn.

Bleeding is a common symptom of gastrointestinal ulceration caused by shock. Hemorrhage has its onset usually within 2 to 10 days after the original insult and often begins without warning. Poor perfusion in the gastrointestinal tract has been credited with allowing intestinal bacteria to enter the bloodstream, thereby contributing to the development of sepsis and shock.[64]

Gastric pH can be monitored by way of a nasogastric tube.[65] With a tube in place, gastric contents can be aspirated and the pH determined. Depending on the pH, antacids can be instilled directly into the stomach through a tube. Frequent pH monitoring is time consuming, and sometimes it is difficult to obtain sufficient aspirate for pH testing. Technologic advances, such as nasogastric tubes with pH sensors on their tips, make this procedure less time consuming and more accurate. Nasogastric tubes, when attached to intermittent suction, also help to diminish the accumulation of hydrogen ions in the stomach. $Histamine_2$ antagonists may be given prophylactically to prevent gastrointestinal ulcerations caused by shock.

Disseminated Intravascular Coagulation

DIC, a complication of septic shock, is characterized by the formation of small clots in the microcirculation. Consumption and depletion of platelets, fibrinogen, and other clotting factors occur, leading to the disruption of the normal clotting process with abnormal bleeding or hemorrhage (see Chapter 7).

Multiple Organ Dysfunction Syndrome

Multiple organ dysfunction syndrome is a particularly life-threatening complication of shock, especially septic shock. Mortality rates vary from 30% to 100%, depending on the number of organs involved. If they are required for long periods, many of the compensatory mechanisms stimulated by shock become the cause of multiple organ failure. Selectively severe vasospasm occurs in the hepatic and mesenteric circulations and the release of endorphins that potentiate the hypotensive effects of vasodilation and release of tumor necrosis factor (TNF) and oxygen free radicals, contributing to failure of multiple organ systems. Impaired oxygen delivery due to hypotension, blood loss, ARDS, and impaired oxygen consumption, as occurs in sepsis and anaphylaxis, contribute to the deadly cycle of cellular necrosis throughout all organ systems. The levels of lactic acid produced by anaerobic metabolism continue to be useful in predicting the development of multiple organ dysfunction syndrome.[66] Interventions for multiple organ failure are focused on support of the affected systems.

In summary, circulatory shock is an acute emergency situation in which body tissues are deprived of oxygen and cellular nutrients or are unable to use these materials in their metabolic processes. Circulatory shock may develop because there is not enough blood in the circulatory system (*i.e.*, hypovolemic shock), blood flow or venous return is obstructed (*i.e.*, obstructive shock), or the tissues are unable to use oxygen and nutrients (*i.e.*, distributive shock). Three types of shock share the basic circulatory pattern of distributive shock: neurogenic shock, anaphylactic shock, and septic shock. Septic shock, which is the most common of these three types, is associated with a severe, overwhelming infection and has a mortality rate of about 50%.

The manifestations of circulatory shock are related to low peripheral blood flow and excessive sympathetic stimulation. The low peripheral blood flow produces thirst, changes in skin temperature, a fall in blood pressure, an increase in heart rate, decreased venous pressure, decreased urine output, and changes in the sensorium. Signs and symptoms, such as changes in skin temperature (*i.e.*, increased in septic shock and decreased in hypovolemic and other forms of shock), may differ with the type of shock. The intense vasoconstriction that serves to maintain blood flow to the heart and brain causes a decrease in tissue perfusion, impaired cellular metabolism, liberation of lactic acid, and eventually, cell death. Whether the shock will be irreversible or the patient will survive is determined largely by changes that occur at the cellular level.

The speed of support to regain perfusion and cellular oxygenation is critical to ensure cellular and patient survival. The treatment of shock is determined by the type of shock. It focuses on correcting or controlling the cause and improving tissue perfusion. In hypovolemic shock, the goal of treatment is to restore vascular volume. In cardiogenic shock, treatment is directed toward reducing the work load of the heart while improving its pumping efficiency. Vasoactive drugs capable of constricting or dilating blood vessels may be used.

The complications of shock result from the deprivation of circulation to vital organs or systems, such as the lungs, kidneys, gastrointestinal tract, and blood coagulation system. Shock lung, or ARDS, produces lung changes that occur with shock. It is characterized by changes in the permeability of the alveolar-capillary membrane with the development of interstitial edema and severe hypoxia that does not respond to oxygen therapy. The renal tubules are particularly vulnerable to ischemia, and acute renal failure is an important complication of shock. Gastrointestinal ischemia may lead to gastrointestinal bleeding and increased permeability to the intestinal bacteria that cause further sepsis and shock. DIC is characterized by formation of small clots in the circulation. It is thought to be caused by sluggish blood flow in the microcirculation or inappropriate activation of the coagulation cascade because of toxins or other products released as a result of the shock state. Multiple organ failure, perhaps the most ominous complication of shock, rapidly depletes the ability of the body to compensate and recover from a shock state.

Circulatory Failure in Children and the Elderly

After you have completed this section of the chapter, you should be able to meet the following objectives:

- Describe the manifestations of heart failure in infants and children
- Cite how the aging process affects heart failure in the elderly
- State how the signs and symptoms of heart failure may differ between younger and older adults

The mechanisms of heart failure in children and the elderly are similar to that of adults. However, the causes and manifestations may differ because of age.

Heart Failure in Infants and Children

As in adults, heart failure in infants and children results from the inability of the heart to maintain the cardiac output required to sustain metabolic demands.[67–69] Congenital heart defects are the most common cause of congestive heart failure during childhood. Surgical correction of congenital heart defects may cause congestive heart failure as a result of intraoperative manipulation of the heart and resection of heart tissue, with subsequent alterations in pressure, flow, and resistance relations.[67] Usually, the heart failure that results is acute and resolves after the effects of the surgical procedure have subsided. Chronic congestive failure is occasionally observed in children with severe chronic anemia, inflammatory heart disease, end-stage congenital heart disease, or cardiomyopathy. Chart 20–3 lists some of the more common causes of heart failure in children. Inflammatory heart disorders (*e.g.*, myocarditis, rheumatic fever, bacterial endocarditis, Kawasaki's disease), cardiomyopathy, and congenital heart disorders are discussed in Chapter 19.

CHART **20-3**
Causes of Heart Failure in Children

Newborn Period

- Congenital heart defects
  - Severe left ventricular outflow disorders
    - Hypoplastic left heart
    - Critical aortic stenosis or coarctation of the aorta
  - Large arteriovenous shunts
    - Ventricular septal defects
    - Ductus arteriosus
  - Transposition of the great vessels
- Heart muscle dysfunction (secondary)
  - Asphyxia
  - Sepsis
  - Hypoglycemia
- Hematologic disorders (*e.g.*, anemia)

Infants 1 to 6 Months

- Congenital heart disease
  - Large arteriovenous shunts (ventricular septal defect)
- Heart muscle dysfunction
  - Myocarditis
  - Cardiomyopathy
- Pulmonary abnormalities
  - Bronchopulmonary dysplasia
  - Persistent pulmonary hypertension

Toddlers, Children, and Adolescents

- Acquired heart disease
  - Cardiomyopathy
  - Viral myocarditis
  - Rheumatic fever
  - Endocarditis
  - Systemic disease
    - Sepsis
    - Kawasaki's disease
    - Renal disease
    - Sickle cell disease
- Congenital heart defects
  - Nonsurgically treated disorders
  - Surgically treated disorders

Manifestations

Many of the signs and symptoms of heart failure in infants and children are similar to those of adults. They include fatigue, effort intolerance, cough, anorexia, and abdominal pain. A subtle sign of cardiorespiratory distress in infants and children is a change in disposition or responsiveness, including irritability or lethargy. Sympathetic stimulation produces peripheral vasoconstriction and diaphoresis. Decreased renal blood flow often results in a urine output of less than 0.5 to 1.0 ml/kg/hour, despite adequate fluid intake.[67] When right ventricular function is impaired, systemic venous congestion develops. Hepatomegaly due to liver congestion is often one of the first signs of systemic venous congestion in infants and children. However, dependent edema or ascites is rarely seen unless the central venous pressure is extremely high. Because of their short, fat necks, jugular venous distention is difficult to detect in infants; it is not a reliable sign until the child is of school age or older.

A third heart sound, or gallop rhythm, is a common finding in infants and children with heart failure. It results from rapid filling of a noncompliant ventricle. However, it is difficult to distinguish at high heart rates.

Most commonly, children develop interstitial edema rather than alveolar pulmonary edema. This reduces lung compliance and increases the work of breathing, causing tachypnea and increased respiratory effort. Older children display use of accessory muscles (*i.e.*, scapular and sternocleidomastoid). Head bobbing and nasal flaring may be observed in infants. Signs of respiratory distress are often the first and most noticeable signal of congestive heart failure in infants and young children. Pulmonary congestion may be mistaken for bronchiolitis or lower respiratory tract infections. The infant or young child with respiratory distress often grunts with expiration. This grunting effort (essentially, exhaling against a closed glottis) is an instinctive effort to increase end-expiratory pressures and prevent collapse of small airways and the development of atelectasis. Respiratory crackles (*i.e.*, rales) are uncommon in infants and usually suggest development of a respiratory tract infection. Wheezes may be heard, particularly if there is a large left-to-right shunt.

Infants with heart failure often have increased respiratory problems during feeding.[22,24] The history is one of prolonged feeding with excessive respiratory effort and fatigue. Weight gain is slow owing to high energy requirements and low calorie intake. Other frequent manifestations of heart failure in infants are excessive sweating (due to increased sympathetic tone), particularly over the head and neck, and repeated lower respiratory tract infections. Peripheral perfusion is generally poor with cool extremities, tachycardia is common (resting heart >150/minute), and respiratory rate is increased (resting rate >50/minute).[22]

Diagnosis and Treatment

Diagnosis of congestive failure in infants and children is based on symptomatology, chest x-ray films, electrocardiographic findings, echocardiographic techniques to assess cardiac structures and ventricular function (*i.e.*, end-systolic and end-diastolic diameters), arterial blood gases to determine intracardiac shunting and ventilation-perfusion inequalities, and other laboratory studies to determine anemia and electrolyte imbalances.

Treatment of congestive failure in infants and children is similar to that in adults. It includes measures aimed at improving cardiac function and eliminating excess intravascular fluid. Oxygen delivery must be supported and oxygen demands controlled or minimized. Whenever possible, the cause of the disorder is corrected (*e.g.*, medical treatment of sepsis and anemia, surgical correction of congenital heart defects). With congenital anomalies that are amenable to surgery, medical treatment is often needed for a time before surgery and is usually continued in the immediate postoperative period. For many children, only medical management can be provided.

Medical management of heart failure in infants and children is similar to that in the adult, although it is tailored to the special developmental needs of the child. Inotropic agents such as digitalis are often used to increase cardiac contractility. Diuretics may be given to reduce preload and vasodilating drugs used to manipulate the afterload. Drug doses must be carefully tailored to control for the child's weight and conditions such as reduced renal function. Daily weighing and accurate measurement of intake and output is imperative during acute episodes of failure.

Most children feel better in the semi-upright position. An infant seat is useful for infants with chronic congestive heart failure. Activity restrictions are usually designed to allow children to be as active as possible within the limitations of their heart disease. Infants with congestive failure often have problems feeding. Small, frequent feedings are usually more successful than larger, less frequent feedings. Severely ill infants may lack sufficient strength to suck and may need to be tube fed.

The treatment of heart failure in children should be designed to allow optimal physical and psychosocial development. It requires the full involvement of the parents, who are often the primary care providers; therefore, parent education and support is essential.

Heart Failure in the Elderly

Congestive heart failure is one of the most common causes of disability in the elderly. The prevalence of heart failure increases with age—from 3% in persons between the ages of 45 and 64 years, to 6% in persons between the ages of 65 and 74 years, to 10% for those 75 years and older.[70] Congestive heart failure is associated with a high mortality rate in the elderly, particularly during the first year after diagnosis.[71] Repetitive readmissions to the hospital are also frequent, accounting for a substantial part of all inpatient Medicare expenditures.[72]

The causes of heart failure in the elderly are similar to those in younger persons. As in younger persons, hypertensive cardiovascular disease and ischemic heart disease are commonly present in elderly persons who develop heart failure. Valvular heart disease and cardiomyopathy, however, are the most frequent causes of heart failure in the elderly. Elderly persons also tend to develop cardiac failure when confronted with stresses that would not produce failure in younger persons. There is no evidence that the cardiovascular changes that occur with aging are sufficient to produce congestive heart failure. Moreover, the effects of heart failure in the elderly are often compounded by other disease conditions, such as hypertension and diabetes.

Manifestations

The manifestations of congestive heart failure in the elderly are similar to those in younger individuals. However, the signs and symptoms are often masked by other disease conditions.[73] Lassitude is a common but nonspecific early symptom of cardiac failure as well as other disease conditions. Nocturia is another early symptom but may be caused by other conditions such as prostatic hypertrophy. Dyspnea on exertion may result from lung disease, lack of exercise, and deconditioning. Lower extremity edema is commonly caused by venous insufficiency.

Among the acute manifestations of congestive heart failure in the elderly are increasing lethargy and confusion, probably the result of impaired cerebral perfusion. Activity intolerance is common. Instead of dyspnea, the prominent sign may be restlessness. Impaired perfusion of the gastrointestinal tract is a common cause of anorexia and profound loss of lean body mass. Loss of lean body mass may be masked by edema.

The elderly also maintain a precarious balance between the managed symptom state and acute symptom exacerbation. During the managed symptom state, they are relatively symptom free while adhering to their treatment regimen. Acute symptom exacerbation, often requiring emergency medical treatment, can be precipitated by seemingly minor conditions such as poor compliance with sodium restriction, infection, or stress. Failure to promptly seek medical care is a common cause of progressive acceleration of symptoms. The most common precipitating cause of acute symptom exacerbation in the hospital is the overzealous administration of intravenous fluids.[70]

Diagnosis and Treatment

The diagnosis of heart failure in the elderly is based on the history, physical examination, chest radiograph, and electrocardiographic findings. However, the presenting symptoms of congestive heart failure often are difficult to evaluate. Poor systemic perfusion may result in cerebrovascular accident, ischemia, confusional states, and symptoms of pulmonary embolism. These may so dominate the picture that underlying congestive failure is overlooked.

Treatment of congestive heart failure in the elderly involves many of the same methods as in younger persons. Activities are restricted to a level that is commensurate with the cardiac reserve. Seldom is bed rest recommended or advised. Bed rest causes rapid deconditioning of skeletal muscles and increases the risk of complications, such as orthostatic hypotension and thromboemboli. Instead, carefully prescribed exercise programs can help to maintain activity tolerance. Even walking around a room is usually preferable to continuous bed rest. Sodium restriction is usually indicated.

Age and disease-related changes increase the likelihood of adverse drug reactions and drug interactions. Drug dosage and the number of drugs that are prescribed should be kept to a minimum. Compliance with drug regimens is often difficult; the simpler the regimen, the more likely it is that the older person will comply. In general, the treatment plan for elderly persons with congestive heart failure must be put in the context of the person's overall needs. An improvement in the quality of life may take precedence over increasing the length of survival.

In summary, the mechanisms of heart failure in children and the elderly are similar to those in adults. However, the causes and manifestations may differ because of age. In children, congestive heart failure is most commonly seen during infancy and immediately after heart surgery. It can be caused by congenital and acquired heart defects and is characterized by fatigue, effort intolerance, cough, anorexia, abdominal pain, and impaired growth. Treatment of congestive heart failure in children includes correction of the underlying cause whenever possible. For congenital anomalies that are amenable to surgery, medical treatment is often needed for a time before surgery and is usually continued in the immediate postoperative period. For many children, only medical management can be provided.

In the elderly, age-related changes in cardiovascular functioning contribute to congestive heart failure but are not in themselves sufficient to cause heart failure. The manifestations of congestive failure are often different and superimposed on other disease conditions; therefore, congestive heart failure is often more difficult to diagnose in the elderly than in younger persons. Because the elderly are more susceptible to adverse drug reactions and have more problems with compliance, the number of drugs that are prescribed is kept to a minimum, and the drug regimen is kept as simple as possible.

REFERENCES

1. Agency for Health Care Policy and Research. (1994). Heart failure: Management of patients with a systolic dysfunction. *Clinical Practice Guidelines—Quick Reference Guide for Clinicians* 11, 1–25.
2. Alpert J.S., Becker P.C. (1993). Mechanisms and management of cardiogenic shock. *Critical Care Clinics* 9 (2), 205–218.
3. Colucci W.C., Braunwald E. (1997). Pathophysiology of heart failure. In Braunwald E. (Ed.). *Heart disease* (5th ed., pp. 394–420). Philadelphia: WB Saunders.
4. Daly P.A., Sole M.J. (1990). Myocardial catecholamines and the pathophysiology of heart failure. *Circulation* 82 (Suppl. I), I35–I43.
5. Mark. A.L. (1995). Sympathetic dysregulation in heart failure: Mechanisms and therapy. *Clinical Cardiology* 18 (3 Suppl. I), I3–I8.
6. Lorell B. (1992). Left ventricular hypertrophy. *Hospital Practice* 27(10), 189–209.
7. Kantner T.R. (1992). ACE inhibitors in congestive heart failure. *Journal of Family Practice* 35, 305–314.
8. Needleman P., Greenwald J.E. (1986). Atriopeptin: A cardiac hormone intimately involved in fluid, electrolyte, and blood-pressure homeostasis. *New England Journal of Medicine* 314 (13), 828.
9. Raine A.E.G., Pil D., Erne P. et al. (1986). Atrial natriuretic peptide and atrial pressure in patients with congestive heart failure. *New England Journal of Medicine* 315 (9), 533.
10. Bonow R.O., Udelson J.E. (1992). Left ventricular diastolic dysfunction as a cause of congestive heart failure. *Annals Internal Medicine* 117 (6), 502–510.
11. Sonnenblick E.H., LeJemtel T.H. (1993). Heart failure: Its progression and treatment. *Hospital Practice* (28)9, 121–130.
12. Androli T.E. (1991). Introduction: Modern aspects of congestive heart failure. *Hospital Practice* 26(4), 7–8.
13. Grossman W. (1991). Diastolic dysfunction in congestive heart failure. *New England Journal of Medicine* 325, 1557–1564.
14. Tresch D.D., McGough M.F. (1995). Heart failure with normal systolic function: A common disorder in older people.
15. Katz A.M. (1991). Energetics and the failing heart. *Hospital Practice* 26(8), 78–90.

16. Iga K., Konishi T, Matsumura T., Miyamoto T, Kujimak G.H. (1994). Markedly enlarged right atrium associated with physical signs of tricuspid regurgitation: A cause of congestive heart failure in the elderly. *Japanese Circulation Journal* 58 (9), 683–689.
17. Nava J.P. (1993). Pathophysiology of edema in congestive heart failure. *Heart Disease and Stroke* July / Aug, 325–329.
18. Mair F.S. (1996). Management of heart failure. *American Family Physician* 54 (1), 245–234.
19. Cohn J.N. (1996). The management of chronic heart failure. *New England Journal of Medicine.* 335 (7), 490–498.
20. Remme W.J. (1993). Congestive heart failure drug therapy: Central or peripheral approach. *Cardiologia* 18 (12 Suppl. 1), 51–59.
21. Moser D.K. (1933). Pharmacologic management of heart failure: Neurohormonal aspects. *Critical Care Clinics of North America* 5 (4), 599–608.
22. The SOLVD Investigators. (1991). Effect of enalapril on survival in patients with reduced left ventricular ejection fractions and congestive heart failure. *New England Journal of Medicine* 325, 293–302.
23. Ryden L. (1992). Heart failure management in the 1990s: The role of linisinopril. *American Journal of Cardiology* 70 (10), 1C–3C.
24. Coraim F.E., Wolner E. (1995). Continuous hemofiltration for the failing heart. *New Horizons* 3 (4), 725–731.
25. Drefus G.D. (1996). Hemopump 31, the sternotomy hemopump: Clinical experience. *Annals of Thoracic Surgery* 61 (1), 323–328.
26. Loisance D.Y., Pouillart F., Benvenuti C., et al. (1996). Mechanical bridge to transplantation: When is too early? When is too late? *Annals of Thoracic Surgery* 61 (1), 388–90.
27. Schigoda M. (1995). Congestive heart failure. In Urban N., Greenlee K., Krumberger J., Winkelman C. (Eds.). *Guidelines for critical care nursing* (pp. 163–175). St. Louis: C.V. Mosby.
28. United Network for Organ Sharing (UNOS). (1993). Statistics for 1991 compiled in 1993. Richmond, VA: UNOS.
29. Rafalowski M. (1991). The heterotropic heart transplant patient: Cardiac monitoring challenges. *Critical Care Nursing* 11, 28–30.
30. Futterman L.G., Lemberg L. (1996). Cardiomyoplasty: A potential alternative to cardiac transplantation. *American Journal of Critical Care* 5 (1), 80–86.
31. Pasternale R.C., Braunwald E. (1991). Acute myocardial infarction. In Wilson J.D. (Eds.). *Harrison's principles of internal medicine* (12th ed.). New York: McGraw-Hill.
32. Califf R.M., Bengton J.R. (1994). Cardiogenic shock. *New England Journal of Medicine* 330 (24), 1724–1730
33. Bone R.C. (1991). The pathogenesis of sepsis. *Annals of Internal Medicine* 115, 457–469.
34. Muehrcke D.D., McCarthy P.M., Foster R.C., Ogella D.A., Borsch J.A., Cosgrove D.M. (1996). Extracorporeal membrane oxygenation post cardiotomy cardiogenic shock. *Annals of Thoracic Surgery* 61 (2), 684–691.
35. Garber P.J., Mathieson A.L., Ducas J., Patton J.N., Geddes J.S., Prewitt R.M. (1995). Thrombolytic therapy for cardiogenic shock: Effect of increased intrathoracic pressure and rapid tPA administration. *Canadian Journal of Cardiology* 11 (1), 30–36.
36. Holmes D.R., Bates E.R., Kleiman N.S., et al. (1995). The GUSTO-I trial experience: Global utilization of streptokinase and plasminogen activator for occluded coronary arteries. *Journal American College Cardiology* 26 (3), 668–674.
37. Hochman J.S., Boland J., Sleeper L.A., et al. (1995). Current spectrum of cardiogenic shock and effect of early revascularization on mortality. *Circulation* 91 (3), 873–881.
38. Guyton A.C., Hall J.E. (1996). *Textbook of medical physiology* (9th ed., pp. 285–293). Philadelphia: W.B. Saunders.
39. Whitman G. (1988). Tissue perfusion. In McKinney M., Packa D., Dunbar S. (Eds.). *ACCN clinical reference for critical-care nursing* (2nd ed., p. 119). New York: McGraw-Hill.
40. Bochner B.S., Lichtenstein L.M. (1991). Anaphylaxis. *New England Journal of Medicine* 324, 1785–1790.
41. Stankiewicz J., Ruta W., Gorski P. (1995). Latex allergy. *International Journal of Occupational Medicine and Environmental Health* 8 (2), 139–148.
42. Leibovici L., Smara Z., Konigsberger H., Drucker M., Askenzi S., Pitlik S.D. (1995). Long-term survival following bacteremia or fungemia. *Journal of the American Medical Association* 274 (10), 897–812
43. Hazinski M.F., Iberti T.J., MacIntyre N.R., et al. (1993). Epidemiology, pathophysiology and clinical presentation of gram-negative sepsis. *American Journal of Critical Care* 2, 224–237.
44. Members of the American College of Chest Physicians/ Society of Critical Care Medicine Consensus Conference Committee. (1992). American College of Chest Physicians/ Society of Critical Care Medicine consensus conference: Definitions of sepsis and organ failure and guidelines for the use of innovative therapies in sepsis. *Critical Care Medicine* 20 (6), 864–874.
45. Parrillo J.E. (1995). Pathogenetic mechanisms of septic shock. *N Engl J Med* 328 (20), 1471–1477.
46. Girardin G., Dayer J.M. (1993). Cytokines and antagonists in septic shock. *Journal Suisse de Medicine* 123 (11), 480–491.
47. Gutierrez G. (1991). Cellular energy metabolism during hypoxia. *Critical Care Medicine* 19, 619–626.
48. Wiessner W.H., Casey L.C., Zbilut J.P. (1995). Treatment of sepsis and septic shock: A review. *Heart and Lung* 24, 380–392.
49. Werdan K., Pilg G. (1996). Supplemental immune globulins in sepsis: A critical appraisal. *Clinical and Experimental Immunology* 104 (Suppl. 1), 83–90.
50. Shands K.N., Schmid G.P., Bruce B.D. (1980). Association of tampon use and *Staphylococcus aureus* and clinical features in 52 cases. *New England Journal of Medicine* 303, 1436.
51. Taylor G., Myers S, Kurth C.D., et al. (1996). Hypertonic saline improves brain resuscitation in pediatric model of head injury and hemorrhagic shock. *Journal of Pediatric Surgery* 31 (1), 65–70.
52. Biro S.P., Ou C., Ryan-McFarlane C., Anderson P.D. (1995). Oxyradical generation after resuscitation of hemorrhagic shock with blood or stroma-free hemoglobin solution. *Artificial Cells, Blood Substitute and Immobilization Biotechnology* 23 (6), 631–645.
53. Shoemaker W.C., Pietzman A.B., Bellamy R., et al. (1996). Resuscitation from severe hemorrhage. *Critical Care Medicine* 24 (2 Suppl.), S12–S23.
54. Bunn H.F. (1995). The role of hemoglobin based blood substitutes in transfusion medicine. *Transfusion Clinique et Biologique* 39 (3), 453–456.
55. Chang F.C., Harrison P.B., Buck R.R., Helman S.D. (1995). PASG: Doesn't it help in management of traumatic shock. *Journal of Trauma* 39 (3), 453–456.
56. Vahedi M.H., Ayuyao A., Parsa M.H., Freeman H.P. (1995). Pneumatic anti-shock garment-associated compartment syndrome in uninjured lower extremities. *Journal of Trauma* 38 (4), 616–618.
57. Kyriakides Z.S., Koukoula A., Paraskevaidis I.A., et al. (1994). Does passive leg raising increase cardiac performance? *International Journal of Cardiology* 44 (3), 288–293.

58. Smith J.J., Kampine J.P. (1980). *Circulatory physiology* (p. 298). Baltimore: Williams & Wilkins.
59. Tuchschmidt J., Oblitas D., Fried J. (1991). Oxygen consumption in sepsis and septic shock. *Critical Care Medicine* 19, 664–671.
60. Jerjes-Sanchez C., Ramrex A., Arraga R., Pimental G. (1993). High does and the rapid infusion of streptokinase for treatment of massive pulmonary thromboembolism. *Archives del Instituto de Cardiolgia de Mexico* 63 (3), 227–234.
61. Krafft P., Fridrich P., Fitygerald R.D., Koc D., Stltzer H. (1996). Effectiveness of nitric oxide inhalation in septic ARDS. *Chest* 109 (2), 486–493.
62. Park J.H., Chang S.H., Lee K.M., Shin S.H. (1996). Protective effect of nitric oxide on endotoxin-induced septic shock. *American Journal of Surgery* 171 (3), 340–345.
63. Mitsuhata H., Shimiqu R., Yokoyama M.M. (1995). Role of nitric oxide in anaphylactic shock. *Journal of Clinical Immunology* 15 (6), 277–283.
64. Fink M. (1991). Gastrointestinal mucosal injury in experimental models of shock, trauma and sepsis. *Critical Care Medicine* 19, 627–641.
65. Collins A.S. (1990). Gastrointestinal complications in shock. *Critical Care Clinics of North America* 2 (2), 269–276.
66. Bakker J., Gris P., Coffernils M., Kahn R.J., Vincent J.L. (1996). Serial lactate levels can predict the development of multiple organ failure following septic shock. *American Journal of Surgery* 171 (2), 221–226.
67. Hazinski F.H. (1992). *Nursing care of the critically ill child* (2nd ed., pp. 156–170). St. Louis: C.V. Mosby.
68. Ruggerie D.P. (1990). Congestive heart failure. In Blumer J.L. (Ed.). *A practical guide to pediatric intensive care* (3rd ed., pp. 104–119). St. Louis: Mosby-Year Book.
69. Behrman R.E., Kliegman R.M., Nelson W.E., Vaughan V.C. (1992). *Nelson's textbook of pediatrics* (14th ed., pp. 1213–1216). Philadelphia: W.B. Saunders.
70. Luchi R.J., Taffet G.E., Teasdale T.A. (1991). Congestive heart failure in the elderly. *Journal of the American Geriatric Society* 39, 810–825.
71. Taffet G.E., Teasdale T.A., Bleyer A.J., et al. (1992). Survival of elderly men with congestive heart failure. *Age and Ageing* 21, 49–55.
72. Vinson J.M., Rich M.W., Sperry J.C., et al. (1990). Early readmission of elderly patients with congestive heart failure. *Journal of the American Geriatric Society* 38, 1290–1295.
73. Alpert M.A. (1984). Cardiac failure in the elderly. *American Family Practice* September, 123.

ADDITIONAL READINGS

Brown A.F. (1995). Anaphylactic shock: Mechanisms and treatment. *Journal of Accident and Emergency Medicine* 12 (2), 89–100.

Exstad B.L. (1994). Oxygen transport goals for resuscitation of critically ill patients. *Journal of Pharmacotherapy* 28 (11), 1273–1284

Francis G.S., Chu C. (1994). Compensatory and maladaptive responses to cardiac dysfunction. *Current Opinion in Cardiology* 9 (3), 280–288.

Proulx F., Fayon M., Farrell C.A., Lacroiz J., Gautheir M. (1996). Epidemiology of sepsis and multiple organ dysfunction syndrome in children. *Chest* 109 (4), 1033–1037.

Hachamovitch R, Chang J.D, Kuntz R.E., Papageorgiou R., Levin M.S., Goldberger M. (1995). Recurrent reversible cardiogenic shock triggered by emotional distress with non obstructive coronary disease. *American Heart Journal* 129 (5), 1026–1028.

Marcus F.I. (1992). Use and toxicity of digitalis. *Heart Disease and Stroke* 1, 27–31.

Pittet D., Hlliger S., Auckenthraler R. (1995). Intravascular device related infections in critically ill patients. *Journal of Chemotherapy* 7 (Suppl. 3), 55–66.

Treasure C.B., Alexander R.W. (1993). The dysfunctional endothelium in heart failure. *Journal of American College of Cardiology* 22 (4 Suppl. A), 129A–134A.

CHAPTER 21

Disorders of Cardiac Conduction and Rhythm

Jill White

Heart muscle is unique among other muscles in that it is capable of generating and rapidly conducting its own action potentials (*i.e.*, electrical impulses). These action potentials result in excitation of muscle fibers throughout the myocardium. Impulse formation and conduction results in weak electrical currents that spread throughout the entire body. When electrodes are applied to various positions on the body and connected to an electrocardiographic machine, an electrocardiogram (ECG) can be recorded. An ECG is a graphic recording of the electrical impulses of the heart.

Cardiac Conduction System

After you have completed this section of the chapter, you should be able to meet the following objectives:

- Describe the cardiac conduction system and relate it to the mechanical functioning of the heart
- Characterize the four phases of a cardiac action potential and differentiate between the fast and slow responses
- Draw an electrocardiogram (ECG) tracing and state the origin of the component parts of the tracing

In certain areas of the heart, myocardial cells have been modified to form specialized cells of the conduction system. Although most myocardial cells are capable of initiating and conducting impulses, it is this specialized conduction system that maintains the pumping efficiency of the heart. Specialized pacemaker cells *generate* impulses at a faster rate than other types of heart tissue, and the conduction tissue *transmits* impulses at a faster rate than other types of heart tissue. Because of these properties, the conduction system generally controls the rhythm of the heart.

The sinoatrial (SA) node has the fastest intrinsic rate (60 to 100 beats per minute) and is normally the *pacemaker* of the heart. It is located in the posterior wall of the right atrium near the entrance of the superior vena cava. Impulses originating in the SA node travel through the atria to the atrioventricular (AV) node (Fig. 21–1). Because of the anatomic location of the SA node, the progression of atrial depolarization occurs in an inferior, leftward, and somewhat posterior direction, and the right atrium is depolarized slightly before the left atrium.[1] There are at least four intraatrial pathways, including Bachmann's bundle, that connect the SA and AV nodes.[2]

The heart essentially has two conduction systems: one controls atrial activity and the other controls ventricular activity. The AV node is located in the posterior septal wall of the right atrium immediately behind the tricuspid valve,[3] and it connects these two systems. Within the AV node, atrial fibers connect with very small junctional fibers of the node itself. The velocity of conduction through these fibers is very slow (approximately one half that of normal cardiac muscle), which greatly delays transmission of the impulse into the AV node.[3] A further delay occurs as the

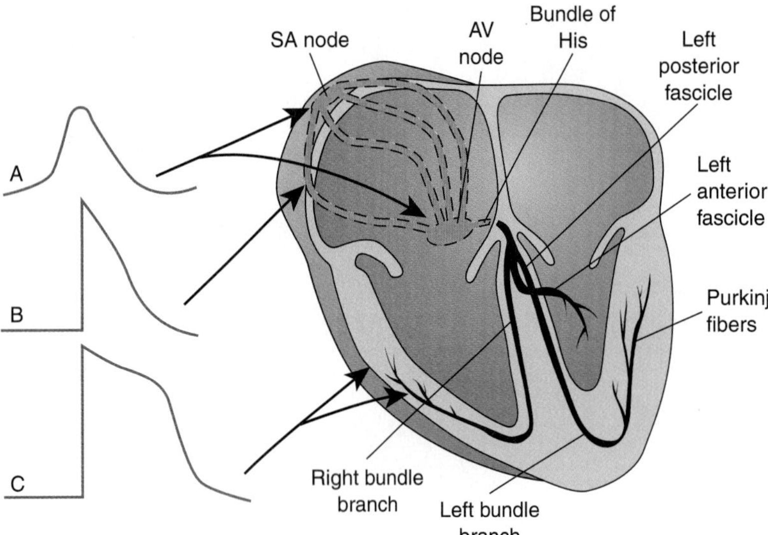

Figure 21–1
Conduction system of the heart and action potentials. (**A**) Action potential of sinoatrial (SA) and atrioventricular (AV) nodes; (**B**) atrial muscle action potential; (**C**) action potential of ventricular muscle and Purkinje fibers.

impulse travels through the AV node into the transitional fibers and into the bundle of His, also called the AV bundle. These delays provide a mechanical advantage whereby the atria complete ejection of blood before initiating ventricular contraction. Under normal circumstances, the AV node provides the only connection between the two conduction systems.[4] The atria and the ventricles would beat independently of each other if the transmission of impulses through the AV node were blocked.

The Purkinje system, which supplies the ventricles, has large fibers that allow for rapid conduction and almost simultaneous excitation of the entire right and left ventricles (0.06 second).[3] This rapid rate of conduction throughout the Purkinje system is necessary for the swift and efficient ejection of blood from the heart. The Purkinje fibers originate in the AV node and proceed to form the bundle of His, which extends through the fibrous tissue between the valves of the heart and into the ventricular system. Because of its proximity to the aortic valve and the mitral valve ring, the His bundle is predisposed to inflammation and deposits of calcific debris that can interfere with impulse conduction.[3,5] The bundle of His penetrates into the ventricles and almost immediately divides into right and left bundle branches that straddle the interventricular septum. The bundle branches move through the subendocardial tissues toward the papillary muscles and then subdivide into the Purkinje fibers, which branch out and supply the outer walls of the ventricles. The main trunk of the left bundle branch extends for approximately 1 to 2 cm before fanning out as it enters the septal area and divides further into two segments: the left posterior and left anterior fascicles.

Action Potentials

Action potentials are electrical currents generated by nerve and muscle cells. They involve the movement or flow of electrically charged ions at the level of the cell membrane and consist of three types of electrical events: the resting membrane potential, depolarization, and repolarization.

During the *resting state,* the membrane is relatively permeable to potassium but much less so to sodium and calcium.[3] Charges of opposite polarity become aligned along the membrane (positive on the outside and negative on the inside) (Fig. 21–2).

Depolarization occurs when the cell membrane suddenly becomes selectively permeable to current-carrying ions such as sodium. Sodium ions enter the cell and result in a sharp rise of intracellular potential to positivity, while potassium ions migrate to the outside of the cell membrane.

Repolarization involves the reestablishment of the resting potential. It is a somewhat slower process and involves the inward flow of electrical charges, and the membrane potential becomes reversed so that the inside becomes negative in relation to the outside.[6] The membrane conductance or permeability for potassium greatly increases, allowing the positively charged potassium ions to move outward across the membrane. This outward movement of potassium removes positive charges from

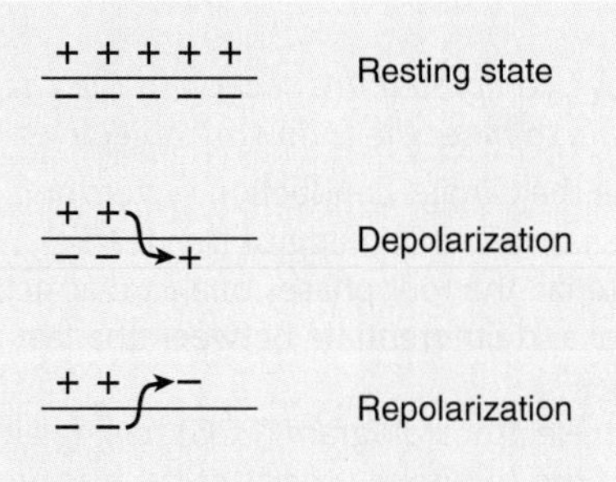

Figure 21–2
The flow of charge during impulse generation in excitable tissue. During the resting state, opposite charges are separated by the cell membrane. Depolarization represents the flow of charge across the membrane, and repolarization denotes the return of the membrane potential to its resting state.

inside the cell, also contributing to the membrane again becoming negative on the inside and positive on the outside. The sodium-potassium membrane pump also assists in repolarization by pumping positively charged sodium ions out across the cell membrane. The sodium-potassium pump helps to preserve the intracellular negativity by moving three sodium ions out of the cell in exchange for two potassium ions.[7]

Phases

The action potential of the cardiac muscle cell is divided into five phases (Fig. 21–3):

Phase 0: rapid depolarization

Phase 1: brief period of repolarization

Phase 2: plateau phase of repolarization

Phase 3: end of repolarization

Phase 4: resting membrane potential

During phase 0, membrane permeability to sodium increases rapidly, resulting in the fast inward movement of current through the fast channels. This rapid influx of sodium produces the rapid electrical spike and overshoot during phase 0 of the action potential.[8] The rapid depolarization that comprises phase 0 is responsible for the QRS complex on the ECG (Fig. 21–4).

Phase 1 occurs at the peak of the action potential and signifies inactivation of the fast sodium channels with an abrupt decrease in sodium permeability. The slight downward slope is believed to be caused by the influx of a small amount of negatively charged chloride ions and efflux of potassium.[9]

Phase 2 represents the plateau of the action potential. If potassium permeability increased to its resting level at this time, as it does in nerve fibers or skeletal muscle, the cell would repolarize rapidly. Instead, potassium permeability is low, allowing the membrane to remain depolarized throughout the phase 2 plateau of the action potential. Contributing to phase 2 is an influx of calcium into the cell through slow channels. Calcium ions entering the muscle during this phase of the action potential play a key role in the contractile process. These unique features of phase 2 plateau in these cells cause the action potential of cardiac muscle to last 20 to 50 times longer than that of skeletal muscle and cause a corresponding increased period of contraction.[2] The phase 2 plateau is believed to be responsible for the ST segment of the ECG.

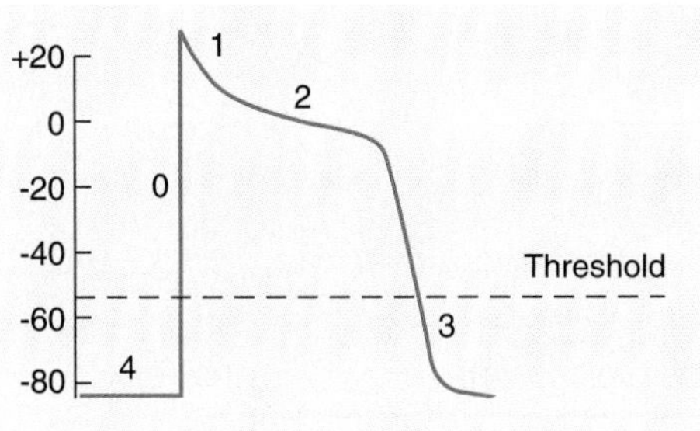

Figure 21–3
Action potential of cardiac muscle cells. In the fast response that occurs in myocardial cells of atrial and ventricular muscle, the phases are identified by numbers: phase 4, resting membrane potential; phase 0, depolarization; phase 1, brief period of repolarization; phase 2, plateau; phase 3, repolarization.

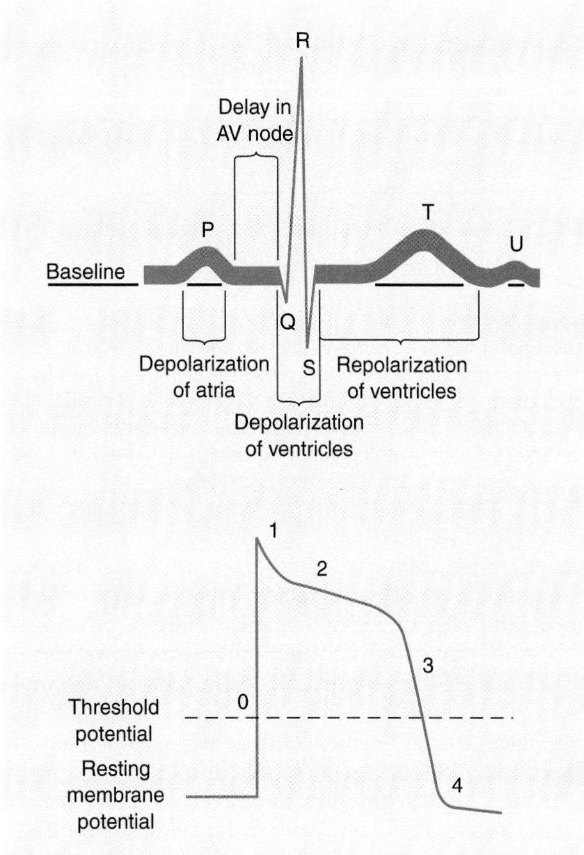

Figure 21–4
Relation between (**A**) the electrocardiogram and (**B**) ventricular action potential.

Phase 3 begins with the downslope of the action potential and represents the repolarization phase. During the phase 3 repolarization period, the slow channels close and the influx of calcium and sodium ceases. There is a sharp rise in potassium permeability. The rapid outward movement of potassium during this phase facilitates the reestablishment of the resting membrane potential. At the conclusion of phase 3, distribution of sodium and potassium returns to the normal resting state. The T wave on the ECG corresponds with phase 3 of the action potential.

Phase 4 is the resting membrane potential. During phase 4, the sodium-potassium pump is activated, whereby sodium is actively transported out of the cell and potassium is moved back into the cell. Phase 4 corresponds to diastole.

There are two main types of action potentials in the heart. The *fast response* occurs in the normal myocardial cells of the atria, the ventricles, and the Purkinje fibers (see Fig. 21–3). The amplitude and the rate of rise of phase 1 are important to the conduction velocity of the

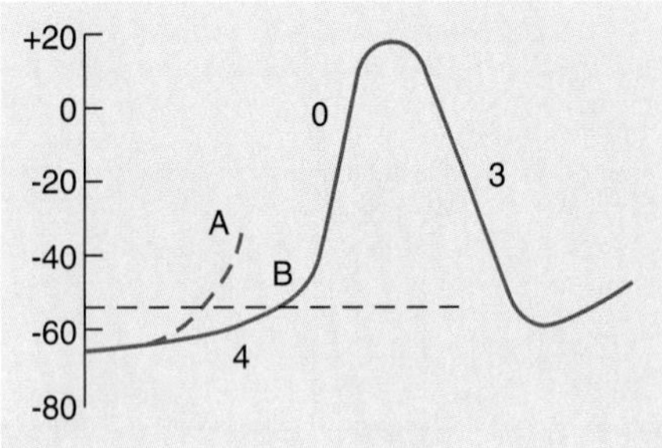

Figure 21–5
Action potential of pacemaker cells. In the sinoatrial and atrioventricular nodes, the slow response is characterized by a slow, spontaneous rise in the phase 4 membrane potential to threshold levels; it has a lesser amplitude and shorter duration than the fast response. Increased automaticity (*A*) occurs when the rate of phase 4 depolarization is increased.

fast response. Myocardial fibers with a fast response are capable of conducting electrical activity at relatively rapid rates (0.5 to 5.0 m/second), thereby providing a high safety factor for conduction.[10] The *slow response*, is found in the SA node, which is the natural pacemaker of the heart, and the conduction fibers of the AV node (Fig. 21–5). Under normal conditions, the slow response, sometimes referred to as the calcium current, does not contribute significantly to depolarization. Its primary role in normal atrial and ventricular cells is the entrance of calcium during systole. The key role of calcium is the excitation-contraction mechanism. The slow response may be the primary mode of depolarization in the presence of hyperkalemia.[2] The hallmark of these pacemaker cells is a spontaneous phase 4 depolarization. The membrane permeability of these cells allows a slow inward leak of current to occur through the slow channels during phase 4. This leak continues until the threshold for firing is reached, at which point the cell spontaneously depolarizes.

The rate of pacemaker cell discharge varies with the resting membrane potential and the slope of phase 4 depolarization. Catecholamines (*i.e.*, epinephrine and norepinephrine) increase the heart rate by increasing the slope or rate of phase 4. Acetylcholine, which is released during vagal stimulation of the heart, decreases the slope of phase 4.

The fast response of atrial and ventricular muscle can be converted to a slow pacemaker response under certain conditions. For example, such conversions may occur spontaneously in individuals with severe coronary artery disease, in areas of the heart where blood supply has been markedly compromised or curtailed. Impulses generated by these cells can lead to ectopic beats and serious arrhythmias.

Refractory Period

The pumping action of the heart requires alternating contraction and relaxation. There is a period in the action potential curve during which no stimuli can generate another action potential (Fig. 21–6). This period is known as the *absolute refractory period*, and it includes phases 0, 1, 2, and part of phase 3. The absolute refractory period is followed by the *relative refractory period*, during which a more intense stimulus is needed to initiate an action potential. The relative refractory period begins when the transmembrane potential in phase 3 reaches the threshold potential level and ends just before the terminal portion of phase 3. After the relative refractory period is a supernormal excitatory period during which a weak stimulus can evoke a response. The supernormal excitatory period extends from the terminal portion of phase 3 until the beginning of phase 4. It is during this period that cardiac dysrhythmias develop.

In skeletal muscle, the refractory period is very short compared with the duration of contraction, such that a second contraction can be initiated before the first is over, resulting in a summated tetanized contraction. In cardiac muscle, the absolute refractory period is almost as long as the contraction, and a second contraction cannot be stimulated until the first is over. The longer length of the absolute refractory period of cardiac muscle is important in maintaining the alternating contraction and relaxation that is essential to the pumping action of the heart and for the prevention of fatal dysrhythmias.

Electrocardiography

The ECG is a recording of the electrical activity of the heart. The electric currents generated by the heart spread through the body to the skin, where they can be sensed by appropriately placed electrodes, amplified, and viewed on an oscilloscope or chart recorder. The deflection points of an ECG are designated by the letters P, Q, R, S, and T. Figure 21–7 depicts the electrical activity of the conduction system on an ECG tracing. The P wave represents the SA node and atrial depolariza-

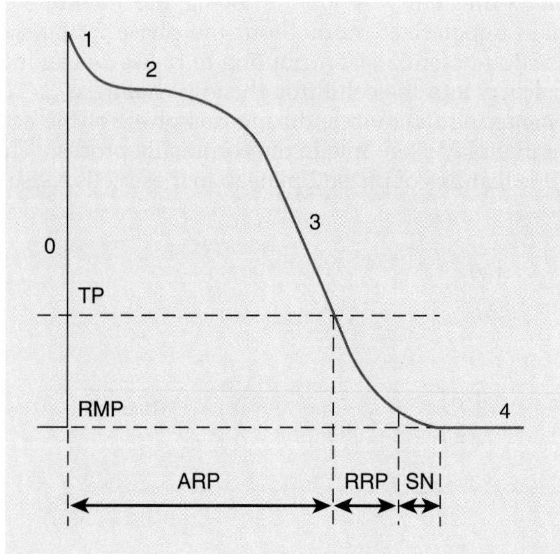

Figure 21–6
Diagram of an action potential of a ventricular muscle cell, showing the resting membrane potential (RMP), absolute refractory period (ARP), relative refractory period (RRP), and supernormal (SN) period.

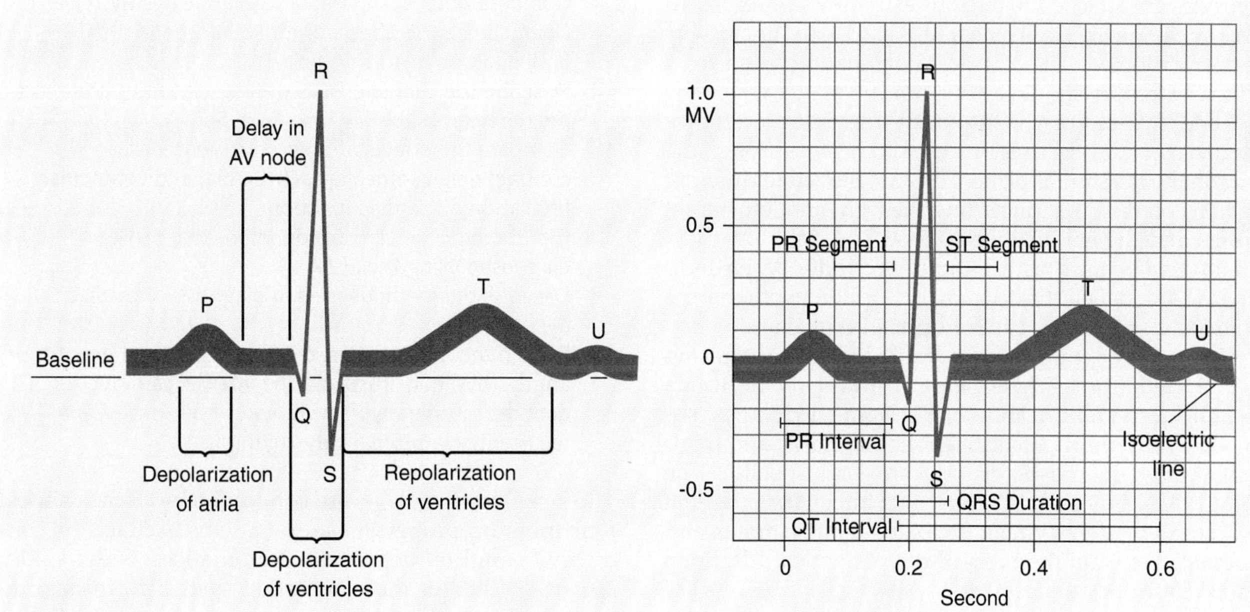

Figure 21–7
Diagram of the electrocardiogram (lead II) and representative depolarization and repolarization of the atria and ventricle. The P wave represents atrial depolarization, the QRS complex ventricular depolarization, and the T wave ventricular repolarization. Atrial repolarization occurs during ventricular depolarization and is hidden under the QRS complex.'

tion; the QRS complex (*i.e.*, beginning of the Q wave to the end of the S wave) represents ventricular depolarization; and the T wave represents ventricular repolarization. The isoelectric line between the P wave and the Q wave represents depolarization of the AV node, bundle branches, and Purkinje system (Fig. 21–8). Atrial repolarization occurs during ventricular depolarization and is hidden in the QRS complex.

The ECG records the potential difference in charge (in millivolts [mV]) that occurs between two electrodes as the depolarization and repolarization waves move through the heart and are conducted to the skin surface. The shape of the recorder tracing is determined by the direction in which the impulse spreads through the heart muscle in relation to electrode placement. A depolarization wave that moves toward the recording electrode registers as a positive, or upward, deflection. Conversely, if the impulse moves away from the recording electrode, the deflection is downward, or negative. When there is no flow of charge between electrodes, the potential is zero, and a straight line is recorded at the baseline of the chart.

The ECG recorder is much like a camera in that it can record different views of the electrical activity of the heart, depending on where the recording electrode is placed. The horizontal axis of the ECG measures time (seconds), and the vertical axis measures the amplitude of the impulse (mV). Each heavy vertical black line represents 0.2 second, and each thin black line represents 0.04 second (see Fig. 21–7). The width of ECG complexes are commonly referred to in terms of duration of time. On the vertical axis, each heavy horizontal line represents 0.5 mV. The connections of the ECG are arranged such that an upright deflection indicates a positive potential and a downward deflection indicates a negative potential. Although the vertical axis determines amplitude in terms of voltage, these values are frequently communicated as millimeters (mm) of positive or negative deflection rather than in volts.

Conventionally, 12 leads are recorded for a diagnostic ECG, each providing a unique view of the electrical forces of the heart from a different position on the body's surface. Six limb leads view the electrical forces as they pass through the heart on the frontal or vertical plane. The

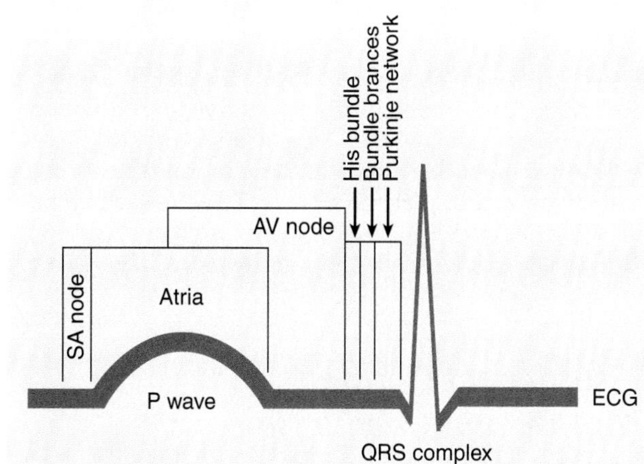

Figure 21–8
Tissues depolarized by a wave of activation commencing in the sinoatrial (SA) node are shown in a series of blocks superimposed on the deflections of the electrocardiogram (ECG). (Katz A.M. [1992]. *Physiology of the heart* [p. 483]. New York: Raven Press)

electrodes are attached to the four extremities or representative areas on the body near the shoulders and lower chest or abdomen. The electrical potential recorded from any one extremity should be the same no matter where the electrode is placed on the extremity. Chest electrodes provide a view of the electrical forces as they pass through the heart on the horizontal plane. They are moved to different positions on the chest, including the right and left sternal borders and the left anterior surface. The right lower extremity lead is used as a ground electrode. When indicated, additional electrodes may be applied to other areas of the body, such as the back or right anterior chest.

The goals of continuous bedside cardiac monitoring have shifted from simple heart rate and dysrhythmia monitoring to identification of ST segment changes, advanced dysrhythmia identification, diagnosis, and treatment. Many diagnostic criteria are lead specific. The monitoring leads selected must maximize the potential for accurately identifying anticipated dysrhythmias and ischemic events on the basis of the patient's underlying clinical situation.

In summary, the rhythmic contraction and relaxation of the heart rely on the specialized cells of the heart's conduction system. Specialized cells in the SA node have the fastest inherent rate of impulse generation and act as the pacemaker of the heart. Impulses from the SA node travel through the atria to the AV node and then to the AV bundle and the ventricular Purkinje system. The AV node provides the only connection between the atrial and ventricular conduction systems. The atria and the ventricles function independently of each other when AV node conduction is blocked.

The action potential of cardiac muscle is divided into five phases: phase 0 represents depolarization and is characterized by the rapid upstroke of the action potential; phase 1 is characterized by a brief period of repolarization; phase 2 consists of a plateau, which prolongs the duration of the action potential; phase 3 represents repolarization; and phase 4 is the resting membrane potential. After an action potential, there is a refractory period during which the membrane is resistant to a second stimulus. During the absolute refractory period, the membrane is insensitive to stimulation. This period is followed by the relative refractory period, during which a more intense stimulus is needed to initiate an action potential. The relative refractory period is followed by a supernormal excitatory period, during which a weak stimulus can evoke a response.

Disorders of Cardiac Rhythm and Conduction

After you have completed this section of the chapter, you should be able to meet the following objectives:

- Describe the possible mechanisms for dysrhythmia generation
- Compare sinus dysrhythmia with atrial dysrhythmia
- Characterize the effects of atrial flutter and atrial fibrillation on heart rhythm
- Describe the characteristics of first-, second-, and third-degree heart block
- Compare the effects of premature ventricular contractions, ventricular tachycardia, and ventricular fibrillation on cardiac function
- Cite the types of cardiac conditions that can be diagnosed using the ECG
- Describe the methods used in diagnosis of cardiac dysrhythmias
- Explain the mechanisms, criteria for use, and benefits of antidysrhythmic drugs and the internal cardioverter defibrillator therapy in treatment of persons with recurrent, symptomatic dysrhythmias

The specialized cells in the conduction system manifest four inherent properties: automaticity, excitability, conductivity, and refractoriness. Automaticity is the ability of certain cells of the conduction system to initiate repeated, spontaneous production of action potentials.[11] Excitability refers to the ability of a cell to respond to external stimuli. These stimuli may be in the form of chemical, mechanical, or electrical input. All cardiac cells have the ability to conduct impulses. It is this ability that allows the heart to function in a synchronous fashion. Refractoriness is a protective mechanism that prevents the cells from responding to repeated rapidly occurring external stimulation.

The term *dysrhythmia* refers to an alteration in cardiac rhythm. An alteration in any of these properties may produce dysrhythmias or conduction defects. There are many causes of altered cardiac rhythms, including congenital defects of the conduction system, degenerative changes, ischemia and myocardial infarction, fluid and electrolyte imbalances, and the effects of drug ingestion. Dysrhythmias are not necessarily pathologic; they can occur in healthy and diseased hearts. Disturbances in cardiac rhythms exert their harmful effects by interfering with the heart's pumping ability. Rapid heart rates reduce the diastolic filling time, causing a subsequent decrease in the stroke volume output and in coronary perfusion while increasing the myocardial oxygen needs. Abnormally slow heart rates may impair the blood flow to vital organs such as the brain.

Mechanisms of Dysrhythmias and Conduction Disorders

The ability of certain cells of the conduction system to spontaneously initiate an impulse or action potential is referred to as *automaticity*. The SA node has an inherent discharge rate of 60 to 100 times per minute. It normally acts as the pacemaker of the heart, because it reaches the threshold for excitation before other parts of the conduction system have recovered sufficiently to be depolarized. If the SA node fires more slowly or the SA node conduction is blocked, another site that is capable of automaticity takes over as pacemaker. Other regions that are capable of automaticity include the atrial fibers that have plateau-type action potentials, the AV node, the bundle of His, and the bundle-branch Purkinje fibers. These pacemakers have a slower rate of discharge than the SA node. The AV node has an inherent firing rate of 40 to 60 times per minute, and the Purkinje system fires at a rate of 30 to 40 times per minute. The SA node may be functioning properly, but because of other precipitating factors, other cardiac cells can assume accelerated properties of automaticity and begin to initiate impulses. These other factors include injury, hypoxia, electrolyte disturbances, enlargement or hypertrophy of the atria or ventricles, and exposure to certain chemicals or drugs.

An *ectopic pacemaker* is an excitable focus outside the normally functioning SA node. These pacemakers can reside in other parts of the conduction system or in the muscle cells of the atria or ventricles. A premature contraction occurs when an ectopic pacemaker initiates a beat. Premature contractions do not follow the normal conduction pathways, they are not coupled with normal mechanical events, and they often render the heart refractory or incapable of responding to the next normal impulse arising in the SA node. They occur without incident in persons with healthy hearts in response to sympathetic nervous system stimulation or other stimulants such as caffeine. In the diseased heart, the premature contraction may lead to more serious dysrhythmias.

Excitability describes the ability of a cell to respond to an impulse and generate an action potential. Myocardial cells that have been injured or replaced by scar tissue do not possess normal excitability. For example, during the acute phase of an ischemic event, involved cells become depolarized. These ischemic cells remain electrically coupled to the adjacent nonischemic area; current from the ischemic zone can induce reexcitation of cells in the nonischemic zone.

Conductivity is the ability to conduct impulses, and *refractoriness* refers to the extent to which the cell is able to respond to an incoming stimulus. The refractory period of cardiac muscle is the interval in the repolarization period during which an excitable cell has not recovered sufficiently to be reexcited. Disturbances in conductivity or refractoriness predispose to dysrhythmias.

An important condition in the development of dysrhythmias is the phenomenon called *reentry*. Under normal conditions, an electrical impulse is conducted through the heart in an orderly, sequential manner. The electrical impulse then dies out and does not reenter adjacent tissue because that tissue has already been depolarized and is refractory to immediate stimulation. However, under certain abnormal conditions, an impulse can reenter an area of myocardium that was previously depolarized and depolarize it again.[12] This activity disrupts the normal conduction sequence. For reentry to occur, there must be areas of slow conduction and unidirectional conduction block (Fig. 21–9). For previously depolarized areas to repolarize adequately enough to conduct an impulse again, slow conduction is necessary. Unidirectional block is necessary to provide a one-way route for the original impulse to reenter, thereby blocking other impulses entering from the opposite direction that might extinguish the reentrant circuit. Reentry requires a triggering stimulus such as an extrasystole. If sufficient time has elapsed for the refractory period in the reentered area to have ended, a self-perpetuating circuitous-type movement can be initiated.

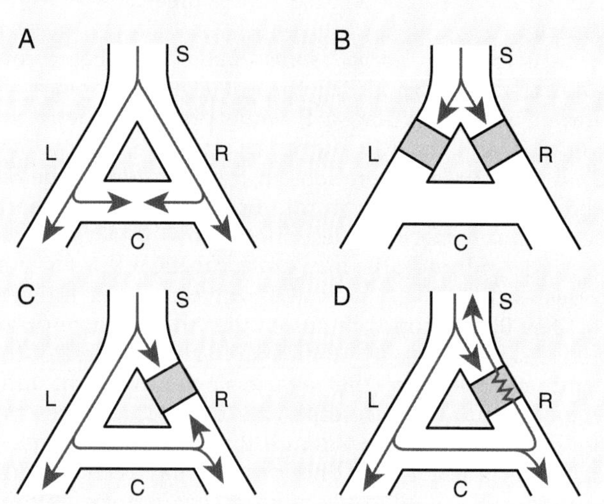

Figure 21–9
The role of unidirectional block in reentry. (**A**) An excitation wave traveling down a single bundle (S) of fibers continues down the left (L) and right (R) branches. The depolarization wave enters the connecting branch (C) from both ends and is extinguished at the zone of collision. (**B**) The wave is blocked in the L and R branches. (**C**) Bidirectional block exists in branch R. The antegrade impulse is blocked, but the retrograde impulse is conducted through and reenters bundle S. (Berne R.M., Levy M.N. [1993]. *Physiology* [3rd ed., p. 385]. St. Louis: C.V. Mosby)

Reentry may occur anywhere in the conduction system. The functional components of a reentry circuit can be large and include an entire specialized conduction system, or it can be microscopic. It can include myocardial tissue, AV nodal cells, or junctional tissue. Factors contributing to the development of a reentrant circuit include ischemia, infarct, and elevated serum potassium levels.[11] Scar tissue interrupts the normally low resistance paths between viable myocardial cells, slowing conduction, promoting asynchronous myocardial activation, and predisposing to unidirectional conduction block. Specially filtered signal-averaged electrocardiography can be used to detect the resultant *late potentials.* Effects of drugs such as epinephrine can produce a shortened refractory period, thereby increasing the likelihood of reentrant dysrhythmias.

Types of Dysrhythmias

Sinus Node Dysrhythmias

In a healthy heart driven by sinus node discharge, the rate ranges between 60 and 100 beats per minute. On the

ECG, a P wave may be observed to precede every QRS complex.

Historically, *normal sinus rhythm* has been considered the "normal" rhythm of a healthy heart. In normal sinus rhythm, a P wave precedes each QRS complex and the RR intervals remain relatively constant over time. Alterations in the function of the SA node lead to changes in rate or rhythm of the heartbeat. *Sinus bradycardia* describes a slow heart rate (<60 beats per minute). In sinus bradycardia, a P wave precedes each QRS. A normal P wave and PR interval (0.12 to 0.20 second) indicates that the impulse originated in the SA node rather than in another area of the conduction system that has a slower inherent rate. Vagal stimulation decreases the firing rate of the SA node and conduction through the AV node to cause a decrease in heart rate. This rhythm may be normal in trained athletes who maintain a large stroke volume and during sleep. Sinus bradycardia may be an indicator of poor prognosis when it occurs in conjunction with acute myocardial infarction, particularly if associated with hypotension.

Years ago, it was believed that sinus rhythm should be regular; that is, all RR intervals should be equal. Today, it is accepted that a more optimal rhythm is *respiratory sinus dysrhythmia*. Respiratory sinus dysrhythmia is a cardiac rhythm characterized by gradually lengthening and shortening of RR intervals. This variation in heart cycles is related to intrathoracic pressure changes that occur with respiration and resultant alterations in autonomic control of the SA node. Inspiration causes acceleration of the heart rate, and expiration causes slowing. Respiratory sinus dysrhythmia accounts for most heart rate variability in healthy individuals. Decreased heart rate variability has been associated with altered health states, including myocardial infarction, congestive heart failure, hypertension, diabetes mellitus, and premature infants.

Sinus tachycardia refers to a rapid heart rate (>100 beats per minute) that has its origin in the SA node. A normal P wave and PR interval should precede each QRS complex. The mechanism of sinus tachycardia is enhanced automaticity related to sympathetic stimulation or withdrawal of vagal tone. Sinus tachycardia is a normal response during fever and exercise and in situations that incite sympathetic stimulation. It may be associated with congestive heart failure, myocardial infarction, and hyperthyroidism. Pharmacologic agents such as atropine, isoproterenol, epinephrine, and quinidine also can cause sinus tachycardia.

Sinus arrest refers to failure of the SA node to discharge and results in an irregular pulse. An escape rhythm develops as another pacemaker takes over. Sinus arrest may result in prolonged periods of asystole and often predisposes to other dysrhythmias. Causes of sinus arrest include disease of the SA node, digitalis toxicity, myocar-

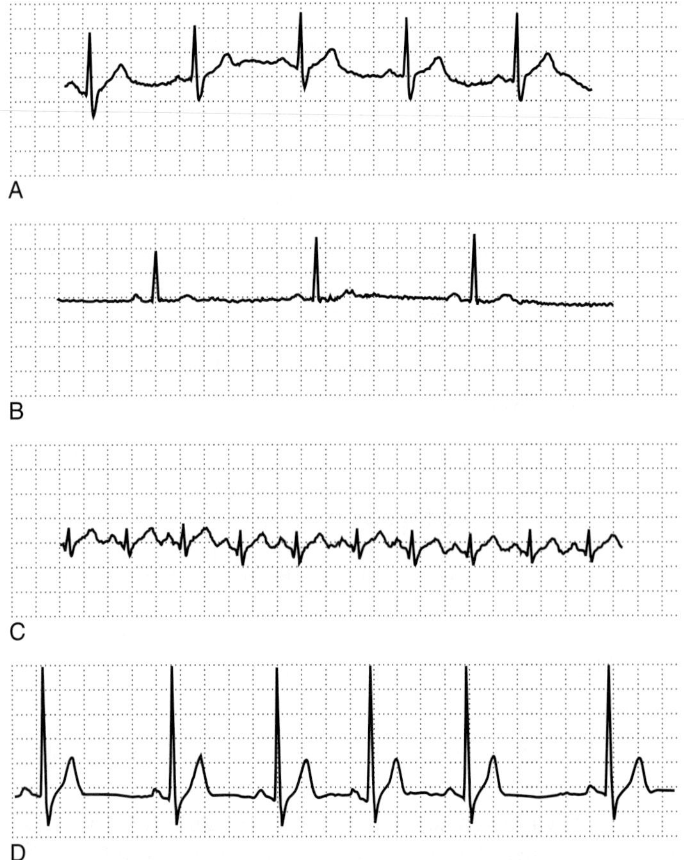

Figure 21–10
Electrocardiographic (ECG) tracings of rhythms originating in the sinus node. **(A)** Normal sinus rhythm (60 to 100 beats/minute). **(B)** Sinus bradycardia (<60 beats/minute). **(C)** Sinus tachycardia (>100 beats/minute). **(D)** Respiratory sinus dysrhythmia, characterized by gradually lengthening and shortening of R-R intervals.

dial infarction, acute myocarditis, excessive vagal tone, quinidine, acetylcholine, and hyperkalemia or hypokalemia.[13] Figure 21–10 illustrates some examples of sinus rhythms and dysrhythmias.

Sick sinus syndrome is a term that describes a number of forms of cardiac impulse formation and intraatrial and AV conduction abnormalities.[14] Some of these types of dysfunction include marked sinus bradycardia, prolonged sinus pauses, and sinoatrial block. The most common use of the term is for a rhythm that consists of periods of bradycardia alternating with tachycardia.[15] The bradycardia is caused by disease of the sinus node (or other intraatrial conduction pathways), and the tachycardia is caused by paroxysmal atrial or junctional dysrhythmias. Individuals with this syndrome often are asymptomatic. Ironically, the development of atrial fibrillation may alleviate symptoms in persons who are symptomatic.[14]

Dysrhythmias That Originate in the Atria

Impulses from the SA node pass through the conductive pathways in the atria to the AV node. *Premature atrial complexes* (PACs) can originate in the atrial conduction pathways or in atrial muscle cells, and they occur before the next expected sinus impulse. This impulse to contract is usually transmitted to the ventricle and back to the SA node. The location of the ectopic focus determines the configuration of the P wave. Generally, the closer the ectopic focus is to the SA node, the more the ectopic complex resembles a normal sinus complex. The retrograde transmission to the SA node often interrupts the timing of the next sinus beat, such that a pause occurs between the two normally conducted beats. In healthy individuals, PACs may be the result of stress, tobacco, or caffeine. They are also associated with myocardial infarction, digitalis toxicity, low serum potassium or magnesium levels, and hypoxia.

Paroxysmal Supraventricular Tachycardia. Paroxysmal supraventricular tachycardia (PSVT), sometimes referred to as paroxysmal atrial tachycardia (PAT), include all tachycardias that originate above the bifurcation of the bundle of His and has a sudden onset and offset. They may be the result of AV nodal reentry, Wolff-Parkinson-White syndrome, or intraatrial or sinus node reentry. Paroxysmal supraventricular tachycardias tend to be recurrent and of short duration.

Atrial Flutter. Atrial flutter is a rapid atrial ectopic tachycardia, with a rate that ranges from 240 to 450 beats per minute. There are two types of atrial flutter.[14] *Type I flutter* is the result of a reentry mechanism in the right atrium and can be entrained and interrupted with atrial pacing techniques. The atrial rate in typical type I flutter is close to 300 beats per minute, but it can range from 240 to 350 beats per minute. The mechanism of *type II flutter* is unknown. The atrial rate in type II flutter ranges between 350 and 450 beats per minute. The ventricular response rate is usually a defined fraction of the atrial rate (i.e., when conduction from the atria to the ventricles is 2:1, an atrial flutter rate of 300 would result in a ventricular response rate of 150 beats per minute). On the ECG, atrial flutter generates a defined sawtooth pattern in leads II, III, and aVF.

Atrial flutter rarely is seen in normal healthy individuals. It may be seen in persons of any age in the presence of underlying atrial abnormalities. Subgroups that are at particularly high risk for developing atrial flutter include children, adolescents, and young adults who have undergone corrective surgery for complex congenital heart diseases.[14]

Atrial Fibrillation. Atrial fibrillation is the result of chaotic current flow within the atria. When the atrial cells cannot repolarize in time for the next incoming stimulus, the ectopic current is rejected by the refractory cells and sent in another direction. These activities result in atrial fibrillation. It is characterized electrocardiographically by grossly disorganized atrial electrical activity that is irregular with respect to rate and rhythm. Conduction through the AV node is disorga-

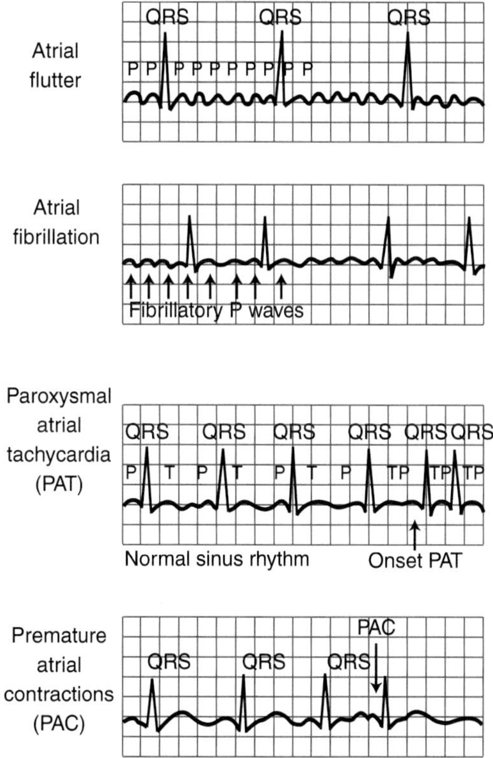

Figure 21–11
Electrocardiographic tracings of atrial dysrhythmias. Atrial flutter (*first tracing*) is characterized by the atrial flutter (P) waves occurring at a rate of 240 to 450 beats per minute. The ventricular rate remains regular because of the conduction of every sixth atrial contraction. Atrial fibrillation (*second tracing*) has grossly disorganized atrial electrical activity that is irregular with respect to rate and rhythm. The ventricular response is irregular, and no distinct P waves are visible. The *third tracing* illustrates paroxysmal atrial tachycardia (PAT), preceded by a normal sinus rhythm. The *fourth tracing* illustrates a premature atrial contraction (PAC).

nized, the peripheral pulse is grossly irregular, and a pulse deficit can be observed. Atrial fibrillation can be seen in persons without any apparent disease, or it may occur in individuals with mitral valve disease, ischemic heart disease, hypertension, and thyrotoxicosis.[15] Atrial fibrillation is the most common atrial dysrhythmia in the elderly. It predisposes individuals to thrombus formation in the atria, with subsequent risk of formation of systemic emboli. Figure 21–11 illustrates the ECG changes that occur with atrial dysrhythmias.

Disorders of Atrioventricular Conduction

Under normal conditions, the AV node provides the only connection for transmission of impulses between the atrial and ventricular conduction systems.[4] Junctional fibers in the AV node have high resistance characteristics, which cause a delay in the transmission of impulses from the atria to the ventricles. This delay provides optimal timing for atrial contribution to ventricular filling, and protects the ventricles from abnormally rapid rates that arise in the atria. Conduction defects of the AV node are most commonly associated with fibrosis or scar tissue in fibers of the conduction system. Conduction defects also may result from medications, including digoxin, β blockers, calcium-channel blockers, and class 1A antiarrhythmics.[16] Additional contributing factors include electrolyte imbalances, inflammatory disease, or cardiac surgery.

Heart Block. Heart block refers to abnormalities of impulse conduction. It may be normal, physiologic (*e.g.*, vagal tone), or pathologic. It may occur in the AV nodal fibers or in the AV bundle (*i.e.*, bundle of His), which is continuous with the Purkinje conduction system that supplies the ventricles. The PR interval on the ECG corresponds with the time it takes for the cardiac impulse to travel from the SA node to the ventricular pathways. Normally, the PR interval ranges from 0.12 to 0.20 second.

First-degree AV block is characterized by a prolonged PR interval (<0.20 second) (Fig. 21–12). The prolonged PR interval indicates delayed AV conduction, but there are no nonconducted sinus impulses. Isolated first-degree heart block is never symptomatic, and temporary or permanent cardiac pacing are not indicated.

Second-degree AV block is characterized by intermittent failure of conduction of one or more impulses from the atria to the ventricles. Second-degree AV block has been divided into two types: type I (*i.e.*, Wenckebach phenomenon or Mobitz type I) and type II (*i.e.*, Mobitz type II). Mobitz type I AV block is characterized by progressive lengthening of the PR interval until an impulse is blocked and the sequence begins again. It is usually associated with an adequate ventricular rate and is rarely symptomatic.[14] In Mobitz type II AV block, an intermittent block of atrial impulses occurs, with a constant PR interval (Fig. 21–12). Mobitz type II AV block is usually associated with organic cardiac disease and frequently progresses to complete heart block. Permanent cardiac pacing usually is indicated.

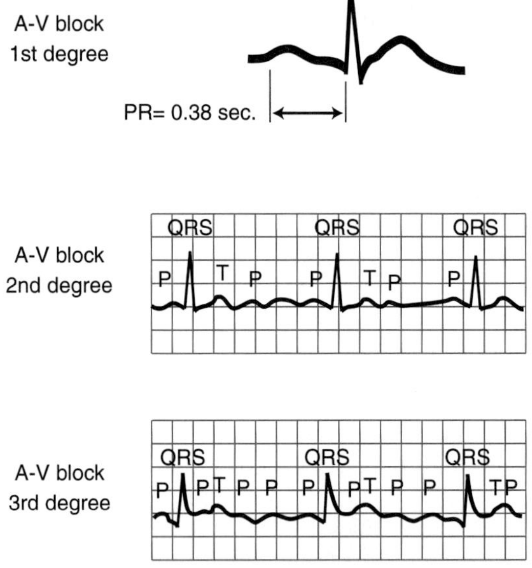

Figure 21–12
Electrocardiographic changes that occur with alterations in atrioventricular (AV) node conduction. The *top tracing* shows the prolongation of the PR interval, which is characteristic of first-degree AV block. The *middle tracing* illustrates Mobitz type II second-degree AV block, in which the conduction of one or more P waves is blocked. In third-degree AV block (*bottom tracing*), complete block in conduction of impulses through the AV node occurs, and the atria and ventricles develop their own rates of impulse generation.

Third-degree, or *complete AV block*, occurs when the conduction link between the atria and ventricles is lost (see Fig. 21–12). The atria continue to beat at a normal rate and the ventricles develop their own rate, which normally is slow (30 to 40 beats per minute). The atrial and ventricular rates are regular but dissociated. Complete heart block causes a decrease in cardiac output with possible periods of syncope, known as a Stokes-Adams attack. Other symptoms include dizziness, fatigue, exercise intolerance, or episodes of acute heart failure. Most persons with complete heart block require a permanent cardiac pacemaker.

Junctional Dysrhythmias

The AV node can act as a pacemaker in the event the SA node fails to initiate an impulse. Junctional rhythms can be transient or permanent, and they generally have a rate of 40 to 60 beats per minute. Junctional fibers in the AV node or bundle also can serve as ectopic pacemakers, producing premature junctional complexes. Another rhythm originating in the junctional tissues is junctional tachycardia. The rate associated with junctional tachycardia ranges from 120 to 200 beats per minute. The P waves may precede, be buried in, or follow the QRS complexes, depending on the site of the originating impulses. The clinical significance of junctional tachycardia is the same as for atrial tachycardias. Catheter ablation therapy has been used successfully to treat some individuals with recurrent or intractable junctional tachycardia.[14]

Ventricular Conduction Defects

The junctional fibers in the AV node join with the bundle of His, which divides to form the right and left bundle branches. The bundle branches continue to divide and form the Purkinje fibers, which supply the walls of the ventricles (see Fig. 21–1). As the cardiac impulse leaves the junctional fibers, it travels through the AV bundle. Next, the impulse moves down the right and left bundle branches that lie beneath the endocardium on either side of the septum, and it spreads out through the walls of the ventricles. Interruption of impulse conduction through the bundle branches is called a *bundle branch block*. These blocks usually do not cause alterations in the rhythm of the heartbeat. Instead, a bundle branch block interrupts the normal progression of depolarization, causing the ventricles to depolarize one after the other because the impulses must travel through muscle tissue rather than through the specialized conductile tissue. This prolonged conduction causes the QRS complex to be wider than the normal 0.08 to 0.12 second. The left bundle branch bifurcates into the left anterior and posterior fascicles. An interruption of one of these fascicles is referred to as a *hemiblock*.

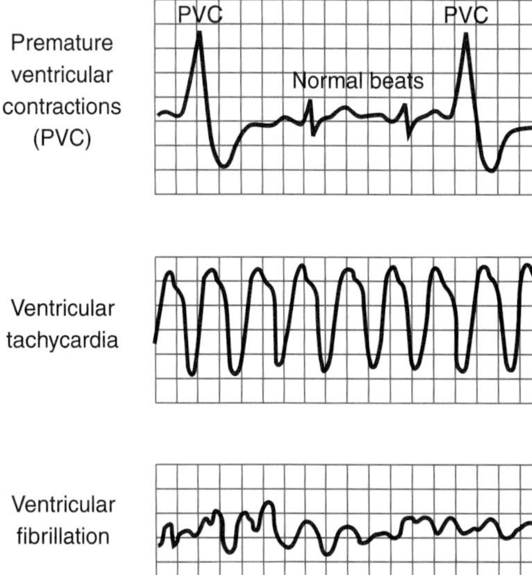

Figure 21–13
Electrocardiographic (ECG) tracings of ventricular dysrhythmias. Premature ventricular contractions (PVCs) (*top tracing*) originate from an ectopic focus in the ventricles, causing a distortion of the QRS complex. Because the ventricle usually cannot repolarize sufficiently to respond to the next impulse that arises in the sinoatrial node, a PVC frequently is followed by a compensatory pause. Ventricular tachycardia (*middle tracing*) is characterized by a rapid ventricular rate of 100 to 250 beats per minute and the absence of P waves. In ventricular fibrillation (*bottom tracing*), there are no regular or effective ventricular contractions, and the ECG tracing is totally disorganized.

Ventricular Dysrhythmias

Dysrhythmias that arise in the ventricles commonly are considered more serious than those that arise in the atria because they afford the potential for interfering with the pumping action of the heart. A *premature ventricular complex* (PVC) is caused by a ventricular ectopic pacemaker. After a PVC, the ventricle usually is not able to repolarize sufficiently to respond to the next impulse that arises in the SA node. This delay is commonly referred to as a *compensatory pause*, which occurs while the ventricle waits to reestablish its previous rhythm (Fig. 21–13). When a PVC occurs, the diastolic volume is usually insufficient for ejection of blood into the arterial system. As a result, PVCs usually do not produce a palpable pulse. In the absence of heart disease, PVCs typically are not clinically significant. The incidence of PVCs is greatest with ischemia, acute myocardial infarction, history of myocardial infarction, hypertrophy, infection, increased sympathetic activity, or increased heart rate.[17] PVCs also can be the result of electrolyte disturbances or medications.

A special pattern of PVC called *ventricular bigeminy* occurs in such a way that each normal beat is followed by or paired with a PVC. This pattern often is an indication of digitalis toxicity or heart disease. The occurrence of frequent PVCs in the diseased heart predisposes to other, more serious dysrhythmias, including ventricular tachycardia and ventricular fibrillation.

Ventricular tachycardia describes a ventricular rate of 100 to 250 beats per minute. This rhythm is dangerous because it causes a reduction in the diastolic filling time to the point at which the cardiac output is severely diminished or nonexistent. The ECG pattern for ventricular tachycardia can vary greatly. Generally, ventricular tachycardia is exhibited electrocardiographically by wide, tall, bizarre-looking QRS complexes that persist longer than 0.12 second (Fig. 21–13).

In *ventricular fibrillation*, the ventricle quivers but does not contract. When the ventricle does not contract, there is no cardiac output, and there are no palpable or audible pulses. The classic ECG pattern of ventricular fibrillation is that of gross disorganization without identifiable waveforms or intervals (Fig. 21–13).

Diagnostic Methods

The diagnosis of disorders of cardiac rhythm and conduction usually is made on the basis of the surface ECG. Further clarification of conduction defects and cardiac dysrhythmias can be done using electrophysiologic studies.

A resting surface ECG records the impulses originating in the heart as they are recorded at the body surface. These impulses are recorded for a limited time and during periods of inactivity. Although there are no complications related to the procedure, errors related to misdiagnosis may result in iatrogenic heart disease.[1] The resting ECG is the first approach to the clinical diagnosis of disorders of cardiac rhythm and conduction, but it is limited to events that occur during the period the ECG is being monitored.

Signal-Averaged Electrocardiogram

Signal-averaged ECG is a special type of ECG that is used to detect ventricular late action potentials that are thought to originate from slow-conducting areas of the myocardium. Ventricular late action potentials are low-amplitude, high-frequency waveforms in the terminal QRS complex, and they persist for tens of milliseconds into the ST segment.[18] These late potentials are detectable from leads of the surface ECG when signal averaging is performed. This technique averages together multiple samples of QRS waveforms and creates a tracing that is an average of all the repetitive signals. The presence of late potentials indicates high risk for development of ventricular tachycardia and sudden cardiac death.

Holter Monitoring

Holter monitoring is one form of long-term monitoring during which a person wears a device that digitally records two or three ECG leads for up to 48 hours. During this time, the person keeps a diary of his or her activities or symptoms, which later are correlated with the ECG recording. Most recording devices also have an event marker button that can be pressed when the individual experiences symptoms, which assists the technician or physician in correlating the diary, symptoms, and ECG changes during analysis. Holter monitoring is useful for documenting dysrhythmias, conduction abnormalities, and ST segment changes.

Intermittent ECG recorders also are used in the diagnosis of dysrhythmias and conduction defects. There are two basic types of recorders that perform this type of monitoring.[19] The first continuously monitors rhythm and is programmed to recognizes abnormalities. In the second variety, the unit does not continuously monitor the ECG and therefore cannot automatically recognize abnormalities. This latter form relies on the person to activate the unit when symptomatic. The data are stored in memory or transmitted transtelephonically to an electrocardiographic receiver, where it is recorded. These types of ECG recordings are useful in persons who have transient symptoms.

Exercise Stress Testing

The exercise stress test elicits the body's response to measured increases in acute exercise.[20] This technique provides information about changes in heart rate, blood pressure, respiration, and perceived level of exercise. It is useful in determining exercise-induced alterations in hemodynamic response and ischemic-type ECG ST segment changes and can detect and classify disturbances in cardiac rhythm and conduction associated with exercise. These changes are indicative of a poorer prognosis in persons with known coronary disease and recent myocardial infarction.

Electrophysiology Studies

An electrophysiologic study involves the passage of two or more electrode catheters into the right side of the heart. These catheters are inserted into the femoral, subclavian, internal jugular, or the antecubital veins and positioned with fluoroscopy into the high right atrium near the sinus node, the area of the His bundle, the coronary sinus that lies in the posterior atrioventricular groove, and into the right ventricle.[21] The electrode catheters are used to stimulate the heart and record intracardiac ECGs. During the study, overdrive pacing, cardioversion, or defibrillation may be necessary to terminate tachycardia induced during the stimulation procedures.

Electrophysiology studies are performed for diagnostic or therapeutic purposes. A diagnostic study is performed to determine a person's potential for dysrhythmia formation. Electrophysiology testing also defines reproducible dysrhythmia induction characteristics and, as a result, can be used to evaluate the therapeutic efficacy of a particular treatment modality. Diagnostic studies can locate dysrhythmia foci for therapeutic intervention as well.

Therapeutic electrophysiology studies are used as interventions. These interventions may include pacing a person out of tachycardia or ablation therapy. Both types of electrophysiology testing may be done repeatedly to test patient responses to drugs, devices such as implantable defibrillators, and surgical interventions used in the treatment of dysrhythmias.

Treatment

The treatment of cardiac rhythm or conduction disorders is directed toward controlling the dysrhythmia, correcting the cause, and preventing more serious or fatal dysrhythmias. Correction may involve simply adjusting an electrolyte disturbance or withholding a medication such as digitalis. Preventing more serious dysrhythmias often involves drug therapy, electrical stimulation, or surgical intervention.

Pharmacologic Treatment

Antidysrhythmic drugs act by modifying disordered formation and conduction of impulses that induce cardiac muscle contraction. These drugs are classified into four major groups according to the drug's effect on the action potential of the cardiac cells. It is important to recognize that although drugs in one category have similar effects on conduction, they may vary significantly in their hemodynamic effects.

Class I drugs act by blocking the fast sodium channels. The drugs effect impulse conduction, excitability, and automaticity to various degrees and therefore have been divided further into three groups: IA, IB, and IC. Class IA drugs (e.g., quinidine, procainamide, disopyramide, moricizine) decrease automaticity by depressing phase 4 of the action potential, decrease conductivity by moderately prolonging phase 0, and prolong repolarization by extending phase 3 of the action potential. Because these drugs are effective in suppressing ectopic foci and in treating reentrant dysrhythmias, they are used for supraventricular and ventricular dysrhythmias.[22] Class IB drugs (*e.g.*, lidocaine, phenytoin, tocainide, mexiletine, aprindine) decrease automaticity by depressing phase 4 of the action potential, have little effect on conductivity, decrease refractoriness by decreasing phase 2, and shorten repolarization by decreasing phase 3. Drugs in this group are used for treating ventricular dysrhythmias only and have little or no effect on myocardial contractility. Class IC drugs (*e.g.*, flecainide, encainide, propafenone, indecainide) decrease conductivity by markedly depressing phase 0 of the action potential but have little effect on refractoriness or repolarization. Drugs in this class are used for life-threatening ventricular dysrhythmias and supraventricular tachycardias.

Class II agents (*e.g.*, propranolol, nadolol, atenolol, timolol, acebutolol, metoprolol, pindolol, esmolol) are β-adrenergic blocking drugs that act by blunting the effect of sympathetic nervous system stimulation on the heart. These drugs decrease automaticity by depressing phase 4 of the action potential; they also decrease heart rate and cardiac contractility. These medications are effective for treatment of supraventricular dysrhythmias and tachydysrhythmias secondary to excessive sympathetic activity, but they are not very effective in treating severe arrhythmias such as recurrent ventricular tachycardia.[23]

Class III drugs (*e.g.*, amiodarone, bretylium, sotalol, *N*-acetylprocainamide [NAPA]) act by extending the action potential and refractoriness. These agents have been used effectively in the treatment of ventricular fibrillation.[22]

Class IV drugs (*e.g.*, verapamil, diltiazem, nifedipine, bepridil, nitrendipine, felodipine, isradipine, nicardipine) act by blocking the slow calcium channels, thereby depressing phase 4 and lengthening phases 1 and 2. By blocking the release of intracellular calcium ions, these agents reduce the force of myocardial contractility, thereby decreasing myocardial oxygen demand. These drugs are used to slow the ventricular response in atrial tachycardias and to terminate reentrant paroxysmal supraventricular tachycardias when the AV node functions as a reentrant pathway.[22]

Two other types of antidysrhythmic drugs, the cardiac glycosides and adenosine, are not included in this classification schema. The cardiac glycosides (*i.e.*, digitalis drugs) slow the heart rate and are used in the management of dysrhythmias such as atrial tachycardia, atrial flutter, and atrial fibrillation. Adenosine, an endogenous nucleoside that is present in every cell, is used for emergency intravenous treatment of paroxysmal supraventricular tachycardia involving the AV node. It interrupts AV node conduction and slows SA node firing.

Electrical Interventions

The correction of conduction defects, bradycardias, and tachycardias can involve the use of an electronic pacemaker, cardioversion, or defibrillation. Electrical interventions can be used in emergency and elective situations. A *pacemaker* is an electronic device that delivers an electrical stimulus to the heart. It is used to initiate heartbeats in situations when the normal pacemaker of the heart is defective or in complete heart block in which the rate of cardiac contraction and consequent cardiac output is inadequate to perfuse vital tissues. *Overdrive pacing* is used to treat recurrent ventricular tachycardia, reentrant atrial or ventricular tachydysrhythmias, and to terminate atrial flutter. A pacemaker may be used as a temporary or a permanent measure. Internal temporary pacing involves the passage, under fluoroscopic or ECG direction, of a venous catheter with electrodes on its tip into the right atrium or ventricle, where it is wedged against the endocardium. External temporary pacing involves the placement of large patch electrodes on the anterior and posterior chest wall. Permanent pacing requires the direct insertion of pacemaker electrodes into the epicardium or the transvenous insertion into the apex of the right ventricle, where the electrode comes in contract with the endocardium.

Defibrillation and synchronized cardioversion are two reliable methods for treating ventricular tachycardia, and defibrillation is the definitive treatment for atrial fibrillation. The discharge of electrical energy that is synchronized with the R wave of the ECG is referred to as *synchronized cardioversion,* and unsynchronized discharge is known as *defibrillation.* The goal of both these techniques is to provide an electrical pulse to the heart in such a way as to completely depolarize the heart during passage of the current. This electrical current interrupts the disorganized impulses, allowing the SA node to regain control of the heart. Defibrillation and synchronized cardioversion can be delivered externally through large patch electrodes on the chest or internally through small paddle electrodes placed directly on the myocardium, patch electrodes sewn into the epicardium, or transvenous wires placed in the right ventricle. Electrical devices that combine antitachycardial pacing, cardioversion, defibrillation, and bradycardial pacing are under investigation.

Ablation and Surgical Interventions

Ablation therapy is employed for treating recurrent life-threatening supraventricular and ventricular tachydysrhythmias. It involves localized destruction, isolation, or excision of cardiac tissue that is considered to be dysrhythmogenic.[24] Ablative therapy may be performed by employing catheter or surgical techniques. Radiofrequency ablation uses radiofrequency energy waves to destroy defective or aberrant electrical conduction pathways. Cryoablation is the direct application of an extremely cold probe to dysrhythmogenic cardiac tissue that causes freezing and necrosis of defective or aberrant electrical conduction pathways.

Additional surgical interventions such as coronary artery bypass surgery, ventriculotomy, and endocardial resection may be used to improve myocardial oxygenation, remove dysrhythmogenic foci, or altered electrical conduction pathways. Coronary artery bypass surgery improves myocardial oxygenation by increasing blood supply to the myocardium. Ventriculotomy involves the removal of aneurysm tissue and the resuturing of the myocardial walls to eliminate the paradoxical ventricular movement and the foci of dysrhythmias. In endocardial resection, endocardial tissue that has been identified as dysrhythmogenic through the use of electrophysiology testing or intraoperative mapping is surgically removed. Ventriculotomy and endocardial resection have been performed with cryoablation or laser ablation as an adjunctive therapy.[25] Other surgical techniques, including transvenous electrocoagulation and laser ablation, are under investigation as potential treatment modalities for recurrent tachycardias.

In summary, disorders of cardiac rhythm arise as the result of disturbances in impulse generation or conduction in the heart. Normal sinus rhythm and respiratory sinus dysrhythmia (i.e., heart rate speeds up and slows down in concert with respiratory cycle) are considered normal rhythms. Cardiac dysrhythmias are not necessarily pathologic; they occur in healthy and in diseased hearts. Sinus dysrhythmias originate in the SA node. They include sinus bradycardia (heart rate <60 beats per minute); sinus tachycardia (heart rate >100 beats per minute); sinus arrest, in which there are prolonged periods of asystole; and sick sinus syndrome, a condition characterized by periods of bradycardia alternating with tachycardia.

Atrial dysrhythmias arise from alterations in impulse generation that occur within the conduction pathways or muscle of the atria. They include atrial premature contractions, atrial flutter (i.e., atrial depolarization rate of 240 to 450 beats per minute), and atrial fibrillation (i.e., grossly disorganized atrial depolarization that is irregular with regard to rate and rhythm). Atrial dysrhythmias often go unnoticed unless they are transmitted to the ventricles.

Alterations in the conduction of impulses through the AV node lead to disturbances in the transmission of impulses from the atria to the ventricles. There can be a delay in transmission (i.e., first-degree heart block), failure to conduct one or more impulses (i.e., second-degree heart block), or complete failure to conduct impulses between the atria and the ventricles (i.e., third-degree heart block). Conduction disorders of the bundle of His, called bundle branch blocks, cause a widening of and changes in the configuration of the QRS complex of the ECG. Because of their potential for interfering with the pumping action of the heart, dysrhythmias that arise in the ventricles usually are considered more serious than those that arise in the atria. A PVC is caused by a ventricular ectopic pacemaker. Ventricular tachycardia is characterized by a ventricular rate of 160 to 250 beats per minute. Ventricular fibrillation (e.g., ventricular rate >350 beats per minute) is a fatal dysrhythmia unless it is successfully treated with defibrillation.

REFERENCES

1. Castellanos A., Kessler K.M., Myerburg R.J. (1994). The resting electrocardiogram. In Schlant R.C., Alexander R.W., O'Rourke R.A., Roberts R., Sonnenblick E.H. (Eds.). *Hurst's the heart* (8th ed., pp. 321–356). New York: McGraw-Hill.
2. Berne R.M., Levy M.N. (1993). *Physiology* (3rd ed., pp. 364–396). St. Louis: C.V. Mosby.
3. Guyton A.C. (1996). *Textbook of medical physiology* (9th ed., pp. 121–160). Philadelphia: W.B. Saunders.
4. Phillips R.E., Feeney M.A. (1990). *The cardiac rhythms* (3rd ed.). Philadelphia: W.B. Saunders.
5. Kernicki J.G., Weiler K.M. (1981). *Electrocardiography for nurses: Physiological correlates*. New York: John Wiley & Sons.
6. Hoffman B.F., Cranefield P.F. (1960). *Electrophysiology of the heart*. New York: McGraw-Hill.
7. Katz A.M. (1992). *Physiology of the heart* (vol. 2). New York: Raven Press.
8. Schlant R.C., Sonnenblick E.H. (1994). Normal physiology of the cardiovascular system. In Schlant R.C., Alexander R.W.. O'Rourke R.A., Roberts R., Sonnenblick E.H. (Eds.). *Hurst's the heart* (8th ed., pp. 113–151.). New York: McGraw-Hill.
9. Braunwald E.B. (1996). *Heart disease: A textbook of cardiovascular medicine* (5th ed., pp. 548–640). Philadelphia: W.B. Saunders.
10. Wit A.L., Friedman P.L. (1975). Basis for ventricular arrhythmias accompanying myocardial infarction. *Archives of Internal Medicine* 135, 459.
11. Kay G.N., Bubien R.S. (1992). *Clinical management of cardiac arrhythmias*. Gaithersburg, MD: Aspen.
12. Moser D.K., Woo M.A. (1994). Recurrent ventricular tachycardia. *Critical Care Clinics of North America* 6 (1), 15–26.
13. Conover M. (1996). *Understanding electrocardiography* (7th ed.). St. Louis: Mosby-Year Book.
14. Myerburg R.J., Kessler K.M., Castellanos A. (1994). Recognition, clinical assessment, and management of arrhythmias and conduction disturbances. In Schlant R.C., Alexander R.W.. O'Rourke R.A., Roberts R., Sonnenblick E.H. (Eds.). *Hurst's the heart* (8th ed., pp. 705–758). New York: McGraw-Hill.
15. Marriott H.J.L. (1988). *Practical electrocardiography* (8th ed.). Baltimore: Williams & Wilkins.
16. Moungey S.J. (1994). Patients with sinus node dysfunction or atrioventricular blocks. *Critical Care Nursing Clinics of North America* 6 (1), 55–68.
17. Bigger Jr. J.T. (1994). Ventricular premature complexes. In Kastor J.A. (Ed.). *Arrhythmias* (pp. 310–325). Philadelphia: W.B. Saunders.
18. Walter P.F. (1994). Technique of signal-averaged electrocardiography. In Schlant R.C., Alexander R.W.. O'Rourke R.A., Roberts R., Sonnenblick E.H. (Eds.). *Hurst's the heart* (8th ed., pp. 893–904). New York: McGraw-Hill.
19. Noble R.J., Zipes D.P. (1994). Long-term continuous electrocardiographic recording. In Schlant R.C., Alexander R.W.. O'Rourke R.A., Roberts R., Sonnenblick E.H. (Eds.). *Hurst's the heart* (8th ed., pp. 873–880. New York: McGraw-Hill.
20. Fletcher G.F., Schlant R.C. (1994). The exercise test. In Schlant R.C., Alexander R.W.. O'Rourke R.A., Roberts R., Sonnenblick E.H. (Eds.). *Hurst's the heart* (8th ed., pp. 423–440). New York: McGraw-Hill.

21. Darling E.J. (1994). Overview of cardiac electrophysiologic testing. *Critical Care Nursing Clinics of North America* 6 (1), 1–13.
22. Morton P.G. (1994). Update on new antiarrhythmic drugs. *Critical Care Clinics of North America* 6 (1), 69–83.
23. Woosley R.L. (1994). Antiarrhythmic drugs. In Schlant R.C., Alexander R.W.. O'Rourke R.A., Roberts R., Sonnenblick E.H. (Eds.). *Hurst's the heart* (8th ed., pp. 775–805). New York: McGraw-Hill.
24. Finkelmeier B.A. (1994). Ablative therapy in the treatment of tachyarrhythmias. *Critical Care Clinics of North America* 6 (1), 103–110.
25. Cox J.L. (1994). Surgical treatment of cardiac arrhythmias. In Schlant R.C., Alexander R.W.. O'Rourke R.A., Roberts R., Sonnenblick E.H. (Eds.). *Hurst's the heart* (8th ed., pp. 863–871). New York: McGraw-Hill.

Respiratory Function

In the early studies of the body, there is almost no mention of the lungs or respiratory passages. Although the pneuma, or "vital spirits," of the body were closely related to the air and vapors of the universe, the lungs and air passages were almost disregarded. It was not until the circulation of blood had been charted that real progress in understanding the respiratory system took place.

A major step in the understanding of respiration began with the work of Robert Boyle (1627–1691), an Irish scholar. Using an air pump, Boyle proved that a candle would not burn and a small bird or mouse could not live inside a jar from which the air had been removed. Scientists at this time believed that when something burned, air lost a mysterious substance called phlogiston. *It was the British clergyman Joseph Priestley (1733–1804) who discovered that a gas made by heating oxide of mercury supported combustion. He called this gas, which later became known as oxygen,* dephlogisticated *air. Priestley showed that a mouse lived longer in a given volume of dephlogisticated air than it did in ordinary air. Antoine Lavoisier (1743–1794), a French chemist, confirmed that oxygen was present in inspired air and carbon dioxide in expired air, and gave oxygen its name. In 1791, just 16 years after Priestley's discovery of oxygen, it was shown that blood contained both oxygen and carbon dioxide. From this point on, a detailed understanding of the respiratory system and its function proceeded rapidly.*

UNIT VI

CHAPTER 22

Control of Respiratory Function

Respiration provides the body with a means of gas exchange. It is the process whereby oxygen from the air is transferred to the blood and carbon dioxide is eliminated from the body. Internal respiration provides for gas exchange at the cellular level. Respiration can be divided into four parts: ventilation, or the movement of air between the atmosphere and the respiratory portion of the lungs; perfusion, or the flow of blood through the lungs; diffusion, or the transfer of gases between the air-filled spaces in the lungs and the blood; and the regulation and control of breathing by respiratory muscles and the nervous system. The discussion in this chapter focuses on the structure and function of the respiratory system as it relates to these aspects of respiration. The function of the red blood cell in the transport of oxygen is discussed in Chapter 8.

Structural Organization of the Respiratory System

After you have completed this section of the chapter, you should be able to meet the following objectives:

- State the difference between the conducting and the respiratory airways
- Trace the movement of air through the airways, beginning in the nose and oropharynx and moving into the respiratory tissues of the lung
- Describe the function of the mucociliary blanket
- Define the term *water vapor pressure* and cite the source of water for humidification of air as it moves through the airways

- Compare the supporting structures of the large and small airways in terms of cartilaginous and smooth muscle support
- Compare the function of the bronchial and pulmonary circulations that supply the lungs
- State the function of the two types of alveolar cells

The respiratory system consists of the air passages and the lungs. Functionally, the respiratory system can be divided into two parts: the conducting airways, through which air moves as it passes between the atmosphere and the lungs, and the respiratory tissues of the lungs, where gas exchange takes place.

The Conducting Airways

The conducting airways consist of the nasal passages, mouth and pharynx, larynx, trachea, bronchi, and bronchioles (Fig. 22–1). The air we breathe is warmed, filtered, and moistened as it moves through these structures. Body heat is transferred from the blood that flows through the air passages; the mucociliary blanket removes foreign materials; and water from the mucous membranes is used to moisten the air.

The conducting airways are lined with a *pseudostratified columnar epithelium* that contains mucus-secreting goblet cells and hairlike projections called *cilia*. The mucus produced by these cells forms the *mucociliary blanket*, a layer that protects the respiratory system and entraps dust and other foreign particles as they move through the conducting airways. The cilia, which constantly are in motion, move the mucociliary blanket with its entrapped particles escalator-fashion toward the oropharynx from where it is expectorated or swallowed.

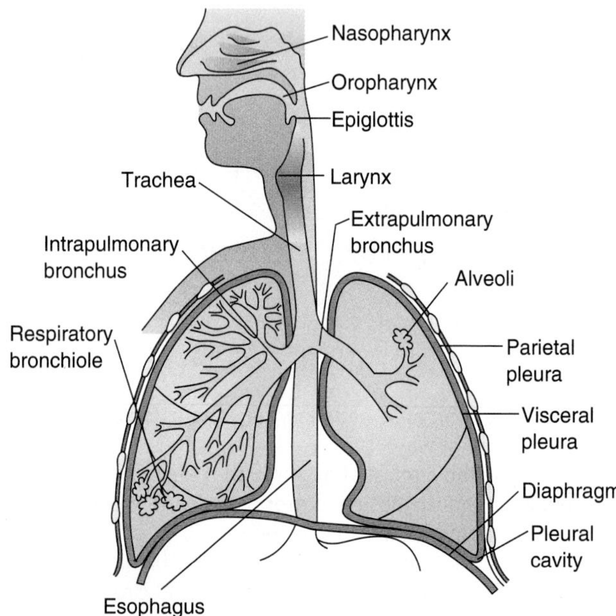

Figure 22–1
Structures of the respiratory system

The function of the mucous escalator in clearing the lower airways and alveoli is optimal at normal oxygen levels and is impaired in situations of low and high oxygen levels. Clearance is stimulated by coughing. It is impaired by drying, such as by heated but unhumidified indoor air during winter. Cigarette smoking also slows down or paralyzes the mucociliary escalator. This slowing allows the residue from tobacco smoke, dust, and other particles to accumulate in the lungs, decreasing the efficiency of this pulmonary defense system. There is also evidence that smoking causes hyperplasia of the goblet cells, with a resultant increase in respiratory tract secretions and increased susceptibility to respiratory tract infections. As discussed in Chapter 24, these changes are thought to contribute to the development of chronic bronchitis and emphysema.

The airways are kept moist by water contained in the mucous layer. Moisture is added to the air as it moves through the conducting airways. The capacity of the air to contain moisture or water vapor without condensation occurring increases as the temperature rises. The body-temperature air in the alveoli usually contains considerably more water vapor than the atmospheric-temperature air that we breathe. The difference between the water vapor contained in the air we breathe and that found in the alveoli is drawn from the moist surface of the mucous membranes that line the conducting airways and is a source of insensible water loss (see Chapter 26). Under normal conditions, about 1 pint of water per day is lost in humidifying the air breathed. This amount is increased during fever caused by the temperature-associated increase in water vapor pressure within the lungs. An increase in the respiratory rate usually accompanies fever, so that more air passes through the airways, withdrawing moisture from its mucosal surface. As a result, respiratory secretions thicken, preventing free movement of the cilia and impairing the protective function of the mucociliary defense system. This is particularly true in persons whose water intake is inadequate.

Nasal Passages

The nose is the preferred route for the entrance of air into the respiratory tract during normal breathing. As air passes through the nasal passages, it is filtered, warmed, and humidified. The outer nasal passages are lined with coarse hairs, which filter and trap dust and other large particles from the air. The upper portion of the nasal cavity is lined with mucous membrane that contains a rich network of small blood vessels; this portion of the nasal cavity supplies warmth and moisture to the air we breathe.

Mouth and Pharynx

The mouth serves as an alternative airway when the nasal passages are plugged or when there is a need for the exchange of large amounts of air, as occurs during exercise. The pharynx is the only opening between the nose and mouth and the lungs. Obstruction of the pharynx leads to immediate cessation of ventilation. Neural control of the tongue and pharyngeal muscles is impaired in coma and certain types of neurologic disease. In these conditions, the tongue falls back into the pharynx and obstructs the airway, particularly if the person is lying on the back. Swelling of the pharyngeal structures caused by injury, infection, or severe allergic reaction also predisposes a person to airway obstruction, as does the presence of a foreign body.

The epiglottis, also referred to as the *glottis*, is a thin, leaf-shaped structure that aids in covering the larynx during the act of swallowing to prevent food and fluids from entering the lungs. When the swallowing mechanism is partially or totally paralyzed, food and fluids can enter the trachea instead of the esophagus when a person attempts to swallow. These substances are not easily removed, and when they are pulled into the lungs, they can cause a serious inflammatory condition called *aspiration pneumonia*.

Larynx

The larynx connects the pharynx with the trachea. The walls of the larynx are supported by cartilaginous structures that prevent collapse during inspiration. The functions of the larynx can be divided into two categories: those associated with speech and those associated with protecting the lungs by preventing the entrance of substances other than air. The larynx is located in a strategic position between the upper airways and the lungs and sometimes is referred to as the "watchdog of the lungs." When confronted with substances other than air, laryngeal muscles contract and close off the airway. At the same time, the cough reflex is initiated as a means of removing the foreign substance from the airway. Paralysis of the laryngeal muscles predisposes a person to aspiration of foreign materials into the lungs.

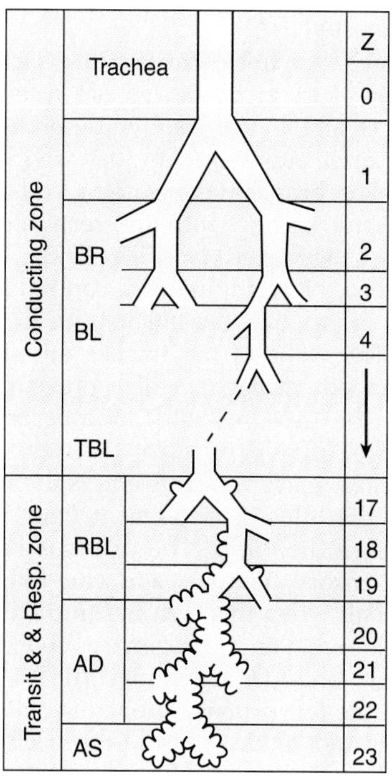

Figure 22–2
Idealization of the human airways. The first 16 generations of branching (Z) make up the conducting airways, and the last seven constitute the respiratory zone (or transitional and respiratory zone). BR, bronchus; BL, bronchiole; TBL, terminal bronchiole; RBL, respiratory bronchiole; AD, alveolar ducts; AS, alveolar sacs. (Weibel, E.R. [1962]. *Morphometry of the human lung* [p. 111]. Berlin: Springer-Verlag)

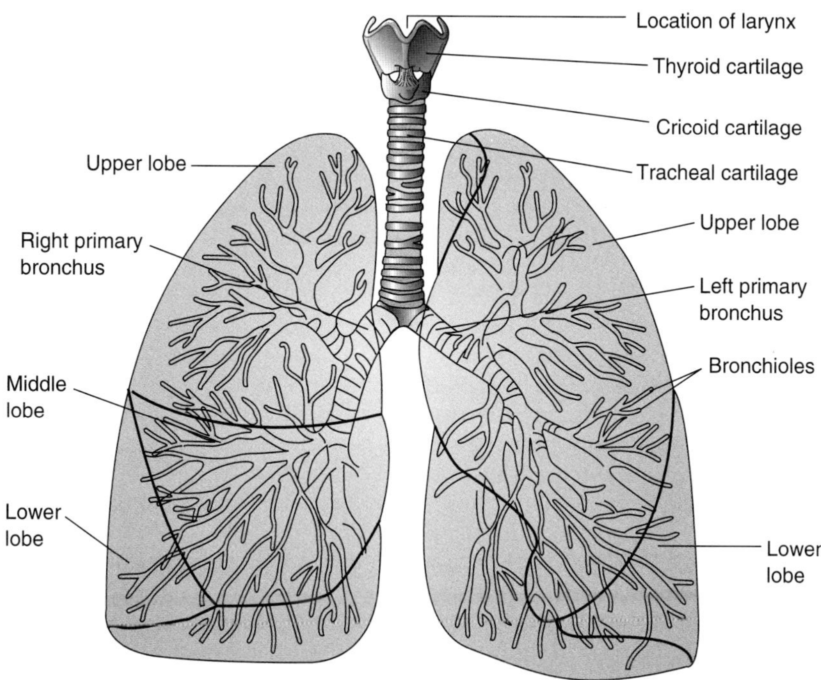

Figure 22–3
Larynx, trachea, and bronchial tree (*anterior view*).

Tracheobronchial Tree

The tracheobronchial tree consists of the trachea, bronchi, and bronchioles and can be viewed as a system of branching tubes. It is similar to a tree whose branches become smaller and more numerous as they divide. There are about 23 levels of branching, beginning with the conducting airways and ending with the respiratory airways, where gas exchange takes place (Fig. 22–2).

The trachea, or windpipe, is a continuous tube that connects the larynx and the major bronchi of the lungs (Fig. 22–3). The walls of the trachea are supported by horseshoe-shaped cartilages, which prevent it from collapsing when the pressure in the thorax becomes negative.

The trachea divides to form the right and the left primary bronchi. Each bronchus enters the lung through a slit called the hilus. The point at which the trachea divides is called the *carina*. The carina is heavily innervated with sensory neurons, and coughing and bronchospasm result when this area is stimulated, as during tracheal suctioning. The right primary bronchus is shorter and wider and continues at a more vertical angle with the trachea than the left primary bronchus, which is longer and narrower and continues from the trachea at a more acute angle. For this reason, when an endotracheal tube is inserted to maintain a patent airway and facilitate ventilation, it is essential to secure the tube properly. If the tube slips into the right main bronchus, it prevents air from entering the left lung, causing it to collapse. Anatomic variations also make it easier for foreign bodies to enter the right main bronchus than to enter the left.

The right and left primary bronchi divide into secondary, or lobular, bronchi, which supply each of the lobes of the lungs. The right middle lobe bronchus is of relatively small caliber and length and sometimes bends sharply near its bifurcation. It is surrounded by a collar of lymph nodes that drain the middle and the lower lobe and is particularly subject to obstruction. The secondary bronchi divide to form the segmental bronchi, which supply the bronchopulmonary segments of the lung. There are ten segments in the right lung and nine segments in the left lung (Fig. 22–4). These segments are identified according to their location in the lung (*e.g.*, the apical segment of the right upper lobe) and are the smallest named units in the lung. Lung lesions such as atelectasis and pneumonia often are localized to a particular bronchopulmonary segment.

The bronchi continue to branch, forming smaller bronchi, until they become the terminal bronchioles, the smallest of the conducting airways. The structure of the primary bronchi is similar to that of the trachea, in that these airways are supported by cartilaginous rings. As the bronchi move into the lungs, the horseshoe-shaped cartilage rings are replaced by irregular plates of cartilage. As these bronchi branch and become smaller, this cartilaginous support becomes thinner and then disappears at the level of the bronchioles. Between the cartilaginous support and the mucosal surface are two crisscrossing layers of smooth muscle that wind in opposite directions (Fig. 22–5). Bronchospasm, or contraction, of these muscles causes narrowing of the bronchioles and impairs air flow.

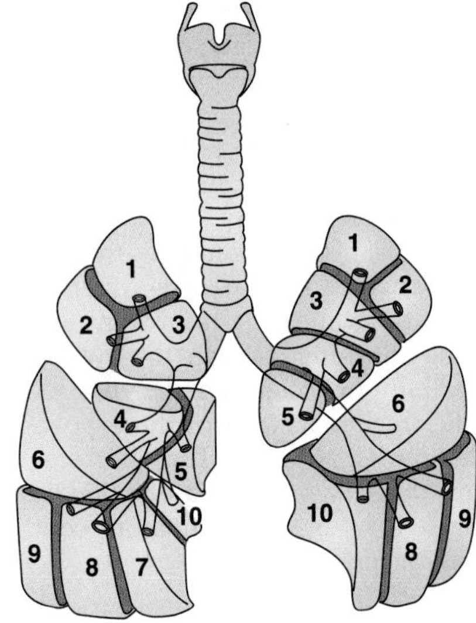

Figure 22–4
Bronchopulmonary segments of the human lung. Left and right upper lobes: (*1*) apical, (*2*) posterior, (*3*) anterior, (*4*) superior, lingular, and (*5*) inferior lingular segments. Right middle lobe: (*4*) lateral and (*5*) medial segments. Lower lobes: (*6*) superior (apical), (*7*) medial-basal, (*8*) anterior-basal, (*9*) lateral-basal, and (*1*) posterior-basal segments. The medial-basal segment (*7*) is absent in the left lung. (Fishman A.P. [1980]. *Assessment of pulmonary function* [p. 19]. New York: McGraw-Hill)

The Lungs

The lungs are soft, spongy, cone-shaped organs located side by side in the chest cavity (see Fig. 22–1). They are separated from each other by the mediastinum (*i.e.*, the space between the lungs) and its contents—the heart, blood vessels, lymph nodes, nerve fibers, thymus gland, and esophagus. The upper part of the lung, which lies against the top of the thoracic cavity, is called the *apex*, and the lower part, which lies against the diaphragm, is called the *base*. The lungs are divided into lobes: three in the right lung and two in the left (see Fig. 22–3).

The lungs are the functional structures of the respiratory system. In addition to their gas exchange function, they inactivate vasoactive substances such as bradykinin; they convert angiotensin I to angiotensin II; and they serve as a reservoir for blood. Heparin-producing cells are particularly abundant in the capillaries of the lung where small clots are trapped.

Respiratory Lobules

The gas exchange function of the lung takes place in the lobules of the lungs. Each lobule is supplied with structures that provide for gas exchange and the circulation of blood (see Fig. 22–5). Gas exchange takes place in the terminal respiratory bronchioles and the alveolar ducts and sacs. Blood enters the lobules through a pulmonary artery and exits through a pulmonary vein. Lymphatic structures surround the lobule and aid in the removal of plasma proteins and other particles from the interstitial spaces.

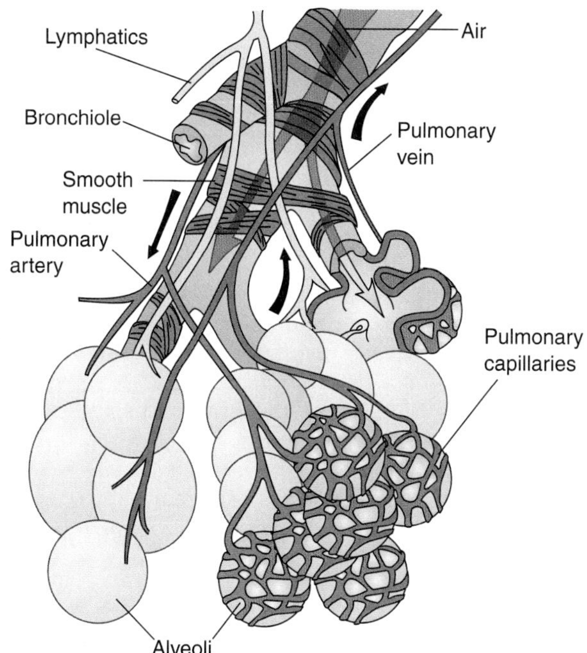

Figure 22–5
Lobule of the lung, showing the bronchial smooth muscle fibers, pulmonary blood vessels, and lymphatics.

The alveolar sacs are cup-shaped, thin-walled structures that are separated from each other by thin alveolar septa. Most of the septa are occupied by a single network of capillaries, so that blood is exposed to air on both sides. There are about 300 million alveoli in the adult lung, with a total surface area of about 50 to 100 m^2. Unlike the bronchioles, which are tubes with their own separate walls, the alveoli are interconnecting spaces that have no separate walls (Fig. 22–6). As a result of this arrangement, there is a continual mixing of air in the alveolar structures. Small holes in the alveolar walls, the pores of Kohn, probably contribute to the mixing of air under certain conditions.

The alveolar structures are composed of two types of cells: type I alveolar cells and the type II alveolar cells (Fig. 22–7). The type I alveolar cells are flat squamous epithelial cells across which gas exchange takes place. The type II alveolar cells produce surfactant, a lipoprotein substance that decreases the surface tension within the alveoli. This action allows for greater ease of lung inflation and helps to prevent the collapse of smaller airways. The alveoli also contain alveolar macrophages, which are responsible for the removal of offending substances from the alveolar epithelium. Available evidence suggests that smoking impairs the function of the macrophages.

Lung Circulation

The lungs are provided with a dual blood supply, the pulmonary and the bronchial circulations. The pulmonary circulation arises from the pulmonary artery and provides for the gas exchange function of the lungs, and the bronchial circulation distributes blood to the conducting airways and supporting structures of the lung.

The bronchial circulation has a secondary function of warming and humidifying incoming air as it moves through the conducting airways. The bronchial arteries arise from the thoracic aorta and enter the lungs with the major bronchi, dividing and subdividing along with the bronchi as they move out into the lung and supplying them and other lung structures with oxygen. The capillaries of the bronchial circulation drain into the bronchial veins, the larger of which empties into the vena cava. The smaller of the bronchial veins empties into the pulmonary veins. This blood is unoxygenated because the bronchial circulation does not participate in gas exchange. As a result, this blood dilutes the oxygenated blood returning to the left side of the heart.

The bronchial blood vessels are the only ones that undergo angiogenesis (*i.e.,* formation of new vessels) and develop collateral circulation when vessels in the pulmonary circulation are obstructed, as in pulmonary embolism. The development of new blood vessels helps to keep lung tissue alive until the pulmonary circulation can be restored.

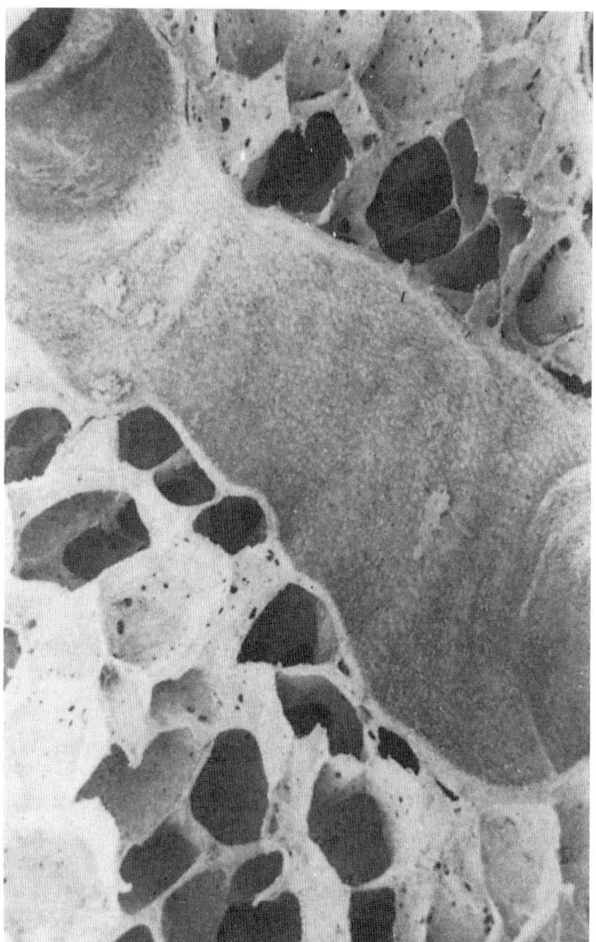

Figure 22–6
Close-up of a cross section of a small bronchus and surrounding alveoli. (Courtesy of Janice A. Nowell, of University of California, Santa Cruz)

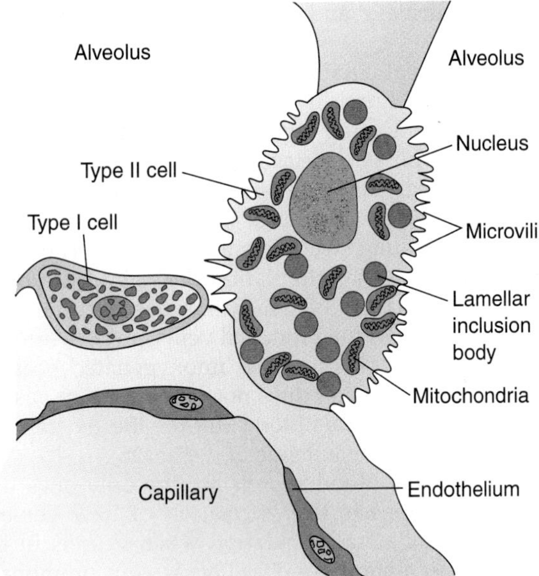

Figure 22–7
Schematic drawing of the two types of alveolar cells and their relation to alveoli and capillaries. Alveolar type I cells comprise most of the alveolar surface. Alveolar type II cells are located in the corner between two adjacent alveoli. Also shown are endothelial cells that line the pulmonary capillaries. (Rhoades R.A., Tanner G.A. [1996]. *Medical physiology* [p. 362]. Boston: Little, Brown)

Pleura

A thin, transparent, double-layered serous membrane, called the pleura, lines the thoracic cavity and encases the lungs. The outer parietal layer lies adjacent to the chest wall, and the inner, visceral layer adheres to the outer surface of the lung. The parietal pleura forms part of the mediastinum and lines the inner wall of the thoracic or chest cavity. A thin film of serous fluid separates the two pleural layers, and this allows the two layers to glide over each other and yet hold together, so there is no separation between the lungs and the chest wall. The pleural cavity is a potential space in which serous fluid or inflammatory exudate can accumulate. The term *pleural effusion* is used to describe an abnormal collection of fluid or exudate in the pleural cavity.

In summary, the respiratory system consists of the air passages and the lungs where gas exchange takes place. Functionally, the air passages of the respiratory system can be structurally divided into two parts: the conducting airways, through which air moves as it passes into and out of the lungs, and the respiratory tissues, where gas exchange actually takes place. The conducting airways include the nasal passages, mouth and nasopharynx, larynx, and tracheobronchial tree. Air is warmed, filtered, and humidified as it passes through these structures.

The lungs are the functional structures of the respiratory system. In addition to their gas exchange function, they inactivate vasoactive substances such as bradykinin; they convert angiotensin I to angiotensin II; and they serve as a reservoir for blood. The lobules, which are the functional units of the lung, consist of the respiratory bronchioles, alveoli, and pulmonary capillaries. It is here that gas exchange takes place. Oxygen from the alveoli diffuses across the alveolar capillary membrane into the blood, and carbon dioxide from the blood diffuses into the alveoli.

The lungs are provided with a dual blood supply: the bronchial circulation distributes blood to the conducting airways and supporting structures of the lung, and the pulmonary circulation provides for the gas exchange function of the lungs. The lungs are encased in a thin, transparent, double-layered serous membrane, called the pleura. The pressure in the pleural space, which is negative in relation to alveolar pressure, prevents the lungs from collapsing.

Exchange of Gases Between the Atmosphere and the Lungs

After you have completed this section of the chapter, you should be able to meet the following objectives:

- Describe the basic properties of gases in relation to their partial pressures and their pressures in relation to volume and temperature
- State the definition of intrathoracic, intrapleural, and intraalveolar pressures, and state how each of these pressures changes in relation to atmospheric pressure during inspiration and expiration
- Define *inspiratory reserve, expiratory reserve, vital capacity*, and *residual volume*
- Describe the method for measuring $FEV_{1.0}$
- State a definition of lung compliance
- Use Laplace's law to explain the need for surfactant in maintaining the inflation of small alveoli
- State the major determinant of airway resistance
- Explain why increasing lung volume (*i.e.*, taking deep breaths) reduces airway resistance

There is nothing mystical about ventilation. It is purely a mechanical event that obeys the laws of physics as they relate to the behavior of gases.

Basic Properties of Gases

The air we breathe is made up of a mixture of gases, mainly nitrogen and oxygen. These gases exert a combined pressure called the *atmospheric pressure*. The pressure at sea level is defined as 1 atmosphere, which is equal to 760 millimeters of mercury (mm Hg) or 14.7 lb per square inch. When measuring respiratory pressures, atmospheric pressure is assigned a value of 0. A respiratory pressure of +15 mm Hg means that the pressure is 15 mm Hg above atmospheric pressure, and a respiratory pressure of −15 mm Hg is 15 mm Hg less than atmospheric pressure. Respiratory pressures often are expressed in centimeters of water (cm H_2O) because of the small pressures involved (1 mm Hg = 1.35 cm H_20).

The pressure exerted by a single gas in a mixture is called *the partial pressure*. The capital letter P followed by the chemical symbol of the gas (PO_2) is used to denote its partial pressure. The law of partial pressures states that the total pressure of a mixture of gases, as in the atmosphere, is equal to the sum of the partial pressures of the different gases in the mixture. If the concentration of oxygen at 760 mm Hg (1 atmosphere) is 20%, its partial pressure is 152 mm Hg (760 × 0.20).

Water vapor is different from other types of gases; its partial pressure is affected by temperature but not atmospheric pressure. The relative humidity refers to the percentage of moisture in the air compared with the amount that the air can hold without causing condensation (100% saturation). Warm air holds more moisture than cold air. This is the reason that precipitation in the form of rain or snow commonly occurs when the relative humidity is high and there is a sudden drop in atmospheric temperature. The air in the alveoli, which is 100% saturated and maintained at body temperature, has a water vapor pressure of 47 mm Hg. The water vapor pressure must be included in the sum of the total pressure of the gases in the alveoli (*i.e.*, the total pressure of the other gases in the alveoli is 760 − 47 = 713 mm Hg).

Air moves between the atmosphere and the lungs because of a pressure difference. According to the laws of physics, the pressure of a gas varies inversely with the volume of its container, provided the temperature remains constant. If equal amounts of a gas are placed in two different-sized containers, the pressure of the gas in the smaller container is greater than the pressure in the larger container. The movement of gases is always from the container with the greater pressure to the one with the lesser pressure. The chest cavity can be viewed as a volume container. During inspiration, the size of the chest cavity increases and air moves into the lungs; during expiration, air moves out as the size of the chest cavity decreases.

Respiratory Pressures

The pressure inside the airways and alveoli of the lungs is called the *intrapulmonary pressure* or *alveolar pressure*. The gases within this area of the lungs are in communication with atmospheric pressure (Fig. 22–8). When the glottis is open and air is not moving into or out of the lungs, as occurs just before inspiration or expiration, the intrapulmonary pressure is 0 or equal to atmospheric pressure.

The pressure in the pleural cavity is called the *intrapleural pressure*. The intrapleural pressure is always negative in relation to alveolar pressure, about −4 mm Hg between breaths when the glottis is open and the alveolar spaces are open to the atmosphere. The lungs and the chest wall have elastic properties, each pulling in the opposite direction. If removed from the chest, the lungs would contract to a smaller size, and the chest wall, if freed from the lungs, would expand. The opposing forces of the chest wall and lungs create a pull against the visceral and parietal layers of the pleura, causing the pressure within the pleural cavity to become negative. During inspiration, the elastic recoil of the lungs increases, causing intrapleural pressure to become more negative than during expiration. Without the negative intrapleural pressure holding the lungs against the chest wall, their elastic recoil properties would cause them to collapse. Although intrapleural pressure is negative in relation to alveolar pressure, it may become positive in relation to atmospheric pressure (*e.g.*, during forced expiration and coughing).

The *intrathoracic pressure* is the pressure within the thoracic cavity. It is essentially equal to intrapleural pressure and is the pressure to which the lungs, heart, and great vessels are exposed. Forced expiration against a closed glottis compresses the air in the thoracic cavity and produces marked increases in intrathoracic pressure and intrapleural pressure.

Ventilation and Lung Volumes

Ventilation is concerned with the movement of gases into and out of the lungs. It depends on a system of open airways and movement of the chest cage by the respiratory muscles.

The Chest Cage and Respiratory Muscles

The lungs and major airways share the chest cavity with the heart, great vessels, and esophagus. The chest cavity is a closed compartment bounded on the top by the neck

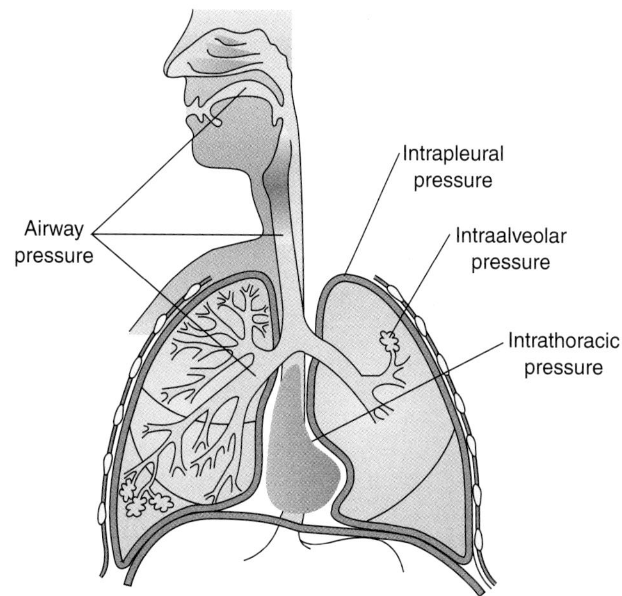

Figure 22–8
Partitioning of respiratory pressures.

muscles and at the bottom by the diaphragm. The outer walls of the chest cavity are formed by 12 pairs of ribs, the sternum, the thoracic vertebrae, and the intercostal muscles that lie between the ribs. Mechanically, the act of breathing depends on the fact that the chest cavity is a closed compartment whose only opening to the exterior is the trachea.

During inspiration, the size of the chest cavity increases, and the intrathoracic pressure becomes more negative. Air is drawn into the lungs because intrathoracic pressure is less than atmospheric pressure. The diaphragm is the principal muscle of inspiration. When the diaphragm contracts, the abdominal contents are forced downward and the chest expands from top to bottom (Fig. 22–9). During normal levels of inspiration, the diaphragm moves about 1 cm, but this can be increased to 10 cm on forced inspiration. The diaphragm is innervated by the phrenic nerve roots, which arise from the cervical level of the spinal cord, mainly from C4 but also from C3 and C5. Paralysis of one side of the diaphragm causes the chest to move up on that side rather than down during inspiration because of the negative pressure in the chest. This is called *paradoxical movement*.

The external intercostal muscles, which also aid in inspiration, connect to the adjacent ribs and slope downward and forward (Fig. 22–10). When they contract, they raise the ribs and rotate them slightly so that the sternum is pushed forward; this enlarges the chest from side to side and from front to back. The intercostal muscles receive their innervation from nerves that exit the central nervous system at the thoracic level of the spinal cord. Paralysis of these muscles usually does not have a serious effect on respiration because of the effectiveness of the diaphragm.

The accessory muscles of inspiration include the scalene muscles and the sternocleidomastoid muscles. The scalene muscles elevate the first two ribs, and the sternocleidomastoid muscles raise the sternum to increase the size of the chest cavity. These muscles contribute little to quiet breathing but contract vigorously during exercise. For the accessory muscles to assist in ventilation, they must be stabilized in some way. For example, persons with bronchial asthma often brace their arms against a firm object during an attack as a means of immobilizing their shoulders so that the attached accessory muscles can exert their full effect on ventilation. The head commonly is bent backward so that the scalene and sternocleidomastoid muscles can elevate the ribs more effectively. Other muscles that play a minor role in inspiration are the alae nasi, which produce flaring of the nostrils during obstructed breathing.

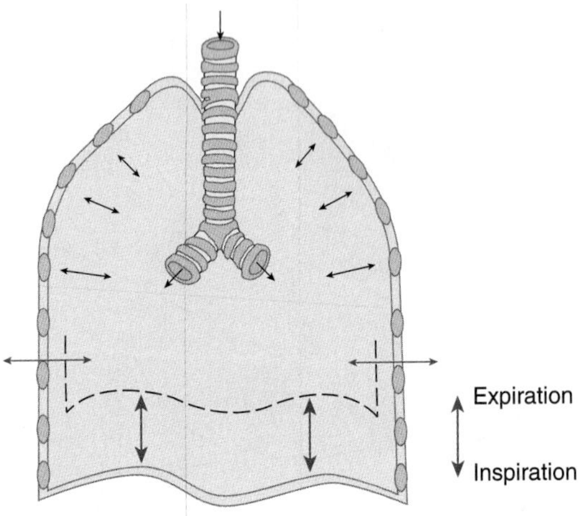

Figure 22–9
Frontal section of the chest showing the movement of the rib cage and diaphragm during inspiration and expiration.

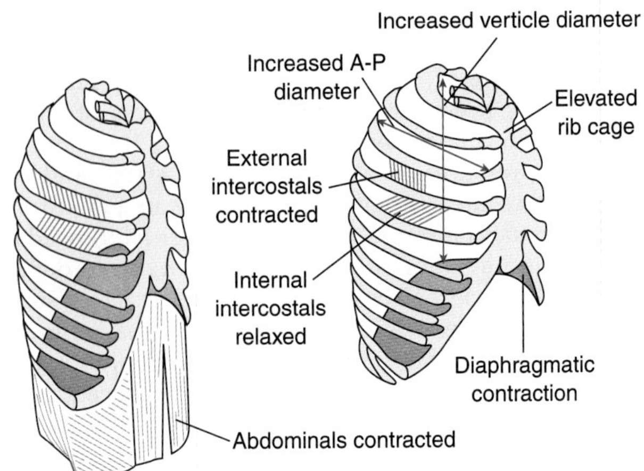

Figure 22–10
Expansion and contraction of the thoracic cage during expiration and inspiration, demonstrating especially diaphragmatic contraction, elevation of the rib cage, and function of the intercostals. (Guyton A.C., Hall J.E. [1996]. *Textbook of medical physiology* [p. 478]. Philadelphia: W.B. Saunders)

During expiration, the elastic components of the chest wall and lung structures that were stretched during inspiration recoil passively, causing the size of the chest cavity to decrease and pressure within the chest cavity to increase. As intrathoracic pressure becomes greater than atmospheric pressure, air moves out of the lungs. When needed, the abdominal and the internal intercostal muscles can be used to increase expiratory effort (see Fig. 22–10). The increase in intraabdominal pressure that accompanies the forceful contraction of the abdominal muscles pushes the diaphragm upward and results in an increase in intrathoracic pressure. The internal intercostal muscles move inward, which pulls the chest downward, increasing expiratory effort.

Lung Volumes

The amount of air that is inhaled or exhaled from various lung volumes can be measured with a spirometer. With the type of spirometer shown in Figure 22–11, the bell, which is inverted over a water bath, moves down during inspiration and up during expiration, causing the pen to move up and down and mark the chart paper. Lung volumes and capacities are summarized in Table 22–1.

Lung volumes can be subdivided into four components: tidal volume, inspiratory reserve volume, expiratory reserve volume, and residual volume. The *tidal volume* (TV), usually about 500 ml, is the amount of air that moves into and out of the lungs during a normal breath. The maximum amount of air that can be inspired in excess of the normal TV is called the *inspiratory reserve volume* (IRV), and the maximum amount that can be exhaled in excess of the normal TV is the *expiratory reserve volume* (ERV). About 1200 ml of air always remains in the lungs after forced expiration; this air is the *residual volume* (RV). The RV increases with age, because there is more trapping of air in the lungs at the end of expiration.

Lung capacities include two or more lung volumes. The *vital capacity* equals the IRV plus the TV plus the ERV and is the amount of air that can be exhaled from the point of maximal inspiration. The *inspiratory capacity* equals the TV plus the IRV. It is the amount of air a person can breathe in beginning at the normal expiratory level and distending the lungs to the maximal amount. The *functional residual capacity* is the sum of the RV and ERV; it is the volume of air that remains in the lungs at the end of normal expiration. The *total lung capacity* is the sum of all the volumes in the lungs. The RV cannot be measured with the spirometer, because this air cannot be expressed from the lungs. It is measured by indirect methods, such

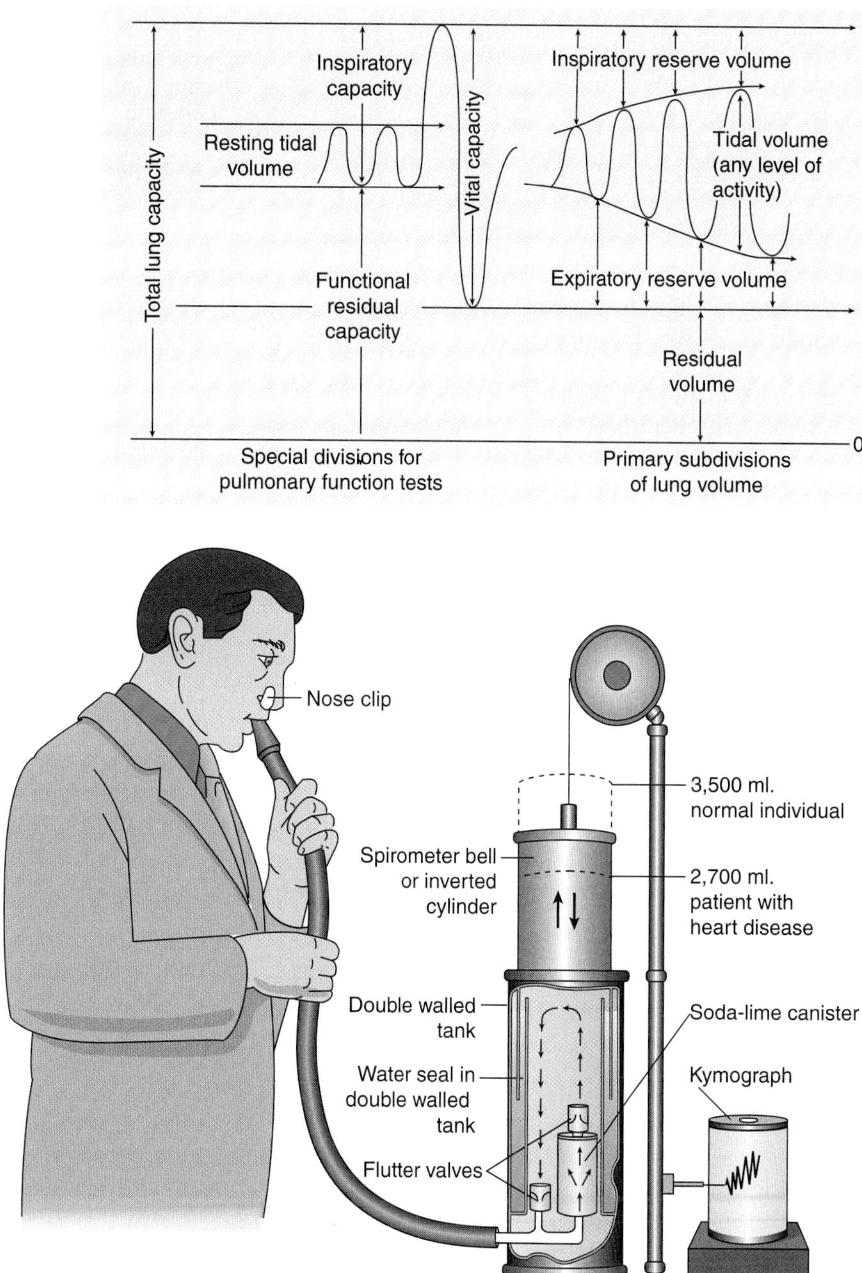

Figure 22–11
Measurement of vital capacity using a spirometer.

TABLE 22-1

Lung Volumes and Capacities

Volume	Symbol	Measurement
Tidal volume (about 500 ml at rest)	TV	Amount of air that moves into and out of the lungs with each breath
Inspiratory reserve volume (about 3000 ml)	IRV	Maximum amount of air that can be inhaled from the point of maximal expiration
Expiratory reserve volume (about 1100 ml)	ERV	Maximum volume of air that can be exhaled from the resting end-expiratory level
Residual volume (about 1200 ml)	RV	Volume of air remaining in the lungs after maximal expiration. This volume cannot be measured with the spirometer; it is measured indirectly using methods such as the helium dilution method, the nitrogen washout technique, or body plethysmography
Functional residual capacity (about 2300 ml)	FRC	Volume of air remaining in the lungs at end-expiration (sum of RV and ERV)
Inspiratory capacity (about 3500 ml)	IC	Sum of IRV and TV
Vital capacity (about 4600 ml)	VC	Maximal amount of air that can be exhaled from the point of maximal inspiration
Total lung capacity (about 5800 ml)	TLC	Total amount of air that the lungs can hold; it is the sum of all the volume components after maximal inspiration. This value is about 20% to 25% less in females than in males.

as the helium dilution methods, the nitrogen washout methods, or body plethysmography.

Pulmonary Function Studies

The previously mentioned lung volumes and capacities are anatomic or static measures, determined by lung volumes and measured without relation to time. The spirometer is also used to measure dynamic lung function (*i.e.*, ventilation with respect to time); these tests often are used in assessing pulmonary function. Pulmonary function is measured for various clinical purposes, including diagnosis of respiratory disease, preoperative surgical and anesthetic risk evaluation, and symptom and disability evaluation for legal or insurance purposes. The tests commonly are used in evaluating dyspnea, cough, wheezing, and abnormal radiologic or laboratory findings.

The *maximum voluntary ventilation* measures the volume of air that a person can move into and out of the lungs during maximum effort lasting for 12 to 15 seconds. This measurement usually is converted to liters per minute. The *forced expiratory vital capacity* (FVC) involves full inspiration to total lung capacity followed by forceful maximal expiration. Obstruction of airways produces a FVC that is lower than that observed with more slowly performed vital capacity measurements. The expired volume is plotted against time. The $FEV_{1.0}$ is the *forced expiratory volume* that can be exhaled in 1 second. The $FEV_{1.0}$ frequently is expressed as a percentage of the FVC. The $FEV_{1.0}$ and FVC are used in the diagnosis of obstructive lung disorders.

The *forced inspiratory vital flow* (FIF) measures the respiratory response during rapid maximal inspiration. Calculation of airflow during the middle half of inspiration ($FIF_{25-75\%}$) relative to the forced midexpiratory flow rate ($FEF_{25-75\%}$) is used as a measure of respiratory muscle dysfunction, because inspiratory flow depends more on effort than does expiration. The pulmonary function tests are summarized in Table 22–2.

Mechanics of Breathing

The respiratory airways and blood vessels are embedded in elastic tissue. When the lungs are inflated, this elastic tissue must be stretched. The degree to which the lung expands depends on the respiratory pressures inflating the lung and on ease of inflation or the stiffness of the lung.

Lung tissue is made up of elastin and collagen fibers that encircle the airways and small blood vessels. The elastin fibers are highly distensible and can be stretched to almost double their resting length. Collagen fibers resist stretching and make lung inflation more difficult. Three terms are used to describe the elastic properties of the lung: *distensibility*, or ease of inflation; *stiffness*, or resistance to stretch; and *elastic recoil*, or the ability of the elastic components of the lung to recoil to their original position. Overstretching the airways, as occurs with emphysema, causes the elastic components of the lung to lose their recoil, making the lung easy to inflate but difficult to deflate because of its inability to recoil.

Lung Compliance

Lung compliance refers to the ease with which the lungs can be inflated. It can be compared with the ease of blowing up a new balloon compared with one that is compliant from having been blown up previously. Specifically, lung compliance (C) describes the change in lung volume (V) that can be accomplished with a given change in respiratory pressure (P).

$$C = V/P$$

The normal compliance of both lungs in the average adult is about 200 ml/cm H_2O pressure. It would take more pressure to move the same amount of air into a noncompliant lung. Compliance is determined by the elastic and collagen fibers of the lung and by its fluid content. In the deflated lung, these fibers are partially contracted. When the lung is inflated, the elastic fibers are stretched out. Lung compliance is decreased in diseases such as interstitial lung disease and pulmonary fibrosis, which cause lung tissues to stiffen and become more difficult to stretch. Pulmonary compliance is increased in elderly persons and in those with emphysema, probably because lung tissues become permanently stretched owing to loss of elastic fibers. Pulmonary congestion and edema produce a reversible decrease in pulmonary compliance.

An important factor in lung compliance is the *surface tension* in the alveoli. The alveoli are lined with a thin film of liquid, and it is at the liquid-air interface that surface tension develops. It arises because the forces that hold the liquid film together are stronger than those that hold the air molecules together. For example, it is surface tension that holds raindrops together. In the alveoli, excess surface tension causes the liquid film to contract, making lung inflation more difficult.

The pressure in the alveoli (which are modeled as spheres with open airways projecting from them) can be predicted using Laplace's law (*i.e.*, pressure = 2 × surface tension/radius). If the surface tension were equal throughout the lungs, the alveoli with the smallest radii would have the greatest pressure, and this would cause them to empty into the larger alveoli (Fig. 22–12). The reason this does not occur is because of special surface tension–lowering molecules, called *surfactant*, that line the inner surface of the alveoli.

Surfactant is a complex mixture of lipoproteins (largely phospholipids) and small amounts of carbohydrates that is synthesized within the type II alveolar cells. The surfactant molecule has two ends: a hydrophobic (water-insoluble) tail and a hydrophilic (water-soluble) group (Fig. 22–13). The hydrophilic group attaches to the fluid molecules, and the hydrophobic tail attaches to the gas molecules, interrupting the intermolecular forces that are responsible for creating the surface tension.

Surfactant exerts four important effects on lung inflation. It lowers the surface tension; it increases lung compliance, or ease of inflation; it provides stability and more even inflation of the alveoli; and it assists in preventing pulmonary edema by keeping the alveoli dry. Without surfactant, lung inflation would be extremely difficult, requiring intrapleural pressures of −20 to −30 mm Hg, compared with the pressures of −3 to −5 mm Hg that normally are needed. Not only does surfactant reduce the surface tension in the alveoli, but it does so more effectively in the small alveoli, which have the greatest tendency to empty into the larger alveoli and collapse. This is because the surfactant molecules are more densely packed in the small alveoli. Their surface tension–reducing properties are therefore greater than in larger alveoli, where the density of the molecules is less. Surfactant also helps to keep the alveoli dry and prevent pulmonary edema. As the surface tension created by the liquid film causes the alveoli to contract, water is pulled out of the pulmonary capillaries

TABLE 22-2

Pulmonary Function Tests

Test	Symbol	Measurement*
Maximal voluntary ventilation	MVV	Maximum amount of air that can be breathed in a given time
Forced vital capacity	FVC	Maximum amount of air that can be rapidly and forcefully exhaled from the lungs after full inspiration. The expired volume is plotted against time.
Forced expiratory volume achieved in 1 second	$FEV_{1.0}$	Volume of air expired in the first second of FVC
Percentage of forced vital capacity	$FEV_{1.0}$/FVC%	Volume of air expired in the first second, expressed as a percentage of FVC
Forced midexpiratory flow rate	$FEF_{25–75\%}$	The forced midexpiratory flow rate determined by locating the points on the volume-time curve recording obtained during FVC corresponding to 25% and 75% of FVC and drawing a straight line through these points. The slope of this line represents the average midexpiratory flow rate.
Forced inspiratory flow rate	$FIF_{25–75\%}$	FIF is the volume inspired from RV at the point of measurement. $FIF_{25–75\%}$ is the slope of a line between the points on the volume pressure tracing corresponding to 25% and 75% of the inspired volume.

*By convention, all the lung volumes and rates of flow are expressed in terms of body temperature and pressure and saturated with water vapor (BTPS), which allows for a comparison of the pulmonary function data from laboratories with different ambient temperatures and altitudes.

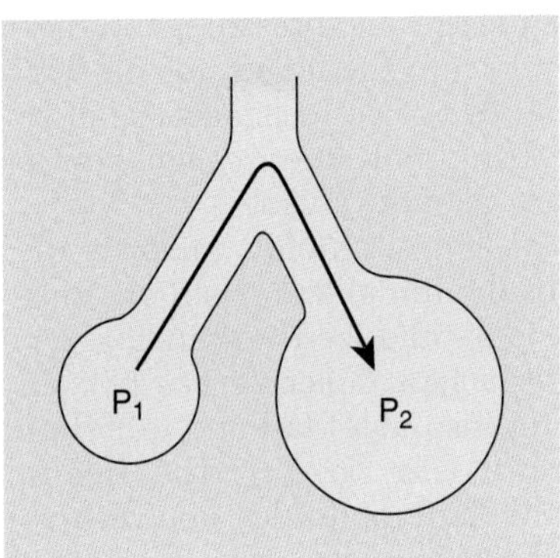

Figure 22–12
Law of Laplace (P =2 T/r, P =pressure, T =tension, r =radius). The effect of the radius on the pressure and movement of gases in the alveolar structures is depicted. Air moves from P_1 with a small radius and higher pressure to P_2 with its larger radius and lower pressure.

into the alveoli. By reducing these surface tension forces, surfactant helps to keep the alveoli dry.

The type II alveolar cells that produce surfactant do not begin to mature until the 26th to 28th week of gestation, and consequently, many premature babies have difficulty producing sufficient amounts of surfactant. This can lead to alveolar collapse and severe respiratory distress. This condition, called *infant respiratory distress syndrome*, is the single most common cause of respiratory disease in premature infants. Surfactant dysfunction is also possible in the adult. This usually occurs as the result of severe injury or infection and can contribute to the development of a condition called *adult respiratory distress syndrome* (see Chapter 24).

Airway Resistance

The volume of air that moves into and out of the air exchange portion of the lungs is directly related to the pressure difference between the lungs and the atmosphere and inversely related to the resistance of the airways.

Airway resistance is the ratio of the pressure driving inspiration or expiration to airflow. The French physician Poiseuille first described the pressure-flow characteristics of laminar flow in a straight circular tube, a correlation that has become known as Poiseuille's law. According to Poiseuille's law, the resistance to flow is inversely related to the fourth power of the radius ($R = 1/r^4$). If the radius is reduced by one half, the resistance increases 16-fold ($2 \times 2 \times 2 \times 2 = 16$).

Airway resistance normally is so small that only small changes in pressure are needed to move large volumes of air into the lungs. For example, the average pressure change that is needed to move a normal breath of 500 ml of air into the lungs is about 1 to 2 cm H_2O. Because the resistance of the airways is inversely proportional to the fourth power of the radius, small changes in airway caliber, such as those caused by pulmonary secretions or bronchospasm, can produce a marked increase in airway resistance. For persons with these conditions to maintain the same rate of air flow as before the onset of increased airway resistance, an increase in driving pressure (*i.e.*, respiratory effort) is needed.

Airway resistance is greatly affected by lung volumes, being less during inspiration than during expiration. This is because elastic-type fibers connect the outside of the airways to the surrounding lung tissues. As a result, these airways are pulled open as the lungs expand during inspiration, and they become narrower as the lungs deflate during expiration (Fig. 22–14). This is one of the reasons that persons with conditions that

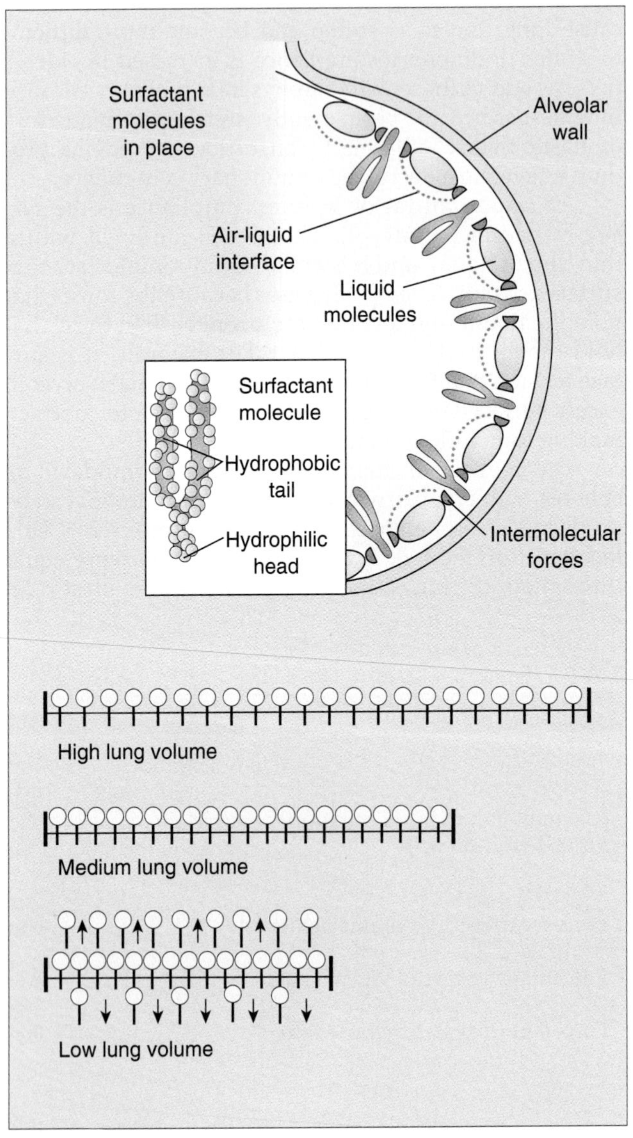

Figure 22–13
(Top) Alveolar wall depicting surface tension resulting from the intramolecular forces in the air–liquid film interface; the surfactant molecule with its hydophobic tail and hydrophilic head; and its function in reducing surface tension by disrupting the intermolecular forces. **(Bottom)** The surface concentration of surfactant molecules at high, medium, and low lung volumes.

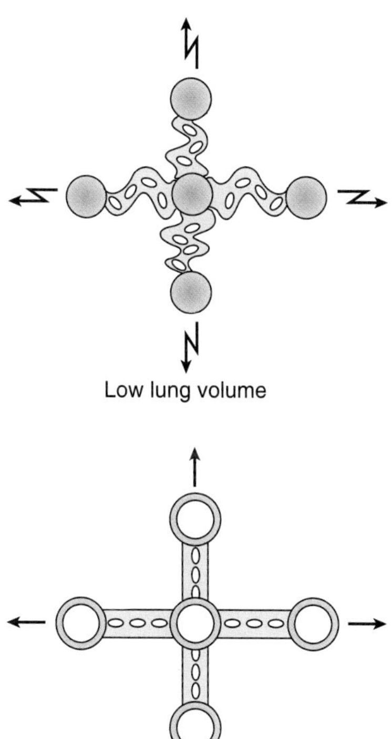

Figure 22–14
Interaction of tissue forces on airways during small and large lung volumes. At small lung volumes the tissue forces tend to fold and place less tension on the airways and they become smaller; during large lung volumes the tissue forces are stretched and pull the airways open.

increase airway resistance, such as bronchial asthma, usually have less difficulty during inspiration than during expiration.

Laminar Versus Turbulent Flow

Airflow can be laminar or turbulent, depending on the rate and pattern of flow. Laminar, or streamlined, airflow occurs at low flow rates in which the air stream is parallel with the sides of the airway. With laminar flow, the air at the periphery must overcome the resistance to flow, and as a result, the air in the center of the airway moves faster. Turbulent flow is disorganized flow in which the molecules of the gas move laterally, collide with one another, and change their velocities. Whether turbulence develops depends on the radius of the airways, the interaction of the gas molecules, and the velocity of airflow. It is most likely to occur when the radius of the airways is large and the velocity of flow is high. Turbulent flow occurs regularly in the trachea. Turbulence of airflow accounts for the respiratory sounds that are heard during chest auscultation (*i.e.,* listening to the chest with a stethoscope).

In the bronchial tree with its many branches, laminar airflow probably occurs only in the very small airways, where the velocity of flow is low. Because the small airways contribute so little resistance, they constitute a silent zone. In small airway disease (*e.g.,* chronic obstructive pulmonary disease), it is probable that considerable abnormalities are present before the usual measurements of airway resistance can detect them.

Airway Compression

Airflow through the collapsible airways in the lungs depends on the distending airway (intrapulmonary) pressures that hold the airways open and the external (intrapleural or intrathoracic) pressures that surround and compress the airways. The difference between these two pressures (*i.e.,* intrathoracic pressure − airway pressure) is called the *transpulmonary pressure.* For airflow to occur, the distending pressure inside the airways must be greater than the compressing pressure outside the airways.

During forced expiration, the transpulmonary pressure is decreased because of a disproportionate increase in the intrathoracic pressure compared with airway pressure. The resistance that air encounters as it moves out of the lungs causes a further drop in airway pressure (Figs. 22–15 and 22–16). If this drop in airway pressure is sufficiently great, the surrounding pressure compresses the collapsible airways (*i.e.,* those that lack cartilaginous support), causing airflow to be interrupted and air to be trapped in the alveoli. Although this type of airway compression usually is seen only during forced expiration in persons with normal respiratory function, it may occur during normal breathing in persons with lung diseases. For example, in conditions that increase airway resistance, such as emphysema, the pressure drop along the smaller airways is magnified, and an increase in intrabronchial pressure is needed to maintain airway patency. Measures such as pursed-lip breathing increase airway pressure and improve expiratory flow rates in persons with chronic obstructive lung disease. This is also the basis for using positive end-expiratory pressure in persons who are on mechanical ventilators. Infants who are having trouble breathing often grunt to increase their expiratory airway pressures and keep their airways open.

Efficiency and the Work of Breathing

The *minute volume,* or total ventilation, is the amount of air that is exchanged in 1 minute. It is determined by the metabolic needs of the body. The minute volume is equal to the TV multiplied by the respiratory rate, which is normally about 6000 ml (*i.e.,* 500 ml TV × respiratory rate of 12 breaths per minute) during normal activity. The efficiency of breathing is determined by matching the TV and respiratory rate in a manner that provides an optimal minute volume while minimizing the work of breathing.

The work of breathing is determined by the amount of effort required to move air through the conducting airways and by the ease of lung expansion (*i.e.,* compliance). Expansion of the lungs is difficult for persons with stiff and noncompliant lungs; they usually find it easier to breathe if they keep their TV low and breathe at a more rapid rate (*i.e.,* 300 × 20 = 6000 ml) to achieve their minute volume and meet their oxygen needs. In

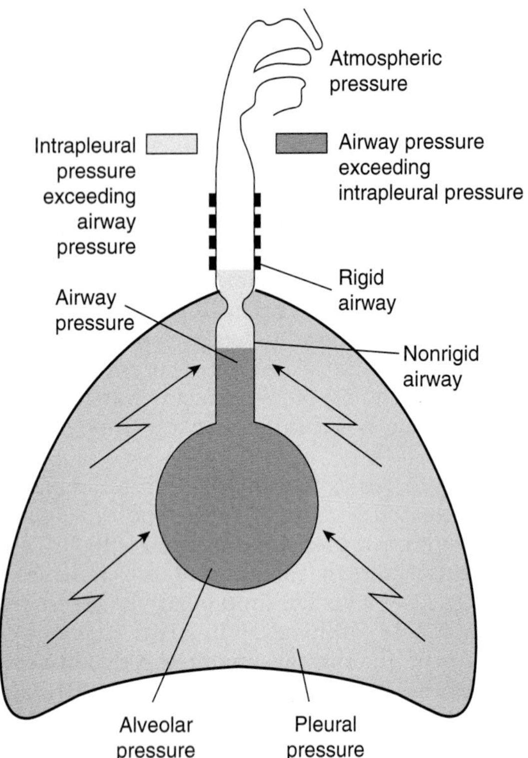

Figure 22–15
Mechanism that limits maximal expiratory flow rate. Forced expiration increases intrapleural pressure, causing airway compression of nonrigid airways where intrapleural pressure exceeds airway pressure.

contrast, persons with obstructive airway disease usually find it less difficult to inflate their lungs but expend more energy in moving air through the airways. As a result, these persons take deeper breaths and breathe at a slower rate (*i.e.*, 600 × 10 = 6000 ml) to achieve their oxygen needs.

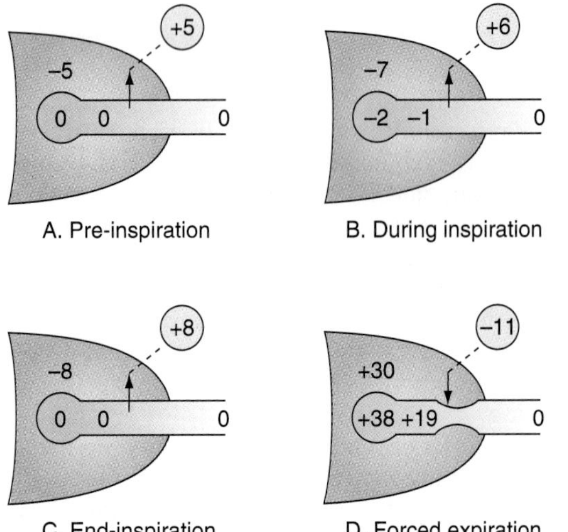

Figure 22–16
Scheme showing why airways are compressed during forced expiration. The pressure difference across the airway is holding it open, except during a forced expiration. (West J.B. [1995]. *Respiratory physiology* [p. 109]. Baltimore: Williams & Wilkins)

In summary, the movement of air between the atmosphere and the lungs follows the laws of physics as they relate to gases. The air in the alveoli contains a mixture of gases, including nitrogen, oxygen, carbon dioxide, and water vapor pressure. With the exception of water vapor, each gas exerts a pressure that is determined by the atmospheric pressure and the concentration of the gas in the mixture. Water vapor pressure is affected by temperature but not atmospheric pressure. Air moves into the lungs along a pressure gradient. The pressure inside the airways and alveoli of the lungs is called intrapulmonary (or alveolar) pressure; the pressure in the pleural cavity is called pleural pressure; and the pressure within the thoracic cavity is called intrathoracic pressure.

Breathing is the movement of gases between the atmosphere and the lungs. It requires a system of open airways and pressure changes resulting from the action of the respiratory muscles in changing the volume of the chest cage. The diaphragm is the principal muscle of inspiration, assisted by the external intercostal muscles. The accessory (*i.e.*, scalene and sternocleidomastoid) muscles elevate the ribs and act as accessory muscles for inspiration. Expiration is largely passive, aided by the elastic recoil of the respiratory muscles that were stretched during inspiration. When needed, the abdominal and internal intercostal muscles can be used to increase expiratory effort. Lung volumes and lung capacities can be measured using a spirometer. Pulmonary function studies are used to assess ventilation with respect to time.

Lung compliance describes the ease with which the lungs can be inflated. It reflects the elasticity of the lung tissue and the surface tension in the alveoli. Surfactant molecules, produced by the type II alveolar cells, reduce the surface tension in the lungs and thereby increase lung compliance. Airway resistance refers to the impediment to flow that the air encounters as it moves through the airways. Minute volume is the amount of air that is exchanged in 1 minute (i.e., respiratory rate and tidal volume) and is determined by the metabolic needs of the body. The efficiency and work of breathing are determined by factors such as impaired lung compliance and airway diseases that increase the work involved to maintain the minute volume.

Exchange and Transport of Gases

After you have completed this section of the chapter, you should be able to meet the following objectives:

- Trace the exchange of gases between the air in the alveoli and the blood in the pulmonary capillaries

- Differentiate between pulmonary and alveolar ventilation
- Explain why ventilation and perfusion must be matched
- Cite the difference between dead air space and shunt
- List four factors that affect the diffusion of gases in the alveoli
- Explain the difference between PO_2 and hemoglobin-bound oxygen and O_2 saturation and content
- Explain the significance of a *shift to the right* and a *shift to the left* in the oxygen-hemoglobin dissociation curve

The primary functions of the lungs are oxygenation of the blood and removal of carbon dioxide. Pulmonary gas exchange is conventionally divided into three processes: ventilation or the flow of gases into and out of the alveoli of the lungs, perfusion or flow of blood in the adjacent pulmonary capillaries, and diffusion or transfer of gases between the alveoli and the pulmonary capillaries. The efficiency of gas exchange requires that alveolar ventilation exists adjacent to perfused pulmonary capillaries.

Ventilation

Ventilation refers to the exchange of gases in the respiratory system. There are two types of ventilation: pulmonary and alveolar. *Pulmonary ventilation* refers to the total exchange of gases between the atmosphere and the lungs; *alveolar ventilation* is the exchange of gases within the gas exchange portion of the lungs. Ventilation requires a system of open airways and a pressure difference that moves air into and out of the lungs. It is affected by body position and lung volume as well as by disease conditions that affect the heart and respiratory system.

Distribution of Ventilation

Body Position. The distribution of ventilation between the top (apex) and bottom (base) of the lung varies with body position, reflecting the weight of the lung and the effects of gravity on intrapleural pressure. In the seated or standing position, gravity exerts a downward pull on the lung, causing intrapleural pressure at the apex of the lung to become more negative than that at the base of lung. As a result, the alveoli at the apex of the lung are more fully expanded and less compliant than those at the base of the lung. The same holds true for lung compliance in the dependent portions of the lung in the supine or lateral position. In the supine position, ventilation in the lowermost (posterior) parts of the lung exceeds that in the uppermost (anterior) parts. In the lateral position (*i.e.*, lying on the side), the dependent lung is best ventilated.

Lung Volume. Distribution of ventilation is also affected by lung volumes. During full inspiration in the seated or standing position, the airways are pulled open and air moves into the more compliant portions of the lower lung. At low lung volumes the opposite occurs. At functional residual capacity, the pleural pressure at the base of the lung exceeds airway pressure compressing the airways so that ventilation is greatly reduced. In contrast, the airways in the apex of the lung remain open and this area of the lung is well ventilated.

Even at low lung volumes, some air remains in the alveoli of the lower portion of the lungs, preventing their collapse. According to the law of Laplace (discussed previously), the pressure needed to overcome the tension in the wall of a sphere or an elastic tube is inversely related to its radius; therefore, the small airways close first, trapping some gas in the alveoli. There may be increased trapping of air in the alveoli of the lower part of the lungs in older persons and in those with lung disease (*e.g.*, emphysema). This condition is thought to result from a loss in the elastic recoil properties of the lungs, so that the intrapleural pressure, created by the elastic recoil of the lung and chest wall, becomes less negative. In these persons, airway closure occurs at the end of normal instead of low lung volumes, trapping larger amounts of air. The air trapping eventually causes an increase in the anteroposterior chest dimensions.

Perfusion

The primary functions of the pulmonary circulation are to perfuse the gas exchange portion of the lung and to facilitate gas exchange. The pulmonary circulation serves several important functions in addition to gas exchange. It filters all the blood that moves from the right to the left side of the circulation; it removes most of the thromboemboli; and it serves as a reservoir of blood for the left side of the heart.

The gas exchange function of the lungs requires a continuous flow of blood through the respiratory portion of the lungs. Deoxygenated blood enters the lung through the pulmonary artery, which has its origin in the right side of the heart and enters the lung at the hilus, along with the primary bronchus. The pulmonary arteries branch in a manner similar to that of the airways. The small pulmonary arteries accompany the bronchi as they move down the lobules and branch to supply the capillary network that surrounds the alveoli (see Fig. 22–5). The meshwork of capillaries in the respiratory portion of the lungs is so dense that the flow in these vessels often is described as being similar to a sheet of blood. The oxygenated capillary blood is collected in the small pulmonary veins of the lobules, and then it moves to the larger veins to be collected in the four large pulmonary veins that empty into the left atrium. The term *perfusion* is used to describe the flow of blood through the pulmonary capillary bed.

The pulmonary blood vessels are thinner, more compliant, and offer less resistance to flow than those in the systemic circulation, and the pressures in the pulmonary system are much lower (*e.g.*, 22/8 mm Hg versus 120/70 mm Hg). The low pressure and low resistance of the pulmonary circulation accommodate the delivery of varying amounts of blood from the systemic circulation without producing signs and symptoms of congestion. The volume in the pulmonary circulation is about 500 ml, with about 100 ml of this volume located in the pulmonary capillary bed. When the output of the right ventricle and input of the left ventricle are equal, pulmonary blood flow remains constant. Small differences between input and output can result in large changes in pulmonary volume if the differences continue for many heartbeats. The movement of blood through the pulmonary capillary bed requires that the mean pulmonary arterial pressure be greater than the mean pulmonary venous pressure. Pulmonary venous pressure increases in left-sided heart failure, allowing blood to accumulate in the pulmonary capillary bed and cause pulmonary edema. Acute pulmonary edema is discussed in Chapter 20.

Distribution of Blood Flow

As with ventilation, the distribution of pulmonary blood flow is affected by body position and gravity. In the upright position, the distance of the upper apices of the lung above the level of the heart may exceed the perfusion capabilities of the mean pulmonary arterial pressure (about 12 mm Hg); therefore, blood flow in the upper part of the lungs is less than that in the base or bottom part of the lungs (Fig. 22–17). In the supine position, the lungs and the heart are at the same level, and blood flow to the apices and base of the lungs becomes more uniform. In this position, blood flow to the posterior or dependent portions (*e.g.*, bottom of the lung when lying on the side) exceeds flow in the anterior or nondependent portions of the lungs. In persons with left-sided heart failure, congestion develops in the dependent portions of the lungs exposed to increased blood flow.

Hypoxia. The blood vessels in the pulmonary circulation undergo marked vasoconstriction when they are exposed to hypoxia. The precise mechanism for this response is unclear. When alveolar oxygen levels drop below 60 mm Hg, marked vasoconstriction may occur, and at very low oxygen levels, the local flow may be almost abolished. In regional hypoxia, as occurs with atelectasis, vasoconstriction is localized to a specific region of the lung. Vasoconstriction has the effect of directing blood flow away from the hypoxic regions of the lungs. When alveolar hypoxia no longer exists, blood flow is restored.

Generalized hypoxia causes vasoconstriction throughout the lung. Generalized vasoconstriction occurs when the partial pressure of oxygen is decreased at high altitudes, or it can occur in persons with chronic hypoxia due to lung disease. Prolonged hypoxia can lead to pulmonary hypertension and increased workload on the right heart. Other active responses of the pulmonary circulation have been described. A low blood pH causes vasoconstriction, especially when alveolar hypoxia is present (*e.g.*, during circulatory shock).

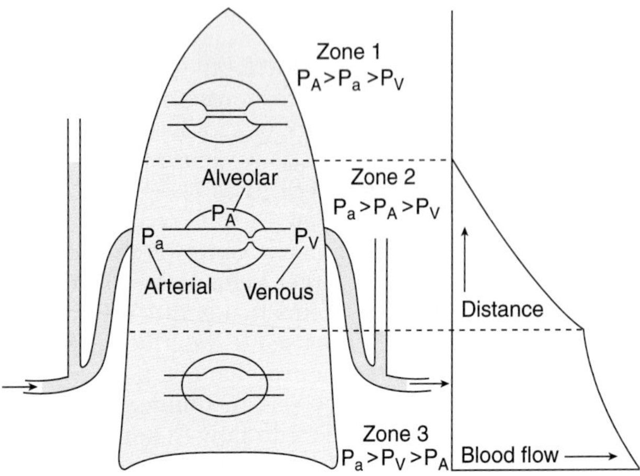

Figure 22–17
The uneven distribution of blood flow in the lung results from different pressures affecting the capillaries, which are affected by body position and gravity. (West J.B. [1995]. *Respiratory physiology* [5th ed., p. 22]. Baltimore: Williams & Wilkins)

Diffusion

There are two types of air movement in the lung, bulk flow and diffusion. Bulk flow occurs in the conducting airways and is controlled by pressure differences between the mouth and that of airways in the lung. Movement of gases in the alveoli and across the alveolar capillary membrane occurs by the process of *diffusion*.

Gas diffusion in the lung can be described by *Fick's law*. Fick's law states that the volume of a gas (Vgas) diffusing across the membrane per unit time is directly proportional to the partial pressure difference of the gas ($P_1 - P_2$), the surface area (SA) of the membrane, and the diffusion coefficient (D) and is inversely proportional to the thickness (T) of the membrane:

$$\text{Vgas} = \frac{P_1 - P_2 \times SA \times D}{T}$$

Several factors influence diffusion of gases in the lung. The administration of high concentrations of oxygen increases the difference in partial pressure between the two sides of the membrane and increases the diffusion of the gas. Diseases that destroy lung tissue (*i.e.*, surface area for diffusion) or increase the thickness of the alveolar-capillary membrane adversely influence the diffusing capacity of the lungs. The removal of one lung, for example, reduces the diffusing capacity by one half. The thickness of the alveolar-capillary membrane and the distance for diffusion are increased in patients with pulmonary edema or pneumonia.

The characteristics of the gas and its molecular weight and solubility constitute the *diffusion coefficient* and determine how rapidly it diffuses through the respiratory membranes. Carbon dioxide diffuses 20 times more rapidly than oxygen because of its greater solubility in the respiratory membranes. The factors that affect alveolar-capillary gas exchange are summarized in Table 22–3. The diffusing capacity of the lung is a measure of the rate of transfer of gases through the alveolar-capillary membrane (measured in milliliters per minute). It is measured using a gas that readily diffuses across the membrane, is easily analyzed, and is affected by the same factors that influence oxygen diffusion. Carbon monoxide, which meets these criteria, commonly is used for this purpose. The test is done by having a person breathe a known concentration of carbon monoxide (usually for a 10-second breathhold). The volume of carbon monoxide that diffuses across the respiratory membranes is calculated from measurements of lung volume and changes in the carbon monoxide content of inspired and expired air. Because blood levels of carbon monoxide usually are zero, there is no "back diffusion" of the gas, and the difference between the inspired and the expired carbon monoxide reflects the diffusion of the gas. The diffusing capacity for oxygen can be calculated using the diffusing capacity of carbon monoxide and known information about the solubility of the two gases. Persons who smoke or are exposed to carbon monoxide may have appreciable amounts of the gas in their lungs, invalidating the test results. The diffusing capacity of the lung is affected by conditions that alter the permeability of the alveolar-capillary membrane and the ability of the red blood cells to bind and transport the gas.

Matching of Ventilation and Perfusion

The gas exchange properties of the lung depend on matching ventilation and perfusion, ensuring that equal amounts of air and blood are entering the respiratory portion of the lungs. Two factors may interfere with the matching of ventilation and perfusion: dead air space and shunt.

Dead Air Space

Not all inspired air reaches the alveoli. Dead space refers to the air that must be moved with each breath but does not participate in gas exchange. The movement of air through dead space contributes to the work of breathing but not to gas exchange.

There are two types of dead space: that contained in the conducting airways, called the *anatomic dead space,* and that contained in the respiratory portion of the lung, called the *alveolar dead space.* The volume of anatomic airway dead space is fixed at about 150 to 200 ml, depending on body size. It constitutes air contained in the nose, pharynx, trachea, and bronchi. The creation of a tracheostomy decreases anatomic dead space ventilation because air does not have to move through the nasal and oral airways. Alveolar dead space, normally about 5 to 10 ml, constitutes alveolar air that does not participate in gas exchange. When alveoli are ventilated but deprived of blood flow, they do not contribute to gas exchange and thereby constitute alveolar dead space.

The physiologic dead space includes the anatomic dead space plus alveolar dead space. In persons with normal respiratory function, physiologic dead space is about the same as anatomic dead space. Only in lung disease does physiologic dead space increase. Alveolar ventilation is equal to the minute ventilation minus the physiologic dead space ventilation.

Shunt

Shunt refers to blood that moves from the right to left side of the circulation without being oxygenated. There are two types of shunts: physiologic and anatomic. In a *physiologic shunt,* there is mismatching of ventilation and perfusion, resulting in not enough ventilation to provide the oxygen needed to oxygenate the blood flowing through the alveolar capillaries. In an *anatomic shunt,* blood moves from the venous to the arterial side of the circulation without moving through the lungs. Anatomic intracardiac shunting of blood because of congenital heart defects is discussed in Chapter 19. Physiologic shunting of blood usually results from destructive lung disease that impairs ventilation or from heart failure that interferes with movement of blood through sections of the lungs.

Mismatching of Ventilation and Perfusion

There are many causes of mismatched ventilation and perfusion, and the most obvious are shown in Figure 22–18. This figure depicts three groups of alveoli with low, normal, and high ventilation-perfusion ratios. The ventilation-perfusion ratio in the center alveoli is normal,

TABLE 22-3

Factors Affecting Alveolar-Capillary Gas Exchange

Factors Affecting Gas Exchange	Examples
Surface area available for diffusion	Removal of a lung or diseases such as emphysema and chronic bronchitis, which destroy lung tissue or cause mismatching of ventilation and perfusion
Thickness of the alveolar-capillary membrane	Conditions such as pneumonia, interstitial lung disease, and pulmonary edema, which increase membrane thickness
Partial pressure of alveolar gases	Ascent to high altitudes where the partial pressure of oxygen is reduced. In the opposite direction, increasing the partial pressure of a gas in the inspired air (*e.g.*, oxygen therapy) increases the gradient for diffusion
Solubility and molecular weight of the gas	Carbon dioxide, which is more soluble in the cell membranes, diffuses across the alveolar-capillary membrane more rapidly than oxygen

resulting in normal gas exchange and oxygen concentrations. Perfusion without ventilation (left) results in a low ventilation-perfusion ratio. This is the type of situation that occurs in atelectasis (see Chapter 24). Ventilation without perfusion (right) results in a high ventilation-perfusion ratio. An example of this type of situation is pulmonary embolism when a blood clot obstructs flow.

The arterial blood leaving the pulmonary circulation reflects mixing of the three alveolar-capillary units. Most of the situations in which ventilation and perfusion are mismatched are less obvious. In lung disease, for example, there may be altered ventilation in one area of the lung and altered perfusion in another area.

Gas Transport

The lungs enable inhaled air to come in contact with blood flowing through the pulmonary capillaries so that exchange of gases between the external environment and the internal environment of the body can take place. The lungs restore the oxygen content of the arterial blood and remove carbon dioxide from the venous blood.

The blood carries oxygen and carbon dioxide in the dissolved state and in combination with hemoglobin. Carbon dioxide is converted to bicarbonate and transported in that form.

The amount of a gas that can dissolve in plasma is determined by two factors: the solubility of the gas in the plasma and the partial pressure of the gas in the alveoli. Oxygen and carbon dioxide dissolve in plasma. The presence of these dissolved gases is similar to the carbon dioxide that is dissolved in a capped bottle of a carbonated drink. In the case of the carbonated drink, the gas is dissolved under increased pressure, which allows more gas to be dissolved. When the bottle cap is removed, the pressure is reduced, and less gas remains in the dissolved state. Tiny bubbles form as the gas moves from the dissolved to the gaseous state.

In the clinical setting, blood gas measurements are used to determine the level of partial pressure (PO_2) and carbon dioxide (PCO_2) in the blood. Arterial blood commonly is used for measuring blood gases. Venous blood is not used, because venous levels of oxygen and carbon dioxide reflect the metabolic demands of the tissues rather than the gas exchange function of the lungs. The PO_2 of arterial blood normally is above 80 mm Hg, and PCO_2 is in the range of 35 to 45 mm Hg. Normally, the arterial blood gases are the same or close to the same as the partial pressure of the gases in the alveoli. The arterial PO_2 is often written PaO_2 and the alveolar PO_2 as PAO_2, with the same types of designations being used for PCO_2. This text uses PO_2 and PCO_2 to designate arterial and alveolar levels of the gases.

Oxygen Transport

Oxygen is transported in two forms: in chemical combination with hemoglobin and in the dissolved state. The hemoglobin in red blood cells serves as a transport vehicle for oxygen. It binds oxygen in the pulmonary capillaries and releases it in the tissue capillaries. As oxygen moves into or out of the red blood cells, it dissolves in the plasma. It is the dissolved form of oxygen that leaves the capillary, crosses cell membranes, and participates in cell metabolism. Only about 1% of the oxygen in the blood is carried in the dissolved state; the remainder is carried in combination with the hemoglobin. The oxygen content of the blood (measured in ml/100 ml blood) includes the oxygen carried by hemoglobin and dissolved oxygen.

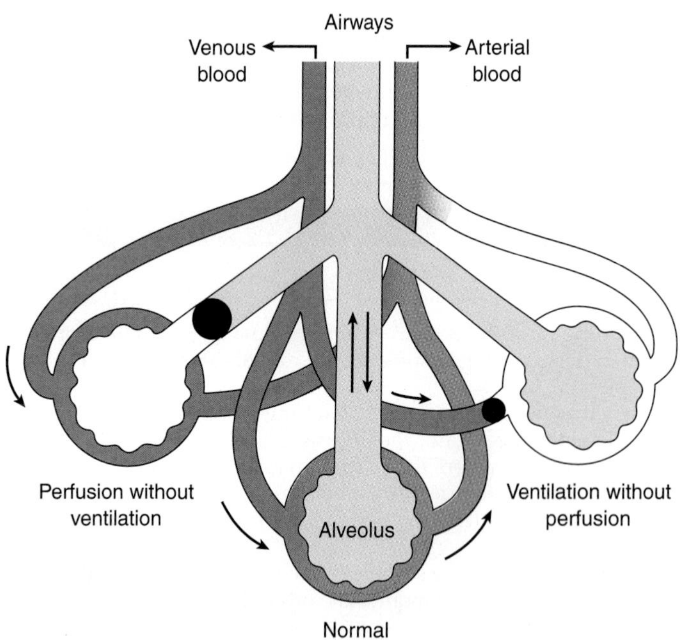

Figure 22–18
Matching of ventilation and perfusion. (**Center**) Normal matching of ventilation and perfusion; (**left**) perfusion without ventilation (*i.e.*, shunt); (**right**) ventilation without perfusion (*i.e.*, dead air space).

Dissolved Oxygen. The partial pressure of oxygen (PO_2) represents the level of dissolved oxygen in plasma. The amount of gas that can be dissolved in a liquid depends on the solubility of the gas and its pressure. The solubility of oxygen in plasma is fixed and very small. For every 1 mm Hg of PO_2 present in the alveoli, 0.003 ml of oxygen becomes dissolved in 100 ml of plasma. This means that at a normal alveolar PO_2 of 100 mm Hg, the blood carries only 0.3 ml of dissolved oxygen in each 100 ml of plasma. This amount is very small compared with the amount that can be carried in an equal amount of blood when oxygen is attached to hemoglobin.

Although the amount of oxygen carried in plasma under normal conditions is small, it can become a lifesaving mode of transport in carbon monoxide poisoning, when most of the hemoglobin sites are occupied by carbon monoxide and are unavailable for transport of oxygen. The use of a hyperbaric chamber, in which 100% oxygen can be administered at high atmospheric pressures, increases the amount of oxygen that can be carried in the dissolved state.

Hemoglobin Transport. Hemoglobin is a highly efficient carrier of oxygen, and about 98% to 99% of the oxygen used by body tissues is carried in this manner. Hemoglobin with bound oxygen is called *oxyhemoglobin,* and when oxygen is removed, it is called *deoxygenated or reduced hemoglobin.* Each gram of hemoglobin carries about 1.34 ml of oxygen when saturated. This means that a person with a hemoglobin of 14 g/100 ml of blood carries 18.8 ml of oxygen per 100 ml of blood. In the lungs, oxygen moves across the alveolar-capillary membrane, through the plasma, and into the red blood cell, where it forms a loose and reversible bond with the hemoglobin molecule. In normal lungs, this process is rapid, so that even with a fast heart rate, the hemoglobin is almost completely saturated with oxygen during the short time it spends in the pulmonary capillaries.

The oxygenated hemoglobin is transported in the arterial blood to the peripheral capillaries, where the oxygen is released and made available to the tissues for use in cell metabolism. As the oxygen moves out of the capillaries in response to the needs of the tissues, the hemoglobin saturation, which is usually about 95% to 97% as the blood leaves the left side of the heart, drops to about 75% as the mixed venous blood returns to the right side of the heart.

Oxygen-Hemoglobin Dissociation. Oxygen that remains bound to hemoglobin cannot participate in tissue metabolism. The efficiency of the oxygen dissociation transport system depends on the ability of the hemoglobin molecule to bind oxygen in the lungs and release it as it is needed in the tissues. The affinity of hemoglobin refers to its capacity to bind oxygen; the hemoglobin binds oxygen more readily when affinity is increased and releases it more readily when affinity is decreased. As described in Chapter 8, the hemoglobin molecule is composed of four polypeptide chains bound to an iron-containing heme group. Because oxygen binds to the iron atom, each hemoglobin molecule can bind four molecules of oxygen. Oxygen binds cooperatively with hemoglobin. After the first molecule of oxygen binds to hemoglobin, the molecule undergoes a change in shape. As a result, the second and third molecules bind more readily, and binding of the fourth molecule is even easier. When oxygen is bound to all four of the heme groups, the hemoglobin molecule is said to be *saturated.* Hemoglobin is *partially saturated* when it contains only one, two, or three molecules of oxygen. In a like manner, unloading of one oxygen molecule enhances the unloading of the next molecule and so on. Thus, the affinity of hemoglobin for oxygen changes with oxygen saturation.

Hemoglobin's affinity for oxygen is influenced by pH, carbon dioxide concentration, and temperature. Hemoglobin binds oxygen more strongly under condition of increased pH (alkalosis), decreased carbon dioxide concentration, and decreased body temperature and releases it more readily under conditions of decreased pH (acidosis), increased carbon dioxide concentration, and fever. Conditions that decrease affinity and favor unloading of oxygen reflect tissue metabolism and need for oxygen. For example, tissue metabolism generates carbon dioxide and metabolic acids. Heat also is a byproduct of tissue metabolism, explaining the effect of fever on oxygen binding.

Red blood cells contain a metabolic intermediate called *2,3-diphosphoglycerate* (2,3-DPG) that also affects oxyhemoglobin affinity. An increase in 2,3-DPG enhances unloading of oxygen from hemoglobin at the tissue level. An increase in 2,3-DPG occurs with exercise and the hypoxia that occurs with high altitude and chronic lung disease.

The relation between the oxygen carried in combination with hemoglobin and the PO_2 of the blood is described by the *oxygen-hemoglobin dissociation* curve, which is shown in Figure 22–19. The x-axis depicts the PO_2; the left y-axis, hemoglobin oxygen saturation, and the right y-axis, oxygen content. There are two important things to remember about the relations among PO_2, oxygen saturation, and oxygen content. First, PO_2 is the dissolved oxygen. It reflects the partial pressure of the gas in the lung (*e.g.*, the PO_2 is about 100 mm Hg when breathing room air but can be increased to 200 mm Hg or higher when breathing oxygen enriched air). Second, it is the oxygen content of the blood rather than the PO_2, or even oxygen saturation, that determines the amount of oxygen carried in the blood and delivered to the tissues. An anemic person has a normal PO_2 and hemoglobin saturation level but decreased oxygen content.

The S-shaped oxygen dissociation curve has a flat top portion representing binding of oxygen by the hemoglobin in the lungs and a steep portion representing its release into the tissue capillaries. The S shape of the curve reflects the effect that oxygen saturation has on the affinity of hemoglobin for oxygen. At about 100 mm Hg PO_2, a plateau occurs, at which point the hemoglobin is about 98% saturated. Increasing the alveolar PO_2 above this level has no further effect on increasing hemoglobin saturation. Even at high altitudes, when the partial pressure of oxygen is considerably decreased, the hemoglobin remains relatively well saturated. At 60 mm Hg PO_2, the hemoglobin is still about 89% saturated.

The steep portion of the dissociation curve—between 60 and 40 mm Hg—represents the removal of oxygen from the hemoglobin as it moves through the tissue capillaries. This portion of the curve is important because it permits considerable transfer of oxygen from hemoglobin to the tissues with only a small drop in PO_2, ensuring a gradient for oxygen to move into body cells. The tissues normally remove about 5 ml of oxygen per 100 ml of blood, and the hemoglobin of mixed venous blood is about 75% saturated as it returns to the right side of the heart. In this portion of the dissociation curve, the rate at which oxygen is released from hemoglobin is largely determined by tissue uptake. During strenuous exercise, for example, the muscle cells may remove as much as 15 ml of oxygen per 100 ml of blood from hemoglobin.

Hemoglobin can be regarded as an oxygen buffer system that regulates oxygen pressure in the tissues. Hemoglobin affinity for oxygen must change with the metabolic needs of the tissues. This change is represented by a shift to the right or left in the dissociation curve, as shown in Figure 22–19. As the curve shifts to the right, the tissue PO_2 is greater for any given of level of hemoglobin saturation. A shift to the right represents reduced affinity of the hemoglobin for oxygen at any given PO_2. It usually is caused by conditions such as fever or acidosis or by an increase in PCO_2, which reflects increased tissue metabolism. High altitude and conditions such as pulmonary insufficiency, heart failure, and severe anemia also cause the oxygen dissociation curve to shift to the right.

A shift to the left in the oxygen dissociation curve represents enhanced affinity of hemoglobin for oxygen and occurs in situations associated with a decrease in tissue metabolism, such as alkalosis, decreased body temperature, and decreased carbon dioxide levels. The degree of shift can be determined by the P_{50}, or the partial pressure of oxygen that is needed to achieve a 50% saturation of hemoglobin. Returning to Figure 22–19, the dissociation curve on the left has a P_{50} of about 20 mm Hg; the normal curve, a P_{50} of 26; and the curve on the right, a P_{50} of 35 mm Hg.

Carbon Dioxide Transport

Carbon dioxide is transported in the blood in three forms: as dissolved carbon dioxide (10%), attached to hemoglobin (30%), and as bicarbonate (60%). Acid-base bal-

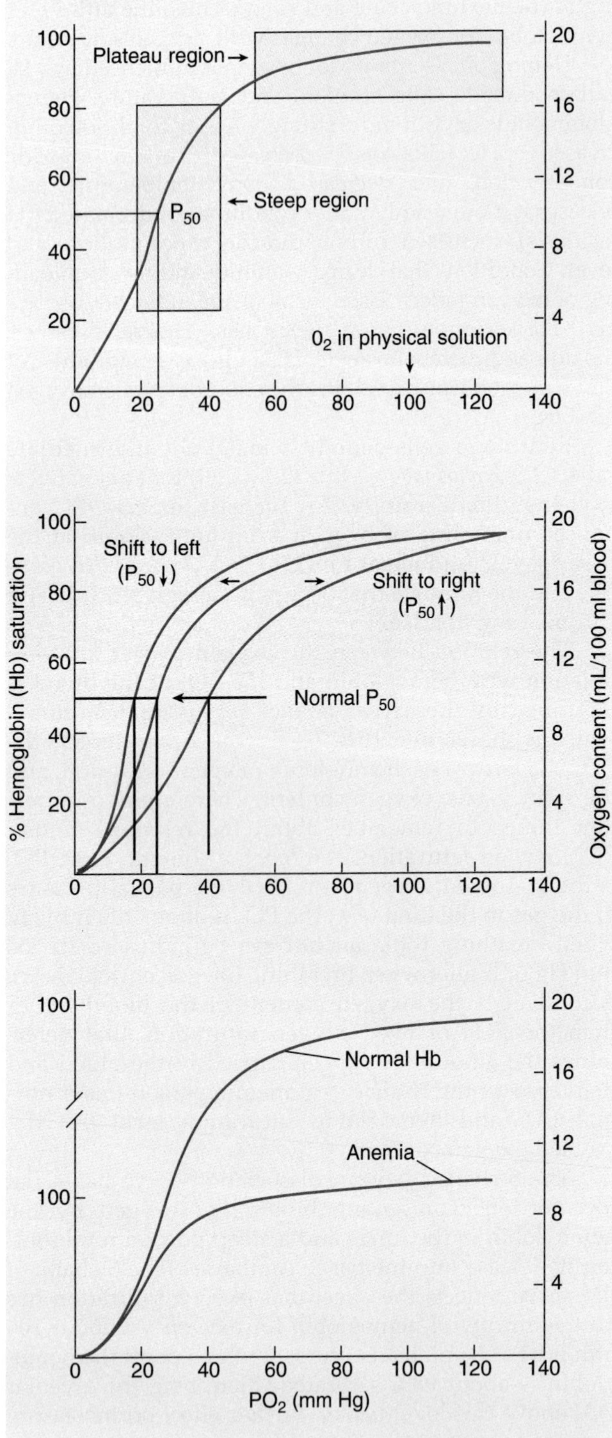

Figure 22–19 Oxygen-hemoglobin dissociation curve. (**Top**) Left boxed area represents the steep portion of the curve where oxygen is released from hemoglobin to the tissues, and the top boxed area the plateau of the curve where oxygen is loaded onto hemoglobin in the lung. P_{50}, partial pressure of oxygen required to saturated 50% of hemoglobin with oxygen. (**Middle**) The effect of body temperature, arterial PCO_2, and pH on hemoglobin affinity for oxygen as indicated by a shift in the curve and position of the P_{50}. A shift of the curve to the right due to an increase in temperature, PCO_2, or decreased pH favors release of oxygen to the tissues. A decrease in temperature, PCO_2, or increase in pH shifts the curve to the left and has the opposite effect. (**Bottom**) Effect of anemia on the oxygen-carrying capacity of blood. The hemoglobin can be completely saturated, but the oxygen content of the blood is reduced. (**Top** and **bottom** adapted from Rhoades R.A., Tanner, G.A. [1996]. *Medical physiology.* Boston: Little, Brown)

ance is influenced by the amount of dissolved carbon dioxide and the bicarbonate level in the blood (see Chapter 27).

As carbon dioxide is formed during the metabolic process, it diffuses out of cells into the tissue spaces and then into the capillaries. Only a small portion of the carbon dioxide is carried in the dissolved state (PCO_2) to the lungs. The PCO_2 of arterial blood is about 40 mm Hg, and the PCO_2 of venous blood is about 45 mm Hg; the difference between the two values represents the amount of dissolved carbon dioxide generated in the tissues. The amount of dissolved carbon dioxide that can be carried in plasma is determined by the partial pressure of the gas and its solubility coefficient (0.03 ml/100 ml/1 mm Hg PCO_2).

Most of the carbon dioxide diffuses in the red blood cell, where it forms carbonic acid or combines with hemoglobin. In the red blood cell, carbon dioxide combines with water to form carbonic acid ($CO_2 + H_2O = H^+ HCO_3^-$). This would be a slow reaction if it were not for an enzyme called *carbonic anhydrase.* Carbonic anhydrase, which increases the reaction between carbon dioxide and water about 5000-fold, is present in large quantities in red blood cells. Carbonic acid (H_2CO_3) readily ionizes in the red blood cell to form bicarbonate (HCO_3^-) and hydrogen (H^+) ions. The hydrogen ion that is generated from the carbonic anhydrase–mediated reaction combines with the hemoglobin, which is a powerful acid-base buffer. The bicarbonate ion that formed from the reaction diffuses into plasma, exchanged for a chloride ion in a bicarbonate-chloride shift. This is made possible by a special bicarbonate-chloride carrier protein in the red blood cell membrane. As a result of the bicarbonate-chloride shift, the chloride content of the red blood cell is greater in venous blood than in arterial blood.

In addition to the carbonic anhydrase–mediated reaction with water, carbon dioxide reacts directly with hemoglobin to form carbaminohemoglobin. The combination of carbon dioxide with hemoglobin is a reversible reaction that involves a loose bond, which allows transport of carbon dioxide from tissues to the lungs, where it is released into the alveoli for exchange with the external environment. The release of oxygen from hemoglobin enhances the binding of carbon dioxide to hemoglobin in the peripheral capillaries; in the lungs, the combination of oxygen with hemoglobin displaces carbon dioxide. Binding with carbon dioxide causes the hemoglobin to become a stronger acid. In the lungs, the highly acidic hemoglobin has a lesser tendency to form carbaminohemoglobin, and carbon dioxide is released from hemoglobin into the alveoli. In the tissues, the release of oxygen from hemoglobin decreases the hemoglobin's acidity, increasing its ability to combine with carbon dioxide and form carbaminohemoglobin.

In summary, the primary functions of the lungs are oxygenation of the blood and removal of carbon dioxide. Pulmonary gas exchange is conventionally divided into three processes: ventilation, or the flow of gases into the alveoli of the lungs; perfusion of blood in the adjacent pulmonary capillaries; and diffusion or transfer of gases between the alveoli and the pulmonary capillaries.

Ventilation refers to the movement of air between the atmosphere and the lungs. Pulmonary ventilation refers to the total exchange of gases between the atmosphere and the lungs, and alveolar ventilation refers to ventilation in the gas exchange portion of the lungs. The distribution of alveolar ventilation and pulmonary capillary blood flow varies with lung volume and body position. In the upright position and at high lung volumes, ventilation is greatest in the lower parts of the lungs. The upright position also produces a decrease in blood flow to the upper parts of the lung, resulting from the distance above the level of the heart and the low mean arterial pressure in the pulmonary circulation.

The diffusion of gases in the lungs is influenced by four factors: the surface area available for diffusion; the thickness of the alveolar-capillary membrane, through which the gases diffuse; the differences in the partial pressure of the gas on either side of the membrane; and the characteristics of the gas. The efficiency of gas exchange requires that there is matching of ventilation and perfusion, so that equal amounts of air and blood enter the respiratory portion of the lungs. Two factors—dead air space and shunt—interfere with matching of ventilation and perfusion and do not contribute to gas exchange. Dead air space occurs when areas of the lungs are ventilated but not perfused. Shunt is the condition under which areas of the lungs are perfused but not ventilated.

The blood transports oxygen to the cells and returns carbon dioxide to the lungs. Oxygen is transported in two forms: in chemical combination with hemoglobin and physically dissolved in plasma (PO_2). Hemoglobin is an efficient carrier of oxygen, and about 98% to 99% of oxygen is transported in this manner. Carbon dioxide is carried in three forms: as carbaminohemoglobin, as dissolved carbon dioxide, and as bicarbonate. Between 70% and 80% of carbon dioxide in plasma is in the bicarbonate or dissolved form.

Control of Breathing

After you have completed this section of the chapter, you should be able to meet the following objectives:

- Compare the neural control of the respiratory muscles, which control breathing, with that of cardiac muscle, which controls the pumping action of the heart
- Describe the function of the chemoreceptors and lung receptors in the regulation of ventilation
- Trace the integration of the cough reflex from stimulus to explosive expulsion of air that constitutes the cough
- Describe the type of periodic breathing known as *Cheyne-Stokes breathing*
- Define *dyspnea* and list three types of conditions in which dyspnea occurs

Unlike the heart, which has inherent rhythmic properties and can beat independently of the nervous system, the muscles that control respiration require continuous input from the nervous system. Movement of the diaphragm, intercostal muscles, sternocleidomastoid, and other accessory muscles that control ventilation are integrated by neurons located in the pons and medulla. These neurons are collectively referred to as the *respiratory center* (Fig. 22–20).

The respiratory center consists of two dense bilateral aggregates of respiratory neurons involved in initiating inspiration and expiration and incorporating afferent impulses into motor responses of the respiratory muscles. The first, or dorsal, group of neurons in the respiratory center is primarily concerned with inspiration. These neurons control the activity of the phrenic nerves that innervate the diaphragm and drive the second, or ventral, group of respiratory neurons. They probably integrate sensory input from the lungs and airways into the ventilatory response. The second group of neurons, which contains inspiratory and expiratory neurons, controls the spinal

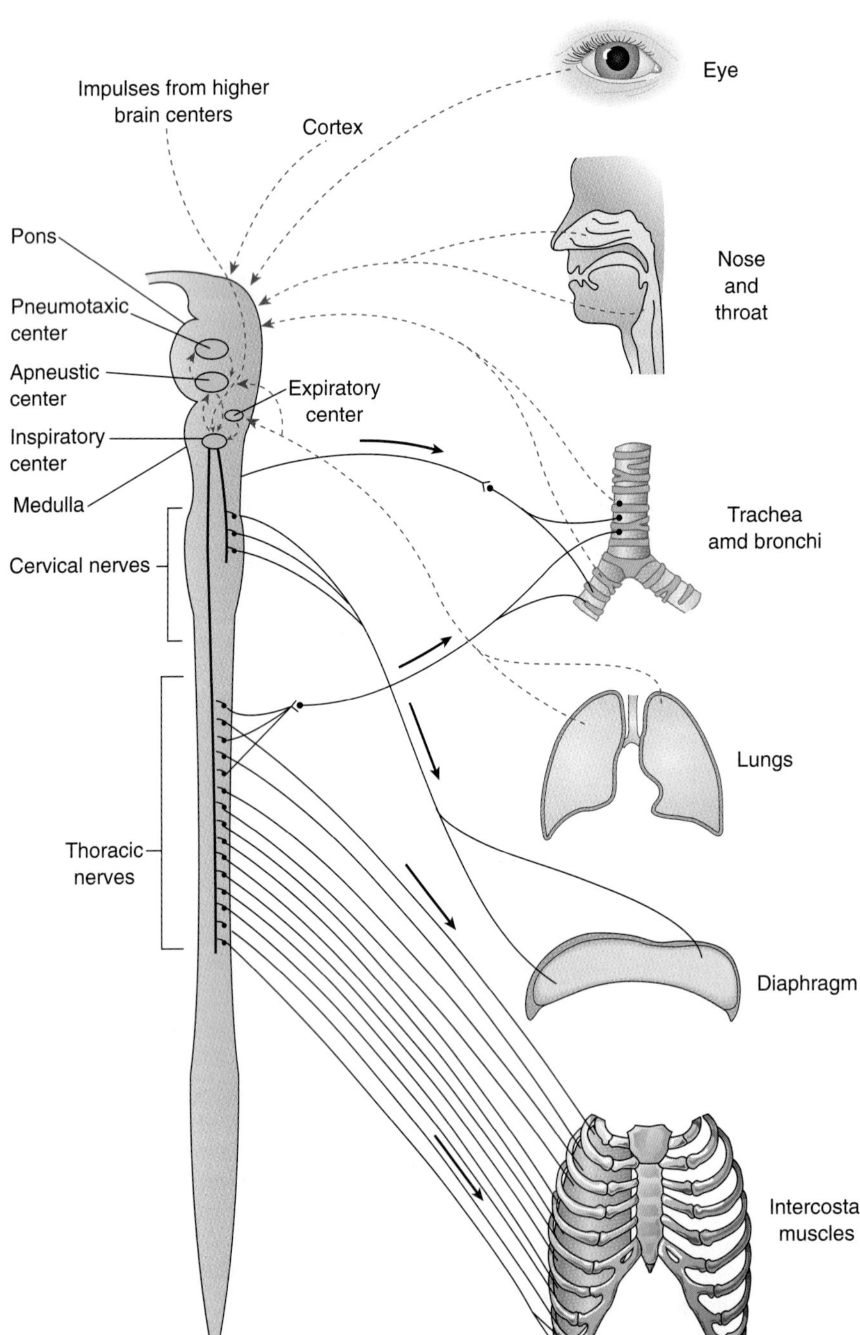

Figure 22–20 Schematic representation of activity in the respiratory center. Impulses traveling over afferent neurons activate central neurons, which activate efferent neurons that supply the muscles of respiration. Respiratory movements can be altered by a variety of stimuli.

motor neurons of the intercostal and abdominal muscles.

The pacemaker properties of the respiratory center result from the cycling of the two groups of respiratory neurons. The pneumotaxic center in the upper pons and apneustic center in the lower pons contribute to the function of the respiratory center in the medulla. The apneustic center has an excitatory effect on inspiration, tending to prolong inspiration. The pneumotaxic center switches inspiration off, assisting in the control of respiratory rate and inspiratory volume. Brain injury that damages the connection between the pneumotaxic and apneustic centers results in an irregular breathing pattern that consists of prolonged inspiratory gasps interrupted by expiratory efforts.

Axons from the neurons in the respiratory center cross in the midline and descend in the ventrolateral columns of the spinal cord. The tracts that control expiration and inspiration are spatially separated in the cord, as are the tracts that transmit specialized reflexes (*i.e.*, coughing and hiccupping) and voluntary control of ventilation. Only at the level of the spinal cord are the respiratory impulses integrated to produce a reflex response. The neural control of ventilation is shown in Figure 22–20.

The control of breathing has automatic and voluntary components. The automatic regulation of ventilation is controlled by input from two types of sensors or receptors: chemoreceptors and lung receptors. Chemoreceptors monitor blood levels of oxygen, carbon dioxide, and pH and adjust ventilation to meet the changing metabolic needs of the body. Lung receptors monitor breathing patterns and lung function. Voluntary regulation of ventilation integrates breathing with voluntary acts such as speaking, blowing, and singing. These acts, initiated by the motor and premotor cortex, cause temporary suspension of automatic breathing. The automatic and voluntary components of respiration are regulated by afferent impulses that come to the respiratory center from a number of sources. Afferent input from higher brain centers is evidenced by the fact that a person can consciously alter the depth and rate of respiration. Fever, pain, and emotion exert their influence through lower brain centers. Vagal afferents from sensory receptors in the lungs and airways are integrated in the dorsal area of the respiratory center. It has been suggested that alterations in the control of automatic and voluntary regulation of breathing may contribute to various forms of sleep apnea (see Chapter 24).

Chemoreceptors

Tissue needs for oxygen and the removal of carbon dioxide are regulated by chemoreceptors that monitor blood levels of these gases. Input from these sensors is transmitted to the respiratory center, and ventilation is adjusted to maintain the arterial blood gases within a normal range.

There are two types of chemoreceptors: central and peripheral. The most important chemoreceptors for sensing changes in blood carbon dioxide content are the *central chemoreceptors.* These receptors are chemosensitive regions located in the medulla near the respiratory center and are bathed in cerebrospinal fluid. Although the central chemoreceptors monitor carbon dioxide levels, the actual stimulus for these receptors is provided by hydrogen ions in the cerebrospinal fluid. This fluid is separated from the blood by the blood-brain barrier, which permits free diffusion of carbon dioxide but not bicarbonate or hydrogen ions. The carbon dioxide combines rapidly with water to form carbonic acid, which dissociates into hydrogen and bicarbonate ions. The carbon dioxide content in the blood regulates ventilation through its effect on the pH of the extracellular fluid of the brain. The central chemoreceptors are extremely sensitive to short-term changes in carbon dioxide. The effect of an increase in plasma carbon dioxide levels on ventilation reaches its peak within a minute or so and then declines if the carbon dioxide level remains elevated. Long-term elevation of the carbon dioxide level prompts a compensatory increase in bicarbonate secretion into the cerebrospinal fluid, which acts as a buffer for the hydrogen ions. Thus, persons with chronically elevated levels of carbon dioxide no longer respond to this stimulus for increased ventilation but rely on the stimulus provided by a decrease in blood oxygen levels.

The *peripheral chemoreceptors* are located in the carotid and aortic bodies, which are found at the bifurcation of the common carotid arteries and in the arch of the aorta, respectively. These chemoreceptors monitor arterial blood oxygen levels. Although the peripheral chemoreceptors also monitor carbon dioxide, they play a much more important role in monitoring oxygen levels. These receptors exert little control over ventilation until the PO_2 has dropped below 60 mm Hg. Hypoxia is the main stimulus for ventilation in persons with chronic hypercapnia. If these patients are given oxygen therapy at a level sufficient to increase the PO_2 above that needed to stimulate the peripheral chemoreceptors, their ventilation may be seriously depressed.

Lung Receptors

Lung and chest wall receptors provide information on the status of breathing is going in terms of airway resistance and lung expansion. There are three types of lung receptors: stretch, irritant, and juxtacapillary (J) receptors. Stretch receptors are located in the smooth muscle layers of the conducting airways. They respond to changes in pressure within the walls of the airways. When the lungs are inflated, these receptors inhibit inspiration and promote expiration (*i.e.*, Hering-Breuer reflex). They are important in establishing breathing patterns and in minimizing the work of breathing by adjusting respiratory rate and tidal volume to accommodate changes in lung compliance and airway resistance.

Irritant receptors have a distribution similar to that of the stretch receptors. They can be mechanically stimulated by increases in airway pressure, changes in lung inflation, and changes in bronchial smooth muscle tone. Stimulation of the irritant receptors leads to airway constriction and a pattern of rapid, shallow breathing. This pattern of breathing probably protects respiratory tissues from the damaging effects of toxic inhalants. It is also thought that the mechanical stimulation of these receptors may ensure more uniform lung expansion by initiating periodic sighing and yawning.

The function of the J receptors is uncertain; it is thought that they sense lung congestion. These receptors may be responsible for the rapid, shallow breathing that occurs with pulmonary edema, pulmonary embolism, and pneumonia.

Cough Reflex

Coughing is a neurally mediated reflex that protects the lungs from accumulation of secretions and from entry of irritating and destructive substances. It is one of the primary defense mechanisms of the respiratory tract.

The cough reflex is initiated by receptors located in the tracheobronchial wall; these receptors are extremely sensitive to irritating substances and to the presence of excess secretions. Afferent impulses from these receptors are transmitted through the vagus to the medullary center, which integrates the cough response.

Coughing itself requires the rapid inspiration of a large volume of air (usually about 2.5 L), followed by rapid closure of the glottis and forceful contraction of the abdominal and expiratory muscles. As these muscles contract, intrathoracic pressures are elevated to levels of 100 mm Hg or more. The rapid opening of the glottis at this point leads to an explosive expulsion of air.

Many conditions can interfere with the cough reflex and its protective function. The reflex is impaired in persons whose abdominal or respiratory muscles are weak. This problem can be caused by disease conditions that lead to muscle weakness or paralysis, by prolonged inactivity, or as an outcome of surgery involving these muscles. Bed rest interferes with expansion of the chest and limits the amount of air that can be taken into the lungs in preparation for coughing, making the cough weak and ineffective. Disease conditions that prevent effective closure of the glottis and laryngeal muscles interfere with accomplishment of the marked increase in intrathoracic pressure that is needed for effective coughing. The presence of a nasogastric tube, for example, may prevent closure of the upper airway structures and may fatigue the receptors for the cough reflex that are located in the area. The cough reflex also is impaired when there is depressed function of the medullary centers in the brain that integrate the cough reflex. Interruption of the central integration aspect of the cough reflex can arise as the result of disease of this part of the brain or the action of drugs that depress the cough center.

Although the cough reflex is a protective mechanism, frequent and prolonged coughing can be exhausting and painful and can exert undesirable effects on the cardiovascular and respiratory systems and on the elastic tissues of the lungs. This is particularly true in young children and elderly persons.

Dyspnea

Dyspnea is a subjective sensation or a person's perception of difficulty in breathing that includes the perception of labored breathing and the reaction to that sensation. The terms *dyspnea, breathlessness,* and *shortness of breath* often are used interchangeably. Dyspnea is observed in at least three major cardiopulmonary disease states: primary lung diseases such as pneumonia, asthma, and emphysema; heart disease that is characterized by pulmonary congestion; and neuromuscular disorders such as myasthenia gravis and muscular dystrophy that affect the respiratory muscles. Although dyspnea commonly is associated with respiratory disease, it also occurs during exercise, particularly in untrained persons.

The cause of dyspnea is unknown. Four types of mechanisms have been proposed to explain the sensation: stimulation of lung receptors; increased sensitivity to changes in ventilation perceived through central nervous system mechanisms; reduced ventilatory capacity or breathing reserve; and stimulation of neural receptors in the muscle fibers of the intercostals and diaphragm and of receptors in the skeletal joints. The first of the suggested mechanisms is stimulation of lung receptors. These receptors are stimulated by the contraction of bronchial smooth muscle, the stretch of the bronchial wall, pulmonary congestion, and conditions that decrease lung compliance. The second category of proposed mechanisms focuses on central nervous system mechanisms that transmit information to the cortex regarding respiratory muscle weakness or a discrepancy between the increased effort of breathing and inadequate respiratory muscle contraction. The third type of mechanism focuses on a reduction in ventilatory capacity or breathing reserve. A reduction in breathing reserve (*i.e.,* maximum voluntary ventilation not being used during a given activity) to less than 65% to 75% usually correlates well with dyspnea. The fourth possible mechanism is stimulation of muscle and joint receptors in the respiratory musculature because of a discrepancy in the tension generated by these muscles and the tidal volume that results. These receptors, once stimulated, transmit signals that bring about an awareness of the breathing discrepancy. Like other subjective symptoms, such as fatigue and pain, dyspnea is difficult to quantify because it relies on a person's perception of the problem.

The most common method for measuring dyspnea is a retrospective determination of the level of daily activity at which a person experiences dyspnea. Several scales are available for this use. One of these uses four grades of dyspnea to evaluate disability. The visual ana-

Breathing Patterns

The act of breathing normally is effortless and does not require conscious thought. In an adult, the normal rate of respiration is about 16 to 18 breaths per minute, with about one breath for every four heartbeats. The rate increases with exercise and other activities that raise the body's metabolism. In normal breathing, expiration is largely passive and accomplished within 4 to 6 seconds.

Respiratory movements are smooth, with equal expansion of both sides of the chest. In men, respiratory movements are primarily diaphragmatic, but in women, there is greater movement of the intercostal muscles. When breathing becomes labored, the accessory muscles of the neck come into play, and the nostrils may flare.

The suffix *-pnea* refers to breathing. *Tachypnea* is rapid breathing, and *hyperpnea* is an increase in the rate and the depth of respiration. Hyperpnea is normal during exercise. *Bradypnea* is an abnormally slow respiratory rate. *Hyperventilation* is ventilation in excess of that needed for normal elimination of carbon dioxide. It is associated with decreased partial pressure of carbon dioxide (PCO_2) in the arterial blood and respiratory alkalosis (see Chapter 29). Hypoventilation is ventilation that is inadequate for alveolocapillary exchange of carbon dioxide and oxygen. Hypoventilation causes an increase in PCO_2 and respiratory acidosis and a decrease in the partial pressure of oxygen (PO_2) in the arterial blood.

Periodic breathing describes a pattern in which there are episodes of apnea, or absence of breathing. *Cheyne-Stokes breathing* is a type of periodic breathing characterized by periods of slowly waxing and waning respirations separated by a period of apnea that lasts as long as 30 seconds. Cheyne-Stokes breathing is thought to be caused by impaired function of the central feedback mechanisms that buffer the respiratory center's response to carbon dioxide. For Cheyne-Stokes respirations to occur, the hyperpneic and apneic phases of the breathing pattern must be long enough for sufficient changes in the carbon dioxide content of the blood to occur. During the hyperpneic phase of Cheyne-Stokes breathing, carbon dioxide levels fall, leading to a decreased stimulus for ventilation and, finally, to apnea. The period of apnea causes carbon dioxide to accumulate in the blood, and this leads to the hyperpneic phase of the respiratory pattern.

Two types of disease conditions predispose to Cheyne-Stokes breathing. One is congestive heart failure, in which there is a great delay in moving blood with its altered carbon dioxide content from the lungs to the chemoreceptors in the brain that control ventilation. The other is impaired function of the brain centers that regulate the feedback mechanisms that control respiration. An area of the brain stem controls the feedback gain of the respiratory center in response to changes in the carbon dioxide level. Cheyne-Stokes respirations may occur in patients who have brain lesions that affect this area. They also occur in healthy persons as an adaptive response to high altitudes, especially during sleep.

Normal

Bradypnea

Tachypnea

Hyperventilation

Cheyne-Stokes

log scale may be used to assess breathing difficulty that occurs with a given activity, such as walking a certain distance. The visual analog scale consists of a line (often 10 cm long) with descriptors such as "easy to breathe" on one end and "very difficult to breathe" on the other. The person being assessed selects a point on the scale that describes his or her perceived dyspnea. It can also be used to assess dyspnea over time.

The treatment of dyspnea depends on the cause. The techniques used clinically to reduce dyspnea include methods to reduce anxiety, breathing retraining, and energy conservation measures.

In summary, the respiratory system requires continuous input from the nervous system. Movement of the diaphragm, intercostal muscles, and other respiratory muscles are controlled by neurons of the respiratory center located in the pons and medulla. The control of breathing has automatic and voluntary components. The automatic regulation of ventilation is controlled by two types of receptors: lung receptors, which protect respiratory structures, and chemoreceptors, which monitor the gas exchange function of the lungs by sensing changes in blood levels of carbon dioxide, oxygen, and pH. There are three types of lung receptors: stretch receptors, which monitor lung inflation; irritant receptors, which protect against the damaging effects of toxic inhalants; and J receptors, which are thought to sense lung congestion. There are two groups of chemoreceptors: central and peripheral. The central chemoreceptors are the most important in sensing changes in carbon dioxide levels and the peripheral chemoreceptors function in sensing arterial blood oxygen levels.

Voluntary respiratory control is needed for integrating breathing and actions such as speaking, blowing, and singing. These acts, which are initiated by the motor and premotor cortex, cause temporary suspension of automatic breathing. The cough reflex protects the lungs from accumulation of secretions and from entry of irritating and destructive substances; it is one of the primary defense mechanisms of the respiratory tract. Dyspnea is a subjective sensation of difficulty in breathing. Alterations in breathing patterns include tachypnea (*i.e.,* rapid breathing), hyperpnea (*i.e.,* increase in the rate and the depth of respiration), bradypnea (*i.e.,* abnormally slow respiratory rate), hyperventilation (*i.e.,* respiration in excess of that needed to maintain a normal level of PCO_2), and hypoventilation (*i.e.,* inadequate ventilation). Periodic breathing is manifested by periods of apnea.

BIBLIOGRAPHY

Berne R.M., Levy M.N. (1995). *Physiology* (3rd ed., pp. 547–599). St. Louis: C.V. Mosby.

Caminiti S.P., Young S.L. (1991). The pulmonary surfactant system. *Hospital Practice* 26 (1A), 87–100.

Carpenter K.D. (1989). Oxygen transport in the blood. *Critical Care Nurse 11* (9), 2033.

Carrieri V.K., Jansen-Bjerklie S. (1984). The sensation of dyspnea: A critical review. *Heart and Lung* 13, 437.

Cormack D.H. (1987). *Ham's histology* (9th ed., pp. 541–563). Philadelphia: J.B. Lippincott.

Fishman A.P. (1980). *Assessment of pulmonary function.* New York: McGraw-Hill.

Guyton A. (1996). *Textbook of medical physiology* (9th ed.). Philadelphia: W.B. Saunders.

Reischman R.R. (1988). Review of ventilation and perfusion physiology. *Critical Care Nurse* 8 (7), 24–28.

Rhoades R.A., Tanner G.A. (1996). *Medical physiology* (pp. 341–414). Boston: Little, Brown.

West J.B. (1995). *Respiratory physiology* (5th ed.). Baltimore: Williams & Wilkins.

CHAPTER 23

Alterations in Respiratory Function: Respiratory Tract Infections, Neoplasms, and Childhood Disorders

Respiratory illnesses represent one of the more common reasons for visits to the physician, admission to the hospital, and forced inactivity among all age groups. The common cold, although not usually serious, results in missed work and school days. Pneumonia is the sixth leading cause of death in the United States, particularly among the elderly and those with compromised immune function. After several decades of decline, the incidence of tuberculosis is rising, and there is increasing resistance to antibiotics and antimicrobial agents by the organisms that cause respiratory tract infections. Lung cancer remains the leading cause of cancer death in the United States.

Respiratory Tract Infections

After you have completed this section of the chapter, you should be able to meet the following objectives:

- Describe the transmission of the common cold from one person to another
- Explain why rest and drinking large amounts of liquids are helpful in treating influenza
- Describe the causes, manifestations, and treatment of acute and chronic sinusitis
- Differentiate among community-acquired pneumonia, hospital-acquired pneumonia, and pneumonia in immunocompromised persons in terms of pathogens, manifestations, and prognosis
- Differentiate between primary tuberculosis and reactivated tuberculosis on the basis of their pathophysiology
- State the mechanism for the transmission of fungal infections of the lung

Respiratory tract infections can involve the upper respiratory tract (*i.e.*, nose, oropharynx, and larynx), the lower respiratory tract (*i.e.*, lower airways and lungs), or the upper and lower airways. The discussion in this section of the chapter focuses on the common cold, influenza, pneumonia, tuberculosis, and fungal infections of the lung. Acute respiratory infections in children are discussed in the last section of the chapter.

The respiratory tract is susceptible to infectious processes caused by many different types of microorganisms. For the most part, the signs and symptoms of respiratory tract infections depend on the function of the structure involved, the severity of the infectious process, and the person's age and general health status.

Viruses are the most frequent cause of respiratory tract infections. They can range from a self-limited cold to life-threatening pneumonia. Moreover, viral infections can damage bronchial epithelium, obstruct airways, and lead to secondary bacterial infections. Each viral species has its own pattern of respiratory tract involvement. The rhinoviruses grow best at 33°C to 35°C and remain strictly confined to the upper respiratory tract.[1] The influenza viruses can infect the upper and lower respiratory tracts. Measles and chickenpox viruses "pass through" the respiratory tract and do not cause respiratory symptoms until secondary viremic spread has occurred. Other microorganisms, such as bacteria (*e.g.*, pneumococci, staphylococci), mycobacteria (*e.g.*, *Mycobacterium tuberculosis*), fungi (*e.g.*, histoplasmosis, coccidioidomycosis, blastomycosis), and opportunistic organisms (*e.g.*, *Pneumocystis carinii*) produce infections of the lung that cause significant morbidity and mortality.

The Common Cold

The common cold is a viral infection of the upper respiratory tract. It occurs more frequently than any other respiratory tract infection. Most adults have 2 to 4 colds per year; the average school child may have up to 10 per year.[2] The condition usually begins with a feeling of dryness and stuffiness affecting mainly the nasopharynx; it is accompanied by excessive production of nasal secretions and lacrimation, or tearing of the eyes. Usually, the secretions remain clear and watery. The mucous membranes of the upper respiratory tract become reddened, swollen, and bathed in secretions. Involvement of the pharynx and larynx causes sore throat and hoarseness. The affected person may experience headache and generalized malaise. In severe cases, there may be chills, fever, and exhaustion. The disease process is usually self-limited, lasting about 7 days.

The viral agent responsible for the common cold varies by season.[2] For example, early fall and late spring are the most common times of outbreaks of colds due to rhinoviruses, which are the most common cause of colds in persons between 5 and 40 years of age. Respiratory syncytial virus tends to cause winter and spring outbreaks, with a peak incidence in January. Parainfluenza type 1 and 2 infections peak in autumn, and parainfluenza type 3 infection peaks in late spring. Adenoviruses and coronaviruses tend to produce epidemics during the winter and spring.

The "cold viruses" are rapidly spread from person to person. The first step in the spreading of the common cold is the shedding of viruses, the area of greatest potential being the nasal mucosa. Studies have shown that colds are spread most frequently in the home or school.[3,4] The fingers are the greatest source of spread, and the nasal mucosa and conjunctival surface of the eyes are the most important portals of entry of the virus. Cold viruses have been found to survive for 3.5 hours on the skin and hard surfaces, such as wood and plastic; survival is poor on facial tissue and porous cloth. The most highly contagious period is during the first 3 days after the onset of symptoms, and the incubation period is about 5 days. Studies suggest that the aerosol spread of colds through coughing and sneezing is much less important than the spread by fingers picking up the virus from contaminated surfaces and carrying it to the nasal membranes and eyes.[5,6] This suggests that careful attention to handwashing is one of the most important preventive measures for avoiding the common cold. Host defenses also influence the development of the common cold. Psychologic stress, which is thought to influence immune function, is reported to increase the risk of developing a cold.[7]

Many over-the-counter (OTC) remedies are available for treating the common cold. Because the common cold is an acute and self-limited illness in persons who are otherwise healthy, treatment with antibiotics and other medications that are potentially harmful is contraindicated. Symptomatic treatment with rest and antipyretic drugs is all that is usually needed. There is some controversy about the use of vitamin C to reduce the incidence and severity of colds and influenza. Several studies have found an association between vitamin C intake and a reduced incidence,[8,9] but others have found that vitamin C had no effect on the number or severity of colds.[10] One study suggested that zinc lozenges decreased the duration of cold symptoms.[11]

Antihistamines are popular OTC drugs because of their action in drying nasal secretions. However, they may dry up bronchial secretions and worsen the cough, and they may cause dizziness, drowsiness, and impaired judgment. As with vitamin C, there is no evidence that they shorten the duration of the cold. Decongestant drugs (*i.e.*, sympathomimetic agents) are available in OTC nasal sprays, drops, and oral cold medications. These drugs constrict the blood vessels in the swollen nasal mucosa and reduce nasal swelling. Rebound nasal swelling can occur with indiscriminate use of nasal drops and sprays. Oral preparations containing decongestants may cause systemic vasoconstriction and elevation of blood pressure when given in doses large enough to relieve nasal congestion, and they should be avoided by persons with hypertension, heart disease, hyperthyroidism, diabetes mellitus, or other health problems.

Rhinitis and Sinusitis

Rhinitis refers to inflammation of the nasal mucosa and sinusitis to inflammation of the paranasal sinuses. The paranasal sinuses are air cells that connect with the nasal cavity through the superior, middle, and inferior nasal conchae (Fig. 23–1). Each sinus is named for the bone in which it occurs—frontal, ethmoid, sphenoid, and maxillary. The maxillary sinus is inferior to the bony orbit and superior to the hard palate, and its opening is located superiorally and medially in the sinus, a location that impedes drainage.[12] The frontal sinuses open into the middle meatus of the nasal cavity. The sphenoid sinus is just anterior to the pituitary fossa behind the posterior ethmoid sinuses, and its paired openings drain into the sphenoethmoidal recess at the top of the nasal cavity. The ethmoid sinuses comprise 3 to 15 air cells on each side, with each maintaining a separate path to the nasal chamber.

The sinus mucosa is similar to that of the respiratory tract and nasal passages. Ciliated mucous membranes help move fluid and microorganisms out of the sinuses and into the nasal cavity. Obstruction of sinus openings by nasal swelling that impairs mucociliary movement is thought to be a major cause of sinus infections. The lower oxygen content in the sinuses facilitates the growth of organisms, impairs local defenses, and alters the function of immune cells.

The most common causes of sinusitis are rhinitis and upper respiratory tract infections. Nasal polyps can also obstruct the sinus opening and facilitate sinus infection. Infections associated with nasal polyps can be self-perpetuating, because constant irritation from infection can cause polyps. Barotrauma caused by changes in barometric pressure, as occurs in airline pilots and flight attendants, may lead to impaired sinus ventilation and clearance of secretions. Swimming, diving, and abuse of nasal decongestants are other causes of sinus irritation and impaired drainage. In about 10% of cases of maxillary sinusitis, the cause is a contiguous dental infection.

The paranasal sinuses are normally sterile. In adults, acute sinusitis most commonly results from infection with *Haemophilus* influenzae or *Streptococcus pneumoniae*.[12,13] In chronic sinusitis, anaerobic organisms, including species of *Peptostreptococcus*, *Fusobacterium*, and *Prevotella*, tend to predominate alone or in combination with aerobes such as the *Streptococcus* species or *Staphylococcus aureus*.

In immunocompromised persons, such as those with the human immunodeficiency virus (HIV) infection, the sinuses may become infected with gram-negative species and opportunistic fungi. In this group, particularly those with leukopenia, the disease may have a fulminant and even fatal course.

Hospital-acquired sinusitis is more often caused by different microbial agents than community-acquired sinusitis. In the hospital, *S. aureus*, *Pseudomonas* species, *Klebsiella* species, and other gram-negative organisms predominate.[13] About 35% to 45% of hospital-acquired infections are polymicrobial.[12] Predisposing factors include irritation from endotracheal tubes, nasogastric tubes, nasal packing, and the use of corticosteroids and other immunosuppressant drugs.

Acute and Chronic Sinusitis

Sinusitis can be classified as acute, subacute, or chronic. Acute suppurative sinusitis is any bacterial infection of the paranasal sinuses that lasts from 1 day to 3 weeks. Subacute sinusitis lasts from 3 weeks to 3 months. Chronic sinusitis lasts beyond 3 months.[12] Persons with chronic sinusitis may have superimposed bouts of acute sinusitis. The epithelial changes that occur during acute and subacute forms of sinusitis are usually reversible, but the mucosal changes that occur with chronic sinusitis are often irreversible.

The symptoms of acute sinusitis are often difficult to differentiate from those of the common cold and allergic rhinitis. They include facial pain, headache, purulent nasal discharge, decreased sense of smell, and fever. A history of preceding common cold, and the presence of purulent rhinitis, pain on bending, unilateral maxillary pain, and pain in the teeth are common findings in maxillary sinusitis.

In persons with chronic sinusitis, the only symptoms may be nasal obstruction, postnasal drip, chronic cough, loss of smell, and unpleasant breath. Sinus pain is often absent; instead, the person may complain of a headache that is dull and constant. Persons who are immunocompromised, such as those with leukemia, aplastic anemia, a bone marrow transplant, primary immunodeficiency disease, or HIV infection, often present with fever of unknown origin, rhinorrhea, or facial edema. Often, other signs of inflammation such as purulent drainage are absent.

Diagnosis and Treatment. The diagnosis of sinusitis is usually based on symptom history and a physical examination that includes inspection of the nose and throat. Headache due to sinusitis needs to be differentiated from other causes of headache. Sinusitis headache is usually exaggerated by bending forward, coughing, or sneezing. Transillumination may be used for detecting fluid in the maxillary or frontal sinus. It is done in a dark room and with a light source such as a light attached to an otoscope. Sinus radiographs and computed tomography (CT) scans may be used. CT scans are usually reserved for diagnosis of chronic sinusitis or to exclude complications. Diagnostic nasal endoscopy,[12] which is done in the office of an otolaryngologist, provides a clear view of the anterior nasal cavity and sinus openings.

Treatment of sinusitis includes appropriate antibiotic therapy, depending on whether the infection is community acquired, hospital acquired, or occurs in an immunocompromised person. The duration of antibiotic therapy is longer for chronic sinusitis than for acute sinusitis. In addition to antibiotic therapy, the treatment of acute sinusitis includes measures to promote adequate drainage by reducing nasal congestion. Oral and

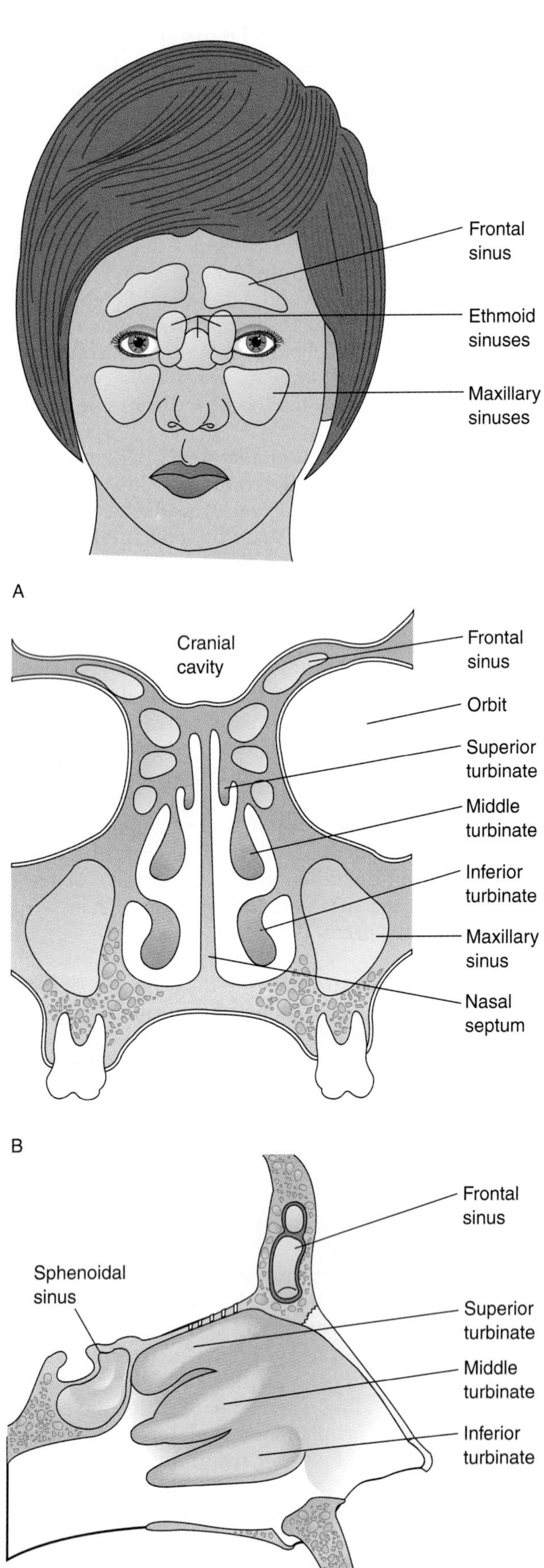

topical decongestants and antihistamines may be used for this purpose. Oral decongestants reduce nasal blood flow, decrease tissue congestion, and facilitate drainage. The use of intranasal decongestants should be limited to 3 to 7 days to prevent rebound vasodilatation. The use of antihistamines is controversial, particularly for acute sinusitis, because they can dry up secretions and thereby decrease drainage. Expectorants such as guaifenesin may be used to thin secretions. Topical corticosteroids may be used to decrease inflammation in persons with allergic rhinitis or sinusitis. Nonpharmacologic measures include saline nasal sprays and steam inhalations.

Surgical intervention directed at correcting obstruction of the ostiomeatal complex may be indicated in persons with chronic sinusitis that is resistant to other forms of therapy. Indications for surgical intervention include obstructive nasal polyps and obstructive nasal deformities.

Complications. Because of the sinuses' proximity to the brain and orbital wall, sinusitis can lead to intracranial and orbital wall complications.[12] Intracranial complications are most commonly seen with infection of the frontal and ethmoid sinuses because of their proximity to the dura and drainage of the veins from the frontal sinus into the dural sinus. Sinusitis is the primary source of infection in as many as two thirds of intracranial abscesses and 5% of community-acquired cases of meningitis.[12] Orbital complications can range from edema of the eyelids to orbital cellulitis and subperiosteal abscess formation. Orbital involvement can result in exophthalmus, edema of the ocular conjunctiva, and visual impairment. Involvement of nerves supplying the extraocular muscles can lead to ophthalmoplegia. In persons with ethmoid sinusitis, infection can extend to the nasolacrimal gland, causing obstruction and tearing.

Allergic Rhinoconjunctivitis

Allergic sinusitis occurs in conjunction with allergic rhinitis. The mucosal changes are the same as those seen in allergic rhinitis. Symptoms usually consist of nasal stuffiness, itching and burning of the nose, frequent bouts of sneezing, recurrent frontal headache, and a watery nasal discharge. Headache located in the frontal area between the eyes and in the frontal area is a common symptom. Allergic rhinitis can lead to polyp formation, and similar polypoid lesions are commonly seen in persons with allergic sinusitis. Treatment consists of oral antihistamines, nasal decongestants, and intranasal cromolyn. Persistent symptoms may be treated with nasal corticosteroids and severe symptoms with oral corticosteroids.[14]

Figure 23–1
Paranasal sinuses. (**A**) Frontal view; (**B**) cross-section of nasal cavity, anterior view; (**C**) lateral wall, left nasal cavity. (Courtesy of Carole Russell Hilmer; C. M. I.)

Influenza

Influenza is a viral infection that can affect the upper and lower respiratory tracts. It usually occurs in epidemics or pandemics. Until the advent of acquired immunodeficiency syndrome (AIDS), it was the last uncontrolled pandemic killer of humans. More persons died in the 1918 and 1919 influenza pandemic than in World War I. In the United States, 10,000 to 20,000 persons die of influenza-related illness during nonpandemic years.[15] Most deaths are caused by pneumonia or exacerbation of cardiopulmonary or other conditions; 80% to 90% of those who die are 65 years of age or older.[16] There are three distinct types of influenza viruses: types A, B, and C. Infection with type A is most common and causes the most severe disease.

The influenza viruses can cause three syndromes: an uncomplicated rhinotracheitis, a respiratory viral infection followed by a bacterial infection, and viral pneumonia. The incubation period for all three syndromes is 1 to 4 days. In the early stages, the symptoms of influenza are often indistinguishable from other viral infections. There is an abrupt onset of fever and chills, malaise, muscle aching, headache, profuse watery nasal discharge, nonproductive cough, and sore throat. One distinguishing feature of an influenza viral infection is the rapid onset, sometimes in as little as 1 to 2 minutes, of profound malaise.[15] The infection causes necrosis and shedding of the serous and ciliated cells that line the respiratory tract, leaving gaping holes between the underlying basal cells and allowing extracellular fluid to escape. This is the reason for the "runny nose" that is characteristic of this phase of the infection. During recovery, the serous cells are replaced more rapidly than the ciliated cells. Mucus is produced, but the ciliated cells are unable to move it adequately; persons recovering from influenza must continue to blow the nose to clear the sinuses and cough to clear the trachea.

The symptoms of uncomplicated rhinotracheitis usually peak by days 3 to 5 and disappear by days 7 to 10. Persons who develop secondary complications generally report that they were beginning to feel better when they experienced a return of symptoms. Complications typically include sinusitis, otitis media, bronchitis, and bacterial pneumonia. The clinical course of influenza pneumonia progresses rapidly. It can cause hypoxemia and death within a few days of onset. The rapid onset is thought to be related to the mode of spread and the absence of an initial rhinotracheitis. If the virus is spread by fingers or large-droplet spray, as from sneezing or coughing, only the upper respiratory tract is involved. Infection of the upper respiratory tract is thought to give the immune system enough time to build the defenses needed to protect against viral pneumonia. When the virus is contained in small droplets, it can bypass the upper respiratory tract and travel directly into the lungs to establish infection.[15]

Treatment

The goals of treatment are designed to limit the infection to the upper respiratory tract. The symptomatic approach, which uses rest, keeping warm, and drinking large amounts of liquids, helps to accomplish this. Rest decreases the oxygen requirements of the body and reduces the respiratory rate and the chance of spreading the virus from the upper to lower respiratory tract. Keeping warm helps maintain the respiratory epithelium at a core body temperature of 37°C (or higher if fever is present), thereby inhibiting viral replication, which is optimal at 35°C. Drinking large amounts of liquids ensures that the function of the epithelial lining of the respiratory tract is not further compromised by dehydration.[15]

Chemoprophylaxis or treatment with influenza-specific antiviral drugs, such as amantadine or rimantadine, is often effective in preventing symptomatic influenza A infections among high-risk groups during an outbreak.[16] It is only effective against influenza A and must be administered throughout the period of risk.

Influenza Immunization

Vaccines are available to protect against influenza infections. Immunization is recommended for high-risk groups who, because of their age or underlying health problems, are unable to cope well with the infection and often require medical attention, including hospitalization. The effectiveness of the influenza vaccine in preventing and lessening the effects of influenza infection depend primarily on the age of the recipient, immunocompetence of the recipient, and the match between the virus strains included in the vaccine and those that circulate during the influenza season.[17] When there is a good match, the vaccine is effective in preventing the illness in about 70% of healthy persons younger than 65 years of age. Under similar circumstances, the vaccine is able to decrease the rate of hospitalization for pneumonia and influenza in elderly persons living in settings other than nursing homes by 30% to 70%.

Several strains of the influenza virus are responsible for epidemics of the disease. These strains undergo small changes over time that affect their antigenicity and the host protection afforded by previous immunization. Influenza's impact is normally greatest when new strains appear against which the population lacks immunity. The formulation of the influenza vaccine must be changed yearly in response to changes in the influenza virus. The Public Health Advisory Committee on Immunization Practices annually updates its recommendations for the composition of the vaccine.

The Immunization Practices Advisory Committee recommends annual immunization using inactivated influenza vaccine to prevent or minimize the effect of influenza infections in any person 6 months of age or older who is at high risk for complications of influenza.[17] Groups at highest risk for complications include persons 65 years of age or older; residents of nursing homes or other chronic-care facilities housing persons of any age with chronic medical conditions; adults or children with chronic disorders of the pulmonary or cardiovascular systems, including children with asthma; adults and children who have required regular medical follow-up or hospitalization during the preceding year because of chronic metabolic diseases (e.g., diabetes mellitus, renal dysfunction, hemoglobinopathies such as sickle cell anemia) or immunosuppression, including immunosuppression caused by medications; and children or teenagers (6 months to 18 years) who are receiving long-term aspirin therapy (because of the risk of developing Reye's syndrome). Immunization is also recommended for groups (*e.g.*, household members, health care workers) who live with or care for persons who are at high risk for developing influenza complications. It is believed that the protection of persons in the high-risk groups can be improved by reducing the chances of exposure to influenza from household contacts and health care providers. Vaccination is contraindicated for persons who have a history of anaphylactic hypersensitivity to egg or other components of the vaccine.

Pneumonias

The term *pneumonia* describes inflammation of parenchymal structures of the lung, such as the alveoli and the bronchioles. An estimated 4 million cases occur annually in the United States, for a rate of 12 cases per 1000 persons per year.[18] Pneumonia is the sixth leading cause of death in the United States and the most common cause of death from infectious disease. Etiologic agents include infectious and noninfectious agents. Although much less common than infectious pneumonia, inhalation of irritating fumes or aspiration of gastric contents can result in severe pneumonia.

Although antibiotics have significantly reduced mortality from pneumonias, these diseases remain an important immediate cause of death of the elderly and persons with debilitating diseases. There have been subtle changes in the spectrum of microorganisms that cause infectious pneumonias, including a decrease in pneumonias caused by *S. pneumoniae* and an increase in pneumonias caused by other microorganisms such as *Pseudomonas, Candida* and other fungi, and nonspecific viruses. Many of these pneumonias occur in persons with impaired immune defenses, including persons who are on immunosuppressant drugs to prevent rejection of a bone marrow or organ transplant. *Pneumocystis carinii*, a virulent type of pneumonia, is associated with AIDS.

Pathogenesis

Bacteria commonly enter the lower airways but do not normally cause pneumonia because of extensive defense mechanisms. When pneumonia does occur, it usually is because of an exceedingly virulent organism, large inoculum, or impaired host defenses. In nonhospitalized persons, bacteria reach the lung by one of four routes: inhalation from the ambient air, aspiration of bacteria from the previously colonized upper airway, direct spread from contiguous infected sites, or hematogenous spread. Critically ill patients may acquire organisms from colonized nasogastric tubes or from an endotracheal tube.

Most of the agents that cause pneumonia and lower respiratory tract infections are aspirated from the tracheobronchial tree or are inhaled into the lung along with the air breathed. Most persons unknowingly aspirate small amounts of organisms that have colonized their upper airways, particularly during sleep. Normally, these organisms do not cause infection because of the small numbers that are aspirated and because of the respiratory tract's defense mechanisms (Table 23–1). After bacteria reach the lower airways they encounter a number of host defenses that prevent them from entering the lung and causing pneumonia. Loss of the cough reflex, damage to the ciliated endothelium that lines the respiratory tract, or impaired immune defenses predispose to colonization and infection of the lower respiratory system. Immune defenses include the bronchial-associated lymphoid tissue, phagocytic cells (*i.e.*, polymorphonuclear cells and macrophages), immunoglobulins (*i.e.*, IgA and IgG), and T-cell–mediated cellular immunity (see Chapter 11). Bacterial adherence also plays a role in colonization of the lower airways. The epithelial cells of critically and chronically ill persons are more receptive to binding organisms that cause pneumonia. Other clinical risk factors for colonization of the tracheobronchial tree include antibiotic therapy that alters the normal bacterial flora, diabetes, smoking, chronic bronchitis, and viral infection.

Until recently, pneumonias have been classified as typical (*i.e.*, bacterial) or atypical (*i.e.*, viral or mycoplasmal) pneumonias. Bacterial pneumonia results from infection by bacteria that multiply extracellularly in the alveoli and cause inflammation and exudation of fluid into the air-filled spaces of the alveoli (Fig. 23–2). They are characterized by chills and fever, severe malaise, purulent sputum, elevated white blood cell counts, and patchy or lobar infiltrates seen on the chest radiograph. Atypical pneumonias produce patchy inflammatory changes that are confined to the alveolar septum and the interstitium of the lung (see Fig. 23–2). They produce less striking symptoms and physical findings than bacterial pneumonia; there is a lack of alveolar infiltration and purulent sputum, leukocytosis, and lobar consolidation on the radiograph.

Because of the overlap in symptomatology and changing spectrum of infectious organisms involved, pneumonias are increasingly being classified as community-acquired and hospital-acquired pneumonias. Persons with compromised immune function constitute a special concern in both categories.

Community-Acquired Pneumonia

The term community-acquired pneumonia is used to describe infections from organisms found in the community rather than in the hospital or nursing home. The definition of community-acquired pneumonia is usually limited to immunocompetent persons because that population is encountered most frequently.[19] Guidelines de-

TABLE 23-1

Respiratory Defense Mechanisms and Conditions That Impair Their Effectiveness

Defense Mechanism	Function	Factors That Impair Effectiveness
Nasopharyngeal defenses	Remove particles from the air; contact with surface lysosomes and immunoglobulins (IgA) protects against infection	IgA deficiency state, hay fever, common cold, trauma to the nose, others
Glottic and cough reflexes	Protect against aspiration into tracheobronchial tree	Loss of cough reflex due to stroke or neural lesion, neuromuscular disease, abdominal or chest surgery, depression of the cough reflex due to sedation or anesthesia, presence of a nasogastric tube (tends to cause adaptation of afferent receptors)
Mucociliary blanket	Removes secretions, microorganisms, and particles from the respiratory tract	Smoking, viral diseases, chilling, inhalation of irritating gases
Pulmonary macrophages	Remove microorganisms and foreign particles from the lung	Chilling, alcohol intoxication, smoking, anoxia

veloped by the American Thoracic Society have divided persons with community-acquired pneumonia into four categories based on severity of illness, presence of coexisting disease and age, and need for hospitalization. The categories are (1) persons younger than 60 years of age, who are without comorbidity and who can be treated on an outpatient basis; (2) persons with comorbidity and who are 60 years of age and older and who can be treated on an outpatient basis; (3) persons with community-acquired pneumonia that require hospitalization but not admission to the intensive care unit; and (4) persons with community-acquired pneumonia who require admission to the intensive care unit.[19]

The most common cause of infection in all categories is *S. pneumoniae*.[18,20,21] Other bacteria commonly encountered in cultures of sputum are *H. influenzae*, *S. aureus*, and gram-negative bacilli.[18] Less common agents are *Moraxella catarrhalis*, *Streptococcus pyrogens*, and *Neisseria meningitis*. *Legionella* species, *Mycoplasma pneumoniae*, and *Chlamydia pneumoniae* (strain TWAR), sometimes called atypical agents, account for 10% to 20% of all cases of pneumonia.[12] The infecting organisms

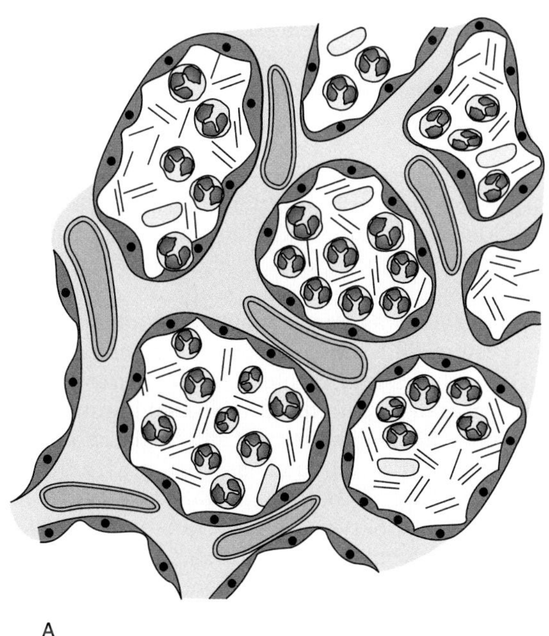

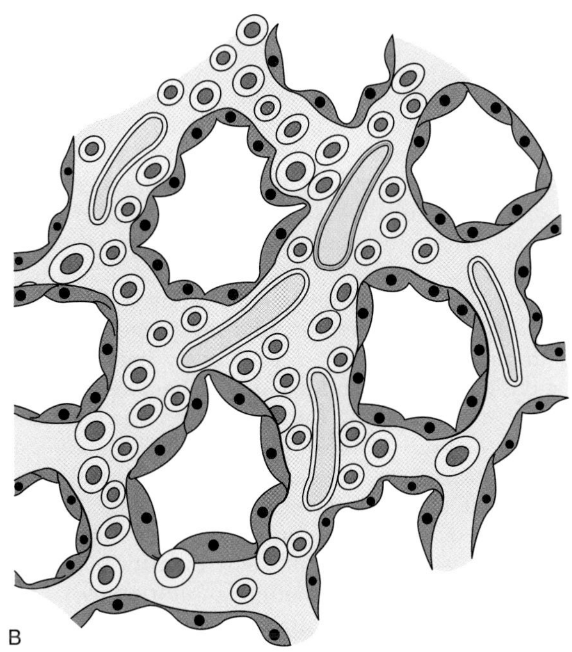

Figure 23–2
Location of inflammatory processes in (**A**) typical and (**B**) atypical forms of pneumonia.

can remain confined to the lungs, as in persons in category one, or they can cause bacteremia and sepsis. The mortality for persons in the first category is low (1% to 2%) compared with category 4, severe community-acquired pneumonia, which requires admission to the intensive care unit and for which the mortality rate can be as high as 50%.

The signs and symptoms of pneumonia vary from fever, general malaise, and cough to signs of severe respiratory compromise that include a respiratory rate above 30 breaths per minute, signs of respiratory failure, and evidence of sepsis syndrome or shock (see Chapter 20).

The type and extent of diagnostic tests depend on the severity of illness. In persons younger than 65 years of age and without coexisting disease, the diagnosis is usually based on history and physical examination, chest radiograph, and knowledge of the current environmental pathogens. Sputum specimens may be obtained for staining procedures and culture. Blood cultures may be done for persons requiring hospitalization. Diagnostic measures may include procedures such as fiberoptic bronchoscopy, which is done to obtain specimens for identifying the pathogen, particularly in severely ill persons and those who are unresponsive to antimicrobial therapy. Thoracentesis may be used to obtain specimens of pleural fluid when the infection extends into the pleural cavity.

Treatment involves the use of appropriate antibiotic therapy. Empiric antibiotic therapy based on knowledge of pathogens affecting certain client populations is often used. The American Thoracic Society has published guidelines for initial treatment of adults with community-acquired pneumonia.[19] These guidelines were published in 1993, and it seems likely that they will be updated as patterns of infection and antibiotic resistance of the organisms change.

Pneumococcal Pneumonia. *S. pneumoniae* remains the most common cause of bacterial pneumonia. In addition to pneumonia, *S. pneumoniae* can also cause meningitis, septicemia, and otitis media. It is among the leading cause of illness and death of young children, persons with other health problems, and the elderly worldwide.

The signs and symptoms of pneumococcal pneumonia vary widely, depending on the age and health status of the infected person. In previously healthy persons, the onset is usually sudden and is characterized by malaise, a severe shaking chill, and fever. The temperature may go as high as 106°F. During the congestive stage, coughing brings up a watery sputum, and breath sounds are limited, with fine crackles. As the disease progresses, the character of the sputum changes; it may be blood tinged or rust colored to purulent. Pleuritic pain, a sharp pain that is more severe with respiratory movements, is common. With antibiotic therapy, fever usually subsides in about 48 to 72 hours, and recovery is uneventful. Elderly persons are less likely to experience marked elevations in temperature; in these persons, the only sign of pneumonia may be a loss of appetite and deterioration in mental status. In the past, *S. pneumoniae* was uniformly susceptible to penicillin. However, penicillin-resistant and multidrug-resistant strains have been emerging in the United States and some communities in other countries.[22]

Pneumococcal pneumonia can be prevented through immunization. A 23-valent pneumococcal vaccine, composed of antigens from 23 types of *S. pneumoniae* is used. The vaccine is recommended for persons 65 years of age or older and for adults and children with chronic illnesses, particularly cardiovascular and pulmonary diseases, diabetes mellitus, and alcoholism, who sustain increased morbidity with respiratory infections. This does not include upper respiratory tract infections, otitis media, or sinusitis in children. Immunization is also recommended for immunocompromised persons 2 years of age or older, including those with sickle cell disease, splenectomy, Hodgkin's disease, multiple myeloma, renal failure, nephrotic syndrome, organ transplantation, and HIV infection. Immunization is recommended for residents in special environments or social settings in which the risk for invasive pneumococcal disease is increased (*e.g.*, Alaskan Natives, certain Native American populations) and for residents of nursing homes and long-term care facilities.

A single dose of pneumococcal vaccine usually confers lifetime immunity. A second dose of vaccine is recommended for persons older than 65 years if 5 years or more have elapsed since the previous vaccine was given and if the person was younger than 65 years at the time of vaccination. Revaccination is also recommended for immunocompromised persons 10 to 64 years of age and those with functional or anatomic asplenia (*i.e.*, sickle cell disease or splenectomy) if more than 5 years have elapsed since the previous dose and after 3 years if the person is younger than 10 years of age.[23]

Legionnaires' Disease. Legionnaires' disease is a form of bronchopneumonia caused by a gram-negative rod, *Legionella pneumophila*.[24,25] The organism is almost ubiquitous in water, particularly in warm, standing water. The disease was first recognized and received its name after an epidemic of severe and, for some, fatal pneumonia that developed among delegates to the 1976 American Legion convention held in a Philadelphia hotel. The spread of infection was traced to a water-cooled air-conditioning system. Although healthy persons can develop the infection, the risk is greatest among persons with chronic diseases or impaired cell-mediated immunity.

Symptoms of the disease typically begin about 2 to 10 days after infection with malaise, weakness, lethargy, fever, and dry cough. Other manifestations include disturbances of central nervous system function, gastrointestinal tract involvement, arthralgias, and elevation in body temperature, sometimes to more than 104°F. The presence of pneumonia along with diarrhea, hyponatremia, and confusion are characteristic of *Legionella* pneumonia. The disease causes consolidation of lung tissues and impairs gas exchange. The mortality rate can be as high as 23% to 30% among previously healthy persons and 80% among immunocompromised persons.[24]

Mycoplasma and Viral Pneumonias. Mycoplasmas and viruses tend to cause atypical or interstitial pneumonias. The mycoplasmas are the smallest free-living agents of disease, having characteristics of viruses and bacteria. The influenza virus is the most common cause of viral pneumonia. Less common offenders are *parainfluenza* and *respiratory syncytial viruses.* Other viruses are sometimes implicated, including measles and chickenpox.

The clinical course among persons with *Mycoplasma* and viral pneumonias varies widely from a mild infection (*e.g.*, influenza A and B, adenovirus) that masquerades as a chest cold to a more serious and even fatal outcome (*e.g.*, chickenpox pneumonia). The symptoms may remain confined to fever, headache, and muscle aches and pains. Cough, when present, is characteristically dry, hacking, and nonproductive. Viruses impair the respiratory tract defenses and predispose to secondary bacterial infections with the development of lobar or bronchopneumonia. Some viruses such as herpes simplex, varicella, and adenovirus may be associated with necrosis of the alveolar epithelium and acute inflammation.

Hospital-Acquired Pneumonia

Hospital-acquired, or nosocomial, pneumonia is defined as a lower respiratory tract infection that was not present or incubating on admission to the hospital. Usually, infections occurring 72 hours or more after admission are considered hospital acquired. Hospital-acquired pneumonia is the second most common cause of hospital-acquired infections and has a mortality rate of 20% to 50%.[26] Persons requiring mechanical ventilation are particularly at risk, as are those with compromised immune function, chronic lung disease, and airway instrumentation, such as endotracheal intubation or tracheotomy.

Ninety percent of infections are bacterial. The organisms are those present in the hospital environment and include *Pseudomonas aeruginosa, S. aureus, Enterobacter* spp, *Klebsiella* spp, *Escherichia coli,* and *Serratia.*[26,27] The organisms that are responsible for hospital-acquired pneumonias are different from those responsible for community-acquired pneumonia, and many of them have developed antibiotic resistance and are more difficult to treat.

Pneumonia in Immunocompromised Persons

Pneumonia in immunocompromised persons may be caused by bacterial, mycobacterial, fungal, protozoal, helminthic, or viral agents. Although almost all types of microorganisms can cause pulmonary infection in immunocompromised persons, certain types of immunologic defects tend to favor certain types of infections. Defects in humoral immunity predispose to bacterial infections against which antibodies play an important role; defects in cellular immunity predispose to infections with viruses, fungi, mycobacteria, and protozoa. Neutropenia and impaired granulocyte function, as occurs in persons with leukemia, chemotherapy, and bone marrow metaplasia, predispose to infections caused by *S. aureus, Aspergillus,* gram-negative bacilli, and *Candida.* The time course of infection often provides a hint to the type of agent involved. A fulminant pneumonia is usually caused by bacterial infection, but an insidious onset probably heralds viral, fungal, protozoal, or mycobacterial infection.

***Pneumocystis carinii* Pneumonia.** *P. carinii* pneumonia is an opportunistic, often fatal form of lung infection seen in debilitated persons and those with impaired immune function, particularly those with impaired cell-mediated immunity. *P. carinii* is a parasite of uncertain classification. Although the terminology applied to protozoa is used to describe the various stages of its life cycle, analysis suggests that it is a fungus. The organism is widely distributed, but it does not produce disease in persons with a healthy immune system.

Pneumocystis pneumonia is seen in persons treated with immunosuppressive or cytotoxic drugs or irradiation for management of organ transplantation or cancer. In the United States, *Pneumocystis* pneumonia develops in 75% to 80% of persons with AIDS.[28,29] It is the most common opportunistic infection in children with AIDS.[30] Because it occurs so regularly in persons with AIDS, it is used as a diagnostic criterion for the disease.

Although the mode of transmission is unknown, *P. carinii* is thought to be airborne. The onset of the disease is abrupt, with high fever, tachypnea, shortness of breath, a mild nonproductive cough, intercostal retractions, and cyanosis. In vulnerable hosts, the disease spreads rapidly throughout the lungs, producing involvement similar to that of adult respiratory distress syndrome (see Chapter 24). The infection produces an initial random and patchy involvement of the lungs. The *P. carinii* trophozoites attach and feed on alveolar epithelial cells but do not invade them. As they divide, some form cup-shaped or boat-shaped cysts that can be detected microscopically. Microscopically, the walls of the involved alveoli become thickened and edematous, and the alveoli become filled with a foamy, protein-rich fluid. As the disease progresses, the gas-exchange function of the lungs becomes severely impaired (Fig. 23–3).

The diagnosis of the disease depends on microscopic methods that use specific stains to identify the organism. Usually, sputum specimens obtained after inhalation of hypertonic saline produced by an ultrasonic nebulizer are required for this purpose. Other methods for obtaining specimens include bronchoalveolar lavage and transbronchial lung biopsy.

Treatment includes the use of trimethoprim-sulfamethoxazole (TMP-SMZ) and pentamidine isethionate. Because of the risk of recurrence, the Centers for Disease Control and Prevention (CDC) recommend that *P. carinii* prophylaxis (*i.e.*, TMP-SMX or alternatively dapsone or aerosolized pentamidine) be provided for all HIV-infected adults who have had an episode of *Pneumocystis* or have a $CD4^+$ T-cell count less than 200/μl or

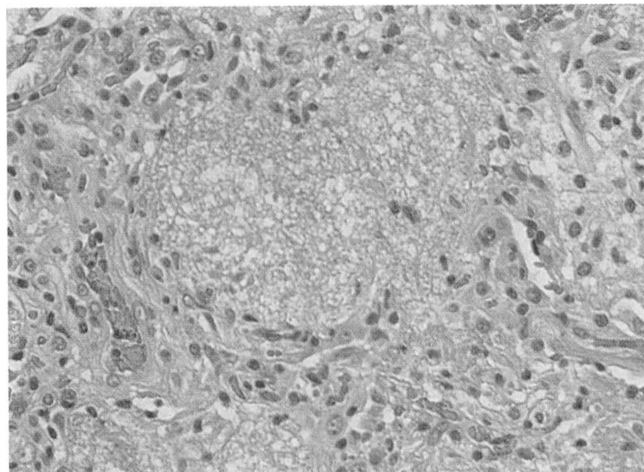
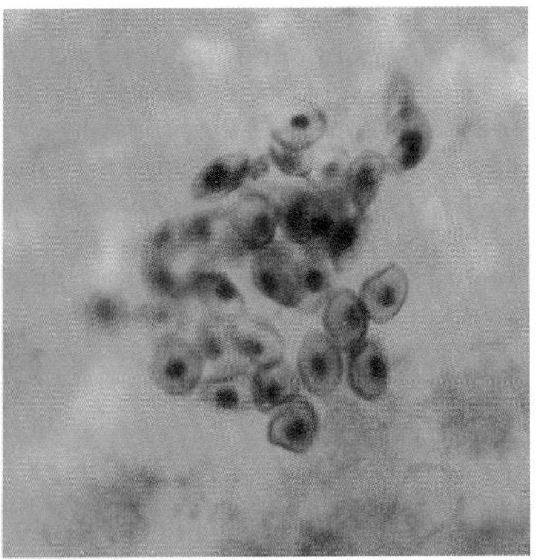

Figure 23–3
Pneumocystis pneumonia. **(A)** The alveoli are filled with a foamy exudate, and the interstitium is thickened and contains a chronic inflammatory infiltrate. **(B)** A centrifuged bronchoalveolar lavage specimen impregnated with silver shows a cluster of Pneumocystis cysts.

less than 20% of total lymphocytes (see Chapters 11 and 13).[31] Because most children with HIV infection develop *P. carinii* pneumonia before the age of 1 year, it is recommended that all infants born to HIV-infected mothers be started on a prophylaxis regimen at 4 to 6 weeks of age, regardless of their $CD4^+$ T-cell count.[30] Infants who are identified as being exposed to HIV after 6 weeks of age should be started on prophylaxis at the time of identification. All HIV-infected infants whose infection status has not been determined should continue prophylaxis until 12 months of age. Treatment is discontinued for infants in whom the infection has been excluded. After 1 year of age, prophylaxis is determined by $CD4^+$ T-cell count.

Tuberculosis

After decades of decline, the incidence of tuberculosis is increasing. The morbidity from tuberculosis has increased 14% from 1985 to 1993.[32] HIV infection has emerged as the most important risk factor for the development of tuberculosis, and the alarming increase in tuberculosis can in part be attributed to the HIV epidemic. Tuberculosis is more common among foreign-born persons from countries with a high incidence of tuberculosis and among residents of high-risk congregate settings such as correctional facilities, drug-treatment facilities, and homeless shelters. Outbreaks of a drug-resistant form of tuberculosis have occurred, complicating the selection of drugs and affecting the duration of treatment.

Tuberculosis is an infectious disease caused by *Mycobacterium tuberculosis. M. tuberculosis* organisms are slender, rod-shaped, acid-fast bacilli. They are similar to other bacterial organisms except for an outer waxy capsule that makes them more resistant to destruction; the organism can persist in old necrotic and calcified lesions and remain capable of initiating growth. The waxy coat also causes the organism to retain red dye when treated with acid in acid-fast staining.[1] *M. tuberculosis* is often referred to as *acid-fast bacillus*. Although tuberculosis can infect practically any organ of the body, the lungs are the most frequently involved. The tubercle bacilli are strict aerobes that thrive in an oxygen-rich environment. This explains their tendency to cause disease in the upper lobe or upper parts of the lower lobe of the lung, where ventilation is greatest.

Two forms of tuberculosis pose a particular threat to humans: *M. tuberculosis hominis* (human tuberculosis) and *M. tuberculosis bovis* (bovine tuberculosis). Human tuberculosis is an airborne infection spread by minute, invisible particles, called *droplet nuclei*, that are harbored in the respiratory secretions of persons with active tuberculosis.[24,25] These droplet nuclei remain suspended in air and are circulated by air currents. They are so small that, when inhaled, they travel directly to the alveoli. Bovine tuberculosis is acquired by drinking milk from infected cows, and it initially affects the gastrointestinal tract. This form of tuberculosis has been virtually eradicated in North America and other developed countries as a result of rigorous controls on dairy herds and the pasteurization of milk.

There has been a recent increase in the United States of atypical mycobacterial infections, including those caused by *M. kansasii* and *M. avium* complex (formerly *M. avium-intracellulare*). These atypical mycobacteria are predominantly opportunistic, causing infection in persons with reduced immunity or preexisting lung disease. The incidence of progressive systemic infection by *M. avium* complex is increasing among persons with AIDS.

Pathogenesis

The tubercle bacillus incites a distinctive chronic inflammatory response referred to as *granulomatous inflammation*. The destructiveness of the disease results from the hypersensitivity response that the bacillus evokes rather than its inherent destructive capabilities. Cell-mediated immunity and hypersensitivity reactions contribute to the evolution of the disease. Tuberculosis can manifest as a primary or reactivated infection.

Primary Tuberculosis. Primary tuberculosis occurs in a person lacking previous contact with the tubercle bacillus. It is typically initiated as a result of inhaling droplet nuclei that contain the tubercle bacillus. After inhalation, the droplet nuclei pass down the bronchial tree without settling on the epithelium and implant in a respiratory bronchiole or alveolus beyond the mucociliary system. Soon after entering the lung, the bacilli are surrounded and engulfed by macrophages. This action is followed by the development of a single, gray-white, circumscribed granulomatous lesion, called a *Ghon's focus,* that contains the tubercle bacilli, modified macrophages, and other immune cells. Within 2 to 3 weeks, the central portion of the Ghon's focus undergoes soft, caseous (cheeselike) necrosis. This occurs at about the time that the tuberculin test result becomes positive, suggesting that the necrosis is caused by the cell-mediated hypersensitivity immune response (see Chapter 12). During this same period, tubercle bacilli, free or within macrophages, drain along the lymph channels to the tracheobronchial lymph nodes of the affected lung and there evoke the formation of caseous granulomas. The combination of the primary lung lesion and lymph node granulomas is called *Ghon's complex* (Fig. 23–4).

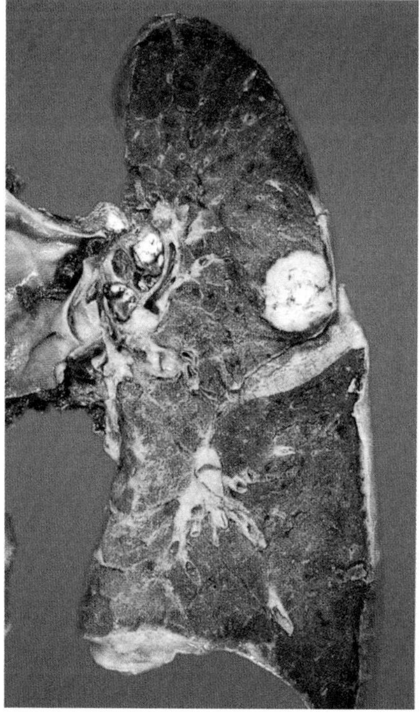

Figure 23–4
Primary tuberculosis. A healed Ghon complex is represented by a subpleural nodule and involved hilar lymph nodes.

The cell-mediated hypersensitivity response plays a dominant role in limiting further replication of the bacilli. The immune response also provides protection against additional tubercle bacilli that may be inhaled at a later time. Infection with HIV, because of its suppression of the cell-mediated immune response, predisposes to a much more severe form of tuberculosis.

When the number of organisms inhaled are small and the body's resistance is adequate, scar tissue forms and encapsulates the primary lesion. In time, most of these lesions become calcified and are visible on a chest x-ray film.

Occasionally, primary tuberculosis may progress, causing more extensive destruction of lung tissue. Often, the granulomatous tissue erodes into a bronchus, and the necrotic inflammatory tissue is discharged into it. An air-filled cavity forms, permitting bronchogenic spread of the disease. Tubercle bacilli also enter the sputum, allowing the person to infect others. In rare instances, tuberculosis may erode into a blood vessel, giving rise to hematogenic dissemination. *Miliary tuberculosis* describes minute lesions resulting from this type of dissemination, and it can involve almost any organ, particularly the brain, meninges, liver, kidney, and bone marrow.

Reactivated Tuberculosis. Reactivated tuberculosis usually results from activation of a previously healed primary lesion. Less commonly, it develops because of reinfection. It often occurs in situations of impaired body defense mechanisms. The partial immunity that follows initial exposure affords protection against reinfection and to some extent aids in localizing the disease should reactivation occur. On the other hand, the hypersensitivity reaction is an aggravating factor in reactivation tuberculosis, as evidenced by the frequency of cavitation and bronchial dissemination. The cavities may coalesce to a size of up to 10 to 15 cm in diameter. Pleural effusion and tuberculous empyema are common as the disease progresses.

Manifestations

Primary tuberculosis is usually asymptomatic, with the only evidence of the disease being a positive tuberculin skin test result and calcified lesions seen on the chest x-ray film. Uncommonly, the immune response is inadequate, and progressive primary tuberculosis develops. The person with progressive primary or reactivation tuberculosis presents with low-grade fevers, night sweats, easy fatigability, anorexia, and weight loss. A cough is initially dry but later becomes productive with purulent and sometimes blood-tinged sputum. Dyspnea and orthopnea develop as the disease advances.

Diagnosis

The most frequently used screening methods for tuberculosis are the tuberculin skin tests and chest x-ray studies. Bacteriologic studies (*i.e.,* acid-fast stain and cultures) of early morning sputum specimens are used to determine the presence of the organism. Multiple specimens often are necessary. Fiberoptic bronchoscopy may be used to obtain bronchial washings for bacteriologic studies. Drug sensitivity studies are done when there is suspicion of a drug-resistant form of the disease. Cultures on solid media may take 6 to 8 weeks, delaying diagnosis. The polymerase chain reaction (PCR) allows rapid detection of *M. tuberculosis* and differentiation from other mycobacteria. A radiometric culture system (Bactec) may allow detection of *M. tuberculosis* in several days.

The tuberculin skin test was introduced by Robert Koch in the late 19th century. The test measures delayed hypersensitivity (*i.e.,* cell-mediated, type IV) that follows exposure to the tubercle bacillus. Persons who become tuberculin positive usually remain so for the remainder of their lives. A positive reaction to the skin test does not mean that a person has active tuberculosis, only that there has been exposure to the bacillus and that cell-mediated immunity to the organism has developed.

The Mantoux test is the standard skin test for the diagnosis of tuberculosis. Multiple-puncture tests are available for population-screening purposes. Because the quantity of tuberculin introduced under the skin using the multiple-puncture technique cannot be precisely controlled, this method of testing should not be used to screen high-risk populations.[32] The Mantoux test involves the intradermal injection of tuberculin (*i.e.,* purified protein derivative standard [PPDS]). The transverse width of induration at the test site is measured after 48 to 72 hours. A 5-mm or larger reaction is considered a positive test result for persons with or at high risk for HIV infections, close contacts of persons with tuberculosis, and persons with radiographic findings consistent with old, healed tuberculosis lesions.[32] In persons who are not immunosuppressed but belong to one of the high-risk groups, such as injecting-drug users, persons with other medical problems that increase the risk of moving from latent to active tuberculosis, residents of high-risk congregate settings, or foreign-born persons from countries with a high prevalence of tuberculosis, a positive reaction is evidenced by a skin elevation of 10 mm or more.[33] An induration of 15 mm is classified as positive in persons who do not belong to either of these groups.[32]

False-positive and false-negative reactions can occur. False-positive reactions often result from cross-reactions with nontuberculosis mycobacteria, such as *M. kansasii* and *M. avium* complex. Because the hypersensitivity response to the tuberculin test depends on cell-mediated immunity, a false-negative test result can occur because of immunodeficiency states that result from HIV infection, immunosuppressive therapy, lymphoreticular malignancies, or aging. This is called *anergy.* In the immunocompromised person, a negative tuberculin test result can mean that the person has a true lack of exposure to tuberculosis or is unable to mount an immune response to the test. Because of the problem with anergy in persons with HIV and other immunocompromised states, the use of control tests is recommended. Three antigens that can be used for control testing are *Candida,* mumps virus, and tetanus toxoid. Most healthy persons in the population have been exposed to these antigens. The CDC recommends the use of control tests with two of these antigens when screening persons with HIV infection for tuberculosis. If a person reacts to at least one of the control antigens, a negative tuberculin test result usually means that the person is not infected with tuberculosis.

A two-step testing procedure, which uses a "boosting" phenomenon, may be used to increase a subsequent tuberculin test in persons who have been infected with tuberculosis.[34] If the first test result of the two-step procedure is negative, a second test is administered 1 week later. If the second test result is negative, the person is considered to be uninfected or anergic. If the second test result is positive, it is assumed to have occurred because of a boosted response. The boosted effect can last for 1 year or longer. Use of the two-step test procedure for employee health or institutional screening can reduce the likelihood that a boosted response in a subsequent test will not be interpreted as a recent infection.

Treatment

Two groups meet the criteria established for the use of antimycobacterial therapy for tuberculosis: persons with active tuberculosis and those who have had contact with cases of active tuberculosis and who are at risk for developing an active form of the disease.

The primary drugs used in the treatment of tuberculosis are isoniazid (INH), rifampin, pyrazinamide, ethambutol, and streptomycin. Isoniazid is remarkably potent against the tubercle bacillus and is probably the most widely used drug for tuberculosis. Although its exact mechanism of action is unknown, it apparently combines with an enzyme that is needed by the isoniazid-susceptible strains of the tubercle bacillus. Resistance to the drug develops rapidly, and combination with other effective drugs delays the development of resistance. Rifampin inhibits RNA synthesis in the bacillus. Although ethambutol and pyrazinamide are known to inhibit the growth of the tubercle bacillus, their mechanisms of action are largely unknown. Streptomycin, the first drug found to be effective against tuberculosis, must be given by injection, which limits its usefulness, particularly in long-term therapy. It remains an important drug in tuberculosis therapy and is used primarily in persons with severe, possibly life-threatening forms of tuberculosis.

Treatment of *active tuberculosis* requires the use of multiple drugs. Tuberculosis is an unusual disease in that chemotherapy is required for a relatively long period of time. The tubercle bacillus is an aerobic organism that multiplies slowly and remains relatively dormant in oxygen-poor caseous material. It undergoes a high rate of mutation and tends to develop a resistance to any one drug. For this reason, multidrug regimens are used for treating persons with active tuberculosis.

Based on the results of several trials, a marked change in chemotherapy for uncomplicated tuberculosis has developed. Short-course programs of therapy (usually for 6 to 9 months) have replaced the earlier 18- to 24-month multidrug regimens. Treatment may need to be prolonged in HIV-infected persons and in persons with drug-resistant strains of *M. tuberculosis*. Prophylactic treatment is used for persons who are infected with *M. tuberculosis* but do not have active disease.[35] This group includes persons with a positive skin test result who have had close contact with active cases of tuberculosis; have converted from a negative to positive skin test result within 2 years; have a history of untreated or inadequately treated tuberculosis; have chest radiographs with evidence of tuberculosis but no bacteriologic evidence of the active disease; have special risk factors such as silicosis, diabetes mellitus, prolonged corticosteroid therapy, immunosuppression therapy, end-stage renal disease, chronic malnutrition from any cause, hematologic or reticuloendothelial cancers; have a positive HIV test result or have AIDS; and are 35 years of age or younger with a positive reaction of unknown duration. These persons harbor a small number of microorganisms and are usually treated with INH.

Outbreaks of multidrug-resistant tuberculosis have posed a problem for the prophylactic treatment of exposed persons, including health care workers.[36] Most exposed persons who have developed active multidrug-resistant tuberculosis were infected with the HIV virus; the fatality rate among these persons is high (72% to 89%). Various treatment protocols are recommended, depending on the type of resistant strain that is identified.

Success of chemotherapy for prophylaxis and treatment of tuberculosis depends on strict adherence to a lengthy drug regimen. This is often a problem, particularly for asymptomatic persons with tuberculosis infections and for poorly motivated groups such as intravenous drug abusers. Directly observed therapy, which requires that a health care worker observe while the person takes the antituberculosis drug, is recommended for some persons and for some types of treatment protocols.

First administered to humans in 1921, the bacille Calmette-Guérin (BCG) vaccine is used to prevent the development of tuberculosis in persons who are at high risk for being infected with the disease. BCG is an attenuated strain of *M. tuberculosis bovis*. The vaccine has been used worldwide to prevent tuberculosis.[37] It is administered only to persons who have a negative tuberculin skin test result. The vaccine, which is given intradermally, produces a local reaction that can last as long as 3 months and may result in scarring at the injection site. Persons who have been vaccinated with BCG usually have a positive tuberculin skin test result that wanes with time and is unlikely to persist beyond 10 years. The vaccine has also been used to increase the immune response in persons with some types of cancers. The CDC recommends that use of the BCG vaccine in the United States be reserved for high-risk groups such as infants and children who reside in settings in which the likelihood of *M. tuberculosis* transmission and infection is high and for health care workers where the risk of transmission of multidrug resistant strains of the bacterium are high. The vaccine is not recommended for children and adults infected with HIV.[37]

Fungal Infections

Although the spores of fungi are constantly present in the air we breathe, only a few reach the lung and cause disease. The most common of these are histoplasmosis, coccidioidomycosis, and blastomycosis. These infections are usually mild and self-limited and are seldom noticed unless they produce local complications or progressive dissemination occurs. The signs and symptoms of these infections commonly resemble those of tuberculosis.

Histoplasmosis

Histoplasmosis is caused by the dimorphic fungus *Histoplasma capsulatum* and is the most common fungal infection in the United States. Skin testing surveys suggest that 18% to 20% of persons in the United States have been infected with the disease.[38] Most cases occur along the major river valleys of the Midwest—the Ohio, the Mississippi, and the Missouri. The organism grows in soil and other areas that have been enriched with bird excreta: old chicken houses, pigeon lofts, barns, and trees where birds roost. The infection is acquired by inhaling the fungal spores that are released when the dirt or dust from the infected areas is disturbed. The spores convert to the parasitic yeast phase when exposed to body temperature in the alveoli. The organisms are then carried to the regional lymphatics and from there are disseminated throughout the body in the bloodstream. They are removed from the circulation by fixed macrophages of the reticuloendothelial system. When delayed hypersensitivity develops (see Chapter 12), the macrophages are usually able to destroy the fungi.

The manifestations of histoplasmosis are strikingly similar to those of tuberculosis. Depending on the host's resistance and immunocompetence, the disease usually takes one of four forms: latent asymptomatic disease, self-limited primary disease, chronic pulmonary disease, or disseminated infection. The average incubation period for the infection is about 14 days. Only 40% of infected persons have symptoms, and only about 10% of these are ill enough to seek the care of a physician.[39]

Latent asymptomatic histoplasmosis is characterized by evidence of healed lesions in the lungs or hilar lymph nodes, accompanied by a positive histoplasmin skin test result (analogous to the tuberculin test). *Primary pulmonary histoplasmosis* occurs in otherwise healthy persons as a mild, self-limited, febrile, respiratory infection. Its symptoms include muscle and joint pains and a nonproductive cough. Erythema nodosum (*i.e.*, subcutaneous nodules) or erythema multiforme (*i.e.*, hivelike lesions) sometimes appears. During this stage of the disease, chest radiographs usually show single or multiple infiltrates.

Chronic histoplasmosis resembles reactivation tuberculosis. Infiltration of the upper lobes of one or both lungs occurs with cavitation. This form of the disease is more common in middle-aged men who smoke and in persons with chronic lung disease. The most common manifestations are productive cough, fever, night sweats, and weight loss. In many persons, the disease is self-limited. In others, there is progressive destruction of lung tissue and dissemination of the disease.

Disseminated histoplasmosis can follow primary or chronic histoplasmosis but most often develops as an acute and fulminating infection in the very old or the very young or in persons with compromised immune function. Although the macrophages of the reticuloendothelial system can remove the fungi from the bloodstream, they are unable to destroy them.[31] Characteristically, this form of the disease produces a high fever, generalized lymph node enlargement, hepatosplenomegaly, muscle wasting, anemia, leukopenia, and thrombocytopenia. There may be hoarseness, ulcerations of the mouth and tongue, nausea, vomiting, diarrhea, and abdominal pain. Often, meningitis becomes a dominant feature of the disease.

Absolute diagnosis of histoplasmosis requires identification of the organism on culture. The infection incites a delayed hypersensitivity immune response, and the histoplasmin skin test is used to test for exposure to the organism. This test result remains positive after the initial infection has occurred and does not indicate whether the disease is of recent or past origin. In addition to the delayed response, the humoral immune system responds to the acute infection by producing antibodies. Although these antibodies are not protective, they serve as markers of infection. These antibodies can be measured by means of the complement fixation (CF) test. An immunodiffusion (ID) test can also be used as a test for the antibodies. The CF and ID tests become positive 2 weeks after the onset of symptoms.

The antifungal drugs amphotericin B and the azoles (*e.g.*, itraconazole, ketoconazole, fluconazole) are used for persons with disease severe enough to require treatment or those with compromised immune function who are at risk for developing disseminated disease. Amphotericin B is given intravenously and is usually the drug of choice in severe disease. The drug can impair kidney and liver function and produce anemia. The azoles are given orally. Treatment is continued until the person's symptoms have resolved and negative cultures have been obtained. This may take 9 months or longer for persons with chronic pulmonary disease.[40]

Coccidioidomycosis

Coccidioidomycosis is a common fungal infection caused by inhaling the spores of *Coccidioides immitis*.[41] The disease resembles tuberculosis, and its mechanisms of infection are similar to those of histoplasmosis. An estimated 100,000 new cases occur annually.[42] It is most prevalent in the southwestern United States, principally in California, Arizona, and Texas. Because of its prevalence in the San Joaquin Valley, the disease is sometimes referred to as "San Joaquin fever" or "valley fever." The *C. immitis* organism lives in soil and can establish new sites in the soil. Events such as dust storms and digging for construction have been associated with increased incidence of the disease.

The disease most commonly occurs as an acute, primary, self-limited pulmonary infection with or without systemic involvement, but in some cases, it progresses to a disseminated disease. About 60% of exposed persons manifest only a positive skin test result (*i.e.*, coccidioidin skin test or spherulin skin test) and are unaware of the infection.[42] In the other 40%, the illness usually resembles influenza. There may be fever, cough, and pleuritic pain, accompanied by erythema multiforme or erythema nodosum. The skin lesions are usually accompanied by arthralgias or arthritis without effusion, particularly of the ankles and knees. The terms "desert bumps" and "desert arthritis" are used to describe these manifestations. The presence of skin and joint manifestations indicates strong host defenses, because persons who have had such manifestations seldom develop disseminated disease. Disseminated disease occurs in 1 of 6000 infected persons and in fewer than 0.5% of persons with symptomatic disease. Commonly affected structures in disseminated disease are the lymph nodes, meninges, spleen, liver, kidney, skin, and adrenals. Meningitis is the most common cause of death. Persons with diabetes, compromised immune function, infants, and members of dark-skinned races tend to localize the disease poorly and are at higher risk for disseminated disease. In HIV-infected persons in endemic areas, coccidioidomycosis is now a common opportunistic infection.

The CF test is commonly used in the diagnosis of coccidioidomycosis. The CF test may be used in following the progress of the disease; an elevated CF titer is considered to indicate the risk of disease dissemination. An immunodiffusion test is also available and may be used as a screening test. Although skin tests are available, they are seldom used to establish a diagnosis. In disseminated disease, anergy often develops, and the test result is negative; in endemic areas, a positive test result can easily have been acquired before the onset of clinical illness.

As with histoplasmosis, the antifungal drugs amphotericin B or the oral azoles are used in the treatment of the disease.

Blastomycosis

Blastomycosis is caused by the organism *Blastomyces dermatitidis*. It is characterized by local suppurative and granulomatous lesions of the lungs and skin. The disease is most commonly found in the South and North Central United States, especially in areas bordering the Mississippi and Ohio River Basins, and the Great Lakes.[43]

The symptoms of acute infection are similar to those of acute histoplasmosis, including fever, cough, aching joints and muscles, and uncommonly, pleuritic pain. In contrast to histoplasmosis, the cough in blastomycosis is often productive, and the sputum is purulent. Acute pulmonary infections may be self-limited or progressive. Persons with overwhelming pulmonary disease may develop diffuse interalveolar infiltrates and evidence of acute respiratory distress syndrome (Chapter 24). Extrapulmonary spread most commonly involves the skin, bones, or the prostate. These lesions may provide the first evidence of the disease.

The diagnosis of blastomycosis is more difficult than that of histoplasmosis. Visualization of the yeast in the sputum after application of 10% potassium hydroxide provides a presumptive diagnosis. When this fails, cultural isolation of the fungus is often attempted. The blastomycin skin test lacked specificity and is no longer available.

Treatment of the progressive or disseminated form of the disease includes the use of amphotericin B, ketoconazole, or fluconazole. Most persons with blastomycosis are identified and treated before the development of overwhelming or fatal disease.[43]

In summary, respiratory infections are the most common cause of respiratory illness. They include the common cold, influenza, pneumonias, tuberculosis, and fungal infections. The common cold occurs more frequently than any other respiratory infection. The fingers are the usual source of transmission, and the most common portals of entry are the nasal mucosa and the conjunctiva of the eye. The influenza virus causes three syndromes: an uncomplicated rhinotracheitis, a respiratory viral infection followed by a bacterial infection, and viral pneumonia.

Pneumonia describes an infection of the parenchymal tissues of the lung. Loss of the cough reflex, damage to the ciliated endothelium that lines the respiratory tract, or impaired immune defenses predispose to pneumonia. Pneumonia is being increasingly classified as community acquired or hospital acquired. Persons with compromised immune function constitute a special concern in both categories. Community-acquired pneumonia involves infections from organisms that are more often present in the community than in the hospital or nursing home. The most common cause of community-acquired pneumonia is *S. pneumoniae.* Hospital-acquired (nosocomial) pneumonia is defined as a lower respiratory tract infection occurring 72 hours or more after admission. Hospital-acquired pneumonia is the second most common cause of hospital-acquired infections. Legionnaires' disease is a form of bronchopneumonia caused by the gram-negative bacillus *Legionella pneumophila.* Viral or atypical pneumonia can occur as a primary infection, such as that caused by influenza virus, or as a complication of other viral infections, such as measles or chickenpox. Viral and atypical pneumonias involve the interstitium of the lung and often masquerade as chest colds. *Pneumocystis carinii* pneumonia is an opportunistic infection that occurs in debilitated persons with impaired immune function, including persons with HIV infection.

Tuberculosis is a chronic respiratory infection caused by *M. tuberculosis,* which is spread by minute, invisible particles called droplet nuclei. After decades of decline, the incidence of tuberculosis is increasing, particularly among HIV-infected persons, foreign-born persons from countries with a high incidence of tuberculosis, and residents of high-risk congregate settings such as correctional facilities, drug-treatment facilities, and homeless shelters. The treatment of tuberculosis has been complicated by outbreaks of drug-resistant forms of the disease. The tubercle bacillus incites a distinctive chronic inflammatory response referred to as granulomatous inflammation. The destructiveness of the disease results from the hypersensitivity response that the bacillus evokes rather than its inherent destructive capabilities. Cell-mediated immunity and hypersensitivity reactions contribute to the evolution of the disease.

Infections caused by the fungi *H. capsulatum* (histoplasmosis), *C. immitis* (coccidioidomycosis), and *B. dermatitidis* (blastomycosis) resemble tuberculosis. These infections are common but seldom serious unless they produce progressive destruction of lung tissue or the infection disseminates outside the lungs.

Cancer of the Lung

After you have completed this section of the chapter, you should be able to meet the following objectives:

- Cite risk factors associated with lung cancer
- Describe the manifestations of lung cancer and list two symptoms of lung cancer that are related to the invasion of the mediastinum
- Define the term *paraneoplastic* and cite three paraneoplastic manifestations of lung cancer
- Characterize the 5-year survival rate for lung cancer

Lung cancer is the leading cause of cancer deaths among men and women in the United States, accounting for 25% of all cancer deaths. In 1997, it was responsible for the deaths of 94,400 men and 66,000 women.[44] The increases in lung cancer incidence and deaths over the past 50 years have coincided closely with the increase in cigarette smoking over the same period. It has been estimated that 85% of lung cancer cases are caused by cigarette smoking. Many studies have shown that the risk of developing lung cancer increases with the number of cigarettes smoked and that the average male smoker is 10 times more likely to develop lung cancer than the nonsmoker. Industrial hazards also contribute to the incidence of lung cancer. A commonly recognized hazard is exposure to asbestos, with the mean risk of lung cancer being significantly greater in asbestos workers than in the general population. Tobacco smoke contributes heavily to the development of lung cancer in persons exposed to asbestos; the risk in this population group is estimated to be 50 to 90 times greater than that for nonsmokers.[1]

Because cancer of the lung is usually far advanced before it is discovered, the prognosis is generally poor. The overall 5-year survival rate is 13% to 15%, a dismal statistic that has not changed over the past 30 years.[45]

Types of Cancers

Bronchiogenic carcinoma, which has its origin in the bronchial or bronchiolar epithelium, constitutes 90% to 95% of all lung cancers. These tumors can be further subdivided into non–small cell lung carcinoma (70% to 75%); small cell lung carcinoma (20% to 25%), and combined patterns (5% to 10%). Bronchiogenic carcinomas are aggressive, locally invasive, and widely metastatic tumors that arise from the epithelial lining of the major bronchi. All varieties of bronchiogenic carcinomas, especially small cell lung carcinoma, have the capacity to synthesize bioactive products and produce paraneoplastic syndromes. These tumors begin as small mucosal lesions that may follow one of several patterns of growth. They may form intraluminal masses that invade the bronchial mucosa and infiltrate the peribronchial connective tissue or they may form large, bulky masses that extend into the adjacent lung tissue. Some large tumors undergo central necrosis and develop local areas of hemorrhage, and some invade the pleural cavity and chest wall and spread to adjacent intrathoracic structures.[1]

There are three types of non–small cell lung carcinomas (NSLC): squamous cell carcinoma (25% to 40%), adenocarcinoma, including bronchioalveolar carcinoma (25% to 40%), and large cell carcinoma (10% to 15%).[1] Squamous cell carcinomas are more common in men than women; are closely associated with a smoking history; and tend to spread centrally into major bronchi and hilar lymph nodes but disseminate outside the thorax later than other types of NSLC.

Adenocarcinoma is the most common type of lung cancer in women and nonsmokers. The association between cigarette smoking is weaker than for squamous cell carcinoma. These tumors may occur as central lesions in the bronchi but are usually more peripherally located, with many arising in relation to peripheral scars. Generally, these tumors grow more slowly than squamous cell carcinomas and produce smaller masses than other types of NSLC. Bronchioalveolar carcinoma, a special category of adenocarcinoma, occurs as two variants: one that forms multifocal mucinous masses and a second that is evidenced by a single tumor that does not elaborate mucin. These tumors have a better prognosis than other bronchiogenic carcinomas. Persons with multifocal lesions have a 20% to 25% 5-year survival rate, and those with localized, single lesions, which are surgically resectable, have a 50% to 70% 5-year survival rate.

Large cell carcinomas constitute a group of neoplasms that are highly anaplastic and difficult to categorize as squamous or adenocarcinoma. They have a poor prognosis because of their tendency to spread to distant sites early in their course. More than one half have spread to the central nervous system at the time of diagnosis, and the 5-year survival rate is 2% to 3%.

The small-cell lung carcinomas (SCLC) are rapidly growing tumors that tend to infiltrate widely, disseminate early in their course, and are rarely resectable. The 2-year survival rate is poor. These tumors are particularly sensitive to chemotherapy and irradiation, and newer protocols have improved the outlook somewhat. The SCLC is one form of cancer that has paraneoplastic properties (see Chapter 5). It has the ability to secrete a host of polypeptide hormones, including adrenocorticotrophic hormone (ACTH), antidiuretic hormone (ADH), parathyroid-like hormone, and gastrin-releasing peptide.

Manifestations

Cancer of the lung develops insidiously, often giving little or no warning of its presence. Because its symptoms are similar to those associated with smoking and chronic bronchitis, they are often disregarded.

The manifestations of lung cancer can be divided into three categories: those due to involvement of the lung and adjacent structures, the effects of local spread and metastasis, and the nonmetastatic paraneoplastic manifestations involving endocrine, neurologic, and connective tissue function. As with other cancers, lung cancer also causes nonspecific symptoms such as anorexia and weight loss.

Effects on the Lung and Adjacent Structures

Lung cancers produce local effects by irritation and obstruction of the airways and invasion of the mediastinum and pleural space. The earliest symptoms are chronic cough, shortness of breath, and wheezing because of airway irritation and obstruction. Hemoptysis (*i.e.,* blood in the sputum) occurs when the lesion erodes blood vessels. Pain receptors in the chest are limited to the parietal pleura, mediastinum, larger blood vessels, and peribronchial afferent vagal fibers. Dull, intermittent, poorly localized retrosternal pain is common in tumors that involve the mediastinum. Pain becomes persistent, localized, and more severe when the disease invades the pleura.

Tumors that invade the mediastinum may cause hoarseness because of the involvement of the recurrent laryngeal nerve and cause difficulty in swallowing because of compression of the esophagus. An uncommon complication called the *superior vena cava syndrome* can occur in some persons with mediastinal involvement. Interruption of blood flow in this vessel usually results from compression by the tumor or involved lymph nodes. The disorder can interfere with venous drainage from the head, neck, and chest wall. The outcome is determined by the speed with which the disorder develops and the adequacy of the collateral circulation.

Tumors adjacent to the visceral pleura often insidiously produce pleural effusion. This effusion can compress the lung and cause atelectasis and dyspnea. It is less likely to cause fever, pleural friction rub, or pain than pleural effusion resulting from other causes.

Metastatic Spread

Metastases already exist in 50% of patients presenting with evidence of lung cancer and develop eventually in 90% of patients. The most common sites of these metastases are the brain, bone, and liver.

Paraneoplastic Disorders

Paraneoplastic disorders are those that are unrelated to metastasis. These include hypercalcemia from secretion of parathyroid-like peptide, Cushing's syndrome from ACTH secretion, diabetes insipidus from inappropriate secretion of ADH, neuromuscular syndromes (*e.g.*, myasthenic syndromes, peripheral neuropathy, polymyositis), and hematologic disorders (*e.g.*, migratory thrombophlebitis, nonbacterial endocarditis, disseminated intravascular coagulation). Neurologic or muscular symptoms can develop 6 months to 4 years before the lung tumor is detected. One of the more common of these problems is weakness and wasting of the proximal muscles of the pelvic and shoulder girdles, with decreased deep tendon reflexes but without sensory changes. Hypercalcemia is seen most often in persons with squamous cell carcinoma, hematologic syndromes in persons with adenocarcinomas, and the remaining syndromes in persons with small cell neoplasms.[1] Manifestations of the paraneoplastic syndrome may precede the onset of other signs of lung cancer and may lead to discovery of an occult tumor.

Diagnosis and Treatment

The diagnosis of lung cancer is based on a careful history and physical examination and other tests such as chest radiography, bronchoscopy, cytologic studies (Papanicolaou's test) of the sputum or bronchial washings, percutaneous needle biopsy of lung tissue, and scalene lymph node biopsy. CT scans, magnetic resonance imaging, and ultrasonography are used to locate lesions and evaluate the extent of the disease. The carcinoembryonic antigen (CEA) is produced by undifferentiated lung tumor cells; high CEA titers usually correlate with extensive disease. This test is often used to follow the progress of the disease and its response to treatment.

Like other types of cancer, lung cancers are classified according to cell type (*i.e.*, squamous cell carcinoma, adenocarcinoma, small cell anaplastic carcinoma, and large cell carcinoma) and staged according to the TNM system (see Chapter 5). These classifications are used for treatment planning.

Treatment methods for lung cancer include surgery, radiotherapy, and chemotherapy.[46–48] These treatments may be used singly or in combination. Surgery is used for the removal of small, localized tumors. It can involve a lobectomy, pneumonectomy, or segmental resection of the lung. Radiation therapy can be used as a definitive or main treatment modality, as part of a combined treatment plan, or for palliation of symptoms. Because of the frequency of metastases, chemotherapy is often used in treating lung cancer. Combination chemotherapy, which uses a regimen of several drugs, is usually employed. Chemotherapy is the treatment of choice for SCLC. Recent advances in the use of combination chemotherapy have improved the outlook for persons with SCLC. National Cancer Institute studies report that 10% of persons with limited-stage disease and 5% of all persons with SCLC treated with combination chemotherapy have survived 10 years or longer.[48]

In summary, cancer of the lung is a leading cause of death among men and women between the ages of 50 and 75, and the death rate is increasing among women. In the United States, the increased death rate has coincided with an increase in cigarette smoking. Industrial hazards, such as exposure to asbestos, increase the risk of developing lung cancer. Of all forms of lung cancer, bronchogenic carcinoma is the most common, accounting for 90% to 95% of cases. Because lung cancer develops insidiously, it is often far advanced before it is diagnosed, a fact that is used to explain the poor 5-year survival rate.

The manifestations of lung cancer can be attributed to the involvement of the lung and adjacent structures, the effects of local spread and metastasis, and the nonmetastatic paraneoplastic manifestations involving endocrine, neurologic, and connective tissue function. As with other cancers, lung cancer causes nonspecific symptoms such as anorexia and weight loss. Treatment methods for lung cancer include surgery, irradiation, and chemotherapy.

Respiratory Disorders in Children

After you have completed this section of the chapter, you should be able to meet the following objectives:

- Trace the development of the respiratory tract through the five stages of embryonic and fetal development
- Cite the function of surfactant in lung function in the neonate
- Cite the possible cause and manifestations of bronchopulmonary dysplasia
- Describe the physiologic basis for sternal and chest wall retractions and grunting, stridor, and wheezing as signs of respiratory distress in infants and small children
- Compare croup, epiglottitis, and bronchiolitis in terms of incidence by age, site of infection, and signs and symptoms
- List the signs of impending respiratory failure in small children

Acute respiratory disease is the most common cause of illness in infancy and childhood, accounting for 50% of illness in children younger than 5 years of age and 30% of illness in children between 5 and 12 years of age.[49] This section focuses on (1) lung development, with an emphasis on the developmental basis for lung disorders in children; (2) respiratory disorders in the neonate; and (3) respiratory infections in children. A discussion of bronchial asthma in children and cystic fibrosis is included in Chapter 24.

Lung Development

Although other body systems are physiologically ready for extrauterine life by as early as 25 weeks of gestation, the lungs require much longer. Immaturity of the respiratory system is a major cause of morbidity and mortality in infants born prematurely. Even at birth, the lungs are not fully mature, and additional growth and maturation continue well into childhood.

Developmental Stages

Lung development may be divided into five stages: embryonic period, glandular period, canicular period, saccular period, and alveolar period.[50–52] The development of the respiratory system begins with the *embryonic period* (weeks 4 to 6 of gestation), during which a rudimentary lung bud branches from the esophagus to begin formation of the airways and alveolar spaces (Fig. 23–5). The lung bud divides into two lung buds that grow laterally; the right bud gives rise to two secondary buds and the left bud to one secondary bud. Consequently, at

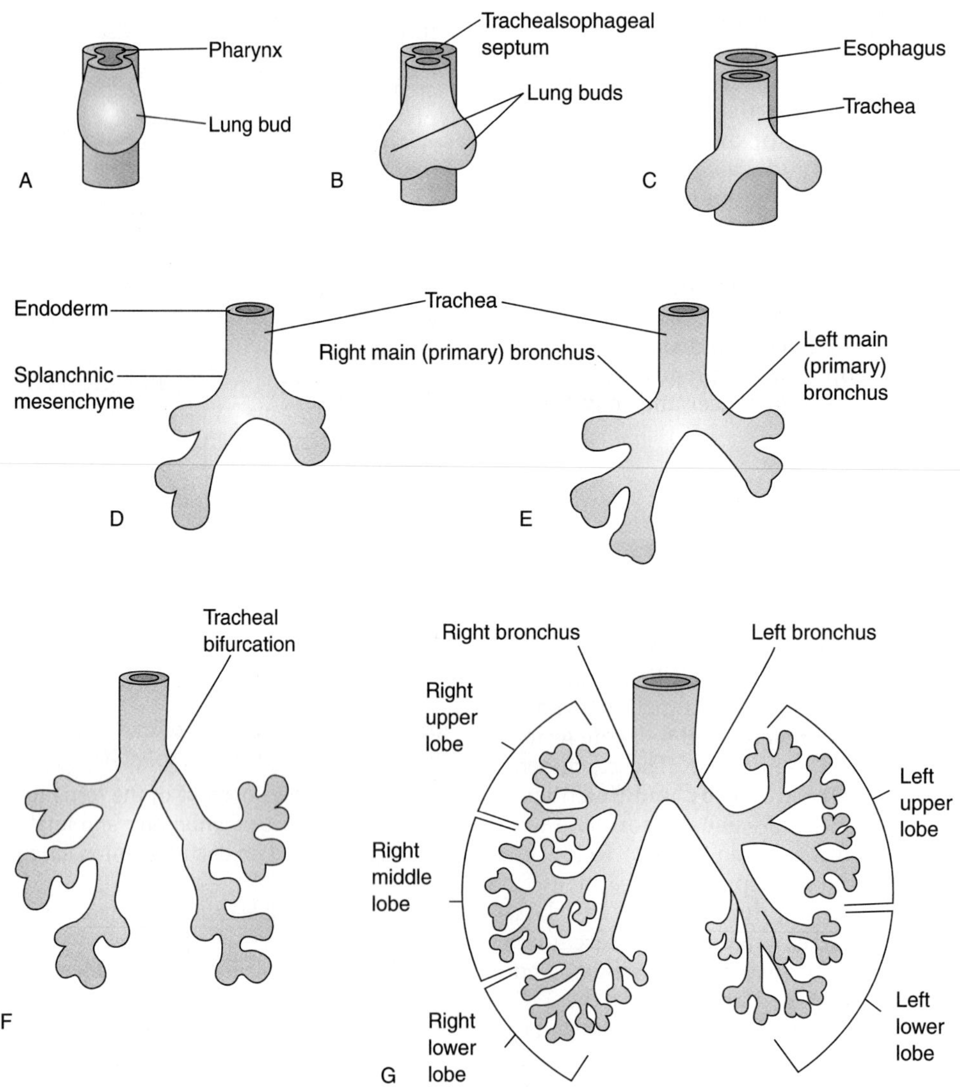

Figure 23–5
Drawings of ventral views illustrating successive stages in the development of the bronchi and lungs. (**A–C**) 4 weeks, (**D, E**) 5 weeks, (**F**) 6 weeks, (**G**) 8 weeks. (Moore K. [1993]. *The developing human* [5th ed.]. Philadelphia: W.B. Saunders)

maturity, there are three main (primary) bronchi and three lung lobes on the right and only two main bronchi and two lung lobes on the left. Each secondary lung bud subsequently undergoes continuous branching. The tertiary (segmental) bronchi (10 in the right lung and 8 or 9 in the left lung) begin to form during the 7th week.

During the *glandular period* (weeks 5 to 16), the lungs resemble a gland. During this period, the conducting airways are formed. At 17 weeks, all of the major elements of the lung have formed except the gas exchange structures. Respiration is not possible because the airways end in blind tubes.

The *canicular period* (weeks 17 to 27) marks the formation of the primitive alveoli. During this period, the lumina of the bronchi and bronchioles become much larger, and the lung tissue becomes more highly vascularized. By the 24th week, each bronchiole has given rise to two or more respiratory bronchioles. Respiration is possible at this time because some primitive alveoli have developed at the ends of the bronchioles.[52]

The *saccular period* (weeks 27 to 35) is devoted to the development of the terminal alveolar sacs, which facilitate gas exchange. During this period, the terminal sacs thin out, and capillaries begin to bulge into the terminal sacs. These thin cells are known as *type I alveolar cells*. By the 25th to 28th week, sufficient terminal sacs are present to permit survival. Before this time, the premature lungs were incapable of adequate gas exchange. It is not so much the presence of the thin alveolar epithelium as it is the adequate matching of pulmonary vasculature to it that is critical to survival.[52] *Type II alveolar cells* begin to develop at about 24 weeks. These cells produce surfactant, a substance capable of lowering the surface tension of the air-alveoli interface (see Chapter 22). By the 28th to 30th week, the amount of surfactant that is available is sufficient to prevent alveolar collapse when breathing begins.

The *alveolar period* (late fetal to early childhood) marks the maturation and expansion of the alveoli. Starting as early as 30 weeks and usually by 36 weeks, the saccular structures become alveoli. Alveolation is characterized by thinning of the pulmonary interstitium and the appearance of a single capillary network, in which one capillary bulges into each terminal alveolar sac. By the late fetal period, the lungs are capable of respiration because the alveolar-capillary membrane is sufficiently thin to allow for gas exchange.

Although transformation of the lungs from glandlike structures to highly vascular alveolilike organs occurs during the late fetal period, mature alveoli do not form for some time after birth. The growth of the lung during infancy and early childhood involves an increase in the number rather than the size of the alveoli. Only one eighth to one sixth of the adult number of alveoli are present at birth. There is a relative slowing of alveolar growth during the first 3 months after birth, and this is followed by a rapid increase in alveolar number during the rest of the first year of life, reaching approximately the adult number of 300 million alveoli by 5 to 6 years of age.

Lung Liquid and Fetal Breathing

The fetal lung is a secretory organ, and fluids and electrolytes are secreted into the potential air spaces. This fluid appears to be important in stimulating alveolar development. For the fetus to complete the transition from intrauterine life to extrauterine life, this fluid must be cleared from the lung soon after birth. Presumably with the onset of labor, the secretion of fluid ceases. During the birth process, pressure on the fetal thorax causes the fluid to be expelled from the mouth and nose. When the lungs expand after birth, the fluid moves into the tissues surrounding the alveoli and is then absorbed into the pulmonary capillaries or removed by the lymphatic system.

Breathing Movements by the Fetus

Fetal breathing movements occur in utero. These movements are irregular in rate and amplitude, ranging from 30 to 70 breaths per minute and become more rapid as gestation advances. Because they are rapid and shallow, these movements do not result in movement of fluid into or out of the fetal lung. These movements are thought to condition the respiratory muscles and stimulate lung development. The breathing movements in the fetus become more rapid in response to an increase in carbon dioxide levels and become slower in response to hypoxia.

Breathing in the Infant and Small Child

The major difference between respiration in the fetus and the neonate is that there is complete separation between gas exchange and breathing movements in the fetus. The gas supply and exchange depend entirely on maternal mechanisms controlling placental circulation. At birth, dependence on the placental circulation is terminated, and the infant must integrate the two previously separate functions of gas exchange and respiratory movements. Within seconds of clamping the umbilical cord, the infant takes its first breath, and rhythmic breathing begins and persists for life.

The Mechanics of Breathing

The diaphragm is the principal muscle of inspiration. When the chest wall is sufficiently stiff, as it is in the adult, contraction of the diaphragm increases chest volume in both the longitudinal and transverse directions. In the adult, the ribs angle downward, from front to back, so that contraction of the external intercostals elevate the rib cage. In contrast to the adult, the chest wall of the neonate is compliant; although this is advantageous during the birth process in that it allows for marked distortion to occur without damaging chest structures, it has implications for ventilation during the postnatal period. Not only is the infant's chest wall compliant, but the diaphragm inserts more horizontally, is flatter, and is less capable of moving downward to increase the volume of the chest cavity.[49] The external intercostals, rather than raising the rib cage, stabilize the chest wall during inspiration.

A striking characteristic of neonatal breathing is the paradoxical inward movement of the upper chest during inspiration, especially during active sleep. This occurs because there is decreased activity of the intercostal muscles during active sleep, which allows the contracting diaphragm to pull the highly compliant chest wall inward. Under circumstances such as crying, the intercostal muscles of the neonate function together with the diaphragm.

Normally, the infant's lungs are also compliant; this is advantageous to the infant with its compliant chest cage, because it takes only small changes in inspiratory pressure to inflate a compliant lung. When respiratory disease develops, lung compliance is reduced and it takes more effort to inflate the lungs. The diaphragm must generate more negative pressure; as a result, the compliant chest wall structures are sucked inward. *Retractions* are abnormal inward movements of the chest wall during inspiration; they may occur intercostally (between the ribs), in the substernal or epigastric area, and the supraclavicular spaces. Because the chest wall of the infant is compliant, substernal retractions become more obvious with small changes in lung function. Retractions can indicate airway obstruction or atelectasis.

Also influencing the effectiveness of ventilation in the neonate is the intrinsic mechanical properties of the diaphragm. Although much uncertainty remains regarding the functioning of the respiratory muscles in the neonate, it seems that these muscles, particularly in the preterm infant, are poorly adapted for high workloads. This is because they contain relatively few fatigue-resistant, slow-twitch, highly oxidative fibers, have low glycogen and fat stores, and can easily become hypoxic.[53]

Airway Resistance

Normal lung inflation requires uninterrupted movement of air through the extrathoracic airways (*i.e.*, nose, pharynx, larynx, and upper trachea) and intrathoracic airways (*i.e.*, bronchi and bronchioles). The neonate (0 to 4 weeks of age) breathes predominantly through the nose and does not adapt well to mouth breathing. Any obstruction of the nose or nasopharynx may increase upper airway resistance and increase the work of breathing.

The airways of the infant and small child are much smaller than those of the adult. Because the resistance to airflow is directly related to the fourth power of the radius (resistance $= 1/\text{radius}^4$), relatively small amounts of mucus secretion, edema, or airway constriction can produce marked changes in airway resistance and airflow (Fig. 23–6). Nasal flaring is a method that infants use to take in more air. This method of breathing increases the size of the nares and decreases the resistance of the small airways.

Normally, the extrathoracic airways in the infant narrow during inspiration and widen during expiration,

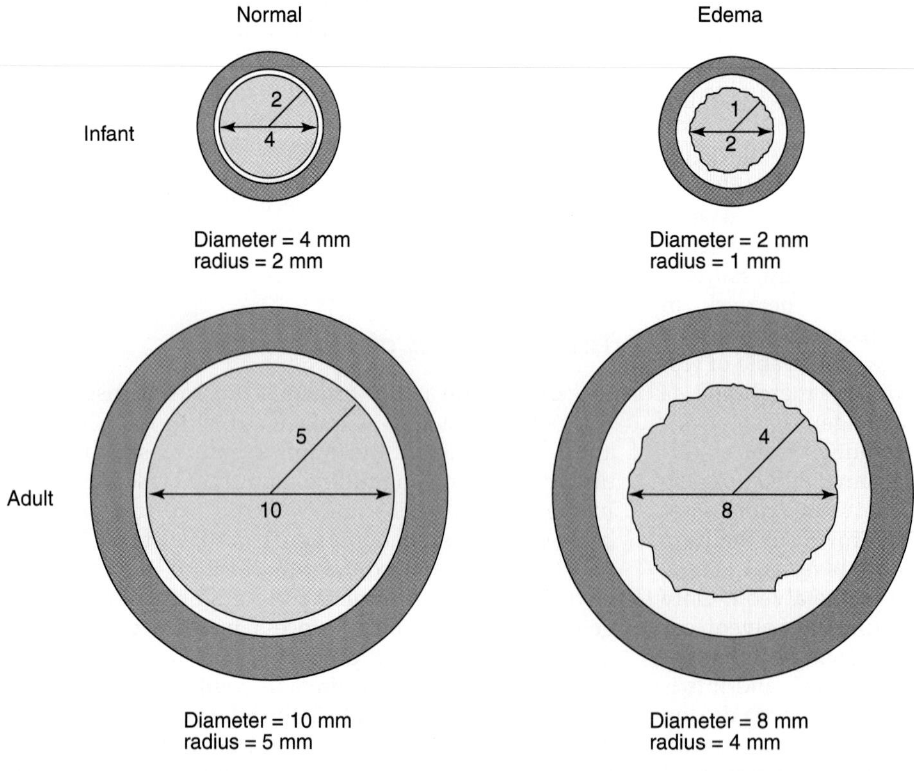

Figure 23–6
Effect of airway swelling on airway radius in infant and adult.

and the intrathoracic airways widen during inspiration and narrow during expiration.[54] This occurs because the pressure inside the extrathoracic airways reflects the intrapleural pressures that are generated during breathing, whereas the pressure outside the airways is similar to atmospheric pressure. Thus, during inspiration, the pressure inside becomes more negative, causing the airways to narrow, and during expiration, it becomes more positive, causing them to widen. In contrast to the extrathoracic airways, the pressure outside the intrathoracic airways is equal to the intrapleural pressure. These airways widen during inspiration as the surrounding intrapleural pressure becomes more negative and pulls them open, and they narrow during expiration as the surrounding pressure becomes more positive.

Lung Volumes and Gas Exchange

The functional residual capacity, which is the air left in the lungs at the end of normal expiration, plays an important role in the gas exchange of the infant. In the infant, the functional residual capacity occurs at a higher lung volume than in the older child or adult.[55] This higher end-expiratory volume results from a more rapid respiratory rate, which leaves less time for expiration. However, the increased residual volume is important to the neonate, because it holds the airways open throughout all phases of respiration; it favors the reabsorption of intrapulmonary fluids; and it maintains more uniform lung expansion and enhances gas exchange. During sleep, the tone of the upper airway muscles is reduced, so that the time spent in expiration is shorter, and the intercostal activity that stabilizes the chest wall is less; this produces a lower end-expiratory volume and less optimal gas exchange during active sleep.[55]

Control Of Ventilation

The fetal blood oxygen (PO_2) levels normally range from 25 to 30 mm Hg, and carbon dioxide (PCO_2) levels range from 45 to 50 mm Hg, independent of any respiratory movements. Any decrease in oxygen levels induces quiet sleep in the fetus with subsequent cessation of breathing movements, both of which lead to a decrease in oxygen consumption. Switching to oxygen derived from the aerated lung at birth causes an immediate increase in PO_2 to about 50 mm Hg; within a few hours, it increases to about 70 mm Hg.[53] These levels, which greatly exceed fetal levels, cause the chemoreceptors (see Chapter 22) to become silent for several days. Although the infant's PO_2 may fluctuate during this critical time, the chemoreceptors do not respond appropriately. It is not until several days after birth that the chemoreceptors "reset" their PO_2 threshold; only then do they become the major controller of breathing. However, the response seems to be biphasic, with an initial hyperventilation followed by a decreased respiratory rate and even apnea. In normal neonates, particularly in preterm infants, breathing patterns and respiratory reflexes depend on the arousal state.[55] Periodic breathing and apnea are characteristic of premature infants and reflect patterns of fetal breathing. The fact that they occur with sleep and disappear during wakefulness underscores the importance of arousal.

Alterations in Breathing

Most lung diseases in children produce decreased lung compliance and manifestations of restrictive lung disease, or they increase airway resistance.

Children with restrictive lung disease breathe at faster rates, and their respiratory excursions are shallow. Grunting is an audible noise emitted during expiration. An expiratory grunt is common as the child tries to raise the functional residual capacity by closing the glottis at the end of expiration. Grunting is a sign of labored breathing that is usually caused by decreased lung compliance or lung volume; it may serve as a compensatory mechanism for lung dysfunction by increasing lung volume and improving arterial oxygenation.

The pressure needed to overcome airway resistance depends on the rate of airflow as it moves into and out of the lungs; the need is greatest during periods of high flow. Because airway resistance increases the work of breathing, children with obstructive disease take slower, deeper breaths. When the obstruction is in the extrathoracic airways, inspiration is more prolonged than expiration, and an inspiratory stridor is commonly heard. When the obstruction is in the intrathoracic airways, expiration is prolonged, and the child makes use of the accessory expiratory muscles.

When obstruction of the extrathoracic airways occurs, as in croup, the pressures distal to the point of obstruction must become more negative to overcome the resistance; this causes collapse of the distal airways, and the increased turbulence of air moving through the obstructed airways produces an audible crowing sound called a *stridor*. With intrathoracic airway obstruction as occurs with bronchiolitis and bronchial asthma, the intrapleural pressure becomes more positive during expiration because of air trapping; this causes collapse of intrathoracic airways and produces an audible *wheezing* or whistling sound during expiration.

Respiratory Disorders in the Neonate

The neonatal period is one of transition from placental dependency to air breathing. This transition requires functioning of the surfactant system, conditioning of the respiratory muscles, and establishment of parallel pulmonary and systemic circulations. Respiratory disorders develop in infants who are born prematurely or who have other problems that impair this transition. Among the respiratory disorders of the neonate are the respiratory distress syndrome (RDS), bronchopulmonary dysplasia (BPD), and persistent fetal circulation (*i.e.*, delayed closure of the ductus arteriosus and foramen ovale).

Respiratory Distress Syndrome

RDS, also known as hyaline membrane disease, is one of the most common causes of respiratory disease in premature infants. In these babies, pulmonary immaturity, together with surfactant deficiency, leads to alveolar collapse. The type II alveolar cells that produce surfactant do not begin to mature until about the 25th to 28th week of gestation, and consequently, many premature babies are born with poorly functioning type II alveolar cells and have difficulty producing sufficient amounts of surfactant. The incidence of RDS is higher among preterm male infants, white infants, infants of diabetic mothers, and those subjected to asphyxia, cold stress, precipitous deliveries, and delivery by cesarean section (when performed before the 38th week of gestation).

Surfactant synthesis is influenced by several hormones, including insulin and cortisol. Insulin tends to inhibit surfactant production; this explains why infants of insulin-dependent diabetic mothers are at increased risk of developing RDS. Cortisol can accelerate maturation of type II cells and formation of surfactant.[56] The reason that premature babies born by cesarean section are presumably at greater risk of developing RDS is because they are not subjected to the stress of vaginal delivery, which is thought to increase the babies' cortisol levels. These observations have led to administration of corticosteroid drugs before delivery to mothers with babies at high risk for developing RDS.[54]

Surfactant reduces the surface tension in the alveoli, thereby equalizing the retractive forces in the large and small alveoli and reducing the amount of pressure needed to inflate and hold the alveoli open.[56] Without surfactant, the large alveoli remain inflated while the small alveoli become difficult to inflate. At birth, the first breath requires high inspiratory pressures to expand the lungs. With normal levels of surfactant, the lungs retain up to 40% of the residual volume after the first breath, and subsequent breaths require far lower inspiratory pressures.[1] With a surfactant deficiency, the lungs collapse between breaths, making the infant work as hard with each successive breath as with the first breath. The airless portions of the lungs becomes stiff and noncompliant. A hyaline membrane forms inside the alveoli as protein- and fibrin-rich fluids are pulled into the alveolar spaces. The fibrin-hyaline membrane constitutes a barrier to gas exchange, leading to hypoxemia and carbon dioxide retention, a condition that further impairs surfactant production.

Infants with RDS present with multiple signs of respiratory distress, usually within the first 24 hours of birth. Central cyanosis is a prominent sign. Breathing becomes more difficult, and retractions occur as the infant's soft chest wall is pulled in as the diaphragm descends. Grunting sounds occur during expiration. As the tidal volume drops because of atelectasis, the respiration rate increases (usually to 60 to 120 breaths/min) in an effort to maintain normal minute ventilation. Fatigue may develop rapidly because of the increased work of breathing. The stiff lung of infants with RDS also increases resistance to blood flow in the pulmonary circulation. As a result, infants with RDS may develop a hemodynamically significant patent ductus arteriosus (see Chapter 19).

Infants with suspected RDS require continuous cardiorespiratory monitoring. Oxygen and carbon dioxide levels can be assessed through an arterial line (umbilical) or by way of transcutaneous oxygen sensor. Treatment includes administration of supplemental oxygen, continuous positive airway pressure by way of nasal prongs, and often includes mechanical ventilation. A neutral thermal environment and prevention of hypoglycemia are recommended.

Surfactant therapy is used to prevent and treat RDS. There are two types of surfactants available in the United States: surfactants prepared from animal sources and synthetic surfactants.[57,58] The surfactants are suspended in saline and administered into the airways, usually through an endotracheal tube. The treatment is often initiated soon after birth in infants who are at high risk for RDS.

Bronchopulmonary Dysplasia

BPD is a chronic pulmonary disease that develops in premature infants who were treated with mechanical ventilation, mainly for RDS. The disorder is thought to be a response of the premature lung to early injury. High inspired oxygen concentration and injury from positive pressure ventilation (*i.e.*, barotrauma) have been implicated. Newer therapies such as administration of surfactants, high-frequency ventilation, and prenatal or postnatal administration of corticosteroids may have altered the severity of BPD, but the condition remains a major health problem.[59,60]

BPD is characterized by chronic respiratory distress, persistent hypoxemia when breathing room air, reduced lung compliance, increased airway resistance, and severe expiratory flow limitation. There is a mismatching of ventilation and perfusion with development of hypoxemia and hypercapnia. Pulmonary vascular resistance may be increased and the infant may develop pulmonary hypertension and cor pulmonale (*i.e.*, right heart failure associated with lung disease).

The infant with BPD may have tachycardia, shall breathing, chest retractions, cough, barrel chest, and poor weight gain and may develop hypoxemia and compensated respiratory acidosis. Clubbing of the fingers occurs in children with severe disease. Infants with right heart failure develop tachycardia, tachypnea, hepatomegaly, and periorbital edema.

The treatment is mechanical ventilation and administration of adequate oxygenation. Weaning from ventilation is accomplished gradually, and some infants may require ventilation at home. Rapid lung growth occurs during the first year of life, and lung function usually improves. Adequate nutrition is essential for recovery of infants with BPD.

Most adolescents and young adults who had BPD during infancy have some degree of pulmonary dysfunction, consisting of airway obstruction, airway hyperreactivity, or hyperinflation.

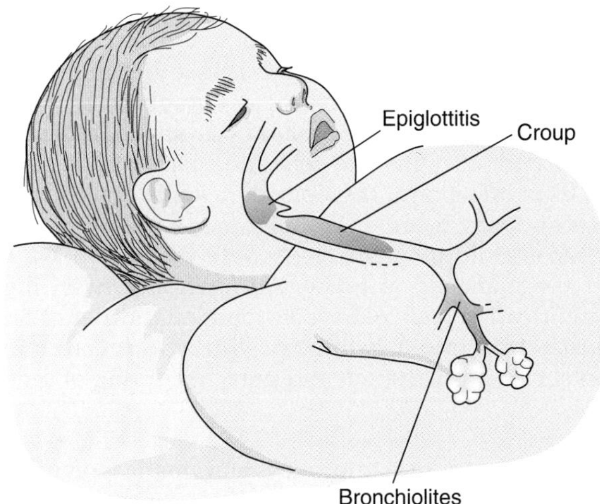

Figure 23–7
Location of airway obstruction in epiglottitis, acute laryngotracheobronchitis (croup), and bronchiolitis. (Courtesy of Carole Russell Hilmer, C. M. I.)

Respiratory Infections in Children

In children, respiratory tract infections are common, and although they are troublesome, they are usually not serious. Frequent infections occur because the immune system of infants and small children has not been exposed to many common pathogens; consequently, they tend to develop infections with each new exposure. Although most such infections are not serious, the small size of an infant or child's airways tends to foster impaired airflow and obstruction. For example, an infection that causes only sore throat and hoarseness in an adult may result in serious airway obstruction in a small child.

Upper Airway Infections

Two serious upper respiratory tract infections are relatively common during early childhood—croup and epiglottitis. Croup is the more common one, and it is usually benign and self-limited. Epiglottitis is a rapidly progressive and life-threatening condition. The site of involvement is illustrated in Figure 23–7, and the characteristics of both infections are described in Table 23–2.

Obstruction of the upper airways because of infection tends to exert its greatest effect during the inspiratory phase of respiration. Movement of air through an obstructed upper airway, particularly the vocal cords in the larynx, causes stridor. Impairment of the expiratory phase of respiration can also occur, causing wheezing. With mild to moderate obstruction, inspiratory stridor is more prominent than expiratory wheezing, because the airways tend to dilate with expiration. When the swelling and obstruction become severe, the airways can no longer dilate during expiration, and both stridor and wheezing occur.

Cartilaginous support of the trachea and the larynx is poorly developed in infants and small children. These structures are soft and tend to collapse when the airway is obstructed and the child cries, causing the inspiratory pressures to become more negative. When this happens, the stridor and inspiratory effort are increased. The phenomenon of airway collapse in the small child is analo-

TABLE 23–2
Characteristics of Epiglottitis, Croup, and Bronchiolitis in Small Children

Characteristics	Epiglottitis	Croup	Bronchiolitis
Common causative agent	*Haemophilus influenzae* type B bacterium	Mainly parainfluenza virus	Respiratory syncytial virus
Most commonly affected age group	2–7 years (peak 3–5 years)	3 months to 5 years	Less than 2 years (most severe in infants younger than 6 months)
Onset and preceding history	Sudden onset	Usually follows symptoms of a cold	Preceded by stuffy nose and other signs
Prominent features	Child appears very sick and toxic Sits with mouth open and chin thrust forward Low-pitch stridor, difficulty swallowing, fever, drooling, anxiety *Danger of airway obstruction and asphyxia*	Stridor and a wet, barking cough Usually occurs at night Relieved by exposure to cold or moist air	Breathlessness, rapid shallow breathing, wheezing, cough, and retractions of lower ribs and sternum during inspiration
Usual treatment	Hospitalization Intubation or tracheotomy Treatment with appropriate antibiotic	Mist tent or vaporizor Administration of oxygen	Supportive treatment, administration of oxygen and hydration

gous to what happens when a thick beverage, such as a milkshake, is drunk through a soft paper straw. The straw collapses when the negative pressure produced by the sucking effort exceeds the flow of liquid through the straw.

Viral Croup. Croup is characterized by an inspiratory stridor, hoarseness, and a barking cough. The British use the term *croup* to describe the cry of the crow or raven, and this is undoubtedly how the term originated.

Viral croup, more appropriately called acute laryngotracheobronchitis, is a viral infection that affects the larynx, trachea, and bronchi. The parainfluenza viruses account for about 75% all cases; the remaining 25% are caused by adenoviruses, respiratory syncytial virus, influenza A and B viruses, and measles virus. Viral croup is generally seen in children 3 months to 5 years of age.[61] The condition may affect the entire laryngotracheal tree, but because the subglottic area is the narrowest part of the respiratory tree in this age group, the obstruction is usually greatest in this area. For example, the subglottic airway in the 1- to 2-year-old child is about 6.5 mm in diameter, and 1 mm of edema can reduce the cross-sectional area by 50%.[61]

Although the respiratory manifestations of croup often appear suddenly, they are usually preceded by upper respiratory infections that cause rhinorrhea (*i.e.*, runny nose), coryza (*i.e.*, common cold), hoarseness, and a low-grade fever. In most children, the manifestation of croup only advances to stridor and slight dyspnea before they begin to recover. The symptoms usually subside when the child is exposed to moist air. For example, letting the bathroom shower run and then taking the child into the bathroom often brings prompt and dramatic relief of symptoms. Exposure to cold air also seems to relieve the airway spasm; often, the severe symptoms are relieved simply because the child is exposed to cold air on the way to the hospital emergency room. Viral croup does not respond to antibiotics; expectorants, bronchodilating agents, and antihistamines are not helpful. The child should be disturbed as little as possible and carefully monitored for signs of respiratory distress.

Airway obstruction may progress in some children. As obstruction increases, the stridor becomes continuous and is associated with nasal flaring with substernal and intercostal retractions. Agitation and crying aggravate the signs and symptoms, and the child prefers to sit up or be held upright. In the cyanotic, pale, or obstructed child, any manipulation of the pharynx, including use of tongue depressor can cause cardiorespiratory arrest and should only be done in a medical setting that has the facilities for emergency airway management. Other treatments may be required when a humidifier or mist tent is ineffective. One method is to administer a racemic mixture of epinephrine (L-epinephrine and D-epinephrine) by positive pressure breathing through a face mask. Establishment of an artificial airway may become necessary in severe airway obstruction.

Spasmodic Croup. Spasmodic croup manifests with symptoms similar to those of acute viral croup. Because the child is afebrile and lacks other manifestations of the viral prodrome, it is thought that it may have an allergic origin. Spasmodic croup characteristically occurs at night and tends to recur with respiratory tract infections. The episode usually lasts several hours and may recur several nights in a row.

Most children with spasmodic croup can be effectively managed at home. An environment of high humidification (*i.e.*, cold-water room humidifier or taking the child into a bathroom with a warm, running shower) lessens irritation and prevents drying of secretions.

Epiglottitis. Acute epiglottitis is a dramatic, potentially fatal condition most often caused by *H. influenzae* type B bacterium. The condition usually occurs in children 2 to 7 years of age, with a peak incidence at about 3.5 years.[61] It is characterized by inflammatory edema of the supraglottic area, including the epiglottis and pharyngeal structures, that comes on suddenly, bringing danger of airway obstruction and asphyxia. Within a matter of hours, epiglottitis may progress to complete obstruction of the airway and death unless adequate treatment is instituted.

The child appears pale, toxic, and lethargic and assumes a distinctive position—sitting up with the mouth open and the chin thrust forward. The child has difficulty in swallowing, a muffled voice, drooling, fever, and extreme anxiety. Moderate to severe respiratory distress is evident. There are inspiratory and sometimes expiratory stridor, flaring of the nares, and inspiratory retractions of the suprasternal notch, supraclavicular, and intercostal spaces. Usually, no other family members are ill with acute respiratory disease.

The child with epiglottitis requires immediate hospitalization. Immediate establishment of an airway by endotracheal tube or tracheotomy is usually needed. If epiglottitis is suspected, the child should never be forced to lie down, because this causes the epiglottis to fall backward and may lead to complete airway obstruction. Examination of the throat with a tongue blade or other instrument may cause cardiopulmonary arrest and should be done only by medical personnel experienced in intubation of small children. It is also unwise to attempt any procedure, such as drawing blood, that would heighten the child's anxiety, because this also could precipitate airway spasm and cause death.

Recovery from epiglottitis is usually rapid and uneventful after an adequate airway has been established and appropriate antibiotic therapy has been initiated. The introduction of *H. influenzae* type B vaccine may reduce the incidence of epiglottitis.

Epiglottitis can occur in adults as well as children. The incidence is low (an estimated 9.7 cases per million persons) but appears to be increasing. In adults, epiglottitis may present with acute respiratory compromise or as a milder form of disease. Although the causative agent or agents have not been identified, *H. influenzae* does not appear to be a primary causative agent in adults. Airway closure is less of a threat in adults; it does occur, however, and provision for emergency tracheotomy should be available.[62]

Lower Airway Infections

Lower airway infections produce air trapping with prolonged expiration. Wheezing results from bronchospasm, mucosal inflammation, and edema. The child presents with increased expiratory effort, increased respiratory rate, and wheezing. If the infection is severe, there are also marked intercostal retractions and signs of impending respiratory failure.

Acute bronchiolitis is a viral infection of the lower airways, most commonly caused by the respiratory syncytial virus.[63] Other viruses, such as adenoviruses, parainfluenza viruses, and rhinoviruses, have also been implicated as causative agents. The infection produces inflammatory obstruction of the small airways and necrosis of the cells lining the lower airways. It occurs during the first 2 years of life, with a peak incidence at approximately 6 months of age.[63] The source of infection is usually a family member with a minor respiratory illness. Older children and adults tolerate bronchiolar edema much better than infants and do not develop the clinical picture of bronchiolitis. Because the resistance to airflow in a tube is related to the fourth power of the radius, even minor swelling of bronchioles in an infant may produce profound changes in airflow.

Most affected infants who develop bronchiolitis have a history of a mild upper respiratory tract infection. These symptoms usually last several days and may be accompanied by fever and diminished appetite. There is then a gradual development of respiratory distress, characterized by a wheezy cough, dyspnea, and irritability. The infant is usually able to take in sufficient air but has trouble exhaling it. Air becomes trapped in the lung distal to the site of obstruction and interferes with gas exchange. Hypoxemia and, in severe cases, hypercapnia may develop. Airway obstruction may produce air trapping and hyperinflation of the lungs or collapse of the alveoli. Babies with acute bronchiolitis have a typical appearance, marked by breathlessness with rapid respirations, a distressing cough, and retractions of the lower ribs and sternum. Crying and feeding exaggerate these signs. Wheezing and rales may or may not be present, depending on the degree of airway obstruction. In infants with severe airway obstruction, wheezing decreases as the airflow diminishes. Generally, the most critical phase of the disease is the first 24 to 72 hours. Cyanosis, pallor, listlessness, and sudden diminution or absence of breath sounds indicate impending respiratory failure. The characteristics of bronchiolitis are described in Table 23–2.

Infants with respiratory distress are usually hospitalized. Treatment is supportive and includes administration of humidified oxygen to relieve hypoxia. Elevation of the head is a position that facilitates respiratory movements and avoids airway compression. Handling is kept at a minimum to avoid tiring. Because the infection is viral, antibiotics are not effective and are given only for a secondary bacterial infection. Dehydration may occur as the result of increased insensible water losses because of the rapid respiratory rate and feeding difficulties, and measures to ensure adequate hydration are needed. Recovery usually begins after the first 48 to 72 hours and is usually rapid and complete.

CHART 23–1
Signs of Respiratory Distress and Impending Respiratory Failure in the Infant and Small Child

Severe increase in respiratory effort, including severe retractions or grunting, decreased chest movement
Cyanosis that is not relieved by administration of oxygen (40%)
Heart rate of 150 per minute or greater and increasing
Bradycardia
Very rapid breathing (rate 60 per minute in the newborn to 6 months or above 30 per minute in children 6 months to 2 years)
Very depressed breathing (rate 20 per minute or below)
Retractions of the supraclavicular area, sternum, epigastrium, and intercostal spaces
Extreme anxiety and agitation
Fatigue
Decreased level of consciousness

Signs of Impending Respiratory Failure

Respiratory problems of infants and small children are often of sudden origin, and recovery is usually rapid and complete. However, children are at risk for the development of airway obstruction and respiratory failure resulting from obstructive disorders or lung infection. The child with epiglottitis is at risk for airway obstruction. The child with bronchiolitis is at risk for respiratory failure resulting from impaired gas exchange. The signs and symptoms of impending respiratory failure are listed in Chart 23–1.

In summary, acute respiratory disease is the most common cause of illness in infancy and childhood, accounting for 50% of illnesses in children younger than 5 years of age and 30% of illnesses in children between 5 and 12 years of age. Although other body systems are physiologically ready for extrauterine life as early as 25 weeks of gestation, the lungs take longer. Immaturity of the respiratory system is a major cause of morbidity and mortality in premature infants.

Lung development may be divided into five stages: embryonic period, glandular period, canicular period, saccular period, and alveolar period. The first three phases are devoted to development of the conducting airways, and the last two phases are devoted to development of the gas exchange portion of the lung. By the 25th to 28th week of gestation, sufficient terminal air sacs are present to permit survival. It is also during this period that type II alveolar cells, which produce surfactant, begin to function. Lung development is incomplete at birth; an infant is born with only one eighth to one sixth the adult number of alveoli. Alveoli continue to be formed during early childhood, reaching the adult number of 300 million alveoli by 5 to 6 years of age.

Children with restrictive lung disease breathe at faster rates, and their respiratory excursions are shallow. An expiratory grunt is common as the child tries to raise the functional residual capacity by closing the glottis at the end of expiration. Obstruction of the extrathoracic airways often produces turbulence of airflow and an audible inspiratory crowing sound called a stridor, and obstruction of the intrathoracic airways produces an audible expiratory wheezing or whistling sound. Respiratory distress syndrome is one of the most common causes of respiratory disease in premature infants. In these babies, pulmonary immaturity, together with surfactant deficiency, leads to alveolar collapse. BPD is a chronic pulmonary disease that develops in premature infants who were treated with mechanical ventilation.

Because of the smallness of the airway of infants and children, respiratory tract infections in these groups are often more serious. Infections that may cause only a sore throat and hoarseness in the adult may produce serious obstruction in the child. Among the respiratory tract infections that affect small children are croup, epiglottitis, and bronchiolitis. Epiglottitis is a life-threatening supraglottic infection that may cause airway obstruction and asphyxia.

REFERENCES

1. Cotran R.S., Kumar V., Robbins S.L. (1994). *Robbins' pathologic basis of disease* (5th ed., pp. 315, 375, 401, 524, 780–832). Philadelphia: W.B. Saunders.
2. Kirkpatrick G.L. (1996). The common cold. *Primary Care* 23 (4), 657–673.
3. Hendley J.A., Gwaltney J.M. Jr., Jordon W.S. (1969). Rhinovirus infections in an industrial population. IV. Infections within the families of employees during two fall peaks of respiratory illness. *American Journal of Epidemiology* 89, 184.
4. Beem M.O. (1969). Acute respiratory illness in nursery school children: A longitudinal study of occurrence of illness and respiratory viruses. *American Journal of Epidemiology* 90, 30.
5. Hendley J.O., Wenzel R.P., Gwaltney J.M. Jr. (1973). Transmission of rhinovirus colds by self-inoculation. *New England Journal of Medicine* 288, 1361.
6. Gwaltney J.M. Jr., Moskalski P.B., Hendley J.O. (1978). Hand-to-hand transmission of rhinovirus colds. *Annals of Internal Medicine* 88, 464.
7. Cohen S., Tyrerell D.A.J., Smith A.P. (1991). Psychological stress and susceptibility to the common cold. *New England Journal of Medicine* 325, 606–612.
8. Anderson T.W., Reid B.W., Beaton G.H. (1974). Vitamin C and the common cold: A double blind study. *Canadian Medical Association Journal* 107, 503–508.
9. Miller J.Z., Nance W.E., Norton J.A., et al. (1977). Therapeutic effect of vitamin C: A co-twin study. *Journal of the American Medical Association* 237, 248–251.
10. Carr B., Einstein R., Lai L.Y., Martin N.G., Starmer G.A. (1981). Vitamin C and the common cold. *Medical Journal of Australia* 2, 411–412.
11. Mossad S.B., Maknin M.L., Medendorp S.V., Mason P. (1996). Zinc gluconate lozenges for treating the common cold. *Annals of Internal Medicine* 125, 81–88.
12. Reuler J.B., Lucas L.M., Kumar K.L. (1995). Sinusitis—A review for generalists. *Western Journal of Medicine* 163, 40–48.
13. Ferguson B.J. (1995). Acute and chronic sinusitis. *Postgraduate Medicine* 97 (5), 45–69.
14. Hollingsworth H.M. (1996). Allergic rhinoconjunctivitis: Current therapy. *Hospital Practice* 31(6), 61–73.
15. Small P.A. Jr. (1990). Influenza: Pathogenesis and host defense. *Hospital Practice* 25 (11A), 51–62.
16. Douglas R.G. (1990). Prophylaxis and treatment of influenza. *New England Journal of Medicine* 322, 443–450.
17. Advisory Committee on Immunization Practices. (1996). Prevention and control of influenza: Recommendations of Advisory Committee on Immunization Practices (ACIP). *Morbidity and Mortality Weekly Report* 45 (RR-5), 1–15.
18. Bartlett J.G., Mundy L.M. (1995). Community-acquired pneumonia. *New England Journal of Medicine* 333 (24), 1618–24.
19. American Thoracic Society. (1993). Guidelines for the initial management of adults with community-acquired pneumonia: Diagnosis, assessment of severity, and initial antimicrobial therapy. *American Review of Respiratory Disease* 148, 1418—1426.
20. Niederman M.S., Sarosi G.A. (1995). Respiratory tract infections. In: George R.B., Light R.W., Matthay M.A., Matthay R.A. *Chest medicine* (3rd ed.). Baltimore: Williams & Wilkins.
21. Mandell L.A. (1995). Community-acquired pneumonia. *Chest* 108, 35S–42S.
22. Centers for Disease Control. (1996). Defining the public health impact of drug-resistant *Streptococcus pneumoniae. Morbidity and Mortality Weekly Report* 45 (RR-1), 1–20.
23. Centers for Disease Control and Prevention. (1996). Prevention of pneumococcal disease: Recommendations of the Advisory Committee on Immunization Practices. *Morbidity and Mortality Weekly Report* 46 (RR-8), 1–24.
24. Yu V.L. (1993). Legionnaires' disease. *Hospital Practice* 28(11), 63–70.
25. Edelstein P.H. (1996). Legionellosis. In: Bennett J.C., Plum F. *Cecil textbook of medicine* (20th ed., pp. 1583–1585). Philadelphia: W.B. Saunders.
26. Bergogne-Bèrèzin E. (1995). Treatment and prevention of nosocomial pneumonia. *Chest* 108, 26S–34S.
27. Craven D.E., Steger K.A. (1995). Epidemiology of nosocomial pneumonia. *Chest* 108 (Suppl.), 1S–15S.

28. Murray J.F., Mills J. (1990). Pulmonary infectious complications of human immunodeficiency virus infection. Part I. *American Review of Respiratory Disease* 141, 1356–1372.
29. Henry S.B., Holzemr W.L. (1992). Critical care management of the patient with HIV infection who has *Pneumocystis carinii. Heart and Lung* 21, 243–249.
30. Centers for Disease Control and Prevention. (1995). 1995 Revised Guidelines for Prophylaxis Against *Pneumocystis carinii* pneumonia for children infected with or perinatally exposed to human immunodeficiency virus. *Morbidity and Mortality Weekly Report* 44 (RR-4), 1–11.
31. Hollander H., Katz M.H. (1997). HIV infection. In: Tierney L.M., McPhee S.J., Papadakis M.A. *Current Diagnosis and Treatment* (36th ed., pp. 1200–1201)/ Norwalk, CT: Appleton & Lange.
32. Centers for Disease Control and Prevention. (1995). Essential components of a tuberculosis prevention and control program: Screening for tuberculosis and tuberculosis infection in high-risk populations. *Morbidity and Mortality Weekly Report* 44 (RR-11), 1–33.
33. American Thoracic Society. (1990). Diagnostic standards and classification of tuberculosis. *American Review of Respiratory Disease* 142, 725–735.
34. Jones S.G. (1996). Tuberculin testing in patients with Human Immunodeficiency Virus/Acquired Immune Deficiency Syndrome. *AACN Clinical Issues* 7 (3), 378–389.
35. Bernardo J. (1991). Tuberculosis: A disease of the 1990s. *Hospital Practice* 25 (10A), 195–222.
36. Centers for Disease Control. (1992). Management of people exposed to multidrug-resistant tuberculosis. *Morbidity and Mortality Weekly Report* 41 (RR-11), 61–71.
37. Centers for Disease Control. (1996). The role of BCG vaccine in the prevention and control of tuberculosis in the United States. *Morbidity and Mortality Weekly Report* 45 (RR-4), 1–19.
38. Dismukes WE. (1996) Histoplasmosis. In: Bennett J.C., Plum F. (Eds). *Cecil textbook of medicine* (20th ed., pp. 1816–1820). Philadelphia: W.B. Saunders.
39. Hammarsten J.E., Hammarsten J.F. (1990). Histoplasmosis: Recognition and treatment. *Hospital Practice* 25 (6A), 95–126.
40. Cleary J.D., Chapman S.W., Clark A., Lucia H. (1995). Fungal infections. In: Young L.Y., Koda-Kimble M.A. (Eds.). *Applied therapeutics: The clinical use of drugs* (6th ed., pp. 16–69). Vancouver, WA: Applied Therapeutics.
41. Galgiani J.N. (1996). Coccidioidomycosis. In: Bennett J.C., Plum F. (Eds). *Cecil textbook of medicine* (20th ed., pp. 1819–1820). Philadelphia: W.B. Saunders.
42. Stevens D.A. (1995). Coccidiomycosis. *New England Journal of Medicine* 332 (16), 1077–1082.
43. Dismukes WE. (1996). Blastomycosis. In: Bennett J.C., Plum F. (Eds). *Cecil textbook of medicine* (20th ed., pp. 1821–1822). Philadelphia: W.B. Saunders.
44. Parker S.L., Tong T., Bolden S., Wingo P. (1997). Cancer Statistics, 1997. *CA: A Cancer Journal for Clinicians*, 4–9.
45. Petty T.L. (1997). Lung cancer. *Postgraduate Medicine* 101 (3), 121–22.
46. Matthay R.A., Carter D.C. (1995). Lung neoplasms. In: George R.B., Light R.W., Matthay M.A., Matthay R.A. (Eds.). *Chest medicine* (3rd ed., pp. 393–422). Baltimore: Williams & Wilkins.
47. Stauffer J.L. (1993). Pulmonary diseases. In Schroeder S.A., Tierney L.M., McPhee S.J., et al. (Eds.). *Current diagnosis and treatment* (pp. 189–201, 229–230, 232–238, 255–261). Norwalk, CT: Appleton & Lange.
48. Lin A.Y., Ihde D.C. (1992). Recent developments in the treatment of lung cancer. *Journal of the American Medical Association 267*, 1661–1664.
49. Zander J., Hazinski M.F. (1992). Pulmonary disorders. In Hazinski M.F. (Ed.). *Nursing care of the critically ill child* (2nd ed., pp. 395–407). Philadelphia: W.B. Saunders.
50. Hanson T., Corbet A. (1991). Lung development and function. In Taeusch H.W., Ballard R.A., Avery M.E. (Eds.). *Shaffer and Avery's diseases of the newborn* (6th ed., pp. 461–469). Philadelphia: W.B. Saunders.
51. Turner B.S. (1990). Embryologic and physiologic basis for neonatal respiration. *AACN Clinical Issues in Critical Care Nursing* 1, 389–398.
52. Moore K. (1988). *The developing human* (4th ed., pp. 207–216). Philadelphia: W.B. Saunders.
53. Davis G.M., Bureau M.A. (1987). Pulmonary and chest wall mechanics in the control of respiration in the newborn. *Clinics in Perinatology* 14, 551–579.
54. Berhrman R.E., Kliegman R. M., Arvin A. (Eds.). (1996). *Nelson textbook of pediatrics* (14th ed., pp. 479–480, 1201–1213). Philadelphia: W.B. Saunders.
55. Oski F.A. (Ed.). (1994). *Principles and practice of pediatrics* (2nd ed., pp. 336–339, 365–370). Philadelphia: J.B. Lippincott.
56. Caminiti S.P., Young S.L. (1991). The pulmonary surfactant system. *Hospital Practice* 26 (1), 87–100.
57. Merenstein G.B. (Chairman). (1991). American Academy of Pediatrics: Committee on Fetus and Newborn: Surfactant replacement therapy for respiratory distress syndrome. *Pediatrics* 87, 946–947.
58. Jobe A.H. (1993). Pulmonary surfactant therapy. *New England Journal of Medicine* 328 (12), 861–868.
59. Abman S.H., Groothius J.R. (1994). Pathophysiology and treatment of bronchopulmonary dysplasia. *Pediatric Clinics of North America* 41 (2), 277–308.
60. Northwood W.B., Moss R.B., Carlisle K.B., et al. (1990). Late pulmonary sequelae of bronchopulmonary dysplasia. *New England Journal of Medicine* 323, 1793–1799.
61. Cressman W.R., Myer C.M. (1994). Diagnosis and management of croup and epiglottis. *Pediatric Clinics of North America* 41 (2), 265–276.
62. Baker A.S., Eavey R.D. (1986). Adult supraglottitis (epiglottitis). *New England Journal of Medicine* 314, 1185.
63. Boron M.E., Zanga J.R. (1996). Bronchiolitis. *Pediatric Clinics of North America* 23 (4), 805–817.

ADDITIONAL READINGS

Cunha B.A., Ortega A.M. (1996). Atypical pneumonia. *Postgraduate Medicine* 99 (1), 123–132.

Dannenberg A.M. (1993). Immunopathogenesis of pulmonary tuberculosis. *Hospital Practice* 28 (1), 51–58.

File T.M., Tan J.S., Plouffe J.F. (1996). Community-acquired pneumonia. *Postgraduate Medicine* 99 (1), 95–107.

Finegold S.M. (1991). Aspiration pneumonia. *Reviews of Infectious Diseases* 13 (Suppl 9), S737–S742.

Garderas J.C. (1996). Rhinitis and sinusitis: Office management. *Mayo Clinic Proceedings* 71, 882–888.

Johnston M.R. (1997). Curable lung cancer. *Postgraduate Medicine* 101 (3), 155–165.

Klein J.O. (1997). Role of nontypeable *Haemophilus influenzae* in pediatric respiratory tract infections. *Pediatric Infectious Disease Journal* 16, S5–S8.

Pramanik A.K., Holtzman R.B., Merritt T.A. (1993). Surfactant replacement therapy for pulmonary diseases. *Pediatric Clinics of North America* 40 (5), 913–936.

Rachelefsky G.S., Slavin R.G., Wald E.R. (1997). Sinusitis: Acute, chronic and manageable. *Patient Care* 31(6), 105–115.

Reichman L.B. (1994). Multidrug-resistant tuberculosis: Meeting the challenge. *Hospital Practice* 29(5), 85–96.

Seierna P.L.E. (1996). Nasal polyps: Relationship to infection and inflammation. *Allergy and Asthma Proceedings* 17 (5), 251–257.

Tuomanen E.I., Austrian R., Masure H.R. (1995). Pathogenesis of pneumococcal infection. *New England Journal of Medicine* 332 (19), 1280–1284.

CHAPTER 24

Alterations in Respiration: Alterations in Ventilation and Gas Exchange

The major function of the lungs is to oxygenate and remove carbon dioxide from the blood as a means of supporting the metabolic functions of body cells. Forty-seven million American children and adults suffer from one or more chronic respiratory diseases that impair ventilation and gas exchange.

Disorders of Lung Inflation

After you have completed this section of the chapter, you should be able to meet the following objectives:

- State the characteristics of pleural pain and differentiate it from other types of chest pain
- Differentiate among the causes and manifestations of spontaneous pneumothorax, secondary pneumothorax, and tension pneumothorax
- Characterize the pathogenesis and manifestations of pleural effusion
- State the difference between a transudate and exudate as it relates to pleural effusion
- Describe the causes and manifestations of atelectasis

Disorders of lung inflation are caused by conditions that produce lung compression or lung collapse. Air entering through the airways inflates the lung, and the negative pressure in the pleural cavity keeps the lung from collapsing. There can be complete collapse of an entire lung as in pneumothorax or collapse of a segment of the lung as in atelectasis.

Disorders of the Pleura

The pleura is a thin, double-layered membrane that encases the lungs. The inner visceral layer lies adjacent to the lung; the outer parietal layer lines the inner aspect of the chest wall, the superior aspect of the diaphragm, and the mediastinum. The visceral and parietal pleurae are separated by a thin layer of serous fluid, and the potential space between these two layers is called the *pleural cavity*. The right and left pleural cavities are separated by the mediastinum, which contains the heart and other thoracic structures.

Both the chest wall and the lungs have elastic properties. Because of these elastic properties, there is a tendency for the chest wall to become larger and move outward and for the lungs to recoil or move inward and collapse (see Chapter 22). As a result of these two opposing forces, the pressure in the pleural cavity becomes negative in relation to alveolar pressure. It is the negative pressure within the pleural cavity that holds the lungs against the chest wall and keeps them from collapsing. Disorders of the pleura include pain, pneumothorax, and pleural effusion.

Pleural Pain

Pain is a frequent symptom of pleuritis or inflammation of the pleura. Pleuritis is common in infectious processes such as viral respiratory infections or pneumonia that extends to involve the pleura. Most commonly the pain is abrupt in onset: the person experiencing it can cite almost to the minute when the pain started. It is usually unilateral and tends to be localized to the lower and lateral part of the chest. Although the pain may radiate to the shoulder or abdomen, it seldom originates from the substernal, paravertebral, or any other central part of the chest. The pain is usually made worse by chest movements, such as deep breathing and coughing, that exaggerate pressure changes within the pleural cavity and increase movement of the inflamed or injured pleural surfaces. Because deep breathing is painful, tidal volumes are usually kept small, and breathing becomes more rapid. Reflex splinting of the chest muscles may occur, causing a lesser respiratory excursion on the affected side.

It is important to differentiate pleural pain from pain produced by other conditions, such as musculoskeletal strain of chest muscles, bronchial irritation, and myocardial disease. Musculoskeletal pain may occur as the result of frequent, forceful coughing. This type of pain is usually bilateral and located in the inferior portions of the rib cage, where the abdominal muscles insert into the anterior rib cage. It is made worse by movements associated with contraction of the abdominal muscles. The pain associated with irritation of the bronchi is generally substernal and dull in character rather than sharp. It is made worse with coughing but is not affected by deep breathing. Myocardial pain, which is discussed in Chapter 19, is usually located in the substernal area and is not affected by respiratory movements.

Although analgesic and narcotic drugs reduce awareness of pleural pain, these agents do not entirely relieve the discomfort associated with deep breathing and coughing. The nonsteroidal antiinflammatory drug (NSAID) indomethacin has been used successfully to relieve pain and facilitate effective coughing.[1]

Pneumothorax

Normally, the pleural cavity is free of air and contains only a thin layer of fluid. When air enters the pleural cavity, it is called *pneumothorax*. Pneumothorax causes partial or complete collapse of the affected lung. Pneumothorax can occur without an obvious cause or injury (*i.e.*, spontaneous pneumothorax) or as a result of direct injury to the chest or major airways (*i.e.*, traumatic pneumothorax). Tension pneumothorax describes a life-threatening condition of excessive pressure within the pleural cavity.

Spontaneous Pneumothorax. Spontaneous pneumothorax occurs when an air-filled bleb, or blister, on the lung surface ruptures. Rupture of these blebs allows atmospheric air from the airways to enter the pleural cavity (Fig. 24–1). Alveolar pressure is normally greater than pleural pressure; if communication develops between alveoli on the lung surface and the pleural space, air flows from the alveoli into the pleural space, causing the involved portion of the lung to collapse as a result of its own recoil. Air continues to flow into the pleural space until a pressure gradient no longer exists or until the decline in lung size causes the leak to seal. Sponta-

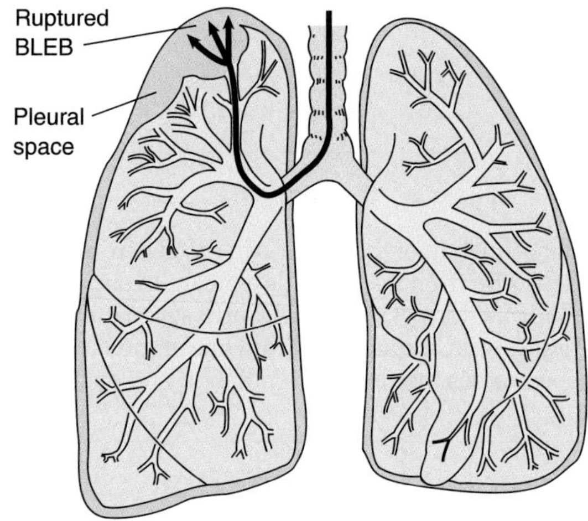

Figure 24–1
Mechanism for development of spontaneous pneumothorax.

neous pneumothoraces can be divided into primary and secondary pneumothoraces.[2] Primary spontaneous pneumothorax occurs in otherwise healthy persons. Secondary spontaneous pneumothorax occurs in persons with underlying lung disease.

What causes the air-filled blebs responsible for *primary spontaneous pneumothorax* and the reasons why they rupture are largely unknown. In primary spontaneous pneumothorax, these blebs are usually located at the top of the lungs. The condition is seen most often in tall young men. It has been suggested that the difference in pleural pressure from the top to the bottom of the lung is greater in tall persons and that this difference in pressure may contribute to the development of blebs. Another factor that has been associated with primary spontaneous pneumothorax is smoking. Disease of the small airways related to smoking probably contributes to the condition.

Secondary spontaneous pneumothoraces are usually more serious because they occur in persons with lung disease. They are associated with many different types of lung conditions that cause trapping of gases and destruction of lung tissue, including asthma, tuberculosis, cystic fibrosis, sarcoidosis, bronchogenic carcinoma, and metastatic pleural diseases. The most common cause of secondary spontaneous pneumothorax is emphysema.

Catamenial pneumothorax occurs in relation to the menstrual cycle and is usually recurrent.[1] Women with the condition usually develop symptoms within 24 to 48 hours of onset of menstrual flow. Although the cause of catamenial pneumothorax is unknown, it has been suggested that air may gain access to the peritoneal cavity during menstruation and then enter the pleural cavity through a diaphragmatic defect. Pleural and diaphragmatic endometriosis have also been implicated as causes of the condition.

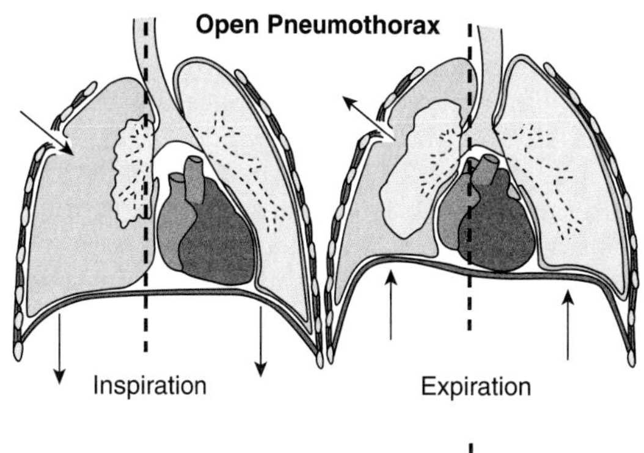

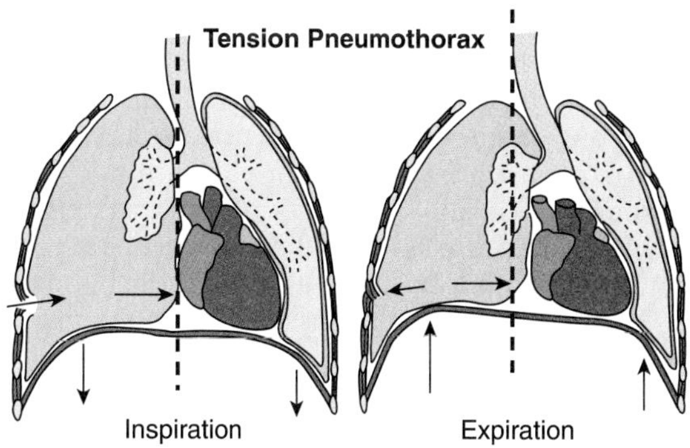

Figure 24–2
Open or communicating pneumothorax (**top**) and tension pneumothorax (**bottom**). In an open pneumothorax, air enters the chest during inspiration and exits during expiration. There may be slight inflation of the affected lung due to a decrease in pressure as air moves out of the chest. In tension pneumothorax, air can enter but not leave the chest. As the pressure in the chest increases, the heart and great vessels are compressed and the mediastinal structures are shifted toward the opposite side of the chest. The trachea is pushed from its normal midline position toward the opposite side of the chest, and the unaffected lung is compressed.

Traumatic Pneumothorax. Traumatic pneumothorax may be caused by penetrating or nonpenetrating injuries. Fractured or dislocated ribs that penetrate the pleura are the most common cause of pneumothorax from nonpenetrating chest injuries. Hemothorax often accompanies these injuries. Pneumothorax may also accompany fracture of the trachea or major bronchus or rupture of the esophagus. Persons with pneumothorax due to chest trauma frequently have other complications and may require chest surgery. Medical procedures such as transthoracic needle aspirations, intubation, and positive-pressure ventilation may occasionally cause pneumothorax. Pneumothorax can occur as a complication of cardiopulmonary resuscitation.

Tension Pneumothorax. Tension pneumothorax occurs when the intrapleural pressure exceeds atmospheric pressure. It is a life-threatening condition and occurs when injury to the chest or respiratory structures permits air to enter but not leave the pleural space (Fig. 24–2). This results in a rapid increase in pressure within the chest with compression atelectasis of the unaffected lung, a shift in the mediastinum to the opposite side of the chest, and compression of the vena cava with impairment of venous return to the heart.[2] Although tension pneumothorax can develop in persons with spontaneous pneumothoraces, it is seen most often in persons with traumatic pneumothoraces.

Manifestations. The manifestations of pneumothorax depend on its size and the integrity of the underlying lung. In spontaneous pneumothorax, manifestations of the disorder include development of pleuritic pain in an otherwise healthy person. There is an almost immediate increase in respiratory rate often accompanied by dyspnea that occurs as a result of the activation of receptors that monitor lung volume. Heart rate is increased. Asymmetry of the chest may occur because of the air trapped in the pleural cavity on the affected side. This asymmetry may be evidenced during inspiration as a lag in the movement of the affected side; the affected side of the chest does not begin to move until the unaffected lung reaches the same degree of inspiration as the lung with the air trapped in the pleural space. Percussion of the chest produces a more hyperresonant sound, and breath sounds are decreased or absent over the area of the pneumothorax. With tension pneumothorax, the structures in the mediastinal space shift toward the opposite side of the chest (see Fig. 24–2). When this occurs, the position of the trachea, normally located in the midline of the neck, deviates with the mediastinum. The position of the trachea can be used as a means of assessing for a mediastinal shift. There may be distention of the neck veins and subcutaneous emphysema (*i.e.*, air bubbles in the subcutaneous tissues of the chest and neck) and clinical signs of shock.

Hypoxemia usually develops immediately after a large pneumothorax, followed by vasoconstriction of the blood vessels in the affected lung, causing the blood flow to shift to the unaffected lung. In persons with spontaneous pneumothorax, this mechanism usually returns oxygen saturation to normal within 24 hours. Hypoxemia is usually more serious in persons with underlying lung disease who develop secondary spontaneous pneumothorax. In these persons, the hypoxemia caused by the partial or total loss of lung function can be life threatening.

Diagnosis and Treatment. Diagnosis of pneumothorax can be confirmed by chest radiograph. Computed tomography (CT) scans may be used. Blood gas analysis may be done to determine the effect of the condition on blood oxygen levels.

The treatment varies with the cause and extent of the disorder. Even without treatment, air within the pleural space usually reabsorbs after the pleural leak seals. In small spontaneous pneumothoraces, the air usually reabsorbs spontaneously, and only observation and follow-up chest radiographs are required. In larger pneumothoraces, the air is removed by needle aspiration or a closed drainage system used with or without an aspiration pump. This type of drainage system allows the air to exit the pleural space through a one-way valve system and prevents air from reentering the chest. This can be effected through a tube submerged in water or a drainage system with a one-way valve and no water. In secondary pneumothorax, surgical closure of the chest wall defect, ruptured airway, or perforated esophagus may be required.

Emergency treatment of tension pneumothorax involves the prompt insertion of a large-bore needle or chest tube into the affected side of the chest along with one-way valve drainage or continuous chest suction to aid in lung reexpansion. Sucking chest wounds, which allow air to pass in and out of the chest cavity, should be treated by promptly, covering the area with an airtight covering (*e.g.*, Vaseline gauze, firm piece of plastic). Chest tubes are inserted as soon as possible.

Because of the risk of recurrence, persons with primary spontaneous pneumothorax should be advised against cigarette smoking, exposure to high altitudes, flying in nonpressurized aircraft, and scuba diving. Injection of a sclerosing agent (*e.g.*, tetracycline) into the pleural space is sometimes used to prevent recurrence.

Pleural Effusion

Pleural effusion refers to a collection of fluid in the pleural cavity. The fluid may be a transudate, exudate, chyle, or blood. Normally, only a thin layer (usually less than 10 to 20 ml) of serous fluid separates the visceral and parietal layers of the pleural cavity. Like fluid developing in other transcellular spaces in the body, pleural effusion occurs when the rate of fluid formation exceeds the rate of its removal (see Chapter 26). Five mechanisms have been linked to the abnormal collection of fluid in the pleural cavity: increased capillary pressure, as in congestive heart failure; increased capillary permeability, which occurs with inflammatory conditions; decreased colloidal osmotic pressure, such as the hypoalbuminemia occurring with liver disease and nephrosis; increased negative intrapleural pressure, which develops with atelectasis; and impaired lymphatic drainage of the pleural space, which results from obstructive processes such as mediastinal carcinoma.

Pleural effusion may involve a transudate or exudate, depending on the protein content of the fluid. A transudate has a protein content of less than 3.0 g/ml, and an exudate has a protein content greater than 3.0 g/ml. Additional characteristics that may be used to define a pleural exudate are a pleural fluid to serum protein ratio greater than 0.5, a pleural fluid lactate dehydrogenase (LDH) level greater than two thirds the upper limit of normal, or a pleural fluid to serum LDH ratio exceeding 0.6.[3] LDH is an enzyme that is released from inflamed and injured pleural tissue; it is easily measured and is a useful marker for diagnosing exudative pleural disorders. Conditions that produce exudative pleural effusions are infections, pulmonary infarction, malignancies, rheumatoid arthritis, and lupus erythematosus.

Noninflammatory collections of serous transudate are called *hydrothorax*. The condition may be unilateral or bilateral. The most common cause of hydrothorax is congestive heart failure. Other causes are renal failure, nephrosis, liver failure, malignancy, and myxedema.

Empyema refers to pus in the pleural cavity; it can be caused by direct spread from adjacent bacterial pneumonia, rupture of a lung abscess into the pleural space, invasion from a subdiaphragmatic infection, or infection associated with trauma.

Chylothorax refers to the presence of chyle in the thoracic cavity. Chyle, a milky fluid containing chylomicrons, is found in the lymph fluid originating in the gastrointestinal tract. The thoracic duct transports chyle to the central circulation. Chylothorax results from trauma, inflammation, or malignant infiltration obstructing chyle transport from the thoracic duct into the central circulation.

Hemothorax is the presence of blood in the thoracic cavity. Bleeding may arise from chest injury, a complication of chest surgery, malignancies, or rupture of a great vessel such as an aortic aneurysm. Hemothorax may be classified as minimal, moderate, or large.[3] A minimal hemothorax involves the presence of 300 to 500 ml of blood in the pleural space. Small amounts of blood are generally absorbed from the pleural space, and a minimal hemothorax generally clears in 10 to 14 days without complication. A moderate hemothorax (500 to 1000 ml blood) fills about one third of the pleural space and may produce signs of lung compression and loss of intravascular volume. It requires immediate drainage and replacement of intravascular fluids. A large hemothorax fills one half or more of one side of the chest; it indicates the presence of 1000 ml or more of blood in the thorax and is usually caused by bleeding from a high-pressure vessel such as an intercostal or mammary artery. It requires immediate drainage and, if the bleeding continues, surgery to control the bleeding. One of the complications of untreated moderate or large hemothorax is fibrothorax—the fusion of the pleural surfaces by fibrin, hyalin, and connective tissue—and in some cases, calcification of the fibrous tissue, which restricts lung expansion.

Manifestations. The manifestations of pleural effusion vary with the cause. Hemothorax may be accompanied by signs of blood loss, and empyema by fever and other signs of inflammation. Fluid in the pleural cavity acts as a space-occupying mass; it causes a decrease in lung volume on the affected side that is proportional to the amount of fluid collected. The effusion causes a mediastinal shift toward the contralateral side with a decrease in lung volume on that side as well. Characteristic signs of pleural effusion are dullness or flatness to percussion and diminished breath sounds. Pleuritic pain usually occurs only when inflammation is present, although a constant type of discomfort may be felt with large effusions. Usually, 2000 ml or more of fluid must be present before dyspnea occurs. A minimum of 250 ml of unilateral fluid accumulation must occur before the condition can be detected on chest radiograph.

Diagnosis and Treatment. Thoracentesis is the aspiration of fluid from the pleural space. It is used to obtain a sample of fluid for diagnosis, or it can be used for therapeutic purposes. The treatment of pleural effusion is directed at the cause of the disorder. With large effusions, thoracentesis may be used to allow reexpansion of the lung. A palliative method of treatment used when pleural effusion is caused by a malignancy is the injection of a sclerosing agent into the pleural cavity; this causes obliteration of the pleural space and prevents the reaccumulation of fluid.

Atelectasis

Atelectasis means imperfect expansion; it refers to the incomplete expansion of a lung or portion of a lung. It can be caused by airway obstruction, lung compression such as occurs in pneumothorax or pleural effusion, or the increased recoil of the lung due to loss of pulmonary surfactant (see Chapter 22). The disorder may be present at birth (*i.e.*, primary atelectasis), or it may develop in the neonatal period or in later life (*i.e.*, acquired or secondary atelectasis).

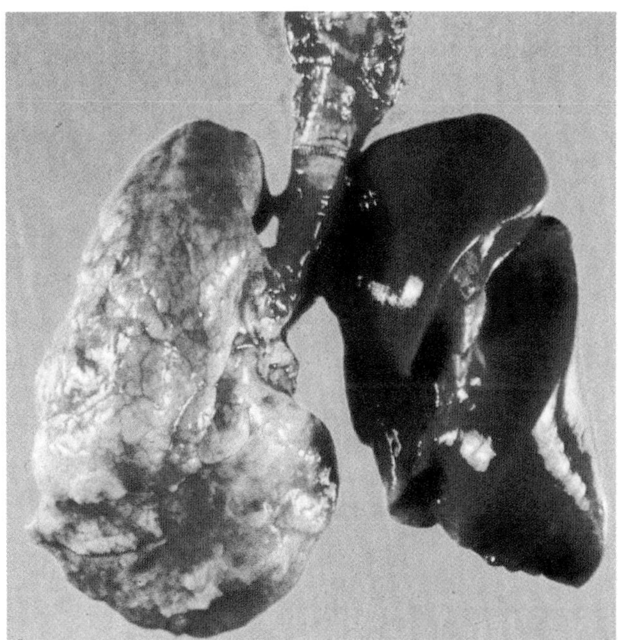

Figure 24–3
Atelectasis. The right lung of an infant (left side of photo) is pale and expanded by air, whereas the left lung is collapsed.

Primary atelectasis of the newborn implies that the lung has never been inflated. It is seen most frequently in premature and high-risk infants (Fig. 24–3). A secondary form of atelectasis can occur in infants who established respiration and subsequently developed impairment of lung expansion. Among the causes of secondary atelectasis in the newborn are the respiratory distress syndrome associated with lack of surfactant and airway obstruction due to aspiration of amniotic fluid or blood. They result in a patchy form of atelectasis.

Acquired atelectasis occurs mainly in adults. It is most commonly caused by airway obstruction and lung compression (Fig. 24–4). Obstruction can be caused by a mucous plug within the airway or by external compression by fluid, tumor mass, exudate, or other matter in the area surrounding the airway. A small segment of lung or an entire lung lobe may be involved in obstructive atelectasis. Complete obstruction of an airway is followed by the absorption of air from the dependent alveoli and collapse of that portion of the lung. Breathing high concentrations of oxygen, such as while on a ventilator, increases the rate at which gases are absorbed from the alveoli and predisposes to atelectasis.

Both chest expansion and breath sounds are decreased on the affected side. There may be intercostal retraction (pulling in of the intercostal spaces) over the involved area during inspiration. If the collapsed area is large, the mediastinum and trachea shift to the affected side. Signs of respiratory distress are proportional to the extent of lung collapse.

The danger of obstructive atelectasis increases after surgery. Anesthesia, pain, administration of narcotics,

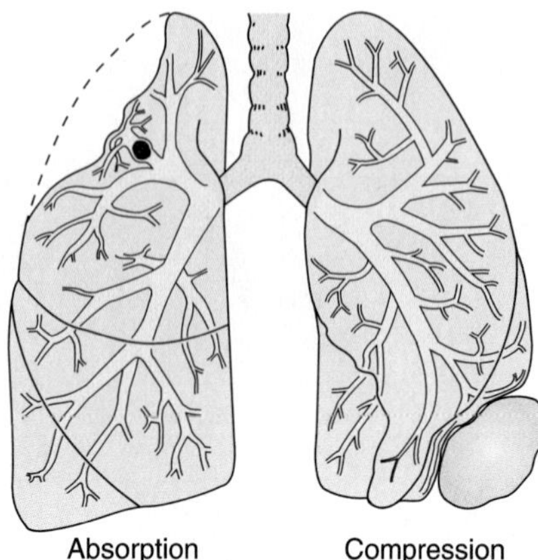

Figure 24–4
Atelectasis caused by airway obstruction and absorption of air from the involved lung area on the *left* and by compression of lung tissue on the *right.*

and immobility tend to promote retention of viscid bronchial secretions and hence airway obstruction. Encouraging a patient to take deep breaths and cough, frequent changes of position, adequate hydration, and early ambulation decrease the likelihood of atelectasis developing.

Another cause of atelectasis is compression of lung tissue. It occurs when the pleural cavity is partially or completely filled with fluid, exudate, blood, a tumor mass, or air. It is most commonly observed in persons with pleural effusion from congestive heart failure or cancer. In compression atelectasis, the mediastinum shifts away from the affected lung.

Manifestations

The clinical manifestations of atelectasis include tachypnea, tachycardia, dyspnea, cyanosis, signs of hypoxemia, diminished chest expansion, absence of breath sounds, and intercostal retractions. Fever and other signs of infection may develop.

Diagnosis and Treatment

The diagnosis of atelectasis is based on signs and symptoms. Chest radiographs are used to confirm the diagnosis. CT scans may be used to designate the exact location of the obstruction.

Treatment depends on the cause and extent of lung involvement. It is directed at reducing the airway obstruction or lung compression and at reinflating the collapsed area of the lung. Ambulation and body positions that favor increased lung expansion are used when appropriate. Administration of oxygen may be needed to treat the hypoxemia. Bronchoscopy may be used as a diagnostic and treatment method.

In summary, disorders of the pleura include pleuritis and pain, pneumothorax, and pleural effusion. Pain is commonly associated with conditions that produce inflammation of the pleura. Characteristically, it is unilateral, abrupt in onset, and exaggerated by respiratory movements. Pneumothorax refers to an accumulation of air in the pleural cavity with the partial or complete collapse of the lung. It can result from rupture of an air-filled bleb on the lung surface or from penetrating or nonpenetrating injuries. A tension pneumothorax is a life-threatening event in which air progressively accumulates within the thorax, collapsing the lung on the injured side and progressively shifting the mediastinum to the opposite side of the thorax, producing severe cardiorespiratory impairment. Pleural effusion refers to the collection of fluid in the pleural cavity. The fluid may be a transudate (*i.e.*, hydrothorax), exudate (*i.e.*, empyema), blood (*i.e.*, hemothorax), or chyle (*i.e.*, chylothorax).

Atelectasis refers to an incomplete expansion of the lung. The disorder may be present at birth (*i.e.*, primary atelectasis), or it may develop in the neonatal period or in later life (*i.e.*, acquired or secondary atelectasis). Primary atelectasis occurs most often in premature and high-risk infants. Acquired atelectasis occurs mainly in adults and is most commonly caused by a mucous plug within the airway or by external compression by fluid, tumor mass, exudate, or other matter in the area surrounding the airway.

Obstructive Airway Disorders

After you have completed this section of the chapter, you should be able to meet the following objectives:

- Describe the physiology of bronchial smooth muscle as it relates to airway disease
- Explain the changes in pulmonary function studies that occur with airway disease
- Characterize the early and late phase responses in the pathogenesis of bronchial asthma and relate them to current methods for treatment of the disorder
- Relate the pathologic changes that occur in bronchial asthma to the production of signs and symptoms
- Explain the distinction between chronic bronchitis and emphysema
- State the chief manifestations of bronchiectasis
- Describe the genetic abnormality responsible for cystic fibrosis and state the disorder's effect on lung function

Obstructive airway disorders are characterized by limitation in expiratory air flow. Bronchial asthma represents a reversible form of airway disease caused by restriction in airway size from bronchospasm, inflammation, and increased airway secretions. Chronic obstructive airway disease can be caused by a variety of airway diseases, including chronic bronchitis, emphysema, bronchiectasis, and cystic fibrosis.

Physiology of Airway Disease

Air moves through the upper airways (*i.e.*, trachea and major bronchi) into the lower or pulmonary airways (*i.e.*, bronchi and alveoli) that are located within the lung. In the pulmonary airways, the cartilaginous layer that provides support for the trachea and major bronchi gradually disappears and is replaced with crisscrossing strips of smooth muscle (see Chapter 22).

The contraction and relaxation of the smooth muscle layer, which is innervated by the autonomic nervous system, controls the resistance to airflow. Parasympathetic stimulation, through the vagus nerve and cholinergic receptors, increases bronchial constriction, and sympathetic stimulation, through β_2-adrenergic receptors, increases bronchodilation. Normally, a slight vagus-mediated bronchoconstrictor tone predominates. When there is need for increased airflow, as during exercise, parasympathetic-mediated bronchoconstrictor tone is inhibited, and the bronchodilator effects of the sympathetic nervous system are stimulated.

Bronchial smooth muscle also responds to inflammatory mediators, such as histamine, that act directly on smooth muscle to produce bronchial constriction and inflammation. During an antigen-antibody response, inflammatory mediators are released by a special type of cell, called the *mast cell*, which is present in the airways. The binding of IgE antibodies to specific receptors on mast cells prepares them for an allergic reaction when antigen appears (see Chapter 12).

Bronchial Asthma

Bronchial asthma is a chronic inflammatory disease of the airways. An estimated 9 to 12 million persons in the United States suffer from bronchial asthma. In the general population, asthma prevalence rates have increased 29% between 1980 and 1987.[4] The disease affects persons of all ages and is the most common cause of chronic illness in children younger than 17 years. There has been a reported increase in incidence and mortality from asthma over the past several decades. One suggested explanation for the growing morbidity and mortality is the increased exposure to indoor "aeroallergens" resulting from tighter houses with more carpets and soft furnishings, which retain dust mites, animal dander, and other allergens.[5]

Pathophysiology

The first Expert Panel of the National Heart, Lung, and Blood Institute's National Asthma Education Program, which met in 1991, defined bronchial asthma as: "(1) airway obstruction that is reversible (but not completely so in some patients) either spontaneously or with treatment; (2) airway inflammation; and (3) increased airway responsiveness to a variety of stimuli."[6] The second Expert Panel, which released its report in 1997, confirmed that asthma results from "complex interactions among inflammatory cells, mediators, and cells and tissue residents in the airway."[6a]

Persons with asthma typically react to low concentrations of agents that do not normally cause symptoms. An asthmatic attack can be triggered by a variety of stimuli. Based on their mechanism of response, these triggers can be divided into two types—bronchospastic or inflammatory.[7] *Bronchospastic triggers* depend on the existing level of airway responsiveness. They do not increase airway responsiveness but produce symptoms in persons who are already predisposed to bronchospasm. Bronchospastic triggers include cold air, exercise, emotional upset, and exposure to bronchial irritants such as cigarette smoke. *Inflammatory triggers* exert their effects through the inflammatory response. They cause inflammation and prime the sensitive airways so they are hyperresponsive to nonallergic stimuli. Many persons with asthma respond to both types of triggers. The mechanisms whereby these two types of triggers produce an asthmatic attack can be further described as the early versus the late response.

The *early response* results in immediate bronchoconstriction on exposure to an inhaled antigen or irritant. Symptoms usually develop within 10 to 20 minutes, and spontaneous recovery occurs within 60 to 90 minutes.[7] The acute response is probably caused by the release of chemical mediators from IgE-coated mast cells. In the case of airborne antigens, the reaction occurs when antigen binds to sensitized mast cells on the mucosal surface of the airways. Although this type of response is caused by inflammatory mediators, it tends to cause bronchospasm but not inflammation of the airways. It can be completely inhibited or reversed by bronchodilators, such as β_2-adrenergic agonists, but not by the antiinflammatory actions of the corticosteroids. The early response is fairly uncommon in persons with severe asthma, probably because it is blocked by the regular use of bronchodilator drugs.

The *late response* usually develops 3 to 5 hours after exposure to an asthmatic trigger.[6,7] The late response involves inflammation and increased airway responsiveness that prolong the attack and cause a vicious cycle of exacerbations. It often follows an early response. Typically, the response reaches a maximum within a few hours and may last for days or even weeks. An initial trigger in the late response causes the release of inflammatory mediators from mast cells, macrophages, and epithelial cells. These substances induce the migration and activation of other inflammatory cells (*e.g.*, basophils, eosinophils, neutrophils), which then produce epithelial injury and edema, changes in mucociliary function and reduced clearance of respiratory tract secretions, and increased airway responsiveness. Responsiveness to cholinergic mediators is often heightened, suggesting changes in parasympathetic control of airway function.[6] Chronic inflammation can lead to airway remodeling, in which case airflow limitations may be only partially reversible.[6a]

Causes of Asthma

A number of factors contribute to an asthmatic attack, including allergens, respiratory tract infections, hyperventilation, cold air, exercise, drugs and chemicals, emotional upsets, and airborne pollutants. Inhalation of allergens is a common cause of asthma. Generally, this form of asthma has its onset in childhood or adolescence and is seen in persons with a family history of atopic allergy (see Chapter 12). Persons with allergic asthma often have other allergic disorders, such as hay fever, hives, and eczema. Attacks are related to exposure to specific allergens.

Respiratory tract infections, especially those caused by viruses, may produce their effects by causing epithelial damage and stimulating the production of IgE antibodies directed toward the viral antigens. In addition to precipitating an asthmatic attack, viral respiratory infections increase airway responsiveness to other asthma triggers that may persist for weeks beyond the original infection.

Exercise-induced asthma occurs in 40% to 90% of persons with bronchial asthma.[8] The cause of exercise-induced asthma is unclear. It has been suggested that during exercise, bronchospasm may be caused by the loss of heat and water from the tracheobronchial tree because of the need for conditioning (*i.e.*, warming and humidification) of large volumes of air.[9] The response is commonly exaggerated when the person exercises in a cold environment; wearing a mask over the nose and mouth often minimizes the attack or prevents it. A proper warm-up period is also important. An attack can usually be prevented by using an inhaled short-acting β_2-adrenergic agonist or antiinflammatory agent (cromolyn, nedocromil) shortly before engaging in exercise.[6a]

Inhaled irritants include tobacco smoke and strong odors. These irritants are thought to induce bronchospasm by way of irritant receptors and a vagal reflex. Passive parenteral smoking has been reported to increase asthma severity in children.[10] High doses of irritant gases such as sulfur dioxide, nitrogen dioxide, and ozone may induce inflammatory exacerbations of airway responsiveness (*e.g.*, smog-related asthma). Occupational asthma is stimulated by fumes and gases (*e.g.*, epoxy resins, plastics, toluene), organic and chemical dusts (*i.e.*, wood, cotton, platinum), and other chemicals (*e.g.*, formaldehyde) in the workplace.[11]

Emotional factors produce bronchospasm by way of vagal pathways. They can act as a bronchospastic trigger, or they can increase airway responsiveness to other triggers through noninflammatory mechanisms.

Several types of drugs and chemicals stimulate asthma. There is a small group of asthmatics in whom aspirin sensitivity is associated with severe asthmatic attacks, presence of nasal polyps, and recurrent episodes of rhinitis. The yellow food dye tartrazine, aspirin, and other NSAIDs, such as aminopyrine, phenylbutazone, ibuprofen, and indomethacin, may provoke attacks. An addition to the list of chemicals that can provoke an asthmatic attack are the sulfites used in food processing and as a preservative added to beer, wine, and fresh vegetables.

Manifestations

Persons with asthma exhibit a wide range of signs and symptoms, from episodic wheezing and feelings of chest tightness to an acute, immobilizing attack. The attacks differ from person to person, and between attacks, many persons are symptom free. Attacks may occur spontaneously or in response to various triggers, respiratory infections, emotional stress, or weather changes. Asthma is often worse at night. Nocturnal asthma attacks usually occur at about 4 AM because of the occurrence of the late response to allergens inhaled during the evening and because of circadian variations in bronchial reactivity.[12]

During an asthmatic attack, the airways narrow because of bronchospasm, edema of the bronchial mucosa, and mucus plugging. Expiration becomes prolonged because of progressive airway obstruction. The amount of air that can be forcibly expired in 1 second ($FEV_{1.0}$) and the peak expiratory flow rate (PEFR) are decreased. A fall in the $FEV_{1.0}$ or PEFR to levels below 25% of the predicted value during an acute asthmatic attack suggests respiratory failure.

Air can become trapped behind the occluded and narrowed airways, causing hyperinflation of the lungs. The functional residual capacity increases, and inspiratory reserve capacity and forced vital capacity (FVC) diminish so that the person breathes close to his or her total lung capacity (see Chapter 22). As a result, more energy is needed to overcome the tension already present in the lungs, and the accessory muscles (*i.e.*, sternocleidomastoid muscles) are used to maintain ventilation and gas exchange. This causes dyspnea and fatigue. Because air is trapped in the alveoli and inspiration is occurring at higher residual lung volumes, the cough becomes less effective.

As the condition progresses, the effectiveness of alveolar ventilation declines, and mismatching of ventilation and perfusion causes hypoxemia and hypercapnia. Pulmonary vascular resistance may increase as a result of the hypoxemia and hyperinflation, causing pulmonary hypertension and increasing the work demands of the right heart.

The physical signs vary with the severity of the attack. A mild attack may produce a slight increase in respiratory rate, with prolonged expiration and mild wheezing. A cough may accompany the wheezing. More severe attacks are associated with use of the accessory muscles, distant breath sounds due to air trapping, and loud wheezing. As the condition progresses, fatigue develops, the skin becomes moist, and anxiety and apprehension are obvious. Dyspnea may be severe, and often the person is able to speak only one or two words before taking a breath. At the point where airflow is markedly decreased, breath sounds become inaudible with diminished wheezing and the cough becomes ineffective despite being repetitive and hacking. This point often marks the onset of respiratory failure.

With increased air trapping, a greater negative intrapleural pressure is needed to inflate the lungs. This negative pressure, which is transmitted to the heart and blood vessels, causes the systolic blood pressure to fall during inspiration, a condition called *pulsus paradoxus*. It can be detected using a blood pressure cuff (see Chapter 19). Detection of pulsus paradoxus suggests that the $FEV_{1.0}$ is reduced to less than 50% of the predicated value.[6]

Diagnosis

Diagnosis of asthma is based on a careful history, physical examination, and laboratory methods. Spirometry provides a means for measuring FVC, $FEV_{1.0}$, PEFR, tidal volume, expiratory reserve, and inspiratory capacity (see Chapter 22). The PEFR is the peak expiratory flow rate that can be generated during a forced expiratory maneuver. It is measured in liters per second.[6]

Small, inexpensive, portable meters that measure PEFR are available. These can be used in clinics and physicians' offices and in the home to provide frequent measures of flow rates. They provide objective measures that can be used as a guide for treatment. Day-night (circadian) variations in asthma and PEFR variability can be used to indicate the severity of bronchial hyperresponsiveness. Peak flow meters are often used to help persons manage their asthma at home. The person's best performance is established using readings that are derived over several weeks. This is often referred to as the individual's *personal best* and is used as a reference to indicate changes in respiratory function.[6] The personal best zones have been adapted to a traffic signal system to make it easier to use and remember. The green (80% to 100% of the personal best) signals an all clear and indicates that the asthma is under control; the yellow (50% to 80%) signals caution and indicates that the asthma is not under sufficient control and additional medication or treatment is needed; and the red signal (50% or less) signals a medical alert and the immediate need for a bronchodilator and the need to consult a health care provider if the person's personal best does not immediately return to the caution range.[6]

The level of airway responsiveness can be measured in the laboratory by inhalation challenge tests using methacholine, a cholinergic agonist, or histamine or testing exposure to a nonpharmacologic agent such as cold air.

Treatment

The Expert Panel of the National Heart, Lung, and Blood Institute's National Asthma Education Program recommends two categories of treatment for asthma: nonpharmacologic and pharmacologic.[6,6a]

Nonpharmacologic Treatment. The nonpharmacologic methods of treatment are aimed at prevention and appropriate early treatment of an asthmatic attack. They include education of the patient and family to avoid bronchial irritants and agents that are known to induce or trigger an attack. A careful history is often needed to identify all the contributory factors.

Relaxation techniques and controlled breathing help to allay the panic and anxiety that aggravate breathing difficulties. The hyperventilation that often accompanies anxiety and panic is known to act as an asthmatic trigger. In a child, measures to encourage independence as it relates to symptom control, along with those directed at helping to develop a positive self-concept, are essential.

When the offending agent cannot be avoided (*e.g.*, house dust mites), a program of desensitization may be undertaken. It involves the injection of selected antigens (based on skin test) to stimulate the production of IgG antibodies that block the IgE response (see Chapter 12).

Pharmacologic Treatment. Pharmacologic treatment is used to prevent or treat reversible airway obstruction and airway hyperresponsiveness because of the inflammatory process. Medications include bronchodilators and antiinflammatory drugs. Some drugs have both bronchodilator and antiinflammatory actions. Two oral leukotriene modifiers, zafirkulast and zileuton, have recently become available for use in the treatment of asthma.[6a] Leukotrienes are inflammatory mediators (see Chapter 11) thought to be involved in bronchoconstriction associated with early- and late-phase responses to allergens. Because these drugs are new, their long-term efficacy is still unknown.

Bronchodilators include β_2-adrenergic agonists, ipratropium, and theophylline. These drugs are most effective for treating asthmatic attacks that are caused by bronchogenic triggers. The *β_2-adrenergic agonists* relax bronchial smooth muscle and relieve congestion of the bronchial mucosa. The drugs are usually administered by inhalation (*i.e.*, metered-dose inhaler [MDI]) or nebulizer. The short-acting β_2-agonists are used for treating acute attacks of asthma but are not recommended for daily use because of concern over safety.[6a] The long-acting β_2-agonists may be used on a regular basis for control of asthma symptoms but should not be used to treat acute symptoms or exacerbations.[6a]

Ipratropium is an anticholinergic drug that blocks postganglionic efferent vagal pathways. It produces bronchodilation by direct action on the large airways and does not change the composition or viscosity of the bronchial mucus. The drug is administered by inhalation to treat acute attacks of asthma.

Theophylline is a bronchodilator that acts by relaxing smooth muscle. It may also augment respiratory muscle activity, reducing muscle fatigue. Theophylline preparations can be administered by the oral or intravenous route. An oral sustained-release form of the drug is available and can be used as an adjuvant to long-term preventative therapy.[6a] Because drug metabolism and elimination vary widely among persons, blood levels are used to determine the proper dosage.

Corticosteroids are used for treating the inflammatory response associated with the late response. Inhaled corticosteroids (*e.g.*, beclomethasone, triamcinolone, budesonide, flunisolide) that are administered by MDI are usually preferred because of minimal systemic absorption and degree of hypothalamic-pituitary-adrenal dysfunction. In severe cases, oral or parenterally administered corticosteroids may be necessary.

The antiinflammatory agents cromolyn and nedocromil are used to prevent an asthmatic attack. The exact mechanism of action is not fully understood. These agents probably stabilize mast cells, thereby preventing release of the inflammatory mediators that cause an asthmatic attack. Cromolyn and nedocromil are used prophylactically to prevent early and late responses. They are of no benefit when taken during an attack. Cromolyn is available as an MDI, a dry powder inhaler, or a solution for use with a nebulizer. Nedocromil is available as an MDI.

The MDI is usually the preferred method for delivery of sympathomimetic, anticholinergic, and corticosteroid drugs. Various extension devices (*i.e.*, spacers) are available to facilitate use and enhance aerosol deposition in the lungs. This is difficult to achieve when the inhaler is held at the level of the mouth. In this position, large droplets tend to be delivered to the oropharynx and throat, rather than moving down into the small airways. Optimal use of the extender requires one inhaler puff just after beginning a slow, deep breath from functional residual capacity, followed by holding the breath in inspiration for 10 seconds.

Nebulizers are specially constructed devices that use a high-pressure gas source to produce an aerosol drug mixture. They use a mouthpiece or mask for drug delivery and are usually powered by portable compressors or hospital gas supplies. Nebulizers can also be placed in mechanical ventilator circuits. Nebulizers are often the method of choice for administration of β-agonist drugs in the initial phase of acute asthma and are used to administer aerosol drugs to children and to persons who have difficulty using the MDI.

Status Asthmaticus and Fatal Asthma

Status asthmaticus is severe, prolonged asthma that is refractory to conventional methods of therapy. The death rate from asthma in the United States from 1980 through 1987 increased 31%, from 1.3 to 1.7 deaths per 100,000 persons.[13] African Americans have asthma-related mortality rates higher than those of whites, especially in young age groups.[13,14]

Most asthma deaths have occurred outside the hospital. Persons at highest risk are those with previous exacerbations resulting in respiratory failure, respiratory acidosis, and the need for intubation. Although the cause of death during an acute asthmatic attack is largely unknown, both cardiac dysrhythmias and asphyxia due to severe airway obstruction have been implicated. Theophylline and β-adrenergic agonists increase myocardial irritability. It has been suggested that an underestimation of the severity of the attack may be a contributing factor. Deterioration often occurs rapidly during an acute attack, and underestimation of its severity may lead to a life-threatening delay in seeking medical attention. Frequent and repetitive use of β-agonist inhalers far in excess of the recommended doses may temporarily blunt symptoms and mask the severity of the condition. Lack of access to medical care is another risk factor associated with asthma-related death. Distance, as in rural areas, or lack of financial resources, as in the uninsured or underinsured, may limit access to emergency care.

Persons who suffer from fatal or near-fatal asthmatic attacks may have impaired perception of dyspnea and its severity.[15] It has been suggested that persons who have had a previous episode of sudden asphyxia be educated in the use of a peak flow meter as a means of determining the severity of their attack rather than relying on their perceptions of dyspnea.[15]

Bronchial Asthma in Children

Asthma is a leading cause of chronic illness in children and is responsible for a significant number of lost school days. It is the most frequent admitting diagnosis in children's hospitals. As many as 10% to 15% of boys and 7% to 10% of girls have asthma at some time during childhood.[16] Asthma may have its onset at any age; 30% of children are symptomatic by 1 year of age, and 80% to 90% are symptomatic by 4 to 5 years of age. Data on inheritance of asthma are most consistent with polygenic or multifactorial determinants. A child with one affected parent has about a 25% risk of developing the disease, and this risk increases to 50% when both parents are affected.

As with adults, asthma in children is commonly associated with an IgE-related reaction.[17,18] It has been suggested that IgE directed against respiratory viruses may be important in the pathogenesis of wheezing illnesses in infants (*i.e.*, bronchiolitis), which often precedes the onset of asthma. One of the suggested contributing factors to development of childhood asthma is exposure during early childhood to dust mite antigens in the home.[19]

The signs and symptoms of asthma in children are fairly typical. Previously well infants and children develop what may seem to be a cold with rhinorrhea, rapidly followed by irritability, cough, tachypnea, and wheezing. The symptoms may progress rapidly and require a trip to the emergency room or hospitalization.[16]

The Expert Panel of the National Heart, Lung, and Blood Institute's National Asthma Education Program has developed guidelines for management of asthma in children.[6a] The Expert Panel recommends that therapy should be initiated when early symptoms occur. For children younger than 5 years of age, symptoms of cough and dyspnea indicate the need for treatment. The antiinflammatory agents cromolyn and nedocromil are recommended as an initial therapy for mild-to-moderate asthma in infants and children. More severe symptoms may require the use of inhaled corticosteroids. Inhaled short-acting β_2-agonists may be used for mild intermittent symptoms or exacerbations. A long-acting β_2-agonist or sustained-release theophylline may be used for persistent asthma in children over 5 years of age.[6a] Theophylline should be considered only if serum concentration levels can be carefully monitored. Sustained-release theophylline may have particularly adverse effects in infants who frequently have febrile illnesses that increase drug levels.[6a] Systemic corticosteroids may be required during an episode of severe disease.

Special delivery systems for administration of inhalation medications are available for infants and small children, including nebulizers with face masks and spacers/holding chambers for use with an MDI. For children younger than 2 years of age, nebulizer therapy is usually preferred. Children between 3 and 5 years of age may begin using an MDI with a spacer/holding chamber. The child's caregiver should be carefully instructed in the appropriate use of these devices. The Expert Panel recommends that adolescents (and younger children when appropriate) be directly involved in developing their asthma management plans. Active participation in physical activities, exercise, and sports should be encouraged.[6a]

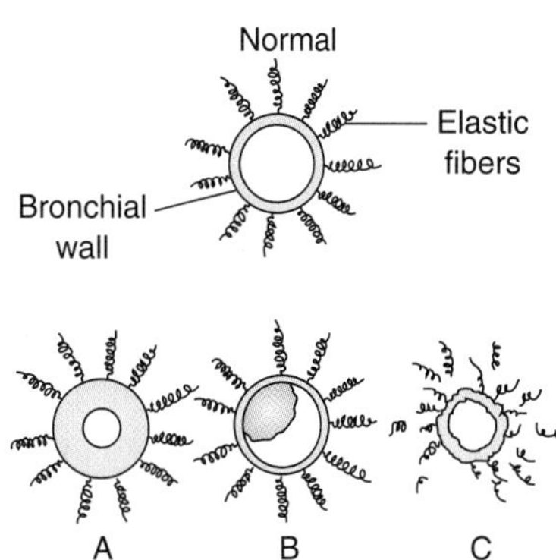

Figure 24–5 ■■■
Mechanisms of airflow obstruction in chronic obstructive lung disease. (**Top**) The normal bronchial airway with elastic fibers that provide traction and hold the airway open. (**Bottom**) Obstruction of the airway caused by (**A**) hypertrophy of the bronchial wall, (**B**) inflammation and hypersecretion of mucus, and (**C**) loss of elastic fibers that hold the airway open.

Chronic Obstructive Pulmonary Disease

The term *chronic obstructive pulmonary disease* (COPD) denotes a group of respiratory disorders characterized by chronic and recurrent obstruction of air flow in the pulmonary airways. About 30 million Americans have some degree of airway obstruction and COPD. In 1992, COPD and other allied conditions were the fourth leading cause of death in the United States, accounting for 91,800 deaths.[20] The death rate from COPD is increasing, especially among older men. Although there are multiple pathways to the development of COPD, the term is commonly associated with emphysema (type A COPD) and chronic bronchitis (type B COPD) because most cases of COPD are caused by these two disorders.

The most common cause of COPD is smoking.[20] The disease is largely preventable. Unfortunately, clinical findings are almost absent during the early stages of COPD, and by the time symptoms appear, the disease is usually far advanced. For smokers with early signs of airway disease, there is hope that early recognition, combined with appropriate treatment and smoking cessation, may prevent the usually relentless progression of the disease. Other risk factors for the development of COPD are exposure to inhaled toxins in the workplace and an inherited deficiency of α_1-antitrypsin.

Pathogenesis

The mechanisms involved in the pathogenesis of COPD are usually multiple and include inflammation, edema, and fibrosis of the bronchial wall; hypertrophy of the submucosal glands and hypersecretion of mucus; and loss of elastic lung fibers and alveolar tissue (Fig. 24–5).[21,22] Inflammation and excess mucus secretion obstruct airflow and cause mismatching of ventilation and perfusion. Loss of alveolar tissue decreases the surface area for gas exchange, and loss of elastic fibers impairs expiratory flow rate and predisposes to airway collapse. The recoil of the elastic fibers that were stretched during inspiration provide the pressure to move air out of the lung during expiration. Because the elastic fibers are attached to the airways, they also provide radial traction to hold the airways open during expiration.

Emphysema

Emphysema, or type A COPD, is characterized by a loss of lung elasticity and abnormal, permanent enlargement of the air spaces distal to the terminal bronchioles with destruction of the alveolar walls and capillary beds without obvious fibrosis (Fig. 24–6).[23] Enlargement of the air spaces results in hyperinflation of the lungs and increased total lung capacity. Two of the recognized causes of emphysema are smoking and an inherited deficiency of α_1-antitrypsin. Smoking stimulates the recruitment of inflammatory cells to the alveoli, enhances the release of elastase from neutrophils, increases elastase activity in macrophages, and activates mast cells, which release mast cell elastases.[24]

Emphysema is thought to result from the breakdown of elastin and other alveolar wall components by enzymes, called *proteases*, that digest proteins. These proteases, particularly elastase, which is an enzyme that digests elastin, are released from polymorphonuclear leukocytes (*i.e.*, neutrophils), alveolar macrophages, and other inflammatory cells. Normally, the lung is protected by an antiprotease enzyme called *α_1-antitrypsin*, and stimuli that increase the number of inflammatory cells in the lung or release elastase also increase α_1-antitrypsin levels. However, with low levels of α_1-antitrypsin, the process of elastic tissue destruction goes unchecked (Fig. 24–7).

There are two commonly recognized types of emphysema: centrilobular and panacinar. The *centrilobu-*

lar type affects the bronchioles in the central part of the respiratory lobule, with initial preservation of the alveolar ducts and sacs (Fig. 24–8). It is the most common type of emphysema and is predominantly seen in male smokers. The *panacinar type* produces initial involvement of the peripheral alveoli and later extends to involve the more central bronchioles. It is the type of emphysema associated with an α_1-antitrypsin deficiency.

A hereditary deficiency in α_1-antitrypsin accounts for about 1% of all cases of COPD and is more common in young persons with emphysema.[25] The type and amount of α_1-antitrypsin that a person has is determined by a pair of codominant genes referred to as *PI* (protein inhibitor) genes. An α_1-antitrypsin deficiency is inherited as an autosomal recessive disorder. There are more than 75 mutations of the gene. One of these, the *PIZ* variant, which occurs in 5% of the population causes the most serious deficiency in α_1-antitrypsin. It is most common in persons of Scandinavian descent and is rare in Jews, Blacks, and Japanese.[25] Homozygotes who carry two defective *PIZ* genes have only about 15% to 20% of the normal plasma concentration of α_1-antitrypsin.[25,26] Almost all persons who develop emphysema before the age 40 years have an α_1-antitrypsin deficiency.

There is evidence that cigarette smoking reduces body stores of α_1-antitrypsin and increases the number of macrophages in the alveolar walls. This influx of macrophages attracts increased numbers of neutrophils. Smoking and repeated respiratory tract infections, which also decrease α_1-antitrypsin levels, contribute to the risk of emphysema in persons with an α_1-antitrypsin deficiency.[26]

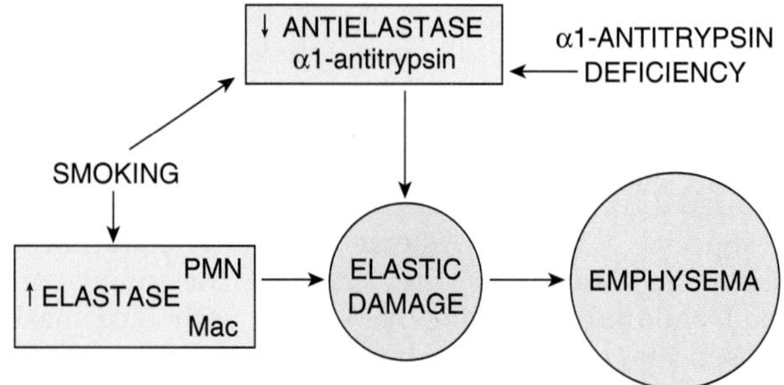

Figure 24–7
Protease-antiprotease mechanisms of emphysema. Smoking inhibits antielastase and favors the recruitment of leukocytes and release of elastase. PMN = polymorphonuclear leukocyte; Mac =alveolar macrophage. (Cotran R.S., Kumar V., & Robbins S.L. [1994]. *Robbins' pathologic basis of disease* [5th ed., p. 686]. Philadelphia: W.B. Saunders)

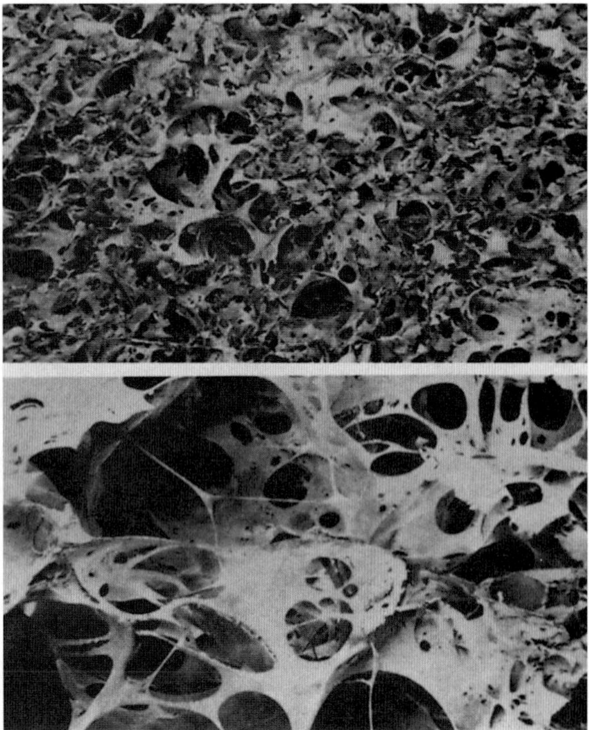

Figure 24–6
Scanning electron micrographs of lung tissue. (**Top**) Normal tissue; (**bottom**) emphysematous tissue (both at same magnification). Note the enlargement of air spaces in the emphysematous lung.

Laboratory methods are available for measuring α_1-antitrypsin levels. A pooled human plasma purified α_1-antitrypsin preparation is available for augmentation therapy. The preparation, which is administered by infusion, has been shown to raise the α_1-antitrypsin levels in the serum and epithelial lining fluid obtained by bronchoalveolar lavage. Because of the considerable expense and difficulties with infusion therapy, attention has focused on alternative routes of administration, including inhalation of a human recombinant DNA preparation of α_1-antitrypsin.[27]

Chronic Bronchitis

In chronic bronchitis, or type B COPD, airway obstruction is caused by inflammation of the major and small airways. There is edema and hyperplasia of submucosal glands and excess mucus excretion into the bronchial tree.[23] A history of a chronic productive cough that has persisted for at least 3 months and for at least 2 consecutive years in the absence of other disease is necessary for diagnosis of chronic bronchitis. Typically, the cough has been present for many years, with a gradual increase in acute exacerbations that produce a frankly purulent sputum. Chronic bronchitis without airflow obstruction is often called *simple bronchitis;* chronic bronchitis with airflow obstruction is called *chronic obstructive bronchitis.* The outlook for persons with simple bronchitis is good, compared with the premature morbidity and mortality associated with chronic obstructive bronchitis.

Chronic bronchitis is seen most commonly in middle-aged men and is associated with chronic irritation from smoking and recurrent infections. In the United States, smoking is the most important cause of chronic bronchitis. Viral and bacterial infections are common and are thought to be a result rather than a cause of

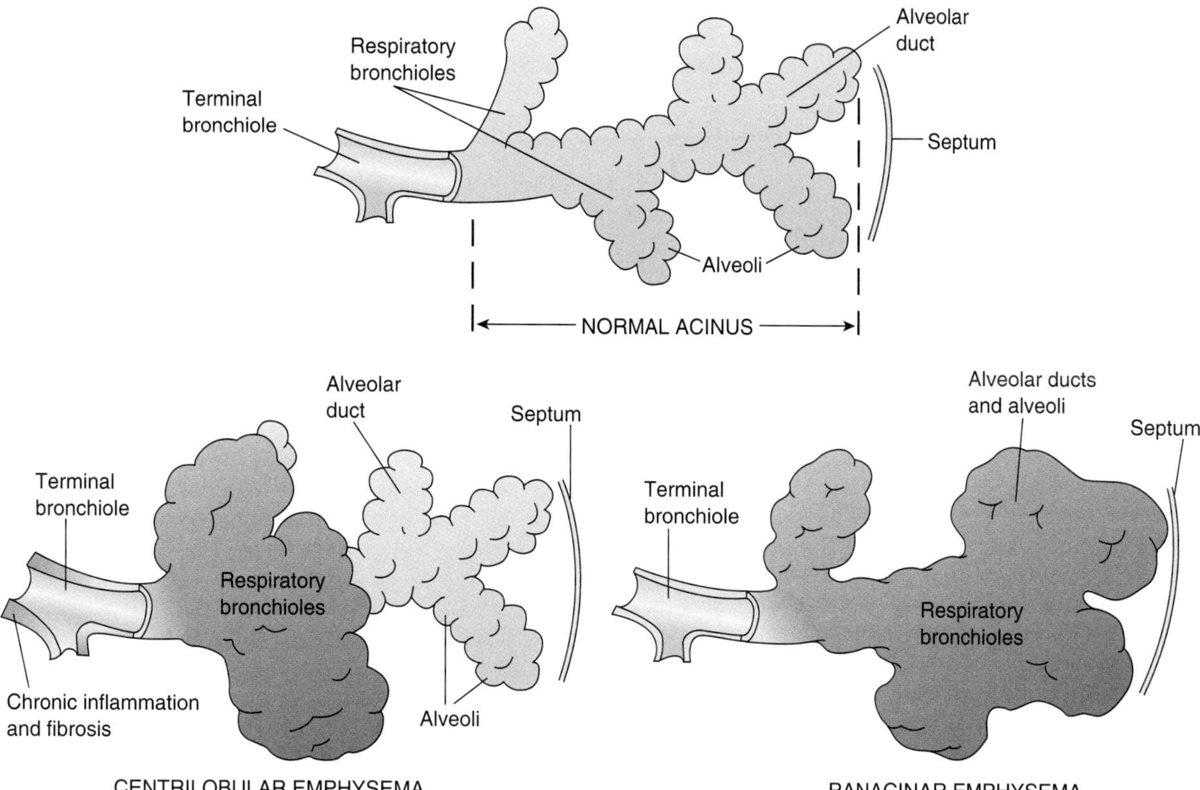

Figure 24–8
Types of emphysema. The acinus is the gas-exchanging structure of the lung distal to the terminal bronchiole. It consists of the terminal bronchiole, respiratory bronchioles, alveolar ducts, alveolar sacs, and alveoli. In centrilobular (proximal acinar) emphysema the respiratory bronchioles are predominantly involved. In paraseptal (distal acinar) emphysema the alveolar ducts are particularly affected. In panacinar (panlobular) emphysema the acinus is uniformly damaged. (Courtesy of Dmitri Karetnikov, artist)

the problem. Chronic asthmatic bronchitis is caused by increased bronchomotor tone and inflammatory triggers that cause bronchial asthma.

Manifestations

The mnemonics "pink puffer" and "blue bloater" have been used to differentiate the clinical manifestations of emphysema and chronic obstructive bronchitis.[27] The important features of these two forms of COPD are described in Table 24–1. In practice, differentiation between the two types is not as vivid as presented here. Persons with COPD often have emphysema and chronic bronchitis.

A major difference between the pink puffers and the blue bloaters is the responsiveness to the hypoxic stimuli. With pulmonary emphysema, there is a proportionate loss of ventilation and perfusion area in the lung. For whatever reason, these persons are pink puffers, or fighters able to struggle and overventilate and thus maintain relatively normal blood gas levels until late in the disease. Chronic obstructive bronchitis is characterized by excessive bronchial secretions and airway obstruction that causes mismatching of ventilation and perfusion. Persons with chronic bronchitis do not compensate by increasing their ventilation; consequently, they develop hypoxemia, cyanosis, and eventually cor pulmonale with peripheral edema. These are the blue bloaters, or nonfighters.

Persons with emphysema have marked dyspnea and struggle to maintain normal blood gas levels with increased ventilatory effort, including prominent use of the accessory muscles. The work of breathing is greatly increased, and eating is often difficult. As a result, there is often considerable weight loss. An increase in the anteroposterior dimensions of the chest because of hyperinflation of the lungs produces the so-called barrel chest that is typical of persons with emphysema. The seated position, which stabilizes chest structures and allows for maximum chest expansion, is preferred. Expiration is often accomplished through pursed lips. With loss of lung elasticity and hyperinflation of the lungs, the airways often collapse during expiration because the

TABLE 24-1

Characteristics of Chronic Bronchitis and Emphysematous Types of Chronic Obstructive Lung Disease

Characteristic	Type A Pulmonary Emphysema ("Pink Puffers")	Type B Chronic Bronchitis ("Blue Bloaters")
Smoking history	Usual	Usual
Age of onset	40 to 50 years of age	30 to 40 years of age; disability in middle age
Clinical features		
Barrel chest (hyperinflation of the lungs)	Often dramatic	May be present
Weight loss	May be severe in advanced disease	Infrequent
Shortness of breath	May be absent early in disease	Predominant early symptom, insidious in onset, exertional
Decreased breath sounds	Characteristic	Variable
Wheezing	Usually absent	Variable
Rhonchi	Usually absent or minimal	Often prominent
Sputum	May be absent or may develop late in the course	Frequent early manifestation, frequent infections, abundant purulent sputum
Cyanosis	Often absent, even late in the disease when there is low PO_2	Often dramatic
Blood gases	Relatively normal until late in the disease process	Hypercapnia may be present Hypoxemia may be present
Cor pulmonale	Only in advanced cases	Frequent Peripheral edema
Polycythemia	Only in advanced cases	Frequent
Prognosis	Slowly debilitating disease	Numerous life-threatening episodes due to acute exacerbations

pressure in the surrounding lung tissues exceeds airway pressure. Pursed-lip breathing increases the resistance to outflow of air, producing a back pressure in the airways sufficient to prevent their collapse. Cough is not a prominent feature in emphysema.

Chronic obstructive bronchitis is characterized by shortness of breath with a progressive decrease in exercise tolerance. As the disease progresses, breathing becomes more labored, even at rest. The expiratory phase of respiration is prolonged, and expiratory rhonchi and rales can be heard on auscultation. In contrast to persons with emphysema, those with chronic obstructive bronchitis do not increase their breathing effort to maintain blood gases. Hypoxemia, hypercapnia, and cyanosis develop, reflecting an imbalance between ventilation and perfusion. Hypoxemia serves as stimulus for increased pulmonary vascular constriction and red blood cell production. As a result, persons with chronic obstructive bronchitis develop pulmonary hypertension, polycythemia, and, eventually, right-sided heart failure with peripheral edema (*i.e.*, cor pulmonale). A common finding in chronic obstructive bronchitis is clubbing of the fingers, a condition in which the tips of the fingers become bulbous, resembling drumsticks.

Although emphysema and chronic bronchitis are diagnosed and treated as specific diseases, most persons with COPD have features of both conditions. Persons with combined forms of COPD characteristically seek medical attention in the fifth or sixth decade of life, complaining of cough, sputum production, and shortness of breath. The symptoms typically have existed to some extent for 10 years or longer. The productive cough usually occurs in the morning. Dyspnea becomes more severe as the disease progresses. Frequent exacerbations of infection and respiratory insufficiency are common, causing absence from work and eventual disability.

The late stages of COPD are characterized by pulmonary hypertension, cor pulmonale, recurrent respiratory infections, and chronic respiratory failure. Death usually occurs during an exacerbation of illness associated with infection and respiratory failure.

Diagnosis

The diagnosis of COPD is based on a careful history and physical examination, pulmonary function studies, chest radiographs, and laboratory tests.

Airway obstruction prolongs the expiratory phase of respiration and affords the potential for impaired gas exchange because of mismatching of ventilation and perfusion. The FVC is the amount of air that can be forcibly exhaled after maximal inspiration. In an adult with normal respiratory function, this should be achieved in 4 to 6 seconds. In patients with chronic lung disease, the time required for FVC is increased, and the $FEV_{1.0}$ and ratio of $FEV_{1.0}$ to FVC are decreased. In severe disease, the FVC is markedly reduced. Lung volume measurements reveal a marked increase in residual volume (RV) and an increase in total lung capacity (TLC) and elevation of the RV to TLC ratio. These and other measurements of expiratory flow are determined by spirometry and are used in the diagnosis of COPD (see Chapter 22).

Treatment

Maintaining or improving physical and psychosocial functioning is an essential part of the treatment plan for persons with COPD. Education of persons with COPD and their families is a key to successful management of the disease.[28] Psychosocial rehabilitation must be individualized to meet the specific needs of persons with COPD and their families. These needs vary with age, occupation, financial resources, social and recreational interest, and interpersonal and family relationships.

A long-term pulmonary rehabilitation program can significantly reduce episodes of hospitalization and add measurably to a person's ability to manage and cope with his or her impairment in a positive way. Breathing exercises and retraining focus on restoring the function of the diaphragm, reducing the work of breathing, and improving gas exchange. Physical conditioning, with a gradual increase in activity, improves exercise tolerance. Work simplification and energy conservation strategies may be needed when impairment is severe. Oxygen therapy is prescribed for selected persons with significant hypoxemia.

Control of Environmental Irritants and Infection. Avoidance of cigarette smoke and other environmental airway irritants is a must. Vocational counseling may be needed if there is occupational exposure. Monitoring of air pollution levels and adjusting activities accordingly aids in controlling shortness of breath. Wearing a cold weather mask often prevents dyspnea and bronchospasm due to cold air and wind exposure.

Respiratory tract infections can prove fatal to persons with severe COPD. A person with COPD should avoid exposure to others with known respiratory tract infections and should avoid attending large gatherings during periods of the year when influenza or respiratory tract infections are prevalent. Immunization for influenza and pneumococcal infections decreases the likelihood of their occurrence. Persons with COPD should be taught to monitor their sputum for signs of infection, so that treatment can be instituted at the earliest sign of infection.

Nutritional Support. Because persons with COPD expend so much effort on breathing, many find it difficult to chew their food and manage the effort of a large meal. This situation, combined with impaired diaphragm descent, air swallowing, and medications that cause anorexia and nausea, impairs nutrition and promotes weight loss. Undernutrition (indicated by a body weight $<90\%$ of ideal weight) affects about 25% of persons with COPD.[28] It is associated with reduced respiratory muscle function and increased mortality. Small, frequent, nutritious, and easily swallowed feedings aid in maintaining good nutrition and preventing weight loss. Carbohydrates can increase carbon dioxide production and arterial carbon dioxide levels, ventilation, and oxygen consumption. However, it is usually not a problem unless a high-carbohydrate diet is followed.[28]

Exercise Training. Appropriate exercise training increases maximum oxygen consumption and reduces the ventilation and heart rate for a given workload consistent with cardiopulmonary conditioning. It also improves the persons sense of well-being. It can include treadmill exercise, riding a stationary bicycle, and stair climbing. In persons with COPD, the use of the upper extremities may lead to dyspnea and altered breathing patterns and increased diaphragmatic work and fatigue.[29] Therefore, exercise training of the upper extremities is often included to improve upper extremity function. Exercise programs should be prescribed by physicians or other health professions who are knowledgeable about pulmonary rehabilitation. While exercising, the use of continuous positive airway pressure to a level sufficient to prevent expiratory airway collapse decreases the work of breathing and allows persons with severe disease to exercise longer.[28]

Breathing Exercises and Retraining. Breathing exercises and retraining are designed to increase respiratory muscle strength and endurance, thereby improving exercise performance. In normal respiration, the diaphragm does 65% of the work of breathing, and the accessory muscles do about 35%.[30] In persons with COPD, the contribution of the diaphragm to the work of breathing is diminished because of loss of lung elasticity, with consequent air trapping, lung distention, and flattening of the diaphragm. Contracting this flattened diaphragm requires greater force generation. To compensate, persons with COPD increasingly use their accessory muscles for breathing. This labored breathing pattern may progress to the point that the diaphragm contributes only about 30% to the effort of breathing, and the accessory muscles carry 70% of the load. Studies have shown that, although respiratory muscles may be weakened in COPD, it is possible to strengthen them through resistive loading inspiratory muscle training.[31] Resistive loading is accomplished by having the person breathe through an inspiratory breathing device that increases the resistance to airflow during inspiration.

Instruction in the use of pursed-lip breathing to prevent airway collapse, abdominal muscle assistance during expiration, and coordination of rib cage and abdominal compartment efforts improve ventilation, relieve fatigue of accessory muscles, and sometimes help prevent dyspnea.

Managing Secretions. The use of water to liquefy secretions in persons with emphysema and chronic bronchitis is controversial, except in situations of dehydration.[28] The use of nebulized water and saline are also of questionable value, as is the use of expectorants such as guaifenesin. Postural drainage and chest percussion are also of limited value for persons with emphysema and chronic bronchitis, except in cases of excessive secretions or a nonproductive cough.[28]

Pharmacologic Treatment. Bronchodilators, including adrenergic drugs, theophylline preparations, and anticholinergic drugs, are probably the most widely prescribed medications for use in the treatment of COPD.

Inhaled β_2-adrenergic agonists have been the mainstay of treatment for COPD for many years. Many of the newer β_2-specific agents have a more specific action than earlier adrenergic drugs and produce fewer cardiac effects. Many adrenergic drugs are available in aerosol form for inhalation, and they are particularly useful in controlling bronchospasm. Because they are convenient and effective, they can be abused by improper administration and overuse.

The anticholinergic agents, ipratropium and nebulized atropine, produce bronchodilation by blocking parasympathetic cholinergic receptors that produce contraction of bronchial smooth muscle. Ipratropium also reduces the volume of sputum without altering its viscosity. Because the drug has a slower onset of action and longer duration of action, it is usually used on a regular basis rather than on an as-needed basis.

Theophylline preparations can be administered orally, rectally, or intravenously. As with bronchial asthma, maintenance therapy with oral theophylline drugs is controversial. However, long-acting theophylline preparations may be used to reduce overnight declines in respiratory function. There is also evidence that theophylline may improve respiratory muscle function, increase mucociliary clearance, and improve central respiratory drive.[28] When theophylline is prescribed, blood levels are used as a guide in arriving at an effective dose schedule.

Although corticosteroid drugs are not routinely prescribed for long-term treatment of COPD, some persons do require them. The corticosteroids are available for local use in aerosol form, minimizing the undesirable effects that often accompany systemic use.

Oxygen Therapy. In advanced cases of COPD, the imbalance between ventilation and perfusion causes hypoxemia. Hypoxemia in which arterial PO_2 levels fall below 55 mm Hg, causes polycythemia and reflex vasoconstriction of the pulmonary vessels, with resultant pulmonary hypertension and further impairment of gas exchange in the lung. Those affected are at risk for developing cor pulmonale.

In severe cases, administration of continuous low-flow (1 to 2 L/min) oxygen to maintain PO_2 levels between 55 and 65 mm Hg decreases dyspnea and pulmonary hypertension and improves neuropsychologic function and activity tolerance. The Nocturnal Oxygen Therapy Trial Group study of persons with advanced disease—particularly those with heart failure associated with COPD—performed at six centers in the United States and Canada showed that oxygen is more effective when given almost continuously (at least 18 hours per day) than when it is given roughly 50% of the time.[32] Persons with COPD may have episodes of hypoxemia at night and during daytime naps. These persons do not, however, experience the daytime hypersomnolence and loud snoring that is usually associated with sleep apnea.[33] Although these persons do not usually experience severe hypoxemia during waking hours and do not meet the criteria for continuous low-flow oxygen therapy, they may benefit from nocturnal oxygen therapy.[33]

The overall goal of oxygen therapy is to maintain a hemoglobin oxygen saturation above 90%. Oxygen is usually administered using a nasal cannulae. Portable oxygen administration units, which allow mobility and the performance of activities of daily living, are usually used. Transtracheal oxygen, delivered by a small-diameter percutaneous catheter placed in the trachea, can be used to increase oxygen delivery and decrease minute ventilation. It is particularly useful in persons with high oxygen requirements.[27,29] It can also be used to increase ambulation by eliminating the need to wear a nasal cannulae. Oxygen administration in persons with severe COPD must be undertaken with a certain amount of caution. The flow rate (in liters per minute) is usually titrated to provide an arterial PO_2 of 55 to 65 mm Hg. Because the ventilatory drive associated with hypoxic stimulation of the peripheral chemoreceptors does not occur until the arterial PO_2 has been reduced to about 60 mm Hg or less, increasing the arterial oxygen above that level tends to depress stimulation for ventilation and often leads to hypoventilation and carbon dioxide retention.

Lung Reduction Surgery. Lung reduction surgery involves the resection of the most distended areas of the lung as a means of improving respiratory function. The procedure is designed to reduce the overall volume of the lung, reshape the configuration of the lung, and improve elastic recoil and its effects on the airways and the diaphragm.[34] Two surgical approaches are used: one in which the chest is opened through a median sternotomy and the other through a thoracoscopic approach.[35] Although, the procedure is still experimental, early results have demonstrated improvement in the 6-minute walk, dyspnea index, and quality of life assessment.[35]

Bronchiectasis

Bronchiectasis is an abnormal dilatation of the large bronchi associated with infection and destruction of the bronchial walls (Fig. 24–9). To be diagnosed as bronchiectasis, the dilatation must be permanent as compared with the reversible bronchial dilatation that sometimes accompanies viral and bronchial pneumonias.

The causes of bronchiectasis include local airway obstruction from conditions such as tumors and foreign bodies; congenital abnormalities associated with abnormal development of the bronchi; lung infection (*e.g.*, tuberculosis, fungal infections, lung abscess); cystic fibrosis, in which airway obstruction is caused by impairment of normal mucociliary function; immunodeficiency states, which predispose to respiratory tract

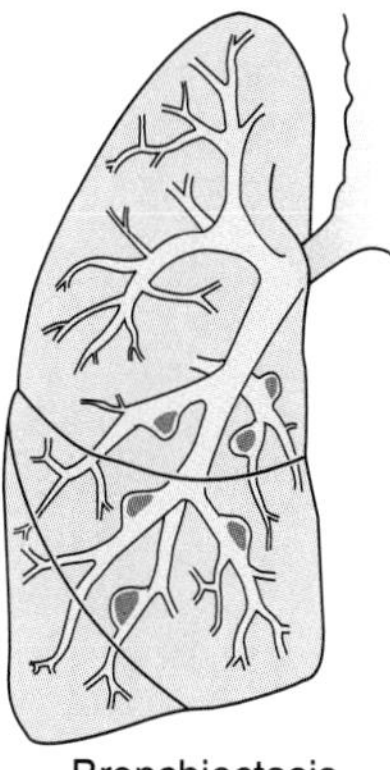

Figure 24–9
Bronchiectasis showing abnormal dilations of the large bronchi that are filled with inflammatory exudate.

infections; and exposure to toxic gases that cause airway obstruction. Two conditions, obstruction and infection, are present in all of these disorders, and both contribute to the development and progression of the disease. Bronchial obstruction causes atelectasis, which results in smooth muscle relaxation and dilatation of the walls of the airways that remain patent. Infection produces inflammation, impairs mucociliary function, and causes weakening and further dilatation of the walls of the bronchioles. Pooling of secretions produces a vicious cycle of chronic inflammation and development of new infections. The disease is primarily a disease of children and young adults. Cystic fibrosis accounts for about half of all cases.[36]

Bronchiectasis is associated with an assortment of abnormalities that profoundly affect respiratory function, including atelectasis, obstruction of the smaller airways, and diffuse bronchitis. Affected persons have fever, recurrent bronchopulmonary infection, coughing, and production of copious amounts of foul-smelling, purulent sputum, and hemoptysis. Weight loss and anemia are common. The physiologic abnormalities that occur in bronchiectasis are similar to those seen in chronic bronchitis and emphysema. As in both of these conditions, chronic bronchial obstruction leads to marked dyspnea and cyanosis.

Treatment consists of early recognition and treatment of infection along with regular postural drainage and chest physical therapy. Persons with this disorder benefit from many of the rehabilitation and treatment measures used for chronic bronchitis and emphysema.

Cystic Fibrosis

Cystic fibrosis is an autosomal recessive exocrine gland disorder involving the mucus-secreting and the eccrine sweat glands. Most of the clinical manifestations of the disease are related to abnormal secretions that result in obstruction of organ passages such as the respiratory airways and pancreatic ducts. About 1 in 2500 of white infants in the United States are born with the disease, and about 5% of persons are asymptomatic carriers.[37] The gene is rare in African Blacks and Asians. Homozygotes (*i.e.*, persons with two defective genes) have all or substantially all of the clinical symptoms of the disease, as compared with heterozygotes who are carriers of the disease but have no recognizable symptoms. The disease is the most common fatal hereditary disorder of whites in the United States and is the most common cause of chronic lung disease in children.

The cystic fibrosis gene was identified on the long arm of chromosome 7.[37,38] In most cases of cystic fibrosis, the mutation consists of the deletion of a single phenylalanine residue from the gene. The gene encodes the production of a single protein, the cystic fibrosis transmembrane conductance regulator (CFTR), which functions in chloride transport across membranes. In cystic fibrosis, chloride transport in airway epithelial cells is diminished. Because of the defective chloride transport, there is a threefold increase in sodium reabsorption. Water moves out of the extracellular fluid with the sodium, causing the exocrine secretions to become exceedingly viscid.

Clinically, cystic fibrosis is manifested by a triad of chronic respiratory disease, pancreatic exocrine deficiency, and elevation of sodium chloride in the sweat. Respiratory manifestations are caused by an accumulation of viscid mucus in the bronchi, impaired mucociliary clearance, and lung infections. Mucus plugs can result in the total obstruction of an airway, causing atelectasis.

Infection and ensuing inflammation are causes of lung destruction in cystic fibrosis. *Staphylococcus aureus* and *Pseudomonas* infections occur. With advanced disease, 80% of persons harbor the *Pseudomonas* organism. New findings suggest that absence of the CFTR predisposes to *Pseudomonas* infections, and once established, *Pseudomonas* is not easily cleared from the lungs, producing a cycle of chronic inflammation, tissue damage, and obstruction.

Pancreatic function is abnormal in about 80% to 90% of affected persons.[39] The pancreatic insufficiency gives rise to malabsorption and steatorrhea. In the newborn, meconium ileus may cause intestinal obstruction.

Early diagnosis and treatment of cystic fibrosis are important in that they may delay the onset of chronic illness. The sweat test, using pilocarpine iontophoresis to collect a sweat sample, remains the standard approach to diagnosis. The test is usually done on sweat obtained from a child's forearm or from an infant's thigh. A small electric current is used to carry the drug pilocarpine, which increases sweat production, into the skin. Sweat is collected using an absorbent paper or gauze sponge and then analyzed in the laboratory. The test is often inaccurate in newborns because the quantity of sweat produced is insufficient for testing. Newborns with cystic fibrosis can be identified by determination of immunoreactive trypsin. The test can be done on blood spots collected for routine metabolic screening. Newborns with cystic fibrosis have elevated blood levels of immunoreactive trypsin, presumably because of secretory obstruction in the pancreas.

Genetic tests can detect carriers of the cystic fibrosis gene. At least 500 mutations of the CFTR gene have been identified; of these, commercially available probes are available for only 70 mutations.[38] Although these 70 mutations account for 90% of all cystic fibrosis, the probes cannot be used to exclude cystic fibrosis in persons without these mutant genes. Even if both genes are abnormal, it is possible for a neutralizing second gene to be present elsewhere. Cystic fibrosis cannot be accurately diagnosed by genetic testing methods unless there are characteristic clinical manifestations or a family history of the disorder.

The treatment of cystic fibrosis usually consists of replacement of pancreatic enzymes, physical measures to improve the clearance of tracheobronchial secretions (*i.e.*, postural drainage and chest percussion), bronchodilator therapy, and prompt treatment of respiratory tract infections. The abnormal viscosity of airway secretions is largely attributed to the presence of polymorphonuclear white blood cells and their degradation products. A purified recombinant human deoxyribonuclease (rhDNase I), an enzyme that breaks down these products, has been developed. Clinical trials have shown that the drug, which is administered by inhalation, can improve pulmonary symptoms and reduce the frequency of respiratory exacerbations. Although many persons benefit from the therapy, the drug is costly, and recommendations for its use are evolving.

Treatment methods to manipulate the increased sodium reabsorption and decreased chloride secretion are being studied. Amiloride, a potassium-sparing diuretic that blocks sodium reabsorption, has been administered in aerosol form. In pilot studies that used the drug, there was a decrease in sputum viscosity and a slowing of the decline of pulmonary function. Agents such as adenosine triphosphate and uridine triphosphate that increase chloride secretion are also being studied.[39]

Progress of the disease is variable. Improved medical management has led to longer survival—to about age 20. Lung transplantation is being used as a treatment for persons with end-stage lung disease. Current hopes reside in the development of gene therapy. The complementary DNA for the CFTR gene has been successfully cloned and introduced into affected epithelial cells in the laboratory. It is hoped that research can develop a method for inserting the gene into cells in the airway lining of persons with cystic fibrosis.

In summary, obstructive ventilatory disorders are characterized by airway obstruction and limitation in expiratory air flow. Bronchial asthma is a chronic inflammatory disorder of the airways, characterized by airway hypersensitivity and episodic attacks of airway narrowing. An asthmatic attack can be triggered by a variety of stimuli. Based on their mechanism of response, these triggers can be divided into two types: bronchospastic or inflammatory. Bronchospastic triggers depend on the level of airway responsiveness. There are two types of responses in persons with asthma: the early response and the late response. The early response results in immediate bronchoconstriction on exposure to an inhaled antigen and usually subsides within 90 minutes. The late response usually develops 3 to 5 hours after exposure to an asthmatic trigger; it involves inflammation and increased airway responsiveness that prolong the attack and cause a vicious cycle of exacerbations.

COPD describes a group of conditions characterized by obstruction to airflow in the lungs. Among the conditions associated with COPD are emphysema, chronic bronchitis, and bronchiectasis. Emphysema, or type A COPD, is characterized by a loss of lung elasticity and abnormal, permanent enlargement of the air spaces distal to the terminal bronchioles, and hyperinflation of the lungs. Chronic bronchitis, or type B COPD, is caused by inflammation of major and small airways and is characterized by edema and hyperplasia of submucosal glands and excess mucus secretion into the bronchial tree. A history of a chronic productive cough that has persisted for at least 3 months and for at least 2 consecutive years in the absence of other disease is necessary for the diagnosis of chronic bronchitis. Emphysema and chronic bronchitis are manifested by eventual mismatching of ventilation and perfusion. As the condition advances, signs of respiratory distress and impaired gas exchange become evident, with development of hypercapnia and hypoxemia.

Bronchiectasis is a form of COPD that is characterized by an abnormal dilatation of the large bronchi associated with infection and destruction of the bronchial walls.

Cystic fibrosis is an autosomal recessive genetic disorder manifested by chronic lung disease, pancreatic exocrine deficiency, and elevation of sodium chloride in the sweat. The disorder is caused by a mutation of the CFTR gene located on the long arm of chromosome 7. The gene functions in chloride transport across membranes; the defect increases sodium reabsorption, causing the exocrine secretions to become exceedingly viscid. Respiratory manifestations are caused by an accumulation of viscid mucus in the bronchi, impaired mucociliary clearance, lung infections, bronchiectasis, and dilatation. Mucus plugs can result in the total obstruction of an airway, causing atelectasis.

Interstitial Lung Diseases

After you have completed this section of the chapter, you should be able to meet the following objectives:

- State the difference between chronic obstructive pulmonary diseases and interstitial lung diseases

- Cite the characteristics of occupational dusts that determine their pathogenicity in terms of the production of pneumoconioses
- Characterize the organ involvement in sarcoidosis

The interstitial lung diseases are a diverse group of lung disorders that produce similar inflammatory and fibrotic changes in the interstitium or interalveolar septum of the lung. They include sarcoidosis, the occupational lung diseases, hypersensitivity pneumonitis, and lung diseases caused by exposure to toxic drugs and radiation. In many cases, no specific cause can be found.[40]

The interstitial lung diseases produce various degrees of inflammation, fibrosis, and disability. The disorders may be acute or insidious in onset; they may be rapidly progressive, slowly progressive, or static in their course. Because they result in a stiff and noncompliant lung, they are commonly classified as fibrotic or restrictive lung disorders. The most common of the interstitial lung diseases are those caused by exposure to occupational and environmental inhalants and sarcoidosis, the cause of which is unknown. Examples of interstitial lung diseases and their causes are listed in Table 24–2.

In contrast to the obstructive lung diseases, which primarily involve the airways of the lung, the interstitial lung disorders exert their effects on the collagen and elastic connective tissue found between the airways and the blood vessels of the lung. Many of these diseases also involve the airways, arteries, and veins. In general, these lung diseases share a pattern of lung dysfunction that includes diminished lung volumes, reduced diffusing capacity of the lung, and varying degrees of hypoxemia.

Current theory suggests that most interstitial lung diseases, regardless of the causes, have a common pathogenesis. It is thought that these disorders are initiated by some type of injury to the alveolar epithelium, followed by an inflammatory process that involves the alveoli and interstitium of the lung. An accumulation of inflammatory and immune cells causes continued damage of lung tissue and the replacement of normal, functioning lung tissue with fibrous scar tissue.

TABLE 24–2

Causes and Examples of Interstitial Lung Diseases

Causes	Examples
Known	
Occupational and environmental inhalants	
Inorganic dusts	Silicosis
	Asbestosis
	Talcosis
	Coal miner's pneumoconiosis
	Berylliosis
Organic dusts	Farmer's lung (moldy hay)
	Pigeon breeder's lung (bird serum, excreta, and feathers)
	Air-conditioner lung (bacteria found in humidifiers and air conditioners)
	Bagassosis (contaminated sugarcane)
Gases, fumes, aerosols	Silo filler's lung (nitrogen dioxide, chlorine, ammonia, phosgene, sulfur dioxide)
Drugs	Cancer therapeutic drugs (*e.g.*, bleomycin), nitrofurantoin, amiodarone, and others
Radiation	External radiation, inhaled radioactive materials
Infections	Widespread tuberculosis
Poisons	Paraquat
Diseases of other organ systems	Chronic pulmonary edema
	Chronic uremia
Unknown	
	Sarcoidosis
	Idiopathic pulmonary fibrosis
	Connective tissue diseases, such as lupus erythematosus, scleroderma, and rheumatoid arthritis

Manifestations

Interstitial lung disease is characterized by an insidious onset of breathlessness that initially occurs during exercise and may progress to the point that the person is totally incapacitated. Typically, a person with a restrictive lung disease breathes with a pattern of rapid, shallow respirations. This tachypneic pattern of breathing, in which the respiratory rate is increased and the tidal volume is decreased, reduces the work of breathing, because it takes less work to move air through the airways at an increased rate than it does to stretch a stiff lung to accommodate a larger tidal volume. A nonproductive cough may occur, particularly with continued exposure to the inhaled irritant. Clubbing of the fingers and toes may develop.

Lung volumes, including vital capacity and TLC, are reduced in interstitial lung disease. In contrast to COPD, in which expiratory flow rates are reduced, the $FEV_{1.0}$ is usually preserved, even though the ratio between the $FEV_{1.0}$ and the FVC may increase. Although resting arterial blood gases are usually normal early in the course of the disease, arterial oxygen levels may fall during exercise, and in cases of advanced disease, hypoxemia is often present, even at rest. In the late stages of the disease, hypercapnia and respiratory acidosis develop. The impaired diffusion of gases that occurs in persons with interstitial lung disease is thought to be caused by an increase in physiologic dead space resulting from unventilated regions of the lung.

Diagnosis and Treatment

The diagnosis of interstitial lung disease requires a careful personal and family history, with particular emphasis on exposure to environmental, occupational, and other injurious agents. Chest radiographs may be used as an initial diagnostic method, and serial chest films are often used in following the progress of the disease. A biopsy specimen for histologic study and culture may be obtained by means of surgical incision or by bronchoscopy using a fiberoptic bronchoscope. In bronchoalveolar lavage, fluid is instilled into the alveoli through a bronchoscope and then removed by suction to obtain inflammatory and immune cells for laboratory study. Gallium lung scans are often used to detect and quantify the chronic alveolitis that occurs in interstitial lung disease. Gallium does not localize in normal lung tissue, but uptake of the radionuclide is increased in interstitial lung disease and other diffuse lung diseases.

The treatment goals for persons with interstitial lung disease focus on identifying and removing the injurious agent, suppressing the inflammatory response, preventing progression of the disease, and providing supportive therapy for persons with advanced disease. Generally, the treatment measures vary with the type of lung disease. Corticosteroid drugs are frequently used to suppress the inflammatory response. Many of the supportive treatment measures used in the late stages of the disease, such as oxygen therapy and measures to prevent infection, are similar to those discussed for persons with COPD.

Occupational Lung Diseases

The occupational lung diseases can be divided into two major groups: the pneumoconioses and the hypersensitivity diseases. The pneumoconioses are caused by the inhalation of inorganic dusts and particulate matter. The hypersensitivity diseases result from the inhalation of organic dusts and related occupational antigens. A third type of occupational lung disease, byssinosis, a disease that affects cotton workers, has characteristics of the pneumoconioses and hypersensitivity lung disease.

Among the pneumoconioses are silicosis, found in hard-rock miners, foundry workers, sandblasters, pottery makers, and workers in the slate industry; coal miner's pneumoconiosis; asbestosis, found in asbestos miners, manufacturers of asbestos products, and installers and removers of asbestos insulation; talcosis, found in talc miners or millers and infants and small children who accidentally inhale powder containing talc; and berylliosis, found in ore extraction workers and alloy production workers. The danger of exposure to asbestos dust is not confined to the workplace. The dust pervades the general environment, because it was used in the construction of buildings and in other applications before its health hazards were realized. It has been mixed into paints and plaster, wrapped around water and heating pipes, used to insulate hair dryers, and woven into theater curtains, hot pads, and ironing-board covers.

Important etiologic determinants in the development of the pneumoconioses are the size of the dust particle, its chemical nature, and its ability to incite lung destruction and the concentration of dust and the length of exposure to it. The most dangerous particles are those in the range of 1 to 5 μm. These small particles are carried through the inspired air into the alveolar structures, whereas larger particles are trapped in the nose or mucous linings of the airways and removed by the mucociliary blanket. Exceptions are asbestos and talc particles, which range in size from 30 to 60 μm but find their way into the alveoli because of their density.

All particles within the alveoli must be cleared by the lung macrophages. Macrophages are thought to transport engulfed particles from the small bronchioles and the alveoli, which have neither cilia nor mucus-secreting cells, to the mucociliary escalator or to the lymphatic channels for removal from the lung. This clearing function is hampered when the function of the macrophage is impaired by factors such as cigarette smoking, consumption of alcohol, and hypersensitivity reactions. This helps to explain the increased incidence of lung disease among smokers exposed to asbestos. In silicosis, the ingestion of silica particles leads to the destruction of the lung macrophages and the release of substances that produce fibrosis. Tuberculosis and other diseases caused by mycobacteria are common in persons with silicosis. Because the macrophages are responsible for protecting the lungs from tuberculosis, the destruction of macrophages accounts for the increased susceptibility of persons with silicosis to tuberculosis.

The concentration of some dusts in the environment strongly influences their effects on the lung. For example, acute silicosis is seen only in persons whose occupations entail intense exposure to silica dust over a short period. It is seen in sandblasters, who use a high-speed jet of sand to clean and polish bricks and the insides of corroded tanks, in tunnelers, and in rock drillers, particularly if they drill through sandstone. Acute silicosis is a rapidly progressive disease, usually leading to severe disability and death within 5 years of diagnosis. In contrast to acute silicosis, which is caused by exposure to extremely high concentrations of silica dust, the symptoms related to chronic, low-level exposure to silica dust often do not begin to develop until after many years of exposure, and then the symptoms are often insidious in onset and slow to progress.

The hypersensitivity occupational lung disorders (*e.g.*, hypersensitivity pneumonitis) are caused by intense and often prolonged exposure to inhaled organic dusts and related occupational antigens. Affected persons have a heightened sensitivity to the antigen. Unlike bronchial asthma, this type of hypersensitivity reaction involves primarily the alveoli. These disorders cause progressive fibrotic lung disease, which can be prevented by the removal of the environmental agent. The most common forms of hypersensitivity pneumonitis are farmer's lung, which results from exposure to moldy hay; pigeon breeder's lung, provoked by exposure to the serum, excreta, or feathers of birds; bagassosis, from contaminated sugar cane; and humidifier or air-conditioner lung, caused by mold in the water reservoirs of these appliances.

Sarcoidosis

Sarcoidosis is a multisystem granulomatous disorder characterized by exaggerated cellular immune response at the sites of involvement. The disease predominantly affects adults younger than 40 years of age,[41] although it can occur in older persons. The annual incidence of sarcoidosis in the United States is about 22,500 cases; it is 10 to 20 times more prevalent among African Americans and whites living in the southeastern part of the country. The cause of sarcoidosis remains obscure. Genetic factors may play a role, although no one gene has been implicated.

Sarcoidosis has variable manifestations and an unpredictable course of progression in which any organ system can be affected. The three systems that most commonly manifest symptoms are the lungs, the skin, and the eyes. More than 40% of persons with sarcoidosis report nonspecific symptoms such as fever, sweating, anorexia, weight loss, fatigue, and myalgia. Although only about 60% of persons with sarcoidosis have respiratory symptoms, almost all have abnormal chest radiographs. In about 25% of cases, the disease is first detected on a routine chest x-ray film. Overall, approximately 50% develop permanent pulmonary abnormalities, and 5% to 15% have progressive pulmonary fibrosis.[42] Sarcoidosis is primarily an interstitial lung disease.

The diagnosis of sarcoidosis is based on history and physical examination, tests to exclude other diseases, chest radiography, and biopsy to obtain conformation of noncaseating granuloma.[41] When treatment is indicated, corticosteroid drugs are used. These agents produce clearing of the lung, as seen on the chest radiograph, and improve pulmonary function, but it is not known whether they affect the long-term outcome of the disease.

In summary, the interstitial lung diseases are characterized by fibrosis and decreased compliance of the lung. They include the occupational lung diseases, lung diseases caused by toxic drugs and radiation, and lung diseases of unknown origin, such as sarcoidosis. These disorders are thought to result from an inflammatory process that begins in the alveoli and extends to involve the interstitial tissues of the lung. Unlike COPDs, which affect the airways, interstitial lung diseases affect the supporting collagen and elastic tissues that lie between the airways and blood vessels. These lung diseases decrease lung volumes, reduce the diffusing capacity of the lung, and cause various degrees of hypoxia. Because lung compliance is reduced, persons with this form of lung disease have a rapid, shallow breathing pattern.

Pulmonary Vascular Disorders

After you have completed this section of the chapter, you should be able to meet the following objectives:

- State the most common cause of pulmonary embolism and the clinical manifestations of the disorder
- Describe the physiology of pulmonary arterial hypertension and three causes of secondary pulmonary hypertension
- Describe the alterations in cardiovascular function that are characteristic of cor pulmonale

As blood moves through the lung, blood oxygen levels are raised, and carbon dioxide is removed. These processes depend on the matching of ventilation (*i.e.*, gas exchange) and perfusion (*i.e.*, blood flow). This section discusses two major problems of the pulmonary circulation, pulmonary embolism and pulmonary hypertension. Pulmonary edema, another major problem of the pulmonary circulation, is discussed in Chapter 20.

Pulmonary Embolism

Pulmonary embolism develops when a bloodborne substance lodges in a branch of the pulmonary artery and obstructs the flow. The embolism may consist of a thrombus, air that has accidentally been injected during intravenous infusion, fat that has been mobilized from the bone marrow after a fracture or from a traumatized fat depot, or amniotic fluid that has entered the maternal circulation after rupture of the membranes at the time of delivery. This discussion is limited to the most common form of pulmonary embolism, thromboembolism.

In the United States, as many as 250,000 hospitalizations and 50,000 deaths occur annually from pulmonary emboli.[43] About 10% of the deaths occur within the first hour, and fewer than 10% of persons who die of pulmonary embolism have been treated for the condition, emphasizing the difficulty encountered in diagnosis.[3]

Almost all pulmonary emboli result from deep vein thrombosis in the lower extremities. Persons at risk for developing venous thrombosis are also at risk for developing thromboemboli. Among the physiologic factors that contribute to venous thrombosis are venous stasis, venous endothelial injury, and hypercoagulability states. Clinical risk factors include prolonged bed rest, trauma, surgery, childbirth, obesity, fractures of the hip and femur, advanced age, myocardial infarction and congestive heart failure, and spinal cord injury. Persons undergoing orthopedic surgery and gynecologic cancer surgery are at particular risk, as are bedridden patients in an intensive care unit.[3] An enlarged fibrillating right atrium often contains thrombosed blood. The presence of thrombosis in the deep veins of the legs or pelvis is often unsuspected until embolism occurs. Venous thrombosis is further discussed in Chapter 16.

The effects of emboli on the pulmonary circulation are related to mechanical obstruction of the pulmonary circulation and neurohumoral reflexes causing vasoconstriction. Obstruction of pulmonary blood flow causes reflex bronchoconstriction in the affected area of the lung, wasted ventilation and impaired gas exchange, and loss of alveolar surfactant. Pulmonary hypertension and right heart failure may develop when there is massive vasoconstriction because of a large embolus. Although small areas of infarction may occur, frank pulmonary infarction is uncommon.

Manifestations

The manifestations of pulmonary embolism depend on the size and location of the obstruction. Chest pain, dyspnea, and increased respiratory rate are the most frequent signs and symptoms of pulmonary embolism. Pulmonary infarction often causes pleuritic pain that changes with respiration; it is more severe on inspiration and less severe on expiration. Moderate hypoxemia without carbon dioxide retention occurs as a result of impaired gas exchange. Small emboli that become lodged in the peripheral branches of the pulmonary artery may exert little effect and go unrecognized. However, repeated small emboli gradually reduce the size of the pulmonary capillary bed, resulting in pulmonary hypertension. Moderate-sized emboli often present with breathlessness accompanied by pleuritic pain, apprehension, slight fever, and cough productive of blood-streaked sputum. Tachycardia is often detected, and the breathing pattern is rapid and shallow. Patients with massive emboli usually present with sudden collapse, crushing substernal chest pain, shock, and sometimes loss of consciousness. The pulse is rapid and weak, the blood pressure is low, the neck veins are distended, and the skin is cyanotic and diaphoretic. Massive pulmonary emboli are often fatal.

Diagnosis and Treatment

Diagnosis of pulmonary embolism is based on blood gas determinations, lung scan (perfusion, ventilation, or both), chest x-ray films, an electrocardiogram (ECG), and in selected cases, angiography. The arterial oxygen tension (PO_2) is almost always decreased when emboli of significant size are present in the lung because of the mismatching of ventilation and perfusion.

The lung scan is a widely used diagnostic test. A perfusion lung scan uses radiolabeled albumin, which is injected intravenously and is distributed in proportion to blood flow in the pulmonary circulation. A scintillation (gamma) camera is used to scan the various lung segments for blood flow. A ventilation scan uses a radiolabeled gas (usually xenon-133).[44] The person inhales the gas by way of a mask and holds his or her breath (for as long as 20 seconds) while a scintillation (gamma) camera scans the lung and records the distribution of the radiolabeled gas. A ventilation scan may be done before a perfusion scan if there is concurrent lung disease. Use of the ventilation-perfusion scans provides a means of evaluating ventilation-perfusion associations in the lung.

The laboratory studies and chest x-ray films are useful in ruling out other conditions that might give rise to similar symptoms. Because emboli can cause an increase in pulmonary vascular resistance, the ECG may be used to detect signs of right heart strain. Angiography involves the passage of a venous catheter through the heart and into the pulmonary artery under fluoroscopy. An embolectomy is sometimes performed during this procedure.

The treatment goals for pulmonary emboli focus on preventing deep vein thrombosis and the development of thromboemboli, protecting the lungs from exposure to thromboemboli when they occur, and in the case of large and life-threatening pulmonary emboli, sustaining life and restoring pulmonary blood flow. Prevention focuses on identification of persons at risk, avoidance of venous stasis and hypercoagulability states, and early detection of venous thrombosis. Early detection of venous thrombosis can be accomplished through the use of compression ultrasonography, impedance plethysmography, and Doppler imaging.[45]

For patients at risk, graded-compression elastic stockings and intermittent pneumatic-compression (IPC) boots can be used to prevent venous stasis. Both of these devices are safe and practical ways to prevent venous thrombosis. IPC boots provide intermittent inflation of air-filled cuffs that prevent venous stasis. Some devices produce sequential gradient compression that moves blood upward in the leg (*i.e.*, pressures of 35, 30, and 20 mm Hg in the ankle, calf, and thigh, respectively).[43]

Pharmacologic prophylaxis involves the use of anticoagulant drugs. Anticoagulant therapy may be used to decrease the likelihood of deep vein thrombosis, thromboembolism, and fatal pulmonary embolism after major surgical procedures.[3] Low-molecular-weight heparin, which can be administered subcutaneously on an outpatient basis, is often used. Warfarin, an oral anticoagulation drug, may be used for persons with long-term risk of developing thromboemboli.

Surgical interruption of the vena cava is often indicated when pulmonary embolism poses a life-threatening risk. There are two surgical procedures for protecting the lung from thromboemboli: venous ligation to prevent the embolus from traveling to the lung and vena caval plication. The plication, done with a suture or by insertion of a clip, filter, or sieve, permits blood to flow while trapping the embolus. Percutaneous transjugular placement of a filter has become the preferred mode of inferior vena caval interruption. Restoration of blood flow in persons with life-threatening pulmonary emboli can be accomplished through the surgical removal of the embolus or emboli. In the case of multiple pulmonary emboli, thrombolytic therapy using streptokinase, urokinase, or recombinant tissue plasminogen activator may be used. It is recommended that the thrombolytic therapy be administered through a peripheral vein rather than through a pulmonary artery, because the latter approach is neither safer nor more effective.[44] Thrombolytic therapy is followed by administration of heparin and then warfarin.

Pulmonary Hypertension

The term *pulmonary hypertension* describes the elevation of pressure in the pulmonary arterial system. The pulmonary circulation is a low-pressure system designed to accommodate varying amounts of blood delivered from the right heart and to facilitate gas exchange. The normal mean pulmonary artery pressure is about 15 mm Hg (28 systolic/8 diastolic). Pulmonary artery hypertension can be caused by an elevation in left atrial pressure, by increased pulmonary blood flow, or by increased pulmonary vascular resistance. Although pulmonary hypertension can develop as a primary disorder, most cases develop secondary to some other condition.

Hypoxia is a common cause of pulmonary hypertension. Unlike the vessels in the systemic circulation, which generally dilate in response to hypoxemia and hypercapnia, the pulmonary vessels constrict. The stimulus for constriction seems to originate in the air spaces in the vicinity of the small branches of the pulmonary arteries. In situations in which certain regions of the lung are hypoventilated, the response is adaptive in that it diverts blood flow away from the poorly ventilated areas to more adequately ventilated portions of the lung. This effect, however, becomes less beneficial as more and more areas of the lung become poorly ventilated. Pulmonary hypertension is a common problem in persons with advanced chronic bronchitis and emphysema. It may also develop at high altitudes in persons with normal lungs. Persons who experience marked hypoxemia during sleep (*i.e.*, those with sleep apnea) often experience marked elevations in pulmonary arterial pressure.

Excessive obliteration or obstruction of the pulmonary vessels can cause pulmonary hypertension. Obliteration of pulmonary vessels can result from vasculitis or connective tissue diseases. In interstitial lung diseases, the fibrotic process may cause obliteration of pulmonary vessels, leading to pulmonary hypertension. Pulmonary emboli are common causes of obstruction. Once initiated, the pulmonary hypertension is self-perpetuating because of hypertrophy and proliferation of vascular smooth muscle.

In conditions such as mitral valve stenosis and left ventricular heart failure, elevation of left atrial pressure is transmitted to the pulmonary circulation and results in a passive elevation of pulmonary arterial pressures. Continued increases in left atrial pressure can lead to medial hypertrophy and intimal thickening of the small pulmonary arteries, causing sustained hypertension.

Increased pulmonary blood flow results from increased flow through left-to-right shunts in congenital heart diseases such as atrial or ventricular septal defects and patent ductus arteriosus. If the high-flow state is allowed to continue, morphologic changes occur in the pulmonary vessels, leading to sustained pulmonary hypertension. The pulmonary vascular changes that occur with congenital heart disorders are discussed in Chapter 19.

Diagnosis is based on radiographic findings, echocardiography, and Doppler ultrasonography. Precise measurement of pulmonary pressures can only be obtained through right heart cardiac catheterization. Treatment measures are directed toward the underlying disorder. Vasodilator therapy may be indicated for some persons.

Primary pulmonary hypertension is a rare, often lethal, form of pulmonary hypertension, the cause of which is unknown. It is characterized by marked intimal fibrosis of the pulmonary arteries and arterioles. The disease can occur at any age, and familial occurrences have been reported. Persons with the disorder usually have a steadily progressive downhill course, with death occurring in 3 to 4 years. The use of the vasodilators hydralazine and diazoxide for the treatment of this form of pulmonary hypertension has met with some degree of success.

Cor Pulmonale

The term *cor pulmonale* refers to heart failure resulting from primary lung disease and longstanding pulmonary hypertension. It involves hypertrophy and the eventual failure of the right ventricle. The manifestations of cor pulmonale include the signs and symptoms of the primary lung disease and the signs of right-sided heart failure (see Chapter 19). The patient has shortness of breath and a productive cough, which becomes worse during periods of heart failure. Failure of the right ventricle and elevation of intrathoracic pressure resulting from airway obstruction cause venous distention and peripheral edema. Plethora (*i.e.*, redness) and cyanosis and warm, moist skin may result from the compensatory polycythemia and desaturation of arterial blood that accompany chronic lung disease. Drowsiness and altered consciousness may occur as the result of carbon dioxide retention. Management of cor pulmonale focuses on the treatment of the lung disease and the heart failure. Low-flow oxygen therapy may be used to reduce the pulmonary hypertension and polycythemia associated with severe hypoxemia due to chronic lung disease.

In summary, pulmonary vascular disorders include pulmonary embolism and pulmonary hypertension. Pulmonary embolism develops when a bloodborne substance lodges in a branch of the pulmonary artery and obstructs blood flow. The embolus can consist of a thrombus, air, fat, or amniotic fluid. The most common form is a thromboemboli arising from the deep venous channels of the lower extremities. Pulmonary hypertension is the elevation of pulmonary arterial pressure. It can be caused by an elevated left atrial pressure, increased pulmonary blood flow, or increased pulmonary vascular resistance secondary to lung disease. The term cor pulmonale describes right heart failure caused by primary pulmonary disease and longstanding pulmonary hypertension.

Impaired Gas Exchange and Respiratory Failure

After you have completed this section of the chapter, you should be able to meet the following objectives:

- Define the terms *hypoxia*, *hypoxemia*, and *hypercapnia*
- Characterize the mechanisms whereby respiratory disorders cause hypoxemia and hypercapnia
- Compare the manifestations of hypoxia and hypercapnia
- Describe the treatment of hypoxia and hypercapnia
- State a general definition for *respiratory failure*
- Describe the pathologic lung changes that occur in adult respiratory distress syndrome and relate them to the clinical manifestations of the disorder

Impaired Gas Exchange

Impaired gas exchange is characterized by inadequate addition of oxygen to the blood and deficient removal of carbon dioxide from the blood. It can result from environmental conditions, lung disease, or neuromuscular problems that impair ventilation or neural control of respiration. The term *hypoxia* refers to a reduction in oxygen supply to the tissues; *hypoxemia*, to a low level of oxygen in the blood; and *hypercapnia* (sometimes referred to as *hypercarbia*), to excess carbon dioxide in the blood. The abbreviation PaO_2 is often used to indicate the partial pressure of oxygen in arterial blood, and PAO_2 is used for the partial pressure of oxygen in alveolar air. The partial pressure of carbon dioxide is designated in a similar way (*i.e.*, $PaCO_2$ arterial; $PACO_2$ alveolar).

In this chapter, the term *hypoxia* is used to describe the reduction in oxygen supply to the tissues and the low level of oxygen in the blood, and the term *hypercapnia* is used to refer to excess carbon dioxide in the blood. Hypoxia and hypercapnia can manifest as acute and chronic conditions, and hypoxia may exist without hypercapnia, or the two conditions may coexist.

Hypoxia

Hypoxia refers to a reduction in tissue oxygenation. It can result from an inadequate amount of oxygen in the air, disease of the respiratory system, alterations in circulatory function, anemia, or the inability of the cells to use oxygen. The focus of the discussion in this chapter is on hypoxia due to respiratory disorders.

Mechanisms

The mechanisms whereby respiratory disorders lead to significant reduction in PO_2 of arterial blood are hypoventilation, diffusion impairment, shunt, and ventilation-perfusion impairment.[22]. A fifth cause of hypoxemia, reduction of the partial pressure of oxygen in the inspired air, only occurs under special circumstances, such as at high altitudes. Often more than one mechanism contributes to hypoxemia in a person with respiratory or cardiac disease.

Hypoventilation. Hypoventilation occurs when the volume of "fresh" air moving into and out of the lung is significantly reduced. Hypoventilation is commonly caused by conditions outside the lung such as depression of the respiratory center (*e.g.*, drug overdose), diseases of the nerves supplying the respiratory muscles (*e.g.*, Gullain-Barré syndrome), disorders of the respiratory muscles (*e.g.*, muscular dystrophy), or thoracic cage disorders (*e.g.*, crushed chest).

Hypoventilation always causes an increase in arterial PCO_2, and it is relieved by the administration of oxygen. The arterial PO_2 falls by 1 mm Hg for every 1 mm Hg rise in PCO_2. Hypoventilation sufficient to double the arterial PCO_2 from 40 to 80 mm Hg decreases PO_2 from 100 to 60 mm Hg.[22]

Impaired Diffusion. Diffusion impairment describes a condition in which oxygen in the alveoli does not equilibrate with that in the pulmonary capillary blood. Impaired diffusion is caused by conditions that alter the thickness or permeability of the alveolar capillary membrane, rather than the time that the blood spends in pulmonary capillaries. Under normal conditions, the alveolar-capillary equilibration of oxygen is rapid, occurring during the first third of the time that blood spends in the pulmonary capillaries. Even under conditions of increased heart rate, as occurs during exercise, there is usually sufficient time for gas exchange to occur.

Conditions that impair diffusion are those that increase the distance from the alveolar gas to the red blood cells or decrease of the permeability of the alveolar capillary membrane to the movement of gases; they include interstitial lung disease, adult respiratory distress syndrome, pulmonary edema, and pneumonia.

Hypoxemia resulting from diffusion impairment can be partially or completely corrected by the administration of 100% oxygen. This occurs because the increase in alveolar oxygen establishes a large alveolar-capillary diffusion gradient that overcomes the resistance of the membrane.

Shunt. Shunt occurs when blood reaches the arterial system without passing through the ventilated portion of the lung. Most shunts, such as those that occur with congenital heart disease, are extrapulmonary. However, a completely unventilated portion of the lung, as occurs with atelectasis, can result in the shunting of blood in the pulmonary circulation. Administration of oxygen usually increases arterial blood gas levels. Because unoxygenated venous blood is being mixed with oxygenated blood, the rise in PO_2 depends on the degree of shunt.

Ventilation-Perfusion Mismatching. Ventilation-perfusion mismatching occurs when areas of the lung are ventilated and not perfused or when areas are perfused and not ventilated. There is some mismatching of ventilation and perfusion even in the normal lung, such as that occurring in the top and bottom of the lung. In disease states, such as COPD, the normal relation between ventilation and perfusion are severely disrupted, causing hypoxemia. The hypoxemia associated with ventilation-perfusion disorders is often exaggerated by conditions such as hypoventilation and decreased cardiac output. For example, sedation can cause hypoventilation in persons with severe COPD, resulting in further impairment of ventilation. Likewise, a decrease in cardiac output because of myocardial infarction can exaggerate the ventilation-perfusion impairment in a person with mild pulmonary edema.

The effects of oxygen administration on arterial PO_2 levels depend on the degree of ventilation-perfusion inequality. Because oxygen administration increases the diffusion gradient in the ventilated portions of the lung, it is usually effective in raising the arterial PO_2.

CHART **24–1**
Signs and Symptoms of Hypoxia

Arterial PO_2 <50 mm Hg	Loss of judgment
Tachycardia	Euphoria
Mild increase in blood pressure	Unruly or combative behavior
Cool and moist skin	Sensory impairment
Confusion	Mental fatigue
Delirium	Drowsiness
Difficulty in problem solving	Stupor and coma (late)
	Hypotension (late)
	Bradycardia (late)

Manifestations

In hypoxia, the blood oxygen level is insufficient to meet the oxidative requirements of body tissues. These tissues vary considerably in their vulnerability to hypoxia; those with the greatest need are the nervous system and heart. The signs and symptoms of hypoxia, which are listed in Chart 24–1, can be grouped into two categories: those resulting from impaired function of vital centers and those resulting from activation of compensatory mechanisms.

Acute hypoxia often produces central nervous system manifestations similar to those of acute alcohol intoxication. There may be personality changes, restlessness, agitated or combative behavior, muscle incoordination, euphoria, impaired judgment, delirium, and eventually, coma. Tachycardia, cool skin (*i.e.*, peripheral vasoconstriction), diaphoresis, and a mild increase in blood pressure result from the recruitment of sympathetic compensatory mechanisms. Although cyanosis may be evident, its presence cannot be relied on. When the hemoglobin concentration is normal, this means that the arterial saturation must be reduced to below 70% and the arterial PO_2 reduced to less than 35 mm Hg before cyanosis develops; it is a late sign of hypoxia. This is especially critical in persons with anemia, because they may be severely hypoxic but lack the hemoglobin necessary for the development of cyanosis. Hypotension and bradycardia often are preterminal events in persons with hypoxia, indicating the failure of compensatory mechanisms.

In conditions of chronic hypoxia, the manifestations may be insidious in onset and attributed to other causes, particularly in chronic lung disease. Decreased sensory function, such as impaired vision or fewer complaints of pain, may be an early sign of worsening hypoxia. This is probably because the involved sensory neurons have the same need for high levels of oxygen as do other parts of the nervous system.

Cyanosis. Cyanosis refers to the bluish discoloration of the skin and mucous membranes that results from an excessive concentration of reduced or deoxygenated hemoglobin in the small blood vessels. It usually is most marked in the lips, nail beds, ears, and cheeks. The degree of cyanosis is modified by the amount of cutaneous pigment, skin thickness, and the state of the cutaneous capillaries. Cyanosis is more difficult to distinguish in persons with dark skin and in areas of the body with increased skin thickness. A concentration of about 5 g/dl of deoxygenated hemoglobin is required in the circulating blood for cyanosis. The absolute quantity of reduced hemoglobin, rather than the relative quantity, is important in producing cyanosis. Persons with anemia and low hemoglobin levels are less likely to exhibit cyanosis (because they have less hemoglobin to deoxygenate), even though they may be relatively hypoxic because of their decreased ability to transport oxygen, than persons who have high hemoglobin concentrations. Someone with a high hemoglobin level because of polycythemia may be cyanotic without being hypoxic.

Cyanosis can be divided into two types: central or peripheral. In central cyanosis, there is an increased amount of deoxygenated hemoglobin or abnormal hemoglobin derivative in the arterial blood, and the mucous membranes and skin are affected. Abnormal hemoglobin derivatives include methemoglobin, in which the nitrite ion reacts with hemoglobin. Because methemoglobin has a low affinity for oxygen, large doses of nitrites can result in cyanosis and tissue hypoxia. Although nitrites are used in treating angina, the therapeutic dose is too small to cause cyanosis. Sodium nitrite is used as a curing agent for meat. In nursing infants, the intestinal flora is capable of converting significant amounts of inorganic nitrate (*e.g.*, from well water) into nitrite ion.[46]

Peripheral cyanosis is caused by slowing of blood flow to an area of the body, with increased extraction of oxygen from the blood. It results from vasoconstriction and diminished peripheral blood flow, as occurs with cold exposure, shock, congestive heart failure, and peripheral vascular disease. Acute arterial obstruction to an extremity, such as with an embolus or arterial spasm (*i.e.*, Raynaud's phenomenon, discussed in Chapter 17), usually presents with pallor and coldness, although there may be cyanosis.

Clubbing of the Fingers. Clubbing of the fingers involves the bulbous enlargement of the distal segment of the digit because of an increase in soft tissue (Fig. 24–10). The condition may be hereditary or acquired. Acquired clubbing of the fingers is associated with various conditions that impair oxygen delivery, including

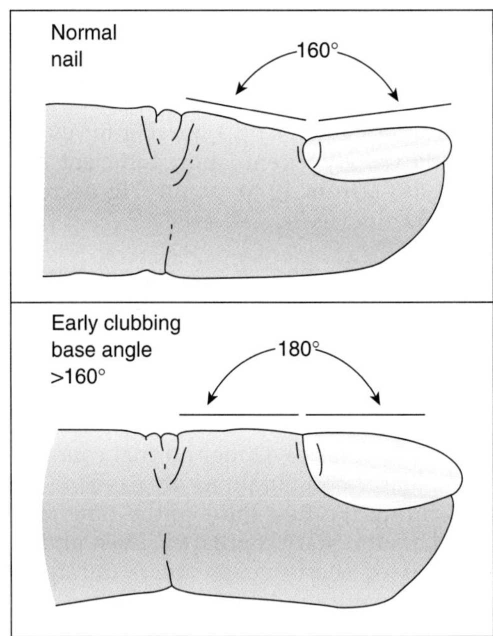

Figure 24–10
Clubbing of the finger. There normally is an obtuse angle of about 160 degrees between the base of the nail and the adjacent dorsal surface of the finger; with clubbing, this angle exceeds 180 degrees.

cyanotic heart disease and chronic lung disease and some gastrointestinal disorders, such as cirrhosis of the liver. Although the mechanisms of clubbing are unclear, it appears to be a response to a substance (presumably one that circulates in the blood) that causes dilation of the vessels of the fingertips.

Compensatory Mechanisms

The body adapts to hypoxia by increased ventilation, pulmonary vasoconstriction, and increased production of red blood cells. Hyperventilation results from the hypoxic stimulation of the chemoreceptors. Increased production of red blood cells results from the release of erythropoietin from the kidneys in response to hypoxia (see Chapter 8). Polycythemia increases the red blood cell concentration and the oxygen-carrying capacity of the blood. Pulmonary vasoconstriction occurs as a local response to alveolar hypoxia; it increases pulmonary arterial pressure and improves the matching of ventilation and blood flow. Other adaptive mechanisms include a shift to the right in the oxygen dissociation curve as a means of increasing oxygen release to the tissues (see Chapter 22). Elevation of intracellular levels of oxidative enzymes increases the efficiency of oxygen use.

Diagnosis and Treatment

Diagnosis of hypoxia is based on clinical observation and diagnostic measures of oxygen levels. The analysis of arterial blood gases provides a direct measure of the oxygen content of the blood and is a good indicator of the lungs' ability to oxygenate the blood. Continuous mixed venous oxygen saturation ($S\bar{v}O_2$) can be monitored using a special type of pulmonary artery catheter.[47] This method, which measures the mixed venous blood that is being returned to the lungs, reflects the use of oxygen by the peripheral tissues. Arterial blood gases and $S\bar{v}O_2$ are often monitored in critically ill patients. Both measurements are invasive and require direct sampling of the patient's blood through a peripheral arterial catheter (for blood gases) or a pulmonary artery catheter (for $S\bar{v}O_2$). Diagnosis of hypercapnia is based on blood gas measurements and end-tidal volume carbon dioxide tension (*i.e.*, capnometry).

There are two noninvasive methods for oxygen assessment: the transcutaneous sensor method and the pulse oximeter.[48] Transcutaneous oxygen monitoring uses an oxygen electrode. The electrode and covering membrane allow oxygen to diffuse through the skin and be measured. The pulse oximeter uses light-emitting diodes and combines plethysmography (*i.e.*, changes in light absorbance and vasodilatation) with spectrophotometry.[48] Spectrophotometry uses a red-wavelength light that passes through oxygenated hemoglobin and is absorbed by deoxygenated hemoglobin and an infrared-wavelength light that is absorbed by oxygenated hemoglobin and passes through deoxygenated hemoglobin. Sensors that can be placed on the ear, finger, toe, or forehead are available. These methods, although not as accurate as the invasive methods, provide a means for monitoring oxygen levels and are useful indicators of respiratory and circulatory status.

The treatment of hypoxia focuses on correcting the problem causing impaired gas exchange and on oxygen administration. Oxygen may be delivered by nasal cannula or mask. It may also be administered directly into an endotracheal or tracheostomy tube. A high-flow administration system is one in which the flow rate and reserve capacity are sufficient to provide all the inspired air. A low-flow oxygen system delivers less than the total inspired air. The oxygen must be humidified as it is being administered. The flow rate (measured in liters per minute) is based on the arterial PO_2. The rate must be carefully monitored in persons with chronic lung disease, because increases in PO_2 above 60 mm Hg are likely to depress the ventilatory drive. There is also the danger of oxygen toxicity with high concentrations of oxygen. Continuous breathing of oxygen at high concentrations can lead to diffuse parenchymal lung injury. Persons with healthy lungs begin to experience respiratory symptoms ranging from cough, sore throat, substernal distress, nasal congestion, and painful inspiration after breathing pure oxygen for 14 to 16 hours.[49]

Hypercapnia

Hypercapnia refers to an increase in the carbon dioxide content of the blood. It is a well-recognized consequence of a number of diseases that involve the lungs and those that involve the neuromuscular, chest wall, circulatory, and neural control components of the respiratory system.

Mechanisms

Lung disease contributes to the retention of carbon dioxide by reducing the effective alveolar ventilation, even when total ventilation is maintained. This occurs because a region of lung is not perfused and gas exchange cannot take place or because an area of the lung is not being ventilated. In persons with chronic lung disease, ventilation-perfusion mismatch is an important factor contributing to hypercapnia. Maintaining a high ventilation rate effectively prevents hypercapnia but also increases the work of breathing.

The carbon dioxide level in the blood, or PCO_2, is proportional to carbon dioxide production and inversely related to alveolar ventilation. In the clinical setting, four factors contribute to hypercapnia: alterations in carbon dioxide production, disturbances in the gas exchange function of the lung, abnormalities in the respiratory function of the chest wall and respiratory muscles, and changes in the neural control of respiration.[50] The diffusing capacity of carbon dioxide is 20 times that of oxygen; therefore, hypercapnia is observed only in situations of hypoventilation sufficient to cause hypoxia.

Increased Carbon Dioxide Production. Changes in the metabolic rate resulting from an increase in activity level, fever, or disease can have profound effects on carbon dioxide production. For example, carbon dioxide production increases 13% for every 1°C increase in temperature above normal.[50] Alveolar ventilation usually rises proportionally with these changes, and hypercapnia occurs only when this increase is inappropriate.

Interest has been focused on the effect of carbohydrate metabolism on carbon dioxide production. The respiratory quotient (RQ), which is the ratio of carbon dioxide production to oxygen consumption (RQ = CO_2 production/O_2 consumption), varies with the type of food metabolized. A characteristic of carbohydrate metabolism is an RQ of 1.0, with equal carbon dioxide being produced and oxygen being consumed. Because fats contain less oxygen than carbohydrates, their oxidation produces less carbon dioxide (RQ = 0.7). The metabolism of pure proteins (RQ = 0.81) results in the production of more carbon dioxide than the metabolism of fat but less than the metabolism of carbohydrates. The type of food that is eaten or the types of nutrients that are delivered through enteral feedings (*i.e.*, through a tube placed in the small intestine) or parenteral nutrition (*i.e.*, through a venous catheter placed in the central vena cava) may influence PCO_2 levels. Portable devices and metabolic carts that use indirect calorimetry to determine the RQ and energy requirements are available for use in the clinical setting.[51]

In persons who receive a high glucose load in association with total parenteral nutrition, the RQ can rise to a level of 1 or more.[25] Persons with adequate respiratory function can increase their alveolar ventilation proportional to the increased PCO_2 production. Hypercapnic respiratory failure can occur in persons who cannot adequately increase their ventilation. It has been suggested that such persons receive a larger proportion of nonprotein calories in the form of fat emulsions because these emulsions are associated with a lower rate of carbon dioxide production.[50]

Disorders of Respiratory Muscle Function. Respiratory muscle fatigue can contribute to carbon dioxide retention in persons with various primary respiratory diseases and in those with neuromuscular disorders. In these persons, respiratory muscle fatigue develops when energy requirements exceed the energy supply. A number of factors increase energy requirements or decrease the energy supply. The energy demands of the respiratory muscles are increased by high levels of ventilation or by factors that increase the work of breathing, such as high levels of airway resistance. The energy supply depends on blood flow and the oxygen content of the blood. Low cardiac output, anemia, and decreased oxygen saturation contribute to a decreased energy supply and increase the likelihood of respiratory muscle fatigue. With malnutrition, the energy stores of the muscles are diminished, and there may be structural changes in the muscle as well. Electrolyte imbalances, especially hypokalemia and hypophosphatemia, contribute to respiratory muscle weakness.[50]

Disorders of Neural Control of Respiration. The respiratory center, which activates the muscles of respiration, is a crucial determinant of ventilation and adequate elimination of carbon dioxide. It is composed of widely dispersed groups of neurons located in the medulla oblongata and pons (see Chapter 22). Carbon dioxide crosses the blood-brain barrier with ease. Carbon dioxide does not stimulate ventilation directly; instead, it does so by reacting with water to form carbonic acid, which dissociates into hydrogen ions that have a potent direct stimulatory effect. The excitation of the respiratory center by carbon dioxide is greatest during the first 1 to 2 days that blood levels are elevated, but it gradually declines over the next 1 to 2 days, decreasing to about one fifth the initial effect.[52] Part of this decline results from renal compensatory mechanisms that readjust the blood pH by increasing blood bicarbonate levels. In persons with respiratory problems that cause chronic hypoxia and hypercapnia, the peripheral chemoreceptors that monitor blood oxygen levels become the driving force for ventilation. Administration of high-flow oxygen to these persons can abolish the input from these peripheral receptors, causing a decrease in alveolar ventilation and a further rise in PCO_2 levels.

Manifestations

Hypercapnia affects the respiratory system, renal function, neural function, cardiovascular function, and acid-base balance. The body adapts to chronic increases in blood levels of carbon dioxide; persons with chronic hypercapnia may not develop symptoms until the PCO_2 is markedly elevated. Elevated levels of PCO_2 are characterized by respiratory acidosis, as discussed in Chapter 27. The body adapts to increased PCO_2 levels by metabolic adjustments, such as renal bicarbonate retention. As long as the pH is in an acceptable range, the main complications result from the associated hypoxia.

Carbon dioxide has a direct vasodilatory effect on many blood vessels and a sedative effect on the nervous system. When the cerebral vessels are dilated, headache develops. The conjunctivae are hyperemic, and the skin flushed. Hypercapnia has nervous system effects similar to those of an anesthetic—hence the term *carbon dioxide narcosis*. There is progressive somnolence, disorientation, and if the condition is untreated, coma. Mild to moderate increases in blood pressure are common. Air hunger and rapid breathing occur when alveolar PCO_2 levels rise to about 60 to 75 mm Hg; as PCO_2 levels reach 80 to 100 mm Hg, the person becomes lethargic and sometimes becomes semicomatose. Anesthesia and death can result when PCO_2 levels reach 100 to 150 mm Hg.[52] The signs and symptoms of hypercapnia are summarized in Chart 24–2.

CHART 24-2
Signs and Symptoms of Hypercapnia

Increased PCO_2
Headache
Conjunctival hyperemia
Flushed skin
Increased sedation
- Drowsiness
- Disorientation
- Coma

Tachycardia
Diaphoresis
Mild to moderate increase in blood pressure

Diagnosis and Treatment

The diagnosis of hypercapnia is based on physiologic manifestations, arterial pH, and blood gas levels. Specific tests of respiratory function are discussed in Chapter 22. Therapy for hypercapnia is directed at decreasing the work of breathing and improving the ventilation-perfusion balance. Intermittent rest therapy, such as nocturnal negative-pressure ventilation, applied to hypercapnic patients with chronic obstructive disease or chest wall disease may be effective in increasing the strength and endurance of the respiratory muscle and improving the PCO_2. Respiratory muscle retraining aimed at improving the respiratory muscles, their endurance, or both has been used to improve exercise tolerance and diminish the likelihood of respiratory fatigue.

TABLE 24-3
Blood Gases in Respiratory Failure Compared with Normal Values

Arterial Blood Gas Value	Normal Value	Respiratory Failure
PO_2	>80 mm Hg	≤50 mm Hg
PCO_2	35–45 mm Hg	≥50 mm Hg

Respiratory Failure

Respiratory failure occurs when the lungs are unable to adequately oxygenate the blood or prevent undue retention of carbon dioxide even at rest. It can develop acutely in persons whose lungs previously had been normal or may be superimposed on chronic disease of the lung or chest wall.

There is no absolute definition of the levels of arterial PO_2 and PCO_2 that indicate respiratory failure. As a general rule, *respiratory failure* refers to a PO_2 level of 50 mm Hg or less and a PCO_2 level greater than 50 mm Hg. These values are not reliable when dealing with persons who have chronic lung disease, because many of these persons are alert and functioning with blood gas levels outside this range. Table 24–3 compares the normal values for blood gases with those of respiratory failure.

Causes

Respiratory failure is not a specific disease. It is associated with a number of disorders in which the lungs fail to deliver sufficient oxygen to the arterial blood or to remove sufficient carbon dioxide. Three types of conditions contribute to the hypoxia in respiratory failure: hypoventilation, impaired diffusion across the alveolocapillary membrane, and mismatching of ventilation and perfusion. These conditions include impaired ventilation caused by upper airway obstruction, weakness or paralysis of the respiratory muscles, chest wall injury, and disease of the pulmonary airways and lungs. The causes of respiratory failure are summarized in Table 24–4; many are discussed in other parts of the text.

Manifestations

Respiratory failure may be seen in previously healthy persons as the result of acute disease or trauma involving the respiratory system, or it may develop in the course of a chronic respiratory disease. The presenting signs and symptoms are different in each of these situa-

TABLE 24-4
Causes of Respiratory Failure

Category of Impairment	Examples
Impaired Ventilation	
Upper airway obstruction	Laryngospasm Foreign-body aspiration Tumor of the upper airways Infection of the upper airways (*e.g.*, epiglottitis)
Weakness or paralysis of the respiratory muscles	Drug overdose Injury to the spinal cord Poliomyelitis Guillain-Barré syndrome Muscular dystrophy Disease of the brain stem
Chest wall injury	Rib fracture Burn eschar
Impaired Matching of Ventilation and Perfusion	Chronic obstructive lung disease Restrictive lung disease Severe pneumonia Atelectasis
Impaired Diffusion	
Pulmonary edema	Left heart failure Inhalation of toxic materials
Respiratory distress syndrome	Respiratory distress syndrome in the neonate Adult respiratory distress syndrome (shock lung)

tions. The common manifestations of respiratory failure are hypoxia and hypercapnia. Various types of respiratory failure are associated with different degrees of hypoxia and carbon dioxide retention. In respiratory disorders that impair diffusion across the alveolocapillary membrane, hypoxia becomes severe, whereas arterial PCO_2 decreases or remains normal because carbon dioxide is more soluble in the alveolocapillary membrane than oxygen. In conditions such as chronic obstructive pulmonary disease, in which respiratory failure is superimposed on lung disease, severe mismatching of ventilation and perfusion often results in both hypoxia and hypercapnia.

Treatment

Treatment of respiratory failure is directed toward correcting the cause and relieving the hypoxia and hypercapnia. A number of treatment modalities are available, including the establishment of an airway, use of bronchodilators, and antibiotics for respiratory infections. Controlled oxygen therapy and mechanical ventilation are used in treating blood gas abnormalities associated with respiratory failure.

When alveolar ventilation is inadequate to maintain PO_2 or PCO_2 levels because of respiratory or neurologic failure, mechanical ventilation may be life saving. A nasotracheal, orotracheal, or tracheotomy tube is inserted into the trachea to provide the patient with the airway needed for mechanical ventilation. There are two basic types of positive-pressure mechanical ventilators: pressure-cycled units and volume-cycled units. The pressure-cycled unit delivers a tidal volume determined by the airway pressure while the flow rate is being controlled. The volume-cycled ventilator delivers a preselected tidal volume while the pressure is monitored. The tidal volume and respiratory rate are adjusted to maintain ventilation at a given minute volume. Ventilators are capable of functioning in assist-control method, in which the ventilator delivers a breath triggered by the patient or independently if such an effort does not occur; an intermittent mandatory ventilation, in which the patient receives periodic positive-pressure ventilation from the ventilator at a preset volume and rate; and pressure-support ventilation, in which the ventilator is set to deliver a set pressure rather than volume to augment each spontaneous respiratory effort.[22,53] Ventilators can also be programed to positive end-expiratory pressure (PEEP) or continuous positive airway pressure (CPAP) in spontaneous breathing patients.

A third type of ventilator (*i.e.*, iron lung, Cuirass, Poncho, and Body Wrap) uses negative pressure to expand the chest. These ventilators do not require an artificial airway. They are not used in the treatment of acute respiratory failure but are occasionally used for persons with chronic neuromuscular disorders who need to be ventilated for months or years.

Adult Respiratory Distress Syndrome

Adult respiratory distress syndrome (ARDS), first described in 1967, is an extreme form of noncardiac pulmonary edema. It is the final common pathway through which many serious localized and systemic disorders produce diffuse lung injury. ARDS affects about 150,000 to 200,000 persons each year; at least 50% to 60% of these persons die, despite the most sophisticated intensive care.

CHART **24-3**
*Conditions in Which Adult Respiratory Distress Syndrome Can Develop**

Aspiration
Gastric acid
Near-drowning

Reaction to Drugs and Toxins
Chlordiazepoxide
Heroin
Methadone
Propoxyphene
Chloroform
Colchicine
Barbiturates
Inhaled gases
- Ammonia
- Phosgene
- Ozone
- Oxygen (high concentrations)
- Smoke

Hematologic Disorders
Multiple blood transfusions
Disseminated intravascular clotting
Exposure to cardiopulmonary bypass

Infectious Causes
Bacterial pneumonia
Fungal and *Pneumocystis carinii* pneumonias
Gram-negative sepsis
Viral pneumonia

Immune Reactions
Anaphylactic shock
Allergic reactions to inhaled substances

Metabolic Disorders
Diabetic ketoacidosis
Uremia

Trauma
Burns
Fat embolus
Heat trauma
Chest trauma and lung injury
Shock

*This list is not intended to be inclusive.

The exact cause of ARDS is unknown. It is thought to result from injury to the microcirculation (*i.e.*, small blood vessels and capillaries) of the lung. Numerous insults are associated with its development. The term *shock lung* (see Chapter 20) has been used to describe the respiratory distress syndrome associated with trauma and hypovolemic or septic shock. It may also result from aspiration of gastric contents, major trauma (with or without fat emboli), sepsis secondary to pulmonary or nonpulmonary infections, acute pancreatitis, hematologic disorders, metabolic events, and reactions to drugs and toxins (Chart 24–3).[54–56]

It is not known whether ARDS results from several distinct pathogenic mechanisms that operate to cause a similar pattern of injury or a similar pattern of injury is triggered by different mechanisms. Many investigators believe that neutrophils play a central role in the pathogenesis of ARDS. Neutrophils can synthesize and release products that are capable of tissue injury, including proteolytic enzymes, toxic oxygen species (free radicals; see Chapter 2), and phospholipid products.

Although a number of conditions may lead to ARDS, they all produce similar pathologic lung changes that include diffuse alveolocapillary injury with increased permeability and decreased surfactant production. The increased permeability of the alveolocapillary membrane permits fluid, protein, and blood cells to move out of the vascular compartment into the interstitium and alveoli of the lung. The resultant pulmonary edema leads to intrapulmonary shunting of blood and profound hypoxia. The mechanism of surfactant abnormality is less well known. It could result from inactivation of surfactant by plasma inhibitors or injury to the surfactant-producing alveolar cells. The type II alveolar cells, which produce surfactant, have the capacity to transport sodium and thereby regulate the clearance of alveolar fluid. When the cells are injured, the clearance of fluid declines, with subsequent flooding of the alveolar space. As these changes take place, the lung stiffens and becomes more difficult to inflate, and the work of breathing increases. Progression of the disease is characterized by formation of hyaline membranes and fibrotic thickening of the alveolar walls, compromising the diffusion of respiratory gases.

Clinically, the syndrome consists of progressive respiratory distress, an increase in respiratory rate, and signs of respiratory failure. Radiologic findings usually show extensive bilateral consolidation of the lung tissue. Severe hypoxia persists despite increased inspired oxygen levels.

The treatment goals in ARDS are to supply oxygen to vital organs and provide supportive care until the condition causing the pathologic process has been reversed and the lungs have had a chance to heal. Assisted ventilation using high concentrations of oxygen may be required to overcome the hypoxia. PEEP breathing, which increases the pressure in the airways during expiration, may be used to assist in reinflating the collapsed areas of the lung and to improve the matching of ventilation and perfusion. There has been interest in the use of NSAIDs (*e.g.*, ibuprofen), surfactant replacement, antioxidant agents, and other blockers of potential mediators of injury. The use of corticosteroid therapy is controversial.

In summary, the lungs enable inhaled air to come in proximity to the blood flowing through the pulmonary capillaries, so that the exchange of gases between the internal environment of the body and the external environment can take place. Hypoxia refers to an acute or chronic reduction in tissue oxygenation. It can occur as the result of hypoventilation, diffusion impairment, shunt, and ventilation-perfusion impairment. Acute hypoxia incites sympathetic nervous system responses such as tachycardia and produces symptoms that are similar to those of alcohol intoxication. In conditions of chronic hypoxia, the manifestations may be insidious in onset and attributed to other causes, particularly in chronic lung disease. The development of cyanosis requires a concentration of 5 g/dl of deoxygenated hemoglobin.

Hypercapnia refers to an increase in carbon dioxide levels. In the clinical setting, four factors contribute to hypercapnia: alterations in carbon dioxide production, disturbance in the gas exchange function of the lungs, abnormalities in respiratory function of the chest wall and respiratory muscles, and changes in neural control of respiration. The manifestations of hypercapnia consist of those associated with the vasodilation of blood vessels, including those in the brain, and depression of the central nervous system (*e.g.*, carbon dioxide narcosis).

Respiratory failure is a condition in which the lungs fail to adequately oxygenate the blood or to prevent undue retention of carbon dioxide. The causes of respiratory failure are many. It may arise acutely in persons with previously healthy lungs, or it may be superimposed in chronic lung disease. Respiratory failure is defined as a PO_2 of 50 mm Hg or less and a PCO_2 of 50 mm Hg or more.

ARDS is an extreme form of noncardiogenic pulmonary edema that results in respiratory failure. The condition can be caused by a number of serious localized and systemic disorders that damage the alveolocapillary membrane of the lung. It results in interstitial edema of lung tissue, an increase in surface tension caused by inactivation of surfactant, collapse of the alveolar structures, a stiff and noncompliant lung that is difficult to inflate, and impaired diffusion of the respiratory gases with severe hypoxia that is resistant to oxygen therapy.

Breathing Disorders

After you have completed this section of the chapter, you should be able to meet the following objectives:

- Define *sleep apnea*
- Compare the respiratory changes that occur in each of the four stages of sleep
- State the signs and symptoms of sleep apnea and differentiate between central and obstructive sleep apnea
- Cite four general causes of hyperventilation syndrome
- State the signs and symptoms of hyperventilation syndrome
- Describe the diagnostic and treatment methods used in sleep apnea and hyperventilation syndrome

Breathing involves the controlled movement of gases into and out of the lungs. It is normally regulated in relation to need, increasing during periods of activity and decreasing during sleep. Two disorders of breathing are sleep apnea and the hyperventilation syndrome.

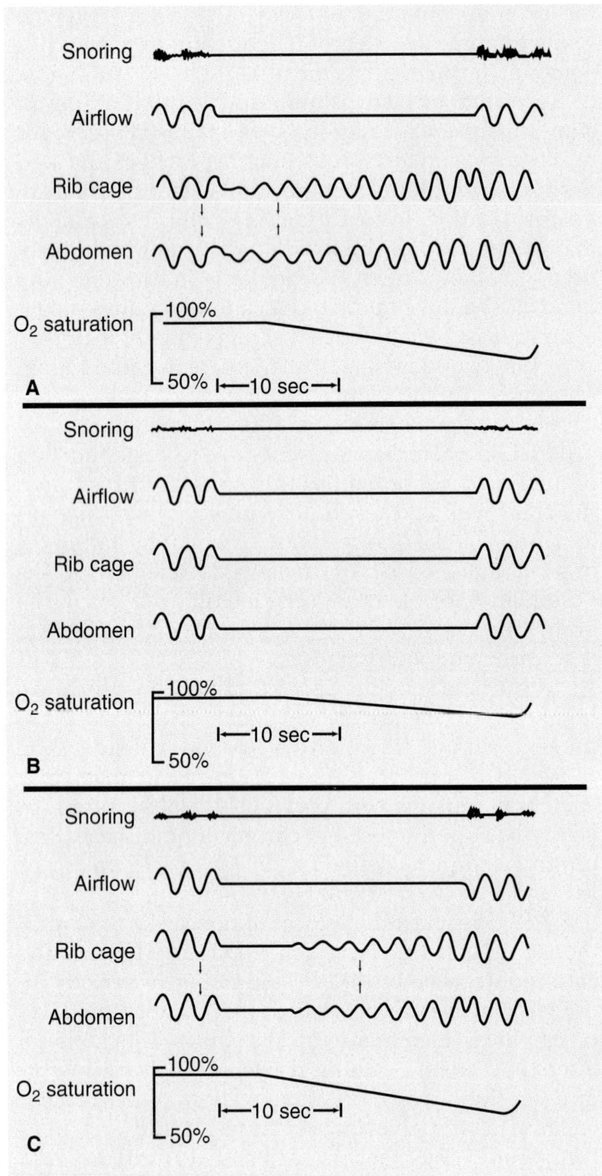

Figure 24–11
Types of sleep apnea. (**A**) Obstructive apnea is characterized by loud intermittent snoring, complete cessation of airflow, paradoxic movement of the chest and abdomen, and moderate to severe oxygen desaturation. (**B**) In central apnea, snoring and simultaneous cessation of airflow and respiratory effort are absent. Only mild to moderate oxygen desaturation usually is present. (**C**) In mixed apnea, an initial central apnea is followed by an obstructive apnea that usually produces moderate to severe oxygen desaturation.

Sleep Apnea

Sleep apnea is the cessation of airflow through the nose and mouth for 10 seconds or longer (Fig. 24–11). The diagnosis of sleep apnea depends on the occurrence of 30 or more apneic periods during 7 hours of sleep.[57] The apneic periods typically last for 15 to 120 seconds, and some persons may have as many as 500 apneic periods per night.

Respiration normally changes during sleep. Stages 1 and 2 of non–rapid eye movement (non-REM) sleep are characterized by a pattern of breathing in which there is cyclic waning and waxing of tidal volume and respiratory rate, which may include brief periods (5 to 15 seconds) of apnea. This pattern is called *periodic breathing*. Although the amount of periodic breathing that occurs during the first two stages of non-REM sleep differs among healthy persons, it is more common in persons older than 40 years.[58] After sleep is stabilized during stages 3 and 4 of non-REM sleep, breathing becomes more regular. During slow-wave sleep, ventilation usually is 1 to 2 L/minute less than during quiet wakefulness; the PCO_2 levels are 2 to 8 mm Hg greater; the PO_2 levels are 5 to 10 mm Hg less; and the pH is 0.03 to 0.05 units less.[59] Control of breathing during non-REM sleep is dominated by automatic (*i.e.*, involuntary reflex) control mechanisms—responses to hypercapnia, hypoxia, and lung inflation are intact and critically important to maintaining ventilation.

During REM sleep, respiration becomes irregular (but not periodic) and may include short periods of apnea. Breathing during REM sleep has many of the features of the voluntary type of control that integrates breathing with voluntary acts such as talking, walking, and swallowing. Automatic control of breathing remains during REM sleep, but its influence is diminished.

All skeletal muscles except the diaphragm undergo a decrease in tone during sleep. This loss of muscle tone is most pronounced during REM sleep. In the awake state, intercostal muscle activity stiffens the rib cage. With the absence of this tone during sleep, the negative intrapleural pressure caused by contraction of the diaphragm can cause paradoxical motion of the rib cage (*i.e.*, the rib cage moves inward during inspiration rather than outward) and a decrease in functional residual capacity. The loss of tone in the upper airways can cause airway obstruction. Negative airway pressure produced by the contraction of the diaphragm brings the vocal cords together, collapses the pharyngeal wall, and sucks the tongue back into the throat. Airway collapse is accentuated in persons with conditions that cause narrowing of the upper airway or weakness of the throat muscles.

Types of Sleep Apnea

Sleep apnea can be classified into three types: obstructive, central, and mixed. Obstructive apnea is caused by the obstruction of the upper airway. With central apnea, the respiratory drive ceases and there is no movement of the rib cage or abdominal muscle. Mixed apnea constitutes a mixture of central and obstructive apnea. Because breathing seems to be controlled by different mechanisms during REM and non-REM sleep, different causes are associated with the different types of sleep apnea. Figure 24–11 shows the variations in airflow and rib cage and abdominal movements in the three types of sleep apnea.

Obstructive Sleep Apnea. Obstructive sleep apnea typically is associated with obesity and disorders that compromise the patency of the airway. Conditions known to predispose to obstructive sleep apnea are male sex, increasing age, obesity, and hypothyroidism. Alcohol and other drugs that depress the central nervous system seem to increase the severity of obstructive apneic episodes. It is most common in middle-aged men. Although androgens are suspected of contributing to the disorder, their mechanism of action is unknown. The pickwickian syndrome, named after the fat boy in Charles Dickens' *The Posthumous Papers of the Pickwick Club*, published in 1837, is characterized by obesity, hypersomnolence, periodic breathing, hypoxemia, and right-sided heart failure.

Obstructive sleep apnea is characterized by loud snoring interrupted by periods of silence. Abnormal gross motor movements during sleep are common. In many cases, the snoring precedes by many years the onset of other signs of sleep apnea. Many persons complain of morning headache and nausea and persistent daytime sleepiness. Hypersomnolence can lead to occupational and driving accidents. Psychologic problems associated with impotence, intellectual deterioration, and depression are also part of the symptom complex. The signs and symptoms of sleep apnea are summarized in Chart 24–4. In children, a decline in school performance may be the only indication of the problem.

In addition to the sleep disturbances, cardiovascular problems are associated with sleep apnea syndromes. A number of cardiac arrhythmias have been observed in persons with sleep apnea. Frequent apneic periods may result in increased pulmonary and systemic blood pressures. In severe cases, pulmonary hypertension, polycythemia, and cor pulmonale may develop.

CHART 24-4
Signs and Symptoms of Sleep Apnea

- Noisy snoring
- Insomnia
- Abnormal movements during sleep
- Morning headaches
- Excessive daytime sleepiness
- Intellectual and personality changes
- Sexual impotence
- Systemic hypertension
- Pulmonary hypertension, cor pulmonale
- Polycythemia

Central Sleep Apnea. Central sleep apnea is associated with disorders that affect the central nervous system and respiratory neurons, such as encephalitis, brain stem infarction, and bulbar poliomyelitis. With central sleep apnea, sleep is difficult to maintain, and several awakenings occur during the night. There may be some daytime fatigue, depression, and impaired sexual functioning. In contrast to persons with obstructive sleep apnea, persons with central sleep apnea are usually of normal weight.

Diagnosis

Sleep apnea usually is suspected from a history of snoring, disturbed sleep, and daytime sleepiness. A definitive diagnosis is accomplished with sleep studies done in a sleep laboratory using polysomnography.[59,60] This procedure consists of electroencephalogram and electro-oculography to determine the sleep stages; monitoring of the airflow; an ECG to detect arrhythmias; impedance pneumography, intercostal electromyography, or esophageal manometry to monitor respiratory effort; and oximetry (ear or finger) or transcutaneous oxygen monitoring to detect changes in oxygen saturation. It is recommended that the evaluation of sleep apnea also include a multiple sleep latency test (MSLT). The MSLT determines the amount of daytime hypersomnolence that is present and excludes narcolepsy, a condition characterized by uncontrolled periods of daytime sleep. The study is begun 1.5 to 2 hours after the person's usual nighttime sleep. Polysomnographic recordings are made during three to five naps spaced 2 hours apart during the day. Special attention is paid to how much time elapses from when the lights go out to the first evidence of sleep. This interval is called *sleep latency*. The MSLT can be used along with nighttime polysomnography to monitor the response to therapy.

Treatment

The treatment of sleep apnea is determined by the type of apnea. Weight loss often is beneficial for persons with obstructive apnea. In many instances, the disordered breathing events are confined to the supine sleeping position, so that training the person to sleep in the lateral position may help to alleviate the problem. The application of CPAP to the nasal airways at night has helped in treating obstructive sleep apnea. This method uses an occlusive nasal mask or a device that fits into the nares, an expiratory valve and tubing, and a blower system to generate positive pressure. The main difficulty with nasal CPAP is that many persons find it unacceptable. Common complaints include dryness of the mouth, claustrophobia, and noise.

Several medications are used in the treatment of sleep apnea. Protriptyline, a nonsedative tricyclic antidepressant that reduces REM sleep, has been used successfully in some persons. Medroxyprogesterone, which is a progestational agent with respiratory stimulant action, may also be used. This drug appears to benefit persons with obesity hypoventilation, mainly by lowering daytime PCO_2, with a subsequent improvement in PO_2. In cases of central sleep apnea, various medications have been used to increase the central respiratory drive, including theophylline, acetazolamide, clomipramine, and medroxyprogesterone.

Several surgical procedures have been used to correct airway obstruction, including nasal septoplasty (*i.e.*, repair of the nasal septum) and uvulopalatopharyngoplasty (*i.e.*, excision of excess soft tissue on the palate, uvula, and posterior pharyngeal wall). Both of these procedures have met with limited success. Severe cases of sleep apnea may require a tracheostomy (*i.e.*, surgical placement of a tube into the trachea for the purpose of maintaining an open airway). The tracheostomy tube remains stoppered during the day and is opened during the night.

Hyperventilation Syndrome

Hyperventilation syndrome involves overbreathing, reduction in PCO_2, and respiratory alkalosis. In 1871, De Costa provided the first account of the syndrome in the medical literature when he reported on the cases of 300 Civil War soldiers affected with the disorder.[61,62] The disorder subsequently has been labeled soldier's heart, irritable heart, De Costa's syndrome, and neurocirculatory asthenia. De Costa noticed that the affected soldier "got out of breath, could not keep up with his comrades, was annoyed with dizziness and palpitation, and with pain in the chest; his accouterments oppressed him, and all through this he appeared well and healthy." The nervous manifestations of the syndrome were "headache, dizziness, and disturbed sleep." Removal from the stress of active duty along with enforced rest reduced the symptoms, but even with removal from active duty, the "irritability of the heart remained."[61]

Causes

The causes of hyperventilation syndrome have been categorized into four groups: organic, physiologic, emotional, and habitual (*i.e.*, faulty breathing habits). Organic causes include drug effects and central nervous system lesions, such as meningitis. Responses to high altitude, heat, and exercise constitute physiologic causes of hyperventilation. Emotional states that predispose to hyperventilation are hysteria, anxiety, depression, and anger. Faulty breathing habits such as rapid and shallow breathing are often linked to emotional states. Although stress may trigger the initial event, anxiety and fear over the symptoms may perpetuate the syndrome. Because the symptoms of hyperventilation syndrome commonly involve the heart and head, the person experiences intense anxiety, often accompanied by a fear of death or of losing control. The condition occurs in children and adults.[63]

Manifestations

Hyperventilation syndrome commonly produces such symptoms as headache, dyspnea, numbness and tingling sensations, dizziness and lightheadedness, chest pain, palpitations, and sometimes, syncope. Many persons complain of dyspnea and of being unable to take a full deep breath. Persons with a full constellation of the syndrome breathe with rapid, shallow breaths marked by irregularity in the depth and rate of respiration. Sighing is common. Those who hyperventilate are primarily thoracic rather than abdominal breathers. They tend to use their upper chest wall intercostal muscles to breathe, which may cause dull aching soreness in the left precordial area, mimicking angina. It has been suggested that the alkalosis associated with hyperventilation syndrome can induce coronary artery spasm in persons with Prinzmetal's angina and in some persons with atherosclerotic coronary artery disease.[64,65] It has also been observed that ST-wave changes can occur with hyperventilation.

Many persons afflicted with hyperventilation syndrome do not have a continuously symptomatic state but rather recurrences of symptoms with or without recognizable provocative stresses. Others have a more chronic form of the disorder in which the respiratory center is reset to enable low levels of PCO_2 to persist despite a normal pH. This may explain the chronicity of the disorder and the ease with which symptoms associated with hyperventilation can be provoked in persons who are chronically hypocapnic. Sympathetic nervous system stimulation provokes a hyperventilatory response and may increase the occurrence of symptoms in persons with chronic hyperventilation problems.

Panic disorder and hyperventilation syndrome have similar manifestations. Hyperventilation has been demonstrated in persons with panic episodes, and panic is a frequent manifestation of hyperventilation. It has been suggested that some persons with either diagnosis have the same disorder and share a biologically and often genetically determined hypersensitivity of a central nervous system alarm system.[66]

Diagnosis and Treatment

A provocative test in which a person deliberately hyperventilates can be done to demonstrate occurrence of the symptoms. Arterial blood gases may be obtained to study the pH and carbon dioxide levels. ECG monitoring is done during the test on persons who have complained of chest pain, and caution should be used when performing the test on persons with known or suspected coronary artery disease.

Treatment focuses on educating the person and his or her family about the disorder, relaxation therapy, and training to overcome faulty breathing patterns. Rebreathing into a paper bag can be used to control the symptoms. For many persons, the realization that they can control their symptoms and nothing is seriously wrong reduces their anxiety and helps them to control the disorder. Adjunctive pharmacologic treatment may be useful in some cases. β-Adrenergic blocking agents lessen the peripheral symptoms of anxiety, such as palpitations and diaphoresis, and may lessen the respiratory stimulatory effect of the catecholamines released during periods of high anxiety.[67]

In summary, sleep apnea involves 30 or more apneic periods characterized by cessation of airflow through the nose and mouth for 10 seconds or longer. It can result from disorders that compromise the patency of the airways during sleep (*i.e.*, obstructive sleep apnea) or that affect the central nervous system and the respiratory center.

Hyperventilation syndrome consists of overbreathing, reduction in PCO_2, and respiratory alkalosis. It can result from organic causes, such as drug effects and central nervous system lesions; physiologic changes caused by heat exposure and exercise; emotional states; or habit. It can cause headache, dizziness, dyspnea, numbness and tingling sensations, lightheadedness, palpitations, and, sometimes, syncope.

REFERENCES

1. Light R.W. (1990). *Pleural diseases* (2nd ed.). Philadelphia: Lea & Febiger.
2. Light R.W. (1995). Diseases of the pleura, mediastinum, chest wall, and diaphragm. In: George R.B., Light R.W., Matthay M.A., Matthay R.A. *Chest medicine* (3rd ed., pp. 501–520), Baltimore: Williams & Wilkins.
3. Stauffer J.L. (1997). Lung. In Tierney L.M., McPhee S.J., Papadakis M.A. *Current medical diagnosis and treatment* (36th ed., pp. 290–303, 314–319). Stamford, CT: Appleton & Lange.
4. Shuttari M.F. (1995). Asthma: Diagnosis and management. *American Family Physician* 52 (8), 2225–2235.
5. Buist A.S., Vollmer W.M. (1994).Preventing death from asthma. *New England Journal of Medicine* 331 (23), 1584– 1585.
6. National Heart, Lung and Blood Institute. (1991). National Asthma Education Program Expert Panel. Guidelines for diagnosis and management of asthma. *Pediatric Asthma Allergy and Immunology* 5 (2), 57–188.

6a. National Asthma Education and Prevention Program. (1997). *Expert Panel report 2: Guidelines for the diagnosis and management of bronchial asthma.* Bethesda, MD: National Institutes of Health. National Heart, Lung, and Blood Institute.

7. Cockcroft D.W. (1990). Airway hyperresponsiveness in asthma. *Hospital Practice* 25 (1A), 111–129.
8. McFadden E.R., Gilbert I.A. (1994). Exercise-induced asthma. *New England Journal of Medicine* 330 (19), 1362–1366.
9. Roberts J.A. (1988). Exercise-induced asthma in athletes. *Sports Medicine* 6, 193–195.
10. Young S., LeSouef P.N., Geelhoed G.C., et al. (1991). The influence of a family history of asthma and parental smoking on airway responsiveness in early infancy. *New England Journal of Medicine* 324, 1168–1173.
11. Chan-Yeung M., Malo J. (1995). Occupational asthma. *New England Journal of Medicine* 333 (2), 107–112.
12. Dubuske D.M. (1994). Asthma: Diagnosis and management of nocturnal symptoms. *Comprehensive Therapy* 20 (11), 628–639.
13. Benatar S.R. (1986). Fatal asthma. *New England Journal of Medicine* 314, 423–428.
14. Macklem P. (1996). Fatal asthma. *Annual Review of Medicine* 47, 161–168.
15. Barnes P.J. (1994). Blunted perception and death from asthma. *New England Journal of Medicine* 330 (19), 1383–1384.
16. Behrman R.E., Kliegman R.M., Arvin A.M. (1996). *Nelson textbook of pediatrics* (14th ed., pp. 628–641). Philadelphia: W.B. Saunders.
17. Moffit J.E., Gearhart J.G., Yates A.B. (1994). Management of asthma in children. *American Family Physician.* 50 (5), 1039–1050.
18. Larsen G.L. (1992). Asthma in children. *New England Journal of Medicine* 326, 1540–1545.
19. Sporik R., Holgate S.T., Platts-Mills T.A.E., et al. (1990). Exposure to house dust mite antigen allergen (*Der p 1*) and the development of asthma in childhood. *New England Journal of Medicine* 323, 502–507.
20. Kochanek K.D., Hudson B.L. (1992). Advance report of final mortality statistics, 1992. *Monthly Vital Statistics Report* 43, 1–73.
21. Silverman E.K., Speizer F.E. (1996). Risk factors for development of chronic obstructive pulmonary disease. *Medical Clinics of North America* 80 (3), 501–523.
22. West J.B. (1992). *Pulmonary pathophysiology: The essentials* (4th ed., pp. 166–171, 181–184). Baltimore: Williams & Wilkins.
23. American Thoracic Society. (1987). Standards for the diagnosis and care of patients with chronic obstructive lung disease (COPD) and asthma. *American Review of Respiratory Disease* 136, 225–228.
24. Kobzik L., Schoen F.J. (1994). In: Cotran R.S., Kumar V., Robbins L. (1994). *Robbins pathologic basis of disease* (5th ed., 673–634). Philadelphia: W.B. Saunders.
25. Rubin E., Farber J.L. (1994). The respiratory system. In Rubin E. (Ed.). *Pathology* (2nd ed., pp. 557–617).
26. Crystal R. (1991). α_1-Antitrypsin deficiency: Pathogenesis and treatment. *Hospital Practice* 26 (2A), 81–94.
27. Stoller J.K., Aboussouan L.S. (1995). Chronic obstructive lung diseases: Emphysema, chronic bronchitis, bronchiectasis, and cystic fibrosis. In George R.B., Light R.W., Matthay M.A., Matthay R.A. (Eds.). *Chest medicine* (3rd ed., pp. 201–246). Baltimore: Williams & Wilkins.
28. Ferguson G.T., Cherniack R.M. (1993). Management of chronic obstructive pulmonary disease. *New England Journal of Medicine* 328, 1017–1022.
29. Celli B.R. (1996). Current thoughts regarding treatment of chronic obstructive pulmonary disease. *Medical Clinics of North America* 80 (3), 589–609.
30. Hodgkin J.E., Balchum O.J., Kass I., et al. (1975). Chronic obstructive airway disease. *Journal of the American Medical Association* 232, 1253–1260.
31. Kim M.J. (1984). Respiratory muscle training: Implications for patient care. *Heart and Lung* 13, 333 339.
32. Nocturnal Oxygen Therapy Group Trial. (1980). Continuous or nocturnal oxygen therapy in hypoxemic chronic

obstructive lung disease. *Annals of Internal Medicine* 93, 391–398.
33. Fletcher E.C., Levin D.C. (1984). Cardiopulmonary hemodynamics during sleep in subjects with chronic obstructive pulmonary disease. *Chest* 85, 6–13.
34. McGraw L.R. (1996). Lung volume reduction surgery: An overview. *Heart and Lung* 26 (2), 131–138.
35. Rogers R.M., Sciurba F.C., Keenan R.J. (1996). Lung reduction surgery in chronic obstructive lung disease. *Medical Clinics of North America* 80 (3), 623–643.
36. Murray J.F. (1991). New presentations of bronchiectasis. *Hospital Practice* 26 (3A), 55–74.
37. Welsh M.J., Smith A.E. (1995). Cystic fibrosis. *Scientific American* 73(6), 52–59.
38. Stern R.C. (1997). The diagnosis of cystic fibrosis. *New England Journal of Medicine* 336 (7), 487–491.
39. Davis P.B. (1994). Evolution in the treatment of cystic fibrosis. *New England Journal of Medicine* 331 (10), 672–673.
40. Reynolds H.V., Matthay R.A. (1995). Diffuse interstitial and alveolar inflammatory diseases. In George R.B., Light R.W., Matthay M.A., Matthay R.A. (Eds). *Chest medicine* (3rd ed., pp. 303–323), Baltimore: Williams & Wilkins.
41. Newman L.S., Rose C.S., Maier L.A. (1997). Sarcoidosis. *New England Journal of Medicine* 336 (7), 1224–1233.
42. Crystal R.G. (1991). Sarcoidosis. In Wilson J.P., Braunwald E., Isselbacher K.J. (Eds.). *Harrison's principles of internal medicine* (pp. 1463–1469). New York: McGraw-Hill.
43. Goldhaber S.Z. (1991). Managing pulmonary embolism. *Hospital Practice* 26 (9A), 37–48.
44. Stratton M.B. (1990). Ventilation-perfusion scintigraphy in diagnosis of pulmonary thromboembolism. *AACN Focus on Critical Care 17*, 287–293.
45. Goldfaber S.Z., Morpurgo M. (1992). Diagnosis, treatment and prevention of pulmonary embolism: Report of the WHO/International Society and Federation of Cardiology Task Force. *Journal of the American Medical Association* 268, 1727–1733.
46. Katzung B.G. (1995). *Basic and clinical pharmacology* (6th ed., p. 176). Stamford, CT: Appleton & Lange.
47. White K.M., Winslow E.H., Clark A., et al. (1990). The physiologic basis for continuous mixed oxygen saturation. *Heart and Lung* 19 (5, part 2), 548–551.
48. Rueden K.T. (1990). Noninvasive assessment of gas exchange in the critically ill patient. *AACN Clinical Issues in Critical Care Nursing* 1, 239–247.
49. Brown L.H. (1990). Pulmonary oxygen toxicity. *Focus on Critical Care* 17 (1), 68–75.
50. Weinberger S.E., Schwartzstein R.M., Weiss J.W. (1989). Hypercapnia. *New England Journal of Medicine* 321, 1223–1230.
51. St. John R.E., Eisenberg P. (1991). Nutrition and use of metabolic assessment in the ventilator-dependent patient. *AACN Clinical Issues in Critical Care Nursing* 2, 453–462.
52. Guyton A.C., Hall J.E. (1996). *Textbook of medical physiology* (9th ed., pp. 527–529, 542–544). Philadelphia: W.B. Saunders.
53. Tobin M.J. (1994). Mechanical ventilation. *New England Journal of Medicine* 330 (15), 1056–1060.
54. Beer D.J. (1992). ARDS: Evolving concepts of a systemic disease. *Hospital Practice* 27, 57–80.
55. Kollef M.H., Schuster D.P. (1995). The acute respiratory distress syndrome. *New England Journal of Medicine* 332 (1), 27–36.
56. Fulkerson W.J., MacIntyre N., Stamler J., Crapo J.D. (1996). Pathogenesis and treatment of adult respiratory distress syndrome. *Archives of Internal Medicine* 156, 29–38.
57. Kales A., Vela-Bueno A., Kales J. (1987). Sleep disorders: Sleep apnea and narcolepsy. *Annals of Internal Medicine* 106, 434.
58. Strollo P.J., Rogers R.M. (1996). Obstructive sleep apnea. *New England Journal of Medicine* 334 (2), 247–268.
59. Berry RA. (1995). Sleep-related breathing disorders. In George R.B., Light R.W., Matthay M.A., Matthay R.A. *Chest medicine* (3rd ed., pp. 247–268). Baltimore: Williams & Wilkins.
60. Kaplan J. (1991). Diagnosis and therapy of sleep-disordered breathing. In Burton G.G., Hodgkin J.E., Ward J.J. (Eds.). *Respiratory care: A guide to clinical practice* (3rd ed., pp. 279–287). Philadelphia: J.B. Lippincott.
61. Krieger M.H. (ed). (1982). *Pathophysiology of Respiration* (p. 265). New York: John Wiley.
62. Magarian G.J. (1982). Hyperventilation syndromes: Infrequently recognized common expression of anxiety and stress. *Medicine (Baltimore)* 61, 219.
63. Herman S.P., Stickler G.B., Lucas A.R. (1981). Hyperventilation syndromes in children and adolescents: Long-term follow-up. *Pediatrics* 67, 183.
64. Mortenson S.A., Vihelmson R., Sande E. (1981). Prinzmetal's variant angina (PVA), circadian variation in response to hyperventilation. *Acta Medica Scandinavica* 644 (Suppl.), 38.
65. Yasue H., Omote S., Takizawa A., et al. (1981). Alkalosis-induced coronary vasoconstriction: Effects of calcium, diltiazem, nitroglycerin and propranolol. *American Heart Journal* 102, 206.
66. Cowley D.S., Roy-Byrne P.P. (1987). Hyperventilation and panic disorder. *American Journal of Medicine* 83, 929.
67. Tavel M.E. (1990). Hyperventilation syndrome: Hiding behind pseudonyms. *Chest* 97, 1285–1288.

ADDITIONAL READINGS

Ball P. (1995). Epidemiology and treatment of chronic bronchitis and its exacerbations. *Chest* 108 (Suppl.), 43S—51S.

Barnes P.J. (1995). Inhaled glucocorticoids for asthma. *New England Journal of Medicine* 332 (13), 868–875.

Breslin E.H. (1996). Respiratory muscle function in patients with chronic obstructive pulmonary disease. *Heart and Lung* 25 (4), 271–285.

Celli B.R., Cosentino A., Fiel S., Petty T.L. (1997). Managing the special problems of chronic lung disease. *Patient Care* 31(7) 15, 87–98.

Garsick E., Schenker M.B., Dosman J.A. (1996). Occupationally induced airways obstruction. *Medical Clinics of North America* 80 (4), 851–878.

Hudgel D.W. (1992). Mechanisms of obstructive sleep apnea. *Chest 101*, 541–549.

Kemper K.J. (1996). Chronic asthma: An update. *Pediatrics in Review* 17 (4), 111–117.

Kleerup E.C., Tashkin D.P. (1995). Outpatient treatment of adult asthma. *Western Journal of Medicine* 163, 49–56.

Martinez F.D., Wright A.L., Taussig L.M., et. al. (1995). Asthma and wheezing in the first six years of life. *New England Journal of Medicine* 332 (3), 133–138.

McFadden E.R. Jr., Rubin L.J. (1997). Primary pulmonary hypertension. *New England Journal of Medicine* 336 (2), 111–118.

Tarpy S.P., Celli B.R. (1995). Long-term oxygen therapy. *New England Journal of Medicine* 333 (11), 710–714.

Undem B.J. (1994). Neural-immunologic interactions in asthma. *Hospital Practice* 29(2), 59–69.

UNIT VII

Renal Function and Fluid and Electrolytes

Throughout the earlier part of the Middle Ages, one of the major concerns of the physician was examination of the urine. Many physicians of this time thought that most diseases could be diagnosed by careful examination of the urine. Numerous illustrations taken from this period show early physicians holding up flasks of urine to study its color, cloudiness, and other properties. It was thought that if the cloudiness was at the top of the urine, the problem was in the head, and if it was at the bottom, the problem was in the legs.

From the 16th century on, anatomists began to acquire a fairly good understanding of the gross structure of the kidney, ureters, and bladder. The first great discovery of the minute structures of the kidney was made by Marcello Malphighi (1628–1694), one of the earliest microscopists, who described the ball-shaped structure of the glomerulus. The work of Malphighi was followed by that of Sir William Bowman (1816–1892), who described the urine collecting capsule of the nephron, Bowman's capsule. Bowman also described the relationship between the glomerulus and the tubules. German pathologist Friedrich Henle (1809–1885) described the long U-shaped loop, called the loop of Henle, that contributes to the concentrating abilities of the kidney. Once the structure of the kidney was established, other scientists began to focus on the chemical composition of urine and on the function of the kidney in the regulation of blood pressure.

CHAPTER 25

Control of Renal Function

It is no exaggeration to say that the composition of the blood is determined not so much by what the mouth takes in as by what the kidneys keep.

Homer Smith, *From Fish to Philosopher*

The kidneys are remarkable organs. Each is smaller than a person's fist, but in a single day the two organs process about 1700 L of blood and combine its waste products into about 1.5 L of urine. As part of their function, the kidneys filter physiologically essential substances, such as sodium and potassium ions, from the blood and selectively reabsorb those substances that are needed to maintain the normal composition of internal body fluids. Substances that are not needed for this purpose or are in excess pass into the urine. In regulating the volume and composition of body fluids, the kidneys perform excretory and endocrine functions. The renin-angiotensin mechanism participates in the regulation of blood pressure and the maintenance of circulating blood volume, and erythropoietin stimulates red blood cell production. The discussion in this chapter focuses on the structure and function of the kidneys, tests of renal function, and the physiologic action of diuretics.

Kidney Structure and Function

After you have completed this section of the chapter, you should be able to meet the following objectives:

- Describe the location and gross structure of the kidney
- Describe the kidney blood supply and mechanisms for regulating blood flow
- Explain the structure and function of the glomerulus and tubular components of the nephron
- Explain the function of sodium in terms of tubular transport mechanisms
- Describe how the kidney produces a concentrated or dilute urine

- Describe the elimination functions of the kidney
- Characterize the function of the juxtaglomerular complex
- Explain the endocrine functions of the kidney

Gross Structure and Location

The kidneys are paired, bean-shaped organs that lie outside the peritoneal cavity in the back of the upper abdomen, one on each side of the vertebral column at the level of the 12th thoracic to 3rd lumbar vertebrae (Fig. 25–1). The right kidney normally is situated lower than the left, presumably because of the position of the liver. In the adult, each kidney is about 10 to 12 cm long, 5 to 6 cm wide, and 2.5 cm deep and weighs about 113 to 170 g. The medial border of the kidney is indented by a deep fissure called the *hilus*. It is here that blood vessels and nerves enter and leave the kidney. The ureters, which connect the kidneys with the bladder, also enter the kidney at the hilus.

The kidney is a multilobular structure, composed of up to 18 lobes. Each lobule is composed of nephrons, which are the functional units of the kidney. Each nephron has a glomerulus that filters the blood and a system of tubular structures that selectively reabsorb and secrete materials in the filtrate as urine is being formed.

On longitudinal section, a kidney can be divided into an outer cortex and an inner medulla (Fig. 25–2).

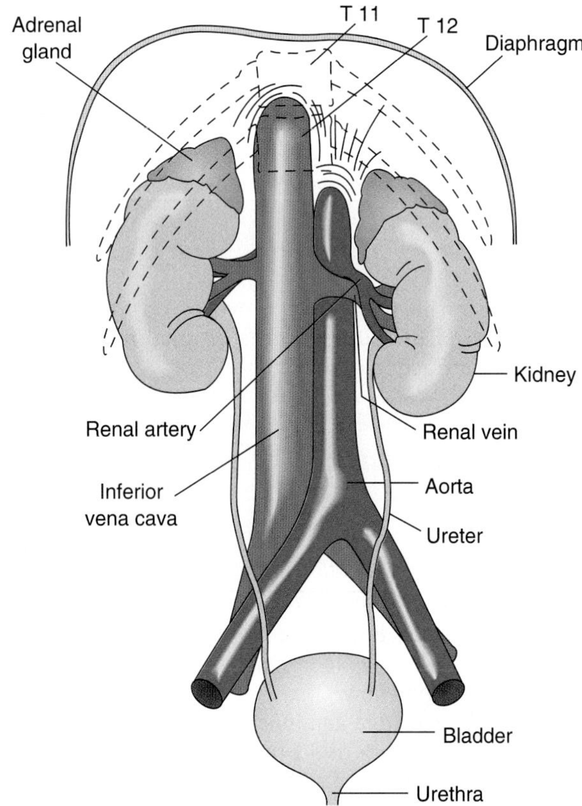

Figure 25–1
Kidneys, ureters, and bladder. (Right kidney is on the left.)

The cortex, which is reddish brown, contains the glomeruli and convoluted tubules of the nephron and blood vessels. The medulla consists of light-colored, cone-shaped masses—the renal pyramids—that are divided by the columns of the cortex (*i.e.*, columns of Bertin) that extend into the medulla. Each pyramid, topped by a region of cortex, forms a lobe of the kidney. The apices of the pyramids form the papillae (*i.e.*, 8 to 18 per kidney, corresponding to the number of lobes), which are perforated by the openings of the collecting ducts. The renal pelvis is a wide, funnel-shaped structure at the upper end of the ureter. It is made up of the calyces or cuplike structures that drain the upper and lower halves of the kidney.

The kidney is ensheathed in a fibrous external capsule and surrounded by a mass of fatty connective tissue, especially at its ends and borders. The adipose tissue protects the kidney from mechanical blows and assists, together with the attached blood vessels and fascia, in holding the kidney in place. Although the kidneys are relatively well protected, they may be bruised by blows to the loin or by compression between the lower ribs and the ilium. Because the kidneys are outside the peritoneal cavity, injury and rupture do not produce the same threat of peritoneal involvement as rupture of organs such as the liver or spleen.

Renal Blood Supply

Each kidney is supplied by a single renal artery that arises on either side of the aorta. As the renal artery approaches the kidney, it divides into five segmental arteries that enter the hilus of the kidney. Within the kidney, each segmental artery branches into several lobular arteries that supply the upper, middle, and lower parts of the kidney. The lobar arteries further subdivide to form the interlobular arteries at the level of the cortical medullary junction (Fig. 25–3). These arteries give off branches, called the arcuate arteries, that arch across the top of the pyramids. Small intralobular arteries radiate from the arcuate arteries to supply the cortex of the kidney. The afferent arterioles that supply the glomeruli arise from the intralobular arteries. Although nearly all the blood flow to the kidneys passes through the cortex, less than 10% is directed to the medulla and only about 1% goes to the papillae. Under conditions of decreased perfusion or increased sympathetic nervous system stimulation, blood flow is redistributed away from the cortex toward the medulla. This redistribution of blood flow decreases glomerular filtration while maintaining the urine concentrating ability of the kidneys, a factor that is important during conditions such as shock.

The nephron is supplied by two capillary systems, the glomerulus and the peritubular capillary network (Fig. 25–4). The glomerulus is a unique high-pressure filtration system located between two arterioles—the afferent and the efferent arterioles—that can selectively dilate or constrict to regulate glomerular capillary pressure. The peritubular capillary network is a low-pressure

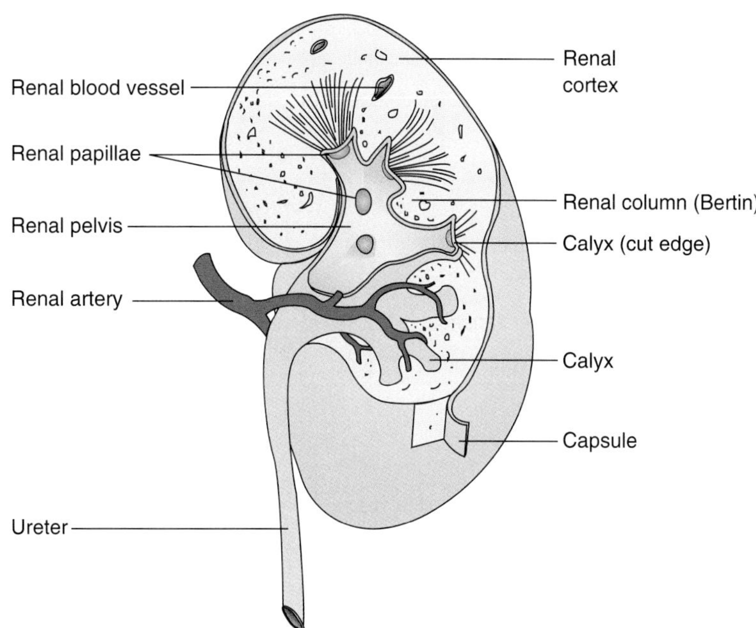

Figure 25–2
Internal structure of the kidney.

reabsorptive system that originates from the efferent arteriole. These capillaries are distributed around all portions of the tubules, an arrangement that permits rapid movement of solutes and water between the tubular lumen and the capillaries. The blood supply for the medullary nephrons are supplied with two types of capillaries: the peritubular capillaries, which are similar to those in the cortex, and the vasa recta, which are long, straight capillaries. The vasa recta accompany the long loops of Henle in the medullary portion of the kidney to assist in exchange of substances flowing in and out of that portion of the kidney. The peritubular capillaries rejoin to form the venous channels by which blood ultimately leaves the kidneys and empties into the inferior vena cava.

The Nephron

Each kidney is composed of more than 1 million tiny, closely packed functional units called *nephrons*. Each nephron consists of a glomerulus, where blood is filtered, and a tubular component. Here water, electrolytes, and other substances needed to maintain the constancy of the internal environment are reabsorbed into the bloodstream while other unneeded materials are secreted into the tubular filtrate for elimination (see Fig. 25–4).

The Glomerulus

The glomerulus consists of compact tufts of capillaries encased in a thin double-walled capsule, called *Bowman's capsule*. Fluid and particles from the blood are filtered through the wall of the glomerulus, into a fluid-filled space within Bowman's capsule, called *Bowman's space*. The mass of capillaries and its surrounding epithelial capsule are collectively referred to as the *renal corpuscle* (Fig. 25–5*A*).

The glomerular capillary membrane is composed of three layers: the capillary endothelial layer, the basement membrane, and the single-celled capsular epithelial layer (see Fig. 25–5*B*). The endothelial layer lines the glomerulus and interfaces with blood as it moves through the capillary. This layer contains many small perforations, called *fenestrations*.

The epithelial layer that covers the glomerulus is continuous with the epithelium that lines Bowman's capsule. The cells of the epithelial layer have unusual octopus-like structures that possess a large number of extensions, or foot processes (*i.e.*, podocytes), which are embedded in the basement membrane (Fig. 25–6). These foot processes form slit pores through which the glomerular filtrate passes. The basement membrane consists of a homogeneous acellular meshwork of collagen fibers,

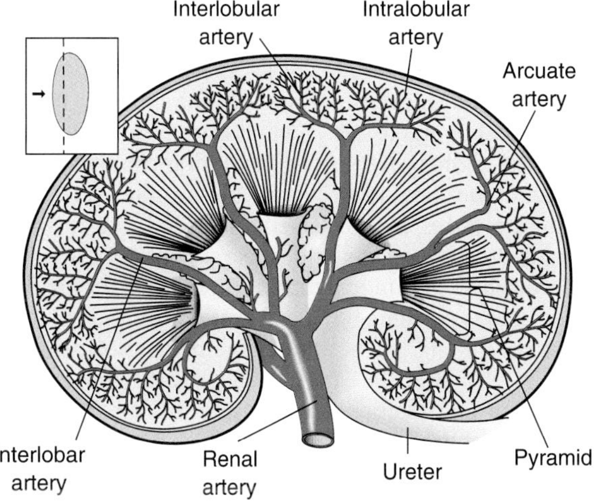

Figure 25–3
Simplified illustration of the arterial supply of the kidney.

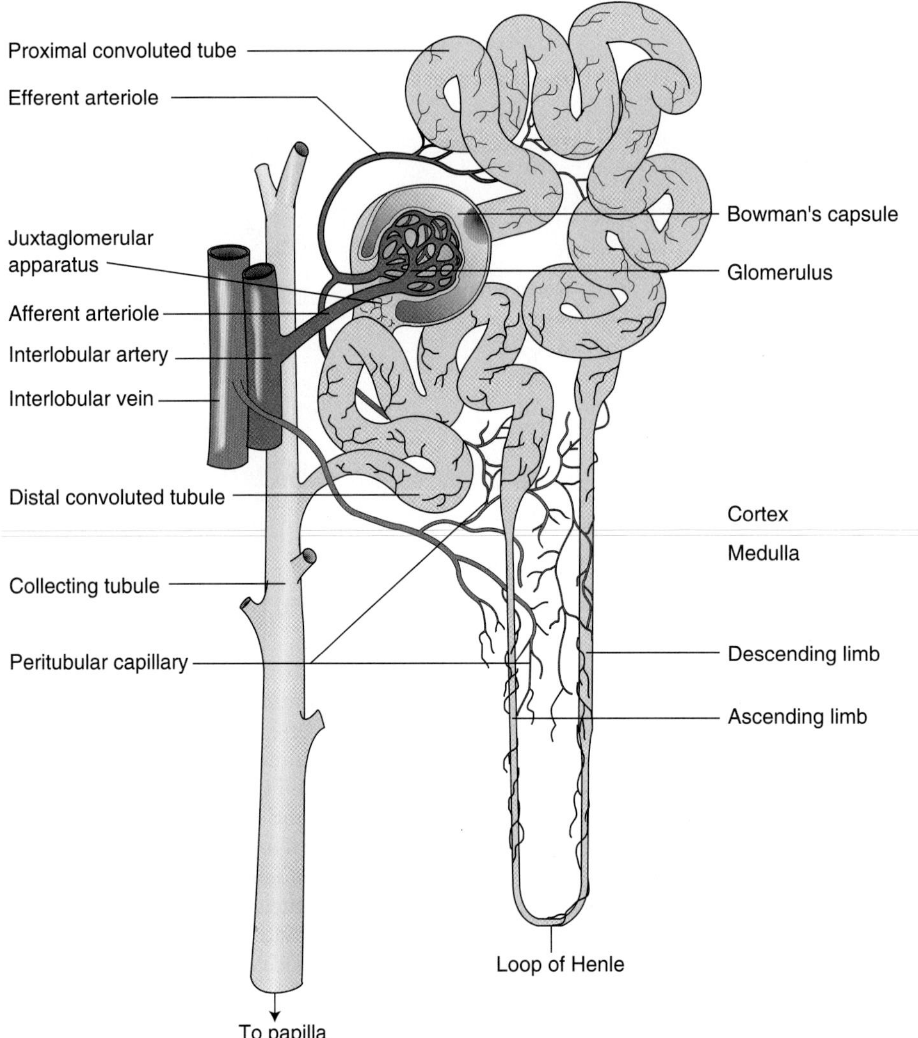

Figure 25–4
Nephron, showing the glomerular and tubular structures along with the blood supply.

glycoproteins, and mucopolysaccharides (see Fig. 25–5C). Because the endothelial and the epithelial layers of the glomerular capillary have porous structures, the basement membrane determines the permeability of the glomerular capillary membrane. The spaces between the fibers that make up the basement membrane represent the pores of a filter and determine the size-dependent permeability barrier of the glomerulus. The size of the pores in the basement membrane normally prevents red blood cells and plasma proteins from passing through the glomerular membrane into the urine filtrate. There is evidence that the epithelium plays a major role in producing the basement membrane components, and it is probable that the epithelial cells are active in forming new basement membrane material throughout life. Alterations in the structure and function of the glomerular basement membrane are responsible for the leakage of proteins and blood cells that occurs in many forms of glomerular disease.

Another important component of the glomerulus is the mesangium. In some areas, the capillary endothelium and the basement membrane do not completely surround each capillary. Instead, the mesangial cells, which lie between the capillary tufts, provide support for the glomerulus in these areas (see Fig. 25–5*B*). The mesangial cells produce an intercellular substance similar to that of the basement membrane. This substance covers the endothelial cells where they are not covered by basement membrane. The mesangial cells possess (or can develop) phagocytic properties and remove macromolecular materials that enter the intercapillary spaces. Mesangial cells also exhibit contractile properties in response to neurohumoral substances and are thought to contribute to the regulation of blood flow through the glomerulus. In normal glomeruli, the mesangial area is narrow and contains only a small number of cells. Mesangial hyperplasia and increased mesangial matrix occur in a number of glomerular diseases.

Tubular Components of the Nephron

The nephron tubule is divided into four segments: a highly coiled segment called the *proximal convoluted tubule,* which drains Bowman's capsule; a thin, looped structure called the *loop of Henle;* a distal coiled portion called the *distal convoluted tubule;* and the final segment called the *collecting tubule,* which joins with several tubules to collect

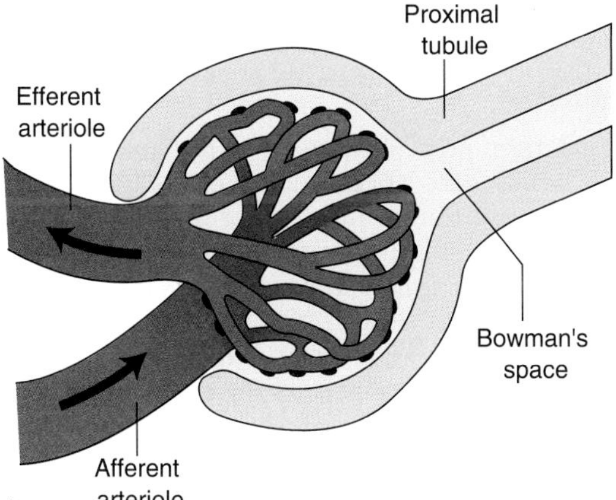

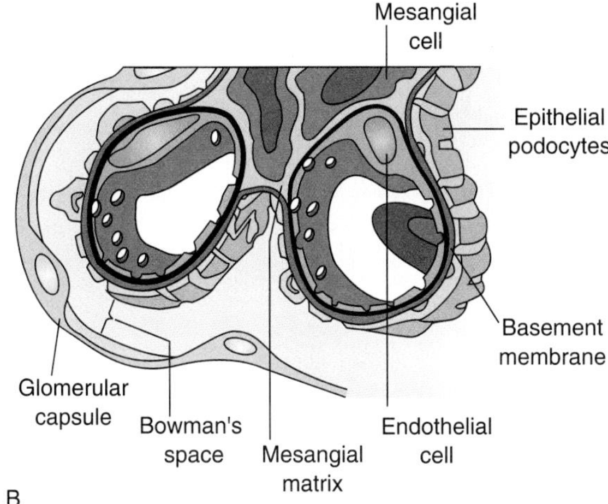

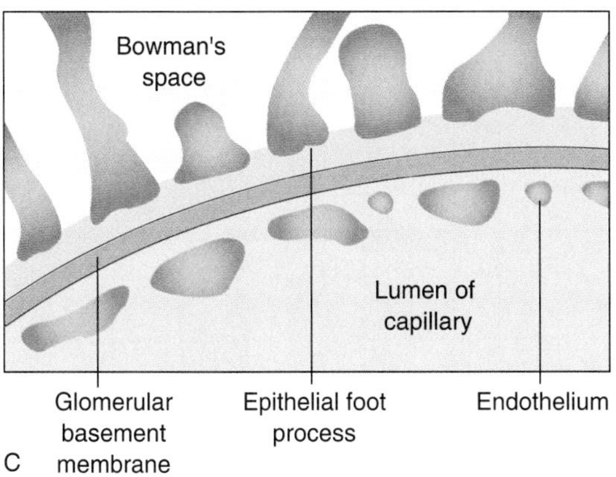

Figure 25–5
Renal corpuscle. (**A**) Structures of the glomerulus. (**B**) Position of the mesangial cells in relation to the capillary loops and Bowman's capsule. (**C**) Cross section of the glomerular membrane, showing the position of the endothelium, basement membrane, and epithelial foot processes.

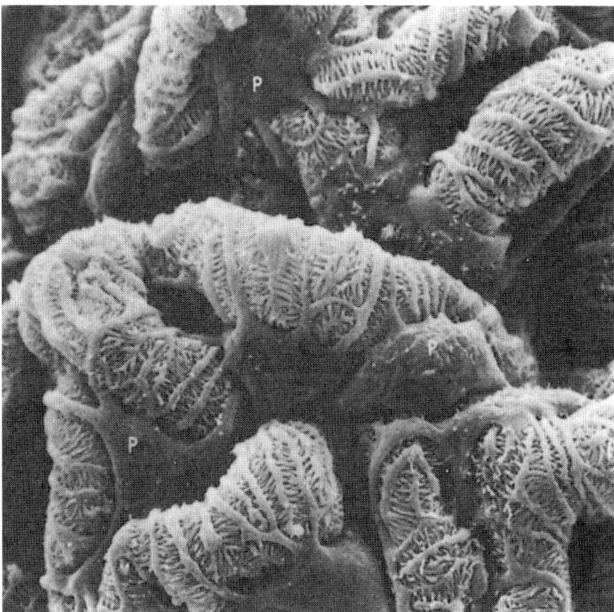

Figure 25–6
Scanning electron micrograph of a glomerulus from the kidney of a normal rat. The visceral epithelial cells, or podocytes (P), extend multiple processes outward from the main cell body to wrap around individual capillary loops. Immediately adjacent pedicels, or foot processes, arise from different podocytes (Original magnification × 4800). (Brenner B.M., Rector F.C. [1981]. *The kidney.* Philadelphia: W.B. Saunders)

the urine filtrate. The filtrate passes through each of these segments before reaching the pelvis of the kidney.

Nephrons can be roughly grouped into two categories. About 85% of the nephrons originate in the superficial part of the cortex and are called *cortical nephrons.* They have short, thick loops of Henle that penetrate only a short distance into the medulla. The remaining 15% are called *juxtamedullary nephrons.* They originate deeper in the cortex and have longer and thinner loops of Henle that penetrate the entire length of the medulla. The juxtamedullary nephrons are largely concerned with urine concentration.

The proximal tubule is a highly coiled structure that dips toward the renal pelvis to become the descending limb of the loop of Henle. The ascending loop of Henle returns to the region of the renal corpuscle, where it becomes the distal tubule. The distal convoluted tubule, which begins at the juxtaglomerular complex, is divided into two segments: the *diluting segment* and the *late distal tubule.* The late distal tubule fuses with the collecting tubule. Like the distal tubule, the collecting duct is divided into two segments: the *cortical collecting tubule* and the *inner medullary collecting tubule.*

Throughout its course, the tubule is composed of a single layer of epithelial cells resting on a basement membrane. The structure of the epithelial cells varies with tubular function. The cells of the proximal tubule have a fine villous structure that increases the surface area for reabsorption; they are also rich in mitochondria, which support active transport processes. The epithelial layer of the thin segment of the loop of Henle has few mitochondria, indicating minimal metabolic activity and active reabsorptive function.

Urine Formation

Urine formation involves the filtration of blood by the glomerulus to form an ultrafiltrate of urine and the tubular reabsorption of electrolytes and nutrients needed to maintain the constancy of the internal environment while eliminating waste materials.

Glomerular Filtration

Urine formation begins with the filtration of essentially protein-free plasma through the glomerular capillaries into Bowman's space. The movement of fluid through the glomerular capillaries is determined by the same factors (*i.e.*, capillary pressure, colloidal osmotic pressure, and capillary permeability) that affect fluid movement through other capillaries in the body (see Chapter 16). The glomerular filtrate has chemical composition similar to plasma, but it contains almost no proteins, because large molecules do not readily cross the glomerular wall. About 125 ml of filtrate is formed each minute. This is called the *glomerular filtration rate* (GFR). This rate can vary from a few milliliters per minute to as high as 200 ml/minute.

The location of the glomerulus between two arterioles allows for maintenance of a high-pressure filtration system. The capillary filtration pressure (about 60 mm Hg) in the glomerulus is about two to three times higher than that of other capillary beds in the body. The filtration pressure and the GFR are regulated by the constriction and relaxation of the afferent and efferent arterioles. Constriction of the efferent arteriole increases resistance to outflow from the glomeruli and increases the glomerular pressure and the GFR. Constriction of the afferent arteriole causes a reduction in the renal blood flow, glomerular filtration pressure, and GFR. The afferent and the efferent arterioles are innervated by the sympathetic nervous system. During periods of strong sympathetic stimulation, as occurs during shock, renal blood flow and the glomerular filtration pressure can be markedly decreased, and urine output can fall almost to zero.

Tubular Reabsorption and Secretion

From Bowman's capsule, the glomerular filtrate moves into the tubular segments of the nephron. In its movement through the lumen of the tubular segments, the glomerular filtrate is changed considerably by the tubular transport of water and solutes. Tubular transport can result in *reabsorption* of substances from the tubular fluid into the blood or *secretion* of substances into the tubular fluid from the blood (Fig. 25–7).

The basic mechanisms of transport across the tubular epithelial cell membrane are similar to those of cell membranes in the body and include active and passive transport mechanisms. Water and urea are passively absorbed along concentration gradients. Sodium, potassium, chloride, calcium, and phosphate ions; urate; glucose; and amino acids are reabsorbed using primary or secondary active transport mechanisms to move across the tubular membrane. Some substances, such as hydrogen, potassium, and urate ions, are secreted into the tubular fluids. Under normal conditions, only about 1 ml of the 125 ml of glomerular filtrate that is formed each minute is excreted in the urine. The other 124 ml is reabsorbed in the tubules. This means that the average output of urine is about 60 ml/hour.

Renal tubular cells have two membrane surfaces through which substances must pass as they are reabsorbed from the tubular fluid. The side of the cell that is in contact with the tubular lumen and tubular filtrate is called the *luminal membrane*. The outside membrane that lies adjacent to the interstitial fluid is called the *basolateral membrane*. In most cases, substances move from the tubular filtrate into the tubular cell along a concentration gradient, but they require facilitated transport

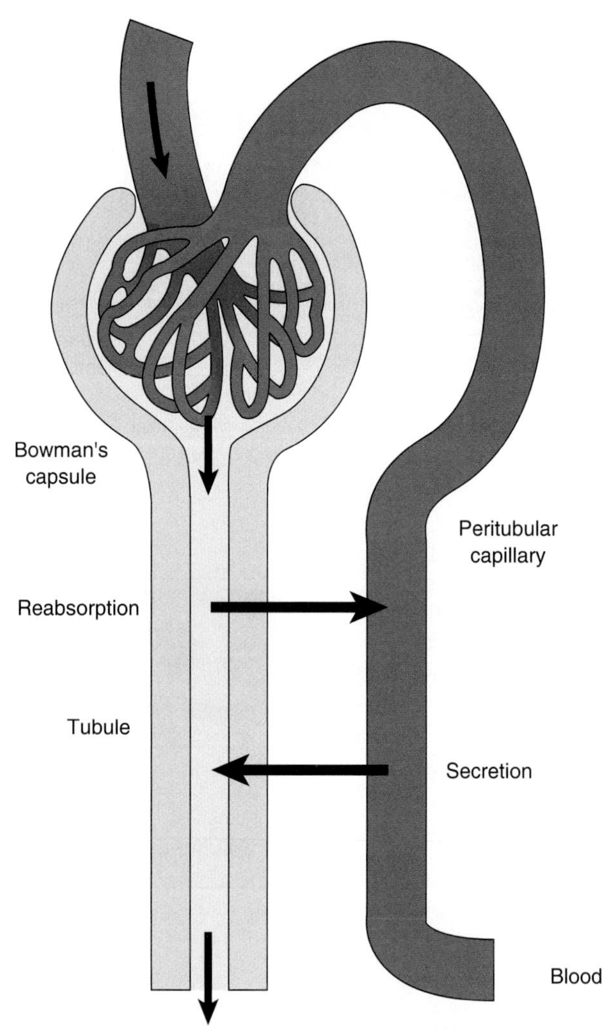

Figure 25–7
Reabsorption and secretion of substances between the renal tubules and peritubular capillaries.

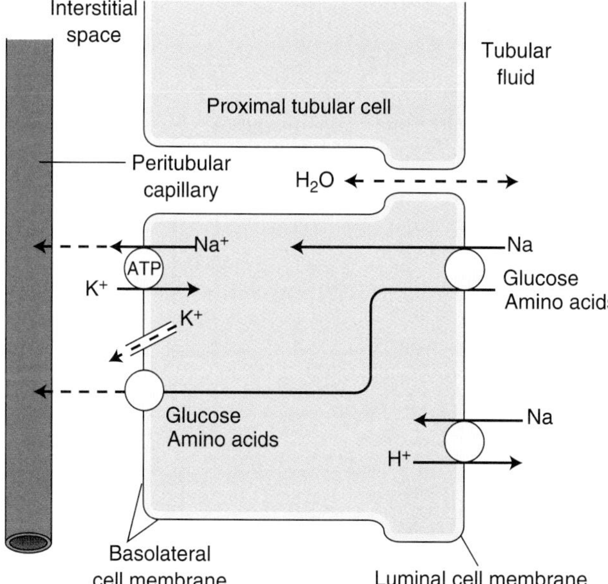

Figure 25–8
Mechanism for secondary active transport or cotransport of glucose and amino acids in the proximal tubule. The energy-dependent sodium-potassium pump on the basal lateral surface of the cell maintains a low intracellular gradient that facilitates the downhill movement of sodium and glucose or amino acids (cotransport) from the tubular lumen into the tubular cell and then into the peritubular capillary.

or carrier systems to move across the basolateral membrane into the interstitial fluid, where they are absorbed into the peritubular capillaries.

With some substances, such as glucose and amino acids, transport is linked to sodium reabsorption. This is called *secondary active transport* or *cotransport* (Fig. 25–8). In secondary active transport, the energy-dependent sodium-potassium ATPase pump on the basolateral side of renal tubular cells maintains a low intracellular sodium concentration that facilitates the downhill (*i.e.*, from a higher to lower concentration) movement of sodium across the luminal membrane. Cotransport uses a carrier system in which the downhill movement of one substance such as sodium is coupled to the uphill movement (*i.e.*, from a lower to higher concentration) of another substance such as glucose or an amino acid. A few substances, such as hydrogen, are secreted into the tubule using countertransport in which the movement of one substance, such as sodium, enables the movement a of second substance in the opposite direction. Sodium ions are the single most abundant cation in the filtrate. The bulk of energy used by the kidney is for active sodium transport mechanisms that facilitate sodium reabsorption and cotransport of other electrolytes and substances such as glucose and amino acids.

Proximal Tubule. About 65% of all reabsorptive and secretory processes that occur in the tubular system take place in the proximal tubule. There is almost complete reabsorption of nutritionally important substances, such as glucose, amino acids, lactate, and water-soluble vitamins. Electrolytes, such as sodium, potassium, chloride, and bicarbonate, are 65% to 80% reabsorbed. As these solutes move into the tubular cells, their concentration within the tubular lumen decreases, providing a concentration gradient for the osmotic reabsorption of water and urea. The proximal tubule is highly permeable to water, and the osmotic movement of water occurs so rapidly that the concentration difference of solutes on either side of the membrane seldom is more than a few milliosmoles.

Many substances, such as glucose, are freely filtered in the glomerulus and reabsorbed by energy-dependent cotransport carrier mechanisms. The maximum amount of substance that these transport systems can reabsorb per unit time is called the *transport maximum*. The transport maximum is related to the number of carrier proteins that are available for transport and is usually sufficient to ensure that all of a filtered substance such as glucose can be reabsorbed rather than being eliminated in the urine. The plasma level at which the substance appears in the urine is called the *renal threshold* (Fig. 25–9). Under some circumstances, the amount of substance filtered in the glomerulus exceeds the transport maximum. For example, when the blood glucose level is elevated in uncontrolled diabetes mellitus, the amount that is filtered in the glomerulus often exceeds the transport maximum (about 320 mg/minute), and glucose spills into the urine.

The Loop of Henle. The loop of Henle is divided into three segments: the thin descending segment, the thin ascending segment, and thick ascending segment. Each

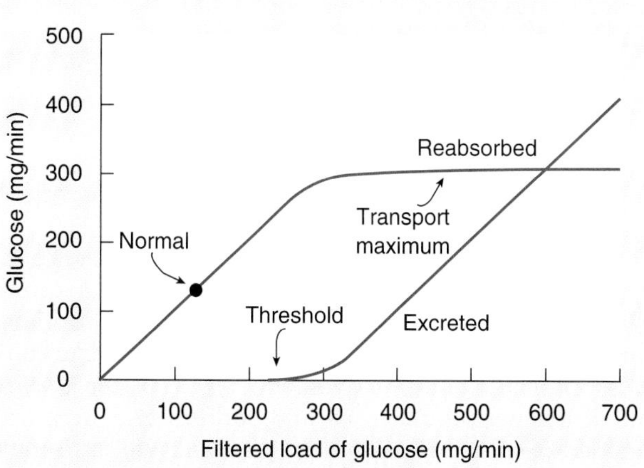

Figure 25–9
Relations among the filtered load of glucose, the rate of glucose reabsorption by the renal tubules, and the rate of glucose excretion in the urine. The *transport maximum* is the maximum rate at which glucose can be reabsorbed from the tubules. The *threshold* for glucose refers to the filtered load of glucose at which glucose first begins to appear in the urine. (Guyton A., Hall J.E. [1996]. *Textbook of medical physiology* [9th ed., p. 335]. Philadelphia: W.B. Saunders)

of these segments has special structural and functional properties.

Fluid that enters the loop of Henle is isosmotic to plasma, but it becomes hypo-osmotic as it moves through the loop. The thin descending limb is highly permeable to water and moderately permeable to urea, sodium, and other ions. The ascending limb, in contrast to the descending limb, is impermeable to water. As fluid moves down the descending limb, water is reabsorbed until the osmolality of the tubular fluid reaches an equilibrium with the interstitial fluid, which is more hypertonic. In the ascending limb, which is impermeable to water, solutes are reabsorbed, but water cannot follow; as a result, the tubular fluid becomes more and more dilute, often reaching an osmolality of 100 mOsm/kg of H_2O as it enters the distal convoluted tubule, compared with the 285 mOsm/kg of H_2O in plasma (Fig. 25–10).

The thick segment of the loop of Henle begins in the ascending limb where the epithelial cells become thickened. As with the thin ascending limb, this segment is impermeable to water. The thick segment contains a Na^+-K^+-2 Cl^- cotransport system. This system involves the cotransport of a positively charged sodium and positively charged potassium ion accompanied by two negatively charged chloride ions (Fig. 25–11). It is here that the loop diuretics exert their action. The gradient for the operation of this cotransport system is provided by the basolateral sodium-potassium pump, which maintains a low intracellular sodium concentration. The repetitive reabsorption of sodium chloride from the thick ascending limb of Henle and continued inflow of new sodium chloride from the proximal tubule into the loop of Henle serves to trap solutes in the medullary interstitium, contributing to the high osmolality in this part of the nephron. About 20% to 25% of the filtered load of sodium, potassium, and chloride are reabsorbed in the thick loop of Henle. Movement of these ions out of the tubule leads to the development of a transmembrane potential that favors the passive reabsorption of small divalent cations such as calcium and magnesium. Inhibition of sodium transport in the thick loop of Henle by loop diuretics causes an increase in urinary excretion of these divalent ions in addition to sodium and chloride.

In about one fifth of the juxtamedullary nephrons, the loops of Henle and special hairpin-shaped capillaries called the *vasa recta* descend into the medullary portion of the kidney. A countercurrent mechanism controls water and solute movement so that water is kept out of the peritubular area and sodium and urea are retained (see Fig. 25–10). The term *countercurrent* refers to a flow of fluids in opposite directions in adjacent structures. There is an exchange of solutes between the adjacent descending and ascending loops of Henle and between the ascending and descending sections of the vasa recta. Because of these exchange processes, a high concentration of the osmotically active particles (about 1200 mOsm/kg of H_2O) collect in the interstitium of this portion of the kidney. It is here, where the kidney interstitium surrounds the collecting tubules, that the presence of these osmotically active particles facilitates

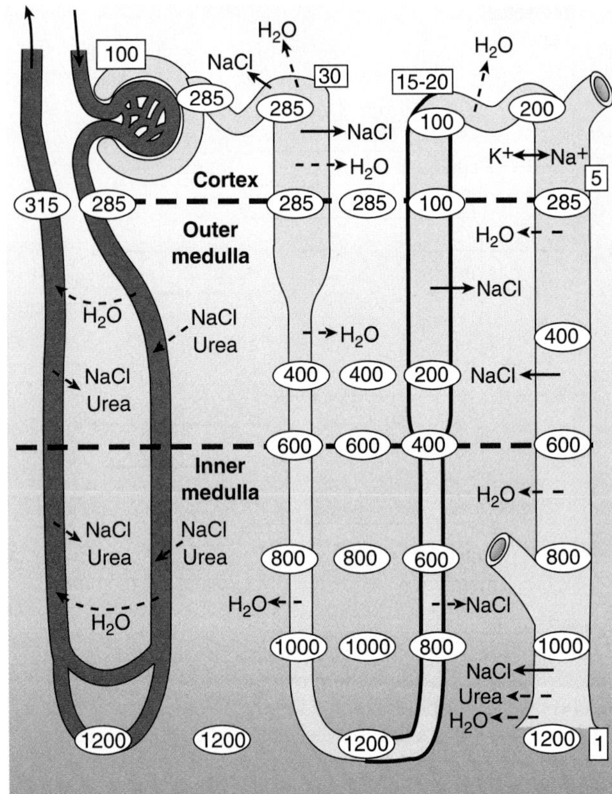

Figure 25–10
Summary of movements of ions, urea, and water in the kidney during production of a maximally concentrated urine (1200 mOsm/kg H_2O). Numbers in ovals give osmolality in mOsm/kg H_2O. Numbers in boxes give the relative amount of water present at each level of the nephron. *Solid arrows* indicate active transport; *dashed arrows* indicate passive transport. The *heavy outlining* along the ascending limb of Henle's loop indicates relative water impermeability. (Rhoades R.A., Tanner G.A. [1996]. *Medical physiology* [p. 441]. Boston: Little, Brown)

the antidiuretic hormone (ADH)–mediated reabsorption of water.

Distal Convoluted Tubule. Like the thick ascending loop of Henle, the distal convoluted tubule is relatively impermeable to water, and reabsorption of sodium chloride from this segment further dilutes the tubular fluid. Sodium reabsorption occurs through a sodium and chloride cotransport mechanism. About 10% of filtered sodium chloride is reabsorbed in this section of the tubule. Unlike the thick ascending loop of Henle, neither calcium nor magnesium are passively absorbed in this segment of the tubule. Instead, calcium ions are actively reabsorbed in a process that is largely regulated by parathyroid hormone and possibly by vitamin D.

The thick ascending loop of Henle, the distal tubule, and cortical collecting tubule are often referred to as the *diluting segment* of the tubule. As solutes are reabsorbed from these segments, the urine becomes more and more dilute, often reaching an osmolar concentration that is equal to or less than that of plasma. This allows excretion of free water from the body.

Late Distal Tubule and Cortical Collecting Tubule. The late distal tubule and the cortical collecting tubule constitute the site where aldosterone exerts its action on sodium and potassium reabsorption. Although responsible for only 2% to 5% of sodium chloride reabsorption, this site is largely responsible for determining the final sodium concentration of the urine. The late distal tubule with the cortical collecting tubule is also the major site for regulation of potassium excretion by the kidney. When the body is confronted with a potassium excess, as occurs with a diet high in potassium content, the amount of potassium secreted at this site may exceed the amount filtered in the glomerulus.

The mechanism for sodium reabsorption and potassium secretion by this section of the kidney is distinct from other tubular segments. This tubular segment is composed of two types of cells, the *principal cells* and the *intercalated cells*. The principal cells reabsorb sodium and water from the lumen filtrate and secrete potassium into the lumen. The intercalated cells reabsorb potassium and secrete hydrogen ions into the lumen. The principal cells use separate channels for transport of sodium and potassium rather than cotransport mechanisms (Fig. 25–12). Aldosterone is thought to exert its effect on sodium and potassium excretion by increasing the number of ion channels and the function of the basolateral sodium-potassium pump.

Medullary Collecting Duct. The epithelium of the inner medullary collecting duct is well designed to resist extreme changes in the osmotic or pH characteristics of tubular fluid, and it is here that the urine becomes highly concentrated, highly diluted, highly alkaline, or highly acidic. During periods of water excess or dehydration, the kidneys play a major role in maintaining water balance.

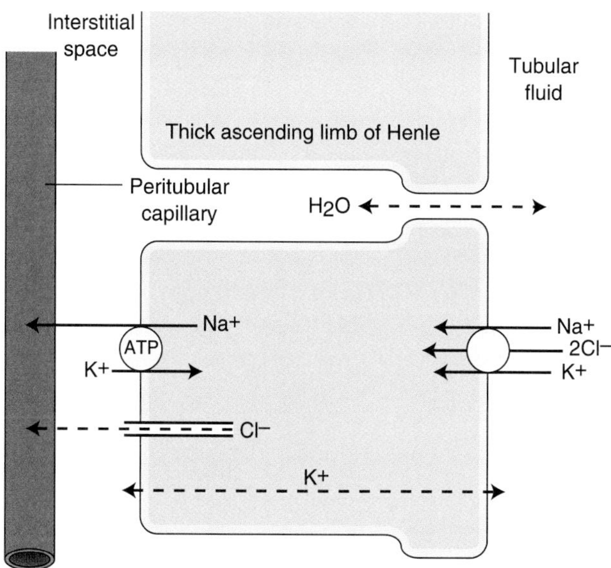

Figure 25–11
Sodium, chloride, and potassium reabsorption in the thick segment of the loop of Henle.

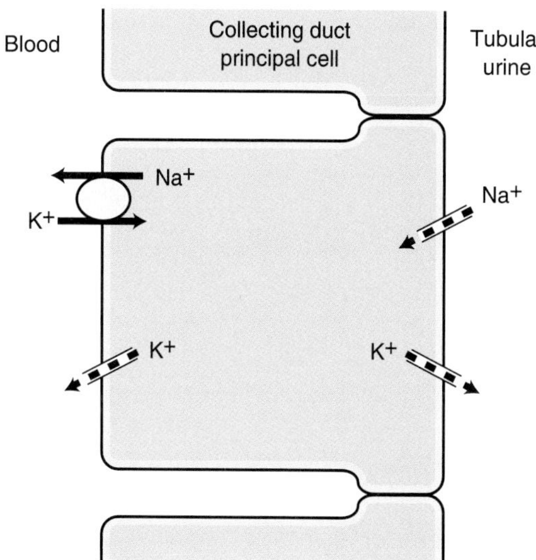

Figure 25–12
Model for ion transport of sodium and potassium by collecting duct principal cells. (Rhoades R.A., Tanner G.A. [1996]. *Medical physiology* [p. 438]. Boston: Little, Brown)

ADH exerts its effect in the medullary collecting duct. ADH maintains extracellular volume by returning water to the vascular compartment and leads to the production of a concentrated urine by removing water from the tubular filtrate. Osmoreceptors in the hypothalamus sense the increase in osmolality of extracellular fluids and stimulate the release of ADH from the posterior pituitary gland (see Chapter 26). The permeability of the collecting ducts to water is determined mainly by the concentration of ADH. In exerting its effect, ADH, also known as vasopressin, binds to vasopressin receptors on the blood side of the tubular cells (Fig. 25–13). Binding of ADH to the vasopressin receptors causes insertion of water channels into the cell membrane on the luminal side of the tubular cells, producing a marked increase in water permeability. After the permeability of the collecting tubules has been established, water moves out of the tubular lumen and into the interstitium of the medullary area, where it enters the peritubular capillaries for return to the vascular system. When the effect of ADH is over, the inserted water channels are removed, the tubular cells lose their water permeability, and a dilute urine is formed.

Regulation of Renal Blood Flow

In the adult, the kidneys are perfused with 1000 to 1300 ml of blood per minute, or 20% to 25% of the cardiac output. This large blood flow is largely needed to ensure a sufficient GFR for the removal of waste products from the blood, rather than for the metabolic needs of the kidney. Feedback mechanisms intrinsic to the kidney normally

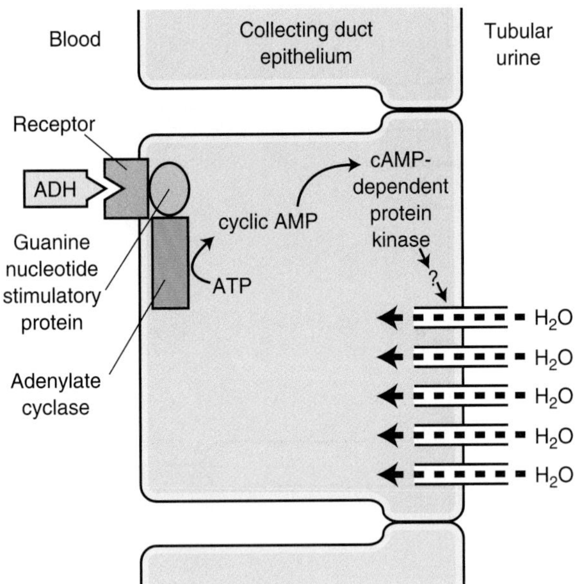

Figure 25–13
Model for the action of antidiuretic hormone (ADH) on the epithelium of the collecting duct. The ADH receptor is on the basolateral side, but the water permeability increase occurs on the luminal side. (Rhoades R.A., Tanner G.A. [1996]. *Medical physiology* [p. 439]. Boston: LIttle, Brown)

keep blood flow and GFR constant despite changes in arterial blood pressure.

Neural and Humoral Control Mechanisms

The kidney is richly innervated by the sympathetic nervous system. Increased sympathetic activity causes constriction of the afferent and efferent arterioles and a fall in renal blood flow. Intense sympathetic stimulation such as occurs in shock and trauma can produce marked decreases in renal blood flow and GFR, even to the extent of causing blood flow to cease altogether.

Several humoral substances, including angiotensin II, ADH, and endothelins, cause vasoconstriction of renal vessels. The endothelins are a group of peptides released from damaged endothelial cells in the kidney and other tissues. Although not thought to be important regulators of renal blood flow during everyday activities, endothelin I, which is released by renal endothelial cells, may play a role in reduction of blood flow in conditions such as postischemic acute renal failure (see Chapter 29).

Other substances such as dopamine, nitric oxide, and prostaglandins (*i.e.*, E_2 and I_2) produce vasodilation. Nitric oxide, a vasodilator produced by the vascular endothelium, appears to be important in preventing excessive vasoconstriction of renal blood vessels and allowing normal excretion of sodium and water. Prostaglandins are a group of mediators of cell function that are produced locally and exert their effects locally. Although prostaglandins do not appear to be of major importance in regulating renal blood flow and GFR under normal conditions, they may protect the kidneys against the vasoconstricting effects of sympathetic stimulation and angiotensin II. Nonsteroidal antiinflammatory drugs that inhibit prostaglandin synthesis may cause reduction in renal blood flow and GFR under certain conditions.

Autoregulation

The constancy of renal blood flow is maintained by a process called autoregulation (see Chapter 16). Normally, autoregulation of blood flow is designed to maintain blood flow at a level consistent with the metabolic needs of the tissues. In the kidney, autoregulation of blood flow must also allow for precise regulation of renal excretion of water and solutes. For autoregulation to occur, the resistance to blood flow through the kidneys must be varied in direct proportion to the arterial pressure. The exact mechanisms responsible for the intrarenal regulation of blood flow are unclear. One of the proposed mechanisms is a direct effect on vascular smooth muscle that causes the blood vessels to relax when there is an increase in blood pressure and to constrict when there is a decrease in pressure. A second proposed mechanism is the juxtaglomerular complex.

The Juxtaglomerular Complex. The *juxtaglomerular complex* is thought to represent a feedback control system that links changes in the GFR with renal blood flow. The juxtaglomerular complex is located at the site where the distal tubule extends back to the glomerulus and then passes between the afferent and efferent arteriole (Fig. 25–14). The distal tubular site that is nearest the glomerulus is characterized by densely nucleated cells called the *macula densa*.

In the adjacent afferent arteriole, the smooth muscle cells of the media are modified as special secretory cells called *juxtaglomerular cells*. These cells contain

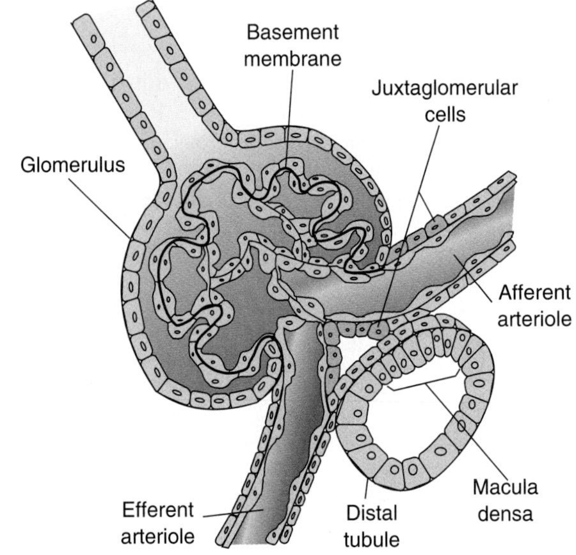

Figure 25–14
Juxtaglomerular apparatus, showing the close contact of the distal tubule with the afferent arteriole, the macula densa, and the juxtaglomerular cells.

granules of inactive renin, an enzyme that functions in the conversion of angiotensinogen to angiotensin. Renin functions by means of angiotensin II to produce vasoconstriction of the efferent arteriole as a means of preventing serious decreases in glomerular filtration rate. The renin-angiotensin system also increases sodium reabsorption by stimulating aldosterone secretion from the adrenal gland.

Because of its location between the afferent and efferent arteriole, the juxtaglomerular complex is thought to play an essential feedback role in linking the level of arterial blood pressure and renal blood flow to the GFR and the composition of the distal tubular fluid. The juxtaglomerular complex monitors the systemic blood pressure by sensing the stretch of the afferent arteriole and it monitors the concentration of sodium chloride in the tubular filtrate as it passes through the macula densa. This information is then used in determining how much renin should be released to keep the arterial blood pressure within its normal range and to maintain a relatively constant GFR.

Effect of Increased Protein and Glucose Load. Although renal blood flow and glomerular filtration are relatively stable under most conditions, two conditions can increase renal blood flow and glomerular filtration. These are an increased amount of protein in the diet and an increase in blood glucose. With ingestion of a high-protein diet, renal blood flow increases 20% to 30% within 1 to 2 hours. Although the exact mechanism for this increase is uncertain, it is thought to be related to the fact that amino acids and sodium are absorbed together in the proximal tubule. As a result, delivery of sodium to the macula densa is decreased, which elicits an increase in renal blood flow through the juxtaglomerular complex feedback mechanism. The resultant increase in blood flow and GFR allows sodium excretion to be maintained at a near-normal level while increasing the excretion of the waste products of protein metabolism such as urea. The same mechanism is thought to explain the large increases in renal blood flow and GFR that occur with high blood glucose levels in persons with uncontrolled diabetes mellitus.

Elimination Functions of the Kidney

Renal Clearance

Renal clearance is the volume of plasma that is completely cleared each minute of any substance that finds its way into the urine. It is determined by the ability of the substance to be filtered in the glomeruli and the capacity of the renal tubules to reabsorb or secrete the substance. Every substance has its own clearance rate, the units of which are always volume of plasma per unit time. It can be determined by measuring the amount of a substance that is excreted in the urine (*i.e.*, urine concentration × urine flow rate in milliliters per minute) and dividing by its plasma concentration. Inulin, a large polysaccharide, is freely filtered in the glomeruli and neither reabsorbed nor secreted by the tubular cells. After intravenous injection, the amount that appears in the urine is equal to the amount that is filtered in the glomeruli (*i.e.*, the clearance rate is equal to the GFR). Because of these properties, inulin can be used as a laboratory measure of the GFR. Some substances, such as urea, are freely filtered in the glomeruli, but the volume that is cleared from the plasma is less than the GFR, indicating that at least some of the substance is being reabsorbed. At normal plasma levels, glucose has a clearance of zero, because it is reabsorbed in the tubules, and none appears in the urine.

Regulation of Sodium and Potassium Elimination

Elimination of sodium and potassium is regulated by the GFR and by humoral agents that control reabsorption. Aldosterone functions in the regulation of sodium and potassium elimination. Atrial natriuretic hormone contributes to the regulation of sodium elimination.

Aldosterone. Sodium reabsorption in the distal tubule and collecting duct is highly variable and depends on the presence of aldosterone, a hormone secreted by the adrenal gland. In the presence of aldosterone, almost all the sodium within the distal tubular fluid is reabsorbed, and the urine essentially becomes sodium free. In the absence of aldosterone, virtually no sodium is reabsorbed from the distal tubule. The remarkable ability of the distal tubular and collecting duct cells to alter sodium reabsorption in relation to changes in aldosterone allows the kidneys to excrete urine with sodium levels that range from a few tenths of a gram to 40 g. Like sodium, potassium is freely filtered in the glomerulus, but unlike sodium, potassium is reabsorbed from and secreted into the tubular fluid. The secretion of potassium into the tubular fluid occurs in the distal tubule and, like that of sodium, is regulated by aldosterone. Only about 70 mEq of potassium is delivered to the distal tubule each day, but the average person consumes this much and more potassium in the diet. Excess potassium that is not filtered in the glomerulus and delivered to the collecting tubule must therefore be secreted (*i.e.*, transported from the blood) into the tubular fluid for elimination from the body. In the absence of aldosterone (as in Addison's disease; see Chapter 26), potassium secretion becomes minimal. In these circumstances, potassium reabsorption exceeds secretion, and blood levels of potassium increase.

Atrial Naturetic Peptide. Atrial natriuretic peptide (ANP), discovered in 1981, is a hormone believed to have an important role in salt and water excretion by the kidney. It is synthesized in muscle cells of the atria of the heart and released when the atria are stretched. The actions of ANP include vasodilation of the afferent and efferent arterioles, which results in an increase in renal blood flow and glomerular filtration rate. ANP inhibits aldosterone secretion by the adrenal gland and it inhibits sodium reabsorption from the collecting tubules through its action on aldosterone and through direct action on the tubular cells. It also inhibits ADH release from the posterior pituitary gland, thereby increasing excretion of water by the kidneys. ANP also has vasodilator properties. Whether these effects are sufficient to produce long-term changes in blood pressure is uncertain.

Regulation of pH

The kidneys regulate body pH by conserving base bicarbonate or eliminating hydrogen ions. Neither the blood buffer systems nor the respiratory control mechanisms for carbon dioxide elimination can eliminate hydrogen ions (H^+) from the body. This is accomplished by the kidneys. The average North American diet results in the liberation of 40 to 80 mmol of hydrogen ions each day. Virtually all the hydrogen ions excreted in the urine are secreted into the tubular fluid by means of tubular secretory mechanisms. The lowest tubular fluid pH that can be achieved is 4.4 to 4.5. The ability of the kidneys to excrete hydrogen ions depends on buffers in the urine that combine with the hydrogen ion. The three major urine buffers are bicarbonate (HCO_3^-), phosphate (HPO_4^-), and ammonia (NH_3). Bicarbonate ions, which are present in the urine filtrate, combine with hydrogen ions that have been secreted into the tubular fluid; this results in the formation of carbon dioxide and water. The carbon dioxide is then absorbed into the tubular cells and bicarbonate is regenerated. The phosphate ion is a metabolic end product that is filtered into the tubular fluid; it combines with a secreted hydrogen ion and is not reabsorbed. Ammonia is synthesized in tubular cells by deamination of the amino acid glutamine; it diffuses into the tubular fluid and combines with the hydrogen ion. An important aspect of this buffer system is that the deamination process increases whenever the body's hydrogen ion concentration remains elevated for 1 to 2 days. These mechanisms for pH regulation are described more fully in Chapter 27.

pH-Dependent Elimination of Organic ions

The proximal tubule actively secretes large amounts of different organic anions. Foreign anions (*e.g.*, salicylates, penicillin) and endogenously produced anions (*e.g.*, bile acids, uric acid) are actively secreted into the tubular fluid. Most of the anions that are secreted use the same transport system, allowing the kidneys to rid the body of many different drugs and environmental agents. Because the same transport system is shared by different anions, there is competition for transport such that elevated levels of one substance tends to inhibit the secretion of other anions. The proximal tubules also possess an active transport system for organic cations that is analogous to that for organic ions.

Uric Acid Elimination

Uric acid is a product of purine metabolism (see Chapter 47). Excessively high blood levels (*i.e.*, hyperuricemia) can cause gout, and excessive levels in the urine can cause kidney stones. Uric acid is freely filtered in the glomerulus and is reabsorbed and secreted into the proximal tubules. Uric acid is one of the anions that uses the previously described anion transport system in the proximal tubule. Tubular reabsorption normally exceeds secretion, and the net effect is removal of uric acid from the filtrate. Although the rate of reabsorption exceeds secretion, the secretory process is homeostatically controlled to maintain a constant plasma level. Many persons with elevated uric acid levels secrete less uric acid than do persons with normal uric acid levels.

Uric acid uses the same transport systems as other anions, such as aspirin, sulfinpyrazone, and probenecid. Small doses of aspirin compete with uric acid for secretion into the tubular fluid and reduce uric acid secretion, and large doses compete with uric acid for reabsorption and increase uric acid excretion in the urine. Because of its effect on uric acid secretion, aspirin is not recommended for treatment of gouty arthritis. Thiazide and loop diuretics (*i.e.*, furosemide and ethacrynic acid) can also cause hyperuricemia and gouty arthritis, presumably through a decrease in extracellular fluid volume and enhanced uric acid reabsorption.

Urea Elimination

Urea is an end product of protein metabolism. The normal adult produces 25 to 30 g/day; the quantity rises when a high-protein diet is consumed, when there is excessive tissue breakdown, or in the presence of gastrointestinal bleeding. With gastrointestinal bleeding, the blood proteins are broken down to form ammonia in the intestine; the ammonia is then absorbed into the portal circulation and converted to urea by the liver before being released into the bloodstream. The kidneys, in their role as regulators of blood urea nitrogen (BUN) levels, filter urea in the glomeruli and then reabsorb it in the tubules. This enables maintenance of a normal BUN, which is in the range of 8 to 25 mg/dl (2.9 to 8.9 mmol/L). During periods of dehydration, the blood volume and GFR drop, and BUN levels increase. The renal tubules are permeable to urea, which means that the longer the tubular fluid remains in the kidneys, the greater is the reabsorption of urea into the blood. Only small amounts of urea are reabsorbed into the blood when the GFR is high, but relatively large amounts of urea are returned to the blood when the GFR is reduced.

Drug Elimination

Many drugs are eliminated in the urine. These drugs are selectively filtered in the glomerulus and reabsorbed or secreted into the tubular fluid. Only drugs that are not bound to plasma proteins are filtered in the glomerulus and therefore able to be eliminated by the kidneys.

Many drugs are weak acids or weak bases and are present in the renal tubular fluid partly as water-soluble ions and partly as nonionized lipid-soluble molecules. The nonionized lipid-soluble form of a drug diffuses more readily through the lipid membrane of the tubule and then back into the bloodstream. The water-soluble ionized form remains in the urine filtrate. The ratio of ionized to nonionized drug depends on the pH of the urine. For example, aspirin is highly ionized in alkaline urine and in this form is rapidly excreted in the urine.

Aspirin is largely nonionized in acid urine and is reabsorbed rather than excreted. Alkaline or acid diuresis may be used to increase elimination of drugs in the urine, particularly in situations of drug overdose.

Endocrine Functions of the Kidney

In addition to their function in regulating body fluids and electrolytes, the kidneys function as an endocrine organ in that they produce chemical mediators that travel through the blood to distant sites where they exert their actions. The kidneys participate in control of blood pressure by way of the renin-angiotensin mechanism, in calcium metabolism by activating vitamin D, and in regulating red blood cell production through the synthesis of erythropoietin.

The Renin-Angiotensin-Aldosterone Mechanism

The renin-angiotensin-aldosterone mechanism plays an important part in short-term and long-term regulation of blood pressure (see Chapter 18).

Renin is synthesized and stored in the juxtaglomerular cells of the kidney. This enzyme is thought to be released in response to a decrease in renal blood flow or a change in the composition of the distal tubular fluid or as the result of sympathetic nervous system stimulation. Renin itself has no direct effect on blood pressure. Rather, it acts enzymatically to convert a circulating plasma protein called *angiotensinogen* to angiotensin I. Angiotensin I, which has few vasoconstrictor properties, leaves the kidneys and enters the circulation; as it is circulated through the lungs, *angiotensin-converting enzyme* catalyzes the conversion of angiotensin I to angiotensin II. Angiotensin II is a potent vasoconstrictor, and it acts directly on the kidneys to decrease salt and water excretion. Both mechanisms have relatively short periods of action. Angiotensin II also stimulates aldosterone secretion by the adrenal gland. Aldosterone acts on the distal tubule to increase sodium reabsorption and exerts a longer-term effect on the maintenance of blood pressure.

Renin also functions by means of angiotensin II to produce constriction of the efferent arteriole as a means of preventing a serious decrease in glomerular filtration pressure.

Erythropoietin

Erythropoietin is a polypeptide hormone that regulates the differentiation of red blood cells in the bone marrow (see Chapter 8). Between 89% and 95% of erythropoietin is formed in the kidneys. The synthesis of erythropoietin is stimulated by tissue hypoxia, which may be brought about by anemia, residence at high altitudes, or impaired oxygenation of tissues due to cardiac or pulmonary disease. Persons with end-stage kidney disease often are anemic because of an inability of the kidneys to produce erythropoietin. This anemia is generally managed by the administration of epoetin-α, a synthetic form of erythropoietin produced through DNA technology, to stimulate erythropoiesis.

Vitamin D

Activation of Vitamin D occurs in the kidneys. Vitamin D increases calcium absorption from the gastrointestinal tract and helps to regulate calcium deposition in bone. It also has a weak stimulatory effect on renal calcium absorption. Although Vitamin D is not synthesized and released from an endocrine gland, it is often considered as a hormone because of its pathway of molecular activation and mechanism of action.

It exists in several forms: natural vitamin D (cholecalciferol), which results from ultraviolet irradiation of the skin, and synthetic vitamin D (ergocalciferol), which is derived from irradiation of ergosterol. The active form of vitamin D is 1,25-dihydroxycholecalciferol. Cholecalciferol and ergocalciferol must undergo chemical transformation to become active: first to 25-hydroxycholecalciferol in the liver and then to 1,25-dihydroxycholecalciferol in the kidneys (see Chapter 44). Persons with end-stage renal disease are unable to transform Vitamin D to its active form and must rely on pharmacologic preparations of the active vitamin (calcitriol) for maintaining mineralization of their bones.

In summary, the kidneys perform excretory and endocrine functions. In the process of excreting wastes, the kidneys filter the blood and then selectively reabsorb those materials that are needed to maintain a stable internal environment. The kidneys rid the body of metabolic wastes, regulate fluid volume, regulate the composition of electrolytes, assist in maintaining acid-base balance, aid in regulation of blood pressure through the renin-angiotensin-aldosterone mechanism and control of extracellular fluid volume, regulate red blood cell production through erythropoietin, and aid in calcium metabolism by activating vitamin D.

The nephron is the functional unit of the kidney. It is composed of a glomerulus, which filters the blood, and a tubular component, where electrolytes and other substances needed to maintain the constancy of the internal environment are reabsorbed into the bloodstream while unneeded materials are secreted into the tubular filtrate for elimination. Urine concentration occurs in the collecting tubules under the influence of ADH. ADH maintains extracellular volume by returning water to the vascular compartment, producing a concentrated urine by removing water from the tubular filtrate.

The GFR is the amount of filtrate that is formed each minute as blood moves through the glomeruli. It is regulated by the arterial blood pressure and renal blood flow in the normal functioning kidney. The juxtaglomerular complex is thought to represent a feedback control system that links changes in the GFR with renal blood flow. Renal clearance is the volume of plasma that is completely cleared each minute of any substance that finds its way into the urine. It is determined by the ability of the substance to be filtered in the glomeruli and the capacity of the renal tubules to reabsorb or secrete the substance.

Tests of Renal Function

After you have completed this section of the chapter, you should be able to meet the following objectives:

- Describe the characteristics of normal urine
- Explain the significance of casts in the urine
- Explain the value of urine specific gravity in evaluating renal function
- Explain the concept of the glomerular filtration rate
- Explain the value of serum creatinine levels in evaluating renal function
- Describe the methods used in cystoscopic examination of the urinary tract, ultrasound studies of the urinary tract, computed tomographic scans, magnetic resonance imaging studies, excretory urography, and renal angiography

The function of the kidneys is to filter the blood, selectively reabsorb those substances that are needed to maintain the constancy of body fluid, and excrete metabolic wastes. The composition of urine and blood provides valuable information about the adequacy of renal function. Radiologic tests, endoscopy, and renal biopsy afford means for viewing the gross and microscopic structures of the kidneys and urinary system.

Urinalysis

Urine is a clear, amber-colored fluid that is about 95% water and 5% dissolved solids. The kidneys normally produce about 1.5 L of urine each day. Normal urine contains metabolic wastes and few or no plasma proteins, blood cells, or glucose molecules.

Urine tests can be performed on a single urine specimen or on a 24-hour urine specimen. First-voided morning specimens are useful for qualitative protein and specific gravity testing. A freshly voided specimen is most reliable. Urine specimens that have been left standing may contain lysed red blood cells, disintegrating casts, and rapidly multiplying bacteria. Table 25–1 describes urinalysis values for normal urine.

Casts are molds of the distal nephron lumen. A gel-like substance called Tamm-Horsfall mucoprotein, which is formed in the tubular epithelium, is the major protein constituent of urinary casts. Casts composed of this gel but devoid of cells are called *hyaline casts*. These casts develop when the protein concentration of the urine is high (as in nephrotic syndrome), urine osmolality is high, and urine pH is low. The inclusion of granules or cells in the matrix of the protein gel leads to the formation of various other types of casts.

The *specific gravity* (or osmolality) of urine varies with its concentration of solutes. Urine specific gravity provides a valuable index of the hydration status and functional ability of the kidneys. Although there are more sophisticated methods for measuring specific gravity, it can be easily measured using an inexpensive piece of equipment called a urinometer. Healthy kidneys can produce a concentrated urine with a specific gravity of 1.030 to 1.040. During periods of marked hydration, the specific gravity can approach 1.000. With diminished renal function, there is a loss of renal concentrating ability, and the urine specific gravity may fall to levels of 1.006 to 1.010 (usual range is 1.010 to 1.025 with normal fluid intake). These low levels are particularly significant if they occur during periods that follow a decrease in water intake (*e.g.*, during the first urine specimen on arising in the morning).

Glomerular Filtration Rate

The GFR provides a gauge of renal function. It can be measured clinically by collecting timed samples of blood and urine. Creatinine, a product of creatine metabolism by the muscle, is filtered by the kidneys but not reabsorbed in the renal tubule. Creatinine values in the blood and urine can be used to measure GFR. The clearance rate for creatinine is the amount that is completely cleared by the kidneys in 1 minute. The formula is expressed as $C = UV/P$, in which C is the clearance rate (ml/minute), U is the urine concentration (mg/dl), V is the urine volume excreted (ml/minute or 24 hours), and P is plasma concentration (mg/dl).

TABLE 25–1
Normal Values for Routine Urinalysis

General Characteristics and Measurements	Chemical Determinations	Microscopic Examination of Sediment
Color: yellow-amber—indicates a high specific gravity and small output of urine Turbidity: clear to slightly hazy Specific gravity: 1.010–1.025 with a normal fluid intake pH: 4.6–4.8—average person has a pH of about 6 (acid)	Glucose: negative Ketones: negative Blood: negative Protein: negative Bilirubin: negative Urobilinogen: 0.1–1 Nitrate for bacteria: negative Leukocyte esterase: negative	Casts negative: occasional hyaline casts Red blood cells: negative or rare Crystals: negative White blood cells: negative or rare Epithelial cells: few

(Fischbach F. [1992]. *A manual of laboratory diagnostic tests* [p. 148]. Philadelphia: J.B. Lippincott)

Normal creatinine clearance is 115 to 125 ml/minute. This value is corrected for body surface area, which reflects the muscle mass where creatinine metabolism takes place. The test may be done on a 24-hour basis, with blood being drawn at the time the urine collection is completed. In another method, two 1-hour urine specimens are collected, and a blood sample is drawn in between.

Blood Tests

Blood tests can provide valuable information about the kidneys' ability to remove metabolic wastes from the blood and to maintain normal electrolyte and pH composition of the blood. Normal blood values are listed in Table 25–2. Serum levels of potassium, phosphate, BUN, and creatinine increase in renal failure. Serum pH, calcium, and bicarbonate levels decrease in renal failure. The effect of renal failure on the concentration of serum electrolytes and metabolic end products is discussed in Chapter 29.

Serum Creatinine

Serum creatinine levels reflect the glomerular filtration rate. Because these measurements are easily obtained and relatively inexpensive, they are often used as a screening measure of renal function. *Creatinine* is a product of *creatine* metabolism in muscles; its formation and release are relatively constant and proportional to the amount of muscle mass present. Creatinine is freely filtered in the glomeruli, is not reabsorbed from the tubules into the blood, and is only minimally secreted into the tubules from the blood; therefore, its blood values depend closely on the GFR.

The normal creatinine value is about 0.7 mg/dl of blood for a woman with a small frame, about 1.0 mg/dl of blood for a normal adult man, and about 1.5 mg/dl of blood (60 to 130 mmol/L) for a muscular man. There is an age-related decline in creatinine clearance in many elderly persons, because muscle mass and the GFR decline with age (see Chapter 29). A normal serum creatinine level usually indicates normal renal function. In addition to its use in calculating the GFR, the serum creatinine level is used in estimating the functional capacity of the kidneys (Fig. 25–15). If the value doubles, the GFR—and renal function—probably has fallen to one half of its normal state. A rise in the serum creatinine level to three times its normal value suggests that there is a 75% loss of renal function, and with creatinine values of 10 mg/dl or more, it can be assumed that about 90% of renal function has been lost.

Blood Urea Nitrogen

Urea is formed in the liver as a byproduct of protein metabolism and eliminated entirely by the kidneys. BUN therefore is related to the GFR but, unlike creatinine, is also influenced by protein intake, gastrointestinal bleeding, and hydration status. Increased protein intake and gastrointestinal bleeding increase urea by means of protein metabolism. In gastrointestinal bleeding, the blood is broken down by the intestinal flora, and the nitrogenous waste is absorbed into the portal vein and transported to the liver, where it is converted to urea. During dehydration, elevated BUN levels result from increased concentration. About two thirds of renal function must be lost before a significant rise in the BUN level occurs.

The BUN is less specific for renal insufficiency than creatinine, but the BUN-creatinine ratio may provide useful diagnostic information. The ratio normally is about 10:1. Ratios greater than 15:1 represent prerenal conditions such as in congestive heart failure and upper gastrointestinal tract bleeding that produce an increase in BUN but not in creatinine. A ratio of less than 10:1 occurs in persons with liver disease and in those who receive a low-protein diet or chronic dialysis, because BUN is more readily dialyzable than creatinine.

TABLE 25–2
Normal Blood Chemistry Levels

Substance	Normal Value
Blood urea nitrogen	8.0–25.0 mg/dl (2.9–8.9 mmol/L)
Creatinine	0.7–1.5 mg/dl (60–130 μmol/L)
Sodium	137–147 mEq/L (137–147 mmol/L)
Chloride	100–106 mEq/L (100–106 mmol/L)
Potassium	3.5–5 mEq/L (3.5–5 mmol/L)
Carbon dioxide (CO_2 content)	24–29 mEq/L (24–29 mmol/L)
Calcium	8.5–10.3 mg/dl (2.1–2.6 mmol/l)
Phosphate	3–4.5 mg/dl (1–1.5 mmol/l)
Uric acid	2.6–7.2 mg/dl (0.154–0.42 mmol/l)
pH	7.35–7.45

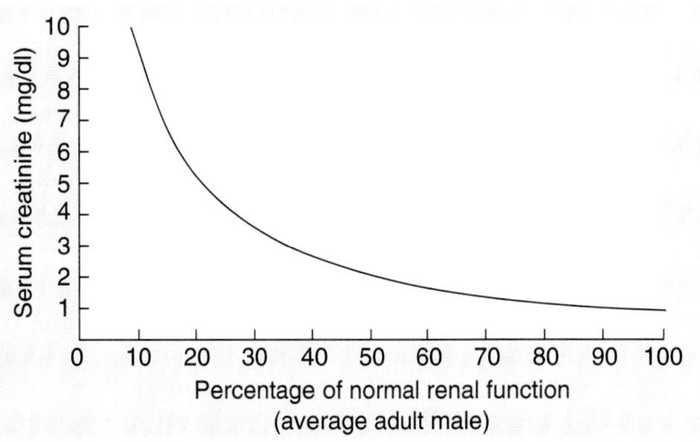

Figure 25–15
Relation between the percentage of renal function and serum creatinine levels.

Cystoscopy

Cystoscopy provides a means for direct visualization of the urethra, bladder, and ureteral orifices. It relies on the use of a cystoscope, an instrument with a lighted lens. The cystoscope is inserted through the urethra into the bladder. Biopsy specimens, lesions, small stones, and foreign bodies can be removed from the bladder. Urethroscopy may be used to remove stones from the ureter and aid in the treatment of ureteral disorders such as ureteral strictures.

Ultrasonography

Ultrasound studies use the reflection of ultrasonic (high-frequency) waves to visualize the deep structures of the body. The procedure is painless and noninvasive and requires no patient preparation. Ultrasonography is used to visualize the structures of the kidneys and has proved useful in the diagnosis of many urinary tract disorders, including congenital anomalies, renal abscesses, hydronephrosis, and kidney stones. It can differentiate a renal cyst from a renal tumor. The use of ultrasonography also enables accurate placement of needles for renal biopsy and catheters for percutaneous nephrostomy.

Radiologic and Other Imaging Studies

Radiologic studies include a simple flat plate (radiograph) of the kidneys, ureters, and bladder that can be used to determine the size, shape, and position of the kidneys and to observe any radiopaque stones that may be in the kidney pelvis or ureters. In excretory urography, or intravenous pyelography, a radiopaque dye is injected into a peripheral vein; the dye is then filtered by the glomerulus and excreted into the urine, and x-ray films are taken as it moves through the kidneys and ureters.

Urography is used to detect space-occupying lesions of the kidneys, pyelonephritis, hydronephrosis, vesicoureteral reflux, and kidney stones. Some persons are allergic to the dye used for urography and may develop an anaphylactic reaction after its administration. Every person undergoing urography studies should be questioned about previous reactions to the dye or to similar dyes. If the test is considered essential in such persons, premedication with antihistamines and corticosteroids may be used. The dye also reduces renal blood flow; acute renal failure can occur, particularly in persons with vascular disease or preexisting renal insufficiency.

Other diagnostic tests include computed tomographic (CT) scans, magnetic resonance imaging (MRI), radionuclide imaging, and renal angiography. CT scans may be used to outline the kidneys and detect renal masses and tumors. MRI is becoming readily available and is used in imaging the kidneys, retroperitoneum, and urinary bladder. It is particularly useful in evaluating vascular abnormalities in and around the kidneys. *Radionuclide imaging* involves the injection of a radioactive material that subsequently is detected externally by a scintillation camera, which detects the radioactive emissions. Radionuclide imaging is used to evaluate renal function and structures, as well as the ureters and bladder. It is particularly useful in evaluating the function of kidney transplants. *Renal angiography* provides x-ray pictures of the blood vessels that supply the kidneys. It involves the injection of a radiopaque dye directly into the renal artery. A catheter usually is introduced through the femoral artery and advanced under fluoroscopic view into the abdominal aorta. The catheter tip is then maneuvered into the renal artery, and the dye is injected. This test is used in evaluating persons suspected of having renal artery stenosis, abnormalities of renal blood vessels, or vascular damage to the renal arteries after trauma.

In summary, urinalysis and blood tests that measure levels of byproducts of metabolism and electrolytes provide information about renal function. Cystoscopic examinations can be used for direct visualization of the urethra, bladder, and ureters. Ultrasonography can be used to determine kidney size, and renal radionuclide imaging can be used to evaluate the kidney structures. Radiologic methods such as excretory urography provide a means by which kidney structures such as the renal calyces, pelvis, ureters, and bladder can be outlined.

Physiologic Action of Diuretics

After you have completed this section of the chapter, you should be able to meet the following objectives:

- Describe the physiologic action of diuretics
- Contrast and compare the actions of osmotic diuretics, loop diuretics, thiazide diuretics, aldosterone antagonists, and carbonic anhydrase inhibitors

Diuresis is the rapid passage of urine through the kidneys. In some disease states, it is desirable to increase urine output through the use of diuretics. Water reabsorption in the kidneys is largely passive and depends on sodium reabsorption. Most diuretics exert their action by interfering with sodium reabsorption. About 70% to 75% of sodium reabsorption takes place in the proximal tubule, 20% to 25% in the loop of Henle, and 2% to 5% in the distal convoluted and collecting tubules (Fig. 25–16). The effectiveness of a diuretic in promoting salt and water excretion depends on the tubular site of action. Because of diuretics' mechanism of action, it is logical to include a discussion of them in this chapter. There are four types of diuretics: osmotic diuretics, inhibitors of sodium transport, aldosterone antagonists, and inhibitors of urine acidification.

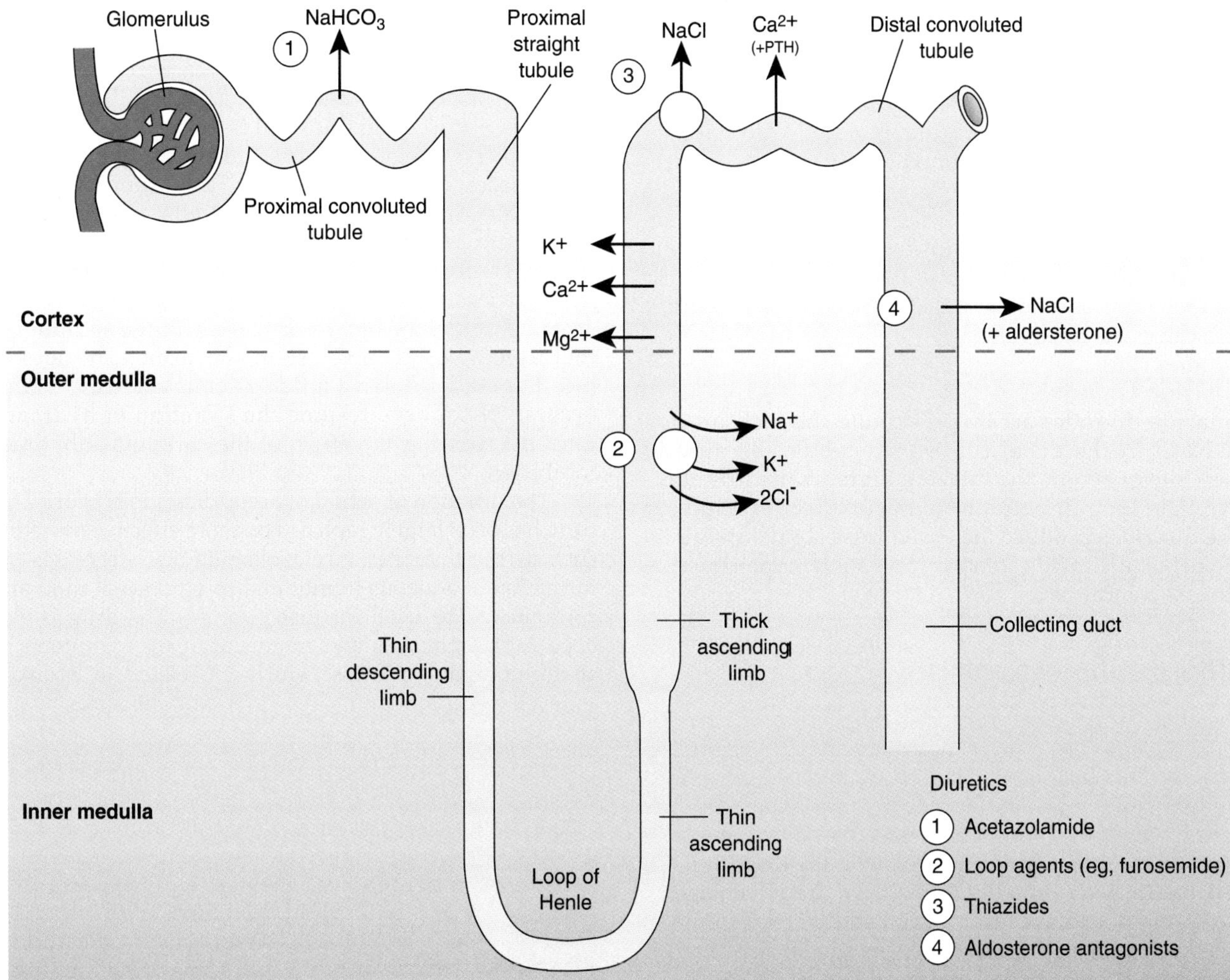

Figure 25–16
Sites of action of diuretics.

Osmotic Diuretics

Osmotic diuretics, such as mannitol, are filtered in the glomerulus but not reabsorbed in the tubules. The proximal tubule and descending limb are freely permeable to water. Because these substances are poorly reabsorbed, they increase the osmolality of the tubular filtrate and cause water diuresis. Because these agents are poorly absorbed, they must be given intravenously rather than orally. The osmotic diuretics increase water elimination in preference to sodium; therefore, they reduce total body water more than cation content and reduce intracellular volume. This effect is used to reduce intracranial pressure in persons with neurologic conditions or intraocular pressure before eye surgery. They are also used to maintain a high urine volume after a hemolytic reaction or the ingestion of toxic substances, such as salicylates or barbiturates, which are excreted in the urine.

Inhibitors of Sodium Transport

Sodium reabsorption occurs in the proximal tubule, the thick ascending loop of Henle, and the distal tubule, where aldosterone regulates sodium and potassium exchange. Diuretics that alter sodium transport can act at any of these levels. About 25% to 30% of sodium is reabsorbed in the thick ascending loop of Henle, about 10% in the distal convoluted tubule, and 2% to 5% is reabsorbed in the late distal and cortical collecting tubule. The effectiveness of a diuretic is determined by its site of action.

Loop Diuretics

Loop diuretics exert their effect in the thick ascending loop of Henle. Because of their site of action, these drugs are the most effective diuretic agents available. These drugs inhibit the coupled Na^+-K^+-$2Cl^-$ transport system on the luminal side of the ascending limb of Henle. By inhibiting this transport system, they reduce the reabsorption of NaCl, decrease potassium reabsorption, and increase calcium and magnesium elimination. Prolonged use can cause significant loss of magnesium in some persons. Because calcium is actively reabsorbed in the distal convoluted tubule, loop diuretics do not usually cause hypocalcemia. Impairment of sodium reabsorption in the loop of Henle causes a decrease in the osmolarity of the interstitial fluid surrounding the collecting ducts and further impedes the kidneys' ability to concentrate urine. The loop diuretics may increase uric acid retention and impair glucose tolerance. These drugs also can cause hypovolemia.

Thiazide Diuretics

Thiazide diuretics act by preventing the reabsorption of NaCl in the distal convoluted tubule. Because of their site of action, the thiazide diuretics are less effective than loop diuretics in terms of effecting diuresis. The thiazides produce increased losses of potassium in the urine, uric acid retention, and some impairment in glucose tolerance.

Aldosterone Antagonists

The aldosterone antagonists, also called *potassium-sparing diuretics,* reduce sodium reabsorption and increase potassium secretion in the late distal tubule and cortical collecting tubule site regulated by aldosterone. Because of their site of action, the aldosterone antagonists have the least effect on diuresis when compared with the loop diuretics and the thiazide diuretics. They have the advantage of increasing potassium reabsorption and thereby eliminating the risk of hypokalemia. These agents also tend to interfere with secretion of hydrogen ions in the collecting duct, in part explaining the metabolic acidosis sometimes seen with the use of these agents.

There are two types of potassium-sparing diuretics: those that act as direct aldosterone antagonists and those that act independently of aldosterone. The first type (*e.g.,* spironolactone) binds to the mineralocoid receptor in the tubule, preventing aldosterone from binding and exerting its effects. The second type (*e.g.,* triamterene, amiloride) does not bind to the receptor, but instead it directly interferes with sodium entry through the sodium-selective ion channel. Because potassium secretion is coupled with sodium reabsorption in this segment of the tubule, these agents are effective potassium-sparing diuretics. These diuretics are used during states of mineralocorticoid excess and because of their effects on potassium excretion. Because the thiazide and aldosterone antagonists affect sodium reabsorption at different tubule sites, combination products of the two agents (*i.e.,* hydrochlorothiazide-triamterene [Dyazide], hydrochlorothiazide-amiloride [Moduretic], hydrochlorothiazide-spironolactone [Aldactazide]) are available. Because of their mechanism of action, these diuretics may cause severe hyperkalemia.

Inhibitors of Urine Acidification

Acetazolamide, a carbonic anhydrase inhibitor, impairs the reaction that converts carbon dioxide and water to bicarbonate and hydrogen ions. Bicarbonate is poorly absorbed in the renal tubules; it instead combines with hydrogen that is secreted into the tubule to form carbon dioxide and water. The carbon dioxide is then reabsorbed into the tubular cells, where it combines with water in a carbonic anhydrase–catalyzed reaction to form bicarbonate and hydrogen ions. When hydrogen ion secretion is blocked by the action of acetazolamide, the bicarbonate ion and the sodium ion that accompany it are lost in the urine. The loss of bicarbonate results in a mild systemic acidosis. As this occurs, the kidneys resume the secretion of hydrogen ions, overcoming the effect of the carbonic anhydrase inhibition.

The duration of action of acetazolamide is short. This drug has been largely replaced by more effective diuretics, such as the thiazides. Acetazolamide also decreases the formation of aqueous humor and cerebrospinal fluid and continues to be used for that purpose. The drug is also used for prophylaxis and treatment of the symptoms of acute mountain sickness, which are related to hypoxia-induced hyperventilation and respiratory alkalosis.

In summary, diuretics are drugs that increase urine output. With the exception of osmotic diuretics, they exert their action by altering sodium transport. Osmotic diuretics are filtered in the glomerulus and reabsorbed in the tubules. They act by increasing the osmolarity of tubular fluid. Inhibitors of urine acidification, such as acetazolamide, prevent bicarbonate reabsorption and the accompanying sodium reabsorption. Loop diuretics block sodium reabsorption in the thick ascending loop of Henle, and thiazide diuretics function in the section of the tubule between the thick ascending loop of Henle and the distal tubule. The potassium-sparing diuretics decrease sodium reabsorption while causing potassium retention.

BIBLIOGRAPHY

Cormack D.H. (1993). *Essential histology* (pp. 322–333). Philadelphia: J.B. Lippincott.

Guyton A. (1996). *Textbook of medical physiology* (9th ed., pp. 315–382). Philadelphia: W.B. Saunders.

Puchett J.B. (1994). Pharmacologic classification and renal actions of diuretics. *Cardiology* 84 (Suppl. 2), 4–13.

Rhoades R.A. (1996). *Medical physiology* (pp. 417–445). Boston: Little, Brown.

Smith H. (1953). *From fish to philosopher* (p. 4). Boston: Little, Brown.

Vander A.J. (1995). *Renal physiology* (5th ed.). New York: McGraw-Hill.

CHAPTER 26

Alterations in Fluid and Electrolytes

Body fluids contain water, electrolytes, proteins, and other substances. The precise regulation of these fluids within a narrow physiologic range is essential to life. The volume and composition of these fluids remain relatively constant in the presence of a wide range of changes in intake and output. Environmental stresses and disease conditions often increase losses, impair intake, and otherwise interfere with mechanisms that regulate body fluid volume, composition, and distribution.

This chapter is divided into four sections: composition and compartmental distribution of body fluids, sodium and water balance, potassium balance, and calcium, phosphate, and magnesium balance. The mechanisms of edema formation are discussed in the section on composition and compartmentalization of body fluids. Because of their effects on fluid and electrolyte balance, disorders of antidiuretic hormone (ADH), including diabetes insipidus and syndrome of inappropriate ADH, are also discussed in this chapter.

Composition and Compartmental Distribution of Body Fluids

After you have completed this section of the chapter, you should be able to meet the following objectives:

- Differentiate the intracellular from the extracellular compartments in terms of distribution and composition of water, electrolytes, and other osmotically active solutes between the intracellular and extracellular compartments
- Relate the concept of a concentration gradient to the processes of diffusion and osmosis
- Describe the control of cell volume and the effect of isotonic, hypotonic, and hypertonic solutions on cell size
- Characterize the distribution of fluids in the extracellular compartment
- Describe factors that control fluid exchange between the vascular and interstitial fluid compartments and relate to the development of edema and third spacing of extracellular fluids
- Describe the manifestations and treatment of edema

Body fluids are distributed between the intracellular and extracellular fluid compartments. The intracellular compartment consists of fluid contained within all of the billions of body cells. It is the larger of the two compartments, containing about two thirds of the body water. The extracellular compartment contains all the fluids outside the body cells, including that in the blood vessels (Fig. 26–1). Extracellular fluids have high concentrations of sodium, chloride, and bicarbonate and low concentrations of potassium, magnesium, calcium, and phosphates. Intracellular fluids have high concentrations of potassium, phosphates, and magnesium and low concentrations of sodium, chloride, and bicarbonate (Table 26–1).

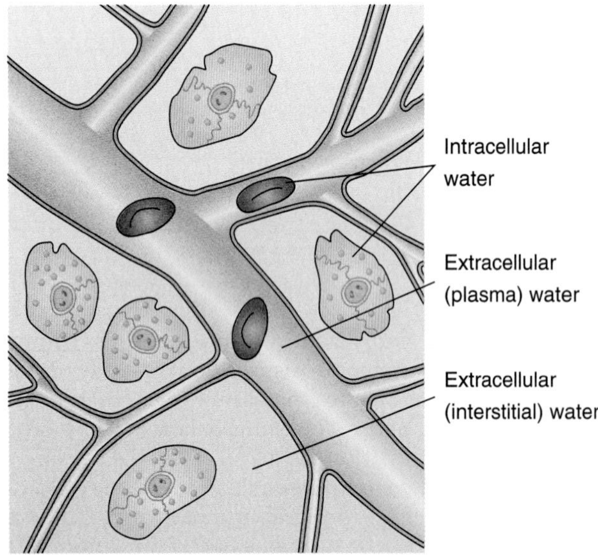

FIGURE 26–1
Distribution of body water. The extracellular space includes the vascular compartment and the interstitial spaces.

TABLE 26–1
Concentrations of Extracellular and Intracellular Electrolytes in Adults

Electrolyte	Extracellular Concentration*	Intracellular Concentration*
Sodium	135–148 mEq/L	10–14 mEq/L
Potassium	3.5–5.0 mEq/L	140–150 mEq/L
Chloride	98–106 mEq/L	3–4 mEq/L
Bicarbonate	24–31 mEq/L	7–10 mEq/L
Calcium	8.5–10.5 mg/dl	< 1 mEq/L
Phosphate/phosphorus	2.5–4.5 mg/dl	4 mEq/kg†
Magnesium	1.8–2.7 mg/dl	40 mEq/kg†

*Values may vary among laboratories, depending on the method of analysis used.
†Values vary among various tissues and with nutritional status.

It is the extracellular levels of electrolytes in the blood or blood serum that are measured clinically. Although blood levels usually are representative of the total body levels of an electrolyte, this is not always the case, particularly with potassium, which is about 28 times more concentrated inside the cell than outside. The cell membrane serves as the primary barrier to the movement of substances between the extracellular and intracellular compartments. Lipid-soluble substances such as gases (*i.e.*, oxygen and carbon dioxide), which dissolve in the lipid bilayer of the cell membrane, pass directly through the membrane. Many ions such as Na^+ and K^+ rely on energy-dependent transport mechanisms such as the Na^+-K^+ membrane pump for movement across the membrane (see Chapter 1). Water crosses the membrane by osmosis using special protein channels.

Introductory Concepts

Dissociation of Electrolytes

Body fluids contain water and electrolytes. Electrolytes are substances that dissociate in solution to form *charged particles*, or *ions*. For example, a sodium chloride (NaCl) molecule dissociates to form a positively charged sodium ion (Na^+) and a negatively charged chloride ion (Cl^-). Particles that do not dissociate into ions such as glucose and urea are called *nonelectrolytes*. Positively charged ions are called *cations* because they are attracted to the cathode of a wet electric cell, and negatively charged ions are called *anions* because they are attracted to the anode. The ions found in body fluids carry one charge (*i.e., monovalent ion*) or two charges (*i.e., divalent ion*). Because of their attraction forces, positively charged cations are always accompanied by negatively charged anions. The distribution of

Measurement Units

The amount of electrolytes and solutes that are in body fluids are expressed as a concentration or amount of solute in a given volume of fluid, such as, milligrams per deciliter (mg/dl), milliequivalents per liter (mEq/L), or millimoles per liter (mmol/L). The *milligrams per deciliter* measurement unit expresses the weight of the solute in one tenths of a liter (dl) or 100 ml of solution. The concentration of electrolytes, such as calcium, phosphate, and magnesium, are often expressed in mg/dl.

The *Milliequivalent* is used to express the charge equivalency for a given weight of an electrolyte. Electroneutrality requires that the total number of cations in the body equal the total number of anions. When cations and anions combine, they do so according to their ionic charge, not according to their atomic weight. Thus, 1 mEq of sodium has the same number of charges as 1 mEq of chloride, regardless of molecular weight (although sodium is positive and chloride is negative). The number of milliequivalents of an electrolyte in a liter of solution can be derived from the following equation:

$$\text{mEq} = \frac{\text{mg/100 mL} \times 10 \times \text{valence}}{\text{atomic weight}}$$

The Système of Internationale (SI) units express electrolyte content of body fluids in *millimoles per liter (mmol/L)*. A millimole is one thousanth of a mole, or the molecular weight of a substance expressed in milligrams. The number of millimoles of an electrolyte in a liter of solution can be calculated using the following equation:

$$\text{mmol/L} = \frac{\text{mEq/L}}{\text{valence}}$$

For monovalent electrolytes such as sodium and potassium, the mmol and mEq values are identical. For example 140 mEq is equal to 140 mmol of sodium.

electrolytes between body compartments is influenced by their electrical charge. However, one cation may be exchanged for another, providing it carries the same charge (*e.g.*, a positively charged hydrogen ion may be exchanged for a positively charged potassium ion), and a negatively charged anion such as bicarbonate may be exchanged for another negatively charged anion such as chloride.

Diffusion and Osmosis

Diffusion. Water and particles in body fluids use the process of diffusion to move between the intracellular and extracellular compartments. *Diffusion* is the movement of charged or uncharged particles along a concentration gradient. All molecules and ions, including water and dissolved molecules, are in constant, random motion. It is the motion of these particles, each colliding with one another, that supplies the energy for diffusion. Because there are more molecules in constant motion in a concentrated solution, particles move from an area of higher concentration to one of lower concentration.

Osmosis. Water molecules also exhibit random motion and have diffusion properties similar to that of solute particles. The diffusion of water across a semipermeable membrane (*i.e.*, one that is permeable to water but impermeable to most solutes) is called *osmosis*. When solutes are added to water, they dilute the water molecules and decrease their activity. Water moves from the side of the membrane with the lesser number of nondiffusible particles to the side with the greater number (Fig. 26–2). As water moves across the semipermeable membrane, it generates a pressure, called the *osmotic pressure*. The osmotic pressure equals the hydrostatic pressure (measured in millimeters of mercury) needed to oppose the movement of water across the membrane.

The osmotic activity that nondiffusible particles exert in drawing water from one side of the semipermeable membrane to the other is measured by a unit called an *osmole*. The osmole is derived from the gram molecular weight of a substance (*i.e.*, 1 gram molecular weight of a nondiffusible and nonionizable substance is equal to 1 osmole). In the clinical setting, osmotic activity usually is expressed in milliosmoles (one thousandth of an osmole) per liter. Each nondiffusible particle, large or small, is equally effective in its ability to pull water through a semipermeable membrane. The osmotic activity of a solution is determined by the number, rather than the size, of the nondiffusible particles.

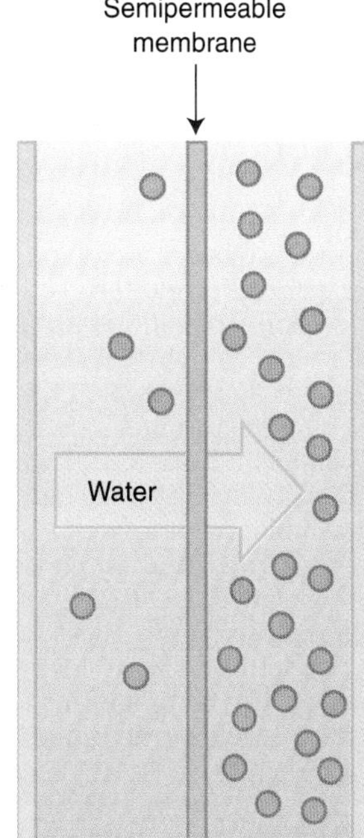

FIGURE 26–2 Movement of water across a semipermeable membrane. Water moves from the side that has fewer nondiffusible particles to the side that has more.

The osmotic activity of a solution may be expressed in terms of its osmolarity or osmolality. *Osmolarity* refers to the osmolar concentration in 1 liter of solution (mOsm/L) and *osmolality* to the osmolar concentration in a kilogram of water (mOsm/kg of H_2O). Osmolarity is usually used when referring to fluids outside the body, but osmolality is used for describing fluids inside the body. Because 1 L of water weighs 1 kg, the terms osmolarity and osmolality are often used interchangeably.

The predominant osmotically active particles in the extracellular fluid are Na^+ and its attendant anions (Cl^- and HCO_3^-), which together account for 90% to 95% of the osmotic pressure. Blood urea nitrogen (BUN) and glucose, which are also osmotically active, account for less than 5% of the total osmotic pressure in the extracellular compartment. This can change, however, as when blood glucose levels are elevated in persons with diabetes mellitus or when BUN levels rise in those with renal failure. Serum osmolality, which normally ranges between 275 and 295 mOsm/kg, can be calculated using the following equation:

$$\text{Osmolality (mOsm/kg)} = 2[\text{Na}^+(\text{mmol/L})] + \frac{\text{Glucose (mg/dl)}}{18} + \frac{\text{BUN (mg/dl)}}{2.8}$$

For example, 1 mOsm of glucose equals 180 mg/L, and 1 mOsm of urea equals 28 mg/L. Ordinarily, the calculated and measured osmolality are within 10 mOsm of one another. The difference between the calculated and measured osmolality is called the *osmolar gap*. An osmolar gap larger than 10 mOsm suggests the presence of an unmeasured, osmotically active substance such as alcohol, acetone, or mannitol.

Urine Osmolality

Urine osmolality reflects the kidneys' ability to produce a concentrated or diluted urine based on serum osmolality and the need for water conservation or excretion. The ratio of urine osmolality to serum osmolality in a 24-hour urine sample normally exceeds 1:1, and after a period of overnight water deprivation, it should be greater than 3:1. A dehydrated person (one who has a loss of water) may have a urine-serum ratio that approaches 4:1. In these persons, urine osmolality may exceed 1000 mOsm/kg H_2O. In those who have difficulty concentrating their urine (e.g., those with diabetes insipidus or chronic renal failure), the urine-serum ratio often is less than or equal to 1:1.

Urine specific gravity compares the weight of urine with that of water, providing an index for solute concentration. Water is considered to be 1.000. A change in specific gravity of 1.010 to 1.020 is an increase of 400 mOsm/kg H_2O. In the sodium-depleted state, the kidneys usually try to conserve sodium; urine specific gravity is normal, and urine sodium and chloride concentrations are low.

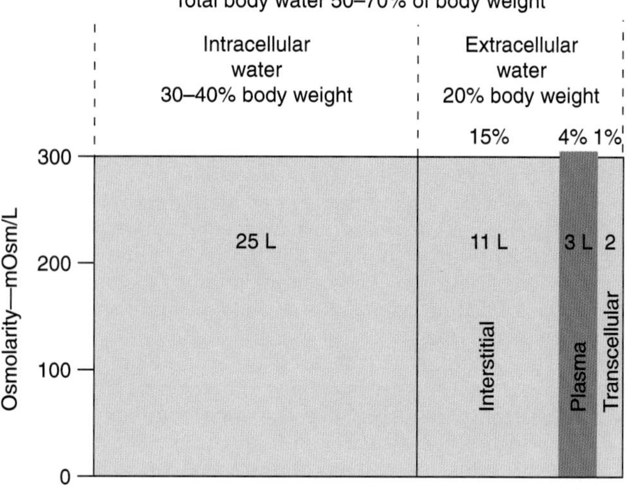

Figure 26–3
Approximate size of body compartments in a 70-kg adult. (Krieger J.N., Sherrard D.J. [1991]. *Practical fluid and electrolytes* [p. 105]. Norwalk, CT: Appleton & Lange)

Compartmental Distribution of Body Fluids

Body water is distributed between the intracellular and extracellular compartments. In the adult, the fluid in the intracellular compartment constitutes 30% to 40% of body weight.[1] The fluid in the extracellular compartment is further divided into two major subdivisions: the plasma compartment, which constitutes about 4% of body weight, and the interstitial fluid compartment, which constitutes about 15% of body weight (Fig. 26–3). Lymph, which is part of extracellular fluid, constitutes another 2% to 3% of body weight.

A third, usually minor, subdivision of the extracellular fluid compartment is the transcellular compartment. It includes the cerebrospinal fluid, and fluid contained within the various body spaces, such as the peritoneal, pleural, and pericardial cavities; the joint spaces; and the gastrointestinal tract. Normally, only about 1% of extracellular fluid is in the transcellular space. This amount can increase considerably in conditions such as ascites, in which large amounts of fluid are sequestered in the peritoneal cavity. When the transcellular fluid compartment becomes considerably enlarged, it is referred to as a *third space*, because this fluid is not easily exchanged with the rest of the extracellular fluid.

Intracellular Fluid Volume

Intracellular volume is regulated by large numbers of proteins and other organic compounds that cannot escape through the cell membrane and by the sodium/potassium ion (Na^+/K^+) membrane pump. Most of these intracellular substances are negatively charged and attract large numbers of positively charged ions, including potassium. All of these substances are osmotically active and would, if left unchecked, pull water into the cell until it ruptured. The reason this does not occur is because the Na^+/K^+

membrane pump continuously removes three Na^+ ions from the cell for every 2 K^+ ions that are moved back into the cell. Situations that impair the function of the Na^+/K^+ pump, such as hypoxia, cause cells to swell because of an accumulation of Na^+ ions.

A change in water content causes cells to swell or shrink. The term *tonicity* refers to the tension or effect that the effective osmotic pressure of a solution with impermeable solutes exerts on cell size because of water movement across the cell membrane. Tonicity is determined solely by those substances that cannot penetrate the cell membrane, thereby, producing an osmotic force that pulls water into or out of the cell and causing it to change size. For example, urea, which is osmotically active and lipid soluble, tends to distribute equally across the cell membrane; when extracellular levels of urea are elevated, intracellular levels are also elevated. Urea is therefore considered to be an ineffective osmole. It is only when extracellular levels of urea change rapidly, as during hemodialysis treatment, that urea affects tonicity.

Solutions to which body cells are exposed can be classified as isotonic, hypotonic, or hypertonic depending on whether they cause cells to swell or shrink (Fig. 26–4). Cells placed in an *isotonic solution,* which has the same effective osmolality as intracellular fluids (*e.g.,* 280 mOsm/L), neither shrink nor swell. When cells are placed in a *hypotonic solution,* which has a lesser osmolality, they swell as water moves into the cell, and when they are placed in a *hypertonic solution,* which has a greater osmolality, they shrink as water is pulled out of the cell.

Extracellular Fluid Volume

Extracellular fluid is divided between the vascular compartment and interstitial fluid compartment. The interstitial water acts as a transport vehicle for gases, nutrients, wastes, and other materials that move

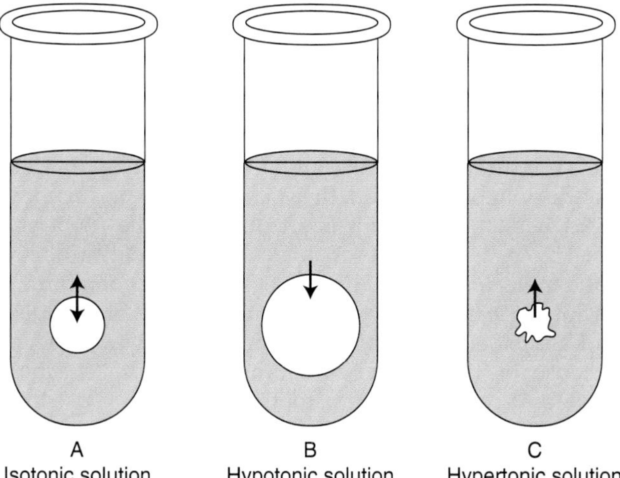

Figure 26–4
Osmosis. (**A**) Red cells undergo no change in size in isotonic solutions. They increase in size in hypotonic solutions (**B**) and decrease in size in hypertonic solutions (**C**).

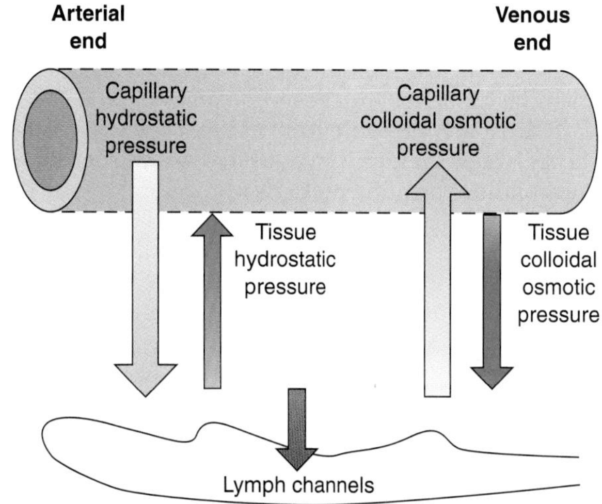

FIGURE 26–5
Exchange of fluid at the capillary level.

between the vascular compartment and body cells. A tissue gel, which is a spongelike material composed of large quantities of mucopolysaccharides, fills the tissue spaces and aids in the even distribution of interstitial fluid. Normally, most of the fluid in the interstitium is in gel form. The tissue gel is supported by collagen fibers that hold the gel in place. The tissue gel, which has a firmer consistency than water, opposes the outflow of water from the capillaries and prevents the accumulation of free water in the interstitial spaces. Interstitial fluid also provides a reservoir from which vascular volume can be maintained during periods of hemorrhage or loss of vascular volume.

Movement of water between the vascular compartment and interstitium is governed by the Starling forces described in Chapter 16. Four forces control the movement of water between the capillary and interstitial spaces: the capillary hydrostatic pressure, which pushes fluid out of the capillary; the capillary colloidal osmotic pressure, which pulls fluids back into the capillary; the tissue hydrostatic pressure, which opposes the pushing of fluids from the capillary into the interstitial spaces; and the tissue colloidal osmotic pressure, which pulls fluid into the interstitial spaces (Fig. 26–5). The term *capillary hydrostatic pressure* is used to describe the pressure pushing water out of the capillary into the interstitial spaces. It is higher at the arterial end of the capillary than at the venous end (*i.e.,* about 30 to 40 mm Hg at the arterial end and 10 to 15 mm Hg at the venous end).[2] Because of this difference, water moves out of the capillaries at their arterial ends and is reabsorbed at their venous ends.

The capillary colloidal osmotic pressure is the osmotic pressure generated by the plasma proteins. The term *colloidal osmotic pressure* differentiates this type of osmotic pressure from the osmotic pressure that develops at the cell membrane from the presence of electrolytes and nonelectrolytes. Because the plasma proteins are the only dissolved substances that do not penetrate the pores of the capillary, it is the dissolved proteins in the plasma and interstitial fluids that are responsible for osmotic pressure at the capillary membrane. The tissue colloidal osmotic pressure and the tissue hydrostatic pressure contribute to movement of water between the capillary and interstitial spaces. The tissue colloidal osmotic pressure contributes to the outward movement of capillary fluid and the hydrostatic pressure to the inward movement of fluid. Normally, the combination of these four forces are such that only a small excess of fluid remains in the interstitial compartment. This excess fluid is removed from the interstitium by the lymph system and returned to the systemic circulation.

Edema

Edema can be defined as palpable swelling produced by expansion of the interstitial fluid volume. Edema does not become evident until the interstitial volume has been increased by 2.5 to 3 L.[3]

Causes. The physiologic mechanisms that contribute to edema formation include increases in capillary filtration pressure, decreases in capillary colloidal osmotic pressure, increases in capillary permeability, and obstruction to lymph flow. The causes of edema are summarized in Chart 26–1.

Increased Filtration Pressure. Increased capillary pressure pushes vascular fluid into the interstitial spaces. Among the factors that increase capillary pressures are decreased resistance to flow through the arterioles and capillary sphincters that supply the capillary bed; increased resistance to outflow at the venous end of the capillary bed; and capillary distention due to increased vascular volume.

Because of the effects of gravity, edema resulting from increased capillary pressure commonly causes fluid to accumulate in the dependent parts of the body, a condition referred to as *dependent edema*. For example, edema of the ankles and feet becomes more pronounced during prolonged periods of standing because of the forces of gravity. The local edema that occurs with urticaria (*i.e.*, hives) and other allergic or inflammatory conditions results from release of histamine and other inflammatory mediators that cause dilation of the precapillary sphincters and arterioles that supply the swollen area. Impaired venous outflow causes capillary pressures to increase. For example, venous thrombosis produces an elevation of venous pressure and edema of the affected part. In right-sided heart failure, blood dams up throughout the entire systemic venous system, causing organ congestion and edema of the dependent extremities. Decreased sodium and water excretion by the kidneys leads to an increase in extracellular volume with an increase in capillary volume and pressure with subsequent movement of fluid into the tissue spaces. The swelling of hands and feet that occurs during hot weather results from vasodilation of superficial blood vessels along with sodium and water retention.

CHART 26-1
Causes of Edema

Increased Capillary Pressure

Arteriolar dilatation
- Allergic responses (e.g., hives, angioneurotic edema)
- Inflammation

Venous obstruction
- Hepatic obstruction
- Heart failure
- Thrombophlebitis

Increased vascular volume
- Heart failure
- Increased levels of adrenocortical hormones
- Premenstrual sodium retention
- Pregnancy
- Environmental heat stress

Effects of gravity
- Prolonged standing

Decreased Colloidal Osmotic Pressure

Decreased production of plasma proteins
- Liver disease
- Starvation or severe protein deficiency

Increased loss of plasma proteins
- Protein-losing kidney diseases
- Extensive burns

Increased Capillary Permeability

Inflammation
Immune responses
Neoplastic disease
Tissue injury and burns

Obstruction of Lymphatic Flow

Infection or disease of the lymphatic structures
Surgical removal of lymph nodes

Decreased Colloidal Osmotic Pressure. Plasma proteins exert the osmotic force needed to move fluid back into the capillary from the tissue spaces. The plasma proteins are a mixture of proteins containing albumin, globulins, and fibrinogen. Albumin, the smallest of the plasma proteins, has a molecular weight of 69,000; the globulins have molecular weights of about 150,000; and fibrinogen has a molecular weight of 400,000. One gram of albumin has about twice as many molecules as 1 g of globulin and almost six times as many molecules as fibrinogen. Because it is the number, rather than the size, of the molecule that contributes to osmotic pressure, 1 g of albumin exerts a much larger effect on colloidal osmotic pressure than the other proteins. The concentration of albumin (about 4.5 g/dl) is greater than the globulins (2.5 g/dl) and fibrinogen (0.3 mg/dl).

Edema develops when plasma protein levels become inadequate because of abnormal losses or inadequate production. Because the plasma proteins are equally distributed throughout the circulatory system, a decrease in plasma colloidal osmotic pressure causes generalized edema, called *anasarca*, that affects dependent and nondependent parts of the body. The glomerulus of the kidney nephron is a network of capillaries. In certain conditions, such as glomerulonephritis, these capillaries become permeable to the plasma proteins, particularly albumin, which is the smaller of the proteins. When this happens, large amounts of albumin are filtered out of the blood and then lost in the urine. An excess loss of plasma proteins also occurs when large areas of skin are injured or destroyed. Edema is a common problem during the early stages of a burn, resulting from capillary injury and loss of plasma proteins.

Plasma proteins are synthesized in the liver. In persons with severe liver failure, impaired synthesis of albumin results in a decrease in colloidal osmotic pressure. Liver disease also contributes to edema formation by causing obstruction to venous flow through the portal circulation and through impaired metabolism of hormones, such as aldosterone, which increase sodium retention. In starvation and malnutrition, edema develops because is a lack of amino acids for use in plasma protein synthesis. In starvation, edema may mask the loss of tissue mass.

Increased Capillary Permeability. When the capillary pores become enlarged or the integrity of the capillary wall is destroyed, capillary permeability is increased. Burn injury, capillary congestion, inflammation, and immune responses increase capillary permeability. After an increase in capillary permeability is established, plasma proteins and other osmotically active particles leak into the interstitial spaces, increasing the tissue colloidal osmotic pressure and contributing to the accumulation of edema fluid.

Obstruction of Lymph Flow. Osmotically active plasma proteins and other large particles that cannot be reabsorbed through the pores in the capillary membrane rely on the lymphatic system for movement back into the circulatory system. Edema due to impaired lymph flow is commonly referred to as *lymphedema*. Malignant involvement of lymph structures and removal of lymph nodes at the time of cancer surgery are common causes of lymphedema. Another cause of lymphedema is infection involving the lymphatic channels and lymph nodes.

Manifestations. The effects of edema are determined largely by its location. Edema of the brain, larynx, or lungs is an acute, life-threatening condition. Swelling of the ankles and feet often is insidious in onset and may or may not be associated with disease. Edema may interfere with movement, limiting motion or making opening of the eyes difficult. At the tissue level, edema increases the distance for diffusion of oxygen, nutrients, and wastes. Edematous tissues usually are more susceptible to injury and to development of ischemic tissue damage, including pressure ulcers. Edema can also compress blood vessels. The skin of a severely swollen finger can act as a tourniquet, shutting off the blood flow to the finger. Edema can also be disfiguring, causing psychologic effects and disturbances in self-concept. Edema often causes a distortion of body features and creates problems in obtaining proper-fitting clothing and shoes.

In chronic edema, the intercellular fibers in the tissue spaces become stretched and lose their elastic recoil so that they no longer are as effective in maintaining the opposing hydrostatic pressure of the interstitial fluid compartment. Less pressure is needed to push fluids into the interstitial spaces. The stretching of fibers in the tissue spaces also makes correction or permanent reversal of edema difficult.

Pitting edema occurs when the accumulation of interstitial fluid exceeds the absorptive capacity of the tissue gel. In this form of edema, the tissue water becomes mobile and can be translocated with pressure exerted by a finger. To test for pitting edema, the observer applies firm finger pressure to the edematous areas. If an indentation remains after the finger has been removed, pitting edema is identified.

Nonpitting edema usually reflects a condition in which serum proteins have accumulated in the tissue spaces and coagulated. The area often is firm and discolored. Brawny edema is a type of nonpitting edema in which the skin thickens and hardens. Nonpitting edema most frequently is seen after local infection or trauma.

Assessment and Treatment. Methods for assessing edema include visual inspection, using finger pressure to determine the degree of pitting, and measurement of the circumference of an extremity (or the abdomen in the case of ascites). Pitting edema is evaluated on a scale of +1 (minimal) to +4 (severe). Daily weight is also a useful index of interstitial fluid gain.

Treatment of edema usually is directed toward maintaining life when the swelling involves vital structures, correcting or controlling the cause, and preventing tissue injury. Diuretic therapy commonly is used to treat edema. Edema of the lower extremities may respond to simple measures such as elevating the feet.

Elastic support stockings and sleeves increase tissue pressure and resistance of the capillary walls to outward movement of fluid and therefore decrease the movement of fluid from the capillary into the tissue spaces. These support devices typically are prescribed for patients with conditions such as lymphatic or venous obstruction and are most efficient if applied before the tissue spaces have filled with fluid—in the morning, for example, before the effects of gravity have caused fluid to move into the ankles.

Serum albumin levels can be measured, as can the colloidal osmotic pressure of the plasma (25.4 mm Hg is normal). Albumin can be administered intravenously to raise the plasma colloidal osmotic pressure when edema is caused by hypoalbuminemia.

Idiopathic Edema. Idiopathic edema is an entity seen almost exclusively in young women of reproductive age. The characteristic feature of idiopathic edema is the occurrence of intermittent and irregularly occurring episodes of edema of the legs, hands, abdomen, breasts, and (rarely) face. The cause is uncertain, but seems to have an orthostatic or postural element with edema beginning in the face or upper part of the body early in the day and progressing to abdomen, legs, and ankles as the day progresses. The edema may cause a weight gain of 4 to 12 pounds by the end of the day.[4] Idiopathic edema is exaggerated by emotional stress, obesity, high carbohydrate and salt intake, heat and humidity, tight-fitting garments, drugs such as nonsteroidal antiinflammatory agents and phenothiazines, and occasionally by the premenstrual state.

One of the methods used in diagnosis of idiopathic edema is the water load test, in which the woman drinks 20 ml of water per 1 kg of body weight over a 15-minute period. She is then asked to urinate, remaining recumbent for the next 4 hours while all urine is collected. The test is repeated the next morning, but the woman remains upright during the 4-hour urine collection period. Women with idiopathic edema retain considerably more water while in the supine than in the upright position. Treatment consists of moderate salt restriction, carbohydrate and calorie restrictions, avoidance of prolonged standing, wearing elastic support stockings, and avoidance of other tight-fitting garments. Smoking should be avoided. In general, diuretics are not recommended, but when one is needed, aldosterone antagonists usually are prescribed.

Fluid Loss From Third Spacing

Third spacing represents the loss of extracellular fluid into the transcellular space. The serous cavities are part of the transcellular compartment (*i.e.*, third space) located in strategic body areas where there is continual movement of body structures—the pericardial sac, the peritoneal cavity, and the pleural cavity. The exchange of extracellular fluid between the capillaries, the interstitial spaces, and the transcellular space of the serous cavity uses the same mechanisms to exchange fluids as capillaries elsewhere in the body. The serous cavities are closely linked with lymphatic drainage systems. The milking action of the moving structures continually forces fluid and plasma proteins back into the circulation, keeping these cavities empty. Any obstruction to lymph flow causes fluid accumulation in the serous cavities.

The prefix *hydro-* may be used to indicate the presence of excessive fluid, as in *hydrothorax*, which means excessive fluid in the pleural cavity. The transudation of fluid into the serous cavities is also referred to as *effusion*. Effusion can contain blood, plasma proteins, and inflammatory cells (*i.e.*, pus), and extracellular fluid.

The accumulation of fluid in the peritoneal cavity is called *ascites*. Because of proximity to the portal circulation, the peritoneal cavity is more susceptible to excess fluid accumulation than are other body cavities. When pressure in the liver sinusoids increases significantly, serum exudes through the capillaries on the surface of the liver and passes into the peritoneal cavity. Congestive heart failure and liver failure are examples of conditions that obstruct hepatic blood flow and cause fluid to move into the peritoneal cavity. Because the portal vein receives blood from the peritoneal surface, portal hypertension creates an increase in the filtration pressure of the capillaries that line the peritoneal cavity, causing fluid to leave the capillaries and leak into the peritoneal cavity. Excess fluid may be aspirated or removed from a serous cavity. The term *paracentesis* refers to puncture of a cavity for removal of fluid. A needle or similar instrument is inserted into the cavity, and the fluid is withdrawn. Analysis of the fluid for the presence of infectious organisms and malignant cells aids in the diagnosis of the disease responsible for the fluid accumulation.

In summary, body fluids are distributed between the intracellular and extracellular compartments of the body. The extracellular fluid compartment contains intravascular fluid, interstitial fluid, and fluid contained in the extracellular spaces, such as the pleural cavity. Body fluids contain water, charged particles called electrolytes, and noncharged particles called nonelectrolytes. Electrolytes and nonelectrolytes move between compartments by diffusion. The movement of water across the semipermeable membranes of the body is controlled by the nondiffusible particles on either side of the membrane in a process called osmosis. Osmosis is regulated by the number, rather than the size, of the nondiffusible particles. The tension or effect that the osmotic pressure of a solution exerts on body cells is called tonicity.

Intracellular volume is largely regulated by the Na+/K+ membrane pump and the tonicity or effective osmolality of the extracellular fluids. Extracellular fluid volume, which is distributed between the vascular and interstitial compartments, is regulated by sodium content of the extracellular fluids. Edema represents an increase in interstitial fluid volume. The physiologic mechanisms that predispose to edema formation are increased capillary pressure, decreased capillary colloidal osmotic pressure, increased capillary permeability, and obstruction of lymphatic flow.

The effect that edema exerts on body function is determined by its location; cerebral edema can be a life-threatening situation, but swollen feet can be a normal discomfort that accompanies hot weather. Fluid can also accumulate in the transcellular compartment—the joint spaces, pericardial sac, the peritoneal cavity, and the pleural cavity. Because this fluid is not easily exchanged with the rest of the extracellular fluid, it is often referred to as third-space fluid.

Sodium and Water Balance

After you have completed this section of the chapter, you should be able to meet the following objectives:

- State the functions and physiologic mechanisms controlling body water and sodium concentration

- Describe the relation between body sodium levels and extracellular fluid volume and between body water and the extracellular sodium concentration
- Describe measures that can be used in assessing sodium concentration and body fluid levels
- Compare and contrast the causes, manifestations, and treatment of isotonic fluid volume deficit, isotonic fluid volume excess, hyponatremia with water excess, and hypernatremia with water deficit
- Describe the causes, manifestations, and treatment of psychogenic polydipsia
- Compare the pathology and manifestations of diabetes insipidus and the syndrome of inappropriate ADH

Body fluid levels depend on water and sodium balance. Water provides about 90% to 93% of volume of body fluids and sodium salts about 90% to 95% of extracellular solutes. Normally, proportionate changes in sodium and water are such that the volume and osmolality of body fluids remain are maintained within a normal range. Alterations of salt and water balance include isotonic contraction or expansion of extracellular fluid volume and alterations in extracellular sodium concentration (Fig. 26–6). Alterations in fluid balance usually result in isotonic contraction or expansion of extracellular fluid volume (*i.e.*, extracellular fluid volume deficit or excess) and disorders of sodium concentration (*i.e.*, hyponatremia or hypernatremia) in the addition or removal of fluid from the intracellular compartment. Disorders of sodium and water balance often accompany other disorders, making differentiation of conditions more difficult.

Water Balance

Water is the main component of body fluids, and the functions of water in the body are many. Water adds to the structure of the body, functions as a transport vehicle, hydrolyzes food in the digestive system, and participates in chemical reactions that occur within body cells.

Total body water varies with age, decreasing from infancy to old age. Because the body is largely water, total body water usually is expressed as a percentage of body weight. In a full-term infant, body water constitutes as much as 75% to 80% of body weight, but body water accounts for only 60% of body weight in an adult. A premature infant has even a greater amount of body

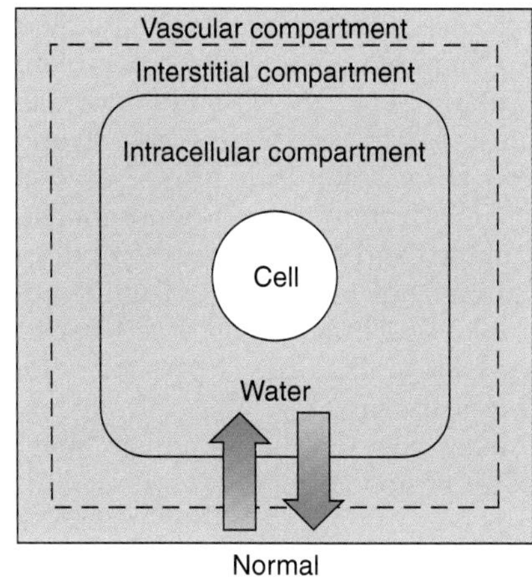

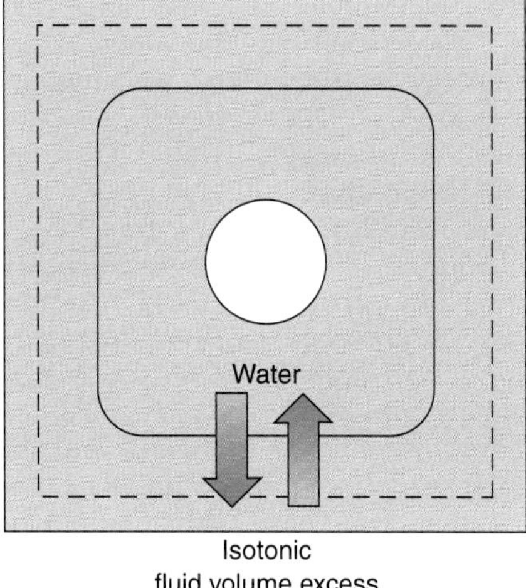

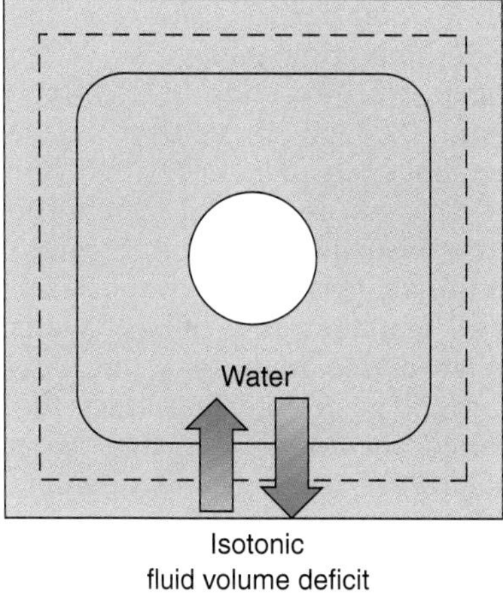

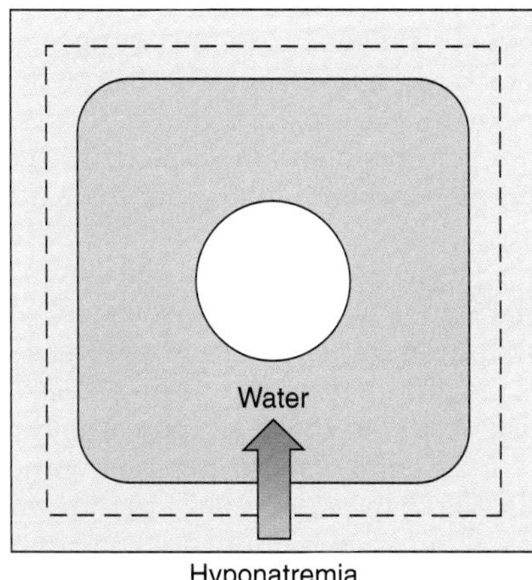

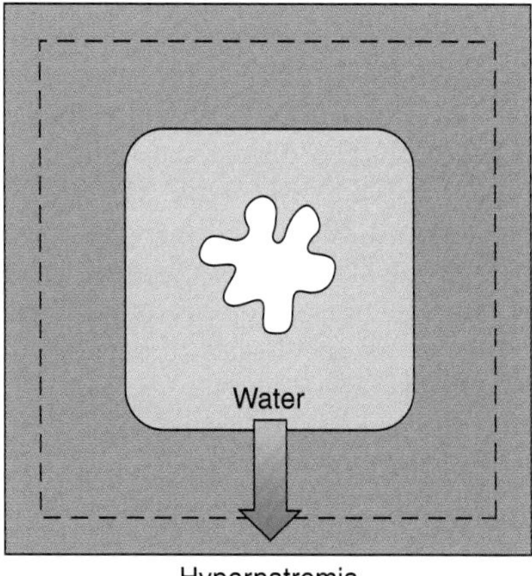

FIGURE 26–6
Effect of isotonic fluid volume excess and and deficit and of hyponatremia and hypernatremia on intracellular fluid volume.

water than a term infant; an elderly person has much less water in relation to body weight than a younger adult. Because fat essentially is water free, obesity decreases the percentage of water that the body contains, sometimes reducing these levels to values as low as 45% of body weight.

Despite its greater body water content, an infant is more likely to develop fluid imbalances than an adult, because an infant has a higher metabolic rate and a larger surface area in relation to its body mass than an older child or an adult. An infant has more difficulty concentrating its urine because its kidney structures are immature. This means that an infant has greater skin and urine losses and that more water is needed for metabolic processes. An infant therefore ingests and excretes greater volumes of water in relation to its size than an adult. An infant may exchange one half of its extracellular fluid volume in a single day, compared with about one sixth of this volume in an adult during the same period. By the third year of life, the percentages and distribution of body water in a young child approach those of an adult.

Gains and Loss

Regardless of age, all healthy persons require about 100 ml of water per 100 calories metabolized for dissolving and eliminating metabolic wastes. This means that a person who expends 1800 calories for energy requires about 1800 ml of water for metabolic purposes. The metabolic rate increases with fever; it rises 12% for every 1°C (7% for every 1°F) increase in body temperature.[2] Fever also increases the respiratory rate, resulting in additional loss of water vapor through the lungs.

The main source of body water gain is through oral intake and oxidation of nutrients. Water is absorbed from the gastrointestinal tract; the water gained in this manner includes that obtained from fluids and ingested foods. Tube feedings and parenterally administered fluids are also a source of water gain. Cellular oxidation of fats and carbohydrates generates water and energy. The quantity gained in this manner varies from 150 to 250 ml, depending on metabolic rate.

Water losses occur through the kidneys, skin, lungs, and gastrointestinal tract. Even when oral or parenteral fluids have been withheld, the kidneys continue to produce urine as a means of ridding the body of metabolic wastes. The urine output that is required to eliminate these wastes is called the *obligatory urine output*. The obligatory urine loss is about 300 to 500 ml/day. Water losses that occur through the skin and lungs are referred to as *insensible water losses* because they occur without a persons awareness. The gains and losses of body water are summarized in Table 26–2.

TABLE 26–2
Sources of Body Water Gains and Losses in the Adult

Gains		Losses	
		Urine	1500 ml
Oral intake		Insensible losses	
As water	1000 ml	Lungs	300 ml
In food	1300 ml	Skin	500 ml
Water of oxidation	200 ml	Feces	200 ml
Total	2500 ml	Total	2500 ml

Mechanisms of Regulation

There are two main physiologic mechanisms that assist in regulating body water levels: thirst and ADH. Thirst is primarily a regulator of water intake and ADH a regulator of water output. Both mechanisms respond to changes in extracellular volume and osmolality.

Thirst. Like appetite and eating, thirst and drinking behavior are two separate entities.[5] Thirst is a conscious sensation or need to obtain and drink fluids high in water content. Drinking consists of the activities that culminate in the ingestion of water or other liquids. Drinking of water or other fluids often occurs as the result of habit or for other reasons that are not necessarily related to thirst.

The hypothalamus plays a central role in the integration of thirst. Sensory neurons, called *osmoreceptors*, which are located in or near the thirst center in the hypothalamus, respond to changes in extracellular osmolality by swelling or shrinking (Fig. 26–7). Thirst normally develops when there is a 0.5% or greater loss of body water. There are two stimuli for true thirst based on water need: cellular dehydration caused by an increase in extracellular osmolality and a decrease in blood volume, which may or may not be associated with a decrease in serum osmolality. Thirst is one of the earliest symptoms of hemorrhage and is often present before other signs of blood loss appear.

A third mechanism, the renin-angiotensin mechanism, contributes to nonosmotic thirst. The renin-angiotensin system is considered a backup system for thirst if other systems should fail. Because it is a backup system, it probably does not contribute to the regulation of normal thirst. However, elevated levels of angiotensin II may lead to thirst in conditions such as chronic renal failure and congestive heart failure, in which renin levels may be elevated. Thirst and elevated renin levels are also found in persons with primary aldosteronism and in those with secondary hyperaldosteronism accompanying anorexia nervosa, hemorrhage, and sodium depletion.

Dryness of the mouth produces a sensation of thirst that is not necessarily associated with the body's state hydration status, such as the thirst a lecturer experiences as the mouth dries out during speaking. Thirst sensation also occurs in those who breathe through their mouths, such as smokers and persons with chronic respiratory disease or hyperventilation syndrome.

Liquids commonly are consumed with meals; more water is consumed when salty foods are ingested. Most persons drink without being thirsty, and water is consumed before it is needed. As a result, thirst is basically

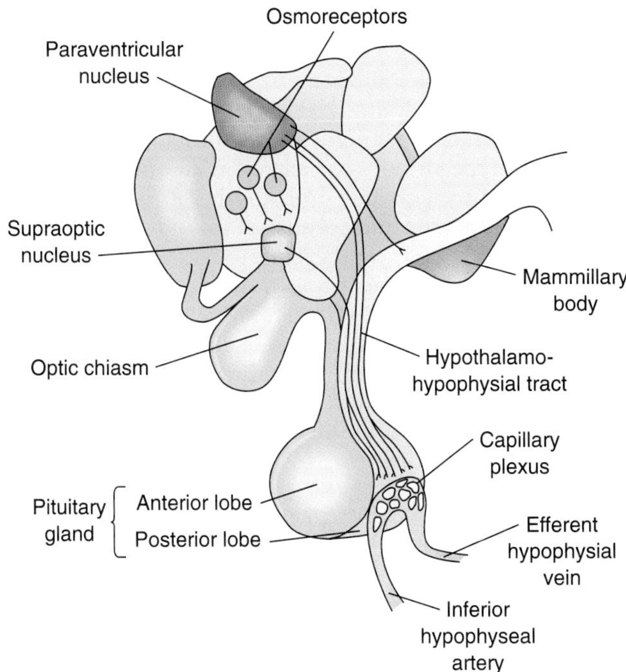

FIGURE 26–7
Sagittal section through the pituitary and anterior hypothalamus. Antidiuretic hormone (ADH) is formed primarily in the supraoptic nucleus and to a lesser extent in the paraventricular nucleus of the hypothalamus. It is then transported down the hypothalamohypophysial tract and stored in secretory granules in the posterior pituitary, where it can be released into the blood. (Rhoades R.A., Tanner G. A. [1996]. *Medical physiology* [p. 449]. Boston: Little, Brown)

an emergency response. It usually occurs only when the need for water has not been anticipated.

Hypodipsia represents a decrease in the ability to sense thirst. There is evidence that thirst is decreased and water intake reduced in elderly persons, despite higher serum sodium and osmolality levels.[6,7] The inability to perceive and respond to thirst is compounded in elderly persons who have had a stroke and may be further influenced by confusion and sensory disturbances.

Polydipsia, or excessive thirst, is normal when it accompanies conditions of water deficit. Increased thirst and drinking behavior can be classified into three categories: symptomatic or true thirst, inappropriate or false thirst that occurs despite normal levels of body water and serum osmolality, and compulsive water drinking. Symptomatic thirst develops when there is a loss of body water and resolves after the loss has been resolved. Among the most common causes of symptomatic thirst are water losses associated with diarrhea, vomiting, diabetes mellitus, and diabetes insipidus. Inappropriate or excessive thirst may persist despite adequate hydration. It is a common complaint in persons with renal failure and congestive heart failure. Although the cause of thirst in these persons is unclear, it may result from increased angiotensin levels. Thirst is also a common complaint in persons with dry mouth caused by decreased salivary function or treatment with drugs with an anticholinergic action (*e.g.,* antihistamines, atropine) that lead to decreased salivary flow. Compulsive water drinking, or psychogenic polydipsia (to be discussed), is usually seen in persons with psychiatric disorders.

Water Output by the Kidney Is Regulated by Antidiuretic Hormone. The reabsorption of water by the kidneys is regulated by ADH, also known as *vasopressin.* ADH is synthesized by cells in three portions of the hypothalamus: the supraoptic, paraventricular, and suprachiasmic nuclei (see Fig. 26–7). ADH from neurons in the supraoptic and paraventricular nuclei is transported along a neural pathway (*i.e.,* hypophysial tract) to the neurohypophysis (*i.e.,* posterior pituitary) and then stored for future release. ADH from the suprachiasmic nuclei, which is released into the cerebrospinal fluid, is not regulated by serum osmolality. It is thought to play a role in nocturnal and circadian patterns of drinking behavior.[8]

ADH exerts its effects through two types of vasopressin (V) receptors V_1 and V_2. The V_2 receptors, located on the tubular cells of cortical collecting duct of the nephron, control water reabsorption by the kidney (see Chapter 25). Binding of ADH to the V_2 receptors increases water reabsorption by increasing the permeability of the collecting duct to water (*i.e.,* the antidiuretic effect). In the absence of ADH, the permeability of the collecting duct to water is very low, and reabsorption of water decreases, leading to polyuria. V_1 receptors, which are located in vascular smooth muscle, cause vasoconstriction—hence the name vasopressin. Although ADH can increase blood pressure through V_1 receptors, this response occurs only when ADH levels are very high.

As with thirst, ADH levels are controlled by volume and osmolar changes in the extracellular fluids. Osmoreceptors in the hypothalamus sense changes in extracellular osmolality and stimulate the production and release of ADH. A small increase in serum osmolality of 1% to 2% is sufficient to cause ADH release. Likewise, stretch receptors in the great veins, atria, and carotid sinus area sense changes in blood volume or blood pressure, and input from these receptors aids in the regulation of ADH release. A blood volume decrease of 10% to 15% produces a maximal increase in ADH levels, and blood pressure reductions of 5% to 10% are needed to increase ADH levels.[9] As with many other homeostatic mechanisms, acute conditions produce greater changes in ADH levels than do chronic conditions; long-term changes in blood volume or blood pressure may exist without affecting ADH levels.

Many stress situations increase the synthesis and release of ADH. Severe pain, nausea, trauma, surgery, certain anesthetic agents, and some analgesic drugs increase ADH levels. Nausea is a potent stimulus of ADH secretion; it can increase ADH levels 10 to 1000 times those required for maximal diuresis.[9] The stimulus is mediated by way of the chemoreceptor trigger zone in the medulla oblongata, which then relays the impulse to the supraoptic and paraventricular nuclei in the hypothalamus. Afferent input from the gastrointestinal tract may also be important in some circumstances. Among the drugs that affect ADH are nicotine, which stimulates its release, and alcohol, which inhibits it (Table 26–3). Two important conditions alter ADH levels: diabetes insipidus and inappropriate secretion of ADH (discussed later).

Sodium Balance

Sodium is the most abundant cation in the body, averaging about 60 mEq/kg of body weight. Most of the body's sodium is in the extracellular fluid compartment (135 to 148 mEq/L), with only a small amount (10 to 14 mEq/L) located in the intracellular compartment. The resting cell membrane is relatively impermeable to sodium. Sodium that enters the cell is transported out of the cell against an electrochemical gradient by the energy-dependent Na^+/K^+ membrane pump.

Sodium functions mainly in regulating extracellular and vascular volume, which is essential for tissue perfusion. As the major cation in the extracellular compartment, Na^+ and its attendant anions (Cl^- and HCO_3^-) account for about 90% to 95% of the osmotic activity in the extracellular fluids. As the base for sodium bicarbonate, sodium is also important in regulating acid-base balance. Sodium contributes to the maintenance of the resting membrane potential and generation of action potentials in excitable tissues.

Gain and Loss

Sodium intake normally is derived from dietary sources. Body needs for sodium usually can be met by as little as 500 mg/day. Dietary intake, which frequently exceeds the amount needed by the body, is often influenced by culture and food preferences rather than need. In the United States, the average salt intake is about 6 to 15 g/day, or 12 to 30 times the daily requirement.

TABLE 26-3

Drugs That Affect Antidiuretic Hormone Levels

Drugs That Decrease ADH Levels/Action	Drugs That Increase ADH Levels/Action
Demeclocycline	Acetaminophen
Ethanol	Analgesics (morphine and meperidine)
Glucocorticoids	Anesthetics (most)
Lithium carbonate	Antipsychotic tranquilizers
Morphine antagonists	Cancer drugs (vincristine and cyclophosphamide)
	Carbamazepine
Phenytoin	Chlorpropamide
Reserpine, chlorpromazine	Clofibrate
	Isoproterenol
	Nicotine
	Phenobarbital
	Thiazide diuretics (chlorothiazide)
	Tricyclic antidepressants

Other sources of sodium are intravenous saline infusions and medications that contain sodium. An often-forgotten source of sodium is the sodium bicarbonate or other sodium-containing home remedies used to treat upset stomach or other ailments. Sodium ingestion in excess of what the kidneys can excrete is an unlikely occurrence in healthy persons, probably because taste keeps this from happening and because of the kidneys' remarkable ability to regulate and excrete excess sodium.

Most sodium losses occur through the kidney. The kidneys are extremely efficient in regulating sodium output, and when sodium intake is limited or conservation of sodium is needed, the kidneys are able to reabsorb almost all the sodium that has been filtered by the glomerulus. This results in an essentially sodium-free urine. Conversely, urinary losses of sodium increase as intake increases.

Usually less than 10% of the usual dietary intake is lost through the skin and gastrointestinal tract. Although the sodium concentration of fluids in the upper part of the gastrointestinal tract approaches that of the extracellular fluid, sodium is reabsorbed as the fluids move through the lower part of the bowel, so that the concentration of sodium in the stool is only about 40 mEq/L. Sodium losses increase with conditions such vomiting, diarrhea, fistula drainage, and gastrointestinal suction that remove sodium from the upper gastrointestinal tract. Irrigation of gastrointestinal tubes with distilled water removes sodium from the gastrointestinal tract, as do repeated tap water enemas.

Sodium losses through the skin can also become extensive. Sweat losses, which are usually negligible, can increase greatly during exercise and periods of exposure to a hot environment. A person who sweats profusely can lose as much as 15 to 30 g of sodium per day. Fortunately, this amount decreases to as little as 3 to 5 g/day with acclimatization to the heat.[2] Loss of skin surface, such as occurs in extensive burns, also leads to excessive skin losses of sodium.

Mechanisms of Regulation

The kidney is the main regulator of sodium. It does this in response to changes in vascular volume. The kidney retains sodium in response to a decrease in circulating blood volume, and it excretes sodium when there is an increase in blood volume. The rate at which the kidney excretes or conserves sodium is regulated in a coordinated manner by the sympathetic nervous system and the renin-angiotensin-aldosterone mechanism. Another possible regulator of sodium excretion by the kidney is atrial natriuretic peptide (ANP), which is released from cells in the atria of the heart. ANP, which is released in response to atrial stretch and overfilling, increases sodium excretion by the kidney (Chapter 25). Although ANP acts at several sites in the kidney to increase sodium excretion, its role in regulating sodium balance remains uncertain.[3]

The Sympathetic Nervous System. The sympathetic nervous system responds to changes in vascular volume by adjusting the glomerular filtration rate and the rate at which sodium is filtered from the blood. Sympathetic activity also increases renin release.

The Renin-Angiotensin-Aldosterone Mechanism. Renin is a small protein enzyme released by the kidney in response to changes in blood pressure and blood flow, glomerular filtration rate, and the amount of sodium in the tubular fluid. Most of the renin that is released leaves the kidney and enters the bloodstream, where it interacts enzymatically to convert a circulating plasma protein called *angiotensinogen* to angiotensin I (see Chapter 16). Angiotensin I is rapidly converted to angiotensin II by the *angiotensin-converting enzyme* in the small blood vessels of the lung. Angiotensin II directly stimulates sodium reabsorption by the renal tubules, and it acts to constrict renal blood vessels, thereby decreasing glomerular filtration and slowing renal blood flow through the kidney so that less sodium is filtered and more is reabsorbed.

Angiotensin II is also a powerful regulator of aldosterone secretion. Aldosterone is a hormone produced by the adrenal cortex that acts at the level of the cortical collecting tubules of the kidneys to increase reabsorption into the blood and increase the elimination of potassium in the urine. Because sodium and potassium are classified as minerals, aldosterone is often referred to as a *mineralocorticoid hormone.*

Four factors are known to stimulate the secretion of aldosterone: angiotensin II, an increase in extracellular potassium levels, a decrease in extracellular sodium levels, and the pituitary adrenocorticotropin hormone (ACTH).[2] Potassium ion concentration and angiotensin II have the greatest influence on aldosterone secretion. The sodium ion, although important, provides a lesser stimulus of aldosterone secretion. ACTH is necessary for aldosterone production, but it has little effect in regulating its secretion.[2]

The pharmacologic inhibition of sodium reabsorption in the cortical collecting tubules can be achieved by blocking the actions of aldosterone (*e.g.,* potassium-sparing diuretics, such as spironolactone, amiloride, and triamterene), by suppressing renin release (*e.g.,* β-adrenergic blocking drugs), or by inhibiting the conversion of angiotensin I to angiotensin II (*e.g.,* angiotensin-converting enzyme inhibitors).

Alterations in Fluid Volume

Alterations in fluid volume represent an isotonic contraction or expansion of extracellular fluids (e.g., water, electrolytes, other solutes). Although these disorders can manifest as isolated conditions, they often occur in combination with other fluid and electrolyte imbalances. For the purposes of this discussion, they are presented as isolated disorders.

Fluid Volume Deficit

Fluid volume deficit is characterized by an decrease in extracellular fluid, including circulating blood volume. The term *isotonic fluid volume deficit,* in which there is proportionate losses in sodium and water, is used to differentiate this type of fluid deficit from water deficit and the hyperosmolar state associated with hypernatremia. Unless other fluid and electrolyte imbalances are present, the concentration of serum electrolytes remain essentially unchanged.

Causes. Isotonic fluid volume deficit can result from impaired intake or excessive losses of body fluids. Fluid intake may be reduced by a lack of access to fluids, impaired thirst, unconsciousness, oral trauma, impaired swallowing, or neuromuscular problems that prevent fluid access. Although access to fluids is taken for granted, for someone with impaired mobility, fluid availability may become a problem.

Fluid volume deficit can result from loss of gastrointestinal fluids, polyuria, sweating due to fever and exercise, and third-space losses. When the effective circulating blood volume is compromised, the condition is often referred to *hypovolemia.*

In a single day, 8 to 10 L of extracellular fluid is secreted into the gastrointestinal tract. Most of it is absorbed in the ileum and proximal colon, and only about 150 to 200 ml per day is eliminated in the feces. Vomiting and diarrhea interrupt the reabsorption process and, in some situations, lead to increased secretion of fluid into the intestinal tract. In Asiatic cholera, death can occur within a matter of hours as the cholera organism causes excessive amounts of fluid to be secreted into the bowel. These fluids are then lost as vomitus or excreted as diarrheal fluid. Gastrointestinal suction, fistulas, and drainage tubes can remove large amounts of fluid from the gastrointestinal tract. Excess sodium and water losses can also occur through the kidney. The kidneys regulate the volume and solute concentration of extracellular fluid, promoting diuresis in conditions of fluid excess and conserving water when extracellular fluid volume is decreased. As a rule of thumb, water follows sodium reabsorption; conditions that increase sodium loss also increase water loss.

Certain forms of kidney disease are characterized by salt wasting due to impaired sodium reabsorption. Fluid volume deficit also can result from osmotic diuresis or injudicious use of diuretic therapy. Glucose in the urine filtrate prevents reabsorption of water by the renal tubules, causing a loss of sodium and water. In *Addison's disease,* a condition of chronic adrenocortical insufficiency, there is unregulated loss of sodium in the urine with a resultant loss of extracellular fluid (see Chapter 35). This is accompanied by increased potassium retention, caused by impaired mineralocorticoid function. The loss of extracellular fluid and low blood volume can lead to circulatory collapse.

The skin acts as an exchange surface for heat and as a vapor barrier to prevent water from leaving the body. Body surface losses of sodium and water increase when there is excessive sweating or when large areas of skin have been damaged. Hot weather and fever increase sweating. In hot weather, water losses through sweating may be increased by as much as 1.5 to 2.0 L/hour.[2] The respiratory rate and sweating usually are increased as body temperature rises. As much as 3 L of water may be lost in a single day as a result of fever. Burns are another cause of excess fluid loss. Evaporative losses range from 0.8 to 2.6 ml/kg for every percent of burn area. In severe burns, this loss can approach a level of 6 to 8 L/day.[10]

Third-space losses cause sequestering of extracellular fluids in an area that is physiologically unavailable to the body—in the serous cavities, extracellular spaces in injured tissues, or lumen of the gut. Because the fluid remains in the body, fluid volume deficit caused by third spacing does not usually cause weight loss.

Manifestations. The manifestations of fluid volume deficit include weight loss and signs and symptoms of loss of extracellular fluids, including vascular fluids (Table 26–4). Hypovolemic shock, which occurs with extreme losses of fluid volume, is discussed in Chapter 20. An acute increase or decrease in body weight is one of the best indicators of a loss or gain in body fluids. One liter of water weighs 1 kg (2.2 lb). A mild extracellular fluid deficit exists when weight loss equals 2% of body weight. In a person who weighs 68 kg (150 lb), this percentage of weight loss equals 1.4 L of water. A moderate deficit equates to a 5% loss in weight and a severe deficit to a 8% or greater loss in weight.[11] To be accurate, weight must be measured at the same time each day with the person wearing the same amount of clothing. Because extracellular fluid is trapped within the body in persons with third-space losses, their body weight may not decrease.

Thirst is a common symptom of fluid deficit, although it is not always present in early stages of isotonic fluid deficit caused by sodium depletion. It develops as the effective circulating volume decreases to a point sufficient to stimulate the thirst mechanism. Urine output usually decreases, and urine osmolality and specific gravity increase during periods of fluid deficit. Although there is an isotonic loss of sodium and water from the vascular compartment, other substances such as hematocrit and BUN become more concentrated.

Arterial and venous volumes decline during periods of fluid deficit, as does filling of the capillary circulation. As the volume in the arterial system declines, the blood pressure decreases and heart rate increases, and the pulse becomes weak and thready. Postural hypotension is an early sign of fluid deficit, characterized by a blood pressure that is at least 10 mm Hg lower when the patient is sitting or standing than when the patient is lying down. When volume depletion becomes severe, signs of shock and vascular collapse appear. On the venous side of the circulation, the veins become less prominent, and venous refill time increases. A simple test to determine venous refill time consists of compressing the distal end of a vein on the dorsal aspect of the hand

TABLE 26–4

Causes and Manifestations of Fluid Volume Deficit

Causes	Manifestation
Inadequate Fluid Intake	**Acute Weight Loss (% Body Weight)**
Oral trauma or inability to swallow	Mild fluid volume deficit: 2%
Inability to obtain fluids (*e.g.*, impaired mobility)	Moderate fluid volume deficit: 2%–5%
Impaired thirst mechanism	Severe fluid volume deficit: 8% or greater
Therapeutic withholding of fluids	**Thirst**
Unconsciousness or inability to express thirst	Increased thirst
Excessive Gastrointestinal Fluid Losses	**Urine Output**
Vomiting	Decreased urine output
Diarrhea	Increased osmolality and specific gravity
Gastrointestinal suction	
Draining gastrointestinal fistula	**Serum Osmolality**
Excessive Renal Losses	Increased serum osmolality
	Increased hematocrit and BUN
Diuretic therapy	
Osmotic diuresis (hyperglycemia)	**Cardiovascular Manifestations**
Adrenal insufficiency (Addison's disease)	Postural hypotension
Salt-wasting kidney disease	Tachycardia, weak, thready pulse
Excessive Skin Losses	Decreased vein filling and increased vein refill time
Fever	Hypotension and shock
Exposure to hot environment	**Extracellular Fluid Loss**
Burns and wounds that remove skin	Depressed fontanelle in an infant
Third-Space Losses	Sunken eyes and soft eyeballs
Intestinal obstruction	**Body Temperature**
Edema	Impaired ability to transfer core heat to environment
Ascites	Increased body temperature
Burns (first several days)	

TABLE 26-5

Causes and Manifestations of Fluid Volume Excess

Causes	Manifestations
Inadequate Sodium and Water Elimination	**Acute Weight Gain (% Body Weight)**
Congestive heart failure	Excess of 5%
Renal failure	**Increased Extracellular Fluid Volume**
Increased corticosteroid levels	Dependent and generalized edema
Hyperaldosteronism	**Increased Vascular Volume**
Cushing's disease	Full and bounding pulse
Liver failure (*e.g.*, cirrhosis)	Venous distention
Excessive Sodium Intake in Relation to Output	Pulmonary edema
Excess dietary intake	Shortness of breath
Excess ingestion of sodium-containing medications or home remedies	Crackles
Excessive administration of sodium-containing parenteral fluids	Dyspnea
Excessive Fluid Intake in Relation to Output	Cough
Excess ingestion of fluid in excess elimination	
Administration of parenteral fluids or blood at excessive rate of volume	

when it is not in the dependent position. The vein is then emptied by "milking" the blood toward the heart. The vein should refill almost immediately when the occluding finger is removed. When venous volume is decreased, as occurs in fluid deficit, venous refill time increases. Capillary refill time is also increased. Capillary refill can be assessed by applying pressure to a fingernail for 5 seconds and then releasing the pressure and observing the time (normally 1 to 2 seconds) that it takes for the color to return to normal.[11]

The amount of fluid in all the body tissues and organs decreases in fluid volume deficit. Although most body spaces are not visible, a decrease in cerebrospinal fluid in the infant causes depression of the anterior fontanelle. Likewise, the eyes assume a sunken appearance and feel softer than normal when the fluid content in the anterior chamber of the eye is decreased.

In terms of temperature regulation, water transports heat from the inner core of the body to the periphery where it can be released into the external environment, and it insulates the body against changes in the external temperature. Body temperature may be elevated in situations of fluid volume deficit. Water adds resiliency to the skin and underlying tissues that is referred to as *skin* or *tissue turgor*. Tissue turgor is assessed by pinching a fold of skin between the thumb and forefinger. The skin should immediately return to its original configuration when the fingers are released. A loss of 3% to 5% of body water in children causes the resiliency of the skin to be lost, and the tissue remains raised for several seconds. Decreased tissue turgor is less predictive of fluid deficit in older persons (≥65 years) because of the loss of tissue elasticity.

Diagnosis and Treatment. Diagnosis of fluid volume deficit is based on a history of conditions that predispose to sodium and water losses, weight loss, and observations of altered physiologic function indicative of decreased fluid volume. Intake and output measurements afford a means for assessing fluid balance. Although these measurements provide insight into the causes of fluid imbalance, they often are inadequate in measuring actual losses and gains, because accurate measurements of intake and output often are difficult to obtain and insensible losses are difficult to estimate.

Treatment of fluid volume deficit consists of fluid replacement and measures to correct the underlying cause. Usually, isotonic electrolyte solutions are used. Acute hypovolemia and hypovolemic shock can cause renal damage; therefore, prompt assessment of the degree of fluid deficit and adequate measures are essential (see Chapter 29).

Isotonic Fluid Volume Excess

Fluid volume excess represents an isotonic expansion of the extracellular fluid compartment that is caused by decreased elimination of sodium and water. Fluid volume excess involves an increase in interstitial and vascular volumes. Although increased fluid volume is usually the result of a disease condition, this is not always true. For example, a compensatory isotonic expansion of body fluids can occur in healthy persons during hot weather as a mechanism for increasing body heat loss.

Causes. Although fluid volume excess can occur as the result of increased sodium intake, it is most commonly caused by a decrease in sodium and water elimination by the kidney, particularly if it is coupled with excess intake. Among the causes of decreased sodium and water elimination are decreased renal function, heart failure, liver failure, and corticosteroid excess (Table 26–5).

Heart failure produces a decrease in renal blood flow and a compensatory increase in sodium and water retention. Liver failure (*e.g.*, cirrhosis of the liver) impairs aldosterone metabolism and alters renal perfusion, leading to increased salt and water retention. Persons with severe congestive heart failure maintain a precarious balance between sodium and water intake and output. Even small increases in sodium intake can precipitate a state of fluid volume excess and a worsening of heart failure. A condition called *circulatory overload* results from an increase in intravascular blood volume; it can occur during infusion of intravenous fluids or transfusion of blood if the amount or rate of administration is excessive. Elderly persons and persons with heart disease require careful observation, because even small amounts of intravenous fluid or blood may overload the circulatory system.

Cushing's syndrome is a condition of glucocorticoid excess (see Chapter 35). Because cortisol, the most active of the glucocorticoids, has weak mineralocorticoid activity, Cushing's disease predisposes to increased sodium retention. The fact that cortisol increases salt and water retention also helps to explain why persons who are being treated with cortisol or related corticosteroid drugs may develop edema and hypertension.

Manifestations. Isotonic fluid volume excess is manifested by an increase in interstitial and vascular fluids. Edema is characteristic of isotonic fluid excess. When the fluid excess accumulates gradually, edema fluid may mask the loss of tissue mass; this often happens in debilitating diseases and in starvation. The edema associated with extracellular fluid excess may be generalized, or it may be confined to dependent areas of the body, such as the legs and feet. The eyelids often are puffy when the person awakens. When excess fluid accumulates in the lungs (*i.e.*, pulmonary edema), there is shortness of breath, complaints of difficult breathing, respiratory rales, and a productive cough (see Chapter 20). An increase in vascular volume causes the pulse to have a full and bounding quality.

Diagnosis and Treatment. Diagnosis of fluid volume excess is usually based a history of factors that predispose to sodium and water retention, weight gain, and manifestations such as edema and cardiovascular symptoms indicative of an expanded extracellular fluid volume.

The treatment of fluid volume excess focuses on providing a more favorable balance between sodium and water intake and output. A sodium-restricted diet is often prescribed as a means of decreasing extracellular sodium levels. Diuretic therapy is commonly used to increase sodium elimination. When there is need for intravenous fluid administration or transfusion of blood components, the procedure requires careful monitoring to prevent fluid overload.

Alterations in Sodium Balance

The normal serum concentration of sodium ranges from 135 to 148 mEq/L (135 to 148 mmol/L). Serum sodium values reflect the sodium concentration (or dilution by extracellular water), expressed in mEq/L or mmol/L, rather than an absolute amount. Sodium dilution occurs when excess water is added to extracellular fluid, reducing its sodium concentration. This can occur because of water retention or because of redistribution of intracellular water to the extracellular fluid. Dehydration increases sodium concentration by decreasing its dilution. This occurs when water is lost from the extracellular compartment in excess of sodium. Because sodium and its attendant anions account for 90% to 95% of the osmolality of extracellular fluids, serum osmolality (normal range 275 to 295 mOsm/kg) generally varies in parallel with serum sodium concentration.

Cells, particularly those in the brain, tend to defend against changes in cell volume caused by increased extracellular osmolality by synthesizing amino acids and other osmotically active organic solutes.[12] Because these solutes cannot cross the cell membrane, they confine their osmotic activity to the intracellular compartment. In contrast to electrolytes and other solutes that disturb cell function and harm cells by altering the resting membrane potential or disrupting metabolic processes when they are present in large amounts, these organic osmoles have unique biochemical properties that allow them to accumulate in high concentrations without disrupting cell structure or function. The generation of these intracellular osmoles begins within 4 to 5 hours and takes several days to become maximally effective.[13]

Hyponatremia

Hyponatremia represents a decrease in serum sodium concentration below 135 mEq/L (135 mmol/L) and serum osmolality of less than 280 mOsm/kg. An artifactual hyponatremia caused by laboratory measurement methods can occur in hyperlipidemic and hyperproteinemic states, because the autoanalyzer equipment used in most clinical laboratories includes excess lipids or proteins in the water volume of the sample, causing an spurious dilution of sodium.

Causes. Hyponatremia can result from a decrease in total body sodium with a lesser decrease in body water, from normal total body sodium content with excess retention of body water, or from an excess in body sodium with an even greater excess in body water. A normal reduction in serum sodium concentration occurs during pregnancy. Serum sodium concentration normally falls by an average of 5 mEq/L and serum osmolality by 10 mOsm/kg within 5 to 8 weeks of pregnancy, and then remain stable for the duration of pregnancy. This change represents a resetting of the osmotic threshold for ADH and an increase in extracellular fluid volume that accompanies pregnancy.[13]

A decrease in serum sodium with a lesser decrease in body water can occur when there is excessive sweating, gastrointestinal losses, and diuresis. Iso-osmotic fluid loss, as in vomiting or diarrhea, does not usually lower serum sodium concentration unless these losses are replaced with disproportionate amounts of orally ingested or parenterally administered water. Excessive sweating in hot weather, particularly during heavy exercise, leads to loss of sodium and water; hyponatremia develops when water rather than electrolyte-containing liquids is used to replace fluids lost in sweating. Another potential cause of sodium loss is repeated tap water enemas or frequent gastrointestinal irrigations with distilled water that removes sodium chloride from the gastrointestinal tract. Salt depletion can also occur with vigorous use of diuretics (Table 26–6).

Hyperglycemia decreases serum sodium concentration. Because sodium is largely an extracellular cation, it becomes diluted as water moves out of cells in response to the osmotic effects of the elevated blood glucose level. There is about a 1.6 mEq/L decrease in serum sodium for every 100 mg/dl rise in serum glucose above the normal level (100 mg/dl).[14] In this case, hyponatremia may occur despite serum hyperosmolality.

Homeostatic mechanisms usually prevent an increase in body water from developing when renal function is adequate and ADH and aldosterone levels are normal. Excess water can be retained, however, when water excretion is reduced because of abnormal kidney function or when ADH levels are elevated. Adrenal insufficiency leads to inadequate levels of aldosterone and decreased reabsorption of sodium by the kidney. Although uncommon, water excess can occur as the result of excessive water intake. Persons with psychogenic polydipsia (discussed later) drink water in excess of what the kidneys can excrete.

Manifestations. The manifestations of hyponatremia are largely related to sodium dilution (Table 26–6). Serum osmolality is decreased and cellular swelling occurs due to the movement of water from the extracellular to intracellular compartment. The manifestations of hyponatremia depend on the rapidity of onset and the severity of the sodium dilution. The signs and symptoms may be acute, as in severe water intoxication, or more insidious in onset and less severe. Because of water movement, hyponatremia causes intracellular hypo-osmolality, which is responsible for many of the clinical manifestations of the disorder.[15] Muscle cramps, weakness, and fatigue reflect the hypo-osmolality of skeletal muscle cells and are often early signs of hyponatremia. If the condition develops slowly, signs and symptoms do not develop until serum sodium levels approach 125 mEq/L (125 mmol/L). The brain and nervous system are the most seriously affected by increases in intracellular water. Progressive neurologic symptoms occur when the serum sodium falls below this level. Symptoms include apathy, lethargy, and headache, which can progress to disorientation, confusion, and gross motor weakness. Gastrointestinal manifestations such as nausea and vomiting, abdominal cramps, and diarrhea may develop.

TABLE 26-6 Causes and Manifestations of Hyponatremia

Causes	Manifestations
Excess Sodium Losses and Replacement With Tap Water or Sodium-Free Losses	**Laboratory Values**
Excess sweating in hot environment or with exercise	Serum sodium level below 135 mEq/L (135 mmol/L)
Gastrointestinal losses	Decreased serum osmolality
Vomiting	Dilution of blood components, including chloride, hematocrit, BUN
Diarrhea	**Nervous System Manifestations**
Diuresis	Movement of water into brain cells and other neurons
Excess Water Intake in Relation to Water Output	Headache
Excess administration of sodium-free parenteral solutions	Depression
Repeated administration of tap water enemas	Personality changes
Kidney disease that impairs water elimination	Confusion
Increased ADH levels	Apprehension, feeling of impending doom
Trauma, stress, pain	Lethargy, weakness
Syndrome of inappropriate ADH	Stupor, coma
Use of medications that increase ADH	**Gastrointestinal Manifestations**
Psychogenic polydipsia	Anorexia, nausea, vomiting
	Abdominal cramps
	Diarrhea
	Increased Intracellular Fluid
	Fingerprint edema

Severe water intoxication is manifested by headache, nausea, vomiting, abdominal cramps, weakness, and stupor. Seizures and coma occur when serum sodium levels reach extremely low levels (<110 mEq/L). These severe effects, which are caused by brain swelling, may be irreversible.[15]

The effect of rapid changes in serum osmolality on the peripheral nervous system often is associated with muscle cramps and depression of deep tendon reflexes. These effects commonly are observed in persons with hyponatremia that occurs during heavy exercise in hot weather.

Fingerprint edema is a sign of excess intracellular water. This phenomenon is demonstrated by pressing the finger firmly over the bony surface of the sternum for 15 to 30 seconds.[11] When excess intracellular water is present, a fingerprint similar to that observed when pressing on a piece of modeling clay is seen.

Diagnosis and Treatment. Diagnosis of hyponatremia is based on laboratory reports of decreased sodium concentration, the presence of conditions that predispose to sodium loss or water retention, and signs and symptoms indicative of the disorder.

The treatment of hyponatremia with water excess focuses on the underlying cause. When hyponatremia is caused by water intoxication, limiting water intake or discontinuing medications that contribute to syndrome of inappropriate ADH may be sufficient. The administration of saline solution orally or intravenously may be needed when hyponatremia is caused by sodium deficiency.

Symptomatic hyponatremia (*i.e.,* neurologic manifestations) is often treated with hypertonic saline solution and a loop diuretic such as furosemide to increase water elimination. This combination allows for correction of serum sodium levels while ridding the body of excess water. There is concern about the rapidity with which serum sodium levels are corrected, particularly in persons with chronic symptomatic hyponatremia. In the case of prolonged water intoxication, brain cells reduce their concentration of organic osmoles as a means of preventing an increase in cell volume. It takes several days for brain cells to restore the organic osmoles lost during hyponatremia.[16] Rapid changes in serum osmolality when brain cells have already undergone volume regulation may shrink brain cells. One of the reported effects of rapid treatment of hyponatremia is a osmotic demyelinating condition called *central pontine myelosis,* which produces serious neurologic sequelae and sometimes causes death.[17]

Hypernatremia

Hypernatremia implies a serum sodium level above 148 mEq/L (148 mmol/L) and a serum osmolality greater than 295 mOsm/kg.

Causes. Hypernatremia represents an imbalance between total body sodium and water balance and can arise when there is excess loss of body water through the urine, gastrointestinal tract, lungs, or skin; a defect in thirst or inability to drink water; or rapid ingestion or infusion of sodium with insufficient time or opportunity for water ingestion (Table 26–7). Hypernatremia almost always follows a loss of body fluids that have a lower than normal concentration of sodium, so that water is lost in excess of sodium. This can result from increased losses from the respiratory tract during fever or strenuous exercise, from watery diarrhea, or when osmotically active tube feedings are given with inadequate amounts of water.

Hypernatremia with an accompanying water deficit stimulates thirst and increases water intake. It is therefore more likely to occur in infants and in persons who cannot express their thirst or obtain water to drink. With hypodipsia, or impaired thirst, the need for fluid intake does not activate the thirst response. Hypodipsia is particularly prevalent among the elderly. In persons with diabetes insipidus, hypernatremia can develop when thirst is impaired or water is unavailable. It is more likely when the condition develops in an unconscious person who is unable to express her or his need for increased water intake. The therapeutic administration of sodium-containing solutions may also cause hypernatremia. For example, the administration of sodium bicarbonate during cardiopulmonary resuscitation increases body sodium levels, because the sodium concentration of each 50-ml ampule of 7.5% sodium bicarbonate contains 892 mEq of sodium.[13] Hypertonic saline solution intended for intraamniotic instillation for therapeutic abortion may inadvertently be injected intravenously, causing hypernatremia. Rarely, salt intake occurs rapidly, as in taking excess salt tablets or during near-drowning in salt water.

Manifestations. The clinical manifestations of hypernatremia with water deficit are similar to those of fluid volume deficit. Body weight is decreased in proportion to the amount of water that has been lost. Because blood plasma is roughly 90% to 93% water, the concentrations of blood cells and other solutes increase as extracellular water decreases. This is also true of hematocrit and BUN levels.

Thirst is an early symptom of water deficit, occurring when water losses are equal to 0.5% of body water. Urine output is decreased and urine osmolality increased because of renal conserving mechanisms. Body temperature frequently is elevated, and the skin becomes warm and flushed. The vascular volume decreases, the pulse rate becomes rapid, and the blood pressure drops.

Unlike isotonic fluid deficit, hypernatremia causes an increase in serum osmolality; this causes water to be pulled out of body cells. As a result, the skin and mucous membranes become dry, and salivation and lacrimation are decreased. The mucous membranes become dry and sticky, and the tongue becomes rough and fissured. Swallowing is difficult. The subcutaneous tissues assume a firm, rubbery texture. Most significantly, water is pulled out of the cells in the central nervous system (CNS), causing decreased reflexes, agitation, headache,

TABLE 26-7 Causes and Manifestations of Hypernatremia

Causes	Manifestations
Excess Water Losses	**Laboratory Values**
Diabetes insipidus	Serum sodium level above 148 mEq/L (148 mmol/L)
Tracheobronchitis	Increased serum osmolality
Watery diarrhea	Increased concentration of hematocrit and blood urea nitrogen
Excessive sweating	**Thirst**
Hypertonic tube feedings	Increased thirst
Decreased Water Intake	**Urine Output**
Oral trauma or inability to express thirst	Oliguria or anuria
Impaired thirst sensation	High urine specific gravity
Withholding water for therapeutic reasons	**Intracellular Dehydration**
Unconsciousness or inability to express thirst	Skin and mucous membranes
Excessive Sodium Intake	Skin dry and flushed
Rapid or excessive administration of sodium-containing parenteral solutions	Mucous membranes dry and sticky
Near-drowning in salt water	Tongue rough and fissured
	Decreased lacrimation and salivation
	Subcutaneous tissue
	Firm and rubbery
	Central Nervous System Manifestations
	Headache
	Agitation and restlessness
	Decreased reflexes
	Maniacal behavior
	Seizures and coma
	Cardiovascular Manifestations
	Tachycardia
	Decreased blood pressure
	Weak and thready pulse

and restlessness. Coma and seizures may develop as hypernatremia progresses.

Diagnosis and Treatment. The diagnosis of hypernatremia is based on laboratory findings and history and physical examination findings indicative of dehydration or excess sodium gain. The treatment of hypernatremia with water deficit consists of replacement therapy, which includes replacing the water and the electrolytes that have been lost. Replacement fluids can be given orally or intravenously. The oral route is preferable. Oral glucose-electrolyte replacement solutions are available for the treatment of infants with diarrhea.[18–20] Until recently, these solutions were only used early in diarrhea illness or as a first step in reestablishing oral intake after parenteral replacement therapy. These solutions are now widely available in grocery stores and pharmacies for use in the treatment of diarrhea and other dehydrating disorders in infants and young children. They are particularly important in developing countries, where the availability of intravenous fluids is limited and diarrhea is a leading cause of death among children.

The composition of oral rehydration solution recommended by the Diarrheal Disease Control Center for the World Health Organization (WHO) contains glucose (2.0 g/L), sodium (90 mEq/L), potassium (20 mEq/L), chloride (80 mEq/L), and bicarbonate (30 mEq/L). It is recommended that ingredients be supplied in preweighed packets. Using teaspoons or other household items for measuring the ingredients is often inaccurate and is not recommended. Glucose is preferred to sucrose (*i.e.*, table sugar), which is a disaccharide and must be broken down before it can be absorbed. Commercially available preparations usually contain less sodium and chloride (*e.g.*, 45 to 50 mEq/L of sodium, 35 to 45 mEq of chloride) than the WHO formulation, with citrate being substituted for bicarbonate. Although cola drinks commonly are recommended as folk remedies for dehydration caused by acute diarrhea, their electrolyte content often is inadequate for replacement purposes, and their high sugar content may complicate the situation by inducing an osmotic diarrhea.[19,21] Sport drinks usually contain more sodium and sugar than the oral rehydration solutions. Intravenous replacement solutions continue to be the treatment of choice for severe fluid deficit.

One of the serious aspects of fluid volume deficit is dehydration of brain and nerve cells. Serum osmolality should be corrected slowly in cases of chronic hypernatremia. This is because brain cells synthesize osmotically active organic solutes to protect against volume changes. These organic solutes serve to produce a gradual increase in intracellular osmolality, allowing osmotic flow of water back into the cell and restoring cell volume. This response begins within 4 to 6 hours of increased serum osmolality and takes several days to become fully effective.[13] Changes in brain water content are greatest during acute hypernatremia but only slightly reduced in chronic hypernatremia. If hypernatremia is corrected too rapidly, before the organic osmoles have had a chance to dissipate, the plasma may become relatively hypotonic in relation to brain cell osmolality. When this occurs, water moves into the brain cells, causing cerebral edema and potentially severe neurologic impairment.

Disorders of Thirst and Antidiuretic Hormone Regulation

Disorders of thirst (*i.e.,* psychogenic polydipsia) and ADH levels (*i.e.,* syndrome of inappropriate ADH and diabetes insipidus) afford the potential for altering body levels of sodium and water.

Psychogenic Polydipsia

Psychogenic polydipsia involves compulsive drinking behavior and is usually seen in persons with psychiatric disorders, most commonly schizophrenia. Persons with the disorder drink large amounts of water and excrete large amounts of urine. The cause of excessive water drinking in these persons is uncertain. It has been suggested that the compulsive water drinking may share the same pathology as the psychosis, because persons with the disorder often increase their water drinking during periods of exacerbation in their psychotic symptoms.[22] The condition may be compounded by antipsychotic medications that increase ADH levels and interfere with water excretion by the kidneys. Cigarette smoking, which is common among persons with psychiatric disorders, also stimulates ADH secretion.

Excessive water ingestion coupled with impaired water excretion (or rapid ingestion at a rate that exceeds renal excretion) in persons with psychogenic polydipsia can lead to water intoxication. The condition is characterized by profound hyponatremia and hypo-osmolality of body fluids sufficient to cause seizures and other neurologic manifestations.

Treatment consists of water restriction and behavioral measures aimed at decreasing water consumption. Measurements of body weight can be used to provide an estimate of water consumption. Medications, such as lithium or demeclocycline, that decrease ADH effects may be prescribed for persons with increased ADH levels.[23] Cases of severe hyponatremia (*i.e.,* those with a serum sodium concentration below 115 mEq/L or signs of water intoxication) are treated with a hypertonic saline solution and measures to control seizures and other neurologic problems. It is recommended that the hypertonic saline solution be infused slowly and only be given until serum sodium levels reach about 120 mEq/L. Exceedingly rapid correction of serum sodium levels can lead to severe neurologic damage.

Syndrome of Inappropriate Antidiuretic Hormone

The syndrome of inappropriate ADH (SIADH) results from a failure of the negative feedback system that regulates the release and inhibition of ADH.[24] In persons with this syndrome, ADH secretion continues even when serum osmolality is decreased; this causes marked retention of water in excess of sodium and dilutional hyponatremia. An increase in the glomerular filtration rate resulting from an increased plasma volume causes further increases in sodium loss by suppressing the renin-angiotensin mechanism. Urine osmolality is high, and serum osmolality is low. Urine output decreases despite adequate or increased fluid intake, and the resultant water retention produces a rapid gain in body weight. Hematocrit and the serum sodium and BUN levels are all decreased because of the expansion of the extracellular fluid volume.

SIADH can be caused by a number of conditions, including lung tumors, chest lesions, and CNS disorders, and by various pharmacologic agents. The first report of SIADH was made in the late 1950s in association with lung cancer. Tumors, particularly bronchogenic carcinomas and cancers of lymphoid tissue, prostate, and pancreas are known to produce and release ADH independent of normal hypothalamic control mechanisms. Other intrathoracic conditions, such as advanced tuberculosis, severe pneumonia, and positive-pressure breathing, also cause SIADH. The suggested mechanism for SIADH in positive-pressure ventilation is activation of baroreceptors (*e.g.,* aortic baroreceptors, cardiopulmonary receptors) that respond to marked changes in intrathoracic pressure. Disease and injury to the CNS can cause direct pressure on or direct involvement of the hypothalamic–posterior pituitary structures. Examples include brain tumors, hydrocephalus, head injury, meningitis, and encephalitis.

Other stimuli, such as pain, stress, and temperature changes, are capable of stimulating ADH release through the limbic system. Drugs induce SIADH in different ways; some drugs are thought to increase hypothalamic production and release, and others are believed to act directly on the renal tubules to potentiate the action of ADH.

SIADH may occur as a transient condition, as in a stress situation, or as a chronic condition, resulting from disorders such as lung tumors. The severity of symptoms usually is proportional to the extent of sodium depletion and water intoxication. Symptoms of mild

SIADH (serum sodium levels of about 130 mEq/L) include headache, anorexia, muscle cramps, general fatigue, and dulling of the sensorium. In severe SIADH (serum sodium levels less than 125 mEq/L), neurologic symptoms of acute water intoxication begin to appear; they include nausea, vomiting, muscle twitching, seizures, and coma.

The treatment of SIADH depends on its severity. In mild cases, treatment consists of fluid restriction. If fluid restriction is not sufficient, diuretics such as mannitol and furosemide (Lasix) may be given to promote diuresis and free-water clearance. Lithium and the antibiotic demeclocycline inhibit the action of ADH on the renal collecting ducts and sometimes are used in treating the disorder. In cases of severe sodium depletion, a hypertonic (3% or 5%) sodium chloride solution may be administered intravenously.

Diabetes Insipidus

Diabetes insipidus means "tasteless diabetes," as opposed to diabetes mellitus, or "sweet diabetes." Diabetes insipidus is characterized by excessive urination of a dilute urine (polyuria) and polydipsia because of a disorder of ADH availability or function. In contrast to psychogenic polydipsia, the polydipsia that occurs with diabetes insipidus is triggered by an increase in serum osmolality rather than compulsive water drinking.

There are two types of diabetes insipidus: *central or neurogenic diabetes insipidus*, which occurs because of a defect in the synthesis or release of ADH, and *nephrogenic diabetes insipidus*, which occurs because the kidneys do not respond to ADH.[25–27] In neurogenic diabetes insipidus, loss of 75% to 80% of ADH-secretory neurons is necessary for clinically important polyuria. Most persons with neurogenic diabetes insipidus have an incomplete form of the disorder and retain some ability to concentrate their urine. Temporary neurogenic diabetes insipidus may follow head injury or surgery near the hypophysial tract. Nephrogenic diabetes insipidus is characterized by impairment of urine-concentrating ability and free-water conservation. It may occur as an genetic trait that affects the V_2 receptor that binds ADH or the protein that forms the water channels in the collecting tubules.[25] Other acquired causes of nephrogenic diabetes insipidus are drugs such as lithium and electrolyte disorders such as potassium depletion or chronic hypercalcemia. Polyuria and polydipsia are common adverse effects of lithium. Lithium and the electrolyte disorders seem to interfere with the postreceptor actions of ADH on the permeability of the collecting ducts.

Persons with diabetes insipidus are unable to concentrate their urine during periods of water restriction; they excrete large volumes of urine, usually 3 to 20 L/day, depending on the degree of ADH deficiency or renal insensitivity to ADH. This large urine output is accompanied by excessive thirst; as long as the thirst mechanism is normal and fluid is readily available, there is little or no alteration in the fluid levels in persons with diabetes insipidus. The danger arises when the condition develops in an unconscious person, because an inadequate fluid intake rapidly leads to hypertonic dehydration and increased serum osmolality.

Diagnosis of diabetes insipidus is based on measurements of ADH along with plasma and urine osmolalities before and after a period of fluid deprivation or hypertonic saline infusion. Persons with neurogenic diabetes insipidus do not increase their ADH levels in response to increased plasma osmolality.

Another diagnostic approach is to conduct a carefully monitored trial of a pharmacologic form of ADH. Persons with nephrogenic diabetes insipidus do not respond to pharmacologic preparations of the hormone. Diagnostic measures for diabetes insipidus include those that exclude psychogenic polydipsia as a reason for the excessive thirst and increased urine output. When central diabetes insipidus is suspected, diagnostic methods such as skull x-ray studies and computed tomographic scanning of the pituitary hypothalamic area are used to determine the cause of the disorder.

The management of central diabetes insipidus consists of treating any underlying disorder and supplying the body with pharmacologic preparations that contain the missing hormone. These preparations cannot be given orally, because they are destroyed in the gastrointestinal tract. Instead, they must be administered parenterally or nasally. The preferred drug for treating chronic diabetes insipidus is desmopressin acetate (DDAVP). Desmopressin, which can be given by intranasal spray, has a duration of action of 8 to 20 hours. Many persons with incomplete neurogenic diabetes insipidus maintain near-normal water balance when permitted to ingest water in response to thirst. Sometimes other drugs are used for persons who can still release ADH. The oral antidiabetic agent chlorpropamide may be used to stimulate ADH release in central diabetes insipidus. Other drugs that are used to treat this form of diabetes insipidus are carbamazepine and clofibrate. In nephrogenic diabetes insipidus, the thiazide diuretics along with a low-sodium diet are the specific form of therapy. These diuretics probably act predominantly by increasing sodium excretion by the kidneys, which lowers the glomerular filtration rate and increases reabsorption of fluid in the proximal tubule.

In summary, regulation of body fluid volume and osmolality depends on water and sodium balance. Body water is distributed between the intracellular and extracellular fluid compartments. Body water levels are regulated by thirst (intake) and by renal mechanisms that control urine concentration (output). Renal mechanisms for concentrating urine are mediated by ADH. As the major cation in the extracellular fluid, sodium controls the osmolality of the extracellular compartment. Sodium intake is mainly derived from dietary source. Sodium elimination is largely regulated by the kidney under the influence of the renin-angiotensin-aldosterone mechanism.

Alterations of salt and water balance include isotonic contraction or expansion of extracellular fluid volume and alterations in extracellular sodium concentration. In general, alterations in sodium balance result in disorders of extracellular fluid volume (i.e., extracellular fluid volume deficit or excess) and alterations in water balance result in disorders of sodium concentration (i.e., hyponatremia or hypernatremia). Isotonic fluid volume deficit is characterized by a reduction in intracellular and extracellular fluids. It causes thirst, a decrease in vascular volume and circulatory function, decreased urine output and increased urine specific gravity, and signs related to loss of fluid from the cellular compartment. Isotonic fluid volume excess can exist as an isotonic expansion of body fluids or as a disproportionate increase in water volume. It is characterized by increases in interstitial and intravascular fluids.

Serum sodium concentration is strongly affected by extracellular water levels; it is increased in water deficit and decreased in water excess. Normal levels of sodium are essential to maintaining the osmolality of the extracellular fluids; many of the manifestations of altered sodium balance are caused by swelling (hyponatremia) or shrinking (hypernatremia) of body cells, including those of the CNS. Hyponatremia results from water volume excess and dilution of extracellular sodium. It is characterized by decreased serum osmolality and cellular swelling. Hypernatremia results from water volume deficit and increased sodium concentration. It causes an increase in serum osmolality and causes water to be pulled out of cells.

Diabetes insipidus is a condition of inadequate ADH levels (i.e., neurogenic diabetes insipidus) or inadequate renal responsiveness to the hormone (i.e., nephrogenic diabetes insipidus); SIADH is a condition of inappropriate secretion of the hormone.

Potassium Balance

After you have completed this section of the chapter, you should be able to meet the following objectives:

- Characterize the distribution of potassium within the body and explain how extracellular potassium levels are regulated in relation to body gains and losses
- State the causes of hypokalemia and hyperkalemia in terms of altered intake, output, and intracellular versus extracellular distribution mechanisms
- Relate the functions of potassium to the manifestations of hypokalemia and hyperkalemia

Regulation of Potassium Balance

Potassium is the second most abundant cation in the body and the major cation in the intracellular compartment. All but about 2% of body potassium is contained within body cells, with intracellular concentration of 140 to 150 mEq/L.[28] The potassium content of extracellular fluid (3.5 to 5.0 mEq/L) is considerably less. Because potassium is an intracellular ion, total body stores of potassium are related to body size and muscle mass. In adults, total body potassium ranges from 50 to 55 mmol/kg of body weight.[29] Potassium content declines with age, mainly as a result of a decrease in muscle mass.

Gains and Losses

Potassium intake is normally derived from dietary sources. In healthy persons, potassium balance usually can be maintained by a daily dietary intake of 50 to 100 mEq. Additional amounts of potassium are needed during periods of trauma and stress. The kidneys are the main source of potassium loss. About 80% to 90% of potassium losses occur in the urine, and the remainder occur in the stool or sweat. Renal losses of potassium are influenced by the urine flow rate, serum sodium concentration, potassium intake, acid-base balance, and aldosterone levels. Potassium is filtered in the glomerulus, reabsorbed with sodium and water in the proximal tubule and with sodium and chloride in the descending limb of Henle, and secreted into the distal tubule and collecting duct for elimination in the urine. The latter mechanism serves to "fine tune" the concentration of potassium in the extracellular fluid.

Mechanisms of Regulation

Serum levels of potassium are mainly regulated by redistribution between the intracellular and extracellular compartments and renal mechanisms that cause potassium to be conserved or eliminated. Normally, it takes 6 to 8 hours to excrete 50% of potassium intake.[13] To avoid a buildup of potassium in extracellular fluids during this time, potassium is temporarily stored in cells such as those of muscle, liver, red cells, and bone. Because potassium is an intracellular ion, serum levels of potassium do not always accurately reflect intracellular levels.

Intracellular-Extracellular Shifts. Precise regulation of potassium movement between the intracellular and extracellular compartments must be extremely efficient, because transfer of even 1% to 2% of potassium into the extracellular compartment can elevate serum potassium levels to dangerously high levels. The movement of potassium into the cell requires the action of the Na^+/K^+ membrane pump. The function of the Na^+/K^+ pump in moving potassium across the cell membrane is facilitated by several hormones, most notably insulin and epinephrine. Extracellular osmolality and pH also influence movement of potassium between the intracellular and extracellular compartments. Tissue injury causes release of intracellular potassium into the extracellular fluid compartment.

Insulin increases movement of potassium into body cells and plays a central role in maintaining normal extracellular-intracellular distribution of potassium. The targets of insulin's action are the same tissues where glucose is stored: the liver, muscle, and adipose tissue. Plasma potassium levels directly affect insulin release.

An increased potassium levels stimulates insulin release, and a low potassium level inhibits insulin release, suggesting a potassium-insulin regulatory feedback mechanism.[30, 31] The catecholamines, particularly epinephrine, facilitate the movement of potassium into muscle tissue. The action of epinephrine on potassium transport is additive to that of insulin.

Acute increases in serum osmolality redistribute potassium out of cells. When serum osmolality increases because of the presence of impermeable extracellular solutes such as mannitol or glucose (without insulin), water leaves the cell. The loss of intracellular water and cell volume increases potassium concentration, causing potassium to diffuse out of the cell. A 1.0 to 1.5 mEq/L increment in serum potassium occurs in response to an acute 10% increase in serum osmolality.[13] A hyperosmolality-induced increase in serum potassium is usually counteracted by the opposing actions of insulin and epinephrine. The reverse condition, hypo-osmolality, usually occurs more slowly and does not affect serum potassium levels.

The hydrogen ion concentration (pH) of the extracellular fluid contributes to compartmental shifts of potassium. In acidosis, hydrogen ions move into the cell as a means of preventing large changes in extracellular pH changes. When a hydrogen ion moves into the cell, another positively charged ion (potassium) must move out into the extracellular fluid. The serum potassium concentration rises 0.6 mEq/L to 0.7 mEq/L for each 0.1 unit fall in serum pH. The pH related shifts in intracellular-extracellular potassium are more pronounced when changes in pH are caused by nonorganic acids (*i.e.*, hyperchloremic acidosis associated with diarrhea and renal failure) in which the companion anion, chloride, cannot permeate the cell membrane and remains outside the cell as a companion for the potassium ion. In contrast, metabolic acidosis due to accumulation of organic acids (*i.e.*, lactic acidosis and ketoacidosis) has little effect on potassium, because the companion anion is able to enter the cell. Although there is increased movement of potassium out of the cell in diabetic ketoacidosis, it is more likely related to the effects of insulin deficiency and the hyperosmolality of the extracellular fluids. Respiratory acidosis and alkalosis cause little change in serum potassium concentration.

Exercise also causes potassium to move from the intracellular to extracellular compartment. Even the clenching and unclenching of the fist during a blood draw can cause potassium to move out of cells. For example, if a person is asked to repeatedly clench and unclench the fist after a tourniquet has been applied to increase venous distention, the action can release potassium into the blood and artificially elevate serum potassium levels.

Renal Regulation. The most important route for eliminating potassium from the body is the kidney. Unlike other electrolytes, the regulation of potassium elimination is controlled by secretion into the tubular fluid rather than through reabsorption. Most of the filtered potassium is reabsorbed in the proximal tubule and loop of Henle. Excess potassium is then secreted to the urine filtrate in cortical collecting tubules as a means of making final adjustments in potassium excretion (see Chapter 25).

Aldosterone plays an essential role in regulating potassium secretion in the cortical collecting tubule. Urinary losses of potassium increase under the influence of aldosterone, while sodium retention is increased. The feedback regulation of aldosterone levels is strongly regulated by serum potassium levels; for example, an increase in potassium ion concentration of less than 1 mEq/L causes aldosterone levels to triple. This increased secretion continues for as long as potassium levels are elevated. There is also a potassium-hydrogen exchange mechanism that secretes potassium in the cortical collecting tubules of the kidney (see Chapter 25). When the extracellular concentration of potassium is elevated, potassium secretion is increased, and hydrogen ion secretion is decreased, causing a decrease in serum pH (*i.e.*, metabolic acidosis). Conversely, when the extracellular concentration of potassium is low, tubular secretion of potassium into the urine is decreased, and hydrogen ion secretion is increased, leading to metabolic alkalosis.

Alterations in Potassium Balance

As the major intracellular cation, potassium is critical to many functions of the cell. Potassium contributes to the maintenance of intracellular osmolality; is necessary for neuromuscular control and the precise regulation of skeletal, cardiac, and smooth muscle activity; influences acid-base balance; and participates in many intracellular enzyme reactions. For example, potassium contributes to the intricate chemical reactions that transform carbohydrates into energy, change glucose into glycogen, and convert amino acids to proteins.

Hypokalemia

Hypokalemia refers to a decrease in serum potassium levels below 3.5 mEq/L (3.5 mmol/L). Because of transcompartmental shifts, temporary changes in serum potassium may occur as the result of movement between the intracellular and extracellular compartments.

Causes. The causes of potassium deficit can be grouped into three categories: inadequate intake; excessive gastrointestinal, renal, and skin losses; and redistribution between the intracellular and extracellular fluid compartments (Table 26–8).

Inadequate Intake. Dietary intake of potassium should be least 10 to 30 mEq/day to compensate for obligatory urine losses.[13] An adult on a potassium-free diet continues to lose about 5 to 15 mEq of potassium daily. Insufficient dietary intake may result from decreased food intake, as during dieting or because of a diet that is low in potassium-containing foods. Dietary intake frequently is impaired at the time potassium losses are increased, such as after surgery or trauma, when new cell formation is

TABLE 26-8 Causes and Manifestations of Hypokalemia

Causes	Manifestations
Inadequate Intake Diet deficient in potassium Inability to eat Administration of potassium-free parenteral solutions **Excessive Renal Losses** Diuretic therapy (except potassium-sparing diuretics) Diuretic phase of renal failure Increased mineralocorticoid levels Cushing's disease Primary hyperaldosteronism Treatment with corticosteroid drugs **Excessive Gastrointestinal Losses** Vomiting Diarrhea Gastrointestinal suction Draining gastrointestinal fistula **Excessive Skin Losses** Heavy sweating in persons acclimated to hot environment **Transcompartmental Shift** Treatment of diabetic ketoacidosis Alkalosis, metabolic or respiratory	**Laboratory Values** Serum potassium level below 3.5 mEq/L (3.5 mmol/L) **Thirst** Increased thirst **Urine Output** Impaired ability of kidneys to concentrate urine Polyuria Urine of low osmolality and specific gravity Nocturia **Gastrointestinal Manifestations** Anorexia, nausea, vomiting Abdominal distention Paralytic ileus **Cardiovascular Manifestations** Postural hypotension Cardiac dysrhythmias Increased sensitivity to digitalis toxicity **Skeletal Muscle Manifestations** Muscle tenderness, paresthesias, muscle cramps Weakness, muscle flabbiness Paralysis **Central Nervous System manifestations** Confusion Depression **Acid-Base Balance** Metabolic alkalosis

needed for wound healing. Elderly persons are particularly likely to develop potassium deficits. Many have poor eating habits as a consequence of living alone; they may have limited income, which makes buying foods high in potassium difficult; they may have difficulty chewing many foods that have a high potassium content because of poorly fitting dentures; or they may have problems with swallowing. Also, many medical problems in elderly persons require treatment with drugs, such as diuretics, that increase potassium losses.

Excessive Losses. The kidneys are the main source of potassium loss. About 80% to 90% of potassium losses occur in the urine, with the remaining losses in the stool and sweat. The kidneys do not have the homeostatic mechanisms needed to conserve potassium during brief periods of insufficient intake. After trauma and in stress situations, urinary losses of potassium are greatly increased, sometimes approaching levels of 150 to 200 mEq/dL (150 to 200 mmol/L). This means that a potassium deficit can develop rather quickly under these conditions if intake is inadequate.

Diuretic therapy (with the exception of potassium-sparing diuretics such as spironolactone) results in additional urinary losses of potassium. Some antibiotics, particularly amphotericin B and gentamicin, are impermeable anions that require the presence of positively charged cations for elimination in the urine; this causes potassium wasting.

Renal losses of potassium are accentuated by aldosterone. *Primary aldosteronism* is caused by a tumor in the cells of the adrenal cortex (in the zona glomerulosa) that secrete aldosterone. Excess secretion of aldosterone by the tumor cells causes severe potassium losses and a decrease in serum potassium levels.

Although potassium losses from the skin and the gastrointestinal tract usually are minimal, these losses can become excessive under certain conditions. For instance, burns increase surface losses of potassium. Losses due to sweating increase in persons who are acclimated to a hot climate, partly because increased secretion of aldosterone during heat acclimatization increases the loss of potassium in urine and sweat.[4] Gastrointestinal losses can also become excessive; this occurs with vomiting and diarrhea and when gastrointestinal suction is being used. The potassium content of liquid stools, for example, is about 40 to 60 mEq/L (40 to 60 mmol/L).[28]

Transcellular Shifts. Because of the high ratio of intracellular to extracellular potassium, a redistribution of potassium from the extracellular to the intracellular compartment can produce a marked fall in serum levels. One cause of potassium redistribution is insulin. After insulin administration, there is increased movement of glucose and potassium into cells. Potent β-adrenergic agonist drugs such as epinephrine and albuterol have a similar effect on potassium distribution.

Manifestations. Manifestations of potassium deficit seldom develop until the serum potassium level has fallen below 3.5 mEq/L (3.5 mmol/L). The signs and symptoms of potassium deficit typically are gradual in onset and for that reason go undetected for a long time. The manifestations of potassium deficit include alterations in renal function, skeletal muscle function, gastrointestinal function, and cardiovascular function, reflecting the crucial role of potassium in cell metabolism and neuromuscular function.

Hypokalemia impairs the kidneys' ability to concentrate urine and leads to increased ammonia production by the kidney. Urine output and serum osmolality are increased, urine specific gravity is decreased, and complaints of polyuria, nocturia, and thirst are common. Increased ammonia production appears to be a compensatory mechanism that occurs in response to a decrease in the cellular pH of renal tubular cells, which occurs as a result of a K^+/H^+ ion exchange that occurs with hypokalemia. As the intracellular pH falls, renal synthesis of ammonia is increased. Because ammonia is obtained through the deamination of amino acids, the nitrogen balance becomes negative, and protein synthesis is impaired. For this reason, children who need proteins for growth and persons who need amino acids for tissue repair are particularly vulnerable to prolonged periods of hypokalemia. Ammonia is converted to urea in the liver. For persons with advanced liver disease, hypokalemia can lead to disturbing elevations in serum ammonia levels.

Hypokalemia causes numerous signs and symptoms associated with gastrointestinal function, including anorexia, nausea, and vomiting. Hypokalemia decreases smooth muscle excitability. Atony of gastrointestinal smooth muscle can cause constipation, decreased peristalsis, intestinal distention, and paralytic ileus.[32] When gastrointestinal symptoms occur gradually and are not severe, they often impair potassium intake and exaggerate the condition.

Potassium deficiency affects vascular smooth muscle and heart function. Postural hypotension is common. Serious cardiac dysrhythmias can result from hypokalemia, and hypokalemia increases the risk of digitalis toxicity. Potassium and digitalis compete for binding to the enzyme (ATPase) that operates the Na^+/K^+ membrane pump. In hypokalemia, more enzyme sites are available for digitalis to bind and exert its action. The dangers associated with digitalis toxicity are compounded in persons who are receiving diuretics that increase urinary losses of potassium.

At least three defects in skeletal muscle function occur with potassium deficiency: alterations in the resting membrane potential, alterations in glycogen synthesis and storage, and impaired ability to increase blood flow during strenuous exercise.[32] Potassium contributes to the resting membrane potential of excitable tissue. As potassium levels decrease, the resting membrane potential becomes more negative (*i.e.*, hyperpolarized), resulting in a decrease in neuromuscular excitability (see Chapter 1). Neuromuscular signs and symptoms appear when serum potassium levels fall to about 2.5 mEq/L (2.5 mmol/L).

Normal concentrations of intracellular potassium are necessary for glycogen synthesis in muscle cells. This means that potassium deficiency can interfere with the electrical activity of skeletal muscle and with muscle metabolism, especially under exercise conditions that rely heavily on anaerobic pathways. The release of potassium from muscle is thought to contribute to the autoregulation of blood flow during exercise. Potassium deficiency can interfere with the release of potassium ions from exercising muscle and can lead to impaired blood flow and consequent ischemic injury to muscle cells during intense physical exercise.[32]

Clinical manifestations of hypokalemia include muscle weakness, fatigue, and cramps, particularly during exercise. Paralysis can occur with severe hypokalemia. Leg muscles, particularly the quadriceps, are most prominently affected. Some persons complain of muscle tenderness and paresthesias rather than weakness. In chronic potassium deficiency, muscle atrophy may contribute to muscle weakness.

In a rare condition called *hypokalemic familial periodic paralysis*, episodes of hypokalemia cause attacks of flaccid paralysis that last 6 to 48 hours if untreated.[3] The paralysis may be precipitated by situations that cause severe hypokalemia by producing an intracellular shift in potassium, such as ingestion of a high-carbohydrate meal or administration of insulin, epinephrine, or glucocorticoid drugs. The paralysis often can be reversed by potassium replacement therapy.

Treatment. When possible, hypokalemia caused by potassium deficit is treated by increasing the intake of foods high in potassium content—meats, dried fruits, fruit juices (particularly orange juice), and bananas. Oral potassium supplements are prescribed for persons whose intake of potassium is insufficient in relation to losses. This is particularly true of persons who are receiving diuretic therapy and those who are taking digitalis.

Potassium may be given intravenously when the oral route is not tolerated or when rapid replacement is needed. Magnesium deficiency may impair potassium correction; in such cases, magnesium replacement is indicated.[33] The rapid infusion of a concentrated potassium solution can cause death resulting from cardiac arrest. Health personnel who assume responsibility for administering intravenous solutions that contain potassium should be fully aware of all the precautions pertaining to their dilution and flow rate.

Hyperkalemia

Hyperkalemia refers to an increase in serum levels of potassium in excess of 5.0 mEq/L (5.0 mmol/L). It seldom occurs in healthy persons, because the body is extremely effective in preventing excess potassium accumulation in the extracellular fluid.

Causes. The three major causes of potassium excess are decreased elimination, excessively rapid administration, and transcellular shift of potassium out of the cell (Table 26–9). Pseudohyperkalemia can occur secondary to release of potassium from intracellular stores after a blood sample has been collected, hemolysis of red blood cells from excessive agitation of blood sample, traumatic venipuncture, or prolonged tourniquet during venipuncture.[34] The most common cause of hyperkalemia is decreased renal function. Chronic hyperkalemia is almost always associated with renal failure or with impaired renal excretion due to aldosterone deficiency. Insufficient aldosterone activity can result from depression of aldosterone release because of a decrease in renin or angiotensin II, adrenal insufficiency (*i.e.*, Addison's disease), or impaired ability of the kidneys to respond to aldosterone. Potassium-sparing diuretics (*e.g.*, spironolactone, amiloride, triamterene) can produce hyperkalemia by means of the latter mechanism. Because of their ability to decrease aldosterone levels, angiotensin-converting enzyme (ACE) inhibitors can also produce an increase in serum potassium levels.

It is difficult to increase potassium intake to the point of causing hyperkalemia when sufficient aldosterone is present and renal function is adequate. An exception to this rule is when potassium solutions are being infused intravenously. In some cases, severe and fatal incidents of hyperkalemia have resulted from the intravenous infusion of potassium. Because the kidneys control potassium elimination, intravenous solutions that contain potassium should never be started until urine output has been assessed and renal function has been deemed to be adequate.

The movement of potassium out of body cells into the extracellular fluids also can lead to elevated serum potassium levels. For example, burns and crushing injuries cause potassium to be liberated into the extracellular fluid. The same injuries often diminish renal function, which contributes to the development of hyperkalemia. Transient hyperkalemia may be induced during extreme exercise or seizures, when muscle cells are permeable to potassium. In a rare autosomal dominant disorder called *hyperkalemic periodic paralysis*, hyperkalemia may cause transient periods of muscle weakness and paralysis after exercise, cold exposure, or other situations that cause potassium to move out of the cells. In contrast to hypokalemic periodic paralysis, the episodes are mild, with a duration of less than 2 hours.[2]

Manifestations. The signs and symptoms of potassium excess are closely related to the alterations in neuromuscular function that accompany potassium deficit. The rise in serum potassium depolarizes cells; although the mechanisms responsible for the altered neuromuscular function observed in hypokalemia and hyperkalemia are different, the end results are similar. The first symptom associated with hyperkalemia typically is pares-

TABLE 26–9 Causes and Manifestations of Hyperkalemia

Causes	Manifestations
Excess Intake and Gain	**Laboratory values**
Excess oral intake	Serum potassium level above 5.0 mEq/L (5.0 mmol/L)
Excess or rapid infusion of potassium-containing parenteral fluids	**Neural and Skeletal Muscle Activity**
Tissue trauma, burns, or crushing injuries that result in massive release of intracellular potassium	Paresthesias
	Weakness and dizziness
	Muscle cramps
Inadequate Renal Losses	**Gastrointestinal Manifestations**
Renal failure	Nausea and vomiting
Adrenal insufficiency (Addisons's disease)	Diarrhea
Treatment with potassium-sparing diuretics	Intestinal colic
Treatment with angiotensin-converting enzyme inhibitors	Gastrointestinal distress
	Cardiac Electrophysiology
	Peaked T waves, depressed ST segment
	Depressed P wave and widening QRS complex
	Cardiac arrest

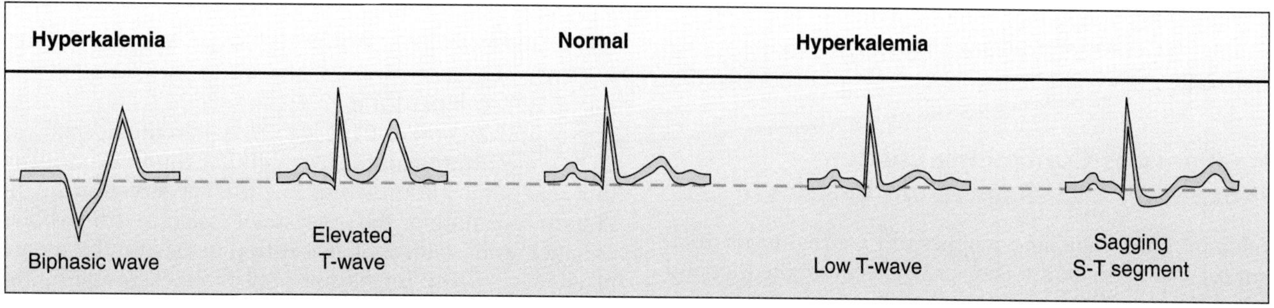

FIGURE 26–8
Electrocardiographic changes with hyperkalemia and hypokalemia.

thesia; this may appear when potassium levels reach 6 mEq/L (6 mmol/L). With serum levels less than 6 mEq/L, symptoms are minor or absent. The most serious effect of hyperkalemia is cardiac arrest. The electrocardiographic changes that occur with alterations in serum potassium levels are described in Figure 26–8.

Treatment. The treatment of potassium excess varies with the severity of the disturbance and focuses on decreasing or curtailing intake or absorption, increasing renal excretion, and increasing cellular uptake.

Decreased intake can be achieved by restricting dietary sources of potassium. The major ingredient in most salt substitutes is potassium chloride, and such substitutes should not be given to patients with renal problems. Increasing potassium output often is more difficult. Patients with renal failure may require hemodialysis or peritoneal dialysis to reduce serum potassium levels. Sodium polystyrene sulfonate, a cation exchange resin, may also be used to remove potassium ions from the colon. The sodium ions in the resin are exchanged for potassium ions, and then the potassium-containing resin is eliminated in the stool. Most emergency methods focus on measures that cause serum potassium to move into the intracellular compartment. Sometimes the intravenous infusion of insulin and glucose is used for this purpose.

In summary, potassium is the major intracellular cation. It contributes to the maintenance of intracellular osmolality, is necessary for normal neuromuscular function, and influences acid-base balance. Potassium is ingested in the diet and eliminated through the kidney. Because potassium is poorly conserved by the kidney, an adequate daily intake is needed. A transcellular shift can produce a redistribution of potassium between the extracellular and intracellular compartments, causing blood levels to increase or decrease.

Hypokalemia represents a decrease in serum potassium levels below 3.5 mEq/L. It can result from inadequate intake, excessive losses, or redistribution between the intracellular and extracellular fluid compartments. The manifestations of potassium deficit include alterations in renal function, skeletal muscle function, gastrointestinal function, and cardiovascular function, reflecting the crucial role of potassium in cell metabolism and neuromuscular function.

Hyperkalemia represents and increase in serum potassium levels greater than 5.0 mEq/L. It seldom occurs in healthy persons, because the body is extremely effective in preventing excess potassium accumulation in the extracellular fluid. The major causes of potassium excess are decreased renal elimination of potassium, excessively rapid intravenous administration of potassium, and transcellular shift of potassium out of the cell to the extracellular compartment. The most serious effect of hyperkalemia is cardiac arrest.

Calcium, Phosphate, and Magnesium Balance

After you have completed this section of the chapter, you should be able to meet the following objectives:

- Describe the associations among intestinal absorption, renal elimination, bone stores, and the functions of vitamin D and parathyroid hormone in regulating calcium, phosphate, and magnesium levels
- State the difference between ionized and bound or chelated forms of calcium in terms of physiologic function
- Describe the mechanisms of calcium gain and loss and relate them to the causes of hypocalcemia and hypercalcemia
- Relate the functions of calcium to the manifestations of hypocalcemia and hypercalcemia
- Describe the mechanisms of phosphate gain and loss and relate them to causes of hypophosphatemia and hyperphosphatemia
- Relate the functions of phosphate to the manifestations of hypophosphatemia and hyperphosphatemia
- Describe the mechanisms of phosphate gain and loss and relate them to the causes of hypomagnesemia and hypermagesemia

- Relate the functions of magnesium to the manifestations of hypomagnesemia and hypermagnesemia

Mechanisms Controlling Calcium, Phosphate, and Magnesium Balance

Calcium, phosphate, and magnesium are the major divalent cations in the body. They are ingested in the diet and absorbed from the intestine, filtered in the glomerulus of the kidney, reabsorbed in the renal tubules, and eliminated in the urine. About 99% of calcium, 85% of phosphate, and 65% of magnesium are found in bone. Most of the remaining calcium (about 1%), phosphate (about 14%), and magnesium (about 45%), are located inside cells. Only a small amount of these three ions are present in extracellular fluid. This small, but vital, amount of extracellular calcium, phosphate, and magnesium is directly or indirectly regulated by parathyroid hormone (PTH) and vitamin D. Calcitonin, a hormone produced by C cells in the thyroid, is thought to act on the kidney and bone to remove calcium from the extracellular circulation. However, the importance of calcitonin on normal day-to-day regulation of calcium has not been established.

Bone is in a dynamic equilibrium with the extracellular calcium and phosphate. Calcium and phosphate found in bone is primarily in the form hydroxyapatite crystal ($3[Ca_3PO_4\}_2] \bullet Ca[OH]_2$). A thin film of water that contains calcium and phosphate in solution surrounds these crystals.[13] Parathyroid hormone increases plasma calcium and phosphate levels by means of osteoclast-mediated bone resorption and diffusional exchange with phosphate and calcium in the surface film. An ionic exchange between positively charged Ca^{2+} and Mg^{2+} ions also occurs at the bone surface such that changes in serum magnesium levels can alter calcium uptake or release.

The extracellular concentrations of calcium and phosphate are reciprocally regulated; when calcium levels are high, phosphate levels are low and vice versa. Normal serum levels of calcium (8.5 to 10.5 mg/dL in adults) and phosphate (2.5 to 4.5 mg/dL in adults) are regulated so that product of the two concentrations ($[Ca^{2+}] \times [PO_4^{2-}]$) is maintained below 60. Maintenance of the calcium × phosphate product within this range is important in preventing crystallization of $CaPO_4$ in bone and tissue.

Vitamin D

The role of vitamin D is to increase plasma levels of calcium and phosphate and maintain conditions favorable for bone mineralization. Vitamin D, although classified as a vitamin, functions as a hormone. Vitamin D_3, the precursor of the active form of vitamin D is synthesized in the skin or obtained from foods in the diet, many of which are fortified with vitamin D. Vitamin D_3 is hydroxylated in the liver to form $25(OH)D_3$ and is transformed into active $1,25(OH)_2D_3$ in the kidney. The activated form of vitamin D, also called calcitriol, increases intestinal absorption of calcium and phosphate, decreases PTH secretion (to decrease resorption of calcium from bone), and increases calcium reabsorption by the kidney.

Parathyroid Hormone

The main function of PTH is to maintain the normal calcium concentration of the extracellular fluids. It performs this function by stimulating calcium conservation by the kidney, promoting the release of calcium from bone, enhancing the intestinal absorption of calcium by means of vitamin D, and increasing phosphate excretion by the kidney. Parathyroid hormone is synthesized in the chief cells of the two pairs of parathyroid glands located on the dorsal surface of the thyroid gland. The main stimulus for PTH secretion is a decrease in plasma calcium levels. Although the secretion of PTH is inhibited by high levels of vitamin D, its action in terms of bone resorption requires normal levels of vitamin D and magnesium.

The activation of vitamin D by the kidney is enhanced by the presence of PTH; it is through the activation of vitamin D that PTH increases intestinal absorption of calcium and phosphate. PTH acts directly on the kidney to increase tubular reabsorption of calcium and magnesium and to increase phosphate elimination. Increased phosphate elimination ensures that calcium released from bone does not produce hyperphosphatemia and increase the risk of calcium phosphate precipitation.

The secretion, synthesis, and action of PTH is influenced by magnesium. Magnesium serves as a cofactor in the generation of cellular energy and function of cellular messenger systems. Magnesium's effect on the synthesis and release of PTH are thought to be mediated through these mechanisms.[35] Severe, prolonged hypomagnesemia markedly inhibits PTH and may be associated with hypocalcemia.

Intestinal Absorption

The absorption of calcium and phosphate from the intestine is increased by vitamin D. The positively charged Ca^{2+} and Mg^{2+} ions compete for reabsorption in the intestine. Factors that increase calcium absorption tend to cause a decrease in magnesium absorption and vice versa.

Renal Elimination

Calcium, phosphate, and magnesium are filtered in the glomerulus, reabsorbed in the renal tubules, and eliminated in the urine. About 60% to 65% of filtered calcium is passively reabsorbed in the proximal tubule, driven by the reabsorption of sodium chloride; 15% to 20% is reabsorbed in the thick ascending limb of Henle, driven by the $Na^+/K^+/2Cl^-$ cotransport system; and 5% to 10% is reabsorbed in the distal convoluted tubule (see Chapter 25). The loop diuretics, which inhibit the $Na^+/K^+/2Cl^-$ cotransporter, decrease calcium reabsorption in the thick ascending loop of Henle. The distal convoluted tubule is an important regulatory site for controlling the amount of calcium that enters the urine. PTH and possibly vitamin D stimulate calcium reabsorption in this segment of the nephron. Other factors that may influence calcium reabsorption in the distal convoluted tubule are phosphate levels and glucose and insulin levels. Thiazide diuretics, which exert their effects in the distal convoluted tubule, enhance calcium reabsorption.[36]

Magnesium is a unique electrolyte in that only about 40% of the filtered amount is reabsorbed in the proximal tubule. The greatest quantity, about 50% of the filtered amount, is passively reabsorbed in the thick ascending loop of Henle. Magnesium reabsorption is decreased in the presence of increased magnesium serum levels, stimulated by PTH, and inhibited by increased calcium levels. The major driving force for magnesium absorption in the thick ascending loop of Henle is the $Na^+/K^+/2Cl^-$ cotransport system (see Chapter 25). Inhibition of this transport system by loop diuretics lowers magnesium reabsorption.

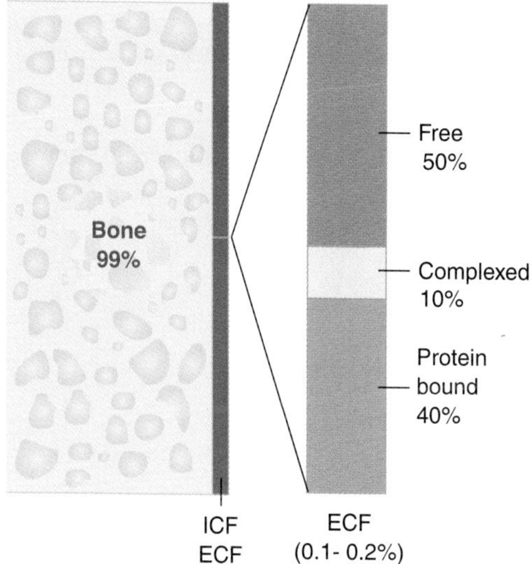

FIGURE 26–9
Distribution of body calcium between the bone and the intracellular and extracellular fluids. The percentages of free, complexed, and protein-bound calcium in extracellular fluids are indicated.

Alterations in Calcium Balance

About 99% of body calcium is found in bone, where it provides the strength and stability for the collagen and ground substance that form the structural matrix of the skeletal system. Only about 0.1% of the remaining calcium is present in the extracellular fluid. The normal serum calcium concentration is about 8.5 to 10.5 mg/dl. The calcium in bone serves as an exchangeable source to maintain extracellular calcium levels.

Gains and Losses

Calcium enters the body through the gastrointestinal tract, is absorbed from the intestine under the influence of vitamin D, is stored in bone, and is excreted by the kidney. The major sources of calcium are milk and milk products. Only about 30% to 50% of dietary calcium is absorbed from the duodenum and upper jejunum; the remainder is eliminated in the stool. There is an influx of calcium of about 150 mg per day into the intestine from the blood. Net absorption of calcium is equal to the amount that is absorbed from the intestine less the amount that moves into the intestine. Calcium balance can become negative when dietary intake (and calcium absorption) is less than intestinal secretion. A dietary intake of less than 400 mg per day can be associated with negative calcium balance.[13]

Extracellular calcium exists in three forms: protein bound, complexed, and ionized. About 40% of serum calcium is bound to plasma proteins and cannot diffuse or pass through the capillary wall to leave the vascular compartment (Fig. 26–9). Most of the nondiffusible calcium is bound to albumin. The total serum calcium level changes with alterations in serum albumin and pH. As a rule, the total serum calcium level is decreased 0.75 to 1.0 mg/dl for every 1 g/dl decrease from normal in the serum albumin level and and by 0.16 mg/dl for each 0.10 unit rise in pH.[13] About 10% of serum calcium is complexed (*i.e.,* chelated) with substances such as citrate, phosphate, and sulfate. This form is not ionized. The remaining 50% of serum calcium is ionized. It is the ionized form of calcium that can leave the vascular compartment and participate in cellular functions.

Ionized calcium serves a number of functions. It participates in many enzyme reactions; exerts an important effect on cell membrane potentials and permeability; is necessary for contraction in skeletal, cardiac, and smooth muscle; participates in the release of hormones, neurotransmitters, and other chemical messengers; influences cardiac contractility and automaticity by way of slow calcium channels; and is essential for blood clotting. The use of calcium-channel–blocking drugs in circulatory disorders demonstrates the importance of the calcium ion in the normal function of the heart and blood vessels. Calcium is required for all but the first two steps of the intrinsic pathway for blood coagulation. Because of its ability to bind calcium, citrate often is used to prevent clotting in blood that is to be used for transfusions.

Hypocalcemia

Hypocalcemia represents a serum calcium level of less than 8.5 mg/dl. Hypocalcemia occurs in many forms of critical illness and has affected as many as 70% to 90% of patients in intensive care units.[37]

Causes. The causes of hypocalcemia can be divided into three categories: impaired ability to maintain and mobilize bone stores, abnormal losses of calcium from the kidney, and increased protein binding so that greater proportions of calcium are in the nonionized form (Table 26–10). A pseudohypocalcemia is caused by hypoalbuminemia. It results in a decrease in protein-bound, rather than ionized, calcium and usually is asymptomatic.[38,39]

Serum calcium exists in a dynamic equilibrium with calcium in bone. The ability to mobilize calcium from bone depends on adequate levels of PTH. Hypocalcemia may develop because of congenital or acquired hypoparathyroidism. An acquired deficiency of PTH may occur after neck surgery, particularly if the surgery

TABLE 26-10

Causes and Manifestations of Hypocalcemia

Causes	Manifestations
Impaired Ability to Mobilize Calcium From Bone	**Laboratory Values**
Hypoparathyroidism	Serum calcium level below 8.5 mg/dl
Resistance to the actions of parathyroid hormone	**Neuromuscular Manifestations**
Hypomagnesemia	Decreased ionized calcium
Decreased Intestinal Absorption	Paresthesias, especially numbness and tingling
Vitamin D deficiency	Skeletal muscle cramps
Impaired ability to activate vitamin D	Abdominal spasms and cramps
Liver disease	Hyperactive reflexes
Kidney disease	Carpopedal spasm
Medications that impair activation of vitamin D (*e.g.*, phenytoin)	Tetany
	Laryngeal spasm
Abnormal Losses	Positive Chvostek's and Trousseau's signs
Renal failure and hyperphosphatemia	**Cardiovascular Manifestations**
Increased Protein Binding or Chelation	Hypotension
Increased pH	Cardiac insufficiency
Increased fatty acids	Failure to respond to drugs that act by calcium-mediated mechanisms
Rapid transfusion of citrated blood	**Bone (Chronic Calcium Deficit)**
Increased Sequestration	Osteomalacia
Acute pancreatitis	Bone pain, deformities, and fractures

involves removal of a parathyroid adenoma, thyroidectomy, and bilateral neck resection for cancer. A transient PTH deficiency may result from parathyroid gland suppression after thyroid surgery. The hypocalcemia may occur immediately or 1 to 2 days after surgery and usually lasts less than 5 days.[11] Suppression of PTH release may occur when vitamin D levels are elevated. The activated form of vitamin D is used to suppress the secondary hyperparathyroidism that occurs in persons with kidney failure. Magnesium deficiency inhibits PTH release and impairs the action of PTH in terms of bone resorption. This form of hypocalcemia is difficult to treat with calcium supplementation alone and requires correction of magnesium deficiency.

There is an inverse relation between calcium and phosphate excretion by the kidneys. Phosphate is retained in renal failure, causing serum calcium levels to decrease and PTH levels to rise. Hypocalcemia and hyperphosphatemia occur when the glomerular filtration rate falls below 25 to 30 ml/minute (normal is 100 to 120 ml/minute).

Only the ionized form of calcium is able to leave the capillary and participate in body functions. A change in pH alters the amount of calcium in the ionized and bound forms. An acid pH decreases binding of calcium to protein, thereby raising the level of ionized calcium, while total serum calcium remains unchanged. An alkaline pH has the opposite effect. Hyperventilation sufficient to cause respiratory alkalosis can produce an effective hypocalcemia with tetany by increasing the protein binding of calcium without altering the total calcium concentrations. Free fatty acids increase binding of calcium to albumin, causing a reduction in ionized calcium. Elevations in free fatty acids sufficient to alter calcium binding may occur during stressful situations that cause elevations of epinephrine, glucagon, growth hormone, and adrenocorticotropic hormone levels. Heparin, β-adrenergic drugs (*i.e.*, epinephrine, isoproterenol, and norepinephrine), and alcohol can also produce elevations in free fatty acids levels sufficient to increase calcium binding.

Hypocalcemia is a common finding in a patient with acute pancreatitis. Inflammation of the pancreas causes release of proteolytic and lipolytic enzymes. It is thought that the calcium ion combines with free fatty acids released by lipolysis in the pancreas, forming soaps and removing calcium from the circulation.

Citrate, which often used as an anticoagulant in blood transfusion, complexes with calcium. Theoretically, excess citrate in donor blood could combine with the calcium in a recipient's blood, producing a sharp drop in ionized calcium. This normally does not occur, because the liver removes the citrate within a matter of minutes. When blood transfusions are administered at a slow rate (<1 L/hour in adults), there is little danger of hypocalcemia caused by citrate binding.[2]

Calcium deficit due to dietary deficiency exerts its effects on bone stores rather than extracellular calcium levels. Deficiency of vitamin D is seldom seen today, because many foods are fortified with vitamin D_3. Vitamin D_3 deficiency is more likely to occur in malabsorption states, such as biliary obstruction, pancreatic insufficiency, and celiac disease, in which the ability to absorb fat and fat-soluble vitamins is impaired. Failure to activate vitamin D_3 is another cause of hypocalcemia. Anticonvulsant medications, particularly phenytoin, can impair initial activation of vitamin D in the liver. The final activation step in activation of vitamin D is impaired in persons with renal failure (see Chapter 29). Fortunately, the activated form of the vitamin D, calcitriol, has been synthesized and is available for use in the treatment of calcium deficit in persons with renal failure.

Manifestations. Hypocalcemia can manifest as an acute or chronic condition. The manifestations of acute hypocalcemia reflect the increased neuromuscular excitability and cardiovascular effects. The severity of the manifestations depends on the underlying cause, rapidity of onset, accompanying electrolyte disorders, and extracellular pH.

Ionized calcium stabilizes neuromuscular excitability by lowering the resting membrane potential, thereby making the cell less sensitive to stimuli.[40] Increased neuromuscular excitability can manifest as paresthesias (*i.e.,* tingling around the mouth and in the hands and feet) and tetany (*i.e.,* muscle spasms of the muscles of the face, hands, and feet). Severe hypocalcemia can lead to laryngeal spasm, seizures, and even death.

Chvostek's and Trousseau's tests can be used to assess for an increase in neuromuscular excitability and tetany. Chvostek's sign is elicited by tapping the face just below the temple at the point where the facial nerve emerges. Tapping the face over the facial nerve causes spasm of the lip, nose, or face when the test result is positive. An inflated blood pressure cuff is used to test for Trousseau's sign. The cuff is inflated to a point where it temporarily occludes the circulation of the hand, usually for 1 to 5 minutes. Contraction of the fingers and hands (*i.e.,* carpopedal spasm) indicates the presence of tetany. Cardiovascular effects of acute hypocalcemia include hypotension, cardiac insufficiency, cardiac dysrhythmias (particularly heart block and ventricular fibrillation), and failure to respond to drugs such as digitalis, norepinephrine, and dopamine that act through calcium-mediated mechanisms.

Chronic hypocalcemia is often accompanied by skeletal manifestations and skin changes. There may be bone pain, fragility, deformities, and fractures. The skin may be dry and scaling, the nails brittle, and hair dry. Development of cataracts is common.

Treatment. Acute hypocalcemia is an emergency situation, requiring prompt treatment. An intravenous infusion containing calcium (*e.g.,* calcium gluconate, calcium gluceptate, calcium chloride) is used when tetany or acute symptoms are present or anticipated because of a decrease in the serum calcium level.

Chronic hypocalcemia is treated with oral intake of calcium. One glass of milk contains about 300 mg of calcium. Oral calcium supplements of carbonate, gluconate, or lactate salts may be used. In some cases, long-term treatment may require the use of vitamin D preparations. The active form of vitamin D is administered when the liver or kidney mechanisms needed for hormone activation are impaired.

Hypercalcemia

Hypercalcemia represents a total serum calcium concentration greater than 10.5 mg/dl. Falsely elevated levels of calcium can result from prolonged drawing of blood with an excessively tight tourniquet. Increased plasma proteins (*e.g.,* hyperalbuminemia, hyperglobulinemia) may elevate the total serum calcium but not affect the ionized calcium concentration.

Causes. A serum calcium excess (*i.e.,* hypercalcemia) results when calcium movement into the circulation overwhelms the calcium regulatory hormones or the ability of the kidney to remove excess calcium ions (Table 26–11). The most common causes of hypercalcemia are increased bone resorption due to neoplasms or hyperparathyroidism. Less frequent causes are prolonged immobilization, increased intestinal absorption of calcium, excessive doses of vitamin D, and the effects of drugs such as lithium and thiazide diuretics. The thiazide diuretics increase calcium reabsorption in the distal convoluted tubule of the kidney. Although the thiazide diuretics seldom cause hypercalcemia, they can unmask hypercalcemia from other causes.[36] Hypercalcemia is a common complication of malignancy, occurring in approximately 10% to 20% of persons with advanced disease.[41] A number of malignant tumors, including carcinoma of the lungs, have been associated with hypercalcemia. Some tumors destroy the bone, but others produce humoral agents that stimulate osteoclastic activity, increase bone resorption, or inhibit bone formation.

Hyperparathyroidism can manifest as a primary disorder caused by hyperplasia of the parathyroid glands or by an adenoma or carcinoma. Seconary hyperparathyroidism involves hyperplasia of the parathyroid glands. It is most commonly seen in persons with chronic renal failure and is caused by continued stimulation of the parathyroid glands because of hypocalcemia and hyperphosphatemia.

Prolonged immobilization and lack of weight bearing cause demineralization of bone and release of calcium into the blood stream.

Intestinal absorption of calcium can be increased by excessive doses of vitamin D or as a result of a condition called the milk-alkali syndrome. The liver functions as the storage site for vitamin D, and 1000 times the normal quantities can be ingested with only a threefold increase in serum levels of the active hormone.[2] The *milk-alkali syndrome* syndrome is caused by excessive ingestion of calcium (often in the form of milk) and absorbable antacids. Because of the advent of nonabsorbable antacids, the condition is seen less frequently than in the past, but it may occur in women who are overzealous in taking calcium preparations for osteoporosis prevention. The condition is thought to be initiated by mild hypercalcemia leading to increased sodium excretion along with

TABLE 26-11

Causes and Manifestations of Hypercalcemia

Cause	Manifestations
Increased Intestinal Absorption	**Laboratory Values**
Excess vitamin D	Serum calcium level above 10.5 mg/dl
Excess calcium in the diet	**Thirst**
Milk-alkali syndrome	Increased thirst
Increased Bone Resorption	**Renal Manifestations**
Increases levels of parathyroid hormone	Polyuria
Malignant neoplasms	Flank pain
Prolonged immobilization	Signs of acute reversible renal insufficiency
Decreased Elimination	Signs of kidney stones
Thiazide diuretics	**Gastrointestinal Manifestations**
Lithium therapy	Anorexia
	Nausea
	Vomiting
	Constipation
	Neuromuscular Manifestations
	Muscle weakness and atrophy
	Ataxia, loss of muscle tone
	Central Nervous System Manifestations
	Lethargy
	Personality and behavioral changes
	Stupor and coma
	Cardiovascular Manifestations
	Hypertension
	Shortening of the QT interval
	Atrioventricular block on electrocardiogram

a decrease in extracellular fluid volume and the glomerular filtration rate. The decreased glomerular filtration rate leads to alkalosis and increased calcium reabsorption by the kidney. Discontinuance of the antacid repairs the alkalosis and increases calcium elimination.

A variety of drugs elevate calcium levels. The use of lithium to treat manic-depressive disorders has caused hypercalcemia and hyperparathyroidism. Thiazide diuretics can increase calcium reabsorption by the kidney. Thiazide diuretics can produce an increase in the total serum calcium concentration of 0.5 to 1.0 mg/dl in otherwise healthy persons.[42] This reflects the indirect effects of hemoconcentration and the direct effects of bone resorption. In most persons, calcium levels return to normal after several weeks of therapy. Thiazide diuretics may cause hypercalcemia in patients with underlying bone disorders and increased bone resorption.

Manifestations. The signs and symptoms associated with calcium excess originate from three sources: neuromuscular activity, resorption of calcium from bone, and exposure of the kidneys to high concentrations of calcium.

Neural excitability is decreased in patients with hypercalcemia. There may be a dulling of consciousness, stupor, weakness, and muscle flaccidity. Behavioral changes may range from subtle alterations in personality to acute psychoses. Acute psychoses are common when calcium levels rise above 16 mg/dl.

Gastrointestinal symptoms include constipation, anorexia, nausea, and vomiting. Pancreatitis is another potential complication of hypercalcemia and is probably related to stones in the pancreatic ducts.

The heart responds to elevated levels of calcium with increased contractility and ventricular dysrhythmias. Digitalis causes these responses to be accentuated.

High calcium concentrations in the urine impair the ability of the kidneys to concentrate urine by interfering with the action of ADH. This causes salt and water diuresis and an increased sensation of thirst. Hypercalciuria also predisposes to the development of renal calculi.

Hypercalcemic crisis describes an acute increase in the serum calcium level.[44] Malignant disease and hyperparathyroidism are major causes of hypercalcemic crisis. In hypercalcemic crisis, polyuria, excessive thirst, volume depletion, fever, altered levels of consciousness, azotemia (*i.e.*, nitrogenous wastes in the blood), and a disturbed mental state accompany other signs of calcium excess. Symptomatic hypercalcemia is associated with a high mortality rate; death often is caused by cardiac arrest.

Treatment. The treatment of calcium excess usually is directed toward rehydration and measures to increase urinary excretion of calcium and inhibiting release of calcium from bone.[43,44] Fluid replacement is needed in situations of volume depletion. The excretion of sodium is accompanied by calcium excretion. Diuretics and sodium chloride can be administered to increase urinary elimination of calcium after the extracellular fluid volume has been restored. Loop diuretics commonly are used rather than thiazide diuretics, which increase calcium reabsorption.

Initial lowering of calcium levels is followed by measures to inhibit bone reabsorption. Drugs that are used to inhibit calcium mobilization include biphosphonates, calcitonin, plicamycin, glucocorticosteroids, and gallium nitrate. The biphosphonates are a relatively new group of drugs that act mainly by inhibiting osteoclastic activity. These agents provide a significant reduction in calcium levels with relatively few side effects. Calcitonin inhibits osteoclastic activity, thereby decreasing resorption. The corticosteroids and plicamycin (Mithramycin) inhibit bone resorption and are used to treat hypercalcemia associated with cancer. The long-term use of plicamycin, an antineoplastic drug, is limited because of its potential for nephrotoxicity and hepatotoxicity. Gallium nitrate is also used in the treatment of severe hypercalcemia associated with malignancy. It is a chemical compound that inhibits bone resorption, although the precise mechanism of action is unclear.

Alterations in Phosphate Balance

Phosphorous is mainly an intracellular anion. It is the fourth most abundant element in the body after carbon, nitrogen, and calcium. Phosphate is essential to many bodily functions. It plays a major role in bone formation; is essential to certain metabolic processes, including the formation of adenosine triphosphate (ATP) and the enzymes needed for metabolism of glucose, fat, and protein metabolism; is a necessary component of several vital parts of the cell, being incorporated into the nucleic acids of DNA and RNA and the phospholipids of the cell membrane; and serves as an acid-base buffer in the extracellular fluid and in the renal excretion of hydrogen ions. Delivery of oxygen by the red blood cell depends on organic phosphates in ATP and 2,3-diphosphoglycerate. Phosphate is also needed for normal function of other blood cells, including the white blood cells and platelets.

About 85% of phosphate is contained in bone, and most of the remainder (14%) is located in cells. Only about 1% is in the extracellular compartment, and of that, only a minute proportion is in the plasma. Extracellular phosphorous exists mainly as phosphate, although laboratory measurements are often reported as elemental phosphorous.[45,46] Most of the intracellular phosphorous (about 90%) is in the organic form (*e.g.*, nucleic acids, phosphoproteins, ATP). Entry of phosphate into cells is enhanced after glucose uptake, because phosphorous is incorporated into the phosphorylated intermediates of glucose metabolism. Cell injury or atrophy leads to a loss of cell components that contain organic phosphate; regeneration of these cellular components results in withdrawal of inorganic phosphate from the extracellular compartment.

Gains and Losses

In the adult, the normal serum phosphate level ranges from 2.5 to 4.5 mg/dl. These values are slightly higher in infants (3.7 to 8.5 mg/dl) and children (4.0 to 5.4 mg/dl), probably because of increased growth hormone and decreased gonadal hormones. Changing the serum phosphate levels to as high as three to four times the normal value does not seem to have an immediate effect on body function.

Phosphate is ingested in the diet and eliminated in the urine. Phosphate is derived from many dietary sources, including milk and meats. About 80% of ingested phosphate is absorbed in the intestine, primarily in the jejunum. Absorption is diminished by concurrent ingestion of substances that bind phosphate, including calcium, magnesium, and aluminum. Renal elimination of phosphate is largely regulated by an overflow mechanism in which the amount of phosphate lost in the urine is directly related to phosphate concentrations in the blood. When serum phosphate levels rise above a critical level, the rate of phosphate loss in the urine reflects the excess serum phosphate levels.

Hypophosphatemia

Hypophosphatemia is commonly defined by a serum phosphorus level of less than 2.5 mg/dl; it is considered severe at concentration of less than 1.0 mEq/L.[46] Hypophosphatemia may occur despite normal body phosphate stores as a result of movement into the intracellular compartment. Serious depletion of phosphate may exist with low, normal, or high serum concentrations.

Causes. The most common causes of hypophosphatemia are depletion of phosphate because of insufficient intestinal absorption, transcompartmental shifts, and increased renal losses (Table 26–12). Often, more than one of these mechanisms is active. Unless food intake is severely restricted, dietary intake and intestinal absorption of phosphorous is usually adequate. Intestinal absorption may be inhibited by administration of glucocorticoids, high dietary levels of magnesium, and hypothyroidism. Prolonged ingestion of antacids may also interfere with intestinal absorption. Antacids that contain aluminum hydroxide, aluminum carbonate, and calcium carbonate bind with phosphate, causing increased phosphate losses in the stool. Because of their

TABLE 26-12

Causes and Manifestations of Hypophosphatemia

Causes	Manifestations
Decreased Intestinal Absorption	**Laboratory Values**
Antacids (aluminum and calcium)	Serum levels below 2.5 mg/dl in adults and 4.0 mg/dl in children
Severe diarrhea	**Neural Manifestations**
Lack of vitamin D	Intention tremor
Increased Renal Elimination	Ataxia
Alkalosis	Paresthesias
Hyperparathyroidism	Hyporeflexia
Diabetic ketoacidosis	Confusion
Renal tubular absorption defects	Stupor and coma
Malnutrition and Intracellular Shifts	Seizures
Alcoholism	**Musculoskeletal Manifestations**
Total parenteral hyperalimentation	Muscle weakness
Recovery from malnutrition	Joint stiffness
Administration of insulin and recovery from diabetic ketoacidosis	Bone pain
	Osteomalacia
	Gastrointestinal Manifestations
	Anorexia
	Dysphagia
	Hemolytic Disorders
	Hemolytic anemia
	Platelet dysfunction with bleeding disorders
	Impaired white blood cell function

ability to bind phosphate, calcium-based antacids are sometimes used therapeutically to decrease phosphate levels in persons with chronic renal failure.

Hypophosphatemia can occur during prolonged courses of glucose administration or hyperalimentation. Glucose administration causes insulin release, with transport of glucose and phosphorous into the cell. The catabolic events that occur with diabetic ketoacidosis also deplete phosphate stores. However, hypophosphatemia does not become apparent until insulin and fluid replacement have reversed dehydration and glucose has started to move back into the cell. Administration of hyperalimentation solutions without adequate phosphorous can cause a rapid influx of phosphorous into the body's muscle mass, particularly if treatment is initiated after a period of tissue catabolism. Because only a small amount of total body phosphorus is in the extracellular compartment, even a small redistribution between the extracellular and intracellular compartments can cause hypophosphatemia even though total phosphate levels have not changed.

Alcoholism is a common cause of hypophosphatemia. The mechanisms underlying hypophosphatemia in the person addicted to alcohol may be related to malnutrition, increased renal excretion rates, or hypomagnesemia. Malnutrition and diabetic ketoacidosis increase phosphate excretion and phosphate loss from the body. Refeeding of malnourished patients increases the incorporation of phosphate into nucleic acids and phosphorylated compounds in the cell. The same thing happens when diabetic ketoacidosis is reversed with insulin therapy. Urinary losses of phosphate may be caused by drugs such as theophylline, corticosteroids, and loop diuretics that increase renal excretion. PTH increases the renal excretion of phosphate.

Respiratory alkalosis due to prolonged hyperventilation can produce hypophosphatemia through decreased levels of ionized calcium from increased protein binding, increased PTH release, and increased phosphate excretion. Clinical conditions associated with hyperventilation include gram-negative septicemia, alcohol withdrawal, heat stroke, and primary hyperventilation.[46]

Manifestations. Many of the manifestations of phosphorous deficiency result from a decrease in cellular energy stores due to deficiency in ATP and impaired oxygen transport due to a decrease in red blood cell 2,3-diphosphoglycerate (see Chapter 24). Hypophosphatemia results in altered neural function, disturbed musculoskeletal function, and hematologic disorders.

Red blood cell metabolism is impaired by phosphate deficiency; the cells become rigid and have increased hemolysis and diminished ATP and 2,3-diphosphoglycerate levels. Chemotaxis and phagocytosis by white blood cells are impaired. Platelet function is also disturbed. Respiratory insufficiency resulting from impaired function of the respiratory muscles can develop in patients with severe hypophosphatemia.

Neural manifestations include intention tremors, paresthesia, hyporeflexia, stupor, coma, and seizures (see Table 26–12). Anorexia and dysphagia can occur. Muscle weakness, which is common in hypophosphatemia, is related to a reduction in 2,3-diphosphoglycerate. Chronic phosphate depletion interferes with mineralization of newly formed bone matrix. In growing children, this process causes abnormal endochondral growth and clinical manifestations of rickets. In adults, the condition leads to joint stiffness, bone pain, and skeletal deformities consistent with osteomalacia (see Chapter 46).

Treatment The treatment of hypophosphatemia is replacement therapy. This may be accomplished with dietary sources high in phosphate (one glassful of milk contains about 250 mg of phosphate) or with oral or intravenous replacement solutions. Phosphate supplements usually are contraindicated in hypercalcemia and renal failure because of increased risk of extracellular calcifications that occur when the calcium × phosphate concentration product exceeds that needed for precipitation of calcium phosphate.

Hyperphosphatemia

Hyperphosphatemia represents a serum phosphorus concentration in excess of 4.5 mg/dl. Growing children normally have serum phosphate levels higher than those of adults.

Causes. Hyperphosphatemia results from failure of the kidneys to excrete excess phosphate, rapid redistribution of intracellular phosphate to the extracellular compartment, and excessive intake of phosphate. The most common cause of hyperphosphatemia is impaired renal function (Table 26–13).

Hyperphosphatemia is a common electrolyte disorder in persons with acute or chronic renal failure and is related to a decrease in glomerular filtration rate. A reduction in glomerular filtration rate to less than 30 to 50 ml/minute results in a reduction of phosphate elimination. PTH deficiency decreases renal losses of phosphate. The increase in phosphate levels in persons with end-stage renal disease occurs despite compensatory increases in PTH. Hypoparathyroidism is another cause of hyperphosphatemia, particularly when it is accompanied by low calcium intake.

Release of intracellular phosphate can result from conditions such as massive tissue injury, heatstroke, potassium deficiency, and seizures. Chemotherapy can raise serum phosphate levels because of the rapid destruction of tumor cells. The administration of excess phosphate-containing antacids, laxatives, or enemas can be another cause of hyperphosphatemia, especially when there is a decrease in vascular volume and a reduced glomerular filtration rate. Phosphate-containing laxatives and enemas predispose to hypovolemia and a decreased glomerular filtration rate by inducing diarrhea, thereby increasing the risk of hypophosphatemia. Serious and even fatal hyperphosphatemia has resulted from administration of Fleets Phospho-Soda enterally[47] or as an enema.

Manifestations. Hyperphosphatemia is associated with a decrease in serum calcium. Plasma calcium levels fall as serum phosphate levels rise; many of the signs and symptoms of a phosphate excess are related to a calcium deficit (see Table 26–13). Ectopic calcifications may develop when the calcium × phosphate concentration product exceeds 60.

Treatment. The treatment of hyperphosphatemia is directed at the cause of the disorder. Dietary restriction of foods that are high in phosphate may be used. Calcium-based phosphate binders are useful in

TABLE 26-13 Causes and Manifestations of Hyperphosphatemia

Causes	Signs and Symptoms
Acute Phosphate Overload	**Laboratory Values**
Phosphate-containing laxatives	Serum levels above 4.5 mg/dL in adults and 5.4 mg/dl in children
Phosphate-containing enemas	Ectopic calcification when Ca × PO_4 >60
Intravenous administration	
	Neuromuscular Manifestations
Intracellular-to-Extracellular Shift	Reciprocal decrease in serum calcium
Massive trauma	Paresthesias
Heat stroke	Tetany
Seizures	
Tumor lysis syndrome	**Cardiovascular Manifestations**
Potassium deficiency	Reciprocal decrease in serum calcium
	Hypotension
Impaired Elimination	Cardiac dysrhythmias
Kidney failure	
Hypoparathyroidism	

chronic hyperphosphatemia. Hemodialysis is used to reduce phosphate levels in persons with end-stage renal disease.

Alterations in Magnesium Balance

Magnesium is the second most abundant intracellular cation. The average adult has about 24 g of magnesium distributed throughout the body.[48] Of the total magnesium content, 50% is stored in bone, 49% is contained in the body cells, and the remaining 1% is dispersed in the extracellular fluids. About 20% to 30% of the extracellular magnesium is protein bound, and only a small fraction of intracellular magnesium (15% to 30%) is exchangeable with the extracellular fluid.[35] The normal serum concentration of magnesium is 1.8 to 2.7 mg/dl.

Only recently has the importance of magnesium to the overall function of the body been recognized. Magnesium acts as a cofactor in many intracellular enzyme reactions. It is essential in all enzyme systems known to be catalyzed by ATP, and profound disruption of cell function occurs in magnesium-deficient tissues. Magnesium is necessary for functioning of the sodium-potassium pump, for protein and deoxyribonucleic acid (DNA) synthesis, DNA and ribonucleic acid (RNA) transcription, and translation of RNA. Magnesium can bind to calcium receptors, and it has been suggested that alterations in magnesium levels may exert their effects through calcium-mediated mechanisms. Magnesium may bind competitively to calcium binding sites, producing the appropriate response; it may compete with calcium for a binding site but not exert an effect; or it may alter the distribution of calcium by interfering with its movement across the cell membrane.

Gains and Losses

Magnesium is ingested in the diet, absorbed from the intestine, and excreted by the kidneys. Intestinal absorption is not closely regulated, and about 25% to 65% of dietary magnesium is absorbed. Magnesium is contained in all green vegetables, grains, nuts, meats, and seafood. Magnesium is also present in much of the ground water in North America. The average dietary intake of magnesium in the United States about 185 to 260 mg for men and 172 to 235 for women, and the Recommended Daily Allowance is 350 mg per day.[49]

Hypomagnesemia

Hypomagnesemia represents a serum magnesium concentration of less than 1.8 mg/dl.[50] It is seen in conditions that limit intake or increase intestinal or renal losses, and it is a common finding in emergency room and critical care patients.

Causes. Magnesium deficiency can result from insufficient intake, excessive losses, or movement between the extracellular and intracellular compartments (Table 26–14). It can result from conditions that directly limit intake, such as malnutrition, starvation, or prolonged maintenance of magnesium-free parenteral nutrition. Other conditions, such as diarrhea, malabsorption syndromes, prolonged nasogastric suction, or laxative abuse, decrease intestinal absorption.[51] Excessive calcium intake impairs intestinal absorption of magnesium by competing for the same transport site.

Another common cause of magnesium deficiency is chronic alcoholism and gastrointestinal losses. Many factors contribute to hypomagnesemia in alcoholism, including low intake and gastrointestinal losses from diarrhea. The effects of hypomagnesemia are exaggerated by other electrolyte disorders, such as hypokalemia, hypocalcemia, and metabolic acidosis. There is also evidence that alcohol inhibits reabsorption of magnesium by the kidney.[48] Although the kidneys are able to defend against hypermagnesemia, they are less able to conserve magnesium and prevent hypomagnesemia. Urine losses are increased in diabetic ketoacidosis,

TABLE 26–14 Causes and Manifestations of Hypomagnesemia

Causes	Manifestations
Impaired Intake or Absorption	**Laboratory Values**
Alcoholism	Serum magnesium level less than 1.8 mg/dl
Malnutrition or starvation	**Neuromuscular Manifestations**
Malabsorption	Personality change
Small bowel bypass surgery	Athetoid or choreiform movements
Parenteral hyperalimentation with inadequate amounts of magnesium	Nystagmus
High dietary intake of calcium without concomitant amounts of magnesium	Tetany
	Positive Babinski's, Chvostek's, Trousseau's signs
Increased Losses	**Cardiovascular Manifestations**
Diuretic therapy	Tachycardia
Hyperparathyroidism	Hypertension
Hyperaldosteronism	Cardiac dysrhythmias
Diabetic ketoacidosis	
Magnesium-wasting kidney disease	

TABLE 26-15
Causes and Manifestations of Hypermagnesemia

Cause	Manifestations
Excess Intake	**Laboratory Values**
Intravenous administration of magnesium for treatment of preeclampsia	Serum values in excess of 2.7 mg/dl
Excess use of oral magnesium-containing medications	**Neuromuscular Manifestations**
Decreased Excretion	Lethargy
Parenchymal renal disease	Hyporeflexia and muscle weakness
Glomerulonephritis	Confusion
Tubulointerstitial kidney disease	Coma
Acute renal failure	**Cardiovascular Manifestations**
	Hypotension
	Cardiac dysrhythmias
	Cardiac arrest

hyperparathyroidism, and hyperaldosteronism. Some drugs increase renal losses of magnesium, including diuretics (particularly loop diuretics), digitalis, aminoglycoside antibiotics, cyclosporine, cisplatin, and amphotericin B.

Relative hypomagnesemia may also develop in conditions that promote movement of magnesium between the extracellular and intracellular compartments, including rapid administration of glucose, insulin-containing parenteral solutions, and alkalosis. Although transient, these conditions can cause serious alteration in body function.

Manifestations. Magnesium deficiency usually occurs in conjunction with hypocalcemia and hypokalemia, producing a number of related neurologic and cardiovascular manifestations. It leads to a reduction in intracellular potassium and impairs the ability of the kidney to conserve potassium. Enhanced potassium efflux and diminished influx occur in magnesium deficiency. Increased efflux occurs through potassium channels in the presence of magnesium deficit, and decreased influx is probably related to impaired activation of the Na^+/K^+ membrane pump than normally pumps sodium out of the cell in exchange for potassium. When hypomagnesemia is present, hypokalemia is unresponsive to potassium replacement therapy.

Magnesium deficit also exerts an effect on extracellular calcium concentration. Hypocalcemia results from decreased PTH levels, probably as a result of impaired function of intracellular mechanisms (*e.g.*, cyclic adenosine monophosphate) that control PTH release and synthesis. There is also evidence that hypomagnesemia decreases the effect of PTH on bone. Hypomagnesemia also decreases the parathyroid-independent calcium-magnesium exchange in bone, leading to increased release of magnesium ions in exchange for increased uptake of calcium from the serum.

Because of its effects on calcium levels, many of the signs and symptoms of hypomagnesemia are similar to those of hypocalcemia. The person may have personality changes, neuromuscular irritability along with tremors, athetoid or choreiform movements, and positive Babinski's, Chvostek's, or Trousseau's signs. Cardiovascular manifestations include tachycardia, hypertension, and ventricular dysrhythmias. Ventricular dysrhythmias, particularly in the presence of digitalis, may be difficult to treat unless magnesium levels are normalized.

Treatment. Hypomagnesemia is treated with magnesium replacement, usually with parenteral administration. Treatment must be continued for several days to replace stored and serum levels. In conditions of chronic intestinal or renal loss, maintenance support with oral magnesium may be required. Patients with any degree of renal failure must be carefully monitored to prevent magnesium excess. Magnesium is often used therapeutically to treat cardiac arrhythmia, myocardial infarct, angina, and pregnancy complicated preeclampsia or eclampsia. Caution to prevent hypermagnesemia is essential.

Hypermagnesemia

Magnesium excess (serum concentration in excess of 2.7 mg/dl). Because of the ability of the normal kidney to excrete magnesium, hypermagnesemia is uncommon.

Causes. When hypermagnesemia does occur, it usually is related to renal insufficiency and the injudicious use of magnesium-containing medications such as antacids, mineral supplements, or laxatives. The elderly are particularly at risk, because they have age-related reductions in renal function and tend to consume more magnesium-containing medications. Hypermagnesemia may also occur in persons with normal renal function who receive magnesium-containing medications. Magnesium sulfate is used to treat toxemia of pregnancy and premature labor; in these cases, careful monitoring for signs of hypermagnesemia is essential (Table 26–15).

Manifestations. Hypermagnesemia affects neuromuscular and cardiovascular function. Because magnesium tends to suppress PTH secretion, hypocalcemia may accompany hypermagnesemia. The signs and symptoms occur only when serum magnesium levels exceed 4.9 mg/dl (2 mmol/L). Deep tendon reflexes begin to decrease as magnesium serum levels exceed 4 mEq/L.[51]

Hypermagnesemia diminishes neuromuscular function, causing hyporeflexia, muscle weakness, and confusion. Magnesium decreases acetylcholine release at the myoneural junction and may cause neuromuscular blockade and respiratory paralysis. Cardiovascular effects are related to the calcium-channel–blocking effects of magnesium. Blood pressure is decreased, and the electrocardiogram shows an increase in the PR interval, a shortening of the QT interval, T wave abnormalities, and prolongation of the QRS and PR intervals. Hypotension due to vasodilation and cardiac dysrhythmias can occur with moderate hypermagnesemia ($<$10 mg/dl), and confusion and coma can occur with severe hypermagnesemia ($>$10 mg/dl). Very severe hypermagnesemia ($>$15 mg/dl) may cause cardiac arrest.

Treatment. The treatment of hypermagnesemia includes cessation of magnesium administration. Calcium is a direct antagonist of magnesium, and intravenous administration of calcium may be used. Peritoneal dialysis or hemodialysis may be required.

In summary, calcium, phosphate, and magnesium are the major cations in the body. Calcium is a major divalent cation. About 99% of body calcium is found in bone; less than 1% is found in the extracellular fluid compartment. The calcium in bone is in dynamic equilibrium with extracellular calcium. Of the three forms of extracellular calcium (i.e., protein-bound, complex, and ionized), only the ionized form can cross the cell membrane and contribute to cellular function. Ionized calcium has a number of functions. It contributes to neuromuscular function, plays a vital role in the blood clotting process, and participates in a number of enzyme reactions. Alterations in ionized calcium levels produce neural effects; neural excitability is increased in hypocalcemia and decreased in hypercalcemia. Phosphate is largely an intracellular anion. It is incorporated into the nucleic acids and ATP.

The most common causes of altered levels of serum phosphate are alterations in intestinal absorption, transcompartmental shifts, and disorders of renal elimination. Phosphate deficit causes signs and symptoms of neural function, disturbed musculoskeletal function, and hematologic disorders. Most of these manifestations result from a decrease in cellular energy stores from a deficiency in ATP and oxygen transport by 2,3-diphosphoglycerate in the red blood cell. Phosphate excess occurs with renal failure and PTH deficit; it is associated with decreased serum calcium levels.

Magnesium is the second most abundant intracellular cation. It acts as a cofactor in many enzyme reactions and affects neuromuscular function in the same manner as the calcium ion. Magnesium deficiency can result from insufficient intake, excessive losses, or movement between the extracellular and intracellular compartments. Hypomagnesemia impairs PTH release and the actions of PTH; it leads to a reduction in intracellular potassium and impairs the ability of the kidney to conserve potassium. The signs and symptoms of hypomagnesemia are therefore similar to those of hypocalcemia. Hypermagnesemia is usually related to renal insufficiency and the injudicious use of magnesium-containing medications such as antacids, mineral supplements, or laxatives. It can cause neuromuscular dysfunction, causing hyporeflexia, muscle weakness, and confusion. Magnesium decreases acetylcholine release at the myoneural junction and may cause neuromuscular blockade and respiratory paralysis.

REFERENCES

1. Krieger J.N., Sherrad D.J. (1991). *Practical fluid and electrolytes* (pp. 104–105). Norwalk, CT: Appleton & Lange.
2. Guyton A., Hall J.E. (1996). *Textbook of medical physiology* (9th ed., pp. 187, 472, 886, 908, 915, 960–962, 915). Philadelphia: W.B. Saunders.
3. Rose B.D. (1994). *Clinical physiology of acid-base and electrolyte disorders* (4th ed., pp. 447, 173–175, 781). New York: McGraw-Hill.
4. Adlaka A., Lobl J.K. (1992). The perplexing case of diurnal edema in a young woman. *Hospital Practice* 27(9), 213–216.
5. Porth C.J.M., Erickson M. (1992). Physiology of thirst and drinking: Implications for nursing practice. *Heart and Lung* 21, 273–284.
6. Rolls B., Phillips P.A. (1990). Aging and disturbances of thirst and fluid balance. *Nutrition Reviews* 48 (3), 137–143.
7. Phillips P.A., Johnson C.L., Gray L. (1993). Disturbed fluid and electrolyte homeostasis following dehydration in elderly people. *Age and Ageing* 22, S26–S33.
8. Toto K.H. (1994). Regulation of Plasma Osmolality. *Critical Care Clinics of North America* 6 (4), 661–674.
9. Robertson G.L. (1983). Thirst and vasopressin function in normal and disordered states of water balance. *Journal of Laboratory and Clinical Medicine* 101 (3), 351.
10. Pruit B.A. (1979). Other complications of burn injury. In Artz C.P., et al. (Eds.). *Burns* (p. 518). Philadelphia: W.B. Saunders.
11. Methaney N.M. (1996). *Fluid and electrolyte balance: Nursing considerations* (3rd ed., pp. 17, 52, 18). Philadelphia: J.B. Lippincott.
12. McManus M.L., Churchwell K.B., Strange K. (1995). Regulation of cell volume in health and disease. *New England Journal of Medicine* 333 (19),1260–1266.
13. Cogan M.G. (1991). *Fluid and electrolytes* (pp. 43, 117–118, 100–111, 112–123, 126, 129–130, 148, 242–251). Norwalk, CT: Appleton & Lange.
14. Katz M.A. (1975). Hyperglycemic-induced hypernatremia—Calculations of expected serum sodium depression. *New England Journal of Medicine* 293, 843.

15. Oh M.S., Carroll H.J. (1992). Disorders of sodium metabolism: Hypernatremia and hyponatremia. *Critical Care Medicine* 20, 94–103.
16. Sterns R.H. (1994). Treating hyponatremia. *Southern Medical Journal* 87 (12), 1283–87.
17. Oh M.S., Kim H., Carroll H.J. (1995). Recommendations for treatment of symptomatic hyponatremia. *Nephron* 70, 143–150.
18. Casteel H.B., Fiedorek S.C. (1990). Oral rehydration therapy. *Pediatric Clinics of North America* 37, 295–311.
19. Behrman R.E., Kliegman R.M., Arvin A.M. (1996). *Nelson Textbook of Pediatrics* (15th ed., pp. 210–214). Philadelphia: W.B Saunders.
20. Meyers A. (1995). Modern management of acute diarrhea and dehydration in children. *American Family Physician* 51 (5), 1103–1015.
21. Weisman Z. (1986). Cola drinks and rehydration in acute diarrhea [letter]. *New England Journal of Medicine* 315, 768.
22. Illowsky B.P., Kirch D.G. (1988). Polydipsia and hyponatremia in psychiatric patients. *American Journal of Psychiatry* 145 (6), 675–683.
23. Vieweg W.V.R. (1994) Treatment strategies for polydipsia-hyponatremia syndrome. *Journal of Clinical Psychiatry* 55 (4), 154–159
24. Batchell J. (1994). Syndrome of inappropriate antidiuretic hormone. *Critical Care Clinics of North America* 69 (4), 687–691.
25. Robertson G.L. (1995). Diabetes insipidus. *Endocrinology and Metabolic Clinics of North America* 24 (3), 549–571.
26. Bell T.N. (1994). Diabetes insipidus. *Critical Care Clinics of North America* 6 (4), 675–685.
27. Holzman E.J., Ausiello D.A. (1994). Nephrogenic diabetes insipidus: Causes revealed. *Hospital Practice* 29(3), 89–104.
29. Knockel J.F. (1987). Etiology and management of potassium deficiency. *Hospital Practice* 22 (1), 153.
28. Bräxmeyer D.L., Keyes J.L. (1996). The pathophysiology of potassium balance. *Critical Care Nurse* 16 (5), 59–71.
30. Tannen R.L. (1996). Potassium disorders. In Kokko J., Tannen R.L. *Fluids and electrolytes* (3rd ed., pp. 116–118). Philadelphia: W.B. Saunders.
31. Williams M.E., Rosa R.M. (1988). Hyperkalemia: Disorders of internal and external potassium balance. *Journal of Intensive Care Medicine* 3, 52–64.
32. Knockel J.P. (1982). Neuromuscular manifestations of electrolyte disorders. *American Journal of Medicine* 72, 521.
33. Whang G., Whang G.G., Ryan M.P. (1992). Refractory potassium repletion: A consequence of magnesium deficiency. *Archives of Internal Medicine* 152, 40.
34. Clark B.A., Brown R.S. (1995). Potassium homeostasis and hyperkalemic syndromes. *Endocrinology and Metabolism Clinics of North America* 24 (3), 753–91.
35. Korbin S.M., Goldfarb S. (1990). Magnesium deficiency. *Seminars in Nephrology* 10 (6), 525–535.
36. Katzung B.G. (1995). *Basic and clinical pharmacology* (6th ed., p. 239). Norwalk, CT: Appleton & Lange.
37. Zaloga G.F. (1992). Hypocalcemia in critically ill patients. *Critical Care Medicine* 20 (2), 251–262.
38. Yucha C.B., Toto K.H. (1994). Calcium and phosphorous derangements. *Critical Care Clinics of North America* 6 (4), 747–765.
39. Reber R.M., Heath H. (1995). Hypocalcemic emergencies. *Medical Clinics of North America* 79 (1), 93–165.
40. Kuffler SW., Nichols JG., Martin AR. (1984). *From neuron to brain* (2nd ed., p. 153). Sunderland, MA: Sinauer.
41. Kaplan M. (1994). Hypercalcemia of malignancy. *Oncology Nursing Forum* 21 (6), 1039.
42. Agus L.S., Wasserstein A., Goldfarb S. (1982). Disorders of calcium and magnesium homeostasis. *American Journal of Medicine* 72, 473.
43. Bilezikian J.P. (1992). Management of acute hypercalcemia. *New England Journal of Medicine* 326 (18), 1196–1203.
44. Edelson G.W., Kleerekoper M. (1995). Hypercalcemic crisis. *Medical Clinics of North America* 79 (1), 79–92.
45. Dennis V.W. (1996). Phosphate disorders. In Kokko J., Tannen R.L. *Fluids and electrolytes* (3rd ed., pp. 359–382). Philadelphia: W.B. Saunders.
46. Hodgson S.F., Hurley D. (1993). Acquired hypophosphatemia. *Endocrinology and Metabolism Clinics of North America* 22 (2), 397–409.
47. Fass R., Do S., Hixson L.J. (1993). Fatal hyperphosphatemia following Fleet phospho-soda in patient with colonic ileus. *American Journal of Gastroenterology* 88 (6), 929.
48. Workman L. (1992). Magnesium and phosphorus: The neglected electrolytes. *ACCN Clinical Issues* 3 (3), 655–663.
49. Altura B.M., Altura B.T. (1995). Magnesium in cardiovascular biology. *Scientific American Science and Medicine* 2(3), 28–37.
50. Toto K., Yucha C.B. (1994). Magnesium: Homeostasis, imbalances, and therapeutic uses. *Critical Care Nursing Clinics of North America* 6 (4), 767–783.
51. Matz. R. (1993). Magnesium deficiencies and therapeutic uses. *Hospital Practice* 28(4), 79–92.

ADDITIONAL READINGS

Al-Ghamdi S.M.G., Cameron E.C., Sutton R.A.L. (1994). Magnesium deficiency: Pathophysiologic and clinical overview. *American Journal of Kidney Diseases* 24 (5), 737–752.

Arieff A.I. (1988). Osmotic failure: Physiology and strategies for treatment. *Hospital Practice* 23 (6), 173.

Ayus J.C., Arieff A.I. (1996). Abnormalities in water metabolism in the elderly. *Seminars in Nephrology* 16 (4), 277–288.

Berry P.L., Belsa C.W. (1990). Hyponatremia. *Pediatric Clinics of North America* 37, 351–363.

Blevins L.S., Wand G.S. (1992). Diabetes insipidus. *Critical Care Medicine* 20, 69–79.

Brem A.S. (1990). Disorders of potassium homeostasis. *Pediatric Clinics of North America* 37, 419–427.

Cannon-Babb M.L., Schwartz A.B. (1986). Drug-induced hyperkalemia. *Hospital Practice* 21 (9), 99.

Friday B.A., Reinhart R.A. (1991). Magnesium metabolism: A case report and literature review. *Critical Care Nurse* 11, 62–71.

Holtzman E.J., Ausiello D.A. (1994). Nephrogenic diabetes insipidus: Causes revealed. *Hospital Practice* (March 15) 89–104.

Khilnani P. (1992). Electrolyte abnormalities in critically ill children. *Critical Care Medicine* 20, 241–250.

Kuhn M.M. (1991). Colloids vs crystalloids. *Critical Care Nurse* 11, 37–51.

Levine M.M., Kleeman C.R. (1987). Hypercalcemia: Pathophysiology and treatment. *Hospital Practice* 22 (7), 93.

Oster J.R. (1994). Hyponatremia: Focus on therapy. *Southern Journal of Medicine* 87 (12), 1195–1202.

Robertson G.L., Harris A. (1989). Clinical use of vasopressin analogs. *Hospital Practice* 24 (10A), 114–139.

Schrier R.W., Briner V.A. (1990). The differential diagnosis of hypernatremia. *Hospital Practice* 25 (9A), 29–37.

Snyder J.D. (1982). From Pedialyte to Popsicles: A look at oral rehydration therapy in the United States. *American Journal of Clinical Nutrition* 35, 157.

Solomon L.R., Lye M. (1990). Hypernatremia in the elderly patient. *Gerontology* 36, 171–179.

Sterns R.H. (1994). Treating hypoglycemia: Why haste makes waste. *Southern Journal of Medicine* 87 (12), 1283–1287.

Streeten D.H.P. (1995). Idiopathic edema. *Endocrinology and Metabolism Clinics* 24 (3), 531–547.

Tannen R.L. (1996). Potassium disorders. In Kokko J.P., Tannen R.L. (Eds.). *Fluids and electrolytes* (3rd ed., pp. 111–171), Philadelphia: W.B. Saunders.

CHAPTER 27

Alterations in Acid-Base Balance

Normal body function depends on acid-base balance being regulated within a narrow physiologic range. The metabolic activities that take place in the body require the precise regulation of pH so that membrane excitability, enzyme systems, and chemical reactions can function in an optimal way. Many conditions, pathologic or otherwise, can alter body pH. This chapter has been organized into two sections: mechanisms of acid-base balance and alterations in acid-base balance.

Mechanisms of Acid-Base Balance

After you have completed this section of the chapter, you should be able to meet the following objectives:

- Characterize an *acid* and a *base*
- Cite the source of metabolic acids
- Describe the three forms of carbon dioxide transport and their contribution to acid-base balance
- Use the Henderson-Hasselbalch equation to calculate pH and compare compensatory mechanisms for regulating pH
- Describe the intracellular and extracellular mechanisms for buffering changes in body pH
- Compare the role of the kidneys and respiratory system in regulation of acid-base balance
- Explain how potassium and hydrogen ions and how bicarbonate and chloride ions interact in pH regulation

Normally, body acids and bases are regulated so that the pH of extracellular body fluids is maintained within a very narrow range of 7.35 to 7.45. This balance is maintained through mechanisms that generate, buffer, and eliminate acids and bases. This section focuses on acid-base chemistry, the production and regulation of metabolic acids and bicarbonate, and calculation of pH.

Acid-Base Chemistry

An *acid* is a molecule that can release a hydrogen (H^+) ion, and a *base* is a molecule that can accept or combine with a H^+ ion. When an acid (HA) is added to water, it dissociates reversibly to form H^+ and anions (*e.g.*, $HA \rightleftharpoons H^+ + A$ [A = anion]). The degree to which an acid dissociates and acts as a H^+ ion donor determines whether it is a strong or weak acid. Strong acids such as sulfuric acid dissociate completely; weak acids such as acetic acid dissociate only to a limited extent. The same is true of a base and its ability to dissociate and accept a H^+ ion. Most of the body's acids and bases are weak acids and bases; the most important are carbonic acid, which is a weak acid derived from carbon dioxide, and bicarbonate, which is a weak base.

The concentration of the H^+ ion in body fluids is low compared with other ions. For example, the sodium ion (Na^+) is present at a concentration approximately 1 million times that of the H^+ ion. Because of its low concentration in body fluids, the H^+ ion is commonly expressed in terms of pH. Specifically, pH represents the negative logarithm (p) of the H^+ ion concentration in equivalents per liter; a pH value of 7.0 implies a hydrogen ion concentration of 10^{-7} equivalents per liter (mEq/L). The pH is inversely related to the H^+ ion concentration; a low pH indicates a high concentration of H^+ ions and a high pH a low concentration of H^+ ions.

The dissociation constant (K) is used to describe the degree to which an acid or base dissociates. The symbol pK_a refers to the negative logarithm of the dissociation constant for an acid. The use of a negative logarithm for the dissociation constant allows pH to be expressed as a positive value. Each acid in an aqueous solution has a characteristic pK_a that varies slightly with temperature and pH. At normal body temperature, the pK_a for the bicarbonate buffer system of the extracellular fluid compartment is 6.1.

Metabolic Acid and Bicarbonate Production

Acids are continuously generated as byproducts of metabolic processes. Physiologically, these acids fall into two groups: the volatile acid carbonic acid (H_2CO_3) and all other nonvolatile or fixed acids.

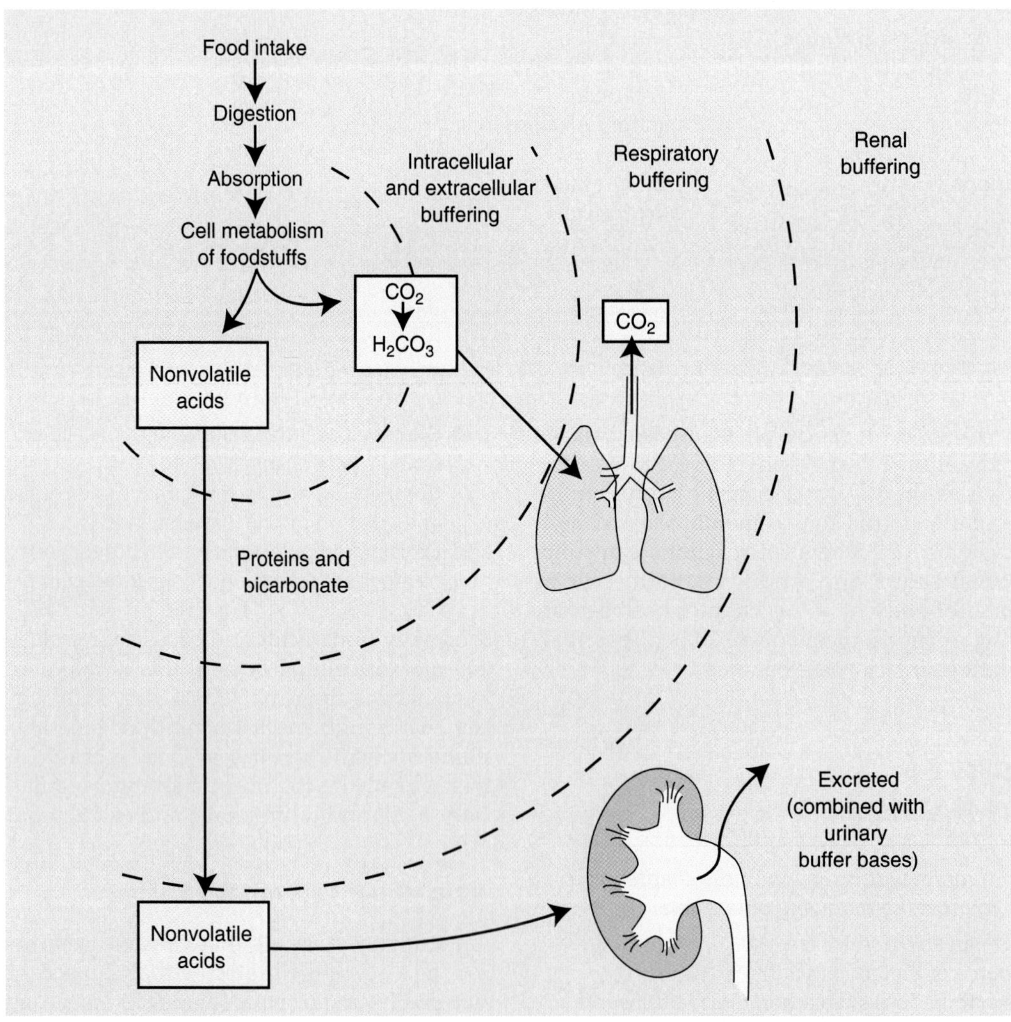

Figure 27–1 ■ ■ ■
The role of intracellular and extracellular buffer, respiratory, and renal mechanisms in maintaining normal blood pH. (Rhoades R.A., Tanner G.A. [1996]. *Medical physiology* [p. 468]. Boston: Little, Brown)

The difference between the two types of acids arises because H_2CO_3 is in equilibrium with the volatile carbon dioxide gas (CO_2), which leaves the body by way of the lungs (Fig. 27–1). The concentration of H_2CO_3 is therefore determined by the lungs and their respiratory capacity. The noncarbonic acids (*e.g.*, sulfuric, hydrochloric, phosphoric) are nonvolatile and are not eliminated by the lungs. Instead, they are buffered by body proteins or extracellular buffers such as bicarbonate and then excreted by the kidney.

Carbon Dioxide and Bicarbonate Production

Body metabolism results in the production of about 15,000 mmol of CO_2 each day.[1] Carbon dioxide is transported in three forms: attached to hemoglobin, as dissolved CO_2, and as bicarbonate (Fig. 27–2). Collectively, dissolved carbon dioxide and bicarbonate constitute about 77% of the carbon dioxide that is transported in the extracellular fluid; the remaining CO_2 travels attached to hemoglobin. Although CO_2 is not an acid, a small percentage of the gas combines with water in the bloodstream to form carbonic acid (H_2CO_3):

$$CO_2 + H_2O \rightleftharpoons H_2CO_3 \rightleftharpoons H^+ + HCO_3^-$$

The reaction between CO_2 and water is catalyzed by an enzyme called *carbonic anhydrase*, which is present in large quantities in red blood cells, renal tubular cells, and other tissues in the body. The rate of the reaction between CO_2 and water is increased about 5000 times by the presence of carbonic anhydrase. Were it not for this enzyme, the reaction would occur too slowly to be of any significance.

Because it is almost impossible to measure H_2CO_3, dissolved CO_2 measurements are commonly substituted when calculating pH. The H_2CO_3 content of the blood can be calculated by multiplying the partial pressure of CO_2 (PCO_2) by its solubility coefficient, which is 0.03. This means that the concentration of H_2CO_3 in venous blood, which normally has a PCO_2 of about 45 mm Hg, is 1.35 mEq/L (45 × 0.03 = 1.35).

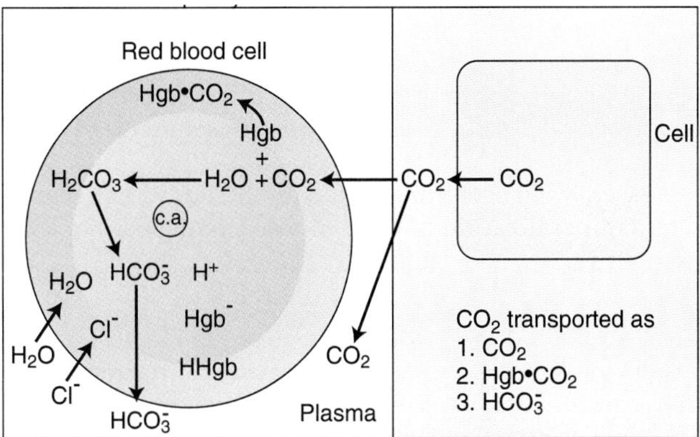

Figure 27–2 Mechanisms of carbon dioxide transport. (Adapted from Guyton A.C., Hall J.E. [1996]. *Textbook of medical physiology* [9th ed.]. Philadelphia: W.B. Saunders)

Production of Metabolic Acids

The metabolism of dietary proteins is the major source of strong inorganic acids—sulfuric acid, hydrochloric acid, and phosphoric acid.[2] Oxidation of the sulfur-containing amino acids (*e.g.*, methionine, cysteine, cystine) results in the production of sulfuric acid. Oxidation of arginine and lysine produce hydrochloric acid and oxidation of phosphorous-containing nucleic acids yield phosphoric acid. Incomplete oxidation of glucose results in the formation of lactic acid, and incomplete oxidation of fats results in the production of ketoacids. The major source of base is the metabolism of amino acids such as aspartate and glutamate and the metabolism of certain organic anions (*e.g.*, citrate, lactate, acetate). Acid production normally exceeds base production, with the net effect being the addition of approximately 1 mmol/kg body weight of nonvolatile acid to the body each day.[2] A vegetarian diet, which contains large amounts of organic anions, results in the net production of base.

Calculation of pH

The serum pH can be calculated using an equation called the *Henderson-Hasselbalch equation*. This equation uses the negative logarithm of the dissociation constant and the logarithm of the bicarbonate to carbon dioxide (HCO_3/CO_2) ratio to calculate pH.

$$pH = pK_a + \log \frac{[HCO_3]}{[CO_2]}$$

It is the ratio rather than the absolute values for bicarbonate and dissolved CO_2 that determines pH (*e.g.*, when the ratio is 20:1, pH = 7.4). Let us consider two examples to emphasize this point. The first situation uses normal serum values, and the second uses increased concentrations of bicarbonate and dissolved CO_2.

Situation 1

$$pH = 6.1 + \log \frac{24 \text{ mEq/L } HCO_3}{1.2 \text{ mEq/L } H_2CO_3}$$

Situation 2

$$pH = 6.1 + \log \frac{48 \text{ mEq/L } HCO_3}{2.4 \text{ mEq/L } H_2CO_3}$$

These examples demonstrate that pH remains relatively stable over a wide range of changes in bicarbonate and dissolved CO_2 concentrations, providing the two concentrations approach a ratio of 20 to 1 (Fig. 27–3). Plasma pH decreases when the ratio is less than 20 to 1, and it increases when the ratio is greater than 20 to 1.

The Henderson-Hasselbalch equation provides the mechanism for calculating pH, and it provides an insight into the physiologic control of acid-base balance. The bicarbonate part of the equation is controlled by the generation of metabolic acids and the availability of bicarbonate to buffer these acids. The H_2CO_3 part of the

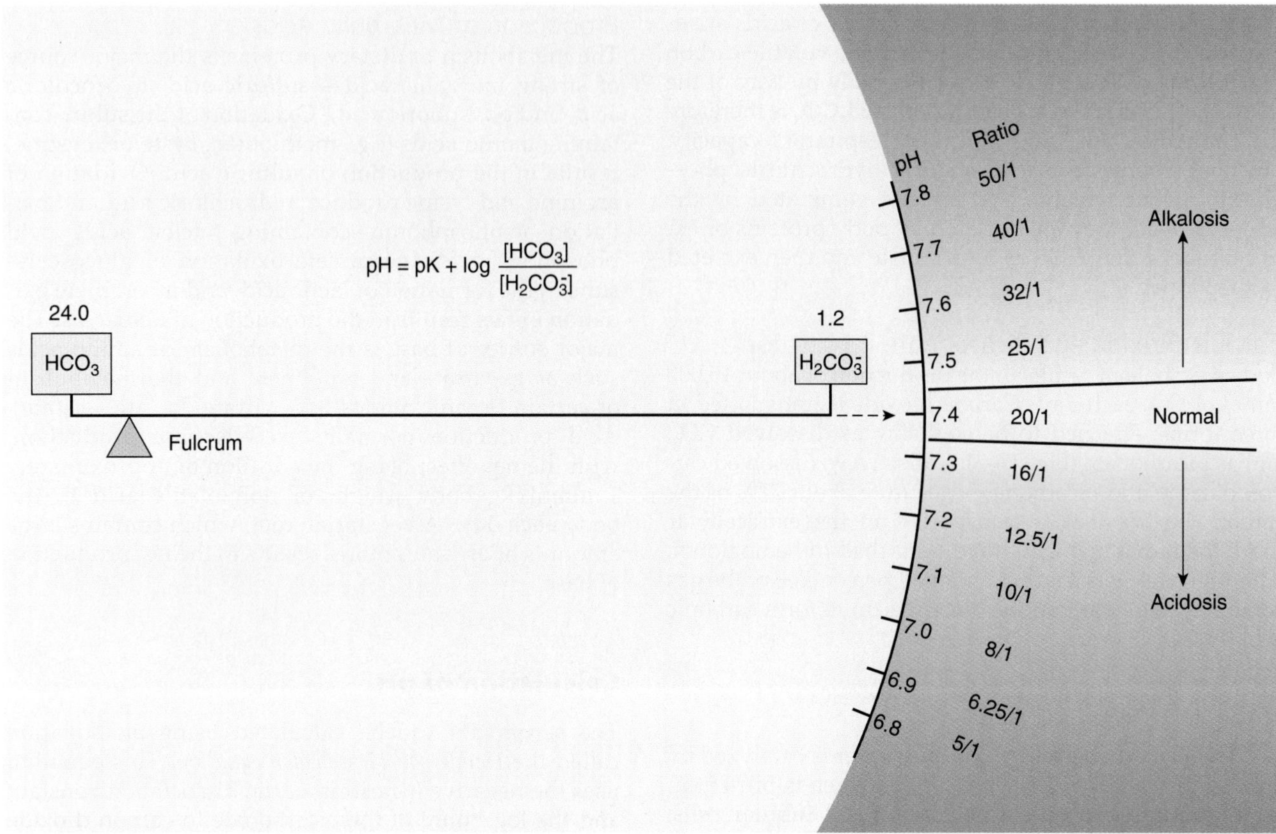

Figure 27–3
The Henderson-Hasselbalch equation expressed as a simple lever. (Adapted from Weisberg H.F. [1962]. *Water, electrolyte, and acid-base balance*. Baltimore: Williams & Wilkins)

equation is regulated by respiration. The equation could be represented as

$$pH = pK_a + \log \frac{[HCO_3] \text{ (controlled by metabolism)}}{[H_2CO_3] \text{ (controlled by respiration)}}$$

The kidney functions in the generation and recycling of bicarbonate and contributes to control of the metabolic part of the equation.

Regulation of pH

The pH of body fluids is regulated by intracellular and extracellular buffering systems that prevent large changes in the extracellular pH from occurring through respiratory mechanisms that eliminate carbon dioxide and by renal mechanisms that conserve bicarbonate and eliminate hydrogen ions. The pH is further influenced by the electrolyte composition of the intracellular and extracellular compartments.

Intracellular and Extracellular Buffer Systems

The moment-by-moment regulation of pH depends on intracellular and extracellular buffer systems. A buffer system consists of a weak acid and the base salt of that acid or of a weak base and its acid salt. In the process of preventing large changes in pH, the system trades a strong acid for a weak acid or a strong base for a weak base.

The two major buffer systems that protect the pH of body fluids are proteins and the bicarbonate buffer system. These buffer systems are immediately available to combine with excess acids or bases and prevent large changes in pH from occurring during the time it takes for respiratory and renal mechanisms to become effective. Bone also represents an important site for buffering of acids and bases. Although difficult to measure, it has been estimated that 40% of acute acid-base buffering occurs in bone.[1] The role of bone buffers is even higher in chronic acid-base disorders. One consequence of bone buffering is the release of calcium from bone and increased renal excretion of calcium. In addition to causing demineralization of bone, it also predisposes to kidney stones.

Protein Buffer Systems. Proteins are the largest buffer system in the body. Proteins are amphoteric, meaning that they can function as acids or bases. They contain many ionizable groups that can release or bind H^+. The protein buffers are largely located within cells, and H^+ ions and CO_2 diffuse across cell membranes for buffering by intracellular proteins. Albumin and plasma globulins are the major protein buffers in the vascular compartment.

Bicarbonate Buffer System. The bicarbonate buffer system uses carbonic acid as its weak acid and bicarbonate as its weak base. It substitutes the weak carbonic acid for a strong acid such as hydrochloric acid ($HCl + NaHCO_3 \rightleftharpoons H_2CO_3 + NaCl$) or the weak bicarbonate base for a strong base such as sodium hydroxide ($NaOH + H_2CO_3 \rightleftharpoons NaHCO_3 + H_2O$). The HCO_3/CO_2 buffer system is particularly efficient system because the buffer components can be readily added or removed from the body.[2,3] Metabolism provides an ample supply of CO_2, which can replace any H_2CO_3 that is lost when excess base is added, and CO_2 can be readily eliminated when excess acid is added. Likewise, the kidney can form new HCO_3 when excess acid is added, and it can excrete HCO_3 when excess base is added.

Plasma Potassium-Hydrogen Exchange. Potassium (K^+) and H^+ ions interact in important ways in the regulation of acid-base balance. Both ions are positively charged, and both ions move freely between the intracellular and extracellular compartments; when excess H^+ ions are present in the extracellular fluid, they move into the intracellular compartment for buffering. When this happens, another cation—in this case potassium—must leave the cell and move into the extracellular fluid. When extracellular potassium levels fall, potassium moves out of the cell and is replaced by hydrogen ions. Thus, alterations in potassium levels can affect acid-base balance, and changes in acid-base balance can influence potassium levels. Potassium shifts tend to be more pronounced in acidemia than alkalemia and are greater in metabolic acidosis than respiratory acidosis.[3,4] Metabolic acidosis caused by an accumulation of nonorganic acids (*e.g.*, hydrochloric acid that occurs in diarrhea, phosphoric acid that occurs in renal failure) produces a greater increase in potassium than does acidosis caused by an accumulation or organic acids (*e.g.*, lactic acid, ketoacids).

An important implication of the potassium and hydrogen transmembrane exchange is its effect on the resting membrane potential of neurons and other excitable tissue. In acidosis, increased levels of extracellular potassium cause the resting membrane potential to become more negative or hyperpolarized such that a greater stimulus is needed for excitation. In alkalosis, a decrease in extracellular potassium cause the resting membrane potential to become less negative so that neurons become more excitable. Changes in neural excitability are further influenced by alterations in ionized calcium (see Chapter 26). In acidosis, the ionized portion of the extracellular calcium is increased, making neurons less excitable, and in alkalosis, the amount of ionized calcium is reduced, making neurons more excitable.

Respiratory Control Mechanisms

The respiratory system provides for the elimination of CO_2 into the air and plays a major role in acid-base regulation. An elevated PCO_2 is a powerful stimulus for ventilation. CO_2 readily crosses the blood-brain barrier and in the process reacts with water to form carbonic acid, which dissociates into H^+ and HCO_3^- ions. It is the H^+ ion that stimulates the respiratory center, causing an increase or decrease in ventilation. The respiratory control of pH is rapid, occurring within minutes, and is maximal within 12 to 24 hours.[1] Although the respiratory response is rapid, it does not completely return the pH to normal. Although CO_2 readily crosses the blood-brain barrier, there is a lag for entry of the HCO_3^- ion. Thus, blood pH and bicarbonate levels drop more rapidly than cerebrospinal fluid (CSF) levels. In metabolic acidosis, for example, there is often a 1- to 3-hour delay in maximal respiratory response.[2] Likewise, when metabolic acid-base disorders are corrected rapidly, the respiratory response may persist because of a delay in CSF adjustments.

In severe ketoacidosis and other forms of metabolic acidosis, the peripheral arterial chemoreceptors in the aortic and carotid bodies, rather than the medullary chemoreceptors in the brain, provide the major stimulus for ventilation. In this case, rapid correction of acidosis by administration of sodium bicarbonate may decrease the respiratory stimulus for ventilation. Because of the delay in HCO_3^- ion entry into the CSF, there may be a drop in the pH of the CSF that occurs simultaneously with a rise in blood pH.

Renal Control Mechanisms

The kidneys regulate acid-base balance by excreting an acidic or an alkaline urine. Excreting an acidic urine reduces the amount of acid in the extracellular fluid, and excreting an alkaline urine removes base from the extracellular fluid. The renal mechanisms for regulating acid-base balance cannot adjust the pH within minutes, as respiratory mechanisms can, but they keep on functioning for days until the pH has returned to normal or near-normal range.

Hydrogen Ion Elimination and Bicarbonate Conservation. The average diet contains acid-generating foods. The strong acids produced by metabolism of these foods combine with buffers, particularly bicarbonate. The kidney must then secrete the excess H^+ ions and restore the HCO_3^- ions. Bicarbonate is freely filtered in the glomerulus (about 4500 mEq/day).[3] Loss of even small amounts of bicarbonate impair the body's ability to buffer its daily load of metabolic acids.

Most of the H^+ ion secretion and retrieval of HCO_3^- takes place in the proximal tubule. The process begins with a coupled Na^+/H^+ transport system in which a H^+ ion is secreted into the tubular fluid and a Na^+ ion is reabsorbed into the tubular cell (Fig. 27–4). The secreted H^+ ion combines with a filtered HCO_3^- ion to yield CO_2 and H_2O. The water is eliminated in the urine, and the CO_2 diffuses into the tubular cell, where it combines with water, in a carbonic anhydrase-mediated reaction to form a HCO_3^- ion and H^+ ion. The HCO_3^- ion is reabsorbed into the blood along with the Na^+ ion; the newly generated H^+ ion is secreted into the tubular fluid to begin another cycle. Normally, only a few of the secreted

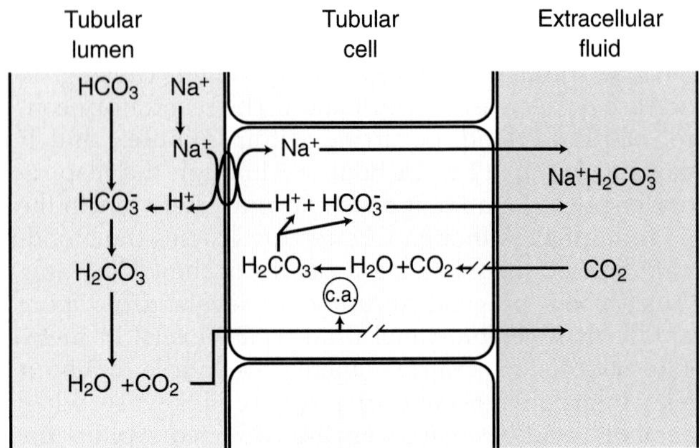

Figure 27–4
Hydrogen ion (H^+) secretion and bicarbonate ion (HCO_3^-) retrieval in a renal tubular cell. Carbon dioxide (CO_2) diffuses from the blood or urine filtrate into the tubular cell, where it combines with water in a carbonic anhydrase–catalyzed reaction that yields carbonic acid (H_2CO_3). The H_2CO_3 dissociates to form H^+ and HCO_3^-. The H^+ is secreted into the tubular fluid in exchange for Na^+. The $Na^+$and HCO_3^- enter the extracellular fluid.

H^+ ions remain in the tubular fluid, because the secretion of H^+ ions is roughly equivalent to the number of HCO_3^- ions that are filtered in the glomerulus.

Tubular Buffering Systems. Because an extremely acidic urine would be damaging to structures in the urinary tract, the pH of the urine is maintained within a range from 4.5 to 8.0. This limits the number of unbuffered hydrogen ions that can be excreted by the kidney. When the number of free H^+ ions secreted into the tubular fluid threatens to cause the pH of the urine to become too acidic, they must be carried in some other form. This is accomplished as H^+ ions combine with intratubular buffers before being excreted in the urine. There are two important intratubular buffer systems: the phosphate buffer system and the ammonia buffer system.

The phosphate buffer system uses HPO_4^{2-} and $H_2PO_4^-$ that are present in the tubular filtrate. The combination of H^+ with HPO_4^{2-} to form $H_2PO_4^-$ allows the kidneys to increase their secretion of H^+ ions (Fig. 27–5). Because they are poorly reabsorbed, the phosphates become more concentrated as they move through the tubules. This system works best when the renal tubular fluid contains a high concentration of H^+ ions.

Another important but more complex buffer system is the ammonia buffer system. Renal tubular cells are able to use the amino acid glutamine to synthesize ammonia (NH_3) and secrete it into the tubular fluid (Fig. 27–6). The H^+ ions then combine with the NH_3 to form an ammonium ion (NH_4^+). The NH_4^+ ions combine with chloride ions (Cl^-), which are present in the tubular fluid, to form ammonium chloride (NH_4Cl), which is then excreted in the urine. The ammonia buffer system allows for elimination of Cl^- and H^+ ions without effecting a change in urine pH. Although most of the negative ions in the tubular fluid are Cl^- ions, only a few Cl^- ions can be transported in direct combination with H^+, because the generation of hydrochloric acid would cause a sharp drop in urine pH. The ammonia buffer system requires large amounts of an enzyme that deaminates the amino acids that are used in ammonia synthesis; it takes 2 or 3 days for the tubular cells to increase enzyme synthesis and for this buffer system to become efficient.

The kidney also participates in gluconeogenesis (*i.e.*, generation of new glucose from sources such as amino acids). The deamination of the amino acid glutamate for use in buffering metabolic acids enables the kidney to increase its production of glucose. This can be particularly effective in situations of starvation and calorie deprivation, when excess ketoacids are formed as the body reverts to using body fats and proteins as fuel sources. In this case, the kidney uses glutamine for generating the ammonia needed for buffering excess metabolic acids and as a substrate for gluconeogenesis and maintenance of blood glucose levels.

Hydrogen and Potassium Ions Compete for Elimination in the Urine. Plasma potassium levels influence renal elimination of H^+ ions and vice versa. When plasma potassium levels fall, there is movement of K^+ ions from body cells into the plasma and a reciprocal movement of H^+ ions from the plasma into body cell. In the kidney, these movements lower the intracellular pH of tubular cells, causing an increase in H^+ secretion. Potassium depletion also stimulates ammonia synthesis by the kidney as a means of buffering the secreted H^+ ions. The result is increased reabsorption of the filtered bicarbonate and development of metabolic alkalosis. An elevation in plasma potassium has the opposite effect. Because of the K^+/H^+ ion exchange that occurs in the kidney, acidosis tends to increase H^+ ion elimination and decrease K^+ ion elimination, with a resultant increase in serum potassium levels. Alkalosis has the opposite effect; it tends to increase K^+ elimination, producing a decrease in serum potassium levels.

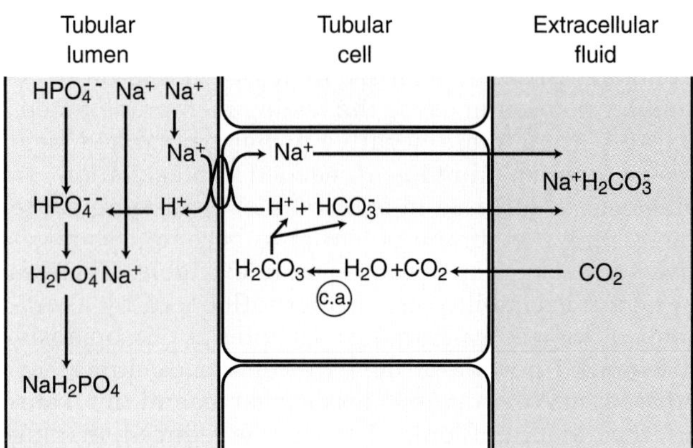

Figure 27–5
The renal phosphate buffer system The mono–hydrogen phosphate ion (HPO_4^{2-}) enters the renal tubular fluid in the glomerulus. A H^+ combines with the HPO_4^{2-} to form $H_2PO_4^-$ and is then excreted into the urine in combination with Na^+. The HCO_3^- moves into the extracellular fluid along with the Na^+ that was exchanged during secretion of the H^+.

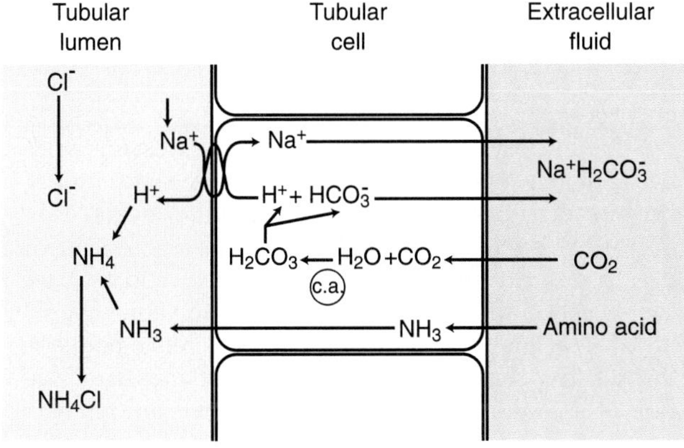

Figure 27–6
The ammonia buffer system in a renal tubular cell. The tubular cell synthesizes ammonia (NH_3) from amino acids. The NH_3 is secreted into the tubular fluid, where it combines with a H^+ to form an ammonium ion (NH_4^+). The ammonium ion combines with chloride for excretion in the urine. The HCO_3^- moves into the extracellular fluid along with the Na^+that was exchanged during secretion of the H^+.

Aldosterone also influences H^+ ion elimination by the kidney. It acts in the collecting duct to indirectly stimulate H^+ ion secretion, while increasing Na^+ ion reabsorption and K^+ secretion. Hyperaldosteronism tends to lead to a decrease in serum potassium levels and increased pH and alkalosis due to increased H^+ ion secretion. Hypoaldosteronism has the opposite effect. It leads to increased potassium levels, decreased H^+ ion secretion, and acidosis.

Influence of Sodium Chloride–Bicarbonate Exchange on pH. Body sodium levels can indirectly influence acid-base balance by way of the chloride–bicarbonate exchange system. Sodium reabsorption in the kidneys requires the reabsorption of an accompanying anion. The two major anions in the extracellular fluid are Cl^- and HCO_3^-.

One of the mechanisms that the kidneys use in regulating the pH of the extracellular fluids is to conserve or eliminate HCO_3^- ions; in the process, it is often necessary to shuffle anions. Chloride is the most abundant anion in the extracellular fluid and can substitute for bicarbonate when an anion shift is needed. As an example, serum HCO_3^- levels normally increase as hydrochloric acid (HCl) is secreted into the stomach after a heavy meal, causing what is called the *postprandial alkaline tide.* Later, as the Cl^- is reabsorbed in the small intestine, the pH returns to normal. *Hypochloremic alkalosis* refers to an increase in pH that is induced by a decrease in serum Cl^- levels. *Hyperchloremic acidosis* occurs when excess levels of Cl^- are present.

Laboratory Tests

Laboratory tests that are used in assessing acid-base balance include those for arterial blood gases and pH, carbon dioxide content and bicarbonate levels, base excess or deficit, and the anion gap. Although useful in determining whether acidosis or alkalosis is present, the pH of the blood as measured by a pH meter or electrode provides little information about the cause of an acid-base disorder.

Carbon Dioxide and Bicarbonate Levels

Arterial blood gases provide a means of assessing the respiratory component of acid-base balance. Arterial blood gases gases are used, because venous blood gases are highly variable, depending on metabolic demands of the various tissues that empty into the vein from where the sample is being drawn. The dissolved CO_2 levels can be determined from arterial blood gas measurements using the PCO_2 and the solubility coefficient for CO_2 (normal arterial PCO_2 is 38 to 42 mm Hg). Arterial blood gases also provide a measure of blood oxygen (PO_2) levels. This can be important in assessing respiratory acid-base disorders. Laboratory measurements of electrolytes include the CO_2 content and bicarbonate levels. However, the CO_2 content that is included in these measurements does not refer to arterial blood gases. Instead, it refers to the total CO_2 content of blood, including that contained in bicarbonate. The CO_2 content is determined by adding a strong acid to a plasma sample and measuring the amount of CO_2 generated. More than 70% of the CO_2 in the blood is in the form of bicarbonate. The serum bicarbonate concentration is then determined from the total CO_2 content of the blood. The normal range of values for venous bicarbonate concentration is 24 mEq/L to 33 mEq/L (24 mmol/L to 33 mmol/L).

Base Excess or Deficit

Base excess or deficit measures the level of all the buffer systems of the blood—hemoglobin, protein, phosphate, and bicarbonate. The base excess or deficit describes the amount of a fixed acid or base that must be added to a blood sample to achieve a pH of 7.4 (normal ± 3.0 mEq/L).[1] For practical purposes, base excess or deficit is a measurement of bicarbonate excess or deficit. A base excess indicates metabolic alkalosis, and a base deficit indicates metabolic acidosis.

Anion Gap

The anion gap describes the difference between the plasma concentration of the major measured cation (Na^+) and the sum of the measured anions (Cl^- and HCO_3^-). This difference represents the concentration of unmeasured anions, such as phosphates, sulfates, organic acids, and proteins (Fig. 27–7). Normally, the anion gap ranges between 8 and 12 mEq/L (a value of 16 mEq is normal if sodium and potassium concentrations are used in the calculation). The anion gap is increased in conditions such as lactic acidosis and ketoacidosis that result from elevated levels of metabolic acids. A low anion gap is found in conditions that produce a fall in unmeasured anions (primarily albumin) or rise in unmeasured cations. The latter can occur in hyperkalemia, hypercalcemia, hypermagnesemia, lithium

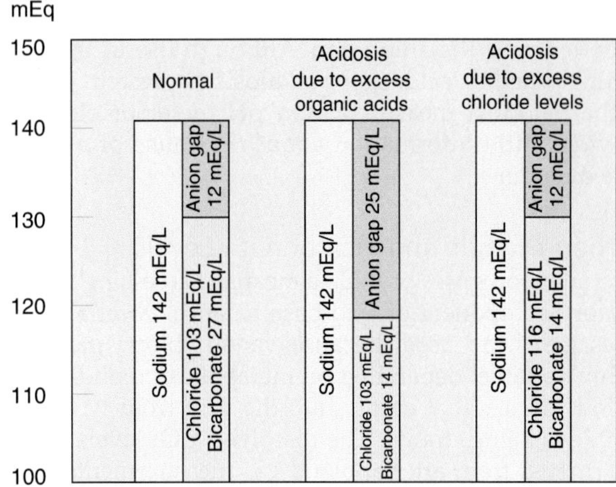

Figure 27–7
The anion gap in acidosis due to excess metabolic acids and excess serum chloride levels. Unmeasured anions such as phosphates, sulfates, and organic acids increase the anion gap because they replace bicarbonate. This assumes there is no change in sodium content.

intoxication, or multiple myeloma, in which an abnormal immunoglobulin is produced.[2]

The anion gap of urine can also be measured. It uses values for the measurable cations (Na^+ and K^+) and measurable anion (Cl^-) to provide an estimate of ammonium (NH_4^+) excretion. Because ammonium is a cation, the value of the anion gap becomes more negative as the ammonium level increases. In normal persons secreting 20 to 40 mmol of ammonium/L, the urine anion gap is close to zero. In metabolic acidosis, the amount of unmeasurable NH_4^+ should increase if renal excretion of H^+ is intact; as a result, the urine anion gap should become more negative.

In summary, normal body function depends on the precise regulation of acid-base balance. The pH of the extracellular fluid is normally maintained within the narrow physiologic range of 7.35 to 7.45. Metabolic processes produce volatile and nonvolatile metabolic acids that must be buffered and eliminated from the body. The volatile acid, H_2CO_3, is in equilibrium with dissolved CO_2, which is eliminated through the lungs. The nonvolatile metabolic acids, most of which are excreted by the kidneys, are derived mainly from protein metabolism and incomplete carbohydrate and fat metabolism. It is the ratio of the bicarbonate ion concentration to dissolved CO_2 (carbonic acid concentration) that determines body pH. When this ratio is 20:1, the pH is 7.4.

The ability of the body to maintain pH within the normal physiologic range depends on respiratory and renal mechanisms and on intracellular and extracellular buffers; the most important of these is the bicarbonate buffer system. The kidney aids in regulation of pH by eliminating H^+ ions or conserving HCO_3^- ions. In the process of eliminating H+ ions, it uses the phosphate and ammonia buffer systems. Body pH is also affected by the distribution of exchangeable cations (K^+ and H^+) and anions (Cl^- and HCO_3^-).

Laboratory tests that are used in assessing acid-base balance include arterial blood gas measurements, carbon dioxide content and bicarbonate levels, base excess or deficit, and the anion gap. The base excess or deficit describes the amount of a fixed acid or base that must be added to a blood sample to achieve a pH of 7.4. The anion gap describes the difference between the plasma concentration of the major measured cation (Na^+) and the sum of the measured anions (Cl^- and HCO_3^-). This difference represents the concentration of unmeasured anions, such as phosphates, sulfates, organic acids, and proteins, that are present.

Alterations in Acid-Base Balance

After you have completed this section of the chapter, you should be able to meet the following objectives:

- Differentiate the terms *acidemia, alkalemia, acidosis,* and *alkalosis*
- Describe a clinical situation involving an acid-base disorder in which primary and compensatory mechanisms might be active
- Define *metabolic acidosis, metabolic alkalosis, respiratory acidosis*, and *respiratory alkalosis*
- Explain the use of the plasma anion gap in differentiating types of metabolic acidosis
- List common causes of metabolic and respiratory acidosis and metabolic and respiratory alkalosis
- Contrast and compare the clinical manifestations and treatment of metabolic and respiratory acidosis and of metabolic and respiratory alkalosis

The terms *acidosis* and *alkalosis* describe the clinical conditions that arise as a result of changes in dissolved CO_2 and HCO_3^- concentration. An *alkali* represents a combination of one or more alkali metals such as sodium or potassium with a highly basic ion such as a hydroxyl ion (OH^-). Sodium bicarbonate ($NaHCO_3$) is the main alkali in the extracellular fluid. Although the definitions differ somewhat, the terms *alkali* and *base* are often used interchangeably. Hence, the term *alkalosis* has come to mean the opposite of acidosis.

Metabolic Versus Respiratory Acid-Base Disorders

There are two types of acid-base disorders: metabolic and respiratory (Fig. 27–8). Metabolic disorders produce an alteration in bicarbonate concentration and result from addition or loss of nonvolatile acid or alkali to or from the extracellular fluid. A decrease in pH due to a reduced bicarbonate is called *metabolic acidosis*, and an elevated pH due to increased bicarbonate levels is called *metabolic alkalosis*. Respiratory disorders involve a disorder in the PCO_2, reflecting an increase or decrease in alveolar ventilation. *Respiratory acidosis* is characterized by a decrease in pH, reflecting an increase in PCO_2. *Respiratory alkalosis* involves an increase in pH, resulting from an increase in alveolar ventilation and a decrease in PCO_2.

Primary Versus Compensatory Mechanisms

Acidosis and alkalosis typically involve a *primary* or initiating event and a *compensatory* state that results from homeostatic mechanisms that attempt to correct or prevent large changes in pH. For example, a person may have a primary metabolic acidosis as a result of overproduction of ketoacids and respiratory alkalosis because of a compensatory increase in ventilation (Fig. 27–9). Compensatory mechanisms adjust the pH toward a more normal level without correcting the underlying cause of the disorder. The respiratory mechanisms, which compensate by increasing or decreasing ventilation, are rapid but seldom able to return the pH to normal, because, as the pH returns toward normal, the respiratory stimulus is lost. The kidneys compensate by conserving HCO_3^- and H^+ ions. It normally takes longer to recruit renal compensatory mechanisms than it does respiratory compensatory mechanisms. Renal mechanisms are more efficient, however, because they continue to operate until the pH has returned to normal or a near-normal value.

Compensatory mechanisms provide a means to control pH when correction is impossible or cannot be immediately achieved. Often, compensatory mechanisms are interim measures that permit survival while the body attempts to correct the primary disorder. Compensation requires the use of mechanisms that are different from those that caused the primary disorder. In other words, the lungs cannot compensate for respiratory acidosis that is caused by lung disease, nor can the kidneys compensate for metabolic acidosis that occurs because of renal failure. The body can, however, use renal mechanisms to compensate for respiratory-induced changes in pH, and it can use respiratory mechanisms to compensate for metabolically induced changes in acid-base balance. Compensatory mechanisms often become more effective with time, and there are differences between the level of pH change that occurs with acute and chronic acid-base disorders. Figure 27–9 is a pH-bicarbonate diagram that can be used to determine the acute or chronic nature of an acid-base disorder and the compensation that has occurred. The diagram shows that a given increase in PCO_2 is associated with a lesser fall in pH in chronic compensated respiratory acidosis than in acute uncompensated respiratory acidosis.

Most of the manifestations of acid-base disorders fall into three categories: those associated with the primary disorder that caused the pH disturbance, those related to the altered pH, and those that occur because of the body's attempt to compensate for the altered pH.

Metabolic Acidosis

Metabolic acidosis involves a primary deficit in base bicarbonate along with a decrease in plasma pH. Metabolic acidosis can result from a decrease in bicarbonate with an increase in the anion gap or from replacement of bicarbonate with chloride ions in which the anion gap remains within normal range.[5] In metabolic acidosis, the body compensates for the decrease in pH by increasing the respiratory rate in an effort to decrease CO_2 and H_2CO_3 levels.

Metabolic acidosis	↓ pH	↓ Bicarbonate
Metabolic alkalosis	↑ pH	↑ Bicarbonate
Respiratory acidosis	↓ pH	↑ Carbon dioxide
Respiratory alkalosis	↑ pH	↓ Carbon dioxide

Figure 27–8
Acid-base disorders and direction of change in pH and serum bicarbonate or carbon dioxide (carbonic acid) levels.

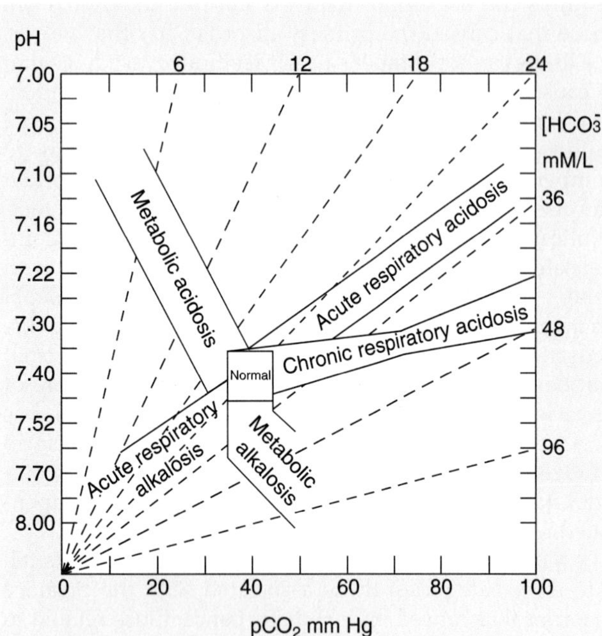

Figure 27–9
Acute and chronic acid-base disorders as determined by PCO_2, bicarbonate, and pH values. (Adapted from Masoro E.J., Siegel P.D. [1977]. *Acid-base regulation: Its physiology, pathophysiology and interpretation of blood gas analysis.* Philadelphia: W.B. Saunders)

Causes

Metabolic acidosis can be caused by one of four mechanisms: increased production of nonvolatile metabolic acids, decreased acid secretion by the kidney, excessive loss of bicarbonate, or an increase in chloride. The causes of metabolic acidosis are summarized in Table 27–1.

Metabolic acids increase when there is accumulation of lactic acid, overproduction of ketoacids, drug and chemical anion ingestion, or an inability of the kidneys to excrete metabolic acids or conserve bicarbonate. The anion gap is often useful in determining the cause of the metabolic acidosis (Chart 27–1). The presence of excess metabolic acids produces an increase in the anion gap as sodium bicarbonate is replaced by the sodium salt of the offending acid (*e.g.*, sodium lactate). When acidosis results from increased chloride levels (*e.g.*, hyperchloremic acidosis), the anion gap remains within normal levels.

Lactic Acidosis. Acute lactic acidosis is one of the most common types of metabolic acidosis. Lactic acidosis develops when there is excess production of lactic acid or diminished lactic acid removal from the blood. Lactic acid is produced by the anaerobic metabolism of glucose. Virtually all tissues can produce lactic acid under appropriate circumstances. Tissues such as red blood cells, intestine, and skeletal muscle do so under normal conditions. The liver and, to a lesser extent, the kidney normally remove lactic acid from the blood and use it for energy or convert it back to glucose.

Most cases of lactic acidosis are caused by inadequate oxygen delivery, as in shock or cardiac arrest.[6] These conditions increase lactic acid production, and they impair lactic acid clearance because of poor liver perfusion. Mortality is high for persons with lactic acidosis because of shock and tissue hypoxia. Excess lactate is also produced with vigorous exercise or grand mal seizures (*i.e.*, convulsions), during which there is a local disproportion between oxygen supply and demand of the contracting muscles.

Lactic acidosis is also associated with disorders in which tissue hypoxia does not appear to be present. It has been reported in patients with leukemia, lymphomas, and other cancers; those with poorly controlled diabetes; and patients with severe liver failure. Mechanisms causing lactic acidosis in these conditions are poorly understood. Some conditions such as neoplasms may produce local increases in tissue metabolism and lactate production or may interfere with blood flow delivery to noncancerous cells. Ethanol produces a slight elevation in lactic acid, but clinically significant lactic acidosis does not occur in alcohol intoxication unless other problems such as liver failure are present. Lactic acidosis may also complicate the severe acidosis that occurs in salicylate poisoning.

Lactic acidosis also occurs in genetic mitochondrial disorders that impair lactate metabolism.[2] One of these disorders, referred to by the acronym MELAS, involves mitochondrial encephalopathy (ME), lactic acidosis (LA), and strokelike episodes (S). Children with the disorder are normal for the first few years of life and then begin to display impaired motor and cognitive development. The mitochondrial defect also leads to short stature, seizure disorders, and multiple strokes. Lowering the serum lactate level of children with severe lactic acidosis may result in marked clinical improvement.

A unique form of lactic acidosis, called D-lactic acidosis, can occur in persons with intestinal disorders that involve the generation and absorption of D-lactic acid (L-lactic acid is the usual cause of lactic acidosis). D-lactic acidosis can occur in persons with jejunoileal bypass, small bowel resection, or short bowel syndrome, in which there is impaired reabsorption of carbohydrate in the small intestine.[1] In these cases, the unabsorbed carbohydrate is delivered to the colon, where it is converted to D-lactic acid by an overgrowth of gram-positive anaerobes. Persons with D-lactic acidosis experience episodic periods of metabolic acidosis often brought on by eating a meal high in carbohydrates. Manifestations include confusion, cerebellar ataxia, slurred speech, and loss of memory. They may complain of feeling (or appear) intoxicated. Treatment includes use of antimicrobial agents to decrease the number of D-lactic acid–producing microorganisms in the bowel along with a low-carbohydrate diet.

Ketoacidosis. Ketoacids (*i.e.*, acetoacetic and β-hydroxybutyric acid), produced in the liver from fatty acids, are the source of fuel for many body tissues. An overproduction of ketoacids occurs when carbohydrate stores are inadequate or when the body cannot use available carbohydrates as a fuel. Under these conditions, fatty acids are

TABLE 27-1
Metabolic Acidosis

Causes	Manifestations
Excess Metabolic Acids (increased Anion Gap)	**Blood pH, HCO_3^-, CO_2**
Excess production of metabolic acids	pH↓
Lactic acidosis	HCO_3↓ (primary)
Diabetic ketoacidosis	Pco_2↓ (compensatory)
Alcoholic ketoacidosis	**Gastrointestinal Function**
Fasting and starvation	Anorexia
Poisoning (*e.g.*, salicylate, methanol, ethylene glycol)	Nausea and vomiting
Impaired elimination of metabolic acids	Abdominal pain
Kidney failure or dysfunction	**Neural Function**
Excess Bicarbonate Loss (Normal Anion Gap)	Weakness
Loss of intestinal secretions	Lethargy
Diarrhea	General malaise
Intestinal suction	Confusion
Intestinal or biliary fistula	Stupor
Increased renal losses	Coma
Renal tubular acidosis	Depression of vital functions
Treatment with carbonic anhydrase inhibitors	**Cardiovascular Function**
Hyperaldosteronism	Peripheral vasodilation
Increased Chloride Levels (Normal Anion Gap)	Decreased heart rate
Excess reabsorption of chloride by the kidney	Cardiac dysrhythmias
Sodium chloride infusions	**Skin**
Treatment with ammonium chloride	Warm and flushed
Parenteral hyperalimentation	**Skeletal System**
	Bone disease (*e.g.*, chronic acidosis)
	Signs of Compensation
	Increased rate and depth of respiration (*i.e.*, Kussmaul breathing)
	Hyperkalemia
	Acid urine
	Increased ammonia in urine

mobilized from adipose tissue and delivered to the liver, where they are converted to ketones. Ketoacidosis develops when ketone production exceeds tissue use.

The most common cause of ketoacidosis is uncontrolled diabetes mellitus, in which an insulin deficiency leads to the release of fatty acids from adipose cells with subsequent production of excess ketoacids (see Chapter 36). Ketoacidosis may also develop as the result of fasting or food deprivation, during which the lack of carbohydrates produces a self-limited state of ketoacidosis. The self-limited nature of ketoacidosis results from low levels of insulin, which suppress the release of fatty acids from fat cells. A ketogenic diet is one that is low in carbohydrate and favors ketoacid production. Over the years, various ketogenic diets have been used for weight reduction; part of the success of these diets derives from symptoms such as anorexia that occur with metabolic acidosis that many of these diets cause.

Ketones are also formed during the oxidation of alcohol, a process that occurs in the liver. A condition called *alcoholic ketoacidosis* can develop in persons who engage in excess alcohol consumption.[7,8] It usually follows prolonged alcohol ingestion, particularly if accompanied by decreased food intake and vomiting that results in using fatty acids as an energy source. The ketoacids responsible for alcoholic ketoacidosis are in part formed as a result of alcohol metabolism. Extracellular fluid volume depletion caused by vomiting and decreased fluid intake, along with alcohol-induced inhibition of antidiuretic hormone (see Chapter 26) often contribute to the acidosis. Ketone formation may be further enhanced by the hypoglycemia that results from alcohol-induced inhibition of glucose synthesis (*i.e.*, gluconeogenesis) by the liver and impaired ketone elimination by the kidneys because of dehydration. Numerous other factors, such as elevations in cortisol, growth hormone, glucagon, and catecholamines,

CHART **27-1**
The Anion Gap in Differential Diagnosis of Metabolic Acidosis

Decreased Anion Gap (<8 mEq/L)

Hypoalbuminemia (decrease in unmeasured anions)
Multiple myeloma (increase in unmeasured cationic IgG paraproteins)
Increased unmeasured cations (hyperkalemia, hypercalcemia, hypermagnesemia, lithium intoxication)

Increased Anion Gap (>12 mEq/L)

Presence of unmeasured metabolic anion
- Diabetic ketoacidosis
- Alcoholic ketoacidosis
- Lactic acidosis
- Starvation
- Renal insufficiency

Presence of drug or chemical anion
- Salicylate poisoning
- Methanol poisoning
- Ethylene glycol poisoning

Normal Anion Gap (8–12 mEq/L)

Loss of bicarbonate
- Diarrhea
- Pancreatic fluid loss
- Ileostomy (unadapted)

Chloride retention
- Renal tubular acidosis
- Ileal loop bladder
- Parenteral nutrition (arginine and lysine)

mediate free fatty acid release and thereby contribute to the development of alcoholic ketoacidosis.

Salicylate Toxicity. Aspirin (acetylsalicylic acid) is rapidly converted to salicylic acid in the body. Salicylate overdose produces serious toxic effects, including death. A fatal overdose can occur with as little as 10 to 30 g in adults and 3 g in children.[1] The diagnosis can only be made with certainty by measurement of serum salicylate concentration. Although aspirin is the most common cause of salicylate toxicity, other salicylate preparations such as methyl salicylate, sodium salicylate, and salicylic acid may be involved.

Increasing doses of aspirin cause a progressively greater risk of toxicity because of the saturation of normal protective mechanisms. At therapeutic levels, much of salicylate is protein bound so that it remains in the vascular compartment; the drug is partially changed in the liver to salicyluric acid, which is less toxic and more rapidly excreted by the kidney than salicylate. With salicylate toxicity, these mechanisms become saturated, and renal elimination is decreased and more salicylate is able to reach the tissues and exert its toxic effects.

A variety of acid-base disturbances occur with salicylate toxicity. The salicylates cross the blood-brain barrier and directly stimulate the respiratory center, causing hyperventilation and respiratory alkalosis. The kidneys compensate by secreting increased amounts of bicarbonate, potassium, and sodium, thereby contributing to the development of metabolic acidosis. Salicylates also interfere with carbohydrate metabolism, which results in increased production of metabolic acids.

One of the treatments for salicylate toxicity is alkalinization of the plasma. Salicylic acid, which is a weak acid, exists in equilibrium with the alkaline salicylate anion. It is the salicylic acid that is toxic because of its ability to cross cell membranes and enter brain cells. The salicylate anion crosses membranes poorly and is less toxic. With alkalinization of the extracellular fluids, the ratio of salicylic acid to salicylate is greatly reduced. This allows cellular salicylic acid to move out of cells into the extracellular fluid along a concentration gradient. The renal elimination of salicylates follows a similar pattern when the urine is alkalinized.

Methanol and Ethylene Glycol Toxicity. Ingestion of methanol and ethylene glycol results in the production of metabolic acids and causes metabolic acidosis. Both produce an osmolar gap because of their small size and osmotic properties (see Chapter 26).

Methanol (wood alcohol) is a component of shellac, varnish, deicing solutions, sterno, and other commercial products. Methanol can be absorbed through the skin or gastrointestinal tract or inhaled through the lungs. A dose as small as 30 ml can be fatal.[5] In addition to metabolic acidosis, methanol produces severe optic nerve and central nervous system toxicity. Organ system damage occurs after a 24-hour period in which methanol is converted to formaldehyde and formic acid.

Ethylene glycol is a component of antifreeze and solvents. It tastes sweet and is intoxicating, factors that contribute to its abuse potential. A lethal dose is about 100 ml. Acidosis occurs as ethylene glycol is converted to oxalic and lactic acid. Manifestations of ethylene glycol toxicity occur in three stages: neurologic symptoms ranging from drunkenness to coma, which appear during the first 12 hours; cardiorespiratory disorders such as tachycardia and pulmonary edema that can follow; and flank pain and renal failure caused by plugging of the tubules with oxalate crystals (from excess oxalic acid production).

Methanol and ethylene glycol are metabolized by way of the enzyme alcohol dehydrogenase into toxic metabolites. This is the same enzyme that is used in the metabolism of ethanol. Because the enzyme has more than a 10 times greater affinity for ethanol, intravenous or oral ethanol is used as an antidote for methanol and ethylene glycol poisoning.[1] Extracellular volume expansion and hemodialysis are also used.

Decreased Renal Function. Renal disease is the most common cause of chronic metabolic acidosis. The *kidneys* normally conserve HCO_3^- and secrete H^+ ions into the urine as a means of regulating acid-base balance. In renal failure, there is loss of glomerular and tubular function, with retention of nitrogenous wastes and metabolic acids. In a condition called *renal tubular acidosis,* glomerular function is normal, but the tubular secretion of H^+ or reabsorption of HCO_3^- is abnormal. Renal tubular acidosis is discussed in Chapter 28.

Increased Bicarbonate Losses. Increased HCO_3^- losses occur with the loss of bicarbonate-rich body fluids or with impaired conservation of HCO_3^- by the kidney.

Intestinal secretions have a high HCO_3^- concentration. Consequently, excessive losses of HCO_3^- ions occur with severe diarrhea; small bowel, pancreatic, or biliary fistula drainage; ileostomy drainage; and intestinal suction. In diarrhea of microbial origin, HCO_3^- is secreted into the bowel to neutralize the metabolic acids produced by the microorganisms causing the diarrhea. Creation of an ileal bladder, which is done for conditions such as neurogenic bladder or surgical removal of the bladder because of cancer, involves the implantation of the ureters into a short, isolated loop of ileum that serves as a conduit for urine collection. With this procedure, contact time between the urine and ileal bladder is normally too short for significant anion exchange, and HCO_3^- is lost in the urine.[1]

Hyperchloremic Acidosis. Hyperchloremic acidosis occurs when Cl^- ion levels are increased. Because Cl^- and HCO_3^- are anions, the HCO_3^- ion concentration decreases when there is an increase in Cl^- ions. Hyperchloremic acidosis can occur as the result of abnormal absorption of chloride by the kidneys or as a result of treatment with chloride-containing medications (*i.e.,* sodium chloride, amino acid–chloride hyperalimentation solutions, and ammonium chloride). Ammonium chloride is broken down into NH_4^+ and Cl^-. The ammonium ion is converted to urea in the liver, leaving the chloride ion free to react with hydrogen to form hydrochloric acid. The administration of intravenous sodium chloride or parenteral hyperalimentation solutions that contain an amino acid–chloride combination can cause acidosis in a similar manner. With hyperchloremic acidosis, the anion gap is within the normal range, but the chloride levels are increased, and bicarbonate levels are decreased.

Manifestations

Metabolic acidosis is characterized by a decrease in pH (<7.35) because of an increase in extracellular H^+ ion concentration and a decrease in HCO_3^- levels (<24 mEq/L). Acidosis typically produces a compensatory increase in respiratory rate with a decrease in PCO_2 and H_2CO_3.

The manifestations of metabolic acidosis fall into three categories: signs and symptoms of the disorder causing the acidosis, alterations in function resulting from the decreased pH, and changes in body function related to recruitment of compensatory mechanisms (see Table 27–1). The signs and symptoms of metabolic acidosis usually begin to appear when the plasma HCO_3^- concentration falls to 20 mEq/L or less. Metabolic acidosis is seldom a primary disorder; it usually develops during the course of another disease. The manifestations of metabolic acidosis are frequently superimposed on the symptoms of the contributing health problem. With diabetic ketoacidosis, which is a common cause of metabolic acidosis, there is an increase in blood and urine glucose and a characteristic smell of ketones to the breath. In metabolic acidosis that accompanies renal failure, blood urea nitrogen levels are elevated, and tests of renal function yield abnormal results.

Changes in pH have a direct effect on body function that can produce signs and symptoms common to most types of metabolic acidosis, regardless of cause. A person with metabolic acidosis often complains of weakness, fatigue, general malaise, and a dull headache. The patient may also have anorexia, nausea, vomiting, and abdominal pain. Tissue turgor is impaired, and the skin is dry when fluid deficit accompanies acidosis. In persons with undiagnosed diabetes mellitus, the nausea, vomiting, and abdominal symptoms may be misinterpreted as being caused by gastrointestinal flu or other abdominal pathology, such as appendicitis. Neural activity becomes depressed as body pH declines. Acidosis directly depresses membrane excitability, and it decreases binding of calcium to plasma proteins so that more free calcium is available to decrease neural activity. As acidosis progresses, the level of consciousness declines, and stupor and coma develop. The skin is often warm and flushed because skin vessels become less responsive to the vasoconstriction input from the sympathetic nervous system.

When the pH falls to 7.0, cardiac contractility and cardiac output decreases, the heart becomes less responsive to the catecholamines (*i.e.,* epinephrine and norepinephrine), and dysrhythmias, including fatal ventricular dysrhythmias, can develop. A decrease in ventricular function may be particularly important in perpetuating of shock-induced lactic acidosis, and partial correction of the acidemia may be necessary before tissue perfusion can be restored.[1]

Metabolic acidosis is also accompanied by signs and symptoms related to the recruitment of compensatory mechanisms. In situations of acute metabolic acidosis, the respiratory system compensates for a decrease in pH by increasing ventilation to reduce PCO_2; this is accomplished through deep and rapid respirations. In diabetic ketoacidosis, this breathing pattern is referred to as *Kussmaul's breathing*. For descriptive purposes, it can be said that Kussmaul's breathing resembles the hyperpnea of exercise—the person breathes as though he or she had been running. There may be complaints of difficult breathing or dyspnea with exertion; with severe acidosis, dyspnea may be present even at rest. Respiratory compensation for acute acidosis tends to be somewhat greater than for chronic metabolic alkalosis.

When kidney function is normal, net acid excretion increases promptly in response to acidosis, and the urine becomes more acid. Net acid excretion may increase 5 to 10 times above normal. Most of the initial acid secretion into the urine is facilitated through use of the phosphate buffer system. Over several days, ammonia production by the kidney increases and becomes the most important mechanism for excreting excess H^+ ions.

Chronic acidemia, as in renal failure, can lead to a variety of skeletal problems, some of which result from the release of calcium and phosphate during bone buffering of excess H^+ ions. Of particular importance is impaired growth in children. In infants and children, acidemia may be associated with a variety of nonspecific symptoms such as anorexia, weight loss, muscle weakness, and listlessness.[1] Muscle weakness and listlessness may result from alterations in muscle metabolism.

Treatment

The treatment of metabolic acidosis focuses on correcting the condition that caused the disorder and restoring the fluids and electrolytes that have been lost from the body. The treatment of diabetic ketoacidosis is discussed in Chapter 36.

The use of supplemental sodium bicarbonate may be indicated in the treatment of some forms of normal anion gap acidosis. However, its use in treatment of increased anion gap types of metabolic acidosis is controversial, particularly in cases of lactic acidosis. In most patients with cardiac arrest, shock, or sepsis, impaired oxygen delivery is the primary cause of lactic acidosis. In these situations, the administration of large amounts of sodium bicarbonate does not improve oxygen delivery and may produce hypernatremia, hyperosmolality, and decreased oxygen release by hemoglobin because of a shift in the oxygen dissociation curve.[5]

Metabolic Alkalosis

Metabolic alkalosis involves a primary excess of base bicarbonate along with an increase plasma pH. It can be caused by a gain in HCO_3^- or loss of H^+ ions. The body compensates for the increase in pH by decreasing the respiratory rate as a means of increasing PCO_2 and H_2CO_3 levels.

Causes

Metabolic alkalosis occurs in conditions that produce ingestion or administration of excess bicarbonate or other alkali (*e.g.*, carbonate, citrate, acetate), increased gastrointestinal or renal loss of hydrogen ions, or volume contraction of the extracellular fluid compartment (Table 27–2).

Most of the body's serum bicarbonate is obtained from CO_2 that is produced during metabolic processes or from recycling or generation of new bicarbonate by the kidney. Usually, bicarbonate production and renal reabsorption are balanced in a manner that prevents alkalosis from occurring. It is only when new bicarbonate is added to the body or excessive amounts of bicarbonate are retained that metabolic alkalosis develops. Excessive alkali ingestion, as in the use of bicarbonate-containing antacids (*e.g.*, Alka-Seltzer) or sodium bicarbonate administration during cardiopulmonary resuscitation, can cause metabolic alkalosis. Other sources of alkali intake are acetate in hyperalimentation solutions, lactate in parenteral solutions such as Ringer's lactate, and citrate used in blood transfusions.

TABLE 27–2 Metabolic Alkalosis

Causes	Manifestations
Excess Gain of Bicarbonate or Alkali	**Blood ph, HCO_3^-, CO_2**
Ingestion or administration of sodium bicarbonate	pH↑
Administration of hyperalimentation solutions containing acetate	HCO_3↑ (primary)
Administration of parenteral solutions containing lactate	PCO_2↓ (compensatory)
Administration of citrate-containing blood transfusions	**Neural Function**
Excess Loss of Hydrogen Ions	Confusion
Vomiting	Hyperactive reflexes
Gastric suction	Tetany
Binge-purge syndrome	Convulsions
Potassium deficit	**Cardiovascular Function**
Diuretic therapy	Hypotension
Hyperaldosteronism	Dysrhythmias
Milk-alkali syndrome	**Respiratory Function**
Increased Bicarbonate Retention	Respiratory acidosis due to decreased respiratory rate
Loss of chloride with bicarbonate retention	**Signs of Compensation**
Volume Contraction	Decreased rate and depth of respiration
Loss of body fluids	Increased urine pH
Diuretic therapy	

Hydrogen, Chloride, and Potassium Ion Loss Associated With Bicarbonate Ion Retention. Hydrogen and chloride losses are associated with increased bicarbonate retention by the kidneys. Cl^- is the major anion in the extracellular fluid, and when it is lost from the body, HCO_3^- is conserved as a replacement anion. The secretion of H^+ ions and reabsorption of HCO_3^- ions are increased by hypercalcemia. A condition called the *milk-alkali syndrome* may develop in persons who consume excessive amounts of milk along with alkaline antacids.

Vomiting, removal of gastric secretion through use of nasogastric suction, and low potassium levels resulting from diuretic therapy are the most common causes of metabolic alkalosis in hospitalized patients. Gastric secretions contain high concentrations of hydrochloric acid and lesser concentrations of potassium chloride. As chloride is taken from the blood and secreted into the stomach, it is replaced by bicarbonate. Under normal conditions, each 1 mEq of H^+ ion that is secreted into the stomach generates 1 mEq of serum HCO_3^-.[10] Normally, the increase in serum HCO_3^- concentration is only transient, because the entry of acid into the duodenum stimulates an equal amount of pancreatic HCO_3^- secretion. Vomiting and gastric suction remove H^+ and Cl^- ions, thereby disrupting balance between acid secretion and HCO_3^- ion generation. The binge-purge syndrome, or self-induced vomiting, is often associated with metabolic alkalosis.[5] Metabolic alkalosis is also associated with low potassium levels caused by certain diuretics (*e.g.*, thiazides, furosemide) and excessive adrenocorticosteroid hormones (*e.g.*, hyperaldosteronism, Cushing's syndrome). In situations of low potassium levels, renal excretion of H^+ ions is increased as the kidneys focus on conserving potassium. The hormone aldosterone increases H^+ ion secretion as it increases Na^+ and HCO_3^- ion reabsorption. In hypoaldosteronism, the concurrent loss of K^+ in the urine serves to perpetuate the alkolosis.

Chronic respiratory acidosis produces a compensatory loss of H^+ and Cl^- ions in the urine along with HCO_3^- retention. When respiratory acidosis is corrected abruptly, as with mechanical ventilation, metabolic alkalosis may develop because of a rapid drop in PCO_2, but the HCO_3 ion concentration, which requires renal elimination, remains elevated.

Volume Contraction Leading to Sustained Metabolic Alkalosis. Sudden decreases in extracellular fluid volume, known as *volume contraction*, produce a decrease in the glomerular filtration rate, activation of the renin-angiotensin-aldosterone mechanism, and a resultant increase in sodium and bicarbonate reabsorption. In vomiting or gastric suction, the loss of hydrochloric acid initiates metabolic alkalosis, but it is the volume contraction from loss of Cl^- and K^+ ions that sustain the alkalosis. In this case, there is aldosterone-mediated increase in Na^+ reabsorption to maintain fluid volume. Na^+ reabsorption requires concomitant anion reabsorption. Because there is a Cl^- deficit, HCO_3^- is reabsorbed along with Na^+, leading to metabolic alkalosis. The loss of K^+ ions leads to a secretion of H^+ ions into the urine, contributing to the development of alkalosis. Volume contraction can also occur in the course of diuretic therapy. Diuretics that block chloride reabsorption in the kidney (i.e., loop and thiazide diuretics) produce a bicarbonate retention through volume contraction and loss of Cl^- ions.

Manifestations

Metabolic alkalosis is characterized by a plasma pH above 7.45, plasma HCO_3^- level above 29 mEq/L (29 mmol/L), and base excess above 3.0 mEq/L (3 mmol/L). Persons with metabolic alkalosis are often asymptomatic or have signs related to volume depletion or hypokalemia. The neurologic signs (e.g., hyperexcitability) occur less frequently with metabolic alkalosis than with other acid-base disorders, because the HCO_3^- ion enters the CSF more slowly than CO_2. When neurologic manifestations do occur, as in acute and severe metabolic alkalosis, they include mental confusion, hyperactive reflexes, tetany, and carpopedal spasm. Metabolic alkalosis also leads to a compensatory hypoventilation with development of various degrees of hypoxemia and respiratory acidosis. Significant morbidity occurs with severe metabolic alkalosis (pH above 7.55), including respiratory failure, dysrhythmias, seizures, and coma.

Treatment

The treatment of metabolic alkalosis is usually directed toward correcting the cause of the condition. A chloride deficit requires correction. Potassium chloride is usually the treatment of choice for metabolic alkalosis when there is an accompanying potassium deficit. When potassium chloride is used as a therapy, the chloride anion replaces the bicarbonate anion, and the administration of potassium corrects the potassium deficit and allows the kidneys to conserve H^+ ions while eliminating the K^+ ions. Fluid replacement with normal saline or one-half normal saline is often used in the treatment of patients with volume contraction alkalosis.

Respiratory Acidosis

Respiratory acidosis involves an increase in PCO_2 and H_2CO_3 along with a decrease in pH. Acute respiratory failure is associated with severe acidosis and only a small change in serum bicarbonate levels. Within 1 day, renal compensatory mechanisms become effective in generating more HCO_3^- ions, and the bicarbonate levels rise. In chronic respiratory acidosis, there is a compensatory increase in bicarbonate levels.

Causes

Respiratory acidosis occurs in conditions that impair alveolar ventilation and cause an accumulation of PCO_2 (Table 27–3). It can occur as an acute or chronic disorder. Because renal compensatory mechanisms take time to

TABLE 27-3

Causes and Manifestations of Respiratory Acidosis

Causes	Manifestations
Depression of Respiratory Center	**Blood pH, CO_2, HCO_3^-**
Drug overdose	pH↓
Head injury	P_{CO_2}↑ (primary)
	HCO_3↓ (compensatory)
Lung Disease	**Neural Function**
Bronchial asthma	Dilation of cerebral vessels and depression of neural function
Emphysema	Headache
Chronic bronchitis	Weakness
Pneumonia	Behavior changes
Pulmonary edema	Confusion
Respiratory distress syndrome	Depression
Airway Obstruction Disorders of Chest Wall and Respiratory Muscles	Paranoia
	Hallucinations
Paralysis respiratory muscles	Tremors
Chest injuries	Paralysis
Kyphoscoliosis	Stupor and coma
Extreme obesity	**Skin**
Treatment with paralytic drugs	Skin warm and flushed
Breathing Air With High CO_2 Content	**Signs of Compensation**
	Acid urine

exert their effects, blood pH can drop sharply in persons with acute respiratory acidosis.

Acute respiratory acidosis can be caused by impaired function of the respiratory center in the medulla (as in narcotic overdose), lung disease, chest injury, weakness of the respiratory muscles, or airway obstruction. Acute respiratory acidosis can also result from breathing air with a high CO_2 content. Almost all persons with acute respiratory acidosis are hypoxemic if they are breathing room air. In many cases, signs of hypoxemia develop before those of respiratory acidosis, because CO_2 diffuses across the alveolar capillary membrane 20 times more rapidly than oxygen.[1]

In many lung disorders, there are some areas of the lung that are more severely compromised in terms of gas-exchange function than others. In these circumstances, the respiratory acidosis or hypoxemia stimulates ventilation so that elimination of CO_2 from the relatively normal areas of the lung is increased, but oxygen uptake from the same area is limited by a hemoglobin saturation that approaches 100%. Chronic respiratory acidosis is a relatively common disturbance in patients with chronic obstructive lung disease (see Chapter 24). In these persons, the persistent elevation of PCO_2 stimulates renal H^+ ion secretion and HCO_3^- reabsorption. The effectiveness of these compensatory mechanisms can often return the pH to near-normal values as long as oxygen levels are maintained within a range that does not unduly suppress chemoreceptor control of respirations.

An acute episode of respiratory acidosis can develop in patients with chronic lung disease who have chronically elevated PCO_2 levels. This is sometimes called *carbon dioxide narcosis*. In these persons, the medullary respiratory center has become adapted to the elevated levels of CO_2 and no longer responds to increases in PCO_2. Instead, the oxygen content of their blood becomes the major stimulus for respiration. If oxygen is administered at a flow rate that is sufficient to suppress this stimulus, the rate and depth of respiration decrease, and the CO_2 content of the blood increases.

Manifestations

Respiratory acidosis is associated with a plasma pH below 7.35 and an arterial PCO_2 above 50 mm Hg. The signs and symptoms of respiratory acidosis depend on the rapidity of onset and on whether the condition is acute or chronic. Because respiratory acidosis is often accompanied by hypoxemia, the manifestations of respiratory acidosis are often intermixed with those of oxygen deficit. Carbon dioxide readily crosses the blood-brain barrier, exerting its effects by changing the pH of brain fluids. Elevated levels of CO_2 produce vasodilation of cerebral blood vessels. Headache, blurred vision, irritability, muscle twitching, and psychologic disturbances can occur with acute respiratory acidosis. If the condition is severe and prolonged, it can cause and increase in cerebral spinal fluid pressure and papilledema. Impaired consciousness, ranging from lethargy to coma, develops as the PCO_2 rises. Paralysis of extremities may occur, and there may be respiratory depression. Less severe forms of acidosis are often accompanied by warm and flushed skin, weakness, and tachycardia.

Treatment

The treatment of acute and chronic respiratory acidosis is directed toward improving ventilation. In severe cases, mechanical ventilation may be necessary. The treatment of respiratory acidosis due to respiratory failure is discussed in Chapter 24.

Respiratory Alkalosis

Respiratory alkalosis involves a decrease in PCO_2 and primary deficit in carbonic acid (H_2CO_3) along with an increase in pH. Because respiratory alkalosis can occur suddenly, a compensatory decrease in bicarbonate level may not occur before respiratory correction has been accomplished. The increase in pH is less in chronic compensated respiratory alkalosis, and the fall in bicarbonate concentration is greater.

Causes

Respiratory alkalosis is caused by hyperventilation or respiratory rate in excess of that needed to maintain normal PCO_2 levels (Table 27–4).

One of the most common causes of respiratory alkalosis is the hyperventilation syndrome, which is characterized by recurring episodes of overbreathing often associated with anxiety (see Chapter 24). Persons suffering from panic attacks frequently present in the emergency room with acute respiratory alkalosis. Other causes of hyperventilation are fever, oxygen deficiency, early salicylate toxicity, and encephalitis. Hypoxemia exerts its effect through the peripheral chemoreceptors. Salicylate toxicity and encephalitis produce hyperventilation by directly stimulating the medullary respiratory center. Hyperventilation can also occur during anesthesia or with use of mechanical ventilatory devices.

Manifestations

Respiratory alkalosis manifests with a decrease in PCO_2 and deficit in H_2CO_3. In respiratory alkalosis, the pH is above 7.45, arterial PCO_2 is below 35 mm Hg, and serum HCO_3^- levels are usually below 24 mEq/L (24 mmol/L).

The signs and symptoms of respiratory alkalosis are associated with hyperexcitability of the nervous system and a decrease in cerebral blood flow. Alkalosis increases protein binding of extracellular calcium. This reduces ionized calcium levels, causing an increase in neuromuscular excitability. A decrease in the CO_2 content of the blood causes constriction of cerebral blood vessels. CO_2 crosses the blood-brain barrier rather quickly; therefore, manifestations of acute respiratory alkalosis are often of sudden onset. The patient often experiences lightheadedness, dizziness, tingling, and numbness of the fingers and toes. These manifestations may be accompanied by sweating, palpitations, panic, air hunger, and dyspnea. Chvostek's and Trousseau's signs may be positive (see Chapter 26), and tetany and convulsions may occur. Because CO_2 provides the stimulus for short-term regulation of respiration, short periods of apnea may occur in persons with acute episodes of hyperventilation.

Treatment

The treatment of respiratory alkalosis focuses on measures to increase the PCO_2. Attention is directed toward correcting the disorder that caused the overbreathing. Rebreathing of small amounts of expired air (breathing into a paper bag) may prove useful in restoring PCO_2 levels in persons with anxiety-produced respiratory alkalosis.

TABLE 27-4

Causes and Manifestations of Respiratory Alkalosis

Causes	Manifestations
Excessive Ventilation	**Blood pH, CO_2, HCO_3^-**
Anxiety and psychogenic hyperventilation	pH ↑
Hypoxia and reflex stimulation of ventilation	PCO_2 ↓ (primary)
Lung disease that reflexly stimulates ventilation	HCO_3 ↓ (compensatory)
Stimulation respiratory center	**Neural Function**
Elevated blood ammonia level	Constriction of cerebral vessels and increased neuronal excitability
Salicylate Toxicity	Dizziness, panic, lightheadedness
Encephalitis	Tetany
Fever	Numbness and tingling of fingers and toes
Mechanical ventilation	Positive Chvostek's and Trousseau's signs
	Seizures
	Cardiovascular Function
	Cardiac dysrhythmias

In summary, acidosis describes a decrease in pH, and alkalosis describes an increase in pH. Acid-base disorders may be caused by alterations in the body's volatile acids (i.e., respiratory acidosis or respiratory alkalosis) or nonvolatile acids (i.e., metabolic acidosis or metabolic alkalosis).

Metabolic acidosis is defined as a decrease in bicarbonate, and metabolic alkalosis is defined as an increase in bicarbonate. Metabolic acidosis is caused by an excessive production and accumulation of metabolic acids or an excessive loss of bicarbonate. Metabolic alkalosis is caused by an increase in bicarbonate or a decrease in H^+ or Cl^- ion levels. Respiratory acidosis reflects an increase in CO_2 levels and is caused by conditions that produce hypoventilation. Respiratory alkalosis is caused by conditions that cause hyperventilation and a reduction in CO_2 levels.

The signs and symptoms of acidosis and alkalosis reflect alterations in body function associated with the disorder causing the acid-base disturbance, the effect of the pH change on body function, and the body's attempt to correct and maintain the pH within a normal physiologic range. In general, neuromuscular excitability is decreased in acidosis and increased in alkalosis.

REFERENCES

1. Rose B.D. (1994). *Clinical physiology of acid-base and electrolyte disorders* (3rd ed., pp. 288, 565, 485, 520–527, 540–557). New York: McGraw-Hill.
2. Koko J.P. (1996). Disorders of fluid balance, electrolyte, and acid-base balance. In Bennett J.C., Plum F. (Eds.). *Cecil textbook of medicine* (20th ed., pp. 525–551). Philadelphia: W.B. Saunders.
3. Rhoades R.A., Tanner G.A. (1996). *Medical physiology* (pp. 465–483). Boston: Little, Brown.
4. Methaney N.M. (1996). *Fluid and electrolyte considerations.* (3rd ed., p. 162). Philadelphia: J.B. Lippincott.
5. Toto R.D., Alpern R.J. (1996). Metabolic acid-base disorders. In Kokko J.P., Tannen R.L. (Eds.). *Fluids and electrolytes* (3rd ed., pp. 201–267). Philadelphia: W.B. Saunders.
6. Mizock B.A., Falk J.L. (1992). Lactic acidosis in critical care. *Critical Care Medicine* 20 (1), 80–93.
7. Duffens K., Marx J.A. (1987). Alcoholic ketoacidosis—A review. *Journal of Emergency Medicine* 5, 399.
8. Wren K.D., Slovis C.M., Minion G.E., Rutkowski R. (1991). The syndrome of alcoholic ketoacidosis. *American Journal of Medicine* 91, 119–128.
9. Arieff A.I. (1991). Indications for use of bicarbonate in patients with metabolic acidosis. *British Journal of Anaesthesiology* 65, 165–177.
10. Gallo J.H., Luke R.G. (1987). Pathophysiology of metabolic acidosis. *Hospital Practice* 22(10), 123–146.
11. Oster J.R. (1987). The binge-purge syndrome: A common albeit unappreciated cause of acid-base and fluid-electrolyte disturbances. *Southern Medical Journal* 80, 58.

ADDITIONAL READINGS

Atkinson D.E., Bourke E. (1987). Metabolic aspects of regulation of systemic pH. *American Journal of Physiology* 252, F947.

Brewer E.D. (1990). Disorders of acid-base balance. *Pediatric Clinics of North America* 37, 429–447.

Duffens K., Marx J.A. (1987). Alcoholic ketoacidosis. *Journal of Emergency Medicine* 5, 399.

Galla J.H., Luke R.G. (1987). Pathophysiology of metabolic alkalosis. *Hospital Practice* 22 (10), 123.

Haber R.J. (1991). A practical approach to acid-base disorders. *Western Journal of Medicine* 155, 146–151.

Hamm L.L., Simon E.E. (1987). Roles and mechanisms of urinary buffer excretion. *American Journal of Physiology* 253, F595–605.

Jenkins J.K., Best T.R., Nicks S.A. (1987). Milk-alkali syndrome with a serum calcium level of 22 mg/dl and J waves on the ECG. *Southern Medical Journal* 80, 1444.

Koch S.M., Taylor R.W. (1992). Chloride ion in intensive care medicine. *Critical Care Medicine* 20, 227–240.

Perez G.O., Oster J.R., Rogers A. (1987). Acid-base disturbances in gastrointestinal disease. *Digestive Disease and Science* 32, 1033–1043.

Salem M.M., Mujais S.K. (1992). Gaps in the anion gap. *Archives of Internal Medicine* 152, 1625–1629.

Williamson J.C. (1995). Acid-base disorders: Classification and management strategies. *American Family Physician* 52 (2), 585–590.

CHAPTER 28

Alterations in Renal Function

More than 20 million North Americans suffer from diseases of the kidneys and urinary tract; about 80,000 die each year because of these diseases. Kidney and urinary tract diseases are a major cause of work loss among men and women: about 10% of America's outpatient visits result from such problems.[1] The number of persons with chronic and disabling kidney disease has increased, in part because recent advances in dialysis and kidney transplantation methods are keeping persons alive who formerly would have died.

The kidneys are subject to many of the same types of disorders that affect other body structures, including developmental defects, infections, altered immune responses, and neoplasms. The kidneys filter blood from all parts of the body, and although many forms of kidney disease originate in the kidneys, referred to as primary kidney disorders, others develop secondary to disorders such as diabetes mellitus and systemic lupus erythematosus.

The discussion in this chapter focuses on congenital disorders of the kidneys, obstructive disorders, urinary tract infections, disorders of glomerular function, tubulointerstitial disorders, and neoplasms of the kidneys. Acute and chronic renal failure are discussed in Chapter 29, and the effects of other disease conditions, such as hypertension, shock, and diabetes mellitus, are discussed in other sections of the book.

Congenital Disorders of the Kidneys

After you have completed this section of the chapter, you should be able to meet the following objectives:

- Cite the effect of urinary obstruction in the fetus
- Define the terms *agenesis*, *dysgenesis*, and *hypoplasia* as they refer to the development of the kidney

- Describe the genetic basis for renal cystic disease, the pathology of the disorder, and its signs and symptoms

About 10% of persons are born with potentially significant malformations of the urinary system. Congenital defects of the kidneys can take several forms: a decrease in the amount of kidney tissue (*i.e.*, agenesis or hypoplasia) or as alterations in the form and position of the kidneys (*i.e.*, kidney displacement or horseshoe kidney). Developmental anomalies of the fetal urinary tract are among the most commonly recognized congenital anomalies. The incidence of lethal anomalies is between 0.3 and 0.7 per 1000 births.[2]

Agenesis and Hypoplasia

The kidneys begin to develop early in the 5th week of gestation and start to function about 3 weeks later. Formation of urine is thought to begin in the 9th to 12th week of gestation; by the 32nd week, the fetal production of urine reaches about 28 ml/hour.[3] Urine is the main constituent of amniotic fluid. The relative amount of amniotic fluid can provide information about the status of fetal renal function.

The term *agenesis* refers to the absence of an organ because of failure to develop. *Dysgenesis* is the failure to develop normally. Unilateral agenesis of the kidneys is relatively common, and many persons with this defect are unaware of it as long as the single kidney functions normally. Dysgenesis or agenesis of both kidneys is relatively rare; when either does occur, it often is accompanied by pulmonary hypoplasia. These defects are incompatible with life, and infants that have them are stillborn or die shortly after birth of pulmonary or renal complications. In renal *hypoplasia*, the kidneys do not develop to normal size. Like agenesis, hypoplasia more commonly affects only one kidney. When both kidneys are affected, there is progressive development of renal failure. In pregnancies that involve babies with nonfunctional kidneys or outflow obstruction of the kidneys, the amount of amniotic fluid is small—a condition called *oligohydramnios*. The cause of fetal death in these babies is thought to be cord compression caused by the oligohydramnios.[2]

Animal experiments have shown that ureteral or bladder outlet obstruction in the fetus causes renal dysgenesis or agenesis and pulmonary hypoplasia. Obstructions in fetal urinary outflow can be diagnosed with ultrasound imaging. In the normal fetus, the kidneys can be visualized as early as 12 weeks. The sensitivity with which fetal obstructive uropathy can be diagnosed is low before 20 weeks and high between 35 and 40 weeks. In utero surgery has been done to relieve outflow obstructions, with the hope of preventing pulmonary hypoplasia and renal dysgenesis. The procedure is experimental, and its success rate is still being determined.[4]

Alterations in Kidney Position and Form

The developmental process can result in kidneys that lie outside their normal position, usually just above the pelvic brim or within the pelvis. Because of the abnormal position, kinking of the ureters and obstruction of urine flow may occur.

One of the most common alterations in kidney form is *horseshoe kidney*. This abnormality occurs in about 1 of every 500 to 1000 persons.[5] In this disorder, the upper or lower poles of the two kidneys are fused, producing a horseshoe-shaped structure that is continuous along the midline of the body anterior to the great vessels. Most horseshoe kidneys are fused at the lower pole. The condition does not cause problems unless there is an associated defect in the renal pelvis or other urinary structures that obstructs urine flow.

Cystic Disease of the Kidney

A renal cyst is a fluid-filled sac or segment of a dilated nephron. The cysts may be single or multiple and can vary in size from microscopic to several centimeters in diameter. Although all types of cysts are not inherited, they are discussed here for convenience.

Renal cystic disease is thought to result from tubular obstructions that increase intratubular pressure or from changes in the basement membrane of the renal tubules that predispose to cystic dilatation. After the cyst begins to form, continued fluid accumulation contributes to its persistent growth. Renal cystic diseases probably exert their effects by compressing renal blood vessels, producing degeneration of functional renal tissue and obstructing tubular flow. There are essentially four types of renal cystic disease: polycystic kidney disease, medullary sponge kidney, acquired cystic disease, and simple kidney cysts (Fig. 28–1).

Simple and Acquired Renal Cysts

Simple cysts are the most common cystic disease of the kidney. These can be single or multiple, unilateral or bilateral, and usually are less than 1 cm in diameter, although they may grow larger. Most simple cysts do not produce signs or symptoms or compromise renal function. When symptomatic, they may cause flank pain, hematuria, infection, and hypertension related to ischemia-produced stimulation of the renin-angiotensin system. They are most common in older persons. Although the cysts are benign, they may be confused clinically with renal cell carcinoma.

Acquired renal cystic disease occurs in persons with end-stage renal failure who have undergone prolonged dialysis treatment. They probably form as a result of tubular obstruction. The cysts may bleed causing hematuria. Tumors, usually adenomas but occasionally adenosarcomas, may develop in the walls of these cysts.

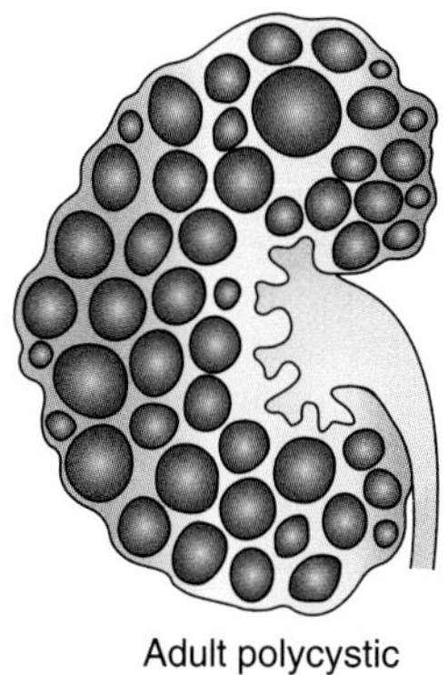

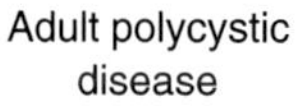

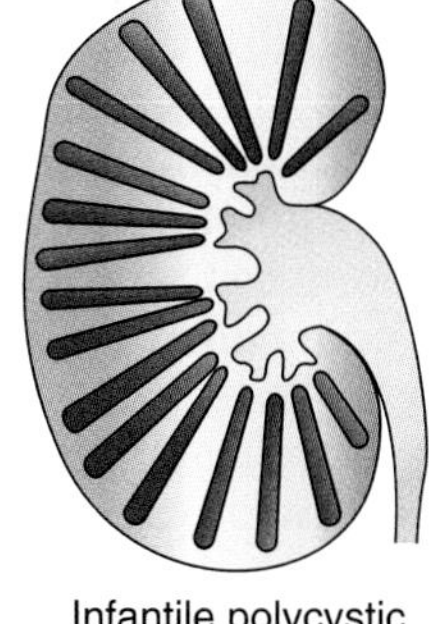

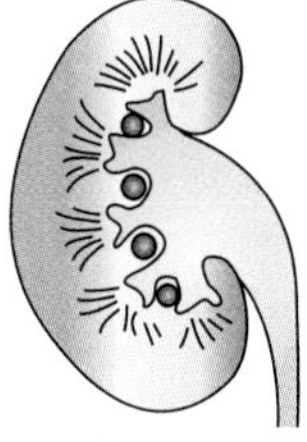

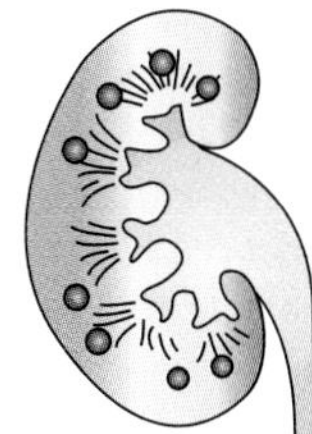

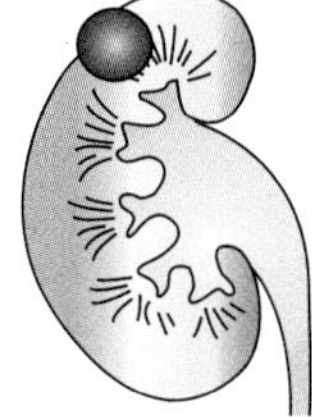

Figure 28–1
Cystic diseases of the kidney. (Courtesy of Dmitri Kartenikov, artist)

Medullary Cystic Disease

There are two major types of medullary cystic disease: medullary sponge kidney and nephronophthisis-medullary cystic disease complex.[6,7] Medullary sponge kidney is characterized by small (<5 mm in diameter), multiple cystic dilations of the collecting ducts of the medulla. The disorder does not cause progressive renal failure; it does, however, produce urinary stasis and predisposes to kidney infections and kidney stones. Symptoms may develop between 30 and 60 years of age when calcification develops in the dilated tubules.

Nephronophthisis-medullary cystic disease complex is a group of related diseases characterized by renal medullary cysts, sclerotic kidneys, and renal failure. About 85% of cases have a hereditary basis. Symptoms usually develop during childhood, and the disorder accounts for 10% to 20% of renal failure in children. Polyuria, polydipsia, and enuresis (bed wetting), which are early manifestations of the disorder, reflect impaired ability of the kidneys to concentrate urine.[7]

Polycystic Kidney Disease

The most common form of renal cystic disease is polycystic kidney disease, which is the result of a hereditary trait. It is one of the most common hereditary diseases in the United States, affecting more than 500,000 Americans.[8] There are two types of inherited polycystic disease: autosomal recessive and autosomal dominant.

Autosomal Recessive Polycystic Kidney Disease. Autosomal recessive polycystic kidney disease is relatively rare. Because the condition is present at birth, it formerly was called *infantile polycystic disease.* The condition is bilateral, and significant renal dysfunction usually is present, accompanied by variable degrees of liver fibrosis and portal hypertension. The disorder can be diagnosed by ultrasonography.

There is no known treatment for the disease, and death often occurs in infancy, often because the large kidneys compress the lungs. Some children may present with less severe kidney problems and more severe liver disease. The disorder is transmitted as a recessive trait, meaning that there is a one in four chance of the parents having another child with the disorder.

Autosomal Dominant Polycystic Kidney Disease. Autosomal dominant polycystic kidney disease, also called adult polycystic kidney disease, affects children and adults in the prime of life and accounts for 10% of persons who require treatment for end-stage renal disease. The disorder is transmitted as a dominant trait, which means that there is a 50% chance of children of an affected parent developing the disorder.

Three mutant genes have been implicated in the disease.[9] A gene called *ADPKD1,* located on chromosome 16, is responsible for most cases. There is a high degree of penetrance for the defect; persons who inherit the gene are likely to develop the disorder. There is considerable variability in gene expression, and many affected persons do not develop clinical symptoms, or if they do, the symptoms occur late in life. A second gene, the *ADPKD2* gene, which is located on chromosome 4, is responsible for a milder form of the disease. Evidence points to a third gene, *ADPKD3,* that also is responsible for the disease.

The pathogenesis of adult polycystic kidney disease is not fully understood. There is tubular dilatation caused by either obstruction or weakening of the tubule structure. Glomerular filtrate collects in the cyst while it is still part of the tubular lumen, or it is secreted into the cyst after it has separated from the tubule. As the fluid accumulates, the cysts gradually increase in size, some of which become as large as 5 cm in diameter. The kidneys of persons with polycystic kidney disease eventually become enlarged because of the presence of multiple cysts (Fig. 28–2). Cysts may also be found in the liver and, less commonly, the pancreas and spleen. Also, there may be a weakness in the walls of the cerebral arteries that

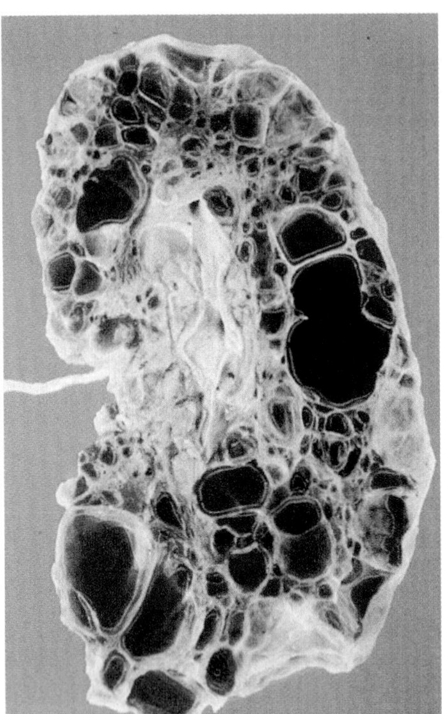

Figure 28–2
Adult polycystic disease. The kidney is enlarged, and the parenchyma is almost entirely replaced by cysts of varying size.

could lead to aneurysm formation. Subarachnoid hemorrhage occurs in about 10% to 15% of persons with polycystic kidney disease.

The manifestations of polycystic kidney disease include pain from the enlarging cysts that may reach debilitating levels, episodes of gross hematuria from bleeding into a cyst, infected cysts from ascending urinary tract infection, and hypertension resulting from compression of intrarenal blood vessels with activation of the renin-angiotensin mechanism. Persons with polycystic kidney disease are also at risk for development of renal cell carcinoma. The progress of the disease is slow, and end-stage renal failure is uncommon before age 40.

The diagnosis of autosomal polycystic kidney disease can be made by radiologic studies, such as excretory urography, and by ultrasonography or computed tomography (CT). Ultrasonography and CT have largely replaced excretory urography because they are better able to detect small cysts. Ultrasonography is particularly useful as a screening test for the disease. It is recommended that first-degree relatives of affected persons be screened for polycystic disease if they are at least 20 years old. The sensitivity of ultrasonography in this age group is about 95%; before that age, false-negative results may occur because the cysts are too small to detect.[3] Persons with a positive family history and no radiologically evident cysts can be further evaluated through gene-linkage analysis.[9] Two related persons who are affected must be included to establish the presence of the defective gene with 99% certainty. It is also possible to diagnosis polycystic kidney disease prenatally using DNA obtained from amniocentesis or chorionic villus sampling.

The treatment of polycystic kidney disease is largely supportive. Control of hypertension and prevention of ascending urinary tract infections are important. The cysts may be surgically removed if the patient has refractory pain.[5] Dialysis and kidney transplantation are reserved for those who progress to end-stage renal disease.

In summary, about 10% of infants are born with potentially significant malformations of the urinary system. These abnormalities can range from bilateral renal agenesis, which is incompatible with life, to hypogenesis of one kidney, which usually causes no problems unless the function of the single kidney is impaired. The developmental process can result in kidneys that lie outside their normal position. Because of the abnormal position, kinking of the ureters and obstruction of urine flow can occur.

Renal cystic disease is a condition in which there is dilatation of tubular structures to form a cyst. Cysts may be single or multiple. Polycystic kidney disease is an inherited form of renal cystic disease; it can be inherited as an autosomal recessive or an autosomal dominant trait. Autosomal recessive polycystic kidney disease is rare and usually presents as severe renal dysfunction during infancy. Autosomal dominant polycystic disease usually does not become symptomatic until later in life, often after age 40.

Obstructive Disorders

After you have completed this section of the chapter, you should be able to meet the following objectives:

- Describe the effects of urinary tract obstruction on renal structure and function
- Cite three theories that are used to explain the formation of kidney stones
- Explain the mechanisms of pain and infection that occur with kidney stones
- Describe methods used in diagnosis and treatment of kidney stones

Urinary obstruction can occur in persons of any age and can involve any level of the urinary tract from the urethra to the renal pelvis (Fig. 28–3). The conditions that cause urinary tract obstruction include developmental defects, calculi (*i.e.,* stones), normal pregnancy, benign prostatic hyperplasia, scar tissue resulting from infection and inflammation, tumors, and neurologic disorders such as spinal cord injury and diabetic neuropathy. The causes of urinary tract obstructions are summarized in Table 28–1.

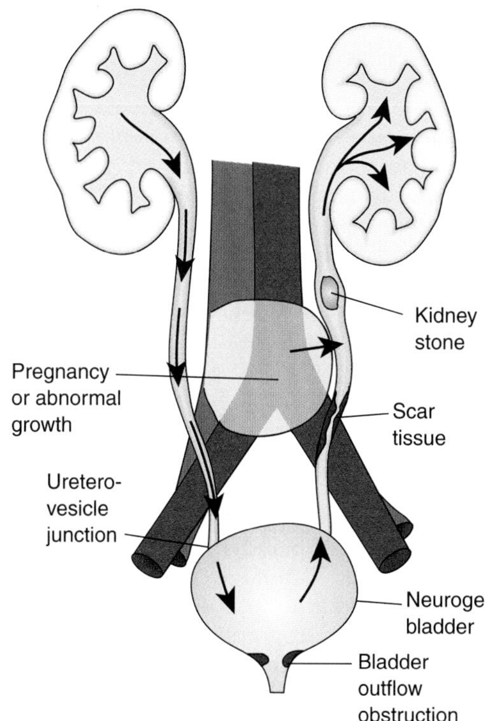

Figure 28–3
Locations and causes of urinary tract obstruction.

Mechanisms of Renal Damage

The destructive effects of urinary obstruction on kidney structures are determined by the degree of obstruction (*i.e.*, partial versus complete, unilateral versus bilateral) and the duration of obstruction. The two most damaging effects of urinary obstruction are stasis of urine, which predisposes to infection and stone formation, and development of a back pressure, which interferes with blood flow and destroys renal tissue.

A common complication of urinary tract obstruction is infection. Stagnation of urine predisposes to infection, which may spread throughout the urinary tract. When present, urinary calculi serve as foreign bodies and contribute to the infection. Once established, the infection is difficult to treat. It often is caused by urea-splitting organisms (*e.g.*, *Proteus*, staphylococci) that increase ammonia production and cause the urine to become alkaline. Calcium salts precipitate more readily in stagnant alkaline urine; urinary tract obstructions also predispose to stone formation.

In situations of marked or complete obstruction, a back pressure develops because of a combination of continued glomerular filtration and impedance to urinary flow. Prolonged or severe partial obstruction causes irreversible kidney damage. Depending on the degree of obstruction, pressure builds up, beginning at the site of obstruction and moving backward from the ureter or renal pelvis into the calices and collecting tubules. Typically, the most severe effects occur at the level of the papillae, because these structures are subjected to the greatest pressure. Damage to the nephrons and other functional components of the kidneys is caused by compression from increased intrapelvic pressure and ischemia from disturbances in blood flow. Experiments have shown recovery of renal function after release of complete obstruction of up to 4 weeks' duration.[10] Irreversible damage can, however, begin as early as 7 days.[10]

Dilatation of the ureters and renal pelvis occurs with prolonged urinary tract obstruction. When the obstruction is in the distal ureter, the increased pressure dilates the proximal ureter, a condition called *hydroureter* (Fig. 28–4). Hydroureter is also a complication of bladder outflow obstruction owing to prostatic hyperplasia (see Chapter 49). With increasing pressure, the ureteral wall becomes severely stretched and loses its ability to undergo peristaltic contractions. In extreme cases, the ureter may become so dilated that it resembles a loop of bowel. *Hydronephrosis* refers to urine-filled dilatation of the renal pelvis and calices. The degree of hydronephrosis depends on the duration, degree, and site of obstruction. Bilateral hydronephrosis occurs only when the obstruction is below the level of the ureters. If the obstruction occurs at the level of the ureters or above, hydronephrosis is unilateral. The kidney eventually is destroyed and appears as a thin-walled shell that is filled with fluid (Fig. 28–5).

Manifestations

The manifestations of urinary obstruction depend on the site of obstruction, the cause, and the rapidity with which the condition developed. Most commonly, the person has pain, signs and symptoms of urinary tract infection, and manifestations of renal dysfunction, such as an impaired ability to concentrate urine. Changes in urine output may be misleading, because output may be normal or even high in cases of partial obstruction.

TABLE **28-1**

Causes of Urinary Tract Obstruction

Level of Obstruction	Cause
Renal pelvis	Renal calculi Papillary necrosis
Ureter	Renal calculi Pregnancy Tumors that compress the ureter Ureteral stricture Congenital disorders of the ureterovesical junction and ureteropelvic junction strictures
Bladder and urethra	Bladder cancer Neurogenic bladder Bladder stones Prostatic hyperplasia or cancer Urethral strictures Congenital urethral defects

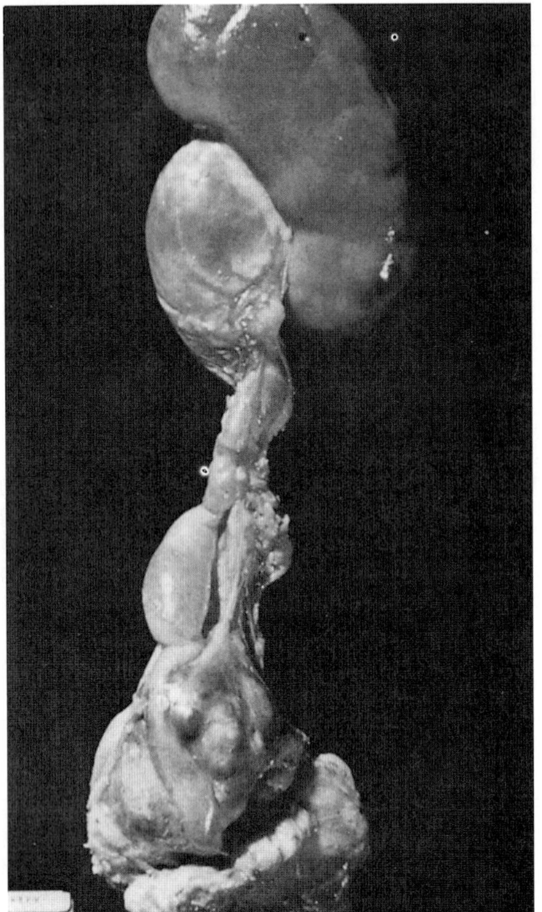

Figure 28–4
Hydroureter caused by ureteral obstruction in a woman with cancer of the uterus.

Pain, which often is the factor that causes a person to seek medical attention, is the result of distention of the bladder, collecting system, or renal capsule. Its severity is most closely related to the rate rather than the degree of distention. Pain most often occurs with acute obstruction, in which the distention of urinary structures is rapid. This contrasts with chronic obstruction, in which distention is gradual and may not cause pain. Instead, gradual obstruction may produce only vague abdominal or back discomfort. When pain occurs, it is related to the site of obstruction. Obstruction of the renal pelvis or upper ureter causes pain and tenderness over the flank area. With lower levels of obstruction, the pain may radiate to the testes in the male or the labia in the female. With partial obstruction, particularly of the ureteropelvic junction, pain may occur during periods of high fluid intake, when a high rate of urine flow causes an acute hydronephrosis. Because of its visceral innervation, ureteral obstruction may produce reflex impairment of gastrointestinal tract peristalsis and motility with abdominal distention and, in severe cases, paralytic ileus.

Hypertension is an occasional complication of urinary tract obstruction. It is more common in cases of unilateral obstruction in which renin secretion is enhanced, probably secondary to impaired renal blood flow. In these circumstances, removal of the obstruction often leads to a reduction in blood pressure. When hypertension accompanies bilateral obstruction, renin levels usually are normal, and the elevated blood pressure probably is volume related. The relief of bilateral obstruction leads to a loss of volume and a fall in blood pressure.[11] In some cases, relieving the obstruction does not correct the hypertension.

Diagnosis and Treatment

Early diagnosis of urinary tract obstruction is important because the condition usually is treatable and a delay in therapy may result in permanent damage to the kidneys. Diagnostic methods vary with the symptoms. For example, a distended bladder suggests prostatic hyperplasia in the male. Radiologic methods commonly are used. The opaque kidney stones often are visible on x-ray films. Excretory urography, CT, and renal scanning using a radiopharmaceutical agent such as gallium may be used. Ultrasonography has proved to be the single most useful noninvasive diagnostic modality for urinary obstruction. Other diagnostic methods, such as urinalysis, are used to determine the extent of renal involvement and the presence of infection.

Treatment of urinary obstruction depends on the cause. Urinary stone removal may be necessary, or surgical treatment of structural defects may be indicated.

Renal Calculi

The most common cause of urinary tract obstruction is urinary calculi. The term *nephrolithiasis* refers to kidney stones. Although stones can form in any part of the urinary tract, most develop in the kidneys. About 1 million North Americans are hospitalized each year with kidney

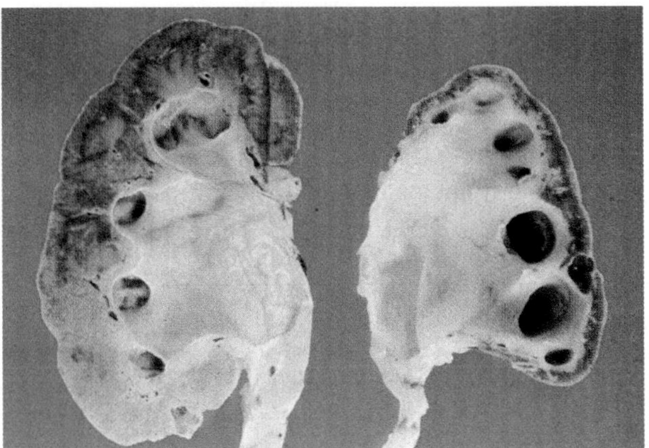

Figure 28–5
Hydronephrosis. Bilateral urinary tract obstruction has led to conspicuous dilatation of the ureters, pelves, and calyces. The kidney on the right shows severe cortical atrophy.

stones, and an equal number are treated for stones without hospitalization.

Kidney stones are crystalline structures made up of materials that the kidneys normally excrete in the urine. They require a nidus, or nucleus, to form and a urinary environment that supports continued precipitation of stone components to grow. It is thought that the urine normally contains substances that inhibit precipitation of stone components.[12]

Three major theories are used to explain stone formation: the saturation theory, the inhibitor deficiency theory, and the matrix theory.[13] One or more of these theories may apply to stone formation in the same person. The saturation theory states that the risk of stone formation is increased when the urine is supersaturated with stone components (*e.g.*, calcium salts, uric acid, magnesium ammonium phosphate, cystine). The inhibitor theory suggests that persons who have a deficiency of endogenous compounds that inhibit stone formation in their urine are at increased risk for stone formation. One such compound has been identified and called *nephrocalcin*.[13] The matrix theory proposes that organic materials, such as mucopolysaccharides derived from the epithelial cells that line the tubules, act as a nidus for stone formation. This theory is based on the observation that organic matrix materials can be found in all layers of kidney stones. It is not known whether the matrix material contributes to the initiation of stone formation or the material is merely entrapped as the stone forms.

Types of Stones

There are four basic types of kidney stones: calcium stones (*i.e.*, oxalate or phosphate), magnesium ammonium phosphate stones, uric acid stones, and cystine stones. The causes and treatment measures for each of these types of renal stones are described in Table 28–2.

Most kidney stones (70% to 80%) are calcium stones—calcium oxalate, calcium phosphate, or a combination of the two materials.[14] Calcium stones usually are associated with increased concentrations of calcium in the blood and urine. Excessive bone resorption caused by immobility, bone disease, hyperparathyroidism, and renal tubular acidosis are all contributing conditions. High oxalate concentrations in the blood and urine predispose to formation of calcium oxalate stones.

Magnesium ammonium phosphate stones, also called *struvite stones*, form only in alkaline urine and in the presence of bacteria that possess an enzyme called urease, which splits the urea in the urine to ammonia and carbon dioxide. The ammonia that is formed takes up a hydrogen ion to become an ammonium ion, increasing the pH of the urine so it becomes more alkaline. Because phosphate levels are increased in alkaline urine and because magnesium is always present in the urine, struvite stones form. These stones enlarge as the bacterial count grows, and they can increase in size until they fill an entire renal pelvis. Because of their shape, they are often called *staghorn stones*. Staghorn stones are almost always associated with urinary tract infections and a persistently alkaline urine.

Uric acid stones develop in conditions of gout and high concentrations of uric acid in the urine. Unlike radiopaque calcium stones, uric acid stones are not visible on x-ray films. Hyperuricosuria may also contribute to calcium stone formation by acting as a nucleus for calcium oxalate stone formation. Cystine stones are rare.

TABLE 28–2

Composition, Contributing Factors, and Treatment of Kidney Stones

Type of Stone	Contributing Factors	Treatment
Calcium (oxalate and phosphate)	Hypercalcemia and hypercalciuria Immobilization Thiazide diuretics Increased fluid intake Hyperparathyroidism Vitamin D intoxication Diffuse bone disease Milk-alkali syndrome Renal tubular acidosis	Treatment of underlying conditions
	Hyperoxaluria Intestinal bypass surgery	Dietary restriction of foods high in oxalate
Magnesium ammonium phosphate (struvite)	Urea-splitting urinary tract infections	Treatment of urinary tract infection Acidification of the urine Increased fluid intake
Uric acid (urate)	Formed in acid urine with pH of about 5.5 Gout High-purine diet	Increased fluid intake Allopurinol for hyperuricuria Alkalinization of urine
Cystine	Cystinuria (inherited disorder of amino acid metabolism)	Increased fluid intake Alkalinization of urine

They are seen in cystinuria, which results from a genetic defect in renal transport of cystine.

Manifestations

Renal colic is the term used to describe the colicky pain that accompanies urinary obstruction caused by kidney stones. The symptoms of renal colic are caused by stones 1 to 5 mm in diameter that can move into the ureter and obstruct flow. Classic ureteral colic is manifested by acute, intermittent, and excruciating pain in the flank and upper outer quadrant of the abdomen on the affected side. The pain may radiate to the lower abdominal quadrant, bladder area, perineum, or scrotum in the male. The skin may be cool and clammy, and nausea and vomiting are common.

Diagnosis and Treatment

Patients with kidney stones often present with acute renal colic, and the diagnosis is based on symptomatology and diagnostic tests, which include urinalysis, abdominal radiographs, and excretory urography. Urinalysis provides information related to hematuria, infection, the presence of stone-forming crystals, and urine pH. At least 90% of stones are radiopaque and are readily visible on a plain x-ray film of the abdomen. Excretory urography uses a contrast medium that is filtered in the glomeruli to visualize the collecting system and the ureters of the kidneys. Retrograde urography, ultrasonography, CT scanning, and magnetic resonance imaging (MRI) may also be used.

Treatment of acute renal colic usually is supportive. Pain relief may be needed during acute phases of obstruction, and antibiotic therapy may be necessary to treat urinary infections. Most stones that are less than 5 mm in diameter pass spontaneously. All urine should be strained during an attack in the hope of retrieving the stone for chemical analysis and determination of type. This information, along with a careful history and laboratory tests, affords the basis for long-term preventive measures.

A major goal of treatment in persons who have passed kidney stones or have had them removed is to prevent their recurrence. Prevention requires investigation into the cause of stone formation using urine tests, blood chemistries, and stone analysis. Underlying disease conditions, such as hyperparathyroidism, are treated. Adequate fluid intake reduces the saturation of stone-forming crystals and needs to be encouraged. Depending on the type of stone that is formed, dietary changes, medications, or both may be used to alter the concentration of stone-forming elements in the urine. For example, persons who form calcium oxalate stones may need to decrease their intake of foods that are high in oxalate (*e.g.*, spinach, Swiss chard, cocoa, chocolate, pecans, peanuts). Thiazide diuretics lower urinary calcium excretion by increasing the fractional absorption of calcium by the kidney so that less remains in the urine and reducing intestinal calcium absorption.

Measures to change the pH of the urine can also influence kidney stone formation. In persons who lose the ability to lower the pH of (or acidify) their urine, there is an increase in the divalent and trivalent forms of urine phosphate that combines with calcium to form calcium phosphate stones. The formation of uric acid stones is increased in acid urine; stone formation can be reduced by raising the pH of urine to 6.0 to 6.5 with potassium alkali salts. Table 28–2 summarizes measures for preventing the recurrence of different types of kidney stones.

In some cases, stone removal may be necessary. Several methods are available for removing kidney stones: ureteroscopic removal, percutaneous removal, and extracorporeal lithotripsy. All these procedures eliminate the need for an open surgical procedure, which is another form of treatment. Struvite stones cannot be passed and require removal; extracorporeal lithotripsy and percutaneous removal can be used to reduce the damage incurred by these stones.

Ureteroscopic removal involves the passage of an instrument through the urethra into the bladder and then into the ureter. The development of high-quality optics has improved the ease with which this procedure is performed and its outcome. The procedure, which is performed under fluoroscopic guidance, involves the use of various instruments for dilating the ureter and for grasping and removing the stone. Preprocedure radiologic studies using a contrast medium (*i.e.*, excretory urography) are done to determine the position of the stone and direct the placement of the ureteroscope.[13]

Percutaneous nephrostomy involves the insertion through the flank of a small-gauge needle into the collecting system of the kidney; the needle tract is then dilated, and an instrument called a *nephroscope* is inserted into the renal pelvis. The procedure is performed under fluoroscopic guidance. Preprocedure radiologic and ultrasound examinations of the kidney and ureter are used in determining the placement of the nephroscope. Stones up to 1 cm in diameter can be removed through this method. Larger stones must be broken up with an electrohydraulic or ultrasonic lithotriptor (*i.e.*, stone breaker).

A nonsurgical treatment called *extracorporeal shock wave lithotripsy*, introduced in Germany in 1980, received U.S. Food and Drug Administration approval in 1984 for treatment of stones primarily in the renal calix and pelvis and the upper third of the ureter. The procedure uses acoustic shock waves to fragment calculi into sandlike particles that are passed in the urine over the next few days. Because of the large amount of stone particles that are generated during the procedure, a ureteral stent (*i.e.*, tubelike device used to hold the ureter open) may be inserted to ensure adequate urine drainage.

In summary, obstruction of urine flow can occur at any level of the urinary tract. Among the causes of urinary tract obstruction are developmental defects, normal pregnancy, infection and inflammation, kidney stones, neurologic defects, and prostatic hypertrophy. Obstructive disorders produce stasis of urine, increasing the risk of infection and calculi formation and resulting in back pressure that is damaging to kidney structures. Kidney stones are a major cause of urinary tract obstruction. There are four types of kidney stones: calcium (*i.e.*, oxalate and phosphate) stones, which are associated with increased serum calcium levels; magnesium ammonium phosphate (*i.e.*, struvite) stones, which are associated with urinary tract infections; uric acid stones, which are related to elevated uric acid levels; and cystine stones, which are seen in cystinuria. A major goal of treatment for persons who have passed kidney stones or have had them removed is to identify stone composition and prevent their recurrence. Treatment measures depend on stone type and include adequate fluid intake to prevent urine saturation, dietary modification to decrease intake of stone forming constituents, treatment of urinary tract infection, measures to change urine pH, and the use of diuretics that decrease the calcium concentration of urine.

Urinary Tract Infections

After you have completed this section of the chapter, you should be able to meet the following objectives:

- Cite the organisms most responsible for urinary tract infections and state why urinary catheters, obstruction, and reflux predispose to infections
- List three physiologic mechanisms that protect against urinary tract infections
- Describe factors that predispose to urinary tract infections in children, sexually active women, pregnant women, and older adults
- Compare the manifestations of urinary tract infections in different age groups, including infants, toddlers, adolescents, adults, and older adults
- Cite measures used in the diagnosis and treatment of urinary tract infections

Urinary tract infections (UTIs) are the second most common type of bacterial infections seen by the physician (respiratory tract infections are first). UTIs can refer to several distinct entities, including asymptomatic bacteriuria, symptomatic infections, lower UTIs such as cystitis, and upper UTIs such as pyelonephritis. Because of their ability to cause renal damage, upper UTIs are considered more serious than lower UTIs.

Bacteria can enter the kidneys through the bloodstream and as an ascending infection from the lower urinary tract. Most infections are of the ascending type. Although the distal portion of the urethra often contains pathogens, the urine formed in the kidneys and found in the bladder normally is sterile or free of bacteria. This is because of the washout phenomenon, in which urine from the bladder normally washes bacteria out of the urethra. When a UTI occurs, the bacteria that have colonized the urethra, vagina, or perineal area often are responsible. *Escherichia coli* is by far the most common urinary pathogen. Other common pathogens include *Proteus, Klebsiella, Enterobacter,* and *Serratia* species.[15,16]

Etiologic Factors

Host-Agent Interactions

Because certain persons seem to be predisposed to developing UTIs, considerable interest has been focused on host-agent interactions and factors that increase the risk of UTI. Studies have shown an increased risk of UTI in persons with urinary obstruction and reflux, in pregnant and nonpregnant women, and in elderly persons.[17] Some conditions, including diabetes mellitus, pregnancy, immunosuppression, and upper urinary tract obstruction, are associated with serious morbidity from UTIs. Instrumentation and urinary catheterization are the most common predisposing factors for nosocomial UTIs.[17]

Host Defenses. In the development of a UTI, host defenses are matched against the virulence of the pathogen. The host defenses of the bladder have several components, including the washout phenomenon, in which bacteria are removed from the bladder and urethra during voiding; the protective mucin layer that lines the bladder and protects against bacterial invasion; and local immune responses. In the ureters, peristaltic movements facilitate the movement of urine from the renal pelvis through the ureters and into the bladder. Immune mechanisms, particularly secretory IgA immunoglobulins, appear to provide an important antibacterial defense. Phagocytic blood cells further assist in the removal of bacteria from the urinary tract.

There has been a growing appreciation of the protective function of the bladder's mucin layer. It is thought that the epithelial cells that line the bladder synthesize protective substances that subsequently become incorporated into the mucin layer that adheres to the bladder wall. One theory proposes that the mucin layer acts by binding water, which then constitutes a protective barrier between the bacteria and the epithelium. Elderly and postmenopausal women produce less mucin than younger women, suggesting that estrogen may play a role in its secretion.

Pathogen Virulence. Investigations are focusing on the adherence properties of the bacteria that infect the urinary tract. These bacteria have fine protein filaments that help them adhere to receptors on the lining of urinary tract structures. These filaments are called *fimbriae* or *pili*. Among the factors that contribute to bacterial virulence, the type of fimbriae that the bacteria possess may be the most important. Bacteria with certain types of fimbriae are associated primarily with cystitis, and those with other types are associated with a high incidence of pyelonephritis. The bacteria associated with pyelonephritis are thought to have fimbriae that bind to carbohydrates that are specific to the surfaces of epithelial cells in this part of the urinary tract.

Obstruction and Reflux

Obstruction and reflux are important contributing factors in the development of UTIs. Any microorganisms that enter the bladder normally are washed out during voiding. When outflow is obstructed, urine remains in the bladder and acts as a medium for microbial growth; the microorganisms in the contaminated urine can then ascend along the ureters to infect the kidneys. The presence of residual urine correlates directly with bacteriuria and with its recurrence after treatment.[18] Another aspect of bladder outflow obstruction and bladder distention is increased intravesicular pressure, which compresses blood vessels in the bladder wall, leading to a decrease in the mucosal defenses of the bladder.

In UTIs associated with stasis of urine flow, the obstruction may be anatomic or functional. Anatomic obstructions include urinary tract stones, prostatic hyperplasia, pregnancy, and malformations of the ureterovesical junction. The latter types of obstruction have been reported in 3% to 21% of children who present with UTIs.[19] Functional obstructions include neurogenic bladder, infrequent voiding, detrusor (bladder) muscle instability, and constipation.

Reflux occurs when urine from the urethra moves into the bladder (*i.e.*, urethrovesical reflux) or from the bladder into the ureters (*i.e.*, vesicoureteral reflux). In women, urethrovesical reflux can occur during activities such as coughing or squatting, in which an increase in intraabdominal pressure causes the urine to be squeezed into the urethra and then to flow back into the bladder as the pressure decreases. This can also happen when voiding is abruptly interrupted. Because the urethral orifice frequently is contaminated with bacteria, the reflux mechanism may cause bacteria to be drawn back into the bladder.

A second type of reflux mechanism, vesicoureteral reflux, occurs at the level of the bladder and ureter. Normally, the distal portion of the ureter courses between the muscle layer and the mucosal surface of the bladder wall, forming a flap. The flap is compressed against the bladder wall during micturition, preventing urine from being forced into the ureter (Fig. 28–6). In persons with vesicoureteral reflux, the ureter enters the bladder at an approximate right angle such that urine is forced into the ureter during micturition. It most commonly is seen in children with UTIs and is believed to result from congenital defects in length, diameter, muscle structure, or innervation of the submucosal segment of the ureter. It is also seen in adults with obstruction to bladder outflow.

Catheter-Induced Infection

Urinary catheters are tubes made of latex or plastic. They are inserted through the urethra into the bladder for the purpose of draining urine. They are a source of urethral irritation and provide a means for entry of microorganisms into the urinary tract.

Catheter-associated bacteriuria remains the most frequent cause of gram-negative septicemia in hospitalized patients. Studies have shown that bacteria adhere to the surface of the catheter and initiate the growth of a biofilm that then covers the surface of the catheter.[15] The biofilm tends to protect the bacteria from the action of antibiotics and makes treatment difficult. A closed drainage system (*i.e.*, closed to air and other sources of contamination) and careful attention to perineal hygiene (*i.e.*, cleaning the area around the urethral meatus) help to prevent infections in persons who require an indwelling catheter. Careful handwashing and early detection and treatment of UTIs are also essential.

Infections in Special Populations

UTIs affect persons of all ages. In infants, they occur more often in boys than in girls. After the first year of life, however, UTIs are more frequent in females because of the shorter length of the urethra and because the vaginal vestibule can be easily contaminated with fecal flora. About 20% of all adult women develop at least one UTI during their lifetime. In men, the longer length of the urethra and the antibacterial properties of the prostatic fluid provide some protection from ascending UTIs until about age 50. After this age, prostatic hypertrophy becomes more common, and with it may come obstruction and UTI.

Urinary Tract Infections in Women

In women, the urethra is short and in close proximity to the vagina and rectum, offering little protection against entry of microorganisms into the bladder. There is a peak incidence of these infections in the 15- to 24-year-old age group, suggesting that hormonal and anatomic changes associated with puberty and sexual activity contribute to UTIs.

The role of sexual activity in the development of urethritis and cystitis is controversial. The well-documented "honeymoon cystitis" suggests that sexual activity may contribute to such infections in susceptible women. The anterior urethra usually is colonized with bacteria; urethral massage or sexual intercourse can force these bacteria back into the bladder. Using a diaphragm and spermicide enhances the susceptibility to infection.[16] A nonpharmacologic approach to the treatment of frequent UTIs associated with sexual intercourse is to increase fluid intake before intercourse and to void soon after intercourse. This procedure uses the washout phenomenon to remove bacteria from the bladder.

UTIs are more common during pregnancy. This is particularly true for women who have bacteriuria during their initial prenatal visit.[20] Normal changes in the functioning of the urinary tract that occur during pregnancy predispose to UTIs. These changes involve the collecting system of the kidneys and include dilatation

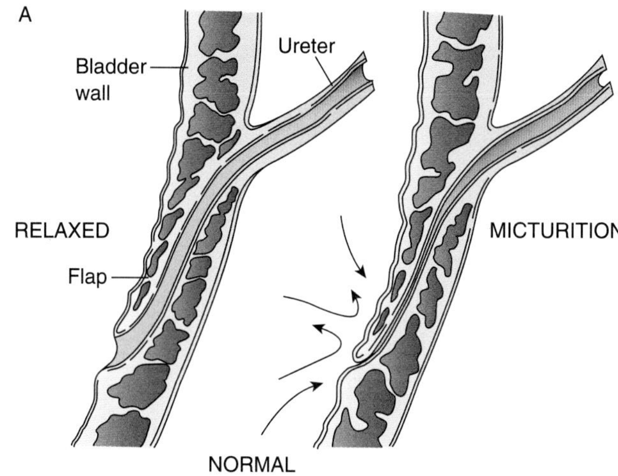

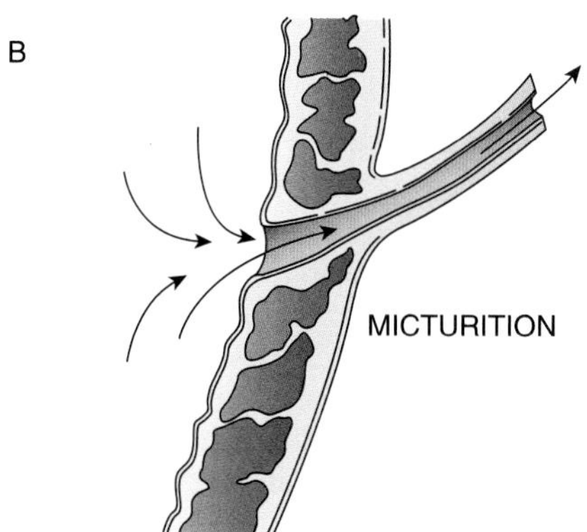

Figure 28–6
Anatomic features of the bladder and kidney in pyelonephritis caused by ureterovesical reflux. Bladder. (**A**) In the normal bladder the distal portion of the intravesical ureter courses between the mucosa and the muscularis of the bladder. A mucosal flap is thus formed. On micturition the elevated intravesicular pressure compresses the flap against the bladder wall, thereby occluding the lumen. (**B**) Persons with a congenitally short intravesical ureter have no mucosal flap, because the entry of the ureter into the bladder approaches a right angle. Thus, micturition forces urine into the ureter. (Courtesy of Dmitri Karetnikov, artist)

of the renal calices, pelves, and ureters that begins during the first trimester and becomes most pronounced during the third trimester. This dilatation of the upper urinary system is accompanied by a reduction in the peristaltic activity of the ureters that is thought to result from the muscle-relaxing effects of progesterone-like hormones and the mechanical obstruction from the enlarging uterus. In addition to the changes in the kidneys and ureters, the bladder becomes displaced from its pelvic position to a more abdominal position, producing further changes in ureteral position.[20]

The complications of UTI during pregnancy include acute pyelonephritis, persistent bacteriuria, chronic pyelonephritis, toxemia of pregnancy, and premature delivery. Evidence suggests that few women become bacteriuric during pregnancy. Rather, it appears that symptomatic UTIs during pregnancy reflect preexisting asymptomatic bacteriuria, and that changes occurring during pregnancy simply permit the prior urinary colonization to lead to symptomatic infection and invasion of the kidneys.[21] About 20% to 40% of women with bacteriuria are detected early in pregnancy, and if not treated, they will develop symptomatic UTIs later in pregnancy.[21] Because bacteriuria may occur as an asymptomatic condition in pregnant women, it is recommended that women be screened for bacteriuria during their first prenatal visit. Women with bacteriuria should be followed closely, and infections should be properly treated to prevent complications.

Urinary Tract Infections in Children

UTIs occur in as many as 5% of female and 1% to 2% of male children.[22] As many as 80% of children with uncomplicated UTIs have recurrences. Children who are at increased risk for bacteriuria or symptomatic UTIs are premature babies discharged from neonatal intensive care units; children with systemic or immunologic disease or urinary tract abnormalities such as neurogenic bladder or vesicoureteral reflux; those with a family history of UTI or urinary tract anomalies with reflux; and girls younger than age 5 with a history of UTI.[22]

Many neonates with UTIs have bacteremia and may show signs and symptoms of septicemia, including fever, hypothermia, apneic spells, poor skin perfusion, abdominal distention, diarrhea, vomiting, lethargy, and irritability. Older infants may present with feeding problems, failure to thrive, diarrhea, vomiting, fever, and foul-smelling urine. Many toddlers present with abdominal pain, vomiting, diarrhea, abnormal voiding patterns, foul-smelling urine, fever, and poor growth. In older children with lower UTIs, the classic features—enuresis, frequency, dysuria, and suprapubic discomfort—are more common. Fever, chills, nausea, vomiting, and flank pain occur in children with upper UTIs.

Diagnosis is based on a careful history of voiding patterns and symptomatology; physical examination to determine fever, hypertension, abdominal or suprapubic tenderness, and other manifestations of UTI; and urinalysis to determine bacteriuria, pyuria, proteinuria, and hematuria. A positive urine culture that is obtained correctly is essential for the diagnosis. Additional diagnostic methods may be needed to determine the cause of the disorder. Urinary symptoms in the absence of bacteriuria suggests vaginitis, urethritis, sexual molestation, the use of irritating bubble baths, pinworms, or viral cystitis. In adolescent girls, a history of dysuria and vaginal discharge makes vaginitis or vulvitis a consideration.

The approach to treatment is based on the clinical severity of the infection, the site of infection (*i.e.*, lower versus upper urinary tract), the risk of sepsis, and the presence of structural abnormalities. The immediate treatment of infants and young children is essential. Most infants with symptomatic UTI and children with clinical evidence of acute upper UTIs require hospitalization and intravenous antibiotic therapy. Children with uncomplicated UTIs usually are treated with antibiotics for 7 to 10 days.

Although most children respond to treatment, severe infection can result in renal scarring, hypertension, and compromised renal function. Children with reflux have a much higher incidence of pyelonephritis and renal scarring than those without reflux.[22]

Urinary Tract Infections in the Elderly

UTIs are relatively common in elderly persons. It has been reported that 5% to 20% of the elderly living at home have bacteriuria. These numbers increase to 15% to 25% for the elderly living in nursing homes or extended-care facilities.[23]

Most of these infections follow invasion of the urinary tract by the ascending route. Several factors predispose elderly persons to UTIs: immobility resulting in poor bladder emptying, bladder outflow obstruction caused by prostatic hyperplasia or kidney stones, bladder ischemia caused by urine retention, senile vaginitis, constipation, and diminished bactericidal activity of urine and prostatic secretions.[24] Added to these risks are other health problems that necessitate instrumentation of the urinary tract. UTIs develop in 1% of ambulatory patients after a single catheterization and within 3 to 4 days in essentially all patients with indwelling catheters.[25]

Elderly persons may not present with the usual symptoms of UTI. Even when symptoms of lower UTIs manifest, they may be difficult to interpret because uninfected elderly persons commonly experience urgency, frequency, and incontinence. Typical signs and symptoms of upper UTIs (*e.g.*, pyelonephritis) include fever, chills, flank pain, and tenderness, but these features may be altered or absent in elderly persons.[23] Sometimes, no symptoms occur until the infection is far advanced.

Manifestations

An acute episode of cystitis or bladder infection is characterized by frequency of urination (sometimes as often as every 20 minutes), lower abdominal discomfort, and burning and pain on urination (*i.e.*, dysuria). There also may be systemic signs of infection, with fever and generalized malaise. If there are no complications, the symptoms disappear within 48 hours. This type of cystitis is mainly a disorder of young women. The symptoms of cystitis may also represent urethritis caused by *Chlamydia trachomatis*, *Neisseria gonorrhoeae*, or herpes simplex virus or vaginitis attributable to *Trichomonas vaginalis* or *Candida* species.

Manifestations of upper urinary tract infections such as acute pyelonephritis include an abrupt onset of shaking chills, moderate to high fever, constant ache in the loin area of the back that is unilateral or bilateral, and signs of cystitis. There may be significant malaise, and the person usually feels ill. Nausea and vomiting may occur along with abdominal pain.

Diagnosis and Treatment

Early diagnosis and treatment of UTI are essential for preventing permanent kidney damage. Screening of high-risk groups and attention to care of patients with indwelling catheters are important measures. Pregnant women and persons with diabetes or renal problems who are at risk for developing UTIs usually can be managed in the physician's office.

The diagnosis of UTI usually is based on symptoms and on examination of the urine for the presence of microorganisms. When necessary, x-ray films, ultrasonography, and CT and renal scans are used to identify contributing factors, such as obstruction.

Bacteriuria, or the presence of bacteria in the urine, often is used in diagnosing UTIs. The source of bacteria in the urine can be contamination of the urine specimen, simple colonization of the urinary tract, or bacterial invasion of urinary structures. Colonization usually is defined as the multiplication of microorganisms in or on a host without apparent evidence of invasiveness or tissue injury. A commonly accepted criterion for diagnosis of a UTI is the presence of more than 100,000 (10^5) organisms per 1 ml of urine. The accuracy of the diagnosis is strengthened if such numbers are found in two consecutive urine specimens and if the bacteria are of a single type. Contaminated urine specimens commonly contain several types of microorganisms.

Care is needed in collecting urine specimens representative of bladder urine. Specimens that are kept for longer than 1 hour must be refrigerated to prevent the contaminating organisms from multiplying. The use of catheterized urine specimens, once common, have largely been replaced with clean-voided specimens. To obtain a clean-voided specimen, the area around the urethra is carefully cleansed and a midstream specimen is obtained by having the person void directly into a sterile container. This method usually is adequate and eliminates the risk of introducing microorganisms into the bladder during insertion of a catheter. In infants and sometimes in other age groups, suprapubic aspiration may be done to obtain a sample of bladder urine.

In addition to the bacterial count, the urine leukocyte count is used. Pyuria ($>$10 leukocytes/μl of uncentrifuged urine) indicates host injury rather than asymptomatic bacterial colonization. Immunofluorescence studies may be done to determine whether the infection involves the upper urinary tract. These tests are expensive and usually are not done routinely. Detailed identification and antibiotic sensitivity tests often are done in cases of chronic infection.

The treatment of UTI is based on the type of infection that is present (lower or upper UTI) and the presence of contributing host-agent factors. Antibiotics typically are used to treat acute infection. Forcing fluids may relieve signs and symptoms, and this approach is used as an adjunct to antibiotic treatment. Most lower UTIs are treated successfully with antimicrobial therapy and increased fluid intake. Acute cystitis usually is treated with a 3-day course of antibiotics, although a longer course of treatment may be needed. Because there is risk of permanent kidney damage with pyelonephritis, these infections are treated more aggressively. Treatment with an appropriate antimicrobial agent usually is continued for 10 to 14 days. Hospitalization may be recommended during the early stages of infection until a response to treatment is observed.

Chronic infection is more difficult to treat. Because it often is associated with obstructive uropathy or reflux flow of urine, diagnostic tests usually are performed to detect such abnormalities. When possible, the condition causing the reflux flow or obstruction is corrected. Most persons with recurrent UTIs are treated with antibiotics for 10 to 14 days in doses sufficient to maintain high urine levels of the drug, and they are examined for obstruction or other causes of infection. Men in particular should be investigated for obstructive disorders or a prostatic focus of infection.

Cranberry juice or blueberry juice has been suggested as a preventative measure for persons with frequent urinary tract infections. These juices contain a substance with biologic activity that can reduce bacterial adhesion to the epithelial lining of the urinary tract.[26] One study demonstrated that the risk of contracting bacteriuria was 42% lower in women who were randomized to the group that drank 300 ml cranberry juice daily compared with women who received a placebo beverage.[27] Although the role of cranberry juice in prevention and treatment of urinary tract infections has been implicated as a folk remedy for decades, these studies provide some of the first explanations related to its effectiveness.

In summary, UTI is the second most common type of bacterial infection seen by health care professionals. Infections can range from simple bacteriuria to severe kidney infections that cause irreversible kidney damage. Predisposition to infection is determined by host defenses and pathogen virulence. Host defenses include washout phenomenon associated with voiding, the protective mucin lining of the bladder, and local immune defenses. Pathogen virulence is enhanced by the presence of fimbriae that facilitate adherence to structures in the urinary tract.

Most UTIs ascend from the urethra and bladder. A number of factors interact in determining the predisposition to development of UTIs, including urinary tract obstruction, urine stasis and reflux, pregnancy-induced changes in urinary tract function, age-related changes in the urinary tract, changes in the protective mechanisms of the bladder and ureters, impaired immune function, and virulence of the pathogen. Urinary tract catheters and urinary instrumentation contribute to the incidence of UTIs. Early diagnosis and treatment of UTI are essential to preventing permanent kidney damage.

Disorders of Glomerular Function

After you have completed this section of the chapter, you should be able to meet the following objectives:

- Describe the two types of immune mechanisms involved in glomerular disorders
- Use the terms *proliferation, sclerosis, membranous, diffuse, focal, segmental*, and *mesangial* to explain changes in glomerular structure that occur with glomerulonephritis
- Relate the proteinuria, hematuria, pyuria, oliguria, edema, hypertension, and azotemia that occur with glomerulonephritis to changes in glomerular structure
- Differentiate the pathology and manifestations of the nephrotic syndrome from those of the nephritic syndrome

The glomeruli are tufts of capillaries that lie between the afferent and efferent arterioles. The capillaries of the glomeruli are arranged in lobules and supported by a stalk consisting of mesangial cells and a basement membrane–like extracellular matrix (Fig. 28–7). The glomerular membrane is composed of three layers: an endothelial layer lining the capillary, a basement membrane, and a layer of epithelial cells forming the outer surface of the capillary and lining Bowman's capsule (see Fig. 25–5, Chapter 25). The epithelial cells are attached to the basement membrane by discrete cytoplasmic extensions, the foot processes (*i.e.*, podocytes). Within the glomeruli, blood is filtered, and the urine filtrate formed. The capillary membrane is selectively permeable: it allows water, electrolytes, and dissolved particles, such as glucose and amino acids, to leave the capillary and enter Bowman's space and prevents larger particles, such as plasma proteins and blood cells, from leaving the blood.

Mechanisms of Glomerular Injury

Glomerulonephritis, an inflammatory process that involves glomerular structures, is the leading cause of chronic renal failure in the United States, accounting for one half of persons who need dialysis. There are many causes of glomerular disease. The disease may occur as a primary condition in which the glomerular abnormality is the only disease present, or it may occur as a secondary condition in which the glomerular abnormality results from another disease, such as vasculitis or systemic lupus erythematosus. An understanding of the various forms of glomerular pathology has emerged only recently. Much of this knowledge can be attributed to advances in immunobiology and electron microscopy, development of animal models, and increased use of renal biopsy during the early stages of glomerular disease.

Although little is known about the causative agents or triggering events that produce glomerular disease, most cases of primary glomerular disease and many cases of secondary disease probably have an immune origin.[5,6] Two types of immune mechanisms have been implicated in the development of glomerular disease: injury resulting from antibodies reacting with fixed glomerular antigens and injury resulting from circulating antigen-antibody complexes that become trapped within the glomerular membrane (Fig. 28–8). Antigens responsible for development of the immune response may be of endogenous origin, such as DNA in systemic lupus erythematosus, or they may be of exogenous origin, such as streptococcal membrane antigens in post-streptococcal glomerulonephritis. Frequently, the source of the antigen is unknown.

The cellular changes that occur with glomerular disease include proliferative, sclerotic, and membranous changes. The term *proliferative* refers to an increase in the cellular components of the glomerulus, regardless of origin; *sclerotic*, to an increase in the noncellular components of the glomerulus, primarily collagen; and *membranous*, to an increase in the thickness of the glomerular capillary wall, often caused by immune complex deposition. Glomerular changes can be *diffuse*, involving all glomeruli and all parts of the glomeruli; *focal*, in which only some glomeruli are affected and others are essentially normal; *segmental*, involving only a certain segment of each glomeruli; or *mesangial*, affecting only the mesangial cell. Figure 28–7 shows changes associated with various types of glomerular disease.

Glomerular disorders are commonly grouped into two categories: nephrotic syndrome, which affects the integrity of the glomerular capillary membrane, and nephritic syndrome, which evokes an inflammatory response within the glomeruli.

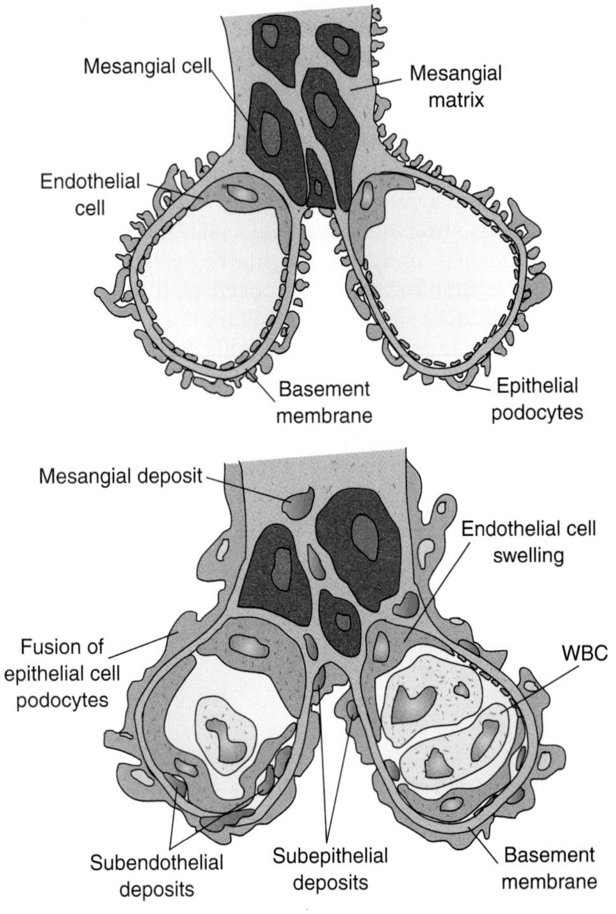

Figure 28–7
Schematic representation of glomerulus. (**A**) Normal; (**B**) localization of immune deposits (mesangial, subendothelial, subepithelial) and changes in glomerular architecture associated with injury. (Whitley K., Keane W.F., & Vernier R.L. [1984]. Acute glomerulonephritis: A clinical overview. *Medical Clinics of North America, 68*(2), 263)

Nephrotic Syndrome

Nephrotic syndrome is not a specific glomerular disease but a constellation of clinical findings that result from increased glomerular permeability to the plasma proteins (Fig. 28–9). It can be caused by a number of other forms of glomerular disease.

Manifestations

The nephrotic syndrome is characterized by massive proteinuria (daily loss $\geq$3.5 g) and lipiduria (*e.g.*, free fat, oval bodies, fatty casts), along with an associated hypoalbuminemia ($<$3 g/dl), generalized edema, and hyperlipidemia (cholesterol $>$300 mg/dl).[28,29] The initiating event in the development of nephrosis is a derangement in the glomerular membrane that causes increased permeability to plasma proteins. The glomerular membrane acts as a size and charge barrier through which the glomerular filtrate must pass. Any increased permeability allows protein to escape from the plasma into the glomerular filtrate.

Generalized edema, which is a hallmark of nephrosis, is caused by a loss of serum albumin below that needed to maintain the colloidal osmotic pressure of the vascular compartment. Other factors, such as increased sodium and water retention, may also play a role in edema formation. Although the largest proportion of plasma protein loss is in albumin, globulins are also lost.

Persons with nephrosis are particularly vulnerable to infections, particularly those caused by staphylococci and pneumococci.[5] This decreased resistance to infection probably is related to loss of immunoglobulins and low-molecular-weight complement components in the urine. The hyperlipidemia that occurs in persons with nephrosis is characterized by elevated levels of triglycerides and cholesterol. These abnormalities are thought

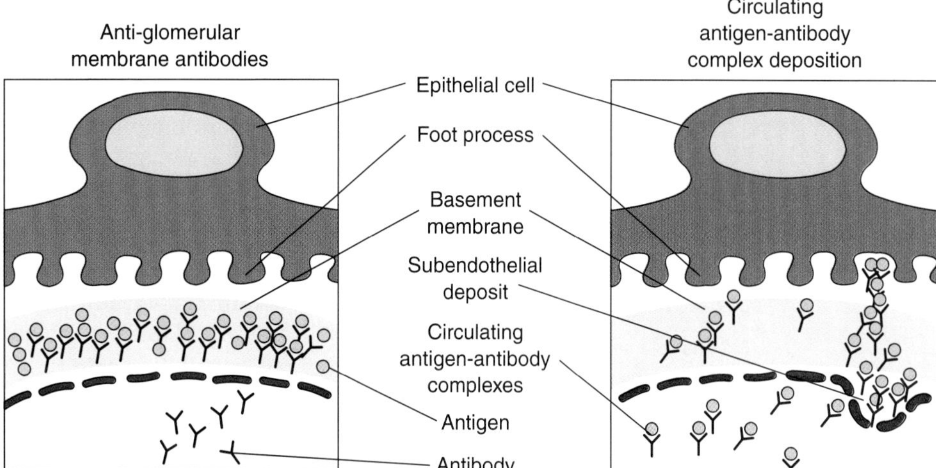

Figure 28–8 Immune mechanisms of glomerular disease.

to be related in part to increased synthesis of lipoproteins in the liver secondary to a compensatory increase in albumin production. Because of the elevated levels of low-density lipoproteins, persons with nephrotic syndrome are at increased risk of developing atherosclerosis. Persons with nephrosis are also at increased risk for thrombotic and thromboembolic complications because of the loss of coagulation and anticoagulation factors.[30]

Causes of Nephrosis

The glomerular derangements that occur with nephrosis can develop as a primary disorder or secondary to changes caused by systemic diseases such as diabetes mellitus and systemic lupus erythematosus. The relative frequency of these causes varies with age. In children younger than 15 years of age, nephrotic syndrome is almost always caused by primary glomerular disease, whereas in adults, it is often a secondary disorder. Among the primary glomerular lesions leading to nephrotic syndrome are minimal change disease, focal sclerosis, membranous glomerulopathy, and membranoproliferative glomerulonephritis.[28,29]

Minimal Change Disease. Minimal change disease is characterized by diffuse loss (through fusion) of foot processes from the epithelial layer of the glomerular membrane. The peak incidence is between 2 and 6 years of age. The cause of minimal change nephrosis is unknown; however, children who develop the disease often have a history of recent upper respiratory infections or of receiving routine immunizations.[5] Although minimal change disease does not progress to renal failure, it can cause significant complications, including predisposition to infection with gram-positive organisms, a tendency toward thromboembolic events, hyperlipidemia, and protein malnutrition. There is usually a dramatic response to corticosteroid therapy.[28]

Focal Sclerosis. Focal sclerosis is characterized by sclerosis (*i.e.*, increased collagen deposition) of some but not all glomeruli, and in the affected glomeruli, only a portion of the glomerular tuft is involved. Focal sclerosis is often an idiopathic syndrome, but it may be associated with heroin abuse, acquired immunodeficiency syndrome, reflux nephropathy, or an idiopathic reaction to nonsteroidal antiinflammatory drugs (NSAIDs).[28] The presence of hypertension and decreased renal function distinguish focal sclerosis from minimal change disease. The disorder is usually treated with corticosteroids. Most persons with the disorder progress to end-stage renal disease within 5 to 10 years.

Membranous Glomerulonephropathies. Membranous glomerulonephropathies are the most common cause of primary nephrosis in adults, most commonly in their fifties or sixties. The disorders are caused by diffuse thickening of the glomerular basement membrane due to deposition of immune complexes. The disorder may be idiopathic or associated with a number of disorders, including autoimmune diseases such as lupus erythematosus, infections such as chronic hepatitis B, metabolic disorders such as diabetes mellitus and thyroiditis, and use of certain drugs such as gold, penicillamine, and captopril.[5,28] Because of the presence of immunoglobulins and complement in the subendothelial deposits, it is thought that the disease represents a chronic antigen-antibody–mediated disorder.

The disorder is treated with corticosteroids. Cytotoxic drugs may be added to the treatment regimen. The progress of the disease is variable; about one half of persons develop a slow but progressive loss of renal function.

Membranoproliferative Glomerulonephritis. With membranoproliferative glomerulonephritis, there is basement membrane thickening and cellular proliferation. The proliferation is primarily of mesangial cells. There are at least two forms of the disorder. Type I is characterized by an increase in mesangial cells and matrix that is interposed between the glomerular base-

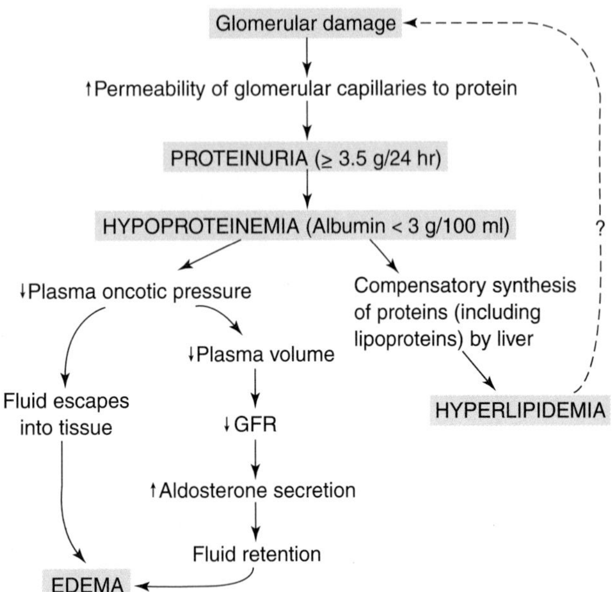

Figure 28–9
Pathophysiology of the nephrotic syndrome. The relationship between hyperlipidemia and glomerular damage (*dashed line*) has been demonstrated in experimental models of certain diseases associated with nephrotic range proteinuria (*e.g.*, focal segmental glomerulosclerosis), but its significance in human renal disease is still somewhat unknown. (*GFR*, glomerular filtration rate)

ment membrane and the endothelial cells. About one third of persons with type I disease have a history of a recent upper respiratory disease.[5] Type II is characterized by the deposition of a dense ribbon-like layer of material in the basement membrane of the glomerulus. Immunoglobulins and complement are present in both types of disorders and suggest an immune etiology. Although corticosteroids and antiplatelet drugs are used in treatment of the disorder, there is no agreement that any form of treatment is beneficial. The disorder usually progresses to end-stage renal disease within a few months or years.

Nephritic Syndrome

The nephritic syndrome is a clinical complex characterized by hematuria with red cell casts, a diminished glomerular filtration rate (GFR), azotemia, oliguria, and hypertension. It is caused by diseases that provoke a proliferative inflammatory response of the endothelial, mesangial, or epithelial cells of the glomeruli. The inflammatory process damages the capillary wall, permitting red blood cells to escape into the urine and producing hemodynamic changes that decrease the GFR. The disorder may result from primary disease of the glomerulus or as a secondary effect of another condition, such as vasculitis or systemic lupus erythematosus. It can be initiated by immune complexes, antiglomerular basement antibodies, cellular mechanisms alone, or bloodborne leukocytes (*i.e.*, neutrophils, monocytes, and lymphocytes). One of the most common primary nephritic disorders is acute proliferative glomerulonephritis. Other causes of the nephritic syndrome are IgA nephropathy and rapidly progressive glomerular nephritis.

Acute Proliferative Glomerulonephritis

The most commonly recognized form of acute nephritic syndrome is diffuse proliferative glomerulonephritis, which follows infections caused by strains of group A β-hemolytic streptococci. Diffuse proliferative glomerulonephritis may also occur after infections by other organisms, including staphylococci and a number of viral agents, such as those responsible for mumps, measles, and chickenpox. With this type of nephritis, the inflammatory response is caused by an immune reaction that occurs when circulating immune complexes become entrapped in the glomerular membrane. Proliferation of the endothelial cells lining the glomerular capillary (*i.e.*, endocapillary form of the disease) and the mesangial cells lying between the endothelium and the epithelium follows (see Fig. 28–7). The capillary membrane swells and becomes permeable to plasma proteins and blood cells. Although the disease is seen primarily in children, adults of any age can also be affected.

The classic case of poststreptococcal glomerulonephritis follows a streptococcal infection by about 10 days to 2 weeks—the time needed for the development of antibodies. Oliguria, which develops as the GFR decreases, is one of the first symptoms. Proteinuria and hematuria follow because of increased glomerular capillary wall permeability. The blood is degraded by materials in the urine, and a cola-colored urine may be the first sign of the disorder. Sodium and water retention give rise to edema, particularly of the face and hands, and hypertension. Important laboratory findings include an elevated streptococcal exoenzyme (antistreptolysin O) titer, a decline in C3 complement (see Chapter 11), and cryoglobulins (*i.e.*, large immune complexes) in the serum.

Treatment for acute poststreptococcal glomerulonephritis is largely symptomatic. The acute symptoms usually begin to subside in about 10 days to 2 weeks, although in some children, the proteinuria may persist for several months. The immediate prognosis is favorable, and about 95% of children recover spontaneously.[5] The outlook for adults is less favorable; about 60% recover completely. In the remainder of cases, the lesions eventually resolve, but there may be permanent kidney damage.

IgA Nephropathy

IgA nephropathy (*i.e.*, Buerger's disease) is usually a primary disorder. It is the most common cause of acute glomerulonephritis in the United States. The disorder tends to present with hematuria and is often preceded by upper respiratory tract infection, gastrointestinal tract symptoms, or a flulike illness. The disorder is characterized by the deposition of IgA and occasionally IgG with complement and fibrin-associated antigens in the mesangium of the glomerulus. Serum IgA levels are elevated and may be helpful in the diagnosis of the disorder.

Gross hematuria usually lasts for 2 to 6 days. About one half of the persons with gross hematuria have a single episode; the remainder have gradual progression of glomerular disease with recurrent episodes of hematuria and mild proteinuria. Progression is usually slow, extending over several decades. Evidence suggests that the daily use of fish oil in the diet may retard the progress of the disease, particularly in persons with mildly impaired renal function.[31]

Rapidly Progressive Glomerulonephritis

Like nephrotic syndrome and nephritic disorders, rapidly progressive glomerulonephritis does not have a single, specific cause. As its name implies, this type of glomerulonephritis is rapidly progressive, often within a matter of months. The disorder occurs by focal and segmental proliferation of glomerular cells and by activation and recruitment of monocytes (macrophages) with formation of crescent-shaped structures that obliterate the Bowman's space. Among the systemic diseases associated with this form of glomerulonephritis are vasculitis, systemic lupus erythematosus, acute poststreptococcal glomerulonephritis (usually in adults), and primary glomerular diseases, such as Goodpasture's syndrome.

Goodpasture's syndrome, which is caused by glomerular basement membrane antibodies (anti-GBM), accounts for about 5% of cases of rapidly progressive glomerulonephritis. It is a rare disease and is associated with a triad of pulmonary hemorrhage, iron deficiency anemia, and glomerulonephritis. All of these manifestations result from anti-GBM antibody deposition in the lungs and glomeruli. The cause of the disorder is unknown, although influenza infection, hydrocarbon solvent exposure, and the presence of HLA-DRw2 and HLA-B7 antigens have been implicated.[28] Treatment includes plasmapheresis to remove circulating anti-GBM antibodies and immunosuppressive therapy (*i.e.*, corticosteroids and cyclophosphamide) to inhibit antibody production.

Chronic Glomerulonephritis

Chronic glomerulonephritis represents the end stage of the many types of glomerulonephritis. Histologically, it is characterized by small kidneys with sclerosed glomeruli. It seldom develops in children with acute poststreptococcal glomerulonephritis and frequently is seen in persons who survive the acute phase of rapidly progressive glomerulonephritis. Some persons who present with chronic glomerulonephritis have no history of glomerular disease.[5] In most cases, chronic glomerulonephritis develops insidiously and is characterized by signs and symptoms of chronic renal failure (see Chapter 29). The disease is progressive but at widely varying rates.

Diabetic Glomerulosclerosis

Diabetic nephropathy, or kidney disease, is a major complication of diabetes mellitus. It affects about 30% of persons with type I diabetes and accounts for 20% of deaths in diabetics younger than 40 years of age.[5] The glomerulus is the most commonly affected structure in diabetic nephropathy, evidenced by three glomerular syndromes: nonnephrotic proteinuria, nephrotic syndrome, and renal failure. Widespread thickening of the glomerular capillary basement membrane occurs in almost all persons with diabetes and can occur without evidence of proteinuria.[5] This is followed by a diffuse increase in mesangial matrix, with mild proliferation of mesangial cells. As the disease progresses the mesangial cells impinge on the capillary lumen, drastically reducing the surface area for glomerular filtration.[32] In nodular glomerulosclerosis, also known as *Kimmelstiel-Wilson syndrome*, there is nodular deposition of hyaline in the mesangial portion of the glomerulus. As the sclerotic process progresses in the diffuse and nodular forms of glomerulosclerosis, there is complete obliteration of the glomerulus, with impairment of renal function.

Although the mechanisms of glomerular changes in diabetes are uncertain, they are thought to represent enhanced or defective synthesis of the basement membrane and mesangial matrix with an inappropriate incorporation of glucose into the noncellular components of these glomerular structures. One hypothesis implicates hemodynamic changes that occur because of increased renal blood flow, increased intracapillary glomerular pressure, and increased GFR that accompanies the need for increased tubular reabsorption of glucose. The increased GFR is associated with microalbuminuria (20 to 200 μg of albumin per minute), which can be used as a method of detecting early changes in glomerular function.[5]

The manifestations of diabetic glomerulosclerosis include recurrent proteinuria with slow but steady progression to renal failure. In many cases, these early changes in glomerular function can be reversed by careful control of blood glucose levels.[32] Inhibition of angiotensin by converting enzyme inhibitors (*e.g.*, captopril) has been shown to have a beneficial effect, possibly by reversing the increased intracapillary glomerular pressure.[6,32]

Hypertensive Glomerular Disease

Renal failure and azotemia occur in 1% to 5% of persons with longstanding hypertension. Hypertension is associated with a number of changes in glomerular structures, including sclerotic changes. As the glomerular vascular structures thicken and perfusion diminishes, the blood supply to the nephron decreases, causing the kidneys to lose some of their ability to concentrate the urine. This may be evidenced by nocturia. Blood urea nitrogen levels may also become elevated, particularly during periods of water deprivation. Proteinuria may occur as a result of changes in glomerular structure.

In summary, diseases of the glomerulus disrupt glomerular filtration and alter the permeability of glomerular capillary membrane to plasma proteins and blood cells. Glomerulonephritis is a term used to describe a group of diseases that cause inflammation and injury of the glomerulus. These diseases disrupt the capillary membrane and cause proteinuria, hematuria, pyuria, oliguria, edema, hypertension, and azotemia. Almost all types of glomerulonephritis are caused by immune mechanisms.

Glomerular pathologies have been grouped into two categories: the nephrotic syndrome, which affects the integrity of the glomerular capillary membrane and is characterized by massive proteinuria, hypoalbuminemia, generalized edema, lipiduria, and hyperlipidemia, and the nephritic syndrome, which evokes an inflammatory response within the glomeruli and is characterized by hematuria with red cell casts in the urine, a diminished GFR, azotemia, oliguria, and hypertension. Both conditions can lead to progressive loss of glomerular function and eventual development of end-stage renal disease. Glomerulosclerosis is a major complication of diabetes mellitus and is thought to be related to increased blood glucose levels and defective synthesis of glomerular structures. Hypertension can also cause damage to the glomeruli.

Tubulointerstitial Disorders

After you have completed this section of the chapter, you should be able to meet the following objectives:

- Cite a definition of tubulointerstitial kidney disease
- Differentiate between the defects in tubular function that occur in proximal and distal tubular acidosis
- Explain the pathogenesis of kidney damage in pyelonephritis
- Explain the vulnerability of the kidneys to injury caused by drugs and toxins

Several disorders affect renal tubular structures, including the proximal and distal tubules. Most also affect the interstitial tissue that surrounds the tubules; the disorders often are called *tubulointerstitial diseases.* These disorders include acute tubular necrosis (see Chapter 29), renal tubular acidosis, pyelonephritis, and the effects of drugs and toxins.

Tubulointerstitial renal diseases may be divided into acute and chronic disorders. The acute disorders are characterized by their sudden onset and by signs and symptoms of interstitial edema; they include acute pyelonephritis and acute hypersensitivity reaction to drugs. The chronic disorders produce interstitial fibrosis, atrophy, and mononuclear infiltrates; most persons are asymptomatic until late in the course of the disease. In the early stages, tubulointerstitial diseases commonly are manifested by fluid and electrolyte imbalances that reflect subtle changes in tubular function. These manifestations can include inability to concentrate urine, as evidenced by polyuria and nocturia; interference with acidification of urine, resulting in metabolic acidosis; and diminished tubular reabsorption of sodium and other substances.[25]

Renal Tubular Acidosis

Renal tubular acidosis refers to a group of tubular disorders that result in acidosis and its subsequent complications, including metabolic bone disease, kidney stones, and growth failure in children. There are two main types of renal tubular acidosis: proximal tubular disorders that affect bicarbonate reabsorption and distal tubular defects that affect the secretion of fixed metabolic acids.[33–35]

The proximal tubule is the site where 90% to 95% of the filtered bicarbonate is reabsorbed. With the onset of impaired tubular bicarbonate absorption, there is a loss of bicarbonate in the urine that reduces plasma bicarbonate levels. The concomitant loss of sodium in the urine that accompanies the bicarbonate loss leads to contraction of the extracellular fluid volume with increased aldosterone secretion and a resultant decrease in serum potassium levels (see Chapter 26). With proximal tubular defects in acid-base regulation, the distal tubular sites for secretion of the fixed acids into the urine continue to function, and the reabsorption of bicarbonate by the proximal cells eventually resumes, albeit at a lower level of serum bicarbonate. Whenever serum levels rise above this decreased level, bicarbonate is lost in the urine. The proximal tubular defect in bicarbonate reabsorption can extend to other substances, such as glucose, amino acids, and phosphate. Defects in calcium and phosphate reabsorption may accentuate bicarbonate losses.

The most common type of distal tubular acidosis usually is a defect in the secretion of hydrogen ions with failure to acidify the urine. Because the secretion of hydrogen ions in the distal tubules is linked to sodium reabsorption, failure to secrete hydrogen ions results in a net loss of sodium bicarbonate in the urine. There is a resultant contraction of fluids in the extracellular fluid compartment, a compensatory increase in aldosterone levels, and development of hypokalemia. The persistent acidosis, which requires buffering by the skeletal system, causes calcium to be released from bone. Increased losses of calcium in the urine lead to increased levels of parathyroid hormone, osteomalacia, bone pain, impaired growth in children, and development of kidney stones.

The treatment of renal tubular acidosis depends on the defect and may require administration of bicarbonate and potassium. The selective use of diuretics may also be indicated.

Pyelonephritis

Pyelonephritis refers to an infection of the kidneys and renal pelvis. In its earliest stages, it is characterized by inflammatory foci that are interspersed throughout the renal interstitium. Small abscesses may form on the surface of the kidneys. In time, the lesions are replaced by scar tissue. There are two forms of pyelonephritis: acute and chronic. Because pyelonephritis affects the tubules and interstitium of the kidneys, it is classified as a tubulointerstitial kidney disease.

Acute pyelonephritis represents an acute suppurative inflammation of renal tubulointerstitial tissues caused by bacterial infection. Infection may occur through the bloodstream or ascend from the bladder. Factors that contribute to the development of acute pyelonephritis are catheterization and urinary tract instrumentation, vesicoureteral reflux, pregnancy, increased susceptibility to infection, and neurogenic bladder.

The onset of acute pyelonephritis typically is abrupt, with chills, fever, headache, back pain, tenderness over the costovertebral angle, and general malaise. It usually is accompanied by symptoms of bladder irritation, such as dysuria, frequency, and urgency. Pyuria occurs but is not diagnostic because it also occurs in lower UTIs. It is possible to determine whether an infection involves the upper or lower urinary tract through detection of the antibody coating on the bacteria. Antibody coating is an immune response that occurs in the kidneys during upper UTIs and is easily detected by the immunofluorescence test. The finding of leukocyte casts in the urine also indicates that the infection is in the kidneys rather than the lower urinary tract.

Acute pyelonephritis is treated with appropriate antimicrobial drugs. Unless obstruction or other complications occur, the symptoms usually disappear within several days. Hospitalization during initial treatment may be necessary. Depending on the cause, recurrent infections are possible.

Chronic pyelonephritis represents a progressive process. There is scarring and deformation of the renal calices and pelvis (Fig. 28–10). The disorder appears to involve a bacterial infection superimposed on obstructive abnormalities or the vesicoureteral reflux. Although the mechanisms by which the urinary obstruction interacts to produce kidney damage in chronic pyelonephritis are unknown, observations suggest that some component of the urine may serve as an antigenic determinant to induce an immune response. One of the suspected urine components is Tamm-Horsfall proteins, which are synthesized in the tubular epithelial cells of the thick ascending loop of Henle and the distal convoluted tubules.[36]

Chronic pyelonephritis may cause many of the same symptoms as acute pyelonephritis, or its onset may be insidious. Loss of tubular function and of the ability to concentrate urine give rise to polyuria and nocturia, and mild proteinuria is common. Severe hypertension often is a contributing factor in the progress of the disease.

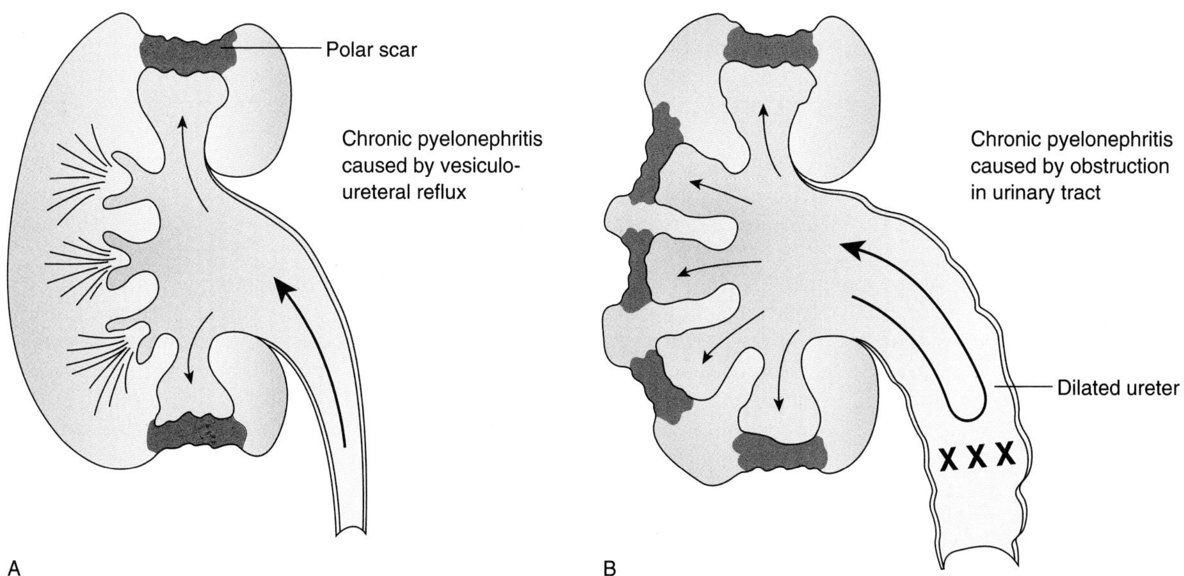

Figure 28–10
The two major types of chronic pyelonephritis. (**A**) Vesicoureteral reflux causes infection of the peripheral compound papillae and, therefore, scars in the poles of the kidney. (**B**) Obstruction of the urinary tract leads to high-pressure backflow of urine that causes infection of all papillae and diffuse scarring of the kidney and thinning of the cortex. (Courtesy of Dmitri Karetnikov, artist)

Chronic pyelonephritis is a significant cause of renal failure. It is thought to be responsible for 11% to 20% of all cases of end-stage renal disease.[5]

Drug-Related Nephropathies

Drug-related nephropathies involve functional or structural changes in the kidneys that occur after exposure to a drug. The kidneys are exposed to a high rate of delivery of any substance in the blood because of their large blood flow and high filtration pressure. The kidneys are also active in the metabolic transformation of drugs and therefore are exposed to a number of toxic metabolites. Some drugs and toxic substances damage the kidneys by causing a decrease in blood flow; others directly damage tubulointerstitial structures; and still others cause damage by producing hypersensitivity reactions.

The tolerance to drugs varies with age and depends on renal function, state of hydration, blood pressure, and the pH of the urine. Because of a decrease in physiologic function, elderly persons are particularly susceptible to kidney damage caused by drugs and toxins. The dangers of nephrotoxicity are increased when two or more drugs capable of producing kidney damage are given at the same time.

Acute drug-related hypersensitivity reactions produce tubulointerstitial nephritis, with damage to the tubules and interstitium. It was initially observed in persons who were sensitive to the sulfonamide drugs; currently, it is most often observed with the use of methicillin and other synthetic antibiotics and with the use of furosemide and the thiazide diuretics in persons sensitive to these drugs. The condition begins about 15 days (range 2 to 40 days) after exposure to the drug.[5] At the onset, there is fever, eosinophilia, hematuria, mild proteinuria, and in about one fourth of cases, a rash. In about 50% of cases, signs and symptoms of acute renal failure develop. Withdrawal of the drug commonly is followed by complete recovery, but there may be permanent damage in some persons, usually in older persons. Drug nephritis may not be recognized in its early stage because it is uncommon.

Chronic analgesic nephritis, which is associated with analgesic abuse, causes interstitial nephritis with renal papillary necrosis. When first observed, it was attributed to phenacetin, a then-common ingredient of over-the-counter medications containing aspirin, phenacetin, and caffeine. Although phenacetin is no longer contained in these preparations, it has been suggested that other ingredients, such as aspirin and acetaminophen, may also contribute to the disorder. How much analgesic it takes to produce papillary necrosis is unknown.

NSAIDs also have the potential for damaging renal structures, including medullary interstitial cells. Prostaglandins (particularly PGI_2 and PGE_2) contribute to regulation of tubular blood flow.[37] The deleterious effects of NSAIDs on the kidney is thought to result from their ability to inhibit prostaglandin synthesis. Persons who are particularly at risk are the elderly because of age-related changes in renal function, persons who are dehydrated or have a decrease in blood volume, and persons with preexisting kidney disease or renal insufficiency.

In summary, tubulointerstitial diseases affect the tubules and the surrounding interstitium of the kidneys. These disorders include renal tubular acidosis, chronic pyelonephritis, and the effects of drugs and toxins. Renal tubular acidosis describes a form of systemic acidosis that results from tubular defects in bicarbonate reabsorption or hydrogen ion secretion. Pyelonephritis, or infection of the kidney and kidney pelvis, can occur as an acute or a chronic condition. Acute pyelonephritis typically is caused by ascending bladder infections or infections that come from the bloodstream; it usually is successfully treated with appropriate antimicrobial drugs. Chronic pyelonephritis is a progressive disease that produces scarring and deformation of the renal calices and pelvis. Drug-induced impairment of tubulointerstitial structure and function usually is the result of hypersensitivity reactions.

Neoplasms

After you have completed this section of the chapter, you should be able to meet the following objectives:

- Characterize Wilms' tumor in terms of age of onset, possible oncogenic origin, manifestations and treatment
- Cite the risk factors for renal cell carcinoma, describe the manifestations, and explain why the 5-year survival rate has been so low

There are two major groups of renal neoplasms: embryonic kidney tumors (*i.e.*, Wilms' tumor), which occur during childhood, and adult kidney cancers.

Wilms' Tumor

Wilms' tumor (*i.e.*, nephroblastoma) is one of the most common solid tumors in young children and usually occurs before age 4.[6] It is a mixed tumor, composed of epithelial and mesenchymal embryonic tissue elements. The tumor seems to be related to a group of cancers that are related to loss of suppressor gene activity (see Chapter 5). Deletions in chromosome 11 have been found in cases of Wilms' tumors.

Wilms' tumor is a solitary mass that occurs in any part of the kidney. It is usually sharply demarcated and variably encapsulated (Fig. 28–11). The tumors grow to a large size, distorting kidney structure. The tumors are usually staged using Wilms' Tumor Study Group classification.[38] Stage I tumors are limited to the kidney and can be excised with capsular surface intact. Stage II

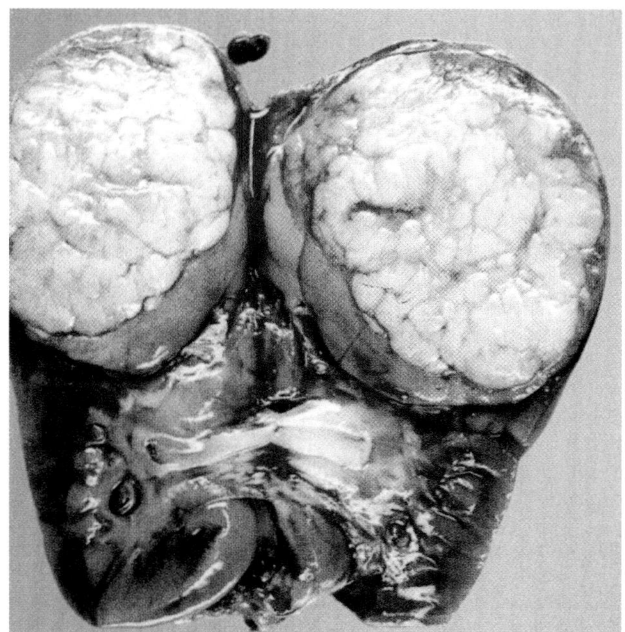

Figure 28–11
Wilms' tumor (nephroblastoma). The bisected kidney of a child with a flank mass reveals a circumscribed, soft, fleshy tumor in the upper pole.

tumors extend into the kidney but can be excised. In stage III, extension of the tumor is confined to the abdomen, and in stage IV, hematogenous metastasis most commonly involves the lung. Bilateral kidney involvement occurs in 5% to 10% of cases.

The common presenting signs are a large abdominal mass and hypertension. About 50% of children have abdominal pain, vomiting, or both.[38] CT scans are used to confirm the diagnosis.

Treatment involves surgery, chemotherapy, and sometimes radiotherapy. Long-term, survival rates have increased to about 90% with an aggressive treatment plan.[7]

Adult Kidney Cancer

Adult kidney cancer accounts for 2% of all cancers. Each year, an estimated 24,000 new cases of kidney cancer are diagnosed, and about 10,300 persons die of this type of cancer.[39] The availability of CT scanning has contributed significantly to earlier diagnosis and more accurate staging of kidney cancers.

Renal cell carcinoma accounts for about 80% to 85% of kidney tumors, with transitional or squamous cell cancers of the renal pelvis accounting for most of the remaining cancers. The cause of renal cell carcinoma remains unclear. It occurs most often in older persons in the sixth to seventh decade. Men are affected twice as frequently as women. Some of these tumors may occur as a result of chronic irritation associated with kidney stones. Epidemiologic evidence suggests a correlation between smoking and kidney cancer. Obesity is also a risk factor, particularly in women. Additional risk factors include hypertension and treatment for hypertension; unopposed estrogen therapy; and occupational exposure to petroleum products, heavy metals, and asbestos. In most cases, renal cancer occurs without evidence of hereditary predisposition.

Kidney cancer is largely a silent disorder during its early stages, and symptoms usually denote advanced disease. Presenting features include hematuria, costovertebral pain, presence of a palpable flank mass, polycythemia, and fever. Hematuria, which occurs in 70% to 90% of cases, is the most reliable sign. It is, however, intermittent and may be microscopic; as a result, the tumor may reach considerable size before it is detected. In about one third of cases, metastases are present at the time of diagnosis.

Kidney cancer is suspected when there are findings of hematuria and a renal mass. Ultrasonography, CT scanning, excretory urography, and renal angiography are used to confirm the diagnosis. MRI with intravenous gadolinium may be used when involvement of the inferior vena cava is suspected.

Surgery (radical nephrectomy with lymph node dissection) is the treatment of choice for all respectable tumors. Nephron-sparing surgery may be done when both kidneys are involved or when the contralateral kidney is threatened by an associated disease such as hypertension or diabetes mellitus. Single-agent and combination chemotherapy have been used with limited success. Interferon and interleukin-2 have been used with some success. The 5-year survival rate for stage I disease ranges from 65% to 85%; 45% to 80% for stage II disease; 15% to 35% for stage III disease; and 0% to 10% for stage IV disease.

In summary, there are two major groups of renal neoplasms: embryonic kidney tumors (*i.e.*, Wilms' tumor) that occur during childhood and adult renal cell carcinomas. Wilms' tumor is the most common malignant tumor of children. The most common presenting signs are a large abdominal mass and hypertension. Treatment is surgery, chemotherapy, and sometimes radiotherapy. The long-term survival rate for children with Wilms' tumor is about 90% with an aggressive plan of treatment.

Adult kidney cancers account for 2% of all cancers. Renal cell carcinoma is the most frequent type of kidney cancer. These tumors are characterized by lack of early warning signs, diverse clinical manifestations, and resistance to chemotherapy and radiotherapy. Because of the lack of early warning signs, the tumors are often far advanced at the time of diagnosis. Diagnostic methods include ultrasonography and CT scans. The treatment of choice is surgical resection. Prognosis depends on the stage of the cancer; the 5-year survival rate for stage I tumors is 65% to 85%, and for stage IV tumors, it is 0% to 10%.

REFERENCES

1. National Kidney Foundation. (1988). Facts about transplantation and kidney and urologic diseases. In *KF news*. New York: National Kidney Foundation.
2. Manning F.A. (1987). Fetal surgery for obstructive uropathy: Rationale considerations. *American Journal of Kidney Diseases* 10, 259–267.
3. Stewart C.L., Jose P.A. (1991). Transitional nephrology. *Urologic Clinics of North America* 18, 143–149.
4. Glassberg K.I. (1988). Summary of the annual meeting of the section of pediatric urology. *Pediatrics* 81, 588.
5. Bennett W.M., Elzinga L.W., Barry J.M. (1992). Polycystic kidney disease: II. Diagnosis and management. *Hospital Practice* 27 (4A), 61–72.
6. Cotran R.S., Kumar V., Robbins S.L. (1994). *Pathologic basis of disease* (4th ed., pp. 1011–1081). Philadelphia: W.B. Saunders.
7. Spargo B.H., Haas M. (1994). The kidney. In: Rubin E., Farber J.L. (Eds.). *Pathology* (2nd ed., pp. 806–864). Philadelphia: J.B. Lippincott.
8. Grantham J.J. (1992). Polycystic kidney disease: I. Etiology and pathogenesis. *Hospital Practice* 27 (3A), 51–59.
9. Martinez J.R., Grantham J.J. (1995). Polycystic kidney disease: Etiology, pathogenesis, and treatment. *Disease-a-Month* 16 (11), 695–765.
10. Tanagho E.A. (1995). Urinary obstruction and stasis. In Tanagho E.A., McAninch J.W. (Eds.). *Smith's general urology* (14th ed., pp. 172–185, 276–304). East Norwalk, CT: Appleton & Lange.
11. Morrison G. (1997). Kidney. In: Tierney L.M., McPhee S.J., Papadakis M.A. (Eds.). *Current medical diagnosis and treatment* (36th ed., pp. 840–849). Stamford, CT: Appleton & Lange.
12. Worchester E.M. (1996). Inhibitors of stone formation. *Seminars in Nephrology* 16 (5), 474–486.
13. Coe F.L., Parks J.H., Asplin J.R. (1992). The pathogenesis and treatment of kidney stones. *New England Journal of Medicine* 327, 1141–1152.
14. Kupin W.L. (1995). A practical approach to nephrolithiasis. *Hospital Practice* 30 (3) 15, 57–66.
15. Stamm W.E., Hooton T.M. (1993). Management of urinary tract infections in adults. *New England Journal of Medicine* 329 (18), 1328–1334.
16. Hooton T.M. (1995). A simplified approach to urinary tract infection. *Hospital Practice* 28 (2) 15, 23–30.
17. Andriole V.T. (1987). Urinary tract infections: Recent developments. *Journal of Infectious Diseases* 156, 865.
18. Lindberg U., Bjure J., Haugstvedt S., et al. (1975). Asymptomatic bacteriuria in schoolgirls: III. Relation between residual urine volume and recurrence. *Acta Paediatrica Scandinavica* 64, 437.
19. Spencer J.R., Schaeffer A.J. (1986). Pediatric urinary tract infections. *Urologic Clinics of North America* 13, 661–672.
20. Krieger J.N. (1986). Complications and treatment of urinary tract infections during pregnancy. *Urologic Clinics of North America* 13, 685–693.
21. Andriole V.T., Patterson T.F. (1991). Epidemiology, natural history, and management of urinary tract infections during pregnancy. *Medical Clinics of North America* 75, 359– 373.
22. Zelikovic I., Adelman R.D., Nancarrow R.A. (1992). Urinary tract infections in children—An update. *Western Journal of Medicine* 157, 554–556.
23. Yoshikawa T.T. (1993). Chronic urinary tract infections in elderly patients. *Hospital Practice* 28 (6), 103–118.
24. Zweig S. (1987). Urinary tract infections in the elderly. *American Family Practice* 35 (5), 123–130.
25. Baldassare J.S., Kaye D. (1991). Special problems of urinary tract infection in the elderly. *Medical Clinics of North America* 75, 375–390.
26. Ofek I., Goldhar J., Jafairi D., Lis H., Adar R., Sharon N. (1991). Anti-*Escherichia coli* adhesin activity of cranberry and blueberry juice. *New England Journal of Medicine* 324, 1599.
27. Avorn J., Monane M., Gurwitz J.H., Glynn R.J., Choodnovskiy I., Lipsitz L.A. (1994). Reduction of bacteria and pyuria after ingestion of cranberry juice. *Journal of the American Medical Association* 271, 751–754.
28. Morrison G. (1997). Kidney. In Tierney L.M., McPhee S.J., Papadakis M.A. (Eds.). *Current medical diagnosis and treatment* (36th ed., pp. 840–849). Norwalk, CT: Appleton & Lange.
29. Vincenti F.G., Amend W.J.C. (1995). Diagnosis of medical renal diseases. In Tanagho E.A., McAninch J.W. (Eds.). *Smith's general urology* (14th ed., pp. 592–603). E. Norwalk, CT: Appleton & Lange.
30. Cameron J.S. (1987). The nephrotic syndrome and its complications. *American Journal of Kidney Diseases* 10, 163–171.
31. Donadeo J.J., Bergstrohl E.J., Offord K.P., et al. (1993). A controlled study of fish oil in IgA nephropathy. *New England Journal of Medicine* 331, 1194.
32. Dunfee T.P. (1995). The changing management of diabetic nephropathy. *Hospital Practice* 30 (5), 45–55.
33. Davidman M., Schmitz P. (1988). Renal tubular acidosis: A pathophysiologic approach. *Hospital Practice* 23 (1), 77–96.
34. Kurtzman N.A. (1987). Renal tubular acidosis: A constellation of syndromes. *Hospital Practice* 22 (11), 173.
35. Arruda J.A.L., Cowell G. (1994). Distal renal tubular acidosis: Molecular and clinical aspects. *Hospital Practice* 29 (1), 75–88.
36. Andriole V.T. (1985). The role of Tamm-Horsfall protein in the pathogenesis of reflux nephropathy and chronic pyelonephritis. *Yale Journal of Biology and Medicine* 58, 91.
37. Palmer B., Hendrich W.L. (1995). Clinical acute renal failure with nonsteroidal anti-inflammatory drugs. *Seminars in Nephrology* 15 (3), 214–227.
38. Sheaver P.D., Wilimas J.A. Neoplasms of the kidney. In: Behrman R.E., Kiegman R.M., Arvin A.M. (Eds). *Nelson textbook of pediatrics* (15th ed., pp. 1463–1464). Philadelphia: W.B. Saunders.
39. Motzer R.J., Bander N.H., Nanus D.M. (1997). Medical progress: Renal-cell carcinoma. *New England Journal of Medicine* 335 (21), 865–875.

ADDITIONAL READINGS

Allen T.D. (1992). Commentary: Voiding dysfunction and reflux. *Journal of Urology* 148, 1706–1707.

Baylis C., Schmidt R. (1996). The aging glomerulus. *Seminars in Nephrology* 16 (4), 265–76.

Davison J.M. (1987). Overview: Kidney function in pregnant women. *American Journal of Kidney Diseases* 14, 248– 252.

Fick G.M., Gabow P.A. (1994). Natural history of autosomal polycystic kidney disease. *Annual Review of Medicine* 45, 23–79.

Hooton T.M., Scholes D., Hughes J.P., et al. (1996). A prospective study of risk factors for symptomatic urinary tract infections in young women. *New England Journal of Medicine* 335 (7), 468–474.

Hooten T.M., Stamm W.E. (1991). Management of uncomplicated urinary tract infections in adults. *Medical Clinics of North America* 75, 339–357.

Klienknecht D. (1995). Interstitial nephritis, the nephrotic syndrome, and chronic renal failure secondary to nonsteroidal anti-inflammatory drugs. *Seminars in Nephrology* 15 (3), 228–235.

Koff A. (1992). Relationship between dysfunctional voiding and reflux. *Journal of Urology* 148, 1703–1705.

Mahnensmith R.L. (1993). Diabetic nephropathy: A comprehensive approach. *Hospital Practice* 28 (3), 129–148.

Mogensen C.E. (1995). Management of early nephropathy in diabetic patients. *Annual Review of Medicine* 46, 79–94.

Richardson K., Gennon C. (1991). Renal function in the preterm neonate: An overview. *Neonatal Network* 10 (4), 17–23.

Ronald A. (1996). Sex and urinary tract infections. *New England Journal of Medicine* 335 (7), 511–512.

Svanborg C. (1993). Resistance to urinary tract infection. *New England Journal of Medicine* 329 (11), 802–803.

Sobel J.D., Reinhart H. (1991). Antibacterial host factors in the urinary tract. *Advances in Internal Medicine* 131–151.

Warren J.W. (1991). The catheter and urinary tract infections. *Medical Clinics of North America* 75, 481–493.

CHAPTER 29

Renal Failure

Susan Gallagher-Lepak

Renal failure is a condition in which the kidneys fail to remove metabolic end products from the blood and to regulate the fluid, electrolyte, and pH balance of the extracellular fluids. The underlying cause may be renal pathology, systemic disease, or urologic defects of nonrenal origin. Renal failure can occur as an acute or a chronic disorder. Acute renal failure is abrupt in onset and often is reversible if recognized early and treated appropriately. In contrast, chronic renal failure is the end result of irreparable damage to the kidneys. It develops slowly, usually over the course of a number of years.

Acute Renal Failure

After you have completed this section of the chapter, you should be able to meet the following objectives:

- List risk factors that predispose to development of acute renal failure
- Define acute renal failure and compare prerenal, intrarenal, and extrarenal forms of the disorder and cite common causes of each
- Describe the clinical manifestations of the oliguric and diuretic phases of acute tubular necrosis

Acute renal failure represents a sudden decrease in renal function sufficient to increase nitrogenous wastes and impair fluid and electrolyte balance. It is a common threat to seriously ill persons in intensive care units. The mortality rate for acute renal failure is high, ranging from 42% to 88%.[1] Although treatment methods such as dialysis and renal replacement methods are effective in correcting life-threatening fluid and electrolyte disorders, the mortality from acute renal failure has not changed substantially during the past 50 years.[2] This is probably because acute renal failure is seen more often in older persons than before and because it is frequently superimposed on the condition that caused the renal failure—heart failure, shock, prostatic hyperplasia, and others. Because of the high mortality rate, it is important that measures be taken to prevent its occurrence. Also, because acute renal failure is potentially reversible, it is important that early signs be recognized so that appropriate treatment measures can be instituted promptly.

The most common indicator of acute renal failure is the accumulation of nitrogenous wastes in the blood. The term *azotemia* is commonly used to describe an abnormally high blood level of nitrogenous wastes (*i.e.*, urea nitrogen, uric acid, and creatinine) related to acute renal failure. Azotemia is largely related to a decrease in the glomerular filtration rate (GFR) and the inability of the kidneys to filter nitrogenous waste products from the blood.

Types of Acute Renal Failure

Acute renal failure can be caused by several conditions, including a decrease in blood flow without ischemic injury; ischemic, toxic, or obstructive tubular injury; or obstruction of urinary tract outflow. The causes of acute renal failure can be categorized as prerenal, postrenal, and intrarenal (Chart 29–1).

Prerenal Failure

Prerenal failure results from impaired renal blood flow that, if sustained, predisposes to tubular necrosis. Prerenal failure is reversible if the cause of renal hypofunction can be identified and corrected before damage to the renal cells occurs. Causes of prerenal failure include severe hemorrhage, profound volume depletion, cardiogenic shock, decreased vascular filling because of increased vascular capacity caused by anaphylaxis or sepsis, and operative procedures associated with interrupted renal blood flow. Elderly persons are particularly at risk because of their predisposition to hypovolemia and high prevalence of renal vascular disorders. Angiotensin-converting enzyme inhibitors reduce the effects of renin on renal blood flow; when combined with diuretics, they may cause prerenal failure in persons with decreased blood flow due to large-vessel or small-vessel renal vascular disease. Prostaglandins have a vasodilatory effect on renal blood vessels. Nonsteroidal antiinflammatory drugs (NSAIDs) reduce renal blood flow through inhibition of prostaglandin synthesis. In some persons with diminished renal perfusion, NSAIDs can precipitate prerenal failure.[3,4]

Normally, the kidneys receive 20% to 25% of the cardiac output. This large blood supply is necessary to maintain the high GFR rates needed to remove metabolic wastes and regulate body fluids and electrolytes. Fortunately, the normal kidney can tolerate relatively large reductions in blood flow before renal cell damage occurs. As renal blood flow is reduced, the GFR drops, and the amount of sodium chloride (and water and other substances) that is filtered by the glomeruli is reduced, and the need for energy-dependent transport mechanisms is reduced (see Chapter 25). As the GFR and urine output approach zero, oxygen consumption by the kidney approximates that required to keep renal tubular cells alive.[5] When blood flow falls below this level, which is usually about 20% of normal, ischemic changes occur. Because of their high metabolic rate, the tubular epithelial cells are most vulnerable to ischemic injury. Improperly treated, prolonged renal hypoperfusion can lead to ischemic tubular necrosis with significant morbidity and mortality.

The GFR is decreased in acute renal failure, and little or no urine is formed. One of the earliest manifestations of prerenal failure is a sharp decrease in urine output. Because a low GFR allows more time for smaller particles such as urea to be reabsorbed into the blood, there is also a disproportionate elevation in the blood urea nitrogen (BUN) to serum creatinine ratio (normally about 10:1). Creatinine, which is larger and nondiffusible, remains in the tubular fluid, and the total amount of creatinine that is filtered, although small, is excreted in the urine.

CHART **29-1**
Causes of Acute Renal Failure

Prerenal
Hypovolemia
- Dehydration
- Loss of gastrointestinal fluid
- Hemorrhage
- Fluid sequestration

Septicemia
- Septic shock

Heart failure
Interruption of renal blood flow caused by surgery or other causes

Intrarenal
Acute tubular necrosis
- Prolonged renal ischemia
- Exposure to nephrotoxic drugs
  - Aminoglycosides (*e.g.*, gentamycin, kanamycin, colistin, others)
  - Radiocontrast agents
  - Nonsteroidal antiinflammatory agents
  - Others
- Exposure to heavy metals (*e.g.*, lead, mercury)
- Exposure to organic solvents (*e.g.*, carbon tetrachloride, ethylene glycol)

Acute glomerulonephritis
Acute pyelonephritis

Postrenal
Ureteral obstruction (*e.g.*, calculi, tumors)
Bladder outlet obstruction (*e.g.*, prostatic hyperplasia, ureteral strictures)

Intrarenal Failure

Intrarenal causes of acute renal failure are categorized according to the primary site of injury: tubular, interstitial, or glomerulus. Injury to the tubules is most common and is often ischemic or toxic in origin. The major causes of intrarenal failure are ischemia associated with prerenal failure, toxic insult to the tubular structures of the nephron, and intratubular obstruction. Intrarenal pathology such as acute glomerulonephritis and acute pyelonephritis are also intrarenal causes of acute renal failure.

Toxic Agents and Obstruction. Common causes of acute tubular damage are nephrotoxic drugs and toxic products of microorganisms responsible for septicemia.[6] The aminoglycoside antibiotics and contrast agents such as those used during cardiac catheterization are the most common nephrotoxic agents implicated in acute tubular necrosis.[2,3,4,7] Several factors contribute to aminoglycoside toxicity, including a decrease in the GFR, preexisting renal disease, hypovolemia, and concurrent administration of other drugs that have a nephrotoxic effect.[2] The risk of renal damage caused by radiopaque contrast media is greatest in elderly persons, in persons with diabetes mellitus, and in persons who, for one reason or another, are susceptible to kidney disease. Allergic drug reactions are common causes of acute interstitial nephritis. Heavy metals (*e.g.*, lead, mercury) and organic solvents (*e.g.*, carbon tetrachloride, ethylene glycol) are other nephrotoxic agents.

Intratubular obstructions are caused by the accumulation of casts and cellular debris that accompanies severe hemolytic reactions or myoglobinuria. Skeletal and cardiac muscles contain myoglobin, which accounts for their rubiginous color. Myoglobin corresponds to hemoglobin in function, serving as an oxygen reservoir within the muscle fibers. Myoglobin normally is not found in the serum or urine. It has a low molecular weight of 17,000; if it escapes into the circulation, it is rapidly filtered in the glomerulus. Myoglobinuria most commonly results from muscle trauma but may result from extreme exertion, hyperthermia, sepsis, prolonged seizures, potassium or phosphate depletion, and alcoholism or drug abuse. Hemoglobin may also escape into the glomerular filtrate when serum levels are markedly increased as a result of a severe hemolytic reaction. Both myoglobin and hemoglobin discolor the urine, which may range from the color of tea to red, brown, or black.

Acute Tubular Necrosis. Acute damage to tubular structures is commonly referred to as *acute tubular necrosis*. The most common cause of acute tubular necrosis is prolonged acute prerenal failure.

The course of acute tubular necrosis usually has four successive phases: onset or initiating phase, oliguric or anuric phase, diuretic phase, and recovery or convalescent phase.[6] The onset or initiating phase is the time from the onset of the precipitating event (*e.g.*, ischemic phase of prerenal failure) until tubular injury occurs. The oliguric phase is represented by a decrease in urine output. Oliguria (urine output <400 ml/day) is more common in postischemic forms of acute tubular necrosis, and nonoliguria (urine output >400 ml/day) is more common in toxic tubular necrosis. When oliguria occurs, it starts shortly after the initiating event and lasts an average of 10 to 14 days.

Formerly, most patients with acute tubular necrosis were oliguric.[8] During the past 2 decades, a nonoliguric form of renal failure has become increasingly prevalent.[7] This is probably the result of new approaches to the treatment of poor cardiac performance and circulatory failure that focus on vigorous plasma volume expansion and the selective use of dopamine, calcium-channel–blocking drugs, and naturetic peptide to improve renal blood flow.[2] Dopamine has renal vasodilator properties and inhibits sodium reabsorption in the proximal tubule, thereby decreasing the work demands of the nephron. Early reports suggest that patients with nonoliguric acute renal failure have a better prognosis than those with the oliguric (classic) form.[8]

The oliguric phase of acute tubular necrosis is characterized by a marked decrease in GFR, causing sudden retention of endogenous metabolites such as urea, potassium, sulfate, and creatinine that normally are cleared by the kidneys. Fluid retention gives rise to edema, water intoxication, and pulmonary congestion. If the period of oliguria is prolonged, hypertension frequently develops and with it signs of uremia. When untreated, uremia's neurologic manifestations progress from neuromuscular irritability to seizures, somnolence, coma, and death. Hyperkalemia usually is asymptomatic until serum levels of potassium rise above 6.0 to 6.5 mEq/L, at which point characteristic electrocardiographic changes and symptoms of muscle weakness are seen. Persons with nonoliguric failure have higher levels of glomerular filtration and excrete more nitrogenous waste, water, and electrolytes in their urine than persons with acute oliguric renal failure. Abnormalities in blood chemistry levels usually are milder and cause fewer complications.

The diuretic phase of acute renal failure typically begins within a few days to 6 weeks after oliguria, indicating that the nephrons have recovered to the point where urine excretion is possible. Diuresis usually occurs before renal function has returned to normal. Consequently, BUN and serum creatinine, potassium, and phosphate levels may remain elevated or continue to rise even though urine output is increased. In some cases, the diuresis may result from impaired nephron function and may cause excessive loss of water and electrolytes. During the convalescent phase, renal function recovers slowly. The GFR usually returns to 70% to 80% of normal within 1 to 2 years. In some cases, mild to moderate kidney damage persists.

Postrenal Failure

Postrenal failure results from obstruction of urine outflow from the kidneys. The obstruction can occur in the ureter (*i.e.*, calculi and strictures), bladder (*i.e.*, tumors or neurogenic bladder), or urethra (*i.e.*, prostatic hypertrophy). Prostatic hyperplasia is the most common underlying problem. Because both ureters must be occluded to produce renal failure, obstruction of the bladder rarely causes acute renal failure unless one of the kidneys is already damaged or a person has only one kidney. The treatment of acute postrenal failure consists of treating the underlying cause of obstruction so that urine flow can be reestablished before permanent nephron damage occurs.

Diagnosis and Treatment

Given the high morbidity and mortality associated with acute renal failure, attention should be focused on prevention. This includes assessment measures to identify persons at risk for developing acute renal failure, including those with preexisting renal insufficiency and diabetes. These persons are particularly at risk for developing acute renal failure due to nephrotoxic drugs such as aminoglycosides and contrast agents or to drugs such as the NSAIDs that alter intrarenal hemodynamics. Elderly persons are susceptible to all forms of acute renal failure because of the effects of aging on renal reserve.

Careful observation of urine output is essential for persons at risk for developing acute renal failure. Urine tests that measure urine osmolality, urinary sodium concentration, and fractional excretion of sodium help differentiate prerenal azotemia, in which the reabsorptive capacity of the tubular cells is maintained, from tubular necrosis, in which these functions are lost. One of the earliest manifestations of tubular damage is the inability to concentrate the urine.

Further diagnostic information that can be obtained from the urinalysis includes evidence of proteinuria, hemoglobinuria, and casts or crystals in the urine. Blood tests for BUN and creatinine provide information regarding the ability to remove nitrogenous wastes from the blood. It is also important to exclude urinary obstruction.

A major concern in the treatment of acute renal failure is identifying and correcting the cause (*e.g.*, improving renal perfusion, discontinuing nephrotoxic drugs). Fluids are carefully regulated in an effort to maintain normal fluid volume and electrolyte concentrations. Adequate caloric intake is needed to prevent the breakdown of body proteins, which increases nitrogenous wastes. Parenteral hyperalimentation may be used for this purpose. Because secondary infections are a major cause of death in persons with acute renal failure, constant effort is needed to prevent and treat such infections.

Dialysis or continuous renal replacement therapy (CRRT) may be indicated when nitrogenous wastes and the water and electrolyte balance cannot be kept under control by other means. Venovenous or arteriovenous CRRT has emerged as a method for treating acute renal failure in patients too hemodynamically unstable to tolerate hemodialysis. An associated advantage of the continuous-replacement therapies is the ability to administer nutritional support. The disadvantages are the need for prolonged anticoagulation and continuous sophisticated monitoring.

In summary, acute renal failure is an acute reversible suppression of kidney function. It is a common threat to seriously ill persons in intensive care units, with a mortality rate of 42% to 88%. Acute renal failure is characterized by an accumulation of nitrogenous wastes in the blood (*i.e.*, azotemia) and alterations in body fluids and electrolytes. Acute renal failure is classified as prerenal, intrarenal, or postrenal in origin. Prerenal failure is caused by decreased blood flow to the kidneys; postrenal failure by obstruction to urine output; and intrarenal failure by disorders within the kidney itself. Intrarenal failure is most often the result of acute tubular necrosis resulting from hypoxia associated with prerenal failure or from exposure of the kidney to nephrotoxic agents.

Acute tubular necrosis typically progresses through four phases: onset or initiating phase, oliguric or anuric phase, diuretic phase, and recovery or convalescent phase. Because of the high morbidity and mortality rates associated with acute renal failure, identification of persons at risk is important to clinical decision making. Acute renal failure is often reversible, making early identification and correction of the underlying cause (e.g., improving renal perfusion, discontinuing nephrotoxic drugs) important. Treatment includes the judicious administration of fluids and dialysis or CRRT.

Chronic Renal Failure

After you have completed this section of the chapter, you should be able to meet the following objectives:

- State the definitions of renal impairment, renal insufficiency, and end-stage renal disease
- List the common problems associated with end-stage renal disease, including fluid and electrolyte imbalances, osteodystrophy, hematologic disorders, alterations in immune function, neurologic manifestations, skin problems, and altered sexual function and explain their physiologic significance
- State the basis for adverse drug reactions in patients with end-stage renal disease
- Describe the scientific principles underlying dialysis treatment, and compare hemodialysis with peritoneal dialysis
- Cite the complications of kidney transplantation
- State the goals for dietary management of persons with end-stage renal disease as they relate to protein restrictions; carbohydrate, fat, and caloric needs; and potassium, sodium, calcium, phosphate, and fluid intake

Unlike acute renal failure, chronic renal failure represents progressive and irreversible destruction of kidney structures. As recently as 30 years ago, many patients with chronic renal failure progressed to the final stages of the disease and then died. The high mortality rate was associated with limitations in the treatment of renal disease and with the tremendous cost of ongoing treatment. In 1972, federal support began for dialysis and transplantation through a Medicare entitlement program. Technologic advances in renal replacement therapy (*i.e.*, dialysis therapy and transplantation) have improved the outcomes for persons with renal disease. In the United States, more than 500,000 persons with end-stage renal disease are living today, a product of continued research and advances in treatment methods.[9]

Chronic renal failure can result from a number of conditions that cause permanent loss of nephrons, including uncontrolled hypertension, urinary tract obstruction and infection, hereditary defects of the kidneys, disorders of the glomeruli, and systemic diseases such as diabetes mellitus and systemic lupus erythematosus. Regardless of cause, chronic renal failure results in progressive deterioration of glomerular filtration, tubular reabsorptive capacity, and endocrine functions of the kidneys. All forms of renal failure are characterized by a reduction in the GFR, reflecting a corresponding reduction in functional nephrons.

The signs and symptoms of renal failure typically occur gradually and do not become evident until the disease is far advanced. This is because of the amazing compensatory ability of the kidneys. As kidney structures are destroyed, the remaining nephrons undergo structural and functional hypertrophy, each increasing its function as a means of compensating for those that have been lost (Fig. 29–1). It is only when the few remaining nephrons are destroyed that the manifestations of renal failure become evident.

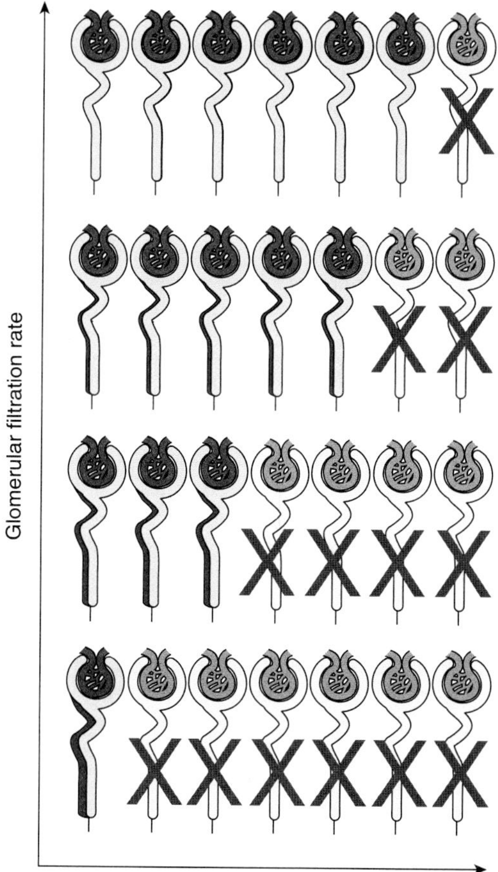

Figure 29–1
Relation of renal function and nephron mass. Each kidney contains 1 million tiny nephrons. A proportional relation exists between the number of nephrons affected by disease and the resulting glomerular filtration rate.

Stages of Progression

The rate of nephron destruction differs from case to case, ranging from several months to many years. The progression of chronic renal failure usually occurs in four stages: diminished renal reserve, renal insufficiency, renal failure, and end-stage renal disease.[10]

Diminished Renal Reserve

Diminished renal reserve occurs when the GFR is about 50% of normal. Serum BUN and creatinine levels are normal, and no symptoms of impaired renal function are evident. Because of the diminished reserve, the risk of developing azotemia increases with an additional renal insult such as that due to nephrotoxic drugs.

Renal Insufficiency

Renal insufficiency represents a reduction in the GFR of about 20% to 50% of normal. During this stage, azotemia, anemia, and hypertension appear. Signs and symptoms of renal insufficiency do not begin to appear until more than one half of the function in both kidneys is lost. This is supported by the fact that many persons survive an entire lifetime with only one kidney. The kidneys initially have tremendous adaptive capabilities. As nephrons are destroyed, the remaining nephrons undergo changes to compensate for those that are lost. In the process, each of the remaining nephrons must filter more solute particles from the blood. Because the solute particles are osmotically active, they cause additional water to be lost in the urine. One of the earliest symptoms of renal failure is *isosthenuria,* which is polyuria that is almost isotonic with plasma.

Conservative treatment during this stage includes measures to retard deterioration of renal function and assist the body in managing the effects of impaired function. Because the kidneys have difficulty eliminating the waste products of protein metabolism, a restricted-protein diet usually produces fewer uremic symptoms and slows progression of renal failure. The few remaining nephrons that constitute the functional reserve of the kidneys can be easily disrupted; at that point, renal failure progresses rapidly.

Renal Failure

Renal failure develops when the GFR is less than 20% to 25% of normal. The kidneys cannot regulate volume and solute composition, and edema, metabolic acidosis, and hypercalcemia develop. Overt uremia may ensue with neurologic, gastrointestinal, and cardiovascular complications.

End-Stage Renal Disease

End-stage renal disease occurs when the GFR is less than 5% of normal. Histologic findings of an end-stage kidney include a reduction in renal capillaries and scarring in the glomeruli. Atrophy and fibrosis are evident in the tubules. The mass of the kidneys usually is reduced. At this final phase of renal failure, treatment with dialysis or transplantation is necessary for survival.

Clinical Manifestations

Azotemia is an early sign of renal failure, usually occurring before other symptoms become evident. Urea is one of the first nitrogenous wastes to accumulate in the blood, and the BUN level becomes increasingly elevated as renal failure progresses. The normal concentration of urea in the plasma is about 26 mg/dl. In renal failure, this level may rise to as high as 800 mg/dl. Creatinine, a byproduct of muscle metabolism, is freely filtered in the glomerulus and is not reabsorbed in the renal tubules. Because creatinine is produced at a relatively constant rate and because any creatinine that is filtered in the glomerulus is lost in the urine rather than being reabsorbed into the blood, serum creatinine can be used as an indirect method for assessing the GFR and the extent of renal damage that has occurred in renal failure (see Chapter 25).

Uremia, which means urine in the blood, is the term used to describe the clinical manifestations of end-stage renal disease. Few symptoms of uremia appear until at least two thirds of the nephrons have been destroyed. Uremia differs from azotemia, which merely indicates the accumulation of nitrogenous wastes in the blood and can occur without symptoms. The uremic state includes signs and symptoms of altered fluid, electrolyte, and acid-base balance; alterations in regulatory functions (*e.g.*, hypertension, anemia, osteodystrophy); and accumulation of waste products (*e.g.*, uremic encephalopathy, peripheral neuropathy, pruritus). At this stage, virtually every organ and structure in the body is affected. The symptoms at the onset of uremia (*e.g.*, weakness, fatigue, nausea, apathy) often are subtle. More severe symptoms include extreme weakness, frequent vomiting, lethargy, and confusion. Without treatment, coma and death follow. These changes are summarized in Table 29–1.

Water, Sodium, Potassium, and Acid-Base Balance

Chronic renal failure can produce dehydration or fluid overload, depending on the pathology of the renal disease. In addition to volume regulation, the ability of the kidneys to concentrate the urine and eliminate or conserve necessary electrolytes is diminished. An early sign of impaired renal function is the inability of the kidneys to regulate the concentration of urine. In renal failure, the specific gravity of the urine becomes fixed (1.008 to 1.012) and varies little from voiding to voiding. Polyuria and nocturia are common.

As renal function declines further, the ability to regulate sodium excretion is reduced. The kidneys normally tolerate large variations in sodium intake (from 1 to 900 mEq) while maintaining normal serum sodium levels. In chronic renal failure, they lose the ability to regulate sodium excretion. There is impaired ability to adjust to a sudden reduction in sodium intake and poor tolerance of an acute sodium overload. Volume depletion with an accompanying decrease in the GFR can occur with a restricted sodium intake or excess sodium loss caused by diarrhea or vomiting. Salt wasting is a common problem in advanced renal failure because of impaired tubular reabsorption of sodium. Increasing sodium intake in persons with chronic renal failure often improves the GFR and whatever renal function remains. In patients with associated hypertension, the possibility of increasing blood pressure or producing congestive heart failure often excludes supplemental sodium intake.

About 90% of potassium excretion is through the kidneys. In renal failure, potassium excretion by each nephron increases as the kidneys adapt to a decrease in the GFR. As a result, hyperkalemia usually does not develop until renal function is severely compromised. Because of this adaptive mechanism, it usually is not necessary to restrict potassium intake in patients with chronic renal failure until the GFR has dropped below 5 ml/minute.[10] In patients with chronic renal failure, hyperkalemia often results from failure to follow dietary potassium restrictions and ingestion of medications that contain potassium or from an endogenous release of potassium, as in trauma or infection.

The kidneys normally regulate blood pH by eliminating hydrogen ions produced in metabolic processes and regenerating bicarbonate. This is achieved through hydrogen ion secretion, sodium and bicarbonate reabsorption, and the production of ammonia, which acts as a buffer for titratable acids (see Chapter 27). With a decline in renal function, these mechanisms become impaired, and metabolic acidosis results. In chronic renal failure, acidosis seems to stabilize as the disease progresses, probably as a result of the tremendous buffering capacity of bone. This buffering action is thought to increase bone resorption and contribute to the skeletal defects present in chronic renal failure.

Calcium, Phosphate, and Bone Metabolism

Abnormalities of calcium, phosphorus, and vitamin D metabolism occur early in the course of chronic renal failure. The regulation of serum phosphate levels requires a daily urinary excretion of an amount equal to that ingested in the diet. With deteriorating renal function, phosphate excretion is impaired, and as a result, serum phosphorus levels rise. At the same time, serum calcium levels, which are inversely regulated in relation to serum phosphorus levels, fall (see Chapter 26). The drop in serum calcium caused by hyperphosphatemia stimulates parathyroid hormone release, with a resultant increase in calcium resorption from bone. Although serum calcium levels are maintained through increased parathyroid function, this adjustment is accomplished at the expense of the skeletal system and other body organs. Most persons with end-stage renal disease develop secondary hyperparathyroidism, the result of chronic stimulation of the parathyroid glands. It has been suggested that other growth factors and suppressors of bone formation (*e.g.*, cytokines) and persistent hypogonadism may be involved in altered bone metabolism seen in persons with end-stage renal disease.[11]

The kidneys control vitamin D activity by converting the inactive form of vitamin D (25-hydroxycholecalciferol) to its active form (1,25-dihydroxycholecalciferol).

TABLE 29-1

Alterations in Body Function That Occur With Chronic Renal Failure

Body System	Change in Function	Manifestation
Body fluids	Compensatory changes in tubular functions	Fixed specific gravity of urine; polyuria and nocturia
	Decreased ability to synthesize ammonia and conserve bicarbonate	Metabolic acidosis
	Inability to excrete potassium	Hyperkalemia
	Inability to regulate sodium excretion	Salt wasting or sodium retention
	Impaired ability to excrete phosphate	Hyperphosphatemia
	Hyperphosphatemia and inability to activate vitamin D	Hypocalcemia and increased levels of parathyroid hormone
Hematologic	Impaired synthesis of erythropoietin and effects of uremia	Anemia
	Impaired platelet function	Bleeding tendencies
Cardiovascular	Activation of renin-angiotensin mechanism, increased vascular volume, and failure to produce vasopressor substances	Hypertension
	Fluid retention and hypoalbuminemia	Edema
	Excess extracellular fluid volume, anemia	Congestive heart failure; pulmonary edema
	Increased metabolic wastes in blood	Uremic pericarditis
Gastrointestinal	Increased metabolic wastes	Anorexia, nausea, vomiting
	Decreased platelet function and increased gastric acid secretion due to hyperparathyroidism	Gastrointestinal bleeding
Neurologic	Fluid and electrolyte imbalance	Headache
	Increase in metabolic acids and other small, diffusible particles, such as urea	Signs of uremic encephalopathy: lethargy, decreased alertness, loss of recent memory, delirium, coma, seizures, asterixis, muscle twitching, and tremulousness
		Signs of neuropathy: restless leg syndrome, paresthesias, muscle weakness, and paralysis
Osteodystrophy	High bone turnover (Osteitis fibrosa)	Muscle weakness
	Hyperphosphatemia	Bone pain and tenderness
	Hypocalcemia	spontaneous fractures
	Low levels of activated vitamin D	
	Secondary hyperparathyroidism	
	Low bone turnover (Osteomalacia)	
	Aluminum intoxication	
Skin	Calcium × phosphate concentration product greater than 60	Extracellular calcifications
	Salt wasting	Dry skin and mucous membranes
	Anemia	Pale, sallow complexion
	Hyperparathyroidism	Pruritus
	High concentration of metabolic end products in body fluids	Uremic frost and odor of urine on skin and breath
Genitourinary	Impaired general health	
	Decreased testosterone	Impotence and loss of libido
	Decreased estrogen	Amenorrhea and loss of libido

With vitamin D deficiency, there is decreased intestinal absorption of calcium and increased secretion of parathyroid hormone. Vitamin D also regulates osteoblast differentiation, thereby affecting bone matrix formation and mineralization.[11]

Renal Osteodystrophy. Renal osteodystrophy is the term used to describe the skeletal complications of end-stage renal disease. The renal osteodystrophies include osteitis fibrosa, osteomalacia, adynamic renal bone disease, and mixed disease that contains features of osteitis and osteomalacia.[11] Inherent to all of these conditions is abnormal reabsorption and defective remodeling of bone (see Chapter 46). The symptoms of renal osteodystrophy, which occur late in the disease, include bone tenderness and muscle weakness. Proximal muscle weakness in the lower extremities is common, making it difficult to get out of a chair or climb stairs.[12] Fractures are more common with osteomalacia and adynamic renal bone disease.

Several factors are thought to contribute to the development of renal osteodystrophy, including elevated serum phosphate levels, decreased serum calcium levels, impaired renal activation of vitamin D, hyperparathyroidism, and aluminum intoxication. Aluminum is minimally absorbed from the gastrointestinal tract and is eliminated by the kidney.[13a] Aluminum toxicity impairs osteoblast and osteoclast function, resulting in defective mineralization of bone.

Osteitis fibrosa, which is the most common type of renal osteodystrophy in North America, is often referred to as *high bone turnover disease.*[12] It is thought to result from hypocalcemia, hyperphosphatemia, and low levels of activated vitamin D, along with impaired regulation of locally produced growth factors and inhibitors. The disorder is characterized by secondary hyperparathyroidism and increased osteoblast and osteoclast numbers and activity. Although the osteoblasts produce excessive amounts of bone matrix, mineralization fails to keep pace, and there is a decrease in bone density and formation of porous and coarse-fibered bone. Cortical bone is affected more severely than cancellous bone. Marrow fibrosis is another component of osteitis fibrosa; it occurs in areas of increased bone cell activity. In advanced stages of the disorder, cysts may develop in the bone, a condition called *osteitis fibrosa cystica.*

Osteomalacia is characterized by decreased numbers of osteoclasts and osteoblasts, a low rate of bone turnover, and an accumulation of unmineralized bone matrix. It is often referred to as *low bone turnover disease.* The most common cause of osteomalacia is aluminum intoxication. Aluminum intoxication causes decreased and defective mineralization of bone by existing osteoblasts and more long-term inhibition of osteoblast differentiation. Aluminum intoxication also inhibits osteoclast function. During the 1970s and 1980s, it was discovered that accumulation of aluminum from water used in dialysis and aluminum salts used as phosphate binders caused osteomalacia and adynamic bone disease.[11] This discovery led to a change in the composition of dialysis solutions and substitution of calcium carbonate for aluminum salts as phosphate binders. As a result, the prevalence of osteomalacia in persons with end-stage renal disease is declining.

A second type of low turnover osteodystrophy is called *adynamic or aplastic renal osteodystrophy.* In persons with adynamic bone disease, bone remodeling is greatly reduced, and the bone surfaces become hypocellular.[11] The disease is associated with an increased fracture rate. It has been suggested that hypersecretion of parathyroid hormone may be necessary to maintain normal rates of bone formation in persons with end-stage renal disease. Thus, this form of renal osteodystrophy is seen more commonly in persons with end-stage renal disease who do not have secondary hyperparathyroidism (*i.e.,* those who have been treated with parathyroidectomy) and have been overtreated with calcium and vitamin D. It is also seen in persons with diabetes mellitus or persons with aluminum intoxication.

Extracellular Calcifications. Soft tissue calcification, or *metastatic calcification* of the cornea, arteries, subcutaneous tissues, and muscle, can occur when the calcium × phosphate concentration product rises higher than 60 (see Chapter 26). This is seen after dialysis has been instituted and usually is associated with a rapid rise in the calcium level, which precedes a fall in the phosphate level. When serum phosphorous levels are high, administration of pharmaceutical preparations of activated vitamin D may increase the calcium × phosphate concentration product, leading to extraskeletal calcifications. Calcium deposits in the eyes cause conjunctivitis and often are evidenced by "band" keratopathy. Calcium deposits in the skin cause intense itching.

Hematologic Function

Chronic anemia is the most profound hematologic alteration that accompanies renal failure. Persons with renal failure experience a gradual reduction in hematocrit as renal function deteriorates. An untreated low hematocrit for a person on hemodialysis may stabilize at about 20%.

The kidneys are the primary site for the production of the hormone *erythropoietin,* which controls red blood cell production. In renal failure, erythropoietin production usually is insufficient to stimulate adequate red blood cell production by the bone marrow. The accumulation of uremic toxins further suppresses red cell production in the bone marrow, and the cells that are produced have a shortened life span. Many persons on maintenance hemodialysis are iron deficient because of blood sampling and accidental loss of blood during dialysis. The manifestations of anemia include pallor, tachycardia, widened pulse pressure, and decreased exercise tolerance. Pharmaceutical preparations of recombinant erythropoietin has increased the well-being of persons with chronic renal failure.

Bleeding disorders manifested by epistaxis, menorrhagia, gastrointestinal bleeding, and bruising of the skin and subcutaneous tissues are common in persons with end-stage renal disease. Although platelet production is normal in number, platelet function is impaired, causing bleeding problems. The problem improves with dialysis but does not completely normalize.

Altered Immune Function

Infection is a common complication and cause of hospitalization and death of patients with chronic renal failure. Immunologic abnormalities decrease the efficiency of the immune response to infection. All aspects of inflammation and immune function may be affected adversely by the high levels of urea and metabolic wastes.[11] This includes a decrease in granulocyte count, impaired humoral and cell-mediated immunity, and defective phagocyte function. The acute inflammatory response and delayed-type hypersensitivity response are impaired. Although persons with end-stage renal disease have normal humoral responses to vaccines, a more aggressive immunization program may be needed. Skin and mucosal barriers to infection may also be defective. In persons who are maintained on dialysis, vascular access devices are common portals of entry for pathogens. Many persons with end-stage renal disease fail to develop fever with an infection, making the diagnosis more difficult.

Cardiovascular Function

Cardiovascular disorders, including hypertension, congestive heart failure, and pericarditis, are common among persons with end-stage renal disease. Atherosclerosis is also accelerated. The most notable abnormality is an elevation in serum triglyceride levels, which is thought to result from decreased removal rather than increased production.

Hypertension commonly is an early manifestation of chronic renal failure. The mechanisms that produce hypertension in end-stage renal disease are multifactorial; they include an increased vascular volume, elevation of peripheral vascular resistance, decreased levels of renal vasodilator prostaglandins, and increased activity of the renin angiotensin system.[13b] Individuals on erythropoietin replacement have increased blood viscosity that can worsen hypertension. *Uremic pericarditis* is a term used to describe pericarditis of unknown origin in persons with end-stage renal disease. It can result from metabolic toxins associated with the uremic state or from dialysis.

Uremic pericarditis is seen less frequently because of the early initiation of dialysis. When it does occur, it usually is related to inadequate dialysis or an infection. It is characterized by sudden onset of pain, usually on the left side of the chest, with respiratory accentuation. Typically, the pericardial fluid is hemorrhagic. Cardiac tamponade may occur (see Chapter 19).

Congestive heart failure and pulmonary edema tend to occur in the late stages of renal failure. Increased extracellular fluid volume resulting from sodium and water retention, proteinuria, and hypoalbuminemia contribute to the disorder.

Gastrointestinal Function

Anorexia, nausea, and vomiting are common in patients with uremia, along with a metallic taste in the mouth that further depresses the appetite. Early-morning nausea is common. Ulceration and bleeding of the gastrointestinal mucosa may develop, and hiccups are common. A possible cause of nausea and vomiting is the decomposition of urea by intestinal flora, resulting in a high concentration of ammonia. Parathyroid hormone increases gastric acid secretion and contributes to gastrointestinal problems. Nausea and vomiting often improve with restriction of dietary protein and after initiation of dialysis and disappear after kidney transplantation.

Neurologic Function

Many persons with chronic renal failure have alterations in peripheral and central nervous system function. Peripheral neuropathy, or involvement of the peripheral nerves, affects the lower limbs more frequently than the upper limbs. It is symmetric and affects sensory and motor function. Neuropathy is caused by atrophy and demyelination of nerve fibers, possibly caused by uremic toxins. Restless legs syndrome is a manifestation of peripheral nerve involvement and can be seen in as many as two thirds of patients on dialysis. This syndrome is characterized by creeping, prickling, and itching sensations that typically are more intense at rest. Temporary relief is obtained by moving the legs. A burning sensation of the feet, which may be followed by muscle weakness and atrophy, is a manifestation of uremia.

The central nervous system disturbances in uremia are similar to those caused by other metabolic and toxic disorders. Sometimes referred to as *uremic encephalopathy*, the condition is poorly understood and may result, at least in part, from an excess of toxic organic acids that alter normal mechanisms, preventing their crossing of the blood-brain barrier. Electrolyte abnormalities, such as sodium shifts, may also contribute. The manifestations are more closely related to the progress of the uremic disorder than to the level of the metabolic end products. Reductions in alertness and awareness are the earliest and most significant indications of uremic encephalopathy. This often is followed by an inability to fix attention, loss of recent memory, and perceptual errors in identifying persons and objects. Delirium and coma occur late in the course; seizures are the preterminal event.

Disorders of motor function commonly accompany the neurologic manifestations of uremic encephalopathy. During the early stages, there often is difficulty in performing fine movements of the extremities; the gait becomes unsteady and clumsy with *tremulousness* of movement. *Asterixis*, dorsiflexion movements of the hands and feet, typically occurs as the disease progresses. It can be elicited by having the person hyperextend his or her arms at the elbow and wrist with the fingers spread apart. If asterixis is present, this position causes side-to-side flapping movements of the fingers.

Skin Integrity

Skin manifestations are common in persons with renal failure. The skin is often pale owing to anemia and may have a sallow, yellow-brown hue. The skin and mucous membranes are often dry, and subcutaneous bruising is common. Skin dryness is caused by a reduction in perspiration owing to the decreased size of sweat glands and the diminished activity of oil glands. Pruritus is common; it results from the high serum phosphate levels and the development of phosphate crystals that occur with hyperparathyroidism. Severe scratching or repeated needlesticks, especially with hemodialysis, break the skin integrity and increase the risk for infection. In the advanced stages of untreated renal failure, urea crystals may precipitate on the skin as a result of the high urea concentration in body fluids. The fingernails may become thin and brittle, with a dark band just behind the leading edge of the nail, followed by a white band. This appearance is known as *Terry's nails.*

Sexual Function

The cause of sexual dysfunction in men and women with chronic renal failure is unclear. The cause probably is multifactorial and may result from high levels of uremic toxins, neuropathy, altered endocrine function, psychologic factors, and medications (*e.g.*, antihypertensive drugs). Alterations in physiologic sexual responses, reproductive ability, and libido are common.

Impotence occurs in as many as 56% of male dialysis patients.[14] Derangements of the pituitary and gonadal hormones, such as decreases in testosterone levels and increases in prolactin and luteinizing hormone levels, are common and cause erectile difficulties and decreased spermatocyte counts. Loss of libido may result from chronic anemia and decreased testosterone levels. Several drugs, such as exogenous testosterone and bromocriptine, have been used in an attempt to return hormone levels to normal.

Impaired sexual function in women is manifested by abnormal levels of progesterone, luteinizing hormone, and prolactin. Hypofertility, menstrual abnormalities, decreased vaginal lubrication, and various orgasmic problems have been described.[15] Amenorrhea is common among women who are on dialysis therapy.

Elimination of Drugs

The kidneys are responsible for the elimination of many drugs and their metabolites. Renal failure and its treatment can interfere with the absorption, distribution, and elimination of drugs. The administration of large quantities of phosphate-binding antacids to control hyperphosphatemia and hypocalcemia in patients with advanced renal failure interferes with the absorption of some drugs. Many drugs are bound to plasma proteins, such as albumin, for transport in the body; the unbound portion of the drug is available to act at the various receptor sites and is free to be metabolized. A decrease in plasma proteins, particularly albumin, that occurs in many persons with end-stage renal disease results in less protein-bound drug and greater amounts of free drug.

In the process of metabolism, some drugs form intermediate metabolites that are toxic if not eliminated. This is true of meperidine (Demerol); it is metabolized to the toxic intermediate normeperidine, which causes excessive sedation, nausea, and vomiting. Some pathways of drug metabolism, such as hydrolysis, are slowed with uremia. In persons with diabetes, for example, insulin requirements may be reduced as renal function deteriorates.[16] Decreased elimination by the kidneys allows drugs or their metabolites to accumulate in the body and requires that drug dosages be adjusted accordingly. Some drugs contain unwanted nitrogen, sodium, potassium, and magnesium and must be avoided in patients with renal failure. Penicillin, for example, contains potassium. Nitrofurantoin and ammonium chloride add to the body's nitrogen pool. Many antacids contain magnesium. Because of problems with drug dosing and elimination, persons with renal failure should be cautioned against the use of over-the-counter remedies.

Treatment

During the past several decades, an increasing number of persons have required renal replacement therapy with dialysis or transplantation. The growing volume is largely attributable to the improvement in treatment and more liberal policies regarding who is treated. Between 1980 and 1992, there was a twofold reported increase in treatment for end-stage renal disease.[17] About 45,000 Americans now begin renal replacement therapy each year, compared with 18,000 new patients during 1980.[18] In 1991, almost 122,000 persons were maintained by dialysis therapy in the United States and another 9900 underwent kidney transplantation operations.[17]

Medical Management

Chronic renal failure can treated by conservative management of renal insufficiency and by renal replacement therapy with dialysis or transplantation. Conservative treatment consists of measures to prevent or retard deterioration in remaining renal function and to assist the body in compensating for the existing impairment. Interventions that have been shown to significantly retard the progression of chronic renal insufficiency include dietary protein restriction and blood pressure normalization. Various interventions are used to compensate for reduced renal function and to correct the resulting anemia, hypocalcemia, and acidosis. These interventions often are used in conjunction with dialysis therapy for patients with renal insufficiency.

A remarkable advance in medical management over the past decade has been the development of recombinant human erythropoietin (rhEPO) to treat profound anemia in patients with end-stage renal disease.[19] Erythropoietin, which is primarily produced by the kidneys, acts on the bone marrow by stimulating erythroblast maturation to maintain the hematocrit level. Since its approval by the Food and Drug Administration in June 1989, rhEPO therapy has been used to maintain hematocrit levels in the range of 28% to 33%, with an upper limit of 36%. Secondary benefits of the therapy, previously attributed to the correction of uremia, include improvement in appetite, energy level, sexual function, skin color, and hair and nail growth, and reduced cold intolerance. The regular use of this medication has reduced the need among dialysis patients for regular blood transfusions to treat anemia. Frequent measurements of hematocrit are necessary. Worsening hypertension and seizures have occurred when the hematocrit was raised too suddenly.[19]

Early treatment of hypocalcemia and hyperphosphatemia is important to prevent or slow long-term bone complications, such as osteodystrophy. Phosphate-binding antacids—calcium carbonate or calcium acetate—are frequently prescribed to decrease absorption of phosphate from the gastrointestinal tract. Phosphate binders work best if taken with meals. Aluminum-containing antacids should be avoided, because they contribute to the development of osteodystrophy. Milk products and other foods high in phosphorus content are restricted in the diet. Activated forms of vitamin D (calcitriol) and calcium supplements often are used to facilitate intestinal absorption of calcium, increase serum calcium levels, and reduce parathyroid hormone levels. Metabolic acidosis, which occurs as a result of the kidneys' inability to appropriately regulate body pH, is treated with sodium bicarbonate.

Treatment of hypertension involves salt and water restriction, and some persons with renal insufficiency need to have antihypertensive medications to control blood pressure.[13] Most persons with renal insufficiency need to take several antihypertensive medications to control blood pressure. A diuretic and a calcium channel blocker, angiotensin-converting enzyme inhibitor, α-adrenergic antagonist, or a β-adrenergic–blocking drug are often prescribed (see Chapter 18). In the later stage of renal failure, dialysis is needed to maintain the extracellular fluid volume.

Dialysis and Transplantation

Dialysis or renal replacement therapy is indicated when advanced uremia or serious electrolyte imbalances are present. The choice between dialysis and transplantation is dictated by age, related health problems, donor availability, and personal preference. Although transplantation often is the treatment preference, dialysis plays a critical role as a treatment method for end-stage renal disease. It is life-sustaining for persons who are not candidates for transplantation or who are awaiting transplantation. There are two broad categories of dialysis: hemodialysis and peritoneal dialysis.

Hemodialysis. The basic principles of hemodialysis have remained unchanged over the years, although new technology has improved the efficiency and the speed of dialysis. A hemodialysis system, or artificial kidney, consists of three parts: a blood compartment, a dialysis fluid compartment, and a cellophane membrane that separates the two compartments. There are several types of dialyzers; all incorporate these parts, and all function in a similar manner.

The cellophane membrane is semipermeable, permitting all molecules except blood cells and plasma proteins to move freely in both directions—from the blood into the dialyzing solution and from the dialyzing solution into the blood. The direction of flow is determined by the concentration of the substances contained in the two solutions. The waste products and excess electrolytes in the blood normally diffuse into the dialyzing solution. If there is a need to replace or add substances, such as bicarbonate, to the blood, these can be added to the dialyzing solution (Fig. 29–2).

During dialysis, blood moves from an artery through the tubing and blood chamber in the dialysis machine and then back into the body through a vein. Access to the vascular system is accomplished through an external arteriovenous shunt (*i.e.*, tubing implanted into an artery and a vein) or, more commonly, through an internal arteriovenous fistula (*i.e.*, anastomosis of a vein to an artery, usually in the forearm). Heparin is used to prevent clotting during the dialysis treatment; it can be administered continuously or intermittently. Problems that may occur during dialysis, depending on the blood flow rate and rate of solute removal, include hypotension, nausea, vomiting, muscle cramps, headache, chest pain, and disequilibrium syndrome.

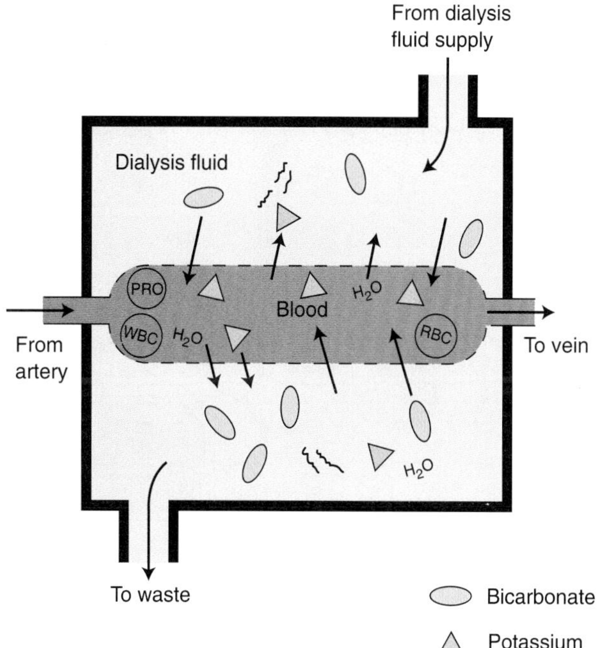

Figure 29–2
Schematic diagram of a hemodialysis system. The blood compartment and dialysis solution compartment are separated by a cellophane membrane. This membrane is porous enough to allow all the constituents, except the plasma proteins and blood cells, to diffuse between the two compartments.

Most persons are dialyzed three times each week for 3 to 4 hours; treatment is determined by kinetic profiles, referred to as KT/V values, which consider dialyzer size, dialysate, flow rate, time of dialysis, and body size. The adequacy of dialysis is a significant predictor of mortality; the clinical standard for hemodialysis is a KT/V of 1.2. [20] Many dialysis centers provide the option for patients to learn how to perform hemodialysis at home.

Peritoneal Dialysis. The same principles of diffusion, osmosis, and ultrafiltration that apply to hemodialysis apply to peritoneal dialysis. The thin serous membrane of the peritoneal cavity serves as the dialyzing membrane. A Silastic catheter is surgically implanted in the peritoneal cavity below the umbilicus to provide access. The catheter is tunneled through subcutaneous tissue and exits on the side of the abdomen (Fig. 29–3). The dialysis process involves instilling a sterile dialyzing solution (usually 2 L) through the catheter over 10 minutes. The solution is then allowed to remain, or dwell, in the peritoneal cavity for a prescribed amount of time, during which the metabolic end products and extracellular fluid diffuse into the dialysis solution. Commercial dialysis solution is available in 1.5%, 2.5%, and 4.25% dextrose concentrations. Solutions with higher dextrose levels increase osmosis, causing more fluid to be removed. At the end of the dwell time, the dialysis fluid is drained out of the peritoneal cavity by gravity into a sterile bag.

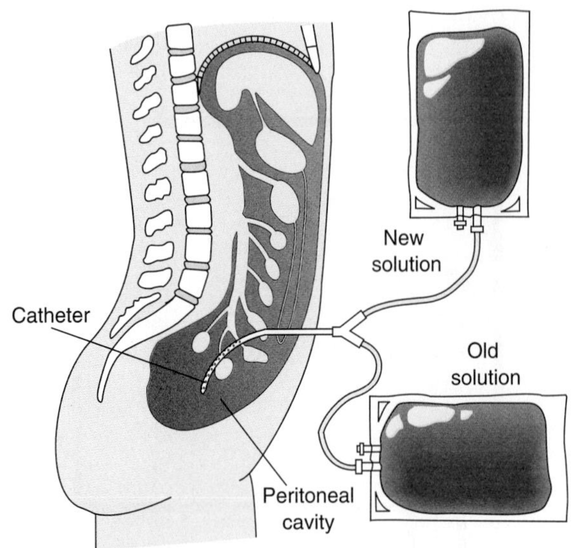

Figure 29–3
Peritoneal dialysis. A semipermeable membrane, richly supplied with small blood vessels, lines the peritoneal cavity. With dialysate dwelling in the peritoneal cavity, waste products diffuse form the network of blood cells into the dialysate.

Peritoneal dialysis can be performed at home or in a center, by an automated or manual system, and on an intermittent or continuous basis—all with variations in the number of exchanges and in dwell time. Individual preference, manual ability, lifestyle, knowledge of the procedure, and physiologic response to treatment influence the dialysis schedule.

The most common method is continuous ambulatory peritoneal dialysis (CAPD). It is a self-care procedure in which the person manages the dialysis procedure and the type of solution (*i.e.*, dextrose concentration) used at home. CAPD involves instilling dialysate into the peritoneal cavity and rolling up the bag and tubing and securing them under clothing during the dwell. After the dwell time is completed (4 to 6 hours during the day), the bag is unrolled and lowered, allowing the waste-containing dialysis solution to drain from the peritoneal cavity into the bag. Each exchange, which involves draining the solution and infusing a new solution, requires about 30 to 45 minutes. Four exchanges usually are performed each day. The continuous rather than intermittent nature of CAPD ensures that the rapid fluctuations in extracellular fluid volume associated with hemodialysis are avoided, and dietary restrictions can be liberalized somewhat.

Potential problems with peritoneal dialysis include infection, catheter malfunction, dehydration caused by excessive fluid removal, hyperglycemia, and hernia. The most serious complication is infection, which can occur at the catheter exit site, in the subcutaneous tunnel, or in the peritoneal cavity (*i.e.*, peritonitis).

Transplantation. Greatly improved success rates have made kidney transplantation the treatment of choice for many patients with chronic renal failure. The availability of donor organs continues to limit the number of transplantations performed each year. Donor organs are obtained from cadavers and living, related donors (*e.g.*, parent, sibling). Transplants from living, nonrelated donors (*e.g.*, spouse) have been used in cases of suitable ABO and tissue compatibility. Of the transplantations performed from 1988 through 1991, 32,932 were from cadaver donors and 6482 were from living donors. The 1-year graft survival rates are about 83% for first-time cadaver-origin transplants; 80% for second-time cadaver-origin transplants; and 79% for subsequent cadaver-origin transplants.[21] The survival rates for grafts from living, related donors tend to be slightly higher. Simultaneous pancreas and kidney transplantation from a single cadaver donor has become an option for persons with end-stage renal disease and diabetes.[22]

The success of transplantation depends primarily on the degree of histocompatibility, adequate organ preservation, and immunologic management. Maintenance immunosuppressive therapy typically consists of corticosteroids, azathioprine, and cyclosporine. Monoclonal antibodies (*e.g.*, OKT-3) and antilymphocyte antibodies may be used as induction therapy.[22] Other immunosuppressive agents are being developed. Because of the increased number of effective immunosuppressive agents that have become available, lower corticosteroid doses are used, resulting in reduced cushingoid effects after transplantation.

Rejection, which is categorized as acute and chronic, can occur at any time. Acute rejection most commonly occurs during the first several months after transplantation and involves a cellular response with the proliferation of T lymphocytes. Chronic rejection can occur months to years after transplantation. Because chronic rejection is caused by cellular and humoral immunity, it does not respond to increased immunosuppressive therapy.

Maintenance immunosuppressive therapy and increased use of immunosuppression to treat rejection predispose the person to a spectrum of infectious complications. Prophylactic antimicrobials are prescribed to decrease the incidence of common infections, such as candidiasis, herpesvirus infections, and *Pneumocystis carinii* pneumonia. Other infections, such as cytomegalovirus infection and aspergillosis, are seen with chronic immunosuppression.

Dietary Management

A major component in the treatment of chronic renal failure is dietary management. The goal of dietary treatment is to provide optimum nutrition while maintaining tolerable levels of metabolic wastes. The specific diet prescription depends on the type and severity of renal disease and on the dialysis modality. Because of the severe restrictions placed on food and fluid intake, these diets may be complicated and unappetizing. After kidney transplantation, a less restrictive diet may be necessary, even when renal function is normal, to control the adverse effects from immunosuppressive medication.

Protein. Restriction of dietary proteins may decrease the progress of renal impairment in persons with advanced renal disease. Proteins are broken down to form nitrogenous wastes, and reducing the amount of protein in the diet lowers the BUN and reduces symptoms. Moreover, a high-protein diet is high in phosphates and inorganic acids. The *Modification of Diet in Renal Disease* (MDRD) study, which was conducted in 15 university hospital outpatient nephrology clinics and included 255 patients between the ages of 18 and 70 years, demonstrated a slower decline in GFR among patients randomized to the very-low-protein diet compared with patients on a low-protein diet.

Considerable controversy exists over the degree of restriction needed. If the diet is too low in protein, protein malnutrition can occur, with a loss of strength, muscle mass, and body weight. Results of the MDRD study indicate that protein requirements can be met by providing 0.6 g of protein per kilogram of body weight per day.[23] At least 60% of protein intake should contain proteins of high biologic value, such as eggs, lean meat, and milk, which are rich in essential amino acids. Proteins with a high biologic value are believed to promote the reuse of endogenous nitrogen, decreasing the amount of nitrogenous wastes that are produced and ameliorating the symptoms of uremia. In reusing nitrogen, the proteins ingested in the diet are broken down into their constituent amino acids and are recycled in the synthesis of protein required by the body. In contrast to proteins with a high biologic value, fewer than half of the amino acids in cereal proteins are reused. Amino acids that are not reused to build body proteins are broken down and form the end products of protein metabolism, such as urea.

Persons who are on peritoneal dialysis require a greater protein intake because of significant protein losses, ranging from 4 to 13 g/day, through dialysis. Even higher protein losses can occur with peritonitis. With kidney transplantation, high doses of prednisone, especially during the immediate postoperative period or during acute rejection episodes, accelerate protein catabolism.[24] Diets with a higher protein content can often help to reverse steroid-induced negative nitrogen balance.[25]

Carbohydrates, Fat, and Calories. With renal failure, adequate calories in the form of carbohydrates and fat are required to meet energy needs. This is particularly important when the protein content of the diet is severely restricted. If sufficient calories are not available, the limited protein in the diet goes into energy production, or body tissue itself is used for energy purposes. Caloric intake for persons on CAPD includes food intake and calories absorbed from the dialysis solution. A 2-L bag of 1.5% dialysate solution equals 105 calories, and a 4.25% solution delivers 289 calories.[26] A 70-kg man on CAPD with an ideal caloric intake of 40 kcal/kg, or 2800 calories, who uses two bags of 1.5% solution and two bags of 4.25% solution per day only needs to ingest about 2000 calories (*i.e.*, 788 calories are from dialysate).

Calories often need to be limited after kidney transplantation, because weight gain is common. Reducing the intake of dietary fats and increasing the percentage of polyunsaturated fats can reduce hyperlipidemia after transplantation.[27]

Potassium. When the GFR falls to extremely low levels and when undergoing hemodialysis therapy, dietary restriction of potassium becomes mandatory. Using salt substitutes that contain potassium or ingesting fruits, fruit juice, chocolate, potatoes, or other high-potassium foods can cause hyperkalemia. Most persons on continuous peritoneal dialysis do not need to limit potassium intake and often may even need to increase intake.

Sodium and Fluid Intake. The sodium and fluid restrictions depend on the kidneys' ability to excrete sodium and water and must be individually determined. Renal disease of glomerular origin is more likely to contribute to sodium retention, whereas tubular dysfunction causes salt wasting. Fluid intake in excess of what the kidneys can excrete causes circulatory overload, edema, and water intoxication. Thirst is a common problem among hemodialysis patients, often resulting in large weight gains between treatments. Increased thirst appears to be related to elevated renin levels and the production of angiotensin II.[28] Inadequate intake, on the other hand, causes volume depletion and hypotension and can cause further decreases in the already compromised GFR. It is common practice to allow a daily fluid intake of 500 to 800 ml, which is equal to insensible water loss plus a quantity equal to the 24-hour urine output.

Exercise

The many medical problems that result from renal failure lead to reductions in physical functioning, energy level, and exercise capacity. Variables that strongly affect rehabilitation include age, diabetic status, and treatment mode. With the initiation of dialysis, younger adults usually have higher activity levels than older adults.[29]

The exercise capacity, as measured by maximal oxygen consumption, for persons treated with hemodialysis or peritoneal dialysis is below that of sedentary healthy persons and those who have had successful kidney transplantations.[30] Suggested causes of reduced exercise capacity include anemia, altered peripheral metabolism of lactate, cardiac changes caused by uremia, and general physical deconditioning. Because of this, some dialysis centers have exercise training programs (*e.g.*, cycling) during hemodialysis treatments.

In summary, chronic renal failure results from the destructive effects of many forms of renal disease. Regardless of the cause, the consequences of nephron destruction in end-stage renal disease are alterations in the filtration, reabsorption, and endocrine functions of the kidneys. The progression of chronic renal failure usually occurs in four stages: diminished renal reserve, renal insufficiency, renal failure, and end-stage renal disease. Renal insufficiency represents a reduction in the GFR of about 20% to 50% of normal; renal failure, a reduction of less than 20% to 25% of normal; and end-stage renal disease, a decrease in GFR of less than 5% of normal.

End-stage renal disease affects almost every body system. It causes an accumulation of nitrogenous wastes (i.e., azotemia), alters sodium and water excretion, and alters regulation of body levels of potassium, phosphate, calcium, and magnesium. It also causes skeletal disorders, anemia, alterations in cardiovascular function, neurologic disturbances, gastrointestinal dysfunction, and discomforting skin changes.

The treatment of end-stage renal disease can be divided into two types: conservative management of renal insufficiency and renal replacement therapy with dialysis or transplantation. Conservative treatment consists of measures to prevent or retard deterioration in remaining renal function and to assist the body in compensating for the existing impairment. Interventions that have been shown to significantly retard the progression of chronic renal insufficiency include dietary protein restriction and blood pressure normalization. The use of activated vitamin D can be used to increase calcium absorption and control secondary hyperparathyroidism. Recombinant human erythropoietin (rhEPO) is used to treat the profound anemia that occurs in persons with end-stage renal disease.

Renal Failure in Children and Elderly Persons

After you have completed this section of the chapter, you should be able to meet the following objectives:

- List the causes of renal failure in children and describe the special problems of children with end-stage renal disease
- State why renal failure is so common in the elderly and describe measures to prevent or delay the onset of end-stage renal disease in this population
- Describe the treatment of end-stage renal disease in children and the elderly

Although the spectrum of renal disease among children and elderly persons is similar to that of adults, several unique issues affecting these groups warrant further discussion.

Chronic Renal Failure in Children

The true incidence of chronic renal failure in infants and children is unknown. The data indicate that 2500 children in the United states who are younger than 20 years begin treatment for chronic renal failure each year; 100 of these children are younger than 2 years of age.[31] The most common cause of chronic renal failure in children is glomerulonephritis and congenital malformations, such as renal hypoplasia or dysplasia, obstructive uropathy, and reflux nephropathy.[31]

Features of renal disease that are marked during childhood include severe growth impairment, developmental delay, delay in sexual maturation, bone abnormalities, and development of psychosocial problems. Critical growth periods occur during the first 2 years of life and during adolescence. Physical growth and cognitive development occur at a slower rate as consequences of renal disease, especially among children with congenital renal disease. Puberty usually occurs at a later age in children with renal failure partly because of endocrine abnormalities. Renal osteodystrophy is more common and extensive in children than in adults because of the presence of open epiphyses. As a result, metaphyseal fractures, bone pain, impaired bone growth, short stature, and osteitis fibrosa cystica occur with greater frequency. Some hereditary renal diseases, such as medullary cystic disease, have patterns of skeletal involvement that further complicate the problems of renal osteodystrophy. Factors related to impaired growth include deficient nutrition, anemia, renal osteodystrophy, chronic acidosis, and cases of nephrotic syndrome that require high-dose corticosteroid therapy.

Success of treatment depends on the level of bone maturation at the initiation of therapy. Nutrition is believed to be the most important determinant during infancy.[32] During childhood, growth hormone is important, and gonadotrophic hormones become important during puberty.[32] The use of parental heights provides a means of assessing growth potential. For many children, catch-up growth is important, because a growth deficit is frequently established during the first months of life.

Recombinant human growth hormone (rhGH) therapy has been used to improve growth in children with end-stage renal disease.[33,34] Success of treatment depends on the level of bone maturation at the initiation of therapy.

All forms of renal replacement therapy can be safely and reliably used for children. Hemodialysis of a premature infant as small as 1500 g has been achieved with only modest difficulties.[35] Children typically are treated with CAPD or transplantation to optimize growth and development. Renal transplantation is considered the best alternative for children.[31,32,34] Early transplantation in young children is regarded as the best way to promote physical growth, improve cognitive function, and foster psychosocial development.[33,36,37] Immunosuppressive therapy in children is similar to that used in adults. All of these immunosuppressive agents have side effects, including increased risk of infection. Corticosteroids, which have been the mainstay of chronic immunosuppressive therapy for decades, carry the risk of hypertension, orthopedic complications (especially aseptic necrosis), cataracts, and growth retardation.

Chronic Renal Failure in Elderly Persons

Adults who are 65 years or older account for about 45% of new patients each year with end-stage renal disease. In particular, the group older than 74 years has shown a four-fold increase in incidence during the past decade.[9] Among elderly persons, the presentation and course of renal failure may be altered because of age-related changes in the kidneys and concurrent medical conditions.

Normal aging is associated with a decline in the GFR and subsequently with reduced homeostatic regulation under stressful conditions. This reduction in GFR makes elderly persons more susceptible to the detrimental effects of nephrotoxic drugs, such as x-ray contrast compounds. The reduction in GFR related to aging is not accompanied by a parallel rise in the serum creatinine level, because the serum creatinine level, which results from muscle metabolism, is significantly reduced in elderly persons because of diminished muscle mass and other age-related changes. Evaluation of renal function in elderly persons should include a measurement of creatinine clearance along with the serum creatinine level. The Cockcoft and Gault equation is gaining popularity as an estimate of renal function with allowance for age.[38] An indirect estimate of creatinine clearance (in ml/minute) is provided by this equation:

$$\text{Creatinine clearance} = \frac{(140 - \text{age}) \times (\text{body weight in kg})}{72 \times \text{serum creatinine in mg/dl}}$$

The equation result should be multiplied by a factor of 0.85 for women.

The prevalence of chronic disease that affects the cerebrovascular, cardiovascular, and skeletal systems is higher in this age group. Because of concurrent disease, the presenting symptoms of renal disease in elderly persons may be less typical than those observed in younger adults. For example, congestive heart failure and hypertension may be the dominant clinical features with the onset of acute glomerulonephritis, whereas oliguria and cola-colored urine are more often the first signs in younger adults.[39] The course of renal failure may be more complicated in older patients with numerous chronic diseases.

Treatment options for chronic renal failure in elderly patients include hemodialysis, peritoneal dialysis, transplantation, and acceptance of death from uremia. The general reduction in T-cell function with age has been suggested as a beneficial effect that increases transplant graft survival.

In summary, there is about a 2% incidence per year of renal failure in children, most frequently resulting from congenital malformations and glomerulonephritis. Problems associated with renal failure in children include growth impairment, delay in sexual maturation, and more extensive bone abnormalities than in adults. Although all forms of renal replacement therapy can be safely and reliably used for children, CAPD or transplantation optimize growth and development.

Adults 65 years of age and older account for close to one half of the new cases of end-stage renal disease each year. Normal aging is associated with a decline in the GFR, which makes elderly persons more susceptible to the detrimental effects of nephrotoxic drugs and other conditions that compromise renal function. Treatment options for chronic renal failure in elderly patients are similar to those for younger persons.

REFERENCES

1. Levy E.M., Viscoli C.M., Horwitz R.I. (1996). The effect of acute renal failure on mortality: A cohort analysis. *Journal of the American Medical Association* 275 (19), 1489–1494.
2. Thadhani R., Pascual M., Bonventre J.V. (1996). Acute renal failure. *New England Journal of Medicine* 334 (22), 1448–1460.
3. Garella S. (1993). Drug-induced renal disease. *Hospital Practice* 28(4), 129–140.
4. Bailie G.R. (1996). Acute renal failure. In Young L.Y., Koda-Kimble M.A. *Applied therapeutics: The clinical use of drugs* (6th ed., chap. 29). Vancouver, WA: Applied Therapeutics.
5. Guyton A., Hall J.E. (1996). *Textbook of medical physiology* (9th ed., pp. 410–418). Philadelphia: W.B. Saunders.
6. Lancaster L. (1990). Renal response to shock. *Critical Care Clinics of North America* 2 (2), 221–233.
7. Anderson R.J. (1993). Prevention and management of acute renal failure. *Hospital Practice* 28(8), 61–75.
8. Myers B.D., Moran S.M. (1986). Hemodynamically mediated acute renal failure. *New England Journal of Medicine* 314, 97–105.
9. Friedman E.A. (1996). End-stage renal disease: An American success story [Commentaries]. *Journal of the American Medical Association* 275 (14), 1118–1822.
10. Cotran R.S., Kumar V., Robbins S.L. (1994). *Robbins' pathologic basis of disease* (5th ed., pp. 932–933). Philadelphia: W.B. Saunders.
11. Brenner B.M., Lazarus J.M. (1991). Chronic renal failure. In Wilson J.D., Braunwald E., Isselbacher K.J., et al. (Eds.). *Harrison's principles of internal medicine* (12th ed., pp. 1150–1156). New York: McGraw-Hill.
12. Hrusks K.A., Teitelbaum S.L. (1995). Renal osteodystrophy. *New England Journal of Medicine* 333 (3), 166–174.

13a. Brunier G.M. (1994). Calcium/phosphate imbalances, aluminum toxicity, and renal osteodystrophy. *American Nephrology Nurses' Association Journal Journal* 21 (4), 171–177.

13b. Preston R.A., Singer I., Epstein M. (1996). Renal parenchymal hypertension. *Archives of Internal Medicine* 156, 602–611.

14. Rickus M.A. (1987). Sexual dysfunction in the female ESRD patient. *American Nephrology Nurses' Association Journal* 14 (3), 185, 186.
15. Foulks C.J., Cushner H.M. (1986). Sexual dysfunction in the male dialysis patient: Pathogenesis, evaluation, and therapy. *American Journal of Kidney Diseases* 8, 211, 212.
16. Rennett W.M., McCarron D.A. (1987). *Pharmacotherapy of renal disease and hypertension* (p. 5). New York: Churchill Livingston.

17. Agodaoa L.Y., Eggers P.W. (1995). Renal replacement therapy in the United States: Data from the United States Renal Data System. *American Journal of Kidney Disease* 25 (1), 119–133.
18. National Institute of Diabetes and Kidney Diseases. Division of Kidney, Urologic, and Hematologic Diseases. (1995). *United States Renal Data System: 1995 annual report*. Bethesda, MD: National Institutes of Health.
19. Lundeen P.A. (1991) Recombinant erythropoietin and chronic renal failure. *Hospital Practice* 26 (4A), 61–69.
20. Renal Physician's Association, Working Committee on Clinical Practice Guidelines. (1993). *Clinical practice guidelines on adequacy of hemodialysis*. Washington, DC: Renal Physician's Association.
21. Suthanthiran M., Strom T.B. (1994). Renal transplantation. *New England Journal of Medicine* 331 (6), 365–376.
22. Pirsch J., Andrews C., Hricik D., et. al. (1996). Pancreas transplantation for diabetes mellitus. *American Journal of Kidney Disease* 27 (3), 444–450.
23. Levey A.S., Adler S., Caggiula A.W., et al. (1996). Effects of dietary protein restriction on the progression of advanced renal disease in the modification of diet in renal disease study. *American Journal of Kidney Diseases* 27 (5), 652–663.
24. Hoy W.E., Sargent J.A., Hall D., et al. (1985). Protein catabolism during the postoperative course after renal transplantation. *American Journal of Kidney Diseases* 5, 187.
25. Cogan M.G., Sargent J.A., Yarbrough S.G., Vincenti F., Amend W.J. (1981). Prevention of prednisone-induced negative nitrogen balance. *Annals of Internal Medicine* 95, 160.
26. Harum P. (1984). Renal nutrition for the renal nurse. *American Nephrology Nurses' Association Journal* 8, 39.
27. Disler P.B., Goldberg R.B., Kuhn L., Meyers A.M., Joffe B.I., Seftel H.C. (1981). The role of diet in the pathogenesis and control of hyperlipidemia after renal transplantation. *Clinical Nephrology* 16, 31.
28. Porth C.M., Erickson M. (1992). Physiology of thirst and drinking: Implication for nursing practice. *Heart and Lung* 21 (3), 275.
29. Carlson D.M., Johnson W.J., Kjellstrand C.M. (1987). Functional status of patients with end-stage renal disease. *Mayo Clinic Proceedings* 62, 340.
30. Painter P., Messer-Rehak D., Hanson P., Zimmerman S.W., Glass N.R. (1986). Exercise capacity in hemodialysis, CAPD, and renal transplant patients. *Nephron* 42, 48.
31. Hanna J.D., Krieg R.J., Scheinman J.I., Chan J.C.M. (1996). Effects of uremia on growth in children. *Seminars in Nephrology* 16 (3), 230–241.
32. Abitbol C., Chan J.C.M., Trachtman H., Strauss J., Greifer I. (1996). Growth in children with moderate renal insufficiency: Measurement, evaluation, and treatment. *Journal of Pediatrics* 129 (2), S3–7.
33. Bereket G., Fine R.N. (1995). Pediatric renal transplantation. *Pediatric Clinics of North America* 42 (6), 1603–1627.
34. Warady B.A., Jabs K. (1995). New hormones in the therapeutic arsenal of chronic renal failure. *Pediatric Clinics of North America* 42 (6), 1551–1577.
35. Nevins T.E., Mauer S.M. (1984). Infant hemodialysis. In Fine R.N., Gruskin A.B. (Eds.). *End-stage renal disease in children* (p. 39). Philadelphia: W.B. Saunders.
36. Fennell R.S., Ruley E.J., Vehaskari M. (1996). Psychosocial aspects of care of the child with moderate renal failure. *Journal of Pediatrics* 129 (2), S8–12.
37. Frawman A.C., Myers J.T. (1994). Cognitive, psychosocial, and physical development in infants and children with end-stage renal disease. *Advances in Renal Replacement Therapy* 1 (1), 49, 54.
38. Levin M.L. (1989). The elderly patient with advanced renal failure. *Hospital Practice* 24 (3A), 35–44.
39. Burkart J.M., Beck L.H. (1990). Renal diseases in the elderly. In Hazzard W.R., Andres R., Bierman E.L., Blass J.P. (Eds.). *Principles of geriatric medicine and gerontology* (2nd ed., p. 565). New York: McGraw-Hill.

ADDITIONAL READINGS

Badr K., Ichikawa I. (1988). Prerenal failure: A deleterious shift from renal compensation to decompensation. *New England Journal of Medicine* 319, 623.

Blumenkrantz M.J., Gahl G.M., Kopple J.D., et al. (1981). Protein loss during peritoneal dialysis. *Kidney International* 19, 593.

Brezis M., Rosen S. (1995). Hypoxia of the renal medulla—Its implication for disease. *New England Journal of Medicine* 332 (10), 647–654.

Burton C., Harris K.P.G. (1996). The role of proteinuria in the progression of chronic renal failure. *American Journal of Kidney Diseases* 27 (6), 756–775.

Chesney R.W., Friedman A.L. (1984). The medical management of chronic renal failure. In Tune B.M., Mendoza S.A. (Eds.). *Pediatric nephrology* (p. 322). New York: Churchill Livingstone.

Coburn J.W., Salusky I.B. (1990). Control of serum phosphorus in uremia. *New England Journal of Medicine* 320, 1140–1142.

Druml W. (1995). Prognosis of acute renal failure. *Nephron* 73 (8), 8–15.

Eckhardt K., Kurtz A. (1992). The biological role, site, and regulation of erythropoietin production. *Advances in Nephrology from the Necker Hospital* 21, 203–233.

Epstein F.H., Brown R.S. (1988). Acute renal failure: A collection of paradoxes. *Hospital Practice* 23 (1), 171.

Evans D., Greenbaum L.A., Ettenger R.B. (1995). Principles of renal replacement therapy in children. *Pediatric Clinics of North America* 42 (6), 1579–1601.

Feldman H.I. (1991). Protein restriction in chronic renal failure. *Hospital Practice* 26 (6), 220–225.

Gutman R.A., Stead W.W., Robinson R.R. (1981). Physical activity and employment status of patients on maintenance dialysis. *New England Journal of Medicine* 304, 310.

Fine L.G. (1991). How much kidney tissue is enough. *New England Journal of Medicine* 325, 1097–1099.

Fraser C.L., Arieff A.I. (1988). Nervous system complications of uremia. *Annals of Internal Medicine* 109, 143.

Giordano C. (1977). The role of diet in renal disease. *Hospital Practice* 12 (11), 115–119.

Harmon WE. (1995). Treatment of children with chronic renal failure. *Kidney International* 47, 951–961.

Hatch F.E. (1990). Reversing the anemia of renal failure. *Hospital Practice* 25 (2A), 25–34.

Health Care Financing Administration. (1987). *U.S. transplant statistics*. Washington, DC: U.S. Department of Health and Human Services.

Ihle B.U., Becker J.A., Whitworth R.A., et al. (1989). The effect of protein restriction on progression of renal insufficiency. *New England Journal of Medicine* 321, 1773–1777.

Klahr S., Schreiner G., Ichikawa I. (1988). The progression of renal failure. *New England Journal of Medicine* 318, 1663, 1657.

Lee D.B., Goodman W.G., Coburn J.W. (1988). Renal osteodystrophy: Some questions on an old disorder. *American Journal of Kidney Diseases* 11, 365.

Levey A.S., Perrone R.D., Madias N.E. (1988). Serum creatinine and renal function. *Annual Review of Medicine* 39, 465.

Malluche H.H., Faugere M.C. (1989). Renal osteodystrophy. *New England Journal of Medicine* 321, 317–319.

McEnery P.T., Stablein D.M., Arbus G., Tejani A. (1992). Renal transplantation in children. *New England Journal of Medicine* 326 (26), 1730.

Morris P.J. (1991). Kidney transplantation, 1960–1990. *Advances in Nephrology* 20, 14.

Nolph K.D., Lindblad A.S., Novak J.W. (1988). Continuous ambulatory peritoneal dialysis. *New England Journal of Medicine* 318, 1595.

Price C.A. (1989). Continuous arteriovenous ultrafiltration: A monitoring guide for nurses. *Critical Care Nurse* 9 (1), 12–19.

Price C.A. (1991). Continuous renal replacement therapy: The treatment of choice for acute renal failure. *American Nephrology Nurses' Association Journal* 18 (3), 239.

Raskin N.H., Fisherman R.A. (1976). Neurological disorders in renal failure. *New England Journal of Medicine* 294, 143, 147.

Sedman A., Friedman A., Boineau F., Strife C.F., Fine R. (1996). Nutritional management of the child with mild to moderate renal failure. *Journal of Pediatrics* 129 (2), S13–17.

Sherwood L.M. (1987). Vitamin D, parathyroid hormone, and renal disease. *New England Journal of Medicine* 316, 1601.

Stapleton S., Wright J. (1992). Continuous arteriovenous hemofiltration: An alternative dialysis therapy in infants. *Neonatal Network* 11 (4), 17–25.

Tolkiff-Rubin N.E., Rubin R.H. (1990). Uremia and host defenses. *New England Journal of Medicine* 322, 770–772.

U.S. Renal Data System. (1991). ESRD in children. *American Journal of Kidney Diseases* 18 (5), 83.

Van Stone J.C. (1983). *Dialysis and the treatment of renal insufficiency* (pp. 1–31). New York: Grune & Stratton.

Walser M., Hill S., Tomalis E.A. (1996). Treatment of nephrotic adults with a supplemental very low-protein diet. *American Journal of Kidney Disease* 128 (3), 354–364.

Zeller K.R. (1991). Low-protein diets in renal disease. *Diabetes Care* 14 (9), 859, 861.

CHAPTER 30

Alterations in Urine Elimination

Although the kidneys control the formation of urine and regulate the composition of body fluids, it is the bladder that stores urine and controls its elimination from the body. Alterations in the storage and expulsion functions of the bladder can result in incontinence, with its accompanying social and hygienic problems, or obstruction of urinary flow, which has deleterious effects on ureteral and, ultimately, renal function. The discussion in this chapter focuses on normal control of urine elimination, urine retention, neurogenic bladder, incontinence, and bladder cancer. Urinary tract infections are discussed in Chapter 28.

Control of Urine Elimination

After you have completed this section of the chapter, you should be able to meet the following objectives:

- Trace the innervation of the bladder from the afferent stretch receptors to reflex control of detrusor muscle contraction and voluntary control of the external sphincter
- Explain the mechanism of low-pressure urine storage in the bladder
- List at least three classes of autonomic drugs and explain their potential effect on bladder function
- Describe at least three urodynamic studies that can be used to assess bladder function

The bladder, also known as the urinary vesicle, is a freely movable organ located behind the pelvic bone in the male and in front of the vagina in the female. It consists of two parts: the fundus, or body, and the neck, or posterior urethra. In the male, the urethra continues anteriorly through the penis. Urine passes from the kidneys to the bladder through the ureters, which are 4 to 5 mm in diameter and about 30 cm long. The ureters enter the bladder bilaterally at a location toward its base and close to the urethra (Fig. 30–1). The triangular area that is bounded by the ureters and the urethra is called the *trigone*. There are no valves at the ureteral openings, but as the pressure of the urine within the bladder rises, the ends of the ureters are compressed against the bladder wall to prevent the backflow of urine.

Bladder Structure

The bladder is composed of four layers. The first is an outer serosal layer, which covers the upper surface and is continuous with the peritoneum. The second is a net-

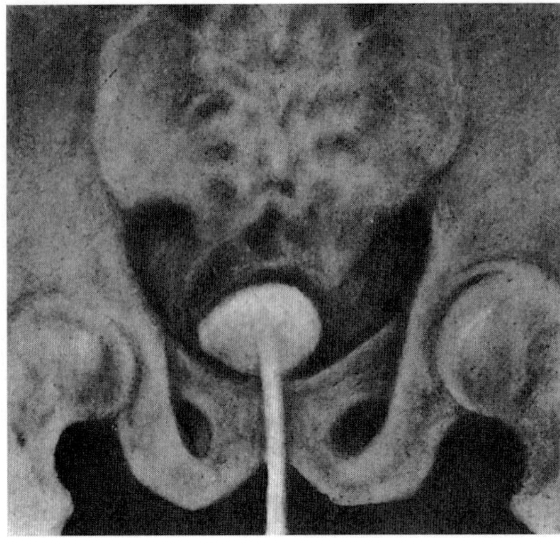

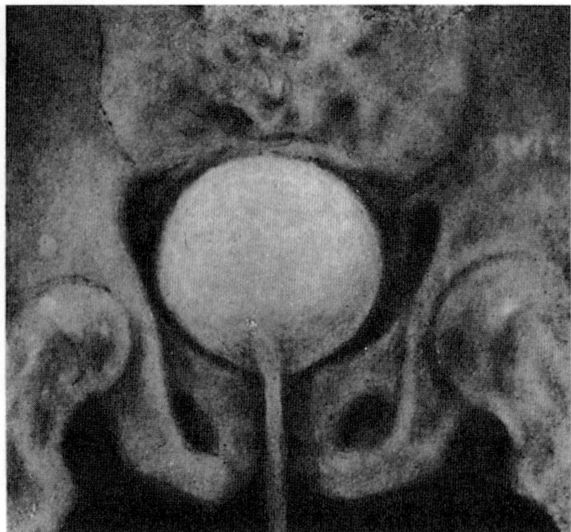

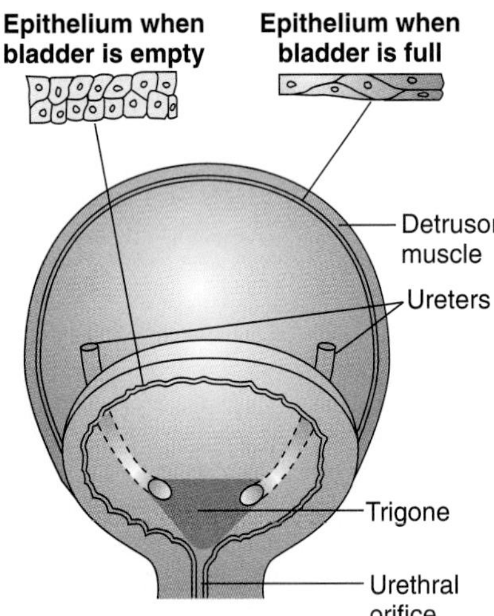

Figure 30–1
(**Top**) Cystogram of male bladder, showing position and filling. (**Bottom**) Diagram of the bladder, showing the detrusor muscle, ureters, trigone area, and urethral orifice. Note the flattening of epithelial cells when the bladder is full and the wall is stretched.

work of smooth muscle fibers called the detrusor muscle. The third is a submucosal layer of loose connective tissue. The fourth is an inner mucosal lining of transitional epithelium.

The tonicity of the urine often is quite different from that of the blood, and the transitional epithelial lining of the bladder acts as an effective barrier to prevent the passage of water between the blood and the bladder contents. The inner elements of the bladder form smooth folds, or rugae. As the bladder expands during filling, these rugae spread out to form a single layer without disrupting the integrity of the epithelial lining.

The detrusor muscle is the muscle of micturition. When it contracts, urine is expelled from the bladder. The abdominal muscles play a secondary role in micturition. Their contraction increases intraabdominal pressure, which further increases intravesicular pressure.

Muscles in the bladder neck, sometimes referred to as the internal sphincter, are a continuation of the detrusor muscle. They run down obliquely behind the proximal urethra, forming the posterior urethra in males and the entire urethra in females. When the bladder is relaxed, these circular muscle fibers are closed and act as a sphincter. When the detrusor muscle contracts, the sphincter is pulled open by the changes that occur in bladder shape. In the female, the urethra (2.5 to 3.5 cm) is shorter than in the male (16.5 to 18.5 cm) and usually affords less resistance to urine outflow.

Another muscle important to bladder function is the external sphincter, a circular muscle composed of striated muscle fibers that surrounds the urethra distal to the base of the bladder. The external sphincter operates as a reserve mechanism to stop micturition when it is occurring and to maintain continence in the face of unusually high bladder pressure. The skeletal muscle of the pelvic floor also contributes to the support of the bladder and the maintenance of continence.

Neural Control of Bladder Function

Innervation of the bladder consists of a peripheral autonomic nervous system reflex that is subject to facilitation or inhibition by higher neurologic centers. There are three main levels of neurologic control for bladder function: the spinal cord reflex centers, the micturition center in the brain stem, and the cortical and subcortical centers.

Spinal Cord Centers

The centers for reflex control of micturition (passage of urine) are located in the sacral (S2 through S4) and thoracolumbar (T11 through L1) segments of the spinal cord (Fig. 30–2). The lower motoneurons (LMNs) for the detrusor muscle of the bladder are located in the sacral segments of the spinal cord; their axons travel to the bladder by way of the pelvic nerve. LMNs for the external sphincter are also located in the sacral segments of the spinal cord. These LMNs receive their control from the motor cortex by way of the corticospinal tract and send impulses to the external sphincter by way of the pudendal nerve. The bladder neck and trigone area of the bladder (because of their different embryonic origin) receive their innervation from sympathetic outflow from the thoracolumbar (T11 to L2) segments of the spinal cord. The seminal vesicles, ampulla of the vas, and vas deferens, also receive sympathetic innervation from the thoracolumbar segments of the cord.

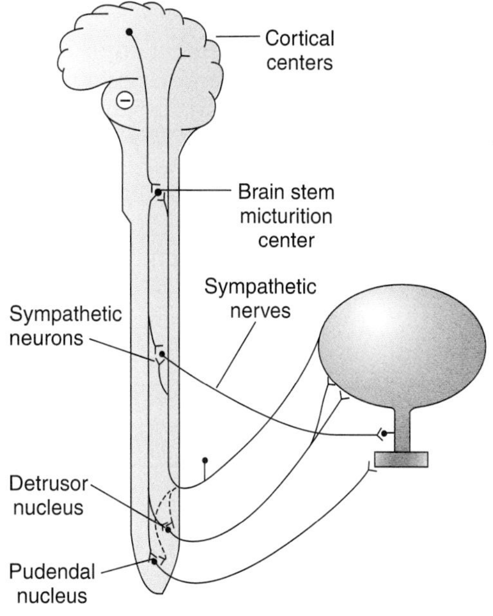

Figure 30–3
Neuronal interactions between lower urinary tract and nervous system. Before micturition, the bladder afferents ascend to the micturition center, which normally is inhibited by higher centers. Efferents from the micturition center descend to the thoracolumbar sympathetic center and the detrusor and pudendal nuclei to coordinate vesical contraction with relaxation of the smooth muscle and striated muscle sphincters. (Krane R.J., & Sirosky M.B. [Eds.][1979]. *Clinical neuro-urology* [p. 145]. Boston: Little, Brown. Used with permission)

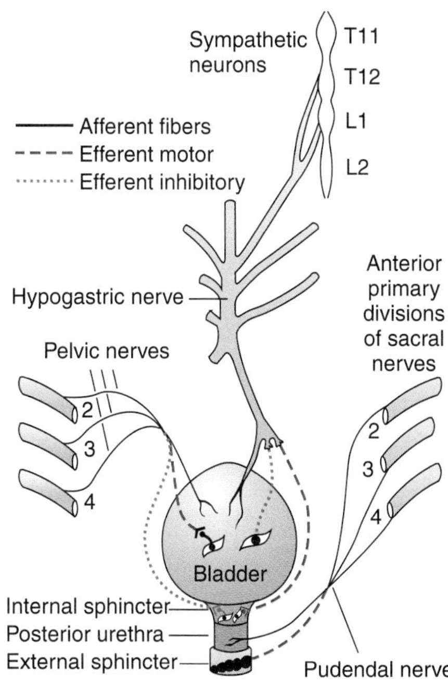

Figure 30–2
Nerve supply to the bladder and the urethra.

The afferent input from the bladder and urethra is carried to the central nervous system by means of fibers that travel with the parasympathetic (pelvic), somatic (pudendal), and sympathetic (hypogastric) nerves. The pelvic nerve carries sensory fibers from the stretch receptors in the bladder wall; the pudendal nerve carries sensory fibers from the external sphincter and pelvic muscles; and the hypogastric nerve carries sensory fibers from the trigone area.

Brain Stem Micturition Center

The immediate coordination of the normal micturition reflex occurs in the micturition center of the brain stem, facilitated by ascending and descending pathways from the reflex centers in the spinal cord (Fig. 30–3). This center is thought to coordinate the activity of the detrusor muscle and the external sphincter. The detrusor motor neurons of the sacral cord do not respond directly to afferent information generated by bladder filling. Instead, bladder emptying occurs only after afferent generation of a brain stem–integrated micturition response.

Cortical and Subcortical Centers

Cortical brain centers enable inhibition of the micturition center in the brain stem and conscious control of urination. Neural influences from the subcortical centers in the basal ganglia, which are conveyed by extrapyramidal pathways, modulate the contractile response. They modify and delay the detrusor contractile response during filling and then modulate the expulsive activity of the bladder to facilitate complete emptying.

Micturition

When the bladder is distended to 150 to 300 ml, the sensation of fullness is transmitted to the spinal cord and then to the cerebral cortex, allowing conscious inhibition of the micturition reflex. During the act of micturition, the detrusor muscle of the bladder fundus and bladder neck contract down on the urine in the fundus of the bladder; the ureteral orifices are forced shut; the bladder neck is widened and shortened as it is pulled up by the globular muscles in the bladder fundus; and the resistance of the internal sphincter in the bladder neck is decreased as urine moves out of the bladder.

In infants and young children, micturition is an involuntary act that is triggered by a spinal cord reflex; when the bladder fills to a given capacity, the detrusor muscle contracts and the external sphincter relaxes. As the bladder grows and increases in capacity, the tonicity of the external sphincter increases. At ages 2 to 3, the child becomes conscious of the need to urinate and can learn to briefly contract the pelvic muscles to maintain closure of the sphincter and delay urination. As the central nervous system continues to mature, inhibition of involuntary detrusor muscle activity takes place. After the child achieves continence, micturition becomes voluntary.

To maintain continence, or retention of urine, the bladder must function as a low-pressure storage system; the pressure within the bladder must remain lower than urethral pressure. To ensure that this condition is met, the increase in intravesicular pressure that accompanies bladder filling is almost imperceptible. An increase in bladder volume from 10 to 400 ml may be accompanied by only a 5 cm H_2O increase in pressure.[1] Sustained elevations in intravesicular pressures (>40 to 50 cm H_2O) often are associated with vesicoureteral reflux (*i.e.*, backward movement of urine from the bladder into the ureter) and the development of ureteral dilatation. Although the pressure within the bladder is maintained at low levels, sphincter pressure remains high (45 to 65 cm H_2O) as a means of preventing loss of urine as the bladder fills.

The *autonomic nervous system* plays a central role in micturition. Both sympathetic and parasympathetic neurotransmitters contribute to the micturition reflex. Parasympathetic innervation of the bladder is mediated by the neurotransmitter acetylcholine. Two types of cholinergic receptors affect various aspects of micturition: nicotinic and muscarinic. Nicotinic receptors are found in the synapses between the preganglionic and postganglionic neurons of the sympathetic and the parasympathetic system, as well as in the neuromuscular end plates of the striated muscle fibers of the external sphincter and pelvic muscles. Muscarinic receptors are found in the postganglionic parasympathetic endings of the detrusor muscle.

Although sympathetic innervation is not essential to the act of micturition, it allows the bladder to store a large volume without the involuntary escape of urine—a mechanism that is consistent with the fight-or-flight function subserved by the sympathetic nervous system. The bladder is supplied with α- and β_2-adrenergic receptors. The β-adrenergic receptors are found in the detrusor muscle; they produce relaxation of the detrusor muscle, increasing the bladder volume at which the micturition reflex is triggered. The α-adrenergic receptors are found in the trigone area, including the intramural ureteral musculature, bladder neck, and internal sphincter. The activation of α receptors produces contraction of these muscles. Sympathetic activity ceases when the micturition reflex is activated. During ejaculation in the male, which is mediated by the sympathetic nervous system, the musculature of the trigone area and that of the bladder neck and prostatic urethra contracts and prevents the backflow of seminal fluid into the bladder.

Because of their effects on bladder function, drugs that selectively activate or block autonomic nervous system outflow or receptor activity can alter urine elimination. Table 30–1 describes the action of drugs that can impair bladder function or can be used in the treatment of micturition disorders. Many of the nonprescription cold preparations contain α-adrenergic agonists and antihistamine agents that have anticholinergic properties. These drugs can cause urinary retention. Many of the antidepressant and antipsychotic drugs also have anticholinergic actions that influence urination.

Diagnostic Methods of Evaluating Bladder Function

Bladder structure and function can be assessed by a number of methods. Reports or observations of frequency, hesitancy, straining to void, and a weak or interrupted stream are suggestive of outflow obstruction. Palpation and percussion provide information about bladder distention.

Physical Examinations

Postvoided residual (PVR) urine volume provides information about bladder emptying. It can be estimated by abdominal palpation and percussion. Catheterization and ultrasonography can be used to obtain specific measurements of PVR. A PVR value of less than 50 ml is considered adequate bladder emptying, and more than 200 ml indicates inadequate bladder emptying.[2]

TABLE 30-1

Bladder Function and Drug Actions

Function	Drug Groups	Examples
Detrusor Muscle		
Increased tone and contraction	Cholinergic drugs (stimulate parasympathetic receptors that cause detrusor muscle contraction)	Bethanechol (Urecholine and others) Neostigmine (Prostigmin)
Inhibition of detrusor muscle relaxation during filling	β-Adrenergic blocking drugs (block β_2 receptors that cause detrusor muscle relaxation)	Propranolol (Inderal)
Decreased tone	Anticholinergic drugs (block parasympathetic receptors that cause detrusor muscle contraction)	Atropine Methantheline (Banthine) Propantheline (Pro-Banthine) Oxybutynin (Ditropan)
	Calcium-channel blocking drugs (may interfere with influx of calcium to support detrusor muscle tone)	Nifedipine (Adalat, Procardia) Virapamil (Calan, Isoptin) Diltiazem (Cardizem)
Internal Sphincter		
Increased tone	α_1-Adrenergic agonists (activate α receptors that cause contraction of muscles of the internal sphincter)	Phenylephrine (generic) Ephedrine (generic) Phenylpropanolamine (generic)
Decreased tone	α_1-Adrenergic blocking drugs	Prazosin (Minipress) Doxazosin (Cardura) Terazosin (Hytrin)
External Sphincter		
Decreased tone	Skeletal muscle relaxants	Baclofen (Lioresal) Dantrolene (Dantrium) Diazepam (Valium)

Pelvic examination is used in women to assess perineal skin condition, perivaginal muscle tone, genital atrophy, pelvic prolapse (*e.g.*, cystocele, rectocele, uterine prolapse), pelvic mass, or other conditions that may impair bladder function. Bimanual examination (*i.e.*, pelvic and abdominal palpation) can be used to assess PVR volume. Rectal examination is used to test for perineal sensation, sphincter tone, fecal impaction, and rectal mass. It is used to assess the contour of the prostate in men.

Laboratory and Radiologic Studies

Urine tests provide information about kidney function and urinary tract infections. The presence of bacteriuria or pyuria suggests urinary tract infection and the possibility of urinary tract obstruction. Blood tests (*i.e.*, blood urea nitrogen and creatinine) provide information about renal function.

Bladder structures can be visualized indirectly by taking x-ray films of the abdomen and by using excretory urography (which involves the use of a radiopaque dye [see Fig. 30–1]), computed tomographic (CT) scanning, magnetic resonance imaging (MRI), or ultrasonography. Cystoscopy enables direct visualization of the urethra, bladder, and ureteral orifices.

Urodynamic Studies

Urodynamic studies are used to study bladder function and voiding problems. Three aspects of bladder function can be assessed by urodynamic studies: bladder, urethral, and intraabdominal pressure changes; characteristics of urine flow; and the activity of the striated muscles of the external sphincter and pelvic floor. Specific urodynamic tests include uroflometry, cystometry, urethral pressure profile, sphincter electromyography, and uroflow studies. It is often advantageous to evaluate several components of bladder function simultaneously.

Uroflometry. Uroflometry measures the flow rate (milliliters per minute) during urination. It commonly is done using a weight-recording device located at the bottom of a commode receptacle unit. As the person being tested voids, the weight of the commode receptacle unit increases. This weight change is electronically recorded and then analyzed using weight (converted to milliliters) and time.

Cystometry. Cystometry is used to measure bladder pressure during filling and voiding. It provides valuable information about total bladder capacity, intravesicular pressures during bladder filling, the ability to perceive bladder fullness and the desire to urinate, the ability of the bladder to contract and sustain a contraction, uninhibited bladder contractions, and the ability to inhibit urination. The test can be done by allowing physiologic filling of the bladder with urine and recording intravesicular pressure throughout a voiding cycle or by filling the bladder with water and measuring intravesicular pressure against the volume of water instilled into the bladder.

Gas cystometry can be used as a substitute for water cystometry. Gas cystometers originally became popular because they were simpler and faster to use, but they have proved less reliable and less informative than water cystometers.[3]

In a normally functioning bladder, the sensation of bladder fullness is first perceived when the bladder contains 100 to 200 ml of urine while bladder pressure remains constant at about 8 to 15 cm H_2O. The desire to void occurs when the bladder is full (normal capacity is about 400 to 500 ml). At this point, a definite sensation of fullness occurs, the pressure rises sharply to 40 to 100 cm H_2O, and voiding occurs around the catheter. Urinary continence requires that urethral pressure exceed bladder pressure. Bladder pressure usually rises 30 to 40 cm H_2O during voiding. If the urethral resistance is high because of obstruction, greater pressures is required, a condition that can be detected by cystometry.

Urethral Pressure Profile. The urethral pressure profile is used to evaluate the intraluminal pressure changes along the length of the urethra with the bladder at rest. It provides information about smooth muscle activity along the length of the urethra. This test can be done using the infusion method (most commonly used), the membrane catheter method, or the microtip transducer. The infusion method involves the insertion of a small double-lumen urethral catheter, then infusing fluid or carbon dioxide into the bladder and measuring the changes in urethral pressure as the catheter is slowly withdrawn.

Sphincter Electromyography. Sphincter electromyography (EMG) allows the activity of the striated (voluntary) muscles of the perineal area to be studied. Activity is recorded using an anal plug electrode, a catheter electrode, adhesive skin electrodes, or needle electrodes. Electrode placement is based on the muscle groups that need to be tested. The test usually is done along with urodynamic tests such as the CMG and uroflow studies.

Ultrasound Bladder Scan. The ultrasound bladder scan provides a noninvasive method for estimating bladder volume. The device measures ultrasonic reflections to differentiate the urinary bladder from the surrounding tissue. A computer system calculates and displays bladder volume. The device can be used to determine the need for catheterization, for evaluation and diagnosis of urinary retention, to measure postvoiding urine volumes, and for facilitating volume-dependent or time-dependent catheterization or toileting programs.

In summary, although the kidneys function in the formation of urine and the regulation of body fluids, it is the bladder that stores and controls the elimination of urine. Micturition is a function of the peripheral autonomic nervous system, subject to facilitation or inhibition from higher neurologic centers. The parasympathetic nervous system controls the motor function of the bladder detrusor muscle and the tone of the internal sphincter; its cell bodies are located in the sacral spinal cord and communicate with the bladder through the pelvic nerve. Efferent sympathetic control originates at the level of segments T11 through L1 of the spinal cord and produces relaxation of the detrusor muscle and contraction of the internal sphincter. Skeletal muscle found in the external sphincter and the pelvic muscles that support the bladder are supplied by the pudendal nerve, which exits the spinal cord at the level of segments S2 through S4. The micturition center in the brain stem coordinates the action of the detrusor muscle and the external sphincter, whereas cortical centers permit conscious control of micturition.

Bladder function can be evaluated using urodynamic studies that measure bladder, urethral, and abdominal pressures; urine flow characteristics; and skeletal muscle activity of the external sphincter.

Alterations in Bladder Function

After you have completed this section of the chapter, you should be able to meet the following objectives:

- State the signs of urine retention
- Differentiate lesions that produce spastic bladder dysfunction from those that produce flaccid bladder dysfunction in terms of the level of the lesions and their effects on bladder function
- Cite the pathology and causes of nonrelaxing external sphincter
- Characterize the cause and manifestations of diabetic bladder neuropathy
- Describe the difference between bladder training methods used for a neurogenic bladder caused by a lesion of the spinal cord micturition reflex center and one caused by a lesion above the level of the reflex center
- Define *incontinence* and list the categories of this condition
- Describe behavioral, pharmacologic, and surgical methods used in treatment of incontinence

Alterations in bladder function include urinary obstruction with retention of urine and urinary incontinence with involuntary loss of urine. Although the two conditions have almost opposite effects on urination, they can have similar causes. Both can result from structural changes in the bladder, urethra, or surrounding organs or from impairment of neurologic control of bladder function.

Urine Retention

In urine retention, urine is produced normally by the kidneys but is retained in the bladder. The condition has a number of causes, including urethral obstruction, impaired innervation of the bladder (*i.e.*, neurogenic bladder), and the effects of drug actions on the control of bladder function. Because it has the potential to produce vesicoureteral reflux and cause kidney damage, urine retention is a serious disorder.

Urethral Obstruction

Major structural urinary obstruction most often results from processes that cause external compression or intrinsic narrowing of the urinary meatus or bladder outlet structures. In males, the most important cause of urinary obstruction is external compression of the urethra caused by the enlargement of the prostate gland (see Chapter 49). External obstructive processes are less common in females. When they do occur, they typically are caused by a cystocele of the bladder (see Chapter 51). Bladder tumors and secondary invasion of the bladder by tumors arising in structures that surround the bladder and urethra can compress the bladder neck or urethra and cause obstruction.

Narrowing of the urethra owing to congenital deformities or scar tissue from injury or infection can also obstruct urine flow. Congenital narrowing of the urinary meatus (*i.e.*, meatal stenosis) is more common in boys, and obstructive disorders of the posterior urethra are more common in girls. Gonorrhea and other sexually transmitted diseases contribute to the incidence of infection-produced urethral strictures.

Constipation and fecal impaction can compress the urethra and produce urethral obstruction. This is a particular problem in elderly persons.

Compensatory Changes

The body compensates for the obstruction of urine outflow with mechanisms designed to prevent urine retention. These mechanisms can be divided into three stages: an irritability stage, a compensatory stage, and a decompensatory stage.[4] The degree to which these changes occur and their effect on bladder structure and urinary function depend on the extent of the obstruction, the rapidity with which it occurs, and the presence of other contributing factors, such as neurologic impairment and infection.

During the early stage of obstruction, the bladder begins to hypertrophy and becomes hypersensitive to afferent stimuli arising from bladder filling. The ability to suppress urination is diminished, and bladder contraction can become so strong that it virtually produces bladder spasm. There is urgency, sometimes to the point of incontinence, and frequency during the day and at night.

With continuation and progression of the obstruction, compensatory changes begin to occur. There is further hypertrophy of the bladder muscle, the thickness of the bladder wall may double, and the pressure generated by detrusor contraction can increase from a normal 20 to 40 cm H_2O to 50 to 100 cm H_2O to overcome the resistance from the obstruction. As the force needed to expel urine from the bladder increases, compensatory mechanisms may become ineffective, causing muscle fatigue before complete emptying can be accomplished. After a few minutes, voiding can again be initiated and completed, accounting for the frequency of urination.

The inner bladder surface forms smooth folds. With continued outflow obstruction, this smooth surface is replaced with coarsely woven structures (*i.e.*, hypertrophied smooth muscle fibers) called *trabeculae*. Small pockets of mucosal tissue, called *cellules*, commonly develop between the trabecular ridges. These pockets form diverticula when they extend between the actual fibers of the bladder muscle (Fig. 30–4). Because the diverticula have no muscle, they are unable to contract and expel their urine into the bladder, and secondary infections caused by stasis are common.

Along with hypertrophy of the bladder wall, there is hypertrophy of the trigone area and the interureteric ridge, which is located between the two ureters. This causes back pressure on the ureters, the development of hydroureters (*i.e.*, dilated, urine-filled ureters), and eventually, kidney damage. Stasis of urine predisposes to urinary tract infections.

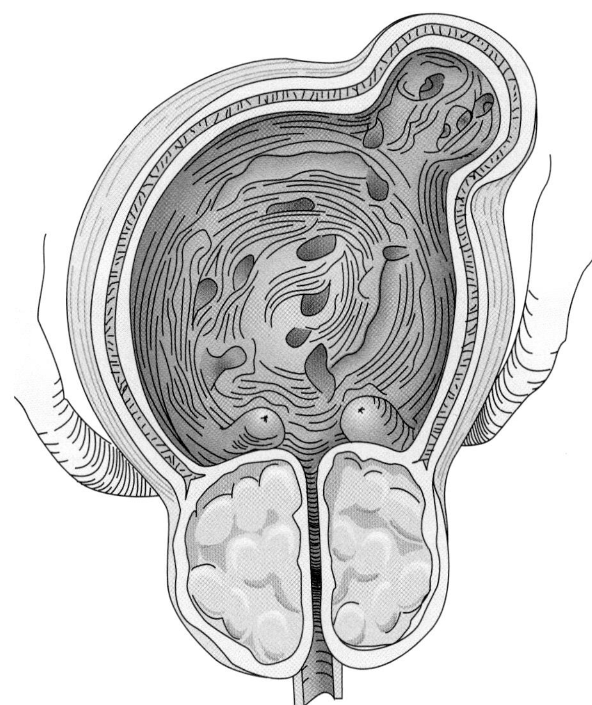

Figure 30–4
Destructive changes of the bladder wall with development of diverticula caused by benign prostatic hypertrophy.

CHART 30-1
Signs of Outflow Obstruction and Urine Retention

Bladder distention
Hesitancy
Straining when initiating urination
Small and weak stream
Frequency
Feeling of incomplete bladder emptying
Overflow incontinence

When compensatory mechanisms are no longer effective, signs of decompensation begin to occur. The period of detrusor muscle contraction becomes too short to completely expel the urine, and residual urine remains in the bladder. At this point, the symptoms of obstruction—frequency of urination, hesitancy, a need to strain to initiate urination, a weak and small stream, and termination of the stream before the bladder is completely emptied—become pronounced. The amount of residual urine may increase up to 1000 to 3000 ml, and overflow incontinence occurs. There may also be acute retention of urine. The signs of urine retention are summarized in Chart 30–1.

Treatment

The immediate treatment of outflow obstruction is directed toward relief of bladder distention. This usually is accomplished through urinary catheterization (discussed later in this chapter). Constipation or fecal impaction should be corrected. Long-term treatment is directed toward correcting the problem causing the obstruction.

Neurogenic Bladder Disorders

The innervation of the bladder can be interrupted at any level and can selectively involve sensory or motor innervation or both. Neurogenic disorders of the bladder commonly are manifested in one of two ways: by spastic bladder dysfunction or by flaccid bladder dysfunction. Spastic bladder dysfunction usually results from neurologic lesions that are above the level of the sacral micturition reflex center, whereas flaccid bladder dysfunction results from lesions at the level of sacral micturition reflexes or peripheral innervation of the bladder. In addition to detrusor muscle dysfunction, disruption of micturition occurs when the neurologic control of external sphincter function is impaired. Some disorders, such as Parkinson's disease, may cause mixed spastic and semiflaccid bladder dysfunction. Table 30–2 describes the characteristics of neurogenic bladder according to the level of the lesion.

TABLE 30-2
Characteristics and Types of Neurogenic Bladder

Level of Lesion	Change in Bladder Function	Common Causes
Sensory cortex, motor cortex or corticospinal tract	Loss of ability to perceive bladder filling; low volume, physiologically normal micturition that occurs suddenly and is difficult to inhibit	Stroke and advanced age
Basal ganglia or extrapyramidal tract	Detrusor contractions are elicited suddenly without warning and are difficult to control; bladder contraction is shorter than normal and does not produce full bladder emptying	Parkinson's disease
Brain stem micturition center or communicating tracts in the spinal cord	Storage reflexes are provoked during filling, and external sphincter responses are heightened; uninhibited bladder contractions occur at a lower volume than normal and do not continue until the bladder is emptied; antagonistic activity occurs between the detrusor muscle and the external sphincter	Spinal cord injury
Sacral cord or nerve roots	Areflexic bladder fills but does not contract; loss of external sphincter tone occurs when the lesion affects the α-adrenergic motoneurons or pudendal nerve	Injury to sacral cord or spinal roots
Pelvic nerve	Increased filling and impaired sphincter control cause increased intravesicular pressure	Radical pelvic surgery
Autonomic peripheral sensory pathways	Bladder overfilling occurs due to a loss of ability to perceive bladder filling	Diabetic neuropathies, multiple sclerosis

Spastic Bladder Dysfunction

The terms *reflex neurogenic bladder, spastic neurogenic bladder, cord bladder,* and *uninhibited bladder* have been variously used to describe a neurogenic disorder that causes spastic bladder dysfunction. This condition can be caused by any neurologic condition above the level of the voiding reflex arc. The degree of spasticity and dysfunction depends on the level and extent of neurologic dysfunction. Common lesions above the level of the brain stem micturition center that affect voiding are stroke, dementia, multiple sclerosis, and brain tumors. Spinal cord lesions are the most important causes of spastic bladder dysfunction. Spinal cord lesions include trauma (*i.e.,* spinal cord injury), herniated intervertebral disk, vascular lesions, multiple sclerosis, tumors, and myelitis.

Uninhibited Neurogenic Bladder. A mild form of reflex neurogenic bladder, sometimes called uninhibited bladder, can develop after a stroke, during the early stages of multiple sclerosis, or as a result of lesions located in the inhibitory centers of the cortex or the pyramidal tract. With this type of disorder, the sacral reflex arc and sensation are retained, the urine stream is normal, and there is no residual urine. Bladder capacity is diminished, however, because of increased detrusor muscle tone and spasticity.

Detrusor-Sphincter Dyssynergia. Depending on the level of the lesion, the coordinated activity of the detrusor muscle and the external sphincter may be affected. Lesions that affect the micturition center in the brain stem or impair communication between this center and spinal cord centers interrupt the coordinated activity of the detrusor muscle and the external sphincter. This is called detrusor-sphincter dyssynergia. Instead of relaxing during micturition, the external sphincter becomes more constricted. This condition can lead to elevated intravesicular pressures and vesicoureteral reflux.

Bladder Dysfunction Caused by Spinal Cord Injury. One of the most common types of spinal cord lesions is spinal cord injury (see Chapter 39).

The immediate and early effects of spinal cord injury on bladder function are quite different from those that follow recovery from the initial injury. During the period immediately after spinal cord injury, a state of spinal shock develops, during which all the reflexes, including the micturition reflex, are depressed. During this stage, the bladder becomes atonic and cannot contract. Catheterization is necessary to prevent injury to urinary structures associated with overdistention of the bladder. Aseptic intermittent catheterization is the preferred method of catheterization. Depression of reflexes lasts for about 1 to 2 months, after which the spinal reflexes return and become hyperactive.

After the acute stage of spinal cord injury, the micturition response changes from a long-tract reflex to a segmental reflex. Because the sacral reflex arc remains intact, stimuli generated by bladder stretch receptors during filling produce frequent spontaneous contractions of the detrusor muscle. This creates a small, hyperactive bladder subject to high-pressure and short-duration uninhibited bladder contractions. Voiding is interrupted, involuntary, or incomplete. Hypertrophy of the trigone develops, often leading to vesicoureteral reflux and renal damage. Dilation of the internal sphincter and spasticity of the perineal muscles innervated by upper motoneurons occur, producing resistance to bladder emptying.

Flaccid Bladder Dysfunction

Detrusor muscle areflexia, or flaccid neurogenic bladder, occurs when there is injury to the micturition center of the sacral cord, the cauda equina, or the sacral roots that supply the bladder. Atony of the detrusor muscle and loss of the perception of bladder fullness permit the overstretching of the detrusor muscle that contributes to weak and ineffective bladder contractions. External sphincter tone and perineal muscle tone are diminished. Voluntary urination does not occur, but fairly efficient emptying can be achieved by increased intraabdominal pressure or manual suprapubic pressure. Among the causes of flaccid neurogenic bladder are meningomyelocele and spina bifida.

Bladder Dysfunction Caused by Peripheral Neuropathies

In addition to central nervous system lesions and conditions that disrupt bladder function, disorders of the peripheral (pelvic, pudendal, and hypogastric) neurons that supply the bladder can occur. These neuropathies can selectively interrupt sensory or motor pathways for the bladder or involve both pathways. One of the most common causes of bladder neuropathies is diabetes mellitus.

Epidemiologic studies indicate that diabetic bladder neuropathy occurs in 43% to 87% of persons with insulin-dependent diabetes, with no age or sex difference.[5] The disorder initially affects the sensory axons of the urinary bladder without involvement of the pudendal nerve. This leads to large residual volumes after micturition, sometimes complicated by infection.[6] There frequently is need for straining, accompanied by hesitation, weakness of the stream, dribbling, and a sensation of incomplete bladder emptying.[7] The chief complications are vesicoureteral reflux and ascending urinary tract infection. Because persons with diabetes are already at risk for developing glomerular disease (see Chapter 28), reflux can have serious effects on kidney function. Treatment consists of client education, including the need for frequent voidings (every 3 hours while awake), use of abdominal compression to effect more complete bladder emptying, and intermittent catherization when necessary.[7] Pharmacologic treatment includes antibiotics for urinary tract infections and cholinergic drugs (*e.g.,* bethanechol).

Nonrelaxing External Sphincter

Another condition that affects the peripheral innervation of micturition is *nonrelaxing external sphincter*.[8] This condition usually is related to a delay in maturation, developmental regression, psychomotor disorders, or locally irritative lesions. Inadequate relaxation of the external sphincter can be the result of anxiety or depression. Any local irritation can produce spasms of the sphincter by means of afferent sensory input from the pudendal nerve; included are vaginitis, perineal inflammation, and inflammation or irritation of the urethra. In men, chronic prostatitis contributes to the impaired relaxation of the external sphincter.

Treatment

The goals of treatment for neurogenic bladder disorders center on preventing bladder overdistention, urinary tract infections, and renal damage that can be life threatening and on reducing the undesirable social and psychologic effects of the disorder. Treatment is based on the type of neurologic lesion that is involved; information obtained through the health history, including fluid intake; report or observation of voiding patterns; presence of other health problems; urodynamic studies when indicated; and the ability of the person to participate in the treatment. Treatment methods include catheterization, bladder training, pharmacologic manipulation of bladder function, and surgery.

Catheterization. Catheterization involves the insertion of a small-diameter latex or silicone tube into the bladder through the urethra. The catheter may be inserted on a one-time basis to relieve temporary bladder distention, left indwelling (*i.e.*, retention catheter), or inserted intermittently. With acute overdistention of the bladder, usually no more than 1000 ml of urine is removed from the bladder at one time. The theory behind this limitation is that removing more than this amount at one time releases pressure on the pelvic blood vessels and predisposes to alterations in circulatory function.

Permanent indwelling catheters sometimes are used when there is urine retention or incontinence in persons who are ill or debilitated or when conservative or surgical methods for the correction of incontinence are not feasible. The use of permanent indwelling bladder catheters in patients with spinal cord injury has been shown to produce a number of complications, including urinary tract infections, urethral irritation and injury, epididymo-orchitis, pyelonephritis, and kidney stones.

Intermittent catheterization is used to treat urine retention or incomplete emptying secondary to various neurologic or obstructive disorders. Properly used, it prevents bladder overdistention and urethral irritation, allows more freedom of activity, and provides periodic distention of the bladder to prevent muscle atony. It often is used with pharmacologic manipulation to achieve continence; when possible, it is learned and managed as a self-care procedure (*i.e.*, intermittent self-catheterization). It may be carried out as an aseptic (sterile) or a clean procedure. Aseptic intermittent catheterization is used in persons with spinal shock and in those who need short-term catheterization.

The clean procedure typically is used for self-catheterization. It is performed at 3- to 4-hour intervals to prevent overdistention of the bladder. The best results are obtained if only 300 to 400 ml is allowed to collect in the bladder between catheterizations. The use of the clean instead of the sterile procedure has been defended on the basis that most urinary tract infections are caused by some underlying abnormality of the urinary tract that leads to impaired mucosal resistance to bacterial infection, the most common cause of which is decreased blood flow because of overdistention.[9] Overdistention has also been shown to decrease the mucin layer that protects the mucosal surface of the bladder.[10]

Bladder Retraining. Bladder retraining differs with the type of disorder. Methods used to supplement bladder retraining includes monitoring fluid intake to prevent urinary tract infections and control urine volume and osmolality, developing scheduled times for urination, and using body positions that facilitate micturition.

Among the considerations when monitoring fluid intake is the need to ensure adequate fluid intake to prevent unduly concentrated urine that may serve to stimulate afferent neurons of the micturition reflex. In hyperreflexive bladder or detrusor-sphincter dyssynergia, the stimulation of afferent nerve endings by irritating constituents of the urine results in increased vesicular pressures, vesicoureteral reflux, and overflow incontinence. Fluid intake must be balanced to prevent bladder overdistention from occurring during the night. Adequate fluid intake is also needed to prevent urinary tract infections, the irritating effects of which increase bladder irritability and the risk of urinary incontinence and renal damage. Developing scheduled times for urinating prevents overdistention of the bladder.

The methods used for bladder retraining depend on the type of lesion. In spastic neurogenic bladder, methods designed to trigger the sacral micturition reflex are used; in flaccid neurogenic bladder, manual methods that increase intravesicular pressure are used. *Trigger voiding methods* include manual stimulation of the afferent loop of the micturition reflex through such maneuvers as tapping the suprapubic area, pulling on the pubic hairs, stroking the glans penis, or rubbing the thighs. *Credé's method*, which is done with the person in a sitting position, consists of applying pressure with four fingers of one hand or both hands to the suprapubic area as a means of increasing intravesicular pressure. The use of Valsalva's maneuver (*i.e.*, bearing down by exhaling against a closed glottis) increases intraabdominal pressure and aids in bladder emptying. This maneuver is repeated until the bladder is empty. For the best results, the patient must cooperate fully with the procedures and, if possible, learn to perform them independently.

Biofeedback methods have been useful for teaching some aspects of bladder control. They involve the use of EMG or cystometry as a feedback signal for training a person to control the function of the external sphincter or raise intravesicular pressure enough to overcome outflow resistance.

Pharmacologic Manipulation. Pharmacologic manipulation includes the use of drugs to alter the contractile properties of the bladder, decrease the outflow resistance of the internal sphincter, and relax the external sphincter. The usefulness of drug therapy often is evaluated during cystometric studies. Anticholinergic drugs, such as propantheline (Pro-Banthine), decrease detrusor muscle tone and increase bladder capacity in persons with spastic bladder dysfunction. Cholinergic drugs that stimulate parasympathetic receptors, such as bethanechol chloride (Urecholine), provide increased bladder tonus and may prove helpful in the symptomatic treatment of milder forms of flaccid neurogenic bladder. Muscle relaxants, such as diazepam (Valium) and baclofen (Lioresal), may be used to decrease the tone of the external sphincter.

Surgical Procedures. Among the surgical procedures used in the management of neurogenic bladder are sphincterectomy or transurethral resection of the bladder neck in men with prostatic hypertrophy, reconstruction of the sphincter, nerve resection of the sacral reflex nerves that cause spasticity or the pudendal nerve that controls the external sphincter, and urinary diversion. Urinary diversion can be done by creating an ileal or a colon loop into which the ureters are anastomosed; the distal end of the loop is brought out and attached to the abdominal wall. Other procedures include the attachment of the ureters to the skin of the abdominal wall or the attachment of the ureters to the sigmoid colon, with the rectum serving as a receptacle for the urine.

Extensive research is being conducted on methods of restoring voluntary control of the storage and evacuation functions of the bladder through the use of implanted electrodes. Single and multiple electrodes can be placed on selected nerves and then coupled to a subcutaneous receiver.

Urinary Incontinence

The Urinary Incontinence Guideline Panel defines urinary incontinence as an involuntary loss of urine that is sufficient to be a problem.[11] This panel was convened by the Agency for Health Care Policy and Research in 1992 and again in 1996 for the purpose of developing specific guidelines to improve the care of persons with urinary incontinence.

Urinary incontinence affects about 13 million Americans. Many body functions decline with age, and incontinence, although not a normal accompaniment of the aging process, is seen with increased frequency in elderly persons. For noninstitutionalized persons older than 60 years of age, the prevalence of urinary incontinence ranges from 15% to 35%, with women affected twice as often as men.[2] The increase in health problems often seen in elderly persons probably contributes to the greater frequency of incontinence. Despite the prevalence of incontinence, most affected persons do not seek help for it, primarily because of embarrassment or because they are not aware that help is available.

TABLE 30-3
Types and Characteristics of Urinary Incontinence

Type	Characteristics
Stress	Involuntary loss of urine associated with activities, such as coughing, that increase intraabdominal pressure
Urge	Involuntary loss of urine associated with strong desire to void
Overflow	Involuntary loss of urine when intravesicular pressure exceeds maximal urethral pressure in the absence of detrusor activity

Incontinence can be caused by a number of conditions. It can occur without the person's knowledge, and at other times, the person may be aware of the condition but be unable to prevent it. The Urinary Incontinence Guideline Panel has identified four main types of incontinence: stress incontinence, urge incontinence, overflow incontinence, and mixed incontinence, which is a combination of stress and urge incontinence.[2] Table 30–3 summarizes the characteristics of stress, urge, and overflow incontinence. The condition may occur as a transient and correctable phenomenon, or it may not be totally correctable and occur with various degrees of frequency. Among the transient causes of urinary incontinence are confusional states; medications that alter bladder function or perception of bladder filling and the need to urinate; diuretics and conditions that increase bladder filling; restricted mobility; and stool impaction.[12]

Stress Incontinence

Stress incontinence is the involuntary loss of urine during coughing, laughing, sneezing, or lifting that increases intraabdominal pressure. The most common cause is hypermobility and significant displacement of the urethra during exertion.

In women, the angle between the bladder and the posterior proximal urethra (*i.e.*, urethrovesical junction) is important to continence. This angle normally is 90 to 100 degrees, with at least one third of the bladder base contributing to the angle when not voiding (Fig. 30–5).[13] During the first stage of voiding, this angle is lost as the bladder descends. In women, diminution of muscle tone associated with normal aging, childbirth, or surgical procedures can cause weakness of the pelvic floor muscles and result in stress incontinence by obliterating the critical posterior urethrovesical angle. In these women, loss of the posterior urethrovesical angle, descent and funneling of the bladder neck, and backward and downward rotation of the bladder occur, so that the

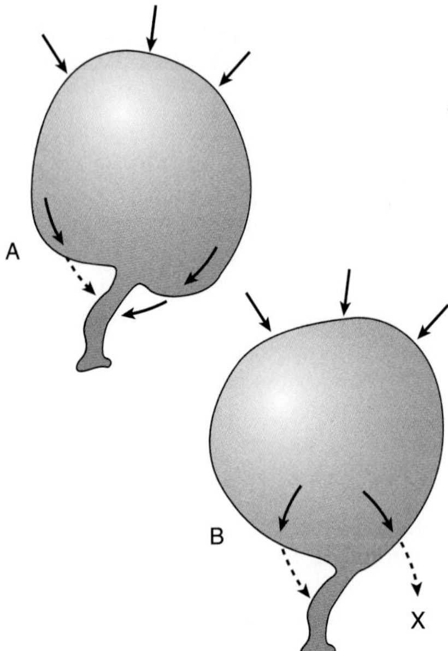

Figure 30–5
Importance of the posterior urethrovesical (PU-V) angle to the continence mechanism. (**A**) In the presence of the normal PU-V angle, sudden changes in intraabdominal pressure are transmitted optimally (indicated by the *arrows* with dotted lines) to all sides of the proximal urethra. In this way, intraurethral pressure is maintained higher than the simultaneously elevated intravesicular pressure. This prevents loss of urine with sudden stress. (**B**) Loss of the PU-V angle results in displacement of the vesicle neck to the most dependent portion of the bladder, preventing the equal transmission of sudden increases in intraabdominal pressure to the lumen of the proximal urethra. Thus, the pressure in the region of the vesicle neck rises considerably more than the intraurethral pressure just beyond it, and stress incontinence occurs. (Green J.T., Jr. [1968]. *Obstetrical and Gynecological Survey, 23*, 603. Reprinted with permission)

bladder and urethra are already in an anatomic position for the first stage of voiding. Any activity that causes downward pressure on the bladder is sufficient to allow the urine to escape involuntarily.

Another cause of stress incontinence is intrinsic urethral deficiency, which may result from congenital sphincter weakness, as occurs with myelomeningocele. It may also be acquired as a result of trauma, prostatectomy, irradiation, or sacral cord lesion. Stress incontinence in men may result from a congenital defect or from trauma or surgery to the bladder outlet, as occurs with prostatectomy. Neurologic dysfunction, as occurs with impaired sympathetic innervation of the bladder neck, pelvic nerve innervation to the intrinsic sphincter, or pudendal nerve innervation to the external sphincter may be a contributing factor. Stress incontinence may occur as a postprostatectomy complication because of sphincter insufficiency or detrusor muscle instability.

Urge Incontinence

Urge, or urgency, incontinence is the involuntary loss of urine associated with a strong desire to void. It often is associated with involuntary and hyperreflexive detrusor contractions. Although hyperreflexive detrusor contractions occur in persons with neurogenic bladder dysfunction (*e.g.*, spastic bladder dysfunction), they can also occur in persons who have no evidence of neurologic dysfunction.

Among the causes of urge incontinence are conditions in which a partial upper motor neuron lesion makes movement difficult, so that the interval between knowing the bladder needs to be emptied and being able to stop it from emptying may be less than the time needed to reach the lavatory. Multiple sclerosis is a common cause of this type of incontinence. Musculoskeletal disorders, such as arthritis and joint instability, may also prevent an otherwise continent person from reaching the toilet in time.

Drugs such as hypnotics, tranquilizers, and sedatives can interfere with the conscious inhibition of voiding, leading to urge incontinence. Diuretics, particularly in elderly persons, increase the flow of urine and may contribute to incontinence, particularly in persons with diminished bladder capacity and in those who have difficulty reaching the toilet. Urinary infections, increased bladder irritability, urgency, and frequency occur in persons of all ages. In elderly persons, these conditions often precipitate incontinence.

Overflow Incontinence

Overflow incontinence is an involuntary loss of urine that occurs when intravesicular pressure exceeds the maximal urethral pressure because of bladder distention in the absence of detrusor activity. It can occur with retention of urine owing to nervous system lesions or obstruction of the bladder neck. With this type of incontinence, the bladder is distended and small amounts of urine are passed, particularly at night. In males, one of the most common causes of obstructive incontinence is enlargement of the prostate gland. Another cause that commonly is overlooked is fecal impaction (*i.e.*, dry, hard feces in the rectum). When a large bolus of stool forms in the rectum, it can push against the urethra and block the flow of urine.

Other Causes of Incontinence

Another cause of incontinence is decreased bladder compliance. This abnormal bladder condition may result from radiation therapy, radical pelvic surgery, or interstitial cystitis. Many persons with this disorder have severe urgency related to bladder hypersensitivity that results in loss of bladder elasticity such that any small increase in bladder volume or detrusor function causes a sharp rise in bladder pressure and severe urgency.

Incontinence may also be caused by factors outside the lower urinary tract, such as the inability to locate, reach, or receive assistance in reaching an appropriate place to void.[14] This may be a particular problem for elderly persons, who may have problems with mobility and manual dexterity or find themselves in unfamiliar surroundings. It occurs when a person cannot find or reach the bathroom or manipulate clothing quickly enough. Failing vision may contribute to the problem. Embarrassment in front of other persons at having to use the bathroom, particularly if the timing seems inappropriate, may cause a person to delay emptying the bladder and may lead to incontinence.

Treatment with drugs such as diuretics may cause the bladder to fill more rapidly than usual, making it difficult to reach the bathroom in time if there are problems with mobility or if a bathroom is not readily available. Night sedation may cause a person to sleep through the signal that normally would waken a person so he or she could get up and empty the bladder and avoid wetting the bed.

Diagnosis and Treatment

Urinary incontinence is a frequent and major health problem. It increases social isolation, frequently leads to institutionalization of elderly persons, and predisposes to infections and skin breakdown.

Urinary incontinence is not a single disease but a symptom with many possible causes. As a symptom, it requires full investigation to establish its cause. This usually is accomplished through a careful history, physical examination, blood tests, and urinalysis. A voiding record (*i.e.*, diary) may be used to determine the frequency, timing, amount of voiding, and other factors associated with the incontinence.[11] Because many drugs affect bladder function, a full drug history is essential. Estimation of PVR volume is recommended for all persons with incontinence. Provocative stress testing is done when stress incontinence is suspected. This test is done by having the person relax and then cough vigorously while the examiner observes for urine loss. The test usually is done in the lithotomy position; if no leakage is observed, it is repeated in the standing position.[11] Urodynamic studies may be needed to provide information about urinary pressures and urine flow rates.

Treatment or management depends on the type of incontinence, accompanying health problems, and the person's age. Exercises to strengthen the pelvic muscles and surgical correction of pelvic relaxation disorders often are used for women with stress incontinence. Noncatheter devices to obstruct urine flow or collect urine as it is passed may be used when urine flow cannot be controlled. Indwelling catheters (discussed earlier in the chapter), although a solution to the problem of urinary incontinence, usually are considered only after all other treatment methods have failed. In some types of incontinence, such as that associated with spinal cord injury or meningomyelocele, self-catheterization provides the means for controlling urine elimination.

Treatment of Stress Incontinence

Stress incontinence can be treated by physiotherapeutic measures, surgery, or a combination of the two. Surgical correction of cystocele and pelvic relaxation disorders may be needed for women.

Active muscle-tensing exercises of the pelvic muscles may prove effective.[15] These exercises were first advocated by Kegel, and they commonly are called *Kegel's exercises*.[16] Two groups of muscles are strengthened: those of the back part of the pelvic floor (*i.e.*, muscles used to contract the anus and control the passing of stool) and the front muscles of the pelvic floor (*i.e.*, muscles used to stop the flow of urine during voiding). In learning the exercises, a woman concentrates on identifying the muscle groups and learning how to control contraction. After this has been accomplished, she can start an exercise program that consists of slowly contracting the muscles, beginning at the front and working to the back while counting to four and then releasing. The exercises can be done while sitting or standing and are usually performed in repetitions of 10, three times each day. A vaginal cone, a tampon-like device, may be used to enhance the benefits of the exercise. The cone is placed in the vagina, and the woman instructed to hold it in place by contracting the proper inner muscles.[14]

The α-adrenergic agonist drugs, such as phenylpropanolamine, increase sympathetic relaxation of the detrusor muscle and internal sphincter tone and may be used in treating stress incontinence.[2] Imipramine, a tricyclic antidepressant agent that has α-adrenergic and anticholinergic properties, has proved useful in some women. Estrogen therapy (oral or vaginal) may be considered as an adjunctive pharmacologic agent for postmenopausal women.

Surgical intervention may be considered when other treatment methods have proved ineffective. Three types of surgical procedures are used: procedures that increase outlet resistance, surgeries that decrease detrusor muscle instability, and operations that remove outflow obstruction to reduce overflow incontinence and detrusor muscle instability.[2]

Noncatheter Devices

Two types of *noncatheter devices* commonly are used in the management of urinary incontinence: one obstructs flow, and the other collects urine as it is passed. Obstruction of urine flow is achieved by compressing the urethra or stimulating the contraction of the pelvic floor muscles. Penile clamps are available that occlude the urethra without obstructing blood circulation to the penis. Clamps must be removed at 3-hour intervals to empty the bladder. Complications such as penile and urethral erosion can occur if clamps are used incorrectly. In females, compression of the urethra usually is accomplished by intravaginal devices.

Surgically implanted artificial sphincters are available for use in males and females.[17] These devices consist of an inflatable cuff that surrounds the proximal urethra. The cuff is connected by tubing to an implanted fluid reservoir and an inflation bulb. Pressing the bulb, which is placed in the scrotum in males, inflates the cuff. It is emptied in a similar manner.

Another method of occluding the bladder outlet in males and females is the use of battery-operated electrodes that cause contraction of the pelvic floor muscles. This treatment is most effective in women with stress incontinence caused by weakness of the pelvic floor muscles. Implantable electrodes have largely been replaced by those that can be worn in the vagina or in the anus.

When urinary incontinence cannot be prevented, various types of urine collection devices or protective pads are used. Men can be fitted with collection devices (*i.e.*, condom or sheath urinals) that are worn over the penis and attached to a container at the bedside or fastened to the body. There are no effective external collection devices for women. Pants and pads usually are used. Dribbling bags (males) and pads (females) in which the urine changes to a nonpourable gel are available for occasional dribbling but are unsuitable for considerable wetting.

Special Needs of Elderly Persons

Urinary incontinence is a common problem in elderly persons. An estimated 15% of community dwelling elders and 50% of institutionalized elders have severe urinary incontinence.[18] Many factors contribute to incontinence in elderly persons, a number of which can be altered.

Pelvic relaxation disorders are more frequent in older than in younger women, and prostatic hypertrophy is more common in older than in younger men. Many elderly persons have difficulty getting to the toilet in time. This can be caused by arthritis that makes walking or removing clothing difficult or by failing vision that makes trips to the bathroom precarious, especially in new and unfamiliar surroundings.

Medication prescribed for other health problems may prevent a healthy bladder from functioning normally. Potent, fast-acting diuretics are known for their ability to cause urge incontinence. Psychoactive drugs, such as tranquilizers and sedatives, may diminish normal attention to bladder clues. Impaired thirst or limited access to fluids predisposes to constipation with urethral obstruction and overflow incontinence and to concentrated and infected urine, which increases bladder excitability.

According to Stanton, "there are two guiding principles in management of incontinence in the elderly. First, growing old does not imply becoming incontinent, and second, incontinence should not be left untreated just because the patient is old."[19] Treatment may involve changes in the physical environment so that the older person can reach the bathroom more easily or remove clothing more quickly. Habit training with regularly scheduled toileting—usually every 2 to 4 hours—often is effective. Many elderly persons who void on a regular schedule can gradually increase the interval between toileting while improving their ability to suppress bladder instability.[20] The treatment plan may require dietary changes to prevent constipation or a plan to promote adequate fluid intake to ensure adequate bladder filling and prevent urinary stasis and symptomatic urinary tract infections.

In summary, alterations in bladder function include urinary obstruction with retention of urine and urinary incontinence with involuntary loss of urine. Urine retention occurs when the outflow of urine from the bladder is obstructed because of urethral obstruction or impaired bladder innervation. Urethral obstruction causes bladder irritability, detrusor muscle hypertrophy, trabeculation and the formation of diverticula, development of hydroureters, and eventually, renal failure.

Neurogenic bladder is caused by interruption in the innervation of the bladder. It can cause spastic bladder dysfunction or flaccid bladder dysfunction, depending on the level of the lesion. Spastic bladder dysfunction usually results from neurologic lesions that are above the level of the sacral micturition reflex center; flaccid bladder dysfunction results from lesions at the level of sacral micturition reflexes or peripheral innervation of the bladder.

Urinary incontinence is the involuntary loss of urine that is sufficient to be a problem. It may manifest as stress incontinence, in which the loss of urine occurs as a result of coughing, sneezing, laughing, or lifting; urge incontinence, characterized by a strong desire to void that often is associated with strong hyperreflexive bladder contraction; or overflow, or reflex, incontinence, which results when intravesicular pressure exceeds the maximal urethral pressure because of bladder distention. Other causes of incontinence include a small, contracted bladder or external environmental conditions that make it difficult to access proper toileting facilities.

The treatment of urinary obstruction, neurogenic bladder, and incontinence requires careful diagnosis to determine the cause and contributing factors. Treatment methods include correction of the underlying cause, such as obstruction due to prostatic hyperplasia; behavior methods that focus on bladder and habit training; exercises to improve pelvic floor function; pharmacologic methods; and the use of catheters and urine collection devices.

Cancer of the Bladder

After you have completed this section of the chapter, you should be able to meet the following objectives:

- Discuss the difference between superficial and invasive bladder cancer in terms of bladder involvement, extension of the disease, and prognosis
- State the most common sign of bladder cancer

Bladder cancer is the most frequent form of urinary tract cancer in the United States, accounting for an estimated 51,600 new cases and 9500 deaths each year.[21] It most commonly occurs in the 50- to 70-year age group and is three times as common in men as in women.[22]

Bladder cancers fall into two major groups: superficial and invasive, according to their natural history.[23]

About 80% of superficial bladder cancers remain confined to the mucosa and submucosa throughout their natural history, whereas most invasive bladder cancers have penetrated the deep bladder layers at the time of presentation and are associated with metastasis and a worse prognosis. About 70% to 75% of bladder cancers present as superficial noninvasive tumors. With traditional methods of therapy (*e.g.*, transurethral resection, electrocautery removal, cystectomy), the long-term survival rate for persons with this type of bladder cancer is more than 80%. These tumors frequently recur, however, and the apparent rate of cure is less than 50%.[23] The remaining 25% to 30% of bladder cancers are highly invasive. These tumors may manifest as in situ lesions that progress rapidly to invasive lesions or as advanced invasive disease. The most common sites of metastasis are the pelvic lymph nodes, lungs, bones, and liver.

Although the cause of bladder cancer is unknown, evidence suggests that its origin is related to local influences, such as carcinogens that are excreted in the urine and stored in the bladder. This includes the breakdown products of aniline dyes used in the rubber and cable industries. Smoking also deserves attention, because it may be responsible for as many as 50% of cases of cancer in men and 33% in women. Chronic bladder infections and bladder stones also increase the risk of bladder cancer. Although earlier studies have suggested an association between bladder cancer and artificial sweeteners such as saccharin and cyclamates, this association has not been proved.

Bladder cancer occurs among persons harboring the parasite *Schistosoma haematobium* in their bladders. It is not known whether the parasite excretes a carcinogen or produces its effects through irritation of the bladder.

Diagnosis and Treatment

The most common sign of bladder cancer is hematuria.[22,23,25] Gross hematuria is a presenting sign in 75% of persons with the disease, and microscopic hematuria is present in most others.[23] Frequency, urgency, and dysuria occasionally accompany the hematuria. Because hematuria often is intermittent, the diagnosis may be delayed. Periodic urine cytology is recommended for all persons who are at high risk for the development of bladder cancer because of exposure to urinary tract carcinogens. Ureteral invasion leading to bacterial and obstructive renal disease and dissemination of the cancer are potential complications and ultimate causes of death. The prognosis depends on the histologic grade of the cancer and the stage of the disease at the time of diagnosis.

Diagnostic methods include cytologic studies, excretory urography, cystoscopy, and biopsy. Ultrasonography, CT scans, and MRI are used as aids for staging the tumor. Cytologic studies performed on biopsy tissues or cells obtained from bladder washings may be used to detect the presence of malignant cells. A technique called *flow cytometry* is helpful in screening persons at high risk for the disease and for monitoring the results of therapy. In flow cytometry, the interaction between fluorochromes or dyes with DNA causes the emission of high-intensity light similar to that produced by a laser.[23] Flow cytometry can be carried out on biopsy specimens, bladder washings, or cytologic preparations. There appears to be a correlation between the DNA content (*i.e.*, ploidy) and the level of differentiation (*i.e.*, grade), depth of invasion (*i.e.*, stage), and response to treatment. The expression of blood group antigens on the surface of bladder cancer cells has proved to be a useful prognostic determinant. Tumors that express the A, B, or H antigens have a better prognosis than tumors that do not express these antigens.[23]

The treatment of bladder cancer depends on the extent of the lesion and the health of the patient. Endoscopic resection usually is done for diagnostic purposes and may be used as a treatment for superficial lesions. Diathermy (*i.e.*, electrocautery) may be used to remove the tumors. Segmental surgical resection may be used for removing a large single lesion. When the tumor is invasive, cystectomy with resection of the pelvic lymph nodes frequently is the treatment of choice. In males, the prostate and seminal vesicles often are removed as well. Until the 1980s, most men who underwent radical cystectomy became impotent.[23] Newer surgical approaches designed to preserve erectile function are now being used. Cystectomy requires urinary diversion, an alternative reservoir, usually created from the ileum (*e.g.*, an ileal loop), that is designed to collect the urine. Traditionally, the ileostomy reservoir drains urine continuously into an external collecting device. Methods of urinary diversion that provide continence and eliminate the need to wear an external collection bag are being explored.[23]

Although a number of chemotherapeutic drugs have been used in the treatment of bladder cancer, no chemotherapeutic regimens for the disease have been established. Perhaps of more importance is the increasing use of intravesicular chemotherapy, in which the cytotoxic drug is instilled directly into the bladder.[22–24] These drugs can be instilled prophylactically after surgical resection of all demonstrable tumor or therapeutically in the presence of residual disease. Among the chemotherapeutic drugs that have been used for this purpose are thiotepa, mitomycin C, and doxorubicin (Adriamycin). The intervesicular administration of *bacillus Calmette-Guérin* (BCG) vaccine, made from a strain of *Mycobacterium bovis* that formerly was used to protect against tuberculosis, causes a significant reduction in the rate of relapse and prolongs relapse-free interval in persons with cancer in situ. The vaccine is thought to act as a nonspecific stimulator of cell-mediated immunity. It is not known whether the effects of BCG are immunologic or include a component of direct toxicity. Several strains of this agent exist, and it is not known which is the most active and least toxic.[23]

In summary, cancer of the bladder is the most common cause of urinary tract cancer in the United States, accounting for about 51,600 new cases and

9500 deaths each year. It most frequently occurs in the 50- to 70-year age group and is twice as common in men as in women. Bladder cancers fall into two major groups: superficial tumors that remain confined to the mucosa and submucosa and invasive cancers that have penetrated the deep bladder layers at the time of presentation and are associated with metastasis and a worse prognosis. Even the superficial tumors tend to recur after removal, and the apparent rate of cure in less than 50%. Although the cause of cancer of the bladder is unknown, evidence suggests that carcinogens excreted in the urine may play a role. Gross hematuria is the most common sign of bladder cancer, occurring in 75% of persons with the disease. Treatment of bladder cancer depends on the cytologic grade of the tumor and the extent of the invasiveness of the lesion.

REFERENCES

1. Berne R.M., Levy M.N. (1993). *Physiology* (3rd ed., p. 726). St. Louis: C.V. Mosby.
2. Fantl J.A., Newman D.K., Colling J., et al. for the Public Health Service, Agency for Health Care Policy and Research. (1996). *Urinary incontinence in adults: Acute and chronic management.* Clinical practice guideline no. 2, 1996 update. AHCPR Publication No. 96–0682. Rockville MD: U.S. Department of Health and Human Services.
3. Tanagho E.A., Schmidt R.A. (1995). Urodynamic studies. In Tanagho E.A., McAninch J.W. (Eds.). *Smith's general urology* (14th ed., pp. 514–535). Los Altos, CA: Lange Medical Publishers.
4. Tanagho E.A., Schmidt R.A. (1995). Urinary obstruction and stasis. In E.A. Tanagho J.W. McAninch (Eds.). *Smith's general urology* (14th ed., pp. 172–185). Los Altos, CA: Lange Medical Publishers.
5. Frimodt-Miller C. (1980). Diabetic cystopathy: Epidemiology and related disorders. *Annals of Internal Medicine* 92 (2), 318.
6. Said G. (1996). Diabetic neuropathy. *Journal of Neurology* 243, 431–440.
7. Bays H.E., Pfiefer M.A. (1988). Peripheral diabetic neuropathy. *Medical Clinics of North America* 72 (6), 1439–1464.
8. Thon W., Altwein J.E. (1984). Voiding dysfunction. *Urology* 23, 323.
9. Lapides J., Diokno A.C., Silber S.J. (1971). Clean, intermittent self-catheterization in treatment of urinary tract disease. *Transactions of the American Association of Genitourinary Surgeons* 63, 92.
10. Perlow D.L., Gikas P.W., Horwitz E.M. (1981). Effects of vesicle overdistention on bladder mucin. *Urology* 18, 380.
11. Urinary Incontinence Guideline Panel. (1992). *Urinary incontinence in adults: Clinical practice guidelines.* APCPR Pub. No 92–0038. Rockville, MD: Agency for Health Care Policy and Research, Public Health Service U.S. Department of Health and Human Services.
12. Gray M., Burns S.M. (1996). Continence management. *Critical Care Clinics of North America* 8 (1), 29–38.
13. Green T.H. (1975). Urinary stress incontinence: Differential diagnosis, pathophysiology, and management. *American Journal of Obstetrics and Gynecology* 122, 368.
14. Boourcier A.P., Jurat J.C. (1995). Nonsurgical therapy for stress incontinence. *Urology Clinics of North America* 22 (3), 613–627.
15. Chutka D.S., Fleming K.C., Evans M.P., Evans J.M., Andrews D.L. (1996). Urinary incontinence in the elderly population. *Mayo Clinic Proceedings* 71, 93–101.
16. Wells T.J., Brink C.A., Kiokno A.C, et al. (1991). Pelvic muscle exercise for stress urinary incontinence in elderly women. *Journal American Geriatric Association* 39, 785–791.
17. Brocklehurst J.C. (1982). Noncatheter devices for urinary incontinence in the elderly. *Medical Instrumentation* 16, 167.
18. Kegel A.H. (1948). Progressive resistance exercises in the functional restoration of the perineal muscles. *American Journal of Obstetrics and Gynecology* 56, 238.
19. Stanton S.L. (1984). Surgical management of female incontinence. In Brocklehurst J.C. (Ed.). *Urology in the elderly* (p. 93). New York: Churchill Livingstone.
20. Rousseau P., Fuentevilla-Clifton A. (1992). Urinary incontinence in the aged. II: Management strategies. *Geriatrics* 47 (6), 37.
21. Parker S.L., Tong T., Bolden S., Wingo P.A. (1997). Cancer statistics, 1997. *CA A Cancer Journal for Clinicians* xx, 4–9.
22. Kelly L.P., Miaskowski C. (1996). An overview of bladder cancer: Treatment and nursing implications. *Oncology Nursing Forum* 23 (3), 459–467.
23. Raghavan D., Shipley W.U., Garnick M.B., et al. (1990). Biology and management of bladder cancer. *New England Journal of Medicine* 322, 1129.
24. Badalament R.A., Schervish E.W. (1996). Bladder cancer. *Postgraduate Medicine* 100 (2), 217–224.

ADDITIONAL READINGS

Burns P.A., Pranikoff K., Nochajski T., et al. (1990). Treatment of stress incontinence with pelvic floor exercise and biofeedback. *Journal of the American Geriatric Society* 38, 314.

Cummings J.M., Houston K. (1994). The treatment of urinary incontinence. *Hospital Practice* 29 (2), 97–107.

Diokno A.C. (1995). Epidemiology and psychosocial aspects of incontinence. *Urologic Clinics of North America* 22 (3), 481–485.

Elbadawi A. (1995). Pathology and pathophysiology of detrusor in incontinence. *Urologic Clinics of North America* 22 (3), 499–511.

Gallo M.M., Gallon P.J., Staskin D.R. (1997). Urinary incontinence: Steps to evaluation, diagnosis, and treatment. *The Nurse Practitioner* 22 (2), 21–44.

Mold J.W. (1996). Pharmacology of urinary incontinence. *American Family Physician* 54 (2), 673–680.

Webb R.J., Lawson A.L., Neal D.E. (1990). Clean intermittent self-catheterization in 172 adults. *British Journal of Urology* 65, 20.

Gastrointestinal Function

The study of the gastrointestinal system aroused none of the philosophical interest that surrounded the elements, humors, and pneuma of Galen's time. During ancient times, the gut was thought merely to provide the chyle that was turned into blood by the liver. Although the structures of the gut had been fairly well described, perhaps owing to observations made during the slaughtering of animals, it was not until the 18th and 19th centuries that the function of the gastrointestinal tract began to unfold.

One of the breakthroughs in gastrointestinal physiology came as the result of an accident. In 1822 William Beaumont (1785–1853), a self-trained surgeon in the United States Army, was called upon to render aid to Alexis St. Martin, a Canadian traveler who had suffered a large gunshot wound to the chest and abdomen. Although not expected to live, young St. Martin rallied and his wounds healed; however, he was left with a permanent fistula that opened to his stomach. Beaumont became intrigued with his patient's unique defect, using this living laboratory to study the process of digestion. He would have St. Martin swallow different types of food and then collect the stomach contents by means of a tube passed into the fistula. Beaumont described the movement of the stomach, and he confirmed the presence of hydrochloric acid and a ferment, later shown to be the result of the protein-breaking enzyme pepsin. Because of an unfortunate accident, both Beaumont and St. Martin gained a place in the history of gastrointestinal physiology.

UNIT VIII

CHAPTER 31

Control of Gastrointestinal Function

The process of digestion and absorption of nutrients requires an intact and healthy gastrointestinal tract epithelial lining that can resist the effects of its own digestive secretions. The process involves movement of materials through the gastrointestinal tract at a rate that facilitates absorption, and it requires the presence of enzymes for the digestion and absorption of nutrients. Structurally, the gastrointestinal tract is a long, hollow tube with its lumen inside the body and its wall acting as an interface between the internal and external environments. The wall does not normally allow harmful agents to enter the body, nor does it permit body fluids and other materials to escape.

The digestive system is an amazing structure. In this system, enzymes and hormones are produced, vitamins are synthesized and stored, and food is dismantled and then reassembled. Nutrients, vitamins, minerals, electrolytes, and water enter the body through the gastrointestinal tract. Wastes are collected and eliminated efficiently.

Although this chapter cannot cover gastrointestinal function in its entirety, it is designed to provide the reader with an overview that is deemed essential to an understanding of subsequent chapters. As a matter of semantics, it should be pointed out that the gastrointestinal tract is also referred to as the *digestive tract*, the *alimentary canal*, and at times, the *gut*. The intestinal portion may also be called the *bowel*. For our purposes, the salivary glands, the liver, and the pancreas, which produce secretions that aid in digestion, are considered accessory organs.

Structure and Organization of the Gastrointestinal Tract

After you have completed this section of the chapter, you should be able to meet the following objectives:

- Describe the physiologic function of the four parts of the digestive system
- List the five layers of the digestive tract and describe their function
- Characterize the function of the intramural neural plexuses in control of gastrointestinal function

In the digestive tract, food and other materials move slowly along its length as they are systematically broken down into ions and molecules that can be absorbed into the body. In the large intestine, unabsorbed nutrients and wastes are collected for later elimination. Although the gastrointestinal tract is located within the body, it is

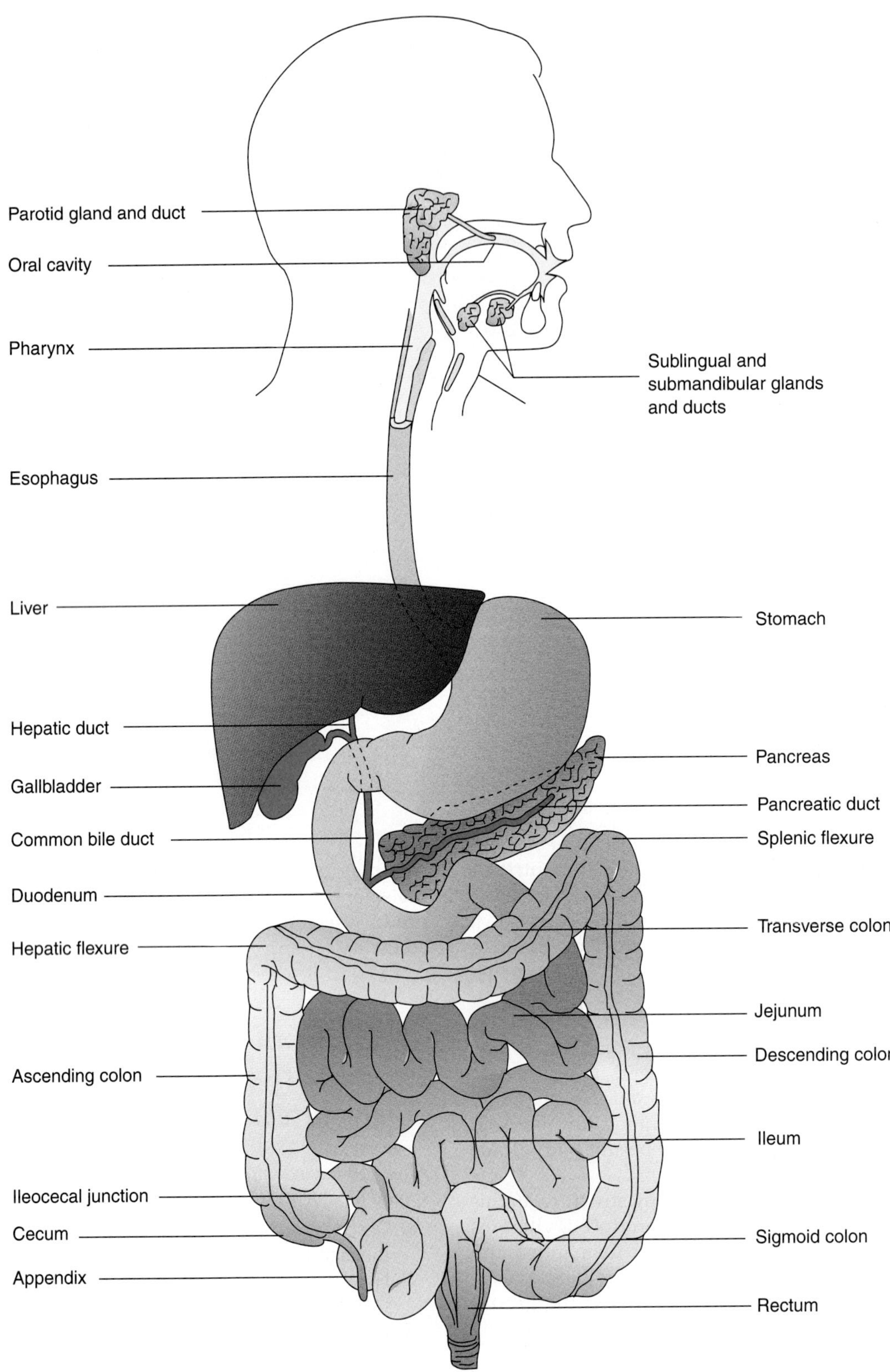

Figure 31–1
The digestive system.

a long, hollow tube, the lumen (*i.e.*, hollow center) of which is an extension of the external environment. Nutrients do not become part of the internal environment until they have passed through the intestinal wall and have entered the blood or lymph channels.

For simplicity and understanding, the digestive system can be divided into four parts (Fig. 31–1). The *upper part*—the mouth, esophagus, and stomach—acts as an intake source and receptacle through which food passes and in which initial digestive processes take place. The *middle portion* consists of the small intestine—the duodenum, jejunum, and ileum. Most digestive and absorptive processes occur in the small intestine. The *lower segment*—the cecum, colon, and rectum—serves as a storage channel for the efficient elimination of waste. The *fourth part* consists of the accessory organs—the salivary glands, liver, and pancreas. These structures produce digestive secretions that help dismantle foods and regulate the use and storage of nutrients. The discussion in this chapter focuses on the first three parts of the gastrointestinal tract. The liver and pancreas are discussed in Chapter 33.

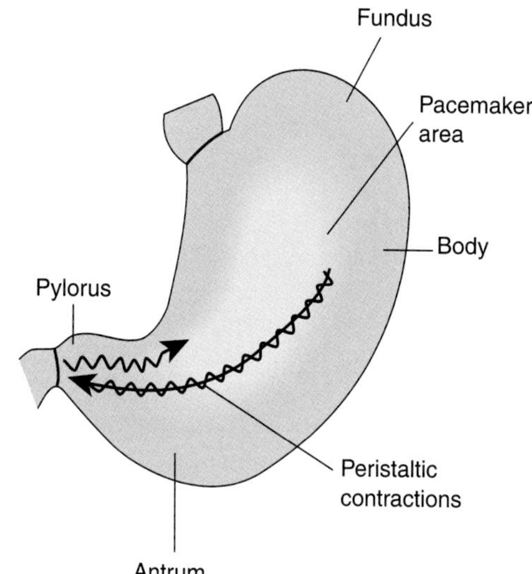

Figure 31–2
Structures of the stomach, showing the pacemaker area and the direction of chyme movement resulting from peristaltic contractions.

Upper Gastrointestinal Tract

The mouth forms the entryway into the gastrointestinal tract for food; it contains the teeth, used in the mastication of food, and the tongue and other structures needed to direct food toward the pharyngeal structures and the esophagus.

The esophagus begins at the lower end of the pharynx. It receives food from the pharynx, and in the process of swallowing, a series of peristaltic contractions moves the food into the stomach. The esophagus is a muscular, collapsible tube, about 25 cm (10 in) long, that lies behind the trachea. The muscular walls of the upper third of the esophagus are skeletal-type striated muscle; these muscle fibers are gradually replaced by smooth muscle fibers until, at the lower third of the esophagus, the muscle layer is entirely smooth muscle.

The upper and lower ends of the esophagus act as sphincters. The upper sphincter is formed by a thickening of the striated muscle; it prevents air from entering the esophagus during respiration. The lower sphincter, which is not identifiable anatomically, occurs at a point 1 cm to 2 cm (0.4 to 0.8 in) from where the esophagus joins the stomach. The lower sphincter prevents gastric reflux into the esophagus.

The stomach is a pouchlike structure that lies in the upper part of the abdomen and serves as a food storage reservoir during the early stages of digestion. Although the luminal volume of the stomach is only about 50 ml, it can increase its volume to almost 1000 ml before intraluminal pressure begins to rise. The esophagus opens into the stomach through an opening called the cardiac orifice, so named because of its proximity to the heart. The part of the stomach that lies above and to the left of the cardiac orifice is called the fundus, the central portion is called the body, the orifice encircled by a ringlike muscle that opens into the small intestine is called the pylorus, and the portion between the body and pylorus is called the antrum (Fig. 31–2). The presence of a true pyloric sphincter is controversial. Whether an actual sphincter exists or not, contractions of the smooth muscle in the pyloric area control the rate of gastric emptying.

Middle Gastrointestinal Tract

The small intestine, which forms the middle portion of the digestive tract, consists of three subdivisions: the duodenum, the jejunum, and the ileum. The duodenum, which is about 22 cm (10 in) long, connects the stomach to the jejunum and contains the opening for the common bile duct and the main pancreatic duct. Bile and pancreatic juices enter the intestine through these ducts. It is in the jejunum and ileum, which together are about 7 m (23 ft) long and must be folded onto themselves to fit into the abdominal cavity, that food is digested and absorbed.

Lower Gastrointestinal Tract

The large intestine, which forms the lower gastrointestinal tract, is about 1.5 m (4.5 to 5 ft) long and 6 cm to 7 cm (2.4 to 2.7 in) in diameter. It is divided into the cecum, colon, rectum, and anal canal. The cecum is a blind pouch that projects down at the junction of the ileum and the colon. The ileocecal valve lies at the upper border of the cecum and prevents the return of feces from the cecum into the small intestine. The appendix arises from the cecum about 2.5 cm (1 in) from the ileocecal valve. The colon is further divided into ascending, transverse, descending, and sigmoid portions. The ascending colon

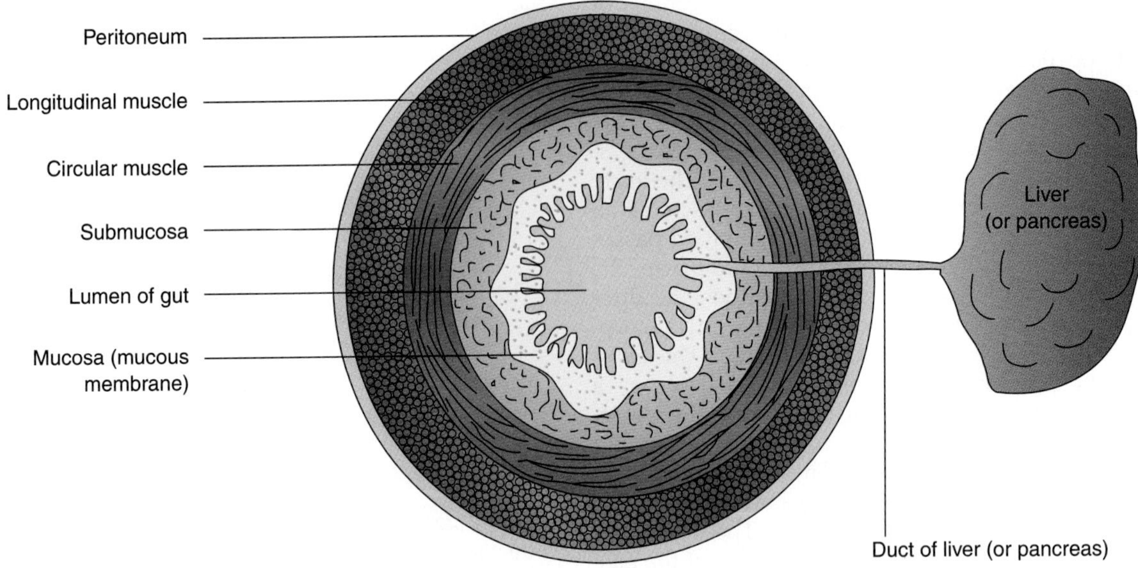

Figure 31–3
Transverse section of the digestive system.

extends from the cecum to the undersurface of the liver, where it turns abruptly to form the right colic (hepatic) flexure. The transverse colon crosses the upper half of the abdominal cavity from right to left and then curves sharply downward beneath the lower end of the spleen, forming the left colic (splenic) flexure. The descending colon extends from the colic flexure to the rectum. The rectum extends from the sigmoid colon to the anus. The anal canal passes between the two medial borders of the levator ani muscles. Powerful sphincter muscles guard against fecal incontinence.

Gastrointestinal Wall Structure

The digestive tract, below the upper third of the esophagus, is essentially a five-layered tube (Fig. 31–3). The inner luminal layer, or *mucosa,* is so named because its cells produce mucus that lubricates and protects the inner surface of the alimentary canal. The epithelial cells in this layer have a rapid turnover rate and are replaced every 4 to 5 days. Approximately 250 g of these cells are shed each day in the stool. Because of the regenerative capabilities of the mucosal layer, injury to this layer of tissue heals rapidly without leaving scar tissue. The *submucosal layer* consists of connective tissue. This layer contains blood vessels, nerves, and structures responsible for secreting digestive enzymes. Movement in the gastrointestinal tract is facilitated by the *circular* and *longitudinal* smooth muscle layers. The outer layer, the *peritoneum,* is loosely attached to the outer wall of the intestine.

The *peritoneum* is the largest serous membrane in the body, having a surface area about equal to that of the skin. The peritoneal membrane is composed of two layers, a thin layer of simple squamous epithelial cells resting on a layer of connective tissue. If the epithelial layer is injured because of surgery or inflammation, there is danger that adhesions (*i.e.,* fibrous scar-tissue bands)

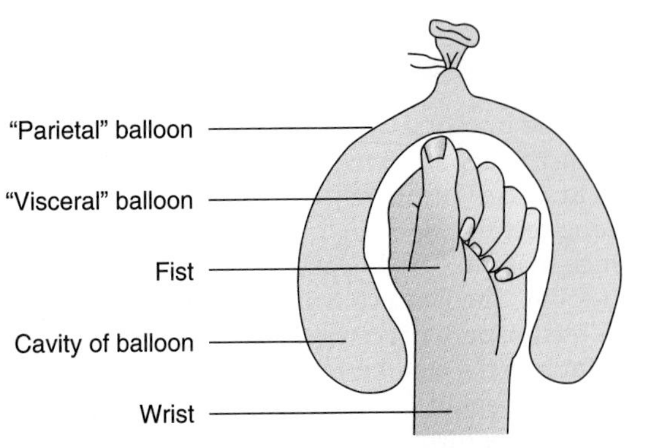

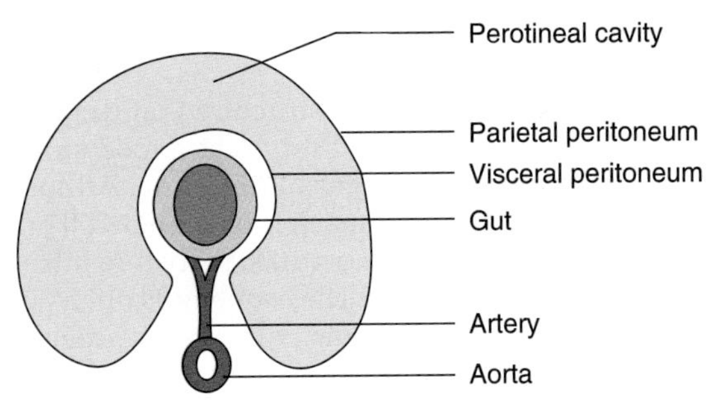

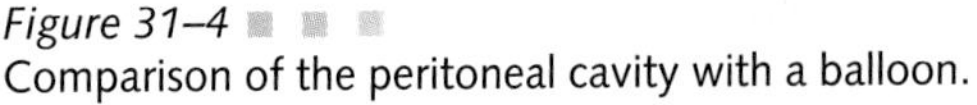
Figure 31–4
Comparison of the peritoneal cavity with a balloon.

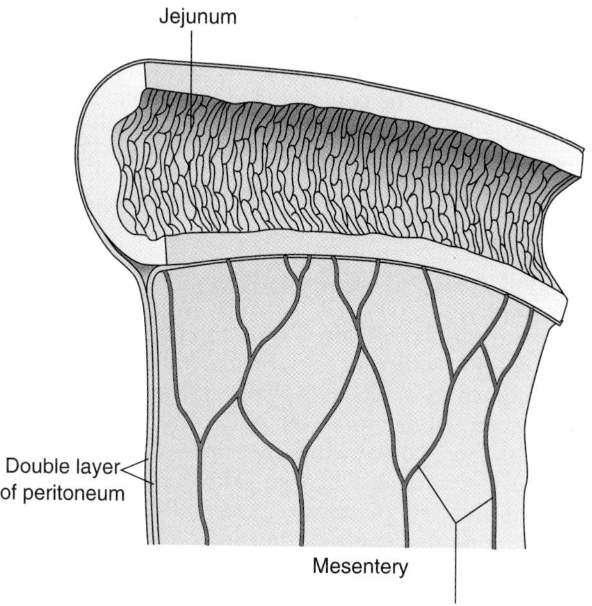

Figure 31–5
The attachment of the mesentery to the small bowel.

may form, causing sections of the viscera to heal together. Adhesions can alter the position and movement of the abdominal viscera.

The *peritoneal cavity* is a potential space formed between what is called the *parietal peritoneum* and the *visceral peritoneum*. The parietal peritoneum comes in contact with and is loosely attached to the abdominal wall, whereas the abdominal organs are in contact with the visceral peritoneum. The two layers of the peritoneum can be compared with a deflated balloon. If one makes a fist into the balloon, the outer surface can be equated with the parietal peritoneum, and the fist interfaces with the visceral peritoneum (Fig. 31–4). In this case, the area within the balloon represents the peritoneal cavity. The connective tissue layer of the peritoneum forms the parietal and the visceral peritoneum, and the smooth, epithelial cell layer of the membrane lines the cavity. The adjacent membrane layers within the peritoneal cavity are separated by a thin layer of serous fluid. This fluid forms a moist and slippery surface that serves to prevent friction between the continuously moving abdominal structures. In certain pathologic states, the amount of fluid in the potential space of the peritoneal cavity is increased, causing a condition called *ascites*.

The jejunum and ileum are suspended by a double-layered fold of peritoneum called the *mesentery* (Fig. 31–5). The mesentery contains the blood vessels, nerves, and lymphatic vessels that supply the intestinal wall. The mesentery is gathered in folds that attach to the dorsal abdominal wall along a short line of insertion, giving a fan-shaped appearance, with the intestines at the edge. A filmy, double fold of peritoneal membrane called the *greater omentum* extends from the stomach to cover the transverse and folds of the intestine (Fig. 31–6). The greater omentum protects the intestines from cold. It always contains some fat, which in obese persons can be

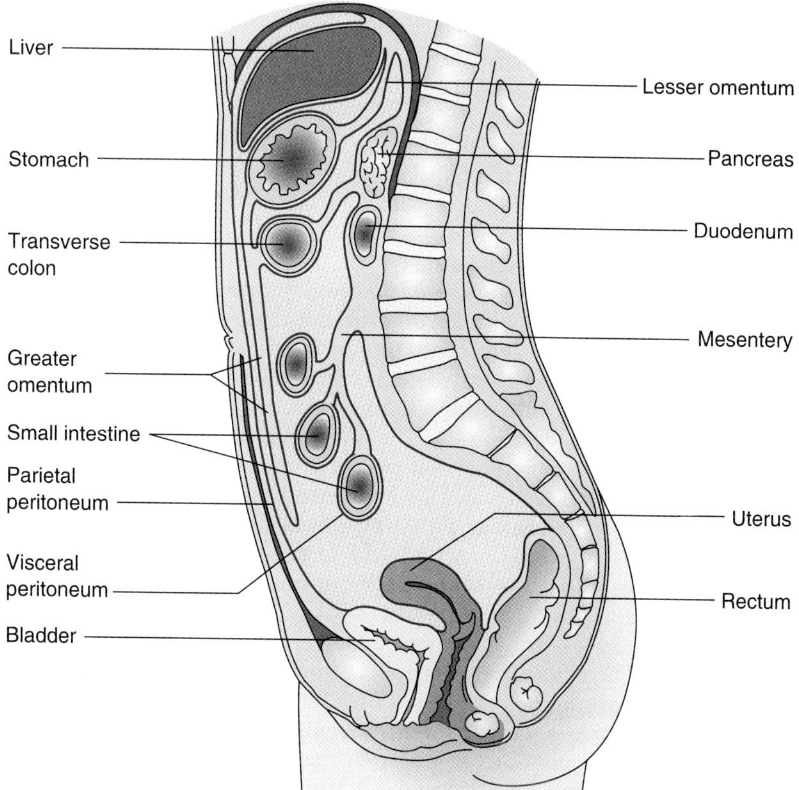

Figure 31–6
Reflections of the peritoneum as seen in sagittal section.

a considerable amount. The omentum also controls the spread of infection from gastrointestinal contents. In the case of infection, the omentum adheres to the inflamed area so that the infection is less likely to enter the peritoneal cavity. The *lesser omentum* extends between the transverse fissure of the liver and the lesser curvature of the stomach.

In summary, the gastrointestinal tract is a long, hollow tube, the lumen of which is an extension of the external environment. The digestive tract can be divided into four parts: an upper part, consisting of the mouth, esophagus, and stomach; a middle part consisting, of the small intestine; a lower part, consisting of the cecum, colon, and rectum; and the accessory organs, consisting of the salivary glands, the liver, and the pancreas. Throughout its length, except for the mouth, throat, and upper esophagus, the gastrointestinal tract is composed of five layers: an inner mucosal layer, a submucosal layer, a layer of circular smooth muscle fibers, a layer of longitudinal smooth muscle fibers, and an outer serosal layer that forms the peritoneum and is continuous with the mesentery.

Motility

After you have completed this section of the chapter, you should be able to meet the following objectives:

- Compare the effects of parasympathetic and sympathetic activity on the motility and secretory function of the gastrointestinal tract
- Differentiate tonic and peristaltic movements in the gastrointestinal tract
- Trace a bolus of food through the stages of swallowing
- Describe the action of the internal and external sphincters in the control of defecation

The motility of the gastrointestinal tract propels food products and fluids along its length, from mouth to anus, in a manner that facilitates digestion and absorption. Except in the pharynx and upper third of the esophagus, smooth muscle provides the contractile force for gastrointestinal motility (the actions of smooth muscle are discussed in Chapter 1). The rhythmic movements of the digestive tract are self-perpetuating, much like the activity of the heart, and are influenced by local, humoral (*i.e.,* bloodborne), and neural influences. The ability to initiate impulses is a property of the smooth muscle itself. Impulses are conducted from one muscle fiber to another.

The movements of the gastrointestinal tract are tonic and rhythmic. The *tonic movements* are continuous movements that last for minutes or even hours. Tonic contractions occur at *sphincters*. The rhythmic movements consist of intermittent contractions that are responsible for mixing and moving food along the digestive tract. *Peristaltic movements* are rhythmic propulsive movements that occur when the smooth muscle layer constricts, forming a contractile band that forces the intraluminal contents forward. During peristalsis, the segment that lies distal to, or ahead of, the contracted portion relaxes, and the contents move forward with ease. Normal peristalsis always moves in the direction from the mouth toward the anus.

Neural Control Mechanisms

Gastrointestinal function is controlled by the enteric nervous system, which is contained within the wall of the gastrointestinal tract, and by the parasympathetic and sympathetic divisions of the ANS. The intramural neurons (*i.e.,* those contained within the wall of the gastrointestinal tract) consist of two networks, the myenteric and submucosal plexuses. These intramural plexuses extend along the length of the gastrointestinal wall. The myenteric (Auerbach's) plexus is located between the outer muscle layers, and the submucosal (Meissner's) plexus is located between the circular muscle and the submucosal layers (Fig. 31–7). The activity of the neurons in the myenteric and submucosal plexuses is regulated by local influences and by input from the ANS. Both plexuses are aggregates of ganglionic cells, most of which receive synaptic input from the vagus nerve. The sympathetic postganglionic fibers synapse directly with the muscle fibers. The myenteric plexus primarily influences motility, and the submucosal plexus affects motility and secretion. Nerve impulses initiated in one ganglionic cell spread through multiple intramural pathways, mainly in a longitudinal direction.

The digestive tract contains two types of afferent fibers: those whose cell bodies are located in the nervous system and those whose cell bodies are within the intramural plexuses. The first group has receptors in the mucosal epithelium and in the muscle layers; their fibers pass centrally in vagal and sympathetic fibers. The second group is located in the intramural plexus and exerts local control over motility.

Efferent parasympathetic innervation to the stomach, small intestine, cecum, ascending colon, and transverse colon occurs by way of the vagus nerve (Fig. 31–8). The remainder of the colon is innervated by parasympathetic fibers that exit the sacral segments of the spinal cord by way of the pelvic nerve. Preganglionic parasympathetic fibers can synapse with intramural plexus neurons, or they can act directly on intestinal smooth muscle. Most parasympathetic fibers are excitatory. Numerous vagovagal reflexes influence motility and secretions of the digestive tract.

Efferent sympathetic innervation of the gastrointestinal tract occurs through the thoracic chain of sympathetic ganglia and the celiac, superior mesenteric, and inferior mesenteric ganglia. The sympathetic nervous system exerts several effects on gastrointestinal function. It controls the extent of mucus secretion by the mucosal glands, reduces motility by inhibiting the activity of intramural plexus neurons, enhances sphincter function, and increases the vascular smooth muscle tone

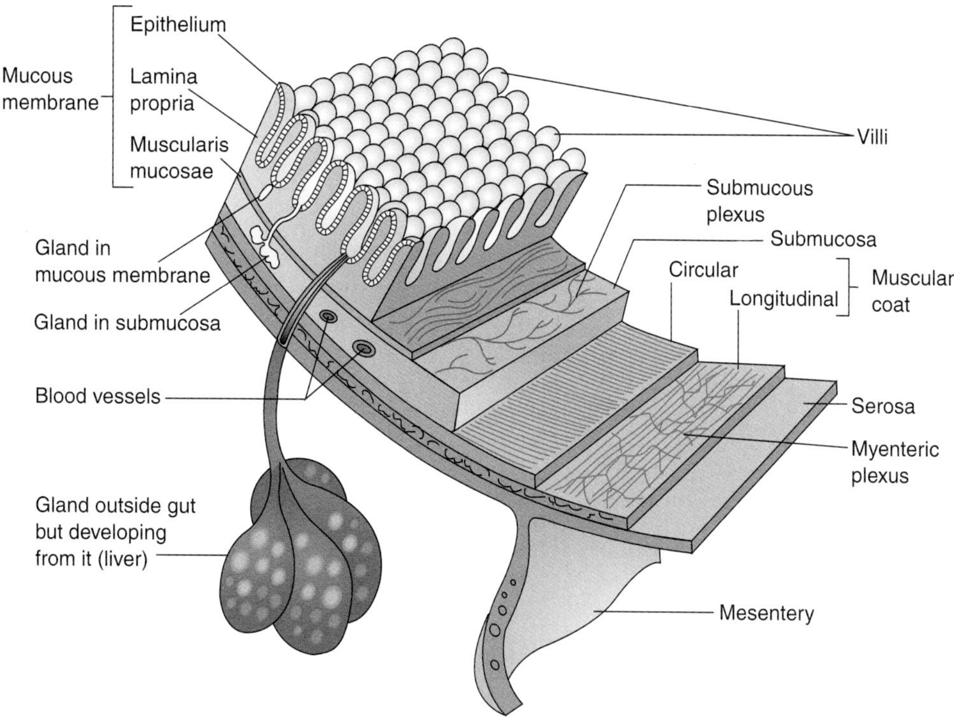

Figure 31–7
Diagram of the four main layers of the wall of the digestive tube: mucosa, submucosa, muscular, and serosa (below the diaphragm).

of the blood vessels that supply the gastrointestinal tract. The effect of the sympathetic stimulation is to block the release of the excitatory neuromediators in the intramural plexuses, inhibiting gastrointestinal motility. Sympathetic control of gastrointestinal function is largely mediated by activity within the intramural plexuses. For example, when gastric motility is enhanced because of increased vagal activity, stimulation of sympathetic centers in the hypothalamus promptly and often completely inhibits motility. The sympathetic fibers that supply the lower esophageal, pyloric, and internal and external anal sphincters are largely excitatory, but their role in controlling these sphincters is poorly understood.

Intramural plexus neurons also communicate with receptors in the mucosal and muscle layers. Mechanoreceptors monitor the stretch and distention of the gastrointestinal tract wall, and chemoreceptors monitor the chemical composition (*i.e.*, osmolality, pH, and digestive products of protein and fat metabolism) of its contents. These receptors can communicate directly with ganglionic cells in the intramural plexuses or with afferent fibers of the sympathetic or parasympathetic nervous system.

Chewing and Swallowing

Chewing begins the digestive process; it breaks the food into particles of a size that can be swallowed, lubricates it by mixing it with saliva, and mixes starch-containing food with salivary amylase. Although chewing is usually considered a voluntary act, it can be carried out involuntarily by a person who has lost the function of the cerebral cortex.

The swallowing reflex is a rigidly ordered sequence of events that results in the propulsion of food from the mouth to the stomach through the esophagus. Although swallowing is initiated as a voluntary activity, it becomes involuntary as food or fluid reaches the pharynx. Sensory impulses for the reflex begin at tactile receptors in the pharynx and esophagus and are integrated with the motor components of the response in an area of the reticular formation of the medulla and lower pons called the *swallowing center.* The motor impulses for the oral and pharyngeal phases of swallowing are carried in the trigeminal (V), glossopharyngeal (IX), vagus (X), and hypoglossal (XII) cranial nerves, and impulses for the esophogeal phase are carried by the vagus nerve. Diseases that disrupt these brain centers or their cranial nerves disrupt the coordination of swallowing and predispose an individual to food and fluid lodging in the trachea and bronchi, leading to risk of asphyxiation or aspiration pneumonia.

Swallowing consists of three phases: an oral, or voluntary phase; a pharyngeal phase; and an esophageal phase. During the oral phase, the bolus is collected at the back of the mouth so the tongue can lift the food upward until it touches the posterior wall of the pharynx. At this point, the second stage of swallowing is initiated. The soft palate is pulled upward, the palatopharyngeal folds are pulled together so that food does not enter the nasopharynx, the vocal cords are pulled together, and the epiglottis is moved so that it covers the larynx. Res-

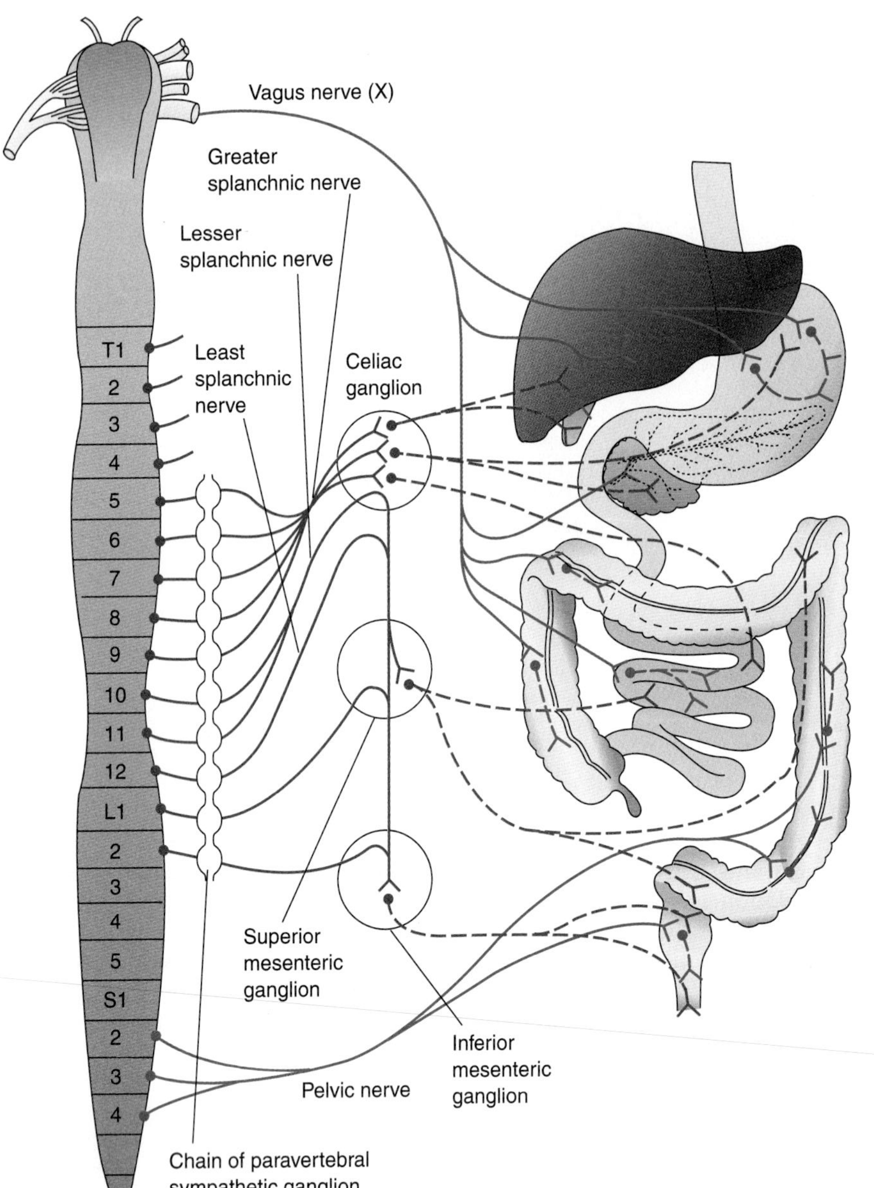

Figure 31–8 The autonomic innervation of the gastrointestinal tract.

piration is inhibited, and the bolus is moved backward into the esophagus by constrictive movements of the pharynx. Although the striated muscles of the pharynx are involved in the second stage of swallowing, it is an involuntary stage.

The third stage of swallowing is the esophageal stage. As food enters the esophagus and stretches its walls, local and central nervous system reflexes that initiate peristalsis are triggered. There are two types of peristalsis—primary and secondary. Primary peristalsis is controlled by the swallowing center in the brain stem and begins when food enters the esophagus. Secondary peristalsis is partially mediated by smooth muscle fibers in the esophagus and occurs when primary peristalsis is inadequate to move food through the esophagus. Peristalsis begins at the site of distention and moves downward. Before the peristaltic wave reaches the stomach, the lower esophageal sphincter relaxes to allow the bolus of food to enter the stomach. The pressure in the lower esophageal sphincter normally is greater than that in the stomach, an important factor in preventing the reflux of gastric contents. The opening of the lower esophageal sphincter is mediated vagally. Increased levels of the parasympathetic neuromediator acetylcholine increase the constriction of the sphincter. The hormone gastrin also increases constriction of the sphincter.

Gastrin provides the major stimulus for stomach acid production, and its action on the lower esophageal sphincter protects the esophageal mucosa when gastric acid levels are elevated.

Gastric Motility

The stomach serves as a reservoir for ingested solids and liquids. Motility of the stomach results in the churning and grinding of solid foods and regulates the emptying of the gastric contents, or chyme, into the duodenum. Peristaltic mixing and churning contractions begin in a pacemaker area in the middle of the stomach and move toward the antrum (see Fig. 31–2). They occur at a frequency of three to five contractions per minute, each with a duration of 2 to 20 seconds. As the peristaltic wave approaches the antrum, it speeds up, and the entire terminal 5 to 10 cm of the antrum contracts, occluding the pyloric opening. Contraction of the antrum reverses the movement of the chyme, returning the larger particles to the body of the stomach for further churning and kneading. Because the pylorus is contracted during antral contraction, the gastric contents are emptied into the duodenum between contractions.

Although the pylorus does not contain a true anatomic sphincter, it does function as a physiologic sphincter to prevent the backflow of gastric contents and allow them to flow into the duodenum at a rate commensurate with the ability of the duodenum to accept them. This is important because the regurgitation of bile salts and duodenal contents can damage the mucosal surface of the antrum and lead to gastric ulcers. Likewise, the duodenum can be damaged by the rapid influx of highly acid gastric contents.

Like other parts of the gastrointestinal tract, the stomach is richly innervated by the enteric nervous system and its connections with the sypathetic and parasympathetic nervous systems. Axons from the intramural plexuses innervate the smooth muscles and glands of the stomach. Parasympathetic innervation is provided by the vagus, and sympathetic innervation by the celiac ganglia. The emptying of the stomach is regulated by hormonal and neural mechanisms. The hormones cholecystokinin and gastric inhibitory peptide, which are thought to control gastric emptying, are released in response to pH and to the osmolar and fatty acid composition of the chyme. Local and central circuitry are involved in the neural control of gastric emptying. Afferent receptor fibers synapse with the neurons in the intramural plexus or trigger intrinsic reflexes by means of vagal or sympathetic pathways that participate in extrinsic reflexes.

Disorders of gastric motility can occur when the rate is too slow or too fast (see Chapter 32). A rate that is too slow causes gastric retention. It can be caused by obstruction or gastric atony. Obstruction can result from the formation of scar tissue in the pyloric area after a peptic ulcer. Another example of obstruction is hypertrophic pyloric stenosis, which can occur in infants with an abnormally thick muscularis layer in the terminal pylorus. Myotomy, or surgical incision of the muscular ring, is usually done to relieve the obstruction. Gastric atony can occur as a complication of visceral neuropathies in diabetes mellitus. Surgical procedures that disrupt vagal activity can also result in gastric atony. Abnormally fast emptying occurs in the dumping syndrome, which is a consequence of certain types of gastric operations. This condition is characterized by the rapid dumping of highly acidic and hyperosmotic gastric secretions into the duodenum and jejunum.

Small Intestine Motility

The small intestine is the major site for the digestion and absorption of food; its movements are mixing and propulsive. Regular peristaltic movements begin in the duodenum near the entry sites of the common duct and the main hepatic duct. A series of local pacemakers maintain the frequency of intestinal contraction. The peristaltic movements (about 12 per minute in the jejunum) become less frequent as they move further from the pylorus, becoming about nine per minute in the ileum.

The peristaltic contractions produce segmentation waves and propulsive movements through the muscles of the small intestine. With segmentation waves, slow contractions of circular muscle occlude the lumen and drive the contents forward and backward. Most of the contractions that produce segmentation waves are local events involving only 1 to 4 cm at a time. They function mainly to mix the chyme with the digestive enzymes from the pancreas and to ensure adequate exposure of all parts of the chyme to the mucosal surface of the intestine, where absorption takes place. The frequency of segmenting activity increases after a meal. Presumably, it is stimulated by receptors in the stomach and intestine.

Propulsive movements occur with synchronized activity in a section 10 to 20 cm long. They are accomplished by contraction of the proximal, or orad, portion of the intestine with the sequential relaxation of its distal, or anal, portion. After material has been propelled to the ileocecal junction by peristaltic movement, stretching of the distal ileum produces a local reflex that relaxes the sphincter and allows fluid to squirt into the cecum.

Motility disturbances of the small bowel are common, and auscultation of the abdomen can be used to assess bowel activity. Inflammatory changes increase motility. In many instances, it is not certain whether changes in motility occur because of inflammation or occur secondary to toxins and unabsorbed materials. Delayed passage of materials in the small intestine can also be a problem. Transient interruption of intestinal motility often occurs after gastrointestinal surgery. Intubation with suction is often required to remove the accumulating intestinal contents and gases until activity is resumed.

Colonic Motility

The storage function of the *colon* dictates that movements within this section of the gut be different from those in the small intestine. Movements in the colon are of two types. First are the segmental mixing movements, called *haustrations,* so named because they occur within sacculations called *haustra*. These movements produce a local digging-type action, which ensures that all portions of the fecal mass are exposed to the intestinal surface. Second are the *propulsive mass movements,* in which a large segment of the colon (≥20 cm) contracts as a unit, moving the fecal contents forward as a unit. Mass movements last about 30 seconds, followed by a 2- to 3-minute period of relaxation, after which another contraction occurs. A series of mass movements lasts for only 10 to 30 minutes and may only occur several times a day. Defecation is normally initiated by the mass movements.

Defecation

Defecation is controlled by the action of two sphincters, the *internal* and *external anal sphincters* (Fig. 31–9). The internal sphincter is controlled by the ANS, and the external sphincter is under the conscious control of the cerebral cortex. The defecation reflex is integrated in the sacral segment of the spinal cord. In this reflex arc, afferent fibers from the rectum communicate with neurons in the sacral cord and with parasympathetic efferent fibers that move back to the bowel (see Fig. 31–7). The efferent signals from this reflex produce increased activity along the entire length of the large bowel. Other actions associated with defecation, such as abdominal pushing movements, are simultaneously integrated in the spinal cord.

To prevent involuntary defecation from occurring, the external anal sphincter is under the conscious control of the cortex. As afferent impulses arrive at the sacral cord, signaling the presence of a distended rectum, messages are transmitted to the cortex. If defecation is inappropriate, the cortex initiates impulses that constrict the external sphincter and inhibit efferent parasympathetic activity. Normally, the afferent impulses in this reflex loop fatigue easily, and the urge to defecate soon ceases. At a more convenient time, contraction of the abdominal muscles compresses the contents in the large bowel, reinitiating afferent impulses to the cord.

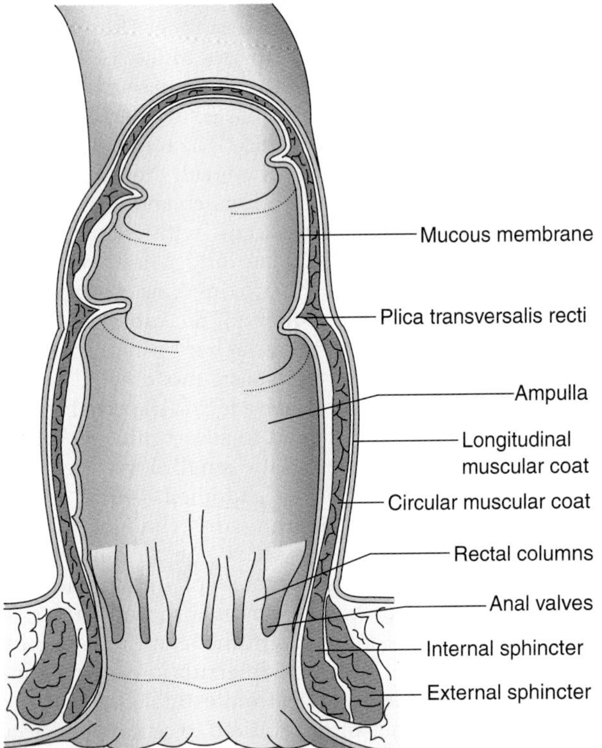

Figure 31–9
Interior of the rectum and anal canal.

In summary, motility of the gastrointestinal tract propels food products and fluids along its length from mouth to anus. Although the activity of gastrointestinal smooth muscle is self-propagating and can continue without input from the nervous system, its rate and strength of contractions are regulated by a network of intramural neurons that receive input from the autonomic nervous system and local receptors that monitor wall stretch and the chemical composition of its luminal contents. Parasympathetic innervation occurs by means of the vagus nerve and nerve fibers from sacral segments of the spinal cord; it increases gastrointestinal motility. Sympathetic activity occurs by way of thoracolumbar output from the spinal cord, its paravertebral ganglia, and celiac, superior mesenteric, and inferior mesenteric ganglia. Sympathetic stimulation enhances sphincter function and reduces motility by inhibiting the activity of intramural plexus neurons.

Secretory Function

After you have completed this section of the chapter, you should be able to meet the following objectives:

- State the source of water and electrolytes in digestive secretions
- Explain the protective function of saliva
- Describe the function of the gastric secretions in the process of digestion
- List three major gastrointestinal hormones and cite their function
- Describe the site of gastric acid and pepsin production and secretion in the stomach
- Describe the function of the gastric mucosal barrier
- Name the secretions of the small and the large intestine

Each day, about 7000 ml of fluid is secreted into the gastrointestinal tract (Table 31–1). About 50 to 200 ml of this

TABLE 31-1

Secretions of the Gastrointestinal Tract

Secretions	Amount Daily (ml)
Salivary	1200
Gastric	2000
Pancreatic	1200
Biliary	700
Intestinal	2000
Total	7100

fluid leaves the body in the stool; the remainder is reabsorbed in the small and large intestines. These secretions are mainly water and have sodium and potassium concentrations similar to those of extracellular fluid. Because water and electrolytes for digestive tract secretions are derived from the extracellular fluid compartment, excessive secretion or impaired absorption can lead to extracellular fluid deficit.

Control of Secretory Function

The secretory activity of the gut is influenced by local, humoral, and neural influences. Neural control of gastrointestinal secretory activity is mediated through the ANS. Secretory activity, like motility, is increased with parasympathetic stimulation and inhibited with sympathetic activity. Many of the local influences, including pH, osmolality, and chyme, consistently act as stimuli for neural and humoral mechanisms.

Gastrointestinal Hormones

The gastrointestinal tract is the largest endocrine organ in the body. It produces hormones that pass from the portal circulation into the general circulation and then back to the digestive tract, where they exert their actions. Among the hormones produced by the gastrointestinal tract are *gastrin, secretin,* and *cholecystokinin* (CCK). These hormones influence motility and the secretion of electrolytes, enzymes, and other hormones. The gastrointestinal tract hormones and their functions are summarized in Table 31–2.

The primary function of gastrin is the stimulation of gastric acid secretion. Gastrin also has a trophic, or growth-producing, effect on the mucosa of the small intestine, colon, and oxyntic (acid-secreting) gland area of the stomach. Removal of the tissue that produces gastrin results in atrophy of these structures. This atrophy can be reversed by the administration of exogenous gastrin.

Secretin is secreted by S cells in the mucosa of the duodenum and jejunum in an inactive form called prosecretin. When an acid chyme with a pH of less than 4.5 to 5.0 enters the intestine, secretin is activated and absorbed into the blood. Secretin causes the pancreas to secrete large quantities of fluid with a high bicarbonate concentration and low chloride concentration.

The primary function of CCK is stimulation of pancreatic enzyme secretion. CCK also regulates gallbladder contraction and gastric emptying. CCK potentiates the action of secretin, increasing the pancreatic bicarbonate response to low circulating levels of secretin. In addition to its effects on the pancreas, CCK secretion stimulates biliary secretion of fluid and bicarbonate.

Two other hormones that contribute to gastrointestinal function are gastric inhibitory peptide and motilin. Gastric inhibitory peptide, which is released from the intestinal mucosa in response to increased concentration of glucose and fats, inhibits gastric acid secretion, gastric motility, and gastric emptying. Motilin, which stimulates intestinal motility and contributes to the control of the interdigestive actions of the intestinal neurons, is released from the upper small intestine.

TABLE 31-2

Major Gastrointestinal Hormones and Their Actions

Hormone	Site of Secretion	Stimulus for Secretion	Action
Cholecystokinin	Duodenum, jejunum	Amino acids	Stimulates contraction of the gallbladder; stimulates secretion of pancreatic enzymes; slows gastric emptying
Gastrin	Antrum of the stomach, duodenum	Vagal stimulation; epinephrine; neutral amino acids; calcium-containing fluids such as milk; and alcohol. Secretion is inhibited by acid contents in the antrum of the stomach (below pH 2.5)	Stimulates secretion of gastric acid and pepsinogen; increases gastric blood flow; stimulates gastric smooth muscle contraction; stimulates growth of gastric mucosa, small intestine and colon mucosa
Secretin	Duodenum	Acid pH or chyme entering duodenum (below pH 3.0)	Stimulates secretion of bicarbonate-containing solution by pancreas and liver

Other neural peptides are found in the neurons of the gut. These include the vasoactive intestinal peptide (VIP), gastrin-releasing peptide (GRP), and the enkephalins. Gastrointestinal muscle is innervated by VIP-containing neurons. VIP mediates relaxation of gastrointestinal smooth muscle and is thought to also cause relaxation of vascular smooth muscle. GRP-containing neurons are located in the gastric mucosa and function in the release of gastrin. The action of the enkephalins, which exert their function through opioid receptors (see Chapter 40), is to slow the transit of material through the gut and inhibit intestinal secretions. The combination of these actions probably accounts for the effectiveness of selected opioid drugs in treating diarrhea.

Histamine and somatostatin are paracrine agents that act at receptors close to the site of release. Somatostatin inhibits gastrin release and gastric acid secretion. Histamine, which is released in response to gastrin, stimulates gastric acid secretion by the parietal cells. Histamine also potentiates the action of gastrin and acetylcholine on gastric acid secretion. $Histamine_2$ antagonists reduce gastric acid secretion by blocking histamine receptors.

Salivary Secretions

Saliva is secreted by the salivary glands. The salivary glands consist of the parotid, submaxillary, sublingual, and buccal glands. Saliva has three functions. The first is protection and lubrication. Saliva is rich in mucus, which protects the oral mucosa and coats the food as it passes through the mouth, pharynx, and esophagus. The sublingual and buccal glands produce only mucus-type secretions. The second function of saliva is its protective antimicrobial action. The saliva cleans the mouth and contains the enzyme lysozyme, which has an antibacterial action. Third, saliva contains ptyalin and amylase, which initiate the digestion of dietary starches. Secretions from the salivary glands are primarily regulated by the ANS. Parasympathetic stimulation increases flow and sympathetic stimulation decreases flow. The dry mouth that accompanies anxiety attests to the effects of sympathetic activity on salivary secretions.

Mumps, or *parotitis,* is an infection of the parotid glands. Although most of us associate mumps with the contagious viral form of the disease, inflammation of the parotid glands can occur in the seriously ill person who does not receive adequate oral hygiene and who is unable to take fluids orally. Potassium iodide increases the secretory activity of the salivary glands, including the parotid glands. In a small percentage of persons, parotid swelling may occur in the course of treatment with this drug.

Gastric Secretions

Two areas of gastric glands in the stomach produce secretions: the oxyntic gland area and the pyloric gland area. The oxyntic gland mucosa is located in the proximal portion of the stomach. It includes the body and fundus of the stomach. The pyloric gland area is located in the distal 20% of the stomach. This area, which is often referred to as the antrum, synthesizes and releases the hormone gastrin. The oxyntic gland area is composed of glands and pits (Fig. 31–10). The surface area and gastric pits are lined with mucus-producing epithelial cells. The base of

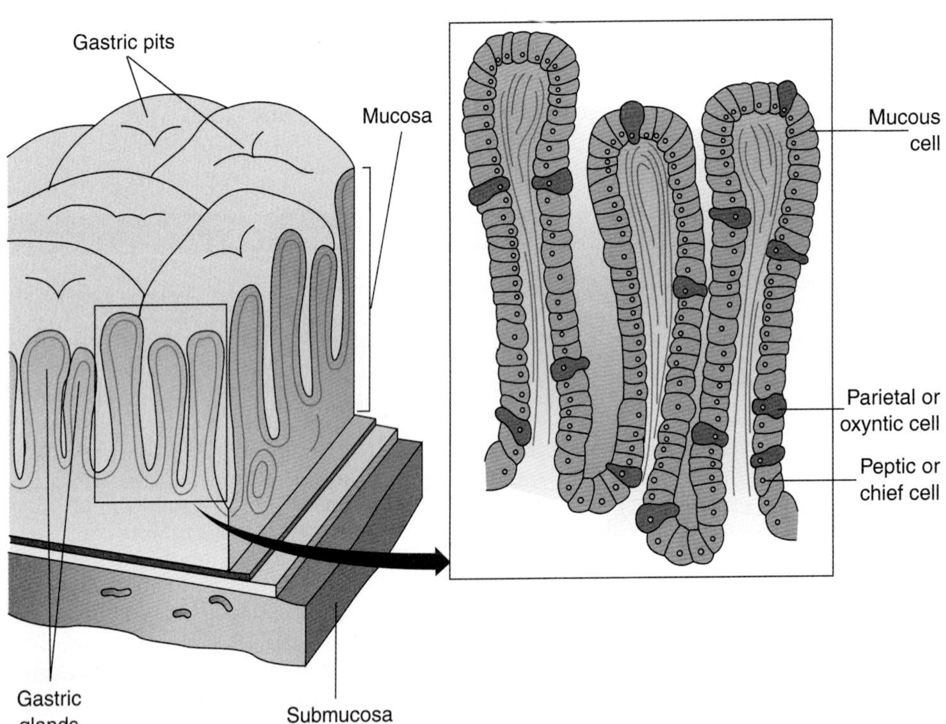

Figure 31–10 Gastric pit from body of the stomach.

the gastric pits contain the chief cells, which secrete hydrochloric acid and intrinsic factor, and the peptic or parietal cells, which secrete large quantities of pepsinogen. There are about 1 billion parietal cells in the stomach; together they produce and secrete about 20 mEq of hydrochloric acid in several hundred milliliters of gastric juice each hour. The pepsinogen that is secreted by the parietal cells is rapidly converted to pepsin when exposed to the low pH of the gastric juices. Gastric intrinsic factor, which is produced by the parietal cells, is necessary for the absorption of vitamin B_{12}.

One of the important characteristics of the gastric mucosa is its resistance to the highly acid secretions that it produces, a property derived from the mucosa's impermeability to hydrogen ions. When the gastric mucosa is damaged by aspirin, indomethacin, ethyl alcohol, or bile salts, this impermeability is disrupted, and hydrogen ions move into the tissue. This is called breaking the mucosal barrier, and substances that alter the permeability are called barrier breakers. As the hydrogen ions accumulate in the mucosal cells, intracellular pH decreases, enzymatic reactions become impaired, and cellular structures are disrupted. The result is local ischemia, vascular stasis, hypoxia, and tissue necrosis. The mucosal surface is further protected by prostaglandins. Aspirin and indomethacin inhibit prostaglandin synthesis, which also impairs the integrity of the mucosal surface.

Parasympathetic stimulation (by the vagus nerve) and gastrin increase gastric secretions. Histamine increases gastric acid secretions. Research and clinical use of the histamine$_2$-receptor antagonists suggest that histamine may be the final common pathway for gastric acid production. Gastric acid secretion and its relation to peptic ulcer are discussed in Chapter 32.

Intestinal Secretions

The *small intestine* secretes digestive juices and receives secretions from the liver and pancreas (see Chapter 33). Mucus-producing glands are concentrated in the duodenum at the site where the contents from the stomach and secretions from the liver and pancreas enter. The secretions of these glands, called *Brunner's glands*, protect the duodenum from the acid content in the gastric chyme and from the action of the digestive enzymes. The activity of Brunner's glands is strongly influenced by autonomic factors. For example, sympathetic stimulation causes a marked decrease in mucus production, leaving this area more susceptible to irritation. Between 75% and 80% of peptic ulcers occur at this site.

In addition to mucus, the intestinal mucosa produces two other types of secretions. The first is a serous fluid (pH 6.5 to 7.5) secreted by specialized cells (*i.e.*, crypts of Lieberkühn) in the intestinal mucosal layer. This fluid, which is produced at the rate of 2000 ml/day, acts as a diluent for absorption. The second type of secretion consists of surface enzymes that aid absorption. These enzymes are the peptidases, or enzymes that separate amino acids, and the disaccharidases, or enzymes that split sugars.

The *large intestine* usually secretes only mucus. ANS activity strongly influences mucus production in the bowel, as in other parts of the digestive tract. During intense parasympathetic stimulation, mucus secretion may increase to the point that the stool contains large amounts of obvious mucus. Although the bowel normally does not secrete water or electrolytes, these substances are lost in large quantities when the bowel becomes irritated or inflamed.

In summary, the secretions of the gastrointestinal tract include saliva, gastric juices, bile, and pancreatic and intestinal secretions. Each day, more than 7000 ml of fluid is secreted into the digestive tract; all but 50 to 200 ml of this fluid is reabsorbed. Water, derived from the extracellular fluid compartment, is the major component of gastrointestinal tract secretions. Neural, humoral, and local mechanisms contribute to the control of these secretions. The parasympathetic nervous system increases secretion, and sympathetic activity exerts an inhibitory effect. In addition to secreting fluids containing digestive enzymes, the gastrointestinal tract produces and secretes hormones, such as gastrin, secretin, and CCK, that contribute to the control of gastrointestinal function.

Digestion and Absorption

After you have completed this section of the chapter, you should be able to meet the following objectives:

- Differentiate digestion from absorption
- Relate the characteristics of the small intestine to its absorptive function
- Explain the function of intestinal brush border enzymes
- Compare the digestion and absorption of carbohydrates, fats, and proteins

Digestion and absorption occur mainly in the small intestine. The stomach is a poor absorptive structure, and only a few lipid-soluble substances, including alcohol, are absorbed from the stomach.

Digestion is the process of dismantling foods into their constituent parts. Digestion requires hydrolysis, enzyme cleavage, and fat emulsification. Hydrolysis is breakdown of a compound that involves a chemical reaction with water. The importance of hydrolysis to digestion is evidenced by the amount of water (7 to 8 L) that is secreted into the gastrointestinal tract daily. The intestinal mucosa is impermeable to most large molecules. Most proteins, fats, and carbohydrates must be broken down into smaller particles before they can be absorbed. Although some digestion of carbohydrates and proteins begins in the stomach, digestion takes place mainly in the small intestine. The hydrolysis of fats to free fatty acids and monoglycerides takes place entirely in the small intestine. The liver, with its production of bile, and the pancreas, which supplies a number of digestive enzymes, play important roles in digestion.

Absorption is the process of moving nutrients and other materials from the external environment of the gastrointestinal tract into the internal environment. Absorption is accomplished by active transport and diffusion. The absorptive function of the large intestine focuses mainly on water reabsorption. A number of substances require a specific carrier or transport system. For example, vitamin B_{12} is not absorbed in the absence of intrinsic factor. Transport of amino acids and glucose occurs mainly in the presence of sodium. Water is absorbed passively along an osmotic gradient.

The distinguishing characteristic of the small intestine is its large surface area, which in the adult is estimated to be about 250 m^2. Anatomic features that contribute to this enlarged surface area are the circular folds that extend into the lumen of the intestine and the villi, which are fingerlike projections of mucous membrane, numbering as many as 25,000, that line the entire small intestine (Fig. 31–11). Each villus is equipped with an artery, vein, and lymph vessel (*i.e.*, lacteal), which bring blood to the surface of the intestine and transport the nutrients and other materials that have passed into the blood from the lumen of the intestine (Fig. 31–12). Fats rely largely on the lymphatics for absorption.

Each villus is covered with cells called *enterocytes* that contribute to the absorptive and digestive functions of the small bowel and goblet cells that provide mucus. The crypts of Lieberkühn are glandular structures that open into the spaces between the villi. The enterocytes have a life span of about 4 to 5 days, and it is believed that replacement cells differentiate from progenitor cells located in the area of the crypts. The maturing enterocytes migrate up the villus and are eventually extruded from the tip.

The enterocytes secrete enzymes that aid in the digestion of carbohydrates and proteins. These enzymes are called *brush border enzymes* because they adhere to the border of the villus structures. In this way they have access to the carbohydrates and protein molecules as they come in contact with the absorptive surface of the intestine. This mechanism of secretion places the enzymes where they are needed and eliminates the need to produce enough enzymes to mix with the entire contents that fill the lumen of the small bowel. The digested molecules diffuse through the membrane or are actively transported across the mucosal surface to enter the blood or, in the case of fatty acids, the lacteal. These molecules are then transported through the portal vein or lymphatics into the systemic circulation.

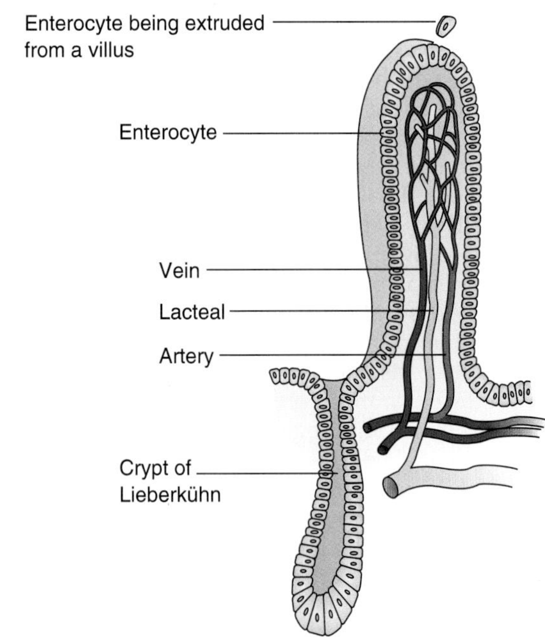

Figure 31–12
A single villus from the small intestine.

Carbohydrate Absorption

Carbohydrates must be broken down into monosaccharides, or single sugars, before they can be absorbed from

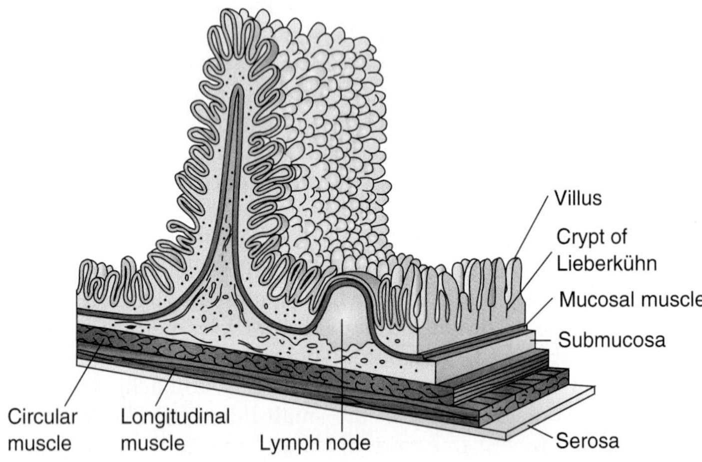

Figure 31–11
The mucous membrane of the small intestine. Note the numerous villi on a circular fold.

TABLE 31-3
Enzymes Used in Digestion of Carbohydrates

Dietary Carbohydrates	Enzyme	Monosaccharides Produced
Lactose	Lactase	Glucose and galactose
Sucrose	Sucrase	Fructose and glucose
Starch	Amylase	Maltose, maltotriase, and α-dextrins
Maltose and maltotriose	Maltase	Glucose and glucose
α-Dextrins	Isomaltase	Glucose and glucose

the small intestine. The average daily intake of carbohydrate in the American diet is about 350 to 400 g. Starch makes up about 50% of this total, sucrose (*i.e.*, table sugar) about 30%, lactose (*i.e.*, milk sugar) about 6%, and maltose about 1.5%.

Digestion of starch begins in the mouth with the action of amylase. Pancreatic secretions also contain an amylase. Amylase breaks down starch into several disaccharides, including maltose, isomaltose, and α-dextrins. The brush border enzymes convert the disaccharides into monosaccharides that can be absorbed (Table 31–3). Sucrose yields glucose and fructose, lactose is converted to glucose and galactose, and maltose is changed to glucose. When the disaccharides are not broken down to monosaccharides, they cannot be absorbed but remain as osmotically active particles in the contents of the digestive system, causing diarrhea. Persons who are deficient in lactase, the enzyme that breaks down lactose, experience diarrhea when they drink milk or eat dairy products.

Fructose is transported across the intestinal mucosa by facilitated diffusion, which does not require energy expenditure. In this case, fructose moves along a concentration gradient. Glucose and galactose are transported by way of a sodium-dependent carrier system that uses adenosine triphosphate (ATP) as an energy source (Fig. 31–13). Water absorption from the intestine is linked to absorption of osmotically active particles, such as glucose and sodium. It follows that an important consideration in facilitating the transport of water across the intestine (and decreasing diarrhea) after temporary disruption in bowel function is to include sodium and glucose in the fluids that are taken. A number of carbonated soft drinks can be used for this purpose.

Fat Absorption

The average adult eats about 60 to 100 g of fat daily, principally as triglycerides containing long-chain fatty acids. These triglycerides are broken down by pancreatic lipase. Bile salts act as a carrier system for the fatty acids and fat-soluble vitamins A, D, E, and K by forming micelles, which transport these substances to the surface of intestinal villi where they are absorbed. The major site of fat absorption is the upper jejunum. Medium-chain triglycerides, with 6 to 10 carbon atoms in their structures, are absorbed better than longer chains of fatty acids because they are more completely hydrolyzed by pancreatic lipase and they form micelles more easily. Because they are easily absorbed, medium-chain triglycerides are often used in the treatment of persons with malabsorption syndrome. The absorption of vitamins A, D, E, and K, which are fat-soluble vitamins, requires bile salts.

Fat that is not absorbed in the intestine is excreted in the stool. *Steatorrhea* is the term used to describe fatty stools. It usually indicates that there are 20 g or more of

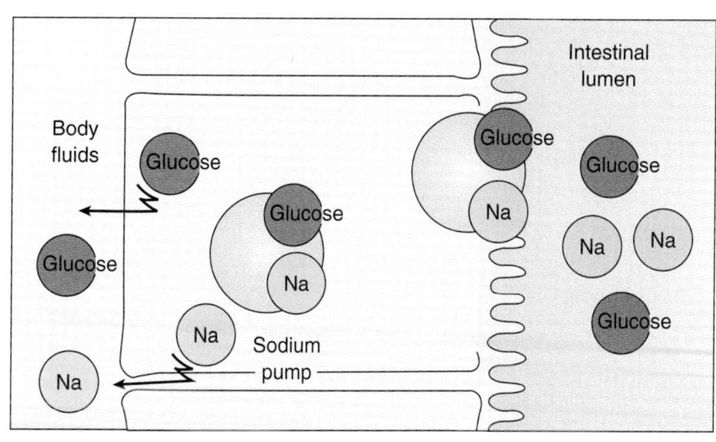

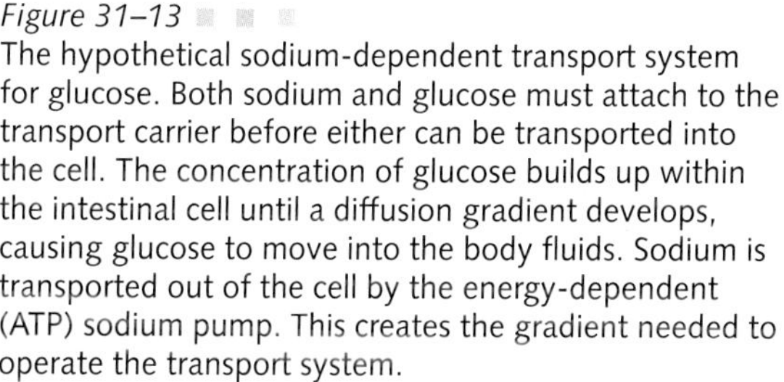
Figure 31–13
The hypothetical sodium-dependent transport system for glucose. Both sodium and glucose must attach to the transport carrier before either can be transported into the cell. The concentration of glucose builds up within the intestinal cell until a diffusion gradient develops, causing glucose to move into the body fluids. Sodium is transported out of the cell by the energy-dependent (ATP) sodium pump. This creates the gradient needed to operate the transport system.

fat in a 24-hour stool sample. Normally, a chemical test is done on a 72-hour stool collection, during which time the diet is restricted to 80 to 100 g of fat per day.

Protein Absorption

Protein digestion begins in the stomach with the action of pepsin. Pepsinogen, the enzyme precursor of pepsin, is secreted by the chief cells in response to a meal and acid pH. Acid in the stomach is required for the conversion of pepsinogen to pepsin. Pepsin is inactivated when it enters the intestine by the alkaline pH.

Proteins are broken down further by pancreatic enzymes, such as trypsin, chymotrypsin, carboxypeptidase, and elastase. As with pepsin, the pancreatic enzymes are secreted as precursor molecules. Trypsinogen, which lacks enzymatic activity, is activated by an enzyme located on the brush border cells of the duodenal enterocytes. Activated trypsin activates additional trypsinogen molecules and other pancreatic precursor proteolytic enzymes. The amino acids are liberated intramurally or on the surface of the villi by brush border enzymes that degrade proteins into peptides that are one, two, or three amino acids long. Similar to glucose, many amino acids are transported across the mucosal membrane in a sodium-linked process that uses ATP as an energy source. Some amino acids are absorbed by facilitated diffusion processes that do not require sodium.

In summary, the digestion and absorption of foodstuffs take place in the small intestine. Digestion is the process of dismantling foods into their constituent parts. Digestion requires hydrolysis, enzyme cleavage, and fat emulsification. Proteins, fats, carbohydrates, and other components of the diet are broken down into molecules that can be transported from the intestinal lumen into the body fluids. Absorption is the process of moving nutrients and other materials from the external environment of the gastrointestinal tract into the internal environment. Brush border enzymes break carbohydrates into monosaccharides that can be transported across the intestine into the bloodstream. The digestion of proteins begins in the stomach with the action of pepsin and is further facilitated in the intestine by the pancreatic enzymes, such as trypsin, chymotrypsin, carboxypeptidase, and elastase. Enzymes that break down proteins are released as proenzymes that are activated in the gastrointestinal tract. The absorption of glucose and amino acids is facilitated by a sodium-dependent transport system. Fat in the diet is broken down by pancreatic lipase into triglycerides containing medium- and long-chain fatty acids. Bile salts form micelles that transport these substances to the surface of intestinal villi, where they are absorbed.

BIBLIOGRAPHY

Berne R.M., Levy M.N. (1993). *Physiology* (3rd ed., pp. 615–716). St. Louis: C.V. Mosby.

Guyton A.C., Hall J.E. (1996). *Textbook of medical physiology* (9th ed., pp. 793–851). Philadelphia: W.B. Saunders.

Johnson L.R. (1997). *Gastrointestinal physiology* (5th ed). St. Louis, CV Mosby.

Johnson L.R. (1992). *Essential of medical physiology* (pp. 449–549). New York: Raven Press.

Rhoades R.A., Tanner G.A. (1996). *Medical physiology* (pp. 487–569). Boston: Little, Brown.

CHAPTER 32

Alterations in Gastrointestinal Function

Gastrointestinal disorders are not cited as the leading cause of death in the United States, nor do they receive the same publicity as heart disease and cancer. However, according to government reports, digestive diseases rank third in the total economic burden of illness, causing considerable human suffering, personal expenditures for treatment, lost working hours, and a drain on the nation's economy. It has been estimated that 20 million Americans, or one of every nine persons in the United States, have digestive disease. Even more important is the fact that proper nutrition or a change in health practices could prevent or minimize many of these disorders.

Manifestations of Gastrointestinal Disorders

After you have completed this section of the chapter, you should be able to meet the following objectives:

- Describe the physiologic mechanisms involved in anorexia, nausea, and vomiting
- Characterize the appearance of blood in vomitus and stool according to the site and extent of bleeding

Several signs and symptoms are common to many types of gastrointestinal disorders. These include anorexia, nausea, vomiting, and gastrointestinal bleeding. Because they occur with so many of the disorders, they are discussed separately as an introduction to the content that follows.

Anorexia, Nausea, and Vomiting

Anorexia, nausea, and vomiting are physiologic responses that are common to many gastrointestinal disorders. These responses are protective to the extent that they signal the presence of disease and, in the case of vomiting, remove noxious agents from the gastrointestinal tract. They can also contribute to impaired intake or loss of fluids and nutrients.

Anorexia is loss of appetite. Several factors influence appetite. One is hunger, which is stimulated by contractions of the empty stomach. Appetite or the desire for food intake is also regulated by the hypothalamus and other associated centers in the brain. Smell plays an important role, as evidenced by the fact that appetite can be stimulated or suppressed by the smell of food. Loss of appetite is associated with emotional situations, such as fear, depression, frustration, and anxiety. Many drugs and disease states cause anorexia. In uremia, for example, the accumulation of nitrogenous wastes in the blood contributes to the development of anorexia. Anorexia is often a forerunner of nausea, and most conditions that cause nausea and vomiting also produce anorexia.

Nausea is an ill-defined and unpleasant subjective sensation. It is conscious recognition of stimulation of the medullary vomiting center. Nausea is usually preceded by anorexia, and stimuli such as foods and drugs that cause anorexia in small doses usually produce nausea when given in larger doses. A common cause of nausea is distention of the duodenum, or upper small intestinal tract. Nausea is frequently accompanied by autonomic responses such as watery salivation and vasoconstriction with pallor, sweating, and tachycardia. Nausea may function as an early warning signal of pathology.

Vomiting, or emesis, is the sudden and forceful oral expulsion of the contents of the stomach. It is usually preceded by nausea. The contents that are vomited are called *vomitus.* Vomiting, as a basic physiologic protective mechanism, limits the possibility of damage from ingested noxious agents by emptying the contents of the stomach and portions of the small intestine. Nausea and vomiting may represent a total-body response to drug therapy, including overdosage, cumulative effects, toxicity, and side effects.

Vomiting appears to involve two functionally distinct medullary centers: the vomiting center and the chemoreceptor trigger zone. The act of vomiting is integrated by the vomiting center, which is located in the dorsal portion of the reticular formation of the medulla near the sensory nuclei of the vagus. The chemoreceptor trigger zone is located in a small area on the floor of the fourth ventricle, where it is exposed to both blood and cerebrospinal fluid. It is thought to mediate the emetic effects of blood-borne drugs and toxins.

The act of vomiting consists of taking a deep breath, closing the airways, and producing a strong, forceful contraction of the diaphragm and abdominal muscles along with relaxation of the gastroesophageal sphincter. Respiration ceases during the act of vomiting. Vomiting may be accompanied by dizziness, lightheadedness, decrease in blood pressure, and bradycardia.

The vomiting center may receive stimuli from the gastrointestinal tract and other organs, from the cerebral cortex, from the vestibular apparatus responsible for motion sickness, and from the chemoreceptor trigger zone activated by many drugs and endogenous and exogenous toxins. Hypoxia exerts a direct effect on the vomiting center, producing nausea and vomiting. This direct effect probably accounts for the vomiting that occurs during periods of decreased cardiac output, shock, environmental hypoxia, and brain ischemia caused by increased intracranial pressure. Inflammation of any of the intraabdominal organs, including the liver, gallbladder, or urinary tract, can cause vomiting because of the stimulation of the visceral afferent pathways that communicate with the vomiting center. Distention or irritation of the gastrointestinal tract also causes vomiting through the stimulation of visceral afferent neurons.

Several neurotransmitters and receptor subtypes are implicated as neuromediators in nausea and vomiting. Dopamine, serotonin (*i.e.,* 5-HT_3), and opioid receptors are found in the gastrointestinal tract and in the vomiting and chemoreceptor trigger zone. Dopamine antagonists such as chlorpromazine (Thorazine) and prochlorperazine (Compazine) depress vomiting caused by stimulation of the chemoreceptor trigger zone. Serotonin is believed to be involved in the nausea and emesis associated with cancer chemotherapy and radiation therapy.[1,2] Serotonin antagonists such as granisetron (Kytril) and ondansetron (Zofran) are effective in treating the nausea and vomiting associated with these stimuli. Motion sickness appears to be a central nervous system (CNS) response to vestibular stimuli. Norepinephrine and acetylcholine receptors are located within the vestibular center. The acetylcholine receptors are thought to mediate the impulses responsible for exciting the vomiting center; norepinephrine receptors may have a stabilizing influence that resists motion sickness. Many of the motion sickness drugs (*e.g.,* dimenhydrinate [Dramamine], meclizine [Antivert and Bonine]) have a strong CNS anticholinergic effects and act on the receptors in the vomiting center and areas related to the vestibular system.

Gastrointestinal Tract Bleeding

Bleeding from the gastrointestinal tract can be evidenced by blood that appears in the vomitus or the feces. It can result from disease or trauma to the gastrointestinal structures, from primary diseases of the blood vessels (*e.g.*, esophageal varices, hemorrhoids), or from disorders in blood clotting.

Hematemesis

Blood in the stomach is usually irritating and causes vomiting. Hematemesis refers to blood in the vomitus. It may be bright red or have a "coffee-ground" appearance because of the action of the digestive enzymes.

Melena

Blood that appears in the stool may range in color from bright red to tarry black. Bright red blood usually indicates that the bleeding is from the lower bowel. When it coats the stool, it is often the result of bleeding hemorrhoids.

The word *melena* means black and refers to the passage of black and tarry stools. These stools have a characteristic odor that is not easily forgotten. Tarry stools usually indicate that the source of the bleeding is above the level of the ileocecal valve, although this is not always the case. Approximately 60 ml of blood are required to produce a single tarry stool; acute blood loss may produce melena for up to 3 days.[3] With hypermotility of the gastrointestinal tract, bright red blood may be present in the stools even though the bleeding is from the upper gastrointestinal tract.

Occult, or hidden, blood can only be detected by chemical means. It can be caused by gastritis, peptic ulcer, or lesions of the intestine. Occult bleeding can be detected by the use of a simple card test for hemoglobin peroxidase. A positive test result can indicate upper or lower gastrointestinal bleeding, dietary peroxidases, or vitamin C.

The blood urea nitrogen (BUN) level is frequently elevated after hematemesis or melena. This results from the breakdown of the blood by the digestive enzymes and the absorption of the nitrogenous end products into the blood. The BUN level usually reaches a peak within 24 hours after the gastrointestinal hemorrhage. It is not elevated when the bleeding is in the colon, because digestion does not take place at this level of the digestive system. An elevation in body temperature may also follow gastrointestinal hemorrhage. It usually occurs within 24 hours and may last for a few days to a few weeks.

In summary, the signs and symptoms of many gastrointestinal tract disorders are manifested by anorexia, nausea, and vomiting. Anorexia, or loss of appetite, may occur alone or may accompany nausea and vomiting. Nausea, which is an ill-defined, unpleasant sensation, signals the stimulation of the medullary vomiting center. It often precedes vomiting and is frequently accompanied by autonomic responses such as salivation and vasoconstriction with pallor, sweating, and tachycardia. The act of vomiting, which is integrated by the vomiting center, involves the forceful oral expulsion of the gastric contents. It is a basic physiologic mechanism that rids the gastrointestinal tract of noxious agents. Disorders that disrupt the integrity of the gastrointestinal tract often cause bleeding, which can be manifested as blood in the vomitus (*i.e.*, hematemesis) or as blood in the stool (*i.e.*, melena).

Disorders of the Esophagus

After you have completed this section of the chapter, you should be able to meet the following objectives:

- Define *dysphagia*, *odynophagia*, and *achalasia*
- Relate the causes of gastroesophageal reflux to measures used in treatment of the disorder
- State the reason for the poor prognosis associated with esophageal cancer

The esophagus is a tube that connects the oropharynx with the stomach. It lies posterior to the trachea and larynx and extends through the mediastinum, intersecting the diaphragm at the level of the 11th thoracic vertebra.

The esophagus functions primarily as a conduit for passage of food from the pharynx to the stomach, and the structures of its walls are designed for this purpose: the smooth muscle layers provide the peristaltic movements needed to move food along its length, and the epithelial layer secretes mucus, which protects its surface and aids in lubricating food. There are sphincters at either end of the esophagus: an upper esophageal sphincter and a lower esophageal sphincter. The upper esophageal, or pharyngoesophageal, sphincter consists of a circular layer of striated muscle, the cricopharyngeal muscle. The lower esophageal, or gastroesophageal, sphincter is a 1- to 2-cm zone of increased pressure that is maintained at a level greater than that of the stomach. The anatomic structure of the lower esophageal sphincter is no different from the rest of the esophagus; however, physiologically, it remains tonically constricted, unlike the middle and upper portions of the esophagus.[4]

Dysphagia

The act of swallowing depends on the coordinated action of the tongue and pharynx. These structures are innervated by cranial nerves V, IX, X, and XII. *Dysphagia* refers to difficulty in swallowing. If swallowing is painful, it is referred to as *odynophagia*. Dysphagia can result from altered nerve function or from disorders that produce narrowing of the esophagus. Lesions of the CNS, such as a stroke, often involve the cranial nerves that control swallowing. Strictures and cancer of the esophagus and strictures resulting from scarring can reduce the size of the esophageal lumen and make swallowing difficult.

In a condition called *achalasia*, the lower esophageal sphincter fails to relax; food that has been swallowed has difficulty passing into the stomach, and the esophagus above the lower esophageal sphincter becomes enlarged. One or several meals may lodge in the esophagus and pass slowly into the stomach over time. There is danger of aspiration of esophageal contents into the lungs when the person lies down. Treatment is mechanical dilatation or surgical procedures to enlarge the sphincter.

Esophageal Diverticulum

A diverticulum of the esophagus is an outpouching of the esophageal wall caused by a weakness of the muscularis layer. An esophageal diverticulum tends to retain food. Complaints that the food stops before it reaches the stomach are common, as are reports of gurgling, belching, coughing, and foul-smelling breath. The trapped food may cause esophagitis and ulceration. Because the condition is usually progressive, correction of the defect requires surgical intervention.

Gastroesophageal Reflux

The term *reflux* refers to backward or return movement. In terms of gastroesophageal reflux, it refers to the backward movement of gastric contents into the esophagus, a condition that causes heartburn. It is probably the most common disorder originating in the gastrointestinal tract. Most persons experience heartburn occasionally as a result of reflux. Such symptoms usually occur soon after eating, are short lived, and seldom cause more serious problems. However, for some persons, persistent heartburn can represent reflux disease with esophagitis.

Reflux esophagitis involves mucosal injury to the esophagus, hyperemia, and inflammation. There is controversy regarding the importance of hiatal hernia (*i.e.*, herniation of the stomach through an enlarged hiatus in the diaphragm) in the pathogenesis of reflux disease.[5] Except in the case of a large hiatal hernia that protrudes into the chest, the defect probably does not play a major role in the pathology of the disorder.[6,7] Instead, it is thought that the condition results from a weak or incompetent lower esophageal sphincter that allows reflux to occur and from factors such as decreased esophageal peristalsis and salivary function that impair clearance of the refluxed acid from the esophagus after it has occurred. Findings indicate that swallowed saliva contributes to acid neutralization and its clearance from the esophagus after reflux.[8] Esophageal acid clearance may be delayed by impaired peristalsis, an abnormality in swallowed saliva, or both.

The most frequent symptom of gastroesophageal reflux is heartburn. It is frequently severe, occurring 30 to 60 minutes after eating. It is often made worse by bending at the waist and recumbency and is usually relieved by sitting upright. The severity of heartburn is not indicative of the extent of mucosal injury; only 30% to 40% of persons who complain of heartburn have mucosal injury.[9] Often, the heartburn occurs during the night. Antacids give prompt, although transient relief. Drinking water or other liquids may afford relief, probably because they wash the irritating gastric contents back into the stomach. Other symptoms include belching and chest pain. The pain is usually located in the epigastric or retrosternal area and often radiates to the throat, shoulder, or back. Because of its location, the pain may be confused with angina. The reflux of gastric contents may also produce respiratory symptoms such as wheezing, chronic cough, and hoarseness.

Complications can result from persistent reflux, producing a cycle of mucosal damage that causes hyperemia, edema, and erosion of the luminal surface. These complications include strictures and a condition called *Barrett's esophagus*.[10] Strictures are caused by a combination of scar tissue, spasm, and edema. They produce narrowing of the esophagus and cause dysphagia when the lumen becomes sufficiently constricted. Barrett's esophagus is characterized by a reparative process in which the squamous mucosa that normally lines the esophagus is gradually replaced by columnar epithelium resembling that in the stomach or intestines.[11] It is associated with increased risk of developing esophageal cancer.

Diagnosis of gastroesophageal reflux depends on history and selective use of diagnostic methods, including radiographic studies using a contrast medium such as barium, esophagoscopy, and 24-hour pH monitoring. Esophagoscopy involves the passage of a flexible fiberoptic endoscope into the esophagus for the purpose of visualizing the lumen of the upper gastrointestinal tract. It also permits performance of a biopsy, if indicated. For the 24-hour pH monitoring, a small tube with a pH electrode is passed through the nose and down into the esophagus. Data from the electrode are recorded in a small, lightweight box worn on a belt around the waist and later are analyzed by computer. The box has a button that the person can press to indicate episodes of heartburn or pain; these can be correlated with episodes of acid reflux.

The treatment of gastroesophageal reflux generally focuses on conservative measures. These measures include avoidance of positions and conditions that increase gastric reflux.[12] Avoidance of large meals and foods that reduce lower esophageal sphincter tone (*e.g.*, fats, chocolate, coffee), alcohol, and smoking is recommended. It is recommended that meals be eaten sitting up and that the recumbent position be avoided for several hours after a meal. Bending for long periods should be avoided, because it tends to increase intraabdominal pressure and cause gastric reflux. Sleeping with the head elevated helps to prevent reflux during the night. This is best accomplished by placing blocks under the head of the bed or by using a wedge-shaped bolster to elevate the head and shoulders by at least 6 inches.

Antacids or a combination of antacids and alginic acid is also recommended for mild disease. Alginic acid produces a foam when it comes in contact with gastric acid; if reflux occurs, the foam rather than acid rises into the esophagus. For some persons, drinking water dilutes the gastric acid and washes it back into the stomach. Histamine$_2$ (H_2)–blocking drugs, which inhibit gastric acid production, are often recommended when additional treatment is needed. A newer drug, omeprazole, acts by inhibiting the gastric proton pump, which regulates the final pathway for acid secretion. This drug may be used for persons who continue to have daytime symptoms, recurrent strictures, or large esophageal ulcerations. Promotility agents (*e.g.*, cisapride, metoclopramide, bethanechol) may be used to increase lower esophageal pressure and enhance esophageal clearance.

Cancer of the Esophagus

Carcinoma of the esophagus accounts for about 6% of all gastrointestinal cancers. This disease is more common in adults older than 50, and the male-to-female ratio is approximately 2:1.[11] Environmental factors that contribute to the development of esophageal cancers include conditions that cause food or drink to remain in the esophagus for prolonged periods and continued exposure to irritants such as alcohol and tobacco. Certain precancerous conditions such as achalasia and a history of caustic injury to the esophagus increase the risk of esophageal cancer, as does Barrett's esophagus.

Dysphagia is by far the most frequent complaint of persons with esophageal cancer. It is apparent first with ingestion of bulky food, later with soft food, and finally with liquids. Unfortunately, it is a late manifestation of the disease. Weight loss, anorexia, fatigue, and pain on swallowing may also occur.

Treatment includes surgical resection, which provides a means of cure when done in early disease and palliation when done in late disease. Irradiation is used as a palliative treatment. Chemotherapy is sometimes used preoperatively to decrease the size of the tumor, and it may be used along with irradiation and surgery in an effort to increase survival.[13]

The prognosis for persons with cancer of the esophagus, although poor, has improved.[13] Even with modern forms of therapy, however, the long-term survival is limited because, in many cases, the disease has already metastasized by the time the diagnosis is made. Better methods of early diagnosis are needed.

In summary, the esophagus is a tube that connects the oropharynx with the stomach; it functions primarily as a conduit for passage of food from the pharynx to the stomach. Dysphagia refers to difficulty in swallowing; it can result from altered nerve function or from disorders that produce narrowing of the esophagus. A diverticulum of the esophagus is an outpouching of the esophageal wall caused by a weakness of the muscularis layer.

Gastrointestinal reflux refers to the backward movement of gastric contents into the esophagus, a condition that causes heartburn. Although most persons experience occasional esophageal reflux and heartburn, persistent reflux can cause esophagitis.

Carcinoma of the esophagus, which accounts for 6% of all cancers, is more common in men older than the age of 50, and the male-to-female ratio is approximately 2:1. It is commonly linked to environmental factors, including conditions that cause food or drink to remain in the esophagus for prolonged periods and continued exposure to irritants such as alcohol and tobacco.

Disorders of the Stomach

After you have completed this section of the chapter, you should be able to meet the following objectives:

- Describe the factors that contribute to the gastric mucosal barrier
- Characterize the proposed role of *Helicobacter pylori* in the development of chronic gastritis and peptic ulcer and cite methods for diagnosing the infection
- Differentiate between the causes and manifestations of acute and chronic gastritis
- Describe the predisposing factors in development of peptic ulcer and cite the three complications of peptic ulcer
- Describe the goals for pharmacologic treatment of peptic ulcer disease
- Cite the etiologic factors in ulcer formation related to Zollinger-Ellison syndrome and stress ulcer
- List risk factors associated with gastric cancer

The stomach is a reservoir for contents entering the digestive tract. It lies in the upper abdomen, anterior to the pancreas, splenic vessels, and left kidney. Anteriorly, the stomach is bounded by the anterior abdominal wall and the left inferior lobe of the liver. While in the stomach, food is churned and mixed with hydrochloric acid and pepsin before being released into the small intestine. Normally, the mucosal surface of the stomach provides a barrier that protects it from the hydrochloric acid and pepsin contained in gastric secretions. Disorders of the stomach include gastritis, peptic ulcer, and gastric carcinoma.

Gastric Mucosal Barrier

The stomach lining usually is impermeable to the acid it secretes, a property that allows the stomach to contain acid and pepsin without having its wall digested. Several factors contribute to the protection of the gastric mucosa, including an impermeable epithelial cell surface covering, mechanisms for the selective transport of hydrogen and bicarbonate ions, and the characteristics of gastric mucus.[14] These mechanisms are collectively referred to as the *gastric mucosal barrier*.

The gastric epithelial cells are connected by tight junctions that prevent acid penetration, and they are covered with an impermeable hydrophobic lipid layer that prevents diffusion of ionized water-soluble molecules. Aspirin, which is nonionized and lipid-soluble in acid solutions, rapidly diffuses across this lipid layer, increasing mucosal permeability and damaging epithelial cells. Gastric irritation and occult bleeding due to gastric irritation occurs in a significant number of persons who take aspirin on a regular basis (Fig. 32–1). Alcohol, which is also lipid soluble, disrupts the mucosal barrier; when aspirin and alcohol are taken in combination, as they often are, there is increased risk of gastric irritation. Bile acids also attack the lipid components of the mucosal barrier and afford the potential for gastric irritation when there is reflux of duodenal contents into the stomach.

Normally, the secretion of hydrochloric acid by the parietal cells of the stomach is accompanied by secretion of bicarbonate ions (HCO_3^-). For every hydrogen ion (H^+) that is secreted, a HCO_3^- is produced and as long as HCO_3^- production is equal to H^+ secretion, mucosal injury does not occur. Changes in gastric blood flow, as in shock, tend to decrease HCO_3^- production. This is particularly true in situations in which decreased blood flow is accompanied by acidosis. Aspirin and the nonsteroidal antiinflammatory drugs (NSAIDs) such as indomethacin and ibuprofen also impair HCO_3^- secretion.

The mucus that protects the gastric mucosa is of two types: water insoluble and water soluble.[13] Water-insoluble mucus forms a thin stable gel that adheres to the gastric mucosal surface and provides protection from the proteolytic (protein-digesting) actions of pepsin. It also forms an unstirred layer that traps bicarbonate, forming an alkaline interface between the luminal contents of the stomach and its mucosal surface. The water-insoluble mucus is washed from the mucosal surface and mixes with the luminal contents; its viscid nature makes it a lubricant that prevents mechanical damage to the mucosal surface. In addition to their effects on mucosal permeability and bicarbonate production, damaging agents such as aspirin and the NSAIDs inhibit and modify the characteristics of gastric mucus.

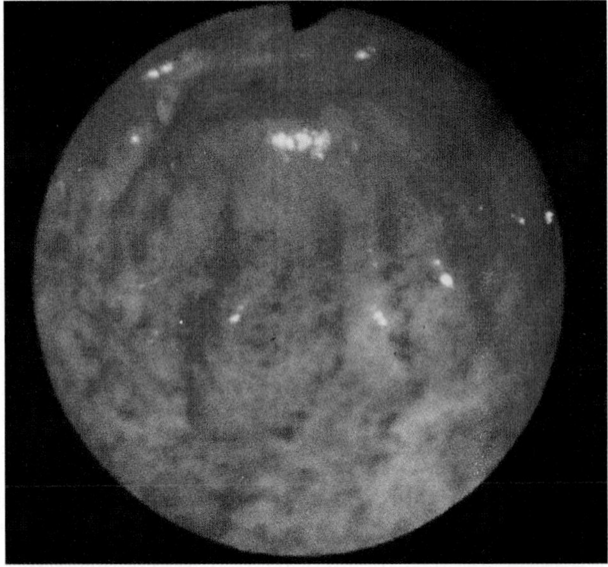

Figure 32–1
Erosive gastritis. This endoscopic view of the stomach in a patient who was ingesting aspirin reveals acute hemorrhagic lesions.

Prostaglandins, chemical messengers derived from cell membrane lipids, play an important role in protecting the gastrointestinal mucosa from injury. The prostaglandins probably exert their effect through improved blood flow, increased bicarbonate ion secretion, and enhanced mucus production. The fact that drugs such as aspirin and the NSAIDs inhibit prostaglandin synthesis may contribute to their ability to produce gastric irritation. Smoking and older age have been associated with reduced gastric and duodenal prostaglandin concentrations; these observations may explain the predisposition to ulcer disease in smokers and older persons.[15]

The S-shaped bacterium called *Helicobacter pylori* (formerly *Campylobacter pylori*) can colonize the mucus-secreting epithelial cells of the stomach and disrupt the barrier.[16,17] The *H. pylori* organisms have multiple flagella, which allow them to move through the mucous layer of the stomach, and they secrete urease, which enables them to produce sufficient ammonia to buffer the acidity of their immediate environment. These properties help to explain why the organism is able to survive in the acidic environment of the stomach. Because the organism adheres only to the mucus-secreting cells of the stomach, it does not usually colonize other parts of the gastrointestinal tract. The exceptions are areas such as Barrett's esophagus and a duodenal ulcer site in which the normal epithelial layer has been replaced with gastric mucosa. The organism produces an enzyme that degrades mucin and has the capacity to interfere with the local protection of the gastric mucosa against acid. It may also produce toxins that directly damage the mucosa and produce ulceration in other ways. The organism contributes to the development of chronic gastritis and peptic ulcer.

Gastritis

Gastritis refers to inflammation of the gastric mucosa. There are many causes of gastritis, most of which can be grouped under the headings of acute or chronic gastritis.

Acute Gastritis

Acute gastritis refers to a transient inflammation of the gastric mucosa. It is most commonly associated with local irritants such as bacterial endotoxins, caffeine, alcohol, and aspirin. Depending on the severity of the disorder, the mucosal response may vary from moderate edema and hyperemia to hemorrhagic erosion of the gastric mucosa.

The complaints of persons with acute gastritis vary. Persons with aspirin-related gastritis can be totally unaware of the condition or may complain only of heartburn or sour stomach. Gastritis associated with excessive alcohol consumption is a different situation;

it often causes transient gastric distress, which may lead to vomiting and, in more severe situations, to bleeding and hematemesis. Gastritis caused by the toxins of infectious organisms, such as the staphylococcal enterotoxins, usually has an abrupt and violent onset, with gastric distress and vomiting ensuing about 5 hours after the ingestion of a contaminated food source. Acute gastritis is usually a self-limiting disorder; complete regeneration and healing usually occur within several days.

Chronic Gastritis

Chronic gastritis is a separate entity from acute gastritis. It is characterized by the absence of grossly visible erosions and the presence of chronic inflammatory changes leading eventually to atrophy of the glandular epithelium of the stomach. The changes may become dysplastic and possibly be transformed into carcinoma. There are two major forms of chronic gastritis: autoimmune gastritis and chronic infectious gastritis. Other factors such as chronic alcohol abuse, cigarette smoking, and chronic use of NSAIDs may contribute to the development of the disease.

Autoimmune gastritis is the least common form of chronic gastritis. It typically involves the fundus and the body of the stomach and is associated with pernicious anemia. This form of chronic gastritis is considered to be of autoimmune origin, and most persons with the disorder have circulating antibodies to parietal cells and intrinsic factor. Autoimmune destruction of the parietal cells leads to hypochlorhydria or achlorhydria, a high intragastric pH, and hypergastrinemia. Because of decreased secretion of intrinsic factor, some persons eventually develop pernicious anemia (see Chapter 8). This type of chronic gastritis is frequently associated with other autoimmune disorders such as Hashimoto's thyroiditis and Addison's disease.

Infectious gastritis is a chronic inflammatory disease of the antrum and body of the stomach caused by *H. pylori* (Fig. 32–2). Colonization with *H. pylori* is common in the general population, and its increasing prevalence with age could explain the increased prevalence of chronic gastritis in the elderly. Although the pathogenesis of *H. pylori*–induced gastritis is unclear, the organism is found attached to the epithelium in areas of chronic gastritis and is absent from uninvolved areas. Chronic infection with *H. pylori* is thought to lead to gastric atrophy and intestinal metaplasia.

Chronic gastritis causes few symptoms related directly to gastric changes. Persons with autoimmune chronic gastritis may develop pernicious anemia. More important is the development of peptic ulcer and increased risk of peptic ulcer and gastric carcinoma. Approximately 2% to 4% of persons with atrophic gastritis eventually develop gastric carcinoma.[11] Evidence demonstrates an association between *H. pylori*–induced gastritis and well-differentiated adenocarcinoma of the antrum and fundus of the stomach.[17]

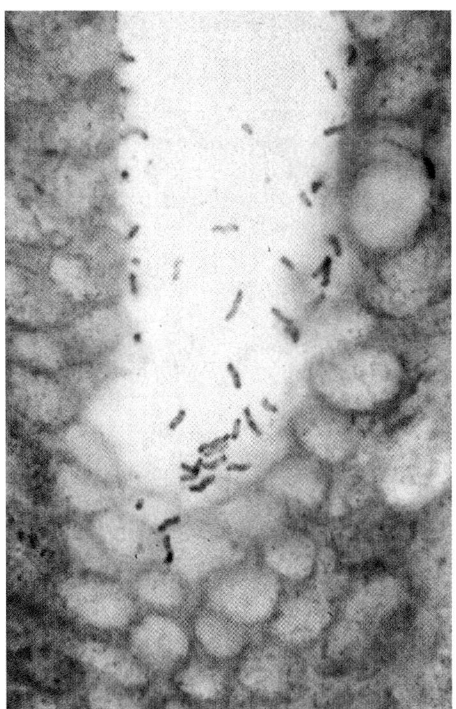

Figure 32–2
Infective gastritis. *H. pylori* appears on silver staining as small, curved rods on the surface of the gastric mucosa.

Peptic Ulcer Disease

Peptic ulcer is a term used to describe a group of ulcerative disorders that occur in areas of the upper gastrointestinal tract that are exposed to acid-pepsin secretions. The most common forms of peptic ulcer are duodenal and gastric ulcers. Two other forms of gastric ulcers, Zollinger-Ellison syndrome and stress ulcers, have different causes and are discussed separately. Peptic ulcer disease, with its remissions and exacerbations, represents a chronic health problem. Ten percent of the population has or will develop peptic ulcer.[17] Duodenal ulcers are two to three times more common than gastric ulcers. Ulcers in the duodenum occur at any age and are frequently seen in early adulthood. Gastric ulcers tend to affect the older age group, with a peak incidence in the sixth and seventh decades. Both types of ulcers affect men three to four times more frequently than women.

Etiology

During the past 20 years, there has been a radical shift in thinking regarding the cause of peptic ulcer. No longer is peptic ulcer thought to result from a genetic predisposition, stress, or dietary indiscretions. Most cases of peptic ulcer are caused by *H. pylori* infection.[18,19] The second most common form of peptic ulcer is from the use of NSAIDs, including aspirin.[19] Much of the familial aggregation of peptic ulcer that was formerly credited with causing peptic ulcer probably was caused by intrafamilial infection with *H. pylori* rather than genetic susceptibility.

***Helicobacter pylori* Infection.** Since its identification in 1982, *H. pylori* has generated worldwide interest. It has been reported that up to 85% to 100% of persons with duodenal ulcer and 70% to 90% of persons with gastric ulcer have *H. pylori* infection and active chronic gastritis.[11] Eradication of the organism can result in resolution of gastritis, with subsequent ulcer healing. Exactly how *H. pylori* and aspirin or NSAIDs lead to ulcer formation is unclear. Although they are independent risk factors, they may act synergistically in causing ulcers and especially in the development of ulcer complications. The risk of complications may be accentuated by the analgesic effects of the drugs that mask the ulcer symptoms.

Nonsteroidal Antiinflammatory Drug-Induced Ulcers. There is a 10% to 20% prevalence of gastric ulcers and a 2% to 5% prevalence of duodenal ulcers among chronic NSAID users. Aspirin appears to be the most ulcerogenic of the NSAIDs. Ulcer development in NSAIDs users is dose dependent, but some risk occurs even with aspirin doses of 325 mg per day.[20] The pathogenesis of NSAID-induced ulcers is thought to involve mucosal injury and inhibition of prostaglandin synthesis.[21] In contrast to peptic ulcer from other causes, NSAID-induced gastric injury is often without symptoms, and life-threatening complications can occur without warning.

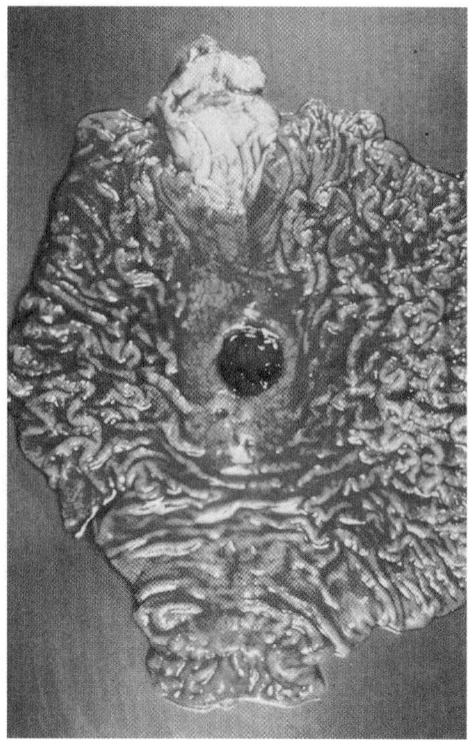

Figure 32–3
Gastric ulcer. The stomach has been opened to reveal a sharply demarcated, deep peptic ulcer on the lesser curvature.

Manifestations and Complications

The clinical manifestations of uncomplicated peptic ulcer focus on discomfort and pain. The pain, which is described as burning, gnawing, or cramplike, is usually rhythmic and frequently occurs when the stomach is empty—between meals and at 1 o'clock or 2 o'clock in the morning. The pain is usually located over a small area near the midline in the epigastrium near the xiphoid and may radiate below the costal margins, into the back or, rarely, to the right shoulder. Superficial and deep epigastric tenderness and voluntary muscle guarding may occur with more extensive lesions. An additional characteristic of ulcer pain is periodicity. The pain tends to recur at intervals of weeks or months. During an exacerbation, it occurs daily for a period of several weeks and then remits until the next recurrence. Characteristically, the pain is relieved by food or antacids.

A peptic ulcer can affect one or all layers of the stomach or duodenum (Fig. 32–3). The ulcer may penetrate only the mucosal surface, or it may extend into the smooth muscle layers. Occasionally, an ulcer penetrates the outer wall of the stomach or duodenum. Spontaneous remissions and exacerbations are common. Healing of the muscularis layer involves replacement with scar tissue; although the mucosal layers that cover the scarred muscle layer regenerate, the regeneration is often less than perfect, which contributes to repeated episodes of ulceration.

The complications of peptic ulcer include hemorrhage, obstruction, and perforation. Hemorrhage is caused by bleeding from granulation tissue or from erosion of an ulcer into an artery or vein. It occurs in 10% to 15% of persons with peptic ulcer. Evidence of bleeding may consist of hematemesis or melena. Bleeding may be sudden, severe, and without warning, or it may be insidious, producing only occult blood in the stool. Acute hemorrhage is evidenced by the sudden onset of weakness, dizziness, thirst, cold moist skin, the desire to defecate, and the passage of loose, tarry, or even red stools and coffee-ground emesis. Signs of circulatory shock develop depending on the amount of blood that is lost.

Obstruction is caused by edema, spasm, or contraction of scar tissue and interference with the free passage of gastric contents through the pylorus or adjacent areas. There is a feeling of epigastric fullness and heaviness after meals. With severe obstruction, there is vomiting of undigested food.

Perforation occurs when an ulcer erodes through all the layers of the stomach or duodenum wall. With perforation, gastrointestinal contents enter the peritoneum and cause peritonitis, or penetrate adjacent structures such as the pancreas. Radiation of the pain into the back, severe night distress, inadequate pain relief from eating foods or taking antacids in persons with a long history of peptic ulcer may signify perforation. Peritonitis is discussed as a separate topic near the end of this chapter.

Diagnosis

Diagnostic procedures for peptic ulcer include history, laboratory findings, radiologic imaging, and endoscopic examination. The history should include careful attention to aspirin and NSAID use. Peptic ulcer should be differentiated from other causes of epigastric pain. Laboratory findings of hypochromic anemia and occult blood in the stools indicate bleeding. X-ray studies with a contrast media such as barium are used to detect the presence of an ulcer crater and to exclude gastric carcinoma.

Endoscopy (*i.e.*, gastroscopy and duodenoscopy) can be used to visualize the ulcer area and obtain biopsy specimens to test for *H. pylori* and exclude malignant disease. Methods for establishing the presence of *H. pylori* include blood tests to obtain serologic titers of *H. pylori* antibodies, urease breath testing using carbon isotope (^{13}C or ^{14}C), or an endoscopic biopsy for urease testing.

Treatment

The treatment of peptic ulcer has changed dramatically over the past several years, with the aim of eradicating the cause and effecting a permanent cure for the disease.[16,17] Previous therapy consisted of acid-neutralizing drugs and acid-inhibiting drugs aimed at relieving symptoms and promoting temporary healing of the ulcer crater. Aspirin and NSAID use should be avoided when possible.

There is no evidence that special diets are beneficial in treating peptic ulcer. Pharmacologic treatment measures are usually aimed at eradicating *H. pylori* and the use conventional ulcer therapy to promote ulcer healing. Medications used in conventional ulcer therapy include mucosal protective agents and agents that reduce gastric acid content.

***Helicobacter pylori* Eradication.** The agents used in eradication of *H. pylori* include combination antibiotic therapy, proton pump inhibitors, and bismuth. The antibiotics that have shown the greatest efficacy against *H. pylori* are clarithromycin, metronidazole, amoxicillin, and tetracycline. Combination regimens that employ two antibiotics and bismuth or proton pump inhibitors are usually required to achieve an acceptable rate of *H. pylori* eradication.

Mucosal Protective Agents. Among the agents that enhance mucosal defenses are sucralfate, bismuth, and prostaglandin analogues. The drug sucralfate, which is a complex salt of sucrose containing aluminum and sulfate, selectively binds to necrotic ulcer tissue and serves as a barrier to acid, pepsin, and bile. Sucralfate also can directly absorb bile salts. The drug is not absorbed systemically. The drug requires an acid pH for activation and should not be administered with antacids or an H_2 antagonist.

Bismuth compounds in a variety of formulations are used to treat dyspepsia, peptic ulcer disease, and diarrhea. The only agent available in the United States is bismuth subsalicylate (Pepto-Bismol). Bismuth promotes ulcer healing through stimulation of mucosal bicarbonate and prostaglandin production. It also has a direct antibacterial effect against *H. pylori*. Bismuth causes a harmless darkening of the stools.

Misoprostol, a prostaglandin analogue, promotes ulcer healing by stimulating mucus and bicarbonate secretion and by modestly inhibiting acid secretion. It is used as a prophylactic agent to prevent NSAID-induced peptic ulcers. The drug causes dose-dependent diarrhea, and because of its stimulant effect on the uterus, it is contraindicated in women of childbearing age.

Agents That Decrease Gastric Acid Content. There are two pharmacologic methods for reducing gastric acid content. The first involves the neutralization of gastric acid through the use of antacids and the second a decrease in gastric acid production through the use of H_2-receptor antagonists or proton pump inhibitors.

Self-prescribed or physician-prescribed antacids represent a large business in the United States, with millions of dollars spent each year for these medications. Essentially three types of antacids are used to relieve gastric acidity: calcium carbonate, aluminum hydroxide, and magnesium hydroxide. Many antacids contain a combination of ingredients, such as magnesium aluminum hydroxide. *Calcium preparations* are constipating and may cause hypercalcemia and the milk-alkali syndrome. There is also evidence that oral calcium preparations increase gastric acid secretion after their buffering effect has been used. *Magnesium hydroxide* is a potent antacid that also has laxative effects. Approximately 5% to 10% of the magnesium in this preparation is absorbed from the intestine; because magnesium is excreted through the kidneys, this formulation should not be used in persons with renal failure. *Aluminum hydroxide* reacts with hydrochloric acid to form aluminum chloride. It combines with phosphate in the intestine, and prolonged use may lead to phosphate depletion and osteoporosis.

Sodium bicarbonate, sometimes used as a home remedy, is not recommended as an antacid. Because of its water solubility, it leaves the stomach rapidly and produces a transient effect, and it tends to cause metabolic alkalosis. It also contains large amounts of sodium. Antacids can decrease the absorption, bioavailability, and renal elimination of a number of drugs; this should be considered when antacids are administered with other medications.

Histamine is the major physiologic mediator for hydrochloric acid secretion. The H_2-receptor antagonists, cimetidine (Tagamet), ranitidine (Zantac), famotidine (Pepcid), and nizatidine (Axid), block gastric acid secretion stimulated by histamine, gastrin, and acetylcholine. The volume of gastric secretion and the concentration of pepsin are also reduced. These drugs are relatively well tolerated. Cimetidine can reduce liver blood flow and interfere with the oxidative metabolism of drugs such as the warfarin-type anticoagulants, phenytoin, propranolol, chlordiazepoxide, diazepam, and theophylline. Cimetidine also binds to androgen receptors and can cause gynecomastia in men and galactorrhea in women.

The proton pump inhibitors, omeprazole and lansoprazole, inhibit the final stage of hydrogen ion secretion by blocking the action of the gastric parietal cell proton pump (H^+/K^+-ATPase).

Surgical Treatment. When the conservative management of peptic ulcer is ineffective, surgical intervention may be indicated. Four types of surgical procedures are done: subtotal gastrectomy, in which 75% to 80% of the stomach is removed, and the remaining portion is attached to the jejunum; parietal cell vagotomy; truncal vagotomy and drainage, in which the vagus nerve trunks are cut and the outlet of the stomach is enlarged; and truncal vagotomy and antrectomy, in which the vagus nerve trunks are cut and the distal 50% of the stomach is removed.

One of the complications following surgery for peptic ulcers is the *dumping syndrome.* It occurs to some extent in about 20% of persons who have this type of operation. It is believed to be caused by the rapid entry of hyperosmolar liquids into the intestine and is characterized by symptoms such as nausea, vomiting, diarrhea, diaphoresis, palpitations, tachycardia, lightheadedness, and flushing that occur while eating or shortly after. It is often followed in about 2 hours by an episode of hypoglycemia, resulting from the rapid absorption of glucose, which acts as a stimulus for insulin release by the β cells of the pancreas. Treatment consists of limiting the diet to small frequent feedings, which are taken without liquids and which are low in simple sugars, because these are the most osmotically active parts of the diet. Symptoms usually diminish with time.

Zollinger-Ellison Syndrome

The Zollinger-Ellison syndrome is a rare condition caused by a gastrin-secreting tumor. In persons with this disorder, gastric acid secretion reaches such levels that ulceration becomes inevitable. The tumors may be single or multiple; although most tumors are located in the pancreas, a few develop in the submucosa of the stomach or duodenum. About two thirds of these tumors are malignant.[22] The increased gastric secretions cause symptoms related to peptic ulcer. Diarrhea may result from hypersecretion or from the inactivation of intestinal lipase and impaired fat digestion that occurs with a decrease in intestinal pH.

The diagnosis of the Zollinger-Ellison syndrome is based on elevated serum gastrin levels and elevated basal gastric acid levels. H_2-receptor blocking drugs are used to control gastric acid secretion. Computed tomography (CT), abdominal ultrasonography, and selective angiography are used to localize the tumor. Surgical removal is indicated when the tumor is malignant and has not undergone metastasis. Gastrectomy surgery and vagotomy may be done in selected cases.

Stress Ulcer

A stress ulcer, sometimes called a *Curling's ulcer,* refers to gastrointestinal ulcerations that develop in relation to major physiologic stress. These lesions occur most often in the gastric fundus and are thought to result from ischemia, tissue acidosis, and bile salts entering the stomach in critically ill persons with decreased gastrointestinal tract motility.[23,24] They are usually manifested by painless upper gastrointestinal tract bleeding. Persons at high risk for developing stress ulcers include those with large surface area burns, trauma, sepsis, acute respiratory distress syndrome, severe liver failure, and major surgical procedures.

Monitoring and maintaining the gastric pH at 3.5 or higher helps to prevent the development of stress ulcers. Antacids, H_2-receptor antagonists, and sucralfate are used in the prevention and treatment of stress ulcers. Prostaglandins may be used to promote ulcer healing.

Cancer of the Stomach

Cancer of the stomach strikes approximately 22,400 persons each year and accounts for 14,000 cancer deaths.[25] It is found more commonly in persons between 50 and 70 years of age. Although its incidence has decreased during the past 50 years, it remains the seventh leading cause of death in the United States.

Among the factors that increase the risk of gastric cancer are a genetic predisposition, carcinogenic factors in the diet (*e.g.,* nitrates, smoked foods), chronic atrophic gastritis, and gastric polyps. Infection with *H. pylori* appears to serve as a cofactor in some types of gastric carcinomas.[11] Between 50% and 60% of gastric cancers occur in the pyloric region or adjacent to the antrum. Compared with a benign ulcer, which has smooth margins and is concentrically shaped, gastric cancers tend to be larger, are irregularly shaped, have irregular margins, and are usually located in the greater curvature of the stomach.

Unfortunately, stomach cancers are often asymptomatic until late in their course. Symptoms, when they do occur, are usually vague and include indigestion, anorexia, weight loss, vague epigastric pain, vomiting, and an abdominal mass. Diagnosis of gastric cancer is accomplished by means of a variety of techniques, including barium x-ray studies, gastroscopy studies with biopsy, and cytologic studies (*e.g.,* Pap smear) of gastric secretions. Cytologic studies can prove particularly useful as routine screening tests for persons with atrophic gastritis or gastric polyps.

Surgery in the form of radical subtotal gastrectomy is usually the treatment of choice.[26] Irradiation and chemotherapy have not proved particularly useful as primary treatment modalities in stomach cancer. These methods are usually employed for palliative purposes or to control metastatic spread of the disease.

In summary, disorders of the stomach include gastritis, peptic ulcer, and cancer of the stomach. Gastritis refers to inflammation of the gastric mucosa. Acute gastritis refers to a transient inflammation of the gastric mucosa; it is most commonly associated with local irritants such as bacterial endotoxins, caffeine, alcohol, and aspirin. Chronic gastritis is characterized by the absence of grossly visible erosions and the presence of chronic inflammatory changes leading eventually to atrophy of the glandular epithelium of the stomach. There are two main types of chronic gastritis: autoimmune gastritis, which involves the fundus and the body of the stomach and is associated with pernicious anemia, and infective gastritis, which is caused by *H. pylori*. Chronic gastritis increases the risk of stomach cancer.

Peptic ulcer is a term used to describe a group of ulcerative disorders that occur in areas of the upper gastrointestinal tract that are exposed to acid-pepsin secretions, most commonly the duodenum and stomach. There are two main causes of peptic ulcer: *H. pylori* and aspirin or NSAID use. *H. pylori* is a S-shaped bacterium that colonizes the mucus-secreting epithelial cells of the stomach. The treatment of peptic ulcer focuses on eradication of *H. pylori*, avoidance of gastric irritation from NSAIDs, and conventional pharmacologic treatment directed at symptom relief and ulcer healing.

The Zollinger-Ellison syndrome is a rare condition caused by a gastrin-secreting tumor, in which gastric acid secretion reaches such levels that ulceration becomes inevitable. Stress ulcers, also called Curling's ulcers, occur in relation to major physiologic stresses such as burns and trauma and are thought to result from ischemia, tissue acidosis, and bile salts entering the stomach in critically ill persons with decreased gastrointestinal tract motility.

Although the incidence of cancer of the stomach has declined during the past 50 years, it remains the seventh leading cause of death in the United States. Because there are few early symptoms with this form of cancer, the disease is often far advanced at the time of diagnosis.

Disorders of the Small and Large Intestines

After you have completed this section of the chapter, you should be able to meet the following objectives:

- State the diagnostic criteria for irritable bowel syndrome
- Compare the characteristics of Crohn's disease and ulcerative colitis
- Relate the use of a high-fiber diet in the treatment of diverticular disease to the etiologic factors for the condition
- Describe the rationale for the symptoms associated with appendicitis
- List the risk factors associated with colorectal cancer and cite the screening methods for detection
- Compare the causes and manifestations of small-volume diarrhea and large-volume diarrhea
- Explain why a failure to respond to the defecation urge may result in constipation
- List five causes of fecal impaction
- Differentiate between mechanical and paralytic intestinal obstruction in terms of cause and manifestations
- List conditions that cause malabsorption by impaired intraluminal malabsorption, mucosal malabsorption, and lymphatic obstruction

There are many similarities in conditions that disrupt the integrity of the small and large intestines. The walls of the small and large intestines consists of five layers (see Chapter 31, Fig. 31–3): an outer serosal layer; a muscularis layer, which is divided into a layer of circular and a layer of longitudinal muscle fibers; a submucosal layer; and an inner mucosal layer, which lines the lumen of the intestine. Among the conditions that cause altered intestinal function are irritable bowel disease, inflammatory bowel disease, diverticulitis, appendicitis, alterations in bowel motility (*i.e.*, diarrhea, constipation, and bowel obstruction), cancer of the colon and rectum, and malabsorption syndrome.

Irritable Bowel Syndrome

The term *irritable bowel syndrome* is used to describe a functional gastrointestinal disorder characterized by a variable combination of chronic and recurrent intestinal symptoms not explained by structural or biochemical abnormalities. There is evidence to suggest that 10% to 20% of people in Western countries suffer from the disorder, although most do not seek medical attention.[27]

The condition is characterized by abdominal pain, altered bowel function, and varying complaints of flatulence, bloatedness, nausea and anorexia, and anxiety or depression. Various stimuli, including stress, alter colonic and small intestine motor activity; it is presumed that the pain symptoms of persons with irritable bowel syndrome are produced by the motor hyperreactivity.[28] Although changes in intestinal activity are normal responses to stress, these responses are exaggerated in persons with irritable bowel syndrome.

Diagnosis of irritable bowel syndrome is based on continuous or recurrent symptoms of at least 3 months' duration consisting of abdominal pain or discomfort relieved by defecation; a change in the frequency or consistency of stool; and the presence of three or more varying patterns of altered defecation that are present at least 25% of the time. These patterns of defecation include altered stool frequency, altered stool form (*i.e.*, hard or loose, watery stool), altered stool passage (*i.e.*, straining, urgency, or feeling of incomplete evacuation), passage of mucus, and bloating or feeling of abdominal discomfort.[29] A history of lactose intolerance should be considered, because intolerance to lactose and other sugars may be a precipitating factor in some persons. The role that psychologic factors play in the cause of the disease is uncertain.

The treatment of irritable bowel syndrome focuses on methods of stress management, particularly those related to symptom production. Reassurance is important.

Usually, no special diet is indicated, although adequate fiber intake is usually recommended. Avoidance of gastrointestinal stimulants such as caffeine-containing beverages may be beneficial.

Inflammatory Bowel Disease

The term *inflammatory bowel disease* is used to designate two inflammatory conditions: Crohn's disease and ulcerative colitis. Although the peak occurrence for both diseases is between 15 and 35 years of age, they occur in all age groups. Ulcerative colitis and Crohn's disease are prominent causes of chronic illness among children and adolescents. There is evidence to suggest that the incidence of ulcerative colitis, which is an inflammatory disorder of the rectum and colon, has reached a plateau, whereas that of Crohn's disease, which can affect the large or small bowel, has increased steadily during the past 20 to 30 years.

The causes of Crohn's disease and ulcerative colitis are largely unknown. The diseases appear to have a familial occurrence, which suggests a hereditary predisposition. There is an increased prevalence of the disease among first-degree relatives and an increased incidence among certain populations, most notably the Ashkenazi Jews.[30] One of the common beliefs is that genetic factors predispose to some form of autoimmune reaction, possibly triggered by some relatively innocuous environmental agent such as a dietary antigen or microbial agent. Although psychogenic factors may contribute to the severity and onset of both conditions, it seems unlikely that they are the primary cause.

Crohn's disease and ulcerative colitis are characterized by remissions and exacerbations of diarrhea, fecal urgency, and weight loss. Acute complications such as intestinal obstruction may develop during periods of fulminant disease. Both diseases may be accompanied by extraintestinal manifestations such as arthritis. Although the two diseases share many common features, they can be differentiated based on clinical, radiologic, endoscopic, and histologic features. The distinguishing characteristics of Crohn's disease and ulcerative colitis are summarized in Table 32–1.

Crohn's Disease

Crohn's disease is a recurrent, granulomatous type of inflammatory response that can affect any area of the gastrointestinal tract from the mouth to the anus. It is a slowly progressive, relentless, and often disabling disease. The disease usually strikes in early adulthood and affects men and women equally. Despite the substantial increase in the prevalence of Crohn's disease in the early 1980s, the distribution of affected sites has not changed substantially. In nearly 40% of persons with disease, the lesions are restricted to the small intestine; in 30%, only the large bowel is affected; and in the remaining 30%, the large bowel and small bowel are affected.[30]

A characteristic feature of Crohn's disease is the sharply demarcated, granulomatous lesions that occur and that are surrounded by normal-appearing mucosal tissue. When the lesions are multiple, they are often referred to as skip lesions, because they are interspersed between what appear to be normal segments of the bowel. All the layers of the bowel are involved, with the submucosal layer affected to the greatest extent. The surface of the inflamed bowel usually has a characteristic "cobblestone" appearance resulting from the fissures and crevices that develop and are surrounded by areas of submucosal edema (Fig. 32–4). There is usually a relative sparing of the smooth muscle layers of the bowel, with marked inflammatory and fibrotic changes of the submucosal layer. The bowel wall, after a time, often becomes thickened and inflexible; its appearance has been likened to a lead pipe or rubber hose. The adjacent mesentery may become inflamed, and the regional lymph nodes and channels may become enlarged.

Crohn's disease is often accompanied by the formation of fistulas, or tubelike passages, that form pathologic connections between different sites in the gastrointestinal tract. They may develop between the bowel and other sites, including the bladder, vagina, urethra, and skin. Perineal fistulas that originate in the ileum are relatively common.[31] Fistulas between segments of the gastrointestinal

TABLE 32–1

Differentiating Characteristics of Crohn's Disease and Ulcerative Colitis

Characteristic	Crohn's Disease	Ulcerative Colitis
Types of inflammation	Granulomatous	Ulcerative and exudative
Level of involvement	Primarily submucosal	Primarily mucosal
Extent of involvement	Skip lesions	Continuous
Areas of involvement	Primarily ileum, secondarily colon	Primarily rectum and left colon
Diarrhea	Common	Common
Rectal bleeding	Rare	Common
Fistulas	Common	Rare
Strictures	Common	Rare
Perianal abscesses	Common	Rare
Development of cancer	Rare	Relatively common

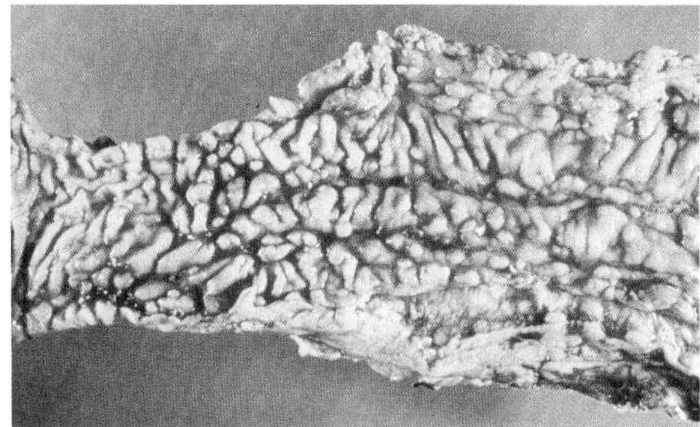

Figure 32–4
Crohn's disease. The mucosal surface of the colon displays a "cobblestone" appearance owing to the presence of linear ulcerations and edema and inflammation of the intervening tissue.

tract may lead to malabsorption, syndromes of bacterial overgrowth, and diarrhea. They can also become infected and cause abscess formation.

The clinical course of Crohn's disease is variable; often, there are periods of exacerbations and remissions, with symptoms being related to the location of the lesions. The principal symptoms include intermittent diarrhea, colicky pain (usually in the lower right quadrant), weight loss, fluid and electrolyte disorders, malaise, and low-grade fever. Because Crohn's disease affects the submucosal layer to a greater extent than the mucosal layer, there is less bloody diarrhea than with ulcerative colitis. Ulceration of the perianal skin is common, largely because of the severity of the diarrhea. The absorptive surface of the intestine may be disrupted; nutritional deficiencies may occur, related to the specific segment of the intestine that is involved. Complications include intestinal obstruction, abdominal abscess formation, and fistula formation.

Fish oil in an enteric-coated preparation has been used to prevent relapses in persons with Crohn's disease.[32] It has been suggested that the oil acts at multiple points in altering the inflammatory process that becomes activated in Crohn's disease, particularly as it relates to the production of messenger molecules of the immune system that attract inflammatory cells.[33]

Ulcerative Colitis

Ulcerative colitis is a nonspecific inflammatory condition of the colon. The disease begins most often in the second and third decade of life, has no sex predilection, and affects whites more often than nonwhites. Unlike Crohn's disease, which can affect various sites in the gastrointestinal tract, ulcerative colitis is confined to the rectum and colon. The disease usually begins in the rectum and spreads proximally, affecting primarily the mucosal layer, although it can extend into the submucosal layer. The length of proximal extension varies. It may involve the entire colon. The inflammatory process tends to be confluent and continuous instead of skipping areas, as it does in Crohn's disease.

Characteristic of the disease are the lesions that form in the crypts of Lieberkühn in the base of the mucosal layer (see Chapter 31, Fig. 31–12). The inflammatory process causes pinpoint mucosal hemorrhages to occur, which in time suppurate and develop into *crypt abscesses*. These inflammatory lesions may become necrotic and ulcerate. Although the ulcerations are usually superficial, they often extend, causing large, denuded areas (Fig. 32–5). As a result of the inflammatory process, the mucosal layer often develops tonguelike projections that resemble polyps and are therefore called *pseudopolyps*. The bowel wall thickens in response to repeated episodes of colitis.

Ulcerative colitis usually follows a course of remissions and exacerbations. The severity of the disease varies from mild to fulminating. Accordingly, the disease has been divided into three types: mild chronic, chronic intermittent, and acute fulminating. The most common form is the mild chronic form of the disease, in which bleeding and diarrhea are mild and systemic signs are minimal or absent. This form of the disease can usually be managed by conservative means. The chronic intermittent form continues after the initial attack. Compared with the milder form, usually more of the colon surface is involved with the chronic intermittent form, and there are more systemic signs and complications. In about 15% of affected persons, the disease assumes a more fulminant course, involves the entire colon, and manifests with severe bloody diarrhea, fever, and acute abdominal pain. These persons are at risk for toxic megacolon and perforation.

Diarrhea, which is the characteristic manifestation of ulcerative colitis, varies according to the severity of the disease. There may be up to 30 to 40 bowel movements a day. Because ulcerative colitis affects the mucosal layer of the bowel, the stools typically contain blood and mucus. Nocturnal diarrhea usually occurs when daytime symptoms are severe. There may be mild

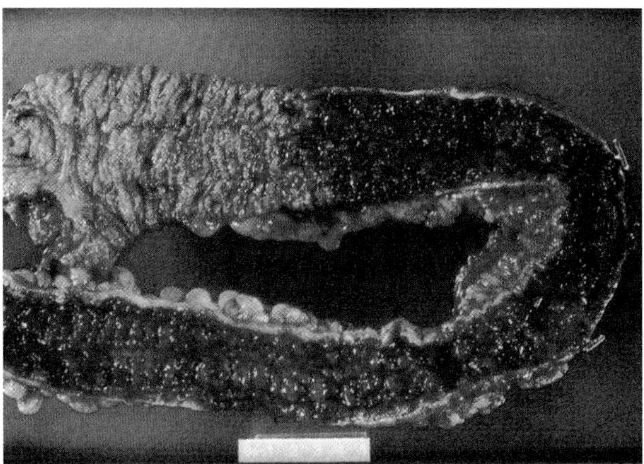

Figure 32–5
Ulcerative colitis. Prominent erythema and ulceration of the colon begin in the ascending colon and are most severe in the rectosigmoid area.

abdominal cramping and fecal incontinence. Anorexia, weakness, and fatigability are common.

Complications

Crohn's disease and ulcerative colitis are associated with a wide variety of complications encompassing the secondary effects of the inflammatory process of the gastrointestinal tract and associated extraintestinal manifestations.

In Crohn's disease, fistulas can develop between the bowel and other sites, including the bladder, vagina, and skin. One potentially life-threatening complication of Crohn's disease and ulcerative colitis is *toxic megacolon*. It is characterized by dilatation of the colon and signs of systemic toxicity. It results from extension of the inflammatory response, with involvement of neural and vascular components of the bowel. Contributing factors include use of laxatives, narcotics, and anticholinergic drugs and the presence of hypokalemia.

A number of extraintestinal manifestations have been identified in persons with Crohn's disease and ulcerative colitis. These include axial arthritis affecting the spine and sacroiliac joints and oligoarticular arthritis affecting the large joints of the arms and legs; inflammatory conditions of the eye, usually uveitis; skin lesions, especially erythema nodosum; stomatitis; and autoimmune anemia, hypercoagulability of blood, and sclerosing cholangitis. Occasionally, these systemic manifestations may herald the recurrence of intestinal disease. In children, growth retardation may occur, particularly if the symptoms are prolonged and nutrient intake has been poor.

Cancer of the colon is one of the feared complications of ulcerative colitis. The risk of developing cancer among persons who have had pancolitis for 10 years or more is 20 to 30 times that of the general population.[11]

Diagnosis and Treatment

The diagnosis of inflammatory bowel disease requires a thorough history and physical examination. Sigmoidoscopy is used for direct visualization of the affected areas and to obtain biopsies. Measures are taken to exclude infectious agents as the cause of the disorder. This is usually accomplished by the use of stool cultures and examination of fresh stool specimens for ova and parasites. In persons suspected of having Crohn's disease, radiologic contrast studies provide a means for determining the extent of involvement of the small bowel and establishing the presence and nature of fistulas. CT scans may be used to detect an inflammatory mass or abscess.

Treatment methods focus on terminating the inflammatory response and promoting healing, maintaining adequate nutrition, and preventing and treating complications. Sulfasalazine (Azulfidine), a poorly absorbed drug with antiinflammatory action, and the corticosteroid drugs are frequently used to treat the acute disease. Sulfasalazine reduces the frequency and severity of recurrent ulcerative colitis. However, no beneficial effect has been demonstrated after acute disease activity has been controlled in Crohn's disease.[34] Unfortunately, hypersensitivity reactions prevent its use in many persons.

The beneficial effects of the sulfasalazine are attributable to one component of the drug: 5-aminosalicylic acid (5-ASA). Other 5-ASA drugs are available in the United States. These agents differ in the segment of the bowel where the drug is released, affording the possibility that drugs released in the small bowel may be more effective in treating Crohn's disease. Topical 5-ASA drugs, given as an enema, also are available. The corticosteroids are used selectively to lessen the acute inflammatory response. These drugs can be given orally, by enema, or in the form of a suppository. Immunosuppressive drugs such as azathioprine and its active derivative, mercaptopurine, may be used to treat persons with refractory Crohn's disease.

The observation that smokers are less likely to develop ulcerative colitis led to investigation of the use of nicotine patches in the treatment of ulcerative colitis.[35] Although the mechanisms of nicotine's action are unclear, some of the results have been promising.[36] Surgical treatment (*i.e.*, removal of the rectum and entire colon) with the creation of an ileostomy or ilioanal anastomosis may be required for those persons with ulcerative colitis who do not respond to conservative methods of treatment.

Nutritional deficiencies are common in Crohn's disease because of diarrhea, steatorrhea, and other malabsorption problems. A nutritious diet that is high in calories, vitamins, and proteins is recommended. Because fats often aggravate the diarrhea, it is recommended that they be avoided. Elemental diets, which are nutritionally balanced but are residue free and bulk free, may be given during the acute phase of the illness. These diets are largely absorbed in the jejunum and allow the inflamed bowel to rest. Total parenteral nutrition (*i.e.*, parenteral hyperalimentation) consists of intravenous administration of hypertonic glucose solutions to which amino acids and fats may be added. This form of nutritional therapy may be needed when food cannot be absorbed from the intestine. Because of the hypertonicity of these solutions, they must be administered through a large-diameter central vein.

Infectious Colitis

Two forms of pathogens have emerged as important causes of infectious colitis: *Clostridium difficile* and *Escherichia coli* serotype O157:H7.

Clostridium difficile Colitis

C. difficile, the agent that causes pseudomembranous colitis associated with antibiotic therapy, has been identified as a common nosocomial pathogen. Treatment with broad-spectrum antibiotics predisposes to disruption of the normal bacterial flora of the colon, leading to colonization by *C. difficile* along with the release of toxins that cause mucosal damage and inflammation. Almost any antibiotic may cause *C. difficile* colitis, but broad-spectrum antibiotics with activity against gram-negative enteric bacteria are the most frequent agents. Broad-spectrum penicillins and cephalosporins are the most common causes.

C. difficile forms heat-resistant spores that persist for months to years in the environment.[37] The spores are resistant to the acid environment of the stomach and convert to vegetative forms in the colon. After antibiotic therapy has made the bowel susceptible to infection, colonization by *C. difficile* occurs by the oral-fecal route. *C. difficile* infection is usually acquired in the hospital where the organism is commonly encountered.

C. difficile infection may involve antibiotic-associated colitis without pseudomembranous formation or pseudomembranous colitis. Fortunately, most cases are not severe and do not involve pseudomembranous formation. The infection commonly manifests with diarrhea that is mild to moderate and is sometimes accompanied by lower abdominal cramping. Symptoms usually begin during or shortly after antibiotic therapy has been initiated, although they can be delayed for weeks. In most cases, systemic manifestations are absent, and the symptoms subside after the antibiotic has been discontinued.

The more severe form of the disease, pseudomembranous *C. difficile* colitis, is characterized by an adherent inflammatory membrane overlying the areas of mucosal injury. It is a life-threatening form of the disease. Persons with the disease are acutely ill, with lethargy, fever, tachycardia, abdominal pain and distention, and dehydration. The smooth muscle tone of the colon may be lost, resulting in toxic dilation of the colon. Prompt therapy is needed to prevent perforation of the bowel.

Diagnostic findings include a history of antibiotic use and laboratory tests that confirm the presence of *C. difficile* toxins in the stool. Treatment includes the immediate discontinuation of antibiotic therapy. Specific treatment aimed at eradicating *C. difficile* is used when symptoms are severe or persistent. Metronidazole is the first drug of choice, with vancomycin being reserved for persons who cannot tolerate metronidazole or do not respond to the drug. Both drugs are given orally.[37] Metronidazole is absorbed from the upper gastrointestinal tract and may cause side effects. Vancomycin is poorly absorbed, and its actions are limited to the gastrointestinal tract.

Escherichia coli O157:H7 Infection

E. coli O157:H7 has become recognized as an important cause of epidemic and sporadic colitis. Attention to the organism was emphasized by the well-publicized outbreak that was associated with undercooked hamburger meat from a national fast-food chain.

E. coli O157:H7 is a strain of *E. coli* found in feces and contaminated milk of healthy dairy and beef cattle, but it has also been found in pork, poultry, and lamb. Infection is usually by foodborne transmission, often by ingesting undercooked hamburger. Person-to-person transmission may occur, particularly in nursing homes, day care settings, and hospitals. The very young and the very old are particularly at risk for the infection and its complications.

The infection may cause no symptoms or cause a variety of manifestations, including acute nonbloody diarrhea, hemorrhagic colitis, hemolytic-uremic syndrome, and thrombotic thrombocytopenic purpura. The infection often presents with abdominal cramping and watery diarrhea and may subsequently progress to bloody diarrhea. The diarrhea commonly lasts 3 to 7 days or longer with 10 to 12 diarrheal episodes per day. Fever occurs in up to one third of the cases.

An important aspect of the disease is the production of toxins and the ability to produce toxanemia. The two complications of the infection, hemolytic-uremic syndrome and thrombotic thrombocytopenic purpura, reflect the effects of toxins. Hemolytic-uremic syndrome is characterized by hemolytic anemia, thrombocytopenia, and renal failure. It occurs predominantly in infants and young children and is the most common cause of acute renal failure in children.[38] It has a mortality rate of 5% to 10%, and one third of survivors are left with permanent disability. Thrombotic thrombocytopenic purpura is manifested by thrombocytopenia, renal failure, fever, and neurologic manifestations. It is often regarded as the severe end of the disease that leads to hemolytic-uremic syndrome plus neurologic problems.

No specific therapy is available for *E. coli* O157:H7 infection. Treatment is largely symptomatic and directed toward treating the effects of complications. Antibiotics have not proved useful and may be harmful, extending the duration of bloody diarrhea.

Because of the seriousness of the infection and its complication, education of the public about techniques for decreasing primary transmission of the infection from animal sources is important. Undercooked meats and unpasteurized milk are sources of transmission. The U.S. Food and Drug Administration recommends a minimal internal temperature of 155°F for cooked hamburger. Food handlers and consumers should be aware of the proper methods for handling uncooked meat to prevent cross contamination of other foods. Particular attention should be paid to hygiene in day care centers and nursing homes, where the spread of infection to the very young and very old may result in severe complications.[38]

Diverticular Disease

Diverticulosis is a condition in which the mucosal layer of the colon herniates through the muscularis layer. Often, there are multiple diverticula, and most occur in the sigmoid colon (Fig. 32–6). Diverticular disease is common in the United States. It is one of the most common disorders of aging, affecting 50% of the population by age 90.[39] Although the disorder is prevalent in the developed countries of the world, it is almost nonexistent in many of the African nations and underdeveloped countries. This suggests that dietary factors (*e.g.*, lack of fiber content), a decrease in physical activity, and poor

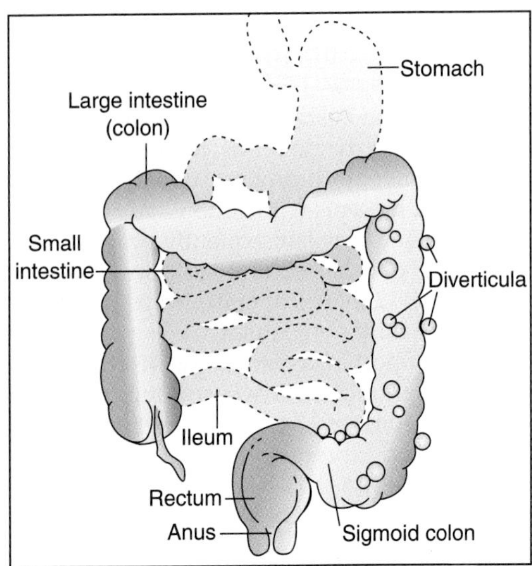

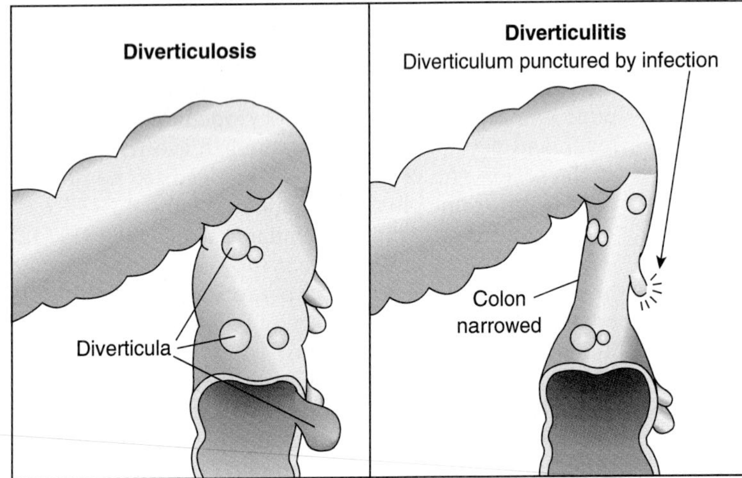

Figure 32–6
(Top) Location of diverticula in the sigmoid colon. **(Bottom left)** Diverticulosis. **(Bottom right)** Diverticulitis. (National Digestive Diseases Information Clearinghouse. [1989]. *Clearinghouse fact sheet: Diverticulosis and diverticulitis.* NIH publication 90–1163. Washington, DC: US Department of Health and Human Services)

bowel habits (*e.g.*, neglecting the urge to defecate), along with the effects of aging, contribute to the development of the disease.

In the colon, the longitudinal muscle does not form a continuous layer, as it does in the small bowel. Instead, there are three separate longitudinal bands of muscle called the *teniae coli.* In a manner similar to the small intestine, bands of circular muscle constrict the large intestine. At each of these constrictive points (about every 2.5 cm), the circular muscle contracts, sometimes constricting the lumen of the bowel so that it is almost occluded. The combined contraction of the circular muscle and the lack of a continuous longitudinal muscle layer causes the unstimulated intestine to bulge outward into pouches called *haustra* (Fig. 32–7). Diverticula develop between the longitudinal muscle bands of the haustra, in the area where the blood vessels pierce the circular muscle layer to bring blood to the mucosal layer. An increase in intraluminal pressure within the haustra provides the force for creating these herniations. The increase in pressure is thought to be related to the volume of the colonic contents. The more scanty the contents, the more vigorous are the contractions and the greater is the pressure within the haustra.

Most persons with diverticular disease remain asymptomatic. The disease is often found when x-ray studies are done for other purposes. When symptoms do

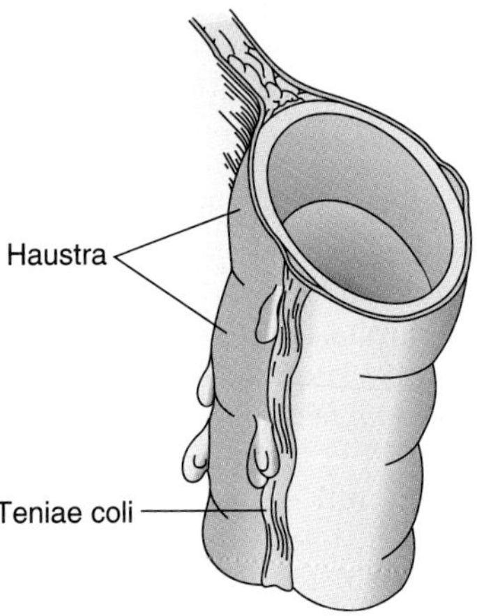

Figure 32–7
A portion of the sigmoid colon, showing the haustra and teniae coli.

occur, they are often attributed to irritable bowel syndrome or other causes. Ill-defined lower abdominal discomfort, a change in bowel habits (*e.g.*, diarrhea, constipation), bloating, and flatulence are common.

Diverticulitis is a complication of diverticulosis in which there is inflammation and gross or microscopic perforation of the diverticulum. One of the most common complaints of diverticulitis is pain in the lower left quadrant, accompanied by nausea and vomiting, tenderness in the lower left quadrant, a slight fever, and elevation in white blood cell count. These symptoms usually last for several days, unless complications occur, and are usually caused by localized inflammation of the diverticuli with perforation and development of a small localized abscess. Complications include perforation with peritonitis, hemorrhage, and bowel obstruction. Fistulas can form, usually involving the bladder (*i.e.*, vesicosigmoid fistula) but sometimes involving the skin, perianal area, or small bowel. Pneumaturia (*i.e.*, air in the urine) is a sign of vesicosigmoid fistula.

The diagnosis of diverticular disease is based on history and presenting clinical manifestations. The disease may be confirmed by barium enema x-ray studies or colonoscopy. Because of the risk of peritonitis, barium enema studies should be avoided in persons who are suspected of having acute diverticulitis. Flat abdominal radiographs may be used to detect complications associated with acute diverticulitis.

The usual treatment for diverticular disease is to prevent symptoms and complications. This includes increasing the bulk in the diet and bowel retraining so that the person has at least one bowel movement each day. The increased bulk promotes regular defecation and increases colonic contents and colon diameter, thereby decreasing intraluminal pressure. Acute diverticulitis is treated by withholding solid food and the use of a broad-spectrum antibiotic. Surgical treatment is reserved for complications.

Appendicitis

Acute appendicitis is extremely common. It is seen most frequently in the 5- to 30-year-old age group, but it can occur at any age. The appendix becomes inflamed, swollen, and gangrenous, and it eventually perforates if not treated. Although the cause of appendicitis is unknown, it is thought to be related to intraluminal obstruction with a fecalith (*i.e.*, hard piece of stool) or to twisting.

Appendicitis usually has an abrupt onset, with pain referred to the epigastric or periumbilical area. This pain is caused by stretching of the appendix during the early inflammatory process. At about the same time that the pain appears, there are one or two episodes of nausea. Initially, the pain is vague, but over a period of 2 to 12 hours, it gradually increases and may become colicky in nature. When the inflammatory process has extended to involve the serosal layer of the appendix and the peritoneum, the pain becomes localized to the lower right quadrant. There is usually an elevation in temperature and a white blood cell count greater than 10,000/mm^3 with 75% or more polymorphonuclear cells. Palpation of the abdomen usually reveals a deep tenderness in the lower right quadrant, which is confined to a small area about the size of the fingertip. It is usually located at about the site of the inflamed appendix. The person with appendicitis often is able to place his or her finger directly over the tender area. Rebound tenderness, which is pain that occurs when pressure is applied to the area and then released, and spasm of the overlying abdominal muscles are common.

Treatment consists of surgical removal of the appendix. Complications include peritonitis, localized periappendiceal abscess formation, and septicemia.

Colorectal Cancer

More than 61,000 persons in the United States die each year of colorectal cancer.[25] It is the second most common site of fatal cancer. The main drawback to successful treatment is the fact that most lesions do not produce symptoms until late in the course of the disease.

Almost all cancers of the colon and rectum are carcinomas. There has been a shift in location of colorectal cancers to the right colon; 25% occur in the cecum and ascending colon, 25% occur in the descending and proximal sigmoid colon, 25% occur in the rectum and distal sigmoid colon, and the remainder are scattered elsewhere.[11]

Etiology and Manifestations

The cause of cancer of the colon and rectum is largely unknown. Its incidence increases with age, as evidenced by the fact that about 80% of persons who develop this form of cancer are older than 50 years. Its incidence is increased among persons with a family history of cancer, persons with ulcerative colitis, and those with familial multiple polyposis of the colon. Genetic and environmental factors are thought to be involved.

Attention has focused on dietary fat intake, refined sugar intake, fiber intake, and the adequacy of such protective micronutrients as vitamins A, C, and E in the diet. It has been hypothesized that a high level of fat in the diet increases the synthesis of bile acids in the liver, which may be converted to potential carcinogens by the bacterial flora in the colon. Bacteroid organisms in particular are suspected of converting bile acids to carcinogens; their proliferation is enhanced by a high dietary level of refined sugars. Dietary fiber is thought to increase stool bulk and thereby dilute and remove potential carcinogens. Refined diets often contain reduced amounts of vitamins A, C, and E, which may act as oxygen free-radical scavengers.

Most colorectal carcinomas arise in preexisting adenomatous polyps. The frequency of polyps increases with age, and the presence of adenomatous polyps is about 20% to 30% before age 40, rising to 40% to 50% after age 60.[11] Men and women are equally affected. The peak incidence of adenomatous polyps precedes by some years the peak for colorectal cancer. Programs that provide careful follow-up for persons with adenomatous polyps and removal of all suspicious lesions have substantially reduced the incidence of colorectal cancer.[11]

Usually, cancer of the colon and rectum is present for a long time before it produces symptoms. Bleeding is a highly significant early symptom, and it is usually the one that causes persons to seek medical care. Other symptoms include a change in bowel habits, diarrhea or constipation and sometimes a sense of urgency or incomplete emptying of the bowel. Pain is usually a late symptom.

The prognosis for persons with colorectal cancer depends largely on the extent of bowel involvement and on the presence of metastasis at the time of diagnosis. This form of cancer can be divided into four categories according to the Duke classification system. A stage A tumor is limited to invasion of the mucosal and submucosal layers of the colon and has a 5-year survival rate of almost 100%. A stage B tumor involves the entire wall of the colon, but without lymph node involvement, and has a 5-year survival rate of 43% to 67%. With a stage C tumor, there is invasion of the serosal layer, with involvement of the regional lymph nodes. The 5-year survival rate is approximately 23%. Stage D colorectal cancer involves far-advanced metastasis.[11]

Recent reports indicate that aspirin may protect against colorectal cancer.[40] An analysis of the incidence of colorectal cancer in the Nurses Health Study showed a decreased incidence in colorectal cancer among women who took 4 to 6 aspirin per week.[41] Although the mechanism of aspirin's action is unknown, it may be related to its effect on prostaglandin synthesis, one or more of which may be involved in signal systems that influence cell proliferation or tumor growth.

Diagnosis and Treatment

Among the methods used in the diagnosis of colorectal cancers are stool occult blood tests and digital rectal examination, usually done during routine physical examinations; x-ray studies using barium (*e.g.*, barium enema); and proctosigmoidoscopy and colonoscopy. Digital rectal examinations are most helpful in detecting neoplasms of the rectum. Rectal examination should be considered a routine part of a good physical examination. The American Cancer Society recommends that all asymptomatic men and women older than 40 years of age should have a digital rectal examination performed annually as a part of their physical examination and that those older than 50 should have an annual stool test for occult blood and a proctosigmoidoscopy examination done every 3 to 5 years, as recommended by their physician.[42]

Almost all cancers of the colon and rectum bleed intermittently, although the amount of blood is small and usually not apparent in the stools. It is therefore feasible to screen for colorectal cancers using commercially prepared tests for occult blood in the stool that are available. This method uses a guaiac-impregnated filter paper. The technique involves preparing two slides per day from different portions of the same stool for 3 to 4 days while the patient follows a high-fiber diet that is free of meat and ascorbic acid. Although the diet is not particularly appealing, this stool test has been shown to be a relatively reliable and inexpensive method of screening for colorectal cancer. Persons with a positive stool occult blood test should be referred to their physicians for further study. Usually, a physical examination, rectal examination, barium enema, and proctosigmoidoscopy or colonoscopy are done.

Proctosigmoidoscopy involves examination of the rectum and sigmoid colon with a hollow, lighted tube that is inserted through the rectum. Polyps can be removed, or tissue can be obtained for biopsy during the procedure.

Colonoscopy provides a means for direct visualization of the rectum and colon. The colonoscope consists of a flexible 4-cm glass bundle that has some 250,000 glass fibers and has a lens at either end to focus and magnify the image. Light from an external source is transmitted by the fiberoptic viewing bundle. Instruments are available that afford direct examination of the sigmoid colon or the entire colon. This method is used for screening persons at high risk for developing cancer of the colon (*e.g.*, those with ulcerative colitis) and for those with symptoms. Colonoscopy is also useful for obtaining a biopsy and for removing polyps. Although this method is one of the most accurate for detecting early colorectal cancers, it is not suitable for mass screening, because it is expensive and time consuming and must be done by a person who is highly trained in the use of the instrument.

The carcinoembryonic antigen (CEA) can be used as a marker for colorectal cancer. However, blood levels are of little screening or diagnostic value because they become elevated only after the tumor has reached considerable size. Moreover, CEA is produced by other types of cancers and noncancerous conditions such as alcoholic cirrhosis, pancreatitis, and ulcerative colitis. This marker is of greatest value for monitoring tumor recurrence in persons after resection of the primary tumor.[11]

The only recognized treatment for cancer of the colon and rectum is surgical removal. Preoperative radiation therapy may be used and has in some cases demonstrated increased 5-year survival rates. Postoperative adjuvant therapy with 5-fluorouracil has had some success. Radiation therapy and chemotherapy are used as palliative treatment methods.

Alterations in Intestinal Motility

The movement of contents through the gastrointestinal tract is controlled by neurons located in the submucosal and myenteric plexuses of the gut (see Chapter 31). The axons from the cell bodies in the myenteric plexus innervate the circular and longitudinal smooth muscle layers of the gut. These neurons receive impulses from local receptors located in the mucosal and muscle layers of the gut and extrinsic input from the parasympathetic and sympathetic nervous systems. As a general rule, the parasympathetic nervous system tends to increase the motility of the bowel, whereas sympathetic stimulation tends to slow its activity.

The colon has sphincters at both ends: the ileocecal sphincter, which separates it from the small intestine, and the anal sphincter, which prevents the movement of feces to the outside of the body. The colon acts as a reservoir for fecal material. Normally, about 400 ml of water, 55 mEq of sodium, 30 mEq of chloride, and 15 mEq of bicarbonate are absorbed each day in the colon. At the same time, about 5 mEq of potassium is secreted into the lumen of the colon. The amount of water and electrolytes that remains in the stool reflects the absorption or secretion that occurs in the colon. The average adult ingesting a typical American diet evacuates about 200 to 300 g of stool each day.

Diarrhea

The usual definition of *diarrhea* is excessively frequent passage of stools. Diarrhea can be acute or chronic. Diarrhea is considered to be chronic when the symptoms persist for 3 weeks in children or adults and 4 weeks in infants. Acute diarrhea affects 500 million children throughout the world and is the leading cause of death of children younger than 4 years of age.[43]

The complaint of diarrhea is a general one and can be related to a number of pathologic and nonpathologic factors. Diarrhea is usually divided into two types: large volume and small volume. Large-volume diarrhea results from an increase in the water content of the stool, and small-volume diarrhea results from an increase in the propulsive activity of the bowel. Some of the common causes of small- and large-volume diarrhea are summarized in Chart 32–1. Often, diarrhea is a combination of these two types.

CHART 32-1
Causes of Large- and Small-Volume Diarrhea

Large-Volume Diarrhea

- Osmotic diarrhea
  - Saline cathartics
  - Dumping syndrome
  - Lactase deficiency
- Secretory diarrhea
  - Failure to absorb bile salts
  - Fat malabsorption
  - Chronic laxative abuse
  - Carcinoid syndrome
  - Zollinger-Ellison syndrome
  - Fecal impaction
  - Acute infectious diarrhea

Small-Volume Diarrhea

- Inflammatory bowel disease
  - Crohn's disease
  - Ulcerative colitis
- Infectious disease
  - Shigellosis
  - Salmonellosis
- Irritable colon

Large-Volume Diarrhea. Large-volume diarrhea can be classified as secretory or osmotic, according to the cause of the increased water content in the feces. Water is pulled into the colon along an osmotic gradient (*i.e.*, osmotic diarrhea) or is secreted into the bowel by the mucosal cells (*i.e.*, secretory diarrhea). The large-volume form of diarrhea is usually a painless, watery type without blood or pus in the stools.

In osmotic diarrhea, water is pulled into the bowel by the hyperosmotic nature of its contents. It occurs when osmotically active particles are not absorbed. In persons with lactase deficiency, the lactose in milk cannot be broken down and absorbed. Magnesium salts, which are contained in milk of magnesia and many antacids, are poorly absorbed and cause diarrhea when taken in sufficient quantities. Another cause of osmotic diarrhea is decreased transit time, which interferes with absorption. This happens in the dumping syndrome, which can occur after surgical treatment of peptic ulcer. Osmotic diarrhea usually disappears with fasting.

Secretory diarrhea occurs when the secretory processes of the bowel are increased. Most acute infectious diarrheas are of this type. Enteric organisms cause diarrhea by several ways. Some are noninvasive but secrete toxins that stimulate fluid secretion (*e.g.*, pathogenic *E. coli* or *Vibrio cholerae*). Others invade and destroy intestinal epithelial cells, thereby altering fluid transport so secretory activity continues while absorption activity is halted.[44] Secretory diarrhea also occurs when excess bile acids remain in the intestinal contents as they enter the colon. This often happens with disease processes of the ileum, because bile salts are absorbed here. It may also occur with bacterial overgrowth in the small bowel, which also interferes with bile absorption. Some tumors, such as those of the Zollinger-Ellison syndrome and carcinoid syndrome, produce hormones that cause increased secretory activity of the bowel.

Small-Volume Diarrhea. Small-volume diarrhea is commonly associated with acute or chronic inflammation or intrinsic disease of the colon, such as ulcerative colitis or Crohn's disease. Diarrhea with vomiting and fever suggests food poisoning, often caused by staphylococcal enterotoxin. Small-volume diarrhea is usually evidenced by frequency and urgency and colicky abdominal pain. It is commonly accompanied by tenesmus (*i.e.*, painful straining at stool), fecal soiling of clothing, and awakening during the night with the urge to defecate.

Diagnosis and Treatment. The diagnosis of diarrhea is based on complaints of frequent stools and a history of accompanying factors such as concurrent illnesses, medication use, and exposure to potential intestinal pathogens. Disorders such as inflammatory bowel disease should be considered. If the onset of diarrhea is related to travel outside the United States, the possibility of traveler's diarrhea must be considered.

Although most acute forms of diarrhea are self-limited and require no treatment, diarrhea can be particularly serious in infants and small children, persons with other illnesses, the elderly, and even previously healthy persons if it continues for any length of time. The replacement of fluids and electrolytes is therefore considered to be a primary therapeutic goal in the treatment of diarrhea.

Oral electrolyte replacement solutions can be given in situations of uncomplicated diarrhea that can be treated at home. Complete oral rehydration solutions contain carbohydrate, sodium, potassium, chloride, and base to replace that lost in the diarrheal stool. The effectiveness of oral rehydration therapy is based on the coupled transport of sodium and glucose or other actively transported small organic molecules (see Chapter 31). Oral rehydration therapy can be particularly effective in treating dehydration associated with diarrheal disease in infants and small children. However, cost may be a factor. The oral rehydration products for infants and children that are available in the United States range in price from $3.50 to $5.00 per liter. In severe cases of diarrhea, a child may require several liters per day. The cost can be a sizable burden on socioeconomically disadvantaged families, which are the same families that are at greatest risk for a poor outcome from diarrhea. Less expensive premeasured packets and recipes for preparing replacement solutions are available. The use of oral rehydration therapy is also labor intensive, requiring frequent feeding, sometimes using a spoon.[45] More importantly, the diarrhea does not promptly cease after oral rehydration has been instituted; this can be discouraging for parents and caregivers who desire early results from their efforts. When oral rehydration is not feasible or adequate, intravenous fluid replacement may be needed.

Evidence suggests that feeding should be continued during diarrheal illness, particularly in children.[46] It is recommended that children who require rehydration therapy because of diarrhea be fed an age-appropriate diet. Starch and simple proteins are thought to provide cotransport molecules (see Chapter 31) with little osmotic activity, increasing fluid and electrolyte uptake by intestinal cells. It has been shown that unrestricted diets do not worsen the course or symptoms of mild diarrhea and can decrease stool output. Although there is little agreement on which foods are best, fatty foods and foods high in simple sugars are best avoided.

Drugs used in the treatment of diarrhea include camphorated tincture of opium (paregoric), diphenoxylate (Lomotil), and loperamide (Imodium), which are opiumlike drugs. These drugs decrease gastrointestinal motility and stimulate water and electrolyte absorption. Adsorbents, such as kaolin and pectin, adsorb irritants and toxins from the bowel. These ingredients are included in many over-the-counter antidiarrheal preparations because they adsorb toxins responsible for certain types of diarrhea. Bismuth subsalicylate (Pepto-Bismol) can be used to reduce the frequency of unformed stools and increase stool consistency, particularly in cases of traveler's diarrhea. The drug is thought to inhibit intestinal secretion caused by enterotoxigenic *E. coli* and cholera toxins. Antibiotics are reserved for persons with identified enteric pathogens.

Constipation

Constipation can be defined as the infrequent passage of stools. The difficulty with this definition arises from the many individual variations of a function that are normal. What is considered normal for one person (*e.g.*, two or three bowel movements per week) may be considered evidence of constipation by another.

Some common causes of constipation are failure to respond to the urge to defecate, inadequate fiber in the diet, inadequate fluid intake, weakness of the abdominal muscles, inactivity and bed rest, pregnancy, hemorrhoids, and gastrointestinal disease. Drugs such as narcotics, belladonna derivatives, diuretics, calcium, iron and aluminum hydroxide, and phosphate gels tend to cause constipation. The sudden onset of constipation may indicate serious disease; one sign of cancer of the colon and rectum is a change in bowel habits.

The treatment of constipation is usually directed toward relieving the cause. A conscious effort should be made to respond to the defecation urge. A time should be set aside after a meal, when mass movements in the colon are most likely to occur, for a bowel movement. Adequate fluid intake and bulk in the diet should be encouraged. Moderate exercise is essential, and persons on bed rest benefit from passive and active exercises. Laxatives and enemas should be used judiciously. They should not be used on a regular basis to treat simple constipation, because they interfere with the defecation reflex and may actually damage the rectal mucosa.

Fecal Impaction

Fecal impaction is the retention of hardened or puttylike stool in the rectum and colon, which interferes with normal passage of feces. If not removed, it can cause partial or complete bowel obstruction. It may occur in any age group but is more common in incapacitated elderly persons. Fecal impaction may result from painful anorectal disease, tumors, or neurogenic disease; use of constipating antacids or bulk laxatives; a low-residue diet; drug-induced colonic stasis; or prolonged bed rest and debility. In children, a habitual neglect of the urge to defecate because it interferes with play may promote impaction.[47]

The manifestations may be those of severe constipation, but frequently there is a history of watery diarrhea and fecal incontinence. This is caused by increased secretory activity of the bowel, representing the body's attempt to break up the mass so that it can be evacuated. The abdomen may be distended, and there may be blood and mucus in the stool. The fecal mass may compress the urethra, giving rise to urinary incontinence. Fecal impaction should be considered in an elderly or immobilized person who develops watery stools with fecal or urinary incontinence.

Digital examination of the rectum is done to assess for the presence of a fecal mass. The mass may need to be broken up and dislodged manually or with the use of a sigmoidoscope. Oil enemas are often used to soften the mass before removal. The best treatment is prevention.

Intestinal Obstruction

Intestinal obstruction designates an impairment of movement of intestinal contents in a cephalocaudal direction. The causes can be categorized as mechanical or paralytic obstruction. Strangulation with necrosis of the bowel may occur and lead to perforation, peritonitis, and sepsis. It is a serious complication and may increase the mortality rate of intestinal obstruction to about 25%.[48]

Mechanical obstruction can result from a number of conditions, intrinsic or extrinsic, that encroach on the patency of the bowel lumen. Major inciting causes include external hernia (*i.e.*, inguinal, femoral, or umbilical) and postoperative adhesions. Less common causes are strictures, tumor, foreign bodies, intussusception, and volvulus. Intussusception involves the telescoping of bowel into the adjacent segment (Fig. 32–8). It is the most common cause of intestinal obstruction in children younger than 2 years of age.[49] The most common form is the intussusception of the terminal ileum into the right colon, but other areas of the bowel may be involved. In most cases, the cause of the disorder is unknown. The condition can also occur in adults when an intraluminal mass or tumor acts as a traction force and pulls the segment along as it telescopes into the distal segment. *Volvulus* refers to a complete twisting of the bowel on an axis formed by its mesentery (Fig. 32–9). Volvulus of the colon accounts for 5% to 10% of large bowel obstruction.[46] Mechanical bowel obstruction may be a simple obstruction, in which there is no alteration in blood flow, or a strangulated obstruction, in which there is impairment of blood flow and necrosis of bowel tissue.

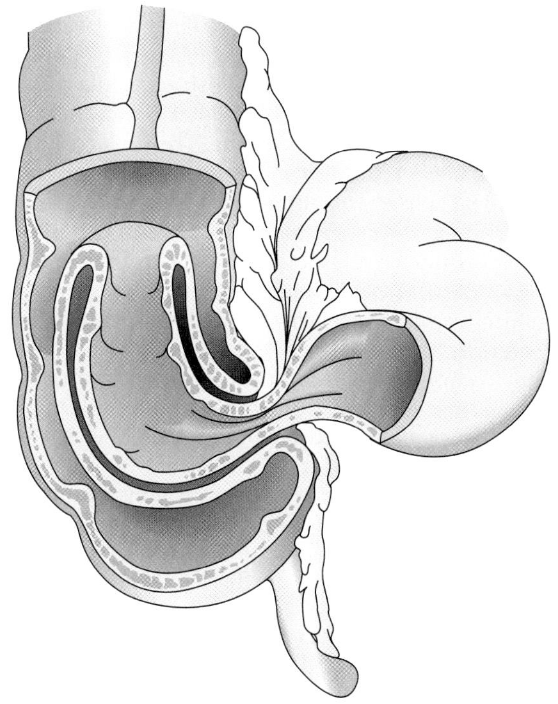

Figure 32–8 ■■■
Intussusception. (From Way L.W. [Ed.]. [1991]. *Current surgical diagnosis & treatment* [p. 1192]. Norwalk, CT: Appleton Lange.)

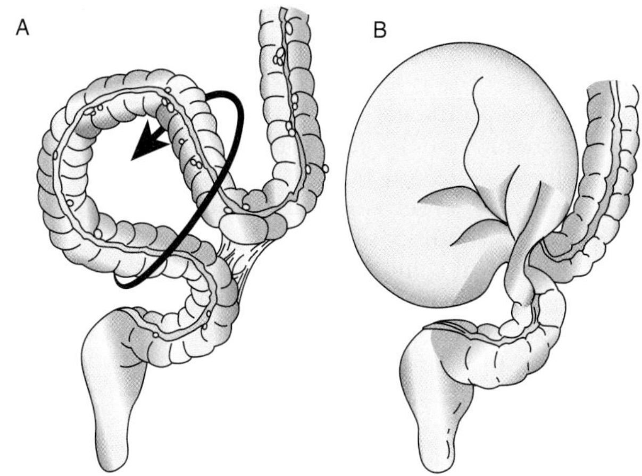

Figure 32–9 ■■■
Volvulus of the sigmoid colon. (From Way L.W. [Ed.]. [1991]. *Current surgical diagnosis & treatment* [p. 664]. Norwalk, CT: Appleton Lange.)

Paralysis, or adynamic, obstruction results from neurogenic or muscular impairment of peristalsis. *Paralytic ileus* is seen most commonly after abdominal surgery. It also accompanies inflammatory conditions of the abdomen, intestinal ischemia, pelvic fractures, and back injuries. It occurs early in the course of peritonitis and can result from chemical irritation caused by bile, bacterial toxins, electrolyte imbalances as in hypokalemia, and vascular insufficiency.

The major effects of both types of intestinal obstruction are abdominal distention and loss of fluids and electrolytes. Gases and fluids accumulate within the area; if untreated, the distention resulting from bowel obstruction tends to perpetuate itself by causing atony of the bowel and further distention. Distention is further aggravated by the accumulation of gases. About 70% of these gases are derived from swallowed air. As the process continues, the distention moves proximally (*i.e.*, toward the mouth), involving additional segments of bowel. Either form of obstruction may eventually lead to strangulation (*i.e.*, interruption of blood flow), gangrenous changes, and ultimately perforation of the bowel. The increased pressure within the intestine tends to compromise mucosal blood flow, leading to necrosis and movement of blood into the luminal fluids. This promotes rapid growth of bacteria within the obstructed bowel. Anaerobes grow rapidly in this favorable environment and produce a lethal endotoxin.

The manifestations of intestinal obstruction depend on the degree of obstruction and its duration. With acute obstruction, the onset is usually sudden and dramatic. With chronic conditions, the onset is often more gradual. The cardinal symptoms of intestinal obstruction are pain, absolute constipation, abdominal distention, and vomiting. With mechanical obstruction, the pain is severe and colicky, in contrast with the continuous pain and silent abdomen of paralytic ileus. There is also borborygmus (*i.e.,* rumbling sounds made by propulsion of gas in the intestine), audible high-pitched peristalsis, and peristaltic rushes. Visible peristalsis may appear along the course of the distended intestine. Extreme restlessness and conscious awareness of intestinal movements are experienced along with weakness, perspiration, and anxiety. Should strangulation occur, the symptoms change. The character of the pain shifts from the intermittent colicky pain caused by the hyperperistaltic movements of the intestine to a severe and steady type of pain. Vomiting and fluid and electrolyte disorders occur with both types of obstruction.

Diagnosis of intestinal obstruction is usually based on history and physical findings. Abdominal x-ray studies reveal a gas-filled bowel.

Treatment depends on the cause and type of obstruction. Most cases of adynamic obstruction respond to decompression of the bowel through nasogastric suction and correction of fluid and electrolyte imbalances. Strangulation and complete bowel obstruction require surgical intervention.

Alterations in Intestinal Absorption

Malabsorption is the failure to transport dietary constituents, such as fats, carbohydrates, proteins, vitamins, and minerals, from the lumen of the intestine to the extracellular fluid compartment for transport to the various parts of the body. It can selectively affect a single component, such as vitamin B_{12} or lactose, or its effects can extend to all the substances absorbed in a specific segment of the intestine. When one segment of the intestine is affected, another may compensate. For example, the ileum may compensate for malabsorption in the proximal small intestine by absorbing substantial amounts of fats, carbohydrates, and amino acids. Similarly, the colon, which normally absorbs water, sodium, chloride, and bicarbonate, can compensate for small intestine malabsorption by absorbing 50% or more of some of the end products of bacterial carbohydrate metabolism.[47]

The conditions that impair one or more steps involved in digestion and absorption of nutrients can be divided into three broad categories: intraluminal maldigestion, mucosal malabsorption, and lymphatic obstruction. Intraluminal maldigestion involves a defect in processing of nutrients within the intestinal lumen. The most common causes are pancreatic insufficiency, hepatobiliary disease, and intraluminal bacterial growth. Mucosal malabsorption is caused by mucosal lesions that impair uptake and transport of available intraluminal nutrients across the mucosal surface of the intestine. They include disorders such as celiac disease, tropical sprue, and Crohn's disease. Lymphatic obstruction interferes with the transport of the products of fat digestion to the systemic circulation after they have been absorbed by the intestinal mucosa. The process can be interrupted by congenital defects, neoplasms, trauma, and selected infectious diseases.

Malabsorption Syndrome

The term *syndrome* implies a common constellation of symptoms arising from multiple causes. Persons with conditions that diffusely affect the small intestine and reduce its absorptive functions share certain common features referred to as *malabsorption syndrome.* Among the causes of malabsorption syndrome are sprue, Crohn's disease, and resection of large segments of the small bowel.

Sprue syndromes result from disturbed small intestine function characterized by impaired absorption. Celiac sprue is an intolerance to dietary gluten found in wheat, barley, and rye. There is convincing evidence that the disorder is caused by an immunologic response to the gliadin fraction of gluten. The condition results in loss of absorptive villi from the small intestine. When the resulting lesions are extensive, they may impair absorption of virtually all nutrients. In about one third of the cases, symptoms begin in childhood. The effects of celiac sprue are usually reversed after removal of all wheat, rye, barley, and oat gluten from the diet. Corn and rice products are not toxic and can be used as substitutes. In a condition called *tropical sprue,* the changes that occur in the villi resemble those seen in celiac sprue. The cause of this disorder is unclear, although administration of folic acid is known to be helpful in treatment.

Persons with intestinal malabsorption usually have symptoms directly referable to the gastrointestinal tract that include diarrhea, steatorrhea, flatulence, bloating, abdominal pain, and cramps. Weakness, muscle wasting, weight loss, and abdominal distention are often present. Weight loss often occurs despite normal or excessive caloric intake. Steatorrheic stools contain excess fat. The fat content causes bulky, yellow-gray, malodorous stools that float in the toilet and are difficult to dispose of by flushing. In a person consuming a diet containing 80 to 100 g of fat each day, excretion of 7 to 9 g of fat indicates steatorrhea.

Along with loss of fat in the stools, there is failure to absorb the fat-soluble vitamins. This can lead to easy bruising and bleeding (*i.e.,* vitamin K deficiency), bone pain, a predisposition to the development of fractures and tetany (*i.e.,* vitamin D and calcium deficiency), macrocytic anemia, and glossitis (*i.e.,* folic acid deficiency). Neuropathy, atrophy of the skin, and peripheral edema may be present. Table 32–2 describes the signs and symptoms of impaired absorption of dietary constituents.

TABLE 32-2

Sites of and Requirements for Absorption of Dietary Constituents and Manifestations of Malabsorption

Dietary Constituent	Site of Absorption	Requirements	Manifestations
Water and electrolytes	Mainly small bowel	Osmotic gradient	Diarrhea Dehydration Cramps
Fat	Upper jejunum	Pancreatic lipase Bile salts Functioning lymphatic channels	Weight loss Steatorrhea Fat-soluble vitamin deficiency
Carbohydrates			
Starch	Small intestine	Amylase Maltase Isomaltase α-dextrins	Diarrhea Flatulence Abdominal discomfort
Sucrose	Small intestine	Sucrase	
Lactose	Small intestine	Lactase	
Maltose	Small intestine	Maltase	
Fructose	Small intestine		
Protein	Small intestine	Pancreatic enzymes (*e.g.*, trypsin, chymotrypsin, elastin)	Loss of muscle mass Weakness Edema
Vitamins			
A	Upper jejunum	Bile salts	Night blindness Dry eyes Corneal irritation
Folic acid	Duodenum and jejunum	Absorptive; may be impaired by some drugs (*i.e.*, anticonvulsants)	Cheilosis Glossitis Megaloblastic anemia
B_{12}	Ileum	Intrinsic factor	Glossitis Neuropathy Megaloblastic anemia
D	Upper jejunum	Bile salts	Bone pain Fractures Tetany
E	Upper jejunum	Bile salts	Uncertain
K	Upper jejunum	Bile salts	Easy bruising and bleeding
Calcium	Duodenum	Vitamin D and parathyroid hormone	Bone pain Fractures Tetany
Iron	Duodenum and jejunum	Normal pH (hydrochloric acid secretion)	Iron-deficiency anemia Glossitis

In summary, disorders of the small and large intestines include irritable bowel syndrome, inflammatory bowel disease, diverticular disease, colorectal cancer, disorders of motility (*i.e.*, diarrhea, constipation, fecal impaction, and intestinal obstruction), and alterations in intestinal absorption.

Irritable bowel disease is a functional disorder characterized by a variable combination of chronic and recurrent intestinal symptoms not explained by structural or biochemical abnormalities. The term inflammatory bowel disease is used to designate two inflammatory conditions: Crohn's disease, which affects the small and large bowel, and ulcerative colitis, which affects the colon and rectum. Both are chronic diseases characterized by remissions and exacerbations of diarrhea, weight loss, fluid and electrolyte disorders, and systemic signs of inflammation. Infectious forms of colitis include *C. difficile*, which is associated with antibiotic therapy, and *E. coli* O157:H7, which is found in undercooked hamburger and unpasteurized milk. Diverticular disease includes diverticulosis, which is a condition in which the mucosal layer of the colon herniates through the muscularis layer, and diverticulitis in which there is inflammation and gross or microscopic perforation of the diverticulum.

Colorectal cancer, the second most common fatal cancer, is seen most commonly in persons older than 50. Most, if not all, cancers of the colon and rectum arise in preexisting adenomatous polyps.

Diarrhea and constipation represent disorders of intestinal motility. Diarrhea, characterized by excessively frequent passage of stools, can be divided into large-volume diarrhea, characterized by an increased water content in the feces, and small-volume diarrhea, associated with intrinsic bowel disease and frequent passage of small stools. Constipation can be defined as the infrequent passage of stools; it is commonly caused by failure to respond to the urge to defecate, inadequate fiber or fluid intake, weakness of the abdominal muscles, inactivity and bed rest, pregnancy, hemorrhoids, and gastrointestinal disease. Fecal impaction is the retention of hardened or puttylike stool in the rectum and colon, which interferes with normal passage of feces. Intestinal obstruction designates an impairment of movement of intestinal contents in a cephalocaudal direction as the result of mechanical or paralytic mechanisms.

Malabsorption results from the impaired absorption of nutrients and other dietary constituents from the intestine. It can involve a single dietary constituent, such as vitamin B_{12}, or extend to involve all of the substances absorbed in a particular part of the small intestine. Malabsorption can result from disease of the small bowel and disorders that impair digestion and can in some cases obstruct the lymph flow by which fats are transported to the general circulation.

Disorders of the Peritoneum

After you have completed this section of the chapter, you should be able to meet the following objectives:

- Describe the characteristics of the peritoneum that increase its vulnerability and protect it against the effects of peritonitis
- Describe the manifestations of peritonitis

Peritonitis

Peritonitis is an inflammatory response of the serous membrane that lines the abdominal cavity and covers the visceral organs. It can be caused by bacterial invasion or chemical irritation. Most commonly, enteric bacteria enter the peritoneum because of a defect in the wall of one of the abdominal organs. The most common causes of peritonitis are perforated peptic ulcer, ruptured appendix, perforated diverticulum, gangrenous bowel, pelvic inflammatory disease, and gangrenous gallbladder. Other causes are abdominal trauma and wounds. Generalized peritonitis, although no longer the overwhelming problem it once was, is still a leading cause of death after abdominal surgery.

The peritoneum has several characteristics that increase its vulnerability to or protect it from the effects of peritonitis. One weakness of the peritoneal cavity is that it is a large, unbroken space that favors the dissemination of contaminants. For the same reason, it has a large surface that permits rapid absorption of bacterial toxins into the blood. The peritoneum is particularly well adapted for producing an inflammatory response as a means of controlling infection. It tends, for example, to exude a thick, sticky, and fibrinous substance that adheres to other structures, such as the mesentery and omentum, and that seals off the perforated viscus and aids in localizing the process. Localization is enhanced by sympathetic stimulation that limits intestinal motility. Although the diminished or absent peristalsis that occurs tends to give rise to associated problems, it does inhibit the movement of contaminants throughout the peritoneal cavity.

One of the most important manifestations of peritonitis is the translocation of extracellular fluid into the peritoneal cavity (through weeping or serous fluid from the inflamed peritoneum) and into the bowel as a result of bowel obstruction. Nausea and vomiting cause further losses of fluid. The fluid loss may encourage development of hypovolemia and shock. The onset of peritonitis may be acute, as with a ruptured appendix, or it may have a more gradual onset, as occurs in pelvic inflammatory disease.

Pain and tenderness are common symptoms. The pain is usually more intense over the inflamed area. The person with peritonitis usually lies still, because any movement aggravates the pain. Breathing is often shallow to prevent movement of the abdominal muscles. The abdomen is usually rigid and sometimes described as boardlike, because of reflex muscle guarding. Vomiting is common. Fever, an elevated white blood cell count, tachycardia, and hypotension are common. Hiccups may develop because of irritation of the phrenic nerve. Paralytic ileus occurs shortly after the onset of widespread peritonitis and is accompanied by abdominal distention. Peritonitis that progresses and is untreated leads to toxemia and shock.

Treatment

Treatment measures for peritonitis are directed toward preventing the extension of the inflammatory response, correcting the fluid and electrolyte imbalances that develop, and minimizing the effects of paralytic ileus and abdominal distention. Surgical intervention may be needed to remove an acutely inflamed appendix or to close the opening in a perforated peptic ulcer. Oral fluids are forbidden. Nasogastric suction, which entails the insertion of a tube placed through the nose into the stomach or intestine, is employed to decompress the bowel and relieve the abdominal distention. Fluid and electrolyte replacement is essential. These fluids are prescribed on the basis of frequent blood chemistry determinations. Antibiotics are given to combat infection. Narcotics are often needed for pain relief.

In summary, peritonitis is an inflammatory response of the serous membrane that lines the abdominal cavity and covers the visceral organs. It can be caused by bacterial invasion or chemical irritation resulting from perforation of the viscera or abdominal organs. It is characterized by severe pain, fluid and electrolyte disorders, paralytic intestinal obstruction, and sepsis. The treatment of peritonitis focuses on preventing the extension of the inflammatory response, correcting the fluid and electrolyte imbalances that develop, and minimizing the effects of bowel obstruction.

REFERENCES

1. Koda-Kimble M.A. (1996). Young L.Y. Nausea and vomiting. In Young L.Y., Koda-Kimble M.A. *Applied therapeutics: The clinical use of drugs* (6th ed., 105–1–105–11). Vancouver, WA: Applied Therapeutics
2. Grélot L., Miller A.D. (1994). Vomiting—Its ins and outs. *NIPS* 9, 142–47.
3. Richter J.M., Isselbacher K.J. (1991). Gastrointestinal bleeding. In Wilson J., Braunwald E., Isselbacher K.J. (Eds.). *Harrison's principles of internal medicine* (12th ed., p. 261). New York: McGraw-Hill.
4. Guyton A.C., Hall J.E. (1996). *Textbook of medical physiology* (9th ed., pp. 803–807). Philadelphia: W.B. Saunders.
5. Mittal R.K., Balaban D.H. (1997). The esophagogastric junction. *New England Journal of Medicine* 336 (13), 924–931.
6. Gelfand G. (1991). Gastroesophageal reflux disease. *Medical Clinics of North America* 75, 923–941.
7. Spiro H.M. (1994). Hiatus hernia and reflux esophagitis. *Hospital Practice* 29 (1), 51–66.
8. Helm J.F., Dodds N.J., Pile L.R., et al. (1984). Effect of esophageal emptying and saliva on clearance of acid from the esophagus. *New England Journal of Medicine* 310, 284–288.
9. Richter J.E. (1992). Gastroesophageal reflux: Diagnosis and management. *Hospital Practice* 27, (1A), 59–66.
10. Crooks G.W., Lichtenstein G.R. (1996). Clinical implications of Barrett's esophagus. *Archives of Internal Medicine* 156, 2174–2180.
11. Kumar V.S., Cotran R.S., Robbins S.L. (1994). *Pathologic Basis of Disease* (5th ed., pp. 755–766, 779–783). Philadelphia: W.B. Saunders.
12. Fass R., Hixson L.J., Ciccolo M.L., et al. (1997). Contemporary medical treatment of gastroesophageal reflux disease. *American Family Physician* 55 (1), 205–212.
13. Ellis F.H., Levitan N., Lo T.C.M. (1991). Cancer of the esophagus. In Hollieb A.I., Fink D.J., Murphy G.P. (Eds.). *Clinical oncology* (pp. 254–262). Atlanta: American Cancer Society.
14. Fromm D. (1987). Mechanisms involved in gastric mucosal resistance to injury. *Annual Review of Medicine* 38, 119.
15. Cryer B., Lee E., Feldman M. (1992). Factors influencing mucosal prostaglandin concentrations: Role of smoking and aging. *Annals of Internal Medicine* 116, 636–640.
16. Lind C.D., Blaser M.J. (1991). *Helicobacter pylori* and duodenal ulcers. *Hospital Practice* 26 (2), 45–63.
17. Pezzi J.S., Shiau Y. (1995). *Helicobacter pylori* and gastrointestinal disease. *American Family Physician* 52 (6), 1717–1723.
18. Rubin R., Farber J.L. (1994). The gastrointestinal tract. In Rubin R., Farber J.L. *Pathology* (2nd ed., pp. 632–648), Philadelphia: J.B. Lippincott.
19. Soll A.H. (1996). Medical treatment of peptic ulcer disease: Practice guidelines. *Journal of the American Medical Association* 275 (8), 622–-629.
20. McQuaid K.R. (1997). Alimentary tract. In Tierney L.M., McPhee S.J., Papadakis M. (Eds). *Current medical diagnosis and treatment* (36th ed., pp. 559–566). Stamford, CT: Appleton & Lange.
21. Wolfe M.M. (1996). NSAIDs and the gastrointestinal mucosa. *Hospital Practice* 31 (12), 37–47.
22. Wolfe M.M., Jensen R.T. (1987). Zollinger-Ellison syndrome. *New England Journal of Medicine* 317, 1200.
23. Zuckerman G.R., Cort D., Schuman R.B. (1988). Stress ulcer syndrome. *Journal of Intensive Care Medicine* 3, 21.
24. Konopad E., Noseworthy T. (1988). Stress ulceration: A serious complication in critically ill patients. *Heart and Lung* 17, 339.
25. Parker S.L., Tong T., Bolden S., et al. (1997). Cancer statistics 1997. *CA Cancer Journal for Clinicians* 47 (1), 8.
26. Lawrence W. (1991). Gastric neoplasms. In Hollieb A.I., Fink D.J., Murphy G.P. (Eds.). *Clinical oncology* (pp. 245–253). Atlanta: American Cancer Society.
27. Dalton C.B., Drossman D.A. (1997). Irritable bowel syndrome. *American Family Physician* 55 (3), 876–212.
28. Drossman D.A., Funch-Jensen P., Janssens J., et al. (1990). Identification of subgroups of functional bowel disorders. *Gastroenterology International* 3, 159–172.
29. Drossman D.A., Thompson W.G. (1992). The irritable bowel syndrome: Review and graduated multicomponent treatment approach. *Annals of Internal Medicine* 116, 1009–1016.
30. Podolsky D.K. (1991). Inflammatory bowel disease (first of two parts). *New England Journal of Medicine* 325, 1008–1016.
31. Podolsky D.K. (1991). Inflammatory bowel disease (second of two parts). *New England Journal of Medicine* 325, 1008–1016.
32. Belluzzi A., Brignola C., Campieri M., et al. (1996). Effect of enteric-coated fish-oil preparation on relapses in Crohn's disease. *New England Journal of Medicine* 334 (24), 1557–1560.
33. Hodgson H.J. (1996). Keeping Crohn's disease quiet. *New England Journal of Medicine* 334 (24), 1599–1600.
34. Elson C.O. (1996). The basis of current and future treatment for inflammatory bowel disease. *The American Journal of Medicine* 100, 656–662.
35. Bonner G.F. (1996). Current medical therapy for inflammatory bowel disease. *Southern Medical Journal* 89 (6), 556–566.
36. Hanauer S.B. (1994). Nicotine for colitis—The smoke has not yet cleared. *New England Journal of Medicine* 330 (12), 856–857.
37. Kelly C.P., Pothoulakis C., LaMont J.T. (1994). *Clostridium difficile* colitis. *New England Journal of Medicine* 330 (4), 257–261.
38. Greenwald D.A., Brandt L.J. (1997). Recognizing *E. coli* O157:H7 infection. *Hospital Practice* 32 (4), 123–140.
39. Van Ness M., Peller C. (1991). Acute diverticular disease: Diagnosis and management. *Hospital Practice* 26 (3A), 83–91.
40. Giovannuncci E., Egan K.M., Hunter D.J., et al. (1995). Aspirin and the risk of colorectal cancer in women. *New England Journal of Medicine* 333 (10), 609–614.
41. Marcus A.J. (1995). Aspirin as prophylaxis against colorectal cancer. *New England Journal of Medicine* 333 (10), 656–657.
42. American Cancer Society (1997). *Cancer facts and figures*. Atlanta: American Cancer Society.

43. Bruckstein A.H. (1988). Acute diarrhea. *American Family Practice* 20, 217.
44. Field M., Rao M.C., Chang E.B. (1989). Intestinal electrolyte transport and diarrheal disease (part 2). *New England Journal of Medicine* 321, 879–883.
45. Avery M.E., Snyder J.D. (1990). Oral therapy for acute diarrhea. *New England Journal of Medicine* 323, 891–894.
46. American Academy of Pediatrics, Subcommittee on Acute Gastroenteritis. (1996). Practice parameter: The management of acute gastroenteritis in young children. *Pediatrics* 424–435.
47. Knauer C.M. (1993). Alimentary tract. In Tierney L.M., McPhee S.J., Papadakis M.A. et al. (Eds.). *Current medical diagnosis and treatment* (pp. 483–484). Norwalk, CT: Appleton & Lange.
48. Schrock T.R. (1991). Large intestine. In Way L.W. (Ed.). *Current surgical diagnosis and treatment* (9th ed., pp. 664, 1192). Norwalk, CT: Appleton & Lange.
49. Wren K. (1989). Fecal impaction. *New England Journal of Medicine* 321, 658–662.
50. Trier J.S. (1988). Intestinal malabsorption: Differentiation of cause. *Hospital Practice* 23, 195.

ADDITIONAL READINGS

Bond J.H. (1997). Screening for colorectal cancer. *Hospital Practice* 32 (1), 59–74.

Foss R., Rosen H.R., Walsh J.H. (1996). Zollinger-Ellison syndrome: Diagnosis and management. *Hospital Practice* 31 (11), 73–79.

Goyal R.K., Hirano K. (1996). The enteric nervous system. *New England Journal of Medicine* 334 (17), 1106–1115.

Gray D.S. (1995). The clinical uses of dietary fiber. *American Family Physician* 51 (2), 419–425.

Hardcastle J.D. (1997). Colorectal cancer. *CA A Cancer Journal for Clinicians* 47 (2), 66–68.

Jessup J.M., Menck H.R., Fremgen A., Winchester D.P. (1997). Diagnosing colorectal carcinoma: Clinical and molecular approaches. *CA A Cancer Journal for Clinicians* 47 (2), 70–92.

Johnson D.A. (1996). Medical therapy of GERD: Current state of the art. *Hospital Practice* 31 (10), 135–147.

Laine L., Peterson W.L. (1994). Bleeding peptic ulcer. *New England Journal of Medicine* 331 (11), 717–727.

Levitt M.D., Suarez F. (1997). A commonsense approach to lactose intolerance. *Patient Care* Apr 15, 185–195.

Markowitz AJ., Winawer S.J. (1997). Management of colorectal polyps. *CA A Cancer Journal for Clinicians* 47 (2), 93–112.

Read N.W., Katsinelos P. (1995). Constipation and incontinence in the elderly. *Journal of Clinical Gastroenterology* 20 (1), 61–70.

Rustgi A.K. (1994). Hereditary gastrointestinal polyposis and nonpolyposis syndromes. *New England Journal of Medicine* 331 (25), 1694–1702.

Swain R. (1995). An update of vitamin B_{12} metabolism and deficiency states. *Journal of Family Practice* 41 (6), 595–600.

Trier J.S. (1993). Diagnosis and treatment of celiac sprue. *Hospital Practice* 28 (4), 41–54.

Worman S., Ganiats T.G. (1995). Hirschsprung's disease: A cause of chronic constipation in children. *American Family Physician* 51 (2), 487–494.

CHAPTER 33

Alterations in Function of the Hepatobiliary System and Exocrine Pancreas

The liver, the gallbladder, and the exocrine pancreas are classified as accessory organs of the gastrointestinal tract. In addition to producing digestive secretions, the liver and the pancreas have other important functions. The endocrine pancreas, for example, supplies the insulin and glucagon needed in cell metabolism, whereas the liver synthesizes glucose, plasma proteins, and blood clotting factors and is responsible for the degradation and elimination of drugs and hormones, among other functions. This chapter focuses on functions and disorders of the liver, the biliary tract and gallbladder, and the exocrine pancreas.

The Liver and Hepatobiliary System

After you have completed this section of the chapter, you should be able to meet the following objectives:

- List the functions of the liver and the signs of disruption of these functions
- State the three ways by which drugs and other substances are metabolized or inactivated in the liver
- Characterize the metabolism of alcohol by the liver and state metabolic mechanisms that can be used to explain liver injury
- Diagram the mechanism of bilirubin formation, transport, and elimination
- Compare hemolytic jaundice and obstructive jaundice with reference to their clinical manifestations
- State the origin of ammonia and describe the function of the liver in terms of its detoxification
- State laboratory tests used to assess for damage to liver cells and impaired functioning of the liver

The liver is the largest internal organ in the body, weighing about 1.3 kg (3 lb) in the adult. It is located below the

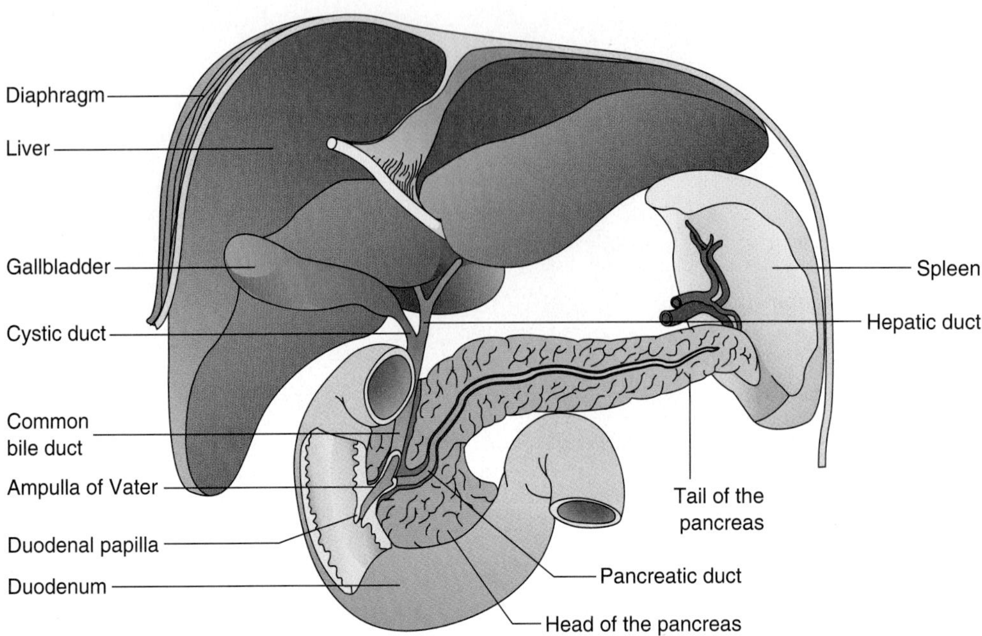

Figure 33–1
The liver and biliary system, including the gallbladder and bile ducts.

diaphragm and occupies much of the right hypochondrium. The falciform ligament, which extends from the peritoneal surface of the anterior abdominal wall between the umbilicus and diaphragm, divides the liver into two lobes, a large right lobe and a small left lobe (Fig. 33–1). There are two additional lobes on the visceral surface of the liver: the caudate and quadrate lobes. Except for the portion that is in the epigastric area, the liver is contained within the rib cage and in healthy persons cannot normally be palpated. The liver is surrounded by a tough fibroelastic capsule called *Glisson's capsule.*

The liver is unique among the abdominal organs in having a dual blood supply—the hepatic artery and the portal vein. About 400 ml of blood per minute enters the liver through the hepatic artery; another 1000 ml per minute enters by way of the valveless portal vein, which carries blood from the stomach, the small and the large intestines, the pancreas, and the spleen (Fig. 33–2). Although the blood from the portal vein is incompletely saturated with oxygen, it supplies about 60% to 70% of the oxygen needs of the liver. The venous outflow from the liver is carried by the valveless hepatic veins, which empty into the inferior vena cava just below the level of the diaphragm. The pressure difference between the hepatic vein and the portal vein is normally such that the liver stores about 200 to 400 ml of blood. This blood can be shifted back into the general circulation during periods of hypovolemia and shock. In congestive heart failure, in which the pressure within the vena cava increases, blood backs up and accumulates in the liver.

The lobules are the functional units of the liver. Each lobule is a cylindrical structure that measures about 0.8 to 2 mm in diameter and is several millimeters long. There are about 50,000 to 100,000 lobules in the liver. Each lobule is organized around a central vein that empties into the hepatic veins and from there into the vena cava. The terminal bile ducts and small branches of the portal vein and hepatic artery are located at the periphery of the lobule. Plates of hepatic cells radiate centrifugally from the central vein like spokes on a wheel (Fig. 33–3). These hepatic plates are separated by wide, thin-walled channels, called *sinusoids,* that extend from the periphery of the lobule to its central vein. There are also small tubular channels, called *bile canaliculi,* that lie between the cell membranes of adjacent hepatocytes. The sinusoids are supplied by blood from the portal vein and hepatic artery. Because the plates of hepatic cells are no more than two layers thick, every cell is exposed to the blood that travels through the sinusoids. The hepatic cells remove substances from the blood and excrete them into the canaliculi. The hepatic cells can also release substances into the blood.

The venous sinusoids are lined with two types of cells: the typical endothelial cells and Kupffer's cells. Kupffer's cells are reticuloendothelial cells that are capable of removing and phagocytizing old and defective blood cells, bacteria, and other foreign material from the portal blood as it flows through the sinusoid. This phagocytic action removes the colon bacilli and other harmful substances that filter into the blood from the intestine.

The bile produced by the hepatocytes flows into the canaliculi and then to the periphery of the lobules, which drain into progressively larger ducts, until it reaches the right and left hepatic ducts. The intrahepatic and extrahepatic bile ducts are often collectively referred to as the *hepatobiliary tree.* These ducts unite to

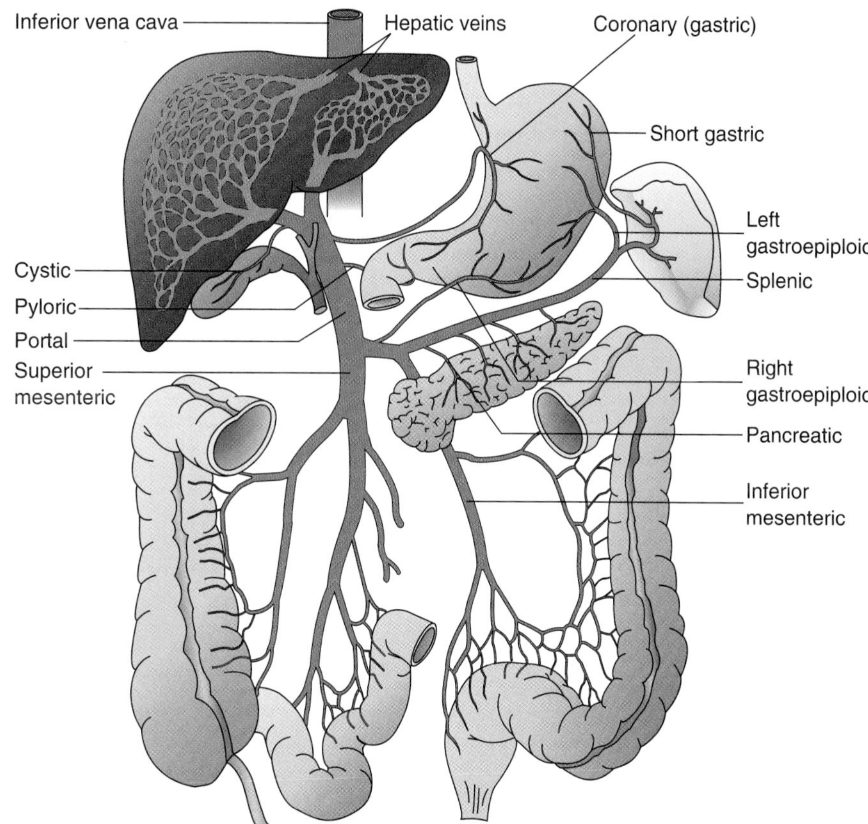

Figure 33–2
The portal circulation. Blood from the gastrointestinal tract, spleen, and pancreas travels to the liver by way of the portal vein before moving into the vena cava for return to the heart.

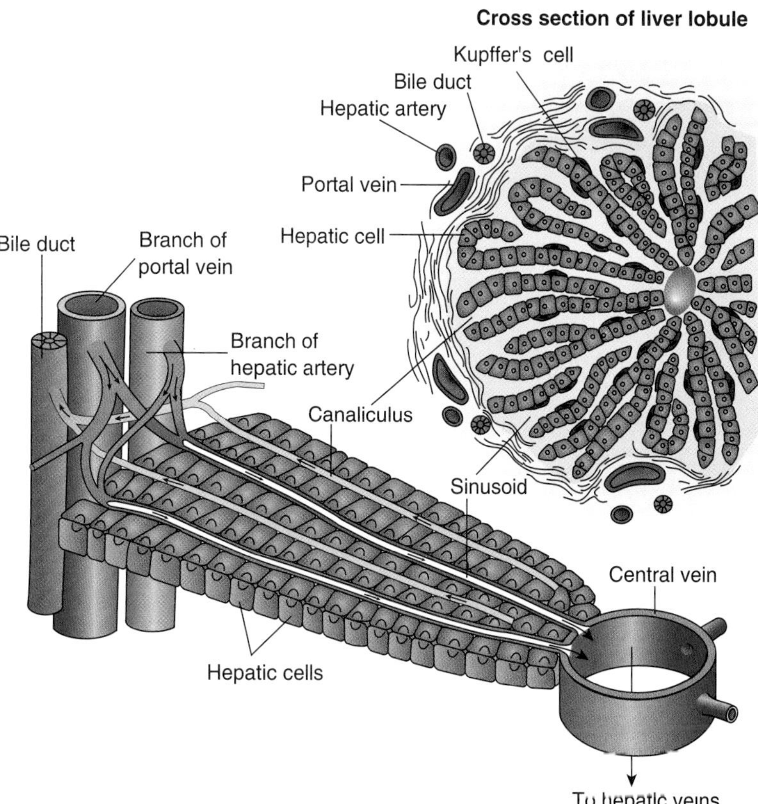

Figure 33–3
A section of liver lobule showing the location of the hepatic veins, hepatic cells, liver sinusoids, and branches of the portal vein and hepatic artery.

form the common duct (see Fig. 33–1). The common duct, which is about 10 to 15 cm long, descends and passes behind the pancreas and enters the descending duodenum. The pancreatic duct joins the common duct in the ampulla of Vater, which empties into the duodenum through the duodenal papilla. Muscle tissue at the junction of the papilla, called the *sphincter of Oddi*, regulates the flow of bile into the duodenum. A second sphincter, the sphincter of Boyden, which is just above the point where the pancreatic duct fuses with the common duct, controls the flow of bile into this area of the common duct. When this sphincter is closed, bile moves back into the gallbladder.

Functions of the Liver

The liver is one of the most versatile and active organs in the body. It produces bile; metabolizes hormones and drugs; synthesizes proteins, glucose, and clotting factors; stores vitamins and minerals; changes ammonia produced by deamination of amino acids to urea; and converts fatty acids to ketones. The liver degrades excess nutrients and converts them into substances essential to the body. It builds carbohydrates from proteins, converts sugars to fats that can be stored, and interchanges protein molecules so that they can be used for a number of purposes. In its capacity for metabolizing drugs and hormones, the liver serves as an excretory organ. In this respect, the bile, which carries the end products of substances metabolized by the liver, is much like the urine, which carries the body wastes filtered by the kidneys. The functions of the liver are summarized in Table 33–1.

Drug and Hormone Metabolism

By virtue of its many enzyme systems that are involved in biochemical transformations and modifications, the liver has an important role in the metabolism of many drugs, hormones, and endogenous substances such as bilirubin. The liver is particularly important in terms of metabolizing lipid-soluble substances that cannot be

TABLE 33–1

Functions of the Liver and Manifestations of Altered Function

Function	Manifestations of Altered Function
Production of bile salts	Malabsorption of fat and fat-soluble vitamins
Elimination of bilirubin	Elevation in serum bilirubin and jaundice
Metabolism of steroid hormones	
Sex hormones	Disturbances in gonadal function, including gynecomastia in the male
Glucocorticoids	Signs of increased cortisol levels (*i.e.*, Cushing's syndrome)
Aldosterone	Signs of hyperaldosteronism (*e.g.*, sodium retention and hypokalemia)
Metabolism of drugs	Decreased drug metabolism
	Decreased plasma binding of drugs owing to a decrease in albumin production
Carbohydrate metabolism	Hyperglycemia may develop when glycogenolysis and gluconeogenesis are impaired
Stores glycogen and synthesizes glucose from amino acids, lactic acid, and glycerol	Abnormal glucose tolerance curve may occur because of impaired uptake and release of glucose by the liver
Fat metabolism	
Formation of lipoproteins	Impaired synthesis of lipoproteins
Conversion of carbohydrates and proteins to fat	
Synthesis, recycling, and elimination of cholesterol	Altered cholesterol levels
Formation of ketones from fatty acid	
Protein metabolism	
Deamination of proteins	
Formation of urea from ammonia	Elevated blood ammonia levels
Synthesis of plasma proteins	Decreased levels of plasma proteins, particularly albumin, which contributes to edema formation
Synthesis of clotting factors (fibrinogen, prothrombin, factors V, VII, IX, X)	Bleeding tendency
Storage of mineral and vitamins	Signs of deficiency of fat-soluble and other vitamins that are stored in the liver
Filtration of blood and removal of bacteria and particulate matter by Kupffer's cells	Increased exposure of the body to colon bacilli and other foreign matter

directly excreted by the kidneys. Because the liver is central to metabolic disposition of virtually all drugs and foreign substances, drug-induced liver toxicity is a potential complication of many medications.

Drug Metabolism. Two major types of reactions are involved in the detoxification and metabolism of drugs and other chemicals: phase 1 reactions, which involve chemical modification or inactivation of a substance, and phase 2 reactions, which involve conversion of lipid-soluble substances to water-soluble derivatives.[1] Often, the two types of reactions are linked. Many phase 1 reactants are not soluble and must therefore undergo a subsequent phase 2 reaction to be eliminated. These reactions, which are called *biotransformations*, are important considerations in drug therapy. A third metabolic pathway involves the detoxification of drug metabolites that contain potentially damaging electrophilic groups.[2]

Phase 1 reactions result in chemical modification of reactive drug groups by oxidation, reduction, hydroxylation, or other chemical reactions. Most drug-metabolizing enzymes are located in the lipophilic membranes of the smooth endoplasmic reticulum of liver cells (see Chapter 1). When these membranes are broken down and separated in the laboratory, they reform into vesicles called *microsomes*. The enzymes in these membranes are often referred to as *microsomal enzymes*. Most oxidative reactions are carried out by a gene superfamily *(CYP)* that has nearly 300 members.[2] These genes code for a group of microsomal isoenzymes that make up the *cytochrome P450 system*. The gene products of many of the *CYP* genes have been identified and traced to the metabolism of specific drugs and to potential interactions among drugs. Each family of genes is responsible for certain drug-metabolizing processes, and each member of the family undertakes specific drug-metabolizing functions. For example, the *CYP3* gene family contains an A subfamily and several genes numbered 1, 2, 3, and so forth. The primary enzyme for the metabolism of erythromycin in humans is P450 3A4.[2]

Many gene members of the P450 system can have their activity induced or suppressed as they undergo the task of metabolizing drugs. For example, drugs such as alcohol and barbiturates can induce certain members to increase enzyme production, accelerating drug metabolism and decreasing the pharmacologic action of the drug and of coadministered drugs that use the same member of the P450 system. In the case of drugs metabolically transformed to reactive intermediates, enzyme induction may exacerbate drug-mediated tissue toxicity. Enzymes in the cytochrome system can also be inhibited by drugs. For example, imidazole-containing drugs such as cimetidine and ketoconazole effectively inhibit the metabolism of testosterone.[1] Environmental pollutants are also capable of inducing P450 gene activity. For example, exposure to benzo[*a*]pyrene, which is present in tobacco smoke, charcoal-broiled meat, and other organic pyrolysis products, is known to induce members of the cytochrome P450 family and alter the rates of metabolism of some drugs.

Phase 2 reactions, which involve the conversion of lipid-soluble derivatives to water-soluble substances, may follow phase 1 reactions or proceed independently. Conjugation, catalyzed by endoplasmic reticulum enzymes that couple the drug with an activated endogenous compound to render it more water soluble, is one of the most common phase 2 reactions. Although many water-soluble drugs and endogenous substances are excreted unchanged in the urine or bile, lipid-soluble substances tend to accumulate in the body unless they are converted to less active compounds or water-soluble metabolites. In general, the conjugates are more soluble than the parent compound and are pharmacologically inactive. Because the endogenous substrates originate in the diet, nutrition plays a critical role in phase 2 reactions.

The third pathway involves a thiol or sulfur-containing substance called glutathione, which is used in detoxifying drugs that form potentially harmful electrophilic groups. The substrate for glutathione is depleted in the detoxification process and must be constantly replenished by compounds from the diet or by cysteine-containing drugs such as *N*-acetylcysteine.[2] The glutathione pathway is central to the detoxification of a number of compounds, including the over-the-counter pain medication acetaminophen (*e.g.*, Tylenol). Acetaminophen metabolism involves a phase 2 reaction. Normally, the capacity of the phase 2 reactants is much greater than that required for metabolizing recommended doses of the drug. However, in situations of acetaminophen overdose, the capacity of the phase 2 system is exceeded and the drug is transformed into toxic metabolites that can cause necrosis of the liver if allowed to accumulate. In this situation, the glutathione pathway plays a critical role in the detoxification of these metabolites. Because the glutathione stores are rapidly depleted, the drug N-acetylcysteine is used as an antidote for acetaminophen overdose. Chronic alcohol ingestion decreases glutathione stores and increases the risk of acetaminophen toxicity.

Hormone Metabolism. In addition to its role in metabolism of drugs and chemicals, the liver is also responsible for hormone inactivation or modification. Insulin and glucagon are inactivated by proteolysis or deamination. Thyroxine and triiodothyronine are metabolized by reactions involving deiodination. Steroid hormones such as the glucocorticoids are first inactivated by a phase 1 reaction and then conjugated by a phase 2 reaction.

Alcohol Metabolism. Alcohol is absorbed readily from the gastrointestinal tract; it is one of the few substances that can be absorbed from the stomach. As a substance, alcohol fits somewhere between a food and a drug. It supplies calories but cannot be broken down or stored as protein, fat, or carbohydrate. As a food, alcohol yields 7.0 kcal/g, compared with the 4.0 kcal/g produced by metabolism of an equal amount of carbohydrate.[3] Between 80% and 90% of the alcohol a person drinks is metabolized by the liver. The rest is excreted through the lungs, kidneys, and skin. The average person can metabolize about 18 g of alcohol per hour; it takes about 2 hours to metabolize one mixed drink.

Alcohol metabolism proceeds simultaneously by three pathways: the alcohol dehydrogenase (ADH) system, located in the cytoplasm of the hepatocytes; the microsomal ethanol-oxidizing system (MEOS), located in the endoplasmic reticulum; and catalase, located in the perxiosomes (see Chapter 1).[4] The ADH and MEOS pathways produce specific metabolic and toxic disturbances, and all three pathways result in the production of acetaldehyde, a very toxic metabolite.[3]

The MEOS pathway, which is located in the smooth endoplasmic reticulum, produces acetaldehyde and free radicals. Prolonged and excessive alcohol ingestion results in enzyme induction and increased activity of the MEOS. One of the most important enzymes of the MEOS, a member of the cytochrome P450 system, also oxidizes a number of other compounds, including various drugs (*e.g.*, acetaminophen, isoniazid), toxins (*e.g.*, carbon tetrachloride, halothane), vitamins A and D, and carcinogenic agents (*e.g.*, aflatoxin, nitrosamines). Increased activity of this system enhances the susceptibility of persons with heavy alcohol consumption to the hepatotoxic effects of industrial toxins, anesthetic agents, chemical carcinogens, vitamins, and acetaminophen.[5]

The metabolic end products of alcohol metabolism (*e.g.*, acetaldehyde, free radicals) are responsible for a variety of metabolic alterations that can cause liver injury. Acetaldehyde, for example, has multiple toxic effects on liver cells and liver function. Age and gender play a role in metabolism of alcohol and production of harmful metabolites. Women appear to be more predisposed to alcohol-induced liver damage than men. The ADH system is depressed by testosterone; women tend to produce greater amounts of acetaldehyde than men.[4] Endogenous and exogenous (*i.e.*, contraceptive agents) female hormones may increase the hepatoxic effects of alcohol through the P450 cytochrome system. Age also appears to effect the alcohol metabolizing abilities of the liver and the resistance to hepatotoxic effects. Liver injury is related to the average amount of daily consumption and the duration of alcohol abuse. Generally, a daily intake of less than 80 g of alcohol in men and 40 g in women seldom results in liver disease.[5]

Alcohol metabolism requires a cofactor, nicotinamide adenine dinucleotide (NAD), that is necessary for many other metabolic processes, including the metabolism of pyruvates, urates, and fatty acids. Because alcohol competes for the use of intracellular cofactors normally needed for other metabolic processes, it tends to disrupt other metabolic functions of the liver. The preferential use of NAD for alcohol metabolism can result in increased production and accumulation of lactic acid in the blood. The increased lactate levels tend to impair uric acid excretion by the kidney, which probably explains why excessive alcohol consumption may aggravate or precipitate gout. Alcohol also appears to stimulate production of uric acid. By reducing the availability of the cofactor NAD, alcohol impairs the liver's ability to form glucose from amino acids and other glucose precursors. Alcohol-induced hypoglycemia can develop when excessive alcohol ingestion occurs during periods of depleted liver glycogen stores. This may become a particular problem for the alcoholic who has been vomiting and has not eaten for several days.

The combination of excess alcohol consumption and starvation can also result in metabolic acidosis from accumulation of lactate and ketoacids. The situation begins with starvation, which causes mobilization of free fatty acids from fat stores. Because of the scarcity of glucose, insulin levels fall, and levels of glucagon, cortisol, and growth hormone rise to promote gluconeogenesis and ketogenesis.

Bile Production

The secretion of bile is essential for digestion of dietary fats and absorption of fats and fat-soluble vitamins from the intestine. The liver produces about 600 to 1200 ml of yellow-green bile daily.[6] Bile contains water, bile salts, bilirubin, cholesterol, and certain products of organic metabolism. Of these, only bile salts, which are formed from cholesterol, are important in digestion. The other components of bile depend on the secretion of sodium, chloride, bicarbonate, and potassium by the bile ducts.

The liver forms about 0.6 g of bile salts daily. Bile salts serve an important function in digestion; they aid in emulsifying dietary fats, and they are necessary for the formation of the micelles that transport fatty acids and fat-soluble vitamins to the surface of the intestinal mucosa for absorption. About 94% of bile salts that enter the intestine are reabsorbed into the portal circulation by an active transport process that takes place in the distal ileum. From the portal circulation, the bile salts pass into the liver, where they are recycled. Normally, bile salts travel this entire circuit about 18 times before being expelled in the feces.[6] This system for recirculation of bile is called the *enterohepatic circulation*.

Bilirubin Elimination

Bilirubin is the substance that gives bile its color. It is formed from senescent red blood cells. In the process of degradation, the hemoglobin from the red blood cell is broken down to form biliverdin, which is rapidly converted to free bilirubin (Fig. 33–4). Free bilirubin, which is insoluble in plasma, is transported in the blood attached to plasma albumin. Even when it is bound to albumin, this bilirubin is still called *free bilirubin*. As it passes through the liver, free bilirubin is released from the albumin-carrier molecule and moved into the hepatocytes. Inside the hepatocyte, free bilirubin is converted to *conjugated bilirubin*, making it soluble in bile. Conjugated bilirubin is secreted as a constituent of bile, and in this form it passes through the bile ducts into the small intestine. In the intestine, about one half of the bilirubin is converted into a highly soluble substance called *urobilinogen* by the intestinal flora. Urobilinogen is absorbed into the portal circulation or excreted in the feces. Most of the urobilinogen that is absorbed is returned to the liver to be reexcreted into the bile. A small amount of urobilinogen,

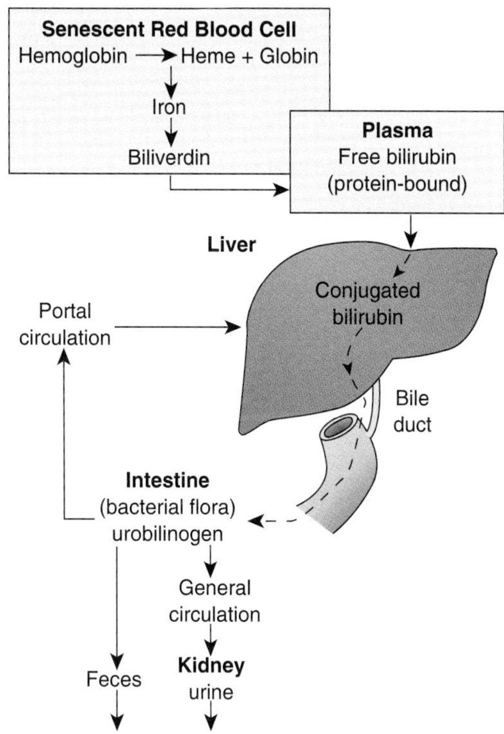

Figure 33–4
The process of bilirubin formation, circulation, and elimination.

about 5%, is absorbed into the general circulation and is then excreted by the kidneys.

Usually, only a small amount of bilirubin is found in the blood; the normal level of total serum bilirubin is 0.1 to 1.2 mg/dl. Laboratory measurements of bilirubin usually measure free and conjugated bilirubin and the total bilirubin. These are reported as the *direct* or conjugated bilirubin and the *indirect* or free bilirubin.

Jaundice. Jaundice (*i.e.,* icterus) results from an abnormally high accumulation of bilirubin in the blood, as a result of which there is a yellowish discoloration to the skin and deep tissues. The normal levels of serum bilirubin are 1.2 mg/dl. Jaundice develops when bilirubin levels rise above 2.0 to 2.5 mg/dl; levels as high as 30 to 40 mg/dl can occur in severe cases.[7] Because normal skin has a yellow cast, the early signs of jaundice are often difficult to detect, especially in persons with dark skin. Bilirubin has a special affinity for elastic tissue. The sclera of the eye, which contains considerable elastic fibers, is usually one of the first structures in which jaundice can be detected.

The four major causes of jaundice are excessive destruction of red blood cells, impaired uptake of bilirubin by the liver cells, decreased conjugation of bilirubin, and obstruction of bile flow in the canaliculi of the hepatic lobules or in the intrahepatic or extrahepatic bile ducts. From an anatomic standpoint, jaundice can be categorized as prehepatic, hepatic, and posthepatic. Chart 33–1 lists the common causes of prehepatic, hepatic, and posthepatic jaundice.

The major cause of *prehepatic jaundice* is excessive hemolysis of red blood cells. Hemolytic jaundice occurs when red blood cells are destroyed at a rate in excess of the liver's ability to remove the bilirubin from the blood. It may follow a hemolytic blood transfusion reaction or may occur in diseases such as hereditary spherocytosis, in which the red cell membranes are defective, or in hemolytic disease of the newborn (see Chapter 8). In prehepatic jaundice, there is normal stool and urine color, mild jaundice, and indirect hyperbilirubinemia, with no bilirubin in the urine.

Intrahepatic or hepatocellular jaundice is caused by disorders that directly affect the ability of the liver to remove bilirubin from the blood or conjugate it so it can be eliminated in the bile. *Gilbert's disease* is inherited as a dominant trait and results in a reduced uptake of bilirubin; the disorder is benign and fairly common. Affected persons have no symptoms other than a slightly elevated unconjugated bilirubin and mild jaundice. Conjugation of bilirubin is impaired whenever liver cells are damaged, when transport of bilirubin into liver cells becomes deficient, or when the enzymes needed to conjugate the bile are lacking. Liver disease, drugs—especially the anesthetic agent halothane—oral contraceptives, estrogen, anabolic steroids, isoniazid, and chlorpromazine are all possible causative factors. Hepatitis and cirrhosis are the most common causes of this form of jaundice. Hepatocellular jaundice usually inter-

CHART **33-1**
Causes of Jaundice

Prehepatic (Excessive Red Blood Cell Destruction)

Hemolytic blood transfusion reaction
Hereditary disorders of the red blood cell
- Sickle cell anemia
- Thalassemia
- Spherocytosis

Acquired hemolytic disorders
Hemolytic disease of the newborn
Autoimmune hemolytic anemias

Intrahepatic

Decreased bilirubin uptake by the liver
Gilbert's disease
Decreased conjugation of bilirubin
Hepatocellular liver damage
- Hepatitis
- Cirrhosis
- Cancer of the liver

Drug-induced cholestasis

Posthepatic (Obstruction of Bile Flow)

Structural disorders of the bile duct
Cholelithiasis
Congenital atresia of the extrahepatic bile ducts
Bile duct obstruction caused by tumors

feres with all phases of bilirubin metabolism—uptake, conjugation, and excretion. It is associated with dark urine and elevated alkaline phosphate. Alkaline phosphatase is produced by the liver and excreted with the bile; when bile flow is obstructed, the blood alkaline phosphatase level becomes elevated.

Posthepatic or obstructive jaundice, also called cholestatic jaundice, occurs when bile flow is obstructed between the liver and the intestine, with the obstruction located at any point between the junction of the right or left hepatic duct and the point where the bile duct opens into the intestine. Among the causes are strictures of the bile duct, gallstones, and tumors of the bile duct or the pancreas. Conjugated and unconjugated bilirubin levels are usually elevated; the stools are clay colored because of the lack of bilirubin in the bile; the urine is dark because of the increased elimination of bilirubin in the urine; and serum levels of alkaline phosphatase are elevated and those of aspartate aminotransferase slightly increased. Blood levels of bilirubin are often elevated in obstructive jaundice. As the bile acids accumulate in the blood, pruritus develops. A history of pruritus preceding jaundice is common in obstructive jaundice.

Protein Synthesis and Conversion of Ammonia to Urea

The liver is an important site for protein synthesis and degradation. Amino acids used for protein synthesis are derived from dietary proteins, metabolic turnover of endogenous proteins (mainly muscle), and direct hepatic synthesis.

Although the muscle contains the greatest amount of protein, the liver has the greatest rate of protein synthesis per gram of tissue. It produces the proteins for its own cellular needs and secretory proteins that are released into the circulation. The most important of these secretory proteins is albumin. The liver produces about 12 g of albumin per day, representing 25% of its total protein synthesis.[8] Albumin contributes significantly to the plasma colloidal osmotic pressure (see Chapter 26) and to the binding and transport of numerous substances, including some hormones, fatty acids, bilirubin, and other anions. The liver also produces other important proteins, such as fibrinogen and the blood clotting factors.

Interconversion of Amino Acids and Ammonia Metabolism. Through a variety of anabolic and catabolic processes, the liver is the major site of amino acid interconversion. Hepatic catabolism and degradation involves two major reactions: transamination and deamination. In transamination, an amino group of an amino acid is transferred to an acceptor substance. As a result of transamination, amino acids can participate in the intermediary metabolism of carbohydrates and lipids. During periods of fasting or starvation, amino acids are used for producing glucose (*i.e.*, gluconeogenesis). Most of the nonessential amino acids are synthesized in the liver by transamination. The process of transamination is catalyzed by aminotransferases, enzymes that are found in high amounts in the liver.

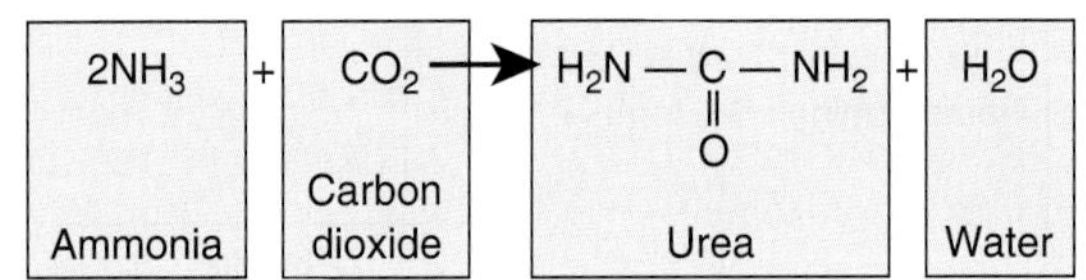

Figure 33–5
Formation of urea from ammonia.

Oxidative deamination results in conversion of amino acids to ketoacids and ammonia. Ammonia is very toxic to body tissues, particularly neurons. The ammonia that is released during deamination is removed from the blood almost immediately and converted to urea, a process in which two amino groups combine with carbon dioxide to form urea (Fig. 33–5). Essentially all urea formed in the body is synthesized in the liver and is then excreted by the kidneys. The average excretion of urea changes with the amount of protein in the diet but averages about 13 g/day. Although urea is mostly excreted by the kidneys, some diffuses into the intestine, where it is converted to ammonia by enteric bacteria. The intestinal production of ammonia also results from bacterial deamination of unabsorbed amino acids and protein derived from the diet, exfoliated cells, or blood in the gastrointestinal tract. This ammonia is absorbed into the portal circulation and transported to the liver, where it is converted to urea before being released into the blood. Intestinal production of ammonia is increased after ingestion of high-protein foods and gastrointestinal bleeding. In advanced liver disease, urea synthesis is often depressed, leading to an accumulation of ammonia and subsequent reduction in blood urea nitrogen (BUN).

Tests of Hepatobiliary Function

The history and physical examination, in most instances, provide clues about liver function. Diagnostic tests help to assess liver function and the extent of liver damage. Laboratory tests are commonly used to assess liver function and confirm the diagnosis of liver disease.

Liver function tests, including serum levels of liver enzymes, are used to assess injury to liver cells, the liver's ability to synthesize proteins, and the excretory functions of the liver.[9,10] Elevated serum enzyme tests usually indicate liver injury earlier than other indicators of liver function. The key enzymes are alanine aminotransferase and aspartate aminotransaminase, which are present in liver cells. Alanine aminotransferase (ALT, formerly known as SGPT) is liver specific, whereas aspartate aminotransferase (AST, formerly SGOT) is derived from organs other than the liver. In most cases of liver damage, there are parallel rises in ALT and AST. The most dramatic rise is seen in cases of acute hepatocellular injury, as occurs with viral hepatitis, hypoxic or ischemic injury, acute toxic injury, or Reye's syndrome.

The liver's synthetic capacity is reflected in measures of serum protein levels and prothrombin time (*i.e.*, synthesis of coagulation factors). Hypoalbuminemia due to depressed synthesis may complicate severe liver disease. Deficiencies of coagulation factor V and vitamin K–dependent factors (II, VII, IX, and X) may occur.

Serum bilirubin, γ-glutamyltransferase (GGT) and alkaline phosphatase (ALP) measure hepatic excretory function. Alkaline phosphatase is present in the membranes between liver cells and the bile duct and is released by disorders affecting the bile duct.[10] GGT is thought to function in the transport of amino acids and peptides into cells; it is a sensitive indicator of hepatobiliary disease.

Ultrasound provides information about the size, composition, and blood flow of the liver. It has largely replaced cholangiography in detecting stones in the gallbladder or biliary tree. Computed tomography (CT) scanning provides information similar to that obtained by ultrasound. Magnetic resonance imaging (MRI) has proved to be useful in some disorders. Selective angiography of the celiac, superior mesenteric, or hepatic artery may be used to visualize the hepatic or portal circulation. A liver biopsy affords a means of examining liver tissue without surgery.

In summary, the hepatobiliary system consists of the liver, gallbladder, and bile ducts. The liver is the largest and, in function, one of the most versatile organs in the body. It is located between the gastrointestinal tract and the systemic circulation; venous blood from the intestine flows through the liver before it is returned to the heart. In this way, nutrients can be removed for processing and storage, and bacteria and other foreign matter can be removed by Kupffer's cells before the blood is returned to the systemic circulation. The liver synthesizes bile salts, fats, glucose, and plasma proteins. Other important functions of the liver include deamination of amino acids, conversion of ammonia to urea, and the interconversion of amino acids and other compounds that are important to the metabolic processes of the body.

The liver also metabolizes drugs, hormones, and alcohol. There are two major types of reactions involved in the detoxification and metabolism of drugs and other chemicals: phase 1 reactions, which involve chemical modification or inactivation of a substance, and phase 2 reactions, which involve conversion of lipid-soluble substances to water-soluble derivatives. Most phase 1 oxidative reactions are carried out by a gene superfamily that codes for the drug-metabolizing enzymes of the cytochrome P450 system. The third pathway involves a thiol or sulfur-containing substance called glutathione, which is used in detoxifying drugs that form potentially harmful electrophilic groups. Because alcohol competes for use of intracellular cofactors normally needed by the liver for other metabolic processes, it tends to disrupt the metabolic functions of the liver. The liver removes, conjugates, and secretes bilirubin into the bile. Jaundice occurs when bilirubin accumulates in the blood. It can occur because of excessive red blood cell destruction, failure of the liver to remove and conjugate the bilirubin, or obstructed biliary flow.

Liver function tests are used to assess injury to liver cells and the liver's ability to synthesize proteins and remove substances from the body.

Alterations in Hepatic and Biliary Function

After you have completed this section of the chapter, you should be able to meet the following objectives:

- Compare hepatitis A, B, C, D, and E in terms of source of infection, incubation period, development of chronic disease, and the carrier state
- Define chronic hepatitis and compare the pathogenesis of chronic autoimmune and chronic viral hepatitis
- Characterize postnecrotic cirrhosis and biliary cirrhosis
- Summarize the three stages of alcoholic cirrhosis
- Describe the physiologic basis for portal hypertension and relate it to the development of ascites, esophageal varices, and splenomegaly
- Characterize hepatic-systemic encephalopathy
- State the reason for the poor prognosis in persons with hepatocellular cancer

The structures of the hepatobiliary system are subject to many of the same pathologic conditions that affect other body systems: inflammation and immune responses, metabolic disorders, toxic injury, and neoplasms. This section focuses on alterations in liver function from hepatitis, cirrhosis, portal hypertension and liver failure, cancer of the liver, and gallbladder disease.

Acute Viral Hepatitis

Hepatitis refers to inflammation of the liver. It can be caused by reactions to drugs and toxins; by infectious disorders such as malaria, infectious mononucleosis, salmonellosis, and amebiasis that cause primary infections of extrahepatic tissues and secondary hepatitis; and by hepatotropic viruses that primarily affect liver cells or hepatocytes.

The known hepatotropic viruses include hepatitis A virus (HAV), hepatitis B virus (HBV), the hepatitis B–associated delta virus (HDV), hepatitis C virus (HCV), and hepatitis E virus (HEV). Although all of these viruses cause acute hepatitis, they differ in the mode of transmission and incubation period; mechanism, degree, and chronicity of liver damage; and ability to evolve to a carrier state. The presence of viral antigens and antigen antibodies can be determined through laboratory tests. Two new viral agents, hepatitis virus F[11] and hepatitis virus G[12] have been identified. However, the mode of transmission and mechanisms of hepatic injury have not been fully elucidated.

Pathogenesis

Hepatotropic viral infection causes various degrees of liver cell injury and necrosis. There are two mechanisms of liver injury in viral hepatitis: direct cellular injury and induction of immune responses against the viral antigens. There is evidence that HDV and HCV are directly cytotoxic, whereas the effects of HBV and possibly HAV are immune mediated.[7]

The mechanisms of injury have been most closely studied in HBV. It is thought that the extent of inflammation and necrosis depends on the individual's immune response. Accordingly, a prompt immune response during the acute phase of the infection would be expected to cause cell injury but at the same time eliminate the virus. Fulminant hepatitis would be explained in terms of an accelerated immune response with severe liver necrosis. This idea has been supported by the observation that persons who survive massive liver damage caused by fulminant hepatitis seldom become carriers. In contrast, persons who respond with a marginal immune response fail to eliminate the virus, and hepatocytes expressing viral antigens persist, leading to low-level continued destruction that is expressed as chronic hepatitis. The carrier state is expressed as a failure of the immune response.

Clinical Manifestations

The clinical manifestations of viral hepatitis range from asymptomatic infection without jaundice to fulminating disease (<1% to 3%) and death in a few days.

The *incubation period* for viral hepatitis ranges from weeks to months, depending on the virus that is involved. Serologic tests are available with which to establish a diagnosis of hepatitis A, B, C, or D. The manifestations of acute hepatitis have been divided into three phases: the preicterus or prodromal period, the icterus period, and the convalescent period.

The *preicterus or prodromal phase* varies from abrupt to insidious, with general malaise, myalgia, arthralgia, easy fatigability, upper respiratory symptoms (nasal discharge and pharyngitis), and severe anorexia out of proportion to the degree of illness. Gastrointestinal symptoms such as nausea, vomiting, and diarrhea or constipation may occur. Abdominal pain is usually mild and felt in the upper right quadrant. Chills and fever may mark an abrupt onset. Upper abdominal pain may occur. In persons who smoke, there may be a distaste for smoking that parallels that of anorexia. Serum levels of AST and ALT show variable increases during the preicterus phase of acute viral hepatitis and precede a rise in bilirubin.

The *icteric phase,* if it appears, is characterized by the development of jaundice (although some persons do not develop jaundice). It may follow the prodromal manifestations by 5 to 10 days or occur at the same time. Jaundice occurs less frequently in persons with hepatitis C. The prodromal symptoms may become worse with the onset of jaundice, followed by progressive clinical improvement. Severe pruritus is common during the icteric phase. The serum bilirubin level typically rises when jaundice appears. Liver tenderness is common. Liver enlargement (*i.e.,* hepatomegaly) and spleen enlargement (*i.e.,* splenomegaly) may occur.

The *convalescent phase* is characterized by a gradual increase in sense of well-being, return of appetite, and disappearance of jaundice. The acute illness usually subsides rapidly over a 2- to 3-week period, with complete clinical recovery by 9 weeks for hepatitis A and by 16 weeks for uncomplicated hepatitis B and C.

HBV and HCV infection can produce a *carrier state* in which the person does not have symptoms but harbors the virus and can therefore transmit the disease. Evidence also indicates a carrier state for HDV infection. There is no carrier state for HAV infection. There are two types of carriers: healthy carriers who have few or no ill effects, and those with chronic disease who may or may not have symptoms. Factors that increase the risk of becoming a carrier are age at time of infection and immune status. The carrier state for infections that occur early in life, as in infants of HBV-infected mothers, may be as high as 90% to 95%, compared with 1% to 10% of infected adults.[7] Other persons at high risk for becoming carriers are those with impaired immunity, those who have received multiple transfusions or blood products, those who are on hemodialysis, and drug addicts.

Diagnosis and Treatment

Diagnosis of viral hepatitis is based on signs and symptoms. An elevation in serum bilirubin often precedes the appearance of jaundice, and the results of enzyme tests that reflect hepatocellular damage, such as the serum ALT and AST, are elevated. Differentiation among the various viruses responsible for hepatitis requires the use of serologic markers.

The treatment of hepatitis is largely symptomatic. Bed rest, which at one time was a mainstay in treatment, has largely been replaced by a more liberal program that permits patients to pace their own activity. Most patients elect to limit activity because of fatigue. Dietary restrictions are usually minimal. If oral intake becomes inadequate, glucose solutions may be administered intravenously. Patients are instructed to avoid strenuous exercise, alcohol, and other hepatotoxic agents.

Hepatitis A

Hepatitis A, formerly called *infectious hepatitis,* is caused by the small, unenveloped, RNA-containing HAV. It is usually a benign, self-limited disease, although it can cause acute fulminant hepatitis and death from liver failure in rare cases. It does not cause chronic hepatitis or induce a carrier state.

Hepatitis A has a brief incubation period (15 to 45 days) and is usually transmitted by the fecal-oral route. The fecal shedding of HAV occurs up to 2 weeks before the development of symptoms and ends as the immunoglobulin M (IgM) levels rise.[7] The disease often occurs sporadically or in epidemics. Drinking contaminated milk or water and eating shellfish from infected waters are fairly common routes of transmission. At special risk

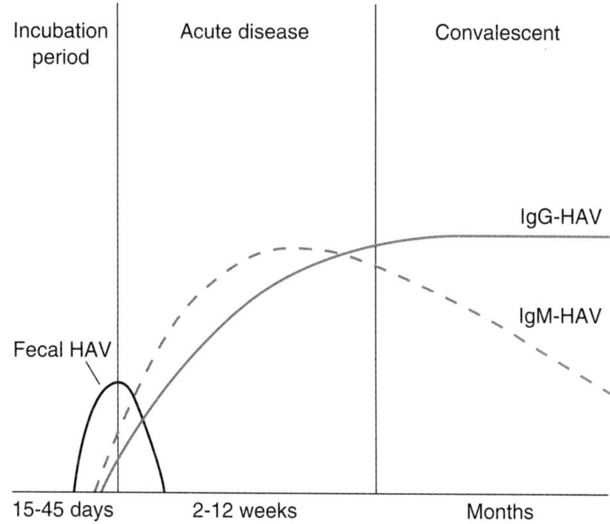

Figure 33–6
The sequence of serologic changes in acute hepatitis A. (Redrawn from Kumar V, Cotran R.S., & Robbins S.L. [1993]. *Basic pathology* [5th ed., p. 532]. Philadelphia: W.B. Saunders)

are persons traveling abroad who have not previously been exposed to the virus. Institutions housing large numbers of persons (usually children) are sometimes stricken with an epidemic of hepatitis A. Oral behavior and lack of toilet training promote viral infection among children attending preschool day care centers, who then carry the virus home to older siblings and parents. Sexual transmission of HAV is common among homosexual men, especially those having oral-anal contact.[13] Hepatitis A is not usually transmitted by transfusion of blood or plasma derivatives, presumably because its short period of viremia usually coincides with clinical illness, so that the disease is apparent, and blood donations are not accepted.

Serologic Markers. Antibodies to HAV (anti-HAV) appear early in the disease and tend to persist in the serum (Fig. 33–6). The IgM antibodies (see Chapter 11) usually appear during the first week of symptomatic disease and begin to decline in a few months. Their presence coincides with a decline in fecal shedding of the virus. Peak levels of IgG antibodies occur after 1 month of illness and may persist for years; they provide long-term protective immunity against reinfection. The presence of IgM anti-HAV is indicative of acute hepatitis A, whereas IgG anti-HAV merely documents past exposure.

Vaccination. A hepatitis A vaccine is available. The vaccine contains formalin-inactivated virus grown in cell culture.[14] The vaccine is intended to replace the use of immune globulin in persons at high risk for hepatitis A exposure. This includes international travelers to regions where sanitation is poor and endemic HAV infections are high, children living in communities with high rates of HAV infection, homosexually active men, and users of illicit drugs. Persons with preexisting chronic liver disease may also benefit from immunization. A public health benefit may also be derived from vaccinating persons with increased potential for transmitting the disease (*e.g.*, food handlers). However, the high cost of the vaccine may limit vaccination. The vaccine is relatively new, and the need for booster doses has not been established. Because the vaccine is of little benefit in prevention of hepatitis in persons with known exposure to hepatitis A, immune globulin is recommended for these persons.

Hepatitis B

Hepatitis B, formerly referred to as *serum hepatitis,* is caused by a double-stranded DNA virus (HBV). The complete virion, also called a *Dane particle,* consists of an outer envelope and an inner nucleocapsid that contains HBV DNA and DNA polymerase (Fig. 33–7). Hepatitis B can produce acute hepatitis, chronic hepatitis, progression of chronic hepatitis to cirrhosis, fulminant hepatitis with massive necrosis, and the carrier state.[7] It also participates in the development of hepatitis D (delta hepatitis).

The Centers for Disease Control and Prevention (CDC) estimate that there are 200,000 to 300,000 new cases of hepatitis B each year and 1 to 1.25 million chronic carriers in the United States.[15] At particular risk of becoming carriers are infants born to hepatitis B–infected mothers. The CDC also estimates that each year in the United States there are 4000 to 5000 deaths from hepatitis B–related cirrhosis and hepatocellular carcinoma. These figures are dwarfed by a much higher frequency of hepatitis B on a global scale. For example, the infection is endemic in regions of Africa and Southeast Asia. Hepatitis B has a longer incubation period and represents a more serious health problem than hepatitis A. The HBV is usually transmitted through inoculation with infected blood or serum. However, the viral antigen can be found in most body secretions and can be spread by oral or sexual contact. In the United States, most persons with hepatitis B acquire the infection as adults or adolescents. The disease is highly prevalent

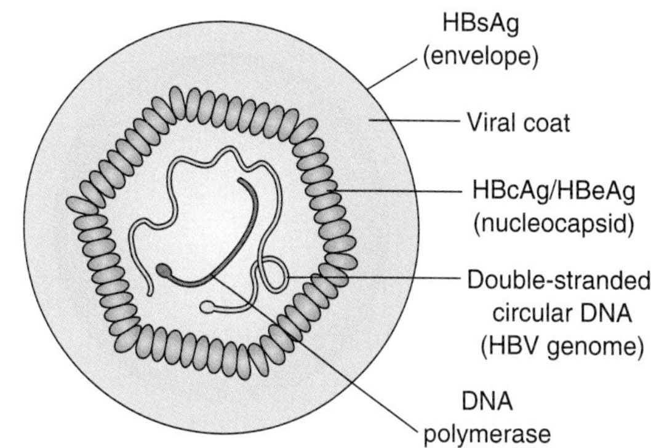

Figure 33–7
The hepatitis B virus. The HBsAg is found in the viral envelope and the HBcAg and HBeAg in the nucleocapsid. The HBV-DNA and DNA polymerase are contained within the core of the virus.

among homosexuals and intravenous drug abusers. Health care workers are at risk owing to blood exposure and accidental needle injuries. Although the virus can be spread through transfusion or administration of blood products, routine screening methods have appreciably reduced transmission through this route. The risk of hepatitis B infection among infants born to HBV-infected mothers ranges from 10% to 85%, depending on the mother's HBV core antigen (HBeAg) status. Infants who become infected have a 90% risk of becoming chronic carriers, and up to 25% will die of chronic liver disease as adults.[15] There is also a high risk of horizontal spread of HBV from mother to child during the first 5 years of life.

Serologic Markers. Three well-defined antigens are associated with the virus: two core antigens, *HBcAg* and *HBeAg*, which are contained in the nucleocapsid, and a third surface antigen, *HBsAg*, which is found in the outer envelope of the virus. These HBV antigens evoke specific antibodies: anti-HBs, anti-HBc, and anti-HBe. These antigens and their antibodies serve as serologic markers for following the course of the disease (Fig. 33–8).

HBsAg is the antigen most routinely measured in blood. It is produced in abundance by infected liver cells and released into the serum. HBsAg is the earliest serologic marker to appear; it appears before the onset of symptoms and is an indicator of acute or chronic infection. The HBsAg level begins to decline after the onset of the illness and is usually undetectable in 3 to 6 months. Persistence beyond 6 months indicates continued viral replication, infectivity, and risk of chronic hepatitis. *Anti-HBs*, a specific antibody to HBsAg, occurs in most individuals after clearance of HBsAg and after successful immunization for hepatitis B. There is usually a delay in appearance of anti-HBs after clearance of HBsAg. During this period of serologic gap, called the *window period*, infectivity has been demonstrated. Development of anti-HBs signals recovery from HBV infection, noninfectivity, and protection from future HBV infection.

HbeAg is thought to be a cleavage product of the viral core antigen; it may be found in the serum as a soluble protein and is an active marker for the disease and shedding of complete virions into the bloodstream. It appears during the incubation period, shortly after the appearance of HBsAg, and is found only in the presence of HBsAg. HBeAg usually disappears before HBsAg. *Anti-HBe* begins to appear in the serum at about the time that HBeAg disappears; its appearance signals the onset of resolution of the acute illness. The clinical usefulness of the antigen and its antibody lies in its predictive value as a marker for infectivity.

HbcAg does not circulate in the blood; therefore, it is not a useful marker for the disease. Although the antigen is not found in the blood, its antibodies *(Anti-HBc)* are the first to be detected. They appear toward the end of the incubation period and persist during the acute illness and for several months to years after that. The initial HBcAg antibody is IgM; it serves as a marker for recent infection and is followed in 6 to 18 months by IgG antibodies. These antibodies are not protective and are detectable in the presence of chronic disease.

The presence of viral DNA (HBV DNA) in the serum is the most certain indicator of hepatitis B infection. It is transiently present during the presymptomatic period and for a brief time during the acute illness. The pres-

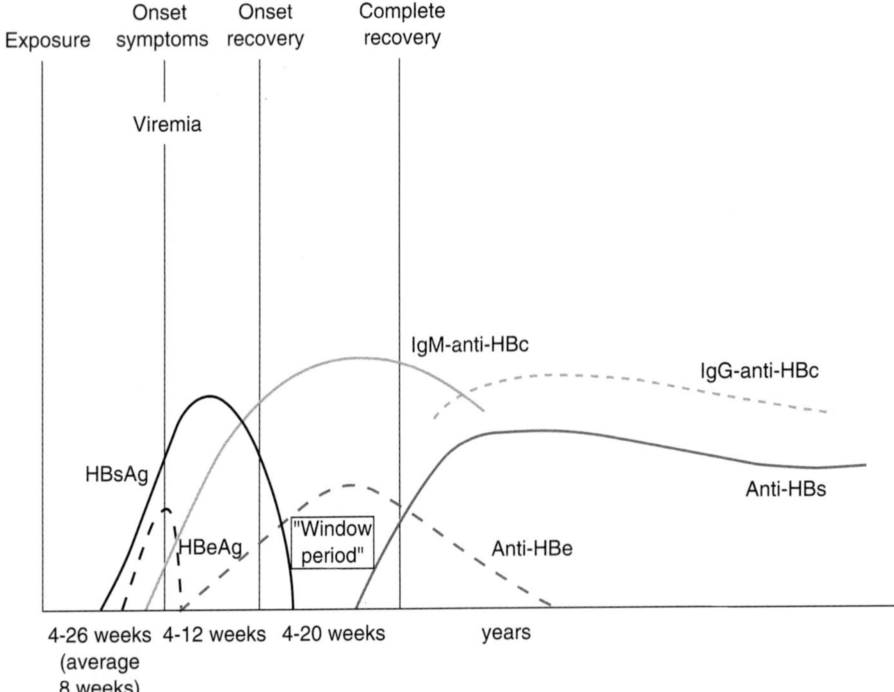

Figure 33–8 The sequence of serologic changes in acute resolving hepatitis B. (Redrawn from Kumar V, Cotran R.S., & Robbins S.L. [1993]. *Basic pathology* [5th ed., p. 533]. Philadelphia: W.B. Saunders]

ence of *DNA polymerase*, the enzyme used in viral replication, is usually transient but may persist for years in persons who are chronic carriers and is an indication of continued infectivity.

Vaccination. There are two forms of protection against infection with HBV: HBV immune globulin and HBV vaccine. Hepatitis B vaccine provides long-term protection against HBV infection.[14] Hepatitis immune globulin may be effective for unvaccinated persons who are exposed to the infection if given within 7 days of exposure. Hepatitis vaccination is recommended for preexposure and postexposure prophylaxis.

The hepatitis B vaccine is produced by recombinant DNA technology. The vaccine is highly recommended for all persons who are at high risk for exposure to the virus, health care workers exposed to blood (required by Occupational Health and Safety Administration regulations), clients and staff of institutions for the developmentally disabled, hemodialysis patients, recipients of certain blood products, household contacts and sexual partners of HBV carriers, adoptees from countries where HBV is endemic, international travelers, injecting drug users, sexually active homosexual and bisexual men, sexually active heterosexual men and women, and inmates of long-term correctional agencies. It is recommended that persons with end-stage renal disease be vaccinated before they require hemodialysis and that universal hepatitis B vaccination of teenagers be implemented in communities where injecting drug use, pregnancy among teenagers, and sexually transmitted diseases are common.[13] The CDC also recommends that all pregnant women be routinely tested for HBsAg during an early prenatal visit and that infants born to HBsAg-positive mothers receive appropriate doses of hepatitis immune globulin and hepatitis B vaccine.[13] The CDC further recommends universal vaccination of infants and children in the United States as a means of controlling spread of the infection.

Hepatitis C

Formerly known as non-A, non-B hepatitis, hepatitis C is caused by a single-stranded RNA virus (HCV) that is distantly related to the viruses that cause yellow fever and dengue fever. Hepatitis C can be transmitted by blood transfusions and blood products. In the United States, 21% of community-acquired cases of acute viral hepatitis result from HCV infection.[16]

The incubation period for HCV infection ranges from 15 to 150 days (average 50 days). Clinical symptoms with acute hepatitis C tend to be milder than those seen in persons with other types of viral hepatitis. Most cases are asymptomatic, and only 25% of persons with posttransfusion hepatitis C develop jaundice. The most alarming aspects of HCV infection is its high rate of persistence and ability to induce chronic hepatitis. Like HBV, HCV causes acute and chronic hepatitis and chronic carrier states and is also a causal agent of hepatocellular cancer.[12] Approximately 60% to 80% of persons infected with HCV after transfusion insidiously develop chronic hepatitis and cirrhosis. In the United States, 3.5 million persons have chronic hepatitis C, and 1000 undergo liver transplantation annually.[17]

Exposure to blood products is the most common mode of transmission.[16,18] Although body secretions may transmit the virus, this form of transmission is less of a risk than with HBV. The HCV virus has been detected in saliva, urine, semen, and ascitic fluid. The high-risk groups for development of HCV are persons who receive blood transfusions, health care workers, intravenous drug abusers, persons on hemodialysis, persons with high-risk sexual behavior, and organ transplant recipients from HCV-positive donors. For mother-to-baby transmission, the risk of transmission correlates with the presence of HCV RNA (a marker for viremia) in the mother's blood. With implementation of HCV testing in blood banks, the risk of HCV infection from blood transfusion has decreased to 0.03%.[16] Only about 5% to 10% of cases of chronic HCV can be traced to contaminated blood products, whereas intravenous drug use accounts for 40% to 50% of cases. Documented cases of HCV infection have occurred from contaminated lots of intravenous immune globulin, prompting the Food and Drug Administration to require that all immune globulin products manufactured through a process that does not include a viral inactivation step be tested for HCV.

Serologic Markers. The development of markers for HAV and HBV infections led to the awareness that about 90% of transfusion-related hepatitis was not caused by either of these viruses. Instead, it was found that the virus was responsible for most cases of non-A, non-B posttransfusion hepatitis. Cloning of the antigenic component of HCV in 1989 led to development of tests to detect antibody to HCV in the serum. With newer antibody testing methods, infection can often be detected as early as 6 to 8 weeks after exposure and as early as 1 to 2 weeks with polymerase chain reaction (PCR) testing methods (see Chapter 10). Unlike hepatitis A and B, antibodies to HCV are not protective, but they serve as markers for the disease. There is no vaccine that protects against HCV infection.

Hepatitis D

HDV, or the delta hepatitis agent, is a defective RNA virus. It can cause acute or chronic hepatitis. Infection depends on concomitant infection with hepatitis B, specifically the presence of HBsAg. Acute hepatitis D occurs in two forms: coinfection that occurs simultaneously with acute hepatitis B and as a superinfection in which hepatitis D is imposed on chronic hepatitis B or hepatitis B carrier state.[19] The delta agent often increases the severity of HBV infection. It can convert mild HBV infection into severe fulminating hepatitis, cause acute hepatitis in asymptomatic carriers, or it can increase the tendency for progression to chronic hepatitis and cirrhosis.

The routes of transmission of hepatitis D are similar to those for hepatitis B. In the United States, infection is largely restricted to persons at high risk for HBV infection, particularly injecting drug users and persons receiving clotting factor concentrates. The greatest risk is in HBsAg carriers; these persons should be informed about the dangers of HDV superinfection.

Hepatitis D is diagnosed by detection of antibody to HDV (anti-HDV) in the serum or HDV RNA in the serum. There is no treatment for hepatitis D. Because the infection is linked to hepatitis B, prevention of hepatitis D should begin with prevention of hepatitis B through vaccination.

Hepatitis E

HEV is an unenveloped, single-stranded RNA virus. It is transmitted by the fecal-oral route and causes manifestations of acute hepatitis that are similar to hepatitis A. It does not cause chronic hepatitis or the carrier state. Its distinguishing feature is the high mortality rate (about 20%) among pregnant women, owing to the development of fulminant hepatitis. The infection occurs primarily in developing countries such as India, other Southeast Asian countries, parts of Africa, and Mexico. The only reported cases in the United States have been in persons who have recently been in an endemic area.

Chronic Hepatitis

Chronic hepatitis is defined as the continuation of hepatitis inflammation and necrosis for longer than 6 months. The causes of chronic hepatitis are diverse and include alcoholic hepatitis, drug-induced hepatitis, hepatitis due to metabolic disorders, and autoimmune hepatitis. Autoimmune hepatitis accounts for only about 10% of chronic hepatitis in the United States, a decrease from previously reported rates that probably does not reflect a true change in incidence but better methods of detecting viral pathogens. All forms of chronic hepatitis target the hepatocyte, whereas other liver diseases such as primary biliary cirrhosis affect the bile ducts.

There are two forms of chronic viral hepatitis: chronic persistent hepatitis and chronic active hepatitis. *Chronic persistent hepatitis* is evidenced by minimal necrosis and a relatively benign course. It is characterized by elevated levels of aminotransferase enzymes (AST and ALT) and alkaline phosphatase. Usually, there are no symptoms, but some persons may experience episodes of malaise, loss of appetite, nausea, and mild jaundice. Although usually benign, chronic persistent hepatitis may progress to chronic active hepatitis. *Chronic active hepatitis* is characterized by progressive liver destruction, often leading to cirrhosis, chronic liver failure, and eventual death. It is associated with highly variable clinical features. About 30% of persons who develop chronic active hepatitis have a history of acute hepatitis. In these persons, the signs and symptoms of acute liver disease persist. The progress of the disease varies. Some persons progress to cirrhosis in a few years, and there is evidence to suggest that some may revert to chronic persistent hepatitis.

Chronic Autoimmune Hepatitis

Chronic autoimmune hepatitis is a chronic inflammatory liver disease of unknown origin, but it is associated with circulating autoantibodies and high serum globulin levels. The pathogenesis of the disorder is one of a genetically predisposed person exposed to an environmental agent that triggers an autoimmune response directed at liver cell antigens.[20] The resulting immune response produces a necrotizing inflammatory response that eventually leads to destruction of liver cells and development of cirrhosis. The factors surrounding the genetic predisposition and the triggering events that lead to the autoimmune response are unclear. Autoimmune hepatitis is mainly a disease of young women, although it can occur at any age and in males or females.

Clinical manifestations of the disorder cover a spectrum that extends from no apparent symptoms to the signs accompanying liver failure. In asymptomatic cases, the disorder may be discovered when abnormal serum enzyme levels are discovered during performance of routine screening tests.

The differential diagnosis includes measures to exclude other causes of liver disease, including hepatitis B and C. A characteristic laboratory finding is that of a marked elevation in serum globulins. A biopsy is used to confirm the diagnosis. Corticosteroid drugs and immunosuppressant drugs are the treatment of choice for this type of hepatitis. Liver transplantation may be the only treatment for end-stage disease.

Chronic Viral Hepatitis

Of the hepatotropic viruses, only three are known to cause chronic hepatitis—HBV, HCV, and HDV. The discovery of specific markers for HBV and HCV infection showed that approximately 70% of all cases of chronic hepatitis result from these viruses.[21] Chronic HDV depends on concurrent infection with HBV. Chronic viral hepatitis is the principal cause of chronic liver disease, cirrhosis, and hepatocellular cancer in the world and now ranks as the chief reason for liver transplantation in adults.[22] The various forms of chronic viral hepatitis are similar in clinical manifestations, biochemical abnormalities, and histologic characteristics that they produce and in their ability to cause cirrhosis.[22]

Chronic Hepatitis B. Chronic hepatitis B accounts for 5% to 10% of chronic liver disease and cirrhosis in the United States.[21,22] HBV is less likely than HCV to progress to chronic infection. Acute HBV resolves in 95% to 98% of otherwise healthy adults. Age at the time of infection is important, because about 90% of infected neonates have a chance of chronic infection. Chronic hepatitis B is characterized by the persistence of HBV DNA and usually by HBeAg in the serum, indicating active viral replication. Many persons are asymptomatic at the time of diagnosis, and elevated serum aminotransferase levels are the first sign of infection.

Chronic Hepatitis C. Chronic hepatitis C accounts for most cases of chronic viral hepatitis. HCV infection becomes chronic in 50% to 75% of cases. Chronic HCV infection often smolders over a period of years, silently destroying liver cells. Clinical and laboratory manifestations do not always reflect the extent of liver damage that has taken place. Most persons with chronic hepatitis C are asymptomatic, and diagnosis usually follows a finding of elevated serum aminotransferase levels, a tender liver, or complaints of fatigue or nonspecific weakness. Because the course of acute hepatitis C is often mild, many persons do not recall the events of the acute infection.

Treatment. There are no simple and effective treatment methods for chronic viral hepatitis. Recombinant interferon-α has been shown to produce remission in some cases of chronic HBV and HCV infection. In hepatitis B, interferon appears to be necessary for HBV-infected liver cells to develop the markers needed for recognition by cytotoxic T cells from the body's immune system. Persons with chronic hepatitis B seem to have developed HBV-infected cells that lack appropriate recognition sites and are hidden from the immune system. Administration of exogenous interferon may serve to unmask the hidden cells, exposing them to cytotoxic T cells. Persons treated with interferon often experience a flare-up of clinical symptoms within weeks to months after treatment is initiated as these hidden cells come under attack.[22] The mechanism of interferon's action in hepatitis C is less clear. The agent has been shown to produce improvement in about 35% to 50% of persons with chronic HCV. However, the disease is often reactivated after treatment is discontinued. Interferon treatment is costly, and side effects are common. There are also questions about the amount of drug that needs to be given and the length of time that treatment needs to be continued.[17]

There has been interest in the use of some nucleoside analogue antiviral drugs such as famciclovir and lamivudine in the treatment of chronic HCV and HBV infection. Both drugs can be given orally and are well tolerated, even after being given for prolonged periods.

Liver transplantation is a treatment option for end-stage liver disease due to viral hepatitis. Liver transplantation has been more successful in patients with hepatitis C than those with hepatitis B. The graft is often reinfected, but the disease seems to progress more slowly.

Cirrhosis

Cirrhosis is characterized by diffuse fibrosis and conversion of normal liver architecture into structurally abnormal nodules.[7,23,24] The fibrous tissue serves to replace normal functioning liver tissue and form constrictive bands that disrupt flow in the vascular channels and biliary duct systems of the liver. The disruption of vascular channels predisposes to portal hypertension and its complications; obstruction of biliary channels and exposure to the destructive effects of bile stasis; and loss of liver cells, to liver failure. Although cirrhosis is usually associated with alcoholism, it can develop in the course of other disorders, including viral hepatitis, toxic reactions to drugs and chemicals, biliary obstruction, and cardiac disease. Cirrhosis also accompanies metabolic disorders that cause the deposition of minerals in the liver. Two of these disorders are hemochromatosis (*i.e.*, iron deposition) and Wilson's disease (*i.e.*, copper deposition).

The classification of cirrhosis is controversial. Some authorities use a morphologic system, classifying the disease as micronodular or macronodular based on the size of the nodules. Other authorities use the cause of the disorder as a means of classification.

The discussion in this chapter focuses on three of the most common types of cirrhosis: postnecrotic cirrhosis, primary biliary cirrhosis, and cirrhosis caused by alcohol abuse. Although each of these types has a different cause, the clinical findings, including portal vein hypertension and eventual liver failure, are much the same.

Postnecrotic Cirrhosis

Postnecrotic cirrhosis is characterized by the replacement of liver tissue with small to large nodules of fibrous tissue, resulting in a markedly deformed and nodular liver. Postnecrotic cirrhosis accounts for 10% to 30% of cases of cirrhosis. It may follow viral hepatitis (type B or type C) or an autoimmune disease, or it may be a toxic response to drugs and other chemicals. It is a predisposing factor in hepatic cancer when it is caused by hepatitis type B.

Primary Biliary Cirrhosis

Primary biliary cirrhosis involves inflammation and scarring of small intrahepatic bile ducts, portal inflammation, and progressive scarring of liver tissue.[25] The disease is seen most commonly in women 30 to 65 years of age and accounts for 2% to 5% of cases of cirrhosis. Familial occurrences of the disease are found between parents and children and among siblings. Abnormalities of cell-mediated and humoral immunity suggest an autoimmune mechanism. Antimitochondrial antibodies are found in 98% of persons with the disease, but their role in the pathogenesis of the disease is unclear.[25,26] Up to 84% of persons with primary biliary cirrhosis have at least one other autoimmune disorder such as scleroderma, Hashimoto's thyroiditis, rheumatoid arthritis, or Sjögren's syndrome.

The disorder is characterized by an insidious onset and progressive scarring and destruction of liver tissue. The liver becomes enlarged and takes on a green hue because of the accumulated bile. The earliest symptoms are unexplained pruritus or itching, weight loss, and fatigue, followed by dark urine and pale stools. Jaundice is a late manifestation of the disorder, as are other signs of liver failure. Serum alkaline phosphatase levels are elevated in persons with primary biliary cirrhosis.

Treatment is largely symptomatic. Bile acid–binding drugs are used as a treatment for itching. Some persons have responded to ultraviolet B light, methyltestosterone, cimetidine, phenobarbital, and prednisone. There is no generally accepted treatment for the underlying disease. Clinical trials using ursodiol, a drug that increases bile flow and decreases the toxicity of bile contents, have shown that the rate of clinical deterioration decreased with the drug. Two other drugs being investigated are colchicine, which acts to prevent leukocyte migration and phagocytosis, and methotrexate, a drug with immunosuppressive properties. However, liver transplant remains the only treatment for advanced disease. Primary biliary cirrhosis does not recur after liver transplantation if appropriate immunosuppression is used.[25]

Primary Sclerosing Cholangitis

Cholangitis involves inflammation of hepatic bile ducts. Primary sclerosing cholangitis is a chronic cholestatic disease of unknown origin that causes destruction and fibrosis of intrahepatic and extrahepatic bile ducts.[27] Bile flow is obstructed (*i.e.*, cholestasis), and the bile retention destroys hepatic structures. The disease is commonly associated with inflammatory bowel disease, occurs more often in men than women, and is seen most commonly in the third to fifth decades of life.[23] Primary sclerosing cholangitis, although much less common than alcoholic cirrhosis, is the fourth leading indication for liver transplantation in adults in the United States.[27]

Most persons with the disorder are initially asymptomatic, with the disorder being detected during routine liver function tests that reveal elevated levels of serum alkaline phosphatase or γ-glutamyltransferase. Alternatively, some persons present with progressive fatigue, jaundice, and pruritus. The later stages of the disease are characterized by cirrhosis, portal hypertension, and liver failure.[27] Ten-year survival rates range from 50% to 75%. Other than measures aimed at symptom relief, the only treatment is liver transplantation.

Alcoholic Liver Disease and Cirrhosis

The spectrum of alcoholic liver disease includes fatty liver disease, alcoholic hepatitis, and cirrhosis. Alcoholic cirrhosis causes 200,000 deaths annually and is the fifth leading cause of death in the United States.[7] Most deaths from alcoholic cirrhosis are attributable to liver failure, bleeding esophageal varices, or kidney failure. It has been estimated that there are 10 million alcoholics in the United States. Only 10% to 15% of alcoholics develop cirrhosis, however, suggesting that other conditions such as genetic and environmental factors contribute to its occurrence.

The metabolism of alcohol leads to chemical attack on certain membranes of the liver, but whether the damage is caused by acetaldehyde or other metabolites is unknown. Acetaldehyde is known to impede the mitochondrial electron transport system, which is responsible for oxidative metabolism and generation of ATP; as a result, the hydrogen ions that are generated in the mitochondria are shunted into lipid synthesis and ketogenesis. Abnormal accumulations of these substances are found in hepatocytes (*i.e.*, fatty liver) and blood. Binding of acetaldehyde to other molecules impairs the detoxification of free radicals and synthesis of proteins. Acetaldehyde also promotes collagen synthesis and fibrogenesis. The lesions of hepatocellular injury tend to be most prevalent in the centrilobular area that surrounds the central vein where the pathways for alcohol metabolism are concentrated.[7] This is the part of the lobule that has the lowest oxygen tension; it is thought that the low oxygen concentration in this area of the liver may contribute to the damage.

Even after alcohol intake has stopped and all alcohol has been metabolized, the processes that damage liver cells continue for many weeks and months.[28] Clinical and chemical effects often become worse before the disease resolves. Usually, the accumulation of fat disappears within a few weeks, and cholestasis and inflammation also subside. However, fibrosis and scarring remain. The liver lobules become distorted as new liver cells regenerate and form nodules.

Although the mechanism by which alcohol exerts its toxic effects on liver structures is somewhat uncertain, the changes that develop can be divided into three stages: fatty changes, alcoholic hepatitis, and cirrhosis.[29] Because these three patterns of hepatocellular injury may occur independently of one another and occur in other types of end-stage liver disease, they are discussed separately.

Fatty Liver. One of the main effects of alcohol is the accumulation of fat within hepatocytes, a condition called *steatosis* (Fig. 33–9). The pathogenesis of fatty liver is not completely understood and can depend on the amount of alcohol consumed, dietary fat content, body stores of fat, hormonal status, and other factors.[23] When alcohol is present, it becomes the preferred fuel for the liver, displacing fuel substrates such as fatty acids. Most of the fat deposited in the liver is derived from the diet. In the fasting state, lipids are derived from endogenous fat stores. Alcohol increases lipolysis and delivery of free fatty acids to the liver. Within the liver, alcohol increases fatty acid synthesis, decreases mitochondrial oxidation of fatty acids, increases production of triglycerides, and impairs the release of lipoproteins.[24]

During the fatty liver stage, the liver becomes yellow and enlarges owing to excessive fat accumulation. There is evidence that ingestion of large amounts of alcohol can cause fatty liver changes even with an adequate diet. For example, young nonalcoholic volunteers had fatty liver changes after 2 days of consuming 18 to 24 oz of alcohol, even though adequate carbohydrates, fats, and proteins were included in the diet.[30] The fatty changes that occur with ingestion of alcohol do not usually produce symptoms and are reversible after the alcohol intake has been discontinued.

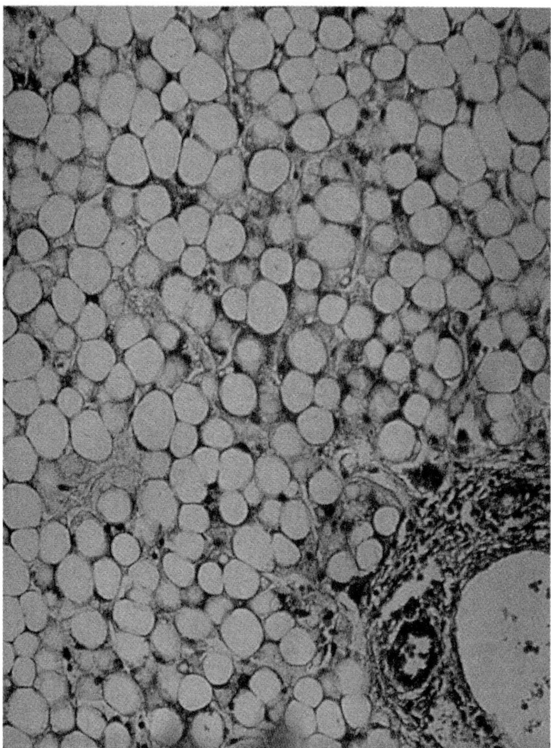

Figure 33–9
Alcoholic fatty liver. A photomicrograph shows the cytoplasm of almost all the hepatocytes to be distended by fat, which displaces the nucleus to the periphery. Note the absence of inflammation and fibrosis.

Alcoholic Hepatitis. Alcoholic hepatitis is the intermediate stage between fatty changes and cirrhosis. It is characterized by inflammation and necrosis of liver cells and is always serious and sometimes fatal. The necrotic lesions are generally patchy but may involve an entire lobe. Although reversible, it is the most common cause of cirrhosis. It is often seen after an abrupt increase in alcohol intake and is common in "spree" drinkers. "Ballooning" of hepatocytes and the toxic effects of the intermediates of alcohol metabolism, such as acetaldehyde, are believed to be contributory factors. This stage is usually characterized by hepatic tenderness, pain, anorexia, nausea, fever, jaundice, ascites, and liver failure, but some individuals may be asymptomatic.

The long-term prognosis depends on whether alcohol consumption ceases. Acute alcoholic hepatitis superimposed on cirrhosis is dangerous, accounting for much of the mortality.[16]

Cirrhosis. With repeated bouts of drinking and hepatitis, liver injury may progress to cirrhosis. The gross appearance of the early cirrhotic liver is one of fine, uniform nodules on its surface. The condition has traditionally been called *micronodular* or *Laennec cirrhosis.* With more advanced cirrhosis, regenerative processes cause the nodules to become larger and more irregular in size and shape. As this happens, the nodules cause the liver to become relobulized through the formation of new portal tracts and venous outflow channels. The nodules may compress the hepatic veins, curtailing blood flow out of the liver and producing portal hypertension, extrahepatic portosystemic shunts, and cholestasis. Cirrhosis designates the onset of end-stage alcoholic liver disease.

Manifestations of Cirrhosis

The manifestations of cirrhosis are variable, ranging from asymptomatic hepatomegaly to hepatic failure. Often there are no symptoms until the disease is far advanced. The most common signs and symptoms of cirrhosis are weight loss (sometimes masked by ascites), weakness, and anorexia. Diarrhea is frequently present, although some persons may complain of constipation. Hepatomegaly and jaundice are also common signs of cirrhosis. There may be abdominal pain because of liver enlargement or stretching of Glisson's capsule. This pain is located in the epigastric area or in the upper right quadrant and is described as dull, aching, and causing a sensation of fullness.

The late manifestations of cirrhosis are related to portal hypertension and liver cell failure. Splenomegaly, ascites, and portosystemic shunts (*i.e.,* esophageal varices, anorectal varices, and caput medusae) result from portal hypertension. Other complications include bleeding due to abnormal clotting factors, thrombocytopenia due to splenomegaly, gynecomastia and feminizing pattern of pubic hair distribution in males because of testicular atrophy, spider angiomas, palmar erythema, and encephalopathy with asterixis and neurologic signs. The manifestations of cirrhosis are discussed in the section that follows and are summarized in Table 33–2.

Portal Hypertension

Portal hypertension is characterized by increased resistance to flow in the portal venous system and sustained portal vein pressure above 12 mm Hg.[31,32] Normally, venous blood returning to the heart from the abdominal organs collects in the portal vein and travels through the liver before entering the vena cava. Portal hypertension can be caused by a variety of conditions that increase resistance to hepatic blood flow, including prehepatic, posthepatic, and intrahepatic obstructions. Prehepatic causes of portal hypertension include portal vein thrombosis and external compression due to cancer or enlarged lymph nodes that produce obstruction to the portal vein before it enters the liver. Posthepatic obstruction is caused by conditions such as thrombosis of the hepatic veins, veno-occlusive disease, and severe right-sided heart failure that impede the outflow of venous blood from the liver. Hepatic veno-occlusive disease is seen most commonly in persons treated with certain cancer chemotherapeutic drugs, hepatic irradiation, or bone marrow transplantation, possibly because of graft-versus-host disease.[23]

TABLE 33-2 Manifestations of Portal Cirrhosis

Primary Alteration in Function	Manifestation
Portal Hypertension	
Development of collateral vessels	Esophageal varices Hemorrhoids Caput medusae (dilated cutaneous veins around the umbilicus)
Portal vein obstruction and decreased levels of serum albumin	Ascites Peripheral edema
Splenomegaly	Anemia Leukopenia Thrombocytopenia
Hepatorenal syndrome	Elevated serum creatinine Azotemia Oliguria
Portal-systemic shunting of blood	Hepatic–systemic encephalopathy
Hepatocellular Dysfunction	
Impaired metabolism of sex hormones	Female: menstrual disorders Male: testicular atrophy, gynecomastia, decrease in secondary sex characteristics Skin disorders: vascular spiders and palmar erythema
Impaired synthesis of plasma proteins	Decreased levels of serum albumin with development of edema and ascites Decreased synthesis of carrier proteins for hormones and drugs
Decreased synthesis of blood-clotting factors	Bleeding tendencies
Failure to remove and conjugate bilirubin from the blood	Jaundice
Impaired bile synthesis	Malabsorption of fats and fat-soluble vitamins
Impaired metabolism of drugs cleared by the liver	Risk of drug reactions and toxicities
Impaired gluconeogenesis	Abnormal glucose tolerance
Decreased ability to convert ammonia to urea	Elevated blood ammonia levels, encephalopathy

Intrahepatic causes of portal hypertension include conditions that cause obstruction of blood flow within the liver. In alcoholic cirrhosis, which is the major cause of portal hypertension, bands of fibrous tissue and fibrous nodules distort the architecture of the liver and increase the resistance to portal blood flow, which leads to portal hypertension. The pathologic consequences of portal hypertension include formation of bypass channels (*i.e.*, portosystemic shunts) from the portal to systemic circulations, splenomegaly, and ascites.

Portosystemic Shunts. With the gradual obstruction of venous blood flow in the liver, the pressure in the portal vein increases, and large, collateral channels develop between the portal and systemic veins that supply the lower rectum and esophagus and the umbilical veins of the falciform ligament that attaches to the anterior wall of the abdomen. The collaterals between the inferior and internal iliac veins may give rise to hemorrhoids. In some persons, the fetal umbilical vein is not totally obliterated; it forms a channel on the anterior abdominal wall (Fig. 33–10). Dilated veins around the umbilicus are called *caput medusae*. Portopulmonary shunts may also develop and cause blood to bypass the pulmonary capillaries, interfering with blood oxygenation and producing cyanosis.

Clinically, the most important collateral channels are those connecting the portal and coronary veins that lead to reversal of flow and formation of thin-walled varicosities in the submucosa of the gastric fundus and esophagus (Fig. 33–11). These thin-walled varicosities are subject to rupture, producing massive and sometimes fatal hemorrhage. Impaired hepatic synthesis of coagulation factors and decreased platelet levels (*i.e.*, thrombocytopenia) due to splenomegaly may further complicate the control of esophageal bleeding. Among persons with cirrhosis and bleeding esophageal varices, a 50% mortality rate is associated with the first hemorrhage.[30]

Treatment of portal hypertension and esophageal varices is directed at prevention of initial hemorrhage, management of acute hemorrhage, and prevention of recurrent variceal hemorrhage. Pharmacologic therapy is used to lower portal venous pressure and prevent initial hemorrhage. Beta adrenergic-blocking drugs (*e.g.*, propranolol) are commonly used for this purpose. These agents reduce portal venous pressure by decreasing splanchnic blood flow and thereby decreasing blood flow in collateral channels.

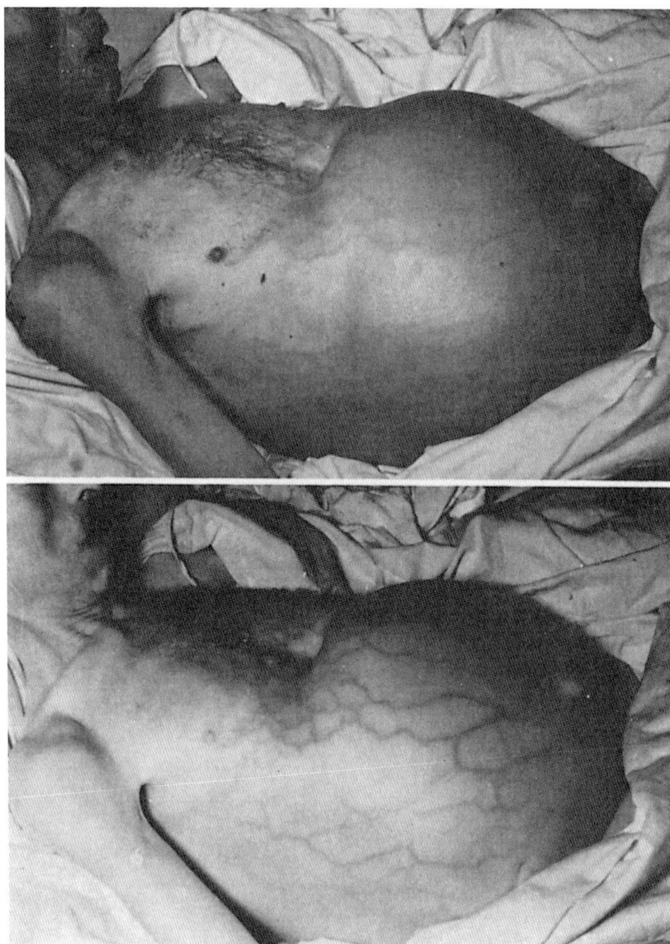

Figure 33–10
Collateral abdominal veins on the anterior abdominal wall in a patient with alcoholic liver disease as recorded by black and white photography (**top**) and infrared photography (**bottom**).

Several methods are used to control acute hemorrhage, including administration of vasopressin or one of its analogues, balloon tamponade, endoscopic injection sclerotherapy, vessel ligation, or esophageal transection. *Vasopressin*, a hormone from the posterior pituitary, constricts the splanchnic arterioles and reduces blood flow and pressure when given intravenously. Because vasopressin can also cause coronary vasoconstriction, nitroglycerin also may be given. *Balloon tamponade* provides compression of the varices and is accomplished through the insertion of a tube with inflatable gastric and esophageal balloons. After the tube has been inserted, the balloons are inflated; the esophageal balloon compresses the bleeding esophageal veins, and the gastric balloon helps to maintain the position of the tube. During *endoscopic sclerotherapy*, the varices are injected with a sclerosing solution that obliterates the vessel lumen.

Prevention of recurrent hemorrhage focuses on lowering portal venous pressure and diverting blood flow away from the easily ruptured collateral channels. Two procedures are commonly used for this purpose, transjugular intrahepatic portosystemic shunt (TIPS) and surgical creation of a portosystemic shunt. With TIPS, a catheter is introduced into the internal jugular vein and then advanced through the inferior vena cava into the right hepatic vein with the assistance of radiologic viewing. After the catheter is in the proper position, the liver tissue is punctured to encounter a main branch of the portal vein, and an expandable metallic shunt is placed between the hepatic vein and the branch of the portal vein.

Surgical portosystemic shunt procedures involve the creation of an opening between the portal vein and a systemic vein. Although these procedures do not improve liver function, they do reduce the pressure within the esophageal veins and prevent esophageal hemorrhage. The three procedures that are done most frequently are portacaval shunt, splenorenal shunt, and partial shunt. In a *portacaval shunt,* an opening is created between the portal vein and the vena cava. A *splenorenal shunt* involves removal of the spleen and anastomosis of the splenic vein to the left renal vein. It is often done when the spleen is enlarged, and it prevents further thrombocytopenia and leukopenia. A *partial shunt* only partially opens a channel between the portal vein and a systemic vein (*e.g.,* partial portacaval shunt). A complication that frequently accompanies the surgical creation of a portosystemic shunt is hepatic encephalopathy, which is thought to result when ammonia and other neurotoxic substances from the gut pass directly into the systemic circulation without going through the liver.

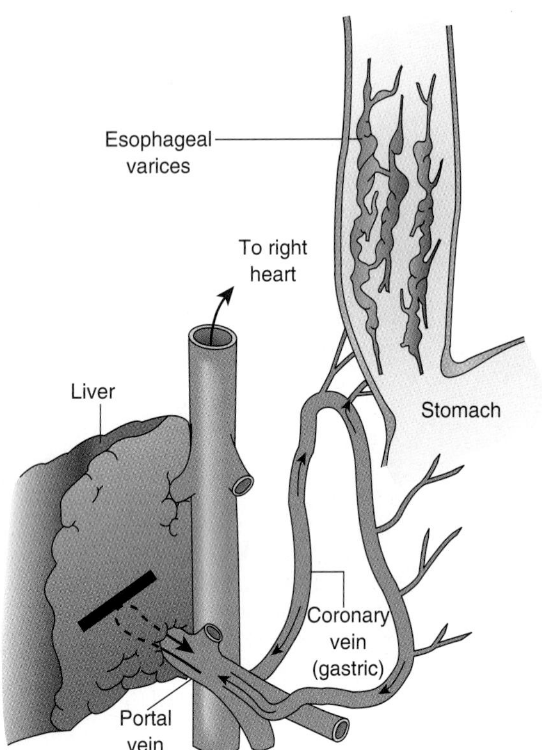

Figure 33–11
Obstruction of blood flow in the portal circulation, with portal hypertension and diversion of blood flow to other venous channels, including the gastric and esophageal veins.

Splenomegaly. The splenomegaly observed in patients with portal hypertension results from the shunting of blood into the splenic vein. This shunting gives rise to hematologic disorders such as anemia, thrombocytopenia, and leukopenia.

Ascites. Ascites occurs when the amount of fluid in the peritoneal cavity is increased, and it is a late-stage manifestation of cirrhosis and portal hypertension.[33] It is not uncommon for persons with advanced cirrhosis to present with an accumulation of 15 L or more of ascitic fluid. Those who gain this fluid often experience abdominal discomfort, dyspnea, and insomnia. Some persons may have difficulty walking or living independently.[34].

Although the mechanisms responsible for the development of ascites are not completely understood, several factors seem to contribute to fluid accumulation, including an increase in capillary pressure due to portal hypertension and obstruction of venous flow through the liver, salt and water retention by the kidney, and decreased colloidal osmotic pressure due to impaired synthesis of albumin by the liver. Diminished blood volume (*i.e.*, underfill theory) and excessive blood volume (*i.e.*, overfill theory) have been used to explain the increased salt and water retention by the kidney. According to the underfill theory, a contraction in the effective blood volume constitutes an afferent signal that causes the kidney to retain salt and water. The effective blood volume may be reduced because of loss of fluid into the peritoneal cavity or because of vasodilation caused by the presence of circulating vasodilating substances. The overfill theory proposes that the initial event in the development of ascites is renal retention of salt and water caused by disturbances within the liver itself. These disturbances include failure of the liver to metabolize aldosterone, causing an increase in salt and water retention by the kidney. Another likely contributing factor in the pathogenesis of ascites is a decreased colloidal osmotic pressure, which limits reabsorption of fluid from the peritoneal cavity (see Chapter 26).

Treatment of ascites usually focuses on dietary restriction of sodium and administration of diuretics. Water intake may also need to be restricted. To counteract the rise in aldosterone, an aldosterone-blocking diuretic, along with another diuretic such as furosemide, is administered. Oral potassium supplements are often given to prevent hypokalemia. The upright position is associated with the activation of the renin-angiotensin-aldosterone system; therefore, bed rest may be recommended for persons with a large amount of ascites. Paracentesis may be done for diagnostic purposes but is seldom done to treat the ascites, because its effects are only temporary and because it may cause a shift in fluid from the vascular compartment to the peritoneal cavity, along with complications such as infection and hemorrhage.

A surgical procedure called a peritoneovenous shunt may be used for severe cases. In this procedure, the peritoneal fluid is shunted from the abdominal cavity through a one-way, pressure-sensitive valve into a silicone tube that is inserted into the superior jugular vein and advanced so that the fluid empties into the superior vena cava. Although effective, these shunts carry considerable risk for complications from conditions such as disseminated intravascular coagulation, bacterial infections, and congestive heart failure.

Liver Failure

Although the liver is among the organs most frequently damaged, only about 10% of hepatic tissue is required for the liver to remain functional. The manifestations of liver failure reflect the various functions of the liver, including hematologic disorders, endocrine disorders, skin disorders, hepatorenal syndrome, and hepatic encephalopathy. *Fetor hepaticus* refers to a characteristic musty, sweetish odor of the breath in the patient in advanced liver failure, resulting from the products of metabolism of the intestinal bacteria.

Hematologic Disorders. Liver failure can cause anemia, thrombocytopenia, coagulation defects, and leukopenia. Anemia may be caused by blood loss, excessive red blood cell destruction, and impaired formation of red blood cells. A folic acid deficiency may lead to severe megaloblastic anemia. Changes in the lipid composition of the red cell membrane increase hemolysis. Because factors V, VII, IX, X, prothrombin, and fibrinogen are synthesized by the liver, their decline in liver disease contributes to bleeding disorders. Malabsorption of the fat-soluble vitamin K contributes further to the impaired synthesis of these clotting factors. Thrombocytopenia often occurs as the result of splenomegaly. The person with liver failure is subject to purpura, easy bruising, hematuria, and abnormal menstrual bleeding and is vulnerable to bleeding from the esophagus and other segments of the gastrointestinal tract.

Endocrine Disorders. The liver metabolizes the sex hormones. Endocrine disorders, particularly disturbances in gonadal function, are common accompaniments of cirrhosis and liver failure. Women may have menstrual irregularities (usually amenorrhea), loss of libido, and sterility. In men the testosterone level usually falls, the testes atrophy, and loss of libido, impotence, and gynecomastia occur. A decrease in aldosterone metabolism may contribute to salt and water retention by the kidney, along with a lowering of serum potassium resulting from increased elimination of potassium.

Skin Disorders. Liver failure brings on numerous skin disorders. These lesions, called variously *vascular spiders, telangiectasia, spider angiomas,* and *spider nevi,* most often are seen in the upper half of the body. They consist of a central pulsating arteriole from which smaller vessels radiate. (Spider angiomas may be seen during pregnancy even when liver function is normal.) *Palmar erythema* is redness of the palms, probably caused by increased blood flow from higher cardiac output. Clubbing of the fingers may be seen in persons with cirrhosis. Jaundice is usually a late manifestation of liver failure.

Hepatorenal Syndrome. The hepatorenal syndrome refers to a functional state of renal failure sometimes seen during the terminal stages of liver failure with ascites. It is characterized by progressive azotemia, increased serum creatinine levels, and oliguria. Although the basic cause is unknown, a decrease in renal blood flow is believed to play a part. Ultimately, when renal failure is superimposed on liver failure, azotemia and elevated levels of blood ammonia occur; this condition is thought to contribute to hepatic encephalopathy and coma.

Hepatic Encephalopathy. Hepatic encephalopathy refers to the totality of central nervous system manifestations of liver failure. It is characterized by neural disturbances ranging from a lack of mental alertness to confusion, coma, and convulsions. A very early sign of hepatic encephalopathy is a flapping tremor called *asterixis.* Various degrees of memory loss may occur, coupled with personality changes such as euphoria, irritability, anxiety, and lack of concern about personal appearance and self. Speech may be impaired, and the patient may be unable to perform certain purposeful movements. The encephalopathy may progress to decerebrate rigidity and then to a terminal deep coma.

Although the cause of hepatic encephalopathy is unknown, the accumulation of neurotoxins, which appear in the blood because the liver has lost its detoxifying capacity, is believed to be a factor. Hepatic encephalopathy develops in about 10% of persons with portosystemic shunts.

One of the suspected neurotoxins is ammonia. A particularly important function of the liver is the conversion of ammonia, a byproduct of protein and amino acid metabolism, to urea. The ammonium ion is produced in abundance in the intestinal tract, particularly in the colon, by the bacterial degradation of luminal proteins and amino acids. The ammonium ion diffuses back into the portal blood and is transported to the liver, where it is converted to urea before entering the general circulation. When the blood from the intestine bypasses the liver or the liver is unable to convert ammonia to urea, ammonia moves directly into the general circulation and from there to the cerebral circulation. Hepatic encephalopathy may become worse after a large protein meal or gastrointestinal tract bleeding. Narcotics and tranquilizers are poorly metabolized by the liver, and administration of these drugs may cause central nervous system depression and precipitate hepatic encephalopathy.

A nonabsorbable antibiotic, such as neomycin, may be given to eradicate bacteria from the bowel and thus prevent this cause of ammonia production. Another drug that may be given is lactulose. It is not absorbed from the small intestine but moves directly to the large intestine, where it is catabolized by colonic bacteria to small organic acids that cause production of large, loose stools with a low pH. The low pH favors the conversion of ammonia to ammonium ions, which are not absorbed by the blood. The acid pH also inhibits the degradation of amino acids, proteins, and blood.

Treatment

The treatment of liver failure is directed toward eliminating alcohol intake when the condition is caused by alcoholic cirrhosis; providing sufficient carbohydrate and calories to prevent protein breakdown; correcting fluid and electrolyte imbalances, particularly hypokalemia; and decreasing ammonia production in the gastrointestinal tract by limiting protein intake.

Liver transplantation is rapidly becoming a realistic form of treatment for many persons with end-stage liver disease.[35] The introduction of cyclosporine in 1980 markedly improved the survival rate of persons with liver transplants. Careful selection of potential recipients and improved preoperative management further contributed to the improved transplantation results. In 1983, the National Institutes of Health Consensus Conference concluded that liver transplantation had become an accepted therapeutic modality, prompting many states and private insurance companies to pay for the procedure. The shortage of donor organs severely limits the number of transplantations that are done, and many persons die each year while waiting for a transplant.[36]

Criteria for liver transplantation include the presence of a chronic liver disease for which all forms of therapy have failed. Conditions for which liver transplantation has been done are metabolic diseases of the liver such as Wilson's disease, primary biliary cirrhosis, chronic active hepatitis, sclerosing cholangitis, and biliary atresia in children. The use of liver transplantation for persons with alcoholic liver disease remains controversial, largely because of the scarcity of donor organs.[37] The agents used to prevent liver transplant rejection—cyclosporine, corticosteroid drugs, and azathioprine—are the same ones used to maintain other whole-organ grafts such as heart and kidney transplants.

Cancer of the Liver

Cancers of the liver include metastatic and primary neoplasms. Metastatic implants from primary cancers arising in areas drained by the portal vein are the most common form of neoplastic involvement of the liver. Although the metastatic lesions may produce gross distortion of liver structure, functional insufficiency is rare because sufficient intervening tissue is spared.

Primary liver tumors are relatively rare in the United States, accounting for about 0.5% to 2% of all cancers. The average age of onset is 60 to 70 years. The two types of primary liver cancer are hepatocellular carcinoma, which arises from the liver cells, and cholangiocarcinoma, which is a primary cancer of bile duct cells.[7]

Three factors are thought to contribute to hepatocellular carcinoma: chronic HBV infection, cirrhosis of the liver, and possible hepatocarcinogens in food. Aflatoxin from moldy peanuts has been implicated. The global distribution of hepatocellular carcinoma is strongly linked to HBV infection. In countries where HBV is endemic, there is a high risk of hepatocellular carcinoma, with an age of onset between 20 to 40 years. In the Western world, where HBV is less common, 85% to 90% of cases of hepatocellular carcinoma are associated with cirrhosis. Cholangiocarcinoma has no association with cirrhosis.

The initial symptoms of liver cancer are weakness, anorexia, weight loss, fatigue, bloating, a sensation of abdominal fullness, and a dull, aching abdominal pain. Ascites, which often obscures weight loss, is common. Jaundice, if present, is usually mild. There may be a rapid increase in liver size and worsening of ascites in persons with preexisting cirrhosis. Usually, the liver is enlarged at the time these symptoms appear, and there is a low fever without apparent cause. Serum α-fetoprotein, a serum protein present during fetal life, normally is barely detectable in the serum after the age of 2 years, but it is present in 60% to 75% of cases of hepatocarcinoma.[7]

Primary cancers of the liver are usually far advanced at the time of diagnosis; the 5-year survival rate is about 1%, and most patients die within 6 months. The treatment of choice is subtotal hepatectomy, if conditions permit.

In summary, the liver is subject to most of the disease processes that affect other body structures, such as vascular disorders, inflammation, metabolic diseases, toxic injury, and neoplasms. Two of the most common liver diseases are hepatitis and cirrhosis. Hepatitis is characterized by inflammation of the liver. Acute viral hepatitis is caused by hepatitis viruses A, B, C, D, and E. Although all these viruses cause acute hepatitis, they differ in terms of mode of transmission, incubation period, mechanism, degree and chronicity of liver damage, and the ability to evolve to a carrier state.

Cirrhosis is characterized by fibrosis and conversion of the normal hepatic architecture into structurally abnormal nodules. There are three types of cirrhosis—postnecrotic, biliary, and alcoholic—of which the most common is alcoholic cirrhosis. Regardless of cause, the manifestations of end-stage cirrhosis are similar and result from portal hypertension and liver failure. Portal hypertension is characterized by increased resistance to flow and increased pressure in the portal venous system; the pathologic consequences of the disorder include ascites, the formation of collateral bypass channels (*e.g.*, esophageal varices) from the portosystemic circulations, and splenomegaly.

Liver failure represents the end-stage of a number of liver diseases and occurs when less than 10% of liver tissue is functional. The manifestations of liver failure reflect the various functions of the liver, including hematologic disorders, endocrine disorders, skin disorders, hepatorenal syndrome, and hepatic encephalopathy. With the introduction of the immunosuppressant agent cyclosporine, liver transplantation is becoming a more realistic form of treatment for end-stage liver disease.

Cancers of the liver include metastatic and primary neoplasms. Metastatic neoplasms are the most common form of liver cancer. Primary liver neoplasms are rare, accounting for only 2% of cancers, and those involving the hepatocytes or liver cells are commonly associated with cirrhosis of the liver.

Gallbladder Disease

After you have completed this section of the chapter, you should be able to meet the following objectives:

- Explain the function of the gallbladder in regulating the flow of bile into the duodenum
- Describe the formation of gallstones
- Describe the clinical manifestations of acute and chronic cholecystitis

The gallbladder is a distensible, pear-shaped, muscular sac located on the ventral surface of the liver. It has a smooth muscle wall and is lined with a thin layer of absorptive cells. The cystic duct joins the gallbladder to the common duct. The function of the gallbladder is to store and concentrate bile. When full, it can hold 20 to 50 ml of bile.

Entrance of food into the intestine causes contraction of the gallbladder and relaxation of the sphincter of Oddi. The stimulus for gallbladder contraction is primarily hormonal. Products of food digestion, particularly lipids, stimulate cholecystokinin release from the mucosa of the duodenum. Cholecystokinin, a gastrointestinal hormone, provides a strong stimulus for gallbladder contraction. The role of other gastrointestinal hormones in bile release is less clearly understood. Passage of bile into the intestine is regulated largely by the pressure within the common duct. Normally, the gallbladder regulates this pressure. It collects and stores bile as it relaxes and the pressure in the common bile duct decreases, and it empties bile into the intestine as the gallbladder contracts and causes an increase in common duct pressure. After gallbladder surgery, the pressure in the common duct changes, causing the common duct to dilate. The flow of bile is then regulated by the sphincters in the common duct.

Two common disorders of the biliary system are *cholelithiasis* (*i.e.*, gallstones) and *cholecystitis* (*i.e.*, inflammation of the gallbladder). At least 10% of adults have gallstones. About twice as many women as men have gallstones, and there is increased prevalence with age—after age 60, 10% to 15% among men and 20% to 40% among women.[38]

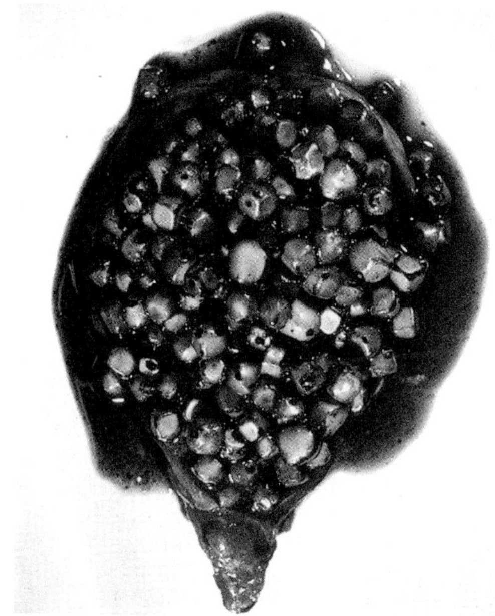

Figure 33–12
Cholesterol gallstones. The gallbladder has been opened to reveal numerous yellow cholesterol gallstones.

Composition of Bile and Formation of Gallstones

Gallstones are caused by precipitation of substances contained in bile, mainly cholesterol and bilirubin. Bile contains bile salts, cholesterol, bilirubin, lecithin, fatty acids, and water and the electrolytes normally found in the plasma. The cholesterol found in bile has no known function; it is assumed to be a byproduct of bile salt formation, and its presence is linked to the excretory function of bile. Normally insoluble in water, cholesterol is rendered soluble by the action of bile salts, which combine with it to form micelles. In the gallbladder, water and electrolytes are absorbed from the liver bile, causing the bile to become more concentrated. Because neither lecithin nor bile salts are absorbed in the gallbladder, their concentration increases along with that of cholesterol; in this way the solubility of cholesterol is maintained.

The bile of which gallstones are formed is usually supersaturated with cholesterol or bilirubinate. About 75% of gallstones are composed primarily of cholesterol; the other 25% are pigment or calcium bilirubinate stones. Many stones have a mixed composition. Figure 33–12 shows a gallbladder with numerous cholesterol gallstones.

Three factors contribute to the formation of gallstones: abnormalities in the composition of bile, stasis of bile, and inflammation of the gallbladder. The formation of cholesterol stones is associated with obesity and occurs more frequently in women, especially women who have had multiple pregnancies or who are taking oral contraceptives. All of these factors cause the liver to excrete more cholesterol into the bile. Estrogen treatment also reduces the synthesis of bile acid in women. Drugs that lower serum cholesterol levels, such as clofibrate, also cause increased cholesterol excretion into the bile. Malabsorption disorders stemming from ileal disease or intestinal bypass surgery, for example, tend to interfere with the absorption of bile salts, which is needed to maintain the solubility of cholesterol. Inflammation of the gallbladder alters the absorptive characteristics of the mucosal layer, allowing excessive absorption of water and bile salts. Cholesterol gallstones are extremely common among Native Americans, which suggests that a genetic component may have a role in gallstone formation. Pigment stones containing bilirubin are seen in persons with hemolytic disease (*e.g.*, sickle cell disease) and hepatic cirrhosis.

Many persons with gallstones have no symptoms. Gallstones cause symptoms when they obstruct bile flow. Small stones not more than 8 mm in diameter pass into the common duct, producing symptoms of indigestion and biliary colic. Larger stones are more likely to obstruct flow and cause jaundice. The pain of biliary colic is generally abrupt in onset and increases steadily in intensity until it reaches a climax in 30 to 60 minutes. The upper right quadrant, or epigastric area, is the usual location of the pain, often with referred pain to the back, above the waist, the right shoulder, and the right scapula or the midscapular region. A few persons experience pain on the left side. The pain usually persists for 2 to 8 hours and is followed by soreness in the upper right quadrant.

Cholecystitis and Cholelithiasis

The term *cholecystitis* refers to acute or chronic inflammation of the gallbladder. Both acute and chronic cholecystitis are associated with cholelithiasis. Acute cholecystitis may be superimposed on chronic cholecystitis.

Acute cholecystitis is almost always associated with complete or partial obstruction of bile flow. It is believed that the inflammation is caused by chemical irritation from the concentrated bile, along with mucosal swelling and ischemia resulting from venous congestion and lymphatic stasis. The gallbladder is usually markedly distended. Bacterial infections may arise secondary to the ischemia and chemical irritation. The bacteria reach the injured gallbladder through the blood, lymphatics, or bile ducts or from adjacent organs. Among the common pathogens are staphylococci and enterococci. The wall of the gallbladder is most vulnerable to the effects of ischemia, as a result of which mucosal necrosis and sloughing occur. The process may lead to gangrenous changes and perforation of the gallbladder.

Manifestations

The signs and symptoms of acute cholecystitis vary with the severity of obstruction and inflammation. Pain, initially similar to that of biliary colic, is characteristic of acute cholecystitis. It is often precipitated by a fatty meal and may initiate with complaints of indigestion. It does not, however, subside spontaneously and responds poorly or only temporarily to potent analgesics. When the inflammation progresses to involve the peritoneum, the pain becomes more pronounced in the right upper quadrant. The right subcostal region is tender, and the muscles that surround the area spasm. About 75% of patients have vomiting, and about 25% have jaundice. Fever and an abnormally high white blood cell count attest to inflammation. Total serum bilirubin, serum transaminase, and alkaline phosphatase levels usually are elevated.

The manifestations of chronic cholecystitis are more vague than those of acute cholecystitis. There may be intolerance to fatty foods, belching, and other indications of discomfort. Often, there are episodes of colicky pain with obstruction of biliary flow caused by gallstones. The gallbladder, which in chronic cholecystitis usually contains stones, may be enlarged, shrunken, or of normal size. The passage of a stone into the common duct causes obstruction of bile flow and may contribute to carcinoma of the gallbladder.

Diagnosis and Treatment

The methods used to diagnose gallbladder disease include oral cholecystography, ultrasonography, and cholescintigraphy.[39,40] *Oral cholecystography* is a radiologic technique that uses oral tablets containing a radiopaque contrast medium, which is absorbed from the gut, excreted in the bile, and becomes concentrated in the gallbladder. The patient must follow a fat-free diet for 1 to 2 days before the test. The dye is taken 10 to 14 hours before the examination; it may produce nausea and vomiting in 5% to 10% of persons and diarrhea in as many as 25%.

Ultrasonography is widely used in diagnosing gallbladder disease and has largely replaced the oral cholecystogram in many medical centers. Its overall accuracy in detecting gallbladder disease is high. In addition to stones, ultrasound methods can detect wall thickening, which indicates inflammation.

Cholescintigraphy, also called a *gallbladder scan,* relies on the ability of the liver to extract a rapidly injected radionuclide, technetium-99m bound to one of several iminodiacetic acids, that is excreted into the bile ducts. Serial scanning images are obtained within several minutes of the injection of the tracer and every 10 to 15 minutes during the next hour. The gallbladder scan is highly accurate in detecting acute cholecystitis. Other methods, such as CT scanning and MRI, are being evaluated for their possible roles in diagnosing gallbladder disease.

Gallbladder disease is usually treated by removing the gallbladder or by dissolving or fragmenting the stones. Laparoscopic cholecystectomy has become the treatment of choice for symptomatic gallbladder disease.[41] The procedure involves insertion of a laparoscope through a small incision near the umbilicus, and surgical instruments are inserted through several stab wounds in the upper abdomen. Although the procedure requires more time than the older open procedure, it usually requires only 1 night in the hospital. A major advantage of the procedure is that patients can return to work in 1 to 2 weeks, compared with 4 to 6 weeks after open cholecystectomy.[38] The gallbladder stores and concentrates bile, and its removal does not usually interfere with digestion.

The bile acids—chenodeoxycholic acid and ursodeoxycholic acid—have proved capable of dissolving gallstones and may be used to treat asymptomatic cholelithiasis.[23] They act by desaturating cholesterol in solution in the bile. For the treatment to be effective, the stones must be predominantly cholesterol and not be calcified. The treatment dissolves most stones within 1 or 2 years. Chenodeoxycholic acid is associated with elevation of low-density lipoproteins (LDL), dose-related diarrhea, and elevated levels of liver enzymes (*i.e.,* ALT and AST). The drug is not recommended for women of childbearing years, because it may adversely affect the fetal liver. Ursodeoxycholic acid appears to have less effect on liver enzymes and produces less diarrhea.

Extracorporeal shock wave lithotripsy uses sound waves to pulverize gallstones so that they can be passed through the bile duct.[42] The procedure is only suitable for radiolucent stones because the shock waves must be focused on each stone. Although not a common complication, stone fragments can become trapped in the bile duct. Adjunctive bile acid therapy is often used to speed dissolution of stone fragments.

Cancer of the Gallbladder

Cancer of the gallbladder is found in approximately 2% of persons operated on for biliary tract disease. The onset of symptoms is usually insidious, and they resemble those of cholecystitis; the diagnosis is often made unexpectedly at the time of gallbladder surgery. Because of their ability to produce chronic irritation of the gallbladder mucosa, it is believed that gallstones play a role in the development of gallbladder cancer. The 5-year survival rate is only about 3%.

In summary, the biliary tract serves as a passageway for the delivery of bile from the liver to the intestine. This tract consists of the bile ducts and gallbladder. The most common causes of biliary tract disease are cholelithiasis and cholecystitis. Three factors contribute to the development of cholelithiasis: abnormalities in the composition of bile, stasis of bile, and inflammation of the gallbladder. Cholelithiasis predisposes to obstruction of bile flow, causing biliary colic and acute or chronic cholecystitis. Cancer of the gallbladder, which has a poor 5-year survival rate, occurs in 2% of persons with biliary tract disease.

Disorders of the Exocrine Pancreas

After you have completed this section of the chapter, you should be able to meet the following objectives:

- Cite the possible causes and describe the manifestations and treatment of acute pancreatitis
- Describe the manifestations of chronic pancreatitis
- State the reason for the poor prognosis in pancreatic cancer

The pancreas lies transversely in the posterior part of the upper abdomen. The head of the pancreas is at the right of the abdomen; it rests against the curve of the duodenum in the area of the ampulla of Vater and its entrance into the duodenum. The body of the pancreas lies beneath the stomach. The tail touches the spleen. The pancreas is virtually hidden because of its posterior position; unlike many other organs, it cannot be palpated. Because of the position of the pancreas and its large functional reserve, symptoms of disease do not usually appear until the disorder is far advanced. This is particularly true of cancer of the pancreas.

The pancreas is an endocrine and exocrine organ. Its function as an endocrine organ is discussed in Chapter 36. The exocrine pancreas is made up of lobules that consist of acinar cells, which secrete digestive enzymes into a system of microscopic ducts. These ducts are terminal branches of larger ducts that drain into the main pancreatic duct, which extends from left to right through the substance of the pancreas (see Fig. 33–1). In most persons, the main pancreatic duct empties into the ampulla of Vater, although in some it empties directly into the duodenum. The pancreatic ducts are lined with epithelial cells that secrete water and bicarbonate and thereby modify the fluid and electrolyte composition of the pancreatic secretions.

The pancreatic secretions contain proteolytic enzymes that break down dietary proteins, including trypsin, chymotrypsin, carboxypolypeptidase, ribonuclease, and deoxyribonuclease. The pancreas also secretes pancreatic amylase, which breaks down starch, and lipase, which hydrolyzes neutral fats into glycerol and fatty acids. The pancreatic enzymes are secreted in the inactive form and become activated in the intestine. This is important, because the enzymes would digest the tissue of the pancreas itself if they were secreted in the active form. The acinar cells secrete a trypsin inhibitor, which prevents trypsin activation. Because trypsin activates other proteolytic enzymes, the trypsin inhibitor prevents subsequent activation of those other enzymes.

Two types of pancreatic disease are discussed in this chapter: acute and chronic pancreatitis and cancer of the pancreas.

Acute Hemorrhagic Pancreatitis

Acute pancreatitis is a severe, life-threatening disorder associated with the escape of activated pancreatic enzymes into the pancreas and surrounding tissues. These enzymes cause fat necrosis, or autodigestion, of the pancreas and produce fatty deposits in the abdominal cavity with hemorrhage from the necrotic vessels. Although a number of factors are associated with the development of acute pancreatitis, most cases result from biliary tract disease (*i.e.*, passed gallstones) or alcohol abuse.[43–45] In the case of biliary tract obstruction due to gallstones, biliary reflux is believed to activate the pancreatic enzymes within the ductile system of the pancreas. The precise mechanisms whereby alcohol exerts its action are largely unknown. Alcohol is known to be a potent stimulator of pancreatic secretions, and it is also known to cause partial obstruction of the sphincter of Oddi. Acute pancreatitis is also associated with hyperlipidemia, hyperparathyroidism, infections (particularly viral), abdominal and surgical trauma, and drugs such as steroids and thiazide diuretics.

The onset of acute pancreatitis is usually abrupt and dramatic, and it may follow a heavy meal or an alcoholic binge. The most common initial symptom is severe epigastric and abdominal pain that radiates to the back. The pain is aggravated when the person is lying supine; it is less severe when the person is sitting and leaning forward. Abdominal distention accompanied by hypoactive bowel sounds is common. An important disturbance related to acute pancreatitis is the loss of a large volume of fluid into the retroperitoneal and peripancreatic spaces and the abdominal cavity. Tachycardia, hypotension, cool and clammy skin, and fever are often evident. Signs of hypocalcemia may develop, probably as a result of the precipitation of serum calcium in the areas of fat necrosis. Mild jaundice may appear after the first 24 hours because of biliary obstruction.

Total serum amylase is the test most frequently used in the diagnosis of acute pancreatitis. Serum amylase levels rise within the first 24 hours after onset of symptoms and remain elevated for 48 to 72 hours. The serum lipase level also becomes elevated during the first 24 to 48 hours but remains elevated for 5 to 14 days. Urinary clearance of amylase is increased. Because the serum amylase level may be elevated as a result of the presence of other serious illnesses, the urinary level of amylase should be measured. The white blood cell count may be increased, and hyperglycemia and an elevated serum bilirubin level may be present.

About 5% of persons with acute pancreatitis die of the acute effects of peripheral vascular collapse. Serious complications include acute respiratory distress syndrome and acute tubular necrosis. Hypocalcemia occurs in about 25% of patients. Age greater than 55 years, an elevated white blood cell count (>16,000/µl), and elevated levels of blood glucose (>200 mg/dl), serum lactate dehydrogenase (>350 IU/L), and AST (>250 IU/L) at the time of diagnosis are associated with a poorer prognosis, as are a fall in hematocrit and serum calcium, increased fluid sequestration (>6 L), an arterial oxygen tension less than 60 mm Hg, and base deficit greater than 4 mEq/L that develop within the first 48 hours.[43]

Plain radiographs of the abdomen may be used for detecting gallstones or abdominal complications. CT scans are useful in detecting an enlarged pancreas.

The treatment consists of measures directed at pain relief, "putting the pancreas to rest," and restoration of lost plasma volume.[43] Meperidine (Demerol) rather than morphine is usually given for pain relief, because it causes fewer spasms of the sphincter of Oddi. Papaverine, nitroglycerin, barbiturates, or anticholinergic drugs may be given as supplements to provide smooth muscle relaxation. Oral foods and fluids are withheld, and gastric suction is instituted to treat distention of the bowel and prevent further stimulation of the secretion of pancreatic enzymes. Intravenous fluids and electrolytes are administered to replace those lost from the circulation and to combat hypotension and shock. Intravenous colloid solutions are given to replace the fluid that has become sequestered in the abdomen and retroperitoneal space. Percutaneous peritoneal lavage has been tried as an early treatment of acute pancreatitis with encouraging results. If a pancreatic abscess develops, it must be drained, usually through the flank.

A *pseudocyst* is a collection of pancreatic fluid in the peritoneal cavity enclosed in a layer of inflammatory tissue. Autodigestion or liquefaction of pancreatic tissue may be the cause. The pseudocyst is most often connected to a pancreatic duct, so that it continues to increase in mass. The symptoms depend on its location; for example, jaundice may occur when a cyst develops near the head of the pancreas, close to the common duct. Pseudocysts may resolve or, if they persist, may require surgical intervention.

Chronic Pancreatitis

Chronic pancreatitis is characterized by progressive destruction of the pancreas. It can be divided into two types: chronic calcifying pancreatitis and chronic obstructive pancreatitis.[7] In chronic calcifying pancreatitis, calcified protein plugs (*i.e.*, calculi) form in the pancreatic ducts. This form is seen most often in alcoholics. Chronic obstructive pancreatitis is associated with stenosis of the sphincter of Oddi. The lesions are prominent in the head of the pancreas. The disease usually is caused by cholelithiasis and is sometimes relieved by removal of the sphincter of Oddi. Chronic pancreatitis is manifested in episodes that are similar, albeit of lesser severity, to those of acute pancreatitis. Patients have persistent, recurring episodes of epigastric and upper left quadrant pain; the attacks are often precipitated by alcohol abuse or overeating. Anorexia, nausea, vomiting, constipation, and flatulence are common. Eventually the disease progresses to the extent that endocrine and exocrine pancreatic functions become deficient. At this point, signs of diabetes mellitus and the malabsorption syndrome (*e.g.*, weight loss, fatty stools [steatorrhea]) become apparent.[46]

Treatment consists of measures to treat coexisting biliary tract disease. A low-fat diet is usually prescribed. The signs of malabsorption may be treated with pancreatic enzymes. When diabetes is present, it is treated with insulin. Alcohol is forbidden because it frequently precipitates attacks. Because of the frequent pain episodes, narcotic addiction is a potential problem in persons with chronic pancreatitis. Surgical intervention is sometimes needed to relieve the pain and usually focuses on relieving any obstruction that may be present. In advanced cases, a subtotal or total pancreatectomy may be necessary.[45]

Cancer of the Pancreas

The incidence of pancreatic cancer has remained fairly stable over the past 25 years. It is the fifth leading cause of cancer death in the United States. The risk of pancreatic cancer increases after the age of 50 years, with most cases occurring between the ages of 65 and 79. Cancer of the pancreas is usually far advanced when diagnosed, and the 5-year survival rate is less than 3%.

The cause of pancreatic cancer is unknown. Smoking appears to be a major risk factor.[47] The incidence of pancreatic cancer is twice as high among smokers than nonsmokers. The second most important factor appears to be diet. A high intake of fat, meat, or both is linked with the disease. A protective effect has been ascribed to a diet containing fresh fruits and vegetables. Diabetes and chronic pancreatitis also are associated with pancreatic cancer, although neither the nature nor the sequence of the possible cause-effect relation has been established.[47,48]

Cancer of the pancreas usually has an insidious onset. Pain, jaundice, or both occur in more than 90% of patients, and along with weight loss, these manifestations constitute the classic presentation of the disease.[48]

Because of the proximity of the pancreas to the common duct and the ampulla of Vater, cancer of the head of the pancreas tends to obstruct bile flow; this causes distention of the gallbladder and jaundice. Jaundice is frequently the presenting symptom of a person with cancer of the head of the pancreas, and it is usually accompanied by complaints of pain and pruritus. Cancer of the body of the pancreas generally impinges on the celiac ganglion, causing pain. The pain usually worsens with ingestion of food or with assumption of the supine position. Cancer of the tail of the pancreas has usually metastasized before symptoms appear.

Ultrasonography and CT scanning are the most frequently used diagnostic methods to confirm the disease. Many tumor markers have been proposed for use in the diagnosis and follow-up of persons with pancreatic cancer. The most extensively studied has been CA 19–9, which is used in many centers. However, because levels are usually normal at the early stages of pancreatic cancer, it cannot be used as a screening method. The level of CA 19–9 is not specific for pancreatic cancer; it also is elevated in other types of gastrointestinal cancers, such as those of the bile duct and colon. Carcinoembryonic antigen is widely used as a marker, but it has low sensitivity and is elevated in many other malignant and benign conditions (see Chapter 5). Percutaneous fine-needle aspiration cytology of the pancreas has been one of the major advances in diagnosis of pancreatic cancer. Unfortunately, the smaller and more curable tumors are most likely missed by this procedure.

Most cancers of the pancreas have metastasized by the time of diagnosis. Surgical resection of the tumor is done when the tumor is localized or as a palliative measure. Radiation therapy may be useful when the disease is not resectable but appears to be localized. The use of irradiation and chemotherapy for pancreatic cancer continues to be investigated.

In summary, the pancreas is an endocrine and exocrine organ. Diabetes mellitus is the most common disorder of the endocrine pancreas, and it occurs independently of disease of the exocrine pancreas. The exocrine pancreas produces digestive enzymes that are secreted in an inactive form and transported to the small intestine through the main pancreatic duct, which usually empties into the ampulla of Vater and then into the duodenum through the sphincter of Oddi. The most common diseases of the exocrine pancreas are acute and chronic forms of pancreatitis and cancer. Acute and chronic types of pancreatitis are associated with biliary reflux and chronic alcoholism. Acute pancreatitis is a dramatic and life-threatening disorder in which there is autodigestion of pancreatic tissue. Chronic pancreatitis causes progressive destruction of the endocrine and exocrine pancreas. It is characterized by episodes of pain and epigastric distress that are similar to but less severe than that which occurs with acute pancreatitis. Cancer of the pancreas has remained relatively stable over the past 25 years. It is usually far advanced at the time of diagnosis, and the 5-year survival rate is less than 3%.

REFERENCES

1. Katzung B.G. (1995). *Basic and clinical pharmacology* (6th ed., pp. 48–59). Norwalk, CT: Appleton & Lange.
2. Lee W.M. (1995). Drug-induced hepatotoxicity. *New England Journal of Medicine* 33 (7), 1118–1127.
3. Alchord J.L. (1995). Alcohol and the liver. *Scientific American Science and Medicine* 2 (2), 16–25.
4. Lieber C.S. (1994). Alcohol and the liver: 1994 update. *Gastroenterology* 106, 1085–1105.
5. Lieber C.S. (1988). Biochemical and molecular basis of alcohol-induced injury to the liver and other tissues. *New England Journal of Medicine* 319, 1639.
6. Guyton A. (1996). *Textbook of medical physiology* (9th ed., pp. 827–829). Philadelphia: W.B. Saunders.
7. Kumar V., Cotran R.S., Robbins S.L. (1994). *Robbins' pathologic basis of disease* (5th ed., pp. 838–841, 843–852). Philadelphia: W.B. Saunders.
8. Podolsky D.K., Isselbacher K.J. (1991). Derangements of hepatic metabolism. In Wilson J.D., Braunwald E., Isselbacher K.J. (Eds.). *Harrison's principles of internal medicine* (12th ed., pp. 1311–1315). Philadelphia: W.B. Saunders.
9. Theal R.M., Scott K. (1996). Evaluating asymptomatic patients with abnormal liver function test results. *American Family Physician* 53 (6), 211–219.
10. Herlong H.F. (1994). Approach to the patient with abnormal liver enzymes. *Hospital Practice* 29 (11), 32–38.
11. Koff R.S. (1994). Solving the mysteries of viral hepatitis. *Scientific American Science and Medicine* 1 (2), 2433.
12. Alter H.J. (1996). The cloning and clinical implications of HGV and HGBV-C. *New England Journal of Medicine* 224 (23), 1536–1537.
13. Lemon S.M. (1985). Type A hepatitis. *New England Journal of Medicine* 313, 1059.
14. Lemon S.M., Thomas D.L. (1997). Vaccines to prevent viral hepatitis. *New England Journal of Medicine* 336 (3), 196–203.
15. Centers for Disease Control. (1991). Hepatitis B virus: A comprehensive strategy for eliminating transmission in the United States through universal childhood vaccination. *Morbidity and Mortality Weekly Reports* 40 (RR-13), 1–25.
16. Sharara A.I., Hunt C.M., Hamilton J.D. (1996). Hepatitis C. *Annuals of Internal Medicine* 125, 658–665.
17. Terrault N., Wright T. (1995). Interferon and hepatitis C. *New England Journal of Medicine* 332 (22), 1509–1511.
18. Bhandari B., Wright T.L. (1995). Hepatitis C: An overview. *Annual Review of Medicine* 46, 309–317.
19. Hoffnagle J.H. (1989). Type D (delta) hepatitis. *Journal of the American Medical Association* 261, 1321–1325.
20. Krawitt E.L. (1996). Autoimmune hepatitis. *New England Journal of Medicine* 334 (14), 897–902.
21. Maddrey W.C. (1994). Chronic viral hepatitis: Diagnosis and management. *Hospital Practice* 29 (2), 117–132.
22. Hoofnagle J.H., DiBisceglie A.M. (1997). The treatment of chronic hepatitis. *New England Journal of Medicine* 336 (5), 347–355.
23. Rubin E., Farber J.L. (1994). Pathology (2nd ed.. pp. 737–745), Philadelphia, J.B. Lippincott.
24. Freidman S.L. (1996). In Bennett J.C., Plum F. *Cecil textbook of medicine* (20th ed., pp. 788–796). Cirrhosis of the liver and its major sequelae. Philadelphia: W.B. Saunders.
25. Kaplan M.M. (1996). Primary biliary cirrhosis. *New England Journal of Medicine* 335 (21), 1570–1580.
26. Gershwin E., Mackay J.R. (1995). New knowledge in primary biliary cirrhosis. *Hospital Practice* 30 (8), 29–36.

27. Lee Y-M., Kaplan M.M. (1995). Primary sclerosing cholangitis. *New England Journal of Medicine* 332 (4),924–932.
28. U.S. Department of Health and Human Services. (1988). *Alcoholic hepatitis: A practical guide for physicians and other health care workers.* DHHS Publication No. (ADM) 88–1547. Washington, DC: Department of Health and Human Services.
29. Lieber C.S., Guadagnini K.S. (1990). The spectrum of alcoholic liver disease. *Hospital Practice* 27 (2A), 51–69.
30. Rubin E., Lieber C.S. (1968). Alcohol-induced hepatic injury in non-alcoholic volunteers. *New England Journal of Medicine* 278, 869–876.
31. Trevillyan J., Carroll P.J. (1997). Management of portal hypertension and esophageal varices in alcoholic cirrhosis. *American Family Physician* 55 (5), 1851–1858.
32. Roberts L.R., Kamath P.S. (1996). Pathophysiology and treatment of variceal hemorrhage. *Mayo Clinic Proceedings* 71, 973–983.
33. Roberts L.R., Kamath P.S. (1996). Ascites and hepatorenal syndrome: Pathophysiology and management. *Mayo Clinic Proceedings* 71, 874–881.
34. Epstein M. (1995). Renal sodium retention in liver disease. *Hospital Practice* 30 (9), 33–41.
35. Starzl T.E., Demetris A.J., Van Thiel D. (1989). Liver transplantation (Part 1). *New England Journal of Medicine,* 321, 1014–1020.
36. Rosen R.H., Shackleton C.R., Martin P. (1996). Indications and timing of liver transplantation. *Medical Clinics of North America* 80 (5), 1069–1102.
37. Knechtle S.J., Flemming M.F., Barry K.L., et al. (1992). Liver transplantation in alcoholic liver disease. *Surgery* 112, 694–701.
38. Johnston D.E., Kaplan M.M. (1993). Pathogenesis and treatment of gallstones. *New England Journal of Medicine* 328, 412–421.
39. Marton K.I. (1988). How to image the gallbladder in suspected cholecystitis. *Annals of Internal Medicine* 109, 722.
40. Health and Policy Committee, American College of Physicians. (1988). How to study the gallbladder. *Annals of Internal Medicine* 109, 752.
41. Birkett D.H. (1993). Laparoscopic cholecystectomy with common duct exploration. *Hospital Practice* 28 (5), 37–44.
42. Chang B., Pamies B.J. (1994). Biliary extracorporeal shockwave lithotripsy: An update. *Hospital Practice* 28 (4), 93–98.
43. Frey C.F., Gerzof S.G., Vennes J.A. (1992). Progress in acute pancreatitis. *Patient Care* 26 (11), 258–290.
44. Steinberg W., Jenner S. (1994). Acute pancreatitis. *New England Journal of Medicine* 330, 1198–1210.
45. Friedman L.S. (1997). Liver, biliary tract, and pancreas. In Tierney L.M., McPhee S.J., Papaakis M.A., et al. (Eds.). *Current medical diagnosis and treatment* (36th ed., pp. 638–643). Norwalk, CT: Appleton & Lange.
46. Steer M.L., Waxman L., Freeman S. (1995). Chronic pancreatitis. *New England Journal of Medicine* 332, 1482.
47. Warshaw A.I., Castillo C.F. (1992). Pancreatic carcinoma. *New England Journal of Medicine* 326, 455–465.
48. Wanebo H.J., Vezeridis M.P. (1996). Pancreatic cancer in perspective. *Cancer* 76 (3), 580–587.

ADDITIONAL READINGS

Alchord J.L. Review of alcoholic hepatitis and its treatment. *American Journal of Gastroenterology* 88, 1822–1829.

Baillie J. (1997). Treatment of acute biliary pancreatitis. *New England Journal of Medicine* 286–87.

Epstein M. (1992). The hepatorenal syndrome—newer perspectives. *New England Journal of Medicine* 327, 1810–1811.

Friedman S.L. (1993). The cellular basis for hepatic fibrosis. *New England Journal of Medicine* 328 (25), 1828–3535.

Koziel M.J. (1996). Immunology of viral hepatitis. *American Journal of Medicine* 100, 98–109.

Lee W.M. (1993). Acute liver failure. *New England Journal of Medicine* 329 (25), 1862–1872.

Mast E.E., Krawczynski K. (1996). Hepatitis E: An overview. *Annual Review of Medicine* 47, 257–266.

Sherman K.E. (1991). Alanine aminotransferase in clinical practice: A review. *Archives of Internal Medicine* 151, 260–265.

Tiollais P., Buendia M.A. (1991). Hepatitis B virus. *Scientific American* Apr, 116–123.

Endocrine Function

By the end of the Middle Ages, a great storehouse of anatomic knowledge existed; however, this repository had been culled from a combination of incomplete observations, religious beliefs, extrapolation from animal structures, and philosophical guesswork. Scientists slavishly adhered to these teachings, many of which were the products of the early Greeks (such as Aristotle and Galen), even though personal experience provided them with contradictory evidence.

The endocrine system fell victim to the outdated theories postulated long before. Even when some of its parts were discovered, their importance went unrecognized. For example, the pituitary gland, first noted in 1524 by Jacob Berengar of Carpi, was considered to be necessary to the cooling function of the brain. The brain was thought to secrete pituita, *phlegm (mucus), and discharge it from the nose as part of its cooling process. The gland received its name from Andreas Vesalius, who referred to it in his text* De Fabrica *(1543) as* glandula pituitam cerebri excipiens, *or the gland that receives the phlegm from the brain. It was not until the late 19th and early 20th centuries that the field of endocrinology had its beginnings. It was then that the importance of the pituitary gland was finally realized, and it was called the master endocrine gland.*

UNIT IX

CHAPTER 34

Mechanisms of Endocrine Control

The endocrine system is involved in all of the integrative aspects of life, including growth, sex differentiation, metabolism, and adaptation to an ever-changing environment. This chapter focuses on general aspects of endocrine function, organization of the endocrine system, hormone receptors and hormone actions, and regulation of hormone levels.

The Endocrine System

After you have completed this section of the chapter, you should be able to meet the following objectives:

- Characterize a hormone
- State a difference between the synthesis of protein hormones and that of steroid hormones
- Describe mechanisms of hormone transport and inactivation
- State the function of a hormone receptor and state the difference between fixed hormone receptors and mobile hormone receptors
- Describe the role of the hypothalamus in regulating pituitary control of endocrine function
- State the major difference between positive and negative feedback control mechanisms

The endocrine system uses chemical substances called *hormones* as a means of regulating and integrating body functions. The endocrine system participates in the regulation of digestion, use, and storage of nutrients; growth and development; electrolyte and water metabolism; and reproductive functions. Although the endocrine system was once thought to consist solely of discrete endocrine glands, it is now known that a number of other tissues release chemical messengers that modulate body processes. The functions of the endocrine system are closely linked with those of the nervous system and the immune system. For example, neurotransmitters such as epinephrine can act as neurotransmitters or as hormones. The functions of the immune system are also closely linked with those of the endocrine system. The immune system responds to foreign agents by means of chemical messengers (*e.g.*, interleukins, interferons) and complex receptor mechanisms (see Chapter 11). The immune system also is extensively regulated by hormones such as the adrenal corticosteroid hormones.

Hormones

Hormones are generally thought of as *chemical messengers* that are transported in body fluids. They are highly specialized organic molecules produced by endocrine organs in response to specific stimuli that exert their action on specific target cells. Hormones do not initiate reactions; they are modulators of systemic and cellular responses. Most hormones are present in body fluids at all times, but in greater or lesser amounts depending on the needs of the body. Hormones can produce a generalized or a localized effect.

A characteristic of hormones is that a single hormone can exert various effects in different tissues, or conversely, a single function can be regulated by several hormones. For example, estradiol, which is produced by the ovary, can act on the ovarian follicles to promote their maturation, on the uterus to stimulate its growth and maintain the cyclic changes in the uterine mucosa, on the mammary gland to stimulate ductal growth, on the hypothalamic-pituitary system to regulate the secretion of gonadotropins and prolactin, and on general metabolic processes to affect adipose tissue distribution. Lipolysis, which is the release of free fatty acids from adipose tissue, is an example of a single function that is regulated by several hormones, including the catecholamines, glucagon, secretin, and prolactin. Table 34–1 lists the major functions and sources of body hormones.

In the past, hormones were described as chemical substances that were released into the bloodstream and transported to distant target sites, where they exerted their action. Although many hormones travel by this mechanism, some hormones and hormone-like substances never enter the bloodstream but instead act locally in the vicinity in which they are released. When they act locally on cells other than those that produced the hormone, the action is called *paracrine*. The action of sex steroids on the ovary is a paracrine action. Hormones can also exert an *autocrine* action on the cell from which it was produced. For example, the release of insulin from pancreatic β cells can inhibit its release from the same cells.

A group of compounds that have a hormonelike action are the eicosanoids, which are derived from polyunsaturated fatty acids in the cell membrane. Among these, *arachidonic acid* is the most important and abundant precursor of the various eicosanoids. The most important of the eicosanoids are the prostaglandins, leukotrienes, and thromboxanes. These fatty acid derivatives are produced by most body cells, are rapidly cleared from the circulation, and are thought to act mainly by paracrine and autocrine mechanisms. Eicosanoid synthesis is often stimulated in response to hormones and serve as mediators of hormone action.

Structural Classification

Hormones have diverse structures ranging from single amino acids to complex proteins and lipids. Hormones are generally divided in three categories according to their structures: amines and amino acids; peptides, polypeptides, and proteins; and steroids. The first category, the amines, includes norepinephrine, epinephrine, and dopamine, which are derived from a single amino acid (*i.e.*, tyrosine), and the thyroid hormones, which are derived from two iodinated tyrosine amino acid residues. The second category, the peptides, polypeptides, and proteins, can be as small as thyroid-releasing hormone, which contains three amino acids, and as large and complex as growth hormone and follicle-stimulating hormone (FSH), which have about 200 amino acids. The third category comprises the steroid hormones, which are derivatives of cholesterol. Table 34–2 presents a listing of hormones according to structure.

TABLE 34-1

Functional Classification of Hormones

Function	Hormone	Major Source
Control of water and electrolyte metabolism	Aldosterone	Adrenal cortex
	Antidiuretic hormone (ADH)	Posterior pituitary
	Calcitonin	C cells, thyroid
	Parathyroid hormone	Parathyroid
	Angiotensin	Kidney
Control of gastrointestinal function	Cholecystokinin	Gastrointestinal tract
	Gastrin	Gastrointestinal tract
	Secretin	Gastrointestinal tract
Regulation of energy, metabolism, and growth	Glucagon	α cells, pancreatic islets
	Insulin	β cells, pancreatic islets
	Growth hormone	Anterior pituitary
	Thyroid hormones	Thyroid gland
Neurotransmitters	Dopamine	CNS
	Epinephrine	Adrenal medulla
	Norepinephrine	Adrenal medulla and nervous system
Reproductive function	Chorionic gonadotropins	Placenta
	Estrogens	Ovary
	Oxytocin	Posterior pituitary
	Progesterone	Ovary
	Prolactin	Anterior pituitary
	Testosterone	Testes
Stress and control of inflammation	Glucocorticoids	Adrenal cortex
Tropic hormones (regulation of other hormone levels)	Adrenocorticotropic hormone (ACTH)	Anterior pituitary
	Follicle-stimulating hormone (FSH)	Anterior pituitary
	Luteinizing hormone (LH)	Anterior pituitary
	Thyroid-stimulating hormone (TSH)	Anterior pituitary

TABLE 34-2

Classes of Hormones Based on Structure

Amines and Amino Acids	Peptides, Polypeptides, and Proteins	Steroids
Epinephrine	Adrenocorticotropic hormone (ACTH)	Aldosterone
Norepinephrine	Angiotensin	Glucocorticoids
Dopamine	Calcitonin	Estrogens
Thyroid hormones	Cholecystokinin	Progesterone
	Erythropoietin	Testosterone
	Follicle-stimulating hormone (FSH)	
	Gastrin	
	Glucagon	
	Growth hormone	
	Insulin	
	Luteinizing hormone (LH)	
	Oxytocin	
	Parathyroid hormone	
	Prolactin	
	Secretin	
	Thyroid-stimulating hormone (TSH)	
	Antidiuretic hormone (ADH)	

Synthesis and Transport

The mechanisms for hormone synthesis vary with hormone structure. Protein and peptide hormones are synthesized and stored in granules or vesicles within the cytoplasm of the cell until secretion is required. The lipid-soluble steroid hormones are released as they are synthesized.

Protein and peptide hormones are synthesized in the rough endoplasmic reticulum in a manner similar to the synthesis of other proteins (see Chapter 1). The appropriate amino acid sequence is dictated by messenger RNAs from the nucleus. Usually, synthesis involves the production of a precursor hormone, which is modified by the addition of peptides or sugar units. These precursor hormones often contain extra peptide units that ensure proper folding of the molecule and insertion of essential linkages. If extra amino acids are present, as in insulin, the precursor hormone is called a *prohormone*. After synthesis and sequestration in the endoplasmic reticulum, the protein and peptide hormones move into the Golgi complex, where they are packaged in granules or vesicles. It is in the Golgi complex that prohormones are converted into hormones.

Steroid hormones are synthesized within the smooth endoplasmic reticulum, and steroid-secreting cells can be identified by their large amounts of smooth endoplasmic reticulum. Certain steroids serve as precursors for the production of other hormones. In the adrenal cortex, for example, progesterone and other steroid intermediates are enzymatically converted into aldosterone, cortisol, or androgens (see Chapter 35).

Hormones that are released into the bloodstream circulate as free molecules or as hormones attached to transport carriers (see Fig. 34–1). Peptide hormones and protein hormones generally circulate unbound in the blood. Steroid hormones and thyroid hormone are carried by specific proteins synthesized in the liver. The extent of carrier binding influences the rate at which hormones leave the blood and enter the cells. The half-life of a hormone—the time it takes for the body to reduce the concentration of the hormone by one half—is positively correlated with its percentage of protein binding. Thyroxine, which is more than 99% protein bound, has a half-life of 6 days. Aldosterone, which is only 15% bound, has a half-life of only 25 minutes. Drugs that compete with a hormone for binding with the transport carrier molecules increase hormone action by increasing the availability of the active unbound hormone. For example, aspirin competes with thyroid hormone for

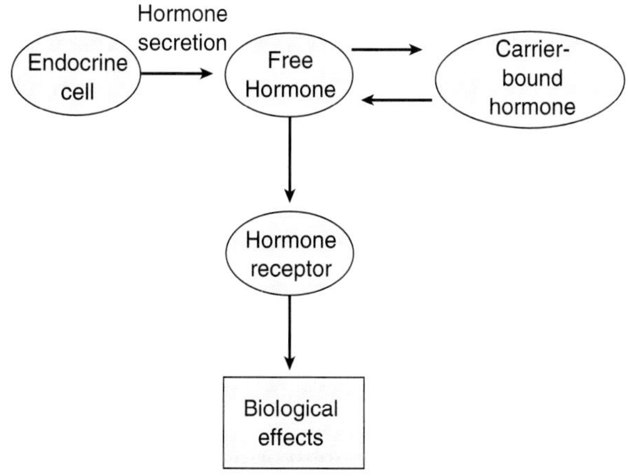

Figure 34–1
Relationship of free and carrier-bound hormone.

binding to transport proteins; when the drug is administered to persons with excessive levels of circulating thyroid hormone (such as during thyroid crisis), serious effects occur.

Metabolism and Rate of Reaction

Hormones secreted by endocrine cells must be continuously inactivated to prevent their accumulation. Intracellular and extracellular mechanisms participate in the termination of hormone function. Some hormones are enzymatically inactivated at receptor sites where they exert their action. Peptide hormones have a short life span and are inactivated by enzymes that split peptide bonds. They are inactivated mainly in the liver and kidneys. Steroid hormones are bound to protein carriers for transport and are inactive in the bound state. Their activity depends on the availability of transport hormones. Unbound adrenal and gonadal steroid hormones are conjugated in the liver, which renders them inactive, and then excreted in the bile or urine. Thyroid hormones are also transported by carrier molecules. The free hormone is rendered inactive by the removal of amino acids (*i.e.*, deamination) in the tissues, and the hormone is conjugated in the liver and eliminated in the bile.

Hormones react at different rates. The neurotransmitters, such as epinephrine, have a reaction time of milliseconds. Thyroid hormone requires days for its effect to occur.

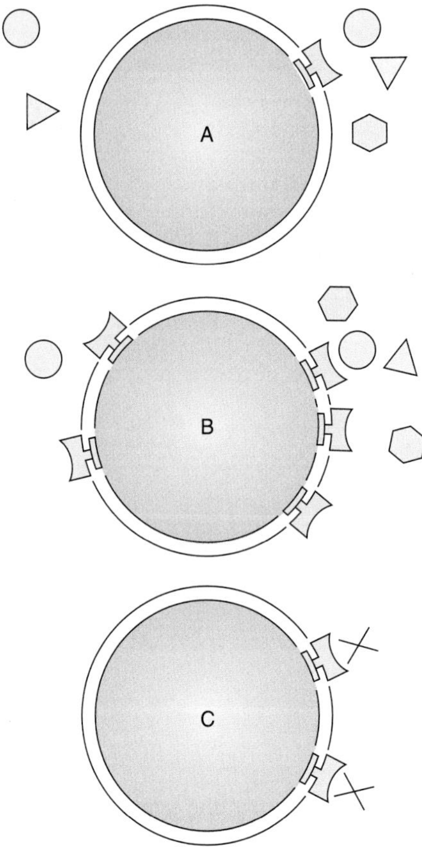

Figure 34–2
(A) The role of cell-surface receptors in mediating the action of hormones. Hormone action is affected by **(B)** the number of receptors that are present and by **(C)** the affinity of these receptors for hormone binding.

Mechanisms of Action

Hormones exert their action by binding to specific receptor sites located on the surfaces of the target cells. The function of these receptors is to recognize a specific hormone and translate the hormonal signal into a cellular response. The structure of these receptors varies in a manner that allows target cells to respond to one hormone and not to others. For example, receptors in the thyroid are specific for the thyroid-stimulating hormone, and receptors on the gonads respond to the gonadotropic hormones.

The response of a target cell to a hormone varies with the *number* of receptors present and with the *affinity* of these receptors for hormone binding. A variety of factors influence the number of receptors that are present on target cells and their affinity for hormone binding (Fig. 34–2).

There are about 2000 to 100,000 hormone receptor molecules per cell. The number of hormone receptors on a cell may be altered for any of several reasons. Antibodies may destroy the receptor proteins. Increased or decreased hormone levels often induce changes in the activity of genes that regulator receptor synthesis. For example, decreased hormone levels often produce an increase in receptor numbers by means of a process called *up-regulation;* this increases the sensitivity of the body to existing hormone levels. Likewise, sustained levels of excess hormone often bring about a decrease in receptor numbers by *down-regulation*, producing a decrease in hormone sensitivity. In some instances, the reverse effect occurs, and an increase in hormone levels appears to recruit its own receptors (*i.e.*, up-regulation), increasing the sensitivity of the cell to the hormone. Obesity has been shown to cause a decrease in the number of insulin receptors on fat cells, and it is speculated that this may influence impaired glucose tolerance in the obese non–insulin-dependent diabetic. Oral hypoglycemic drugs, the sulfonylureas, cause an increase in the number of insulin receptors on body cells.

The affinity of receptors for binding hormones is also affected by a number of conditions. For example, the pH of the body fluids plays an important role in the affinity of insulin receptors. In ketoacidosis, a lower pH reduces insulin binding.

Some hormone receptors are located on the surface of the cell and act through second-messenger mechanisms, and others are located within the cell, where they modulate the synthesis of enzymes, transport proteins, or structural proteins. The receptors for thyroid hormones, which are found in the nucleus, are thought to be directly associated with one or more of the chromosomes. Chart 34–1 lists hormones that act through the two types of receptors.

CHART 34-1
Hormone–Receptor Interactions

Fixed Messenger Interactions

Glucagon
Insulin
Epinephrine
Parathyroid hormone
Thyroid-stimulating hormone (TSH)
Andrenocorticotropic hormone (ACTH)
Follicle-stimulating hormone (FSH)
Luteinizing hormone (LH)
Antidiuretic hormone (ADH)
Secretin

Mobile Hormone–Carrier–Nuclear Interactions

Estrogens
Testosterone
Progesterone
Adrenal cortical hormones
Thyroid hormones

Surface Receptors. Because of their low solubility in the lipid layer of cell membranes, peptide hormones and catecholamines cannot readily cross the cell membrane. Instead, these hormones interact with surface receptors in a manner that incites the generation of an intracellular signal or message. The intracellular signal system is considered to be the *second messengers*, and the hormone is considered to be the first messenger (Fig. 34–3). For example, the first messenger glucagon binds to surface receptors on liver cells to incite glycogen breakdown by way of the second messenger system.

The most widely distributed second messenger is cyclic adenosine monophosphate (cAMP). cAMP is formed from cellular ATP by the enzyme adenylate cyclase, a membrane-bound enzyme that is located on the inner aspect of the cell membrane. Adenylate cyclase is functionally coupled to various cell surface receptors by the regulatory actions of G proteins (see Chapter 1). A second messenger similar to cAMP is cyclic GMP, derived from guanine monophosphate. As a result of binding to specific cell receptors, many peptide hormones incite a series of enzymatic reactions that produce an almost immediate increase in cAMP. Some hormones act to decrease cAMP levels and have an opposite effect.

In some cells, binding of hormones or neurotransmitters to surface receptors acts directly rather than through a second messenger to open ion channels in the cell membrane. The influx of ions serves as an intracellular signal to convey the hormonal message to the cell interior. In many instances, activation of hormone receptors results in the opening of calcium channels. The increasing cytoplasmic concentration of calcium may result in direct activation of calcium-dependent enzymes or calcium-calmodulin complexes with their attendant effects.

Intracellular Receptors. A second type of receptor mechanism is involved in mediating the action of hormones such as the steroid and thyroid hormones, which are transported in body fluids attached to carrier proteins (see Fig. 34–3). These hormones are lipid soluble and pass freely through the cell membrane. They then attach to intracellular receptors and form a hormone-receptor complex that functions as a second messenger. For many hormones, this second messenger is unknown. The hormone-messenger complex activates or suppresses intracellular mechanisms such as gene activity, with subsequent production or inhibition of messenger RNA and protein synthesis.

Control of Hormone Levels

Hormone secretion varies widely over a 24-hour period. Some hormones, such as growth hormone and adrenocorticotrophic hormone (ACTH), have diurnal fluctuations that vary with the sleep-wake cycle. Others, such as the female sex hormones, are secreted in a complicated cyclic manner. The levels of hormones such as insulin and antidiuretic hormone (ADH) are regulated by feedback mechanisms that monitor the amount of organic and inorganic substances in the body. The levels of many of the hormones are regulated by feedback mechanisms that involve the hypothalamic-pituitary–target cell system.

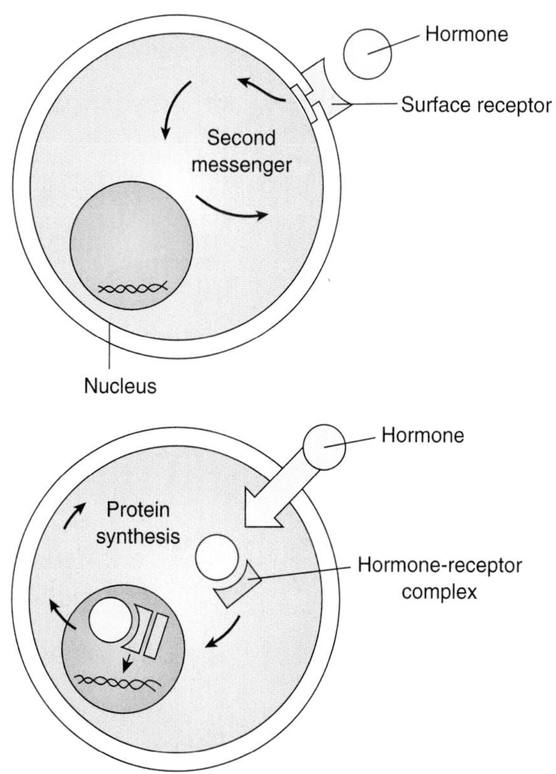

Figure 34–3
The two types of hormone–receptor interactions: the membrane receptor (**top**) and the intracellular mobile receptor (**bottom**).

Hypothalamic-Pituitary Regulation

Because the integration of body function relies on input from the nervous system and the endocrine system, it seems logical that input from the nervous system would participate in the regulation of hormone levels. The hypothalamus and the pituitary (*i.e.*, hypophysis) act as links between the central nervous system and many of the endocrine-mediated functions of the body. These two structures are connected by blood flow in the hypophyseal portal system, which begins in the hypothalamus and drains into the anterior pituitary gland, and by the nerve axons that connect the supraoptic and paraventricular nuclei of the hypothalamus with the posterior pituitary gland (Fig. 34–4). Embryologically, the anterior pituitary gland developed from glandular tissue and the posterior pituitary developed from neural tissue.

The synthesis and release of anterior pituitary hormones are largely regulated by the action of releasing or inhibiting hormones from the hypothalamus, which is the coordinating center of the brain for endocrine, behavioral, and autonomic nervous system function. It is at the level of the hypothalamus that emotion, pain, body temperature, and other neural input are communicated to the endocrine system (Fig. 34–5). The posterior pituitary hormones, ADH and oxytocin, are synthesized in the cell bodies of neurons in the hypothalamus that have axons that travel to the posterior pituitary. The release and function of ADH are discussed in Chapter 26.

The pituitary gland has been called the "master gland" because its hormones control the functions of many target glands and cells. Hormones produced by the anterior pituitary control body growth and metabolism (*i.e.*, growth hormone), function of the thyroid gland (*i.e.*, thyroid-stimulating hormone), glucocorticoid hormone levels (*i.e.*, ACTH), function of the gonads (*i.e.*, FSH and luteinizing hormone [LH]), and breast growth and milk production (*i.e.*, prolactin). Melanocyte-stimulating hormone, which controls pigmentation of the skin, is produced by the pars intermedia of the pituitary gland.

Feedback Regulation

The level of many of the hormones in the body is regulated by negative feedback mechanisms. The function of this type of system is similar to that of the thermostat in a heating system. In the endocrine system, sensors detect a change in the hormone level and adjust hormone secretion so that body levels are maintained within an appropriate range. When the sensors detect a decrease in hormone levels, they initiate changes that cause an increase in hormone production; when hormone levels rise above the set point of the system, the sensors cause hormone production and release to decrease. For example,

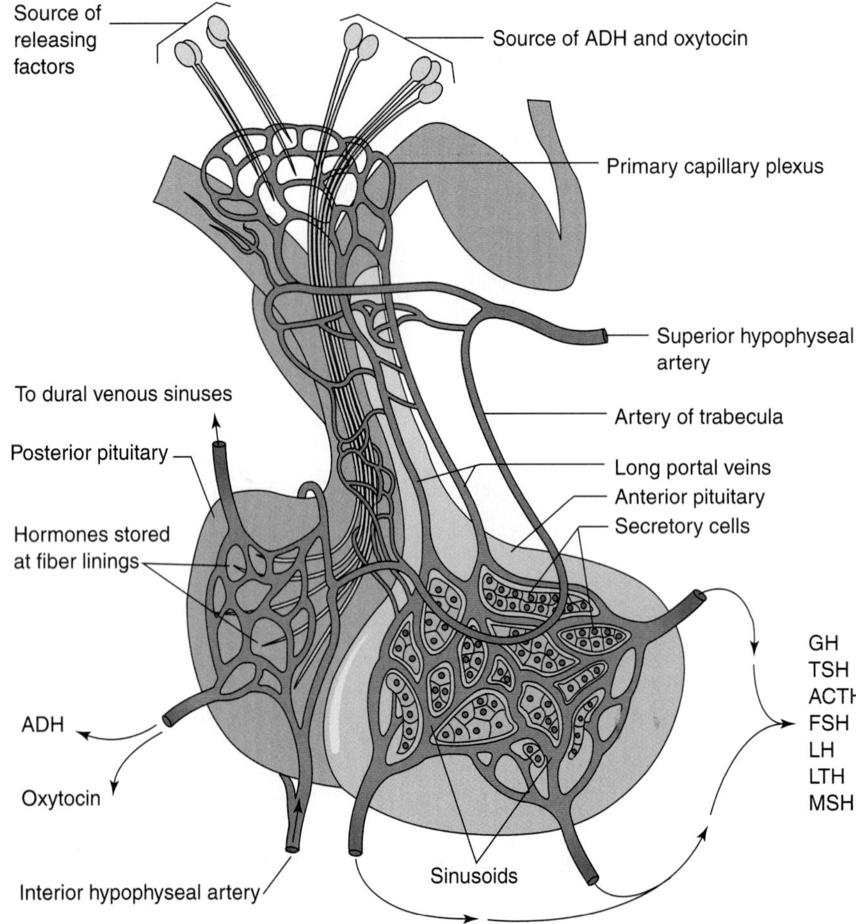

Figure 34–4 The hypothalamus and the anterior and posterior pituitary. The hypothalamic releasing or inhibiting hormones are transported to the anterior pituitary by way of the portal vessels. ADH and oxytocin are produced by nerve cells in the supraoptic and paraventricular nuclei of the hypothalamus and then transported through the nerve axon to the posterior pituitary, where they are released into the circulation.

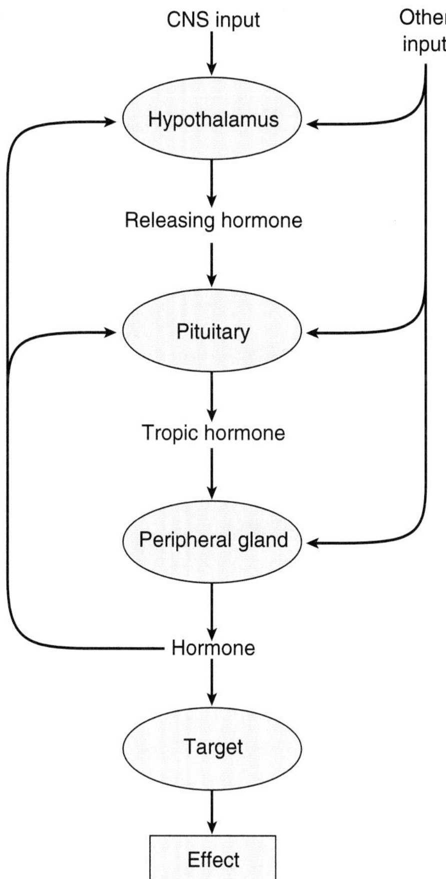

Figure 34–5
Hypothalamic–pituitary control of hormone levels.

an increase in thyroid hormone is detected by sensors in the hypothalamus or anterior pituitary gland, and this causes a reduction in the secretion of thyroid-stimulating hormone (TSH), with a subsequent decrease in the output of thyroid hormone from the thyroid gland. The feedback loops for the hypothalamic-pituitary feedback mechanisms are illustrated in Figure 34–6.

Exogenous forms of hormones (given as drug preparations) can influence the normal feedback control of hormone production and release. One of the most common examples of this influence occurs with the administration of the adrenocortical hormones, which causes suppression of the hypothalamic-pituitary–target cell system that regulates the production of these hormones.

Although the levels of most hormones are regulated by negative feedback mechanisms, a small number are under positive feedback control, in which rising levels of a hormone cause another gland to release a hormone that is stimulating to the first. There must, however, be a mechanism for shutting off the release of the first hormone, or its production would continue unabated. An example of such a system is that of the female ovarian hormone estradiol. Increased estradiol production during the follicular stage of the menstrual cycle produces increased gonadotropin (FSH) production by the anterior pituitary gland. This stimulates further increases in estradiol levels until the demise of the follicle, which is the source of estradiol, results in a fall in gonadotropin levels.

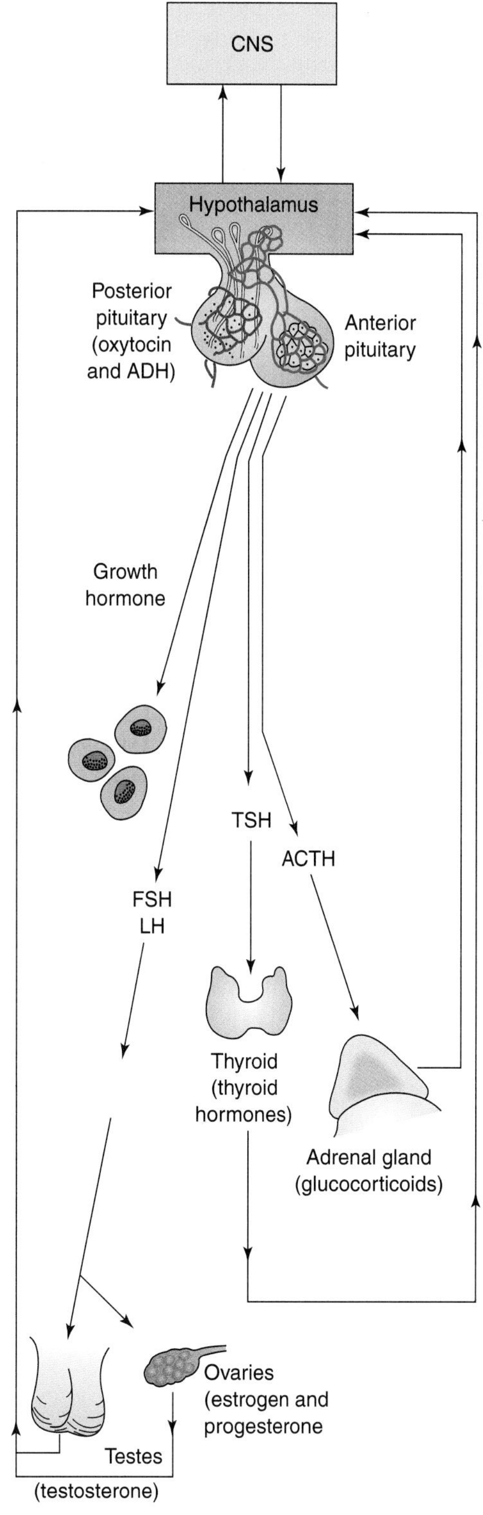

Figure 34–6
Control of hormone production by hypothalamic–pituitary–target cell feedback mechanism. Hormone levels from the target glands regulate the release of hormones from the anterior pituitary by means of a negative feedback system.

In addition to positive and negative feedback mechanisms that monitor changes in hormone levels, some hormones are regulated by the the level of the substance they regulate. For example, insulin levels are normally regulated in response to blood glucose levels and aldosterone in response to body levels of sodium and potassium. Other factors such as stress, environmental temperature, and nutritional status can alter feedback regulation of hormone levels.

In summary, the endocrine system acts as a communications system that uses chemical messengers, or hormones, for the transmission of information from cell to cell and from organ to organ. Hormones act at the level of the cell membrane, which has surface receptors that are specific for the different types of hormones. Many of the endocrine glands are under the regulatory control of other parts of the endocrine system. The hypothalamus and the pituitary gland form a complex integrative network that joins the nervous system and the endocrine system; this central network controls the output from many of the other glands in the body.

General Aspects of Altered Endocrine Function

After you have completed this section of the chapter, you should be able to meet the following objectives:

- Describe the mechanisms of endocrine hypofunction and hyperfunction and differentiate primary from secondary endocrine disorders
- Characterize the basis for immunoassay methods of measuring hormone levels

Hypofunction and Hyperfunction

Disturbances of endocrine function can usually be divided into two categories: hypofunction and hyperfunction. *Hypofunction* of an endocrine gland can occur for a variety of reasons. Congenital defects can result in the absence or impaired development of the gland or the absence of an enzyme needed for hormone synthesis. The gland may be destroyed by a disruption in blood flow, infection, inflammation, autoimmune responses, or neoplastic growth. There may be a decline in function with aging, or the gland may atrophy as the result of drug therapy or for unknown reasons. Some endocrine-deficient states are associated with receptor defects: hormone receptors may be absent, the receptor binding of hormones may be defective, or the cellular responsiveness to the hormone may be impaired. It is suspected that in some cases a gland may produce a biologically inactive hormone or that an active hormone may be destroyed by circulating antibodies before it can exert its action.

Hyperfunction is generally associated with excessive hormone production. This can result from excessive stimulation and hyperplasia of the endocrine gland or from a hormone-producing tumor of the gland. An ectopic tumor can produce hormones; for example, certain bronchogenic tumors produce hormones such as ADH and ACTH.

Primary and Secondary Disorders

Endocrine disorders can generally be divided into primary and secondary groups. *Primary defects* in endocrine function originate within the target gland responsible for producing the hormone. In *secondary disorders* of endocrine function, the target gland is essentially normal, but its function is altered by defective levels of stimulating hormones or releasing factors from the hypothalamic-pituitary system. For example, adrenalectomy produces a primary deficiency of adrenocorticosteroid hormones. Removal or destruction of the pituitary gland eliminates ACTH stimulation of the adrenal cortex and brings about a secondary deficiency.

Diagnostic Methods

Several techniques are available for assessing endocrine function and hormone levels. One technique measures the effect of a hormone on body function. Measurement of blood glucose, for example, reflects insulin levels and is an indirect method of assessing insulin availability. Another method is to measure hormone levels.

Blood Tests

Hormones circulating in the plasma were first detected by bioassays using the intact animal or a portion of tissue from the animal. At one time, female rats or male frogs were used to test women's urine for the presence of human chorionic gonadotropin, which is produced by the placenta during pregnancy. Unfortunately, most bioassays lack the precision, sensitivity, and specificity to measure low concentrations of hormones in plasma, and they are inconvenient to perform.

Blood hormone levels provide information about hormone blood levels at a specific time. For example, blood insulin levels can be measured along with blood glucose after administration of a challenge dose of glucose to measure the time course of change in blood insulin levels.

Real progress in measuring plasma hormone levels came more than 30 years ago with the use of competitive binding and the development of radioimmunoassay (RIA) methods. This method uses a radiolabeled form of the hormone and a hormone antibody that has been prepared by injecting an appropriate animal with a purified form of the hormone. The unlabeled hormone in the sample being tested competes with the radiolabeled hormone for attachment to the binding sites of the antibody. Measurement of the radiolabeled hormone-antibody complex then provides a means of arriving at a measure of hormone level in the sample. Because hormone binding is competitive, the amount of radiolabeled hormone-antibody complex that is formed decreases as the amount of unlabeled hormone in the sample is increased. RIA has several disadvantages, including limited shelf-life of the radiolabeled hormone and increasing the cost for the disposal of radioactive waste.

Nonisotope methods have been developed in which the antigen of the hormone being measured is linked to an enzyme-activated label (*e.g.*, fluorescent label, chemiluminescent label) or latex particles that can be agglunated with an antigen and measured. The enzyme-linked immunosorbent assays (ELISA) use antibody-coated plates and an enzyme-labeled reporter antibody. Binding of the hormone to the enzyme-labeled reporter antibody produces a colored reaction that can be measured using a spectrophotometer.

Urine Tests

Measurements of urinary hormone or hormone metabolite excretion are often done on a 24-hour urine sample and provide a better measure of hormone levels during that period than hormones measured in an isolated blood sample. The advantages of a urine test include the fact that urine samples are relatively easy to obtain and do not require blood sampling. The disadvantages are that reliably timed urine collections are often difficult to obtain. For example, a person may be unable to urinate at specific timed intervals, and urine samples may be accidentally discarded or inaccurately preserved. Because many urine tests involve the measure of a hormone metabolite rather than the hormone itself, drugs or disease states that alter hormone metabolism may interfere with the test result. Some urinary hormone metabolite measurements include hormones from more than one source and are of little value in measuring hormone secretion from a specific source. For example, urinary 17-ketosteroids are a measure of adrenal and gonadal androgens.

Stimulation and Suppression Tests

Stimulation tests are used when hypofunction of an endocrine organ is suspected. A trophic or stimulating hormone can be administered to test the capacity of an endocrine organ to increase hormone product. The capacity of the target gland to respond is measured by an increase in the appropriate hormone. For example, the function of the hypothalamic-pituitary-thyroid system could be evaluated through stimulation tests using thyrotropin-releasing factor and thyroid-stimulating hormone (TSH). Failure to effect an increase in thyroid hormone after a stimulation using thyrotropin-releasing factor suggests inadequate production of TSH, and failure to effect an increase in thyroid hormone after stimulation with TSH suggests a defect in production of thyroid hormone by the thyroid gland.

Suppression tests are used to determine if negative feedback control mechanisms are intact. For example, a glucocorticoid hormone can be administered to persons suspected of having hypercortisolism to assess the capacity to inhibit corticotropin-releasing hormone.

In summary, endocrine disorders are the result of hypofunction or hyperfunction of an endocrine gland. They can occur as a primary defect in hormone production by a target gland or as a secondary disorder resulting from a defect in the hypothalamic-pituitary system that controls a target gland's function. Laboratory tests measure hormone levels or assess the effect of a hormone on body function (*e.g.*, assessment of insulin function through blood sugar).

BIBLIOGRAPHY

Giffin J.E., Sergio R.O. (Eds.). (1992). *Textbook of endocrine physiology* (2nd ed.). New York: Oxford University Press.

Greenspan F.S., Baxter J.D. (1994). *Basic and clinical endocrinology* (4rd ed.). Norwalk, CT: Appleton & Lange.

Guyton A.C., Hall J.E. (1996). *Textbook of medical physiology* (9th ed., pp. 925–932), Philadelphia: W.B. Saunders.

Hanley R.M., Steiner A.L. (1989). The second-messenger system for peptide proteins. *Hospital Practice* 24 (8A), 59–70.

Rhoades R.A., Tanner G.A. (1996). *Medical physiology* (pp. 633–53). Boston: Little, Brown.

CHAPTER 35

Alterations in Endocrine Control of Growth and Metabolism

Growth Disorders

After you have completed this section of the chapter, you should be able to meet the following objectives:

- State the effects of a deficiency in growth hormone
- Differentiate genetic short stature from constitutional short stature
- State the mechanisms of short stature in hypothyroidism, poorly controlled diabetes mellitus, treatment with adrenal glucocorticosteroid hormones, malnutrition, and psychosocial dwarfism
- List three causes of tall stature
- Explain why children with isosexual precocious puberty are tall-statured children but short-statured adults
- Relate the functions of growth hormone to the manifestations of acromegaly

Several hormones are essential for normal body growth and maturation, including growth hormone (GH), insulin, thyroid hormone, and androgens. In addition to its actions on carbohydrate and fat metabolism, insulin plays an essential role in growth processes. Children with diabetes, particularly those with poor control, often fail to grow normally even though GH levels are normal. When levels of thyroid hormone are lower than normal, bone growth and epiphyseal closure are delayed. Androgens such as testosterone and dihydrotestosterone exert anabolic growth effects through their actions on protein synthesis. Glucocorticoids at excessive levels inhibit growth, apparently because of their antagonistic effect on GH secretion.

Growth Hormone

Also called *somatotropin*, GH is a 191–amino-acid polypeptide hormone synthesized and secreted by special cells in the anterior pituitary called somatotropes. For many years it was thought that GH was produced primarily during periods of growth. However, this has proved to be incorrect, because the rate of GH production in adults is almost as great as in children. GH is necessary for growth and contributes to the regulation of metabolic functions.[1,2] All aspects of cartilage growth are stimulated by GH; one of the most striking effects of GH is on linear bone growth, resulting from its action on the epiphyseal cartilage plates of long bones. The width of bone increases because of enhanced periosteal growth; visceral and endocrine organs, skeletal and cardiac muscle, skin, and connective tissue all undergo increased growth in response to GH. In many instances, the increased growth of visceral and endocrine organs is accompanied by enhanced functional capacity. For example, increased growth of cardiac muscle is accompanied by an increase in cardiac output.

In addition to its effects on growth, GH facilitates the rate of protein synthesis by all of the cells of the body; it enhances fatty acid mobilization and increases the use of fatty acids for fuel; and it maintains or increases blood glucose levels by decreasing the use of glucose for fuel. GH has an initial effect of increasing insulin levels. However, the predominant effect of prolonged GH excess is to increase glucose levels despite an insulin increase, because GH induces a resistance to insulin in the peripheral tissues, inhibiting the uptake of glucose by muscle and adipose tissues.

Many of the effects of GH depend on a family of peptides called *insulin-like growth factors* (IGF), also called *somatomedins,* which are produced mainly by the liver. GH cannot directly produce bone growth; instead it acts indirectly by causing the liver to produce IGF. These peptides act on cartilage and bone to promote their growth. At least four insulin-like growth factors have been identified; of these, IGF-1 (somatomedin C) appears to be the more important in terms of growth, and it is the one that is usually measured in laboratory tests.[1] The IGFs have been sequenced and have structures that are similar to proinsulin. This undoubtedly explains the insulin-like activity of the IGF and the weak action of insulin on growth.

GH is carried unbound in the plasma and has a half-life of about 20 to 50 minutes. The secretion of GH is regulated by two hypothalamic hormones: growth hormone–releasing hormone (GH-RH), which increases GH release, and somatostatin, which inhibits GH release. Somatostatin is also produced by delta cells in the islets of Langerhans in the pancreas, where it influences glucagon and insulin release. These hypothalamic influences (*i.e.,* GH-RH and somatostatin) are tightly regulated by neural, metabolic, and hormonal factors. The secretion of GH fluctuates over a 24-hour period, with peak levels occurring 1 to 4 hours after onset of sleep (*i.e.,* during sleep stages 3 and 4). The nocturnal sleep bursts, which account for 70% of daily GH secretion, are greater in children than in adults.[3]

GH secretion is stimulated by hypoglycemia, fasting, starvation, increased blood levels of amino acids (particularly arginine), and stress conditions such as trauma, excitement and emotional stress, and heavy exercise. GH is inhibited by increased glucose levels, free fatty acid release, cortisol, and obesity. Impairment of secretion, leading to growth retardation, is not uncommon in children with severe emotional deprivation.

Short Stature

Short stature is a condition in which the attained height is well below the fifth percentile or linear growth is below normal for age and sex. Short stature, or growth retardation, has a variety of causes, including chromosomal abnormalities such as Turner's syndrome (see Chapter 4), GH deficiency, hypothyroidism, and panhypopituitarism. Other conditions known to cause short stature include protein-calorie malnutrition, chronic diseases such as renal failure and poorly controlled diabetes mellitus, malabsorption syndromes, and certain therapies such as corticosteroid administration. Emotional disturbances can lead to functional endocrine disorders causing psychosocial dwarfism. The causes of short stature are summarized in Chart 35–1.

Two forms of short stature, genetic short stature and constitutional short stature, are not disease states but variations from population norms. Genetically short children tend to be well proportioned and to have a height close to the mean height of their parents. *Constitutional short stature* is a term used to describe children (particularly boys) who have moderately short stature, thin build, delayed skeletal and sexual maturation, and absence of other causes of decreased growth.

Catch-up growth is a term used to describe an abnormally high growth rate that occurs as a child approaches normal height for age. It occurs after the initiation of therapy for GH deficiency and hypothyroidism and the correction of chronic diseases. *Psychosocial dwarfism* in-

CHART 35–1
Causes of Short Stature

Variants of Normal

Genetic short stature
Constitutional short stature

Endocrine Disorders

- Growth hormone deficiency
  - Primary growth hormone deficiency
    - Idiopathic growth hormone deficiency
    - Pituitary agenesis
  - Secondary growth hormone deficiency
    - Hypothalamic-pituitary tumors
    - Postcranial radiation
    - Head injuries
    - Brain infections
    - Hydrocephalus
  - Biologically inactive growth hormone production
- Hypothyroidism
- Diabetes mellitus in poor control
- Glucocorticoid excess
  - Endogenous (Cushing's disease)
  - Exogenous (glucocorticoid drug treatment)

Chronic Illness and Malnutrition

Renal failure
Nutritional deprivation
Malabsorption syndrome

Functional Endocrine Disorders

Psychosocial dwarfism

Chromosomal Disorders

Turner's syndrome

volves a functional hypopituitarism and is seen in some emotionally deprived children. These children usually present with poor growth, potbelly, and poor eating and drinking habits. Typically, there is a history of disturbed family relationships in which the child has been severely neglected or disciplined. Often, the neglect is confined to one child in the family. GH function usually returns to normal after the child is removed from the constraining environment. The diagnosis depends on improvement in behavior and catch-up growth. Family therapy is usually indicated, and foster care may be necessary.

Accurate measurement of height is an extremely important part of the physical examination of children. Completion of the developmental history and growth charts is essential. Growth curves and growth velocity studies are also needed. Diagnosis of short stature is not made on a single measurement but is based on actual height and on velocity of growth and parental height.

The diagnostic procedures for short stature include tests to exclude nonendocrine causes. If the cause is hormonal, extensive hormonal testing procedures are initiated. Usually, GH and IGF levels are determined. Tests can be performed using insulin (to induce hypoglycemia), levodopa, and arginine, all of which stimulate and evaluate GH reserve. Because administration of such agents can result in false-negative responses, two or more tests are usually performed. If a prompt rise in GH is realized, the child is considered normal. Levels of IGF usually reflect those of GH and may be used to indicate GH deficiency. Radiologic films are used to assess bone age, which is most often delayed. The size and shape of the sella turcica (*i.e.*, depression in the sphenoid bone that contains the pituitary gland) are studied to determine if a pituitary tumor exists. After the cause of short stature has been determined, treatment can be initiated.

There are several forms of GH deficiency. Children with idiopathic GH deficiency lack GH-RH but have adequate somatotropes, whereas children with pituitary tumors or agenesis of the pituitary lack somatotropes. The term *panhypopituitarism* refers to conditions that cause a deficiency of all of the anterior pituitary hormones. In a rare condition called *Laron-type dwarfism*, GH levels are normal or elevated, but there is a hereditary defect in IGF receptors. Congenital GH deficiency is associated with normal birth length, followed by a decrease in growth rate that can be identified by careful measurement during the first year and that becomes obvious by 1 to 2 years of age.[4] Persons with classic GH deficiency have normal intelligence, short stature, obesity with immature facial features, and some delay in skeletal maturation. Puberty is often delayed, and males with the disorder have microphallus, especially if the condition is accompanied by gonadotropin-releasing hormone (Gn-RH) deficiency. In the neonate, GH deficiency can lead to hypoglycemia and seizures; if adrenocorticotrophic hormone (ACTH) deficiency is also present, the hypoglycemia is often more severe. Acquired GH deficiency develops in later childhood; it may be caused by a hypothalamic-pituitary tumor, particularly if it is accompanied by other pituitary deficiencies.

When short stature is caused by a GH deficiency, GH replacement therapy is the treatment of choice. GH is species specific, and only human GH is effective in humans. GH was previously obtained from human cadaver pituitaries but now is produced by recombinant DNA technology and is available in adequate supply. In 1985, the National Hormone and Pituitary Program halted the distribution of human GH derived from cadaver pituitaries in the United States after receiving reports that three recipients died of Creutzfeldt-Jakob disease. The disease, which is caused by a neurotropic virus, was thought to be transmitted by cadaver GH preparations. GH is administered subcutaneously in multiple weekly doses during the period of active growth.

Children with short stature due to Turner's syndrome and chronic renal insufficiency are also treated with GH. GH therapy is considered for children with short stature but without GH deficiency.[5–7] Several studies suggest that short-term treatment with GH increases rate of growth in these children.[7] However, the effect of GH on adult height is not yet known, and the frequency of adverse effects is uncertain. There are concerns about misuse of the drug to produce additional growth in children with normal GH function who are of near-normal height. Guidelines for use of the hormone continue to be established.

There are two categories of GH deficiency in adults: those in whom GH deficiency was present in childhood and those who acquired a GH deficiency during adulthood, mainly as the result of hypopituitarism resulting from a pituitary tumor or its treatment.[8] A small number of persons with GH deficiency have been treated with GH, with significant improvement in overall functional status. GH levels decline with aging, and there has been interest in the effects of declining GH levels in the elderly. However, there has been no evidence that GH treatment increases the functional capacity in the elderly.

Tall Stature

Just as there are children who are short for their age and sex, there are also children who are tall for their age and sex. Normal variants of tall stature include genetic tall stature and constitutional tall stature. Children with exceptionally tall parents tend to be taller than children with short parents. The term *constitutional tall stature* is used to describe a child who is taller than his or her peers and is growing at a velocity that is within the normal range for bone age. Other causes of tall stature are genetic or chromosomal disorders such as Marfan's syndrome or XYY syndrome (see Chapter 4). Endocrine causes of tall stature include sexual precocity because of early onset of estrogen and androgen secretion and excessive GH.

Exceptionally tall children (*i.e.*, genetic tall stature and constitutional tall stature) can be treated with sex hormones—estrogens in girls and testosterone in boys—to effect early epiphyseal closure. Such treatment is undertaken only after full consideration of the risks involved. To be effective, such treatment must be instituted 3 to 4 years before expected epiphyseal fusion.

GH excess occurring before puberty and before the fusion of the epiphyses of the long bones results in *gigantism.* Excessive secretion of GH by somatotrope adenomas causes gigantism in the prepubertal child. It occurs when the epiphyses are not fused and high levels of IGF stimulate excessive skeletal growth. Fortunately, the condition is rare because of early recognition and treatment of the adenoma.

Isosexual Precocious Puberty

Precocious sexual development may be idiopathic or may be caused by gonadal, adrenal, or hypothalamic tumors. *Isosexual precocious puberty* is defined as early activation of the hypothalamic-pituitary-gonadal axis, resulting in the development of appropriate sexual characteristics and fertility. Sexual development is considered precocious and warrants investigation when it occurs before 8 years of age for girls and before 9 years of age for boys. Benign and malignant tumors of the central nervous system (CNS) can cause precocious puberty. These tumors are thought to remove the inhibitory influences normally exerted on the hypothalamus during childhood.[9] CNS tumors are found more often in boys with precocious puberty than in girls. In girls, most cases are idiopathic.

Diagnosis of precocious puberty is based on physical findings of early thelarche (*i.e.,* beginning of breast development), adrenarche (*i.e.,* beginning of augmented adrenal androgen production), and menarche (*i.e.,* beginning of menstrual function) in girls. The most common sign in boys is early genital enlargement. Radiologic findings may indicate advanced bone age. Persons with precocious puberty are usually tall for their age as children but are short as adults because of the early closure of the epiphyses. Computed tomography (CT) or magnetic resonance imaging (MRI) may be used to exclude intracranial lesions.

Depending on the cause of precocious puberty, the treatment may involve surgery, medication, or no treatment. The treatment of choice is administration of a long-acting Gn-RH agonist.[9] Constant levels of the hormone cause a decrease in pituitary responsiveness to Gn-RH, leading to decreased secretion of gonadotropic hormones and sex steroids. Parents often need education, support, and anticipatory guidance in dealing with their feelings and the child's physical needs and in relating to a child who appears older than his or her years.

Acromegaly

When GH excess occurs in adulthood or after the epiphyses of the long bones have fused, a condition known as *acromegaly* develops. Acromegaly is a chronic and debilitating disorder of body growth and metabolic derangements in the adult caused by excess levels of GH. The mean age at the time of diagnosis is about 40 for men and 45 for women.[10] Most cases of acromegaly are caused by pituitary adenoma.

The disorder usually has an insidious onset, and symptoms are often present for a considerable period before a diagnosis is made. When the production of excessive GH occurs after the epiphyses of the long bones have closed, as in the adult, the person cannot grow taller, but the soft tissues continue to grow. Enlargement of the small bones of the hands and feet and in the membranous bones of the face and skull results in a pronounced enlargement of the hands and feet, a broad and bulbous nose, a protruding lower jaw, and a slanting forehead (Fig. 35–1). The teeth become splayed, causing a disturbed bite and difficulty in chewing. The cartilaginous structures in the larynx and respiratory tract also become enlarged, resulting in a deepening of the voice and tendency to develop bronchitis. Vertebral changes often lead to kyphosis, or hunchback. Bone overgrowth often leads to arthralgias and degenerative arthritis of the spine, hips, and knees. Virtually every organ of the body is increased in size. Enlargement of the heart and accelerated atherosclerosis may lead to an early death.

The metabolic effects of excess levels of GH include alterations in fat and carbohydrate metabolism. Increased levels of GH have a diabetogenic effect. GH acts as an insulin antagonist; in excess, it decreases carbohydrate use and impairs glucose uptake into cells. This leads to glucose intolerance, which stimulates the beta cells of the pancreas to produce additional insulin. GH also enhances the ability of the beta cells to respond to

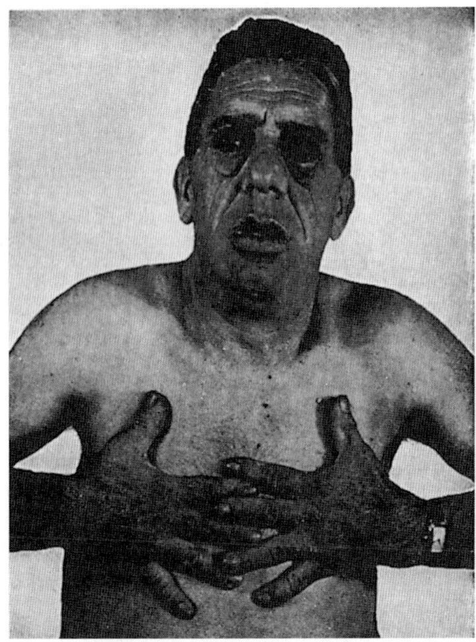

Figure 35–1
Acromegaly, showing protrusion of the lower jaw, heavy lips, and "spade" hands.

insulinogenic stimuli. Long-term elevation of GH results in overstimulation of the beta cells, causing them to "burn out" and predisposing to development of diabetes mellitus. Impaired glucose tolerance occurs in as many as 50% to 70% of persons with acromegaly; overt diabetes mellitus develops in a small number of these.[3]

The pituitary gland is located in the pituitary fossa of the sphenoid bone (*i.e.*, sella turcica), which lies directly below the optic nerve. Almost all persons with acromegaly have a recognizable adenohypophysial tumor. Enlargement of the pituitary gland eventually causes erosion of the surrounding bone, and because of its location, this can lead to headaches, visual field defects resulting from compression of the optic nerve, and palsies of cranial nerves III, IV, and VI. Compression of other pituitary structures can cause secondary hypothyroidism, hypogonadism, and adrenal insufficiency. Other manifestations include excessive sweating with an unpleasant odor, oily skin, heat intolerance, moderate weight gain, muscle weakness and fatigue, menstrual irregularities, and decreased libido. Hypertension is relatively common. Paresthesias may develop because of nerve entrapment and compression caused by excess soft tissue and accumulation of subcutaneous fluid.

Acromegaly often develops insidiously, and only a small number of persons (about 13%) seek medical care because of changes in appearance.[10] The diagnosis of acromegaly is facilitated by the typical features of the disorder: enlargement of the hands and feet and coarsening of facial features. Laboratory tests to detect elevated levels of GH not suppressed by a glucose load are used to confirm the diagnosis. CT and MRI scans can detect and localize the pituitary lesions. Because most of the effects of GH are mediated by IGF-1, IGF-1 levels may provide information about disease activity.

The goals of treatment in acromegaly are rapid normalization of GH to prevent or reverse progression of the disorder; prevention or reversal of the pressure effects of the tumor on structures surrounding the sella turcica; and preservation or restoration of normal pituitary function. Pituitary tumors can be removed surgically using the transsphenoidal approach, or if that is not possible, a transfrontal craniotomy.[11] Radiation therapy may be used, but GH levels do not return to normal for several years after therapy. Radiation therapy also significantly increases the risk of hypopituitarism, hypothyroidism, hypoadrenalism, and hypogonadism.

Octreotide acetate, a long-acting analogue of somatostatin, has been effective in the medical management of acromegaly. However, the medication must be given subcutaneously three times each week for effective dosing. Bromocriptine, a long-acting dopamine antagonist, reduces GH levels and has been used with some success in the medical management of acromegaly. However, high doses are often required, and side effects may be troublesome.

In summary, a number of hormones are essential for normal body growth and maturation, including GH, insulin, thyroid hormone, and androgens. GH exerts its growth effects through a group of IGFs. GH also exerts an effect on metabolism and is produced in the adult and in the child. Its metabolic effects include a decrease in peripheral use of carbohydrates and an increased mobilization and use of fatty acids.

In children, alterations in growth include short stature, isosexual precocious puberty, and tall stature. Short stature is a condition in which the attained height is well below the fifth percentile or the linear growth velocity is below normal for a child's age or sex. Short stature can occur as a variant of normal growth (*i.e.*, genetic short stature or constitutional short stature) or as the result of endocrine disorders, chronic illness, malnutrition, emotional disturbances, or chromosomal disorders. Short stature resulting from GH deficiency can be treated with human GH preparations. Isosexual precocious puberty defines a condition of early activation of hypothalamic-pituitary-gonadal axis (*i.e.*, before 8 years of age in girls and 10 years of age in boys), resulting in the development of appropriate sexual characteristics and fertility. It causes tall stature during childhood but results in short stature in adulthood because of the early closure of the epiphyses. Tall stature describes the condition in which children are tall for their age and sex. It can occur as a variant of normal growth (*i.e.*, genetic tall stature or constitutional tall stature) or as the result of a chromosomal abnormality or GH excess. GH excess in adults results in acromegaly, which involves proliferation of bone, cartilage, and soft tissue along with the metabolic effects of excessive hormone levels.

Thyroid Disorders

After you have completed this section of the chapter, you should be able to meet the following objectives:

- Characterize the synthesis, transport, and regulation of thyroid hormone
- Diagram the hypothalamic-pituitary-thyroid feedback system
- Describe tests in diagnosis and management of thyroid disorders
- Relate the functions of thyroid hormone to hypothyroidism and hyperthyroidism
- Describe the effects of congenital hypothyroidism
- Characterize the manifestations and treatment of myxedematous coma and thyroid storm

Control of Thyroid Function

The thyroid gland is a shield-shaped structure located immediately below the larynx in the anterior middle portion of the neck. The thyroid gland is composed of a large number of tiny saclike structures called follicles

(Fig. 35–2). These are the functional cells of the thyroid. Each follicle is formed by a single layer of epithelial (follicular) cells and is filled with a secretory substance called *colloid,* which consists largely of a glycoprotein-iodine complex called *thyroglobulin.*

The thyroglobulin that fills the thyroid follicles is a large glycoprotein molecule that contains 140 tyrosine amino acids. In the process of thyroid synthesis, iodine is attached to these tyrosine amino acids. Both thyroglobulin and iodide (I^-) are secreted into the colloid of the follicle by the follicular cells.

The thyroid is remarkably efficient in its use of iodide. A daily absorption of 100 to 200 μg of dietary iodide is sufficient to form normal quantities of thyroid hormone. In the process of removing iodide from the blood and storing it for future use, iodide is pumped into the follicular cells against a concentration gradient. As a result, the concentration of iodide within the normal thyroid gland is about 40 times that in the blood.

Once inside the follicle, most of the iodide is oxidized by the enzyme peroxidase in a reaction that facilitates combination with a tyrosine molecule to form *monoiodotyrosine* and then *diiodotyrosine* (Fig. 35–3). In time, two diiodotyrosine residues become coupled to form *thyroxine* (T_4), or a monoiodotyrosine and a diiodotyrosine become coupled to form *triiodothyronine* (T_3). Only T_4 (90%) and T_3 (10%) are secreted into the circulation. There is evidence that T_3 is the active form of the hormone and that T_4 is converted to T_3 before it can act physiologically.

Thyroid hormones are bound to thyroid-binding globulin and other plasma proteins for transport in the blood. Only the free hormone enters cells and regulates the pituitary feedback mechanism. Protein-bound thyroid hormone forms a large reservoir that is slowly drawn on as free thyroid hormone is needed. There are three major thyroid-binding proteins: thyroid hormone–binding globulin (TBG), thyroxine-binding prealbumin (TBPA), and albumin. More than 99% of T_4 and T_3 are carried in the bound form. TBG carries about 70% of T_4 and T_3; TBPA binds about 10% of circulating T_4 and lesser amounts of T_3; and albumin binds about 15% of circulating T_4 and T_3.[12]

A number of disease conditions and pharmacologic agents can decrease the amount of binding protein in the plasma or influence the binding of hormone. Congenital TBG deficiency is an X-linked trait that occurs in 1 of every 2500 live births.[12] Corticosteroid medications and systemic disease conditions such as protein malnutrition, nephrotic syndrome, and cirrhosis decrease TBG concentrations. Medications such as phenytoin, salicylates, and diazepam can affect the binding of thyroid hormone to normal concentrations of binding proteins.

The secretion of thyroid hormone is regulated by the hypothalamic-pituitary-thyroid feedback system (Fig. 35–4). In this system, thyrotropin-releasing hormone (TRH), which is produced by the hypothalamus, controls the release of thyroid-stimulating hormone (TSH) from the anterior pituitary gland. TSH increases the overall activity of the thyroid gland by increasing the thyroglobulin breakdown and release of thyroid hormone from follicles into the bloodstream, activating the iodide pump, increasing the oxidation of iodide and the

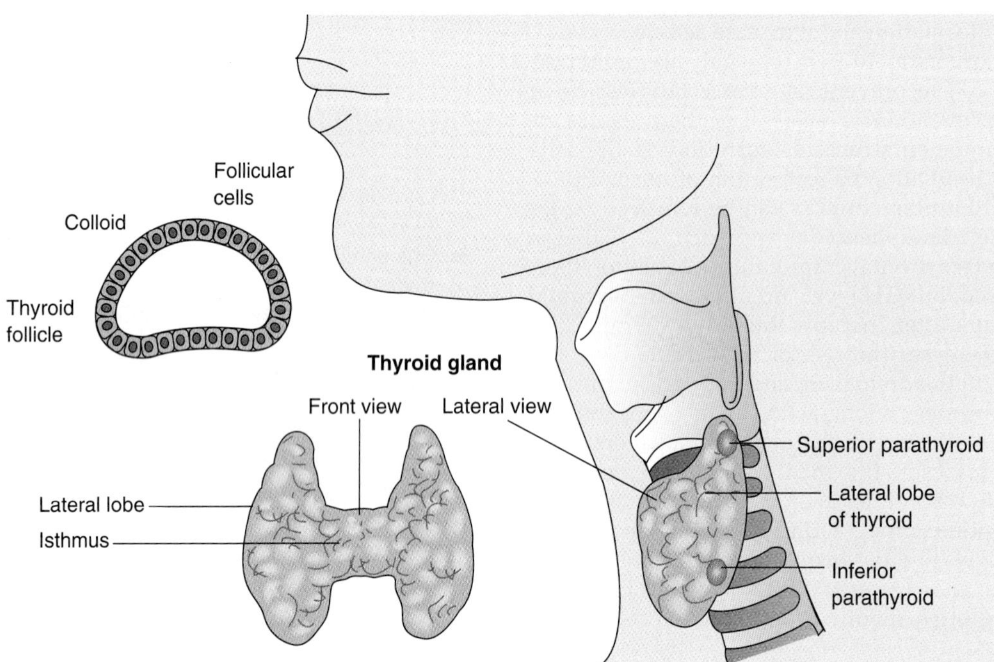

Figure 35–2
The thyroid gland and the follicular structure.

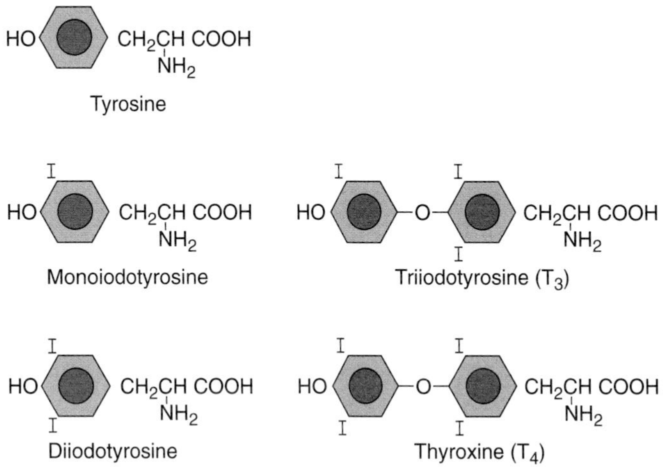

HO–(ring)–$CH_2CH(NH_2)COOH$
Tyrosine

Monoiodotyrosine

Triiodotyrosine (T_3)

Diiodotyrosine

Thyroxine (T_4)

Figure 35–3
Chemistry of thyroid hormone production.

coupling of iodide to tyrosine, and increasing the number and the size of the follicle cells. The effect of TSH on the release of thyroid hormones occurs within about 30 minutes, but the other effects require days or weeks.

Increased levels of thyroid hormone act in the feedback inhibition of TRH or TSH. High levels of iodide (*e.g.*, from iodide-containing cough syrup or kelp tablets) also cause a temporary decrease in thyroid activity that lasts for several weeks, probably through a direct inhibition of TSH on the thyroid. Cold exposure is one of the strongest stimuli for increased thyroid hormone production and is probably mediated through TRH from the hypothalamus. Various emotional reactions can also affect the output of TRH and TSH and therefore indirectly affect secretion of thyroid hormones.

Actions of Thyroid Hormone

All the major organs in the body are affected by altered levels of thyroid hormone. Thyroid hormone has two major functions; it increases metabolism and protein synthesis, and it is necessary for growth and development in children, including mental development and attainment of sexual maturity.

Metabolic Rate. Thyroid hormone increases the metabolism of all body tissues except the retina, spleen, testes, and lungs. The basal metabolic rate can increase by 60% to 100% above normal when large amounts of thyroxine are present.[1] As a result of this higher metabolism, the rate of glucose, fat, and protein use increases. Lipids are mobilized from adipose tissue, and the

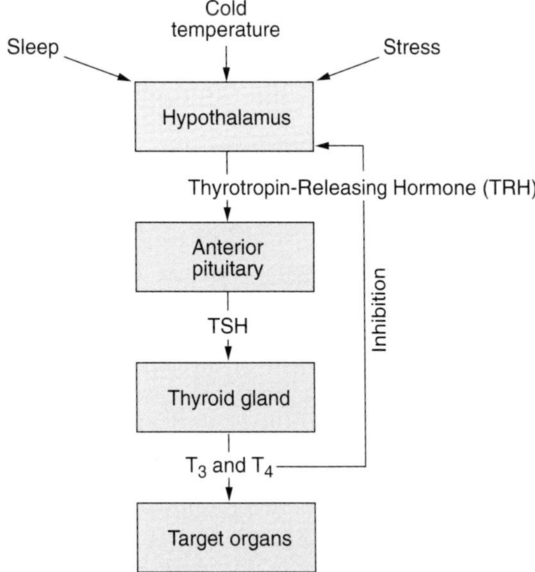

Figure 35–4
The hypothalamic–pituitary–thyroid feedback system, which regulates the body levels of thyroid hormone.

catabolism of cholesterol by the liver is increased. Blood levels of cholesterol are decreased in hyperthyroidism and increased in hypothyroidism. Muscle proteins are broken down and used as fuel, probably accounting for some of the muscle fatigue that occurs with hyperthyroidism. The absorption of glucose from the gastrointestinal tract is increased. Because vitamins are essential parts of metabolic enzymes and coenzymes, an increase in metabolic rate "speeds up the use" of vitamins and tends to cause vitamin deficiency.

Cardiovascular Function. Cardiovascular and respiratory functions are strongly affected by thyroid function. With an increase in metabolism, there is a rise in oxygen consumption and production of metabolic end products, with an accompanying increase in vasodilatation. Blood flow to the skin, in particular, is augmented as a means of dissipating the body heat that results from the higher metabolism. Blood volume, cardiac output, and ventilation are all increased as a means of maintaining blood flow and oxygen delivery to body tissues. Heart rate and cardiac contractility are enhanced as a means of maintaining the needed cardiac output. On the other hand, blood pressure is likely to change little, because the increase in vasodilatation tends to offset the increase in cardiac output.

Gastrointestinal Function. Thyroid hormone enhances gastrointestinal function, causing an increase in motility and production of gastrointestinal secretions that often results in diarrhea. An increase in appetite and food intake accompanies the higher metabolic rate that occurs with increased thyroid hormone levels. At the same time, weight loss occurs because of the increased use of calories.

Neuromuscular Effects. Thyroid hormone produces marked effects on neural control of muscle function and tone. Slight elevations in hormone levels cause skeletal muscles to react more vigorously, and a drop in hormone levels causes muscles to react more sluggishly. In the hyperthyroid state, a fine muscle tremor is present. The cause of this tremor is unknown, but it may represent an increased sensitivity of the neural synapses in the spinal cord that control muscle tone.

In the infant, thyroid hormone is necessary for normal brain development. The hormone enhances cerebration; in the hyperstate, it causes extreme nervousness, anxiety, and difficulty in sleeping.

Evidence suggests a strong interaction between thyroid hormone and the sympathetic nervous system. Many of the signs and symptoms of hyperthyroidism suggest overactivity of the sympathetic division of the autonomic nervous system, such as tachycardia, palpitations, and sweating. Tremor, restlessness, anxiety, and diarrhea also may reflect autonomic nervous system imbalances. Drugs that block sympathetic activity have proved to be valuable adjuncts in the treatment of hyperthyroidism because of their ability to relieve some of these undesirable symptoms.

Tests of Thyroid Function

Various tests aid in the diagnosis of thyroid disorders. Measures of T_3, T_4, and TSH have been made available through immunoassay methods. The free T_4 test measures the unbound portion of thyroxin that is free to enter cells to produce its effects. The resin uptake test is an inverse test of thyroid-binding globulin. The test involves adding radiolabeled T_3 or T_4 to a serum sample and allowing it to compete with the T_3 or T_4 in the sample for binding sites on the thyroid-binding globulin. The mixture is then added to a thyroid hormone–binding resin and the resin assayed for uptake of the labeled T_3 or T_4. A high resin test indicates that the serum sample contains low amounts of thyroid-binding globulin or high thyroxine levels. TSH levels are used to differentiate between primary and secondary thyroid disorders. T_3, T_4, and free T_4 levels are low in primary hypothyroidism, and the TSH level is elevated.[13]

The radioiodine (^{123}I) uptake test measures the ability of the thyroid gland to remove and concentrate iodine from the blood. Thyroid scans (*i.e.*, ^{123}I, ^{99m}Tc-pertechnetate) can be used to detect thyroid nodules and determine the functional activity of the thyroid gland. Ultrasonography can be used to differentiate cystic from solid thyroid lesions, and CT and MRI scans are used to demonstrate tracheal compression or impingement on other neighboring structures.

Alterations in Thyroid Function

An alteration in thyroid function can represent a hypofunctional or a hyperfunctional state. The manifestations of these two altered states are summarized in Table 35–1. Disorders of the thyroid may represent a congenital defect in thyroid development, or they may develop later in life, with a gradual or sudden onset.

Goiter is an increase in the size of the thyroid gland. It can occur in hypothyroid, euthyroid, and hyperthyroid states. Goiters may be diffuse, involving the entire gland without evidence of nodularity, or they may contain nodules. Diffuse goiters usually become nodular. Goiters may be toxic, producing signs of extreme hyperthyroidism, or *thyrotoxicosis*, or they may be nontoxic. Diffuse nontoxic and multinodular goiters are the result of compensatory hypertrophy and hyperplasia of follicular epithelium from some derangement that impairs thyroid hormone output.

The degree of thyroid enlargement is usually proportional to the extent and duration of thyroid deficiency. Multinodular goiters produce the largest thyroid enlargements and are often associated with thyrotoxicosis. When sufficiently enlarged, they may compress the esophagus and trachea, causing difficulty in swallowing, a choking sensation, and inspiratory stridor. Such lesions may also compress the superior vena cava, producing distention of the veins of the neck and upper

TABLE 35-1 Manifestations of Hypothyroid and Hyperthyroid States

Level of Organization	Hypothyroidism	Hyperthyroidism
Basal metabolic rate	Decreased	Increased
Sensitivity to catecholamines	Decreased	Increased
General features	Myxedematous features	Exophthalmos
	Deep voice	Lid lag
	Impaired growth (child)	Decreased blinking
Blood cholesterol levels	Increased	Decreased
General behavior	Mental retardation (infant)	Restlessness, irritability, anxiety
	Mental and physical sluggishness	Hyperkinesis
	Somnolence	Wakefulness
Cardiovascular function	Decreased cardiac output	Increased cardiac output
	Bradycardia	Tachycardia and palpitations
Gastrointestinal function	Constipation	Diarrhea
	Decreased appetite	Increased appetite
Respiratory function	Hypoventilation	Dyspnea
Muscle tone and reflexes	Decreased	Increased, with tremor and fibrillatory twitching
Temperature tolerance	Cold intolerance	Heat intolerance
Skin and hair	Decreased sweating	Increased sweating
	Coarse and dry skin and hair	Thin and silky skin and hair
Weight	Gain	Loss

extremities, edema of the eyelids and conjunctiva, and syncope with coughing.

Hypothyroidism

Hypothyroidism can occur as a congenital or an acquired defect. The absence of thyroid function at birth is called *cretinism*. When the condition occurs later in life, it is called *myxedema*. The term *cretin* hardly seems appropriate for describing the normally developing infant in whom replacement thyroid hormone therapy was instituted shortly after birth.

Congenital Hypothyroidism

Congenital hypothyroidism is a common cause of preventable mental retardation. It affects about 1 of 4000 infants.[14] Hypothyroidism in the infant may result from a congenital lack of the thyroid gland or from abnormal biosynthesis of thyroid hormone or deficient TSH secretion. With congenital lack of the thyroid gland, the infant usually appears normal and functions normally at birth, because hormones have been supplied in utero by the mother.

Thyroid hormone is essential for normal brain development and growth, almost half of which occurs during the first 6 months of life. If untreated, congenital hypothyroidism causes mental retardation and impairs growth. Long-term studies show that closely monitored T_4 supplementation begun in the first 6 weeks of life results in normal intelligence.[15,16] Fortunately, neonatal screening tests have been instituted to detect congenital hypothyroidism during early infancy. Screening is usually done in the hospital nursery. In this test, a drop of blood is taken from the infant's heel and analyzed for T_4 and TSH.

Transient congenital hypothyroidism has become more frequently recognized since the introduction of neonatal screening.[16] It is characterized by high TSH levels and low thyroid hormone levels. The fetal and infant thyroids are sensitive to iodine excess. Iodine crosses the placenta and mammary glands and is readily absorbed by infant skin. Transient hypothyroidism may be caused by maternal ingestion of substances such as potassium iodide for asthma, povidone-iodine used as a disinfectant (*i.e.,* vaginal douche or skin disinfectant, in the nursery). The use of iodine-containing radiographic contrast media may be another cause of excess iodine exposure. Antithyroid drugs such as propylthiouracil, methimazole, and carbimazole also cross the placenta and block fetal thyroid function.

Congenital hypothyroidism is treated by hormone replacement. Evidence indicates that it is important to normalize T_4 levels as rapidly as possible, because a delay is accompanied by poorer psychomotor and mental development. Dosage levels are adjusted as the child grows.[9] Infants with transient hypothyroidism can usually have the replacement therapy withdrawn at 6 to 12 months. When early and adequate treatment regimens are followed, the risk of mental retardation in infants detected by screening programs is essentially nonexistent.[9]

Myxedema

When hypothyroidism occurs in older children or adults, it is called *myxedema.* Myxedema implies the presence of a nonpitting mucous type of edema caused by an accumulation of a hydrophilic mucopolysaccharide substance in the connective tissues throughout the body. The hypothyroid state may be mild, with only a few signs and symptoms, or it may progress to a life-threatening condition called *myxedematous coma.* It can result from destruction or dysfunction of the thyroid gland (*i.e.,* primary hypothyroidism), or it can be a secondary disorder caused by impaired hypothalamic or pituitary function.

Primary hypothyroidism is much more common than secondary hypothyroidism. It may result from thyroidectomy (*i.e.,* surgical removal) or ablation of the gland with radiation. Certain goitrogenic agents, such as lithium carbonate (*i.e.,* used in the treatment of manic-depressive states) and the antithyroid drugs propylthiouracil and methimazole in continuous dosage can block hormone synthesis and produce hypothyroidism with goiter. Large amounts of iodine (*i.e.,* ingestion of kelp tablets or iodide-containing cough syrups or administration of iodide-containing radiographic contrast media) can also block thyroid hormone production and cause goiter, particularly in persons with autoimmune thyroid disease. Iodine deficiency, which can cause goiter and hypothyroidism, is rare in the United States because of the widespread use of iodized salt and other iodide sources.

The most common cause of hypothyroidism is *Hashimoto's thyroiditis,* an autoimmune disorder in which the thyroid gland may be totally destroyed by an immunologic process. It is the major cause of goiter and hypothyroidism in children. Hashimoto's thyroiditis is predominantly a disease of women, with a female-to-male ratio of 5:1.[17] The course of the disease varies. At the onset, only a goiter may be present. In time, hypothyroidism usually becomes evident. Although the disorder generally causes hypothyroidism, a hyperthyroid state may develop midcourse in the disease. The transient hyperthyroid state is caused by leakage of preformed thyroid hormone from damaged cells of the gland.

Myxedema affects almost all of the organ systems in the body. The manifestations of the disorder are largely related to two factors: the hypometabolic state resulting from thyroid hormone deficiency and myxedematous involvement of body tissues. Although the myxedema is most obvious in the face and other superficial parts, it also affects many of the body organs and is responsible for many of the manifestations of the hypothyroid state (Fig. 35–5).

The hypometabolic state associated with myxedema is characterized by a gradual onset of weakness and fatigue, a tendency to gain weight despite a loss of appetite, and cold intolerance. As the condition progresses, the skin becomes dry and rough and acquires a pale yellowish cast, which primarily results from carotene deposition, and the hair becomes coarse and brittle. There is loss of the lateral one third of the eyebrows. Gastrointestinal motility is decreased, producing constipation, flatulence, and abdominal distention. Nervous system involvement is manifested in mental dullness, lethargy, and impaired memory.

As a result of myxedematous fluid accumulation, the face takes on a characteristic puffy look, especially around the eyes. The tongue is enlarged, and the voice is hoarse and husky. Myxedematous fluid can collect in the interstitial spaces of almost any organ system. Pericardial or pleural effusion may develop. Mucopolysaccharide deposits in the heart cause generalized cardiac dilatation, bradycardia, and other signs of altered cardiac function. The signs and symptoms of hypothyroidism are summarized in Table 35–1.

Diagnosis of hypothyroidism is based on history, physical examination, and laboratory tests. A low serum

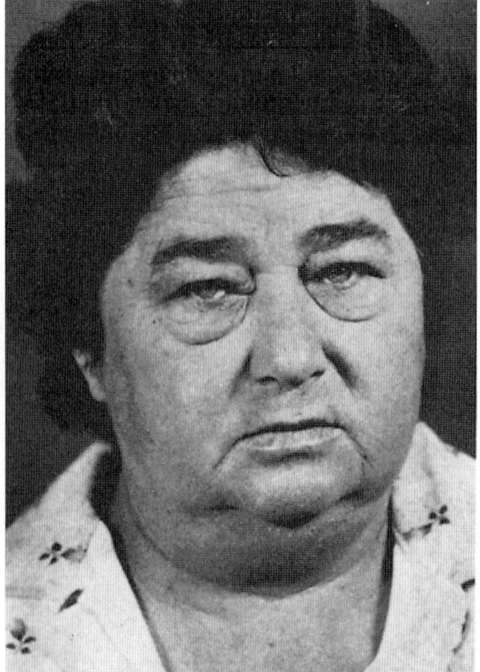

Figure 35–5
Patient with myxedema. (Courtesy of Dr. Herbert Langford. (From Guyton A. [1981]. *Medical physiology* [6th ed., p. 941]. Philadelphia: W.B. Saunders. Reprinted by permission)

T_4, low resin T_3, and elevated TSH levels are characteristic of primary hypothyroidism. The tests for antithyroid antibodies may be done when Hashimoto's thyroiditis is suspected. In secondary hypothyroidism, a TRH stimulation test is helpful in differentiating pituitary from hypothalamic disease.

Hypothyroidism is treated by replacement therapy with synthetic preparations of T_3, T_4, or a mixture of T_3 and T_4. Thyroid hormones obtained from domestic animals are also available.

Myxedematous Coma

Myxedematous coma is a life-threatening, end-stage expression of hypothyroidism. It is characterized by coma, hypothermia, cardiovascular collapse, hypoventilation, and severe metabolic disorders that include hyponatremia, hypoglycemia, and lactic acidosis. It occurs most often in elderly women who have chronic hypothyroidism from a spectrum of causes.[18] The fact that it occurs more frequently in winter months suggests that cold exposure may be a precipitating factor. The severely hypothyroid person is unable to metabolize sedatives, analgesics, and anesthetic drugs, and buildup of these agents may precipitate coma.

Treatment includes aggressive management of precipitating factors; supportive therapy such as management of cardiorespiratory status, hyponatremia, and hypoglycemia; and thyroid replacement therapy. Prevention is preferable to treatment and entails special attention to high-risk populations, such as women with a history of Hashimoto's thyroiditis. These persons should be informed about the signs and symptoms of severe hypothyroidism and the need for early medical treatment.

Hyperthyroidism

Hyperthyroidism, or *thyrotoxicosis*, results from excessive delivery of thyroid hormone to the peripheral tissue. The most common cause of hyperthyroidism is Graves' disease, which is accompanied by exophthalmos (*i.e.*, bulging of the eyeballs) and goiter. Other causes of hyperthyroidism are multinodular goiter, adenoma of the thyroid, and occasionally, ingestion of an overdose of thyroid hormone. Thyroid crisis, or storm, is an acutely exaggerated manifestation of the hyperthyroid state.

Many of the manifestations of hyperthyroidism are related to the increase in oxygen consumption and the increased use of metabolic fuels associated with the hypermetabolic state and to the increase in sympathetic nervous system activity that occurs. The fact that many of the signs and symptoms of hyperthyroidism resemble those of excessive sympathetic nervous system activity suggests that the thyroid hormone may heighten the sensitivity of the body to the catecholamines or that thyroid hormone may act as a pseudocatecholamine. With the hypermetabolic state, there are frequent complaints of nervousness, irritability, and fatigability. Weight loss is common despite a large appetite. Other manifestations include tachycardia, palpitations, shortness of breath, excessive sweating, muscle cramps, and heat intolerance. The person appears restless and has a fine muscle tremor. Even in persons without exophthalmos, there is an abnormal retraction of the eyelids and infrequent blinking such that they appear to be staring. The hair and skin are usually thin and have a silky appearance. The signs and symptoms of hyperthyroidism are summarized in Table 35–1.

The treatment of hyperthyroidism is directed toward reducing the level of thyroid hormone. This can be accomplished with eradication of the gland with radioactive iodine, through surgical removal of part or all of the thyroid gland, or the use of drugs that decrease thyroid function and thereby the effect of the thyroid hormone on the peripheral tissues. Eradication of the thyroid with radioactive iodine is used more frequently than surgery.[19] The β-adrenergic blocking drug propranolol is often administered to block the effects of the hyper~ thyroid state on sympathetic nervous system function. It is given in conjunction with other antithyroid drugs such as propylthiouracil and methimazole. These drugs prevent the thyroid gland from converting iodine to its organic (hormonal) form in the thyroid and block the conversion of T_4 to T_3 in the tissues. Iodinated contrast agents (iopanoic acid and ipodate sodium) may be given orally to block thyroid hormone synthesis and release as well as the peripheral conversion of T_4 and T_3. These agents may be used in treatment of thyroid storm or in persons who are intolerant of propylthiouracil or methimazole.

Graves' Disease

Graves' disease is a state of hyperthyroidism, goiter, and exophthalmos. The onset is usually between the ages of 20 and 40, and women are five times more likely to develop the disease than men. Graves' disease is an autoimmune disorder characterized by abnormal stimulation of the thyroid gland by thyroid-stimulating antibodies that act through the normal TSH receptors. It may be associated with other autoimmune disorders such as myasthenia gravis and pernicious anemia. The disease is associated with HLA-DR3 and HLA-B8, and a familial tendency is evident.

The exophthalmos is thought to result from a separate antibody called *exophthalmos-producing factor*, causing lymphocytic infiltration of the extraocular muscles. The ophthalmopathy of Graves' disease can cause severe eye problems, including paralysis of the extraocular muscles, involvement of the optic nerve with some visual loss, and corneal ulceration because the lids do not close over the protruding eyeball. The exophthalmos usually tends to stabilize after treatment of the hyperthyroidism. Unfortunately, not all of the ocular changes are reversible. Figure 35–6 depicts a woman with Graves' disease.

Thyroid Storm

Thyroid storm, or crisis, is an extreme and life threatening form of thyrotoxicosis, rarely seen today because of improved diagnosis and treatment methods. When it

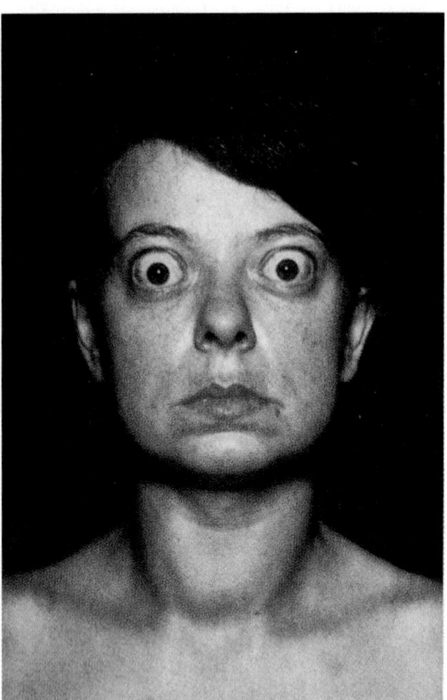

Figure 35–6
Graves' disease. A young woman with hyperthyroidism presented with a mass in the neck and exophthalmos.

does occur, it is seen most often in undiagnosed cases or in persons with hyperthyroidism who have not been adequately treated. It is often precipitated by stress such as an infection (usually respiratory), by diabetic ketoacidosis, by physical or emotional trauma, or by manipulation of a hyperactive thyroid gland during thyroidectomy. Thyroid storm is manifested by a very high fever, extreme cardiovascular effects (*i.e.*, tachycardia, congestive failure, and angina), and severe CNS effects (*i.e.*, agitation, restlessness, and delirium). The mortality rate is high.

Thyroid storm requires rapid diagnosis and implementation of treatment. Peripheral cooling is initiated with cold packs and a cooling mattress. For cooling to be effective, the shivering response must be prevented. General supportive measures to replace fluids, glucose, and electrolytes are essential during the hypermetabolic state. A β-adrenergic blocking drug, such as propranolol, is given to block the undesirable effects of thyroxine on cardiovascular function.[20] Glucocorticoids are used to correct the relative adrenal insufficiency resulting from the stress imposed by the hyperthyroid state and to inhibit the peripheral conversion of T_4 to T_3. Propylthiouracil or methimazole may be given to block thyroid synthesis. Aspirin increases the levels of free thyroid by displacing the hormones from their protein carriers and should not be used during thyroid storm.

In summary, thyroid hormones play a role in the metabolic process of almost all body cells and are necessary for normal physical and mental growth in the infant and small child. Alterations in thyroid function can manifest as a hypostate or a hyperstate. Hypothyroidism can occur as a congenital or an acquired defect. When it is present at birth, it is called cretinism; when it occurs later in life, it is called myxedema. Congenital hypothyroidism leads to mental retardation and impaired physical growth unless treatment is initiated during the first months of life. Hypothyroidism leads to a decrease in metabolic rate and an accumulation of a mucopolysaccharide substance within the intercellular spaces; this substance attracts water and causes a mucous type of edema called myxedema. Hyperthyroidism causes an increase in metabolic rate and alterations in body function similar to those produced by enhanced sympathetic nervous system activity. Graves' disease is characterized by the triad of hyperthyroidism, goiter, and exophthalmos.

Disorders of Adrenal Cortical Function

After you have completed this section of the chapter, you should be able to meet the following objectives:

- Describe the function of the adrenal cortical hormones and their feedback regulation
- State the underlying cause of the adrenogenital syndrome
- Relate the functions of the adrenal cortical hormones to Addison's disease (*i.e.*, adrenal insufficiency) and Cushing's syndrome (*i.e.*, cortisol excess)

Control of Adrenal Cortical Function

The adrenal glands are small, bilateral structures that weigh about 5 g each and lie retroperitoneally at the apex of each kidney (Fig. 35–7). The medulla, or inner, portion of the gland secretes epinephrine and norepinephrine and is part of the sympathetic nervous system.

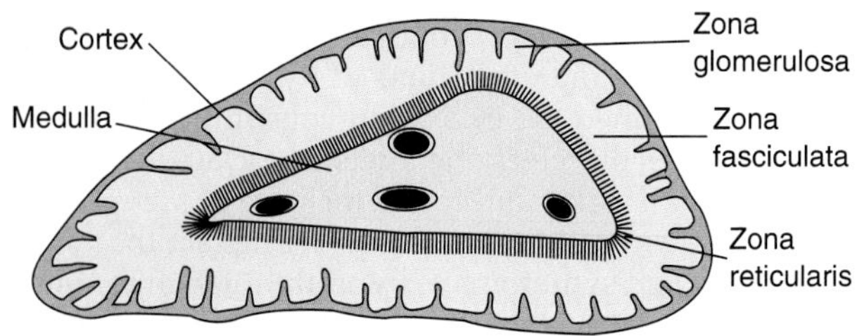

Figure 35–7
The adrenal gland, showing the medulla and the three layers of the cortex. The zona glomerulosa is the outer layer of the cortex and is primarily responsible for mineralocorticoid production. The middle layer, the zona fasciculata, and the inner layer, the zona reticularis, produce the glucocorticoids and the adrenal sex hormones.

The cortex forms the bulk of the adrenal gland and is responsible for secreting three types of hormones: the glucocorticoids, the mineralocorticoids, and the adrenal sex hormones. Because the sympathetic nervous system also secretes epinephrine and norepinephrine, adrenal medullary function is not essential for life, but adrenal cortical function is. The total loss of adrenal cortical function is fatal in 4 to 14 days if untreated.[1] This section of the chapter describes the synthesis and function of the adrenal cortical hormones and the effects of adrenal cortical insufficiency and excess.

Biosynthesis, Transport, and Metabolism

More than 30 hormones are produced by the adrenal gland. Of these hormones, aldosterone is the principal mineralocorticoid, cortisol (hydrocortisone) is the major glucocorticoid, and androgens are the chief sex hormones. All of the adrenal cortical hormones have a similar structure in that all are steroids and are synthesized from acetate and cholesterol; the glucocorticoid drugs are often called steroids. Each of the steps involved in the synthesis of the various hormones requires a specific enzyme (Fig. 35–8). The secretion of the glucocorticoids and the adrenal androgens are controlled by the ACTH secreted by the anterior pituitary gland.

Cortisol and the adrenal androgens are secreted in an unbound state and bind to plasma proteins for transport in the circulatory system. Cortisol binds largely to corticosteroid-binding globulin and to a lesser extent to albumin. It has been suggested that the pool of protein-bound hormones may extend the duration of their action by delaying metabolic clearance.[21]

The main site for metabolism of the adrenal cortical hormones is the liver, where they undergo a number of metabolic conversions before being conjugated and made water soluble. They are then eliminated in the urine or bile.

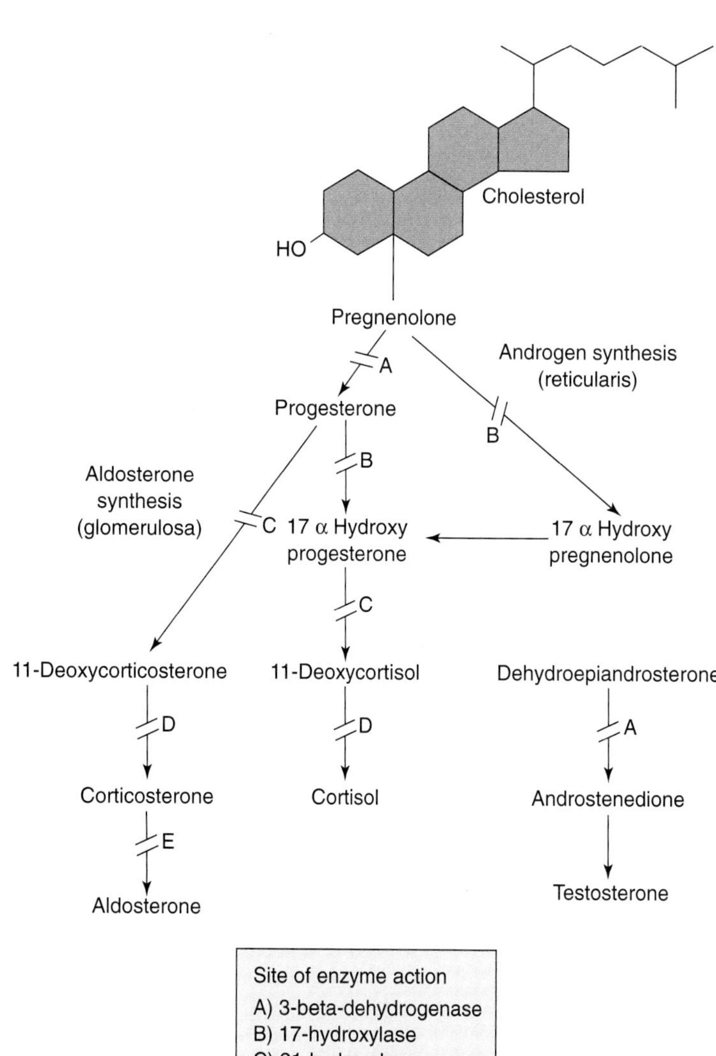

Figure 35–8
Predominant biosynthetic pathways of the adrenal cortex. Critical enzymes in the biosynthetic process include 11-beta-hydroxylase and 21-hydroxylase. A deficiency in one of these enzymes blocks the synthesis of these hormones dependent on that enzyme and routes the precursors into alternative pathways.

Adrenal Sex hormones

The adrenal sex hormones are synthesized primarily by the zona reticularis and the zona fasciculata of the cortex (see Fig. 35–8). These sex hormones probably exert little effect on normal sexual function. There is evidence, however, that the adrenal sex hormones contribute to the pubertal growth of body hair, particularly pubic and axillary hair in women. They may also play a role in the steroid hormone economy of the pregnant woman and the fetal-placental unit.

Mineralocorticoids

The mineralocorticoids play an essential role in regulating potassium and sodium levels and water balance. They are produced in the zona glomerulosa, the outer layer of cells of the adrenal cortex. Aldosterone secretion is regulated by the renin-angiotensin mechanism and by blood levels of potassium. Increased levels of aldosterone promote sodium retention by the distal tubules of the kidney while increasing urinary losses of potassium. The influence of aldosterone on fluid and electrolyte balance is discussed in Chapter 29.

Glucocorticoids

The glucocorticoid hormones, mainly cortisol, are synthesized in the zona fasciculata and the zona reticularis of the adrenal gland. The blood levels of these hormones are regulated by negative feedback mechanisms of the hypothalamic-pituitary-adrenal (HPA) system (Fig. 35–9). In the same manner that other pituitary hormones are controlled by releasing factors from the hypothalamus, the corticotropin-releasing factor (CRF) is important in controlling the release of ACTH. Cortisol levels increase as ACTH levels rise and decrease as ACTH levels fall. There is considerable diurnal variation in ACTH levels, which reach their peak in the early morning (around 6 to 8 AM) and decline as the day progresses. This appears to be due to rhythmic activity in the CNS, which causes bursts of CRF secretion and, in turn, ACTH secretion. This diurnal pattern is reversed in people who work during the night and sleep during the day. The rhythm may also be changed by physical and psychological stresses, endogenous depression, manic-depressive psychosis, and liver disease or other conditions that affect cortisol metabolism. One of the earliest signs of Cushing's syndrome, a disorder of cortisol excess, is the loss of diurnal varation in CRF and ACTH secretion.

The glucocorticoids perform a necessary function in response to stress and are essential for survival. When produced as part of the stress response, these hormones aid in regulating the metabolic functions of the body and in controlling the inflammatory response. The actions of cortisol are summarized in Table 35–2. Many of the antiinflammatory actions attributed to cortisol result from the administration of pharmacologic levels of the hormone.

Metabolic Effects. Cortisol stimulates glucose production by the liver, promotes protein breakdown, and causes mobilization of fatty acids. As body proteins are broken down, amino acids are mobilized and transported to the liver, where they are used in the production of glucose (*i.e.*, gluconeogenesis). Mobilization of fatty acids converts cell metabolism from the use of glucose for energy to the use of fatty acids instead. As glucose production by the liver rises and peripheral glucose use falls, a moderate resistance to insulin develops. In persons with diabetes and those who are diabetes prone, this has the effect of raising the blood sugar level.

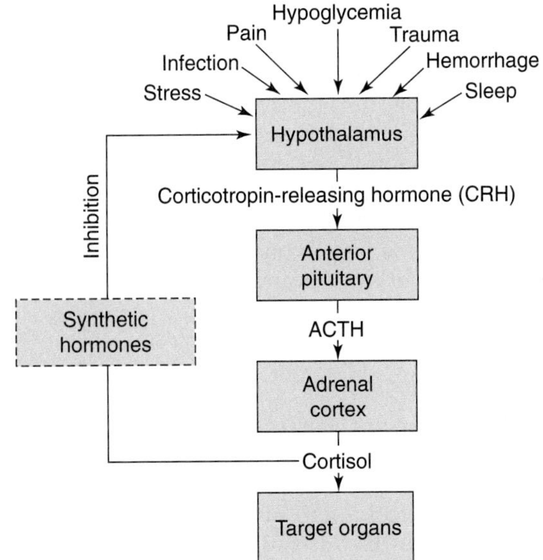

Figure 35–9
The hypothalamic–pituitary–adrenal (HPA) feedback system that regulates glucocorticoid (cortisol) levels. Cortisol release is regulated by ACTH. Stress exerts its effects on cortisol release through the HPA system and the corticotrophin-releasing factor (CRF), which controls the release of ACTH from the anterior pituitary gland. Increased cortisol levels incite a negative feedback inhibition of ACTH release. Pharmacologic doses of synthetic steroids inhibit ACTH release by way of the hypothalamic CRF.

Psychologic Effects. The glucocorticoid hormones appear to be involved directly or indirectly in emotional behavior. Receptors for these hormones have been identified in brain tissue, which suggests that they play a role in the regulation of behavior.[22] Persons treated with adrenal cortical hormones have displayed behavior ranging from mildly aberrant to psychotic.

Immunologic and Inflammatory Effects. Cortisol influences multiple aspects of immunologic function and inflammatory responsiveness. Large quantities of cortisol are required for an effective antiinflammatory action. This is achieved by the administration of pharmacologic rather than physiologic doses of synthetic cortisol. The increased cortisol blocks inflammation at an early stage by decreasing capillary permeability and stabilizing the lysosomal membranes so that inflammatory mediators are not released. Cortisol suppresses the immune response by reducing humoral and cell-mediated immunity. With this lessened inflammatory response comes a reduction in fever. During the healing

TABLE 35-2

Actions of Cortisol

Major Influence	Effect on Body
Glucose metabolism	Stimulates gluconeogenesis Decreases glucose use by the tissues
Protein metabolism	Increases breakdown of proteins Increases plasma protein levels
Fat metabolism	Increases mobilization of fatty acids Increases use of fatty acids
Antiinflammatory action (pharmacologic levels)	Stabilizes lysosomal membranes of the inflammatory cells, preventing the release of inflammatory mediators Decreases capillary permeability to prevent inflammatory edema Depresses phagocytosis by white blood cells to reduce the release of inflammatory mediators Suppresses the immune response Causes atrophy of lymphoid tissue Decreases eosinophils Decreases antibody formation Decreases the development of cell-mediated immunity Reduces fever Inhibits fibroblast activity
Psychic effect	Tends to contribute to emotional stability
Permissive effect	Facilitates the response of the tissues to humoral and neural influences, such as that of the catecholamines, during trauma and extreme stress

phase, cortisol suppresses fibroblast activity and thereby lessens scar formation. Cortisol also inhibits prostaglandin synthesis, which may account in large part for its antiinflammatory actions.

Suppression of Adrenal Function

A highly significant aspect of long-term therapy with pharmacologic preparations of the adrenal cortical hormones is adrenal insufficiency on withdrawal of the drugs. The deficiency results from suppression of the HPA system. Chronic suppression causes atrophy of the adrenal gland, and the abrupt withdrawal of drugs can cause acute adrenal insufficiency. Recovery to a state of normal adrenal function may be prolonged, requiring up to 12 months.

Tests of Adrenal Function

Several diagnostic tests can be sued to evaluate adrenal cortical function and the HPA system. Blood levels of cortisol, aldosterone, and ACTH can be measured using radioimmunoassay methods. A 24-hour urine specimen measures the excretion of 17-ketosteroids, 17-ketogenic steroids, and 17-hydroxycorticosteroids. These metabolic end products of the adrenal hormones and the male androgens provide information about alterations in the biosynthesis of the adrenal cortical hormones. Suppression and stimulation tests afford a means of assessing the state of the HPA feedback system. For example, a test dose of ACTH can be given to assess the response of the adrenal cortex to pituitary stimulation. Similarly, administration of dexamethasone, a synthetic glucocorticoid drug, provides a means of measuring negative feedback suppression of ACTH. Adrenal tumors and ectopic ACTH-producing tumors are generally unresponsive to ACTH suppression by dexamethasone. Metyrapone (Metopirone) blocks the final step in cortisol synthesis, resulting in the production of 11-dehydroxycortisol, which does not inhibit ACTH. This test measures the ability of the pituitary to release ACTH.

Congenital Adrenal Hyperplasia

Congenital adrenal hyperplasia (CAH) or the adrenogenital syndrome, describes a congenital disorder caused by an autosomal recessive trait in which a deficiency exists in any of the five enzymes necessary for the synthesis of cortisol. A common characteristic of all types of CAH is a defect in the synthesis of cortisol that results in increased levels of ACTH and adrenal hyperplasia. The increased levels of ACTH overstimulate the pathways for production of adrenal androgens. Mineralocorticoids may be produced in excessive or insufficient amounts, depending on the precise enzyme deficiency. Male and female infants are affected. Males are seldom diagnosed at birth, unless they have enlarged genitalia or lose salt and manifest adrenal crisis; in female infants, an increase in androgens is responsible for creating the virilization syndrome of ambiguous genitalia with an enlarged clitoris, fused labia, and urogenital sinus (Fig. 35–10). In male and female children, other secondary sex characteristics are normal, and fertility is unaffected if appropriate therapy is instituted.

The two most common enzyme deficiencies are the 21-hydroxylase and 11-β-hydroxylase deficiencies. The clinical manifestations of both deficiencies are largely determined by the functional properties of the steroid

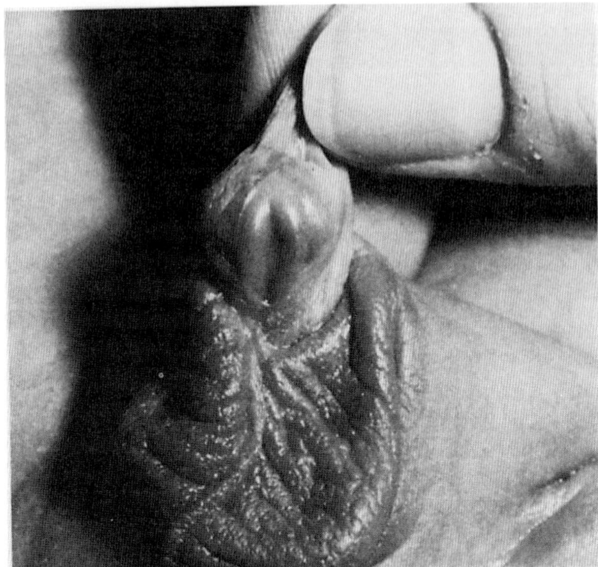

Figure 35–10
Female infant with congenital adrenal hyperplasia demonstrating virilization of the genitalia. Note the enlarged clitoris and the fused labia, which resembles a scrotal sac. (Hurwitz L.S. [1980]. Nursing implications of selected endocrine disorders. *Nursing Clinics of North America, 15*[3], 528. Reprinted with permission)

intermediates and the completeness of the block in the cortisol pathway.

A spectrum of 21-hydroxylase deficiency states exists, ranging from simple virilizing CAH to a complete salt-losing enzyme deficiency.[23] Simple virilizing CAH impairs the synthesis of cortisol, and steroid synthesis is shunted to androgen production. Persons with these deficiencies usually produce sufficient aldosterone or aldosterone intermediates to prevent signs and symptoms of mineralocorticoid deficiency. The salt-losing form is accompanied by deficient production of aldosterone and its intermediates. This results in fluid and electrolyte disorders after the fifth day of life, including hyponatremia, hyperkalemia, vomiting, dehydration, and shock.

The 11-β-hydroxylase deficiency is rare and manifests a spectrum of severity. Affected persons have excessive androgen production and impaired conversion of 11-deoxycorticosterone to corticosterone. The overproduction of 11-deoxycorticosterone, which has mineralocorticoid activity, is responsible for the hypertension that accompanies this deficiency. Diagnosis of adrenogenital syndrome depends on the precise biochemical evaluation of metabolites in the cortisol pathway and on clinical signs and symptoms.

Medical treatment of adrenogenital syndrome includes oral or parenteral cortisol replacement. Fludrocortisone acetate, a mineralocorticoid, may also be given to children who are salt losers. Depending on the degree of virilization, reconstructive surgery during the first 2 years of life is indicated to reduce the size of the clitoris, separate the labia, and exteriorize the vagina. Surgery has provided excellent results and does not impair sexual function.

Adrenal Insufficiency

There are two forms of adrenal insufficiency: primary and secondary. Primary adrenal insufficiency, or Addison's disease, is caused by destruction of the adrenal gland. Secondary adrenal insufficiency results from a disorder of the HPA system.

Primary Adrenal Insufficiency

In 1855, Thomas Addison, an English physician, provided the first detailed clinical description of primary adrenal insufficiency, now called Addison's disease. Addison's disease is a relatively rare disorder in which all the layers of the adrenal cortex are destroyed. Autoimmune destruction is the most common cause of Addison's disease in the United States. Tuberculosis is an infrequent cause in the United States but common where tuberculosis is more prevalent. Rare causes include metastatic carcinoma, fungal infection (particularly histoplasmosis), cytomegalovirus, amyloid disease, and hemochromatosis. Bilateral adrenal hemorrhage may occur in persons taking anticoagulants, during open heart surgery, and during birth or major trauma. Adrenal insufficiency can be caused by acquired immuno-deficiency syndrome (AIDS), in which the adrenal gland is destroyed by a variety of opportunistic infectious agents.[24] The use of the term *Addison's disease* is reserved for adrenal insufficiency due to adrenocortical disease in which adrenocortical hormones are deficient and ACTH levels are elevated because of feedback stimulation.

Addison's disease, like insulin-dependent diabetes mellitus, is a chronic metabolic disorder that requires lifetime hormone replacement therapy. The adrenal cortex has a large reserve capacity, and the manifestations of adrenal insufficiency do not usually become apparent until about 90% of the gland has been destroyed.[10] These manifestations are primarily related to mineralocorticoid deficiency, glucocorticoid deficiency, and hyperpigmentation resulting from elevated ACTH levels. Although lack of the adrenal androgens exerts few effects in men because the testes produce these hormones, women have sparse axillary and pubic hair. The manifestations of adrenal insufficiency are summarized in Table 35–3.

Mineralocorticoid deficiency causes increased urinary losses of sodium, chloride, and water, along with decreased excretion of potassium. The result is hyponatremia, loss of extracellular fluid, decreased cardiac output, and hyperkalemia. There may be an abnormal appetite for salt. Orthostatic hypotension is common. Dehydration, weakness, and fatigue are common early symptoms. If loss of sodium and water is extreme, cardiovascular collapse and shock ensue. Because of a lack of glucocorticoids, the person with Addison's disease has poor tolerance to stress. This deficiency causes hypoglycemia, lethargy, weakness, fever, and gastroin-

TABLE 35-3

Manifestations of Adrenal Cortical Insufficiency and Excess

Parameter	Adrenal Cortical Insufficiency	Glucocorticoid Excess
Electrolytes	Hyponatremia* Hyperkalemia*	Hypokalemia
Fluids	Dehydration* (*e.g.*, elevated BUN)	Edema
Blood pressure	Hypotension* Shock* Orthostatic hypotension	Hypertension
Musculoskeletal	Muscle weakness* Fatigue*	Muscle wasting Fatigue
Hair and skin	Skin pigmentation	Easy bruisability Hirsutism, acne, and striae (abdomen and thighs)
Inflammatory response	Low resistance to trauma, infection, and stress	Decrease in eosinophils, lymphocytopenia
Gastrointestinal	Nausea, vomiting* Abdominal pain*	Possible gastrointestinal bleeding
Glucose metabolism	Hypoglycemia*	Impaired glucose tolerance Glycosuria Elevated blood sugar
Emotional	Depression and irritability	Emotional lability to psychosis
Other	Menstrual irregularity Decreased axillary and pubic hair in women	Oligomenorrhea Impotence in the male Centripetal obesity (moon face and buffalo hump)

*Occurs with acute adrenal insufficiency.

testinal symptoms such as anorexia, nausea, vomiting, and weight loss.

Hyperpigmentation results from elevated levels of ACTH. The skin looks bronzed or suntanned in exposed and unexposed areas, and the normal creases and pressure points tend to become especially dark. The gums and oral mucous membranes may become bluish black. This hyperpigmentation becomes more pronounced during periods of stress. The amino acid sequence of ACTH is strikingly similar to that of melanocyte-stimulating hormone; hyperpigmentation occurs in about 98% of persons with Addison's disease and is helpful in distinguishing the primary and secondary forms of adrenal insufficiency.

Secondary Adrenal Insufficiency

Secondary adrenal insufficiency can occur as the result of hypopituitarism or because the pituitary gland has been surgically removed. However, a far more common cause than either of these is the rapid withdrawal of glucocorticoids that have been administered therapeutically. These drugs suppress the HPA system, with resulting adrenal cortical atrophy and loss of cortisol production. This suppression continues long after drug therapy has been discontinued and can be critical during periods of stress or when surgery is performed.

Acute Adrenal Crisis

Acute adrenal crisis is a life-threatening situation. If Addison's disease is the underlying problem, exposure to even a minor illness or stress can precipitate nausea, vomiting, muscular weakness, hypotension, dehydration, and vascular collapse. The onset of adrenal crisis may be sudden, or it may progress over a period of several days. The symptoms may occur suddenly in children with salt-losing forms of the adrenogenital syndrome. Massive bilateral adrenal hemorrhage causes an acute fulminating form of adrenal insufficiency. Hemorrhage can be caused by meningococcal septicemia (*i.e.*, Waterhouse-Friderichsen syndrome), adrenal trauma, anticoagulant therapy, adrenal vein thrombosis, or adrenal metastases.

Adrenal insufficiency is treated with hormone replacement therapy that includes a combination of glucocorticoids and mineralocorticoids. For acute adrenal insufficiency, cortisol is given intravenously, followed by rapid infusion of saline and glucose. The daily regulation of the chronic phase of Addison's disease is usually accomplished with oral cortisol, and higher doses are given during periods of stress. Because persons with the disorder are likely to have episodes of hyponatremia and hypoglycemia, they need to have a regular schedule for meals and exercise.

Glucocorticoid Hormone Excess

The term *Cushing's syndrome* refers to the manifestations of hypercortisolism from any cause.[24,25] Three important forms of Cushing's syndrome result from excess glucocorticoid production by the body. One is a *pituitary form*, which results from excessive production of ACTH by a tumor of the pituitary gland; it accounts for about two thirds of the disease cases, and because this form of the disease was the one originally described by Cushing, it is called Cushing's disease. The second form is the *adrenal form,* caused by a benign or malignant adrenal tumor. The third form is *ectopic Cushing's,* caused by a nonpituitary ACTH-secreting tumor. Certain extrapituitary malignant tumors such as small cell carcinoma of the lung may secrete ACTH or, rarely, CRF and produce Cushing's syndrome. Cushing's syndrome can also result from long-term therapy with one of the potent pharmacologic preparations of glucocorticoids; this form is called *iatrogenic Cushing's syndrome.*

The major manifestations of Cushing's syndrome represent an exaggeration of the many actions of cortisol (see Table 35–3). Altered fat metabolism causes a peculiar deposition of fat characterized by a protruding abdomen; subclavicular fat pads or "buffalo hump" on the back; and a round, plethoric "moon face." There is muscle weakness, and the extremities are thin because of protein breakdown and muscle wasting. In advanced cases, the skin over the forearms and legs becomes thin, having the appearance of parchment. Purple striae, or stretch marks, from stretching of the catabolically weakened skin and subcutaneous tissues are distributed over the breast, thighs, and abdomen. Osteoporosis may develop because of destruction of bone proteins and alterations in calcium metabolism, resulting in back pain, compression fractures of the vertebrae, and rib fractures. As calcium is mobilized from bone, renal calculi may develop.

Derangements in glucose metabolism are found in about 75% of patients, with clinically overt diabetes mellitus occurring in about 20%.[17] The glucocorticoids possess mineralocorticoid properties; this causes hypokalemia as a result of excessive potassium excretion and hypertension resulting from sodium retention. Inflammatory and immune responses are inhibited, resulting in increased susceptibility to infection. Cortisol increases gastric acid secretion, which may provoke gastric ulceration and bleeding. An accompanying increase in androgen levels causes hirsutism, mild acne, and menstrual irregularities in women. Excess levels of the glucocorticoids may give rise to extreme emotional lability, ranging from mild euphoria and absence of normal fatigue to grossly psychotic behavior.

Diagnosis of Cushing's syndrome depends on the finding of cortisol hypersecretion. The determination of 24-hour excretion of cortisol in urine provides a reliable and practical index of cortisol secretions.[26] One of the prominent features of Cushing's syndrome is loss of the diurnal pattern of cortisol secretion. Cortisol determinations are often made on three blood samples: one taken in the morning, one in late afternoon or early evening, and a third drawn the following morning after a midnight dose of dexamethasone. Measurement of the plasma levels of ACTH, 24-hour urinary 17-ketosteroids, 17-ketogenic steroids, and 17-hydroxycorticosteroids and suppression or stimulation tests of the HPA system are often made. Skull x-ray films and intravenous pyelograms, which outline the shadows of the kidneys and adrenal glands, may be done. CT scans afford a means for locating adrenal or pituitary tumors.

Untreated, Cushing's syndrome produces serious morbidity and even death. The choice of surgery, irradiation, or pharmacologic treatment is largely determined by the cause of the hypercortisolism. The goal of treatment for Cushing's syndrome is to remove or correct the source of hypercortisolism without causing any permanent pituitary or adrenal damage. Transsphenoidal removal of a pituitary adenoma or a hemihypophysectomy is the preferred method of treatment for Cushing's disease. This allows removal of only the tumor rather than the entire pituitary gland. After successful removal, the person must receive cortisol replacement therapy for 6 to 12 months or until adrenal function returns. Patients may also receive pituitary irradiation therapy, but the full effects of treatment may not realized for 3 to 12 months.[26] Unilateral or bilateral adrenalectomy may be done in the case of adrenal adenoma. When possible, ectopic ACTH-producing tumors are removed. Pharmacologic agents that block steroid synthesis (*i.e.,* ketoconazole, metyrapone, and aminoglutethimide) may used to treat persons with ectopic tumors that cannot be resected.

In summary, the adrenal cortex produces three types of hormones: mineralocorticoids, glucocorticoids, and adrenal sex hormones. The mineralocorticoids along with the renin-angiotensin mechanism aid in controlling body levels of sodium and potassium. The glucocorticoids have antiinflammatory actions and aid in regulating glucose, protein, and fat metabolism during periods of stress. These hormones are under the control of the HPA system. The adrenal sex hormones exert little effect on daily control of body function, but they probably contribute to the development of body hair in women. The adrenal genital syndrome describes a genetic defect in the cortisol pathway resulting from a deficiency of one of the enzymes needed for its synthesis. Depending on the enzyme involved, the disorder causes virilization of female infants and, in some instances, fluid and electrolyte disturbances because of impaired mineralocorticoid synthesis.

Chronic adrenal insufficiency is called Addison's disease. It can be caused by destruction of the adrenal gland or by dysfunction of the HPA system. Adrenal insufficiency requires replacement therapy with cortical hormones. Acute adrenal insufficiency is a life-threatening situation.

Cushing's syndrome refers to the manifestations of excessive cortisol levels. This syndrome may be a result of pharmacologic doses of cortisol, a pituitary or adrenal tumor, or an ectopic tumor that produces ACTH. The clinical manifestations of Cushing's syndrome reflect the very high level of cortisol that is present.

REFERENCES

1. Guyton A. (1996). *Medical physiology* (9th ed., pp. 936–945, 957–969). Philadelphia: W.B. Saunders.

2. Ganong W.F. (1993). *Medical physiology* (16th ed., pp. 61–74, 287–301). Norwalk, CT: Appleton Lange.
3. Tyrell B.J., Findling J.W., Aron D.W. (1994). Hypothalamus and pituitary. In Greenspan F.S., Baxter J.D. (Ed.). *Basic and clinical endocrinology* (4th ed., pp. 64–87). Norwalk, CT: Appleton & Lange.
4. Styne D.M. (1994). Growth. In Greenspan F.S., Baxter J.D. (Ed.). *Basic and clinical endocrinology* (4th ed., pp. 128–157). Norwalk, CT: Appleton & Lange.
5. Neely E.K., Rosenfeld R.G. (1996). Use and abuse of human growth hormone. *Annual Review of Medicine* 45, 407–420.
6. Allen D.B., Blizzard R.M., Rosenfeld R.G. (1995). The use—and misuse—of growth hormone. *Patient Care* 29 (2), 41–57.
7. Cuttler L., Silvers J.B., Singh J., et al. (1996). Short stature and growth hormone therapy. *JAMA* 276 (7), 531–537.
8. Inzucchi S.E. (1997). Growth hormone in adults: Indications and implications. *Hospital Practice* 31 (1), 79–96.
9. Wheeler M.D., Styne D.M. (1990). Diagnosis and management of precocious puberty. *Pediatric Clinics of North America* 37, 1255–1271.
10. Melmed S. (1990). Acromegaly. *New England Journal of Medicine* 322, 966–977.
11. Romeo J.H. (1996). Hyper- and hypofunction of the anterior pituitary. *Nursing Clinics of North America* 31 (4), 769–778.
12. Greenspan F.S. (1994). The thyroid gland. In Greenspan F.S., Baxter J.D. (Ed.). *Basic and clinical endocrinology* (4th ed., pp. 160–216). Norwalk, CT: Appleton & Lange.
13. Hoekelman R.A. (1992). Screening for congenital hypothyroidism. *Pediatric Annals* 21 (6), 372–373.
14. Glorieux J., Dussault J.H., Morissette J., et al. (1985). Follow-up at ages 5 and 7 years on mental development in children with hypothyroidism detected in the Quebec Screening Program. *Journal of Pediatrics* 107, 913.
15. New England Congenital Hypothyroid Collaborative. (1985). Neonatal hypothyroid screening: Status of patients at 6 years of age. *Journal of Pediatrics* 107, 915.
16. Guters A. (1992). Congenital hypothyroidism. *Pediatric Annals* 21, 17–28.
17. Cotran R.S., Kumar V., Robbins S.L. (1994). *Pathologic basis of disease* (5th ed., pp. 1150–1153). Philadelphia: W.B. Saunders.
18. Gavin L.A. (1990). Thyroid crisis. *Medical Clinics of North America* 75, 179–193.
19. Hennessey J.V. (1996). Diagnosis and management of thyrotoxicosis. *American Family Physician* 54 (4), 1315–1324.
20. Franklyn J.A. (1994). The management of hyperthyroidism. *New England Journal of Medicine* 330 (24), 1731–1738.
21. Aron D.C., Tyrell B. (1994). Glucocorticoids and adrenal androgens. In Greenspan F.S., Baxter J.D. (Ed.). *Basic and clinical endocrinology* (4th ed., pp. 307–42). Norwalk, CT: Appleton & Lange.
22. McEwan B.S. (1978). Influences of the adrenocortical hormone on pituitary and brain function. *Monographs on Endocrinology* 12, 467.
23. Cutler G.B., Laue L. (1996). Congenital adrenal hyperplasia due to 21-hydroxylase deficiency. *New England Journal of Medicine* 323 (26), 1806–1813.
24. Oelker W. (1996). Adrenal insufficiency. *New England Journal of Medicine* 335 (16), 1206–1212.
25. Utiger R.D. (1997). Treatment, and retreatment of Cushing's disease. *New England Journal of Medicine* 336 (3), 215–217.
26. Orth D.N. (1995). Cushing's syndrome. *New England Journal of Medicine* 332 (12), 791–803.

ADDITIONAL READINGS

Bahn R.S., Heufelder A.E. (1993). Pathogenesis of Graves' ophthalmopathy. *New England Journal of Medicine* 329 (300), 1668–1674.

Brent G.A. (1994). The molecular basis of thyroid hormone action. *New England Journal of Medicine* 331 (13), 847–853.

Daylan C.M., Daniels G.H. (1996). Chronic autoimmune thyroiditis. *New England Journal of Medicine* 335 (2), 89–105.

Gumowski J., Loughran M. (1996). Diseases of the adrenal gland. *Nursing Clinics of North America* 31 (4), 747–768.

Rusterholtz A. (1996). Interpretation of diagnostic laboratory tests in selected endocrine disorders. *Nursing Clinics of North America* 31 (4), 715–724.

Strief M.M., Pachucki-Hyde L.C. (1996). Management of the patient with thyroid disease. *Nursing Clinics of North America* 31 (4), 779–796.

Winger J.M., Hornick T. (1996). Age-related changes in the endocrine system. *Nursing Clinics of North America* 31 (4), 827–844.

Toft A.D. (1994). Thyroxine therapy. *New England Journal of Medicine* 331 (3), 174–180.

CHAPTER 36

Diabetes Mellitus

Safak Guven and Julie Kuenzi

Diabetes mellitus is a chronic health problem affecting more than 16 million persons in the United States. The direct and indirect costs of diabetes are $2 billion per year (1992 data). The disease affects persons in all age groups and from all walks of life. It is more prevalent among African Americans (9.6%) and Hispanic Americans (10.9) compared with whites (6.2%).[1] The acute complications of diabetes are the most common causes of medical emergencies resulting from metabolic disease. Diabetes is the leading risk factor in coronary heart disease and stroke, and it is the leading cause of blindness, end-stage renal disease, and a major contributor to lower extremity amputations.

Hormonal Control of Blood Glucose

After you have completed this section of the chapter, you should be able to meet the following objectives:

- Characterize the actions of insulin with reference to glucose, fat, and protein metabolism
- Explain what is meant by a counterregulatory hormone and describe the actions of glucagon, epinephrine, growth hormone, and the adrenocortical hormones in regulation of blood glucose levels

The body uses glucose, fatty acids, and other substrates as fuel to satisfy its energy needs. Although the respiratory and circulatory systems combine efforts to furnish the body with the oxygen needed for metabolic purposes, it is the liver, in concert with the endocrine pancreas, that controls the body's fuel supply.

The pancreas is made up of two major tissue types: the acini and the islets of Langerhans (Fig. 36–1). The acini secrete digestive juices into the duodenum, and the islets of Langerhans secrete hormones into the blood. Each islet is composed of *beta cells* (β cells) that secrete insulin, *alpha cells* (α cells) that secrete glucagon, and *delta cells* that secrete somatostatin. Insulin lowers blood sugar concentration by facilitating the movement of glucose into body tissues. Glucagon maintains blood glucose by increasing the release of glucose from the liver into the blood. Somatostatin inhibits the release of insulin and glucagon. Somatostatin also decreases gastrointestinal activity after ingestion of food. By decreasing gastrointestinal activity, somatostatin is thought to extend the time during which food is absorbed into the blood, and by inhibiting

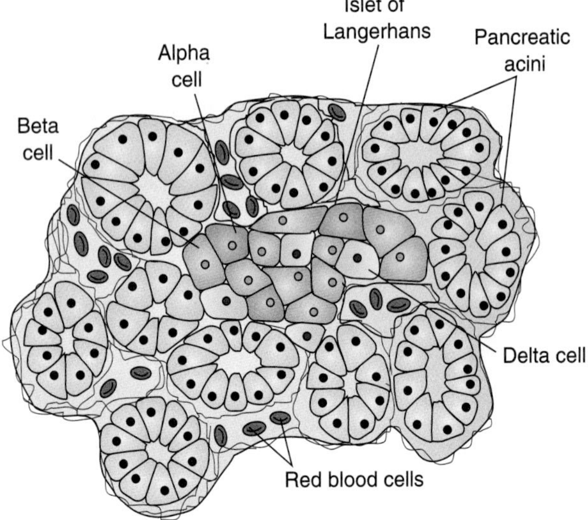

Figure 36–1
Islet of Langerhans in the pancreas. (Guyton A.C., Hall J.E. [1996]. *Textbook of medical physiology* [9th ed., p. 972]. Philadelphia: W.B. Saunders.)

insulin and glucagon, it is thought to extend the use of absorbed nutrients by the tissues.[2]

Blood Glucose

Body tissues obtain glucose from the blood. In nondiabetic persons, fasting blood glucose levels are tightly regulated between 80 to 90 mg/dl. After a meal, blood glucose levels rise, and insulin is secreted in response to this rise in glucose. About two thirds of the glucose that is ingested with a meal is removed from the blood and stored in the liver as glycogen. Between meals, the liver releases glucose as a means of maintaining blood glucose within its normal range.

Glucose is an optional fuel for tissues such as muscle, adipose tissue, and the liver, which largely use fatty acids and other fuel substrates for energy. Glucose that is not needed for energy is stored as glycogen or converted to fat. When tissues such as those in the liver and skeletal muscle become saturated with glycogen, the additional glucose is converted into fatty acids and then stored as triglycerides in fat cells. When blood glucose levels fall below normal, as they do between meals, glycogen is broken down by a process called *glycogenolysis*, and glucose is released. Glycogen stored in the liver can be released into the bloodstream. However, skeletal muscle lacks the enzyme glucose-6-phosphatase that allows glucose to be broken down sufficiently so it can pass through the cell membrane and enter the bloodstream, limiting its use to the muscle cell. In addition to mobilizing its glycogen stores, the liver synthesizes glucose from amino acids, glycerol, and lactic acid in a process called *gluconeogenesis*. Glucose metabolism is discussed more fully in Chapter 54.

In contrast to muscle, liver, and other body tissues, the brain and nervous system relies almost exclusively on glucose for its energy needs. Because the brain can neither synthesize nor store more than a few minutes' supply of glucose, normal cerebral function requires a continuous supply from the circulation. Severe and prolonged hypoglycemia can cause brain death, and even moderate hypoglycemia can result in substantial brain dysfunction.[2] The body maintains a system of *counterregulatory mechanisms* to counteract hypoglycemia-producing situations and ensure brain function and survival. The physiologic mechanisms that prevent or correct hypoglycemia include the actions of the counter-

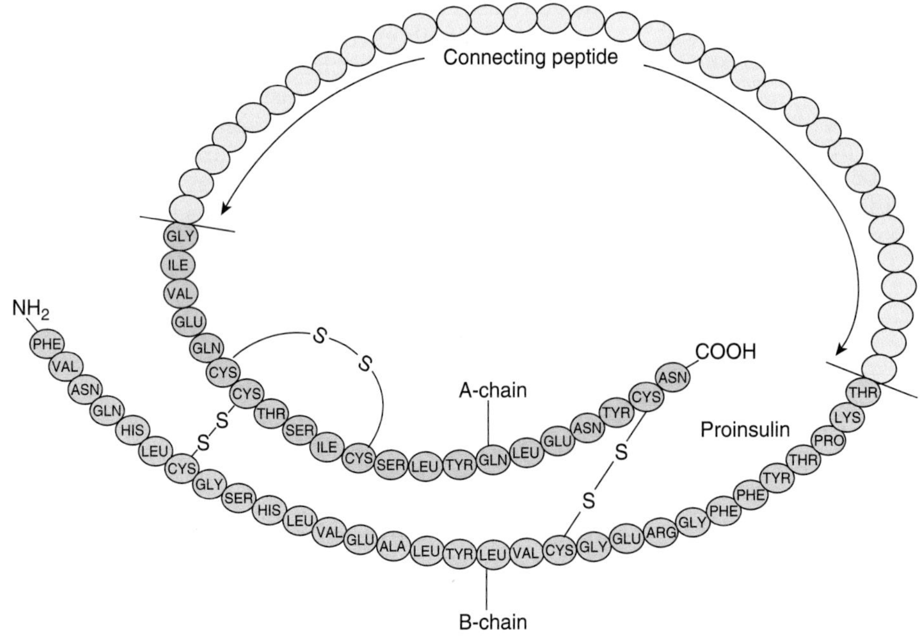

Figure 36–2
Structure of proinsulin. With removal of the connecting peptide (C-peptide), proinsulin is converted to insulin.

regulatory hormones: glucagon, the catecholamines, growth hormone, and the glucocorticoids.

Glucose Regulating Hormones

Insulin

Insulin is produced by the pancreatic β cells in the islets of Langerhans. The actions of insulin are threefold: it promotes glucose uptake by target cells and provides for glucose storage, it prevents fat and glycogen breakdown, and it inhibits gluconeogenesis and increases protein synthesis (Chart 36–1).

The active form of the hormone is composed of two polypeptide chains—an A chain and a B chain (Fig. 36–2). The two chains emerge with the appropriate linkage required for biologic activity from a single chain called *proinsulin*. In converting proinsulin to insulin, enzymes in the β cell cleave proinsulin at specific sites to form two substances: active *insulin* and a biologically inactive *C-peptide (connecting peptide) chain* that joined the A and B chains before they were separated. Active insulin and the inactive C-peptide chain are packaged into secretory granules and released simultaneously from the β cell. The C-peptide chains can be measured clinically, and this measurement can be used to study β-cell activity. For example, injected (exogenous) insulin in a person with type 2 diabetes would provide few or no C-peptide chains, whereas insulin (endogenous) secreted by the β cells would be accompanied by the secretion of C-peptide chains.

The release of insulin from the pancreatic β cells is regulated by blood glucose levels, increasing as blood glucose levels rise and decreasing when blood glucose levels decline. Glucose enters β cells by means of the membrane glucose transporter (GLUT2); is phosphorylated by an enzyme called *glucokinase*, then undergoes glycolysis, and is eventually oxidized to CO_2 and water. During this process, Ca^{2+} ions are recruited, which leads to movement of the secretory granules to the cell membrane and release of insulin from the β cell. Secretion of insulin occurs in an oscillatory (*i.e.*, pulsatile) fashion. After exposure to glucose, which is a nutrient secretagogue, a *first-phase release* of stored preformed insulin occurs, followed by a *second-phase release* of newly synthesized insulin (Fig. 36–3).[3] Diabetes may result from dysregulation or deficiency in any of the steps involved in this process (*e.g.*, β-cell failure, impaired function of the glucose transporters, intracellular metabolic defects, glucokinase deficiency). Serum insulin levels begin to rise within minutes after a meal, reach a peak in about 3 to 5 minutes, and then return to baseline levels within 2 to 3 hours. The glucose tolerance test, described later in this chapter, uses a glucose challenge as an indirect measure of the body's ability to secrete insulin and remove glucose from the blood.

Insulin secreted by the β cells enters the portal circulation and travels directly to the liver, where about 50% is used or degraded. Insulin, which is rapidly bound to peripheral tissues or destroyed by the liver or kidneys,

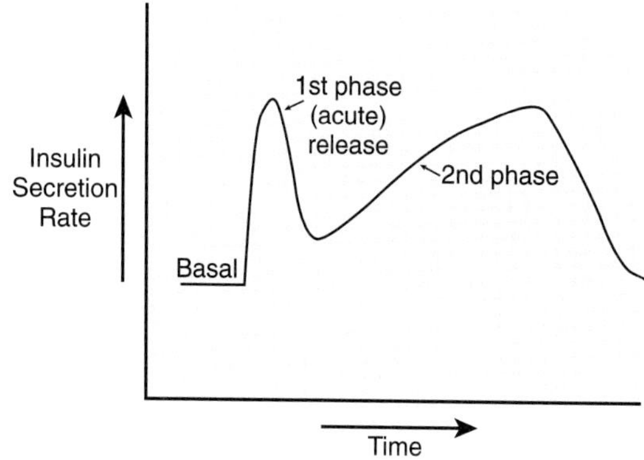

Figure 36–3
Biphasic insulin response to a constant glucose stimulus. The peak of the first phase in humans is 3 to 5 minutes; the second phase begins at 2 minutes and continues to increase slowly for at least 60 minutes or until the stimulus stops. (From Ward W.K., Beard J.C., Halter J.B., Pfeifer M.A., Porte D. Jr. [1984]. Pathology of insulin secretion in non-insulin-dependent diabetes mellitus. *Diabetes Care* 7:491–502. Used with permission.)

has a half-life of about 15 minutes once it is released into the general circulation.

Although several hormones are known to increase blood glucose levels, insulin is the only hormone known to have a direct effect in lowering blood glucose levels. Insulin lowers the concentration of blood glucose by facilitating its transport into skeletal muscle and adipose tissue. An insulin receptor and a specific glucose transporter are involved. This transporter removes insulin from the blood and shuttles it across the cell membrane

CHART **36-1**
Actions of Insulin on Glucose, Fats, and Proteins

Glucose
- Increases glucose transport into skeletal muscle and adipose tissue
- Increases glycogen synthesis
- Increases gluconeogenesis

Fats
- Increases glucose transport into fat cells
- Increases fatty acid transport into adipose cells
- Increases triglyceride synthesis
- Inhibits adipose cell lipase
- Activates lipoprotein lipase in capillary walls

Proteins
- Increases active transport of amino acids into cells
- Increases protein synthesis by increasing transcription of messenger RNA and accelerating protein synthesis by ribosomal RNA
- Decreases protein breakdown by enhancing the use of glucose and fatty acids as fuel

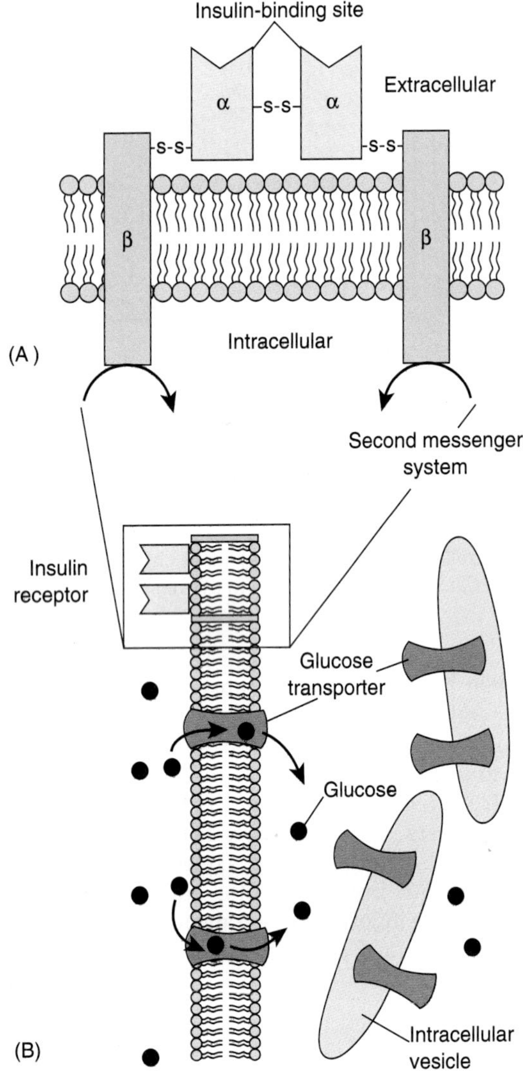

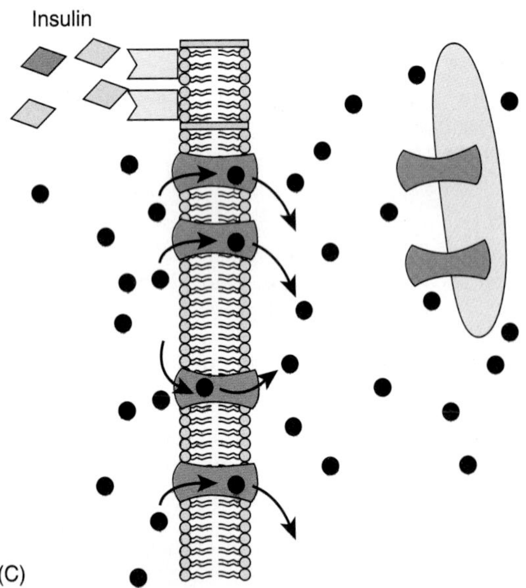

Figure 36-4

Mechanism of glucose transport. (**A**) Structure of insulin receptor. The α subunits on the outside of the cell membrane are linked to the β subunits in the membrane. Binding of insulin to the α subunits activates an intracellular second messenger system, which controls the function of the glucose transporter system depicted in **B** and **C**. (**B**) Glucose transporter (GLUT 4) in skeletal and adipose tissue. The situation that might exist in the fasting state when most glucose transporters are located in inactive cellular sites. (**C**) The situation following a meal when glucose and insulin levels are high and glucose transporters have been inserted into the cell membrane to facilitate glucose movement out of the blood, across the cell membrane, and into the cell. (Modified from Rhoades R.A. Tanner G.A. [1996]. *Medical physiology.* Boston: Little, Brown)

into cells at a faster rate than would occur by diffusion alone. Considerable research has revealed a family of glucose transporters, commonly called GLUT1, GLUT2, and so on. In skeletal muscle and adipose tissue, the function of insulin is to promote the translocation of the glucose transporter from an inactive intracellular site into the cell membrane (Fig. 36–4).[4] Although liver cells do not require insulin for glucose transport, a rise in insulin levels does cause an increase in the hepatic uptake of glucose and its conversion to glycogen. Insulin also decreases the breakdown of glycogen within the liver and in muscle tissue.

Fat is the most efficient form of fuel storage. It provides 9 kcal/g of stored energy, compared with the 4 kcal/g provided by carbohydrates and proteins. Insulin acts to promote fat storage by increasing the transport of glucose into fat cells. It also facilitates triglyceride synthesis from glucose within fat cells and inhibits the intracellular breakdown of stored triglycerides.

Insulin also inhibits protein breakdown and increases protein synthesis by increasing the active transport of amino acids into body cells. Insulin inhibits gluconeogenesis, or the building of glucose from new sources, mainly amino acids. When sufficient glucose and insulin are present, protein breakdown is minimal because the body is able to use glucose and fatty acids as a fuel source. In children and adolescents, insulin is needed for normal growth and development.

Glucagon

Glucagon, a small protein molecule produced by the pancreatic α cells of the islets of Langerhans, maintains blood glucose between meals and during periods of fasting. Like insulin, glucagon travels by way of the portal vein to the liver, where it exerts its main action. Unlike insulin, glucagon secretion is inhibited by glucose. The actions of glucagon are opposite to those of insulin. Glucagon stimulates glycogenolysis and gluconeogenesis, increases lipolysis and the output of ketones by the liver, and enhances the uptake of amino acids by the liver (Chart 36–2).

CHART 36-2
Actions of Glucagon on Glucose, Fats, and Proteins

Glucose

Promotes the breakdown of glycogen into glucose phosphate
Increases gluconeogenesis

Fats

Enhances lipolysis in adipose tissue, liberating glycerol for use in gluconeogenesis
Activates adipose cell lipase
Enhances lipolysis in adipose tissue, liberating fatty acids

Proteins

Increases breakdown of proteins into amino acid for use in gluconeogenesis
Increases transport of amino acids into hepatic cells
Increases conversion of amino acids into glucose precursors

It has been suggested that abnormalities in glucagon secretion contribute to the elevation of blood glucose levels observed in diabetes mellitus. Unger suggested that it is the ratio of insulin to glucagon, rather than the absolute amount of either hormone, that determines blood glucose levels.[5] According to theory, it is the unopposed action of glucagon, brought about by a lack of insulin in persons with uncontrolled diabetes, which leads to increased production of glucose by the liver.

Catecholamines

The catecholamines, epinephrine and norepinephrine, help to maintain blood glucose levels during periods of stress. The actions of epinephrine are summarized in Chart 36–3. Epinephrine inhibits insulin release and promotes glycogenolysis by stimulating the conversion of muscle and liver glycogen to glucose. Muscle glycogen cannot be released into the blood; nevertheless, the mobilization of these stores for muscle use conserves blood glucose for use by other tissues such as the brain and the nervous system. During periods of exercise and other types of stress, epinephrine inhibits insulin release from the β cells and thereby decreases the movement of glucose into muscle cells. The catecholamines also increase lipase activity and thereby increase mobilization of fatty acids; this process conserves glucose. The blood glucose–elevating effect of epinephrine is an important homeostatic mechanism during periods of hypoglycemia.

CHART 36-3
Actions of Epinephrine on Glucose and Fat Metabolism

Mobilizes glycogen stores
Decreases movement of glucose into body cells
Inhibits insulin release from beta cells
Mobilizes fatty acids from adipose tissue

Growth Hormone

Growth hormone has many metabolic effects. It increases protein synthesis in all cells of the body, mobilizes fatty acids from adipose tissue, and antagonizes the effects of insulin. Growth hormone decreases cellular uptake and use of glucose, thereby increasing the level of blood glucose, sometimes to as much as 50% to 100% of normal.[2] The increased blood glucose level stimulates further insulin secretion by the β cells. The secretion of growth hormone normally is inhibited by insulin and increased levels of blood glucose. During periods of fasting, when both blood glucose levels and insulin secretion fall, growth hormone levels increase. Exercise, such as running and cycling, and various stresses, including anesthesia, fever, and trauma, increase growth hormone levels.

Chronic hypersecretion of growth hormone, as occurs in acromegaly (see Chapter 35), can lead to glucose intolerance and the development of diabetes mellitus. In persons who already have diabetes, moderate elevations in growth hormone levels that occur during periods of stress and periods of growth in children can produce the entire spectrum of metabolic abnormalities associated with poor regulation, despite optimized insulin treatment.

Glucocorticoid Hormones

The glucocorticoid hormones, which are synthesized in the adrenal cortex along with other corticosteroid hormones, are critical to survival during periods of fasting and starvation. They stimulate gluconeogenesis by the liver, sometimes producing a 6- to 10-fold increase in hepatic glucose production. These hormones also moderately decrease tissue use of glucose. In predisposed persons, the prolonged elevation of glucocorticoid hormones can lead to hyperglycemia and the development of diabetes mellitus. In persons with diabetes, even transient increases in cortisol can complicate control.

There are several steroid hormones with glucocorticoid activity; the most important of these is cortisol, which accounts for about 95% of all glucocorticoid activity.[2] Cortisol levels increase during periods of stress, such as that produced by infection, pain, trauma, surgery, prolonged and strenuous exercise, and acute anxiety. Hypoglycemia is a potent stimulus for cortisol secretion. The control of cortisol secretion is discussed in Chapter 35.

In summary, energy metabolism is controlled by a number of hormones, including insulin, glucagon, epinephrine, growth hormone, and the glucocorticoids. Of these hormones, only insulin has the effect of lowering the blood glucose level. Insulin's blood glucose–lowering action results from its ability to increase the transport of glucose into body cells and decrease hepatic production and release of glucose into the bloodstream. Other hormones—glucagon, epinephrine, growth hormone, and the glucocorticoids—maintain or increase blood glucose concentrations and are referred to as counterregulatory hormones. Glucagon and epinephrine promote glycogenolysis. Glucagon and the glucocorticoids increase gluconeogenesis. Growth hormone decreases the peripheral use of glucose. Insulin has the effect of decreasing lipolysis and the use of fats as a fuel source; glucagon and epinephrine increase fat use.

Diabetes Mellitus

After you have completed this section of the chapter, you should be able to meet the following objectives:

- Compare the distinguishing features of type 1 and type 2 diabetes mellitus, list causes of other specific types of diabetes, and cite the criteria for gestational diabetes
- Relate the physiologic functions of insulin to the manifestations of diabetes mellitus
- Compare blood glucose regulation during exercise in persons without diabetes and those with type 1 diabetes, and relate this to the increased risk for development of hypoglycemia in a person with type 1 diabetes
- List five principles for diet management in persons with diabetes
- Characterize the actions of oral hypoglycemic agents in terms of the lowering of blood glucose
- Describe the clinical manifestations of diabetic ketoacidosis and their physiologic significance
- Describe the clinical condition resulting from the nonketotic hyperosmolar state
- Name and describe the types (according to duration of action) of insulin
- Describe the clinical manifestations of insulin-induced hypoglycemia and state how these may differ in elderly persons
- Describe and compare the Somogyi effect and the dawn phenomenon
- Describe alterations in physiologic function that accompany diabetic peripheral neuropathy, retinopathy, and nephropathy
- Describe the causes of foot ulcers in persons with diabetes mellitus
- Explain the relation between diabetes mellitus and infection

The term *diabetes mellitus* means "the running through of sugar." Reports of the disorder can be traced back to the first century A.D., when Aretaeus the Cappadocian described the disorder as a chronic affection characterized by intense thirst and voluminous honey-sweet urine: "the melting down of flesh into urine."[6] It was the discovery of insulin by Banting and Best in 1921 that transformed the once-fatal disease into a manageable chronic health problem.

Diabetes is a disorder of carbohydrate, protein, and fat metabolism resulting from an imbalance between insulin availability and insulin need. It can represent an absolute insulin deficiency, impaired release of insulin by the pancreatic β cells, inadequate or defective insulin receptors, or the production of inactive insulin or insulin that is destroyed before it can carry out its action. A person with uncontrolled diabetes is unable to transport glucose into fat and muscle cells; as a result, the body cells are starved, and the breakdown of fat and protein is increased.

Classification and Etiology

Although diabetes mellitus is clearly a disorder of insulin availability, it is probably not a single disease. A revised system for the classification of diabetes was developed in 1997 by the Expert Committee on the Diagnosis and Classification of Diabetes Mellitus.[7] The intent of the revised system, which replaces the 1979 classification system, was to move away from a system that focused on the type of pharmacologic treatment used in management of diabetes to one based on disease etiology.[7] The revised system continues to include type 1 and type 2 diabetes, but uses Arabic rather than Roman numerals and eliminates the use of "insulin-dependent" and "noninsulin-dependent" diabetes mellitus (Table 36–1). Included in the classification system are the categories of gestational diabetes (*i.e.*, diabetes that develops during pregnancy) and other specific types of diabetes, many of which occur secondary to other conditions (*e.g.*, Cushing's syndrome, hematochromatosis, pancreatitis, acromegaly). The revised classification system also includes a system for diagnosing diabetes according to stages of glucose intolerance.

Type 1 Diabetes Mellitus

Type 1 diabetes mellitus is characterized by autoimmune destruction of pancreatic β cells. Type 1 diabetes is subdivided into two types: type 1A, immune-mediated diabetes, and type 1B, idiopathic diabetes. In the United States and Europe, about 10% to 20% of persons with diabetes have type 1 diabetes; most of them have immune-mediated, type 1A, diabetes mellitus.[8]

Type 1A diabetes is characterized by autoimmune destruction of cells. This type of diabetes, formerly called juvenile diabetes, occurs more commonly in young persons but can occur at any age. Type 1 diabetes is a catabolic disorder characterized by an absolute lack of insulin, an elevation in blood glucose, and a breakdown of body fats and proteins. One of the actions of insulin is the inhibition of lipolysis (*i.e.*, fat breakdown) and release of free fatty acids from fat cells. In the absence of insulin, ketosis develops when these fatty acids are released from fat cells and converted to ketones in the liver. The absolute lack of insulin in persons with type 1 diabetes mellitus means that they are particularly prone to develop ketoacidosis. Because of the loss of the first-

TABLE 36-1
Etiologic Classification of Diabetes Mellitus

Type	Subtypes	Etiology of Glucose Intolerance
I. Type 1*	*(β-Cell destruction, usually leading to absolute insulin deficiency)*	
	A. Immune-mediated	Autoimmune destruction of β-cells
	B. Idiopathic	Unknown
II. Type 2*	*(May range from predominantly insulin resistance with relative insulin deficiency to a predominantly secretory defect with insulin resistance)*	
III. Other specific types	A. Genetic defects of β-cell function**	
	1. Chromosome 12, HNF-1α (formerly MODY 3)	Regulates HNF-4α expression; reduces insulin response of β-cell to glucose
	2. Chromosome 7, glucokinase (formerly MODY 2).	Defect in signaling insulin secretion due to defect in glucokinase generation
	3. Chromosome 20, HNF-4α (formerly MODY 1)	Transcription factor; reduces insulin response of β-cell to glucose
	B. Genetic defects in insulin action**	
	1. Type A insulin resistance	Mutation in insulin receptor
	2. Leprechaunism 3. Rabson-Mendenhall syndrome	Pediatric syndromes that have mutations in insulin receptor
	4. Lipoatrophic diabetes	Postreceptor defect in signal transduction
	C. Diseases of the exocrine pancreas**	
	1. Pancreatitis 2. Trauma / pancreatectomy 3. Neoplasms 4. Cystic fibrosis	Conditions of the exocrine pancreas that result in loss or destruction of insulin-producing β-cells
	D. Endocrinopathies**	
	1. Acromegaly 2. Cushing's syndrome 3. Glucogonoma 4. Hyperthyroidism 5. Somatostatinoma	Diabetogenic effects of excess hormone levels
	E. Drug- or chemical-induced**	
	1. Vacor	Toxic destruction of β-cells
	2. Pentamide (intravenous)	Toxic destruction of β-cells
	3. Nicotinic acid	Impaired insulin action
	4. Glucocorticosteroids	Increased glucose synthesis; insulin resistance
	5. Thyroid hormone	Impaired insulin action
	6. Diazoxide	Impaired insulin secretion
	7. β-Adrenergic agonists	Increased hepatic glucose output
	β-Adrenergic blockers	Impaired insulin secretion and sensitivity
	8. Thiazide diuretics	Impaired insulin secretion due to potassium loss
	9. Phenytoin (Dilantin)	Direct inhibition of insulin secretion
	10. α-Interferon	Production of islet cell antibodies
	F. Infections**	
	1. Congenital rubella 2. Cytomegalovirus	β-cell injury followed by an autoimmune reaction
	G. Uncommon forms of immune-mediated diabetes**	
	1. "Stiff-man" syndrome	Autoimmune disorder of CNS with immune-mediated β-cell destruction
	2. Anti-insulin receptor antibodies	Destruction of insulin receptors
	H. Other genetic syndromes sometimes associated with diabetes**	
	1. Down's syndrome 2. Klinefelter's syndrome 3. Turner's syndrome	Disorders of glucose tolerance related to defects associated with chromosomal abnormalities
IV. Gestational diabetes X mellitus (GDM)	*(Any degree of glucose intolerance with onset or first recognition during pregnancy)*	Combination of insulin resistance and impaired insulin secretion

*Patients with any form of diabetes may require insulin treatment at some stage of their disease. Such use of insulin does not, of itself, classify the patient.

**Not inclusive.

(Adapted from The Expert Committee on the Diagnosis and Classification of Diabetes Mellitus. [1997]. Report of the Expert Committee on the Diagnosis and Classification of Diabetes Mellitus. *Diabetes Care* 70[7], 1183–1197)

phase insulin (preformed insulin) response, all persons with type 1A diabetes require exogenous insulin replacement to reverse the catabolic state, control blood glucose levels, and prevent ketosis.

It has been suggested that immune-mediated type 1 diabetes results from a genetic predisposition (*i.e.*, diabetogenic genes), a hypothetical triggering event that involves an environmental agent that serves to incite an immune response, and immunologically mediated β-cell destruction.[9,10] Much evidence has focused on the inherited major histocompatibility complex (MHC) genes that encode three human leukocyte antigens (HLA-DP, -DQ, and -DR) found on the surface of body cells (see Chapter 11). Susceptibility to type 1 diabetes has also been associated with HLA-DR3 and -DR4. It appears that what is inherited as part of the HLA genotype in persons with type 1 diabetes is a susceptibility to an abnormal immune response that affects β cells. On the other hand, resistance to the development of type 1 diabetes has been traced to other HLA subtypes: DR11, DR15, and DQB1.[11–13] Type 1 diabetes-associated autoantibodies exist years before the onset of hyperglycemia. There are two major types of autoantibodies: islet cell autoantibodies (ICA) and insulin autoantibodies (IAA). Islet cell antibodies are present in 70% to 80% of persons with newly diagnosed type 1 diabetes and insulin autoantibodies in 50%. When there is an absence of both of these autoantibodies, the risk of developing type 1 diabetes is nil.[14] In addition to the MHC genes on chromosome 6, an insulin gene regulating β-cell replication and function has been identified on chromosome 11.

The fact that type 1 diabetes is thought to result from an interaction between genetic and environmental factors has led to research into methods directed at prevention and early control of the disease. These methods include the identification of genetically susceptible persons and early intervention in newly diagnosed persons with type 1 diabetes. After the diagnosis of type 1 diabetes, there often is a short period of β-cell regeneration, during which symptoms of diabetes disappear and insulin injections are not needed. Immune interventions designed to interrupt the destruction of β cells before development of type 1 diabetes are being investigated in the Diabetes Prevention Trial, which is trying to find a way to prevent complete and irreversible β-cell failure.

The classification of idiopathic type 1 diabetes is used to describe those cases of β-cell destruction in which no evidence of autoimmunity is present. Only a small number of persons with type 1 diabetes fall into this category; most are of African or Asian descent. Type 1B diabetes is strongly inherited. Persons with the disorder have episodic ketoacidosis—varying degrees of insulin deficiency with periods of absolute insulin deficiency that may come and go.

Type 2 Diabetes Mellitus

Type 2 diabetes mellitus describes a condition of fasting hyperglycemia that occurs despite the availability of insulin. In contrast to type 1 diabetes, type 2 diabetes is not associated with HLA markers or autoantibodies. Most persons with type 2 diabetes are older and overweight. The metabolic abnormalities that contribute to hyperglycemia in persons with type 2 diabetes include impaired insulin secretion, peripheral insulin resistance, and increased hepatic glucose production. Insulin resistance initially stimulates insulin secretion from the β cells in the pancreas to overcome the increased demand to maintain a normoglycemic state. In time, the insulin response by the β cells declines because of exhaustion. This results in elevated postprandial blood glucose levels. During the evolutionary phase, an individual with type 2 diabetes may become insulinopenic because of β-cell failure.

The insulin resistance and increased glucose production in obese persons with type 2 diabetes may stem from an increased concentration of free fatty acids (FFA). There are three explanations for this. First, FFAs act at the level of the β cell to stimulate more insulin secretion. Second, they act at the level of the peripheral tissues to inhibit glucose uptake, phosphorylation, and glycogen storage through a reduction in muscle glycogen synthetase activity. Third, a FFA-mediated increase in insulin delivery to the liver through the portal vein counteracts the FFA-mediated stimulation of hepatic glucose production.[14–16] An increase in FFA that occurs in obese individuals with a genetic predisposition to type 2 diabetes may eventually lead to β cell exhaustion and an inability to secrete insulin. The resultant decrease in insulin secretion causes hepatic overproduction of glucose and peripheral underutilization of glucose (Fig. 36–5).[14–16]

About 80% of persons with type 2 diabetes are overweight. The presence of obesity and the type of obesity are important considerations in the development of type 2 diabetes. It has been found that persons with upper-body obesity are at greater risk for developing type 2 diabetes than persons with lower-body obesity (see Chapter 54). Obese persons have increased resistance to the action of insulin and impaired suppression of glucose production by the liver, resulting in both hyperglycemia and hyperinsulinemia. The increased insulin resistance has been attributed to increased visceral (intraabdominal) fat detected on CT scan. In addition to increased insulin resistance, insulin release from β cells in response to glucose is impaired. Over time, insulin resistance may improve with weight loss, to the extent that many persons with type 2 diabetes can be managed with a weight-reduction program and exercise.

Twenty-five centers in the United States are participating in the Diabetes Prevention Program. The main goal of the this study is to prevent or delay the onset of type 2 diabetes in persons at high risk because they have impaired glucose tolerance.[17,18]

Other Specific Types

The category labeled *other specific types of diabetes,* formerly known as secondary diabetes, describes diabetes that is associated with certain other conditions and syndromes. Such diabetes can occur with pancreatic disease or the removal of pancreatic tissue and with endocrine diseases, such as acromegaly, Cushing's syndrome, or pheochromo-

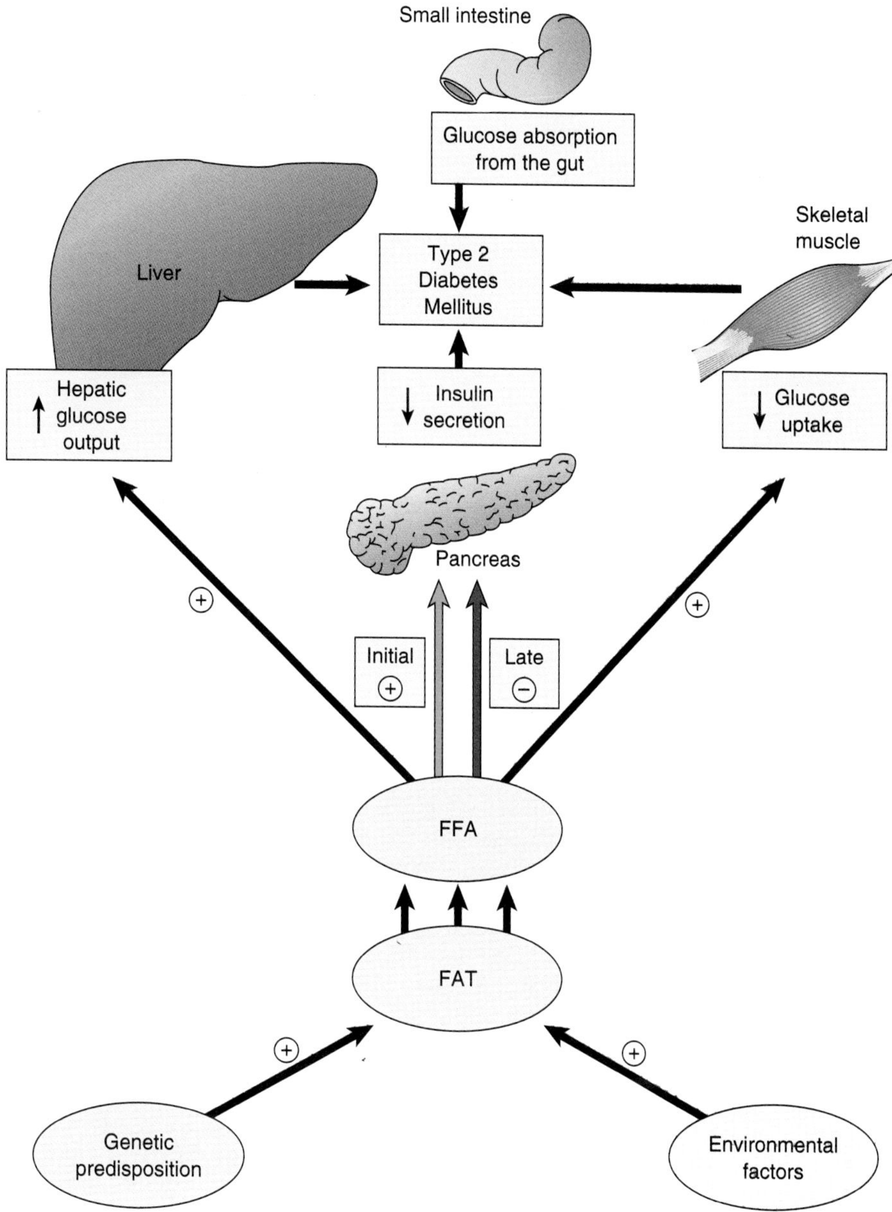

Figure 36–5 Pathogenesis of type 2 diabetes mellitus. FFA = free fatty acids.

cytoma. Endocrine disorders that produce hyperglycemia do so by increasing the hepatic production of glucose or decreasing the cellular use of glucose. Several specific types of diabetes are associated with monogenetic defects in β cell function. These specific types of diabetes, which resemble type 2 diabetes but occur at an earlier age (generally before age 25), were formerly referred to as maturity-onset diabetes of the young (MODY).

Environmental agents that have been associated with altered pancreatic β-cell function include viruses (*e.g.*, mumps, congenital rubella, coxsackievirus) and chemical toxins. Among the suspected chemical toxins are the nitrosamines, which are sometimes found in smoked and cured meats. The nitrosamines are related to streptozocin, which is used to induce diabetes in experimental animals, and to the rat poison Vacor, which can produce diabetes when ingested by humans.

Several diuretics—thiazides and loop diuretics—elevate blood glucose. These diuretics increase potassium loss, which is thought to impair insulin release. Other drugs known to cause hyperglycemia are diazoxide, glucocorticoids, levodopa, oral contraceptives, sympathomimetics, phenothiazines, phenytoin, and total parenteral nutrition (*i.e.*, hyperalimentation). Drug-related increases in blood glucose usually are reversed after the drug has been discontinued.

TABLE 36–2

National Diabetes Data Group for Interpretation of Fasting Plasma Glucose and Oral Glucose Tolerance Test with Use of Venous Plasma or Serum Using a 75-g Carbohydrate Load

Test	Normal	Impaired Fasting Glucose (IFG)†	Impaired Glucose Tolerance (IGT)†,‡	Diabetes†,‡	Gestational Diabetes§ (100-g Glucose load)
Fasting Plasma Glucose*	<110 (6.1)	≥110 (6.1) – <126 (7.0)		≥126 (7.0)	≥105
Glucose Tolerance test* (hours after glucose load)					
0.5					
and/or					
1					≥190
2	<140 (7.8)		≥140–≤200 (7.8–11.1)	≥200 (11.1)	≥165
3					≥145

*Values are given in mg/dl; values in parentheses are in mM.
†In nonpregnant individuals.
‡For diagnosis of diabetes in children, fasting value is required to be ≥140 mg/dl in addition to 1- and 2-hour elevations of glucose tolerance test.
§Criteria of O'Sullivan and Mahan, 1964.[48] (WHO Study Group recommendations omit values between fasting and 2 hours.)
(The Expert Committee on the Diagnosis and Classification of Diabetes Mellitus [1997]. Report of the Expert Committee on the Diagnosis and Classification of Diabetes Mellitus. *Diabetes Care* 20(7), 1183–1199.)

Gestational Diabetes

Gestational diabetes mellitus (GDM) refers to glucose intolerance of various degrees that occurs in 2% to 5% of pregnancies. It most frequently affects women with a family history of diabetes; glycosuria; with a history of stillbirth or spontaneous abortion, fetal anomalies in a previous pregnancy, or a previous large- or heavy-for-date baby; and who are obese, of advanced maternal age, or have had five or more pregnancies. However, because these risk factors fail to identify about 50% of persons with GDM, the American Diabetes Association (ADA) recommends that all pregnant women be screened for glucose tolerance. The ADA Clinical Practice Recommendations suggest that pregnant women who have not been identified as having glucose intolerance before the 24th week have a screening load glucose tolerance test between the 24th and 28th week of pregnancy. On the other hand, women who are considered to be low-risk (age <25 years, normal body weight, have no family history of diabetes, not members of a high-risk ethnic/racial group such as Hispanic, Native American, Asian, African American) may not need to be screened.[7] This test consists of 50 g of glucose given without regard to the last meal and followed in 1 hour by a venous blood sample for glucose concentration.[19] If the blood glucose level is greater than 140 mg/dl, then a 100-g, 3-hour glucose tolerance test is indicated to establish the diagnosis of GDM. The test should be performed after an overnight fast (see Table 36–2).

Diagnosis and careful medical management are essential, because women with GDM are at higher risk for complications of pregnancy, mortality, and fetal abnormalities. Fetal abnormalities include macrosomia (*i.e.*, large body size), hypoglycemia, hypocalcemia, polycythemia, and hyperbilirubinemia.

Treatment of GDM includes close observation of mother and fetus, because even mild hyperglycemia has been shown to be detrimental to the fetus. Maternal fasting and postprandial blood glucose levels should be measured regularly. Fetal surveillance depends on the degree of risk for the fetus. The frequency of growth measurements and determinations of fetal distress depends on available technology and gestational age. All women with GDM require nutritional guidance. If dietary management alone does not achieve a fasting blood glucose level equal to or less than 105 mg/dl or a 2-hour postprandial blood glucose equal to or less than 120 mg/dl, the Third International Workshop on GDM recommends therapy with human insulin. Oral antidiabetic agents are teratogenic and not recommended in pregnancy. Self-monitoring of blood glucose levels is essential. Nutrition is also the cornerstone of therapy. The nutrition plan should provide the necessary nutrients for maternal and fetal health, result in normoglycemia and proper weight gain, and prevent ketosis.

Women with GDM are at increased risk of developing diabetes 5 to 10 years after delivery. Women in whom GDM is diagnosed should be followed after delivery to detect diabetes early in its course. These women should be evaluated during their first postpartum visit with a 2-hour oral glucose tolerance test with a 75-g glucose load.[19]

Stages of Glucose Intolerance

Included in the report of the Expert Committee on the Diagnosis and Classification for Diabetes Mellitus are recommendations for changes in the stages of glucose intolerance (Table 36–2). The revised criteria have retained the former category of impaired glucose tolerance and have added a new category of impaired fasting blood glucose (IFG). The categories of IFG and IGT refer to a metabolic stage intermediate between normal glucose homeostasis and diabetes.[7] A fasting blood glucose <110 mg/dl or a 2-hour oral glucose tolerance test <140 mg/dl is considered normal.[7] IFG is defined as a fasting blood glucose ≥110 mg/dl but <126 mg/dl.[7] IGT reflects abnormal blood glucose measurements (≥ 140 mg/dl but < 200 mg/dl) 2 hours following an oral glucose load.[7] Approximately 5% of persons with IFG and IGT will progress to diabetes each year.[20] IFG and IGT may be associated with increased risk of atherosclerotic heart disease. Calorie restriction and weight reduction are important in overweight persons in this class.

Manifestations

Diabetes mellitus may have a rapid or an insidious onset. In type 1 diabetes, signs and symptoms often arise suddenly. Type 2 diabetes often develops more insidiously; its presence may be detected during a routine medical examination or when a patient seeks medical care for other reasons.

The most commonly identified signs and symptoms of diabetes are referred to as the three "polys"—*polyuria* (*i.e.,* excessive urination), *polydipsia* (*i.e.,* excessive thirst), and *polyphagia* (*i.e.,* excessive hunger). These three symptoms are closely related to the hyperglycemia and glycosuria of diabetes. Glucose is a small, osmotically active molecule. When blood glucose levels are sufficiently elevated, the amount of glucose filtered by the glomeruli of the kidney exceeds the amount that can be reabsorbed by the renal tubules; this results in glycosuria accompanied by large losses of water in the urine. Thirst results from the intracellular dehydration that occurs as blood glucose levels rise and water is pulled out of body cells, including those in the thirst center. Cellular dehydration also causes dryness of the mouth. This early symptom may be easily overlooked in type 2 diabetes, in which there is a gradual increase in blood glucose without accompanying signs of ketoacidosis. Polyphagia usually is not present in persons with type 2 diabetes. In type 1 diabetes, it probably results from cellular starvation and the depletion of cellular stores of carbohydrates, fats, and proteins.

Weight loss despite normal or increased appetite is a common occurrence in a person with uncontrolled type 1 diabetes. The cause of weight loss is twofold. First, loss of body fluids results from osmotic diuresis. Vomiting may exaggerate the fluid loss in ketoacidosis. Second, body tissue is lost because the lack of insulin forces the body to use its fat stores and cellular proteins as sources of energy. In terms of weight loss, there often is a marked difference between type 2 diabetes and type 1 diabetes. Weight loss is a frequent phenomenon in persons with uncontrolled type 1 diabetes, whereas many persons with uncomplicated type 2 diabetes have problems with obesity.

Other signs and symptoms of hyperglycemia include recurrent blurred vision, fatigue, paresthesias, and skin infections. In type 2 diabetes, these often are the symptoms that prompt a person to seek medical treatment. Blurred vision develops as the lens and retina are exposed to hyperosmolar fluids. Lowered plasma volume produces weakness and fatigue. Paresthesias reflect a temporary dysfunction of the peripheral sensory nerves. Chronic skin infections are common in persons with type 2 diabetes. Hyperglycemia and glycosuria favor the growth of yeast organisms. Pruritus and vulvovaginitis resulting from candidal infections are common initial complaints in women with diabetes.

Diagnosis and Management

The diagnosis of diabetes mellitus in nonpregnant adults is based on fasting blood glucose levels, random blood glucose tests, or the results of a glucose challenge test. Self-monitoring of capillary blood glucose can be performed by persons with diabetes to manage their disease. Glycosylated hemoglobin is used to evaluate the level of achievement of metabolic control. Treatment plans for diabetes usually involve diet, exercise, and antidiabetic agents. Weight loss and dietary management may be sufficient to control blood glucose levels in persons with type 2 diabetes.

Blood Tests

Fasting Blood Glucose Test. The fasting blood glucose has been suggested as the preferred diagnostic test because of ease of administration, convenience, patient acceptability, and cost.[7] Glucose levels are measured after food has been withheld for 8 to 12 hours. If the fasting plasma glucose level is higher than 126 mg/dl on one occasion, diabetes is diagnosed. A fasting plasma glucose level below 110 mg/dl is normal. A level between 110 mg/dl and 126 mg/dl is significant and should *not* be accepted as diagnostic without confirmation by a 75-g glucose tolerance test (see Table 36–2).

Random Blood Glucose. A random blood glucose concentration that is unequivocally elevated (>200 mg/dl) in the presence of classic symptoms of diabetes such as polydipsia, polyphagia, polyuria, and blurred vision is diagnostic of diabetes mellitus at any age.

Glucose Tolerance Test. The oral glucose tolerance test is an important screening test for diabetes. The test measures the body's ability to store glucose by removing it from the blood. In men and women, the test measures the plasma glucose response to 75 g (1.75 g/kg of ideal body weight) of concentrated glucose solution at selected intervals, usually 1 hour and 2 hours. In pregnant women, a glucose load of 100 g is given (see the Gestational Diabetes section) with an additional 3-hour plasma glucose determination. In persons with normal glucose tolerance, blood glucose levels return to normal within 2 to 3 hours after ingestion of a glucose load, in which case it can be assumed that sufficient insulin is present to allow glucose to leave the blood and enter body cells. Because a person with diabetes lacks the ability to respond to an increase in blood glucose by releasing adequate insulin to facilitate storage, blood glucose levels rise above those observed in normal persons and remain elevated for longer periods (see Table 36–2).

Capillary Blood Tests and Self-Monitoring of Capillary Blood Glucose Levels. Technologic advances have provided the means for monitoring blood glucose levels by using a drop of capillary blood. This procedure has provided health professionals with a rapid and economical means for monitoring blood glucose and has given persons with diabetes a way of maintaining near-normal blood glucose levels through self-monitoring. These methods use a drop of capillary blood obtained by pricking the finger with a special needle or small lancet. Small trigger devices make use of the lancet virtually painless. The drop of capillary blood is placed on or absorbed by a reagent strip, and glucose levels are determined electronically using a glucose meter or visually using a color chart.

Glycosylated Hemoglobin Test. This test measures the amount of glycosylated hemoglobin (*i.e.*, hemoglobin into which glucose has been incorporated) in the blood. Hemoglobin normally does not contain glucose when it is released from the bone marrow. During its 120-day lifespan in the red blood cell, hemoglobin normally becomes glycosylated to form glycohemoglobins A_{1a} and A_{1b} (2% to 4%) and A_{1c} (4% to 6%). In uncontrolled diabetes or diabetes with hyperglycemia, there is an increase in the level of hemoglobin A_{1c}. The ADA recommends initiating corrective measures for a hemoglobin A_{1c} level greater than 8%.[21] Because glucose entry into the red blood cell is not insulin dependent, the rate at which glucose becomes attached to the hemoglobin molecule depends on blood glucose. Glycosylation is essentially irreversible, and the level of glycosylated hemoglobin present in the blood provides an index of blood glucose levels over the previous 2 to 3 months.

Urine Tests

The ease, accuracy, and convenience of self-administered blood glucose monitoring techniques have made urine testing obsolete for most persons with diabetes. Urine tests only reflect urine glucose levels; they are influenced by such factors as the renal threshold for glucose, fluid intake and urine concentration, urine testing methodologies, and some drugs. Because of these factors, the ADA recommends that all persons who use insulin should self-monitor their blood glucose, not urine glucose.[22] Unlike glucose tests, urine ketone determinations remain an important part of monitoring diabetic control, particularly in persons with type 1 diabetes who are at risk for developing ketoacidosis.

Dietary Management

Diet therapy usually is prescribed to meet the specific needs of each person with diabetes. Goals and principles of diet therapy differ between type 1 and type 2 diabetes, as well as for lean and obese persons.

Integral to diabetes management is a prescribed plan for nutrition therapy.[23–25] Therapy goals include maintenance of near-normal blood glucose levels, achievement of optimal lipid levels, adequate calories to maintain and attain reasonable weights, prevention and treatment of chronic diabetes complications, and improvement of overall health through optimal nutrition.

A coordinated team effort, including the person with diabetes, is needed to individualize the nutrition plan. The diabetic diet has undergone marked changes over the years, particularly in the recommendations for distribution of calories among carbohydrates, proteins, and fats (Table 36–3). There is no longer a specific diabetic or ADA diet but rather a dietary prescription based on nutrition assessment and treatment goals. Evaluating the effectiveness of the meal plan requires monitoring metabolic parameters such as blood glucose, glycosylated hemoglobin, lipids, blood pressure, body weight, and quality of life. Self-management education is essential for the person with diabetes to facilitate understanding

TABLE 36-3 Historical Perspective of Nutritional Recommendations

	Distribution of Calories		
Year	% Carbohydrate	% Protein	% Fat
Before 1921		Starvation diets	
1921	20	10	70
1950	40	20	40
1971	45	20	35
1986	up to 60	12–20	<30
1994	*	10–20	*,†

*Based on nutritional assessment and treatment goals.
†Less than 10% of calories from saturated fats.
(American Diabetic Association. [1997]. Nutritional recommendations and principles for people with diabetes mellitus. *Diabetes Care* 20. [Suppl.], S14–S17)

of the associations among food, exercise, medication, and blood glucose. For a person with type 1 diabetes, the usual food intake is assessed and used as a basis for adjusting insulin therapy to fit with the person's lifestyle. Eating consistent amounts and types of food at specific and routine times is encouraged. Home blood glucose monitoring is used to fine tune the plan. Newer forms of therapy, such as multiple daily insulin injections and the use of an insulin pump provide many options.

The registered dietitian plays an essential role in the diabetes care team and is able to select from a variety of methods such as carbohydrate counting, food exchanges, healthy food choices, and total available glucose to tailor the meal plan to meet individual needs. Simpler recommendations have been associated with improved client understanding and dietary adherence. Carbohydrate counting uses product label information that is easily available to persons with diabetes. Regardless of food source, total grams of carbohydrate are counted, placing an emphasis on the nutrient that most affects blood glucose control.

Most persons with type 2 diabetes are overweight. Nutrition therapy goals focus on achieving glucose, lipid, and blood pressure goals, and weight loss if indicated. Mild to moderate weight loss (5 to 10 kg or 10 to 20 pounds) has been shown to improve diabetes control, even if desirable weight is not achieved.[26,27]

Nutrition therapy is tailored in terms of other dietary components. Because diabetes is a risk factor for cardiovascular disease, it is prudent to recommend less than 10% of daily calories be obtained from saturated fat and that dietary cholesterol be limited to 300 mg or less. Periodic fasting lipid panels may identify concomitant lipid disorders. If lipid disorders are identified, appropriate modifications according to the National Cholesterol Program Step II diet guidelines should be considered. For example, with low-density lipoprotein (LDL) cholesterol elevation, a diet with less than 7% of total calories from saturated fat, with less than 30% of daily calories obtained from fat, and with a cholesterol intake of less than 200 mg/day is recommended. For persons with diabetic nephropathy, some studies suggest lowering the intake of protein to 10% of daily calories. Recommendations for dietary sodium are the same as for the general population: 2400 to 3000 mg/day as a baseline; less than 2400 mg/day if mild to moderate hypertension is present; and less than 2000 if severe hypertension or nephropathy exists. The ADA provides literature with more detailed information on diet therapy and patient education. Included is the method of calculating individual meal plans. Registered dietitians are valuable resources to the nurse, physician, and person with diabetes and should be included in diet management.

Exercise

The benefits of exercise include cardiovascular fitness and psychologic well-being. For many persons with type 2 diabetes, the benefits of exercise inclulde a decrease in body fat, better weight control, and improvement in insulin sensitivity. The resulting improvement in glucose tolerance may free them from the use of antidiabetic drugs. Exercise is so important in diabetes management that a planned program of regular exercise usually is considered an integral part of the therapeutic regimen for every person with diabetes.

For persons without diabetes, the uptake of glucose into the exercising muscle increases 7- to 20-fold during short-term exercise, and blood glucose levels are maintained by an adrenergically induced decrease in insulin release from β cells and increased breakdown of liver glycogen stores mediated by counterregulatory hormones. When exercise is prolonged for more than 2 hours, the exercising muscles obtain the greater amount of their energy from fatty acids, and glucose release from the liver is derived from gluconeogenesis.

The beneficial effects of exercise are accompanied by an increased risk of hypoglycemia. Although muscle uptake of glucose increases significantly, the ability to maintain blood glucose levels is hampered by failure to suppress the absorption of injected insulin and activate the counterregulatory mechanisms that maintain blood glucose. Not only is there an inability to suppress insulin levels, but insulin absorption may increase. This increased absorption is more pronounced when insulin is injected into the subcutaneous tissue of the exercised muscle, but it occurs even when insulin is injected into other body areas. Even after exercise ceases, the lowering effect on blood glucose levels continues. In some persons with type 1 diabetes, the symptoms of hypoglycemia occur many hours after cessation of exercise. This may occur because subsequent insulin doses (in persons using multiple daily insulin injections) are not adjusted to accommodate the exercise-induced decrease in blood glucose. The cause of hypoglycemia in persons who do not administer a subsequent insulin dose is unclear. It may be related to the fact that the liver and skeletal muscles increase their uptake of glucose after exercise as a means of replenishing their glycogen stores or that the liver and skeletal muscles are more sensitive to insulin during this time. Persons with diabetes should be aware that delayed hypoglycemia can occur after exercise and that they may need to alter their insulin dose, their carbohydrate intake, or both.

Although of benefit to persons with diabetes, exercise must be weighed on the risk-benefit scale. The goal of exercise is safe participation in activities consistent with an individual's lifestyle. As with nutrition guidelines, exercise recommendations need to individualized. Considerations include hypoglycemia, hyperglycemia, ketosis, cardiovascular ischemia and dysrhythmias (particularly silent ischemic heart disease), exacerbation of proliferative retinopathy, and lower extremity injury. For those with chronic diabetes, the complications of vigorous exercise can be harmful and cause eye hemorrhage and other problems. For persons with type 1 diabetes who exercise during periods of poor control (*i.e.*, when blood glucose is elevated, exogenous insulin levels are low, and ketonemia exists), blood glucose and ketone levels rise to even higher levels because the stress of exercise is superimposed on preexisting insulin deficiency and increased counterregulatory hormone activity.[28–31]

Because most sporadic exercise has only transient benefits, a regular exercise or training program is the most beneficial. It is better for cardiovascular conditioning and can maintain a muscle-fat ratio that enhances peripheral insulin receptivity.

Antidiabetic Agents

There are two categories of antidiabetic agents: oral medications and injectable insulin. Persons with type 2 diabetes have increased hepatic glucose production; decreased peripheral use of glucose; decreased use of ingested carbohydrates; and over time, impaired insulin secretion from the pancreas. It is not surprising that the oral antidiabetic agents used in the treatment of type 2 diabetes attack each one of these areas and sometimes both. If good glycemic control cannot be achieved with a combination of oral agents, insulin can be used with the oral agents or by itself. Because persons with type 1 diabetes are deficient in insulin, they are in need of exogenous insulin replacement therapy from the start.

Oral Antidiabetic Agents. Oral antidiabetic agents approved by the U.S. Food and Drug Administration (FDA) fall into four categories: sulfonylureas, biguanides, α-glucosidase inhibitors, and thiazolidinediones (Fig. 36–6).

Sulfonylureas. The sulfonylureas were discovered accidentally in 1942, when scientists noticed that one of the sulfonamide drugs being developed at the time caused hypoglycemia. These drugs reduce blood glucose by stimulating the release of insulin from β cells in the pancreas and increasing the sensitivity of peripheral tissues to insulin. These agents are effective only when some residual β-cell function remains. Sulfonylurea receptors

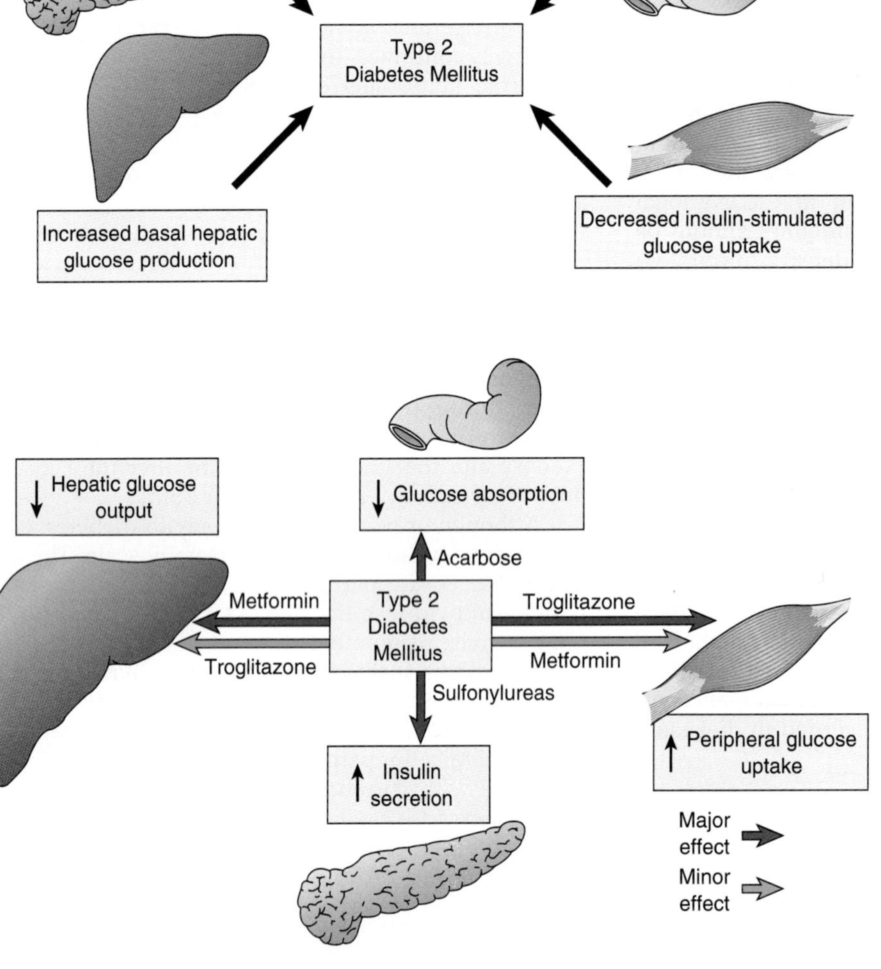

Figure 36–6 (**Top**) Mechanisms of elevated blood glucose in type 2 diabetes. (**Bottom**) Action sites of oral hypoglycemic agents and mechanisms of lowering blood glucose in type 2 diabetes mellitus.

in β cells of the pancreas are linked to potassium/ATP channels; when the drug attaches to the receptors, these channels close, and a coupled reaction leads to an influx of calcium. The influx of calcium triggers secretion of insulin from the β cells.[32]

The sulfonylureas are used in the treatment of type 2 diabetes and cannot be substituted for insulin in persons with type 1 diabetes, who have an absolute insulin deficiency. Slight modifications in the basic structure of the members of this drug group produce agents that have similar qualitative actions but markedly different potencies. The sulfonylureas are traditionally grouped into two generations. The first generation of drugs includes tolbutamide, acetohexamide, tolazamide, and chlorpropamide. The second generation of drugs—glyburide, glipizide, and glimepiride—are considerably more potent than the earlier drugs. These preparations differ in dosage and duration of action (Table 36–4).

Because the sulfonylureas increase the rate at which glucose is removed from the blood, it is important to recognize that they can cause hypoglycemic reactions. This problem is more common in elderly persons with impaired hepatic and renal function who are taking the longer-acting sulfonylureas.[33]

Biguanides. Metformin is the most significant agent in this group. The biguanides are older oral antidiabetic drugs. Phenformin, the earlier form of the drug was used extensively in the 1960s but was removed from the U.S. market in 1977 because of the occurrence of lactic acidosis in persons treated with it. After more than a decade of use in Europe, Canada, and other countries, metformin was approved by the FDA in 1995. Unlike its precursor, phenformin, metformin rarely results in lactic acidosis (0.03 cases per 1000 patients). Metformin inhibits hepatic glucose production and increases the sensitivity of peripheral tissues to the actions of insulin.[34] This medication does not stimulate insulin secretion, which explains the absence of hypoglycemia. Secondary benefits of metformin therapy include weight loss and improved lipid profiles.[35] Whereas the primary action of the sulfonylurea drugs is to increase insulin secretion, metformin exerts its beneficial effects on glycemic control through increased peripheral use of glucose and decreased hepatic glucose production (main effect).[36] To decrease the risk of lactic acidosis, metformin is contraindicated in persons with elevated serum creatinine levels (>1.5 mg/dl in men), clinical and laboratory evidence of hepatic disease, and any condition associated with hypoxemia or dehydration.

α-Glucosidase Inhibitors. In type 2 diabetes patients, sulfonylureas, biguanides, or both may have beneficial effects on fasting plasma glucose levels. However, postprandial hyperglycemia persists in more than 60% of patients and probably accounts for sustained increases in glycosylated hemoglobin levels. An alternative approach to the problem of postprandial hyperglycemia is the use of drugs such as acarbose, an inhibitor of α-glucosidase, which is a small intestine brush border enzyme that breaks down complex carbohydrates. Acarbose delays the absorption of carbohydrates from the gut and blunts the postprandial increase in plasma glucose and insulin levels.[37]

Thiazolidinediones. The thiazolidinediones are analogues of ciglitazone. Troglitazone received FDA approval in 1997. This medication is mainly an insulin sensitizer and reduces insulin resistance. It also suppresses hepatic glucose output. The mechanism of action is complex and not fully understood. Its action is associated with binding of nuclear receptors that regulate gene transcription associated with increases in GLUT1 and GLUT4 glucose transporters in muscle and fat cells. Additional effects are decreases in plasma free fatty acids, triglycerides, and a decrease in blood pressure.[38]

Insulin. Insulin-dependent diabetes mellitus requires treatment with insulin. Insulin is destroyed in the gastrointestinal tract and must be administered by injection. All insulin is measured in units, and the international unit of insulin is defined as the amount of insulin required to lower the blood glucose of a fasting 2-kg rabbit from 145 mg to 120 mg/dl. Most types of insulin are available in U-100 strength (*i.e.*, 100 units of insulin/1 ml) strength. Insulin preparations are categorized according to onset, peak, and duration of action. There are three principal

TABLE 36-4

Sulfonylurea Preparations: Duration of Action and Dosages

Sulfonylurea Preparations	Dosage Range (mg)	Duration of Action (hr)
First Generation		
Tobutamide (Orinase)	500–3000	6–12
Tolazamide (Tolinase)	100–1000	12–24
Acetohexamide (Dymelor)	250–2000	12–24
Chlorpropamide (Diabinase)	100–750	60–90
Second Generation		
Glyburide (Diabeta, Micronase)	1.25–20.0	24
Glipizide (Glucotrol)	2.50–40.0	24
Glimepiride (Amaryl)	1.0–8.0	24

TABLE 36–5

Activity Profile of Human Insulin Preparations in the United States

Type of Insulin	Onset (hr)	Peak (hr)	Duration (hr)
Short-acting			
Lispro (Humalog)	0.25*	0.5–1.5	3.0
Regular	0.5–1.0	2.0–3.0	4.0–6.0
Intermediate-acting			
NPH	1.5–4.0	4.0–8.0	12.0–16.0
Lente	2.5–4.0	4.0–8.0	16.0–20.0
Long-acting			
Ultralente human	4.0–10.0	12.0–16.0	20.0–30.0

*The times listed are variable, with marked differences from one injection to another because of multiple factors that affect insulin kinetics.

types of insulin: short acting, intermediate acting, and long acting (Table 36–5).

Insulin regimens that call for two or three daily injections of rapid-acting insulin or rapid-acting insulin mixed with intermediate-acting insulin are the most common. Lispro (Humalog) has a more rapid onset, peak, and duration of action than the classic short-acting regular insulin.[39] These regimens provide a blood glucose level that is within a more normal physiologic range than that provided by the once-daily injection.

During the past several decades, many pharmaceutical companies have entered the insulin-manufacturing market. After much research, human insulin has become available, providing an alternative to previous forms of insulin that were obtained from bovine and porcine sources. The manufacture of human insulin uses recombinant DNA. Beef insulin differs from human insulin by three amino acids, and pork insulin differs by only one amino acid. Many persons with diabetes develop antibodies to beef and pork insulin. Improvements in the purification techniques for insulin extracted from animal pancreases have made it possible to reduce or eliminate many of the contaminants that could incite antibody formation. Synthetic human insulin is widely available and is commonly used. A change from pork or beef to human insulin should be carefully monitored, because hypoglycemia can occur because of increased receptivity to the human insulin.

Two intensive treatment regimens—multiple daily injections and continuous subcutaneous infusion of insulin (CSII)–closely simulate the normal pattern of insulin secretion by the body.[39] With each method, a basal insulin level is maintained, and bolus doses of short-acting insulin are delivered before meals. The choice of management is determined by the patient in collaboration with the health care team.

Multiple Daily Injections. With multiple daily injections, the basal insulin requirements are met by long-acting insulin (Ultralente) or by intermediate-acting insulin (Lente or NPH) administered once or twice daily.[40] Boluses of short-acting insulin are used before meals. The development of convenient injection devices (*e.g.*, pen injector) has made it easier for persons with diabetes to comply with the multiple doses of Lispro or Regular insulin that are administered before meals.

Continuous Subcutaneous Insulin Infusion. With the CSII method, the basal insulin requirements are met by continuous infusion of subcutaneous insulin whose rate can be varied to accommodate diurnal variations. The CSII technique involves the insertion of a small needle into the subcutaneous tissue of the abdomen. Tubing from the needle is connected to a syringe set into a small infusion pump worn on a belt or in a jacket pocket. The computer-operated pump then delivers one or more set basal amounts of insulin. In addition to the basal amount delivered by the pump, a bolus amount of insulin may be delivered when needed (*e.g.*, before a meal) by pushing a button. Self-monitoring of blood glucose levels is a necessity when using this method of management. Each basal and bolus dose is determined individually and programmed into the infusion pump computer. Only persons who are highly motivated to do frequent blood glucose tests and to make daily insulin adjustments are candidates for this method of treatment. Although the pump's safety has been proven, strict attention must be paid to signs of hypoglycemia. However, investigations have found CSII therapy to be associated with a marked and sustained reduction in the rate of severe hypoglycemia.[41] Ketotic episodes caused by pump failure and infections at the needle site are possible complications.

Persons lacking the behavioral, mental, or physical abilities to undertake an intensive diabetes management program should not be considered for this form of therapy. Candidate selection is crucial to the successful use of the insulin pump. Use of an insulin pump requires an intensive therapy program that is best implemented with the support of a diabetes health care team (Chart 36–4). The diabetologist, nurse educator, and dietitian are key team members; a social worker or

CHART **36-4**
Elements of an Intensive Diabetes Therapy Program

Multiple-component insulin regimen
Balance of food intake, activity, and insulin dose
Daily home blood glucose monitoring
Use of predetermined algorithms to adjust food intake or supplement insulin
Individualized target blood glucose levels
Frequent contact between patient and staff
Patient education and motivation
Psychological support
Objective assessment (glycosylated hemoglobin level)

(Modified from Hirsch I.B. [1995]. Implementation of intensive diabetes therapy for IDDM. *Diabetes Reviews* 3 (2), 288–307)

psychologist and exercise physiologist are helpful additions to the team.[42]

Pancreas Transplantation

Pancreas transplantation is being performed with increased frequency and success rates for the treatment of diabetes. When successful, pancreas transplants can restore carbohydrate metabolism to normal or nearly normal. Worldwide, more than 5000 pancreas transplants were performed between 1966 and 1993, with most of these occurring in the last 7 years of this period. Between 1987 and 1990, the 1- and 3-year survival rates were 91% and 80%, respectively, and the graft survival rates (with total freedom from insulin therapy) were 72% and 57%, respectively.[43]

Persons with pancreas transplants require immunosuppression, usually achieved with a combination of cyclosporine, azathioprine, and prednisone, to prevent transplant rejection. This procedure may be considered for persons who need a kidney transplant and require immunosuppression for that purpose.[43]

Pancreas transplantation is not a lifesaving procedure. It does, however, afford the potential for significantly improving the quality of life. The most serious problems are the requirement for immunosuppression and the need for diagnosis and treatment of rejection. Investigators are looking for methods of transplanting islet cells and protecting the cells from destruction without the use immunosuppressive drugs.[44]

Acute Complications

The three major acute complications of diabetes are diabetic ketoacidosis, hyperglycemic hyperosmolar nonketotic syndrome, and hypoglycemia.

Diabetic Ketoacidosis

Diabetic ketoacidosis (DKA) occurs when ketone production by the liver exceeds cellular use and renal excretion. DKA most commonly occurs in a person with type 1 diabetes, in whom the lack of insulin leads to mobilization of fatty acids from adipose tissue because of the unsuppressed adipose cell lipase activity that breaks down triglycerides into fatty acids and glycerol. The increase in fatty acid levels leads to ketone production by the liver (Fig. 36–7). It can occur at the onset of the disease, often before the disease has been diagnosed. For example, a mother may bring a child into the hospital with reports of lethargy, vomiting, and abdominal pain, unaware that the child has diabetes. Stress increases the release of gluconeogenic hormones and predisposes the person to the development of ketoacidosis. DKA often is preceded by physical or emotional stress, such as infection, pregnancy, or extreme anxiety. In clinical practice, ketoacidosis also occurs with the omission or inadequate use of insulin.

The three major metabolic derangements in DKA are hyperglycemia, ketosis, and metabolic acidosis. The definitive diagnosis of DKA consists of hyperglycemia (blood glucose levels >250 mg/dl), low bicarbonate (<15 mEq/L), and low pH (<7.3) with ketonemia (positive at 1:2 dilution) and moderate ketonuria (Chart 36–5).[45] Hyperglycemia leads to osmotic diuresis, dehydration, and a critical loss of electrolytes. Hyperosmolality of extracellular fluids from hyperglycemia leads to a shift of water and potassium from the intracellular to the extracellular compartment. Extracellular sodium concentration is frequently low or normal despite enteric water losses because of the intracellular-extracellular fluid shift. This dilutional effect is referred to as *pseudohyponatremia*. Serum potassium levels may be normal or elevated, despite total potassium depletion resulting from protracted polyuria and vomiting. Metabolic acidosis is caused by the excess ketoacids that require buffering by bicarbonate ions; this leads to a marked decrease in serum bicarbonate levels.

Compared with an insulin reaction, DKA usually is slower in onset, and recovery is more prolonged. The person typically has a history of 1 or 2 days of polyuria, polydipsia, nausea, vomiting, and marked fatigue, with eventual stupor that can progress to coma. Abdominal pain and tenderness may be experienced without abdominal disease. The breath has a characteristic fruity smell because of the presence of the volatile ketoacids. Hypotension and tachycardia may be present because of a decrease in blood volume. A number of the signs and symptoms that occur in DKA are related to compensatory mechanisms. The heart rate increases as the body compensates for a decrease in blood volume, and the rate and depth of respiration increase (*i.e.*, Kussmaul's respiration) as the body attempts to prevent further decreases in pH. Metabolic acidosis is discussed further in Chapter 27.

The goals in treating DKA are to improve circulatory volume and tissue perfusion, decrease serum glucose, correct the acidosis, and correct electrolyte imbalances.[45] These objectives usually are accomplished through the administration of insulin and intravenous fluid and electrolyte replacement solutions. Because insulin resistance accompanies severe acidosis, low-dose insulin therapy is

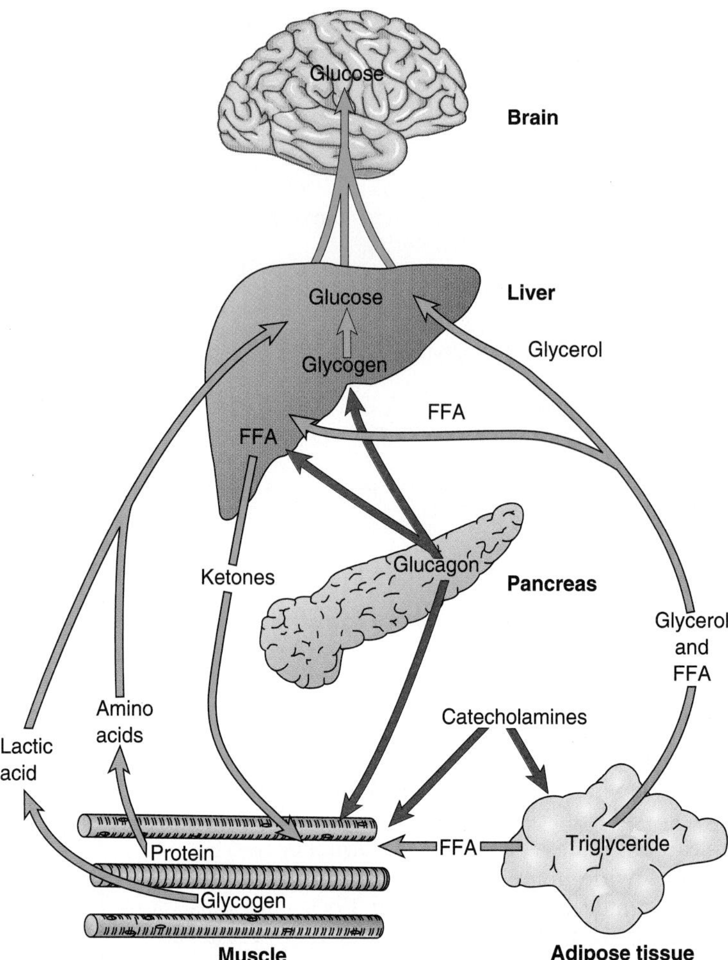

Figure 36–7
Mechanisms of diabetic ketoacidosis. Diabetic ketoacidosis is associated with very low insulin levels and extremely high levels of glucagon, catecholamines, and other counterregulatory hormones. Increased levels of glucagon and the catecholamines (*red arrows*) lead to mobilization of substrates (*blue arrows*) for gluconeogenesis and ketogenesis by the liver (*green arrows.*) Gluconeogenesis in excess of that needed to supply glucose for the brain and other glucose-dependent tissues produces a rise in blood glucose levels. Mobilization of free fatty acids (FFA) from triglyceride stores in adipose tissue leads to accelerated ketone production and ketosis.

used. An initial loading dose of regular insulin often is given intravenously, followed by continuous low-dose infusion. Frequent laboratory tests are used to monitor blood glucose and serum electrolyte levels and to guide fluid and electrolyte replacement. It is important to replace fluid and electrolytes and correct pH while bringing the blood glucose concentration to a normal level. Too rapid a drop in blood glucose may cause hypoglycemic symptoms and cerebral edema. A sudden change in the osmolality of extracellular fluid occurs when blood glucose is lowered rapidly, and this can cause cerebral edema. Serum potassium levels often fall as acidosis is corrected and extracellular potassium moves into the intracellular compartment; at this time, it may be necessary to add potassium to the intravenous infusion. Identification and treatment of the underlying cause, such as infection, are also important. With the better understanding of pathogenesis of DKA and more uniform agreement on diagnosis and treatment, the mortality rate has been reduced to less than 5%.

Hyperglycemic Hyperosmolar (HHNK) Syndrome

HHNK coma is characterized by plasma osmolarity of 310 mOsm/L or more, blood glucose in excess of 600 mg/dl of blood, the absence of ketoacidosis, and depression of the sensorium.[46]

HHNK syndrome may occur in various conditions, including type 2 diabetes, acute pancreatitis, severe infection, myocardial infarction, and treatment with oral or parenteral nutrition solutions. It is seen most frequently in persons with type 2 diabetes. Two factors appear to contribute to the hyperglycemia that precipitates the condition: an increased resistance to the effects of insulin and an excessive carbohydrate intake.

In hyperosmolar states, the increased serum osmolarity has the effect of pulling water out of body cells, including brain cells. The condition may be complicated by thromboembolic events arising because of the high serum osmolality. The most prominent manifestations are dehydration, neurologic signs and symptoms, polyuria, and thirst (Chart 36–6). The neurologic signs include grand mal seizures, hemiparesis, Babinski's reflexes, aphasia, muscle fasciculations, hyperthermia, hemianopia, nystagmus, and visual hallucinations. The onset of HHNK syndrome often is insidious, and because it occurs most frequently in older persons, it may be mistaken for a stroke.

The treatment of HHNK syndrome requires judicious medical observation and care, because water moves

CHART 36-5
Signs and Symptoms of Diabetic Ketoacidosis

Onset 1 to 24 hours
Laboratory findings
- Blood glucose greater than 250 mg/dl
- Ketonemia and presence of ketones in the urine
- Decreased plasma pH (less than 7.3) and bicarbonate (less than 15 mEq/L)

Dehydration caused by hyperglycemia
- Warm, dry skin
- Dry mucous membranes
- Tachycardia
- Weak, thready pulse
- Acute weight loss
- Hypotension

Ketoacidosis
- Anorexia, nausea, and vomiting
- Odor of ketones on the breath
- Depression of the central nervous system
  - Lethargy and fatigue
  - Stupor
  - Coma
- Abdominal pain

Compensatory responses
- Rapid, deep respirations (Kussmaul's respiration)

back into brain cells during treatment, posing a threat of cerebral edema. Extensive potassium losses that have also occurred during the diuretic phase of the disorder require correction. Because of the problems encountered in the treatment and the serious nature of the disease conditions that cause HHNK syndrome, the prognosis for this disorder is less favorable than that for ketoacidosis.

CHART 36-6
Signs and Symptoms of Hyperglycemic Hyperosmolar Syndrome

Onset insidious; 24 hours to 2 weeks
Laboratory findings
- Blood glucose greater than 600 mg/dl
- Serum osmolarity 300 mOsm/L or greater

Severe dehydration
- Dry skin and mucous membranes
- Extreme thirst

Neurologic manifestations
- Depressed sensorium lethargy to coma
- Neurologic deficits
  - Positive Babinski's sign
  - Paresis or paralysis
  - Sensory impairment
  - Hyperthermia
  - Hemianopia

Seizures

Hypoglycemia

Hypoglycemia, or an insulin reaction, occurs from a relative excess of insulin in the blood and is characterized by below-normal blood glucose levels. It occurs most commonly in persons treated with insulin injections, but prolonged hypoglycemia can also result from some oral hypoglycemic agents.

Hypoglycemia generally has a rapid onset and progression of symptoms (Chart 36–7). The signs and symptoms of hypoglycemia can be divided into two categories: those caused by altered cerebral function and those related to activation of the autonomic nervous system. Because the brain relies on blood glucose as its main energy source, hypoglycemia produces behaviors related to altered cerebral function. Headache, difficulty in problem solving, disturbed or altered behavior, coma, and seizures may occur. At the onset of the hypoglycemic episode, activation of the parasympathetic nervous system often causes hunger. The initial parasympathetic response is followed by activation of the sympathetic nervous system; this causes anxiety, tachycardia, sweating, and constriction of the skin vessels (*i.e.*, the skin is cool and clammy). Although different persons respond in different ways to an insulin reaction, each person usually has the same individual pattern of response during each insulin reaction.

There is wide variation in the manifestation of signs and symptoms; not every person with diabetes manifests all or even most of the symptoms. The signs and symptoms of hypoglycemia are more variable in children and in elderly persons. Elderly persons may not display the typical autonomic responses associated with hypoglycemia but frequently develop signs of impaired function of the central nervous system, including men-

CHART 36-7
Signs and Symptoms of Insulin Reaction

Sudden onset
Laboratory findings
- Blood glucose less than 53 mg/dl

Impaired cerebral function (caused by decreased glucose availability for brain metabolism)
- Feeling of vagueness
- Headache
- Difficulty in problem solving
- Slurred speech
- Impaired motor function
- Change in emotional behavior
- Seizures
- Coma

Autonomic nervous system responses
- Hunger
- Anxiety
- Hypotension
- Sweating
- Vasoconstriction of skin vessels (skin is pale and cool)
- Tachycardia

tal confusion. Some persons develop hypoglycemic unawareness. Unawareness of hypoglycemia should be suspected in persons who do not report symptoms when their blood glucose concentration is less than 50 to 60 mg/dl. This occurs most commonly in persons who have a longer duration of diabetes and glycosylated hemoglobin levels within the normal range.[47,48] Some medications, such as β-adrenergic–blocking drugs, interfere with the sympathetic response normally seen in hypoglycemia.

Many factors precipitate an insulin reaction in a person with type 1 diabetes, including error in insulin dose, failure to eat, increased exercise, decreased insulin need after removal of a stress situation, and a change in insulin site. Alcohol decreases liver gluconeogenesis, and a person with diabetes needs to be cautioned about its potential for causing hypoglycemia, especially if it is consumed in large amounts or on an empty stomach.

The most effective treatment of an insulin reaction is the immediate ingestion of a concentrated carbohydrate source, such as sugar, honey, candy, or orange juice. Alternative methods for increasing blood glucose may be required when the person having the reaction is unconscious or unable to swallow. Glucagon may be given intravenously, intramuscularly, or subcutaneously. Glucagon acts by hepatic glycogenolysis to raise blood sugar. The liver contains only a limited amount of glycogen (about 75 g); glucagon is ineffective in persons whose glycogen stores have been depleted. Some persons report becoming nauseated after glucagon administration, which could also be in response to the severe hypoglycemia. A small amount of glucose gel (available in most pharmacies) may be inserted into the buccal pouch when glucagen is unavailable. Monosaccharides such as glucose, which can be absorbed directly into the bloodstream, work best for this purpose. It is important not to overtreat hypoglycemia and cause hyperglycemia.

Treatment usually consists of an initial administration of 15 to 20 g of glucose, which can be repeated as necessary. Complex carbohydrates can be administered after the acute reaction has been controlled. In situations of severe or life-threatening hypoglycemia, it may be necessary to administer glucose (20 to 50 ml of a 50% solution) intravenously.

Somogyi Effect and Dawn Phenomenon

The *Somogyi effect* describes a cycle of insulin-induced posthypoglycemic episodes. In 1924, Joslin and his associates noticed that hypoglycemia was associated with alternate episodes of hyperglycemia.[49] It was not until 1959 that Somogyi presented the results of his 20 years of studies, which confirmed the observation that "hypoglycemia begets hyperglycemia." In a person with diabetes, insulin-induced hypoglycemia produces a compensatory increase in blood levels of catecholamines, glucagon, cortisol, and growth hormone. These counterregulatory hormones cause blood glucose to become elevated and produce some degree of insulin resistance. The cycle begins when the increase in blood glucose and insulin resistance are treated with larger insulin doses. The hypoglycemic episode often occurs during the night or at a time when it is not recognized, rendering the diagnosis of the phenomenon more difficult. Figure 36–8 shows the events that occur with the Somogyi effect.

Research suggests that even rather mild insulin-associated hypoglycemia, which may be asymptomatic, can cause hyperglycemia in those with type 1 diabetes through the recruitment of counterregulatory mechanisms, although the insulin action does not wane. A concomitant waning of the effect of insulin (*i.e.*, end of the duration of action), when it occurs, exacerbates posthypoglycemic hyperglycemia and accelerates its development. These findings may explain the labile nature of the disease in some persons with diabetes. Measures to prevent hypoglycemia and the subsequent activation of counterregulatory mechanisms include a redistribution of dietary carbohydrates and an alteration in insulin dose or method of administration.[50]

The *dawn phenomenon* is characterized by increased levels of fasting blood glucose or insulin requirements or both between 5 and 9 AM without antecedent hypoglycemia. It occurs in persons with type 1 diabetes or type 2 diabetes. It has been suggested that a change in the normal circadian rhythm for glucose tolerance, which usually is higher during the later part of the morning, is altered in persons with diabetes.[51] Growth hormone has been suggested as a possible factor. When the dawn phenomenon occurs alone, it may produce only mild hyperglycemia, but when it is combined with the Somogyi effect, it may produce profound hyperglycemia.

Chronic Complications

The chronic complications of diabetes include neuropathies, disorders of the microcirculation (*i.e.*, nephropathies and retinopathies), macrovascular complications, and foot ulcers. These disorders occur in the insulin-independent tissues of the body—tissues that do not require insulin for glucose entry into the cell. This probably means that intracellular glucose concentrations in

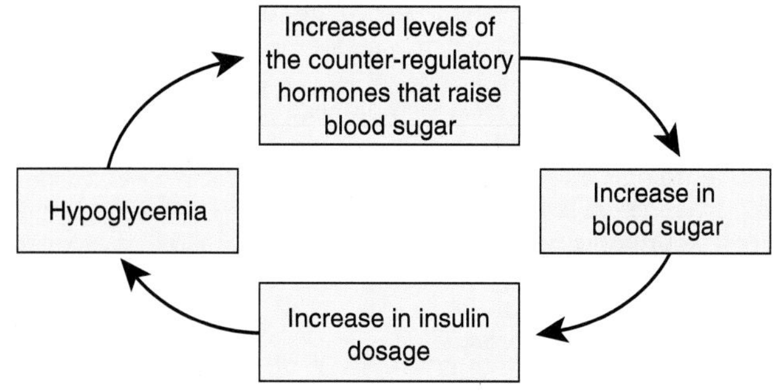

Figure 36–8
Cycle of events that occur with the Somogyi phenomenon.

many of these tissues approach or equal those in the blood. The level of chronic glycemia is the best established concomitant factor associated with diabetic complications.[52] The Diabetes Control and Complications Trial (DCCT),[53] which was conducted with 1441 persons with type 1 diabetes, has demonstrated that the incidence of retinopathy, nephropathy, and neuropathy can be reduced by intensive diabetic treatment.[54]

Theories of Pathogenesis

The interest among researchers in explaining the causes and development of chronic lesions in a person with diabetes has led to a number of theories. Several of these theories have been summarized to prepare the reader for understanding specific chronic complications.[55]

Polyol Pathway. A polyol is an organic compound that contains three or more hydroxyl groups. The polyol pathway refers to the intracellular mechanisms responsible for changing the number of hydroxyl units on a glucose molecule. In the sorbitol pathway, glucose is transformed first to sorbitol and then to fructose. Although glucose is readily converted to sorbitol, the rate at which sorbitol can be converted to fructose and then metabolized is limited. Sorbitol is osmotically active, and it has been hypothesized that the presence of excess intracellular amounts may alter cell function in those tissues that use this pathway (*e.g.*, lens, kidneys, nerves, blood vessels). In the lens, for example, the osmotic effects of sorbitol cause swelling and opacity. Increased sorbitol is also associated with a decrease in myoinositol and reduced adenosine triphosphatase activity. The reduction of these compounds may be responsible for the peripheral neuropathies caused by Schwann cell damage.

Formation of Abnormal Glycoproteins. Glycoproteins, or what could be called glucose proteins, are normal components of the basement membrane in smaller blood vessels and capillaries. It has been suggested that the increased intracellular concentration of glucose associated with uncontrolled blood glucose levels in diabetes favors the formation of abnormal glycoproteins. These abnormal glycoproteins are thought to produce structural defects in the basement membrane of the microcirculation and to contribute to eye, kidney, and vascular complications.

Problems With Tissue Oxygenation. Proponents of the tissue oxygenation theories suggest that many of the chronic complications of diabetes arise because of a decrease in oxygen delivery in the small vessels of the microcirculation. Among the factors believed to contribute to this inadequate oxygen delivery is a defect in red blood cell function that interferes with the release of oxygen from the hemoglobin molecule. In support of this theory is the finding of a twofold to threefold increase in glycosylated hemoglobin (HbA_{1c}) in some persons with diabetes. In glycosylated hemoglobin, a glycoprotein is substituted for valine in the β chain, causing a high affinity for oxygen. The red blood cell 2,3-diphosphoglycerate (2,3-DPG) concentration declines during the acidotic and recovery phases of DKA. The glycolytic intermediate 2,3-DPG reduces the hemoglobin affinity for oxygen. An increase in glycosylated hemoglobin and a decrease in 2,3-DPG increase the hemoglobin's affinity for oxygen, and less oxygen is released for tissue use.

Peripheral Neuropathies

Although the incidence of peripheral neuropathies is high among persons with diabetes, it is difficult to document exactly how many are affected by these disorders because of the diversity in clinical manifestations and because the condition often is far advanced before it is recognized. Results of the DCCT study showed that intensive therapy can reduce the incidence of clinical neuropathy by 60% compared with conventional therapy.[56,57]

Two types of pathologic changes have been observed in connection with diabetic peripheral neuropathies. The first is a thickening of the walls of the nutrient vessels that supply the nerve, leading to the assumption that vessel ischemia plays a major role in the development of these neural changes. The second finding is a segmental demyelinization process that affects the Schwann cell. This demyelinization process is accompanied by a slowing of nerve conduction. Research on the sorbitol pathway suggests that the formation and accumulation of sorbitol or the reduction of myoinositol within Schwann cells may lead to injury and impair nerve conduction.

It appears that the diabetic peripheral neuropathies are not a single entity. The clinical manifestations of these disorders vary with the location of the lesion. Although there are several methods for classifying the diabetic peripheral neuropathies, a simplified system divides them into somatic and autonomic disturbances (Chart 36–8). In addition to the discomforts associated with the loss of sensory or motor function, lesions in the somatic or the peripheral nervous system predispose a person with diabetes to other complications. The loss of feeling, touch, and position sense increases the risk of falling. Impairment of temperature and pain sensation increases the risk of serious burns and injuries to the feet. Defects in vasomotor reflexes can lead to dizziness and syncope when the person moves from the supine to the standing position. Incomplete emptying of the bladder because of impaired innervation predisposes the person to urinary stasis and bladder infection and increases the risk of renal complications (see Chapter 28).

In the male, disruption of sensory and autonomic nervous system function can cause impotence. Diabetes is the leading physiologic cause of impotence, and it occurs in both type 1 diabetes and type 2 diabetes. Of the 5 million men with diabetes in the United States, 30% to 60% suffer from impotence.[55]

CHART **36-8**
Classification of Diabetic Peripheral Neuropathies

Somatic

Polyneuropathies (bilateral sensory)
- Paresthesias, including numbness and tingling
- Impaired pain, temperature, light touch, two-point discrimination, and vibratory sensation
- Decreased ankle and knee-jerk reflexes

Mononeuropathies
- Involvement of a mixed nerve trunk that includes loss of sensation, pain, and motor weakness

Amyotrophy
- Associated with muscle weakness, wasting, and severe pain of muscles in the pelvic girdle and thigh

Autonomic

Impaired vasomotor function
- Postural hypotension

Impaired gastrointestinal function
- Gastric atony
- Diarrhea, often postprandial and nocturnal

Impaired genitourinary function
- Paralytic bladder
- Incomplete voiding
- Impotence
- Retrograde ejaculation

Cranial nerve involvement
- Extraocular nerve paralysis
- Impaired pupillary responses
- Impaired special senses

Nephropathies

Diabetic nephropathy is the leading cause of end-stage renal disease, accounting for 36% of new cases. The most common kidney lesions in persons with diabetes are those that affect the glomeruli. Diabetes affects the arterioles as well, causing arteriolar sclerosis; it also increases the susceptibility to pyelonephritis and papillary sclerosis. The term *diabetic nephropathy* is used to describe the combination of lesions that often occur concurrently in the diabetic kidney. In the United States, 33% of all persons who seek renal replacement therapy (see Chapter 29) have diabetes.[58]

Not all persons with diabetes develop clinically significant nephropathy; for this reason, attention is focusing on risk factors for the development of this complication. Among the suggested risk factors are genetic and familial predisposition, kidney and glomerular enlargement, poor glycemic control, and capillary and systemic hypertension.[59] Diabetic nephropathy occurs in family clusters, suggesting a family predisposition, although this does not exclude the possibility of environmental factors shared by siblings.[60] Kidney enlargement, nephron hypertrophy, and hyperfiltration occur early in the disease, suggesting increased work of the kidneys in reabsorbing excessive amounts of glucose. One of the first manifestations of diabetic nephropathy is an increase in urinary albumin excretion (*i.e.*, microalbuminuria), which is easily assessed by laboratory methods. Microalbuminuria is defined as a urine protein loss between 30 and 300 mg/day. The risk of microalbuminuria increases abruptly with hemoglobin A_{1c} levels above 8.1% (Fig. 36–9).[61] Hypertension places increased stress on the arteriolar and capillary structures of the kidneys.

Various glomerular changes may occur in persons with diabetic nephropathy, including capillary basement membrane thickening, diffuse glomerular sclerosis, and nodular glomerulosclerosis. Changes in the capillary basement membrane take the form of thickening of basement membranes along the length of the glomeruli. Diffuse glomerulosclerosis consists of thickening of the basement membrane and the mesangial matrix. It is found in most persons with diabetes of more than 10 years' duration.[62] Nodular glomerulosclerosis, also called intercapillary glomerulosclerosis or *Kimmelstiel-Wilson disease*, is a form of glomerulosclerosis that involves the development of nodular lesions in the glomerular capillaries of the kidneys, causing impaired blood flow with progressive loss of kidney function and, eventually, renal failure. Nodular glomerulosclerosis is thought to occur only in persons with diabetes. This syndrome is encountered in 10% to 35% of persons with diabetes and is a major cause of morbidity and mortality.[62] Changes in the basement membrane in diffuse glomerulosclerosis and Kimmelstiel-Wilson syndrome allow plasma proteins to escape in the urine, causing

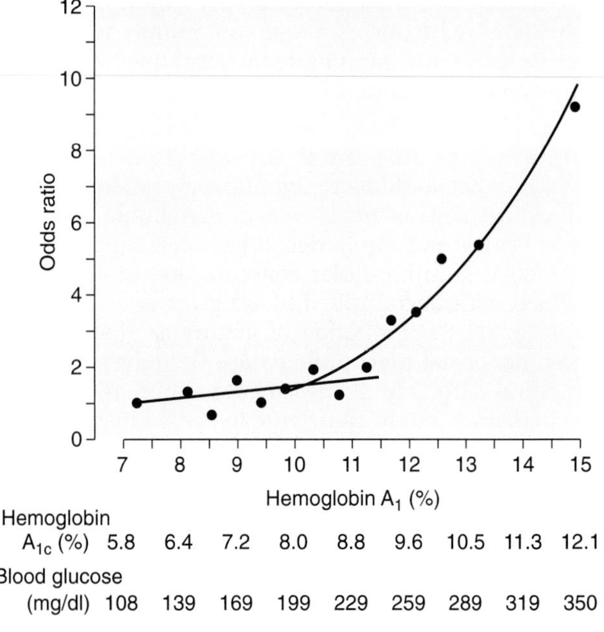

Figure 36–9
Relationship between mean hemoglobin A_1 and the risk of microalbuminuria in patients with type 2 diabetes mellitus. (Krolewski A.S., Laffel L.M.B., Krowelski M. et al. [1995]. Glycosylated hemoglobin and the risk of microalbuminuria in patients with insulin-dependent diabetes mellitus. *New England Journal of Medicine* 332(19):1251–1255)

proteinuria, the development of hypoproteinemia (*i.e.,* decreased levels of plasma proteins), and edema. Glomerular disorders of the kidneys are further discussed in Chapter 28.

Retinopathies

Diabetes is the leading cause of acquired blindness in the United States. Although persons with diabetes are at increased risk for developing cataracts and glaucoma, retinopathy is the most common pattern of eye disease. Diabetic retinopathy is characterized by abnormal retinal vascular permeability, microaneurysm formation, neovascularization and associated hemorrhage, scarring, and retinal detachment (see Chapter 42). Twenty years after the onset of diabetes, nearly all persons with type 1 diabetes and more than 60% of persons with type 2 diabetes have some degree of retinopathy. Diabetic retinopathy is estimated to be the most frequent cause of newly diagnosed blindness among Americans between the ages of 20 and 74 years.[63]

Because of the risk of retinopathy, it is important that persons with diabetes have regular eye examinations. Persons with diabetes should have an initial examination for retinopathy shortly after the diagnosis of diabetes is made. The recommendation for follow-up examinations is based on the type of examination that was done and the findings of that examination. Persons with persistently elevated glucose levels or proteinuria should be examined yearly.[64] Women who are planning a pregnancy should be counseled on the risk of development or progression of diabetic retinopathy. Women with diabetes who become pregnant should be followed closely throughout pregnancy. This does not apply to women who develop gestational diabetes, because such women are not at risk for developing diabetic retinopathy.[63]

Persons with macular edema, moderate to severe nonproliferative retinopathy, or any proliferative retinopathy should receive the care of an ophthalmologist. Methods used in the treatment of diabetic retinopathy include the destruction and scarring of the proliferative lesions with laser photocoagulation. The diabetic retinopathy study demonstrated that photocoagulation may delay or prevent visual loss in more than 50% of eyes with proliferative retinopathy.[65,66]

Macrovascular Complications

Diabetes mellitus is a major risk factor for coronary artery disease, cerebrovascular disease, and peripheral vascular disease. The prevalence of these macrovascular complications is increased twofold to fourfold in persons with diabetes.[67]

Multiple risk factors for macrovascular disease, including obesity, hypertension, hyperglycemia, hyperinsulinemia, hyperlipidemia, altered platelet function, and elevated fibrinogen levels, frequently are found in persons with diabetes. The prevalence of coronary artery disease, stroke, and peripheral vascular disease is substantially increased in persons with diabetes, even in the absence of these risk factors. There appear to be differences between type 1 and type 2 diabetes in terms of duration of disease and the development of macrovascular disease. In persons with type 2 diabetes, macrovascular disease may be present at the time of diagnosis. In type 1 diabetes, the attained age and the duration of diabetes appear to correlate with the degree of macrovascular disease.[68] The reason for these discrepancies has been attributed to the impaired glucose tolerance that exists before actual diagnosis of type 2 diabetes.

Diabetic Foot Ulcers

Foot problems are common among persons with diabetes and may become severe enough to cause ulceration, infection, and eventually, a need for amputation. Foot problems have been reported as the most common complication leading to hospitalization among persons with diabetes. In a controlled study of 854 outpatients with diabetes followed in a general medical clinic, foot problems accounted for 16% of hospital admissions over a 2-year period and 23% of total hospital days.[68] More than one half of all nontraumatic amputations of lower extremities in the United States are reported among persons with diabetic foot problems.[69] In persons with diabetes, lesions of the feet represent the effects of neuropathy and vascular insufficiency. About 60% to 70% of persons with diabetic foot ulcers have neuropathy without vascular disease, 15% to 20% have vascular disease, and 15% to 20% have neuropathy and vascular disease.[70] Approximately 54,000 amputations are performed each year for persons with diabetes.

Persons with sensory neuropathies have impaired pain sensation and often are unaware of the constant trauma to the feet caused by poorly fitting shoes, improper weight bearing, hard objects or pebbles in the shoes, or infections such as athlete's foot. Neuropathy prevents persons from detecting pain; they are unable to adjust their gait to avoid walking on an area where pressure is causing trauma and necrosis. Common sites of trauma are the back of the heel, the plantar metatarsal area, or the great toe, where weight is borne during walking (Fig. 36–10). Motor neuropathy with weakness of the intrinsic muscles of the foot may result in increased weight bearing over the metatarsal heads.

Because of the constant risk of foot problems, it is important that persons with diabetes wear shoes that have been fitted correctly and inspect their feet daily, looking for blisters, open sores, and fungal infection (*e.g.,* athlete's foot) between the toes. If their eyesight is poor, a family member should do this for them. In the event a lesion is detected, prompt medical attention is needed to prevent serious complications. Specially designed shoes have been demonstrated to be effective in preventing relapses in persons with previous ulcerations.[71] Smoking should be avoided, because it causes vasoconstriction and contributes to vascular disease. Because cold produces vasoconstriction, appropriate foot coverings should be used to keep the feet warm and dry. Toenails should be cut straight across to prevent in-

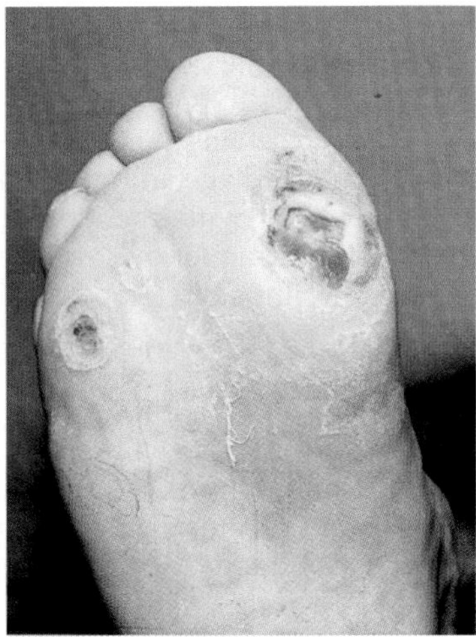

Figure 36–10
Neuropathic ulcers occur on pressure points in areas with diminished sensation in diabetic polyneuropathy. Pain is absent (and therefore the ulcer may go unnoticed).

grown toenails. The toenails often are thickened and deformed, requiring the services of a podiatrist.[72,73]

Infections

Although not specifically an acute or a chronic complication, infections are common concerns of a person with diabetes. Certain types of infections occur with increased frequency in persons with diabetes: soft tissue infections of the extremities, osteomyelitis, urinary tract infections and pyelonephritis, candidal infections of the skin and mucous surfaces, and tuberculosis. Controversy exists about whether infections are more common in persons with diabetes or whether infections seem more prevalent because they often are more serious in persons with diabetes.

Suboptimal response to infection in a person with diabetes is caused by the presence of chronic complications, such as vascular disease and neuropathies, and by the presence of hyperglycemia and altered neutrophil function. Sensory deficits may cause a person with diabetes to ignore minor trauma and infection, and vascular disease may impair circulation and delivery of blood cells and other substances needed to produce an adequate inflammatory response and effect healing. Pyelonephritis and urinary tract infections are relatively common in a person with diabetes, and it has been suggested that these infections may bear some relation to the presence of a neurogenic bladder or nephrosclerotic changes in the kidneys. Hyperglycemia and glycosuria may influence the growth of microorganisms and increase the severity of the infection. Diabetes and elevated blood glucose levels may also impair host defenses such as the function of neutrophils and immune cells.

In summary, diabetes mellitus is a disorder of carbohydrate, protein, and fat metabolism resulting from an imbalance between insulin availability and insulin need. The disease can be classified as type 1 diabetes, in which there is destruction of β cells and an absolute insulin deficiency, or type 2 diabetes, in which there is a lack of insulin availability or effectiveness. Type 1 diabetes can be further subdivided into type 1A immune-mediated diabetes, which is thought to be caused by autoimmune mechanisms, and type 1B idiopathic diabetes, for which the cause is unknown. Other specific types of diabetes include secondary forms of carbohydrate intolerance, which occur secondary to some other condition, such as pancreatic disorders, which destroy β cells, or endocrine diseases such as Cushing's syndrome, which cause increased production of glucose by the liver and decreased use of glucose by the tissues. Gestational diabetes develops during pregnancy, and although glucose tolerance often returns to normal after childbirth, it indicates an increased risk for developing diabetes.

The diagnosis of diabetes mellitus is based on clinical signs of the disease, fasting blood glucose levels, random plasma glucose measurements, and results of the glucose tolerance test. In persons with type 1 diabetes, self-monitoring provides a means of maintaining near-normal blood glucose levels through frequent testing of blood glucose and adjustment of insulin dosage. Glycosylation involves the irreversible attachment of glucose to the hemoglobin molecule; the measurement of glycosylated hemoglobin provides an index of blood glucose levels over several months.

The treatment of diabetes includes diet, exercise, and in many cases, the use of an antidiabetic agent. Dietary management focuses on maintaining a well-balanced diet, controlling calories to achieve and maintain an optimum weight, and regulating the distribution of carbohydrates, proteins, and fats. Two types of antidiabetic agents are used in the management of diabetes: injectable insulin and oral diabetic drugs. Type I diabetes requires treatment with injectable insulin. Oral diabetic drugs include the sulfonylureas, biguanides, α-glucosidase inhibitors, and the thiazolidinediones. These drugs require a functioning pancreas and may be used in the treatment of type 2 diabetes. The benefits of exercise include cardiovascular fitness and psychologic well-being. Many persons with type 2 diabetes benefit from a decrease in body fat, better weight control, and an improvement in insulin sensitivity. In persons with type 1 diabetes, the benefits of exercise are accompanied by a risk of hypoglycemia. The metabolic disturbances associated with diabetes affect almost every body system. The acute complications of diabetes include DKA, HHNK coma, and hypoglycemia. The chronic complications of diabetes affect the non–insulin-dependent tissues, including the retina, blood vessels, kidneys, peripheral nervous system, and feet.

REFERENCES

1. National Diabetes Information Clearinghouse (1996), Bethesda MD. *Diabetes Care* 13, 1.
2. Guyton A., Hall J.E. (1996). *Medical physiology* (9th ed., pp. 971–983). Philadelphia: W.B. Saunders.
3. Ward W.K., Beard J.C., Halter J.B., Pfeifer M.A., Porte D. Jr. (1984). Pathology of insulin secretion in non-insulin diabetes mellitus. *Diabetes Care* 7, 791–502.
4. Rhoades R.A., Tanner G.A. (1996). *Medical Physiology* (pp. 707–719). Boston: Little, Brown.
5. Unger R.H. (1985). The essential role of glucagon in pathogenesis of diabetes mellitus. *Lancet* 1, 14.
6. Waif S.O. (Ed.). (1980). *Diabetes mellitus*. Indianapolis: Eli Lilly.
7. Expert Committee on the Diagnosis and Classification of Diabetes Mellitus. (1997). Report of the Expert Committee on the Diagnosis and Classification of Diabetes Mellitus. *Diabetes Care* 20 (7), 1183–1199.
8. Karam J.H., Solber P.R., Forsham P.H. (1991). Pancreatic hormones and diabetes mellitus. In Greenspan F.S. (Ed.). *Basic clinical endocrinology* (3rd ed., pp. 592–650). East Norwalk, CT: Appleton & Lange.
9. Eisenbarth G.S. (1986). Type I diabetes mellitus: A chronic autoimmune disease. *New England Journal of Medicine* 314, 1360.
10. Skyler J.S., Rabinovitch A. (1987), Etiology and pathogenesis of insulin dependent diabetes mellitus. *Pediatric Annals* 16, 682.
11. Atkinson M.A., Mcclaren N.K. (1994). The pathogenesis of insulin-dependent diabetes mellitus (review). *New England Journal of Medicine* 331 (21), 1428–1436.
12. Todd J.A., Bain S.C. (1992). A practical approach to identification of susceptibility genes for IDDM. *Diabetes* 41, 1049–1034.
13. MacLaren N.K., Riley W., Skordin N., et al. (1988). Inherited susceptibility to insulin dependent diabetes is associated with HLA DR 1, while DR 5 is protective. *Autoimmunity* 1, 197–205.
14. Bloomgarden Z.T. (1996). American Diabetic Association scientific sessions, 1995: IDDM: treatment and prevention. *Diabetes Care* 19 (1), 96–98.
15. Boder G. (1997). Role of fatty acids in the pathogenesis of insulin resistance and NIDDM. *Diabetes Care* 1, 3–11.
16. Boder G., Chen X., Run J., et al. (1995). Effects of fat on glucose uptake and utilization in patients with noninsulin dependent diabetes. *Journal of Clinical Investigation* 96, 1261–1268.
17. Fujimoto W.Y. (1996). Can NIDDM be prevented: the Diabetes Prevention Project. *Practical Diabetology* 15 (3), 10–15.
18. DeFonzo R.A., Goodman A.M., and the Multicenter Metformin Study Group (1995). Efficacy of metformin in patients with noninsulin-dependent diabetes mellitus. *New England Journal of Medicine* 333, 541–549.
19. American Diabetes Association. (1991). Gestational diabetes mellitus [position paper]. *Diabetes Care* 14 (Suppl. 2), 5–6.
20. National Diabetes Data Group. (1989). Impaired glucose tolerance in the American population. *Diabetes Care* 12, 464–474.
21. American Diabetes Association (1997). Standards of medical care for patients with diabetes mellitus. *Diabetes Care* 20 (Suppl. 1), S5–S13.
22. American Diabetes Association. (1992). Urine glucose and ketone determinations (position paper). *Diabetes Care* 15 (Suppl. 2), 38–39.
23. Wheeler M.L. (1997). A brave new world for nutrition and diabetes. *Diabetes Care* 20 (1), 109–110.
24. Gregory R.P., Davis D.L. (1997) Use of carbohydrate counting for meal planning in type I diabetes. *Diabetes Educator* 20 (5), 406–409.
25. American Diabetes Association. (1997). Nutrition recommendations and principles for persons with diabetes mellitus. *Diabetes Care* 20 (Suppl. 1), S-4–S17.
26. McCullock D.K., Mitchell R.D., Ambler J., Tattersall R.B. (1983). Influence of imaginative teaching of diet on compliance and metabolic control in insulin-dependent diabetes. *British Medical Journal* 287, 1857–1862.
27. Nuttall F.Q. (1993). Carbohydrate and dietary management of individuals with insulin-requiring diabetes. *Diabetes Care* 16, 1039–1062.
28. Yomonouchi K., Shinozaki T., Chikada, K., et al. (1995). Daily walking combined with diet therapy is a useful means for obese NIDDM patients not only to reduce body weight but also to improve insulin sensitivity. *Diabetes Care* 18 (6), 775–778.
29. Pergeghin G., Price T.G., Peterson K.F., et al. (1996). Increased glucose transport-phosphorylation and muscle glycogen syntheses after exercise training in insulin-resistant subjects. *New England Journal of Medicine* 335 (18), 1357–1362.
30. Monsen J.E., Remm E.B., Stampfer M.J. (1991). Physical activity and residence of non-insulin dependent diabetes mellitus in women. *Lancet* 338, 774–778.
31. American Diabetes Association (1996). Diabetes mellitus and exercise (position statement). *Diabetes Care* 19 (Suppl. 1), S30.
32. Iwamoto Y., Kosaka K., Kuzuya T., Akanuma Y., Shigeta Y., Kaneko T. (1996). Effects of troglitazone. *Diabetes Care* 19 (2), 151–155.
33. Gilman A.G., Rall T.W., Nies A.S., et al. (1990). *Goodman and Gilman's the pharmacologic basis of therapeutics* (8th ed., pp.1484–1487). New York: Pergamon Press.
34. Johnson A.B., Webster J.M., Sum C.F., et al. (1993). The impact of metformin therapy on hepatic glucose production and skeletal muscle glycogen synthase activity in overweight type II diabetic patients. *Metabolism* 42, 1217–1222.
35. DeFronzo R.A., Barzilain N., Simonson D.C. (1991). Mechanism of metformin action in obese and lean non-diabetic subjects. *Journal Clinical Endocrinology and Metabolism* 73, 1294–1301.
36. Bailey C.J., Turner R.C. (1996). Metformin. *New England Journal of Medicine* 334, 574–579.
37. Chiasson J.L., Josse R.G., Hunt J.A., et al. (1994). The efficacy of acarbose in treatment of patients with noninsulin-dependent diabetes mellitus. *Annals of Internal Medicine* 121 (12), 928–935.
38. Nolan J.J., Luduik B., Berber P., et al. (1994). Improvements in glucose tolerance and insulin resistance in obese subjects treated with troglitazone. *New England Journal of Medicine* 331, 1188–1193.
39. Torlone E., Pampanelli S., Lalli C., et al. (1996). Effects of the short-acting insulin analog (Lys [B25] Pro [B29]) on postprandial blood glucose control in IDDM. *Diabetes Care* 19 (9), 945–952.
40. Zinman B. (1989). The physiologic replacement of insulin. *New England Journal of Medicine* 321, 363–370.

41. Bode B.W., Steed R.D., Davidson P. (1996). Reduction in severe hypoglycemia with long-term continuous subcutaneous insulin infusion in type I diabetes. *Diabetes Care* 19 (4), 324–327.
42. Hirsch I.B. (1995). Implementation of intensive diabetes therapy for IDDM. *Diabetes Reviews* 3 (2), 288–307.
43. Robertson R.P. (1992). Pancreatic and islet cell transplantation for diabetes–cures or curiosities. *New England Journal of Medicine* 327, 1861–1868.
44. Lacy P.E. (1995). Islet cell transplantation for insulin-dependent diabetes. *Hospital Practice* June 15, 41–45.
45. Kitabachi A.E., Wall B.M. (1995). Diabetic ketoacidosis. *Medical Clinics of North American* 79 (1), 9–35.
46. Karam J.H. (1997). Diabetes mellitus and hypoglycemia. In Tierney L. M., McPhee S.J., Papadakis M.A., et al. (Eds.). *Current medical diagnosis and treatment* (36th ed., pp. 1102–1103). East Norwalk, CT: Appleton & Lange.
47. Bolli G.B., Fanelli C.G. (1995). Unawareness of hypoglycemia [editorial]. *New England Journal of Medicine* 333 (26), 1771–1772.
48. Cryer P.E., Fisher J.N., Shamoon H. (1994). Hypoglycemia. *Diabetes Care* 17 (7), 734–755.
49. Somogyi M. (1957). Exacerbation of diabetes in excess insulin action. *American Journal of Medicine* 26, 169.
50. Bolli G.B., Gotterman I.S., Campbell P.J. (1984). Glucose counterregulation and waning of insulin in the Somogyi phenomenon (posthypoglycemic hyperglycemia). *New England Journal of Medicine* 311, 1214.
51. Bolli G.B., Gerich J.E. (1984). The Dawn phenomenon—a common occurrence in both non-insulin and insulin dependent diabetes mellitus. *New England Journal of Medicine* 310, 746–750.
52. Strowing S.M., Raskin P. (1995). Glycemic control and complication of diabetes. *Diabetes Reviews* 3 (2), 337–357.
53. The Diabetes Control and Complications Trial Research Group. (1993). The effect of intensified treatment of diabetes on the development and progression of long-term complications in insulin-dependent diabetes mellitus. *New England Journal of Medicine* 329, 977–955.
54. Cloch C.M., Lee D.A. (1995). Prevention and treatment of the complications of diabetes mellitus. *The New England Journal of Medicine* 332 (18), 1210–1217.
55. Carlin B.W. (1988). Impotence and diabetes. *Metabolism* 37, 19.
56. Said G. (1996). Diabetic neuropathy: An update. *Neurology* 243, 431–440.
57. Vinik A.I., Milicevik Z. (1996). Recent advances in the diagnosis and treatment of diabetic neuropathy. *The Endocrinologist* 6 (6), 443–461.
58. Viberti G., Yip-Messent J., Morocutti A. (1992). Diabetic nephropathy. *Diabetes Care* 15, 1216–1222.
59. Hostetter T.H. (1992). Diabetic nephropathy. *Diabetes Care* 15, 1205–1211.
60. Sequist E.R., Goetz F.C., Rich S., et al. (1989). Familial clustering of diabetic kidney disease. *New England Journal of Medicine* 320, 1161–1165.
61. Krolewski A.S., Laffel L.M.B., Krolewski M., et al. (1995). Glycosylated hemoglobin and the the risk of microalbuminuria in patients with insulin-dependent diabetes mellitus. *New England of Journal of Medicine* 332 (19), 1251–1255.
62. Kumar V., Cotran R.S., Robbins S.L. (1992). *Basic pathology* (5th ed., pp. 576–577). Philadelphia: W.B. Saunders.
63. Singer D.E., Nathan, D.M., Fogel, H.A., et al. (1992). Screening for diabetic retinopathy. *Annals of Internal Medicine* 116, 660–671.
64. American Academy of Ophthalmology. (1992). Screening for diabetes retinopathy (Guide~ lines of the American College of Physicians, American Diabetes Association). *Diabetes Care* 15 (Suppl. 2), P16–P18.
65. Browner W.S. (1986). Preventable complications of diabetes mellitus. *Western Journal of Medicine* 145, 701.
66. Klein R., Klein, B.E.K., Moss S.E. (1996). Relation of glycemic control to diabetic microvascular complications in diabetes mellitus. *Annals of Internal Medicine* 124 (1), 90–96.
67. American Diabetes Association. (1992). Role of cardiovascular risk factors in prevention and treatment of macrovascular disease in diabetes (consensus statement). *Diabetes Care* 15 (Suppl. 2), 68–74.
68. Smith D., Weinberger M., Katz B. (1987). A controlled trial to increase office visits and reduce hospitalizations of diabetic patients. *Journal of General Internal Medicine* 2, 232–238.
69. Reiber G.E. (1992). Diabetes foot care. *Diabetes Care* 15 (Suppl. 1), 29–31.
70. Grunfeld, C. (1991). Diabetic foot ulcers: Etiology, treatment, and prevention. *Advances in Internal Medicine* 37, 103–133.
71. Levin ME. (1995) Preventing amputation in the patient with diabetes. *Diabetes Care* 18 (10), 1383–1394.
72. Uccioli L., Faglia F., Monticone G., et al. (1995). Manufactured shoes in the prevention of diabetes foot ulcers. *Diabetes Care* 18 (10), 1376–1378.
73. Levin M.E., O'Neal L.W., Bowker J.H. (1995). *The Diabetic Foot* (5th ed.). St. Louis: C.V. Mosby.

ADDITIONAL READINGS

American Diabetes Association (1997). Standards of medical care for patients with diabetes mellitus. *Diabetes Care* 20 (Suppl 1), S5–S13.

Amiel S. (1993). Reversal of unawarenss of hypoglycemia (Editorial). *New England Journal of Medicine* 329 (12), 876–877.

Baily C.J., Turner R.C. (1996). Metformin. *New England Journal of Medicine* 334 (9),574–579.

Bode B.W., Steed R.D., Davidson P. (1996). Reduction in hypoglycemia with long-term continuous subcutaneous insulin infusion in type I diabetes. *Diabetes Care* 19 (4), 324–327.

Boder G., Chen X. (1994). Mechanisms of fatty acids induced inhibition of glucose uptake. *Journal of Clinical Investigation* 93, 2438–2446.

DeVenciana M., Major C.A., Morgan , et al. (1995). Postprandial versus preprandial blood glucose monitoring in women with gestational diabetes mellitus requiring insulin. *New England Journal of Medicine*. 333, 1237–1241.

Dorhnorst A., Girling J.C. (1995). Management of gestational diabetes mellitus. *New England Journal of Medicine* 333 (19), 1281–1282.

Iwamoto Y., Kosaka K., Kuzuka K., et. al., (1996). Effect of combination troglitazone and sulfonylureas in patients with type 2 diabetes who were poorly controlled on sulfonylurea therapy alone. *Diabetes Medicine* 13, 365–370.

Nathan D.M. (1996). The pathophysiology of diabetic complications: How much does the glucose hypothesis explain. *Annals of Internal Medicine* 124 (1), 86–89.

Remuzzi G., Paggenenti P., Mauer S.M. (1994). Pancreas and kidney/pancreas transplants: Experimental medicine or real improvement? *Lancet* 343, 27–31.

Alterations In Neural Function

For centuries, the nervous system was ignored or even deemed unimportant. Aristotle (384–332 BC), the great Greek philosopher, decreed that the heart was the seat of the soul whereas the brain—which he assumed was composed largely of water—simply cooled it. Although Galen (AD 130–200) was able to show that the spinal cord was essential to many sensations and movements, his experiments were conducted only on animals. Not until the 1500s, when the Flemish anatomist Andreas Vesalius (1514–1564) dissected "the heads of executed criminals... still warm," was the overarching importance of the human brain and spinal cord established.

Investigations continued with scientists debating whether the brain should be considered as a whole or as consisting of separate areas, each responsible for specific functions. Progress in brain research took an impressive, if accidental leap, in 1848, when an explosion at a railroad work site in Vermont shot an iron rod into the left cheek of Phineas Gage, through his brain, and out the top of his head. Gage survived the accident, but it became clear to all who knew him that he had changed greatly. Formerly a conscientious, hard-working man, he became fitful, obstinate, foul-mouthed, and capricious. Gage died in 1860 and an autopsy showed destruction of the left lobe of his brain and damage to his right lobe. Scientists concluded that his personality change was the result of the grievous damage to the frontal lobes, an observation that supported the then-emerging concept that different parts of the brain serve different functions.

UNIT X

CHAPTER 37

Organization and Control of Neural Function

Edward W. Carroll and Robin L. Curtis

The nervous system, in coordination with the endocrine system, provides the means by which cell and tissue functions are integrated into a solitary, surviving organism. It controls skeletal muscle movement and helps to regulate cardiac and visceral smooth muscle activity. The nervous system makes possible the reception, integration, and perception of sensory information; it provides the substratum necessary for intelligence, anticipation, and judgment; and it facilitates adjustment to an ever-changing external environment. No part of the nervous system functions separately from other parts. In the human, who is a thinking and feeling creature, the effects of emotion can exert a strong influence on neural and hormonal control of body function. However, alterations in neural and endocrine function, particularly at the biochemical level, can also exert a strong influence on psychologic behavior. This chapter is divided into four parts: nervous tissue cells, the development and organization of the nervous system, neuronal communication, and the autonomic nervous system.

Nervous Tissue Cells

After you have completed this section of the chapter, you should be able to meet the following objectives:

- Differentiate between the central and peripheral nervous systems

- List the three parts of a neuron and describe their structure and function
- Name the supporting cells in the central nervous system and peripheral nervous system and state their functions
- Describe the energy requirements of nervous tissue

The nervous system can be divided into two parts: the central nervous system (CNS) and the peripheral nervous system (PNS). The CNS consists of the brain and spinal cord, which are located within the protected confines of the axial skeleton in the cranium and spinal column. The PNS is located outside these structures. The basic design of the nervous system provides for the concentration of computational and control functions within the CNS. In this design, the PNS functions as an input-output system for relaying input to the CNS and for transmitting output messages that control effector organs, such as muscles and glands.

Nervous tissue contains two types of cells: neurons and supporting cells. The *neurons* are the functional cells of the nervous system. Neurons exhibit membrane excitability and conductivity and secrete neurotransmitters and hormones, such as epinephrine and antidiuretic hormone. The *supporting cells,* such as Schwann cells in the PNS and the glial cells in the CNS, protect the nervous system and supply metabolic support for the neurons.

Neurons

The functioning cells of the nervous system are called neurons. Neurons have three distinct parts: the cell body with its cytoplasm-filled processes, the dendrites, and the axons (Fig. 37–1). These processes form the functional connections, or synapses, with other nerve cells, with receptor cells, or with effector cells. The axonal processes are particularly designed for rapid communication with other neurons and the many body structures that are innervated by the nervous system. Afferent, or sensory, neurons transmit information from the PNS to the CNS. Efferent, or motor neurons, carry information away from the CNS. Interspersed between the afferent and efferent neurons is a network of interconnecting neurons that modulate and control the body's response to changes in the internal and external environments.

The *cell body,* or *soma,* of a neuron contains a large, vesicular nucleus with one or more distinct nucleoli and a well-developed rough endoplasmic reticulum. The nucleus has the same DNA code content that is present in other cells of the body. The nucleoli, which are composed of particular portions of several chromosomes, produce RNAs associated with protein synthesis. The cytoplasm contains large masses of ribosomes that are prominent in most neurons. These acidic RNA masses, which are involved in protein synthesis, stain as dark *Nissl* bodies with basic histologic stains (see Fig. 37–1).

The *dendrites* (*i.e.,* treelike) are multiple, branched extensions of the nerve cell body; they conduct information toward the cell body and are the main source of information for the neuron. The dendrites and cell body are studded with synaptic terminals that communicate with axons and dendrites of other neurons (Fig. 37–2).

The *axon* is a long efferent process that projects from the cell body and carries impulses away from the cell. There is usually only one axon for each nerve cell. Most axons undergo multiple branching, resulting in many axonal terminals. The cytoplasm of the cell body extends to fill the dendrites and the axon (see Fig. 37–1). The proteins and other materials that are used by the axon are synthesized in the cell body and then flow down the axon through its cytoplasm.

The cell body of the neuron is equipped for a high level of metabolic activity. This is necessary because the cell body must synthesize the cytoplasmic and membrane constituents required to maintain the function of the axon and its terminals. Some of these axons extend for a distance of 1 to 1.5 m and have a volume that is sometimes 200 to 500 times greater than the cell body itself. Two axonal transport systems, one slow and one rapid, move molecules from the cell body through the cytoplasm of the axon to its terminals. Replacement proteins and nutrients slowly diffuse from the cell body, where they are synthesized, down the axon, moving at the rate of about 1 mm/day. Other molecules, such as some of the neurosecretory granules or their precursors, are conveyed by a rapid, energy-dependent active transport system, moving at the rate of about 400 mm/day. In many instances, membrane-bound vesicles containing neurosecretory granules (*e.g.,* neurotransmitters, neuromodulators, neurohormones) are moved to the axon synaptic terminals by the active transport process. For example, rapid axonal transport carries antidiuretic hormones and oxytocin from hypothalamic neurons through their axons to the posterior pituitary, where the hormones are released into the blood. A reverse rapid (*i.e.,* retrograde) axonal transport system moves materials, including target cell messenger molecules, from axonal terminals back to the cell body.

Supporting Cells

Supporting cells of the nervous system, the Schwann and satellite cells of the PNS and the several types of glial cells of the CNS, provide the neurons with protection and metabolic support. The supporting cells segregate the neurons into isolated metabolic compartments, which are required for normal neural function. Together with the tightly joined endothelial cells of the capillaries in the CNS, these supporting cells contribute to what is called the *blood-brain barrier.* This term is used to emphasize the impermeability of the nervous system to large or potentially harmful molecules.

The many-layered myelin wrappings of Schwann cells of the PNS and the oligodendroglia of the CNS provide the myelin sheath segments that serve to increase the velocity of nerve impulse conduction in axons having larger diameters. Myelin has a high lipid content, which gives it a whitish color, and the name *white matter*

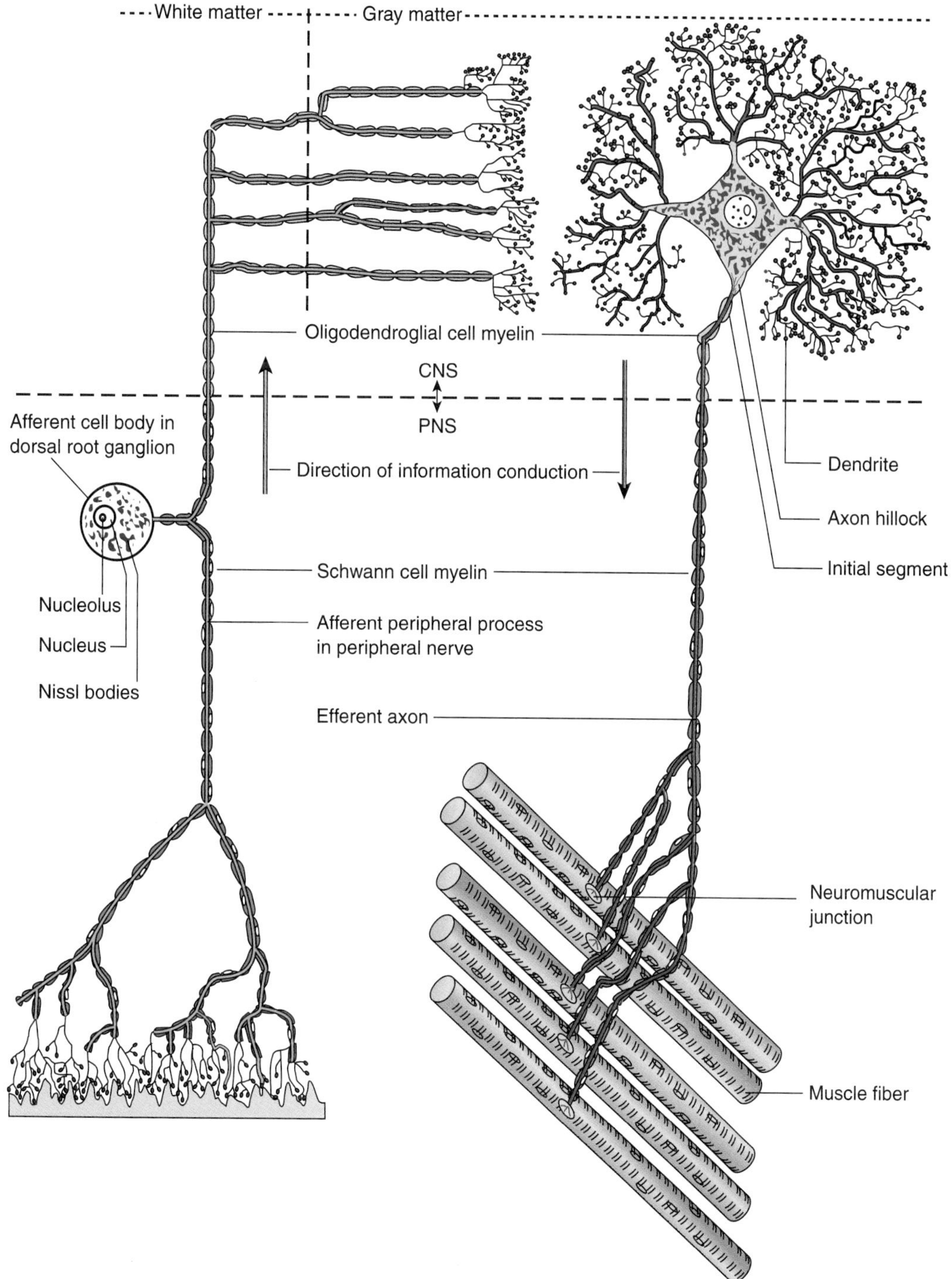

Figure 37–1
Afferent and efferent neurons.

is given to the masses of myelinated fibers of the spinal cord and brain. In addition to its role in increasing conduction velocity, the myelin sheath is essential for the survival of large neuronal processes, perhaps by the secretion of neurotrophic compounds. In some pathologic conditions, such as multiple sclerosis in the CNS and Guillain-Barré syndrome in the PNS, the myelin may degenerate or be destroyed, leaving a section of the axonal process without myelin but with nearby Schwann or oligodendroglial cells. Unless remyelination takes place, the axon will eventually die.

There are essentially no glycogen stores in the cytoplasm of the neuron. The major source of glucose for neurons and their processes is by diffusion from the supporting cells, including Schwann and oligodendroglial cells, and from the vascular system. The metabolic inter-

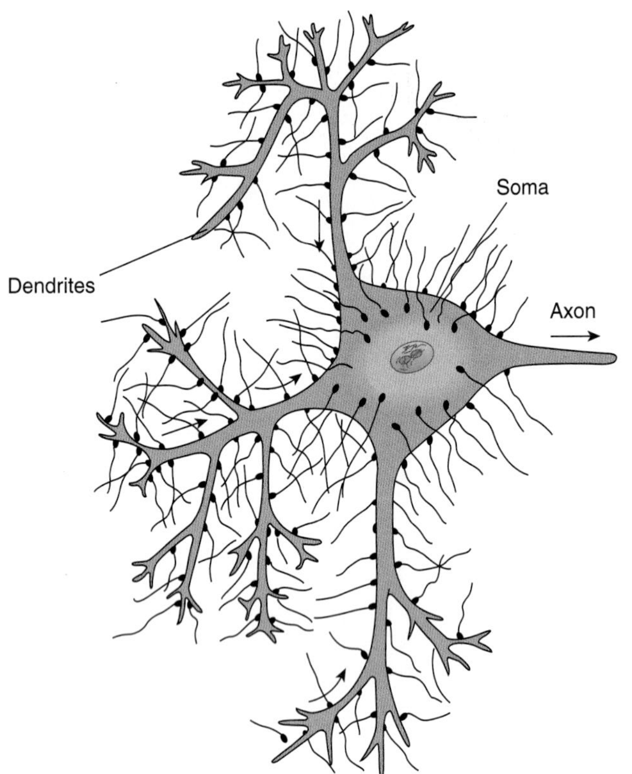

Figure 37–2
A typical motor neuron, showing presynaptic terminals on the neuronal soma and dendrites. Notice the single axon. (Guyton A.C., Hall J.E. [1996]. *Textbook of medical physiology* [p. 559]. Philadelphia: W.B. Saunders)

vention of these supporting cells is essential for the long-term survival of the neuron and its processes.

Supporting Cells of the Peripheral Nervous System

The two types of supporting cells of the PNS are the satellite and Schwann cells. Normally, the nerve cell bodies in the PNS are collected into *ganglia,* such as the dorsal root and autonomic ganglia. Each of the cell bodies and processes of the peripheral nerves is surrounded, or enclosed, in cellular sheaths of supporting cells. The cells that surround the ganglion cells are called *satellite cells.* The satellite cells secrete a basement membrane that protects the cell body from the diffusion of large molecules.

The processes of the larger nerves, the axons of the afferent and efferent neurons, are surrounded by the cell membrane and cytoplasm of Schwann cells, which are close relatives of the satellite cells. The Schwann cell surrounds the nerve process and then twists many times around the process in jelly-roll fashion (Fig. 37–3). Schwann cells line up along the neuronal process, and each of these cells forms its own discrete myelin segment. The end of each myelin segment attaches to the cell membrane of the axon by means of sealed junctions. Successive Schwann cells are separated by short extracellular fluid gaps called the *nodes of Ranvier,* where the myelin is missing and voltage-gated sodium channels are concentrated (Fig. 37–4). The nodes of Ranvier increase nerve conduction by allowing the impulse to jump from node to node through the extracellular fluid in a process called *saltatory conduction.* In this way, the impulse can travel more rapidly than it could if it were required to move systematically along the entire nerve process. This increased conduction velocity greatly reduces reaction time, or time between the application of a stimulus and the subsequent motor response. The short reaction time is of particular importance in peripheral nerves with long distances (sometimes 1 to 1.5 m) for conduction between the CNS and distal effector organs.

Each of the end-to-end series of Schwann cells is enclosed within a continuous tube of basement membrane, which is surrounded by a multilayered, collagen-rich *endoneurial tube* (Fig. 37–5). These endoneurial tubes are bundled together with blood vessels into small bundles or clusters of nerves called *fascicles,* which are surrounded by a collagenous *perineurial sheath.* Usually, several fascicles are further surrounded by the heavy, protective *epineurial sheath* of the peripheral nerve. The protective layers that surround the peripheral nerve processes are continuous with the connective tissue capsule of the sensory nerve endings and the connective tissue that surrounds the effector structures, such as the skeletal muscle cell. Centrally, the connective tissue layers continue along the dorsal and ventral roots of the nerve and fuse with the meninges that surround the spinal cord and brain. The endoneurial tube does not penetrate the CNS.

The endoneurial sheath is essential to the regeneration of peripheral axons. This sheath provides a collage-

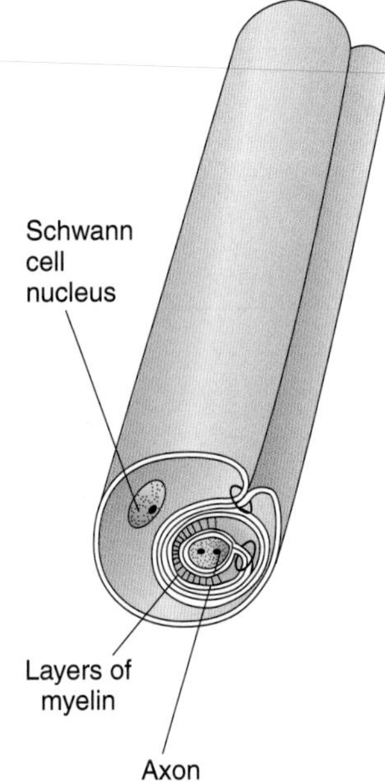

Figure 37–3
The Schwann cell migrates down a larger axon to a bare region, settles down, and encloses the axon in a fold of its plasma membrane. It then rotates around and around, wrapping the axon in many layers of plasma membrane, with most of the Schwann cell cytoplasm squeezed out. The resultant thick, multiple-layered coating around the axon is called myelin.

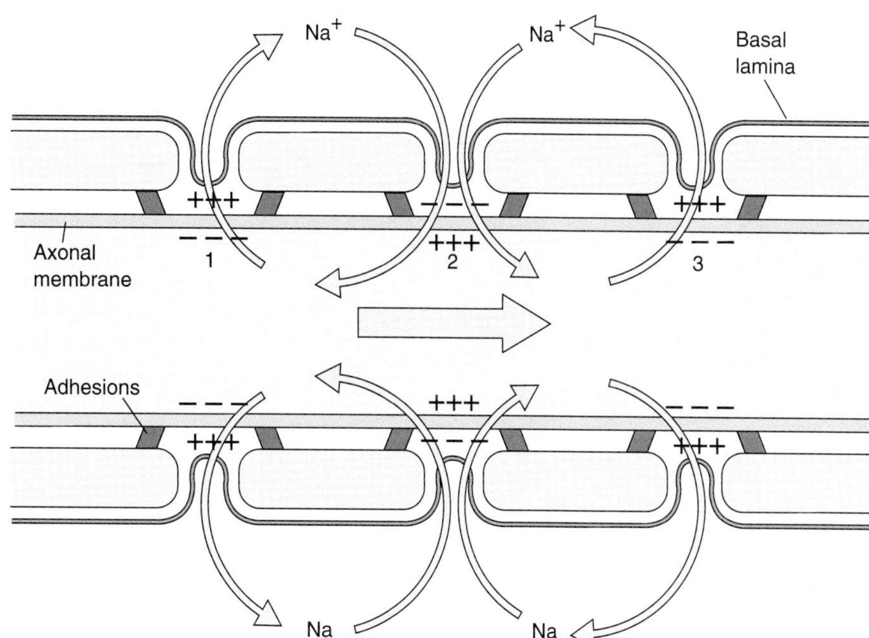

Figure 37–4
Schematic drawing of a longitudinal section of myelinated axon in the peripheral nervous system. Schwann cells insulate the axon, decreasing ion flow through the membrane. Action potentials occur at the nodes of Ranvier, which are unmyelinated areas of the basal lamina between the Schwann cells. The impulses jump from node to node in a process called saltatory conduction, which greatly increases the velocity of conduction. (1) represents the trailing hyperpolarized region behind the action potential, (2) the hypopolarized region at the action potential, and (3) the leading hyperpolarized area ahead of the action potential. The Schwann cell adhesions (*red*) to the plasma membrane of the axon block the leakage of current under the myelin.

nous tube through which a regenerating axon can again reach its former target. The entire ganglion is protected by a heavy collagenous layer, which also surrounds the large bundles of neural processes in the PNS, called the epineurial sheath. The absence of these tubular collagenous structures is thought to be a major factor in the limited axonal regeneration of CNS nerves compared with those of the PNS.

Supporting Cells of the Central Nervous System

The supporting cells of the CNS consist of the oligodendroglia, astroglia, microglia, and the ependymal cells. The *oligodendroglial cells* form the myelin for the CNS. Instead of forming a myelin covering for a single axon, these cells reach out with several processes, each wrapping around and forming a multilayered myelin segment around several different axons (Fig. 37–6). The coverings of the nerve axons in the CNS also function in speeding the velocity of nerve conduction in a manner similar to that of the peripheral myelinated fibers.

A second type of glial cell, the *astroglia,* is particularly prominent in the gray matter, or more central portion of the brain. These large cells have many processes, some reaching to the surface of the capillaries, others reaching

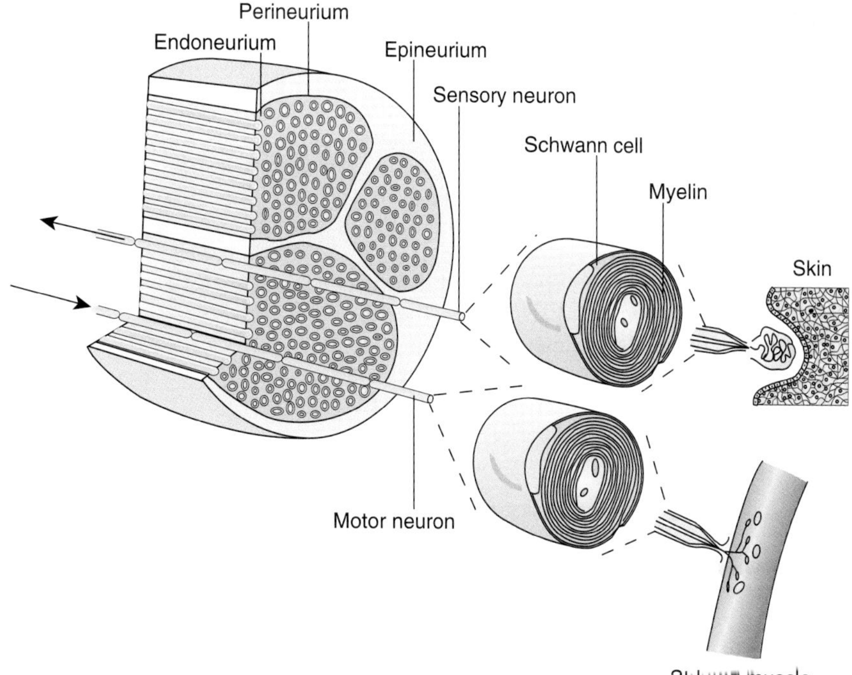

Figure 37–5
Section of a peripheral nerve containing axons of both afferent (sensory) and efferent (motor) neurons.

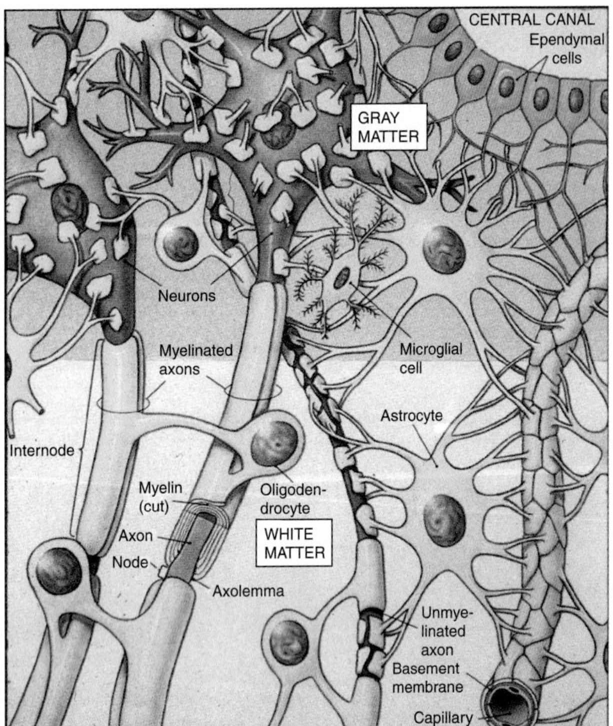

Figure 37–6
The histology of neural tissue in the CNS. (**Top**) Diagrammatic view of relationships between the major glial elements and cell bodies of CNS neurons. (**Bottom**) A comparable view that shows the relationships between and axons inside the CNS. (From Martini F.H. [1995]. *Fundamentals of anatomy and physiology* [3rd ed.]. Englewood Cliffs, NJ: Prentice-Hall)

to the surface of the nerve cells, and still others filling most of the intercellular space of the CNS. The astrocytic linkage between the blood vessels and the neurons may provide a transport mechanism for the exchange of oxygen, carbon dioxide, and metabolites. The astrocytes also have an important role in sequestering cations such as calcium and potassium from the intercellular fluid. The astrocytes are capable of filling their cytoplasm with microfibrils (*i.e.*, fibrous astrocytes), and masses of these cells form the special type of scar tissue called *gliosis* that develops in the CNS when tissue is destroyed.

A third type of glial cell, the *microglia,* is a small phagocytic cell that is available for cleaning up debris after cellular damage, infection, or cell death. The fourth type of cell, the *ependymal cells* form the lining of the neural tube cavity, the ventricular system. In some areas, these cells combine with a rich vascular network to form the choroid plexus, where production of the cerebrospinal fluid (CSF) takes place.

Metabolic Requirements of Nervous Tissue

Nervous tissue has a great need for metabolic energy. Although the brain comprises only 2% of the body's weight, it receives about 15% of the resting cardiac output and consumes 20% of its oxygen. Despite its substantial energy requirements, the brain cannot store oxygen, nor can it engage in anaerobic metabolism. An interruption in the blood or oxygen supply to the brain rapidly leads to clinically observable signs and symptoms. In the absence of oxygen, brain cells continue to function for about 10 seconds. Unconsciousness occurs almost simultaneously when cardiac arrest occurs, and the death of brain cells begins within 4 to 6 minutes. Interruption of blood flow also leads to the accumulation of metabolic byproducts that are toxic to neural tissue.

Glucose is the major fuel source for the nervous system, but neurons have no provisions for storing glucose. Ketones can provide for limited temporary energy requirements; however, these sources are rapidly depleted. Unlike muscle cells, neurons have no glycogen stores and must rely on glucose from the blood or the glycogen stores of supporting glial cells. Persons receiving insulin for diabetes may experience signs of neural dysfunction and unconsciousness (*i.e.*, insulin reaction or shock) when blood glucose drops as a result of insulin excess (see Chapter 36).

In summary, nervous tissue is composed of two types of cells: neurons and supporting cells. Neurons are composed of three parts: a cell body, which controls cell activity; the dendrites, which conduct information toward the cell body; and the axon, which carries impulses from the cell body. The supporting cells consist of Schwann and satellite cells of the PNS and the glial cells of the CNS. The supporting cells protect and provide metabolic support for the neurons and aid in segregating them into isolated compartments, which is necessary for normal neuronal function. The function of the nervous system demands a high amount of metabolic energy. Glucose is the major fuel for the nervous system. The brain comprises only 2% of body weight but receives of the 15% of the resting cardiac output.

Nerve Cell Communication

After you have completed this section of the chapter, you should be able to meet the following objectives:

- Describe the function of ion channels and relate this to the different phases of an action potential
- Differentiate electrical from chemical synapses
- Describe the interaction of the presynaptic and postsynaptic terminals
- Relate excitatory and inhibitory postsynaptic potentials to the process of spatial and temporal summation of membrane potentials
- Briefly describe how neurotransmitters are synthesized, stored, released, and inactivated

Neurons are characterized by the ability to communicate with other neurons and body cells through pulsed electrical signals called *impulses*. An impulse, or action potential, represents the lateral, or lengthwise, movement of electrical charge along the axon membrane.

This phenomenon is based on the rapid flow, sometimes called *conductance,* of charged ions through the membrane in a progressive manner. In excitable tissue, ions such as sodium, potassium, and calcium move through membrane channels, carrying the electrical charges that are involved in the initiation and transmission of such impulses.

Action Potentials

The cell membranes of excitable tissue, including neurons, contain ion channels that are responsible for generating action potentials. These membrane channels are guarded by voltage-dependent gates that open and close with changes in the membrane potential. There are separate voltage-gated channels for the sodium, potassium, and calcium ions. Each type of ion channel has a characteristic membrane potential that opens and closes its channels. There are also ligand-gated channels that respond to chemical messengers such as neurotransmitters.

Nerve signals are transmitted by action potentials that are abrupt, pulselike changes in the membrane potential that last a few ten thousandths to a few thousandths of a second. Action potentials can be divided into three phases: the resting or polarized state, depolarization, and repolarization (Fig. 37–7).

The *resting phase* is the undisturbed period of the action potential during which the membrane is impermeable to the flow of current-carrying ions. During this period, the membrane is said to be polarized because of the large separation of charge (*i.e.,* positive on the outside and negative on the inside). The resting membrane potential for large nerve fibers is about −90 mV. However, in small neurons and in many neurons in the CNS, the resting membrane potential is often as little as −40 to −60 mV. The resting phase of the membrane potential continues until some event causes the membrane to increase its permeability to sodium.

The *threshold potential* represents the membrane potential at which neurons or other excitable tissue are stimulated to fire. In large nerve fibers, the sodium channels open at about −60 mV, which is the threshold for initiation of an action potential. When this threshold potential is reached, the gatelike structures in the membrane open widely in an all-or-none manner. Under ordinary circumstances, the threshold stimulus is sufficient to open large numbers of these channels, triggering massive depolarization of the membrane—the action potential.

Depolarization is characterized by the flow of electrically charged ions. During the depolarization phase the membrane suddenly becomes permeable to sodium ions; the rapid inflow of sodium ions produces local currents that travel through the adjacent cell membrane, and this causes the sodium channels in this part of the membrane to open. In neurons, the sodium ion gate remains open for only about a quarter of a millisecond and closes quickly. During this phase of the action potential the inside of the membrane becomes positive (about +30 to +45 mV).

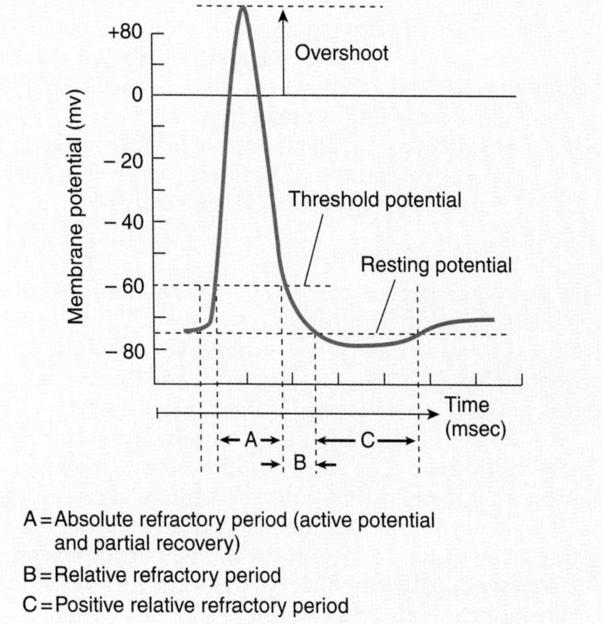

Figure 37–7
Time course of the action potential recorded at one point of an axon with one electrode inside and one on the outside of the plasma membrane. The rising part of the action potential is called the spike. The rising phase plus approximately the first half of the repolarization phase is equal to the absolute refractory period (A). The portion of the repolarization phase that extends from the threshold to the resting membrane potential represents the relative refractory period (B). The remaining portion of the repolarization phase to the resting membrane potential is equal to the negative after potential (C). Hyperpolarization is equal to the positive relative refractory period.

Repolarization is the phase during which the polarity of the resting membrane potential is reestablished. This is accomplished with closure of the sodium channels and opening of the potassium channels. The outflow of positively charged potassium ions across the cell membrane returns the membrane potential to negativity. The sodium-potassium pump gradually reestablishes the resting ionic concentrations on each side of the membrane. The membrane of an excitable cell must be sufficiently repolarized before it can be reexcited. In the process of repolarization, the membrane remains refractory (*i.e.,* does not fire) until the repolarization is about one-third complete. This period, which lasts about one half of a millisecond, is called the *absolute refractory period.* There is an additional portion of the recovery period during which the membrane can be excited, although only by a stronger-than-normal stimulus. This period is called the *relative refractory period.*

Synaptic Transmission

Neurons communicate with each other through structures known as *synapses.* There are two types of synapses:

electrical and chemical. Electrical synapses permit the passage of current carrying ions through small openings called *gap junctions* that penetrate the cell junction of adjoining cells. The gap junctions allow an action potential to pass directly and quickly from one neuron to another. Gap junctions can communicate in either direction. They may couple neurons that form a close functional relation into circuits where this is required.

Chemical Synapses

The more common type of synapse is the chemical synapse. Chemical synapses involve special presynaptic and postsynaptic membrane structures, separated by a synaptic cleft (Fig. 37–8). The presynaptic terminal secretes one and often several chemical messenger molecules (*i.e.*, neurotransmitters or neuromodulators) into the synaptic cleft. The most rapid acting of these, the neurotransmitters, diffuse into and unite with receptors on the postsynaptic membrane, and this causes excitation or inhibition of the postsynaptic neuron by producing hypopolarization or hyperpolarization of the postsynaptic membrane, respectively.

Hypopolarization increases the excitability of the postsynaptic neuron by bringing the membrane potential closer to the threshold potential so that a smaller stimulus is needed to cause the neuron to fire. Such a synapse is called *excitatory*. *Hyperpolarization* brings the membrane potential further from the threshold potential and has the opposite effect. It has an *inhibitory* effect and decreases the likelihood that an action potential will be generated. Synapses fall into two main classes: excitatory or inhibitory, depending on the type of receptors on the postsynaptic membrane.

In contrast to an electrical synapse, a chemical synapse serves as a rectifier, permitting only one-way communication. The one-way conduction is a particularly important characteristic of chemical synapses. It is this specific transmission of signals to discrete and highly localized areas of the nervous system that allow it to perform the myriad functions of sensation, motor control, and memory. Consider for a moment, what would happen if this one-way communication system were to be disrupted.

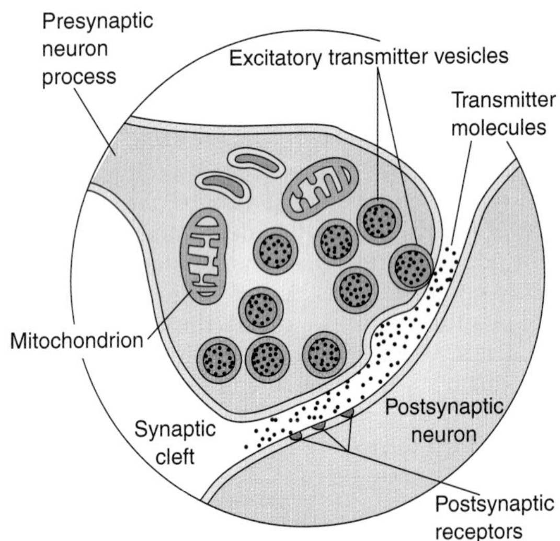

Figure 37–8
Synapse, showing the presynaptic and postsynaptic neuronal surfaces.

Chemical synapses are the slowest component in progressive communication through a sequence of neurons such as in a spinal reflex. In contrast to the conduction of electrical action potentials, each successive event at the chemical synapse—transmitter secretion, diffusion across the synaptic cleft, interaction with postsynaptic receptors, and generation of a subsequent action potential in the postsynaptic neuron—consumes time. On the average, conduction across a chemical synapse requires approximately 0.3 milliseconds.

A neuron's cell body and dendrites are covered by thousands of synapses, any or many of which can be active at any moment in time. Because of this rich synaptic input, each neuron resembles a little integrator in which there are many circuits of neurons that interact with each other. It is the complexity of these interactions that gives the system its intelligence in terms of the subtle integrations involved in producing behavioral responses. It is also what makes the prediction of stimulus-response associations difficult in the absence of a millisecond-to-millisecond knowledge of the excitatory and inhibitory activity that takes place on the surfaces of each neuron in a functional circuit. It is amazing, with billions of these little integrators capable of becoming involved in such a response, that predictions are possible at all. It is even more astounding that the basic microcircuitry involved in the nervous system is reproduced reliably during the development of each new organism.

There are many types of chemical synapses. Axons can synapse with dendrites (*axodendritic*), with the cell body (*axosomatic*), or to other axons (*axoaxonic*). Dendrites can synapse with axons (*dendroaxonic*), other dendrites (*dendrodendritic*), or the soma of other neurons (*dendrosomatic*). There are *somatoaxonic* synapses. Synapses occurring between the soma of neighboring neurons (*somasomatic*) are uncommon except in some efferent nuclei. The mechanism of communication between the *presynaptic* and the *postsynaptic* neuron is similar in all types of synapses; the action potential sweeps into the axonal terminals of the afferent neuron and triggers the rapid release of neurotransmitter molecules from the axonal, or presynaptic, surface. Conversion of action potentials into neurotransmitter release is called *coupling*, and although it is not completely understood, it is believed that the release of calcium ions is involved.

Excitatory and Inhibitory Postsynaptic Potentials

Many CNS neurons possess thousands of synapses on their dendritic or somatic surfaces, each of which can produce partial excitation or inhibition of the postsynaptic neuron. When the combination of a neurotransmitter with a receptor site causes partial depolarization of the postsynaptic membrane, it is called an *excitatory postsynaptic potential* (EPSP). In other synapses, the combination of a transmitter with a receptor site is inhibitory in the sense that the combination of the transmitter with the receptor site causes the local nerve membrane to become hyperpolarized and less excitable. Then it is called an *inhibitory postsynaptic potential* (IPSP).

An action potential does not begin in the membrane adjacent to the synapse. It begins in the *initial segment* (axon hillock) of the axon, just before the first myelin segment, at which point the axon is more excitable than the rest of the neuron. The local currents resulting from any one EPSP (sometimes called a *generator potential*) are usually insufficient to pass threshold and cause depolarization of the axon's initial segment. However, if several EPSPs occur simultaneously, the area of depolarization can become large enough and the currents at the initial segment can become strong enough to exceed the threshold potential and initiate a conducted action potential. This summation of depolarized areas is called *spatial summation.* The EPSPs can also summate and cause an action potential if they come in close temporal relation to each other. This temporal aspect of the occurrence of two or more EPSPs is called *temporal summation.*

IPSPs can also undergo spatial and temporal summation with each other and with EPSPs, reducing the effectiveness of the latter by a roughly algebraic summation. If the sum of EPSPs and IPSPs keeps the depolarization at the initial segment below threshold levels, the generation of an action potential does not occur.

The spatial and temporal summation required in the distribution and timing of synaptic activity serves as a sensitive and complicated switch requiring just the right combination of incoming activity before the cell releases its own message in the form of the action potential. The frequency of action potentials in the axon is an all-or-none language (*i.e.,* digital language), which can vary only as to the presence or absence of such impulses and their frequency. Action potentials permit rapid communication over distances, but it is the rich capacity for integration of excitatory and inhibitory synaptic bombardment of the soma and dendrites that gives the neuron and the nervous system the capability for complexity, memory, and intelligence.

Messenger Molecules

Neurotransmitters are the chemical messenger molecules of the nervous system. The process of neurotransmission involves the synthesis, storage, and release of a neurotransmitter; the reaction of the neurotransmitter with a receptor; and termination of the receptor action (Fig. 37–9). New research methods, including staining techniques and the use of radiolabeled antibodies, have allowed scientists to study and gain answers in each of these areas.

The nervous system and the endocrine system use chemical molecules as messengers. As more information is obtained about the chemical messengers of both systems, the distinction between the nervous system and the endocrine system becomes somewhat blurred. Many neurons, such as those in the adrenal cortex, secrete transmitters that are released into the bloodstream, and it has been found that other neurons possess receptor

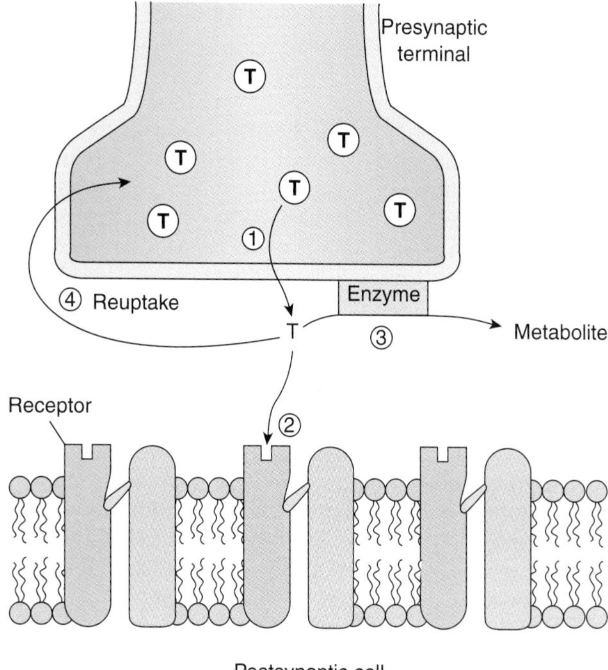

Figure 37–9
Schematic illustration of (1) neurotransmitter (T) release, (2) binding of transmitter to receptor, (3) degradation of transmitter, and (4) reuptake of transmitter into the presynaptic terminal. (Rhoades R.A., Tanner G.A. [1996]. *Medical physiology* [p. 46]. Boston: Little, Brown)

sites for hormones. Many hormones have turned out to be neurotransmitters. Vasopressin (also known as antidiuretic hormone), a peptide hormone released from the posterior pituitary gland, acts as a hormone in the kidney and as a neurotransmitter for nerve cells in the hypothalamus. More than a dozen of these cell-to-cell and bloodborne messengers are known to be capable of relaying signals in the nervous system or in the endocrine system.

Neurotransmitters are synthesized in the cytoplasm of the axon terminal. The synthesis of transmitters may require one or more enzyme-catalyzed steps (*i.e.,* one for acetylcholine and three for norepinephrine). The various types of neurons are limited in terms of the type of transmitter they can synthesize by their enzyme systems.

After synthesis, the transmitter molecules are stored in the axon terminal in tiny membrane-bound sacs called *synaptic vesicles.* There may be thousands of vesicles in a single terminal, each containing 10,000 to 100,000 molecules of transmitter. The vesicle protects transmitters from enzyme destruction within the nerve terminal. The arrival of an impulse at a nerve terminal causes a large number of transmitter molecules to be released into the synaptic space.

Neurotransmitters exert their actions through specific proteins, called *receptors,* embedded in the postsynaptic membrane. These receptors are tailored precisely to match the size and shape of the transmitter. In each case, the interaction between a transmitter and receptor results in a specific physiologic response. The action of a transmitter is determined by the type of receptor it binds to. For example, acetylcholine is excitatory when it is released at a myoneural junction, and it is inhibitory when it is released at the sinoatrial node in the heart. Receptors are named according to the type of neurotransmitter they interact with. For example, the term *cholinergic receptor* is used to indicate a receptor that binds acetylcholine. Some neurotransmitters act as modulators of neural action rather than initiators or inhibitors.

Rapid removal of a transmitter, once it has exerted its effects on the postsynaptic membrane, is necessary to maintain precise control of neural transmission. A transmitter that has been released can undergo one of three fates. It can be broken down into inactive substances by enzymes, it can be taken back up into the presynaptic neuron in a process called *reuptake,* or it can diffuse away into the intercellular fluid until its concentration is too low to influence postsynaptic excitability. Acetylcholine, for example, is rapidly broken down by acetylcholinesterase into acetic acid and choline, with the choline being taken back into the presynaptic neuron for reuse in acetylcholine synthesis. The catecholamines are largely taken back into the neuron in an unchanged form for reuse. The catecholamines can also be degraded by enzymes in the synaptic space or by enzymes in the nerve terminals.

Neurotransmitters tend to be small molecules that incorporate a positively charged nitrogen atom; they include amino acids, peptides, and monoamines. Amino acids are the building blocks of proteins and are present in body fluids. Peptides are low-molecular-weight molecules that yield two or more amino acids on hydrolysis. They include substance P and the endorphins and enkephalins, which are involved in pain sensation and perception (see Chapter 40). A monoamine is an amine molecule containing one amino group (NH_2). Serotonin, dopamine, norepinephrine, and epinephrine are monoamines that are synthesized from amino acids. Fortunately, the nervous system is protected by the blood-brain barrier from circulating amino acids and other molecules that could act in an unregulated manner as neurotransmitters.

There is still much to be learned about the role of certain amino acids and peptides as neurotransmitters. For example, several amino acids (especially, glutamic acid and aspartic acid) appear to exert powerful excitatory effects on synaptic transmission; they are often called *excitatory amino acids.* Glycine, another amino acid, is known to have strong inhibitory effects. One of the most common inhibitory transmitters is gamma-aminobutyric acid (GABA). This amino acid is unique in that it is synthesized almost exclusively in the brain and spinal cord. It has been established that almost one third of all synapses use GABA. With the inclusion of amino acids as neurotransmitters comes the puzzling idea that the same amino acid can function as a neurotransmitter and as a building block for protein synthesis.

The actions of most neurotransmitters are localized in specific clusters of neurons with axons that project to highly specific brain regions. As more has been learned about the location and mechanism of action of the various neurotransmitters, it has become apparent that many disease conditions have their origin in altered neurotransmitter responses. In some cases, there is evidence of degeneration or dysfunction of the neurons producing the neurotransmitters; in others, there is an apparent alteration in the postsynaptic response to the neurotransmitter. For example, the neurons containing dopamine are concentrated in regions of the midbrain known as the *substantia nigra* and *ventral tegmentum.* Many of these dopamine-containing neurons project their axons to areas of the forebrain that are thought to be involved in regulation of emotional behavior. Other dopamine fibers terminate in regions near the middle of the brain called the *corpus striatum.* These latter fibers seem to play an essential role in the performance of complex motor movements. Degeneration of the dopamine fibers in this area of the brain leads to the tremor and rigidity that are characteristic of Parkinson's disease. Some forms of mental illness, such as schizophrenia, are thought to involve abnormal release or responses to neurotransmitters in the brain. Pharmacologic methods of supplying neurotransmitters (*e.g.,* in Parkinson's disease) or modifying their actions (*e.g.,* with psychoactive drugs) are used to treat some of these disorders. Undoubtedly, more specific treatment methods will become available as more is learned about the transmission of neural information.

Other classes of messenger molecules are released from axon terminals in addition to or instead of neurotransmitters. Neuromodulator molecules apparently react with postsynaptic receptors to produce slower and longer lasting changes in membrane excitability. This has the effect of making the action of the faster-acting neurotransmitter molecules more or less effective. Some of the peptide molecules may fall into the modulator category.

Neurohumoral mediators reach the target cell through the bloodstream and produce an even slower action than the neuromodulators. Neurotrophic or growth factors are required to maintain the long-term survival of the postsynaptic cell and are secreted by axon terminals independent of an action potential. Examples include lower motor neurons (LMNs) to muscle cell trophic factors and neuron-to-neuron trophic factors in sequential chains of CNS, sensory systems. Trophic factors from the target cell that can enter the axon terminal and are essential to the long-term survival of the presynaptic neuron have also been demonstrated. Target cell to neuron trophic factors probably have great significance in establishing specific neural connections during normal embryonic development.

In summary, neurons are characterized by the ability to communicate with other neurons and body cells through pulsed electrical signals called action potentials. The cell membranes of neurons contain ion channels that are responsible for generating action potentials. These channels are guarded by voltage-dependent gates that open and close with changes in the membrane potential. Action potentials are divided into three parts: the resting membrane potential, during which the membrane is polarized but no electrical activity occurs; the depolarization phase, during which sodium channels open and allow rapid inflow of the sodium ions that generate the electrical impulse; and the repolarization phase, during which the membrane is permeable to the potassium ion allowing for the efflux of potassium ions and return of resting membrane potential. The membrane threshold represents the membrane potential at which the sodium channels open, heralding the onset of an action potential. Once initiated, an action potential travels rapidly along the cell's axonal membrane to trigger transmitter release with the next neuron in the sequence.

Synapses are structures that permit communication between neurons. There are electrical and chemical synapses. Electrical synapses consist of gap junctions between adjacent cells that allow action potentials to move rapidly from one cell to another. Chemical synapses involve special presynaptic and postsynaptic structures, separated by a synaptic cleft. They rely on chemical messengers, released from terminals on the presynaptic neuron, that cross the synaptic cleft and then interact with receptors on the postsynaptic neuron.

Neurotransmitters are chemical messengers that control neural function; they selectively cause excitation or inhibition of action potentials. There are three major types of neurotransmitters: amino acids such as glutamic acid and GABA, peptides such as the endorphins and enkephalins, and monoamines such as epinephrine and norepinephrine. Neurotransmitters interact with cell membrane receptors to produce an excitatory or inhibitory action. Neuromodulators are chemical messengers that react with membrane receptor to produce slower and longer-acting changes in membrane permeability. Neurotrophic or growth factors, also released from presynaptic terminals, are required to maintain the long-term survival of postsynaptic neurons.

Developmental Organization of the Nervous System

After you have completed this section of the chapter, you should be able to meet the following objectives:

- Cite the significance of the hierarchy of control levels of the CNS
- Use the segmental approach to explain the development of the nervous system and the organization of the postembryonic nervous system
- Define the terms *afferent, efferent, ganglia, association neuron, cell column,* and *tract*
- State the origin and destination of nerve fibers contained in the dorsal and ventral roots
- State the type of structures that are innervated by general somatic afferent, general visceral afferent, special somatic afferent, general visceral efferent, pharyngeal efferent, and general somatic efferent neurons

The development of the nervous system can be traced far back into evolutionary history. In the course of its development, newer functional features and greater complexity resulted from the modification and enlargement of more primitive structures. For a moving organism, rapid reaction to environmental danger, to potential food sources, or to a sexual partner was required for the survival of the species.

The front, or rostral, end of the CNS became specialized as a means of sensing the external environment and controlling reactions to it. In time, the ancient organization, which is largely retained in the spinal cord segments, was expanded in the forward segments of the nervous system. Of these, the most forward segments have undergone the most radical modification and have developed into the forebrain: the diencephalon and the cerebral hemispheres. The dominance of the front end of the CNS is reflected in a hierarchy of control levels—brain stem over spinal cord and forebrain over brain stem. Because the newer functions were added onto the outside of older functional systems and because the newer functions became concentrated at the rostral end of the nervous system, they are much more vulnerable to injury.

These three principles—no part of the nervous system functions independently of the other parts, newer systems control older systems, and the newer systems are more vulnerable to injury—form a basis for understanding many of the manifestations of injury or disease of the nervous system.

Embryonic Development

The nervous system appears very early in embryonic development. The early development of the nervous system is essential because it influences the development and organization of many other body systems, including the axial skeleton, skeletal muscles, and sensory organs such as the eyes and ears. During later fetal life and thereafter, the nervous system provides communication, signal processing, and integrative and memory functions by means of electrochemical and chemical secretory functions of neurons. The early induction and later lifelong communication functions of the nervous system are at the center of the integrity, survival, and individuality of each person.

During the second week of development, there are two layers of embryonic tissue, the endoderm and ectoderm. At the beginning of third week, the ectoderm begins to invaginate and migrate between the two layers, forming a third layer called the *mesoderm* (see Fig. 37–8). The mesoderm along the entire midline of the embryo forms a specialized rod of embryonic tissue called the *notocord*. The notochord and adjacent mesoderm provides the necessary induction signal for the overlying ectoderm to differentiate and form a thickened structure called the *neural plate:* the primordium of the nervous system. The neural plate develops an axial groove (*i.e.,* neural groove) that sinks into the underlying mesoderm; its walls fuse across the top, forming a hollow ectodermal tube called the *neural tube*. This process, which is called *closure,* occurs during the latter third and fourth weeks of gestation and is vital to the survival of the embryo. In the process of development, the neural tube develops into the CNS; the notochord becomes the foundation around which the vertebral column ultimately develops, and the surface ectoderm separates from the neural tube and fuses over the top to become the outer layer of skin. Closure of the neural tube begins at the cervical and high thoracic levels and zippers rostrally toward the cephalic end of the embryo and caudally toward the sacrum. The last locations for completion of closure are at the rostral-most end of the brain (*i.e.,* anterior neuropore, 25 days) and at the lumbosacral region (*i.e.,* posterior neuropore, 27 days).

As the neural tube closes, ectodermal cells called *neural crest cells* migrate away from the dorsal surface of

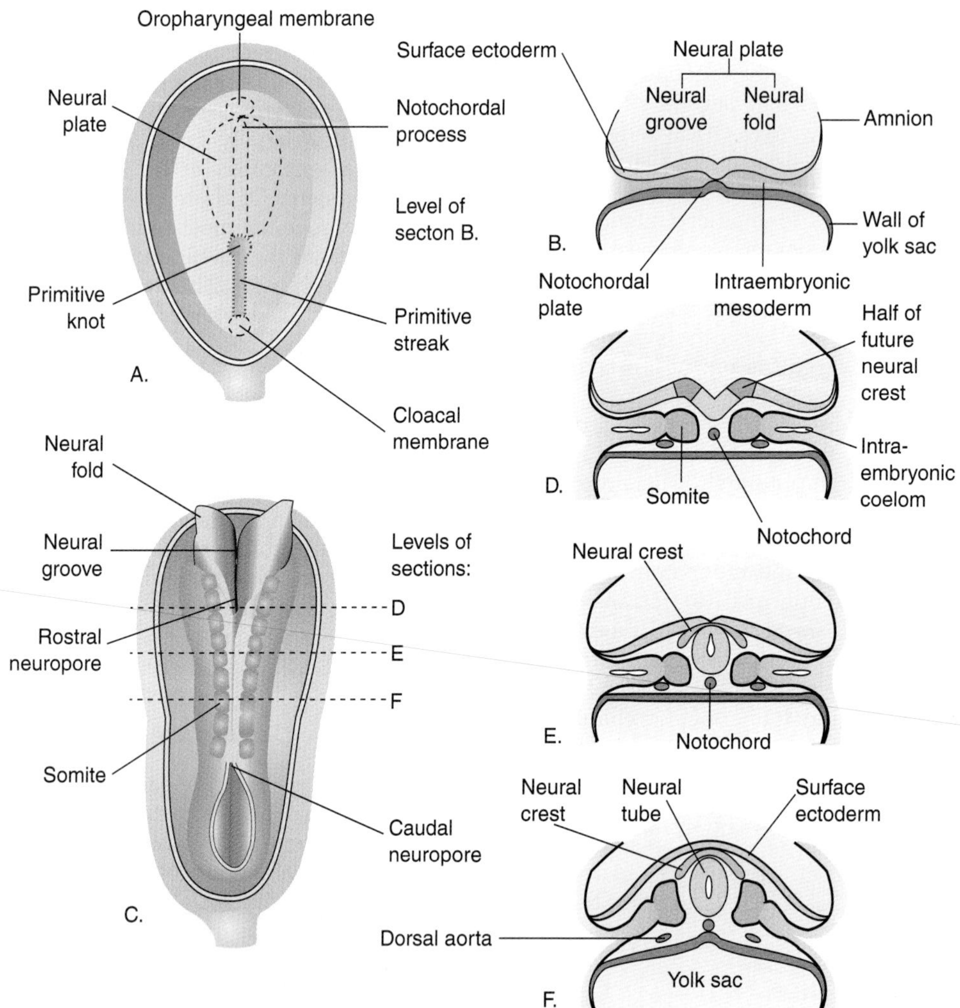

Figure 37–10
Diagram showing formation of the neural crest and folding of the neural tube. (**A**) Dorsal view of an embryo of about 18 days, exposed by removing the amnion. (**B**) Transverse section of this embryo shows the neural plate and early development of the neural groove. The developing notochord is also shown. (**C**) Dorsal view of an embryo of about 22 days. The neural folds have fused opposite the somites but are widely spread out at both ends of the embryo. The rostal and caudal neuropores are indicated. (**D, E, F**) Transverse sections of this embryo at the levels shown in **C,** illustrating formation of the neural tube and its detachment from the surface ectoderm. Some neuroectodermal cells are not included in the neural tube but remain between it and the surface ectoderm as the neural crest. These cells first appear as paired columns on the dorsolateral aspect of the neural tube, but they soon become broken up into a series of segmented masses. (Moore K.L., Persaud T.V.M. [1993]. *The developing human.* [5th ed., p. 386] Philadelphia: W.B. Saunders)

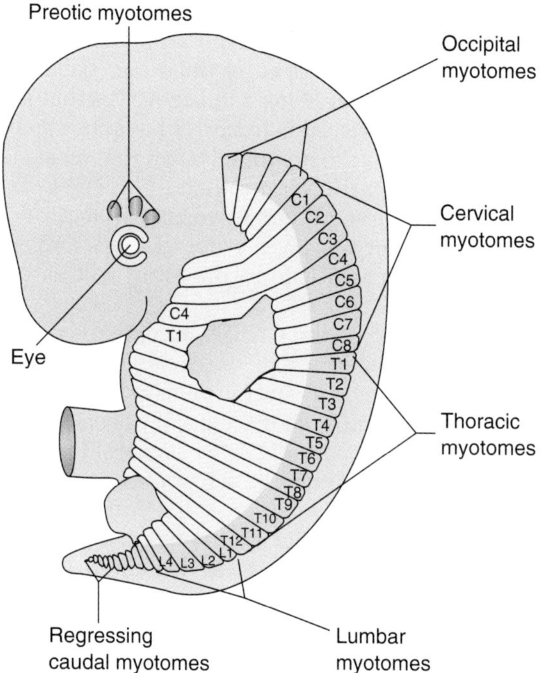

Figure 37–11
The developing muscular system in a 6-week-old embryo. The segmental muscle masses, or myotomes, which give rise to most skeletal muscles, reflect the basic segmental organization of the body and head. Efferent cranial nerves innervating the myotomes of the head are as follows: preotic myotomes (nerves III, IV, and VI) and the occipital myotomes (XII). (Moore K.L., Persaud T.V.M. [1993]. *The developing human* [5th ed., p. 372]. Philadelphia: W.B. Saunders)

the forming neural tube to become the progenitors of the neurons and supporting cells of the PNS (Fig. 37–10). Some of these cells gather into clumps, or ganglia, at the sides of each spinal cord segment (*i.e., dorsal root ganglia*) and most brain segments (*i.e., cranial ganglia*). Neurons of these ganglia become the afferent or sensory neurons of the PNS. Other neural crest cells become the pigment cells of the skin or contribute to the formation of the meninges, many of the structures of the face, and the peripheral ganglion cells of the autonomic nervous system. The latter include cells of the adrenal cortex.

In the process of development, the more rostral part of the embryonic neural tube—approximately 10 segments—undergoes extensive modification and enlargement to form the brain (Fig. 37–11). In the early embryo, three swellings, or primary vesicles, develop, subdividing these 10 segments into the prosencephalon, or forebrain, which contains the first two segments; the mesencephalon, or midbrain, which develops from segment 3; and the rhombencephalon, or hindbrain, which develops from segments 4 to 10 (Fig. 37–12).

The 10 brain segments represent modifications of the spinal cord neural tube and are often called, collectively, *the brain stem.* The brain stem does not include later developed outgrowths—the cerebral hemispheres, the optic nerve and retina, and the cerebellum. The central canal of the prosencephalon develops two pairs of lateral outpouchings that carry the neural tube with them: the optic cup, which becomes the optic nerve and retina, and the telencephalic vesicles, which become the olfactory bulbs and the cerebral hemispheres. The central canal of the neural tube extends into the cerebral hemispheres as enlarged CSF-filled cavities, the first and second (lateral) ventricles. The remaining neural tube of these three segments is called the *diencephalon;* it develops into the thalamus and hypothalamus. The neurohypophysis (posterior pituitary) grows as a midline ventral outgrowth at the junctions of segments 1 and 2. A dorsal outgrowth, the pineal body, develops between segments 2 and 3, the diencephalic-mesencephalic junction.

Each of these brain segments, except for segment 2, retains some portion of the basic segmental organization of the nervous system. The evolutionary development of the brain is reflected in the cranial and upper cervical paired segmental nerves. This reflects the prototype or original pattern: a segmented neural tube, each segment of which has multiple paired branches containing a grouping of particular component axons. One segment would have paired branches to body muscles and another set to visceral structures, and so on. The classic pattern of the spinal nerve organization, which consists of a pair of dorsal and a pair of ventral roots, is a later evolutionary development that has not occurred in the cranial nerves. Consequently, the cranial nerves, which are arbitrarily numbered 1 through 12, retain the ancient pattern with more than one cranial nerve branching from a single segment. The truly segmental nerve pattern of the cranial nerves is further clouded by the loss

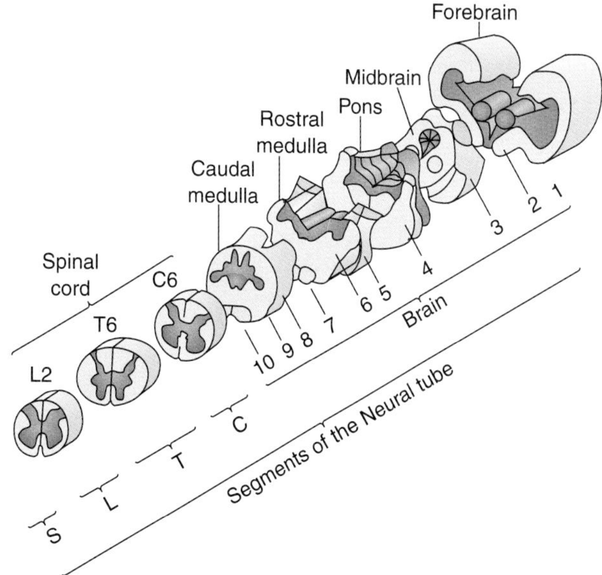

Figure 37–12
The adult human central nervous system. The dorsal (*vertical hatching*) and ventral (*horizontal hatching*) horns of the gray matter are surrounded by the white matter that contains the longitudinal tracts. Numbers indicate segmental divisions of the neural tube.

of all branches from segment 2 and most of the branches from segment 1. The second cranial nerve, also called the optic nerve, is not a segmental nerve branch. Rather, it is a brain tract connecting the retina (modified brain) with the first forebrain segment from which it developed.

Soma and Viscera. All body tissues and organs have developed from the three layers of tissue (*i.e.*, endoderm, ectoderm, and mesoderm) that were present during third week of embryonic life. On cross section, the body is organized into the soma and viscera (Fig. 37–13). The soma, or body wall, includes all of the structures derived from the embryonic ectoderm, such as the epidermis of the skin and the CNS. The mesodermal connective tissues of the soma include the dermis of the skin, skeletal muscle, bone, and the outer lining of the body cavity (*i.e.*, parietal pleura and peritoneum). The nervous system innervates all of the more internal structures constituting the *viscera*, including the great vessels derived from the intermediate mesoderm, the urinary system, and the gonadal structures. The viscera also includes the inner lining of the body cavities, such as the visceral pleura and peritoneum, and the mesodermal tissues that surround the entoderm-lined gut and its derivative organs (*e.g.*, lungs, liver, pancreas).

Segmental Organization

The early pattern of segmental development is presented as a framework for understanding the nervous system. In the process of development, the basic organizational pattern of the body is that of a longitudinal series of segments, each repeating the same fundamental pattern (Fig. 37–14). Although the early muscular, skeletal, vascular, and excretory systems and the nerves that supply these somatic and visceral structures have the same segmental pattern, it is the nervous system that most clearly retains this organization in postnatal life. The CNS and its associated peripheral nerves consist of about 43 segments, 33 of which form the spinal cord and spinal nerves, and 10 of which form the brain and its cranial nerves.

Each segment of the CNS is accompanied by two pairs (one member of a pair on each side) of bundled nerve fibers, or *roots:* a ventral pair and a dorsal pair. The paired dorsal roots connect a pair of *dorsal root ganglia* and their corresponding CNS segment. These ganglia contain the afferent nerve cell bodies, each of which has two axonlike processes—one that ends in a peripheral receptor and the other that enters the central neural segment. The axonlike process that enters the central neural segment communicates with a neuron called an *input association (IA) neuron.* Somatic afferents transmit information from the soma to somatic IA neurons, and visceral afferents transmit information from the viscera to visceral IA neurons. The paired ventral roots of each segment are bundles of axons that provide efferent (motor) output to effector sites such as muscle and glandular cells of the body segment.

On cross section, the hollow embryonic neural tube can be divided into a central canal, or ventricle, that contains the CSF and the wall of the tube. The latter develops into an inner gray cellular portion, functionally divided into longitudinal columns of neurons called the *cell*

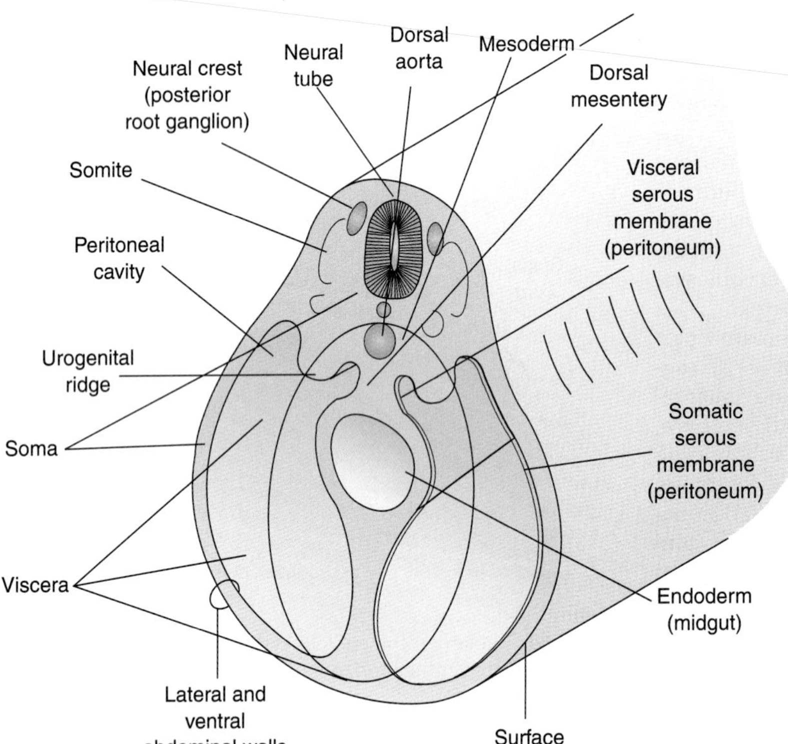

Figure 37–13
Cross section of a human embryo, illustrating the development of the somatic and visceral structures.

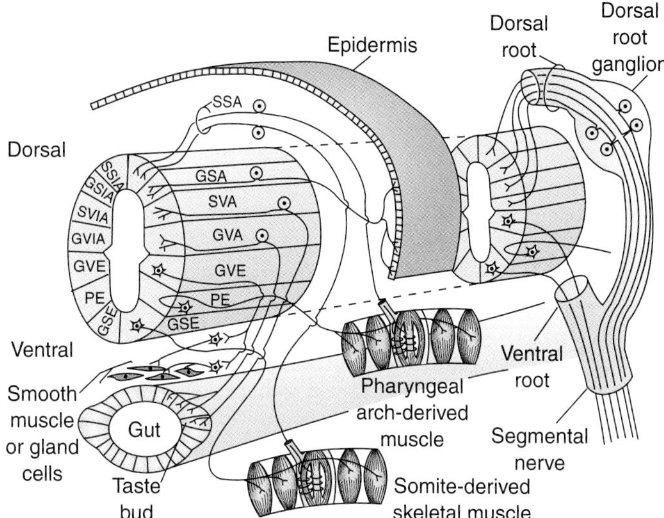

Figure 37–14
Cell columns of the central nervous system. The columns in the dorsal horn contain input association neurons: special sensory (SSIA), general sensory (GSIA), special visceral (SVIA), and general visceral (GVIA). The ventral horn contains the efferent neurons; the general visceral efferent (GVE), pharyngeal efferent (PE), and general somite efferent (GSE).

columns, that contains nerve cell bodies, and an outer white matter region that contains longitudinal tract systems of the CNS made up of nerve cell processes. The dorsal half of the gray matter is called the *dorsal horn.* It contains sensory IA neurons that receive afferent information from the dorsal roots. The ventral portion, or *ventral horn,* contains efferent neurons that communicate by way of the ventral roots with effector cells of the body segment. Many of the CNS neurons develop axons that grow longitudinally as tract systems that communicate among neighboring and distal segments of the neural tube.

Cell Columns

The complexity of the organizational structure of the nervous system is somewhat simplified by a pattern in which PNS and CNS neurons are repeated as parallel cell columns running lengthwise along the nervous system. In this organizational pattern, afferent neurons, dorsal horn cells, and ventral horn cells are organized as a series of 11 cell columns. A box of 22 colored beverage straws (a set of 11 straws on each side of the midline) can be used to represent the cell columns. In this model, each lateral half of the nervous system (right and left sides) is represented in mirror fashion by one set of 11 colored straws. If these straws were cut crosswise (equivalent to a transverse section through the nervous system) at several places along their length, the spatial relations among the different colored straws would be repeated in each section.

The cell columns on each side can be further grouped according to their location in the PNS: four in the dorsal ganglia that contain sensory neurons; four in the dorsal horn that contain the sensory IA neurons; and three in the ventral horn that contain motor neurons. Each column of dorsal root ganglia projects to its particular column of IA neurons in the dorsal horn. The IA neurons distribute afferent information to local reflex circuitry and more rostral and elaborate segments of the CNS. The ventral horns contain *output association (OA) neurons* and LMNs. The lower motor neurons provide the final circuitry for organizing efferent nerve activity.

Between the IA neurons and the OA neurons are networks of small internuncial neurons or interneurons that are arranged in complex circuits. The internuncial neurons provide the discreteness, appropriateness, and intelligence of responses to stimuli. Most of the billions of CNS cells in the spinal cord and brain gray matter are internuncial neurons.

Dorsal Horn Cell Columns. There are four columns of afferent (sensory) neurons in the dorsal root ganglia that directly innervate four corresponding columns of input association neurons in the dorsal horn. These columns are categorized as special and general afferents: special somatic afferent, general somatic afferent, special visceral afferent, and general visceral afferent.

Special somatic afferent fibers are concerned with internal sensory information such as joint and tendon sensation (*i.e.,* proprioception). The *general somatic afferents* innervate the skin and other somatic structures; they respond to stimuli such as those that produce pressure or pain. The general somatic afferent IA column cells relay the sensory information to protective and other reflex circuits and project the information to the forebrain, where it is perceived as painful, warm, cold, and such. The special somatic afferent IA column cells relay their information to local reflexes concerned with posture and movement. These neurons also relay information to the cerebellum, contributing to coordination of movement, and to the forebrain, contributing to experience. Afferents innervating the labyrinth and derived auditory end organs of the inner ear also belong to the special soma category.

Special visceral afferent cells innervate specialized gut-related receptors, such as the taste buds and receptors of the olfactory mucosa. Their central processes communicate with special sensory input association column neurons that project to reflex circuits to produce salivation, chewing, swallowing, and other responses. The forebrain projection fibers from these association cells provide the sensations of taste (*i.e.*, gustation) and smell (*i.e.*, olfaction). *General visceral afferent* neurons innervate visceral structures such as the gastrointestinal tract, urinary bladder, heart and great vessels; they project to the general visceral IA column, which relays to vital reflex circuits and sends information to the forebrain regarding visceral sensations such a stomach fullness, bladder pressure, and sexual experience.

Ventral Horn Cell Columns. The ventral horn contains three separate longitudinal cell columns: general visceral efferent, pharyngeal efferent, and general somatic efferent. Each of these cell columns contain OA and efferent neurons. The OA neurons coordinate and integrate the function of the efferent motor neuron cells of its column.

General visceral efferent neurons transmit the efferent output of the autonomic nervous system and are called *preganglionic neurons.* The general visceral efferents are structurally and functionally divided into the sympathetic and parasympathetic nervous system, and their axons project through the segmental ventral roots to innervate smooth and cardiac muscle and glandular cells of the body, most of which are in the viscera. In the viscera, three additional neural crest–derived cell columns are present on each side of the body. These become the postganglionic neurons of the autonomic nervous system. For the sympathetic nervous system, the columns are the paravertebral or sympathetic chain ganglia and the prevertebral series of ganglia (*e.g.*, celiac ganglia) associated with the dorsal aorta. For the parasympathetic system, these become the enteric plexus in the wall of the gut-derived organs and a series of ganglia in the head.

Pharyngeal efferent neurons innervate the branchial arch skeletal muscles: the muscles of mastication, facial expression, head turning, and muscles of the pharynx and larynx.

The *general somatic efferent* column neurons supply the somite-derived muscles of the body and head, which include the skeletal muscles of the body, limbs, tongue, and extrinsic eye muscles (see Fig. 37–14). These efferent neurons transmit the commands of the CNS to peripheral effectors—the skeletal muscles. They are the "final common pathway neurons" in the sequence leading to motor activity. They are often called *LMNs* because they are under the control of higher levels of the CNS, including precise control by *upper motor neurons* (UMNs).

Longitudinal Tracts

The gray matter of the cell columns in the CNS is surrounded by bundles of myelinated axons (*i.e.*, white matter) and unmyelinated axons that travel longitudinally along the length of the neural axis. This white matter can be divided into three layers: inner, middle, and outer (Fig. 37–15). The inner, or *archi,* layer contains short fibers that project for a maximum of about five segments before reentering the gray matter. The middle, or *paleo,* layer projects six or more segments. The archi-layer and the paleo-layer fibers have many branches, or *collaterals,* that enter the gray matter of intervening segments. The outer, or *neo,* layer contains large-diameter axons that can travel the entire length of the nervous system (Table 37–1). The term *suprasegmental* refers to higher levels of the CNS, such as the brain stem and cerebrum and structures above a given CNS segment. Paleo- and neo-level fibers have suprasegmental projections.

The longitudinal layers are arranged in bundles, or fiber tracts, which contain axons that have the same destination, origin, and function. These longitudinal tracts are named systematically to reflect their origin and destination; the origin is named first, and the destination is named second. For example, the *spinothalamic tract* originates in the *spinal* cord and terminates in the *thalamus.* The *corticospinal* tract originates in the cerebral *cortex* and ends in the *spinal* cord.

Inner Layer. The inner layer of white matter contains the axons of neurons of the gray matter that connect with neighboring segments of the nervous system. The axons of this layer permit the pool of motor neurons of several segments to work together as a functional unit. They also allow the afferent neurons of one segment to trigger reflexes that activate motor units in neighboring and in the same segments. In terms of evolution, this is the oldest of the three layers, and it is sometimes referred to as the archi-level layer. It is the first of the longitudinal layers to become functional, and it appears to be limited to reflex types of movements. Reflex movements of the fetus (*i.e.*, quickening) that begin during the

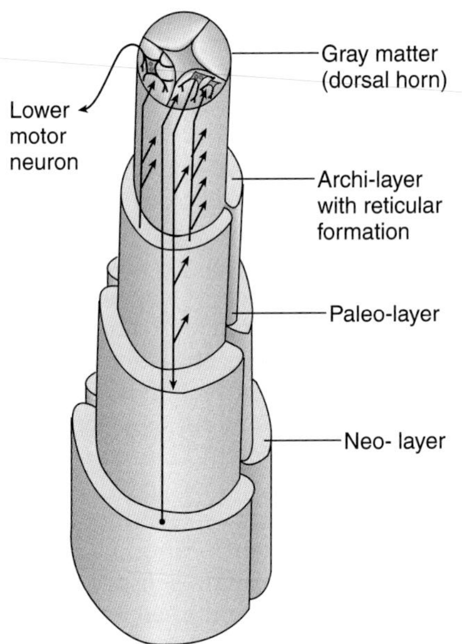

Figure 37–15
The three concentric subdivisions of the tract systems of the white matter. Migration of neurons into the archi layer converts it into the reticular formation of the white matter.

TABLE 37-1

Characteristics of the Concentric Subdivisions of the Longitudinal Tracts in the White Matter of the Central Nervous System

Characteristics	Archi-Level Tracts	Paleo-Level Tracts	Neo-Level Tracts
Segmental span	Intersegmental (<5 segments)	Suprasegmental (≥5 segments)	Suprasegmental
Number of synapses	Multisynaptic	Multisynaptic but fewer than archi-level tracts	Monosynaptic with target structures
Conduction velocity	Very slow	Fast	Fastest
Examples of functional systems	Flexor withdrawal reflex circuitry	Spinothalamic tracts	Corticospinal tracts

fifth month of intrauterine life involve the inner archi-level layer.

The inner layer of the white matter differs from the other two layers in one important aspect. Many neurons in the embryonic gray matter migrate out into this layer, resulting in a rich mixture of neurons and local fibers called the *reticular formation.* The circuitry of most reflexes is contained in the reticular formation. In the brain stem, the reticular formation becomes quite large and contains major portions of vital reflexes, such as those controlling respiration, cardiovascular function, swallowing, and vomiting, to mention a few. A functional system called the *reticular activation system* operates in the lateral portions of the reticular formation of the medulla, pons, and especially the midbrain. The convergence of information from all sensory modalities, including those of the somesthetic, auditory, visual, and visceral afferent nerves, bombards the neurons of this system. The reticular activation system has descending and ascending portions. The descending portion communicates with all spinal segmental levels through paleo-level reticulospinal tracts and serves to facilitate many of the cord-level reflexes. For example, it speeds reaction time and stabilizes postural reflexes. The ascending portion, sometimes called the *centrencephalic system,* accelerates brain activity, particularly thalamic and cortical activity. This is reflected by the appearance of awake brain-wave patterns. Sudden stimuli result in protective and attentive postures and cause increased awareness.

Middle Layer. The middle layer of the white matter contains most of the major fiber tract systems required for sensation and movement. It contains the ascending spinoreticular and spinothalamic tracts. This system consists of larger-diameter and longer suprasegmental fibers, which ascend to the brain stem and are largely functional at birth. In terms of evolutionary development, these tracts are quite old, and this layer is sometimes called the paleo layer. It facilitates many of the primitive functions, such as the "auditory startle reflex," which occurs in response to loud noises. This reflex consists of turning the head and body toward the sound, dilating the pupils of the eyes, catching of the breath, and quickening of the pulse.

Outer Layer. The outer layer of the tract systems is the newest of the three layers in terms of evolutionary development, and it is sometimes called the neo layer. It becomes functional at about the second year of life, and it includes the pathways needed for bladder training. Myelination of the neo-layer suprasegmental tracts, which include many of the pathways required for delicate and highly coordinated skills, is not complete until sometime around the fifth year of life. This includes the development of tracts needed for fine manipulative skills, such as the finger-thumb coordination required for the use of many tools and the toe movements needed for acrobatics. These are the most recently evolved systems and, being on the outside of the brain and spinal cord, these tracts are the most vulnerable to injury. When these outer tracts are damaged, the paleo and archi tracts often remain functional, and rehabilitation methods can result in effective use of the older systems. Delicacy and refinement may be lost, but basic function remains. For example, an important outer system, or neosystem, the corticospinal system, permits the fine manipulative control required for writing. If this is lost, paleo-level systems remaining intact permit the grasping and holding of objects. The hand can still be used to perform its basic function but the individual manipulation of the fingers is permanently lost.

Collateral Communication Pathways. Axons in the archi and paleo layers characteristically possess many collateral branches, which move into the gray cell columns or synapse with fibers of the reticular formation as the axon passes each succeeding CNS segment. Should a major axon be destroyed at some point along its course, these collaterals provide multisynaptic alternative pathways that bypass the local damage. Neo-level tracts do not possess these collaterals but are instead highly discrete about the target neurons with which they communicate. Because of their discreteness, damage to the neo tracts causes permanent loss of function. Damage to the archi or paleo systems is usually followed by slow return of function, presumably through the collateral connections. For example, the surgical section of pathways carrying pain impulses (*i.e.*, spinothalamic paleo-level tracts) can be used for temporary relief of intractable pain. The pain experience usually returns after some weeks or months. When it does return, it is often poorly localized and sometimes more unpleasant than it was initially. Consequently, this surgical procedure, which is called a tractotomy, is usually reserved for persons who are not expected to survive for longer than a few months.

The development of the nervous system can be traced far back into evolutionary history. The CNS develops from the ectoderm of the early embryo by formation of a hollow tube that closes along its longitudinal axis and sinks below the surface of its longitudinal axis. The cavity of the tube forms the ventricles of the brain and spinal canal, and the side wall develops to form the brain stem and spinal cord. The brain stem and spinal cord are subdivided into the dorsal horn, which contains neurons that receive and process incoming or afferent information, and the ventral horn, which contains efferent motor neurons that handle the final stages of output processing. The PNS develops from ectodermal cells called neural crest cells that migrate away from the dorsal surface of the forming neural tube.

Throughout life, the organization of the nervous system retains many patterns that were established during early embryonic life. The segmental pattern of early embryonic development is retained in the fully developed nervous system. Each one of the 43 or more body segments is connected to corresponding CNS or neural tube segments by segmental afferent and efferent neurons. Afferent neuronal processes enter the CNS by way of the dorsal root ganglia and the dorsal roots. Afferent neurons of the dorsal root ganglia are of four types: general somatic afferent, special somatic afferent, general visceral afferent, and special visceral afferent. Each of these afferent neurons synapse with their appropriate input association neurons in the cell columns of the dorsal horn (e.g., general somatic afferents synapse with neurons in the general somatic afferent IA cell column). Efferent fibers from motoneurons in the ventral horn exit the CNS in the ventral roots. General somatic efferent neurons are LMNs that innervate somite-derived skeletal muscles, and general visceral efferent neurons are preganglionic fibers that synapse with postganglionic fibers that innervate visceral structures. This pattern of afferent and efferent neurons, which is generally repeated in each segment of the body, forms parallel cell columns running lengthwise through the CNS and PNS.

Longitudinal communication between CNS segments is provided by neurons that send the axons into nearby segments by means of the innermost layer of the white matter, the ancient archi-level system of fibers. These cells provide coordination between neighboring segments. Neurons have invaded this layer, and the mix of these cells and axons, called the reticular formation, is the location of much of the important reflex circuitry of the spinal cord and the brain stem. Paleo-level tracts, which are located outside this layer, provide the longitudinal communication between more distant segments of the nervous system; this layer includes most of the important ascending and descending tracts. The recently evolved neo-level systems, which become functional during infancy and childhood, travel on the outside of the white matter and provide the means for very delicate and discriminative function. The outside position of the neo tracts and their lack of collateral and redundant pathways make them the most vulnerable to injury.

The Spinal Cord

After you have completed this section of the chapter, you should be able to meet the following objectives:

- Describe the longitudinal and transverse structures of the spinal cord
- Trace an afferent and efferent neuron from its site in the periphery through its entrance or exit into the spinal cord
- Explain muscle tone and posture using the myotatic or stretch reflex

In the adult, the spinal cord is located in the upper two thirds of the spinal canal of the vertebral column (Fig. 37–16). It extends from the foramen magnum at the base of the skull to a cone-shaped termination, the conus medullaris, which is usually located at the level of the first or second lumbar vertebra in the adult. From this point, the dorsal and ventral roots angle downward from the cord, forming what is called the *cauda equina,* or horse's tail. The filum terminale, which is composed of nonneural tissues and the pia mater, continues caudally and attaches to the second sacral vertebra. The spinal cord and the dorsal and ventral roots are covered with a connective tissue sheath, the *pia mater,* which carries the vascular supply to the white and gray matter of the cord.

The spinal cord is oval or rounded on transverse section. The internal gray matter has the appearance of a butterfly or letter H (see Fig. 37–16). Some of the neurons that make up the gray matter of the cord have processes or axons that leave the cord, enter the peripheral nerves, and supply tissues such as autonomic ganglia or skeletal muscles. The white matter of the cord that surrounds the gray matter contains nerve fiber tracts or descending axons that transmit information between segments of the cord or from higher levels of the CNS, such as the brain stem or cerebrum.

The extensions of the gray matter that form the letter H are called the horns. Those that extend posteriorly are called the *dorsal horns,* and those that extend anteri-

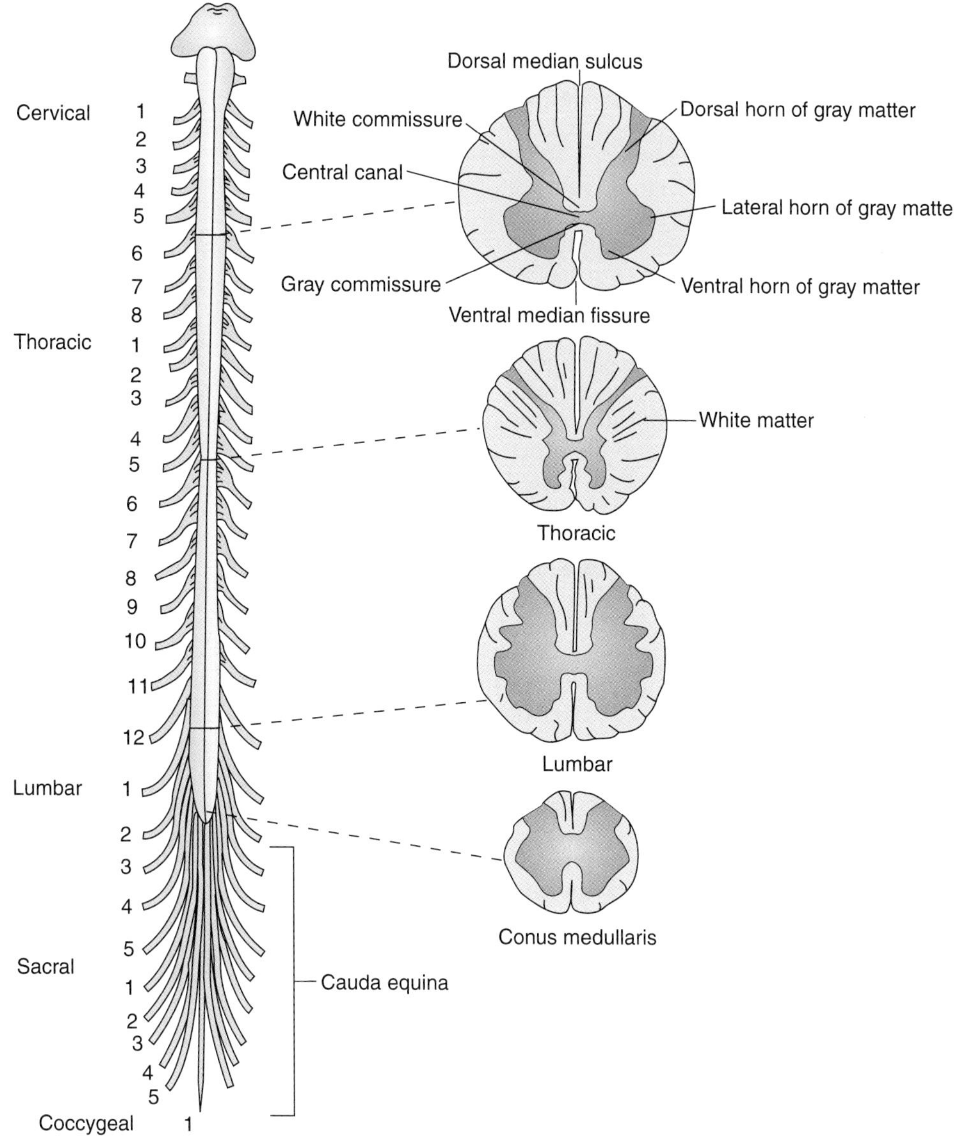

Figure 37–16
Cross-sectional views of the spinal cord, showing regional variations in gray matter and increasing white matter as the cord ascends.

orly are called the *ventral horns.* The dorsal horns contain input association neurons that receive afferent impulses through the dorsal roots and other connecting neurons. The ventral horns contain output association neurons and the efferent LMNs that leave the cord by way of the ventral roots.

The spinal cord contains many small internuncial neurons that surround the efferent motoneurons and synapse with the cell body or dendrites of the efferent cells. Action potentials of these internuncial neurons exert excitatory or inhibitory effects on the LMNs, and if the sum of the action potentials passes threshold, LMN action potentials are triggered. Although some CNS systems communicate directly with the LMNs, almost all LMN activity is controlled by systems communicating through excitatory or inhibitory internuncial neurons. These internuncial neurons represent the final stage of communication between elaborate CNS neuronal circuits and transmission of information to the skeletal muscle cells of the motor unit.

A central portion of the cord, which connects the dorsal and ventral horns and surrounds the central canal, is called the *intermediate gray matter.* In the thoracic area, the small, slender projections that emerge from the intermediate gray matter are called the *intermediolateral columns of the horns.* These columns contain the visceral output association neurons and the efferent neurons of the sympathetic nervous system.

The amount of gray matter in the cord is proportional to the amount of tissue innervated by a given segment of the cord (see Fig. 37–16). Larger amounts of gray matter are present in the lower lumbar and upper sacral segments, which supply the lower extremities, and in cervical segment 5 to thoracic segment 1, which supply the upper limbs. The volume of white matter in the spinal cord also increases progressively toward the brain, because more and more ascending fibers are added and because the number of descending axons is greater.

The spinal cord and the dorsal and ventral roots are covered by a connective tissue sheath, the pia mater, which also contains the blood vessels that supply the white and gray matter of the cord (Fig. 37–17). On the lateral sides of the spinal cord, extensions of the pia mater, the denticulate ligaments, attach the sides of the spinal cord to the bony walls of the spinal canal. Thus, the cord is suspended by both the denticulate ligaments and the segmental nerves. A fat- and vessel-filled epidural space intervenes between the spinal dura mater and the inner wall of the spinal canal. Each vertebral body has two pedicles that extend posteriorally and support the laterally oriented transverse processes of the neural laminae, which arch medially and fuse together to continue as the spinal processes.

The gaps between the vertebrae and their body parts are filled with tough ligaments. A gap, the intervertebral foramen, occurs between each two succeeding pedicles, allowing for exit of the segmental nerves and passage of blood vessels. The spinal cord lives within the protective confines of this series of concentric flexible tissue and body sheaths. The supporting structures of the spinal cord are discussed further in Chapter 39.

The location of the spinal cord in relation to the vertebral column results in a disparity between the positions of each succeeding cord segment and the exit of its dorsal and ventral nerve roots through the corresponding intervertebral foramina (Fig. 37–18). This disparity becomes more pronounced at the more caudal levels. The arachnoid and its enclosed subarachnoid space, which is filled with CSF, do not close down on the filum terminale until they reach the second sacral vertebra. This results in the formation of a pocket of CSF, the dural *cisterna spinalis,* which extends from about the second lumbar vertebra to the second sacral vertebra. Because there is an abundant supply of spinal fluid and

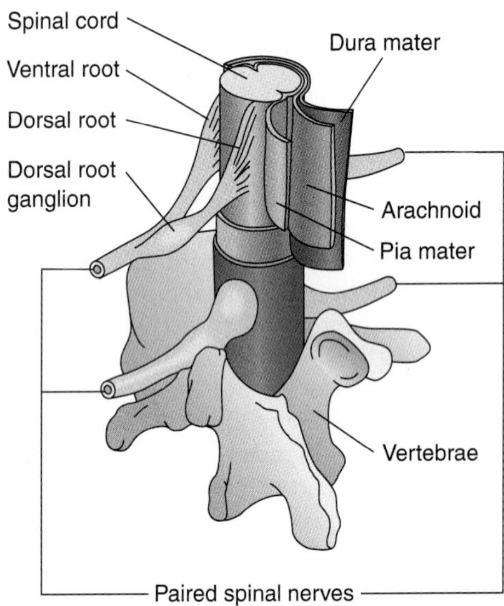

Figure 37–17
Spinal cord and meninges.

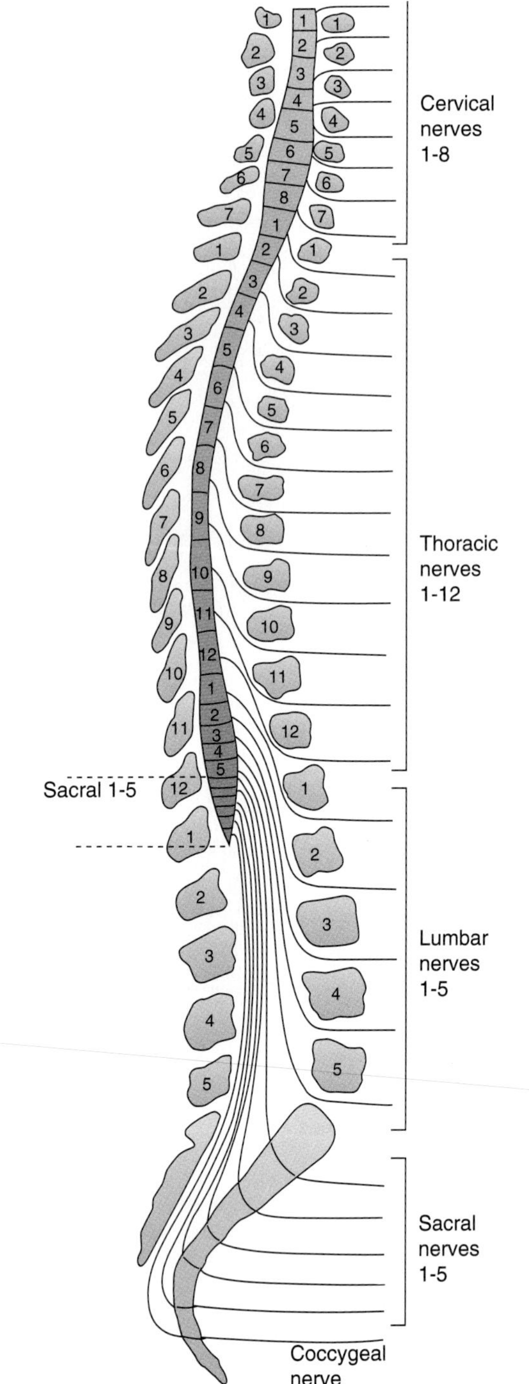

Figure 37–18
Relation of segments of the spinal cord and spinal nerves to the vertebral column.

the spinal cord does not extend this far, the area is often used for sampling the CSF. A procedure called a spinal tap, or puncture, can be done by inserting a special type of needle into the dural sac at the level of L3 or L4. The spinal roots, which are covered with pia mater, are in relatively little danger of trauma from the needle used for this purpose.

Spinal Nerves

The peripheral nerves that carry information to and from the spinal cord are called *spinal nerves*. There are 32 or more pairs of spinal nerves (*i.e.*, 8 cervical, 12 thoracic, 5 lumbar, 5 sacral, and 2 or more coccygeal); each pair is named for the segment of the spinal cord from which it exits. Because the first cervical (C1) spinal nerve exits the spinal cord just above the first cervical vertebra, the nerve is given the number of the bony vertebra just below it. The numbering is changed for all lower levels, however. An extra cervical nerve, the C8 nerve, exits above the T1 vertebra, and each subsequent nerve is numbered for the vertebra just above its point of exit (see Fig. 37–18).

Each spinal cord segment communicates with its corresponding body segment through the paired segmental spinal nerves (Fig. 37–19). Each spinal nerve, along with blood vessels that supply the spinal cord, enters the spinal canal through an intervertebral foramen, where it divides into two branches, or roots. One of the branches enters the dorsolateral surface of the cord (*i.e.*, dorsal root), carrying the axons of afferent neurons into the CNS. The other branch leaves the ventrolateral surface of the cord (*i.e.*, ventral root), carrying the axons of efferent neurons into the periphery. These two branches or roots fuse at the intervertebral foramen, forming the mixed spinal nerve—mixed because it has afferent and efferent axons.

After emerging from the vertebral column, the mixed spinal nerve divides into two branches: a small dorsal primary ramus and a larger ventral primary ramus (Fig. 37–20). The thoracic and upper lumbar spinal nerves also give rise to a third branch (*i.e.*, ramus communicans) that contains sympathetic axons supplying the blood vessels, the genitourinary system, and the gastrointestinal system. The dorsal ramus contains sensory fibers from the skin and motor fibers to muscles of the back. The anterior primary ramus contains motor fibers that innervate the skeletal muscles of the anterior body wall and the legs and arms.

The spinal nerves do not go directly to skin and muscle fibers; instead, they form complicated nerve networks called *plexuses*. A plexus is a site of intermixing nerve branches. A number of spinal nerves enter a plexus and connect with other spinal nerves before exiting from the plexus. The nerves that emerge from a plexus form smaller and smaller branches that supply the skin and muscles of the various parts of the body. There are four major plexuses of the PNS: the cervical plexus, the brachial plexus, the lumbar plexus, and the sacral plexus (Fig. 37–21).

Spinal Reflexes

A reflex is defined as a highly reliable relation between a stimulus and a motor response. Its anatomic basis consists of an afferent neuron, the connection or synapse with CNS interneurons that communicate with the effector neuron that innervates a muscle or organ. Reflexes are essentially "wired in" to the CNS in that normally they are always ready to function; with training, most reflexes can be modulated to become parts of more complicated movements. A reflex may involve neurons within a single cord segment (*i.e.*, segmental reflexes), several or many segments (*i.e.*, intersegmental reflexes), or structures in the brain (*i.e.*, suprasegmental reflexes). Two important types of spinal motor reflexes are discussed in this chapter: the myotatic and the withdrawal reflex.

Myotatic or Stretch Reflex. The myotatic or stretch reflex controls muscle tone and helps maintain posture. Specialized sensory nerve terminals in skeletal muscles and tendons relay information on muscle stretch and

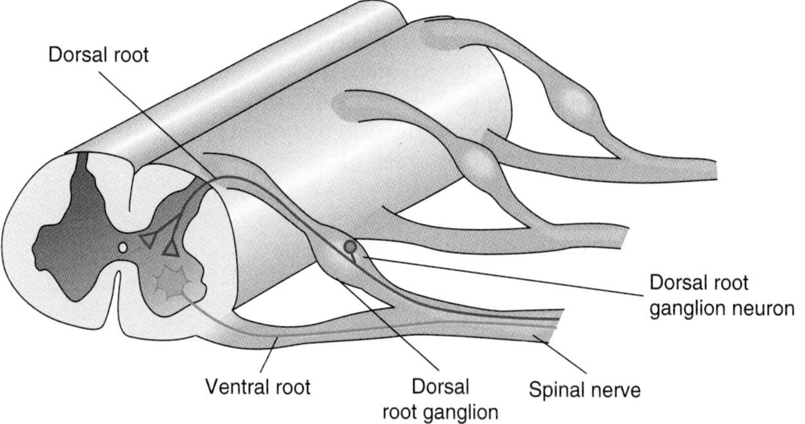

Figure 37–19
In the diagram of two segments of the spinal cord, three dorsal roots enter the dorsal lateral surface of the cord, and three ventral roots exit. The dorsal root ganglion contains dorsal root ganglion cells, whose axons bifurcate: one process enters the spinal cord in the dorsal root, and the other extends peripherally to supply the skin and muscle of the body. The ventral root is formed by axons from motor neurons in the spinal cord.

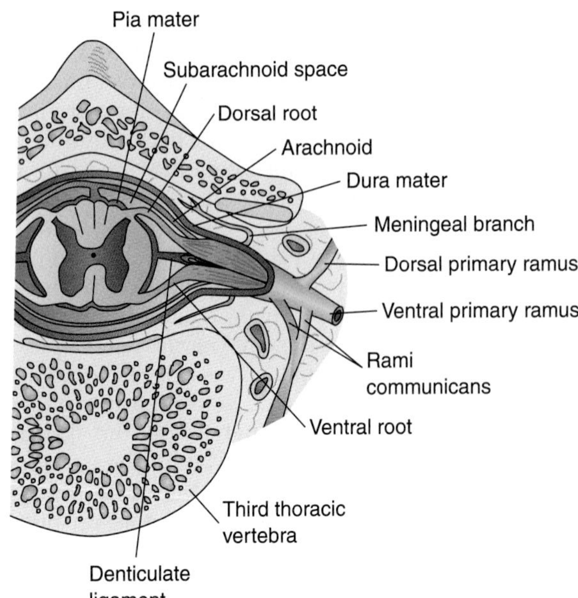

Figure 37–20
Cross section of vertebral column at the level of the third thoracic vertebra, showing the meninges, the spinal cord, and the origin of a spinal nerve and its branches or rami.

joint tension to the CNS. This information, which drives postural reflex mechanisms, is also relayed to the thalamus and the sensory cortex and is experienced as *proprioception*, a sense of the body itself. To provide this information, the muscles and their tendons are supplied with two types of sensory receptors: muscle spindle receptors and Golgi tendon organs. The muscle spindles, which are distributed throughout the belly of a muscle, provide information about muscle length and rate of stretch. The Golgi tendons organs are located in muscle tendons and transmit information about muscle tension.

Essentially all skeletal muscles contain large numbers of specialized stretch receptor apparatus called *muscle spindles* (Fig. 37–22). These consist of a group of specialized, miniature, skeletal muscle fibers (i.e., *intrafusal fibers*) that are encased in a connective tissue capsule and attached to the muscle fibers (i.e., *extrafusal fibers*) of a skeletal muscle. There are two types of intrafusal fibers: nuclear bag fibers, named for the large amount of nuclei in their middle, and nuclear chain fibers, in which the nuclei are arranged in a single row. These fibers are supplied by two types of afferent endings: large-diameter primary, or type Ia, and smaller secondary, or type II fibers. The type Ia fibers, which are stimulated by the rate and amount of stretch, have endings that wind in a helical fashion around the middle of the spindle intrafusal fibers, where there are no contractile elements. The endings of the type II fibers, which are only stimulated by the degree of stretch, are wound around the contractile elements of the intrafusal fibers, located near the end of the spindle.

The extrafusal fibers and the intrafusal fibers are innervated by motoneurons that reside in the ventral horns of the spinal cord. The extrafusal fibers are innervated by large alpha motoneurons that produce contraction of the muscle. The intrafusal fibers are innervated by two types of gamma motoneurons: dynamic gamma axons with endings on the nuclear bag fibers and static gamma axons that innervate the nuclear chain fibers. The interfusal fibers are equipped to monitor dynamic and static changes in muscle function.

The intrafusal muscle fibers in a spindle function as "skinniness" receptors. When a skeletal muscle is stretched, the spindle and its infrafusal fibers are stretched and therefore become more slender. Increased slenderness of the intrafusal fibers results in an increased firing rate of its afferent fibers at a rate proportional to the degree of

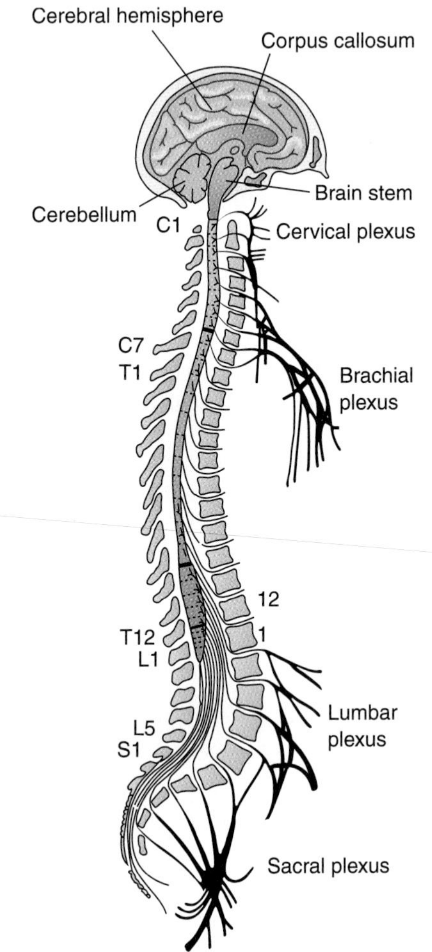

Figure 37–21
Drawing of the brain and cord in situ. The brain is shown in the median plane. Although not illustrated, the first cervical vertebra articulates with the base of the skull. The letters along the vertebral column indicate cervical, thoracic, lumbar, and sacral vertebrae. The cord ends at the upper border of the second lumbar vertebra. (Gardner E. [1975]. *Fundamentals of neurology* [2nd ed., p. 35]. Philadelphia: W.B. Saunders)

spindle stretch and therefore of extrafusal muscle length. Axons of the spindle afferent neurons enter the spinal cord through the dorsal root and have several branches, including one that terminates in the segment of entry and one that ascends the dorsal column of the cord to the medulla of the brain stem. The segmental branch makes a connection, among several others, that passes directly to the anterior gray matter of the spinal cord and establishes monosynaptic contact with each of the LMNs that have motor units in the muscle containing the spindle receptor, producing an opposing muscle contraction. This single synapse, or monosynaptic connection, is the only known instance of direct afferent-to-efferent reflex in the nervous system. Another segmental branch of the same afferent neuron innervates an internuncial neuron that is inhibitory to motor units of antagonistic muscles. Inhibition of these muscle units assists further in opposing muscle stretch.

Branches of the afferent axon also ascend the spinal cord, sending collateral branches into the dorsal horn of the adjacent segments influencing reflex function at each level. The intersegmental reflexes are particularly important in coordinating hand, leg, neck, and limb movements. Ascending fibers from the stretch reflex ultimately provide information about muscle length to the cerebellum and cerebral cortex.

The role of afferent spindle fibers is to inform the CNS of the status of muscle length. When a skeletal muscle lengthens or shortens against tension, a feedback mechanism needs to be available for readjustment such that the spindle apparatus remains sensitive to moment-to-moment changes in muscle stretch, even while changes in muscle length are occurring. This is accomplished by the gamma motoneurons that adjust spindle fiber length to match the length of the extrafusal muscle fiber. Descending fibers of motor pathways synapse with and simultaneously activate both alpha and gamma motoneurons so that the sensitivity of the spindle fibers is coordinated with muscle movement.

When a muscle is supporting body weight, the stretch reflex operates continuously, producing a continuous resistance to passive stretch, which is referred to as *muscle tone*. This resistance to stretch can be assessed by observing muscle tone or the "floppiness" of a relaxed muscle. If the stretch reflex is not operating within normal limits, this usually indicates that the reflex pathway has suffered damage or that the excitability of the ventral horn LMN pool of the muscle is abnormal. Reduced excitability of the stretch reflex results in decreased muscle tone or *hypotonia* that can range from postural weakness to total flaccid paralysis. It can result from reduced function of descending

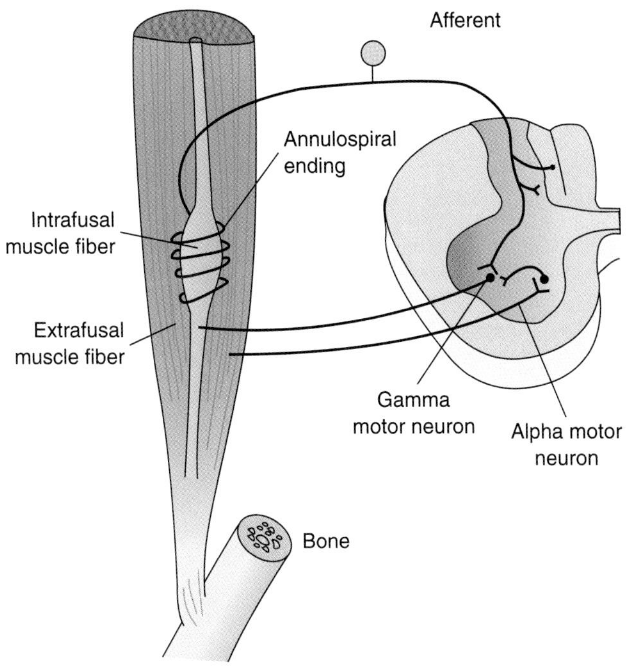

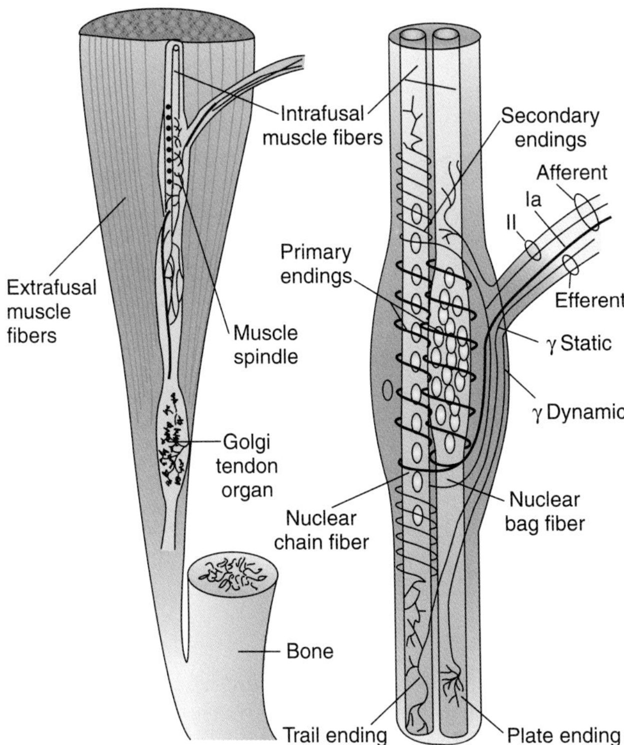

Figure 37–22
(**Top**) Spinal cord innervation of muscle spindle and Golgi tendon organ. Cell bodies from both the alpha motoneurons that innervate the extrafusal muscle fibers and the gamma (γ) fibers that innervate the intrafusal fibers reside in the ventral horns of the spinal cord and are activated by the same afferent systems. (**Bottom**) Golgi tendon organ and extrafusal muscle fibers (*left*) and the nuclear bag fiber and nuclear chain fiber of the interfusal fibers of the muscle spindle (*right*). (Modified from Rhoades R.A., Tanner G.A. [1996]. *Medical physiology*. [p. 94]. Boston: Little, Brown)

facilitory systems or from damage to the stretch receptor or motor unit. *Hypertonia* can result from excessive descending facilitation or to changes in segmental circuitry, such as occurs some weeks after an UMN lesion (*i.e.,* spasticity) or after damage to the portions of the basal ganglia (*i.e.,* rigidity). Under these conditions of greatly increased stiffness (*i.e.,* resistance to passive stretch), movement becomes difficult or impossible.

The muscle tone in the agonist and antagonist muscles around a joint provides for a fixed, stable situation. Central control over the gamma LMN mechanism permits increases or decreases in muscle tone in anticipation of changes in the muscle force required to oppose ongoing conditions, such as when weight is about to be lifted. If a centrally programmed movement such as pitching a ball is to occur, the CNS through its coordinated control of the muscle's alpha LMNs and spindle's gamma LMNs can suppress the stretch reflex so the muscle can produce its greatest range of motion. Without this programmed adjustability of the stretch reflex, any movement is immediately opposed and prevented. All reflex and learned movement patterns involve programmed control of gamma efferents, resulting in continuous readjustments of stretch reflex sensitivity in agonists, antagonists, and synergists as the movement progresses.

The status of the stretch reflex can be determined by assessing muscle tone and deep tendon reflexes, as shown in Box 37–1.

Inverse Myotatic Reflex. The *inverse myotatic reflex,* most prominent in antigravity extensor muscles, reduces the strength of alpha LMN-driven muscle contraction when the force generated by the muscle threatens the integrity of the muscle or tendon. This protective reflex, which involves two or more synapses in its path, has a very high threshold and activates inhibitory interneurons in the ventral horn that decrease the firing rate of alpha LMNs. Type II muscle spindle afferents in the Golgi tendon apparatus and nociceptive afferents from the connective tissue of muscle and tendon unit drive this high-threshold, protective reflex. The inverse myotatic reflex also has a contralateral component. If, for example, the inverse myotatic reflex produced relaxation of the quadriceps in one leg, the cross component would produce contraction in the quadriceps of the other leg. The inverse myotatic reflex provides postural stability to ambulatory movements. For example, when the inverse myotatic reflex produces relaxation of antigravity muscles (with flexion) of one leg as we walk, the cross component produces contraction and extension of the opposite leg.

In persons with spastic paralysis, the inverse myotatic reflex becomes hyperactive and produces what is called the *clasp-knife reaction.* If an examiner were to passively flex the lower limb of such a person at the knee, increasing resistance would be encountered. This resistance would continue to increase until, at some point, it would abruptly cease and the leg could then be passively flexed. Similar signs are seen in spastic upper limbs.

Assessment of Deep Tendon Reflexes

The status of the stretch reflex can be determined by assessing muscle tone and deep tendon reflexes. Clinically, muscle tone is evaluated by asking a person to relax while supporting the limb except at the joint that is being examined. The distal part of the extremity is then moved passively around the joint. Normally, there is a mild resistance to movement. A method for assessing muscle stretch excitability is to tap the tendon of a muscle briskly with a reflex hammer, which is normally immediately followed by a sudden contraction or *muscle jerk,* as illustrated. The stretch reflex has been "tricked" by the sudden tug on the tendon. A synchronous burst of afferent Ia nerve activity from the many spindles in the muscle results in essentially simultaneous firing of a large number of lower motor neuron units. The stretch reflex was tricked into responding, as though the muscle had been suddenly stretched. These muscle jerk reflexes are called *deep tendon reflexes* (DTRs). They are usually checked at the wrists, elbows, knees, and Achilles tendons.

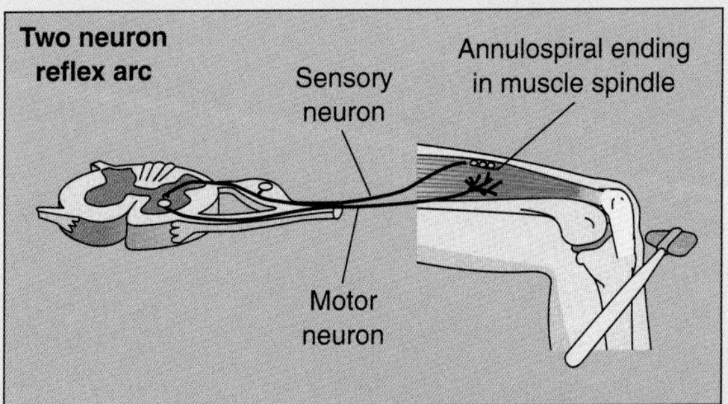

Testing the stretch reflex with a reflex hammer.

The DTRs can provide much information in a brief period. A normal range DTR indicates that the afferent peripheral process in the peripheral muscle and nerves is normal; the dorsal root ganglion function is normal; the dorsal root function is normal; and the dorsal, intermediate, and ventral horns are functioning appropriately, as are the ventral root and lower motor neuron cell body and axon. It also means that the neuromuscular synapse is functioning normally; the muscle fibers are capable of normal contraction; and suprasegmental input is normal. Using this method of assessment, it is possible to test the function of many spinal nerves and spinal cord segments and some of the cranial nerves and brain stem segments in a short time. If abnormality of excitability is detected, further tests are required to determine the nature and location of the pathologic process.

Withdrawal Reflex. The *withdrawal reflex* is stimulated by a tissue-threatening or -damaging (nociceptive) stimulus and quickly moves the body part away from the offending stimulus, usually by flexing a limb part (Fig.

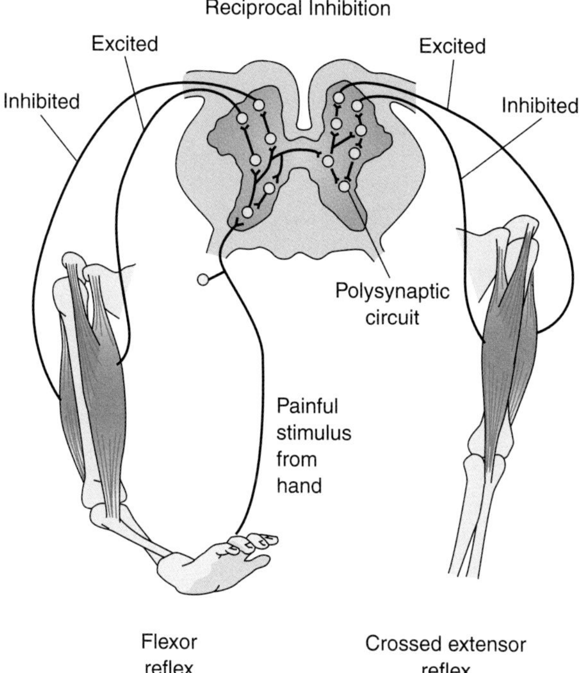

Figure 37–23
Withdrawal reflex response, indicating the flexor reflex, the crossed extensor reflex, and the reciprocal inhibition. (Guyton A.C., Hall J.E. [1996]. *Textbook of medical physiology* [9th ed., p. 559]. Philadelphia: W.B. Saunders)

37–23). The withdrawal reflex is powerful reflex, taking precedence over other reflexes associated with locomotion. Any of the major joints may be involved, depending on the site of afferent stimulation. All of the joints of an extremity (*e.g.*, finger, wrist, elbow, shoulder) typically are involved. This complex, polysynaptic reflex also shifts postural support to the opposite side of the body with a crossed extensor reflex and simultaneously alerts the forebrain to the offending stimulus event. The withdrawal reflex can also produce contraction of muscles other than the extremities. For example, irritation of the abdominal viscera may cause contraction of the abdominal muscles.

In summary, In the adult, the spinal cord is located in the upper two thirds of the spinal canal of the vertebral column. The spinal cord is oval or rounded on transverse section. The internal gray matter has the appearance of a butterfly or letter H. The dorsal horns receive afferent information from dorsal root and other connecting neurons. The ventral horns contain the output association neurons and efferent LMNs that the leave the cord by the ventral roots.

There are 32 or more pairs of spinal nerves (i.e., 8 cervical, 12 thoracic, 5 lumbar, 5 sacral, and 2 or more coccygeal) that communicate with their corresponding body segments. Each spinal nerve, along with blood vessels that supply the spinal cord, enters the spinal canal through an intervertebral foramen, where it divides into two branches, or roots, one of which enters the dorsolateral surface of the cord (i.e., dorsal root), carrying the axons of afferent neurons into the CNS. The other leaves the ventrolateral surface of the cord (i.e., ventral root), carrying the axons of efferent neurons into the periphery. These two roots fuse at the intervertebral foramen, forming the mixed spinal nerve—mixed because it has afferent and efferent axons.

A reflex provides a highly reliable relation between a stimulus and a motor response. Its anatomic basis consists of an afferent neuron, the connection or synapse with CNS neurons that communicates with the effector neuron, and the effector neuron that innervates a muscle or organ. Reflexes are essentially "wired in" to the CNS in that normally they are always ready to function; with training, most reflexes can be modulated to become parts of more complicated movements.

Two important types of spinal motor reflexes are the myotatic or stretch reflex and the withdrawal reflex. The myotatic reflex controls muscle tone and is important in maintaining posture. The withdrawal reflex is stimulated by any tissue-threatening or -damaging stimulus and quickly moves the body part away from the offending stimulus. Hundreds of reflexes are available, including stepping, gagging, swallowing, and inspiration. All of these are polysynaptic and complex, except for the disynaptic inverse myotatic reflex and monosynaptic stretch reflex.

The Brain

After you have completed this section of the chapter, you should be able to meet the following objectives:

- List the structures of the hindbrain, midbrain, and forebrain and describe their functions
- Name the cranial nerves and cite their location and function
- State the characteristics of the dominant and nondominant hemispheres of the brain
- Describe the characteristics of the cerebral spinal fluid and trace its passage through the ventricular system
- Contrast and compare the blood-brain and CSF-brain barriers

The brain is divided into three regions: the hindbrain, the midbrain, and the forebrain. The hindbrain includes the medulla oblongata, the pons, and its dorsal outgrowth, the cerebellum. The midbrain includes two pairs of dorsal enlargements, the superior and inferior colliculi. The forebrain, which consists of two hemispheres and is covered by the cerebral cortex, contains masses of gray matter, the basal ganglia, and rostral end of the neural tube, the diencephalon with its adult derivatives—the thalamus and hypothalamus.

An important concept is that the more rostral, recently developed parts of neural tube gain dominance or control over regions and functions at lower levels. They do not replace the more ancient circuitry but merely dominate it. After damage to the more vulnerable parts of the forebrain, as occurs with brain death, a *brain stem organism* remains capable of respiration and survival if environmental temperature is regulated and if nutrition and other aspects of care are provided. However, all aspects of intellectual function, experience, perception, and memory are usually permanently lost. The organization of content in this section moves from the more ancient circuity of the hindbrain to the more dominant and recently developed structures of the forebrain.

Hindbrain

The term *brain stem* is often used to include the hindbrain, pons, and midbrain. These regions of the neural tube have the organization of spinal cord segments, except that more of the longitudinal cell columns are present, reflecting the increased complexity of the cranial segmental nerves. In the brain stem, the structure and function of the reticular formation has been greatly expanded with networks controlling basic breathing, eating, and locomotion functions located in the medulla and pons, with the higher-level integrative aspects of these functions located in the midbrain. It is surrounded on the outside by the long tract systems that connect the forebrain with lower parts of the CNS (Fig. 37–24).

Medulla

The medulla oblongata represents the caudal five segments of the brain part of the neural tube; the cranial nerve branches entering and leaving it have functions similar to the spinal segmental nerves. The ventral horn area in the medulla is quite small, but the dorsal horn is enlarged, processing a great amount of the information pouring through the cranial nerves. The segmental peripheral nerve components of the medulla can be divided into those that leave the neural tube ventromedially (*i.e.,* hypoglossal and abducens cranial nerves) and those that exit dorsolaterally (*i.e.,* vagus, spinal accessory, glossopharyngeal, and vestibulocochlear cranial nerves). Because pathologic signs and symptoms reflect the spatial segregation of brain stem components, neurologic syndromes resulting from trauma, tumors, aneurysms, and cerebrovascular accidents are often classified as ventral or dorsolateral syndromes.

The general somatic efferent LMNs of the lower segments of the medulla supply the extrinsic and intrinsic muscles of the tongue by means of the *hypoglossal nerve,* or cranial nerve XII (Table 37–2). Damage to the hypoglossal nerve results in partial or total denervation and therefore weakness or paralysis of tongue muscles. When the tongue is protruded, it deviates toward the damaged and therefore weaker side because of the greater protrusion strength on the normal side. The axons of the hypoglossal nerve leave the medulla adjacent to two long, longitudinal ridges along the medial undersurface of the medulla, called the *pyramids,* which contain the corticospinal fibers, most of which cross to descend in the lateral column to the opposite side of the spinal cord. Lesions of the ventral surface of the caudal

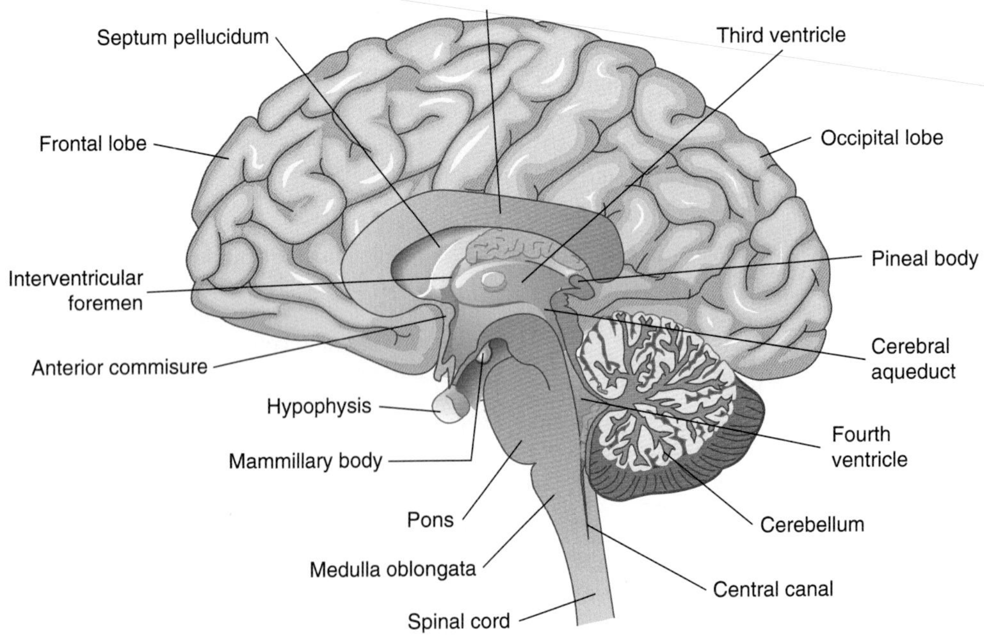

Figure 37–24
Midsagittal section of the brain.

TABLE 37-2
The Segmental Nerves and Their Components

Segment and Nerve	Component	Innervation	Function
1. Forebrain			
I. Olfactory	SVA	Receptors in olfactory mucosa	Reflexes, olfaction (smell)
2. II. Optic nerve		Optic nerve and retina (part of brain system, not a peripheral nerve)	
3. Midbrain			
V. Trigeminal (V_1) ophthalmic division			
	SSA	Muscles: upper face: forehead, upper lid	Facial expression, proprioception
	GSA	Skin, subcutaneous tissue; conjunctiva; frontal/ethmoid sinuses	Somesthesia Reflexes (blink)
III. Oculomotor	GVE	Iris sphincter Ciliary muscle	Pupillary constriction Accommodation
	GSE	Extrinsic eye muscles	Eye movement, lid movement
4. Pons			
V. Trigeminal (V_2) maxillary division			
	SSA	Muscles: facial expression	Proprioception
	GSA	Skin, oral mucosa, upper teeth, hard palate, maxillary sinus	Reflexes (sneeze), somesthesia
V. Trigeminal (V_3) mandibular division			
	SSA	Lower jaw, muscles: mastication	Proprioception, jaw jerk
	GSA	Skin, mucosa, teeth, anterior 2/3 tongue	Reflexes, somesthesia
	PE	Muscles: mastication tensor tympani tensor veli palantini	Mastication: speech Protects ear from loud sound Tenses soft palate
IV. Trochlear	GSE	Extrinsic eye muscle	Moves eye down and in
5. Caudal Pons			
VIII. Vestibular, cochlear (vestibulocochlear)	SSA	Vestibular end organs Organ of Corti	Reflexes, sense of head position Reflexes, hearing
VII. Facial nerve, intermedius portion			
	GSA	External auditory meatus	Somesthesia
	GVA	Nasopharynx	Gag reflex: sensation
	SVA	Taste buds anterior 2/3 tongue	Reflexes: gustation (taste)
	GVE	Nasopharynx Lacrimal, sublingual, submandibular glands	Mucous secretion, reflexes Lacrimation, salivation
Facial nerve	PE	Muscles: facial expression, stapedius	Facial expression Protects ear from loud sounds
VI. Abducens	GSE	Extrinsic eye muscle	Lateral eye deviation
6. Middle Medulla			
IX. Glossopharyngeal			
	SSA	Stylopharyngeus muscle	Proprioception
	GSA	Posterior external ear	Somesthesia
	SVA	Taste buds posterior 1/3 tongue	Gustation (taste)
	GVA	Oral pharynx	Gag reflex: sensation
	GVE	Parotid gland; pharyngeal mucosa	Salivary reflex: mucous secretion
	PE	Stylopharyngeus muscle	Assists swallowing
7,8,9,10. Caudal Medulla			
X. Vagus			
	SSA	Muscles: pharynx, larynx	Proprioception
	GSA	Posterior external ear	Somesthesia

(continued)

TABLE 37-2
The Segmental Nerves and Their Components *(continued)*

Segment and Nerve	Component	Innervation	Function
7,8,9,10. Caudal Medulla			
X. Vagus	SVA	Taste buds, pharynx, larynx	Reflexes, gustation
	GVA	Visceral organs (esophagus to midtransverse colon, liver, pancreas, heart, lungs)	Reflexes, sensation
	GVE	Visceral organs as above	Parasympathetic efferent
	PE	Muscles: pharynx, larynx	Swallowing, phonation, emesis
XII. Hypoglossal	GSE	Muscles of tongue	Tongue movement, reflexes
Spinal Segments			
C1–C4 Upper Cervical XI. Spinal assessory	PE	Muscles: sternocleidomastoid, trapezius	Head, shoulder movement
Spinal nerves	SSA	Muscles of neck	Proprioception, DTRs
	GSA	Neck, back of head	Somesthesia
	GSE	Neck muscles	Head, shoulder movement
C5–C8 Lower Cervical	SSA	Upper limb muscles	Proprioception, DTRs
	GSA	Upper limbs	Reflexes, somesthesia
	GSE	Upper limb muscles	Movement, posture
T1–L2 Thoracic, Upper Lumbar	SSA	Muscles: trunk, abdominal wall	Proprioception
	GSA	Trunk, abdominal wall	Reflexes, somesthesia
	GVA	All of viscera	Reflexes and sensation
	GVE	All of viscera	Sympathetic reflexes, vasomotor control, sweating, piloerection
	GSE	Muscles: trunk, abdominal wall, back	Movement, posture, respiration
L2–S1 Lower Lumbar, Upper Sacral	SSA	Lower limb muscles	Proprioception, DTRs
	GSA	Lower trunk, limbs, back	Reflexes, somesthesia
	GSE	Muscles: trunk, lower limbs, back	Movement, posture
S2–S4 Lower Sacral	SSA	Muscles: pelvis, perineum	Proprioception
	GSA	Pelvis, genitalia	Reflexes, somesthesia
	GVA	Hindgut, bladder, uterus	Reflexes, sensation
	GVE	Hindgut, visceral organs	Visceral reflexes, defecation, urination, erection
S5–Co2 Lower Sacral, Coccygeal	SSA	Perineal muscles	Proprioception
	GSA	Lower sacrum, anus	Reflexes, somesthesia
	GSE	Perineal muscles	Reflexes, posture

Afferent (sensory) components: SSA; special afferent; GSA; general afferent; SVA, special visceral afferent; GVA, general visceral afferent.
Efferent (motor) components: GVE, general visceral efferent (autonomic nervous system); PE, pharyngeal efferent; GSE, general somatic efferent.
DTRs, deep tendon reflexes.

medulla result in the syndrome of *alternating hypoglossal hemiplegia*, characterized by signs of ipsilateral (*i.e.*, same side) denervation of the tongue and contralateral (*i.e.*, opposite side) weakness or paralysis of both the upper and lower extremities.

The *vagus nerve*, or cranial nerve X, has several afferent (sensory) and efferent (motor) components. General somatic afferents innervate the external ear and special visceral afferents innervate the pharyngeal taste buds. Sensory and motor components of the nerve innervate the pharynx, the gastrointestinal tract (from the laryngeal pharynx to the midtransverse colon), the heart, spleen, and lungs. Initiation of many essential reflexes and normal functions depend on intact vagal innervation. For example, 80% of the fibers of the vagus are afferents, some of which are involved in vomiting and hiccup reflexes and in ongoing feedback during swallowing and speech. The unilateral loss of vagal function can result in slowed gastrointestinal motility, a permanently husky voice, and deviation of the uvula away from the damaged side. Bilateral loss of vagal function can seriously damage reflex maintenance of cardiovascular and respiratory reflexes. Swallowing may become difficult, and in some cases, paralysis of laryngeal structures causes life-threatening airway obstruction.

The sternocleidomastoid, a powerful head-turning muscle, and the trapezius muscle, which elevates the shoulders, are innervated by the *spinal accessory nerve,* or cranial nerve XI, with LMNs in the upper four cervical spinal segments. Intermediate rootlets from these segmental levels combine and enter the cranial cavity through the foramen magnum and then exit through the jugular foramen with cranial nerves IX and X. Loss of spinal accessory nerve function results in drooping of the shoulder on the damaged side and weakness when turning the head to the opposite side.

The dorsolateral *glossopharyngeal nerve,* or cranial nerve IX, contains the same components as the vagus nerve but for a more rostral segment of the gastrointestinal tract and the pharynx. This nerve provides the special visceral sensory innervation of the taste buds of the oral pharynx and the back of the tongue; the afferent innervation of the oral pharynx and the baroreceptors of the carotid sinus; the efferent innervation of the otic ganglion, which controls the salivary function of the parotid gland; and the efferent innervation of the stylopharyngeal muscle of the pharynx. This cranial nerve is seldom damaged, but when it is, anesthesia of the ipsilateral oral pharynx develops because of dry mouth resulting from reduced salivation.

The special sensory afferent *vestibulocochlear nerve,* or cranial nerve VIII, formerly called the *auditory nerve,* is attached laterally at the junction of the medulla oblongata and the pons, often called the caudal pons. It consists of two distinct fiber divisions, both of which are sensory: the cochlear division, which arises from cell bodies in the cochlea in the inner ear and transmits impulses related to the sense of hearing, and the vestibular division, which arises from two ganglia that innervate cell bodies in utricle, saccule, and semicircular canals and transmits impulses related to head position and movement of the body through space. Irritation of the cochlear division results in tinnitus (*i.e.,* ringing of the ears); destruction of the nerve results in nerve deafness (in contrast to conduction deafness caused by disease of the middle ear); injury to the vestibular division leads to vertigo, nystagmus, and some postural instability (see Chapter 43).

Another segmental branch of the caudal pons, the *facial nerve,* or cranial nerve VII, and its intermediate component (the intermedius) contain both afferent and efferent functional components. The intermedius nerve, which contains the general somatic afferent, special visceral afferent, general visceral afferent, and general visceral efferent neurons, innervates the nasopharynx and taste buds of the palate, the forward two thirds of the tongue, the submandibular and sublingual salivary glands, the lacrimal glands, and mucous membranes of the nose and roof of the mouth. Loss of this branch of the facial nerve can lead to eye dryness with risk of corneal scarring and blindness. The pharyngeal efferent LMNs of the facial nerve proper innervate muscles that control facial expression, such as wrinkling of the brow and smiling. Unilateral loss of facial nerve function results in flaccid paralysis of the muscles of one half of the head, a condition called *Bell's palsy.* The facial nerve passes through a bony tunnel behind the middle ear cavity. In some cases, Bell's palsy has been attributed to inflammatory reactions involving the facial nerve in or near this bony tunnel. Because such injuries result from pressure caused by edematous tissue, the integrity of the endoneurial tube is retained, and regeneration with full recovery of all muscles generally occurs within several months.

Another segmental nerve branch of the caudal pons, the *abducens nerve,* or cranial nerve VI, sends LMNs out ventrally on either side of the pyramids and then forward into the orbit to innervate the lateral rectus muscle of the eye. As the name indicates, the abducens nerve abducts the eye (lateral or outward rotation); peripheral damage to them results medial strabismus, which is a weakness or loss of eye abduction (see Chapter 42).

Pons

The pons (meaning bridge) develops from the fifth neural tube segment. The central canal of the spinal cord, which remains small but is greatly enlarged in the pons and rostral medulla, forms the fourth ventricle (see Fig. 37–24). An enlarged area on the ventral surface of the pons contains the pontine nuclei, which receive information from all parts of the cerebral cortex. The axons of these neurons form a massive bundle that swings around the lateral side of the fourth ventricle to enter the cerebellum. The reticular formation of the pons is large and contains the circuitry for masticating food and manipulating the jaws during speech.

The *trigeminal nerve,* or cranial nerve V, which has sensory (*i.e.,* general somatic afferent) and motor (*i.e.,* pharyngeal efferent) subdivisions, exits the brain stem laterally on the forward surface of the pons. The trigeminal is the main sensory nerve conveying the modalities of pain, temperature, touch, and proprioception to the superficial and deep regions of the face. The regions innervated include the skin of the anterior scalp and face, the conjunctiva and orbit, the meninges, the paranasal sinuses, and the mouth, including the teeth and the anterior two thirds of the tongue. The LMNs of the trigeminal nerve innervate skeletal muscles involved with mastication and also contribute to swallowing and speech, movements of the soft palate, and tension of the tympanic membrane through the tensor tympani muscle. The latter apparently has a protective reflex function, dampening movement of the middle ear ossicles during high-intensity sound.

Cerebellum

The cerebellum is located in the posterior fossa of cranium superior to the pons (see Fig. 37–24). It is separated from the cerebral hemispheres by a fold of dura mater, the tentorium cerebelli. The cerebellum consists of a small unpaired median portion, called the *vermis,* and two large lateral masses, the *cerebellar hemispheres.* In contrast to the brain stem with its external white matter and internal gray nuclei, the cerebellum, like the cerebrum, has an outer cortex of gray matter overlying the white matter. Next to the fourth ventricle, several masses of gray matter, called the deep cerebellar nuclei, border the roof of the fourth ventricle. Cells of the cerebellar cortex and deep nuclei interact, and axons from the latter send information to many regions, particularly to the motor cortex by means of a thalamic relay. The synergistic (*i.e.,* temporal and spatial smoothing) functions of the cerebellum participate in all movement of limbs, trunk, head, larynx, and eyes, whether the movement is part of a voluntary movement or of a highly learned semiautomatic or automatic movement. During highly skilled movements, the motor cortex sends signals to the cerebellum, informing it about the movement that is to be performed. The cerebellum makes continuous adjustments, resulting in smoothness of movement, particularly during the delicate maneuvers. Highly skillful movement requires extensive motor training, and there is considerable evidence that many of these learned movement patterns involve cerebellar circuits.

The cerebellum receives proprioceptor input from the vestibular system; feedback from the muscles, tendons, and joints; and indirect signals from the somesthetic, visual, and auditory systems that provide background information for ongoing movement. The sensory input from a given area of the body arrives at the same area in the cerebellum as input from the motor cortex that controls the motor units in that body area. In this way, the cerebellum is able to assess continuously the status of each body part—position, rate of movement, and forces, such as gravity, that are opposing movement. The cerebellum compares what is actually happening with what is intended to happen; it then transmits appropriate corrective signals back to the motor system, instructing it to increase or decrease the activity of certain muscle groups and regulating their contractions so that smooth and accurate movements are performed.

One of the functions of the cerebellum is the dampening of muscle movement. All body movements are basically pendular (*i.e.,* swinging to and fro). As movement begins, momentum develops and must be overcome before the movement can be stopped. Because of momentum, all movements have a tendency to overshoot if they are not dampened. Within the intact cerebellum, automatic signals stop movement precisely at the intended point. In providing for this type of control, the cerebellum uses proprioceptive information to predict the future position of moving parts of the body and the rapidity with which the limb is moving, as well as the projected time course of the movement. This allows the cerebellum to inhibit agonist muscles and excite antagonist muscles when movement approaches the intended target.

Midbrain

The midbrain develops from the fourth segment of the neural tube, and its organization is similar to that of a spinal segment. The central canal is reestablished as the cerebral aqueduct, connecting the fourth ventricle with the third ventricle (see Fig. 37–24). Two general somatic efferent cranial nerves, the *oculomotor nerve,* or cranial nerve III, and the *trochlear nerve,* or cranial nerve IV, exit the midbrain.

Massive fiber bundles of the cerebral peduncles pass from the forebrain to the pons along the ventral surface of the midbrain. On the dorsal surface, four "little hills," the superior and inferior colliculi, are areas of cortical formation. The inferior colliculus is involved in directional turning and, to some extent, in experiencing the direction of sound sources. The superior colliculus is an essential part of the reflex mechanisms that control conjugate eye movements when the visual environment is surveyed.

The ventral central gray matter (*i.e.,* ventral horn) contains the general somatic efferent LMNs that innervate most of the skeletal muscles that move the optic globe about and raise the eyelids. These axons leave the midbrain through the *oculomotor nerve,* or cranial nerve III. This nerve also contains general visceral efferents, the parasympathetic LMNs that control pupillary constriction and ciliary muscle focusing of the lens. Damage to the ventrally exiting cranial nerve III and to the adjacent cerebral peduncle, which includes the corticospinal axon system on one side, results in paralysis of eye movement combined with contralateral hemiplegia. A small group of cells in the ventral part of the caudal central gray matter contains the general visceral efferent LMNs that innervate the superior oblique eye muscles that move the upper part of the eye downward and toward the nose when the eye is adducted, or turned inward. Developmentally, cranial nerve IV is a component of the pontine segment, but in the adult, it exits the dorsal surface of the midbrain as the *trochlear* or cranial nerve IV and decussates (crosses over) before exiting the brain stem. Lesions involving the trochlear cranial nerve are unusual. The diplopia, or double vision, resulting from such lesions affects downward gaze to the side opposite the denervated muscle. Walking downstairs becomes particularly difficult. The trochlear nerve–innervated superior oblique muscle has as its major function intorsion of the optic globe; to avoid diplopia, the person usually carries the head tilted to the side of damage.

Forebrain

The forebrain is the most rostral part of the brain; it consists of the telencephalon, or "end brain," and the dien-

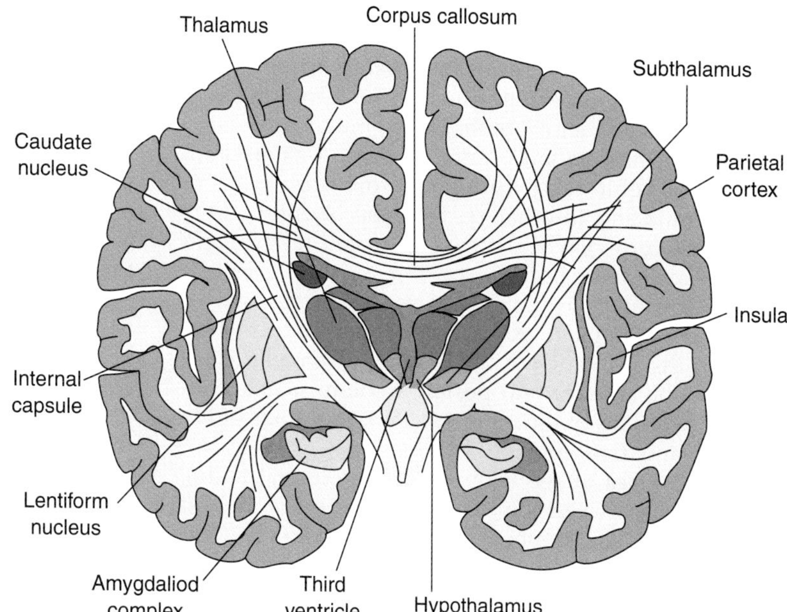

Figure 37–25
Frontal section of the brain passing through the third ventricle, showing the thalamus, subthalamus, hypothalamus, internal capsule, corpus callosum, basal ganglia (caudate nucleus, *lenticular nucleus*), amygdaloid complex, insula, and parietal cortex.

cephalon, or "between brain." The diencephalon forms the core of the forebrain, and the telencephalon forms the cerebral hemispheres.

Diencephalon

The three most forward brain segments form an enlarged dorsal horn and ventral horn with a narrow, deep, enlarged central canal—the third ventricle—separating the two sides. This region is called the *diencephalon*. The dorsal horn part of the diencephalon is the thalamus and subthalamus, and the ventral horn part is the hypothalamus (Fig. 37–25).

The *optic nerve,* or cranial nerve II, and retina are outgrowths of the diencephalon from the region of the optic chiasm. The structure and function of the optic nerve are presented in Chapter 42.

The thalamus consists of two large, egg-shaped masses, one on either side of the third ventricle. The thalamus is divided into several major parts, and each part is divided into distinct nuclei, which are the major relay stations for information going to and from the cerebral cortex. All sensory pathways have direct projections to thalamic nuclei, which convey the information to restricted areas of the sensory cortex. The coordination and integration of peripheral sensory stimuli occur within the thalamus, and there is some crude interpretation of highly emotion-laden auditory experiences that not only occur but can be remembered. For example, a person can recover from a deep coma in which cerebral cortex activity is minimal and remember some of what was said at the bedside.

The thalamus also plays a role in relaying critical information regarding motor activities to and from selected areas of the motor cortex. There are two neuronal circuits that are significant in this regard. One is the pathway from the cerebral cortex to the pons and cerebellum and then, by way of the thalamus, back to the motor cortex. The second is the feedback circuit that travels from the cortex to the basal ganglia, then to the thalamus, and from the thalamus back to the cortex. The subthalamus also contains movement control systems related to the basal ganglia.

Through its connections with the ascending reticular activating system, the thalamus processes neural influences that are basic to cortical excitatory rhythms (*i.e.,* those recorded on the electroencephalogram) and that are essential to sleep-wakefulness cycles and to the process of attending to stimuli. In addition to their cortical connections, the thalamic nuclei have connections with each other and with neighboring nonthalamic brain structures such as the limbic system. Through their connections with the limbic system, some thalamic nuclei are involved in the relation between stimuli and their emotional responses.

The ventral horn portion of the diencephalon is the hypothalamus, which borders the third ventricle and includes a ventral extension, the neurohypophysis (*i.e.,* posterior pituitary). The hypothalamus is the area of master-level integration of homeostatic control of the body's internal environment. Maintenance of blood gas concentration, water balance, food consumption, and major aspects of endocrine and autonomic nervous system control require hypothalamic function.

The internal capsule is a broad band of projection fibers that lies between the thalamus medially and the basal ganglia laterally (see Fig. 37–25). The internal capsule contains all of the fibers that connect the cerebral cortex with deeper structures, including the basal ganglia, thalamus, midbrain, pons, medulla, and spinal cord.

Cerebral Hemispheres

The two cerebral hemispheres are lateral outgrowths of the diencephalon. The cerebral hemispheres contain the lateral ventricles (*i.e.,* ventricles I and II), which are con nected with the third ventricle of the diencephalon by a small opening called the interventricular foramen (*i.e.*, foramen of Monro). Axons of the *olfactory nerve*, or cranial nerve I, terminate in the most ancient portion of the cerebrum—the olfactory bulb, where initial processing of olfactory information occurs. Projection axons from the olfactory bulb relay through the olfactory tracts to the thalamus and to other parts of the cerebral cortex (*i.e.*, orbital cortex), where olfactory-related reflexes and olfactory experience occur.

The corpus callosum is a massive commissure, or bridge, of myelinated axons that connect the cerebral cortex of the two sides of the brain. Two smaller commissures, the anterior and posterior commissures, connect the two sides of the more specialized regions of the cerebrum and diencephalon.

The surfaces of the hemispheres are lateral (side), medial (area between the two sides of the brain), and basal (ventral). The cerebral cortex exposed to view laterally is the recently evolved six-layered neocortex. The surface of the hemispheres contains many ridges and grooves. The ridge between two grooves is called a *gyrus*, and the groove is called a *sulcus* or *fissure*. The cerebral cortex is arbitrarily divided into lobes named after the bones that cover them: the frontal, parietal, temporal, and occipital lobes (Fig. 37–26).

Basal Ganglia

A section through the cerebral hemispheres reveals the surface of the cerebral cortex, a subcortical layer of white matter made up of masses of myelinated axons, and deep masses of gray matter: the basal ganglia that border the lateral ventricle. The basal ganglia lie on either side of the internal capsule, just lateral to the thalamus. The *basal ganglia* comprise the comma-shaped caudate (tailed) nucleus, the shield-shaped putamen, and the globus pallidus (*i.e.*, pale globe). The term *striatum* (*i.e.*, striped body) refers to the caudate plus the putamen. The globus pallidus and putamen make up the lentiform (lens-shaped) nucleus.

The basal ganglia supply axial and proximal unlearned and learned postures and movements, which enhance and add gracefulness to UMN-controlled manipulative movements. These background movement functions are called *associated movements*. Intact and functional basal ganglia provide the swinging of the arms during walking and running and the follow-through movements that accompany throwing a ball or swinging a club. As with the motor cortex, the nuclei on the left side control movement on the right side of the body, and vice versa. Circuits connecting the premotor cortex and supplementary motor cortex, the basal ganglia, and parts of the thalamus provide associated movements that accompany highly skilled behaviors. Parkinson's disease, Huntington's chorea, some forms of cerebral palsy, among other dysfunctions involving the basal ganglia result in a frequent or continuous release of abnormal postural or axial and proximal movement patterns. If damage to the basal ganglia is localized to one side, the movements occur on the opposite side of the body. These automatic movement patterns stop only in sleep, but in some conditions, the movements are so violent that getting to sleep becomes difficult.

Frontal Lobe

The frontal lobe extends from the frontal pole to the central sulcus (*i.e.*, fissure) and is separated from the temporal lobe by the lateral sulcus. The frontal lobe can be subdivided rostrally into the frontal pole and laterally into the superior, middle, and inferior gyri, which continue on the undersurface over the eyes as the orbital cortex. These areas are associated with the medial thalamic nuclei, which are also related to the limbic system. In general terms, the prefrontal cortex appears to be

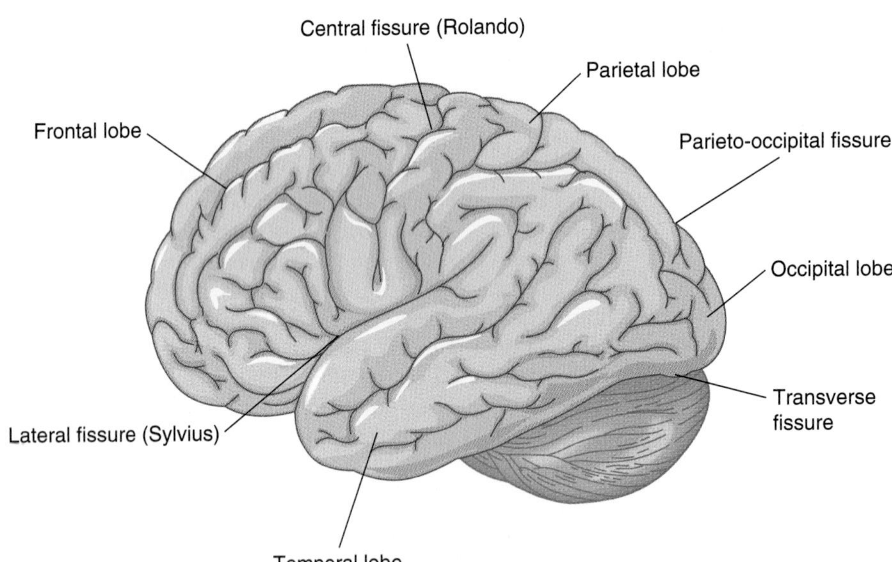

Figure 37–26 Lateral aspect of the left cerebral and cerebellar hemispheres.

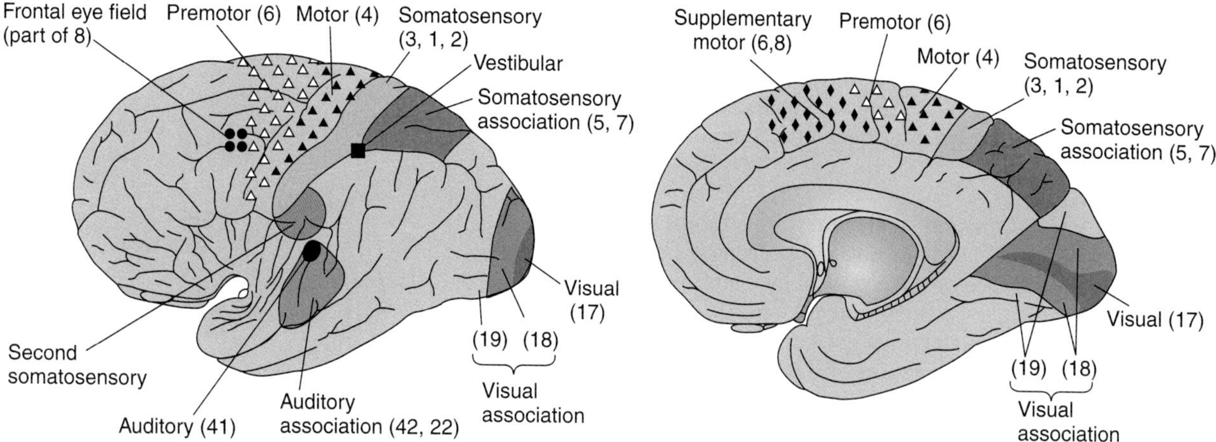

Figure 37–27
Motor and sensory areas of the cerebral cortex. (**Left**) The lateral view of the left (dominant) side is drawn as though the lateral sulcus had been pried open, exposing the insula. (**Right**) The diagram represents the areas in a brain that has been sectioned in the median plane. (Reproduced by permission from Nolte J. [1981]. *The human brain.* St. Louis: C.V. Mosby)

involved in anticipation and prediction of consequences of behavior. This "future-oriented" region is particularly depressed by many drugs, including alcohol.

The precentral gyrus (area 4), adjacent to the central sulcus, is the primary motor cortex (M1) (Fig. 37–27). This area of the cortex provides precise movement control for distal flexor muscles of the hands and feet and of the phonation apparatus required for speech. The frontal cortex just rostral to the precentral gyrus is called the *premotor* or *motor association cortex*. This region (area 8 and rostral area 6) is involved in the planning of complex learned movement patterns, and damage to these areas results in dyspraxia or apraxia. Such patients can manipulate a screwdriver, for instance, but cannot use it to loosen a screw. The primary motor cortex and the association motor cortex are connected with lateral thalamic nuclei, through which they receive feedback information from the basal ganglia and cerebellum. On the medial surface of the hemisphere, the premotor area includes a *supplementary motor cortex* involved in the control of bilateral movement patterns requiring great dexterity.

Parietal Lobe

The parietal lobe of the cerebrum lies behind the central sulcus (*i.e.,* postcentral gyrus) and above the lateral sulcus. The strip of cortex bordering the central sulcus is called the primary somatosensory cortex (areas 3, 1, 2), or S1, because it receives very discrete sensory information from the lateral nuclei of the thalamus. Just behind the primary sensory cortex is a region of the somesthetic association cortex (areas 5 and 7), which is connected with the thalamic nuclei and with the primary sensory cortex. This region is necessary for somesthetic perception (*i.e.,* appreciation of the meaningfulness [gnosis] of integrated sensory information from various sensory systems), especially with reference to perception of "where" the stimulus is in space and with relation to body parts. Localized lesions of this region can result in the inability to recognize the meaningfulness of an object (*i.e.,* agnosia). With the patient's eyes closed, a screwdriver can be felt and described in terms of shape and texture, but the person cannot integrate the sensory information required to identify it as a screwdriver (*i.e.,* astereognosis). The somesthetic functions of the sensory cortex are further discussed in Chapter 40.

Temporal Lobe

The temporal lobe lies below the lateral sulcus and merges with the parietal and occipital lobes. It includes the temporal pole and three primary gyri: superior, middle, and inferior. It is separated from the limbic areas on the ventral surface by the collateral or rhinal sulcus. The primary auditory cortex (area 41) involves the part of the superior temporal gyrus that extends into the lateral sulcus (see Fig. 37–27). This area is particularly important for fine discrimination from sound entering the opposite ear. It receives auditory input projections by way of the inferior colliculus of the midbrain and a ventral-lateral thalamic nucleus. The more exposed part of the superior temporal gyrus involves the auditory association or perception area (area 22). The gnostic aspects of hearing (e.g., the meaning of a certain sound pattern) require the function of this area. The remaining portion of the temporal cortex has a less well-defined function but is apparently important in long-term memory recall, particularly perception and memory for complex sensory patterns such as geometric figures and faces (*i.e.,* recognition of "what" or "who" the stimulus is). Irritation or stimulation can result in vivid hallucinations of long-past events. These higher-order temporal and parietal cortical regions are connected with a large, recently evolved dorsal lateral thalamic nuclear complex.

The cortices of the frontal, parietal, and temporal lobes surrounding the older cortex of the *insula,* located deep in the lateral fissure, represent the most recently evolved parts of the cerebral cortex. These areas contain primary and association functions for motor control and somesthesias for the lips and tongue and for audition; they are particularly involved in speech mechanisms.

Occipital Lobe

The occipital lobe is located posterior to the temporal and parietal lobes and is only arbitrarily separated from them. The medial surface of the occipital lobe contains a deep sulcus extending from the limbic lobe to the occipital pole, the *calcarine sulcus*, which contains the primary visual cortex (area 17). Stimulation of this cortex causes the experience of bright lights (phosphenes) in the visual field. Just superior and inferior and extending onto the lateral side of the occipital pole is the association cortex for vision (areas 18 and 19). This area is closely connected with the primary visual cortex and with complex nuclei of the thalamus. The integrity of the association cortex is required for gnostic visual function—the meaningfulness of visual experience, including experiences of color, motion, depth perception, pattern, form, and location in space.

The neocortical areas of the parietal lobe, between the somesthetic and the visual cortices, have a function in relating the texture, or "feel," and location of an object with its visual image. Between the auditory and visual association areas, the parieto-occipital region is necessary for relating the sound and image of an object or person.

Limbic System

The medial aspect of the cerebrum is organized as three concentric bands of cortex: the limbic system, which surrounds the connection between the lateral and third ventricle (*i.e.*, interventricular foramen). The

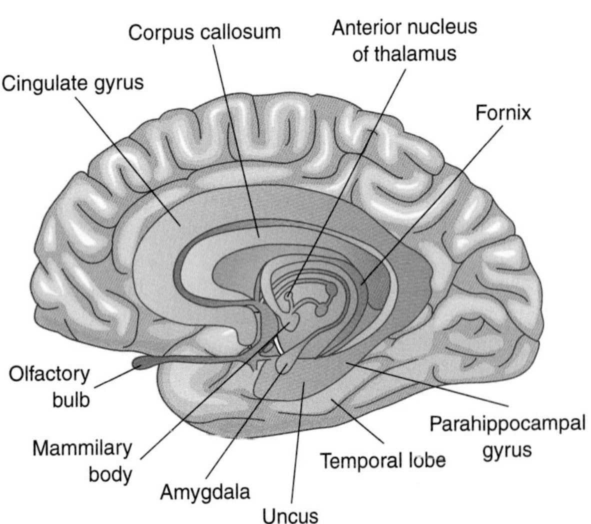

Figure 37–28
The limbic system includes the limbic cortex (cingulate gyrus, parahippocampal gyrus, uncus) and associated subcortical structures (thalamus, hypothalamus, amygdala).

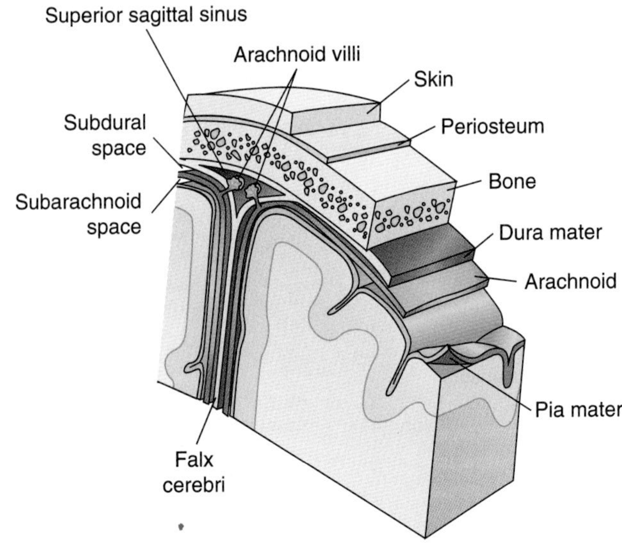

Figure 37–29
The cranial meninges. Arachnoid villi, shown within the superior sagittal sinus, are one site of cerebrospinal fluid absorption into the blood.

innermost band just above and below the cut surface of the corpus callosum is folded out of sight but is an ancient, three-layered cortex ending as the hippocampus in the temporal lobe. Just outside the folded area is a band of transitional cortex, which includes the cingulate and the parahippocampal gyri (Fig. 37–28). This limbic lobe has reciprocal connections with the medial and the intralaminar nuclei of the thalamus, with the deep nuclei of the cerebrum (*e.g.*, amygdaloid nuclei, septal nuclei) and with the hypothalamus. In general, this region of the brain is involved in emotional experience and in the control of emotion-related behavior. Stimulation of specific areas in this system can lead to feelings of dread, high anxiety, or exquisite pleasure. It can also result in violent behaviors, including attack, defense, or explosive and emotional speech.

Cerebral Dominance

Cerebral dominance refers to the fact that control of certain learned forms of behavior is exerted primarily by one of the two cerebral hemispheres. Handedness, perception of language, performance of speech, and appreciation of spatial relations are primarily expressions of one or the other hemisphere. By convention, speech is used to designate the dominant hemisphere. The dominant hemisphere has a major role in verbal and analytic abilities; the nondominant hemisphere has a lesser role in these functions and a major role in nonverbal and spatial abilities. In most persons, even left-handed persons, the left hemisphere is the dominant hemisphere for speech. Although it is assumed that the dominance of speech and handedness are assigned to the same hemisphere, this is not always the case. In clinical practice, communication dominance is a determinant of cerebral dominance. Because there is substantial overlap, the concept of strict lateralization may not be appropriate other than in primary sensory areas.

The interhemispheric communication pathways are largely undeveloped at birth. The communication between the two hemispheres increases with age and is fairly well developed by the second or third year of life. Cerebral dominance probably develops gradually throughout childhood. This explains why a child with an injury to the normally dominant hemisphere can be trained to become left-handed and proficient in speech, but an older person with similar deficits finds such learning difficult or impossible.

Meninges

Inside the skull and vertebral column, the brain and spinal cord are loosely suspended and protected by several connective tissue sheaths called the *meninges* (Fig. 37–29). The surfaces of the spinal cord, brain, and segmental nerves are covered with a delicate connective tissue layer called the *pia mater* (*i.e.,* delicate mother). The surface blood vessels and those that penetrate the brain and spinal cord are encased in this protective tissue layer. A second very delicate, nonvascular, and waterproof layer, called the *arachnoid* because of its spider-web appearance, encloses the entire CNS (Fig. 37–30). The CSF is contained within the subarachnoid space. Immediately outside the arachnoid is a continuous sheath of strong connective tissue, the *dura mater* (*i.e.,* tough mother), which provides the major protection for the brain and spinal cord carried within it. The cranial dura often splits into two layers, and the outer layer serves as the periosteum of the inner surface of the skull.

The inner layer of the dura forms two major folds. The first, a longitudinal fold called the *falx cerebri*, separates the cerebral hemispheres and fuses with a second transverse fold, called the *tentorium cerebelli* (Fig. 37–31). The latter acts as a hammock, supporting the occipital lobes above the cerebellum. The tentorium forms a tough septum, which separates the cranial cavity into the anterior and middle fossae, which contain the cerebral hemispheres, from the posterior fossa, which lies inferior to it and contains the brain stem and cerebellum. The tentorium attaches to the petrous portion of the temporal bone and the dorsum sellae of the cranial floor, with a semicircular gap, or *incisura*, formed at the midline to permit the midbrain to pass forward from the posterior fossa. The resultant compartmentalization of the cranial cavity is the basis for the commonly used terms *supratentorial* (*i.e.,* above the tentorium) and *infratentorial* (*i.e.,* below the tentorium). The cerebral hemispheres and the diencephalon are supratentorial structures, and the pons, cerebellum, and medulla are infratentorial structures.

The strong folds of the inner dura, the tentorium, and falx cerebri normally support and protect the brain, which floats in the CSF within the enclosed space. Dur-

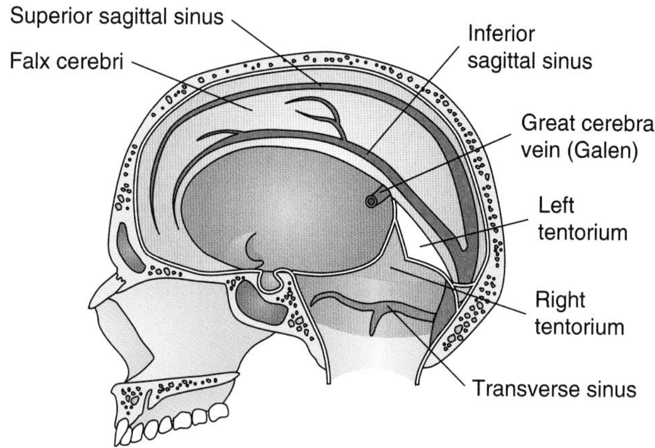

Figure 37–31
Cranial dura mater. The skull is open to show the falx cerebri and the right and left portions of the tentorium cerebelli, as well as some of the cranial venous sinuses.

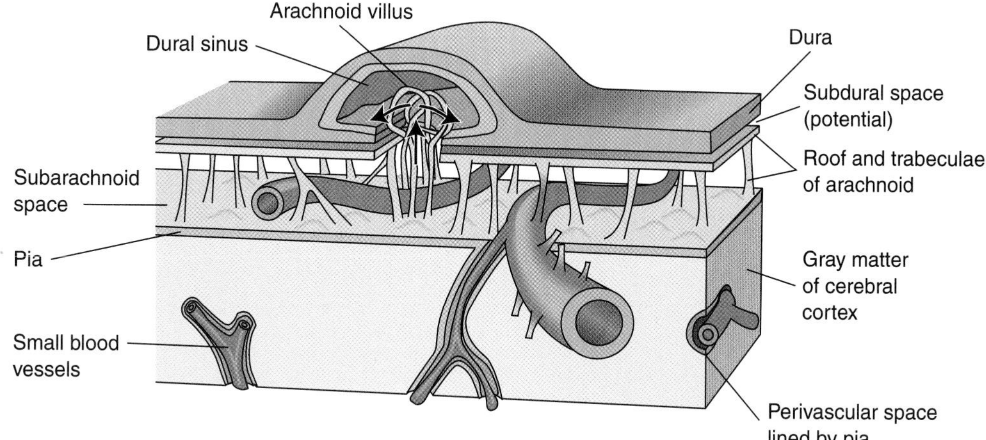

Figure 37–30
Schematic diagram of the three connective tissue membranes (pia, arachnoid, and dura) constituting the meninges of the central nervous system. Cerebrospinal fluid is resorbed (*arrows*) by way of the arachnoid villi projecting into the dural sinuses.

ing extreme trauma, however, the sharp edges of these folds can damage the brain. Space-occupying lesions such as enlarging tumors or hematomas can squeeze the brain against these edges or through the incisura (*i.e.*, herniation) of the tentorium. As a result, brain tissue can be compressed, contused, or destroyed, often causing permanent deficits (see Chapter 38).

Ventricular System and Cerebrospinal Fluid

The ventricular system is a series of CSF-filled cavities within the brain (Fig. 37–32). The lining of the ventricles and central canal of the spinal cord, called the *ependymal lining*, undergoes great expansion in the roof of the lateral, third and fourth ventricles, with multiple foldings and an especially rich blood supply called the *choroid plexuses*, which are the source of 90% of the CSF. The other 10% of the CSF is produced by the remainder of the ependymal lining of the ventricles and central canal of the spinal cord. The choroid plexuses total only 2 to 3 g of tissues, or approximately 0.25% of the brain weight. The surface of the choroid epithelium facing the CSF contains many microvilli, from which about 500 ml of CSF are secreted each day. The total volume in the ventricular system is only about 150 ml, meaning that the CSF is completely replaced several times each day.

The CSF is an ultrafiltrate of blood plasma, composed of 99% water with other constituents, making it close to the composition of the brain extracellular fluid (Table 37–3). The functions of the CSF are twofold. It provides a supporting and protective fluid within which the brain and spinal cord float, and it provides a relatively constant ionic environment that serves as a medium for diffusion of nutrients, electrolytes, and metabolic end-products between the extracellular fluid surrounding CNS neurons and glia. Filling the ventricles, the CSF supports the mass of the brain. Because it fills the subarachnoid space surrounding the CNS, a physical force delivered to the cranial or spinal skeleton is to some extent diffused and cushioned.

TABLE 37–3

Composition of Cerebrospinal Fluid Compared With Plasma

Substance	Plasma	Cerebrospinal Fluid
Protein mg/dl	7500.00	20.00
Na^+mEq/L	145.00	141.00
CL^-mEq/L	101.00	124.00
K^+mEq/L	4.50	2.90
HCO^-mEq/L	25.00	24.00
pH	7.4	7.32
Glucose mg/dl	92.00	61.00

The CSF produced in the ventricles must flow through the interventricular foramen, the third ventricle, the cerebral aqueduct, and the fourth ventricle to exit from the neural tube. Three openings, or *foramina*, allow the CSF to pass into the subarachnoid space. Two of these, the *foramina of Luschka*, are located at the lateral corners of the fourth ventricle. The third, the medial *foramen of Magendie*, is located in the midline at the caudal end of the fourth ventricle (see Fig. 37–32). About 30% of the CSF passes down into the subarachnoid space that surrounds the spinal cord, mainly on its dorsal surface, and moves back up to the cranial cavity along its ventral surface.

Reabsorption of CSF into the vascular system occurs along the sides of the superior sagittal sinus in the anterior and middle fossa. To reach this area, the CSF must

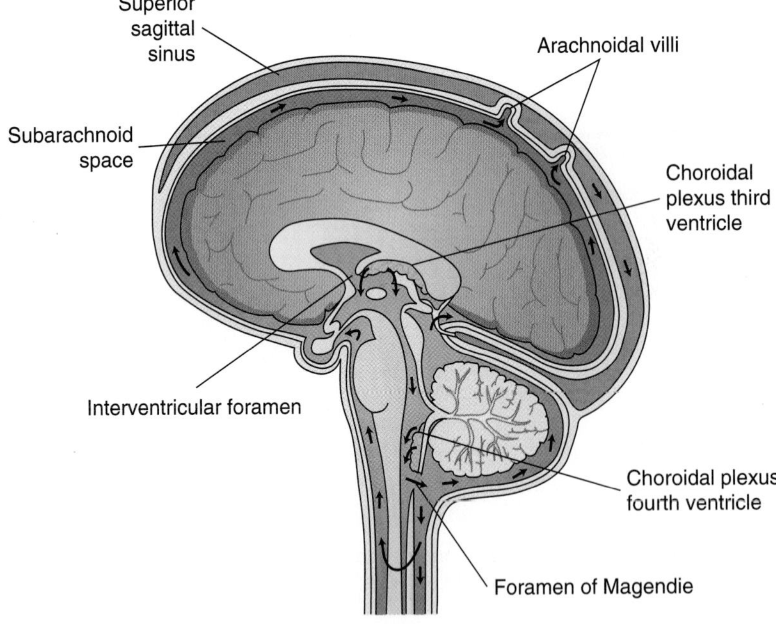

Figure 37–32 The flow of cerebrospinal fluid from the time of its formation from blood in the choroid plexuses until its return to the blood in the superior sagittal sinus. Plexuses in the lateral ventricles are not illustrated.

pass along the sides and ventral surface of the medulla and pons and then through the tentorial incisura or opening that surrounds the midbrain. Some of the CSF exits the posterior fossa ventrally, along the sides of the basilar artery rostrally and through a CSF cistern between the midbrain peduncles (*i.e.*, basilar cistern). The major part of the flow continues along the sides of the hypothalamus to the region of the optic chiasma and then laterally and superiorly along the lateral fissure and over the parietal cortex to the superior sagittal sinus region. Here the waterproof arachnoid has protuberances, the *arachnoid villi*, which penetrate the inner dura and venous walls of the superior sagittal sinus.

The reabsorption of CSF into the vascular system occurs by way of a pressure gradient. The normal CSF pressure is about 150 mm H_2O. The microstructures of the arachnoid villi are such that if the CSF pressure falls below approximately 50 mm H_2O, the passageways collapse, and reverse flow is blocked. The arachnoid villi function as one-way valves, permitting CSF outflow into the blood but not allowing blood to pass into the arachnoid spaces.

Blood-Brain and Brain–Cerebrospinal Fluid Barriers

Maintenance of a chemically stable environment is essential to the function of the brain. In most regions of the body, extracellular fluid undergoes small fluctuations in pH and concentrations of hormones, amino acids, and potassium ions during routine daily activities such as eating and exercising. If the brain were to undergo such fluctuations, the result would be uncontrolled neural activity, because some substances such as amino acids act as neurotransmitters and ions such as potassium influence the threshold for neural firing. Two barriers, the blood-brain barrier and the CSF-brain barrier, provide the means for maintaining the stable chemical environment of the brain. Only water, carbon dioxide, and oxygen enter the brain with relative ease; the transport of other substances between the brain and the blood is slow. The site of the barrier is the endothelial cells of the cerebral capillaries in the blood-brain barrier and the choroid epithelium in the CSF-brain barrier.

Blood-Brain Barrier

The blood-brain barrier depends on the unique characteristics of the brain capillaries. The endothelial cells of brain capillaries are joined by continuous tight junctions. In addition to the endothelial cell junctions, the brain capillaries are almost completely surrounded by processes of supporting cells of the brain, called astrocytes. The blood-brain barrier permits passage of essential substances while excluding unwanted materials. Reverse transport systems remove materials from the brain. Large molecules such as proteins and peptides are largely excluded from crossing the blood-brain barrier. Acute cerebral lesions, such as trauma and infection, increase the permeability of the blood-brain barrier and alter brain concentrations of proteins, water, and electrolytes.

The blood-brain barrier prevents many drugs from entering the brain. Most highly water-soluble compounds are excluded from the brain, especially molecules with high ionic charge such as many of the catecholamines. In contrast, many lipid-soluble molecules cross the lipid layers of the blood-brain barrier with ease. Some drugs, such as the antibiotic chloramphenicol, are highly lipid soluble and therefore enter the brain readily. Other medications have a low solubility in lipids and enter the brain slowly or not at all. Alcohol, nicotine, and heroin are very lipid soluble and rapidly enter the brain. Some substances that enter the capillary endothelium are converted by metabolic processes to a chemical form incapable of moving into the brain.

The cerebral capillaries are much more permeable at birth than in adulthood, and the blood-brain barrier develops during the early years of life. In severely jaundiced infants, bilirubin can cross the immature blood-brain barrier, producing kernicterus and brain damage (see Chapter 8). In adults, the mature blood-brain barrier prevents bilirubin from entering the brain, and the nervous system is not affected.

Cerebrospinal Fluid–Brain Barrier

The ependymal lining cells of the choroid plexus are linked together by tight junctions, forming a blood-CSF barrier to diffusion of many molecules from the blood plasma of choroid plexus capillaries to the CSF. Water is transported through the choroid epithelial cells by osmosis. Oxygen and carbon dioxide move into the CSF by diffusion, resulting in partial pressures roughly equal to those of plasma. The high sodium and low potassium contents of the CSF are actively regulated and kept relatively constant. Lipids and nonpeptide hormones diffuse through the barrier rather easily, but most large molecules, such as proteins, peptides, many antibiotics, and other medications, do not normally get through. The choroid epithelium uses energy in the form of ATP to actively secrete many components into the CSF, including proteins; sodium ions; a number of micronutrients such as vitamins C, B_6 (pyridoxine), and folates; and ribonucleosides and deoxyribonucleosides. Because the resultant CSF has a relatively high sodium content, the negatively charged chloride and bicarbonate diffuse into the CSF along an ionic gradient. The choroid also generates bicarbonate from carbon dioxide in the blood. The generation of bicarbonate is important to the regulation of the pH of the CSF.

Mechanisms exist that facilitate the transport of other molecules such as glucose without energy expenditure. Ammonia, a toxic metabolite of neuronal activity, is converted to glutamine by astrocytes. Glutamine moves by facilitated diffusion through the choroid epithelium into the plasma. This exemplifies a major function of the CSF, that of providing a means of removal of toxic waste products from the CNS. Because the brain and spinal cord have no lymphatic channels, the CSF serves this function.

There are several specific areas of the brain where the blood-CSF barrier does not exist. One area is at the caudal end of the fourth ventricle (*i.e.*, area postrema), where specialized receptors for the carbon dioxide level of the CSF influence respiratory function. Another area consists of the walls of the third ventricle, which permit hypothalamic neurons to monitor blood glucose levels reflected in CSF glucose levels. This mechanism permits hypothalamic centers to respond to these blood glucose levels, contributing to hunger and eating behaviors.

In summary, in the process of development, the most rostral part of the embryonic neural tube develops to form the brain. The brain can be divided into three parts: hindbrain, midbrain, and forebrain. The hindbrain, consisting of the medulla oblongata, pons, and cerebellum, contains the neuronal circuits required for eating, breathing, and locomotive functions required for survival. Cranial nerves XII, XI, X, IX, VIII, VII, VI, and V are located in the hindbrain. The midbrain contains cranial nerves III and IV. The forebrain is the most rostral part of the brain; it consists of the diencephalon and the telencephalon. The dorsal horn part of the diencephalon is the thalamus and subthalamus, and the ventral horn part is the hypothalamus. The cerebral hemispheres are the lateral outgrowths of the diencephalon. Although there may be considerable overlap, one of the hemispheres is the more dominant hemisphere; it has a major role in verbal and analytic abilities. The less dominant hemisphere has a major role in nonverbal and spatial abilities.

The cerebral hemispheres are arbitrarily divided into lobes—the frontal, parietal, temporal, and occipital lobes—named after the bones of the skull that cover them. The prefrontal premotor area and primary motor cortex are located in the frontal lobe; the primary sensory cortex and somesthetic association area are in the parietal cortex; the primary auditory cortex and the auditory association area are in the temporal lobe; and the primary and association visual cortex are in the occipital cortex. The limbic system, which is involved in emotional experience and release of emotional behaviors, is located in the medial aspect of the cerebrum. These cortical areas are reciprocally connected with underlying thalamic nuclei through the internal capsule. Thalamic involvement is essential for normal forebrain function.

The brain is enclosed and protected by the pia mater, arachnoid, and dura mater. The protective CSF in which the brain and spinal cord float isolates them from minor and moderate trauma. The CSF is secreted into the ventricles, circulates through the ventricular system, passes outside to surround the brain, and is reabsorbed into the venous system through the arachnoid villi. The CSF-brain barrier and the blood-brain barrier protect the brain from substances in the blood that would disrupt brain function.

The Autonomic Nervous System

After you have completed this section of the chapter, you should be able to meet the following objectives:

- State the function of the autonomic nervous system
- Compare the sensory and motor components of the autonomic nervous system with those of the CNS
- Compare the anatomic location and functions of the sympathetic and parasympathetic nervous systems
- Describe the neurotransmitter synthesis and release, degradation, and receptor function in the sympathetic and parasympathetic nervous systems

The ability to maintain homeostasis and perform the activities of daily living in an ever-changing physical environment is largely vested in the autonomic nervous system (ANS). The ANS functions at the subconscious level and is involved in regulating, adjusting, and coordinating vital visceral functions such as blood pressure and blood flow, body temperature, respiration, digestion, metabolism, and elimination. The ANS is strongly affected by emotional influences and is involved in many of the expressive aspects of behavior. Blushing, pallor, palpitations of the heart, clammy hands, and dry mouth are several emotional expressions that are mediated through the ANS. Biofeedback and relaxation exercises have been used for modifying the subconscious functions of the ANS.

As with the somatic nervous system, the ANS is represented in both the CNS and the PNS. Traditionally, the ANS has been defined as a general efferent system innervating visceral organs. The efferent outflow from the ANS has two divisions: the sympathetic nervous system and parasympathetic nervous system. The afferent input to the ANS is provided by visceral afferent neurons, generally not considered to be part of the ANS.

The functions of the sympathetic nervous system include maintaining body temperature and adjusting blood flow and blood pressure to meet the changing needs of the body that occur with activities of daily living, such as moving from the supine to the standing position. The sympathoadrenal system can also discharge as a unit when there is a critical threat to the integrity of the individual—the fight or flight response. During a stress situation, the heart rate accelerates; the blood pressure rises; blood flow shifts from the skin and gastrointestinal tract to the skeletal muscles and brain; blood sugar increases; the bronchioles and pupils dilate; the sphincters of the stomach and intestine and the internal sphincter of the urethra constrict; and the rate of secretion of exocrine glands that are involved in digestion diminishes. Emergency situations often require vasoconstriction and shunting of blood away from the skin and into the muscles and brain, a mechanism that provides for a reduction in blood flow should a wound occur and preservation of vital functions needed for survival. Sympathetic function is often summarized as catabolic in that its actions predominate during periods of pronounced energy expenditure, such as when survival is threatened.

In contrast to the sympathetic nervous system, the functions of the parasympathetic nervous system are concerned with conservation of energy, resource replenishment and storage (*i.e.*, anabolism), and maintenance of organ function during periods of minimal activity. The parasympathetic nervous system slows heart rate, stimulates gastrointestinal function and related glandular secretion, promotes bowel and bladder elimination, and contracts the pupil, protecting the retina from excessive light during periods when visual function is not vital to survival. The two divisions of the ANS are generally viewed as having opposite and antagonistic actions (*i.e.*, if one activates, the other inhibits a function). Exceptions are functions, such as sweating and regulation of arteriolar blood vessel diameter, that are controlled by a single division of the ANS, in this case the sympathetic nervous system.

The sympathetic and parasympathetic nervous systems are continually active. The effect of this continual or basal (baseline) activity is referred to as *tone.* The tone of an effector organ or system can be increased or decreased and is usually regulated by a single division of the ANS. For example, vascular smooth muscle tone is controlled by the sympathetic nervous system. Increased sympathetic activity produces local vasoconstriction from increased vascular smooth muscle tone, and decreased activity results in vasodilatation due to decreased tone. In structures such as the sinoatrial node and atrioventricular node of the heart, which are innervated by both divisions of the ANS, one division predominates in controlling tone. In this case, the tonically active parasympathetic nervous system exerts a constraining or braking effect on heart rate, and when parasympathetic outflow is withdrawn, similar to releasing a brake, the heart rate increases. The increase in heart rate that occurs with vagal withdrawal can be further augmented by sympathetic stimulation. Table 37–4 describes the responses of effector organs to sympathetic and parasympathetic impulses.

Autonomic Efferent Pathways

The outflow of both divisions of the ANS follow a two-neuron pathway. The first motor neuron, called the *preganglionic neuron,* lies in the intermediolateral cell column in the ventral horn of the spinal cord or its equivalent location in the brain stem. The second motoneuron, called the *postganglionic neuron,* synapses with a preganglionic neuron in an autonomic ganglion located in the PNS. The two divisions of the ANS differ in terms of location of preganglionic cell bodies, relative length of preganglionic fibers, general function, nature of peripheral responses, and preganglionic and postganglionic neuromediators (see Table 37–4). This two-neuron outflow pathway and the interneurons in the autonomic ganglia that add further modulation to ANS function are features distinctly different from the arrangement in somatic motor innervation.

Most visceral organs are innervated by both sympathetic and parasympathetic fibers. Exception are structures such as blood vessels and sweat glands that have input from only one division of the ANS. The fibers of the sympathetic nervous system are distributed to effectors throughout the body, and as a result, sympathetic actions tend to be more diffuse than those of the parasympathetic nervous system, in which there is a more localized distribution of fibers. The preganglionic fibers of the sympathetic nervous system may traverse a considerable distance and pass through several ganglia before synapsing with postganglionic neurons, and their

TABLE 37-4

Characteristics of the Sympathetic and Parasympathetic Nervous Systems

Characteristic	Sympathetic Outflow	Parasympathetic Outflow
Location of preganglionic cell bodies	Thoracic 1–12, lumbar 1 and 2	Cranial nerves: III, VII (intermedius), IX, X; sacral segments 2, 3, and 4
Relative length of preganglionic fibers	Short—to paravertebral chain of ganglia or to aortic prevertebral of ganglia	Long—to ganglion cells near or in the innervated organ
General function	Catabolic—mobilizes resources in anticipation of challenge for survival (preparation for "fight-or-flight" response)	Anabolic—concerned with conservation, renewal, and storage of resources
Nature of peripheral response	Generalized	Localized
Transmitter between preganglionic terminals and postganglionic neurons	Acetylcholine (ACh)	ACh
Transmitter of postganglionic neuron	ACh (sweat glands and skeletal muscle vasodilator fibers); norepinephrine (NE) (most synapses); NE and epinephrine (secreted by adrenal gland)	ACh

terminals make contact with a large number of postganglionic fibers. In some ganglia, the ratio of preganglionic to postganglionic cells may be 1:20; because of this, the effects of sympathetic stimulation are diffuse. There is considerable overlap, and one ganglion cell may be supplied by several preganglionic fibers. In contrast to the sympathetic nervous system, the parasympathetic nervous system has its postganglionic neurons located very near or within the organ of innervation. Because the ratio of preganglionic to postganglionic communication is often 1:1, the effects of the parasympathetic nervous system are much more circumscribed.

Sympathetic Nervous System

The neurons of the sympathetic nervous system are located primarily in the thoracic and upper lumbar segments (T1 to L2) of the spinal cord; hence, the sympathetic nervous system is often referred to as *thoracolumbar division* of the ANS. These preganglionic neurons, which are located primarily in the ventral horn intermediolateral cell column, have axons that are largely myelinated and relatively short. The postganglionic neurons of the sympathetic nervous system are located in the paravertebral ganglia of the sympathetic chain of ganglia that lie on either side of the vertebral column or in prevertebral sympathetic ganglia such as the celiac ganglia (Fig. 37– 33). In addition to postganglionic efferent neurons, the sympathetic ganglia contain neurons of the internuncial, short-axon type, similar to those associated with complex circuitry in the brain and spinal cord. Many of these inhibit and others modulate preganglionic to postganglionic transmission. The full significance of these modulating circuits awaits further investigation.

The axons of the preganglionic neurons leave the spinal cord by way of the ventral root of the spinal nerves (T1 to L2), enter the ventral primary rami, and leave the spinal nerve through white rami of the rami communicantes to reach the paravertebral ganglionic chain (Fig. 37–34). Within the sympathetic chain of ganglia, preganglionic fibers may synapse with neurons of the ganglion it enters, pass up or down the chain and synapse with one or more ganglia, or pass through the chain and move outward through a splanchnic nerve to terminate in one of the prevertebral ganglia (*i.e.*, celiac, superior mesenteric, or inferior mesenteric) that are scattered along the dorsal aorta and its branches.

Preganglionic fibers from the thoracic segments of the cord pass upward to form the cervical chain connecting the inferior, middle, and superior cervical sympathetic ganglia with the rest of the sympathetic chain at lower levels. Postganglionic sympathetic axons of the cervical and lower lumbosacral chain ganglia spread further through nerve plexuses along continuations of the great arteries. Cranial structures, particularly blood vessels, are innervated by the spread of postganglionic axons along the external and internal carotid arteries into the face and the cranial cavity. The sympathetic fibers from T1 generally pass up the sympathetic chain into the head; those from T2 pass into the neck; those from T1 to T5 pass to the heart: those from T3, T4, T5, and T6 pass to the thoracic viscera; those from T7, T8, T9, T10, and T11 pass to the abdominal viscera; and those from T12, L1, L2, and L3 pass to the kidneys and pelvic organs. Many of the preganglionic fibers from the fifth to the last thoracolumbar segment pass through the paravertebral ganglia to continue as the splanchnic nerves. Most of these fibers do not synapse until they reach the celiac or superior mesenteric ganglion; others pass to the adrenal medulla.

The adrenal medulla, which is part of the sympathetic nervous system, contains postganglionic sympathetic neurons that secrete sympathetic neurotransmitters directly into the bloodstream. Some of the postganglionic fibers, all of which are unmyelinated, from the paravertebral ganglionic chain reenter the segmental nerve through unmyelinated branches called *gray rami* of all segmental nerves and are then distributed to all parts of the body wall in the spinal nerve branches. These fibers innervate the sweat glands, piloerector muscles of the hair follicles, all of the blood vessels of the skin and skeletal muscles, and the CNS itself.

Parasympathetic Nervous System

The preganglionic fibers of the parasympathetic nervous system, also referred to as the *craniosacral division* of the ANS, originate in some segments of the brain stem and sacral segments of the spinal cord (see Fig. 37–33). The central regions of origin are the midbrain, pons, medulla oblongata, and the sacral part of the spinal cord. The midbrain outflow passes through the oculomotor (III) cranial nerve to the ciliary ganglia that lies in the orbit behind the eye; it supplies the pupillary sphincter muscle of the eye and the ciliary muscles that control lens thickness for accommodation. Caudal pontine outflow comes from preganglionic fibers of the intermedius component of the facial (VII) nerve complex, which synapse in the submandibular ganglia, supplying the submandibular and sublingual glands, and the pterygopalatine ganglia, supplying the lacrimal and nasal glands. The medullary outflow develops from cranial nerves VII, IX, and X. Fibers in the glossopharyngeal (IX) nerve synapse in the otic ganglia, which supply the parotid salivary glands. About 75% of parasympathetic efferent fibers are carried in the vagus (X) nerve. The vagus nerve provides parasympathetic innervation for the heart, trachea, lungs, esophagus, stomach, small intestine, proximal half of the colon, liver, gallbladder, pancreas, kidneys, and upper portions of the ureters.

The sacral preganglionic axons leave the S2 to S4 segmental nerves by gathering into the pelvic nerves, also called the *nervi erigentes.* The pelvic nerves leave the sacral plexus on each side of the cord and distribute their peripheral fibers to the bladder, uterus, urethra, prostate, distal portion of the transverse colon, descending colon and rectum. The sacral parasympathetic fibers also supply the venous outflow from the external genitalia to facilitate erectile function.

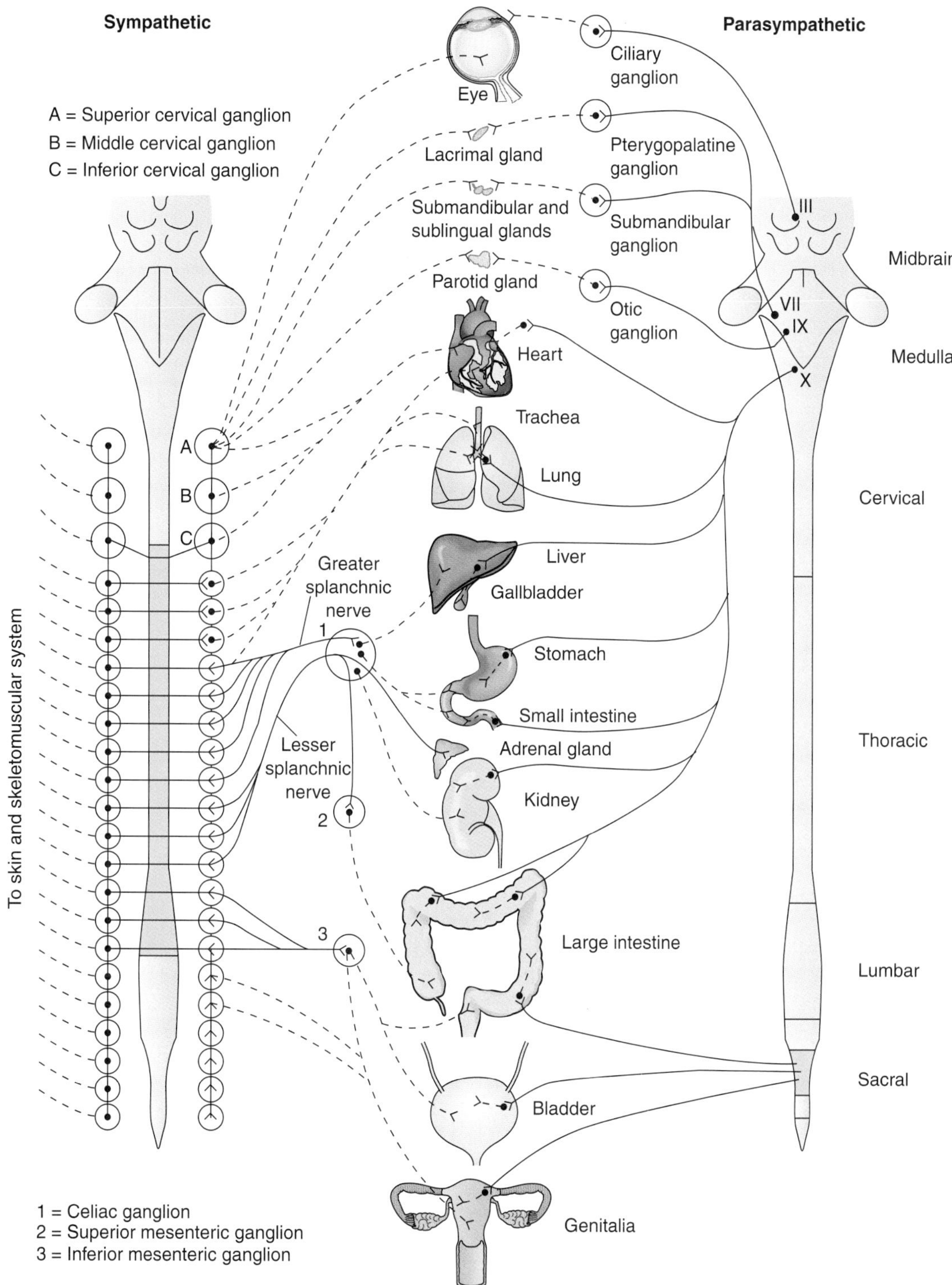

Figure 37–33
The autonomic nervous system. The involuntary organs are depicted with their parasympathetic innervation (craniosacral) indicated on the right and sympathetic innervation (thoracolumbar) on the left. Preganglionic fibers are *solid lines;* postganglionic fibers are *dashed lines.* For purposes of illustration, the sympathetic outflow to the skin and skeletomuscular system is shown separately (to the far left); effectors include sweat glands, pilomotor muscles and blood vessels of the skin, and blood vessels of the skeletal muscles and bones. (Modified from Heimer L. [1983]. *The human brain and spinal cord: Functional neuroanatomy and dissection guide.* New York: Springer-Verlag)

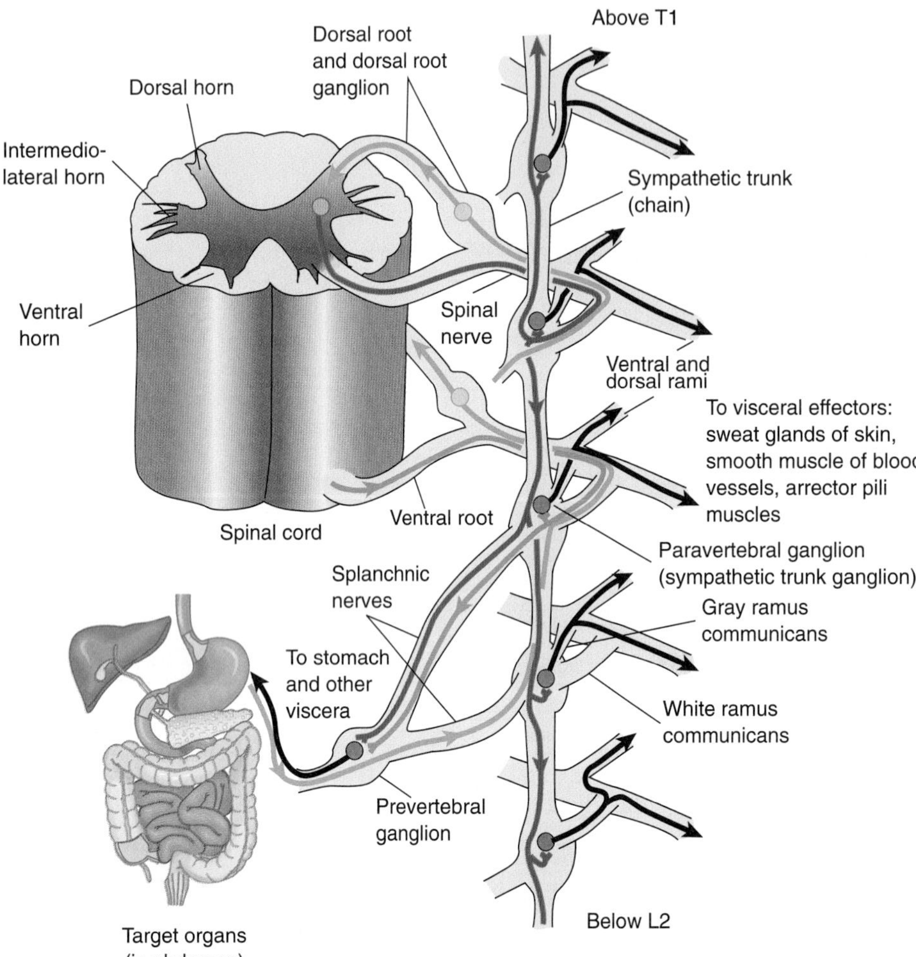

Figure 37–34 Sympathetic pathways. Sympathetic fibers leave the spinal cord by way of the ventral root of the spinal nerves, enter the ventral primary rami and pass through the white rami to the prevertebral or paravertebral ganglia of the sympathetic chain, where they synapse with postganglionic neurons. Some postganglionic fibers from the paravertebral ganglia reenter the segmental nerves through the gray rami and are then distributed in the spinal nerve branches. Other postganglionic neurons travel directly to their destination in the various effector organs. General visceral afferents carry information from the effector organs through the white rami to the dorsal root ganglia and into the dorsal horn of the spinal cord.

With the exception of cranial nerves III, VII, and IX that synapse in discrete ganglia, the long parasympathetic preganglionic fibers pass uninterrupted to short postganglionic fibers located in the organ wall. In the walls of these organs, postganglionic neurons send axons to smooth muscle and glandular cells that modulate their functions.

The gastrointestinal tract has its own intrinsic network of ganglionic cells located between the smooth muscle layers, called the *enteric* (intramural) *plexus,* which controls local peristaltic movements and secretory functions. This network of parasympathetic postganglionic neurons and interneurons runs from the upper portion of the esophagus to the internal anal sphincter. Local afferent sensory neurons respond to mechanical and chemical stimuli and communicate these influences to motor fibers in the enteric plexus. The number of neurons in the enteric neural network (10^8) is so large that it approximates that of the spinal cord. It is thought that this enteric nervous system is capable of independent function without control from CNS fibers. The CNS has a modulating role, by way of preganglionic innervation of the plexus, converting local peristalsis to longer-distance movements, thereby speeding the transit of intestinal contents.

Central Integrative Pathways

General visceral afferent fibers accompany the sympathetic and parasympathetic outflow into the spinal and cranial nerves, bring chemoreceptor, pressure, organ capsule stretch, and nociceptive information from organs of the viscera to the brain stem, thoracolumbar cord, and sacral cord. Local reflex circuits relating visceral afferent and autonomic efferent activity are integrated into a hierarchic control system in the spinal cord and brain stem. Progressively greater complexity in the responses and greater precision in their control occur at each higher level of the nervous system. Most visceral reflexes contain contributions from the lower motoneurons that innervate skeletal muscles as part of their response patterns. The distinction between purely visceral and somatic reflex hierarchies becomes less and less meaningful at the higher levels of hierarchic control and behavioral integration.

For most autonomic-mediated functions, the hypothalamus serves as the major control center. The hypothalamus, which has connections with the cerebral cortex, the limbic system, and the pituitary gland, is in a prime position to receive, integrate, and transmit information to other areas of the nervous system. The neurons concerned with thermoregulation, thirst, and feeding behaviors are found in the hypothalamus. The hypothalamus is also the site for integrating neuroendocrine function. Hypothalamic releasing and inhibiting hormones control the secretion of anterior pituitary hormones (*i.e.*, thyroid-stimulating hormone, corticotropin, growth hormone, luteinizing hormone, follicle-stimulating hormone, and prolactin). The supraoptic nuclei of the hypothalamus are involved in water metabolism through synthesis of antidiuretic hormone and its release from the posterior pituitary gland (see Chapter 26). Oxytocin, which causes contraction of the pregnant uterus and milk letdown during breast-feeding, is synthesized in the hypothalamus and released from the posterior pituitary gland in a manner similar to that of antidiuretic hormone.

Organization of many life-support reflexes occurs in the reticular formation of the medulla and pons. These areas of reflex circuitry, often called *centers,* produce complex combinations of autonomic and somatic efferent functions required for the respiration, gag, cough, sneeze, swallow, and vomit reflexes, as well as for the more purely autonomic control of the cardiovascular system. At the hypothalamic level, these reflexes are integrated into more general response patterns such as rage, defensive behavior, eating, drinking, voiding, and sexual function. Forebrain and especially limbic system control of these behaviors involves inhibiting or facilitating release of the response patterns according to social pressures during learned emotion-provoking situations.

Reflex adjustments of cardiovascular and respiratory function occur at the level of the brain stem. A prominent example is the carotid sinus baroreflex. Increased blood pressure in the carotid sinus increases the discharge from afferent fibers that travel by way of the ninth cranial nerve to cardiovascular centers in the brain stem. These centers increase the activity of descending efferent vagal fibers that slow heart rate, while inhibiting sympathetic fibers that increase heart rate and blood vessel tone. One of the striking features of ANS function is the rapidity and intensity with which it can change visceral function. Within 3 to 5 seconds, it can increase heart rate to about twice its resting level. Bronchial smooth muscle tone is largely controlled by way of parasympathetic fibers carried in the vagus nerve. These nerves produce mild to moderate constriction of the bronchioles.

Other important ANS reflexes are located at the level of the spinal cord. As with other spinal reflexes, these reflexes are modulated by input from higher centers. When there is loss of communication between the higher centers and the spinal reflexes, as occurs in spinal cord injury, these reflexes function in an unregulated manner (see Chapter 39). There is uncontrolled sweating, vasomotor instability, and reflex bowel and bladder function.

Autonomic Neurotransmission

The generation and transmission of impulses in the ANS occur in the same manner as transmission in other neurons. There are self-propagating action potentials with transmission of impulses across synapses and other tissue junctions by way of neurohumoral transmitters. However, the somatic motoneurons that innervate skeletal muscles divide into many branches, with each branch innervating a single muscle fiber; in contrast, the distribution of postganglionic fibers of the ANS forms a diffuse neural plexus at the site of innervation. The membranes of the cells of many smooth muscle fibers are connected by conductive protoplasmic bridges, called *gap junctions,* that permit rapid conduction of impulses through whole sheets of smooth muscle, often in repeating waves of contraction. Autonomic neurotransmitters released near a limited portion of these fibers provide a modulating function extending to a large number of effector cells. The muscle layers of the gut and of the bladder wall are examples. In some instances, isolated smooth muscle cells are individually innervated by the ANS; the piloerector cells that elevate the hair on the skin during cold exposure are an example.

The main neurotransmitters of the autonomic nervous system are acetylcholine and the catecholamines, epinephrine and norepinephrine. Acetylcholine is released at all of the sites of preganglionic transmission in the autonomic ganglia of sympathetic and parasympathetic nerve fibers and at the sites of postganglionic transmission in parasympathetic nerve endings. It is also released at sympathetic nerve endings that innervate the sweat glands and cholinergic vasodilator fibers found in skeletal muscle. Norepinephrine is released at most sympathetic nerve endings. The adrenal medulla, which is a modified prevertebral sympathetic ganglion, produces epinephrine along with small amounts of norepinephrine. Dopamine, which is an intermediate compound in the synthesis of norepinephrine, also acts as a neurotransmitter. It is the principal inhibitory transmitter of internuncial neurons in the sympathetic ganglia. It also has vasodilator effects on renal, splanchnic, and coronary blood vessels when given intravenously and is sometimes used in the treatment of shock (see Chapter 20).

A considerable number of neurons secreting peptide molecules have been identified in ANS ganglia, especially in the enteric plexus and in postganglionic ANS terminals of the sympathetic and parasympathetic systems. Many of these are secreted by internuncial neurons or as additional or "cotransmitters" by preganglionic and postganglionic neurons. Binding at postsynaptic neuropeptide receptors usually does not result in action potentials; instead, it alters the membrane potential or receptor numbers producing long-term (minutes to hours) changes in responsiveness to the neurotransmitter. For example, dual secretion of norepinephrine and neuropeptide Y in some sympathetic vasoconstrictor terminals results in longer vasomotor constriction. Similarly, some parasympathetic postganglionic aceylcholine-secreting neurons can secrete vasoactive intestinal peptide (VIP) as a cotransmitter that potentiates postsynaptic actions. Many neuropeptides involved in peripheral ANS function are under active investigation, including substance P, cholecystokinin, somatostatin, and neurotensin.

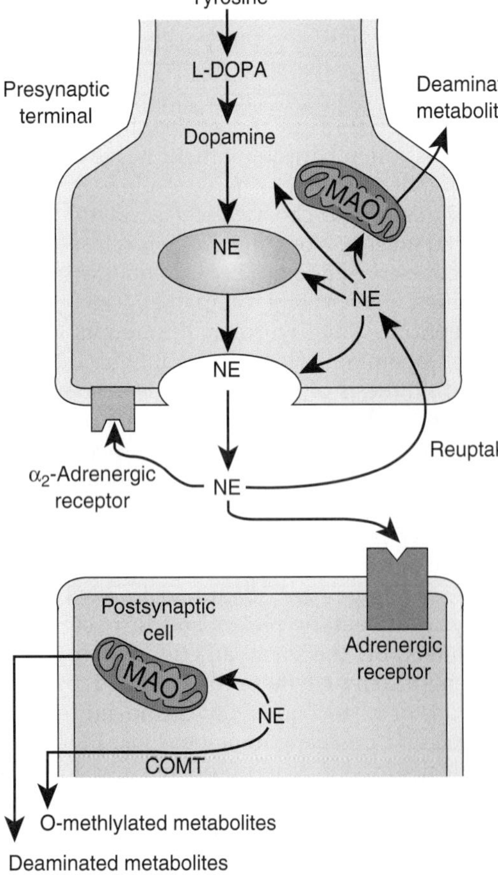

Acetylcholine and Cholinergic Receptors

Acetylcholine is synthesized in the cholinergic neurons from choline and acetyl coenzyme A (acetyl CoA) (Fig. 37–35). After acetylcholine is secreted by the cholinergic nerve endings, it is rapidly broken down by the enzyme acetylcholinesterase. The choline molecule is transported back into the nerve ending, where it is used again in the synthesis of acetylcholine.

Receptors that respond to acetylcholine are called *cholinergic receptors.* There are two types of cholinergic receptors: muscarinic and nicotinic. Muscarinic receptors are present on the innervational targets of postganglionic fibers of the parasympathetic nervous system and the sweat glands, which are innervated by the sympathetic nervous system. Nicotinic receptors are found in autonomic ganglia and the end plates of skeletal muscle. Acetylcholine has an excitatory effect on muscarinic and nicotinic receptors except for those in the heart and lower esophagus, where it has an inhibitory effect. The drug atropine is a antimuscarinic or muscarinic cholinergic-blocking drug that prevents the action of acetylcholine at excitatory and inhibitory muscarinic receptor sites. Because it is a muscarinic-blocking drug, it exerts little effect at nicotinic receptor sites.

Catecholamines and Adrenergic Receptors

The catecholamines, which include norepinephrine, epinephrine, and dopamine, are synthesized in the axoplasm of sympathetic nerve terminal endings from the amino acid tyrosine (see Fig. 37–35). In the process of catecholamine synthesis, tyrosine is hydroxylated (*i.e.,* has a hydroxyl group added) to form DOPA, DOPA is decarboxylated (*i.e.,* has a carboxyl group removed) to form dopamine, and dopamine is hydroxylated to form norepinephrine. In the adrenal gland, an additional step occurs during which norepinephrine is methylated (*i.e.,* a methyl group is added) to form epinephrine.

Each of the steps in sympathetic neurotransmitter synthesis requires a different enzyme, and the type of neurotransmitter that is produced depends on the type of enzymes that are available in a nerve terminal. For example, the postganglionic sympathetic neurons that supply blood vessels synthesize norepinephrine, but postganglionic neurons in the adrenal medulla produce epinephrine or norepinephrine. Epinephrine accounts for about

Figure 37–35
Schematic illustration of cholinergic parasympathetic (**A**) and noradrenergic sympathetic (**B**) neurotransmitter synthesis, release, receptor binding, neurotransmitter degradation, and metabolite transport back into the presynaptic neuron (acetylcholine) and reuptake (norepinephrine). (Adapted from Rhoades R.A., Tanner G.A. [1996]. *Medical physiology.* Boston: Little, Brown)

80% of the catecholamines released from the adrenal gland. The synthesis of epinephrine by the adrenal medulla is influenced by the glucocorticoid secretion from the adrenal cortex. These hormones are transported by way of a intraadrenal vascular network from the adrenal cortex to the adrenal medulla, where they cause the sympathetic neurons to increase their production of epinephrine through increased enzyme activity. Thus, any stress situation sufficient to evoke increased levels of glucocorticoids also increases epinephrine levels.

As the catecholamines are synthesized, they are stored in vesicles. The final step of norepinephrine synthesis occurs in these vesicles. When an action potential reaches an axon terminal, the neurotransmitter molecules are released from the storage vesicles. The storage vesicles provide a means for concentrated storage of the catecholamines and protect them from the cytoplasmic enzymes that degrade the neurotransmitters.

In addition to neuronal synthesis, there is a second major mechanism for replenishment of norepinephrine in sympathetic nerve terminals. This mechanism consists of the active recapture or reuptake of the released neurotransmitter into the nerve terminal. Between 50% and 80% of the norepinephrine that is released during an action potential is removed from the synaptic area by an active reuptake process. This process terminates the action of the neurotransmitter and allows it to be reused by the neuron. The remainder of the released catecholamines diffuse into the surrounding tissue fluids or are degraded by two special enzymes: catechol-O-methyltransferase (COMT), which is diffusely present in all tissues, and monoamine oxidase (MAO), which is found in the nerve endings themselves. Some drugs, such as the tricyclic antidepressants, are thought to increase the level of catecholamines at the site of nerve endings in the brain by blocking the reuptake process. Others, such as the MAO inhibitors, decrease the enzymatic degradation of the neurotransmitters and increase their levels.

The catecholamines can cause excitation or inhibition of smooth muscle contraction, depending on the site, dose, and type of receptor present. Norepinephrine has potent excitatory activity and low inhibitory activity. Epinephrine is potent as both an excitatory agent and an inhibitory agent.

The excitatory or inhibitory responses of organs to sympathetic neurotransmitters are mediated by interaction with special structures in the cell membrane called *receptors.* In 1948, Ahlquist proposed the terms *alpha* and *beta* for the receptor sites where catecholamines produce their excitatory (α) and inhibitory (β) effects.

In vascular smooth muscle, excitation of α receptors causes vasoconstriction, and excitation of β receptors causes vasodilatation. Endogenously and exogenously administered norepinephrine produces marked vasoconstriction of the blood vessels in the skin, kidneys, and splanchnic circulation that are supplied with α receptors. The β receptors are most prevalent in the heart, the blood vessels of skeletal muscle, and the bronchioles. Blood vessels in skeletal muscle have α and β receptors. In these vessels, high levels of norepinephrine produce vasoconstriction; low levels produce vasodilatation. The low levels are thought to have a diluting effect on norepinephrine levels in the arteries of these blood vessels so that the beta effect predominates. In vessels with few receptors such as those that supply the brain, norepinephrine has little effect.

α-Adrenergic receptors have been further subdivided into α_1 and α_2 receptors and β-adrenergic receptors into β_1 and β_2 receptors. Beta$_1$ receptors are found primarily in the heart and can be selectively blocked by β_1-receptor blockers. Beta$_2$ receptors are found in the bronchioles and in other sites that have beta-mediated functions. The α_1 receptors are found primarily in postsynaptic effector sites; they mediate responses in vascular smooth muscle. The α_2 receptors are mainly located presynaptically and can inhibit the release of norepinephrine from sympathetic nerve terminals. The α_2 receptors are abundant in the CNS and are thought to influence the central control of blood pressure.

The various classes of adrenergic receptors provide a mechanism by which the same adrenergic neurotransmitter can have many discretely different effects on differing effector cells. This mechanism also permits neurotransmitters carried in the bloodstream, whether from neuroendocrine secretion by the adrenal gland or from subcutaneous or intravenous administered drugs, to produce the same effects.

The catecholamines that are produced and released from sympathetic nerve endings are referred to as *endogenous neuromediators.* Sympathetic nerve endings can also be activated by *exogenous* forms of these neuromediators, which reach the nerve endings by way of the bloodstream after being injected into the body or being administered by mouth. These drugs mimic the action of the neuromediators and are said to have a *sympathomimetic* action. Other drugs can selectively block the receptor sites on the neurons and temporarily prevent the neurotransmitter from exerting its action.

In summary, the ANS regulates, adjusts, and coordinates the visceral functions of the body. The ANS, which is divided into the sympathetic and parasympathetic systems, is an efferent system. It receives its afferent input from visceral afferent neurons. The ANS has CNS and PNS components. The outflow of the sympathetic and parasympathetic nervous system follows a two-neuron pathway, which consists of a preganglionic neuron located within the CNS and a postganglionic neuron located outside the CNS. Sympathetic fibers leave the CNS at the thoracolumbar level, and the parasympathetic fibers leave at the craniosacral level. In general, the sympathetic and parasympathetic nervous systems have opposing effects on visceral function—if one excites, the other inhibits. The hypothalamus serves as the major control center for most ANS functions; local reflex circuits relating visceral afferent and autonomic efferent activity are integrated in a hierarchic control system in the spinal cord and brain stem.

The main neurotransmitters for the ANS are acetylcholine and the catecholamines, epinephrine and norepinephrine. Acetylcholine is the transmitter for all preganglionic neurons, for postganglionic parasympathetic neurons, and for selected postganglionic sympathetic neurons. The catecholamines are the neurotransmitters for most postganglionic sympathetic neurons. The neurotransmitters exert their target action through specialized cell surface receptors—cholinergic receptors that bind acetylcholine and adrenergic receptors that bind the catecholamines. The cholinergic receptors are divided into nicotinic and muscarinic receptors, and adrenergic receptors are divided into α and β receptors. Different receptors for the same transmitter at various sites in the same tissue or in other tissues results in differences in tissue responses to the same transmitter. This arrangement also permits the use of pharmacologic agents that act at specific receptor types.

BIBLIOGRAPHY

Bear M.F., Connors M.A., Paradise M.A. (1996). *Neuroscience* (pp. 167–169). Baltimore: Williams & Wilkins.

Carlson B.M. (1994). *Human embryology and developmental biology* (pp. 204–240). St. Louis: C.V. Mosby.

Conn P.H. (Ed.). (1995). *Neuroscience in medicine* (pp. 172–175). Philadelphia: J.B. Lippincott.

Cooper J.R., Bloom F.E., Roth R.H. (1996). *The biochemical basis of neuropharmacology* (7th ed., pp. 44–81, 126–162, 226–292, 410–451). New York: Oxford University Press.

Gartner L.P., Hiatt J.L. (1997). *Color textbook of histology* (pp. 155–185). Philadelphia: W.B. Saunders.

Guyton A.C., Hall J.E. (1996). *Textbook of medical physiology* (9th ed.). Philadelphia: W.B. Saunders.

Haines D.E. (Ed.). (1997). *Fundamental neuroscience* (pp. 115–121, 126–127, 146–148, 443–454). New York: Churchill Livingston.

Parent A. (1996). *Carpenter's human neuroanatomy* (9th ed., pp. 186–192, 268–292, 748–756). Baltimore: Williams & Wilkins.

Paximos G. (1990). *The human nervous system* (pp. 91–123). New York: Academic Press.

Rhoades R.A., Tanner G.A. (1996). *Medical physiology* (pp. 91–127). Boston: Little, Brown.

CHAPTER 38

Disorders of Brain Function

Sheila M. Curtis and Carol M. Porth

The brain is protected from external forces by the rigid confines of the skull and the cushioning afforded by the cerebrospinal fluid (CSF). The metabolic stability required by its electrically active cells is maintained by a number of regulatory mechanisms, including the blood-brain barrier and autoregulatory mechanisms that ensure its blood supply. Nonetheless, the brain remains remarkably vulnerable to injury by ischemia, trauma, tumors, degenerative processes, and metabolic derangements.

Mechanisms and Manifestations of Brain Injury

After you have completed this section of the chapter, you should be able to meet the following objectives:

- Differentiate cerebral hypoxia from cerebral ischemia and focal from global ischemia

- Differentiate cytotoxic, vasogenic, and interstitial cerebral edema
- Characterize the role of excitatory amino acids as a common pathway for neurologic disorders
- State the determinants of intracranial pressure (ICP) and describe compensatory mechanisms used to prevent large changes in ICP when there are changes in brain, blood, and CSF volumes
- Draw a pressure-volume curve and explain the relation between a change in intracranial volume and ICP
- Explain the causes of tentorial herniation of the brain and its consequences
- Compare the causes of communicating and noncommunicating hydrocephalus
- Define *consciousness* and trace the rostral to caudal progression of consciousness in terms of pupillary changes, respiration, and motor function as the effects of brain dysfunction progress to involve structures in the diencephalon, midbrain, pons, and medulla
- State two criteria for the diagnosis of brain death

Mechanisms of Injury

Injury to brain tissue can result from a number of conditions, including trauma, tumors, stroke, metabolic derangements, and degenerative disorders. Brain damage resulting from these disorders involves several common pathways, including the effects of ischemia, excitatory amino acid injury, cerebral edema, and injury due to increased intracranial pressure. In many cases, the mechanisms of injury are interrelated.

Hypoxic and Ischemic Injury

The energy requirements of the brain are provided mainly by adenosine triphosphate (ATP); the ability of the cerebral circulation to deliver oxygen in sufficiently high concentrations to facilitate metabolism of glucose and generate ATP is essential to brain function. Although the brain makes up only 2% of the body weight, it receives one sixth of the resting cardiac output and accounts for 20% of the oxygen consumption.[1] It follows that deprivation of oxygen or blood flow can have a deleterious effect on brain structures.

By definition, *hypoxia* denotes a deprivation of oxygen with maintained blood flow; *ischemia* is a situation of greatly reduced or interrupted blood flow. Hypoxia is usually seen in conditions such as exposure to reduced atmospheric pressure, carbon monoxide poisoning, severe anemia, and failure to oxygenate the blood. Because hypoxia indicates decreased oxygen levels in the tissue, it produces a generalized depressant effect on the brain.

The cellular pathophysiology of hypoxia and ischemia are quite different, and the brain tends to have different sensitivities to the two conditions. Contrary to popular belief, hypoxia is fairly well tolerated, particularly in situations of chronic hypoxia. Neurons are capable of substantial anaerobic metabolism and fairly tolerant of pure hypoxia; it commonly produces euphoria, listlessness, drowsiness, and impaired problem solving. Unconsciousness and convulsions may occur when hypoxia is sudden and severe. However, the effects of severe hypoxia (*i.e.*, anoxia) on brain function are seldom seen, because the condition rapidly leads to cardiac arrest and ischemia.

Ischemia can be *focal*, as in stroke, or *global*, as in cardiac arrest. Persons with global ischemia have no collateral circulation during the ischemic event. In contrast, collateral circulation may provide low levels of blood flow during focal ischemia. The residual perfusion may provide sufficient substrates to maintain a low level of metabolic activity, thereby preserving membrane integrity. At the same time, the delivery of glucose under anaerobic conditions may result in additional lactic acid production and worsening of lactic acidosis.[2]

Global Ischemia. Global ischemia occurs when blood flow is inadequate to meet the metabolic needs of the entire brain, as in cardiac arrest or circulatory shock. The result is a spectrum of neurologic disorders. Unconsciousness occurs within seconds of severe global ischemia, such as that resulting from complete cessation of blood flow, as in cardiac arrest, or with marked decrease in blood flow, as in serious cardiac dysrhythmias. If circulation is restored immediately, consciousness is quickly regained. However, if blood flow is not promptly restored, severe pathologic changes take place. Energy sources, glucose and glycogen, are exhausted in 2 to 4 minutes, and cellular ATP stores are depleted in 4 to 5 minutes. About 50% to 75% of the total energy requirement of neuronal tissue is spent on mechanisms for maintenance of ionic gradients across the cell membrane (*e.g.*, sodium-potassium pump), resulting in fluxes of sodium, potassium, and calcium ions (Table 38–1).[3] Excessive influx of sodium results in neuronal and interstitial edema. The influx of calcium initiates a cascade of events, including release of intracellular and nuclear enzymes that cause cell destruction. When ischemia is sufficiently severe or prolonged, infarction or death of all the cellular elements of the brain occurs.

TABLE 38–1 Pathophysiologic Consequences of Impaired Cerebral Perfusion

Consequences	Timing
Depletion of oxygen	10 sec
Depletion of glucose	2–4 min
Conversion to anaerobic metabolism	2–4 min
Exhaustion of cellular ATP	4–5 min
Consequences	
Efflux of potassium	
Influx of sodium	
Influx of calcium	

(Richmond T.S. [1997]. Cerebral resuscitation after global brain ischemia: Linking research to practice. *AACN Clinical Issues* 8 [2], p. 173)

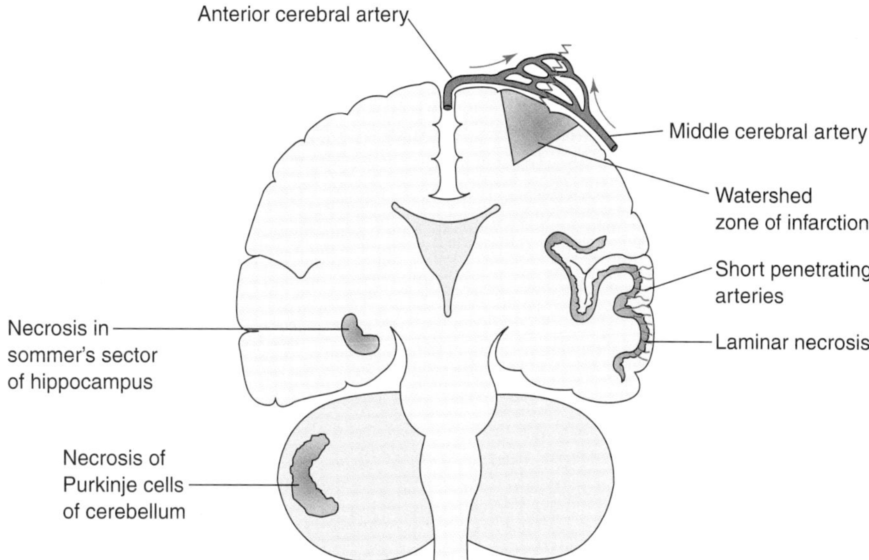

Figure 38–1 Consequences of global ischemia. A global insult induces lesions that reflect the vascular architecture (watershed infarcts, laminar necrosis) and the sensitivity of individual neuronal systems (pyramidal cells of Sommer's section, Purkinje cells). (Courtesy of Dmitri Karetnikov, artist)

The pattern of global ischemia reflects the anatomic arrangement of the cerebral vessels and the sensitivity of various brain tissues to oxygen deprivation (Fig. 38–1).[4] Selective neuronal sensitivity to a lack of oxygen is most apparent in the Purkinje cells of the cerebellum and neurons in Sommer's sector of the hippocampus.

The anatomic arrangement of blood vessels predisposes to two types of injury: watershed infarcts and laminar necrosis. Watershed infarcts are concentrated in anatomically vulnerable border zones between the overlapping territories supplied by the major cerebral arteries, notably the middle, anterior, and posterior cerebral arteries. The overlapping territory at the distal ends of these vessels form extremely vulnerable areas in terms of ischemia, called *watershed zones*. During events such as severe hypotension, these territories undergo a profound lowering of blood flow, predisposing to infarction of brain tissues. As a consequence, areas of the cortex that are supplied by the major cerebral arteries usually regain function on recovery of adequate blood flow; however, infarctions may occur in the watershed boundary strips, resulting in severe neurologic deficits.[4]

Laminar necrosis occurs in areas supplied by the penetrating arteries. The gray matter of the cerebral cortex receives its major blood supply through short penetrating arteries that emerge at right angles from larger vessels in pia mater and then form a cascade as they repeatedly branch, forming a rich capillary network. An abrupt loss of arterial blood pressure markedly diminishes flow through these capillary channels. Because of the branching arrangement of these vessels, the necrosis that develops is laminar and is most severe in the deeper layers of the cortex.

Although the threshold for ischemic neuronal injury is unknown, there is a period during which neurons can survive if blood flow is reestablished. Unfortunately, brain injury may not be reversible if the duration of ischemia is such that the threshold of injury has been reached. Even after circulation has been reestablished, damage to blood vessels and changes in blood flow can prevent return of adequate tissue perfusion. This period of postischemic hypoperfusion is thought to be associated with mechanisms such as desaturation of venous blood, capillary and venular clotting, or sludging of blood.[2] Because of sludging, blood viscosity increases, and there is increased resistance to blood flow. There is evidence of immediate vasomotor paralysis of the surface conducting blood vessels due to extracellular acidosis, followed by ischemic vasoconstriction.

Hypermetabolism due to increased circulating catecholamines has also been implicated as a contributing factor in postischemic hypoperfusion. Catecholamine release results in an increased cerebral metabolic rate and increased need for all energy-producing substrates, which the damaged brain is unable to maintain.

The neurologic deficits that result from global ischemia injury vary widely. If the period of nonflow or low flow is minimal, the neurologic damage is usually minimal to nonexistent. When the period is extensive or resuscitation is lengthy, the early neurologic picture is that of fixed and dilated pupils, abnormal motor posturing, and coma.[5] If the brain recovers, there is gradual improvement in neurologic status, although cognitive defects usually persist and can prevent a return to the preischemic functioning level.

An exception to this time frame is the circumstance of cold-water drowning in which the person, especially a child, is submerged in cold water for longer than 10 minutes.[6] Hypothermia develops and reduces the cerebral metabolic requirements for oxygen; it subsequently serves as a protective mechanism for the neurons. In this case, recovery can be rapid and remarkable, and resuscitation efforts should not be discontinued precipitously.

Treatment of global ischemia is aimed at providing oxygen to the troubled brain and decreasing the metabolic needs of brain tissue during the nonflow state.

Methods that decrease brain temperature as a means of decreasing brain metabolism have shown promise.[3] Normovolemic hemodilution may be used to overcome sludging of cerebral blood flow during reperfusion. Because both hypoglycemia and hyperglycemia adversely affect outcome in persons suffering from global ischemia, control of blood glucose within a range of 100 to 200 mg/dl has been advocated.[3,7] Although several pharmacologic agents have been advocated as a means of preventing brain damage in global ischemia, none have proven to be highly effective. In the past, barbiturates were used as a means of decreasing brain metabolism. However, the beneficial effects of barbiturates are minimal unless administered before the anticipated ischemia (*e.g.*, before neurosurgery, pediatric drowning).[2] Interest has focused on pharmacologic agents that could minimize injury from free radicals and excitatory amino acids.

Injury From Excitatory Amino Acids

In many neurologic disorders, injury to neurons may be caused by overstimulation of receptors for specific amino acids such as glutamate and aspartate that act as excitatory neurotransmitters.[8] These neurologic conditions range from acute insults such as stroke, hypoglycemic injury, and trauma to chronic degenerative disorders such as Huntington's disease and possibly Alzheimer's dementia. The term *excitotoxicity* has been coined for the final common pathway for neuronal cell injury and death associated with excessive activity of the excitatory neurotransmitters and their receptor-mediated functions.

Glutamate is the principal excitatory neurotransmitter in the brain, and its interaction with specific receptors is responsible for many higher-order functions, including memory, cognition, movement, and sensation.[8] Many of the actions of glutamate are coupled with receptor-operated ion channels. Glutamate channels are large, complex proteins that bridge the plasma membrane and contain a central pore or channel that, when open, permits ions to diffuse across the cell membrane. One subtype in particular, called the glutamate N-methyl-D-aspartate (NMDA) receptor, has been implicated in causing CNS injury. This subtype of glutamate receptor opens a large-diameter calcium channel that permits calcium and sodium ions to enter the cell and allows potassium ions to exit, resulting in prolonged (seconds) action potentials. The uncontrolled opening of NMDA receptor–operated channels produce an increase in intracellular calcium and leads to a series of calcium-mediated processes called the *calcium cascade*. Activation of the calcium cascade leads to the release of intracellular enzymes that cause protein breakdown, free radical formation, lipid peroxidation, fragmentation of DNA, and nuclear breakdown.

The intracellular concentration of glutamate is about 16 times that of the extracellular concentration.[8] Normally, extracellular concentrations of glutamate are tightly regulated, with excess amounts removed and actively transported into astrocytes and neurons. During prolonged ischemia, these transport mechanisms become immobilized, causing extracellular glutamine to accumulate. In the case of cell injury and death, intracellular glutamine is released from the damaged cells, causing injury to surrounding cells.

The first sign of glutamate toxicity, which develops within minutes of exposure to excessive amounts of glutamate, is neuronal swelling from the increased amounts of sodium and water entering the cell. The effects of acute toxicity do not necessarily lead to cell death; they are reversible if excess glutamate can be removed or if its effects can be blocked. Later signs of glutamate toxicity result from the effects of excessive levels of intracellular calcium. Neurons die within several hours after exposure to glutamate, at least partly depending on extracellular calcium levels and the inability of the nervous system to remove glutamate from the extracellular spaces.

Central nervous system (CNS) neurons can be divided into two major categories: macroneurons and microneurons. Macroneurons are large cells with long axons that leave the local network of intercommunicating neurons to send action potentials to other regions of the nervous system at distances of centimeters to meters (*e.g.*, upper motoneurons that communicate with lower motoneurons that control leg movement). Microneurons are very small cells that are intimately involved in local circuitry. Their axons transmit action potentials to other members of the same local network. In contrast to macroneurons, which number in the thousands, microneurons account for most of the many billions of CNS neurons.

Many macroneurons use glutamate as a neurotransmitter in their excitatory communication with microneurons. Macroneurons synapse on the postsynaptic excitatory amino acid receptors of the microneurons. It is the microneuron network that provides the analytic, integrative, and learning circuitry that is the basis for the higher-order function of the CNS. The microneurons of the cerebral cortex and hippocampus are particularly vulnerable to excessive stimulation of the glutamate NMDA receptors and the neurotoxic effects of increased intracellular calcium levels. Because of their increased vulnerability, many of the small interneurons that make up essential parts of the complex control and memory functions of the brain are selectively damaged, even if the remainder of the brain survives the insult. This pattern may account for the long-term effects of brain insult, which frequently include subtle and noticeable reductions in cognitive and memory functions.

Research is being directed toward attenuating or preventing the accumulation and injurious effects of excitatory amino acids. The pharmacologic methods being explored block the synthesis or release of excitatory amino acid transmitters; block the NMDA receptors; stabilize the membrane potential to prevent initiation of the calcium cascade using lidocaine and certain barbiturates; and specifically block certain intracellular proteases, endonucleases, and lipases that are known to be cytotoxic.[9–11] Animal studies and human clinical trials are underway, looking for methods of preventing brain damage from excitatory amino acids. Under investigation is the use of the drug riluzole in the treatment of amyotrophic lateral sclerosis (see Chapter 39). This drug acts presynaptically to inhibit glutamine release. Nimodipine, a calcium channel blocker that acts at the level of the NMDA receptor–operated channels, is being investigated for use in subarachnoid hemorrhage and AIDS dementia.[8]

Increased Intracranial Volume and Pressure

The brain is enclosed within the rigid confines of the skull or cranium, making it particularly susceptible to increases in increased intracranial pressure (ICP). Increased ICP is a common pathway for brain injury from different types of insults and agents. Excessive ICP can obstruct cerebral blood flow, destroy brain cells, displace brain tissue as in herniation, and otherwise damage delicate brain structures.

The cranial cavity contains blood (about 10%), brain tissue (about 80%), and CSF (about 10%) within the rigid confines of a nonexpandable skull.[12] Each of these three volumes contributes to the ICP, which normally is maintained within a range of 0 to 15 mm Hg when measured within the lateral ventricles. The volumes of each of these components can vary slightly without causing marked changes in ICP. This is because small increases in the volume of one component can be compensated for by a decrease in the volume of one or both of the other two components.[13] This association is called the *Monro-Kellie hypothesis*. Normal fluctuations in ICP occur with respiratory movements and activities of daily living such as straining, coughing, and sneezing.

Abnormal variation in intracranial volume with subsequent changes in ICP can be caused by a volume change in any of the three intracranial components. For example, an increase in tissue volume can result from a brain tumor, brain edema, or bleeding into brain tissue. An increase in blood volume develops when there is vasodilatation of cerebral vessels or obstruction of venous outflow. Excess production, decreased absorption, or obstructed circulation of CSF affords the potential for an increase in the CSF component. When the change in volume is caused by a brain tumor, it tends to occur slowly and is usually localized to the immediate area, whereas the increase resulting from head injury usually develops rapidly.

According to the modified Monro-Kellie hypothesis, reciprocal compensation occurs among the three intracranial compartments.[12] Of the three intracranial volumes, tissue volume is relatively restricted in the ability to undergo change; CSF and blood volume are the most able to compensate for changes in ICP. Initial increases in ICP are buffered by a translocation of CSF to the spinal subarachnoid space and increased reabsorption of CSF. The compensatory ability of the blood compartment is limited by the small amount of blood that is in the cerebral circulation. The cerebral blood vessels contain less than 10% of the intracranial volume, most of which is contained in the low pressure venous system. As the volume-buffering capacity of this compartment becomes exhausted, venous pressure increases and cerebral blood volume and ICP rise. Also, cerebral blood flow is highly controlled by autoregulatory mechanisms, which affect its compensatory capacity. Conditions such as ischemia and elevated PCO_2 levels produce vasodilation of the cerebral blood vessels in an attempt to increase cerebral blood flow. A decrease in PCO_2 has the opposite effect; for this reason, hyperventilation is sometimes used in the treatment of ICP.

Cerebral Compliance and the Impact of ICP. The impact of increases in blood, brain tissue, or CSF volumes on ICP varies among individuals and depends on the amount of increase that occurs, the effectiveness of compensatory mechanisms, and the compliance of brain tissue. Compliance represents the ratio of change in volume to the resulting change in pressure (*i.e.*, compliance = change in volume/change in pressure).[12] The effect of intracranial volume changes (*i.e.*, horizontal axis) on ICP changes (*i.e.*, vertical axis) are depicted in Figure 38–2.[12] The shape of the curve demonstrates effects of intracranial volume changes on ICP. The ICP remains constant from point A to point B when volume is added to the intracranial space. Because the compensatory mechanisms are adequate, compliance is high in this area of the curve, and there is little change in ICP. From points B to C, the compensatory mechanisms become less efficient; compliance decreases, and ICP begins to rise. At points C to D, the compensatory mechanisms have been exceeded such that even small changes in volume produce large changes in ICP.

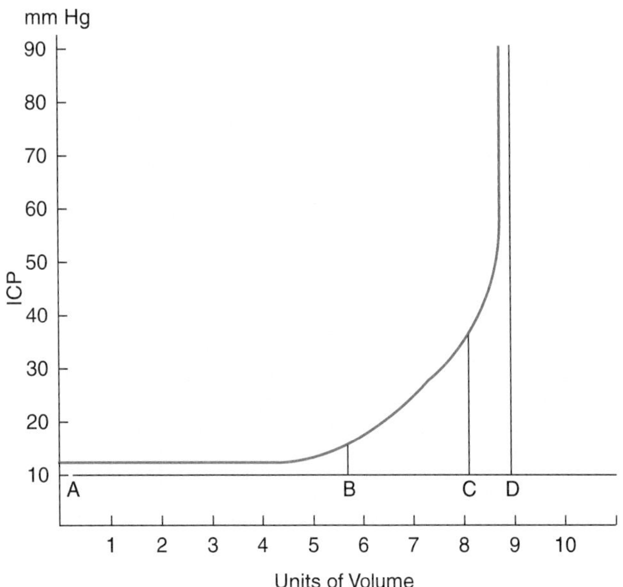

Figure 38–2
Pressure–volume curve. From point A to just before B, the ICP remains constant although there is an addition of volume (compliance is high). At point B, even though the ICP is within normal limits, compliance begins to change, as evidenced by the slight rise in ICP. From points B to C, the ICP rises with an increase in volume (low compliance). From points C to D, ICP rises significantly with each minute increase in volume (compliance is lost).

Impact of ICP on Cerebral Perfusion Pressure. The cerebral perfusion pressure (CPP), which represents the difference between the mean arterial blood pressure (MABP) and the ICP (*i.e.*, CPP = MABP − ICP), is the pressure perfusing the brain. Cerebral perfusion pressure is determined by the pressure gradient between the internal carotid artery and the subarachnoid veins. The MABP and ICP are frequently monitored in persons with brain conditions that increase ICP and impair brain perfusion. Normal CPP ranges from 70 to 100 mm Hg. Brain ischemia develops at levels below 50 to 70 mm Hg.[12] When the pressure in the cranial cavity approaches or exceeds the mean arterial pressure, tissue perfusion becomes inadequate, cellular hypoxia results, and if maintained, neuronal death may occur. The highly specialized cortical neurons are the most sensitive to oxygen deficit; a decrease in the level of consciousness is one of the earliest and most reliable signs of increased ICP. The continued cellular hypoxia leads to general neurologic deterioration; the level of consciousness may deteriorate from alertness through confusion, lethargy, obtundation, stupor, and coma.

One of the late reflexes seen with a marked increase in ICP is the CNS ischemic response, which is triggered by ischemia of the vasomotor center in the brain stem. Neurons in the vasomotor center respond directly to ischemia by producing a marked increase in mean arterial blood pressure, sometimes to levels as high as 270 mm Hg, accompanied by a widening of the pulse pressure and reflex slowing of the heart rate. These three signs, sometimes called the *Cushing reflex*, are important but late indicators of increased ICP.[14] They result from a severely increased ICP that compresses the blood flow to the brain stem. If the increase in blood pressure initiated by the CNS ischemic reflex is greater than the pressure surrounding the compressed vessels, blood flow is reestablished. The ischemic reflex is a last ditch effort by the nervous system to maintain the cerebral circulation. The Cushing reflex is seldom seen in modern clinical settings since the advent of ICP monitoring.

Brain Herniation

The brain is protected by the nonexpandable skull and supporting septa, the falx cerebri and the tentorium cerebelli, that divide the intracranial cavity into fossae or compartments that normally protect against excessive movement. The falx cerebri is a sickle-shaped septum that separates the two hemispheres. The tentorium cerebelli divides the cranial cavity into anterior and posterior fossae (see Fig. 38–2).[15] This inflexible dural sheath extends posteriorly from the bony petrous ridges and anterior to the clinoid process, sloping downward and outward from its medial edge to attach laterally to the occipital bone. Extending posteriorly into the center of the tentorium is a large semicircle opening called the *incisura* or *tentorial notch*. The temporal lobe rests on the tentorial incisura, and the midbrain occupies the anterior portion of the tentorial notch. The cerebellum is closely opposed to the dorsum of the midbrain and fills the posterior part of the notch. Other important anatomic associations exist among the anterior cerebral, internal carotid, posterior communicating, and the posterior and superior cerebellar arteries and the incisura (Fig. 38–3B). The oculomotor (cranial nerve III) emerges from the medial-lateral surface of each peduncle just caudal to the tentorium.

Brain herniation is displacement of brain tissue under the falx cerebri or through the tentorial notch or incisura of the tentorium cerebelli. A rising ICP created by the increased volume causes displacement of the cerebral tissue toward a less-dense area. The different types of herniation syndromes are based on the area of the brain that has herniated and the structure under which it has been pushed (see Fig. 38–3C). They are commonly divided into two broad categories, supratentorial and infratentorial, based on whether they are located above or below the tentorium.

Supratentorial Herniations. Three major patterns of supratentorial herniation were described by Plum and Posner in their classic work: cingulate or across the falx cerebri, uncal or lateral, and central or transtentorial.[15] Each herniation syndrome has distinguishing features in the early phases, but as the forced downward displacement on the pons and medulla continues, clinical signs become similar. Any of the supratentorial herniation syndromes can compress vascular and CSF flow, which can further complicate the neurologic manifestations of brain lesions. Downward displacement of the brain in any of the supratentorial herniation syndromes can cause brain stem herniation, in which the medulla herniates into the foramen magnum, which is the opening between the cranial cavity and the vertebral canal. Death is immediate and caused by medullary compression.

Cingulate herniation involves displacement of the cingulate gyrus and hemisphere beneath the sharp edges of the falx cerebri to the opposite side of the brain. Displacement of the falx can compress the local blood supply and brain tissue, causing ischemia and edema, which further increase ICP levels. Little is known about the specific signs and symptoms that permit its recognition.

Uncal herniation occurs when a lateral mass pushes the brain tissue centrally and forces the medial aspect of the temporal lobe, which contains the uncus and hippocampal gyrus, under the edge of the tentorial incisura, into the posterior fossa. The diencephalon and midbrain are compressed and displaced to the opposite side in uncal herniations. Cranial nerve III (oculomotor) and the posterior cerebral artery are frequently caught between the uncus and the tentorium. The oculomotor nerve controls pupillary constriction. The entrapment of this nerve results in ipsilateral pupillary dilatation, which is usually an early sign of uncal herniation. Consciousness may be unimpaired because the reticular activating system (RAS) has not yet been affected. Deterioration, however, may proceed rather rapidly—making it important

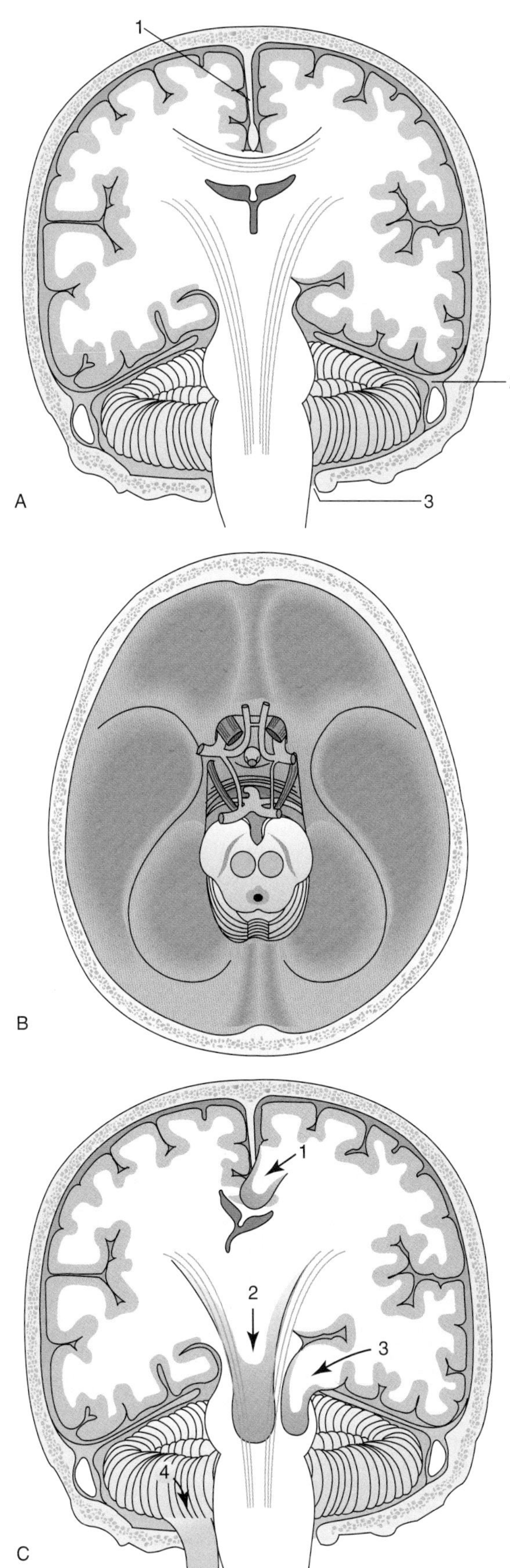

to recognize the distinguishing early features of lateral herniations.

As central and lateral herniations progress, there are changes in motor strength and coordination of voluntary movements because of compression of the descending motor pathways. It is not unusual for initial changes in motor function to occur on the side of the damage because of compression of the contralateral cerebral peduncles. This may result in a false localizing sign of hemiparesis on the same side as cranial nerve III, rather than on the opposite side, where the motor nerves have crossed over as would be expected. As the condition progresses, bilateral positive Babinski responses and respiratory changes (*e.g.,* Cheyne-Stokes, ataxic patterns) occur. Decorticate and decerebrate posturing may develop, followed by dilated, fixed pupils, flaccidity, and respiratory arrest.

Central or transtentorial herniation involves the downward displacement of the cerebral hemispheres, basal ganglia, diencephalon, and midbrain through the tentorial incisura. The diencephalon may be compressed tightly against the midbrain with such force that edema and hemorrhage result. It may or may not be associated with uncal herniation. In the early diencephalic stage, central herniation is manifested by a clouding of consciousness, with bilaterally small pupils (about 2 mm in diameter) with a full range of constriction and with motor responses to pain that are purposeful or semipurposeful (localizing) and often asymmetric. The clouding of consciousness is caused by pressure on the RAS in the upper midbrain, which is responsible for wakefulness. The pressure interferes with RAS function, and central herniations are first evidenced by changes in the level of consciousness.

As the herniation progresses to the late diencephalic stage, painful stimulation results in decorticate posturing, which may be asymmetric (Fig. 38–4), and there is a waxing and waning of respirations with periods of apnea (*i.e.,* Cheyne-Stokes respirations). With midbrain involvement, the pupils are fixed and midsize (about 5 mm in diameter), reflex adduction of the eyes is impaired, and pain elicits cerebrate posturing. Respirations change from Cheyne-Stokes breathing to neurogenic hyperventilation in which the frequency of ventilation may exceed 40 breaths per minute because of uninhibited stimulation of the inspiratory and expiratory centers. Progression to involve the pons and medulla produces fixed, midsized pupils, although with loss of reflex abduction and adduc-

Figure 38–3
Supporting septa of the brain and patterns of herniation. (**A**) The falx cerebri [1], tentorium cerebelli [2], foramen magnum [3]. (**B**) The location of the insicura or tentorial notch in relation to the cerebral arteries and oculomotor nerve. (**C**) Herniation of the cingulate gyrus under the falx cerebri [1], central or transtentorial herniation [2], herniation of the temporal lobe into the tentorial notch [3], and infratentorial herniation of the cerebellar tonsils [4]. (Courtesy of Carole Hilmer, C.M.I.)

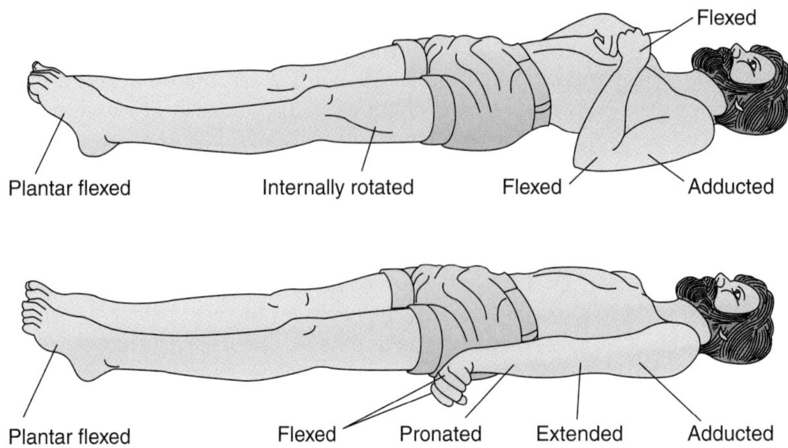

Figure 38–4
Abnormal rigidity. (**Top**) Decorticate rigidity. In decorticate rigidity, the upper arms are held tightly to the sides, with elbows, wrists, and fingers flexed. The legs are extended and internally rotated. The feet are plantar flexed. This posture implies a destructive lesion of the corticospinal tracts within or very near the cerebral hemispheres. When rigidity is unilateral, this is the posture of chronic spastic hemiplegia. (**Bottom**) Decerebrate rigidity. In decerebrate rigidity, the jaws are clenched and the neck extended. The arms are adducted and stiffly extended at the elbows, with forearms pronated, wrists and fingers flexed. The legs are stiffly extended at the knees, with the feet plantar flexed. Decerebration is caused by a lesion in the diencephalon, midbrain, or pons, although severe metabolic disorders, such as hypoxia or hypoglycemia, may also produce it.

tion of the eyes and with no motor response or only leg flexion on painful stimulation.

Infratentorial Herniation. Infratentorial herniation results from increased pressure in the infratentorial compartment. It often progress rapidly and can cause death, because it is likely to involve the lower brain stem centers that control vital cardiopulmonary functions. Herniation may occur superiorly (upward) through the tentorial incisura or interiorly (downward) through the foramen magnum.

Upward displacement of brain tissue can cause blockage of the aqueduct of Sylvius and lead to hydrocephalus and coma. Downward displacement of the midbrain through the tentorial notch or the cerebellar tonsils through the foramen magnum can interfere with medullary functioning and cause cardiac or respiratory arrest. In cases of preexisting ICP, herniation may occur when pressure is released from below, such as in a lumbar puncture. If the CSF pathway is blocked and fluid cannot leave the ventricles, the volume expands, and fluid is displaced downward through the tentorial notch. The expanding volume causes all function at a given level to cease as destruction progresses in a rostral to caudal direction. The result of this displacement is brain stem ischemia and hemorrhage extending from the diencephalon to the pons. If the lesion expands rapidly, displacement and obstruction occur quickly, leading to irreversible infarction and hemorrhage.

Cerebral Edema

Cerebral edema, or brain swelling, is an increase in tissue volume secondary to abnormal fluid accumulation. There are three types of brain edema: interstitial, vasogenic, and cytotoxic.[12] Interstitial edema is associated with an increase in sodium and water content of the periventricular white matter. Vasogenic edema results from an increase in the extracellular fluid that surrounds brain cells. Cytotoxic edema involves the actual swelling of brain cells themselves. Brain edema may or may not increase ICP. The impact of brain edema depends on the brain's compensatory mechanisms and the extent of the swelling.

Interstitial Edema. Interstitial edema involves movement of the CSF across the ventricular wall so there is water and sodium in the periventricular white matter. It is most commonly seen in noncommunicating hydrocephalus.

Vasogenic Edema. Vasogenic edema occurs with conditions such as tumors, prolonged ischemia, hemorrhage, brain injury, and infectious processes (*e.g.*, meningitis) that impair function of the blood-brain barrier and allow transfer of water and protein into the interstitial space. When brain injury occurs, the blood-brain barrier is disrupted and increased permeability occurs. There is almost free diffusion across the capillary membranes. Vasogenic edema occurs primarily in the white matter of the brain, possibly because the white matter is more compliant than the gray matter and offers less resistance to fluid accumulation. Vasogenic edema can displace a cerebral hemisphere and can be responsible for various types of herniation. The functional manifestations of vasogenic edema include focal neurologic deficits, disturbances in consciousness, and severe intracranial hypertension.

Cytotoxic Edema. Cytotoxic edema involves an increase in fluid within the intracellular space, chiefly the gray matter, although the white matter may be involved. Cytotoxic edema can result from hypoosmotic states such as water intoxication or severe ischemia that impairs the function of the sodium-potassium membrane pump. This causes rapid accumulation of sodium within the cell, followed by water moving along the osmotic gradient. Major changes in cerebral function, such as stupor and coma, occur with cytotoxic edema. The edema associated with ischemia may be severe enough to produce cerebral infarction with necrosis of brain tissue.

Abnormal conditions such as hypoxia, acidosis, and brain trauma may also result in cytotoxic edema, causing neuronal cell damage and possible death. If normal blood flow in the brain falls to abnormally low levels, cellular hypoxia results in reduced energy (ATP) production and depletion of energy stores. A low-energy state reduces the function of the membrane ion pumps. Low blood flow also results in the inadequate removal of anaerobic metabolic end products such as lactic acid, producing extracellular acidosis. The altered osmotic conditions result in water entry and cell swelling. Depending on the nature of the insult, cellular edema can occur in the vascular endothelium or smooth muscle cells, astrocytes, the myelin-forming processes of oligodendrocytes, or neurons. If blood flow is reduced to low levels for extended periods or to extremely low levels for a few minutes, cellular edema can cause the cell membrane to rupture, allowing the escape of intracellular contents into the surrounding extracellular fluid. This leads to damage of neighboring cells.

Cytotoxic edema is a slowly progressive process. When neurons are involved in this cytopathic process, presynaptic and postsynaptic elements become hypopolarized. Presynaptic hypolarization opens voltage-gated calcium channels, producing increased levels of free intracellular calcium and the release of neurotransmitters. The gradual change in membrane potentials brings the presynaptic and postsynaptic neurons into the threshold range, resulting in electrical hyperactivity; this process continues until there is insufficient energy for recovery to the threshold potential, at which time the cells fall into electrical silence. This progression suggests possible mechanisms of seizure generation, loss of neuronal function, and eventual cell death.

Treatment. Although cerebral edema is viewed as a pathologic process, it does not necessarily disrupt brain function unless it increases the ICP. The localized edema surrounding a brain tumor often responds to corticosteroid therapy (*e.g.*, dexamethasone); but use of these drugs on generalized edema is controversial. The mechanism of action of the corticosteroid drugs in the treatment of cerebral edema is unknown, but in therapeutic doses, they seem to stabilize cell membranes and scavenge free radicals. Osmotic diuretics (*e.g.*, mannitol) may be useful in the acute phase of vasogenic and cytotoxic edema when hypoosmolarity is present.

Hydrocephalus

Enlargement of the CSF compartment occurs with hydrocephalus, which is defined as an abnormal increase in CSF volume within any part or all of the ventricular system. The two causes of hydrocephalus are decreased absorption or overproduction of CSF. There are two types of hydrocephalus: noncommunicating and communicating.

Noncommunicating or *obstructive hydrocephalus* occurs when obstruction within the ventricular system prevents the CSF from reaching the arachnoid villi. CSF flow can be obstructed by congenital malformations, from tumors encroaching on the ventricular system, and by inflammation or hemorrhage. The ependyma (*i.e.*, lining of ventricles and CSF-filled spaces) is particularly sensitive to viral infections, particularly during embryonic development; ependymitis is believed to be the cause of congenital aqueductal stenosis.[4]

Communicating hydrocephalus results from impaired reabsorption of CSF from the arachnoid villi into the venous system. Decreased absorption can result from a block in the CSF pathway to the arachnoid villi or a failure of the villi to transfer the CSF to the venous system. It can occur if too few villi are formed, if postinfective (meningitis) scarring occludes them, or if the villi become obstructed with fragments of blood or infectious debris. Adenomas of the choroid plexus can cause an overproduction of CSF. This form of hydrocephalus is much less common than that resulting from decreased absorption of CSF.

Similar pathologic patterns occur with noncommunicating and communicating types of hydrocephalus. The cerebral hemispheres become enlarged, and the ventricular system is dilated beyond the point of obstruction. The gyri on the surface of the brain become less prominent and the white matter is reduced in volume. The presence and extent of the ICP is determined by fluid accumulation and the type of hydrocephalus, the age at onset, and the rapidity and extent of pressure rise. Acute hydrocephalus is usually manifested by increased ICP. Slowly developing hydrocephalus is less likely to produce an increase in ICP, but it may produce deficits such as progressive dementia and gait changes. Computed tomography (CT) scans are used to diagnose all types of hydrocephalus. The usual treatment is a shunting procedure, which provides an alternative route for return of CSF to the circulation.

When hydrocephalus develops in utero or before the cranial sutures have fused in infancy, the ventricles expand beyond the point of obstruction, the cranial sutures separate, the head expands, and there is bulging of the fontanels (Fig. 38–5). Because the skull is able to expand, signs of increased ICP are usually absent and intelligence is usually spared. Seizures are common, and in severe cases, optic nerve atrophy leads to blindness. Weakness and uncoordinated movement are common. Surgical placement of a shunt allows for diversion of excess CSF fluid, preventing extreme enlargement of the head. Before surgical shunting procedures were available, the weight and size of the enlarged head made ambulation difficult.

In contrast to hydrocephalus that develops in utero or during infancy, head enlargement does not occur in adults, and increases in ICP depend on whether the condition developed rapidly or slowly. Acute-onset hydrocephalus in adults is usually marked by symptoms of increased ICP, including headache and vomiting, followed by papilledema. If the obstruction is not relieved, mental deterioration eventually occurs. The pressure of CSF is not always elevated, and the syndrome of low-pressure hydrocephalus may go undetected. Treatment includes surgical shunting for noncommunicating hydrocephalus. In communicating hydrocephalus, attempts to clear the arachnoid villi of exudate may be made, and if this is unsuccessful, surgical shunting may be required.

Manifestations of Brain Injury

Brain injury is manifested by alterations in sensory and motor function and by changes in the level of consciousness. Focal injury commonly causes alterations in sensory function (Chapter 40) or motor function (Chapter 39); more global injury tends to result in altered levels of consciousness. Severe injury that seriously compromises brain function may result in brain death.

Consciousness

Consciousness is the state of awareness of self and the environment and of being able to become oriented to new stimuli.[14] The state of consciousness involves arousal and wakefulness and content or cognition, which includes the sum of cognitive functions. Arousal and wakefulness rely on an intact ascending RAS in the brain stem to act as the alerting or awakening element of consciousness. The content and cognitive aspects of consciousness are determined by a functioning cerebral cortex.

Reticular Formation. The reticular formation is a diffuse, primitive system of interlacing nerve cells and fibers that receive input from multiple sensory pathways (Fig. 38-6). Anatomically, the reticular formation constitutes the central core of the brain stem, extending from the medulla through the pons to the midbrain, which is continuous caudally with the spinal cord and rostrally with the subthalamus, the hypothalamus, and the thalamus.[16,17] A unique characteristic of neurons in the reticular formation is their widespread system of collaterals, which make extensive synaptic contacts and travel long distances in the CNS. Along with this widespread distribution of converging contacts, there is a loss of specificity, because many afferent signals contribute to the efferent output of reticular formation neurons.[17]

Ascending fibers of the reticular formation, known as the *ascending reticular activating system* (ARAS), relay activating information to all parts of the cerebral cortex. The flow of information in the ARAS activates the hypothalamic and limbic structures that regulate emotional and behavioral responses such as those that occur in response to pain, and they exert facilitory effects on cortical neurons. Other examples of ARAS activity include the alerting responses to loud noises or a splash of water on the face. Without cortical activation, a person is less able to detect specific stimuli, and the level of consciousness is reduced. The pathways for the ARAS travel through the midbrain, and lesions of the midbrain can

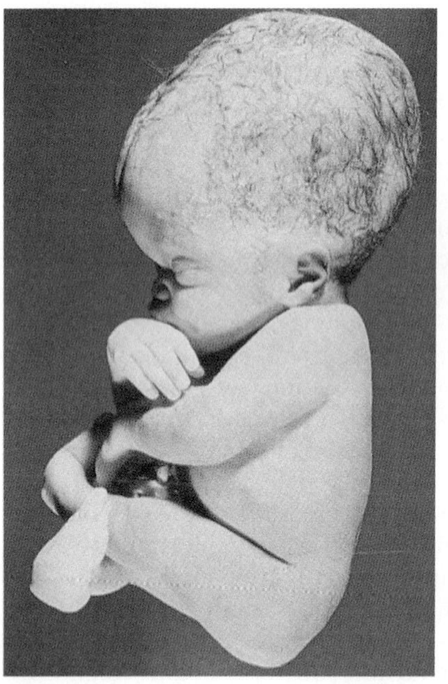

A

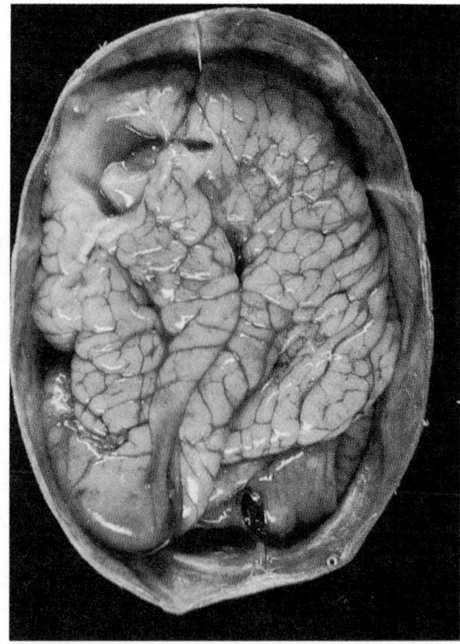

B

Figure 38–5
Congenital hydrocephalus. (**A**) Hydrocephalus occurring before the fusion of the cranial sutures causes pronounced enlargement of the head. (**B**) Removal of the calvarium demonstrates an atrophic and collapsed cerebral cortex.

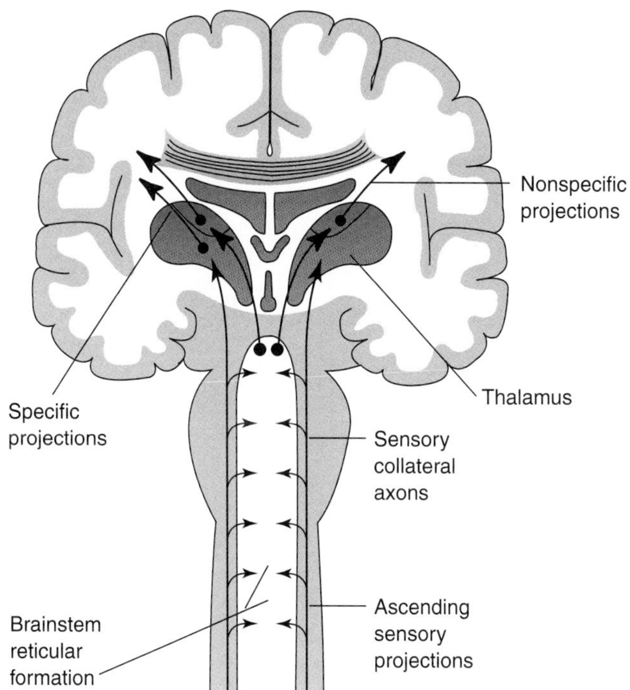

Figure 38–6
The brain stem reticular formation and reticular activating system. Ascending sensory tracts send axon collateral fibers to the reticular formation. These give rise to fibers synapsing in the nonspecific nuclei of the thalamus. From there the nonspecific thalamic projections influence widespread areas of the cerebral cortex and limbic system. (Rhoades R.A., & Tanner G.A. [1996]. *Medical physiology.* Boston: Little, Brown)

interrupt ARAS activity leading to altered levels of consciousness and coma.

Fibers from the RAS also project to the hypothalamus, to the autonomic nervous system, and to motor systems. The hypothalamus plays a predominant role in maintaining homeostasis through integration of somatic, visceral, and endocrine functions. Inputs from the reticular formation, vestibulospinal projections, and other motor systems are integrated to provide a continuously adapting background of muscle tone and posture to facilitate voluntary motor actions. Reticular formation neurons that function in regulation of cardiovascular, respiratory, and other visceral functions are intermingled with those that function in the maintenance of other reticular formation functions. Cardiovascular neurons are located primarily in the medulla and those that influence respiratory rhythms are located in the medulla and pons.

Levels of Consciousness. Level of consciousness reflects an orientation to person, place, and time. A fully conscious person is totally aware of her or his surroundings.[18] Levels of consciousness exist on a continuum that includes consciousness, confusion, delirium, obtundation, stupor, and coma.[19] Stupor and coma are signs of advanced brain failure. As with failure of other body systems, a wide spectrum of conditions can injure the brain and cause progressive deterioration of consciousness and coma. Table 38–2 describes the various states of consciousness.

Deterioration of brain function from supratentorial lesions tends to follow a rostral to caudal progression, which is observed as the brain initially compensates for the injury and subsequently decompensates with the loss of autoregulation and cerebral perfusion. Subtentorial (brain stem) lesions may lead to an early, sometimes abrupt disturbance in consciousness without any orderly rostrocaudal progression of neurologic signs.

The cerebral hemispheres are most susceptible to damage, and the most frequent sign of brain dysfunction is altered level of consciousness and change in behavior. As brain structures in the diencephalon, midbrain, pons, and medulla are affected, additional motor and pupillary signs become evident. Hemodynamic and respiratory instability are the last signs to occur, because their regulatory centers are located low in the medulla.

Disruptions affecting the diencephalon, midbrain, pons, and medulla usually cause a predictable pattern of change in the level of consciousness. The highest level of consciousness is seen in an alert person who is oriented to person, place, and time and is totally aware of the surroundings. The first symptoms of diminution in level of consciousness are decreased concentration, agitation,

TABLE 38-2

Descending Levels of Consciousness and Their Characteristics

Level of Consciousness	Characteristics
Confusion	Disturbance of consciousness characterized by impaired ability to think clearly and with customary repetition, and to perceive, respond to, and remember current stimuli; also disorientation
Delirium	State of disturbed consciousness with motor restlessness, transient hallucinations, disorientation, and sometimes delusions
Obtundation	Disorder of decreased alertness with associated psychomotor retardation
Stupor	A state in which the person is not unconscious but exhibits little or no spontaneous activity
Coma	A state of being unarousable and unresponsive to external stimuli or internal needs; often determined by the Glasgow Coma Scale

(Data from Bates D. [1993]. The management of medical coma. *Journal of Neurology, Neurosurgery, and Psychiatry* 56, 590)

dullness, and lethargy. With further deterioration, the person becomes obtunded and may respond only to vigorous shaking. Early respiratory changes include yawning and sighing, with progression to Cheyne-Stokes breathing. These signs are indicative of bilateral hemisphere damage with a danger of tentorial herniation. Although the pupils may respond briskly to light, the full range of eye movements is seen only when the head is passively rotated from side to side (*i.e.*, oculocephalic reflex or "doll's-head eye" maneuver) or when the caloric test (*i.e.*, instillation of hot or cold water into the ear canal) is done to elicit nystagmus. In the doll's-head eye test, the eyes move in the direction of rotation rather than rolling in the opposite direction, as occurs normally (see Chapter 41). There is some combative movement and purposeful movement in response to pain. As coma progresses, the bulboreticular facilitory area becomes more active as fewer inhibitory signals descend from the basal ganglia and cerebral cortex. This results in decorticate posturing (see Fig. 38–4).

With progression continuing in a rostral to caudal direction, the midbrain becomes involved. Respirations change from Cheyne-Stokes breathing to neurogenic hyperventilation in which the frequency of ventilation may exceed 40 breaths per minute because of uninhibited stimulation of the inspiratory and expiratory centers. The pupils become fixed in midposition and no longer respond to stimuli. Muscle excitability increases, producing a condition called *decerebrate posturing* (see Fig. 38-4), in which the arms are rigid and extended with the palms of the hands turned away from the body.

As coma advances to involve the pons, the pupils remain in midposition and fixed, and the decerebrate posturing continues. Breathing becomes apneustic, with sighs evident in midinspiration and with prolonged inspiration and expiration because of excessive stimulation of the respiratory center.

With medullary involvement, the pupils remain fixed in midposition. Respiration become ataxic (*i.e.*, totally uncoordinated and irregular). Apnea may occur because of the loss of responsiveness to carbon dioxide stimulation. Complete ventilatory assistance should be considered for any person with atactic breathing. Because the medulla has bulboreticular neurons but not facilitory neurons, the hyperexcitability that gave rise to decorticate and decerebrate posturing disappears, giving way to flaccidity.

In progressive brain deterioration, the person's neurologic capabilities appear to deteriorate in stepwise fashion. Similarly, as neurologic function returns, there appears to be stepwise progress to higher levels of consciousness. An assessment tool called the *Glasgow Coma Scale* is often used to describe levels of coma. This scale uses three aspects of neurologic function—eye opening, verbal response, and motor response—to arrive at a numeric score that represents the level of coma (Table 38–3).[19,20] It has been suggested that, although the Glasgow Coma Scale is effective in measuring coma outcome, it is not a reliable measure for monitoring changes in levels of consciousness, particularly in the middle range of scores.[21]

TABLE 38-3

The Glasgow Coma Scale

Test	Score*
Eye Opening (E)	
Spontaneous	4
To call	3
To pain	2
None	1
Motor Response (M)	
Obeys commands	6
Localizes pain	5
Normal flexion (withdrawal)	4
Abnormal flexion (decorticate)	3
Extension (decerebrate)	2
None (flaccid)	1
Verbal Response (V)	
Oriented	5
Confused conversation	4
Inappropriate words	3
Incomprehensible sounds	2
None	1

*GSC Score =E + M + V. Best possible score = 15; worse possible score = 3.

Brain Death

Brain death is defined as the irreversible loss of function of the brain, including the brain stem.[22,23] With advances in scientific knowledge and technology that have provided the means for artificially maintaining ventilatory and circulatory function, the definition of death has had to be reexamined. In 1968, criteria for irreversible coma were published by a Harvard Medical School Ad Hoc Committee.[24] Advances in treatment, including the development of effective artificial cardiopulmonary support for brain-injured persons, have created a need for reevaluation of the determination of death. The definitive criteria for brain death that are followed in the United States were proposed in 1981 by the President's Commission for the Study of Ethical Problems in Medicine and Biomedical and Behavioral Research.[25] According to these criteria, a diagnosis of death requires cessation of all brain functions, including those of the brain stem, and irreversibility.[26]

In 1995, the Quality of Standards Subcommittee of the American Academy of Neurology published the clinical parameters for determining brain death and procedures for testing persons older than 18 years of age.[23] According to these parameters "brain death is the absence of clinical brain function when the proximate cause is known and demonstrably irreversible."[23]

Clinical examination must disclose at least the absence of responsiveness, brain stem reflexes, and respiratory effort. Brain death is a clinical diagnosis, and a repeat evaluation at least 6 hours later is recommended.[23] Longer periods of observation of absent brain activity are required in cases of drug overdose (*e.g.*, barbiturates, other CNS depressants), drug toxicity (*e.g.*, neuromuscular blocking drugs, aminoglycoside antibiotics), neuromuscular diseases such as myasthenia gravis, hypothermia, and shock. Medical circumstances may require use of confirmatory tests. In the United States, electroencephalographic (EEG) testing is used to establish brain death. EEG testing should reveal no electrical activity during at least 30 minutes of recording that adheres to the minimal technical criteria for EEG recording in suspected brain death as adopted by the American Electroencephalographic Society, including 16-channel EEG instruments. Other confirmatory tests include conventional angiography (*i.e.*, no intracerebral filling at the level of the carotid bifurcation or circle of Willis), transcranial Doppler ultrasonography, technetium-99m hexamethylpropylene-amineoxime brain scan (*i.e.*, no uptake of isotope in brain parenchyma), and somatosensory evoked potentials.

Medical documentation should include cause and irreversibility of the condition, absence of brain stem reflexes and motor responses to pain, absence of respiration with PCO_2 of 60 mm Hg or more, and the justification for use of confirmatory tests and their results.[23] Brain stem reflexes that are assessed include the pupillary reaction to light, corneal reflexes, the gag or swallowing reflex, and the oculovestibular reflex. Adequate testing for apnea is important. An acceptable method is ventilation with pure oxygen or an oxygen and carbon dioxide mixture for 10 minutes before withdrawal from the ventilator, followed by passive flow of oxygen. This method allows blood levels of carbon dioxide to rise without hazardously lowering the oxygen content of the blood. If respiratory reflexes are intact, the hypercarbia that develops should stimulate ventilatory effort within 30 seconds when the carbon dioxide tension (PCO_2) is greater than 60 mm Hg. A 10-minute period of apnea is usually sufficient to attain this level of PCO_2. Spontaneous breathing efforts indicate that the brain stem is functioning.

Irreversibility implies that brain death cannot be reversed. Some conditions such as drug and metabolic intoxication can cause cessation of brain functions that are completely reversible, even when they produce clinical cessation of brain functions and EEG silence. This needs to be excluded before declaring that a person is brain dead. The brains of infants and small children have increased resistance to damage and may recover substantial function after exhibiting unresponsiveness. Particular caution needs to be used when applying neurologic criteria to determine death in children younger than 5 years.[25]

Persistent Vegetative State

Advances in the care of brain-injured persons during the past several decades has resulted in survival of many persons who would previously have died. Unfortunately, some of these persons remain in what is often called the *persistent vegetative state*. The vegetative state is characterized by loss of all cognitive functions and the unawareness of self and surroundings. Reflex and vegetative functions remain.[22,27] Persons in the vegetative state must be fed and require full nursing care.

The criteria for diagnosis of vegetative state include the absence of awareness of self and environment and an inability to interact with others; the absence of sustained or reproducible voluntary behavioral responses; lack of language comprehension; sufficiently preserved hypothalamic and brain stem function to maintain life; bowel and bladder incontinence; and variably preserved cranial nerve (*e.g.*, pupillary, oculocephalic, gag) and spinal cord reflexes.[28] The diagnosis of persistent vegetative state requires that the condition has continued for at least 1 month.

In summary, many of the agents that cause brain damage do so through common pathways, including hypoxia or ischemia, accumulation of excitatory neurotransmitters, increased ICP, and cerebral edema. Deprivation of oxygen (*i.e.*, hypoxia) or blood flow (*i.e.*, ischemia) can have deleterious effects on the brain structures. Ischemia can be focal, as in stroke, or global. Global ischemia occurs when blood flow is inadequate to meet the metabolic needs of the brain, as in cardiac arrest. In many neurologic disorders, neuron injury may be caused at least in part by overstimulation of receptors for specific amino acids such as glutamate and aspartate that act as excitatory neurotransmitters. Many of the actions of the excitatory neurotransmitters are coupled with glutamate NMDA receptor–operated ion channels that control the calcium entry into neurons. Increased intracellular calcium leads to activation of intracellular enzymes that cause protein breakdown, free radical formation, lipid peroxidation, fragmentation of DNA, and nuclear breakdown. Neurons of the cerebral cortex and hippocampus have large numbers of special glutamate NMDA receptors and are particularly vulnerable to injury through this mechanism.

The contents of the cranial cavity, which are enclosed in the rigid confines of the skull, consist of brain tissue, blood, and CSF. The collective volumes of these three intracranial components determine ICP. A variation in volume of any of these components can cause the ICP to rise, affecting cerebral function. Compensatory mechanisms protect the brain from small variations in the volume. Large variations, however, exceed the compensatory mechanisms and may lead to hypoxia, brain herniation, and death. Disorders of cerebral volumes and pressure include increases in brain tissue (*i.e.*, neoplasms), increased extracellular fluid and edema, and increased CSF (*i.e.*, hydrocephalus). Brain herniation is the displacement of brain tissue under the tough dural folds of the falx cerebri or past the incisura or notch of the tentorium cerebelli. Brain herniation is commonly divided into two broad categories, supratentorial and infratentorial, based on location of the herniation.

Brain edema represents an increase in tissue volume from abnormal fluid accumulation. There are three types of brain edema: vasogenic, which results from an increase in extracellular fluid; cytotoxic, which involves the actual swelling of brain cells; and interstitial, which involves an increase in fluid of the periventricular white matter.

Consciousness is a state of awareness of self and environment. It exists on a normal continuum of wakefulness and sleep and a pathologic continuum of wakefulness and coma. Consciousness depends on the normal functioning of the reticular activating system. Coma usually follows a rostral to caudal progression with characteristic changes in levels of consciousness, pupillary response, muscle tone, and respiratory activity occurring as the diencephalon through the medulla are affected.

Brain death is defined as the irreversible loss of function of the brain, including that of the brain stem. Clinical examination must disclose at least the absence of responsiveness, brain stem reflexes, and respiratory effort. Brain death is a clinical diagnosis, and a repeat evaluation at least 6 hours later is recommended. Confirmatory tests include EEG testing, conventional angiography, transcranial Doppler ultrasonography, technetium-99m hexamethylpropyleneamineoxime brain scan, and somatosensory evoked potentials. The vegetative state is characterized by loss of all cognitive functions and the unawareness of self and surroundings. Reflex and vegetative functions remain.

Cerebrovascular Disease

After you have completed this section of the chapter, you should be able to meet the following objectives:

- List the major vessels in the cerebral circulation and state the contribution of the internal carotid arteries, the vertebral arteries, and the circle of Willis to the cerebral circulation
- Explain autoregulation of cerebral blood flow
- Explain the substitution of "brain attack" for stroke in terms of making a case for early diagnosis and treatment
- Compare the pathology of ischemic and hemorrhagic stroke
- Explain the significance of transient ischemic attacks, the ischemic penumbra, and watershed zones of infarction and how these conditions relate to ischemic stroke
- List the manifestations of stroke and the major vessel involved
- Cite the most common cause of subarachnoid hemorrhage and state the complications associated with subarachnoid hemorrhage
- Describe the alterations in cerebral vasculature that occur with arteriovenous malformations
- Describe the progression of motor deficits that occurs as a result of stroke
- Characterize problems of speech and language that can result from stroke
- Cite the characteristics of the denial or hemiattention syndrome

Cerebrovascular disease encompasses a number of disorders involving vessels in the cerebral circulation. These disorders include stroke and transient ischemic attacks (TIAs), aneurysmal subarachnoid hemorrhage, and arteriovenous malformations.

Cerebral Circulation

Anatomy and Physiology

The blood flow to the brain is supplied by the two internal carotid arteries anteriorly and the vertebral arteries posteriorly (Fig. 38–7). The internal carotid artery, a terminal branch of the common carotid artery, branches into several arteries: ophthalmic, posterior communicating, anterior cerebral, and middle cerebral (Fig. 38–8). Most of the arterial blood within the internal carotid arteries is distributed by way of the anterior and middle cerebral arteries. The anterior cerebral arteries supply the medial surface of the cerebrum and the anterior half of the thalamus, the corpus striatum, part of the corpus callosum, and the internal capsule. The posterior cerebral arteries supply the remaining occipital and inferior regions of the temporal lobes.

The middle cerebral artery passes laterally, supplying the insula, and then emerges on the lateral cortical surface, supplying the inferior frontal gyrus, the motor and premotor frontal cortex concerned with delicate face and hand control. It is the major vascular source for the primary and association somesthetic cortex for the face and hand and the superior temporal gyrus with the primary and association auditory cortex. It also is a major source of supply for the genu and the posterior limb of the internal capsule and much of the basal ganglia. The middle cerebral artery is functionally a continuation of the internal carotid; emboli of the internal carotid most frequently become lodged in branches of the middle cerebral artery. The consequences of ischemia of these areas may be most devastating, resulting in damage to the fine manipulative skills of the face or upper limb and to receptive and expressive communication functions. Occlusion of the local branches of the artery result in more restricted deficits.

The distal branches of the internal carotid and vertebral arteries communicate at the base of the brain through the *circle of Willis;* this anastomosis of arteries can provide continued circulation if blood flow through one of the main vessels is disrupted. Without collateral input, cessation of blood flow in cerebral arteries may result in neural damage, because metabolic needs of electrically active cells of the brain can no longer be met.

The two vertebral arteries arise from the subclavian artery and enter the foramina in the transverse spinal processes at the level of the sixth cervical vertebra and continue upward through the foramina of the upper six vertebrae; they wind behind the atlas and enter the skull through the foramen magnum and

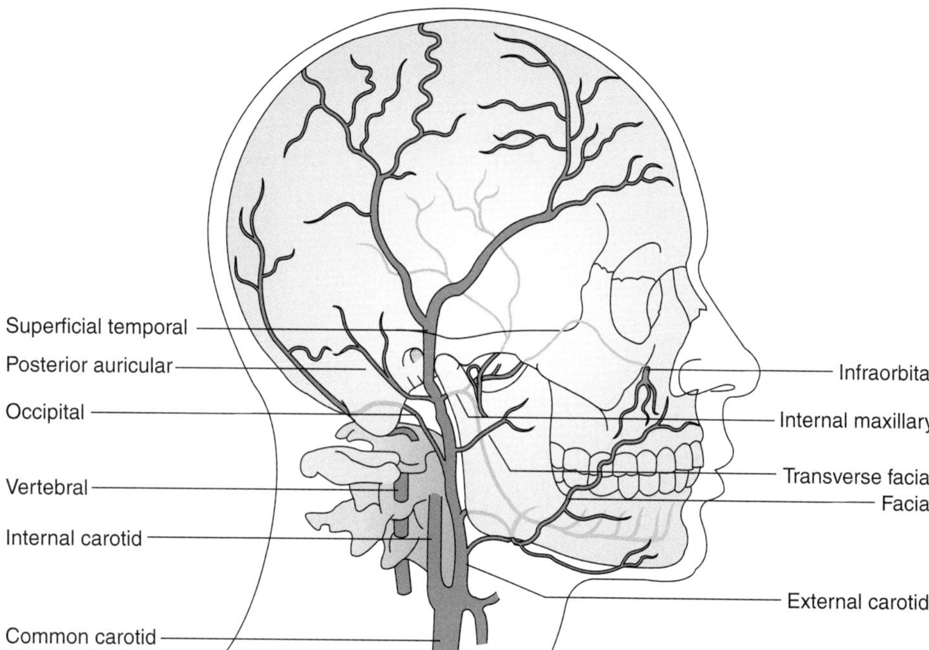

Figure 38–7
Branches of the right external carotid artery. The internal carotid artery ascends to the base of the brain. The right vertebral artery is also shown as it ascends through the transverse foramina of the cervical vertebrae.

unite to form the basilar artery. Branches of the basilar and vertebral arteries supply the medulla, pons, cerebellum, midbrain, and caudal part of the diencephalon. Because the vertebral arteries supply the basic life support reflexes that are located in these areas of the brain, interruption of blood flow in the carotid arteries may result in severe coma, although not necessarily death.

The cerebral blood is drained by two sets of veins that empty into the dural venous sinuses: the deep (great) cerebral venous system and the superficial venous system. The deep system is well protected, in contrast to the superficial cerebral veins that travel through the pia mater on the surface of the cerebral cortex. These vessels connect directly to the sagittal sinuses within the falx cerebri by way of bridging veins. They travel through the CSF-filled subarachnoid space and penetrate the arachnoid and then the dura to reach the dural venous sinuses. This system of sinuses returns blood to the heart primarily by way of the internal jugular veins. Alternate routes for venous flow also exist; for example, venous blood may exit through the emissary veins that pass through the skull and through veins that traverse various foramina to empty into extracranial veins.

The intracranial venous system has no valves. The direction of flow depends on gravity or the relative pres-

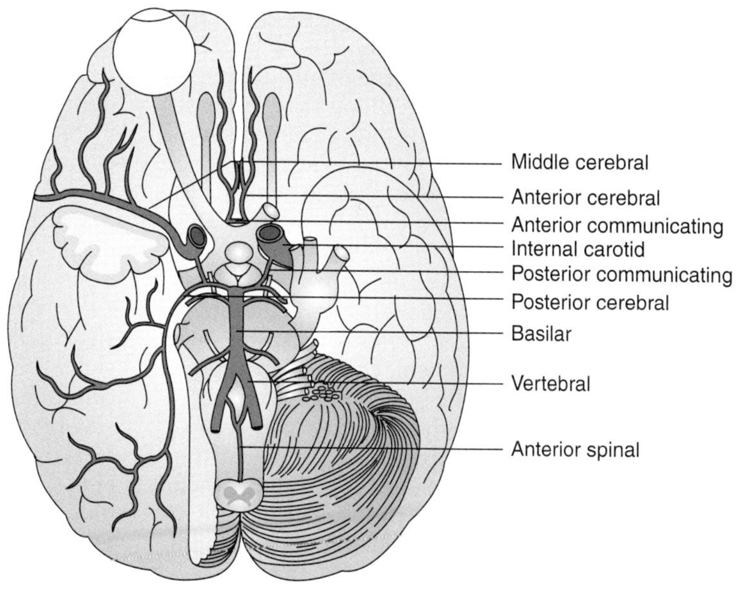

Figure 38–8
The circle of Willis as seen at the base of a brain removed from the skull.

sure in the venous sinuses compared with that of the extracranial veins. Increases in intrathoracic pressure, as can occur with coughing or performance of a Valsalva maneuver, produce a rise in central venous pressure that is reflected back into the internal jugular veins and to the dural sinuses. This briefly raises the ICP.

Regulation of Cerebral Blood Flow

The blood flow to the brain is maintained at about 750 ml/minute or one sixth of the resting cardiac output. The regulation of blood flow to the brain is largely controlled by autoregulatory or local mechanisms that respond to the metabolic needs of the brain. Cerebral autoregulation has been classically defined as the ability of the brain to maintain constant cerebral blood flow despite changes in systemic arterial pressure. The autoregulation of cerebral blood flow is efficient within a mean arterial blood pressure range of about 60 to 140 mm Hg. If blood pressure falls below 60 mm Hg, cerebral blood flow becomes severely compromised, and if it rises above the upper limit of autoregulation, blood flow increases rapidly and overstretches the cerebral vessels. In persons with hypertension, this autoregulatory range shifts to a higher level. Autoregulation has been further defined as the ability of the cerebral cortex to adjust cerebral blood flow to satisfy its metabolic needs. Although total cerebral blood flow remains relatively stable throughout marked changes in cardiac output and arterial blood pressure, regional blood flow may change markedly in response to local changes in metabolism.

At least three metabolic factors affect cerebral blood flow: carbon dioxide concentration, hydrogen ion concentration, and oxygen concentration. Increased carbon dioxide concentration and increased hydrogen ion concentration increase cerebral blood flow; decreased oxygen concentration also increases blood flow. Carbon dioxide, by way of the hydrogen ion concentration, provides a potent stimulus for control of cerebral blood flow—a doubling of the carbon dioxide pressure (PCO_2) in the blood results in a doubling of cerebral blood flow. Other substances that alter the pH of the brain produce similar changes in cerebral blood flow. Because increased hydrogen ion concentration greatly depresses neural activity, it is fortunate that blood flow increases to wash the hydrogen ions and other acidic materials away from the brain tissue.[13] Profound extracellular acidosis also induces vasomotor paralysis; in which case, cerebral blood flow may depend entirely on the system arterial blood pressure.

The deep cerebral blood vessels appear to be completely controlled by autoregulation. However, the superficial and major cerebral blood vessels are innervated by the sympathetic nervous system. Under normal physiologic conditions, the sympathetic nervous system exerts little effect on superficial cerebral blood flow, because local regulatory mechanisms are so powerful that they compensate almost entirely for the effects of sympathetic stimulation. However, when local mechanisms fail, sympathetic control of cerebral blood pressure becomes important. For example, when the arterial pressure rises to very high levels during strenuous exercise or in other conditions, the sympathetic nervous system constricts the large and intermediate-sized superficial blood vessels as a means of protecting the smaller, more easily damaged vessels. Sympathetic reflexes are believed to cause vasospasm in the intermediate and large arteries in some types of brain damage, such as that caused by rupture of a cerebral aneurysm.

Stroke (Brain Attack)

Stroke is a vascular disorder that injures brain tissue. Stroke remains one of the leading causes of mortality and morbidity in the United States. Each year, 500,000 Americans are afflicted with stroke, and approximately 150,000 of these persons survive, many with at least some degree of neurologic impairment.[29] The term *brain attack* has become a popular substitute for stroke, with the intent of equating stroke with a heart attack in terms of the timetable associated with the development of neurologic deficits and the need for prompt emergency treatment.[30]

There are two main types of strokes: ischemic stroke and hemorrhagic stroke. Ischemic strokes are caused by an interruption of blood flow in a cerebral vessel and are the most common type of stroke, accounting for 70% to 80% of all strokes. Hemorrhagic strokes, which account for the smallest percentage, are caused by bleeding into brain tissue. This type of stroke is usually caused by hypertension, aneurysms, arteriovenous malformations, head injury, or blood dyscrasias and has a much higher fatality rate than ischemic strokes.

Risk Factors

Among the risk factors for stroke are age, sex, race, hypertension, high cholesterol levels, cigarette smoking, and diabetes mellitus.[29,31] Other risk factors include prior stroke, sickle cell disease, polycythemia, moderate to increased levels of alcohol use, cocaine and illicit drug use, obesity, sedentary lifestyle, previous ischemic episodes, and heart disease. The incidence of stroke increases with age, with a 1% per year increased risk for persons 65 to 74 years of age; the incidence of stroke is about 19% greater in men than women; and African Americans have a 60% greater risk of death and disability from stroke than whites.[29] Heart disease, particularly atrial fibrillation and other conditions that predispose to clot formation on the wall of the heart or valve leaflets predisposes to cardioembolic stroke. Polycythemia and sickle cell disease (during sickle cell crisis) predispose to clot formation in the cerebral vessels. Alcohol can contribute to stroke in several ways: induction of cardiac arrhythmias and defects in ventricular wall motion that lead to cerebral embolism, induction of hypertension, enhancement of blood coagulation disorders, and reduction of cerebral blood flow.[32]

Another cause of stroke is cocaine. Cardiovascular events begin soon after cocaine use and include increased blood pressure, heart rate, body temperature, and metabolic rate. Cocaine also causes vasospasm and enhances the platelet response. The reported ages of persons with cocaine stroke have ranged from newborn (*i.e.,* from maternal cocaine used) to 48 years of age. Ischemic and hemorrhagic strokes have been reported. The mechanisms of cocaine-related stroke vary. In some persons, stroke was associated with hemorrhage from aneurysms or arteriovenous malformations; and in other cases, it was associated with thrombotic lesions.[33,34]

Elimination or control of risk factors for cerebrovascular disease (*e.g.,* use of tobacco, control of blood lipids, reduction of hypertension) offers the best opportunity to prevent cerebral ischemia from cerebral atherosclerosis. Early detection and treatment offer significant advantages over waiting until a serious event has occurred.

Ischemic Stroke

Ischemic strokes are caused by cerebrovascular obstruction by thrombosis or emboli. Various methods have been used to classify ischemic cerebroocclusive vascular disease. One classification system, largely defined by results from brain imaging and vascular studies, identifies six major subtypes: atherosclerotic large cerebral artery disease; nonatherosclerotic large cerebral artery disease; penetrating artery disease (*i.e.,* lacunar strokes); cardioembolic strokes; stroke of undetermined origin; and miscellaneous causes of stroke (*i.e.,* sickle cell or migraine related). The reported incidence for large cerebral artery stroke is about 16%; for cardioembolic stroke, 19%; for penetrating artery stroke, 27%, and for stroke of undetermined origin, 40%.[35]

Like the occurrence of angina that precedes a heart attack, stroke may be preceded by TIAs. Similar to a heart attack, the area of brain damage involved in a stroke is often characterized by a penumbra of ischemic but potentially viable tissue surrounding the infarcted area.

Transient Ischemic Attacks. TIAs are characterized by focal ischemic cerebral neurologic deficits that last for less than 24 hours (usually less than 1 to 2 hours). The causes of TIAs are multiple and include atherosclerotic disease of cerebral vessels and emboli. TIAs are important because they may provide warning of impending stroke. Diagnosis may permit surgical or medical intervention and prevent extensive damage. Overall, the risk of a stroke varies. There is about a 4% to 8% risk of stroke within 1 month of a TIA, a 12% to 13% risk during the first year, and 24% to 29% risk over 5 years.[36]

The signs and symptoms of TIA depend on the cerebral vessel that is involved. There is often numbness and mild weakness on one side of the body. The forearm, hand, and angle of the mouth are commonly affected areas with middle cerebral involvement. There may be transient visual disturbances such as graying-out, blurring, or fogging of vision if the posterior cerebral artery is affected. When the carotid artery is involved, the symptoms reflect ischemia to the same-side eye or brain. Brief global aphasia may occur in transient ischemia of the left hemisphere. Vertebasilar TIAs often include vestibulocerebellar symptoms (*i.e.,* ataxia, dizziness, and vertigo), abnormalities of eye movements (*i.e.,* diplopia), and unilateral or bilateral motor or sensory symptoms. Isolated vertigo or dizziness is seldom caused by TIAs, as is confusion, amnesia, or seizures.[36]

Prompt evaluation of a TIA is important in preventing stroke. Hospitalization may be needed to expedite evaluation and lessen the danger of stroke. Diagnostic methods include CT scans, cerebrovascular arterial imaging, and cardiac imaging. Assessment for risk factors such as cigarette smoking, hypertension, and heart disease is also important.

Treatment of a TIA depends on the type and the location of the ischemia-producing lesion and is usually designed to prevent stroke. Pharmacologic treatment includes the use of aspirin and other antiplatelet drugs (*i.e.,* dipyridamole or ticlopidine). Anticoagulants, such as warfarin, are often used for prevention of cardioembolic strokes. In some cases, ischemia may be caused by focal loss of cerebral autoregulation, and blood flow to the area of the brain involved can be particularly sensitive to any rise or fall in blood pressure. Dehydration and relative hypotension should be avoided. In persons with hypertension, the judicious use of medication to lower blood pressure may be indicated. However, care must be taken to avoid rapid decreases in blood pressure or hypotensive episodes.

Surgical treatment using endarterectomy (*i.e.,* arterial surgery to remove atherosclerotic plaque) may be used for persons with obstructive carotid lesions. Indications for carotid endoartectomy include one or more TIAs or a mild stroke within the past 6 months and carotid stenosis of more than 70%, although the procedure may be beneficial in persons with less obstruction or in persons with progressive stroke.[37] A procedure called an *extracranial-intracranial bypass operation* involves redirecting of blood flow from an artery in the scalp through the cranium and into the arteries that supply the brain. This procedure remains controversial but may be beneficial for vertebrobasilar disease.[36]

Thrombic Stroke. Thrombi are the most common cause of ischemic strokes, usually occurring in atherosclerotic blood vessels. In the cerebral circulation, atherosclerotic plaques are found most commonly at arterial bifurcations. Common sites of plaque formation include larger vessels of the brain, notably the origin of the internal carotid origin, vertebral arteries, and junctions of the basilar and vertebral arteries. Atherosclerotic thrombosis usually occurs gradually over several days, during which CNS symptoms may plateau and then deteriorate further. In most cases, only one region supplied by a single cerebral artery is affected. Usually, thrombotic strokes are seen in older persons and are frequently accompanied by evidence of arteriosclerotic heart disease. The thrombotic stroke is not associated with activity and may occur in a person at rest. Consciousness may or may not be lost, and improvement may be rapid.

Lacunar Infarcts. Lacunar infarcts are small (1.5 to 2.0 cm) to very small (3 to 4 mm) infarcts located in the deeper noncortical parts of the brain or in the brain stem. They are found in the territory of single deep penetrating arteries supplying the internal capsule, basal ganglia, or brain stem. They result from occlusion of the smaller branches of large cerebral arteries, commonly the middle cerebral and posterior cerebral arteries and less commonly the anterior cerebral, vertebral, or basilar arteries. In the process of healing, lacunar infarcts leave behind small cavities, or lacuna.

Six basic causes of lacunar infarcts have been proposed: embolism, hypertension, small-vessel occlusive disease, hematologic abnormalities, small intracerebral hemorrhages, and vasospasm. Because of their size and location, lacunar infarcts do not usually cause profound deficits such as aphasia or apractic agnosia of the minor hemisphere. Instead, they often produce syndromes such as pure motor hemiplegia, pure sensory hemiplegia, and dysarthria with the clumsy hand syndrome.

Cardiogenic Embolic Stroke. An embolic stroke is caused by a moving blood clot. It usually affects the smaller cerebral vessels, often at bifurcations. The most frequent site of embolic strokes is the middle cerebral artery distribution, probably because it offers the path of least resistance. Although most cerebral emboli originate in a thrombus in the left heart, they may also originate in an atherosclerotic plaque in the carotid arteries. The embolus travels quickly to the brain and becomes lodged in a small artery through which it cannot pass. Embolic stroke usually has a sudden onset with immediate maximum deficit.

Various cardiac conditions predispose to formation of emboli that produce embolic stroke, including rheumatic heart disease, atrial fibrillation, recent myocardial infarction, ventricular aneurysm, and bacterial endocarditis. Advances in the diagnosis and treatment of heart disease can be expected to alter favorably the incidence of embolic stroke.

Ischemic Penumbra in Evolving Stroke. During the evolution of a stroke, there is usually a central core of dead or dying cells, surrounded by an ischemic area of minimally surviving cells called the *penumbra* (*i.e.*, halo). Brain cells of the penumbra receive marginal blood flow, and their metabolic activities are altered; although the area undergoes an "electrical failure," the structural integrity of brain cells has been maintained.[38] Whether the cells of a penumbra continue to survive depends on the successful return of adequate circulation, the volume of toxic products released by the neighboring dying cells, the degree of cerebral edema, and alterations in local blood flow. If the toxic products of dead tissue result in cell death in the penumbra, the core of dead or dying tissue enlarges, and the volume of surrounding ischemic tissue increases.

Hemorrhagic Stroke

The most frequently fatal stroke is a hemorrhage into the brain substance. With rupture of a blood vessel, hemorrhage into the brain tissue occurs, resulting in edema, compression of the brain contents, or spasm of the adjacent blood vessels. The most common predisposing factor is hypertension. Other causes of hemorrhage are aneurysm, trauma, erosion of the vessels by tumors, arteriovenous malformations, coagulopathies, vasculitis, and drugs. A cerebral hemorrhage occurs suddenly, usually when the person is active. Vomiting commonly occurs at the onset, and headache sometimes occurs. Focal symptoms depend on which vessel is involved. In the most common situation, hemorrhage into the internal capsule results in contralateral hemiplegia, with initial flaccidity progressing to spasticity. The hemorrhage and resultant edema exert great pressure on the brain substance, and the clinical course progresses rapidly to coma and frequently to death.

Acute Manifestations of Stroke

The specific manifestations of stroke are determined by the cerebral artery that is affected, by the area of brain tissue that is supplied by that vessel, and the adequacy of the collateral circulation (Table 38–4). The manifestations may include loss of consciousness, cognitive and motor disorders, specific motor or sensory impairment, aphasia, and hemineglect syndrome. Certain classic syndromes are expected, but in the clinical situation, they frequently overlap one another.

Diagnosis

Accurate diagnosis of stroke is based on a complete history and thorough physical and neurologic examination. A careful history, including documenting TIAs, their rapidity of onset, and focal symptoms and those of any coexisting diseases, can help to determine the type of stroke that is involved.

CT scans and magnetic resonance imaging (MRI) have become important tools in diagnosing stroke and in differentiating cerebral hemorrhage from intracranial lesions that mimic stroke. Arteriography can demonstrate the site of the vascular abnormality and afford visualization of most intracranial vascular areas. Magnetic resonance angiography (MRA) has improved the reliability of noninvasive techniques and is extremely useful for screening and follow-up; it is not useful in guiding invasive therapeutic decisions.

Two other types of imaging, positron emission tomography (PET) and single-photon emission computed tomography (SPECT), are used to study the distribution of blood flow and metabolic activity of the brain. PET and SPECT involve the detection of photons emitted from radionuclides. The radionuclides used for these two tests are very short-lived (minutes), and they emit radioactive energy as they move through the circulation. The use of PET makes it possible to define the location

TABLE 38-4 Signs and Symptoms of Stroke by Involved Cerebral Artery

Cerebral Artery	Brain Area Involved	Signs and Symptoms*
Anterior cerebral	Infarction of the medial aspect of one frontal lobe if lesion is distal to communicating artery; bilateral frontal infarction if flow in other anterior cerebral artery is inadequate	Paralysis of contralateral foot or leg; impaired gait; paresis of contralateral arm; contralateral sensory loss over toes, foot, and leg; problems making decisions or performing acts voluntarily; lack of spontaneity, easily distracted; slowness of thought; aphasia depends on the hemisphere involved; urinary incontinence; cognitive and affective disorders
Middle cerebral	Massive infarction of most of lateral hemisphere and deeper structures of the frontal, parietal, and temporal lobes; internal capsule; basal ganglia	Contralateral hemiplegia (face and arm); contralateral sensory impairment; aphasia; homonymous hemianopsia; altered consciousness (confusion to coma); inability to turn eyes toward paralyzed side; denial of paralyzed side or limb (hemiattention); possible acalculia, alexia, finger agnosia and left-right confusion; vasomotor paresis and instability
Posterior cerebral	Occipital lobe; anterior and medial portion of temporal lobe	Homonymous hemianopia and other visual defects such as color blindness, loss of central vision, and visual hallucinations; memory deficits, perseveration (repeated performance of same verbal or motor response)
	Thalamus involvement	Loss of all sensory modalities; spontaneous pain; intentional tremor; mild hemiparesis; aphasia
	Cerebral peduncle involvement	Oculomotor nerve palsy with contralateral hemiplegia
Basilar and vertebral	Cerebellum and brain stem	Visual disturbance such as diplopia, dystaxia, vertigo, dysphagia, dysphonia

*Dependent on hemisphere involved and adequacy of collaterals.

and size of strokes by providing data on cerebral blood flow and volume and brain cell metabolism. SPECT provides metabolic and flow-related information, without the cost and complexity of regular PET scanning.

The introduction of several Doppler ultrasound techniques has facilitated the noninvasive evaluation of cerebral circulation. Emitted signals may be uninterrupted (*i.e.,* continuous-wave Doppler) or intermittent (*i.e.,* pulsed-wave Doppler). The flow characteristics of all vessels within the depth of field is demonstrated on the continous-wave Doppler; the pulsed-wave Doppler samples flow at any depth. Use of these methods has increased because of low cost, ease of application, safety features, continuous technical advances, improved imaging quality, and increased reliability.[38]

Treatment of Stroke

The treatment of acute ischemic stroke has changed markedly in the past decade, with an emphasis on salvaging of brain tissue and minimizing long-term disability. The realization that there is a "window of opportunity" during which ischemic but viable brain tissue can be salvaged has led to the use of thrombolytic agents in the early treatment of ischemic stroke. Although the emergent treatment of hemorrhagic stroke has been less dramatic, continued efforts to reduce disability have been promising.

Investigation into the use of thrombolytic therapy for stroke was first attempted in the late 1960s and early 1970s, but it was quickly abandoned because of hemorrhagic complications.[30] Because these studies were done before CT scans, exclusion of persons with hemorrhagic stroke was difficult. Patients were also treated many hours after stroke, at which time cerebral blood vessels may have been weakened by the death of brain tissue. The interest in thrombolytic therapy has increased because of the development of new thrombolytic agents and the availability of diagnostic scanning methods that are able to differentiate between ischemic and hemorrhagic stroke.

Thrombolytic agents include streptokinase, urokinase, recombinant tissue-type plasminogen activator (rtPA), *p*-anisolylated lys-plasminogen-streptokinase activator complex, and prourokinase (see Chapter 7). A subcommittee of the Stroke Council of the American Heart Association has developed guidelines for the use of thrombolytic therapy for acute stroke.[39–41] These guidelines recommend that persons with suspected stroke be admitted to a skilled care facility (*i.e.*, intensive care unit or acute stroke unit) that permits close observation, frequent neurologic assessment, and cardiovascular monitoring. The diagnosis of ischemic stroke can be established through the use of CT scanning before administration of thrombolytic therapy, and therapy can be instituted within 3 hours of onset of symptoms. A number of conditions, including use of oral anticoagulant medications, a history of gastrointestinal bleeding, recent myocardial infarction, previous stroke or head injury within 3 months, surgery within the past 14 days, and a blood pressure greater than 200/120 mm Hg are considered contraindications for thrombolytic therapy.[40]

The successful treatment of stroke depends on education of the public, paramedics, and health care professionals in emergency care facilities about the need for early diagnosis and treatment. As with heart attack, the message should be "do not wait to decide if the symptoms subside but seek immediate treatment." Effective medical and surgical procedures may preserve brain function and prevent disability.

Longer-term treatment is aimed at preventing complications and promoting the fullest possible recovery of function. During the acute phase, proper positioning and range of motion exercises are essential. Early rehabilitation efforts include all members of the rehabilitation team—physician, nurse, speech therapist, physical therapist, and occupational therapist, and the family.

Aneurysmal Subarachnoid Hemorrhage

Aneurysmal subarachnoid hemorrhage represents bleeding into the subarachnoid space, caused by a ruptured cerebral aneurysm. Bleeding into the subarachnoid space can extend well beyond the site of origin, flooding the basal cistern, ventricles, and spinal subarachnoid space.[42] Aneurysmal subarachnoid hemorrhages occur most frequently between ages 30 and 60 and are seldom seen in children. The mortality and morbidity of aneurysmal subarachnoid hemorrhage is high. About 50% of persons who suffer from the hemorrhage die within 3 months, and one half of the survivors have serious disability.[43]

An aneurysm is a bulge at the site of a localized weakness in the muscular wall of an arterial vessel. Most aneurysms are small saccular aneurysms called *berry aneurysms* (Fig. 38–9). They usually occur in the anterior circulation and are found at bifurcations and other junctions of vessels such as those in the circle of Willis. There is angiographic evidence that these aneurysms enlarge with time and produce weakening of the vessel wall, often to the extent that only a thin fibrous vessel wall remains. The probability of rupture increases with the size of the aneurysm; aneurysms larger than 10 mm in diameter have a 50% chance of bleeding per year.[1] Rupture often occurs with acute increases in ICP. Large aneurysms may also cause chronic headache, neurologic deficits, or both. For example, giant aneurysms of the internal carotid artery may cause persistent headache and ptosis because of pressure on the third cranial nerve. Small aneurysms may go unnoticed; intact aneurysms are frequently found at autopsy as an incidental finding.[1]

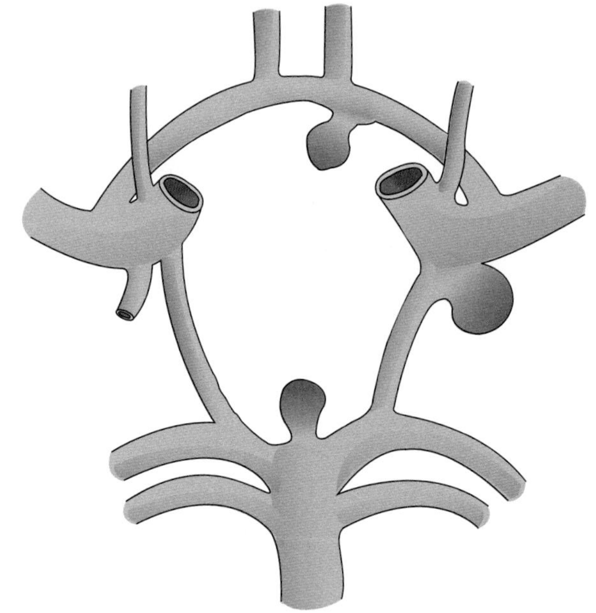

Figure 38–9
Locations of berry aneurysms.

The cause of aneurysms is unknown. Intracranial aneurysms are thought to arise from a congenital defect in the media of the involved vessels, particularly at bifurcations. Considerable evidence supports the role of genetic factors in the pathogenesis of intracranial aneurysms. Family history seems to be a significant risk factor. Persons with two or more family members who have had aneurysms and are between 35 and 65 years are particularly at risk.[1] Persons with heritable connective tissue disorders such as autosomal dominant polycystic kidney disease, Ehlers-Danlos syndrome, neurofibromatosis type I, and Marfan's syndrome are at particular risk.[44] There is also evidence linking age and environmental factors with the development of aneurysms. For example, intracranial aneurysms are rare in children, and although the mean age for subarachnoid hemorrhage is around 50 years, the incidence of hemorrhage increases with age. Of the various environmental factors that may predispose to aneurysmal subarachnoid hemorrhage, cigarette smoking and hypertension appear to constitute the greatest risk.

Subarachnoid hemorrhage is a dreaded complication of cerebral aneurysm. When it occurs, the onset of subarachnoid aneurysmal rupture is often heralded by a sudden and severe headache, described as "the worst headache of my life." Other manifestations of subarachnoid hemorrhage include signs of meningeal irritation such as nuchal rigidity (*i.e.*, neck stiffness) and photophobia; cranial nerve deficits, especially cranial nerve II, and sometimes IV and IV (*i.e.*, diplopia and blurred vision); stroke syndrome; loss of consciousness; increased ICP; and pituitary dysfunction. Bleeding into the subarachnoid space causes meningeal irritation with the resulting signs of headache and nuchal rigidity. The optic nerves are ensheathed in meninges, and meningeal irritation causes photophobia. Occasionally, nausea and vomiting accompany the presenting symptoms. In other cases, there may be no focal neurologic findings. If bleeding is severe, headache may be accompanied by collapse and loss of consciousness. Depending on the course of the bleeding, the headache subsides slowly over a matter of days. Hypertension is a frequent finding and may be the result of the hemorrhage. Cardiac dysrhythmias and noncardiac edema result from massive release of catecholamines triggered by the subarachnoid hemorrhage.

About 50% of persons who suffer from subarachnoid hemorrhage have a history of atypical headaches occurring days to weeks before the onset of hemorrhage, suggesting the presence of a small leak.[44,45] These headaches are characterized by sudden onset and are often accompanied by nausea, vomiting, and dizziness. Persons with these symptoms may be mistakenly diagnosed as having tension or migraine headaches.

The complications of aneurysmal rupture include rebleeding, vasospasm with cerebral ischemia, hydrocephalus, hypothalamic dysfunction, and seizure activity. Rebleeding and vasospasm are the most severe and most difficult to treat. Rebleeding, which has its highest incidence on the first day after the initial rupture, results in further and usually catastrophic neurologic deficits.

Vasospasm is a dreaded complication of aneurysmal rupture. The condition is difficult to treat and is associated with a high incidence of morbidity and mortality. Although the description of aneurysm-associated vasospasm is relatively uniform, its proposed mechanisms are controversial. Usually, the condition develops 3 to 10 days (peak, 7 days) after aneurysm rupture and involves a focal narrowing of the cerebral artery or arteries that can be visualized on arteriography. The neurologic status gradually deteriorates as blood supply to the brain in the region of the spasm is decreased; this can usually be differentiated from the rapid deterioration seen in rebleeding. Vasospasm is treated by attempting to maintain adequate cerebral perfusion pressure by use of vasopressor drugs or administration of large amounts of intravenous fluids to increase intravascular volume and produce hemodilution to maintain vessel patency and prevent sludging of blood flow. There is risk of rebleeding from this therapy. Early surgery may provide some protection from vasospasm. Endovascular techniques, including balloon dilatation, have been developed to mechanically treat narrowed arterial segments. Nimodipine, a drug that blocks calcium channels and that selectively acts on cerebral blood vessels, may be used to prevent or treat vasospasm.

Another complication of aneurysm rupture is the development of hydrocephalus. It is thought to result from obstruction of the arachnoid villi of the CSF system, which are responsible for reabsorption of CSF. The lysis of blood in the subarachnoid space causes the protein content of the CSF to increase, thereby preventing diffusion of CSF across the arachnoid villi, plugging the system and resulting in hydrocephalus. Occasionally, hydrocephalus can be medically managed by the use of osmotic diuretics, but if neurologic deterioration is significant, surgical placement of a shunt is indicated. Hydrocephalus is diagnosed by serial CT scans, by the increasing size of the ventricles, and by the clinical signs of increased ICP.

The diagnosis of subarachnoid hemorrhage and intracranial aneurysms is made by clinical presentation, CT scan, lumbar puncture, and angiography. The CT scan is the most commonly used diagnostic method for subarachnoid hemorrhage. Lumbar puncture may be used to detect blood in the CSF, but the procedure has a risk of rebleeding and brain herniation. Among the methods used for diagnosis of intracranial aneurysms are conventional angiography, MRA, and helical (spiral) CT angiography. Conventional angiography is the definitive diagnostic tool for detecting the aneurysm. This procedure involves the injection of a contrast into an artery so the vessel can be visualized using fluoroscopic or x-ray methods; defects such as vasospasm can be detected. MRA does not require the intravascular administration of contrast. Helical CT angiography has the advantage of screening for new aneurysms in persons with ferromagnetic clips for whom the use of MRI is contraindicated.

The course of treatment after aneurysm rupture depends on the extent of neurologic deficit. Persons with less severe deficits, with or without headache and no neurologic deficits, may undergo cerebral arteriography and early surgery, usually within 24 to 72 hours. A procedure involving craniotomy and *clipping* is often used. In this procedure, a specially designed silver clip is inserted and tightened around the neck of the aneurysm. This procedure offers protection from rebleeding and may permit removal of the hematoma. Some persons with subarachnoid hemorrhage are managed medically for 10 days or more in an attempt to improve their clinical status before surgery. The use of endovascular techniques such as balloon embolization and platinum coil electrothrombosis is evolving.

Arteriovenous Malformations

Arteriovenous malformations are congenital abnormal communications between arterial and venous channels that result from failure in development of the capillary network in the embryonic brain (Fig. 38–10). As the child's brain grows, the malformation acquires additional arterial contributions that enlarge to form a tangled collection of thin-walled vessels that shunt blood directly from the arterial to the venous circulation. About 90% of arteriovenous malformations are in the cerebral hemispheres; one half are superficial, and the others are buried more deeply.

The hemodynamic effects of arteriovenous malformations are twofold.[46] First, blood is shunted from the high-pressure arterial system to the low-pressure venous system without the buffering advantage of the

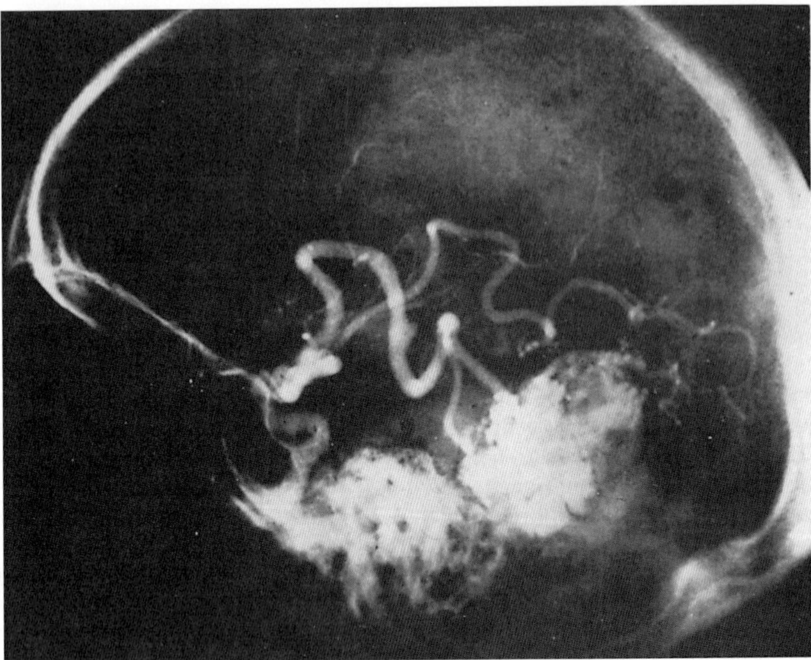

Figure 38–10
Arteriovenous malformations consist of dilated arterial and venous channels with the apex pointing toward the lateral ventricle.

capillary network. The draining venous channels are exposed to high levels of pressure, predisposing them to rupture and hemorrhage. Second, impaired perfusion affects the cerebral tissue adjacent to the arteriovenous malformation. The elevated arterial and venous pressures and lack of a capillary circulation impair cerebral perfusion by producing a high-flow situation that diverts blood away from the surrounding tissue. Clinically, this is evidenced by slowly progressive neurologic deficits. The diversion of blood to the arteriovenous malformation has been referred to as a vascular *steal phenomenon.*

The major clinical manifestations of arteriovenous malformations are hemorrhage, seizures, headache, and progressive neurologic deficits. Arteriovenous malformations are the third most common cause of intracranial bleeding, after aneurysm and spontaneous intracerebral hemorrhage.[46] Bleeding from the malformations is most common between 10 and 30 years of age and is rare after age 60, with males being affected more often than females.[1] In about 65% of cases, bleeding occurs into brain tissue and in the subarachnoid space; in about 25% of cases, it is confined to the subarachnoid space; and in the remainder, it occurs only in brain tissue. Seizures occur as an initial symptom in 20% and 50% of cases. Headaches are often severe, and persons with the disorder may describe them as being throbbing and synchronous with their heart beat. Other less common symptoms include visual symptoms (*i.e.,* diplopia and hemianopia), hemiparesis, mental deterioration, and speech deficits. Definitive diagnosis is often obtained through cerebral angiography.

Treatment methods include surgical excision, embolization, proton beam therapy, and Nd:YAG laser therapy. Because of the nature of the malformation, each of these methods is accompanied by some risk of complications. If the arteriovenous malformation is accessible, surgical excision is usually the treatment of choice. Embolization, which is performed on large arteriovenous malformations, is accomplished by insertion of a catheter into the carotid or vertebral circulation to allow a substance such as Silastic spheres, Gelfoam, or metallic pellets to form emboli and gradually obliterate blood flow in the arteriovenous malformation. Proton beam therapy, a form of radiation therapy, may be recommended when the lesion is incompletely removed or when the lesion is considered inoperable. When the proton beam is directed into the arteriovenous malformation, it causes a thickening of its vascular elements. The ND:YAG laser, which is still considered experimental, permits photocoagulation of the arteriovenous malformations.

Long-Term Disabilities

Stroke and cerebrovascular disorders often involve long-term disabilities, including motor deficits, language and speech problems, and a condition called the hemineglect syndrome. Although there are many other disorders of motor, sensory, and perceptual function, they are considered beyond the scope of this text.

Motor Deficits

After a stroke affecting the corticospinal tract such as the motor cortex, posterior limb of the internal capsule, or medullary pyramids, there is profound weakness on the contralateral side. It is characterized by a decrease or absence of normal muscle tone, immediate loss of fine manipulative skills, and a tendency of the affected limbs to move as a whole. A slight corticospinal lesion may be indicated by clumsiness in carrying out fine movements of the fingers (*e.g.,* buttoning, sewing) rather than obvious weakness. There is a tendency toward foot drop, outward rotation of the leg, and dependent edema in the affected extremities. Putting the extremities through passive range of motion exercises helps to maintain the joint function and to prevent edema, shoulder subluxation (*i.e.,* incomplete dislocation), and muscle atrophy. The smooth sequential movement of the exercises may also help to reestablish motor patterns.

When the corticospinal tract has been affected, muscle tone gradually returns after a few weeks and then spasticity begins to replace the initial flaccidity within 6 to 8 weeks. Spasticity involves an increase in the tone of affected muscles and usually an element of weakness. Because of the distribution of muscle hypertonia with spasticity, the flexor muscles are usually more strongly affected in the upper extremities and the extensor muscles more strongly affected in the lower extremities. Various mechanisms, including disinhibition of segmental and suprasegmental reflexes and reorganization of segmental circuitry, appear to contribute to spasticity. Altered limb posture may be manifested by shoulder adduction, forearm pronation, finger flexion, and knee and hip extension. If no voluntary movement or movement on command appears within a few months, function will probably not return to that extremity. Passive range of motion exercises should be continued, and positioning should be directed toward keeping all the joints in functional positions.

Language and Speech Problems

Communication is a complex process by which ideas and feelings are exchanged; it is accomplished by means of various behavioral patterns, gestures, expressions, and symbols. Communication involves memory, reasoning, and emotions, as well as speech and language. Two key aspects of communication are language and speech. *Language* involves higher-order integrative functions of the forebrain. It is used to communicate thoughts and feeling through the use of symbolic formulations, such as words or numbers, and information is transmitted vocally or graphically. *Speech* involves the mechanical act of articulating language, the "motor act" of verbal expression.[47] Speech depends on the functional integrity of the peripheral musculature involved and its control by upper motoneurons and lower motoneurons.

Disorders of language and speech generally fall into three categories: disturbances of the central processing mechanisms of language, which result in aphasia; dysfunction of the larynx, pharynx, palate, tongue, lips, or mouth that results in dysarthria; and apraxia of speech, in which the person is unable to program a sequence of the volitional movements needed for speech despite the absence of motor deficits.[48] Some persons exhibit elements of all three components of speech and language disorders. Aphasia may be localized above the tentorium; dysphonia may be localized at other levels as well.

Dysarthria. Dysarthria is imperfect articulation of speech sounds or changes in voice pitch or quality. It is caused by disturbed motor control resulting from damage to the nervous system. A person with dysarthria may demonstrate an inability to articulate while still retaining language ability.

Aphasia. Aphasia is a general term that encompasses varying degrees of inability to comprehend, integrate, and express language. The most common cause is a vascular lesion of the middle cerebral artery of the dominant hemisphere (*i.e.,* the hemisphere responsible for mediation of language). The left hemisphere is dominant in about 95% of right-handed and 70% of left-handed persons. The cerebral hemispheres usually function similarly in controlling opposite sides of the body. However, some functions, such as body language, are controlled by the dominant hemisphere but require the simultaneous action of both hemispheres. Language dominance by one hemisphere does not occur before 1 to 2 years of age. Because the other hemisphere appears to take over, unilateral lesions occurring during childhood usually result in only transient language disorders.

Aphasia can be categorized as receptive or expressive. Most aphasias are partial, and a thorough speech evaluation is needed to determine the type and extent of language disorder and appropriate therapy.

Receptive aphasia represents a sensory agnosia or the inability to comprehend spoken words (*i.e.,* Wernicke's aphasia) and often written words. Two major forms of the disorder are auditory-receptive aphasia and visual-receptive aphasia. In *auditory-receptive aphasia,* auditory acuity remains intact, but the person is unable to understand the spoken word. In *visual-receptive aphasia,* understanding of written language is impaired (*i.e.,* dyslexia, alexia). *Alexia* may occur with visual object agnosia, such as difficulty in recognizing or naming objects (*i.e.,* anomia) or colors (*i.e.,* color anomia). Sometimes, the ability to read numbers is retained, although the person is unable to read letters or words. Lesions of the posterior temporal or lower parietal lobe (areas 22 or 39) are associated with receptive aphasia lesions.

One of the most common characteristics of aphasia is distorted spontaneous or conversational speech. This has been classified as fluent (*i.e.,* many words) or nonfluent (*i.e.,* few words). *Receptive aphasia* has been classified as fluent aphasia. The term *fluent* refers to the characteristics of the speech generated but not to its content or the ability of the person to comprehend what is being said. Fluent speech requires little or no effort, is articulate, and is of increased quantity. There are three categories of fluent aphasia: Wernicke's, anomic, and conductive aphasia. *Wernicke's aphasia* is characterized by an inability to comprehend the speech of others and of oneself. Wernicke's aphasia sometimes includes reading and writing. *Anomic aphasia* is speech that is nearly normal except for the difficulty the person has with selected words. *Conduction aphasia* is inappropriate word use despite good comprehension. Conduction aphasia (*i.e.,* disconnection syndrome) results from destruction of the fiber system under the insula that connects Wernicke's and Broca's areas.

Expressive or nonfluent aphasia (apraxia of speech) is characterized by an inability to translate thoughts or ideas into meaningful speech or writing. Speech production is limited and often poorly articulated. The person may be able, with difficulty, to utter two or three words, especially those with an emotional overlay. If Broca's area, or the precentral gyrus of the dominant frontal lobe, is affected, automatic speech appears to be intact, but neologisms (*i.e.*, invented words), paraphasic errors (*e.g.*, "weathery winter"), and cursing are common. The person seems to be aware of communication problems but is unable to correct them. This often leads to frustration, anger, and depression. Expressive aphasia is associated with lesions of Broca's area of the dominant frontal lobe (areas 44 and 45) and associated with abnormal programming of the motor function of language (*i.e.*, motor speech ataxia).

Denial or Hemiattention

Because of an inability to analyze and interpret incoming sensory information caused by the disruptive lesion of the brain and the internal production of abnormal signals, a high percentage of persons with stroke have a form of denial of illness and a denial of one half of the body and environment on that side of the body (*i.e.*, hemiattention). Such persons are unaware of the deficit. For example, a person with left hemiplegia may raise the right arm when asked, but when asked to raise the left arm, he or she may say, "I just did." Spatial orientation is often impaired, and patients have difficulty localizing stimuli, their own limbs, and objects in space. Affected persons may totally disregard stimuli coming from the involved side of the body, even though they can see and hear. The affected side of the body may go unattended and ungroomed (*i.e.*, hemineglect). The person may wash or shave only the unaffected side of the body. When asked to draw a picture of themselves, these persons often draw a person with only one arm and leg. The condition is more common in persons with strokes that affect the nondominant side of the brain, usually the right hemisphere, which is more involved with spatial orientation, body image, and inductive modes of reasoning.

In summary, a stroke, or "brain attack," is a sudden, severe deficit in neurologic function caused by a focal vascular occlusion. It is the third leading cause of death in the United States and a major cause of disability. Uncontrolled hypertension is a significant risk factor for the development of stroke. The most serious effect of global ischemia occurs in brain tissues supplied by the most distal branches of the cerebral arteries in territories called watershed zones. These territories receive less blood, with profound lowering of blood flow, such as in severe hypotension, predisposing to infarction of brain tissues. Stroke can result from hemorrhage, embolus, or thrombus. The effects of stroke depend on the location of the blood vessel that is involved and can include motor, sensory, and speech manifestations. Treatment is primarily symptomatic, involving the combined efforts of the health care professionals in the rehabilitation team, the patient, and the family.

A subarachnoid hemorrhage involves bleeding into the subarachnoid space. Most subarachnoid hemorrhages are the result of a ruptured cerebral aneurysm. Fifty percent of persons with subarachnoid hemorrhage do not survive the initial hemorrhage. Presenting symptoms include headache, nuchal rigidity, photophobia, and nausea. Complications include rebleeding, vasospasm, and hydrocephalus.

Arteriovenous malformations are congenital abnormal communications between arterial and venous channels that result from failure in development of the capillary network in the embryonic brain. The vessels in the arteriovenous malformations may enlarge to form a space-occupying lesion, become weak and predispose to bleeding, and divert blood away from other parts of the brain; they can cause brain hemorrhage, seizures, headache, and other neurologic deficits.

Trauma, Infections, and Neoplasms

After you have completed this section of the chapter, you should be able to meet the following objectives:

- Differentiate primary and secondary brain injuries due to head trauma
- Describe the mechanism of brain damage in coup-contrecoup injuries
- List the constellation of symptoms involved in the postconcussion syndrome
- Compare the manifestations of mild, moderate, and severe head injury
- Differentiate among the location, manifestations, and morbidity of epidural, subdural, and intracerebral hematoma
- List the sequence of events that occur with meningitis
- Describe the symptoms of encephalitis
- List the major categories of brain tumors and interpret the meaning of benign and malignant as related to brain tumors
- Describe the general manifestations of brain tumors
- List the methods used in diagnosis and treatment of brain tumors

Head Injury

The brain is enclosed within the protective confines of the rigid bony skull. Although the skull affords protection for the tissues of the CNS, it also provides the potential for development of ischemic and traumatic brain injuries. This is because it cannot expand to accommodate the increase in volume that occurs when there is swelling or bleeding within its confines. The bony structures themselves can cause injury to the nervous system. Fractures of the skull can compress sections of the nervous system, or they can splinter and cause penetrating wounds.

The term *head injury* is used to describe all structural damage to the head and has become synonymous with brain injury.[49] In the United States, head injury is the leading cause of death among persons younger than 24 years of age. The main causes of head injury are road accidents, falls, and assaults, and the most common cause of fatal head injuries is road accidents involving vehicles and pedestrians.[50]

Head injuries can involve both closed injuries and open wounds. Skull fractures can be divided into three groups: simple, depressed, and basilar. A *simple or linear* skull fracture is a break in the continuity of bone. A *comminuted* skull fracture refers to a splintered or multiple fracture line. When bone fragments are embedded into the brain tissue, the fracture is said to be *depressed.* A fracture of the bones that form the base of the skull is called a *basilar* skull fracture.

Radiologic examination usually is needed to confirm the presence and extent of a skull fracture. This evaluation is important because of the possible damage to the underlying tissues. The ethmoid cribriform plate, through which the olfactory fibers enter the skull, represents the most fragile portion of the neurocranium and is shattered in basal skull fractures. A frequent complication of basilar skull fractures is leakage of CSF from the nose (*i.e.,* rhinorrhea) or ear (*i.e.,* otorrhea); this occurs because of the proximity of the base of the skull to the nose and ear. This break in protection of the brain becomes a probable source of infection of the meninges or of brain substance. There may be lacerations to the vessels of the dura, with resultant intracranial bleeding. Damage to the cranial nerves (I, II, III, VII, VIII) may also result from basilar skull fractures if the fracture is in the vicinity of the foramina magnum from which the cranial nerves exit the skull.

Types of Brain Injuries

The effects of traumatic head injuries can be divided into two categories: primary or direct injuries, in which damage is caused by impact, and secondary injuries, in which damage results from the subsequent brain swelling, intracranial hematomas, infection, cerebral hypoxia, and ischemia.

Primary head injuries include concussion, contusion, and laceration. Even if there is no break in the skull, a blow to the head can cause severe and diffuse brain damage. Such closed injuries vary in severity and can be classified focal or diffuse. Focal injuries include contusion, laceration, and hemorrhage. Diffuse injuries include concussion, contusion, diffuse axonal injury (formerly known as shearing lesion), and hypoxic brain injury.

Ischemia is considered to be the most common cause of secondary brain injury. It can cause the hypoxia and hypotension that occur during the resuscitation process or the impairment of regulatory mechanisms by which cerebrovascular responses maintain an adequate blood flow and oxygen supply.[51,52] Insults that occur immediately after injury or in the course resuscitation efforts are important determinants of the outcome from severe brain injury. More than 25% of severe head injury patients suffer one or more secondary insults during the time between injury and resuscitation, indicating the need for improved airway management and circulatory status.[51] The significance of secondary injuries depends on the extent of damage caused by the primary injury. Certain secondary injuries have been discussed, such as increased ICP, cerebral edema, and brain herniation.

In mild head injury, there may be momentary loss of consciousness without demonstrable neurologic symptoms or residual damage, except for possible residual amnesia. Microscopic changes can usually be detected in the neurons and glia within hours of injury. *Concussion* is defined as a momentary interruption of brain function with or without loss of consciousness. Although recovery usually takes place within 24 hours, mild symptoms, such as headache, irritability, insomnia, and poor concentration and memory, may persist for months. This is known as the *postconcussion syndrome.* Because these complaints are vague and subjective, they are sometimes regarded as being of psychologic origin. An organic basis for the postconcussion syndrome is strongly suspected. Postconcussion syndrome can have a significant effect on activities of daily living and return to employment. Persons with postconcussion syndrome may need cognitive retraining or psychologic support.

Moderate head injury is characterized by a longer period of unconsciousness and may be associated with focal manifestations such as hemiparesis, aphasia, and cranial nerve palsy. In this type of injury, many small hemorrhages and some swelling of brain tissue occur. A *contusion* or bruising of brain tissue often can be visualized on CT scan, whereas a concussion cannot be visualized except microscopically. Contusions are often distributed along the rough, irregular inner surface of the brain and are more likely to occur in the frontal or temporal lobes, resulting in cognitive and motor deficits.

Severe head injury involves more extensive damage to brain structures and a deeper level of coma than moderate head injury. In severe head injury, primary damage to the brain is often instantaneous and irreversible, resulting from shearing and pressure forces that cause diffuse axonal injury, disruption of blood vessels, and tissue damage. It is often accompanied by neurologic deficits such as hemiplegia. Severe head injuries often occur with injury to other parts of the body such as the extremities, chest, and abdomen. Blood may extravasate into the brain; if the contusion is severe, the blood may accumulate as in intracranial hemorrhage. Similarly, when laceration of the brain directly under the area of injury occurs, especially if the skull is fractured, hemorrhage may be sufficiently extensive to form a hematoma.

Although the skull and CSF provide protection for the brain, they can also contribute to trauma. A form of brain injury that can cause concussion or contusion from bouncing of the brain in the closed confines of the rigid skull is called a *coup-contrecoup injury*. The brain is thrown against one side of the skull (coup) in one continuous motion, which causes damage immediately below the site of impact (Fig. 38–11). The brain then rebounds and strikes the opposite side of the skull (contrecoup), which causes injury in regions of the brain opposite the side of impact. This movement occurs because the brain floats freely in the CSF while the brain stem is stable. As the brain strikes the rough surface of the cranial vault, brain tissue, blood vessels, nerve tracts, and other structures are bruised and torn.

Hematomas

Hematomas result from vascular injury and bleeding. Depending on the anatomic position of the ruptured vessel, bleeding can occur within any of several compartments, including the epidural, subdural, and subarachnoid spaces or into the brain itself (intracerebral hematoma).

Epidural Hematoma. Epidural hematomas are usually caused by head injury in which the skull is fractured. An epidural (extradural) hematoma is one that develops between the inner table of the bones of the skull and the dura (Fig. 38–12). It usually results from a tear in an artery, most often the middle meningeal, which is located under the thin temporal bone. Because bleeding is arterial in origin, rapid compression of the brain occurs. Epidural hematoma is more common in a young person because the dura is not so firmly attached to the skull surface as it is in an older person; as a consequence, the dura can be easily stripped away from the inner surface of the skull, allowing the hematoma to form.

Typically, a person with an epidural hematoma presents with a history of head injury and a brief period of unconsciousness followed by a lucid period in which consciousness is regained, followed by rapid progression to unconsciousness. The lucid interval does not always occur, but when it does, it is of great diagnostic value. With rapidly developing unconsciousness, there are focal symptoms related to the area of the brain involved. These symptoms can include ipsilateral (same side) pupil dilatation and contralateral (opposite side) hemiparesis. If the hematoma is not removed, the condition progresses, with increased ICP, tentorial herniation, and death. Prognosis is excellent, however, if the hematoma is removed before loss of consciousness occurs.

Subdural Hematoma. A subdural hematoma develops in the area between the dura and the arachnoid (subdural space) and is usually the result of a tear in the small bridging veins that connect veins on the surface of the cortex to dural sinuses. The bridging veins pass from the pial vessels through the CSF-filled subarachnoid space, penetrate the arachnoid and the dura, and empty into the intradural sinuses. These veins are readily snapped in head injury when the brain moves suddenly in relation to the cranium (Fig. 38–13). Bleeding can occur between the dura and arachnoid (*i.e.,* subdural hematoma) or into the CSF-filled subarachnoid space

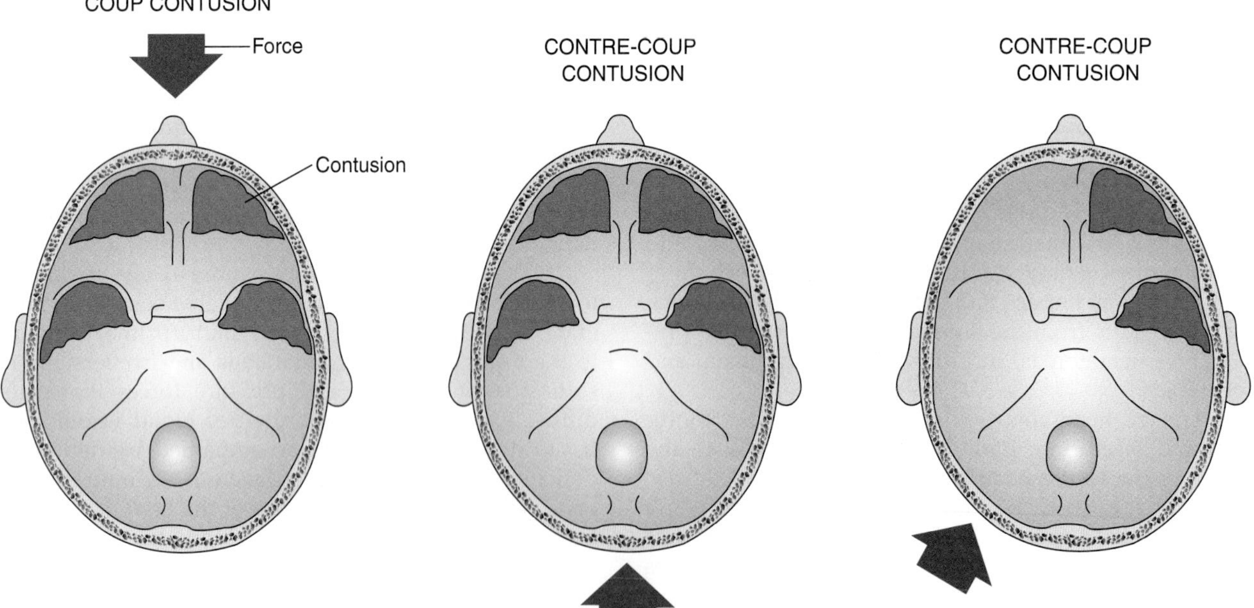

Figure 38–11
Mechanisms of cerebral contusion. The cerebral hemispheres float in the cerebrospinal fluid. Rapid deceleration or, less commonly, acceleration of the skull causes the cortex to impact forcefully into the anterior and middle fossa. The position of a contusion is determined by the direction of the force and the intracranial anatomy. (Courtesy of Dmitri Karetnikov, artist)

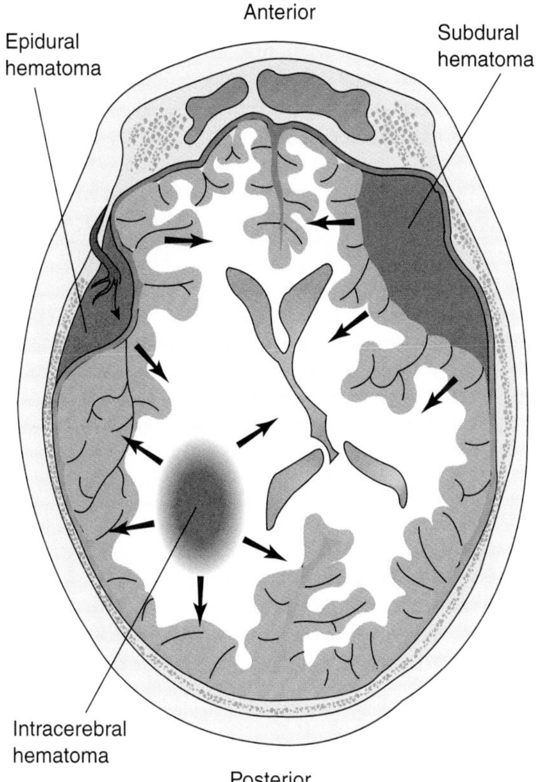

Figure 38–12
Location of epidural, subdural, and intracerebral hematomas.

(*i.e.*, subarachnoid hematoma). Subdural hematoma develops more slowly than an epidural hematoma because the tear is in the venous system, whereas epidural hematomas are arterial.

Subdural hematomas are classified as acute, subacute, or chronic. This classification system is based on the approximate time intervals before the appearance of symptoms. Symptoms of acute hematoma are seen within 24 hours of the injury, whereas subacute hematoma does not produce symptoms until 2 to 10 days after injury. Symptoms of chronic subdural hematoma may not arise until several weeks after the injury. These

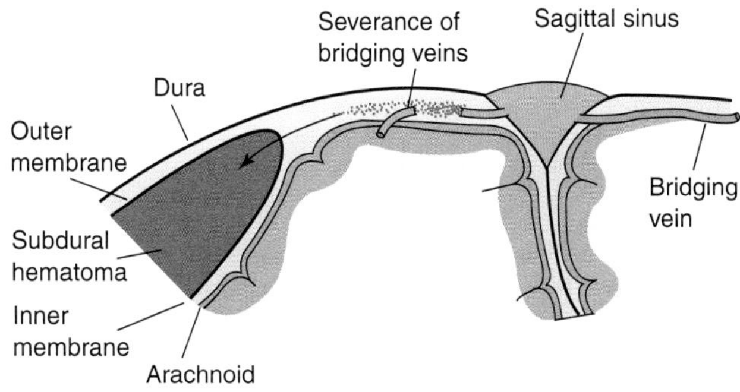

Figure 38–13
Mechanism of bleeding in subarachnoid hematoma. (Courtesy of Dmitri Karetnikov, artist)

classifications are based partially on pathologic considerations.

Acute subdural hematomas progress rapidly and have a high mortality rate because of the severe secondary injuries related to edema and increased ICP. The high mortality rate has been associated with uncontrolled ICP increase, loss of consciousness, decerebrate posturing, and delay in surgical removal of the hematoma.[36] The clinical picture is similar to that of epidural hematoma, except that there is usually no lucid interval. In subacute hematoma, there may be a period of improvement in the level of consciousness and neurologic symptoms, only to be followed by deterioration if the hematoma is not removed.

Symptoms of chronic subdural hematoma develop weeks after a head injury, so much later that the person may not remember having had a head injury. This is especially true of older persons with fragile vessels and whose brain has shrunk away from the dura. Seepage of blood into the subdural space may occur slowly. Because the blood in the subdural space is not absorbed, fibroblastic activity begins, and the hematoma becomes encapsulated. Within this encapsulated area, the blood cells are slowly lysed, and a fluid with a high osmotic pressure is formed. This creates an osmotic gradient, with fluid from the surrounding subarachnoid space being pulled into the area; the mass increases in size, exerting pressure on the cranial contents. In some instances, the clinical picture is less defined, with the most prominent symptom being a decreasing level of consciousness indicated by drowsiness, confusion, and apathy. The person may also have headache. Morbidity and mortality are highest with acute subdural hematoma compared with epidural and intracerebral hematoma.

Intracerebral Hematoma. Intracerebral hematoma can result from head injury. This type of bleeding occurs in the brain tissue itself. Blood often leaks into the CSF, causing the same problems as a bridging vein bleed, but the phenomenon is more rapid because of the arterial origin. The severe motion that the brain undergoes can cause bleeding within brain tissue, or a contusion can coalesce into a hematoma (see Fig. 38–12). Intracerebral hematoma occurs more frequently in older persons and alcoholics whose brain vessels are more friable. Intracerebral hematomas can occur in any lobe of the brain but are most common in the frontal or temporal lobes. There can be one hematoma or many.

The signs and symptoms produced by an intracerebral hematoma depend on its size and location within the brain. Signs of increased ICP can be manifested if the hematoma is large and encroaching on vital structures. A hematoma in the temporal lobe can be dangerous because of the potential for lateral herniation.

Treatment of an intracerebral hematoma can be medical or surgical. For a large hematoma with a rapidly deteriorating neurologic condition, surgery to evacuate the clot is generally indicated. Surgery may not be needed in someone who is neurologically stable despite neurologic deficits; in this case, the hematoma may resolve much like a contusion.

Infections

Infections of the CNS may be classified according to the structure involved: the meninges, meningitis; the brain parenchyma, encephalitis; the spinal cord, myelitis; and the brain and spinal cord, encephalomyelitis. They may also be classified by the type of invading organism: bacterial, viral, or other. In general, the pathogens enter the CNS through the bloodstream by crossing the blood-brain barrier or by direct invasion through skull fracture, a bullet hole, or rarely, contamination during surgery or lumbar puncture.

Meningitis

Meningitis is an infection of the pia mater, the arachnoid, and the CSF-filled subarachnoid space. Inflammation spreads rapidly because of CSF circulation around the brain and spinal cord. The inflammation usually is caused by an infection, but chemical meningitis can occur. There are two types of acute infectious meningitis: acute pyogenic meningitis (usually bacterial) and acute lymphocytic (usually viral) meningitis.[53] Factors responsible for the severity of meningitis include virulence factors of the pathogen, host factors, brain edema, and permanent neurologic sequelae.

Bacterial Meningitis. In the United States, the incidence of bacterial meningitis is approximately 3 to 10 cases per 100,000 persons, and two thirds of cases are children younger than 5 years of age. The most common pyogenic infectious agents are *Haemophilus influenzae, Neisseria meningitidis* (*i.e.,* the meningococcus), *Streptococcus pneumoniae,* and *Escherichia coli.* In children younger than 5 years, the most common agent of infection is *H. influenzae* serotype b; above that age, infection with *S. pneumoniae* is most common. The meningococcus can reside asymptomatically in the throat and nasopharynx, and this infection has the highest incidence among children and young adults. Epidemics occur in situations such as the military, where the recruits must reside in close contact. The very young and the very old are at highest risk for pneumococcal meningitis. Meningitis due to *E. coli* occurs most often in the neonate, especially if there is a neural tube defect. Risk factors associated with contracting meningitis include head trauma with basilar skull fractures, otitis media, sinusitis or mastoiditis, neurosurgery, dermal sinus tracts, systemic sepsis, or immunocompromise.

The most common symptoms of acute pyogenic meningitis are fever and chills; headache; back, abdominal, and extremity pains; and nausea and vomiting. A petechial rash is found in most persons with meningococcal meningitis. These petechiae vary from pinhead size to large ecchymoses or even areas of skin gangrene that sloughs if the person survives. Other types of meningitis may also produce a petechial rash. Persons infected with *H. influenzae* or *S. pneumoniae* may present with difficulty in arousal and seizures, whereas those with *N. meningitidis* infection may present with delirium or coma.[53] The development of brain edema, hydrocephalus, or increased cerebral blood flow can increase ICP.

Meningeal signs (*i.e.,* photophobia and nuchal rigidity), such as those seen in subarachnoid hemorrhage can also be exhibited. Two assessment techniques can help determine whether meningeal irritation is present. Kernig's sign is resistance to extension of the leg while the person is lying with the hip flexed at a right angle. Brudzinski's sign is elicited when flexion of the neck results in flexion of the hip and knee. These postures are caused by stretching of the inflamed meninges from the lumbar level to the head. Stretching of the inflamed meninges is extremely painful, producing resistance to stretching.

Lumbar puncture (*i.e.,* spinal tap) yields a cloudy and purulent CSF under increased pressure. The CSF typically contains large numbers of polymorphonuclear neutrophils (up to 90,000/mm^3), increased protein content, and reduced sugar content. Bacteria can be seen on smears and can be easily cultured with appropriate media.

Arthritis, cranial nerve damage (especially the eighth nerve, with resulting deafness), and hydrocephalus may occur as complications of pyogenic meningitis. As the pathogens enter the subarachnoid space, they cause inflammation, characterized by a cloudy, purulent exudate. Thrombophlebitis of the bridging veins and dural sinuses may develop, followed by congestion and infarction in the surrounding tissues. Ultimately, the meninges thicken, and adhesions form. These adhesions may impinge on the cranial nerves, giving rise to cranial nerve palsies, or may impair the outflow of CSF, causing hydrocephalus.

In the pathophysiology of bacterial meningitis, the bacterial organisms replicate and undergo lysis in the CSF, releasing endotoxins or cell wall fragments. These substances initiate the release of inflammatory mediators (*i.e.,* cytokines), which set the stage for a complex but coordinated sequence of events by which neutrophils bind to cerebral endothelial cells of the blood-brain barrier, damage these cells by the release of toxic oxygen products (*i.e.,* free radicals), and move fluid across the capillary wall. Experimental evidence strongly suggests that inflammatory mediators released into the CSF impair the blood-brain barrier to the extent that pathogens, neutrophils, and albumin cross the endothelial wall into the CSF.

Although antibiotic therapy was introduced approximately 50 years ago, morbidity and mortality remain high for bacterial meningitis. The mortality rate for *S. pneumoniae* infection remains between 20% and 30%, and neurologic sequelae such as deafness affect one half of the survivors.[54] This has important implications for the growth and development of children. Elucidation of some of the pathophysiologic molecular mechanisms involved in meningitis has important implications and has stimulated the investigation of more effective approaches to therapy.[55–57]

Rapidly acting antibiotic therapy is essential. However, high concentrations of bacterial fragments (*e.g., H. influenzae* lipopolysaccharide, *S. pneumoniae* cell wall fragments) have the potential for exacerbating the abnormalities of the blood-brain barrier and the inflammatory process within the CSF. Adjunctive glucocorticoid therapy, especially that given before antibiotic therapy, can reduce inflammation and decrease the neurologic sequelae.[56] More clinical investigations are needed to study these and other adjunctive agents such as nonsteroidal antiinflammatory drugs, phosphodiesterase inhibitors, and monoclonal antibodies that show promise of decreasing the morbidity and mortality rates associated with bacterial meningitis.[54,55] In bacterial meningitis, prompt therapy is essential to prevent death and minimize serious sequelae. Persons who have been exposed to someone with meningococcal meningitis should be treated prophylactically.

Viral Meningitis. Viral meningitis manifests in much the same way as bacterial meningitis, but the course is less severe, and the CSF findings are markedly different. There are lymphocytes in the fluid rather than polymorphonuclear cells, the protein content is only moderately elevated, and the sugar content is usually normal. The acute viral meningitides are self-limited and usually require only symptomatic treatment. Viral meningitis can be caused by many different viruses, including mumps, coxsackie, Epstein-Barr virus, and herpes simplex type 2. In many cases, the virus cannot be identified.

Encephalitis

Generalized infection of the parenchyma of the brain or spinal cord usually is caused by a virus, but it may also be caused by bacteria, fungi, and other organisms. Less frequent causes of encephalitis are toxic substances such as ingested lead and vaccines for measles, mumps, and rabies, which cause postvaccination encephalitis. Encephalitis caused by human immunodeficiency virus infection is discussed in Chapter 13.

The pathologic picture of encephalitis includes local necrotizing hemorrhage, which ultimately becomes generalized, with prominent edema. There is progressive degeneration of nerve cell bodies. The histologic picture, although rather general, demonstrates some specific characteristics. For example, the poliovirus selectively destroys the cells of the anterior horn of the spinal cord.

Encephalitis, like meningitis, is characterized by fever, headache, and nuchal rigidity. Patients experience a wide range of neurologic disturbances, such as lethargy, disorientation, seizures, dysphagias, focal paralysis, delirium, and coma. The nervous system is subjected to invasion by many viruses, such as arbovirus, poliovirus, and rabies virus. The mode of transmission may be the bite of a mosquito (*i.e.,* arbovirus), a rabid animal (*i.e.,* rabies virus), or ingestion (*i.e.,* poliovirus). A common cause of encephalitis in the United States is herpes simplex virus. Diagnosis of encephalitis is made by clinical history and presenting symptoms, in addition to traditional CSF studies.

Brain Tumors

Brain tumors account for 2% of all cancer deaths. The American Cancer Society reports that there are more than 17,600 new cases and more than 13,200 deaths from brain and CNS cancers each year.[38] Another 17,000 to 18,000 patients (18% of all cancer patients) develop metastases to the brain from other sites. More adults die each year of brain tumors than of Hodgkin's disease or multiple sclerosis.[58] In children, brain tumors are second only to leukemia as a cause of death from cancer, and they kill about 1600 children and young adults annually.

Types of Tumors

For most neoplasms, the term *malignant* is used to describe the lack of cell differentiation, the invasive nature of the tumor, and its ability to metastasize. In the brain, however, even a well-differentiated and histologically benign tumor may grow and cause death because of its location.

Brain tumors can be divided into three types: primary intracranial tumors of CNS tissue (*e.g.,* neurons, neuroglia), primary intracranial tumors that originate within the skull cavity but are not derived from the brain tissue itself (*e.g.,* meninges, pituitary gland, pineal gland), and metastatic tumors. Primary intracranial neoplasms of CNS origin can be classified according to the site of origin and histologic type (Chart 38–1).

Collectively, the neoplasms of astrocyte origin are the most common type of primary brain tumor in the adult. Astrocytomas fall into three clinicopathologic groups: astrocytomas, including glioblastoma multiforme; brain stem glioma; and pilocytic astrocytomas.[1]

Astrocytomas of the cerebral hemispheres are commonly divided into three grades of increasing pathologic anaplasia and rapidity of progression: astrocytoma, anaplastic astrocytoma, and glioblastoma multiforme (see Chapter 5 for a discussion of cell differentiation and anaplasia). Together, these tumors account for approximately 80% of all glial tumors in adults. They are most common in middle age, with the anaplastic astrocytomas having a peak incidence in the sixth decade.

Glioblastoma multiforme is commonly used as a synonym for highly malignant forms of astrocytoma (grades III and IV). Astrocytomas have a marked tendency to become more anaplastic with time, so that a tumor beginning as an astrocytoma may develop into a glioblastoma. Brain stem gliomas occur in the first two decades of life and account for about 20% of brain tumors in this age group.[1]

Pilocytic astrocytomas are distinguished from other astrocytomas by their cellular appearance and their benign behavior. Typically, they occur in children and young adults and are usually located in the cerebellum, but they can also be found in the floor and walls of the

CHART 38-1
Types of Brain Tumors

Tumors of the Neuroglia
- Astrocytoma
  - Glioblastoma multiforme
  - Brain stem glioma
  - Pilocytic astrocytomas
- Oligodendrocytes
  - Oligodendroglioma
- Ependymal cells
  - Ependymona
- Mixed gliomas

Tumors of Neural Cells
- Neuroblastoma
- Ganglion cell tumors
- Tumors of primitive cells
  - Medulloblastoma

Tumors of Non-neural Tissue
- Meningioma and tumors of related tissue
- Pineal tumors
- Pituitary tumors
- Developmental tumors
  - Hemangioblastoma and tumors of blood vessel origin
  - Craniopharyngiomas

Metastatic Tumors

third ventricle, the optic chiasm and nerves, and occasionally in the cerebral hemispheres.

Oligodendrogliomas comprise about 5% of glial tumors. They are most common in middle life and are found in the cerebral hemispheres.[1]

Ependymomas are derived from the single layer of epithelium that lines the ventricles and spinal canal. Although they can occur at any age, they are most likely to occur in the first two decades of life and most frequently affect the fourth ventricle; they constitute 5% to 10% of brain tumors in this age group.[1] The spinal cord is the most common site for ependymomas occurring in middle age.

Meningiomas develop from the meningothelial cells of the arachnoid and are outside the brain. They comprise about 20% of primary brain tumors and generally have their onset in the middle or later years of life.[1] Meningiomas are slow-growing, well-circumscribed, and often highly vascular tumors. They are usually benign, and complete removal is possible if the tumor does not involve vital structures. Pituitary adenomas comprise 12% to 14% of brain tumors; they are usually nonmalignant.[1]

Etiology

Although a number of chemical and viral agents can cause brain tumors in laboratory animals, there is no evidence that these agents directly cause brain cancer in humans. Cranial irradiation and exposure to some chemicals may lead to an increased incidence of astrocytomas and meningiomas. There may also be a hereditary factor. Sixteen percent of persons with primary brain tumors have a family history of cancer. Childhood tumors are considered to be developmental in origin.

Manifestations

Intracranial tumors give rise to focal disturbances in brain function and increased ICP. Focal disturbances occur because of brain compression, tumor infiltration, disturbances in blood flow, and brain edema.

Tumors may be located intraaxially (*i.e.*, within brain tissue) or extraaxially (*i.e.*, outside brain tissue). Disturbances in brain function are generally greatest with fast-growing, infiltrative, intraaxial tumors because of compression, infiltration, and necrosis of brain tissue. Extraaxial tumors, such as meningiomas, may reach a large size without producing signs and symptoms. Cysts may form within tumors and contribute to brain compression. Cerebral edema is usually of the vasogenic type, which develops around brain tumors and is characterized by increased brain water and expanded extracellular fluid. The edema is thought to result from increased permeability of tumor capillary endothelial cells.

Because the volume of the intracranial cavity is fixed, brain tumors cause a generalized increase in ICP when they reach sufficient size. Tumors can obstruct the flow of CSF in the ventricular cavities and produce hydrocephalic dilatation of the proximal ventricles and atrophy of the cerebral hemispheres. Complete compensation of ventricular volumes can occur with very slow-growing tumors, but with rapidly growing tumors, increased ICP is an early sign. Depending on the location of the tumor, brain displacement and herniation of the uncus or cerebellum may occur. The clinical manifestations of brain tumors depend on the size and location of the tumor. General signs and symptoms include headache, nausea, vomiting, mental changes, papilledema, visual disturbances (*e.g.*, diplopia), alterations in sensory and motor function, and seizures.

The brain itself is insensitive to pain. The headache that accompanies brain tumors results from compression or distortion of pain-sensitive dural or vascular structures. It may be felt on the same side of the head as the tumor but is more commonly diffuse in nature. In the early stages, the headache, which is caused by irritation, compression, and traction on the dural sinuses or blood vessels, is mild and occurs in the morning when the person awakens. It usually disappears after the person has been up for a short time. The headache becomes more constant as the tumor enlarges and is often worsened by coughing, bending, or sudden movements of the head.

Vomiting occurs with or without preceding nausea and is a common symptom of increased ICP and brain stem compression. Direct stimulation of the vomiting center, which is located in the medulla, may contribute to the vomiting that occurs with brain tumors. The vomiting may be projectile in nature. Vomiting caused by brain tumor is usually unrelated to meals and is often associated with headache. Papilledema (*i.e.*, edema of the optic disk) results from increased ICP and obstruction of the CSF pathways. It is associated with decreased visual acuity, diplopia, and deficits in the visual fields. Visual defects associated with papilledema are often the reason that persons with brain tumor seek medical care.

Personality and mental changes are common with brain tumors. Persons with brain tumors are often irritable initially and later become quiet and apathetic. They may become forgetful, seem preoccupied, and appear to be psychologically depressed. Because of the mental changes, a psychiatric consultation may be sought before a diagnosis of brain tumor is made.

Focal signs and symptoms are determined by the location of the tumor. Tumors arising in the frontal lobe may grow to large size, increase the ICP, and cause signs of generalized brain dysfunction before focal signs are recognized. Tumors that impinge on the visual system cause visual loss or visual field defects long before generalized signs develop. Certain areas of the brain have a relatively low threshold for seizure activity; tumors arising in relatively silent areas of the brain may produce focal epileptogenic discharges. Temporal lobe tumors often produce seizures as their first symptom. Hallucinations of smell or hearing and déjà vu phenomenon are common focal manifestations of temporal lobe tumors. Brain stem tumors commonly produce upper and lower motoneuron signs, such as weakness of facial muscles and ocular palsies that occur with or without involvement of sensory or long motor tracts. Cerebellar tumors often cause ataxia of gait.

Diagnosis and Treatment

Diagnostic procedures for brain tumor include physical and neurologic examinations, visual field and funduscopic examination, CT scans and MRI, skull x-ray films, technetium pertechnetate brain scans, electroencephalography, and cerebral angiography. Physical examination is used to assess motor and sensory function. Because the visual pathways travel through many areas of the cerebral lobes, detection of visual field defects can provide information about the location of tumors. A funduscopic examination is done to detect papilledema. CT scanning has become the screening procedure of choice for diagnosing and localizing brain tumors and other intracranial masses. MRI scans can be diagnostic when a clinically suspected tumor is not detected by CT scanning. Skull x-ray films are used to detect calcified areas within a neoplasm or erosion of skull structures due to tumors. About 75% of persons with a brain tumor have an abnormal electroencephalogram; in some cases, the results of the test can be used to localize the tumor. Cerebral angiography can be used to locate a tumor and visualize its vascular supply, information that is important when planning surgery. MRI angiography can be used to distinguish vascular masses from tumors.

The three general methods for treatment of brain tumors are surgery, irradiation, and chemotherapy.[59] Surgery is part of the initial management of virtually all brain tumors; it establishes the diagnosis and achieves tumor removal in many cases. The development of microsurgical neuroanatomy, the operating microscope, the fusion of imaging systems with resection techniques, advanced stereotactic and ultrasound technology, and intraoperative monitoring of evoked potentials have improved the effectiveness of surgical resection.[59] However, removal may be limited by the location of the tumor and its invasiveness. Stereotactic surgery uses three-dimensional coordinates and CT and MRI to localize a brain lesion precisely. Ultrasound technology has been used for localizing and removing tumors. The ultrasonic aspirator, which combines a vibrating head with suction, permits atraumatic removal of tumors from cranial nerves and important cortical areas. Intraoperative monitoring of evoked potentials is an important adjunct to some types of surgery. For example, evoked potentials can be used to monitor auditory, visual, speech, or motor responses during surgery done under local anesthesia.

Most malignant brain tumors respond to external irradiation. Irradiation can increase longevity and sometimes can allay symptoms when tumors recur. The treatment dose depends on the tumor's histologic type, radioresponsiveness, and anatomic site and on the level of tolerance of the surrounding tissue. Radiation therapy is avoided in treating children younger than 2 years of age because of the long-term effects, which include developmental delay, panhypopituitarism, and secondary tumors.[59]

The use of chemotherapy for brain tumors is somewhat limited by the blood-brain barrier. Chemotherapeutic agents can be administered intravenously, intraarterially, intrathecally (*i.e.*, into the spinal canal), or intraventricularly. A promising area of improved delivery of chemotherapeutic agents is the use of biodegradable anhydrous wafers impregnated with a drug and implanted into the tumor at the time of surgery. These wafers are constructed so they release the drug over a period of many months.[60]

In summary, although the skull and the CSF provide protection for the brain, they can also contribute to brain injury through compression and bone splinters that occur with skull fracture and coup-contrecoup injuries. Head injuries may result from penetration or impact, with each type affecting the brain and supporting structures in different ways. Head injuries can be classified as direct, resulting from the immediate effects of injury, skull fracture, concussion, or contusion, or as secondary, resulting from edema, hemorrhage, or infection. Secondary injury may result from epidural, subdural, or intracerebral hematoma formation.

Infections of the CNS may be classified according to the structures involved (*e.g.*, meningitis, encephalitis) or the type of organism causing the infection. The damage caused by infection may predispose to hydrocephalus, seizures, or other neurologic defects.

Brain tumors account for 2% of all cancer deaths and are the second most common type of cancer in children. Brain tumors can arise primarily from intracranial structures, and tumors from other parts of the body often metastasize to the brain. Primary brain tumors can arise from any structure within the cranial cavity. Most begin in brain tissue, but the pituitary, the pineal region, and the meninges are also sites of tumor development. Brain tumors cause focal disturbances in brain function and increase the ICP. Focal disturbances result from brain compression, tumor infiltration, disturbances in blood flow, and cerebral edema. The clinical manifestations of brain tumor depend on the size and location of the tumor. General signs and symptoms include headache, nausea, vomiting, mental changes, papilledema, visual disturbances, alterations in motor and sensory function, and seizures. Diagnostic tests include physical examination, visual field testing and funduscopic examination, CT scans, MRI studies, skull x-ray films, brain scans, electroencephalography, and cerebral angiography. Treatment includes surgery, irradiation, and chemotherapy.

Seizure Disorders

After you have completed this section of the chapter, you should be able to meet the following objectives:

- Explain the difference between *seizure activity* and *epileptic seizure*
- State four or more causes of seizures other than epilepsy
- Differentiate between the origin of seizure activity in partial and generalized forms of epilepsy and compare the manifestations of simple partial seizures with those of complex partial seizures and major and minor motor seizures
- Characterize status epilepticus

Seizures, sometimes called convulsions, are paroxysmal motor, sensory, or cognitive manifestations of spontaneous, abnormally synchronous discharges of collections of neurons in the cerebral cortex of the brain. This uncontrolled neuronal activity causes signs and symptoms that vary according to the location of the originating focus of seizure activity, involvement of surrounding neurons, and spread to other parts of the brain. These signs and symptoms can include strange sensations and perceptions (*i.e.*, hallucinations), unusual or repetitive muscle movements, autonomic visceral activity, and the onset of a confusional state or loss of consciousness. The neuronal hyperexcitability that results in a seizure occurs regardless of the discrete functions of individual neurons. However, its manifestations depend on the particular population of nerve cells involved.

About 2 million persons in the United States are subject to recurrent seizures. Seizure activity is the most common disorder encountered in pediatric neurology, and among adults, its incidence is exceeded only by cerebrovascular disorders. Age of onset can be a clue to the type or cause of seizure. When there is no other known cause, seizures may be caused by vulnerability of the developing nervous system to seizure activity. In most persons, the first seizure episode occurs before 20 years of age. After 20 years of age, a seizure is most often caused by a structural change, trauma, tumor, or stroke.

Etiology

A seizure is not a disease but a symptom of an underlying CNS dysfunction. Seizures may occur during almost all serious illnesses or injuries affecting the brain, including infections, tumors, drug abuse, vascular lesions, congenital deformities, and brain injury.

Many theories have been proposed to explain the initiation of the abnormal brain activity that occurs with seizures. Seizures may be caused by alterations in cell membrane permeability or distribution of ions across the neuronal cell membranes. Another cause may be decreased inhibition of cortical or thalamic neuron activity or structural changes that alter the excitability of neurons. Neurotransmitter imbalances such as an acetylcholine excess or γ-aminobutyric acid (GABA, an inhibitory neurotransmitter) deficiency have been proposed as a cause.

Everyone has a seizure threshold that, when exceeded, can result in seizure activity. Whether seizure activity occurs depends on the individual's seizure threshold and the extent to which it has been altered by pathologic processes. Some individuals have a low seizure threshold and are more likely to experience them, even in response to benign stimuli. The role of genetic or familial predisposition to seizures and *interictal* (*i.e.*, between seizures) alterations in EEG tracings remain under active investigation. The incidence of certain types of seizure activity is statistically higher in families with a genetic predisposition toward cerebral dysrhythmia, but evidence of cerebral dysrhythmia is not invariably associated with clinical manifestations of a primary seizure disorder.

The terms *seizure disorder* or *epileptic syndrome* are often used interchangeably, although most clinicians prefer seizure disorder because of the negative connotations still associated with the term epilepsy. A seizure disorder can be defined as a syndrome in which there is a tendency to have recurrent, paroxysmal seizure activity without evidence of a reversible metabolic cause. It is a chronic condition for which long-term medication may be appropriate.

Provoked and Unprovoked Seizures

Clinically, seizures may be categorized as unprovoked (*i.e.*, primary or idiopathic) or provoked (*i.e.*, secondary or acute symptomatic).[61] Provoked or symptomatic seizures include febrile seizures, seizures precipitated by systemic metabolic conditions, and those that follow a primary insult to the CNS. Unprovoked or idiopathic seizures are those for which no identifiable cause can be determined.

The most common subgroup of seizures under the category of provoked seizures is that of febrile seizures in children. They are associated with a high fever, usually with a temperature higher than 104°F. In the United States, 2% to 5% of children experience a febrile seizure before the age of 5 years. Of these, approximately 30% have one recurrence, and only one half of those have a third recurrence. Because the risks of treatment (*e.g.*, side effects of medications used to control seizures) often exceed the benefits, anticonvulsant medications may be avoided in these cases.[62]

Seizures precipitated by systemic or metabolic disturbances and by primary CNS insult also fall into the category of provoked seizures. Transient systemic metabolic disturbances may precipitate seizures. Examples include electrolyte imbalances, hypoglycemia, hypoxia, hypocalcemia, and alkalosis. Toxemia of pregnancy, water intoxication, uremia, and CNS infections such as meningitis may also precipitate a seizure. The rapid withdrawal of sedative-hypnotic drugs, such as alcohol or barbiturates, is another cause of seizures. Approximately 5% to 10% of those who suffer a CNS insult, such as occurs with cerebral bleeding, edema, or neuronal damage, experience a seizure at the time. Treatment of the immediate cause of these seizures often results in their disappearance. Long-term prophylactic treatment with anticonvulsant medications remains controversial in these situations.

Multiple episodes or frequent recurrences of apparently unprovoked seizures are considered a seizure disorder or epilepsy, the less preferred term. These persons are evaluated to determine and possibly treat the underlying dysfunction. In these cases, anticonvulsant therapy may be prescribed to keep seizure activity under control.

CHART 38-2
Classification of Epileptic Seizures

Partial Seizures

Simple partial seizures (no impairment of consciousness)
- With motor symptoms
- With sensory symptoms
- With autonomic signs
- With psychic symptoms

Complex partial seizures (impairment of consciousness)
- Simple partial onset followed by impaired consciousness
- Impairment of consciousness at onset

Partial seizures evolving to secondarily generalized seizures
- Simple partial leading to generalized seizures
- Complex partial leading to generalized seizures

Unclassified Seizures

Classification not possible due to inadequate or incomplete data

Generalized Seizures

Absence seizures (typical or atypical)
Atonic seizures
Myoclonic seizures
Clonic seizures
Tonic
Tonic-clonic seizures

(Adapted from Commission on Classification and Terminology of the International League Against Epilepsy [1981]. *Epilepsia 22,* 489)

Classification

Although a knowledge of the cause is important, seizure management is usually directed toward identifying the seizure type and controlling seizure occurrence. Two classification systems are in use. The first is based on seizure type and the second on the concept of epilepsies and epileptic syndromes.[61] Both systems were developed by the International League Against Epilepsy, and both are based on clinical manifestations and EEG activity. The first, the International Classification of Epileptic Seizures is based on symptoms during the seizure. It divides seizures into two broad categories: partial seizures, in which the seizure begins in a specific or focal area of one cerebral hemisphere, and generalized seizures, which involve virtually simultaneous onset in both cerebral hemispheres (Chart 38–2).[62,63]

The second classification system is the International Classification of Epilepsies and Epileptic Syndromes.[64] This system maintains the dichotomy of partial and generalized seizures but substitutes the term localized-related for partial seizures. The system further divides epilepsies into idiopathic, symptomatic, and cryptogenic (*i.e.*, suspected to be symptomatic despite absence of definitive proof of an underlying cause). The system also has categories for seizures of undetermined origin such as neonatal seizures and a category of special syndromes such as febrile seizures.

Partial Seizures

Partial or focal seizures are the most common type of seizures among newly diagnosed cases in all groups older than 10 years of age. Partial seizures can be subdivided into three major groups: simple partial (*i.e.*, consciousness is not impaired), complex partial (*i.e.*, impairment of consciousness), and secondarily generalized partial seizures. These categories are primarily based on current neurophysiologic theories related to seizure propagation and the extent of involvement of the brain's hemispheres.

Simple Partial Seizures. Simple partial seizures usually involve only one hemisphere and are not accompanied by loss of consciousness or responsiveness. These seizures have also been referred to as elementary partial seizures, partial seizures with elementary symptoms, or focal seizures. The 1981 Commission on Classification and Terminology of the International League Against Epilepsy classified simple partial seizures according to motor signs, sensory symptoms, autonomic manifestations, and psychic symptoms.

The observed clinical signs and symptoms depend on the area of the brain where the abnormal neuronal discharge is taking place. If the motor area of the brain is involved, the earliest symptom is motor movement corresponding to the location of onset on the contralateral side of the body. The motor movement may remain localized or may spread to other cortical areas, with sequential involvement of body parts in an epileptic type "march," known as a Jacksonian seizure. If the sensory portion of the brain is involved, there may be no observable clinical manifestations. Sensory symptoms correlating with the location of seizure activity on the contralateral side of the brain may involve somatic sensory disturbance (*i.e.*, tingling and crawling sensations) or special sensory disturbance (*i.e.*, visual, auditory, gustatory, or olfactory phenomena). When abnormal cortical discharge stimulates the autonomic nervous system, flushing, tachycardia, diaphoresis, hypotension or hypertension, or pupillary changes may be evident.

The term *prodrome* or *aura* has traditionally meant a sensory warning sign of impending seizure activity or the onset of seizure that affected persons could describe because they were conscious. The aura itself is now considered part of the seizure.[44] Because consciousness is maintained and only a small portion of the brain is involved, an aura is a simple partial seizure. Simple partial seizures may progress to complex partial seizures or generalized tonic-clonic seizures that result in unconsciousness. Therefore, the aura in simple partial seizure may be considered a warning sign of impending complex partial seizures.

Complex Partial Seizures. Complex partial seizures involve impairment of consciousness and often arise from the temporal lobe. The seizure begins in a localized area of the brain but may rapidly progress to involve both hemispheres. These seizures also may be referred to as temporal lobe seizures or psychomotor seizures.

Complex partial seizures are often accompanied by automatisms. Automatisms are repetitive, nonpurposeful activity such as lip smacking, grimacing, patting, or rubbing clothing. Confusion during the postictal state (*i.e.*, after a seizure) is common. Hallucinations and illusional experiences such as *déjà vu* (*i.e.*, familiarity with unfamiliar events or environments) or *jamais vu* (*i.e.*, unfamiliarity with a known environment) have been reported. There may be overwhelming fear, uncontrolled forced thinking or a flood of ideas, and feelings of detachment and depersonalization. A person with a complex partial seizure disorder is sometimes misunderstood and believed to require hospitalization for a psychiatric disorder.

Secondarily Generalized Partial Seizures. During these seizures, the ictal neuronal discharge spreads, involving deeper structures of the brain, such as the thalamus or the reticular formation. Discharges spread to both hemispheres, resulting in progression to tonic-clonic seizure activity. These seizures may start as simple or complex partial seizures. The aura, or peculiar sensations that precede the seizure, is usually the result of partial seizure activity.

Generalized-Onset Seizures

Generalized-onset seizures are the most common type in young children. These seizures are classified as primary or generalized when clinical signs, symptoms, and supporting EEG changes indicate involvement of both hemispheres. The clinical symptoms include unconsciousness and involve varying bilateral degrees of symmetric motor responses without evidence of localization to one hemisphere.

These seizures are divided into four broad categories: absence seizures (typical and atypical), atonic (akinetic) seizures, myoclonic seizures, and major motor (formerly grand mal) seizures, characterized by tonic, clonic, or tonic-clonic activity.[63]

Absence Seizures. Absence seizures are a generalized, nonconvulsive epileptic event and are expressed mainly as disturbances in consciousness. Absence seizures typically occur only in children and cease in adulthood or evolve to generalized motor seizures. Children may present with a history of school failure that predates the first evidence of seizure episodes. Although typical absence seizures have been characterized as a blank stare, motionlessness, and unresponsiveness, motion occurs in many cases of absence seizures. This motion takes the form of automatisms such as lip smacking, mild clonic motion (usually in the eyelids), increased or decreased postural tone, and autonomic phenomena. There is often a brief loss of contact with the environment. The seizure usually lasts only a few seconds, and then the person is able to resume normal activity immediately. The manifestations are often so subtle that they may pass unnoticed.

Atypical absence seizures are similar to typical absence seizures except for greater alterations in muscle tone and less abrupt onset and cessation. In practice, it is difficult to distinguish typical from atypical absence seizures without benefit of supporting EEG findings. However, it is important for the clinician to distinguish between complex partial and absence seizures, because the drugs of choice are different. Medications that are effective for partial seizures may increase the frequency of absence seizures.

Atonic Seizures. In akinetic or atonic seizures, there is a sudden, split-second loss of muscle tone leading to slackening of the jaw, drooping of the limb, or falling to the ground. These seizures are also known as *drop attacks*.

Myoclonic Seizures. Myoclonic seizures involve brief involuntary muscle contractions induced by stimuli of cerebral origin. A myoclonic seizure involves bilateral jerking of muscles, generalized or confined to the face, trunk, or one or more extremities. Tonic seizures are characterized by a rigid, violent contraction of the muscles, fixing the limbs in a strained position. Clonic seizures consist of repeated contractions and relaxations of the major muscle groups.

Tonic-Clonic Seizures. Tonic-clonic seizures, formerly called *grand mal seizures,* are the most common major motor seizure. Frequently, a person has a vague warning (probably a simple partial seizure) and experiences a sharp tonic contraction of the muscles with extension of the extremities and immediate loss of consciousness. Incontinence of bladder and bowel is common. Cyanosis may occur from contraction of airway and respiratory muscles. The tonic phase is followed by the clonic phase, which involves rhythmic bilateral contraction and relaxation of the extremities. At the end of the clonic phase, the person remains unconscious until the RAS begins to function again. This is called the *postictal phase.* The tonic-clonic phases last approximately 60 to 90 seconds.

Unclassified Seizures

Unclassified seizures are those that cannot be placed in one of the previous categories. These seizures are observed in the neonatal and infancy periods. Determination of whether the seizure is focal or generalized is not possible. Unclassified seizures are difficult to control with medication.

Diagnosis and Treatment

The diagnosis of seizure disorders is based on a thorough history and neurologic examination, including a full description of the seizure. The physical examination and laboratory studies helps exclude any metabolic disease (*e.g.,* hyponatremia) that could precipitate seizures. Skull radiographs and CT or MRI scans are used to identify structural defects. One of the most useful diagnostic tests is the electroencephalogram, which is used to record changes in the brain's electrical activity. It is used to support the clinical diagnosis of epilepsy, to provide a guide for prognosis, and to assist in classifying the seizure disorder.

The first rule of treatment is to protect the person from injury during a seizure, preserve brain function by aborting or preventing seizure activity, and treat any underlying disease. Persons with epilepsy should be advised to avoid situations that could be dangerous or life threatening if seizures occur. Treatment of the underlying disorder may reduce the frequency of seizures.

After the underlying disease is treated, the aim of treatment is to bring the seizures under control with the least possible disruption in lifestyle and minimum side effects from medication. During the past 25 years, the therapy for epilepsy has changed drastically because of an improved classification system, the ability to measure serum anticonvulsant levels, and the availability of potent new anticonvulsant drugs. With proper drug management, 60% to 80% of persons with epilepsy can obtain good seizure control.

Anticonvulsant Medications. More than 18 drugs are available in the United States for the treatment of epilepsy.[65] This group includes three antiepileptic drugs that were approved for use in the United States during the past 3 years.

Drugs used as first-line therapy for seizure disorders are carbamazepine, phenytoin, ethosuximide, valproate, phenobarbital, primidone, and clonazepam.[65,66] Carbamazepine and phenytoin are the drugs of choice in treating partial seizures. They are also used for tonic-clonic seizures resulting from partial seizures. Ethosuximide is the drug of choice for absence seizures, but it is not effective for tonic-clonic seizures that progress from partial seizures. Valproate is helpful for persons with many of the minor motor seizures and tonic-clonic seizures. Valproate and ethosuximide can be used together. Phenobarbital is used for tonic-clonic seizures, as is primidone. Primidone also is prescribed for simple and complex partial seizures. Absence and myoclonic seizures can be treated with clonazepam. Atonic seizures are highly resistant to therapy. Each of the three new drugs—Gabapentin, lamotrigine, and felbamate—is approved for use in adults who have partial seizures alone or with secondarily generalized (grand mal) seizures.[67]

Women of childbearing age require special consideration concerning fertility, contraception, and pregnancy. Many of the drugs interact with oral contraceptives; some affect hormone function or decrease fertility. For women with epilepsy who become pregnant, antiseizure drugs increase the risk of congenital abnormalities and other perinatal complications.[65]

Whenever possible, a single drug should be used in epilepsy therapy. Monotherapy eliminates drug interactions and additive side effects. Determining the proper dose of the anticonvulsant drug is often a long and tedious process, which can be very frustrating for the person with epilepsy. Consistency in taking the medication is essential. Anticonvulsant drugs should never be discontinued abruptly; the dose should be decreased slowly to prevent seizure recurrence. The most frequent cause of recurrent seizures is patient noncompliance with drug regimens. Ongoing education and support are extremely important in the management of seizures. The psychosocial implications of a diagnosis of epilepsy continue to have a large impact on those affected with the disorder.

The neurologist and primary care physician must work together when a person on anticonvulsant medication becomes ill and must take additional medications. Some drugs act synergistically, and others interfere with the actions of anticonvulsant medications. This situation needs to be carefully monitored to avoid overmedication or interference with successful seizure control.

Surgical Therapy. Surgical treatment may be an option for persons with epilepsy that is refractory to drug treatment.[68] With the use of modern neuroimaging and surgical techniques, a single epileptogenic lesion can be identified and removed without leaving a neurologic deficit. The most common surgery consists of removal of the amygdala and anterior part of the hippocampus and entorhinal cortex, as well as a small part of the temporal pole, leaving the lateral temporal neocortex intact. Another surgical procedure involves partial removal of the corpus callosum to prevent spread of a unilateral seizure to a generalized seizure. Modern epilepsy surgery requires a multidisciplinary team of highly skilled surgeons and specialists working together in an epilepsy center. Most procedures require only a few hours in the operating room and a few days' stay in the hospital postoperatively. However, surgery for epilepsy is still in its early stages and is considered as a treatment modality for only a limited numbers of persons with epilepsy.

Generalized Convulsive Status Epilepticus

Seizures that do not stop spontaneously or occur in succession without recovery are called *status epilepticus.* There are as many types of status epilepticus as there are types of seizures. Tonic-clonic status epilepticus is a medical emergency and, if not promptly treated, may lead to respiratory failure and death.

The disorder occurs most frequently in the young and old. Morbidity and mortality is highest in elderly persons and persons with acute symptomatic seizures, such as those related to anoxia or cerebral infarction.[69] About one third of patients have no history of a seizure disorder, and in another one third, status epilepticus occurs as an initial manifestation of epilepsy.[69] If status epilepticus is caused by neurologic or systemic disease, the cause needs to be identified and treated immediately, because the seizures probably will not respond until the underlying cause has been corrected.

Treatment consists of appropriate life-support measures. Medications are given to control seizure activity. Intravenously administered diazepam or lorazepam are considered first-line therapy for the condition. The prognosis is related to the underlying cause more than to the seizures themselves.

In summary, seizures are caused by spontaneous, uncontrolled, paroxysmal, transitory discharges from cortical centers in the brain. Seizures may occur as a reversible symptom of another disease condition or as a recurrent condition called epilepsy. Epileptic seizures are classified as partial or generalized seizures. Partial seizures have evidence of local onset, beginning in one hemisphere. They include simple partial seizures, in which consciousness is not lost, and complex partial seizures, which begin in one hemisphere but progress to involve both. Generalized seizures involve both hemispheres and include unconsciousness and rapidly occurring widespread bilateral symmetric motor responses. They include minor motor seizures such as absence, akinetic seizures, and major motor or grand mal seizures. Control of seizures is the primary goal of treatment and is accomplished with anticonvulsant medications. Anticonvulsant medications interact with each other and need to be monitored closely when more than one drug is used.

Dementias

After you have completed this section of the chapter, you should be able to meet the following objectives:

- State the criteria for a diagnosis of dementia
- Compare the causes associated with Alzheimer's disease, dementia, Pick's disease, Creutzfeldt-Jakob disease, the Wernicke-Korsakoff syndrome, and Huntington's disease
- Describe the changes in brain tissue that occur with Alzheimer's disease
- Use the three stages of Alzheimer's disease to describe its progress
- Cite the difference between Wernicke's disease and the Korsakoff component of the Wernicke-Korsakoff syndrome
- State the pros and cons for the presymptomatic use of genetic testing for Huntington's disease

Dementia is a syndrome of intellectual deterioration severe enough to interfere with occupational or social performance. It involves disturbances in memory, language use, perception, and motor skills and interrupts the ability to learn necessary skills, solve problems, think abstractly, and make judgments. Depression is the most common treatable illness that may masquerade as dementia, and it must be excluded when a diagnosis of dementia is considered (see Chapter 58). This is important, because cognitive functioning usually returns to baseline levels after depression is treated. Dementia can be caused by any disorder that permanently damages large association areas of the cerebral hemispheres, including Alzheimer's disease, multi-infarct dementia, Pick's disease, Creutzfeldt-Jakob disease, Wernicke-Korsakoff syndrome, and Huntington's chorea.

Alzheimer's Disease

Dementia of the Alzheimer's type occurs in middle or late life and accounts for 50% to 70% of all cases of dementia. The disorder affects approximately 4 million Americans and may be the fourth leading cause of death in the United States.[70] The risk of developing Alzheimer's disease increases with age and occurs in nearly half of persons 85 years old and older. As the elderly population in the United States continues to increase, the number of persons with Alzheimer's-type dementia is also expected to increase.

Pathophysiology

Alzheimer's disease is characterized by cortical atrophy and loss of neurons, particularly in the frontal and temporal lobes (Fig. 38–14). With significant atrophy, there is ventricular enlargement (*i.e.*, hydrocephalus) from the loss of brain tissue.

The major microscopic features of Alzheimer's disease are the presence of amyloid-containing neuritic plaques and neurofibrillary tangles.[4] The neurofibrillary tangles, found within the cytoplasm of abnormal neurons, consist of fibrous proteins that are wound around each other in a helical fashion. These tangles are resistant to chemical or enzymatic breakdown, and they persist in brain tissue long after the neuron in which they arose has died and disappeared. The senile plaques are patches or flat areas composed of clusters of degenerating nerve terminals arranged around a central core of β-amyloid peptide (BAP). These plaques are found in areas of the cerebral cortex that are linked to intellectual function. BAP is a fragment of a much larger membrane-spanning amyloid precursor protein (APP). The function of APP is unclear, but it appears to be associated with the cytoskeleton of nerve fibers. Normally, the degradation of APP involves cleavage in the middle of the BAP portion of the molecule, with both fragments being lost in the extracellular fluid. In Alzheimer's disease, the APP molecule is cut at both ends of the BAP segment, thereby releasing an intact BAP molecule that accumulates in neuritic plaques as amyloid fibrils.

It is important to recognize that some plaques and tangles can be found in the brains of older persons who do not show cognitive impairment. The number and distribution of the plaques and tangles appear to contribute to the intellectual deterioration that occurs with Alzheimer's disease. In persons with the disease, the plaques and tangles are found throughout the neocortex, with relative sparing of the primary sensory cortex, and in the hippocampus and amygdala.[1] Hippocampal function in particular may be compromised by the pathologic changes that occur in Alzheimer's disease. The hippocampus is crucial to information processing, acquisition of new memories, and retrieval of old memories. The development of neurofibrillary tangles in the entorhinal cortex and superior portion of the hippocampal gyrus interferes with cortical input and output, thereby isolating the hippocampus from the remainder of the cortex and rendering it functionless.[71]

Neurochemically, Alzheimer's disease has been associated with a decrease in the level of choline acetyltransferase activity in the cortex and hippocampus. This enzyme is required for the synthesis of acetylcholine, a neurotransmitter that is associated with memory. The reduction in choline acetyltransferase is quantitatively related to the numbers of neuritic plaques and severity of dementia. Unfortunately, attempts to increase brain levels of acetylcholine or its precursors in persons with Alzheimer's disease have been unsuccessful. Initial trials using choline and lecithin, the precursors of acetylcholine, have failed to demonstrate any improvement in memory.

It is likely that Alzheimer's disease is caused by several factors that interact differently in different persons. Progress on the genetics of inherited early-onset Alzheimer's disease shows that mutations in at least three genes—amyloid precursor protein *(APP)*, a gene on chromosome 21; presenilin-1 *(PS1)*, a gene on chromosome 14; and presenilin-2 *(PS2)*, a gene on chromosome 1—can cause Alzheimer's disease in certain families.[72,73] The *APP* gene is associated with an autosomal dominant form of early onset Alzheimer's disease. Persons with Down syndrome (trisomy 21) develop the pathologic changes of Alzheimer's disease and a comparable decline in cognitive functioning at a relatively young age. Virtually all persons with Down syndrome who survive past the age of 50 develop the full-blown pathologic features of dementia. Because the *APP* gene

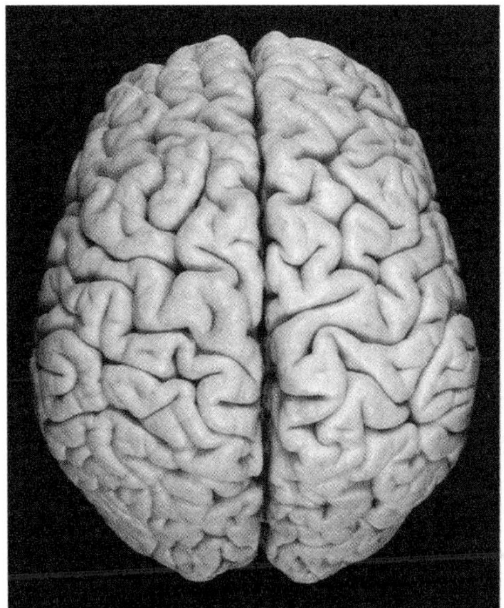

A

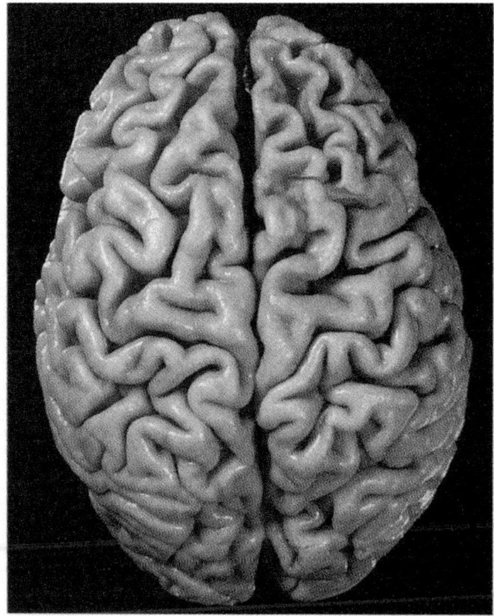

B

Figure 38–14
Alzheimer disease. (**A**) Normal brain. (**B**) The brain of a patient with Alzheimer disease shows cortical atrophy, characterized by slender gyri and prominent sulci.

is located on chromosome 21, it is thought that the additional dosage of the gene product in trisomy 21 predisposes to accumulation of BAP.[4] A second gene, an allele of the apolipoprotein E gene, APOE ϵ4, has been identified as a risk factor for late-onset Alzheimer's disease.

Manifestations

Alzheimer's-type dementia follows an insidious and progressive course. Major symptoms include loss of memory, disorientation, impaired abstract thinking and impulse control, and changes in personality and affect.[74] Three stages of Alzheimer's dementia have been identified, each characterized by progressive degenerative changes (Chart 38–3). The *first stage,* which may last for 2 to 4 years, is characterized by a subjective memory deficit that is often difficult to differentiate from the normal forgetfulness that occurs in the elderly. Although most elderly forget unimportant events and details, persons with Alzheimer's disease randomly forget important and unimportant details. They forget where things are placed, get lost easily, and have trouble remembering appointments. Recent memory and remote memory are affected. Mild changes in personality, such as a flat affect, lack of spontaneity, and loss of a previous sense of humor, occur during this stage.

As the disease progresses, the person with Alzheimer's disease enters the *second or confusional stage* of dementia. This stage may last several years and is marked by a more global impairment of cognitive functioning. During this stage, there are changes in higher cortical functioning needed for language, spatial relationships, and problem solving. Depression may occur in persons who are aware of their deficits. There is extreme confusion, disorientation, lack of insight, and inability to carry out the activities of daily living. Personal hygiene is neglected, and language becomes impaired because of difficulty in remembering and retrieving words. Wandering, especially in the late afternoon or early evening, becomes a problem. The *sundown syndrome,* which is characterized by confusion, restlessness, agitation, and wandering, may become a daily occurrence late in the afternoon. Some persons may become hostile and abusive toward family members. Persons who enter this stage can no longer live alone and should be assisted in making decisions about supervised placement with family members or friends or in a community-based facility.

Stage 3 is the *terminal stage.* It is usually relatively short (1 to 2 years) compared with the other stages, but it has been known to last for as long as 10 years.[75] The person becomes incontinent, apathetic, and unable to recognize family or friends. It is usually during this stage that the sufferer is institutionalized.

CHART 38-3
Stages of Alzheimer's Disease

Stage 1

Memory loss
Lack of spontaneity
Subtle personality changes
Disorientation to time and date

Stage 2

Impaired cognition and abstract thinking
Restlessness and agitation
Wandering, "sundown syndrome"
Inability to carry out activities of daily living
Impaired judgment
Inappropriate social behavior
Lack of insight, abstract thinking
Repetitive behavior
Voracious appetite

Stage 3

Emaciation, indifference to food
Inability to communicate
Urinary and fecal incontinence
Seizures

(Matteson M.A., McConnell E.S. [1988]. *Gerontological nursing* [p. 251]. Philadelphia: J.B. Lippincott)

Diagnosis and Treatment

Alzheimer's disease is essentially a diagnosis of exclusion. There are no peripheral biochemical markers or tests for the disease. The diagnosis can be confirmed only by microscopic examination of tissue obtained from a cerebral biopsy or at autopsy. The diagnosis is based on clinical findings. Guidelines for the early recognition and assessment of Alzheimer's disease have been published by the Agency for Health Care Policy and Research (AHCPR).[75] A diagnosis of Alzheimer's disease requires the presence of dementia established by clinical examination and documented by results of a mini-mental state examination, Blessed dementia test, or similar mental status test; no disturbance in consciousness; onset between ages 40 and 90 years, most often after age 65; and absence of systemic or brain disorders that could account for the memory or cognitive deficits.[75] Brain imaging, CT scan, or MRI is done to exclude other brain disease. Metabolic screening should be done for known reversible causes of dementia such as vitamin B_{12} deficiency, thyroid dysfunction, and electrolyte imbalance.

There is no specific treatment for Alzheimer's dementia. Drugs are used primarily to control depression, agitation, or sleep disorders. Two major goals of care are maintaining the person's socialization and providing support for the family. Self-help groups that provide support for family and friends have become available, with support from the Alzheimer's Disease and Related Disorders Association. Day care and respite centers are available in many areas to provide relief for caregivers.

Although there is no current drug therapy that is curative for Alzheimer's disease, some show promise in terms of slowing the progress of the disease. The use of pharmacologic agents such as tacrine (Cognex) and donepizil (Aricept) has been approved for symptomatic therapy in Alzheimer's disease.[76] There is also interest in the use of agents such as antioxidents (*e.g.,* vitamin E), antiinflammatory agents, and estrogen replacement therapy in women to prevent or delay the onset of the disease.

Other Types of Dementia

Multi-infarct Dementia

Dementia associated with cerebrovascular disease does not result directly from atherosclerosis, but rather it is caused by multiple infarctions throughout the brain—hence the name *multi-infarct dementia.* About 20% to 25% of dementias are vascular in origin, and the incidence is closely associated with hypertension.[74] Other contributing factors are arrhythmias, myocardial infarction, peripheral vascular disease, diabetes mellitus, and smoking. The usual onset is between the ages of 55 and 70 years. The disease differs from Alzheimer's dementia in its presentation and tissue abnormalities. The onset may be gradual or abrupt, and there may be focal neurologic symptoms related to local areas of infarction.

Pick's Disease

Pick's disease is a rare form of dementia characterized by atrophy of the frontal, temporal, and parietal lobes of the brain. The neurons in the affected areas contain cytoplasmic inclusions called Pick bodies.

The average age at onset of Pick's disease is 38 years. The disease is more common in women than men. Behavioral manifestations may be noticed earlier than memory deficits, taking the form of a striking absence of concern and care, a loss of initiative, echolalia (*i.e.,* automatic repetition of anything said to the person), hypotonia, and incontinence. The course of the disease is relentless, with death ensuing within 2 to 10 years. The immediate cause of death usually is infection.

Creutzfeldt-Jakob's Disease

Creutzfeldt-Jakob's disease is a rare, transmissible form of dementia thought to be caused by an infective protein agent called a *prion.* The pathogen is resistant to chemical and physical methods commonly used for sterilizing medical and surgical equipment. The disease has reportedly been transmitted through corneal transplants and human growth hormone obtained from cadavers. The National Hormone and Pituitary Program halted the distribution of human pituitary hormone in 1985 after reports that three young persons who had received the hormone had died of Creutzfeldt-Jakob disease.[77] Because of the uncertainty and dangers surrounding the transmission of Creutzfeldt-Jakob disease, it is recommended that persons who received human-derived growth hormone refrain from blood, tissue, or organ donation.[12]

Creutzfeldt-Jakob's disease causes degeneration of the pyramidal and extrapyramidal systems and is most readily distinguished by its rapid course. Affected persons are usually demented within 6 months of onset. The disease is uniformly fatal, with death often occurring within months, although a few persons may survive for several years.[1] The early symptoms consist of abnormalities in personality and visual-spatial coordination. Extreme dementia and myoclonus follow as the disease progresses.

Wernicke-Korsakoff Syndrome

Wernicke-Korsakoff syndrome results from chronic alcoholism. Wernicke's disease is characterized by weakness and paralysis of the extraocular muscles, nystagmus, ataxia, and confusion. The affected person may also have signs of peripheral neuropathy. The person has an unsteady gait and complains of diplopia. There may be signs attributable to alcohol withdrawal such as delirium, confusion, and hallucinations. This disorder is caused by a deficiency of thiamine (vitamin B_1), and many of the symptoms are reversed when nutrition is improved with supplemental thiamine.

The Korsakoff component of the syndrome involves severe impairment of recent memory. There is often difficulty in dealing with abstractions, and the person's capacity to learn is defective. Confabulation (*i.e.,* recitation of imaginary experiences to fill in gaps in memory) is probably the most distinctive feature of the disease. Polyneuritis is also common. Unlike Wernicke's disease, Korsakoff's psychosis does not improve significantly with treatment.

Huntington's Disease

Huntington's disease is a rare, hereditary disorder characterized by chronic progressive chorea, psychologic changes, and dementia. Although the disease is inherited as an autosomal dominant disorder, symptoms do not usually develop until after 30 years of age.[13] By the time the disease has been diagnosed, the person has often passed the gene on to his or her children.

Huntington's disease produces localized death of brain cells. The first and most severely affected neurons are the caudate nucleus and putamen of the basal ganglia. The neurochemical changes that occur with the disease are complex. The neurotransmitter GABA is an inhibitory neurotransmitter in the basal ganglia. Postmortem studies have shown a decrease of GABA and GABA receptors in the basal ganglia of persons dying of Huntington's disease. Likewise, the levels of acetylcholine, an excitatory neurotransmitter in the basal ganglia, are reduced in persons with Huntington's disease. The dopaminergic pathway of the nigrostriatal system, which is affected in parkinsonism, is preserved in Huntington's disease, suggesting that an imbalance in dopamine and acetylcholine may contribute to manifestations of the disease.

Depression and personality changes are the most common early psychologic manifestations; memory loss is often accompanied by impulsive behavior, moodiness, antisocial behavior, and a tendency to emotional outbursts.[78] Other early signs of the disease are lack of initiative, loss of spontaneity, and inability to concentrate. Fidgeting or restlessness may represent early signs of dyskinesia, followed by choreiform and some dystonic posturing. Eventually, progressive rigidity and akinesia (rather than chorea) develop in association with dementia.

There is no cure for Huntington's disease. The treatment is largely symptomatic. Drugs may be used to treat the dyskinesias and behavioral disturbances.

Study of the genetics of Huntington's disease led to the discovery that the gene for the disease is located on chromosome 4.[4] The discovery of a marker probe for the gene locus has enabled testing that can predict whether a person will develop the disease. The testing procedure requires obtaining DNA samples from the person at risk and from several relatives to determine which member of the gene pair travels with the marker probe for the Huntington's gene in a particular family. DNA for determining the genotype can be obtained from the blood of a consenting person, from amniotic fluid, or from frozen brain tissue from a diseased person.[13] Presymptomatic testing raises many ethical questions, including that of providing a person with knowledge that he or she is carrying a gene that will eventually lead to prolonged physical and mental deterioration.

In summary, cognitive disorders can be caused by any disorder that permanently damages large association areas of the cerebral hemispheres, including Alzheimer's disease, multi-infarct dementia, Pick's disease, Creutzfeldt-Jakob's disease, Wernicke-Korsakoff syndrome, and Huntington's disease. Multi-infarct dementia is associated with vascular disease and Pick's disease with atrophy of the frontal and temporal lobes. Creutzfeldt-Jakob disease is a rare, transmissible form of dementia. Wernicke-Korsakoff syndrome results from chronic alcoholism. Huntington's disease is a rare, hereditary disorder characterized by chronic and progressive chorea, psychologic change, and dementia.

By far the most common cause of dementia (50% to 70%) is Alzheimer's disease. The condition is a major health problem among the elderly. It is characterized by cortical atrophy and loss of neurons, the presence of neuritic plaques, granulovacuolar degeneration, and cerebrovascular deposits of amyloid. The disease follows an insidious and progressive course that begins with memory impairment and terminates in an inability to recognize family or friends and the loss of control over bodily functions. The particular tragedy of Alzheimer's disease and other related dementias is that they dissolve the mind and rob the victim of humanity. Simultaneously, these disorders devastate the lives of spouses and other family members, who must endure an insidious loss of the person and a valued relationship.

REFERENCES

1. Cotran R.S., Kumar V., Robbins S.L. (1994). *Robbin's pathologic basis of disease* (5th ed, p. 3). Philadelphia: W.B. Saunders.
2. Meyer F.B. (1992). Brain metabolism, blood flow, and ischemic thresholds. In Awad I.A. (Ed.). *Neurosurgical topics: Cerebrovascular occlusive disease and brain ischemia* (pp. 1–24). Cleveland: AANS.
3. Richmond T.S. (1997). Cerebral resuscitation after global brain ischemia: Linking research to practice. *AACN Clinical Issues* 8 (2), 171–181.
4. Rubin E., Farber J.L. (1994). Pathology (2nd ed. pp. 1349—1437), Philadelphia: J.B. Lippincott.
5. Neatherlin J.S., Brillhardt B. (1988). Glasgow coma scores in the patient postcardiopulmonary resuscitation. *Journal of Neuroscience Nursing* 20 (2), 104.
6. Martin T.G. (1986). Drowning and near-drowning. *Hospital Medicine* 22 (7), 53.
7. Sieber F.E., Traystman R.J. (1992). Special issues: Glucose and the brain. *Critical Care Medicine* 20 (1), 104–116.
8. Lipton S.A., Rosenberg P.A. (1994). Excitatory amino acids as a final common pathway in neurologic disorders. *New England Journal of Medicine* 330 (9), 613–622.
9. Feurerstein G., Hunter J., Barone F.C. (1992). Calcium blockers and neuroprotection. In Marangos P.J., Lal H. (Eds.). *Advances in neuroprotection: Emerging strategies in neuroprotection* (p. 129). Boston: Birkhauser.
10. Sauer D., Massiu L., Allegrini P.R., Amacker H., Schmutz M., Fagg G.E. (1992). Excitotoxicity, cerebral ischemia, and neuroprotection by competitive NMDA receptor antagonists. In Marangos P.J., Lal H. (Eds.). *Advances in neuroprotection: Emerging strategies in neuroprotection* (pp. 93–105). Boston, Birkhauser.
11. Meldrum B. (1992). Excitatory amino acids and neuroprotection. In Marangos P.J., Lal H. (Eds.). *Advances in neuroprotection: Emerging strategies in neuroprotection* (p 106). Boston: Birkhauser.
12. Hickey J.V. (1996). *The clinical practice of neurological and neurosurgical nursing* (4th ed., pp. 295–327). Philadelphia: Lippincott.
13. Lang E.W., Chestnut R.M. (1995). Intracranial pressure and cerebral perfusion pressure in severe head injury. *New Horizon* 3 (3), 400–409.
14. Guyton A.C., Hall J.E. (1996). *Textbook of medical physiology* (9th ed., pp 217, 783). Philadelphia: W.B. Saunders.
15. Plum F., Posner J.B. (1980). *The diagnosis of stupor and coma* (3rd ed.). Philadelphia: F.A. Davis.
16. Conn P.M. (1995). *Neuroscience in medicine* (pp. 232–235), Philadelphia: J.B. Lippincott.
17. Rhoades R.A., Tanner G.A. (1996). *Medical physiology* (pp. 132–133), Boston: Little, Brown.
18. Samuels M.A. (1993). The evaluation of comatose patients. *Hospital Practice* 28 (3), 165–181.
19. Bates D. (1993). The management of medical coma. *Journal of Neurology, Neurosurgery, and Psychiatry* 56, 589–598.
20. Ingersoll G.L., Leyden D.B. (1987). The Glasgow coma scale for patients with head injuries. *Critical Care Nursing* 7 (5), 26.
21. Knight R.L. (1986). The Glasgow coma scale: Ten years later. *Critical Care Nursing* 6 (3):65.
22. Segatore M., Way C. (1992). The Glasgow coma scale: Time for change. *Heart and Lung* 21 (6), 548–557.
23. Wijdicks E.F.M. (1995). Determining brain death in adults. *Neurology* 45, 1003–1011.
24. Quality Standards Subcommittee of American Academy of Neurology. (1995). Practice parameters for determining brain death in adults. *Neurology* 45, 1012–1014.
25. Beecher H.K. (1968). A definition of irreversible coma: Report of the Ad Hoc Committee of the Harvard Medical School to examine the definition of brain death. *Journal of the American Medical Association* 237, 337–340.
26. Presidents Commission for the Study of Ethical Problems in Medicine and Biomedical and Behavioral Research. (1981). Guidelines for determination of death. *Neurology* 32, 395–399.

27. Celesia G.G. (1993). Persistent vegetative state. *Neurology* 43, 1457–1458.
28. Quality Standards Subcommittee of American Academy of Neurology (1995). Practice parameters: Assessment and management of patients with persistent vegetative state. *Neurology* 45, 1015–1018.
29. American Heart Association. (1996). *Heart stroke facts.* Dallas: American Heart Association.
30. Macabasco A.C., Hickman J.L. (1995). Thrombolytic therapy for brain attack. *Journal of Neuroscience Nursing* 27 (3), 138–149.
31. Bronner L.L., Kaner D.S., Manson J.E. (1995). Primary prevention of stroke. *New England Journal of Medicine* 333 (21), 1392–1400.
32. Gorelick P.B. (1987). Alcohol and stroke. *Current Concepts in Cerebrovascular Disease* 21 (5), 21.
33. Levine S.R., Welch K.M.A. (1987). Cocaine and stroke. *Current Concepts in Cerebrovascular Disease* 22 (5), 25.
34. Blank-Reid C. (1996). How to have a stroke at an early age: The effects of crack, cocaine and other illicit drugs. *Journal of Neuroscience Nursing* 28 (1), 19–27.
35. Chimowitz M.L. (1992). Clinical spectrum and natural history of cerebrovascular occlusive disease. In Awad IA (Ed.). *Neurosurgical topics: Cerebrovascular occlusive disease and brain ischemia* (pp. 117–134). Cleveland: AANS.
36. American Heart Association Ad Hoc Committee. (1994). Guidelines for management of transient ischemic attacks. *Circulation* 89, 2950–2965.
37. American Heart Association Ad Hoc Committee. (1995). Guidelines for carotid endartectomy. *Stroke* 26, 188–121.
38. Zambramski J.M., Anson J.A. (1992). Diagnostic evaluation of ischemic cerebrovascular disease. In Awad I.A. (Ed.). *Neurosurgical topics: Cerebrovascular occlusive disease and brain ischemia* (pp. 73–101). Cleveland: AANS.
39. Adams H.P. (Chair). (1994). Guidelines for the management of patients with acute ischemic stroke: A statement for healthcare professionals from a special writing group of the Stroke Council, American Heart Association. *Stroke* 25 (9), 1901–1914.
40. Adams H.P. (Chair). (1996). Guidelines for thrombolytic therapy of acute stroke: A supplement to the guidelines for the management of patients with acute ischemic stroke: A statement for healthcare professionals from the Special Writing Group of the Stroke Council, American Heart Association. *Circulation* 94, 1167–1174.
41. Albers G.W. (1997). Management of acute ischemic stroke: An update for primary care physicians. *Western Journal of Medicine* 166, 253–262.
42. Cook H.A. (1991). Aneurysmal subarachnoid hemorrhage: Neurosurgical frontiers and nursing challenges. *AACN Clinical Issues in Critical Care* 2:665–675.
43. Schievink W.I. (1997). Intracranial aneurysms. *New England Journal of Medicine* 336 (1), 28–39.
44. Mayberg M.R. (Chair). (1994). Guidelines for the management of aneurysmal subarachnoid hemorrhage: A statement for healthcare professionals from a Special Writing Group of the Stroke Council, American Heart Association. *Stroke* 25 (11), 2315--2327.
45. Sawin P.D., Loftus C.M. (1997). Diagnosis of spontaneous subarachnoid hemorrhage. *American Family Physician,* 55 (1), 145–155.
46. McNair N. (1988). Arteriovenous malformations. *Critical Care Nursing* 8 (4), 35–40.
47. Bronstein K.S., Popovich J.M., Stewart-Amidei C. (1991). Promoting stroke recovery: A research based approach for nurses (p. 200). St. Louis: C.V. Mosby.
48. Gresham G.E., Duncan P.W., Stason W.B., et al. (1995). *Post-stroke rehabilitation: Clinical practice guidelines,* no. 16. AHCPR publication No. 95–0662. Rockville, MD: U.S. Department of Health and Human Services, Public Health Services, Agency for Health Care Policy and Research.
49. White R.J., Likavec M.J. (1992). The diagnosis and initial management of head injury. *New England Journal of Medicine* 327 (21), 1507–1511.
50. Jennett B. (1996). Epidemiology of head injury. *Journal of Neurology, Neurosurgery, and Psychiatry* 60, 362–369.
51. Chestnut R.M. (1995). Secondary brain insults after head injury: Clinical perspectives. *New Horizons* 3 (3), 366–375.
52. Teasdale G.M. (1995). Head injury. *Journal of Neurology, Neurosurgery, and Psychiatry* 58, 526–539.
53. Weinstein L. (1985). Bacterial meningitis: Specific etiologic diagnosis on the basis of distinctive epidemiologic, pathogenetic, and clinical features. *Medical Clinics of North America* 69 (2), 219.
54. Quagliarello V., Scheld M. (1992). Bacterial meningitis: Pathogenesis, pathophysiology, and progress. *New England Journal of Medicine* 327, 864–872.
55. Saez-Llorens X., McCracken G.H. (1991). Mediators of meningitis: Therapeutic implications. *Hospital Practice* 26 (1A), 68–77.
56. Odio C.M., Faingelzight I., Paris M., et al. (1991). The beneficial effects of early dexamethasone administration in infants and children with bacterial meningitis. *New England Journal of Medicine* 324, 1525–1531.
57. Parker S.L., Tong T., Bolden S., Wingo P. (1997). Cancer statistics, 1997. *CA Cancer Journal for Clinicians* 47 (1), 8–9.
58. Black P.M. (1991). Brain tumors (second of two parts). *New England Journal of Medicine* 324, 1555–1564.
59. Black P.M. (1991). Brain tumors (first of two parts). *New England Journal of Medicine* 324, 1471–1476.
60. Ransohoff J., Koslow M., Cooper P.R. (1991). Cancer of the central nervous system and pituitary. In Hollieb A.I., Fink D.J., Murphy G.P. (Eds.). *American Cancer Society textbook of clinical oncology* (pp. 229–237). Atlanta: American Cancer Society.
61. Mosewich R.K., So E.L. (1996). The clinical approach to classification of seizures and epileptic syndromes. *Mayo Clinic Proceedings* 71, 405–441.
62. Freeman J.M. (1992). What have we have learned from febrile seizures? *Pediatric Annals* 21 (6), 355–361.
63. Commission on Classification and Terminology of the International League Against Epilepsy. (1981). Proposal for revised clinical and electroencephalographic classification of epileptic seizures. *Epilepsia* 22, 489–501.
64. Commission on Classification and Terminology of the International League Against Epilepsy. (1989). Proposal for revised classification of epilepsies and epileptic syndromes. *Epilepsia* 30, 389–399.
65. Schachter S.C., Yerby M.S. (1997). Management of epilepsy. *Postgraduate Medicine* 101 (2), 133–153.
66. Brodie M.J., Dichter M.A. (1996). Antiepileptic drugs. *New England Journal of Medicine* 334 (3), 168–175.
67. Dichter M.A., Brodie M.J. (1996). New antiepileptic drugs. *New England Journal of Medicine* 334 (24), 1583–1589.
68. Engel J. (1996). Surgery for seizures. *New England Journal of Medicine* 334 (10), 647–652.
69. Cascino G.D. (1996). Generalized convulsive status epilepticus. *New England Journal of Medicine* 71, 787–792.
70. Morrison-Borgorad M., Phelps C., Buckholtz N. (1996). Alzheimer disease research comes of age. *Journal of the American Medical Association* 277 (10), 837–840.
71. Hyman B.T., Van Hoesen G.W., Kromer I., et al. (1986). Understanding the memory loss in Alzheimer's disease.

American Journal of Alzheimer's Care and Related Disorders 1, 18.
72. van Duijn C.M. (1996). Epidemiology of the dementias: recent developments and new approaches. *Journal of Neurology, Neurosurgery, and Psychiatry* 60, 478–488.
73. Lendon C.L., Ashall F., Goate A.M. (1996). Exploring the etiology of Alzheimer's disease using molecular genetics. *Journal of the American Medical Association* 277, 825–831.
74. Matteson M.A., McConnell E.S. (1988). *Gerontological nursing* (pp. 249–254). Philadelphia: J.B. Lippincott.
75. U.S. Department of Health and Human Services. (1996). *Recognition and initial assessment of Alzheimer's disease and related disorders* (AHCPR Publication No. 97-0702). Washington D.C.: Public Health Service, Agency for Health Care Policy and Research.
76. Morris J.C. (1997). Alzheimer's disease: A review of clinical assessment and management issues. *Geriatrics* 52 (Suppl 2), S22–25.
77. Rappaport E.B. (1987). Iatrogenic Creutzfeldt-Jakob disease. *Neurology* 37, 1520.
78. Martin J.B. (1987). Huntington's disease: Pathogenesis and management. *New England Journal of Medicine* 315, 1267.

ADDITIONAL READINGS

Albers G.W. (1997). Management of acute ischemic stroke. *Western Journal of Medicine* 166, 253–262.

Annegers J.F., Rocca W.A., Hauser W.A. (1996). Causes of epilepsy: Contributions of the Rochester Epidemiology Project. *Mayo Clinic Proceedings* 71, 570–575.

Barnett H.J.M., Eliasziw M., Meldrum H.E. (1995). Drugs and surgery in the prevention of ischemic stroke. *New England Journal of Medicine* 332 (4), 238–248.

Bricker M.E. (1996). Cardioembolic stroke. *American Journal of Medicine* 100, 465–473.

Bonstein K.S. (1996). Epidemiology and classification of brain tumors. *Critical Care Nursing Clinics of North America* 7 (1), 79–88.

Brummel-Smith K. (1995). Management of the poststroke patient. *Hospital Practice* 30 (2), 43–51.

Chestnut R.M. (1995). Medical management of severe head injury: Present and future. *New Horizon* 3 (3), 581–593.

Costa P.T. Jr., Williams T.F., Albert M.S, et al. for the Agency for Health Care Policy and Research. (1996). *Recognition and initial assessment of Alzheimer's disease and related dementias.* Clinical Practice Guideline No. 19, AHCPR Publication No. 96–0702. Rockville, MD: U.S. Department of Health and Human Services, Public Health Service.

Cummings J.L. (1993) The mental status examination. *Hospital Practice* 28 (5), 56–68.

Davis M., Lucatorto M. (1992). The false localizing signs of increased intracranial pressure. *Journal of Neuroscience Nursing* 24 (5), 245–550.

Feinberg W.M. (1994). Guidelines for management of transient ischemic attacks. *Heart Disease and Stroke* Sept/Oct, 275–283.

Fischer M. (1997). Characterizing the target of acute stroke therapy. *Stroke* 28 (4), 866–872.

Fishman RA. (1975). Brain edema. *New England Journal of Medicine* 293 (14), 706.

Miller J.D. (1993). Head injury. *Journal of Neurology, Neurosurgery, and Psychiatry* 56, 440–447.

Working Goup on Emergency Brain Resuscitation. Emergency brain resuscitation. *Annals of Internal Medicine* 122, 622–627.

Zupanc M.L. (1996). Update on epilepsy in pediatric patients. *Mayo Clinic Proceedings* 71, 899–916.

CHAPTER 39

Alterations in Motor Function

Robin Curtis and Sylvia McDonald

Effective motor function requires that muscles move and that the mechanics of their movement be programmed in a manner that provides for smooth and coordinated movement. In some cases, purposeless and disruptive movements can be almost as disabling as relative or complete absence of movement. This chapter addresses control of motor function, alterations in function of the neuromuscular unit, alterations in pyramidal or extrapyramidal function, and spinal cord injury. Although motor function relies on continuous input from sensory neurons, the focus of this chapter is on the efferent output that controls movement. Spinal cord injury is presented as an example of a condition that affects multiple motor systems.

Control of Motor Function

After you have completed this section of the chapter, you should be able to meet the following objectives:

- Define a *motor unit* and characterize its mechanism of controlling muscle movement
- Define the function of the following muscle types: extensors, flexors, adductors, abductors, rotators, agonists, antagonists, and synergists
- Contrast the functions of the pyramidal and extrapyramidal systems
- Construct a movement model for voluntary muscle movement that begins in the motor cortex and terminates in the muscle fibers of a motor unit

Movement begins in utero at about 21 weeks of gestation with the quickening of the fetus, and the capability for some coordinated movement is present at birth. Maturation of the spinal cord and brain circuitry during the first year or two of life allows the child to defy the force of gravity and learn to sit, then stand, and in rapid sequence, master the skills of walking, running, jumping, and climbing.

Motor Function

Motor function, whether it involves walking, running, or precise finger movements, requires movement and maintenance of posture. Posture can be described as the active muscular resistance to the displacement of the body by gravity or acceleration.[1] The two functions are intricately related, and it is virtually impossible to successfully perform one without the other. Purposeful movement of the hands and feet is accomplished only by first placing the body and the arm or leg in a stable posture and appropriate position. The structures that control posture and movement are located throughout the neuromuscular system. The system consists of the neuromuscular unit, which includes the motoneurons, the myoneural junction, and the muscle fibers; the spinal cord, which contains the basic reflex circuitry for posture and movement; and the descending pathways from the brain stem circuits, the cerebellum, basal ganglia, and the motor cortex.

Muscle Groups

Skeletal muscle is composed of muscle cells, or fibers, which contain the interacting actin and myosin filaments that generate the contractile force required for movement (see Chapter 1). In terms of function, muscles can be classified as *extensors,* muscles that increase the angle of a joint, or *flexors,* muscles that decrease the angle of a joint. In the legs, groups of extensor muscles work together to resist gravity and function to maintain the upright posture and provide locomotion power. In general, flexor muscle groups assist gravity, participate in withdrawal reflexes, and provide the more delicate aspects of manipulation. Other muscle groups act roughly in pairs: *adductors* versus *abductors,* which move a part toward or away from the midline of the body, and *rotators,* which work in pairs to rotate a part of the limb, the trunk, or the head around each part's longitudinal axis. Many muscles participate in more than one of these functions.

Coordinated movement requires the action of two or more muscle groups: *agonists,* which promote a movement; *antagonists,* which oppose it; and *synergists,* which assist the agonist muscles by stabilizing a joint or contributing additional force to the movement. Some simple types of movement require only a burst of energy from an agonist muscle group. Other types of movements, such as self-terminated actions, require a smooth sequence of movements: agonist, antagonist, and co-contraction of agonist and antagonist to stop and stabilize the end of the movement. Agonist and antagonist contractions are programmed by higher brain centers to fit the situation. Simple movements are programmed before they start so that the movement proceeds from start to finish without modification. Self-terminated movements are more complex and are programmed to start and are then modified as they proceed.

The Motor Unit

The neurons that control motor function are referred to as *motoneurons* or sometimes as *alpha motoneurons.* A motor unit consists of one motoneuron and the group of muscle fibers it innervates within a muscle. The motoneurons supplying a motor unit are located in the ventral horn of the spinal cord and are called lower motoneurons (LMNs). The synapse between an LMN and the muscle fibers of a motor unit is called the *neuromuscular junction.* Upper motoneurons (UMNs), which exert control over LMNs, project from the motor strip in the cerebral cortex to the ventral horn and are fully contained within the central nervous system (CNS) (Fig. 39–1).

Axons of the LMNs exit the spinal cord at each segment to innervate skeletal muscle cells, including those of the limbs, back, abdomen, and chest. Each LMN undergoes multiple branching, making it possible for a single LMN to innervate 10 to 2000 muscle cells. In general, large muscles—those containing hundreds or thousands of muscle cells and providing gross motor movement—have large motor units. This sharply contrasts with those that control the hand, tongue, and eye movements, for which the motor units are small and permit very discrete control.

Basic to the understanding of motor control is the concept of the motor unit—the LMN and the muscle fibers it innervates—functioning as a unit. All muscles contain thousands of muscle fibers and are innervated by fewer LMNs. When the LMN develops an action potential, all of the muscle fibers in the motor unit it innervates develop action potentials, causing them to contract simultaneously. Thus, an LMN and the muscle fibers it innervates function as a single unit—the basic unit of motor control. All neurally controlled motor functions involve the differential use of combinations of motor units in agonist and antagonist muscle around a joint, manipulating the resultant joint angle. Movement involves some joints being held stable and the joint angle of other joints being changed.

Most skeletal muscle groups fall into three categories based on differences in the chemistry of their contractile proteins and their source of energy. The first type, the slow-twitch fibers, have many mitochondria, depend on bloodborne oxygen for energy, and are slow to fatigue. The second type, the fast-twitch fatigable fibers, depend on muscle glycogen stores that can be rapidly depleted. The third type, the fast-twitch fatigue-resistant fibers, rely on both mechanisms for energy. The antigravity postural muscles that use slow-twitch fibers are slow to fatigue. Muscles used for more rapid movements such as jumping and throwing are rich in large, powerful, but rapidly fatiguing fast-twitch motor units.

Most muscles contain motor units with most or all of these muscle fiber types, but the proportions may vary with muscle function. For example, postural muscles and delicate distal flexor muscles are predominantly slow-type fibers, whereas the large, proximal limb muscles such as the gastrocnemius are mixed, with many fast-twitch fatigable and fast-twitch fatigue-resistant fiber motor units that can provide brief, high power.

The muscle fiber members for each motor unit are uniform as to muscle fiber type. Thus, motor units usually fall into the same categories of slow-twitch, fast-

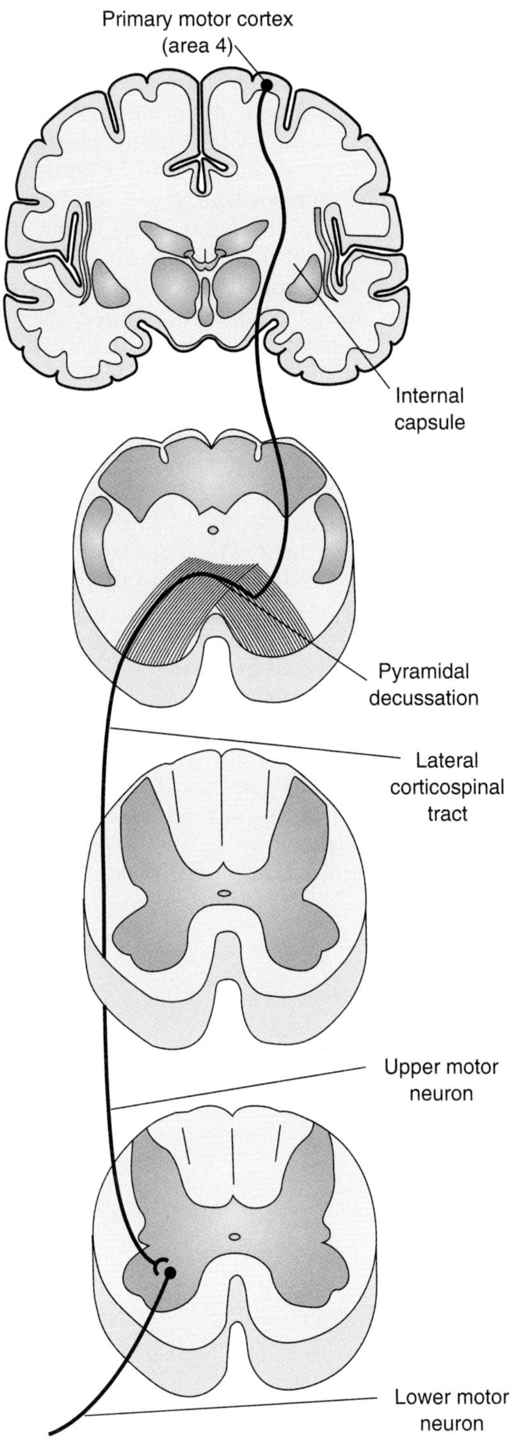

Figure 39–1
The corticospinal tract. The long axons of motoneurons originating in the primary motor cortex descend through the telencephalon via the internal capsule and traverse the brain stem in a ventral path through the cerebral peduncles and the pyramids. The axons cross in the lower medulla (pyramidal decussation) to the opposite side and continue as the corticospinal tract in the spinal cord, where they synapse on motoneurons and interneurons in the ventral horns. (Modified from Kandel E.R., & Schwartz J.H. *Principles of neural science* [2nd ed]. New York: Elsevier, 1985.)

twitch fatigable, and fast-twitch fatigue-resistant. The group of LMNs in the spinal cord ventral horn that have muscle fibers in a particular muscle are called a motoneuron pool. When reflex or descending systems activate such a pool, the first motor units to fire are the slow-twitch units. With stronger activation, the fast-twitch fatigue-resistant units begin firing, and the last to be recruited are the fast-twitch fatigable units.

The motor system is designed to minimize participation of the forebrain in details of movements, permitting the forebrain to specialize in the planning and motor learning required for precise control of motor function. The recruitment order of slow before fast, fatigue-resistant before fast fatigable motor units provides the automatic sequence for increasing muscle contraction power and for initial, delicate control.

The Motor Cortex

Delicate, skillful, intentional movement of distal and especially flexor muscles of the limbs and the speech apparatus is initiated and controlled from the motor cortex located in the posterior part of the frontal lobe. It consists of the primary, premotor, and supplementary motor cortex (Fig. 39–2).[2,3] These areas receive information from the thalamus and somesthetic cortex and, indirectly, from the cerebellum and basal ganglia. The *primary motor cortex* (area 4), also called the *motor strip*, is located on the rostral surface and adjacent portions of the central sulcus. The primary motor cortex controls discrete muscle movement sequences and is the first level of descending control for precise movements. Discrete lesions within the most posterior part of the primary motor cortex can result in profound weakness in specific distal flexor muscle groups and permanent inability to perform delicate manipulative motor patterns on the opposite side of the body or face. Lesions restricted to the more anterior part of the motor strip result in weakness of larger limb, girdle, and axial muscles.

The *premotor cortex* (areas 6 and 8), which is located just anterior to the primary motor cortex, sends some fibers into the corticospinal tract but mainly innervates the primary motor strip. A movement pattern to accomplish a particular objective, such as throwing a ball or picking up a fork, is programmed by the prefrontal association cortex and associated thalamic nuclei. The "program" for the movement pattern includes the muscle contractional sequences for complex distal manipulation and for the larger preparative and supportive actions of whole limb and limb girdle muscles.

The *supplementary motor cortex,* which contains representations of all parts of the body, is located on the medial surface of the hemisphere (areas 6 and 8) in the premotor region. It contains representation of all parts of the body. It is intimately involved in the performance of complex skillful movements that involve both sides of the body. Bilateral lesions cause long-lasting loss (*i.e.,* akinesis) of movements involving both hands or both feet and can result in long-term loss of speech (*i.e.,* mutism).

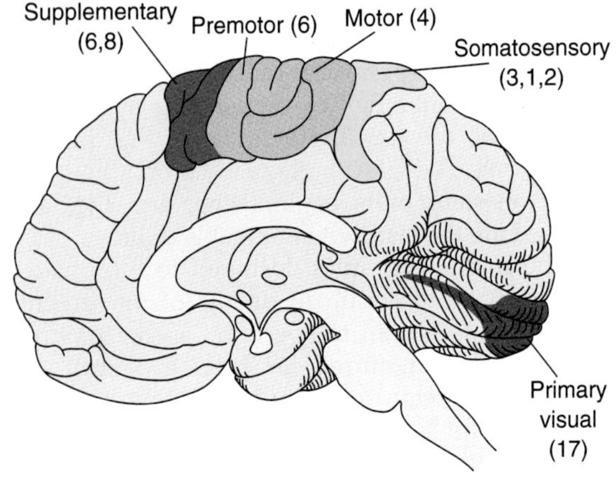

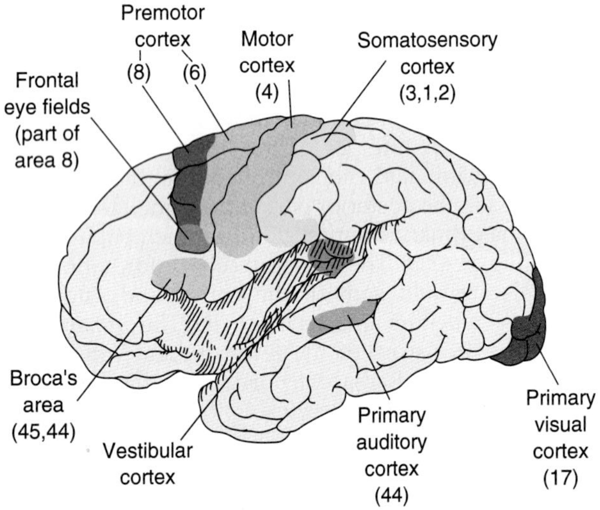

Figure 39–2
Primary motor cortex. (**Top**) The location of the primary, premotor, and supplementary cortex on the medial surface of the brain. (**Bottom**) The location of the primary and premotor cortex on the lateral surface of the brain. (Courtesy of Carole Russell Hilmer, C.M.I.)

The neurons in the primary motor cortex are arranged in a somatotopic array or distorted map of the body called the *motor homunculus* (Fig. 39–3). This map, which shows the degree of representation of the neurons that control voluntary movement of a particular body part, was prepared by Penfield and Rasmussen.[4] The mapping was done by electrically stimulating the brain of persons who were undergoing brain surgery. The body parts that require the greatest dexterity have the greatest cortical areas devoted to them. More than one half of the primary motor cortex is concerned with controlling the muscles of the hands, of facial expression, and muscles of speech.[2]

The primary motor cortex is very thick. It contains many layers of pyramid-shaped output neurons that project to the same side of the cortex (*i.e.,* premotor and somesthetic areas), project to the opposite side of the cortex, or descend to subcortical structures such as the basal ganglia and thalamus. The large pyramidal cells located in the fifth layer project to the brain stem and spinal cord. The axons of these UMNs project through the subcortical white matter and internal capsule to the deep surface of the brain stem, through the ventral bulge of the pons, and to the ventral surface of the medulla, where they form a ridge or pyramid (see Fig. 39–1). At the junction between the medulla and cervical spinal cord, 80% or more of the UMN axons cross the midline to form the lateral *corticospinal* tract in the lateral white matter of the spinal cord. This tract extends throughout the spinal cord, with roughly 50% of the fibers terminating in the cervical segments, 20% in the thoracic segments, and 30% in the lumbosacral segments. Most of the remaining uncrossed fibers travel down the ventral column of the cord, mainly to cervical levels, where they cross and innervate contralateral LMNs.

Monosynaptic innervation of LMNs by UMNs of the primary motor cortex only occurs for the most distal muscles involved with delicate manipulative skills, such as those of the hands and fingers, tongue, mouth, and pharynx. For LMNs of other muscles, the connection is multisynaptic and less discrete. As the UMN axons pass along their long pathways, collateral branches move out and innervate regions of the basal ganglia, the thalamus, the brain stem, and nuclei that project into the cerebellum. The cerebellum matches the temporal smoothness aspect of the ongoing movement against very rapid proprioceptive feedback from the actual movement and sends error signals back to the thalamus and motor

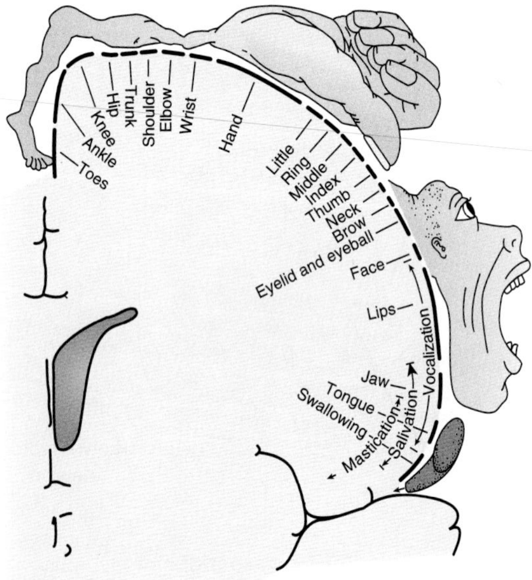

Figure 39–3
Representation of the relative extent of motor cortical area 4 devoted to muscles of the various body regions. Medial surface is at the left, lateral fissure is at the right, with pharyngeal and laryngeal muscle representation extending toward the insula. (Penfield E., & Rasmussen T. [1968]. *The cerebral cortex in man: A clinical study of localization of function.* New York: Macmillan)

cortex for corrective modifications of the ongoing movement. Similarly, sensory feedback to the basal ganglia results in error-correcting feedback for supportive and background aspects of the movement. Slower sensory feedback from the somesthetic cortex permits error correction on the next trial. Ongoing error correction becomes less and less important for well-learned movements that can proceed without sensory feedback.

Movement Model

The performance of skilled motor movements can be represented by the movement model depicted in Figure 39–4. This model involves the use of a repertoire of inherited and learned neural interactions that contribute skill, grace, and temporal smoothness to the movement.

A movement sequence, such as moving a body part to a precise point in three-dimensional space involves the higher-order functions of the primary motor, premotor, and supplementary motor cortex. The plan is programed into a sequence of component actions, a learned function performed by the premotor cortex. Complex bilateral movements require the function of the supplementary motor cortex, with the precise control of distal muscle movements being provided by the primary motor cortex. Descending axons from the motor cortex project to the brain stem or spinal cord, where they directly or indirectly innervate LMNs that supply the muscle fibers. The basal ganglia provide the axial and proximal support required for the movement. Continuous sensory feedback from the involved muscles and from all sensory systems are matched against the model, and adjustments for errors in timing or in sequence are continuously relayed from the cerebellum, the basal ganglia, and the primary sensory cortex back to the motor cortex. The programmed movement, which is continuously corrected and adjusted, progresses until the precise goal is accomplished.

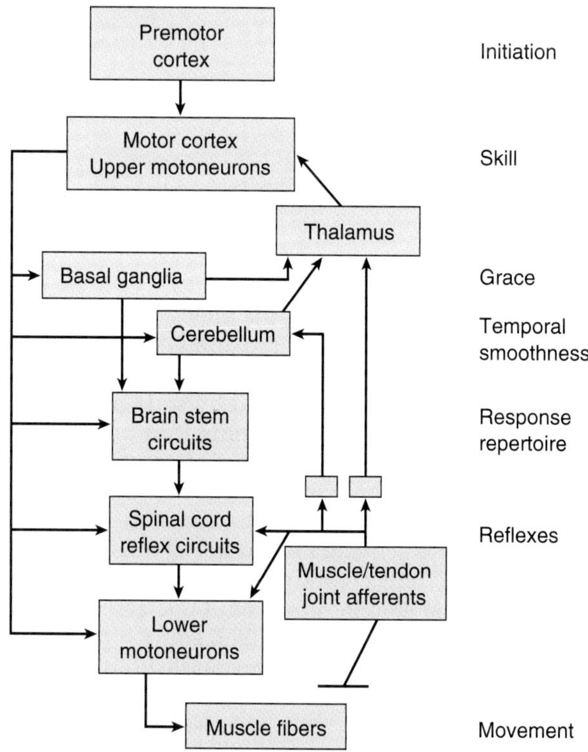

Figure 39–4
Diagram of neural pathways for control of motor function.

The efficiency of the entire motor system depends on optimally functioning motor units on a background of muscle tone provided by the stretch reflex and vestibular system input to maintain stable postural support. The program for motor function involves parallel processing and ongoing interactive communication between these functions. A highly skilled movement is beautiful to behold, but it can be easily damaged or distorted because of the necessary complexity of its control.

Pyramidal and Extrapyramidal Systems

By convention, motor tracts are often classified as belonging to one of two motor systems: the *pyramidal* and *extrapyramidal systems.* The pyramidal system consists of the motor pathways originating in the motor cortex and terminating in the brain stem (*i.e.*, corticobulbar fibers) and the spinal cord (*i.e.*, corticospinal fibers). The corticospinal fibers traverse the ventral surface of the medulla in a bundle called the *pyramid* before decussating or crossing to the opposite side of the brain at the medulla–spinal cord junction, hence the name *pyramidal system.* Other fibers from the cortex and basal ganglia also project to the brain stem reticular formation and reticulospinal systems, following a more ancient pathway to LMNs of proximal and extensor muscles. These fibers do not decussate in the pyramids, hence the name *extrapyramidal system.*

The pyramidal and extrapyramidal systems have different effects on muscle tone. The pyramidal system is largely excitatory; it provides control of delicate muscle movement. The extrapyramidal system provides the more crude, background supportive movement patterns. In terms of actual function, the pyramidal and extrapyramidal systems do not function independently, but the concept of two separate systems is helpful in understanding motor function. After severe damage to the pyramidal system, the crude movements and slurred speech that remain result from extrapyramidal system function.

Disorders of Motor Function

Disorders of motor function include skeletal muscle weakness and paralysis, which result from lesions in the voluntary motor pathways, including the UMNs of the corticospinal and corticobulbar tracts or the LMNs that leave the CNS and travel by way of the peripheral nerve to the muscle. Muscle tone, which is a necessary component of muscle movement, is a function of the muscle spindle (myotatic) system (see Chapter 37) and the extrapyramidal system, which monitors and buffers input to the LMNs by way of the multisynaptic pathways.

Disorders of Muscle Tone

Muscle tone is the normal tension in a muscle as evidenced by the resistance to passive movement around a joint. Disorders of skeletal muscle tone are characteristic of many nervous system pathologies. Any interruption of the myotatic reflex circuit by peripheral nerve injury, pathology of the neuromuscular junction and of skeletal muscle fibers, damage to the corticospinal system, or injury to the spinal cord or spinal nerve root results in disturbance of muscle tone. Muscle tone may be described as less than normal (*i.e., hypotonia*), absent (*i.e., flaccidity*), or excessive (*i.e., hypertonia, rigidity, spasticity,* or *tetany*). The latter three terms are extremes of hypertonia that include other distinguishing features.

Paresis and Paralysis

The word *plegia* is Greek for a blow, a stroke, or paralysis. Terms used to describe the extent and anatomic location of motor damage are *paralysis,* meaning loss of movement, and *paresis,* implying weakness or incomplete loss of muscle function. The term *plegia* is substituted for paresis if the abnormality is more severe. *Monoparesis* or *monoplegia* results from the destruction of pyramidal UMN innervation of one limb; *hemiparesis or hemiplegia,* both limbs on one side; *diparesis or diplegia* or *paraparesis or paraplegia,* both upper or lower limbs; and *tetraparesis or tetraplegia,* also called *quadriparesis or quadriplegia,* all four limbs (Fig. 39–5). Paresis or paralysis can be further designated as of upper motoneuron origin or lower motoneuron origin.

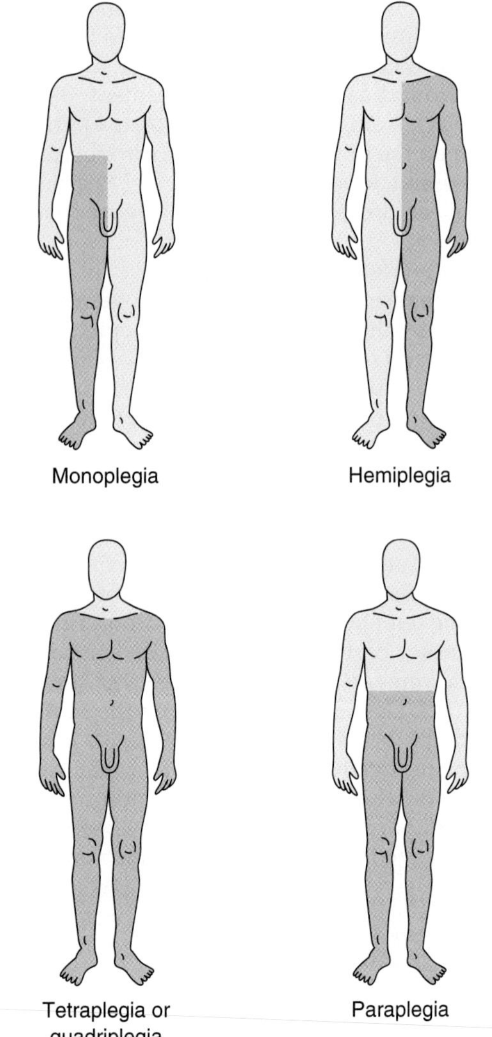

Figure 39–5
Areas of the body affected by monoplegia, hemiplegia, tetra- or quadriplegia, and paraplegia. The *shaded area* shows the extent of motor and sensory loss.

Upper Motoneuron Lesions

An UMN lesion can involve the motor cortex, the internal capsule, or other brain structures through which the corticospinal or corticobulbar tracts descend, or the spinal cord. When the lesion is at or above the level of the pyramids, paralysis affects structures on the opposite side of the body. In UMN disorders involving injury to the L1 level or above, there is an immediate profound weakness and loss of fine skilled voluntary lower limb movement, reduced bowel and bladder control, and diminished sexual functioning, followed by an exaggeration of muscle tone. With UMN damage above C5, upper limb movement is also affected.

With UMN lesions, the LMN spinal reflexes remain intact, but communication and control from higher brain centers are lost. Descending excitatory influences from the pyramidal system and some descending inhibitory influences from other cortical regions are lost after injury, resulting in immediate weakness accompanied by the loss of control of delicate skilled movements. After several weeks, this weakness becomes converted to hypertonicity or spasticity which is manifested by increased resistance to passive movement (*i.e.,* stiffness) of a joint in which the initial resistance to movement quickly fades away. The spasticity is often greatest in the flexor muscles of the upper limbs and extensor muscles of the lower limbs. Sometimes, a lesion of the pyramidal tract is less severe and results in a relatively minor degree of weakness. In this case, the finer and more skilled movements are most severely impaired.

Clonus is the rhythmic contraction and alternate relaxation of a limb that is caused by suddenly stretching a muscle and gently maintaining it in the stretched position. It is seen in the hypertonia of spasticity associated with UMN lesions. It is caused by an oscillating stimulation of the muscle spindles that occurs when the spindle fibers are activated by an initial muscle stretch. This results in reflex contraction of the muscle and unloading of the spindle fibers with decreased afferent activity. The reduced spindle fiber activity causes the muscle to relax, which causes the spindle fiber to stretch again, and the cycle starts over.

Lower Motoneuron Lesions

In contrast to UMN lesions in which the spinal reflexes remain intact, LMN disorders disrupt communication between the muscle and all neural input from spinal cord reflexes, including the stretch reflex, which maintains muscle tone.

Infection or irritation of the cell body of the LMN or its axon can lead to hyperexcitability, which causes spontaneous contractions of the muscle units. These can be observed as twitching and squirming movements on the muscle surface, a condition called *fasciculations.* Toxic agents, such as the tetanus toxin of *Clostridium tetani,* produce extreme hyperexcitability of the LMN, which results in continuous firing at maximum rate. The resultant sustained contraction of the muscles is called *tetany.* Tetany of muscles on both sides of a joint produces immobility or tetanic paralysis. When a virus, such as the poliomyelitis virus, attacks an LMN, it first irritates the LMN, causing fasciculations to occur. These fasciculations are often followed by death of LMNs. Weakness and severe muscle wasting or denervation atrophy result. If muscles are totally denervated, total weakness and total loss of reflexes, called *flaccid paralysis,* occurs.

With complete LMN lesions, the muscles of the affected limbs, bowel, bladder, and genital areas become atonic, and it is impossible to elicit contraction by stretching the tendons. One of the outstanding features of LMN lesions is the profound development of muscle atrophy. Damage to LMN with or without spinal cord damage, often called *peripheral nerve injury,* may occur at any level of the spinal cord. For example, a C7 peripheral nerve injury leads to LMN hand weakness only. All segments below the level of injury that have intact LMNs manifest UMN signs. Usually, injury to the spinal cord at the T12 level or below results in LMN injury and flaccid paralysis to all areas below the level of injury. This occurs because the spinal cord ends at the T12 to L1 level, and from this level, the spinal roots of the LMNs continue caudally in the vertebral canal as part of the cauda equina.

In summary, motor function involves the neuromuscular unit, spinal cord circuitry, brain stem neurons, the cerebellum, the basal ganglia, and the motor cortex. A motor unit consists of one LMN and the group of muscle fibers it innervates within the muscle. Delicate, skillful, intentional movement of distal and especially flexor muscles of the limbs and the speech apparatus is initiated and controlled from the motor cortex located in the posterior part of the frontal lobe. It consists of the primary, premotor, and supplementary motor cortex. These areas receive information from the thalamus and somesthetic cortex and, indirectly, from the cerebellum and basal ganglia. The UMNs in the motor cortex send their axons through the subcortical white matter and internal capsule and the deep surface of the brain stem to the ventral surface to the opposite side of the medulla, where they form a pyramid before crossing the midline to form the lateral corticospinal tract in the spinal cord. Skillful movement patterns are planned in the prefrontal cortex, a sequential model is organized in the premotor cortex, and it is carried out by the primary motor cortex. If the UMN system is severely damaged, delicate and skillful movement is lost, but crude movement still can be made using extrapyramidal systems.

Alterations in musculoskeletal function include weakness resulting from lesions of voluntary UMN pathways of the corticobulbar and corticospinal tracts and the LMN of the peripheral nerves. Muscle tone is maintained through the combined function of the muscle spindle system and the extrapyramidal system that monitors and buffers UMN innervation of the LMNs. Hypotonia is a condition of less than normal muscle tone, and hypertonia or spasticity is a condition of excessive tone. Paresis refers to weakness in muscle function, and paralysis refers to a loss of muscle movement. UMN lesions produce spastic paralysis, and LMN lesions produce flaccid paralysis. Damage to the UMNs of the corticospinal and corticobulbar tracts is a common component of stroke.

Skeletal Muscle and Peripheral Nerve Disorders

After you have completed this section of the chapter, you should be able to meet the following objectives:

- Describe muscle atrophy and differentiate between disuse and degenerative atrophy
- Explain the causes of muscle atrophy
- Describe the pathology associated with Duchenne's muscular dystrophy
- Relate the clinical manifestations of myasthenia gravis to its cause
- Trace the steps in regeneration of an injured peripheral nerve
- Describe the manifestation of peripheral nerve root injury due to a ruptured intervertebral disk
- Compare the cause and manifestations of peripheral mononeuropathies with peripheral polyneuropathies

Skeletal Muscle Disorders

Disorders of skeletal muscle groups involve atrophy and dystrophy. *Atrophy* describes a decrease in muscle mass. *Muscular dystrophy* is a primary disorder of muscle tissue and is characterized by defect in the muscle fibers.

Muscle Atrophy

Maintenance of muscle strength requires relatively frequent movements against resistance. Reduced use results in muscle atrophy, which is characterized by a reduction in the diameter of the muscle fibers because of a loss of protein filaments. When a normally innervated muscle is not used for long periods, the muscle cells shrink in diameter, and although the muscle cells do not die, they lose much of their contractile protein and become weakened. This is called *disuse atrophy*, and it occurs with conditions such as immobilization and chronic illness.

The most extreme examples of muscle atrophy are found in persons with disorders that deprive muscles of their innervation. This form is called *denervation atrophy*. During early embryonic development, outgrowing skeletal nerves innervate partially mature muscle cells. If the developing muscle cells are not innervated, they do not mature and eventually die. In the process of innervation, randomly contracting muscle cells become enslaved by the innervating neurons, and from then on, the muscle cell contracts only when stimulated by that particular neuron. If the LMN dies or its axon is destroyed, the skeletal muscle cell is again free of neural domination. When this happens, it begins to have temporary spontaneous contractions, called *fibrillations*, of its own. It also begins to lose its contractile proteins and, after several months, if not reinnervated, it degenerates.

If a peripheral motor neuron is crushed and its endoneurial tube remains intact, regenerating axons can grow down the connective tissue tube to reinnervate the muscle cell. If the nerve is cut, however, scar tissue between the cut ends of the endoneurial tube reduces the likelihood of reinnervation by the original axon, and muscle cell loss is likely to occur. If some intact LMN axons remain within the muscle, nearby denervated muscle cells apparently emit what is called a *trophic signal*, probably a chemical messenger, that signals intact axons to sprout and send outgrowing collaterals into the denervated area and recapture control of some of the denervated muscle fibers. The degree of axonal regeneration that occurs after injury to an LMN depends on the amount of scar tissue that develops at the site of injury and how quickly reinnervation occurs. If reinnervation occurs after the muscle cell has degenerated, no recovery is possible. Peripheral nerve section usually results in some loss of muscle cell function, which is experienced as weakness. Collateral sprout reinnervation results in enlarged motor units and therefore in a reduction in the precision of muscle control after recovery.

Muscular Dystrophy

Muscular dystrophy is a term applied to a number of genetic disorders that produce progressive deterioration of skeletal muscles because of mixed muscle cell hypertrophy, atrophy, and necrosis. They are primary diseases of muscle tissue and probably do not involve the nervous system. As the muscle undergoes necrosis, fat and connective tissue replace the muscle fibers, which increases muscle size and results in muscle weakness. The increase in muscle size resulting from connective tissue infiltration is called *pseudohypertrophy*. The muscle weakness is insidious in onset but continually progressive, varying with the type of disorder.

The most common form of the disease is *Duchenne's muscular dystrophy*, which has an incidence of about 3 cases per 100,000 persons. Duchenne's muscular dystrophy is inherited as a recessive single gene defect on the X chromosome and is transmitted from the mother to her male offspring (see Chapter 4).[5] A spontaneous (mutation) form may occur in females. Another form of dystrophy, *Becker's muscular dystrophy*, is similarly X-linked but manifests later in childhood or adolescence and has a slower course. The Duchenne's muscular dystrophy mutation results in a defective form of a very large protein associated with the muscle cell membrane, which fails to provide the normal attachment site for the contractile proteins. Regeneration of new muscle cells produces more defective cells.

In Duchenne's muscular dystrophy, the postural muscles of the hip and shoulder are affected first, and the child usually has no problems until about 3 years of age, when frequent falling begins to occur. Imbalances between agonist and antagonist muscles lead to abnormal postures and the development of contractures and joint immobility. Wheelchairs are usually needed at about 9 to 10 years of age.[6] Death from respiratory and cardiac muscle involvement usually occurs in young adulthood. About 70% of deaths result from respiratory causes alone.[6]

Observation of the child's voluntary movement and a complete family history provide important diagnostic data for the disease. Muscle biopsy, which shows a mixture of muscle cell degeneration and regeneration and reveals fat and scar tissue replacement; electromyograms; and serum levels of the enzyme creatine kinase (formerly called creatine phosphokinase), which leaks out of damaged muscle fibers, can be used to confirm the diagnosis. Gene probes are being developed for carrier detection and prenatal diagnosis.[7]

Management of the disease is directed toward maintaining ambulation and preventing deformities. Passive stretching, correct or counter posturing, and splints help to prevent deformities. Precautions should be taken to avoid respiratory infections. Although there have been exciting advances in identifying the gene and gene product involved in Duchenne's muscular dystrophy, there is no known cure.

Disorders of the Neuromuscular Junction

The transmission of impulses at the neuromuscular junction is mediated by the release of the neurotransmitter *acetylcholine* from the axon terminals. Acetylcholine binds to specific receptors in the end-plate region of the muscle fiber surface to cause muscle contraction. Studies suggest that there are more than 1 million binding sites per motor end-plate.[1]

Acetylcholine is active in the neuromuscular junction for only a brief period, during which an action potential is generated in the innervated muscle cell. Some of the transmitter diffuses out of the synapse, and the remaining transmitter is rapidly inactivated by an enzyme called *acetylcholinesterase*. This enzyme splits the acetylcholine molecule into choline and acetic acid. The choline is then transported back into the nerve terminal and reused in the synthesis of acetylcholine. The rapid inactivation of acetylcholine allows repeated muscle contractions and gradations of contractile force.

A number of drugs and agents can alter neuromuscular function by changing the release, inactivation, or receptor binding of acetylcholine. Curare acts on the postjunctional membrane of the motor end-plate to prevent the depolarizing effect of the neurotransmitter. Blocking of neuromuscular transmission by curare-type drugs is used during many types of surgical procedures to facilitate relaxation of involved musculature. Drugs such as physostigmine and neostigmine inhibit the action of acetylcholinesterase and allow acetylcholine released from the motoneuron to accumulate. These drugs are used in the treatment of myasthenia gravis. Toxins from the botulism organism produce paralysis by blocking acetylcholine release. Spores from the botulism organism may be found in soil-grown foods that are not cooked at temperatures of at least 100°C in home-canning procedures.

The organophosphates (*e.g.*, Malathion, parathion) that are used in some insecticides bind acetylcholinesterase to prevent the breakdown of acetylcholine. They produce excessive and prolonged acetylcholine action with a depolarization block of cholinergic receptors, including those of the neuromuscular junction.[8] The organophosphates are well absorbed from the skin, lungs, gut, and conjunctiva of the eye, making them particularly effective as insecticides but also potentially dangerous to humans. Malathion and certain other organophosphates are rapidly metabolized to inactive products in humans and are considered safe for sale to the general public. The sale of other insecticides, such as parathion, which is not effectively metabolized to inactive products, have been banned. Other organophosphate compounds were developed as nerve gases during World War I with similar and, if absorbed in high concentrations, lethal effects from depolarization block and loss of respiratory muscle function.

Myasthenia Gravis

Myasthenia gravis is a disorder of transmission at the neuromuscular junction that affects communication between the motoneuron and the innervated muscle cell. The incidence of myasthenia gravis in the United States is 50 to 125 cases per million persons.[9] The disease may occur at any age, but the peak incidence occurs between 20 and 30 years of age, and the disease is about three times more common in women than men. A smaller second peak occurs in later life and affects men more often than women. The disorder appears transiently and lasts for days to weeks in about 10% of infants born to mothers with myasthenia gravis.

Myasthenia gravis is thought to result from a decrease in acetylcholine receptor sites at the neuromuscular junction that leads to decreased muscle function. Evidence indicates that the reduction in acetylcholine receptors results from an autoimmune response.[9,10] Autoantibodies binding to acetylcholine receptors are found in most persons with the disease. This receptor antibody is thought to cause receptor degradation and inhibition of receptor synthesis. The exact mechanism that triggers the autoimmune response is unknown but is thought to be related to abnormal T-lymphocyte characteristics. About 75% of persons with myasthenia gravis also have thymic abnormalities, such as a thymoma (*i.e.*, thymus tumor) or thymic hyperplasia (*i.e.*, increased thymus weight from an increased number of thymus cells).[9]

The primary clinical manifestations of myasthenia gravis are weakness of the eye muscles, with ptosis (*i.e.*, drooping of the upper eyelids) and diplopia caused by weakness of the extraocular muscles. Neuromuscular and eyelid weakness can be checked after giving instructions to have the affected person firmly close his or her eyes. Normally, eyelashes are not seen with firm eye closure. In persons with myasthenia gravis, the eyelid muscles are weakened and the eyelashes often remain visible.[11] Extraocular muscle weakness can be tested by having the person maintain an upward gaze for 2 to 3 minutes while observations for eye muscle fatigue are being made.

The clinical course varies. The disease may progress from ocular muscle weakness to generalized weakness, including respiratory weakness. Chewing and swallowing may be difficult, and persons with the disease often choose to eat soft puddings and cereals rather than meats and hard fruit. Masticatory weakness can be checked by having the person repetitively open and close the jaw against resistance.[11] Weakness in limb movement is usually more pronounced in proximal than in distal parts of the extremity, so that climbing stairs and lifting objects are difficult. As the disease progresses, the muscles of the lower face are affected, causing speech impairment. When this happens, the person often supports the chin with one hand to assist in speaking. In most persons, symptoms are least evident when arising in the morning, but they grow worse with effort and as the day proceeds. General muscle weakness can be assessed by having the person continuously maintain a position such as holding the arms overhead or extending the fingers.

Cranial nerve weakness and progressive muscle fatigue after exertion without sensory symptoms, changes in consciousness, or autonomic dysfunction are early signs of myasthenia gravis. Because the disease is relatively uncommon, it frequently goes undiagnosed until generalized weakness occurs.

Diagnosis. The diagnosis of myasthenia gravis is based on history and physical examination, the anticholinesterase test, repetitive nerve stimulation, assay for anti–acetylcholine-receptor antibodies, and single-fiber electromyography. The anticholinesterase test uses drugs that inhibit the enzyme acetylcholinesterase. Edrophonium (Tensilon), a short-acting acetylcholinesterase inhibitor, is commonly used for the test. The drug, which is administered intravenously, decreases the breakdown of acetylcholine at the myoneural junction by the enzyme acetylcholinesterase. When weakness is caused by myasthenia gravis, a dramatic transitory improvement in muscle function occurs. Repetitive nerve simulation uses electrophysiologic measurements to demonstrate a decremental response to repeated 2- or 3-Hz stimulation of motor nerves. A radioimmunoassay test can be used to detect the presence of acetylcholine receptor antibodies circulating in the blood.

An advance in diagnostic methods for myasthenia gravis is the single-fiber electromyography, which is available in many medical centers. Single-fiber electromyography detects delayed or failed neuromuscular transmission in muscle fibers supplied by a single nerve fiber.

Treatment. Treatment methods include the use of pharmacologic agents; immunosuppressive therapy, including corticosteroid drugs; management of myasthenic crisis; thymectomy; and plasmapheresis or intravenous immunoglobulin. Pharmacologic treatment with reversible anticholinesterase drugs inhibits the breakdown of acetylcholine at the neuromuscular junction by acetylcholinesterase. Pyridostigmine (Mestinon, Regonol) and neostigmine (Prostigmin) are the drugs of choice. Corticosteroid drugs, which suppress the immune response, are used in cases of a poor response to anticholinesterase drugs and thymectomy. Immunosuppressant drugs (*e.g.*, azathioprine, cylosporine) may also be used, often in combination with plasmapheresis.

Plasmapheresis removes antibodies from the circulation and provides short-term clinical improvement. It is used primarily to stabilize the condition of persons in myasthenic crisis or for short-term treatment in persons undergoing thymectomy. Intravenous immunoglobulin also produces improvement in persons with myasthenia gravis. Although the effect is temporary, it may last for weeks to months. The indications for its use are similar to those for plasmapheresis. The mechanism of action of intravenous immunoglobulin is unknown. Intravenous immunoglobulin therapy is very expensive, which limits its use.

Thymectomy, or surgical removal of the thymus, may be used as a treatment for myasthenia gravis. Because the mechanism whereby surgery exerts its effect is unknown, the treatment is controversial. Thymectomy is performed in persons with thymoma, regardless of age, and in persons 50 to 60 years of age or older with recent onset of moderate disease.

Myasthenia Crisis. Persons with myasthenia gravis may develop a sudden exacerbation of symptoms and weakness known as *myasthenia crisis.* This usually occurs during a period of stress, such as infection, emotional upset, pregnancy, alcohol ingestion, cold, or after surgery. Many times, no primary cause can be identified. However, myasthenic crisis resulting from the need for more medication is virtually indistinguishable from cholinergic crisis resulting from too much medication. In the case of too much medication, cholinergic crisis is often accompanied by nausea, vomiting, pallor, sweating, salivation, colic, diarrhea, miosis, or bradycardia from the muscarinic effects of the anticholinesterase drugs. Whatever the cause, prompt medical treatment is needed. To determine whether the crisis was precipitated by the disease process or by cholinergic drugs, the Tensilon test is used. If the crisis is myasthenic, the symptoms will improve. Provision for respiratory support should be available in either case.

Peripheral Nerve Disorders

The peripheral nervous system consists of the motor and sensory nerves of the cranial and spinal nerves, the peripheral parts of the autonomic nervous system, and peripheral ganglia. A peripheral neuropathy is any primary disorder of the peripheral nerves. The result is usually muscle weakness, with or without atrophy and sensory changes. The disorder can involve a single nerve (*i.e.*, mononeuropathy) or multiple nerves (*i.e.*, polyneuropathy).

Unlike the nerves of the CNS, peripheral nerves are fairly strong and resilient. They contain a series of connective tissue sheaths that enclose their nerve fibers. An outer fibrous sheath called the *epineurium* surrounds the medium-sized to large nerves; inside, a sheath called the *perineurium* invests each bundle of nerve fibers, and within each bundle, a delicate sheath of connective tissue known as the *endoneurium* surrounds each nerve fiber (see Chapter 37, Fig. 37–5). Small peripheral nerves lack the epineurial covering. Within its endoneurial sheath, each nerve fiber is invested by a segmented sheath of Schwann cells. The Schwann cells produce the myelin sheath that surrounds the peripheral nerves. Each Schwann cell, however, can only myelinate one segment of a single axon—the one that it covers—so that myelination of an entire axon requires the participation of a long line of these cells.

Peripheral Nerve Injury and Repair

Neurons exemplify the general principle that the more specialized the function of a cell type, the less able it is to regenerate. In neurons, cell division ceases by the time of birth, and from then on, the cell body of a neuron is unable to divide and replace itself. Although the entire neuron cannot be replaced, it is often possible for the dendritic and axonal cell processes to regenerate as long as the cell body remains viable.

When a peripheral nerve is destroyed by a crushing force or by a cut that penetrates the nerve, the portion of the nerve fiber that is separated from the cell body rapidly undergoes degenerative changes, whereas the central stump and cell body of the nerve are often able to survive (Fig. 39–6). Because the cell body synthesizes the material required for nourishing and maintaining the axon, it is likely that the loss of these materials results in the degeneration of the separated portion of the nerve fibers.

After injury, the Schwann cells that are distal to the site of damage are also able to survive, but their myelin degenerates in a process called *wallerian degeneration.* The Schwann cells assist other phagocytic cells in the area in the cleanup of the debris caused by the degenerating axon and myelin. As they remove the debris, the Schwann cells multiply and fill the empty endoneurial tube. At this point, nothing further happens, unless a

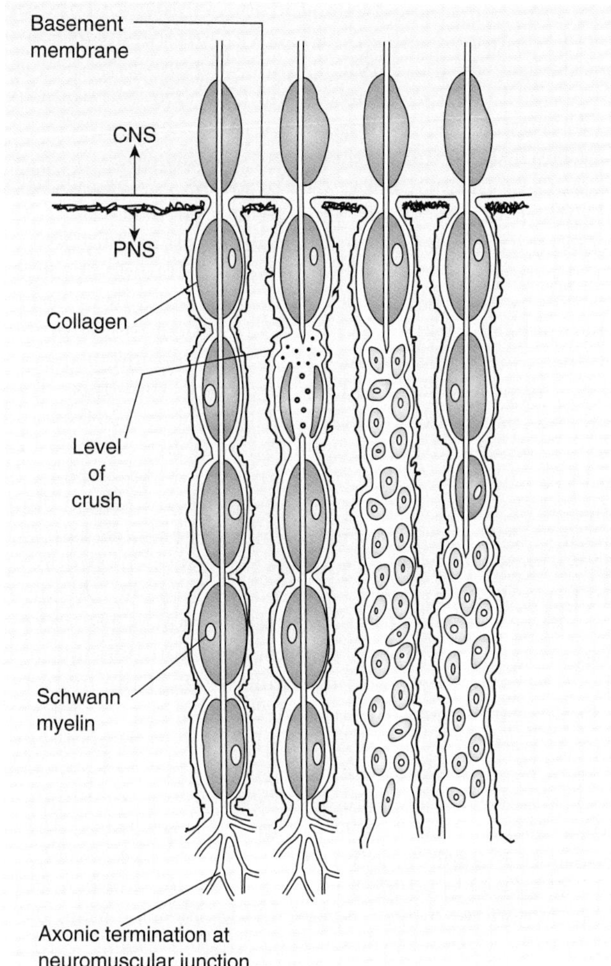

Figure 39–6
Sequential stages in efferent axon degeneration and regeneration within its endoneurial tube, following peripheral nerve crush injury.

regenerating nerve fiber penetrates into the endoneurial tube, in which case the Schwann cells reform the myelin segments around the fiber.

Meanwhile, the cell body of the neuron responds to the loss of part of its nerve fiber by shifting into a phase of greatly increased protein and lipid synthesis. It does this by dispersing the masses of ribosomes, which stain as Nissl granules. They cease to be stainable and disappear in a process called *chromatolysis.* In the process, the nucleus moves away from the axonal side of the cell body, as though displaced by the active synthetic apparatus of the cells. These changes reach their height within about 10 days of injury and continue until regrowth of the nerve fiber ceases.

In the process of regeneration, the injured nerve fiber develops one or more new branches from the proximal nerve stump that grow into the developing scar tissue. If a crushing injury has occurred and the endoneurial tube is intact through the trauma area, the outgrowing fiber will grow back down this tube to the structure that was originally innervated by the neuron. If, however, the injury involves the severing of a nerve, the outgrowing branch must come in contact with its original endoneurial tube if it is to be reunited with its original target structure. The rate of outgrowth of regenerating nerve fibers is about 1 mm to 2 mm per day; the recovery of conduction to a target structure depends on regrowth into the appropriate endoneurial tube and on the distance involved. It can take weeks or months for the regrowing fiber to reach the end-organ and communicative function to be reestablished. More time is required for the Schwann cells to form new myelin segments and for the axon to recover its original diameter and conduction velocity.

The successful regeneration of a nerve fiber in the peripheral nervous system depends on many factors. If a nerve fiber is destroyed relatively close to the neuronal cell body, the chances are that the nerve cell will die, and if it does, it will not be replaced. If a crushing type of injury has occurred, partial or often full recovery of function occurs. Cutting-type trauma to a nerve is an entirely different matter. Connective scar tissue forms rapidly at the wound site, and when it does, only the most rapidly regenerating axonal branches are able to get through to the intact distal endoneurial tubes. A number of scar-inhibiting agents have been used in an effort to reduce this hazard but have met with only moderate success. In another attempt to improve nerve regeneration, various types of tubular implants have been placed to fill longer gaps in the endoneurial tube.

Perhaps the most difficult problem is the alignment of the proximal and distal endoneurial tubes so that a regenerating fiber can return down its former tube and innervate its former organ. This problem is similar to realigning a large telephone cable that has been cut so that all the wires are reconnected exactly as before the separation. Microscopic alignment of the cut edges during microsurgical repair results in improved success. An efferent nerve fiber that formerly innervated a skeletal muscle regrows down an endoneurial tube formerly occupied by an afferent fiber, reaches the former sensory area, and then its cell body eventually dies. A sensory fiber that grows down an endoneurial tube that connects with a skeletal muscle fiber undergoes the same fate. If, however, these fibers grow down endoneurial tubes that innervate the appropriate type of target organ, reinnervation and function may return, even though the fibers have changed places. Under the best of conditions, a 50% regeneration to the appropriate organ is considered a success after a peripheral nerve has been severed. Even so, considerable function can return with that amount of innervation.

Peripheral Nerve Root Injury

Herniated Intervertebral Disk. Although back problems are commonly attributed to a herniated disk, most acute back problems are caused by other less serious conditions. It has been reported that 90% of persons with acute lower back problems of less than 3 months' duration recover spontaneously.[14] Thus, the current trend in treatment of acute back problems is to focus on

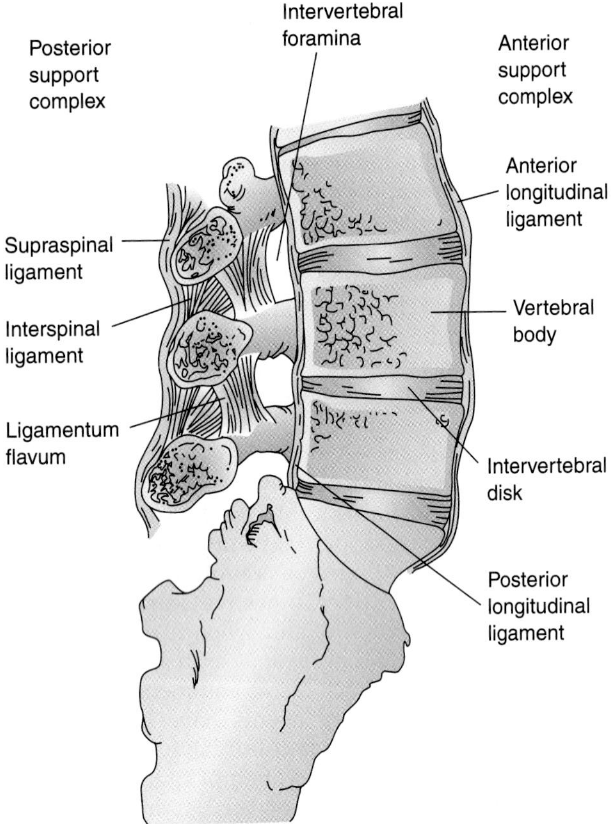

Figure 39–7
Soft tissue supporting structures of the spine. Two basic soft tissue units constitute each spinal segment: the anterior support complex, formed by the anterior and posterior longitudinal ligaments, the disk, and the annulus; and the posterior support complex, formed by the supraspinal ligament and interspinal ligament, the ligamentum flavum, and the facet capsules. The intravertebral foramen forms the passageway through which a spinal nerve root travels as it passes from the spinal canal to the periphery.

improvement in activity tolerance rather than exclusively on the pain associated with the problem.[14] Persons with signs of a herniated disk are evaluated for the problem.

The intervertebral disk is considered the most critical component of the load-bearing structures of the spinal column (Fig. 39–7). The intervertebral disk consists of a soft, gelatinous center called the *nucleus pulposus,* which is encircled by a strong, ringlike collar of fibrocartilage called the *annulus fibrosus*. The structural components of the disk make it capable of absorbing shock and changing shape while allowing movement. With dysfunction, the nucleus pulposus can be squeezed out of place and herniate through the annulus fibrosus, a condition referred to as a *herniated* or *slipped disk* (Fig. 39–8).

The cervical and lumbar regions are the most flexible area of the spine and most easily injured. Usually, herniation occurs at the lower levels of the lumbar spine, where the mass being supported and the bending of the vertebral column are greatest. About 90% to 95% of lumbar herniations occur in the L4 or L5 to S1 regions. With herniations of the cervical spine, the most frequently involved levels are C6 to C7 and C5 to C6.[12] Men suffer from herniated disks more frequently than women.

The intervertebral disk can become dysfunctional because of trauma, the effects of aging, or degenerative disorders of the spine. This results in movement between the articulating vertebral segments and the loss of the elastic properties of the disk itself. Trauma accounts for 50% of disk herniations. Trauma results from activities such as lifting while in the flexed position, slipping, falling on the buttocks or back, or suppressing a sneeze. With aging, the gelatinous center of the disk dries out and loses much of its elasticity, causing it to fray and tear.[13] Degenerative processes such as osteoarthritis or ankylosing spondylitis predispose to malalignment of the vertebral column. The anterior longitudinal ligament, which extends along the anterior (ventral) surface of the spinal column, is so strong that nucleus pulposus protrusion anteriorly is rare (see Fig. 39–7). A corresponding posterior longitudinal ligament is less strong and weakest laterally. The most common herniation is directed posteriorly and obliquely toward the intervertebral foramen and its contained spinal nerve root and dorsal root ganglion (Fig. 39–8). The consequent compression and irritation causes spontaneous firing of sensory afferents and severe pain locally because of injured tissue and pain referred to the area of dermatomal distribution of the spinal nerve root.

The level at which a herniated disk occurs is important. When the injury occurs in the lumbar area, only the cauda equina is irritated or crushed. Because these elongated dorsal and ventral roots contain endoneurial tubes of connective tissue, regeneration of the nerve fibers is likely. However, several weeks or months are

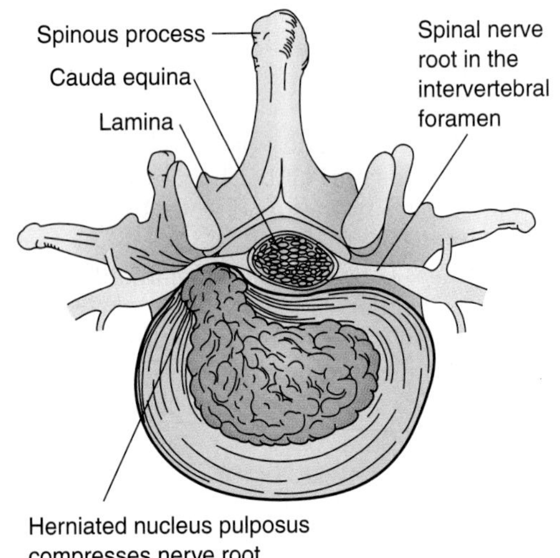

Figure 39–8
A prolapsed (herniated) intervertebral disk. The soft central portion of the disk is protruding into the vertebral canal, where it exerts pressure on a spinal nerve root.

required for full recovery to occur because of the distance to the innervated muscle or skin of the lower limbs.

The posterior longitudinal ligament is strongest along the midline so that nucleus pulposus displacement into the spinal canal, possibly compressing or damaging the spinal cord itself is uncommon. When it does occur, the axons of the ventral white column, including those of the spinothalamic system, are irritated, causing referred pain that can be experienced for many lower segments on the opposite side of the body. Sometimes the entire spinal segment can be damaged, resulting in functional transection of the spinal cord at that skeletal level.

The signs and symptoms of a slipped disk are localized to the area of the body innervated by the nerve roots. Pain is the first and most common symptom of a herniated disk. The nerve roots of L4, L5, S1, S2, and S3 give rise to a syndrome of back pain that spreads down the back of the leg and over the sole of the foot. The pain from a herniated disk is intensified by coughing, sneezing, straining, stooping, standing, and jarring motions that occur during walking or riding. Motor and sensory symptoms may also occur because of nerve root compression. Slight motor weakness may occur, although major weakness is rare. The most common sensory deficits from spinal nerve root compression are paresthesias and numbness, particularly of the leg and foot. Knee and ankle reflexes may also be diminished or absent.

A herniated disk must be differentiated from other causes such as traumatic injury or fracture of the vertebral column, tumor, infection, cauda equina syndrome, or other conditions that cause back pain.[14] Diagnostic measures include history and physical examination. Neurologic assessment includes testing of muscle strength and reflexes. The straight leg test is done in the supine position and is performed by passively raising the person's leg. Normally, it is possible to raise the leg about 90 degrees without causing discomfort of the hamstring muscles. The test result is positive if pain is produced when the leg is raised to 60 degrees or less. Other diagnostic methods include radiographs of the back, magnetic resonance imaging (MRI), computed tomography (CT), myelography and CT-myelography. Myelography and MRI and CT are usually reserved for persons suspected of having more complex causes of back pain.

Treatment is usually conservative and consists of analgesic medications and education on how to protect the back. Pain relief can usually be provided using nonsteroidal antiinflammatory drugs (NSAIDs), although short-term use of opioid pain medications may be required for severe pain. Muscle relaxants such as diazepam, cyclobenzaprine, carisoprodol, or methocarbamol may be used on a short-term basis. Bed rest, once the mainstay of conservative therapy, is now understood to be ineffective for acute pain. Instruction in the correct mechanics for lifting and methods of protecting the back is important. Conditioning exercises of the trunk muscles, particularly back extensors may be recommended for persons with acute low back problems, particularly if the problem persists. Surgical treatment may be indicated when there is documentation of herniation by some imaging procedure, consistent pain, or consistent neurologic deficit that has failed to respond to conservative therapy.

Mononeuropathies

Mononeuropathies are usually caused by localized conditions such as trauma, compression, or infections that affect a single spinal nerve, plexus, or peripheral nerve trunk. Fractured bones may lacerate or compress nerves; excessively tight tourniquets may injure nerves directly or produce ischemic injury; and infections such as herpes zoster may affect a single segmental afferent nerve distribution. Recovery of nerve function is usually complete after compression lesions and incomplete or faulty after nerve transection.

Carpal Tunnel Syndrome. Carpal tunnel syndrome is an example of a compression-type mononeuropathy

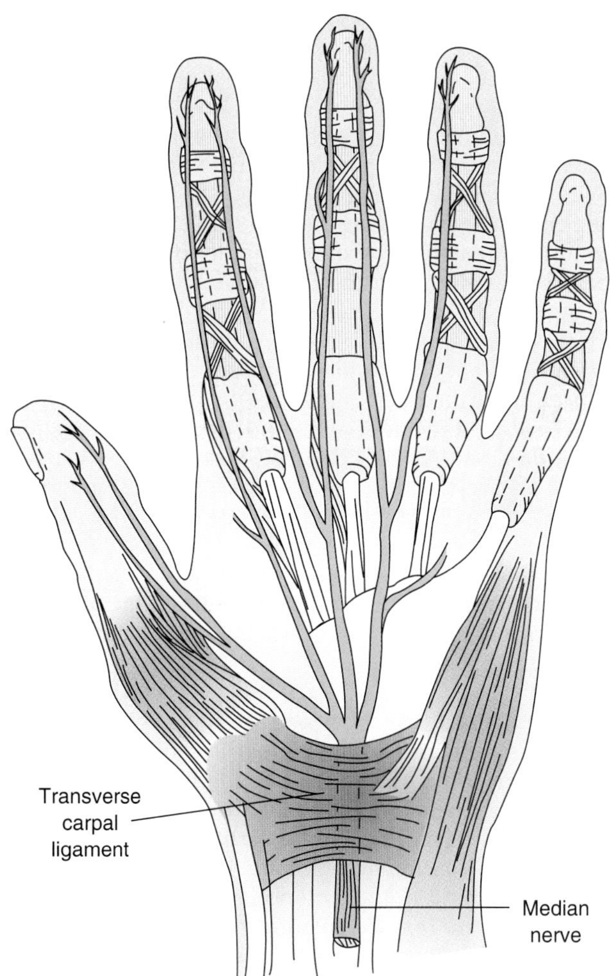

Figure 39–9
Carpal tunnel syndrome: compression of the median nerve by the transverse carpal ligament. (Courtesy Carole Russell Hilmer, C.M.I.)

that is relatively common. It is caused by compression of the median nerve as it travels with the flexor tendons through a canal made by the carpal bones and transverse carpal ligament (Fig. 39–9). The condition can be caused by a variety of conditions that produce a reduction in the capacity of the carpal tunnel (*i.e.*, bony or ligament changes) or increase in the volume of the tunnel contents (*i.e.*, inflammation of the tendons, synovial swelling, or tumors).[12] Carpal tunnel syndrome can be a feature of many systemic diseases such as rheumatoid arthritis, hyperthyroidism, acromegaly, and diabetes mellitus.[15,16] The condition can result from wrist injury; it can occur during pregnancy and use of birth control drugs; and it is seen in persons with repetitive use of the wrist (*i.e.*, flexion-extension movements and stress associated with pinching and gripping motions).

Carpal tunnel syndrome is characterized by pain, paresthesia, and numbness of the thumb and first two and one-half digits of the hand; pain in the wrist and hand, which worsens at night; atrophy of abductor pollicis muscle; and weakness in precision grip. All of these abnormalities may contribute to clumsiness of fine motor activity.

Diagnosis is usually based on hypoesthesia confined to median nerve distribution, a positive Tinel's sign, and a positive Phalen's sign. Tinel's sign describes the development of a tingling sensation radiating into the palm of the hand that is elicited by light percussion over the median nerve at the wrist. The Phalen test is performed by having the person hold the wrist in complete flexion for about a minute; if numbness and paresthesia along the median nerve are reproduced or exaggerated, the test result is considered to be positive. Electromyography and nerve conduction studies are often done to confirm the diagnosis and exclude other causes of the disorder.

Treatment includes avoidance of use, splinting, and antiinflammatory medications. Measures to decrease the causative repetitive movements should be initiated. Splints may be confined to nighttime use. When splinting is ineffective, corticosteroids may be injected into the carpal tunnel to reduce inflammation and swelling. Surgical intervention consists of operative division of the volar carpal ligaments as a means of relieving pressure on the medial nerve.

Polyneuropathies

Polyneuropathies lead to symmetric sensory, motor, or mixed sensorimotor deficits. The condition is characterized by demyelination or axonal degeneration of peripheral nerves. Typically, the longest axons are involved first, with symptoms beginning in the distal part of the extremities. If the autonomic nervous system is involved, there may be postural hypotension, constipation, and impotence. Polyneuropathies can result from immune mechanisms (*e.g.*, Guillain-Barré syndrome), toxic agents (*e.g.*, arsenic polyneuropathy, lead polyneuropathy, alcoholic polyneuropathy), and metabolic diseases (*e.g.*, diabetes mellitus, uremia). Different causes tend to affect axons of different diameters and to affect sensory, motor, or autonomic neurons to different degrees.

Guillain-Barré Syndrome. Guillain-Barré syndrome is a subacute polyneuropathy. The manifestations of the disease involve an infiltration of mononuclear cells around the capillaries of the peripheral neurons, edema of the endoneurial compartment, and demyelination of ventral spinal roots. The annual incidence of Guillain-Barré is about 1 case per 50,000 persons and is more common with increasing age.[17] About 80% to 90% of persons with the disease achieve a spontaneous recovery.

The cause of Guillain-Barré syndrome is unknown. About two thirds of cases follow an infection that is mundane and of viral origin. There is an association with preceding gastrointestinal tract infection caused by *Campylobacter jejuni*. A widely studied outbreak of the disorder followed the swine flu vaccination program of 1976 and 1977. It has been suggested that an altered immune response to peripheral nerve antigens contributes to the development of the disorder.

The disorder is characterized by progressive ascending muscle weakness of the limbs, producing a symmetric flaccid paralysis. Symptoms of paresthesia and numbness often accompany the loss of motor function. The rate of disease progression varies, and there may be disproportionate involvement of the upper or lower extremities. Paralysis may progress to involve the respiratory muscles; about 20% of persons with the disorder require ventilatory assistance.[17] Autonomic nervous system involvement that causes postural hypotension, arrhythmias, facial flushing, abnormalities of sweating, and urinary retention is common.

Guillain-Barré syndrome is usually a medical emergency. There may be a rapid development of ventilatory failure and autonomic disturbances that threaten circulatory function. Treatment includes support of vital functions and prevention of complications such as skin breakdown and thrombophlebitis. Clinical trials have shown the effectiveness of plasmapheresis in decreasing morbidity and shortening the course of the disease. Treatment is most effective if initiated early in the course of the disease. High-dose intravenous immunoglobulin therapy has also proved effective.[18]

In summary, the motor unit consists of the LMN, the neuromuscular junction, and the skeletal muscle that the nerve innervates. Disorders of the neuromuscular unit include muscular dystrophy, myasthenia gravis, and peripheral nerve disorders. Muscular dystrophy is a term used to describe a number of disorders that produce progressive deterioration of skeletal muscle. Muscle necrosis is followed by fat and connective tissue replacement. The disease usually affects children. One form, Duchenne's muscular dystrophy, is inherited as a sex-linked trait and transmitted by the mother to her offspring. Myasthenia gravis is a disorder of the neuromuscular junction, most likely resulting from a deficiency of functional acetylcholine receptors, which causes weakness of the skeletal muscles. Because the disease affects the neuromuscular junction, there is no loss of sensory function. The most common manifestations are weakness of the eye muscles, with ptosis and diplopia. Weakness of the jaw muscles can make chewing and swallowing difficult. Usually, the proximal muscles and extremities are involved, making it difficult to climb stairs and lift objects. Myasthenia crisis, which involves a sudden and transient weakness, may occur and necessitate mechanical ventilatory assistance.

Disorders of peripheral nerves include mononeuropathies and polyneuropathies. Mononeuropathies involve a single spinal nerve, plexus, or peripheral nerve trunk. Carpal tunnel syndrome, a mononeuropathy, is caused by compression of the medial nerve that passes through the carpal tunnel in the wrist. Polyneuropathies produce symmetric sensory, motor, and mixed sensorimotor deficits. A number of conditions, including immune mechanisms, toxic agents, and metabolic disorders, are implicated as causative agents in polyneuropathies. Guillain-Barré syndrome is a subacute polyneuropathy of uncertain origin. It causes progressive ascending motor, sensory, and autonomic nervous system manifestations. Respiratory involvement may occur and necessitate mechanical ventilation.

Disorders of the Basal Ganglia and Cerebellum

After you have completed this section of the chapter, you should be able to meet the following objectives:

- Describe the functional organization of the basal ganglia and communication pathways with the thalamus and cerebral cortex
- State the possible mechanisms responsible for the development of Parkinson's disease and characterize the manifestations and treatment of the disorder
- Relate the functions of the cerebellum to production of vestibulocerebellar ataxia, decomposition of movement, and cerebellar tremor

Disorders of the Basal Ganglia

The basal ganglia are a group of deep, interrelated subcortical nuclei that play an essential role in control of movement. The basal ganglia receive indirect input from the cerebellum and from all sensory systems, including vision, and direct input from the motor cortex. They appear to organize inherited and highly learned and rather automatic movement programs, especially those affecting the trunk and proximal limbs. The movements are released when commanded by the motor cortex, contributing *gracefulness* to cortically initiated and controlled skilled movements. The function of the basal ganglia is not limited to motor functions. They also are involved in cognitive and perception functions.

Disorders of the basal ganglia comprise a complex group of motor disturbances characterized by involuntary movements, alterations in muscle tone, and disturbances in body posture. Unlike disorders of the motor cortex and corticospinal (pyramidal) tract, lesions of the basal ganglia disrupt movement but do not cause paralysis. Because of these and other differences, the basal ganglia and associated structures are often referred to as the *extrapyramidal system.*

Functional Organization of the Basal Ganglia

The structural components of the basal ganglia include the caudate nucleus, putamen, and the globus pallidus in the forebrain. The caudate and putamen are collectively referred to as the *neostriatum* and the putamen and the globus pallidus form a wedge-shaped region called the *lentiform nucleus.* Two other structures, the subthalamic nucleus of the diencephalon and the substantia nigra of the midbrain are considered part of the basal ganglia (Fig. 39–10). The dorsal part of the substantia nigra contains cells that use dopamine as a neurotransmitter and are rich in a black pigment called *melanin.* The high concentration of melanin gives the structure a black color, hence the name *substantia nigra.* The axons of the substantia nigra form the nigrostriatal pathway, which supplies dopamine to the striatum. The dopamine released from the substantia nigra regulates the overall excitability of the striatum and release of other neurotransmitters.

The basal ganglia have input structures that receive afferent information from outside structures, internal circuits that connect the various structures of the basal

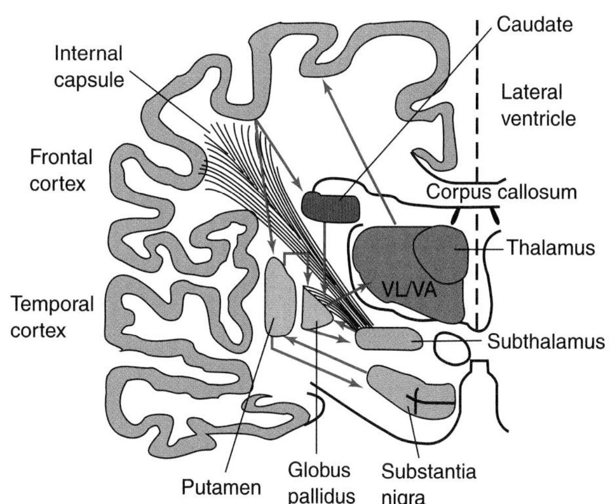

Figure 39–10
Basal ganglia.

ganglia, and output structures that deliver information to other brain centers. The neostriatum represents the major input structure for the basal ganglia. Virtually all areas of the cortex and afferents from the thalamus project to the neostriatum. The output areas of the basal ganglia, including the lateral globus pallidus, have ascending and descending components. The major ascending output is transmitted to thalamic nuclei, which process all incoming information that is transmitted to the cerebral cortex. Descending output is directed to the midbrain, brain stem, and spinal cord. The output functions of the basal ganglia are mainly inhibitory. Looping circuits from specific cortical areas pass through the basal ganglia to modulate the excitability of specific thalamic nuclei and control the cortical activity involved in highly learned, automatic, and stereotyped motor functions.

Each region of the cerebral cortex is interconnected with a corresponding region of the ventral row of thalamic nuclei. For the motor and premotor cortex, these nuclei are the ventral lateral (VL) and the ventral anterior (VA) nuclei. The cortex-to-thalamus (corticothalamic) and thalamus-to-cortex (thalamocortical) feedback circuitry are excitatory and, if unmodulated, would produce hyperactivity of the cortical area, causing stiffness and rigidity of the face, body, and limbs and, if alternating, a continuous tremor (*i.e.,* tremor at rest). The excitability of the thalamic nuclei in this reciprocal circuit is regulated by other thalamic afferents, many of which depress thalamic excitability.

For many semiautomatic stereotyped movements, thalamic excitability is modulated through inhibition by the basal ganglia. The basal ganglia form a major component of an inhibitory loop from each specific cortical region. Discrete inhibitory cortex-to-basal ganglia and thalamus-to-cortex loops modulate the function of all cerebral cortex regions. These modulatory loops exist for the prefrontal, limbic, premotor, motor, sensory, and parietal higher-order areas of the cerebral cortex. Abnormalities of the modulatory loop that influence motor function have such dramatic results that the role of the basal ganglia has often been relegated to that of the modulation of movement patterns.

The most is known about the inhibitory basal ganglia loop involved in modulating cortical motor control. This loop regulates release of stereotyped movement patterns that add efficiency and gracefulness to precise and delicate cortically controlled movements. These movements include inherited patterns that add efficiency, balance, and gracefulness to motion, such as the swinging of the arms during walking and running, and the highly learned automatic postural and follow-through movements of throwing a ball or swinging a bat. The basic repertoire of many of these complex movement patterns is built into brain stem circuitry under gene control. Individual differences limit the extent to which learning and practice can enhance their perfection. Thus, not everyone can become an accomplished ballerina or gymnast.

There are four functional pathways involving the basal ganglia: a dopamine pathway from the substantia nigra to the striatum; a γ-aminobutyric acid (GABA) pathway from the striatum to the globus pallidus and substantia nigra; acetylcholine-secreting neurons, which are important in networks within the neostriatum; and multiple general pathways from the brain stem that secrete norepinephrine, serotonin, enkephalin, and several other neurotransmitters in the basal ganglia and in the cerebral cortex. These pathways provide a balance of inhibitory and excitatory activity. GABA functions as an inhibitory neurotransmitter, and GABAergic neurons participate in the negative feedback loop from the cortex through the basal ganglia and back to the cortex. Dopamine also functions as an inhibitory neurotransmitter. There are multiple glutamine pathways that provide excitatory signals that balance the large number of inhibitory signals transmitted by GABAergic and dopaminergic neurons.

Within the cortex-to-basal ganglia and thalamus-to-cortex loop are two pathways that normally balance each other (Fig. 39–11).[19] One permits cortical disinhibition of the thalamus, and the other permits increased inhibition of the thalamus. Cortical release of a stereotyped movement pattern requires withdrawal of the inhibitory influence of the globus pallidus on the thalamus. The circuit involves cortical facilitation (glutaminergic action) of the neostriatum, which is inhibitory (GABAergic) to the internal segment of the globus pallidus, which is inhibitory (GABAergic) to the thalamus. Activation of a motor cortex movement pattern involves disinhibition of the thalamus, thereby potentiating cortical activity. The second circuit involves globus pallidus inhibition (GABAergic) and cortical facilitation of the subthalamic nucleus, which is excitatory (glutaminergic) to the internal segment of the globus pallidus. Increased activity in this circuit increases the inhibitory function of the globus pallidus. Pathologic movement regulation results from damaged function of one or both of these circuits. For example, destruction of the subthalamic nucleus by a stroke results in loss of thalamic inhibition, with a consequent release of violent, flailing (ballistic) limb movements on the contralateral side of the body.

An additional modulating circuit involves a neostriatal inhibitory projection (GABAergic) on the substantia nigra. The substantia nigra projects dopaminergic axons back on the neostriatum. A deficiency in the dopaminergic projection of this modulating circuit is implicated in Parkinson's syndrome. The function of the neostriatum also involves local cholinergic interneurons, and their destruction is thought to be related to the choreiform movements of Huntington's chorea, another basal ganglia-related syndrome (see Chapter 38). Precisely how these transmitter-related abnormalities affect the functional microcircuitry of the basal ganglia circuit remains to be elucidated. However, some progress has been made in supplying decreased or missing transmitters, reducing at least temporarily the severity of several extrapyramidal diseases.

Movement Disorders

Reduced function of the basal ganglia loop results in *hyperkinesis*, or release of movement patterns at inap-

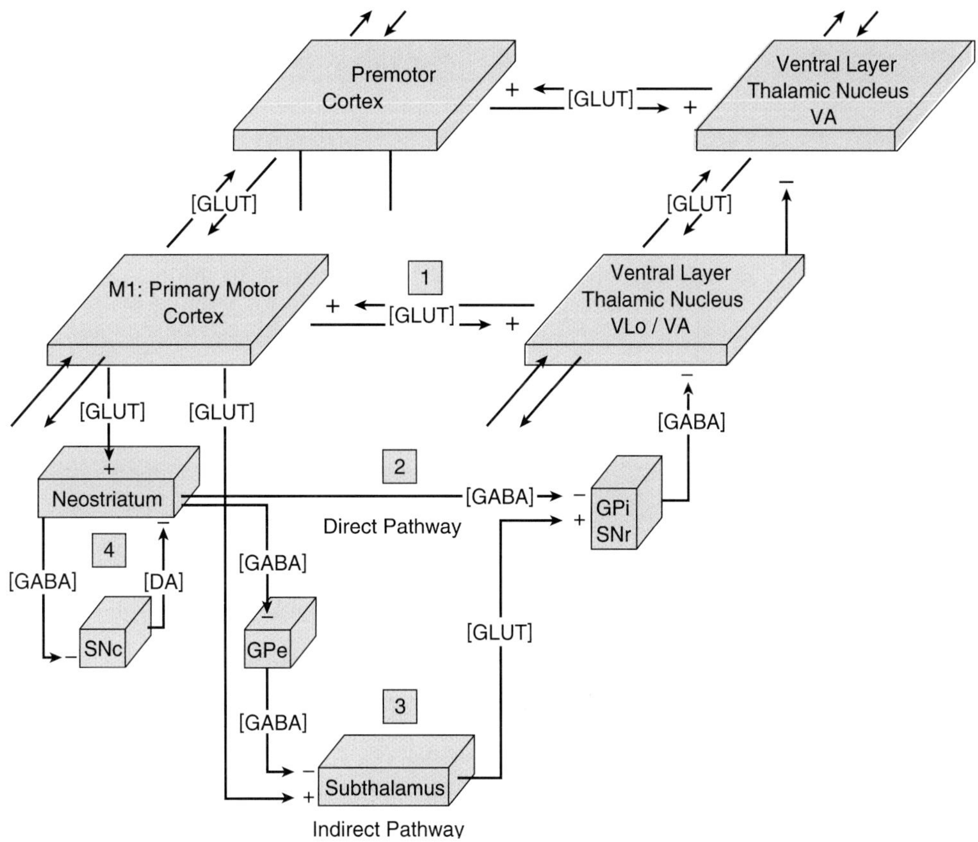

Figure 39–11
Diagram of neurotransmitters involved in function of the basal ganglia. (1) Excitatory cortico–thalamo–cortical loop: Facilitates UMN activity; modulated by cortico–basal ganglia–thalamic loops. (2) Direct pathway: Releases response patterns by reducing pallidal inhibition. (Disinhibitory cortico–neostriato–pallido–thalamo–cortical loop.) (3) Indirect pathway: Increases pallidal inhibition of the release of response patterns. (Inhibitory cortico–subthalamo–pallido–thalamo–cortical loop.) (4) Neostriatal excitability modulatory loop: Regulates level of neostriatal excitability. (Neostriato–nigro–striatal loop.) (R.L. Curtis, PhD)

propriate times or sometimes continuously. Pathologically released patterns that are often disabling include rigidity and movement disorders. These movement patterns are not under cortical control and are often called *involuntary movement*. Destruction of the corticospinal system does not eliminate the extrapyramidal movements. These movements are lost during sleep, although they may make getting to sleep difficult.

Descending pathways to the LMNs involved in basal ganglia–related movements involve the corticospinal systems and other descending systems. Although these signs are always on the side of the body opposite to basal ganglia damage, in metabolic or toxic abnormalities the signs are usually bilateral.

Rigidity and Bradykinesia. Basal ganglia–derived *rigidity* involves a strong resistance to movement that decreases to a stiffness after the movement does get underway. In some instances, forcing a rigid joint to turn is met with a series of sudden releases followed by renewed resistance, a phenomenon called *cog-wheel rigidity.*

Hyperfunction of the basal ganglia inhibitory loop results in excessive inhibition of cortical function, producing *bradykinesia or hypokinesis*. The results are slowness in beginning movement, a reduced range and force of the movement ("poverty of movement"), reduced or absence of emotional responses, including emotion-related facial expressions, and a loss of the balance and grace-producing movements and postures associated with skilled motion. An example of hypokinesis is seen in the severely affected persons with the parkinsonian syndrome.

Involuntary Movements. Involuntary movements include tremor, tics, choreiform movements, athetoid movements, and ballism. These disorders are summarized in Table 39–1).

Tremor is caused by involuntary, oscillating contractions of opposing muscle groups around a joint. It is

TABLE 39-1

Involuntary Movements Disorders Associated With Extrapyramidal Disorders

Movement Disorder	Characteristics
Tremor	Rhythmic oscillating contractions or movements of whole muscles or major portions of a muscle. They can occur as resting tremors, which are prominent at rest and decrease or disappear with movement; intention tremors, which increase with activity and become worse when the target is reached; and postural tremors, which appear when the affected part is maintained in a stabilized position.
Tics	Irregularly occurring brief, repetitive, stereotyped, coordinated movements such as winking, grimacing, or shoulder shrugging
Chorea	Brief, rapid, jerky, and irregular movements that are coordinated and graceful. The face, head, and distal limbs are most commonly involved. They often interfere with normal movement patterns.
Athetosis	Continuous slow, wormlike, twisting and turning motions of a limb or body that most commonly involve the face and distal extremities and are often associated with spasticity
Ballismus	Involve violent sweeping, flinging-type limb movements, especially on one side of the body (hemiballismus)
Dystonia	Abnormal maintenance of posture results from a twisting, turning motion of the limbs, neck, or trunk. Motions are similar to athetosis but involve larger portions of the body. They can result in grotesque and twisted postures.
Dyskinesias	Rhythmic, repetitive, bizarre movements that chiefly involve the face, mouth, jaw, or tongue, causing grimacing, pursing of the lips, protrusion of the tongue, opening and closing of the mouth, and deviations of the jaw. The limbs are affected less often.

(From Bates B. [1991]. *A guide to physical examination and history taking* [5th ed., pp. 554–556]. Philadelphia: J.B. Lippincott)

usually fairly uniform in frequency and amplitude. Certain tremors are considered physiologic in that they are transitory and normally occur under conditions of increased muscle tone, as in highly emotional situations, or they may be related to muscle fatigue or to reduced body temperature (*i.e.,* shivering). Toxic tremors are produced by hyperexcitability related to endotoxic conditions such as in thyrotoxicosis. The tremor of Parkinson's disease is caused by degenerative changes in the basal ganglia.

Tics involve sudden and irregularly occurring contractions of whole muscles or major portions of a muscle. These are particularly evident in the muscles of the face, but can occur elsewhere.

Choreiform movements are sudden, jerky, and irregular but are coordinated and graceful. They can involve the distal limb, face, tongue, or swallowing muscles. Choreiform movements are accentuated by movement and by environmental stimulation; they often interfere with normal movement patterns. The word *chorea* originated from the Greek word meaning to dance. There may be grimacing movements of the face, raising of the eyebrows, rolling of the eyes, and curling, protrusion and withdrawal of the tongue. In the limbs, the movements are largely distal; there may be piano playing–type movements with alternating extension and flexion of the fingers. The shoulders may be elevated and depressed or rotated. Movements of the face or limbs may occur alone or, more commonly, in combination.

Athetoid movements are relatively continuous, wormlike twisting and turning of the joints of a limb or body. These result from continuous and prolonged contraction of agonist and antagonistic muscle groups. These are normal, smooth, and useful movements, except in extrapyramidal diseases, when they occur continuously in a nonrhythmic, often irregular sequence.

The term *ballismus* originated from a Greek word meaning to jump around. Ballistic movements are violent sweeping, flinging motions, especially of the limbs on one side of the body (*i.e.,* hemiballismus). They may occur as the result of a small vascular accident involving the subthalamic nucleus on the opposite side of the brain.

Dystonia refers to the abnormal maintenance of a posture resulting from a twisting, turning movement of the limbs, neck, or trunk. These postures often result from simultaneous opposing movements, producing a paralysis (*i.e.,* nonmovement). Long-sustained simultaneous hypertonia across a joint can result in degenerative changes and permanent fixation in unusual postures. These effects can occur as untoward reactions to some of the antipsychotic medications. *Spasmodic torticollis,* the most common type of dystonia, affects the muscles of the neck and shoulder. The condition, which is caused by bilateral and simultaneous contraction of the neck and shoulder muscles, results in unilateral head turning or head extension, sometimes limiting rotation. Elevations of the shoulder commonly accompany the spasmodic movements of the head and neck. Immobility of the cervical vertebrae eventually can lead to degenerative fixation in the twisted posture. Torsional spasm involving the trunk can also occur.

Dyskinesias are rhythmic, repetitive, bizarre movements. They frequently involve the face, mouth, jaw, and tongue, causing grimacing, pursing of the lips, or protrusion of the tongue. The limbs are affected less often. Tardive dyskinesia is an untoward reaction that can develop with long-term use of some of the antipsychotic medications.

Parkinson's Disease

Parkinson's disease is a degenerative disorder of basal ganglia function that results in variable combinations of slowness (bradykinesia), increased muscle tonus (rigidity), rest tremor, and impaired autonomic postural responses. About 1.5 million persons in the United States are affected by Parkinson's disease.[20] It usually begins after age 50; most cases are diagnosed in the sixth and seventh decade of life. Up to 1% of the population older than 60 years may be affected with the disease.[20]

Pathology. Parkinson's disease is characterized by progressive destruction of the nigrostriatal pathway, with subsequent reduction in striatal concentrations of dopamine. Usually, there has been an 80% loss of dopamine in the striatum at the time that symptoms become clinically apparent.[21] Secondary degenerative changes occur in the striatum, particularly in the putamen.

The pathologic changes that occur in Parkinson's disease can result from other degenerative and disease conditions. The most common form of parkinsonism is idiopathic Parkinson's disease (*i.e.,* paralysis agitans), named after James Parkinson, who first described the disorder in 1817. In the idiopathic form of the disease, dopamine depletion results from degeneration of the dopamine nigrostriatal system. Parkinsonism can also develop as a postencephalitic syndrome, as a side effect of therapy with antipsychotic drugs that block dopamine receptors, as a toxic reaction to a chemical agent, or as an outcome of severe carbon monoxide poisoning. Symptoms of parkinsonism may also accompany conditions such as cerebral vascular disease, brain tumors, or degenerative neurologic diseases that structurally damage the nigrostriatal pathway. The national attention given Muhammad Ali, former world heavyweight boxing champion and 1960 Olympic gold medal winner, as he lighted the Olympic torch for the 1996 Summer Games in Atlanta, not only served as a recognition of one person's remarkable courage in coping with the disease, but also as a reminder that Parkinson's disease may have multiple causes, including repeated head trauma.[22]

Postencephalitic parkinsonism was a particular problem in the 1930s and 1940s as a result of an outbreak of lethargic encephalitis (*i.e.,* sleeping sickness) that occurred in 1914 to 1918. Drug-induced parkinsonism can follow taking antipsychotic drugs in high doses (*e.g.,* phenothiazines, butyrophenones). These drugs block dopamine receptors and dopamine output by the cells of the substantia nigra. Of interest in terms of research was the development of Parkinson's disease in several persons who had attempted to make a narcotic drug and instead synthesized a compound called *MPTP* (1-methyl-phenyl,2,3,6-tetrahydropyridine).[22] This compound selectively destroys the dopaminergic neurons of the substantia nigra. This incident prompted investigations into the role of toxins that are produced by the body as a part of metabolic processes and those that enter the body from outside sources in the pathogenesis of Parkinson's disease. One theory is that the autooxidation of catecholamines such as dopamine during melanin synthesis injures neurons in the substantia nigra. There is increasing evidence that the development of Parkinson's disease may be related to oxidative metabolites of this process and the inability of neurons to render these products harmless. MPTP is an inhibitor of the mitochondrial electron transport system that functions in the inactivation of these metabolites, suggesting that it may produce Parkinson's disease in a manner similar to the naturally occurring disease.[23]

Manifestations. Parkinson's disease often begins insidiously, with slow movement, weakness, and resting tremor. Resting tremor is an initial symptom in 50% to 75% of persons with the disease. The tremor affects the distal segments of the limbs, mainly the hands and feet; head, neck, face, lips, and tongue; or jaw. It is characterized by rhythmic, alternating flexion and contraction movements (four to six beats per minute) that resemble the motion of rolling a pill between the thumb and forefinger. The tremor is usually unilateral, occurs when the limb is supported and at rest, and disappears with movement and sleep. The tremor eventually progresses to involve both sides of the body. The tremor is gradually followed by rigidity, which is most evident on passive joint movement, and involves jerky, cogwheel-type or ratchet-like movements that require considerable energy to perform. Flexion contractions may develop as a result of the rigidity.

In addition to tremor, there is slowness in initiating and performance of voluntary movements (*i.e.,* bradykinesia) and difficulty in sudden, unexpected stopping of voluntary movements. Unconscious associative movements occur in a series of disconnected steps rather than in a smooth, coordinated manner. Persons with Parkinson's disease have difficulty initiating walking and difficulty turning. While walking, they may freeze in place and feel as if their feet are glued to the floor, especially when moving through a doorway or preparing to turn.

When they walk, they lean forward to maintain their center of gravity and take small, shuffling steps without swinging their arms, and they have difficulty in changing their stride. Loss of postural reflexes predispose them to falling, often backward.

Emotional and voluntary facial movements become limited and slow as the disease progresses, and facial expression becomes stiff and masklike. There is loss of the blinking reflex and a failure to express emotion. The tongue, palate, and throat muscles become rigid; the person may drool because of difficulty in moving the saliva to the back of the mouth and swallowing it. The speech becomes slow and monotonous, without modulation and poorly articulated.

Because the basal ganglia also influence the autonomic nervous system, persons with Parkinson's disease often have excessive and uncontrolled sweating, sebaceous gland secretion, and salivation. Autonomic symptoms such as lacrimation, dysphagia, orthostatic hypotension, thermal regulation, constipation, impotence, and urinary incontinence may be present, especially late in the disease. Other advanced-stage Parkinson's manifestations are falls, fluctuations in motor function, neuropsychiatric disorders, and sleep disorders.

Dementia is an important feature associated with Parkinson's disease. It occurs in approximately 15% to 20% of persons with the disease and develops late in the course of the disease.[24] The mental state of some persons with Parkinson's disease may be indistinguishable from that seen in Alzheimer's disease.[25] It has been suggested that many of the brain changes in both diseases may result from degeneration of acetylcholine-containing neurons in a region of the brain called the *nucleus basalis of Meynert,* which is the main source of cholinergic innervation of the cerebral cortex. Persons with Parkinson's disease also have other neurochemical disturbances that can account for some of the features of dementia. Parkinson's disease is usually slowly progressive over several decades, but the rate of progression varies from 2 to 30 years.[20] There are several stages in the progression of Parkinson's disease. The symptoms are usually noticed first on one side of the body and progress to bilateral involvement, with early postural changes beginning 1 to 2 years after onset. The tremor often begins in one or both hands and then becomes generalized. Postural changes and gait disturbances continue to become more pronounced, until the person has significant disability and requires constant care.

Drug Treatment. The approach to treatment of parkinsonism must be highly individualized, including nonpharmacologic and pharmacologic methods. Nonpharmacologic interventions offer group support, education, daily exercise, and adequate nutrition.

Pharmacologic treatment is usually determined by the severity of symptoms. Antiparkinson drugs act by increasing the functional ability of the underactive dopaminergic system, or they reduce the excessive influence of excitatory cholinergic neurons. Drugs that increase dopamine levels include levodopa and levodopa with the decarboxylase inhibitor (carbidopa), amantadine (Symmetrel), bromocriptine (Parlodel), and selegiline. Because dopamine transmission is disrupted in Parkinson's disease, there is a preponderance of cholinergic activity, which be decreased with the use of anticholinergic drugs.

Dopamine does not cross the blood-brain barrier. Administration of *levodopa,* a precursor of dopamine that does cross the blood-brain barrier, has yielded significant improvement in clinical symptoms of Parkinson's disease and remains the most effective drug for treatment. The evidence of decreased dopamine levels in the striatum in Parkinson's disease led to the administration of large doses of the synthetic compound levodopa, which is absorbed from the intestinal tract, crosses the blood-brain barrier, and is converted to dopamine by centrally acting dopa decarboxylase. Unfortunately, only 1% to 3% of administered levodopa enters the brain unaltered; the remainder is metabolized outside the brain, predominantly by decarboxylation to dopamine, which cannot cross the blood-brain barrier. This means that large doses of levodopa are needed when the drug is used alone, and this leads to many side effects. However, when levodopa is given in combination with carbidopa, a decarboxylase inhibitor, the peripheral metabolism of levodopa is reduced, plasma levels of levodopa are higher, the plasma half-life is longer, more dopa is available for the entry into the brain, and a smaller dose is needed.

A later adverse effect of levodopa treatment is the "on-off phenomenon," in which frequent, abrupt, and unpredictable fluctuations in motor performance occur during the day.[26] These fluctuations include periods of dyskinesia (the on response) and periods of bradykinesia (the off response). Some fluctuations reflect the timing of drug administration, in which case the on response coincides with peak drug levels and the off response with low drug levels.

Amantadine (Symmetrel) was introduced as an antiviral agent for prophylaxis of A_2 influenza and was unexpectedly found to cause symptomatic improvement of persons with parkinsonism. Although the exact mechanism of action remains to be elucidated, it may augment release of dopamine from the remaining intact dopaminergic terminals in the nigrostriatal pathway of persons with Parkinson's disease. It is used to treat persons with mild symptoms, but no disability. *Bromocriptine* (Parlodel) and *pergolide* (Permax) are dopamine agonists that act to directly stimulate dopamine receptors. These drugs are used as adjunctive therapy in Parkinson's disease. They are often used for persons who have become refractory to levodopa or have developed an on-off phenomenon.

Selegiline (Deprenyl) is a monoamine oxidase B inhibitor that inhibits the metabolic breakdown of dopamine. Selegiline may be used as adjunctive treatment to reduce mild on-off fluctuations in the responsiveness of persons who are receiving levodopa. It has been proposed that in inhibiting dopamine metabolism and the generation of destructive metabolites, selegiline may also delay the progression of the disease. Early results from the Deprenyl and Tocopherol Antioxidative Trial of Parkinson's Disease (DATATOP) suggest that selegiline delays the progression of disability in persons with Parkinson's disease.[27]

Anticholinergic drugs are thought to restore a "balance" between reduced dopamine and uninhibited cholinergic neurons in the striatum.[24] They are more useful in alleviating tremor and rigidity than bradykinesia. The anticholinergic drugs lessen the tremors and rigidity and afford some improvement of function. However, their potency seems to decrease over time, and increasing the dosage merely increases side effects such as blurred vision, dry mouth, bowel and bladder problems, and some mental changes.

Surgical Treatment. When medical therapy is ineffective in controlling symptoms, pallidectomy performed by stereotactic surgery may be explored. With this surgical procedure, part of the globus pallidum in the basal ganglia is destroyed using an electrical stimulator. Brain mapping is done during the surgery to identify and prevent injury to sensory and motor tracts.

Autotransplantation of adrenal medullary tissue into the caudate has been used with limited success. Results of this procedure have been contradictory, and this approach is highly controversial.

Disorders of the Cerebellum

The functions of the cerebellum, or "little brain," are essential for smooth, coordinated, skillful movement. The cerebellum influences voluntary and automatic aspects of movement. It does not initiate activity, but it is responsible for smoothing the temporal and spatial aspects of rapid movement anywhere in the body.

The signs of cerebellar dysfunction can be grouped into three classes: vestibulocerebellar disorders, cerebellar ataxia or decomposition of movement, and cerebellar tremor. These disorders occur on the side of cerebellar damage, whether because of congenital defect, vascular accident, or growing tumor. The abnormality of movement occurs whether the eyes are open or closed. Visual monitoring of movement cannot compensate for cerebellar defects.

Damage to the part of the cerebellum associated with the vestibular system leads to difficulty or inability to maintain a steady posture of the trunk, which normally requires constant readjusting movements. This is seen as an unsteadiness of the trunk, called *truncal ataxia,* and it can be so severe that standing is not possible. The ability to fix the eyes on a target can also be affected. Constant conjugate readjustment of eye position, called *nystagmus,* results and makes reading extremely difficult, especially when the eyes are deviated toward the side of cerebellar damage.

Cerebellar ataxia and tremor are different aspects of defects in the smooth, continuously correcting functions. Cerebellar dystaxia or, if severe, ataxia includes a *decomposition of movement;* each succeeding component of a complex movement occurs separately instead of being blended into a smoothly proceeding action. Because ethanol specifically affects cerebellar function, persons who are inebriated often walk with a staggering and unsteady gait. Rapid alternating movements such as supination-pronation-supination of the hands is jerky and performed slowly (*i.e.,* dysdiadochokinesia). Reaching to touch a target breaks down into small sequential components, each going too far, followed by overcorrection. The finger moves jerkily toward the target, misses, corrects in the other direction, and misses again, until the target is finally reached. This is called *over-and-under reaching,* and the general term is *dysmetria.*

Cerebellar tremor is a rhythmic back-and-forth movement of a finger or toe that worsens as the target is approached. The tremor results from the inability of the damaged cerebellar system to maintain ongoing fixation of a body part and to make smooth, continuous corrections in the trajectory of the movement; overcorrection occurs, first in one direction and then the other. Often, the tremor of an arm or leg can be detected during the beginning of an intended movement. The common term for cerebellar tremor is *intention tremor.* Cerebellar function as it relates to tremor can be assessed by asking a person to touch one heel to the opposite knee, to gently move the toes along the back of the opposite shin, or to move the hand so as to touch the nose with a finger.

Cerebellar function can also affect the motor skills of chewing and swallowing (*i.e.,* dysphagia) and of speech (*i.e.,* dysarthria). Normal speech requires smooth control of respiratory muscles and highly coordinated control of the laryngeal, lip, and tongue muscles. Cerebellar dysarthria is characterized by slow, slurred speech of continuously varying loudness. Rehabilitative efforts directed by speech therapists include learning to slow the rate of speech and to compensate as much as possible through the use of less-affected muscles.

In summary, alterations in coordination of muscle movements and abnormal muscle movements result from disorders of the cerebellum and basal ganglia. The basal ganglia organize basic movement patterns into more complex patterns and release them when commanded by the motor cortex, contributing gracefulness to cortically initiated and controlled skilled movements. Disorders of the basal ganglia are characterized by involuntary movements, alterations in muscle tone, and disturbances in posture. These disorders include tremor, tics, hemiballismus, chorea, athetosis, dystonias, and dyskinesias.

Parkinsonism, a disorder of basal ganglia, is characterized by destruction of the nigrostriatal pathway, with a subsequent reduction in striatal concentrations of dopamine. This results in an imbalance between the inhibitory effects of dopaminergic basal ganglia functions and an increase the excitatory cholinergic functions. The disorder is manifested by combinations of slowness of movement (*i.e.,* bradykinesia), increased muscle tonus (*i.e.*, rigidity), rest tremor, gait disturbances, and impaired autonomic postural responses. The disease is usually slowly progressive over several decades, but the rate of progression varies from 2 to 30 years. The tremor often begins in one or both hands and then becomes generalized. Postural changes and gait disturbances continue to become more pronounced, resulting in significant disability.

The function of the cerebellum is essential for smooth, coordinated movements. Cerebellar disorders include vestibulocerebellar dysfunction, cerebellar ataxia, and cerebellar tremor.

Upper Motoneuron Disorders

After you have completed this section of the chapter, you should be able to meet the following objectives:

- Relate the pathologic UMN and LMN changes that occur in amyotrophic lateral sclerosis to the manifestations of the disease
- Explain the significance of demyelination and plaque formation in multiple sclerosis
- Describe the manifestations of multiple sclerosis
- Relate the structures of the vertebral column to mechanisms of spinal cord injury
- Explain how loss of UMN function contributes to the muscle spasms that occur after recovery from spinal cord injury
- State the effects of spinal cord injury on ventilation and communication, the autonomic nervous system, cardiovascular function, sensorimotor function, and bowel and bladder function

Amyotrophic Lateral Sclerosis

Amyotrophic lateral sclerosis (ALS), also known as *Lou Gehrig's disease* after the famous New York Yankee baseball player, is a devastating neurologic disorder that selectively affects motor function. There are about 5000 new cases of ALS in the United States each year. ALS is primarily a disorder of middle life, affecting persons between 40 and 60 years of age, with men developing the disease nearly twice as often as women. The disease typically follows a progressive course, with a mean survival period of 2 to 5 years from the onset of symptoms.

Pathophysiology

ALS affects the UMNs (*i.e.*, large pyramidal and Betz cells) contained in the cerebral cortex and the cell bodies of the LMNs contained in the brain stem and anterior horn cells of the spinal cord.[28] The fact that the disease is more extensive in the distal parts of the affected tracts in the lower spinal cord rather than the proximal parts suggests that affected neurons first undergo degeneration at their distal terminals and that the disease proceeds in a centripetal direction until ultimately the parent nerve cell dies.[29] A remarkable feature of the disease is that the entire sensory system, the regulatory mechanisms of control and coordination of movement, and the intellect remain intact. The neurons for ocular motility and the parasympathetic neurons in the sacral spinal cord are also spared.

The death of LMNs leads to denervation, with subsequent shrinkage of musculature and muscle fiber atrophy. It is this fiber atrophy, called *amyotrophy*, which appears in the name of the disease. The loss of nerve fibers in lateral columns of the white matter of the spinal cord along with fibrillary gliosis imparts a firmness or sclerosis to this CNS tissue; the term *lateral sclerosis* designates these changes.

The cause of LMN and UMN destruction in ALS is uncertain. One form of the disease, familial ALS, which accounts for 5% to 10% of cases, has been mapped to a gene for superoxide dismutase on chromosome 21.[30,31] This enzyme functions in the prevention of free radical formation (see Chapter 2). There is no linkage of this gene to the more common type of ALS, sporadic ALS, for which there is no family history of the disease. One theory suggests that sporadic ALS may be caused by an untoward reaction to an environmental agent that causes glutamine, an excitatory neurotransmitter, to accumulate to toxic concentrations in the neural synapse, causing neuronal death. Another theory of pathogenesis is that sporadic ALS is caused by an autoimmune process.

Manifestations

The symptoms of ALS may be referable to UMN or LMN involvement. Manifestations of UMN lesions include weakness, spasticity or stiffness, and impaired fine motor control. Dysphagia (*i.e.*, difficulty swallowing), dysarthria (*i.e.*, impaired articulation of speech), and dysphonia (*i.e.*, difficulty making the sounds of speech) may result from brain stem LMN involvement or from dysfunction of UMNs descending to the brain stem. Manifestations of LMN destruction include fasciculations, weakness, muscle atrophy, and hyporeflexia. Muscle cramps involving the distal legs is often an early symptom. The most common clinical presentation is slowly progressive weakness and atrophy in distal muscles of one upper extremity. This is followed by regional spread of clinical weakness, reflecting involvement of neighboring areas of the spinal cord. Eventually, UMNs and LMNs involving multiple limbs and the head are affected. In the more advanced stages, muscles of the palate, pharynx, tongue, neck, and shoulders become involved, causing impairment of chewing, swallowing, and speech. Dysphagia with recurrent aspiration and weakness of the respiratory muscles produce the most significant acute complications of the disease. Death usually results from involvement of cranial and respiratory musculature.

Currently, there is no treatment that influences the progress of ALS. Rehabilitation measures assist persons with the disorder to manage their disability, and respiratory and nutritional support allow persons with the disorder to survive longer than would otherwise have been the case. An investigational antiglutamate drug, riluzole, designed to decrease glutamate accumulation and slow disease progression in persons with sporadic ALS, is being tested.[32]

Multiple Sclerosis

Multiple sclerosis, a demyelinating disease of the CNS, is a major cause of neurologic disability among young and middle-aged adults. Estimates of the total number of cases of multiple sclerosis in the United States range from 250,000 to 350,000.[33,34] The incidence of multiple sclerosis among women is almost double that among men. Approximately two thirds of persons with multiple sclerosis experience their first symptoms between 20 and 40 years of age. Sometimes, a diagnosis may be delayed until the fourth or fifth decade because symptoms were short lasting or were not bothersome enough to warrant medical attention. In these cases, a detailed medical history usually reveals that symptoms did appear previously.

In approximately 60% of the cases, the disease is characterized by exacerbations and remissions over many years in several different sites in the CNS. Initially, there is normal or near-normal neurologic function between exacerbations. As the disease progresses, there is less improvement between exacerbations and increasing neurologic dysfunction.

Pathophysiology

Multiple sclerosis is caused by demyelination of white matter in the brain, spinal cord, and optic nerve. Demyelinated nerve fibers display a variety of conduction abnormalities, ranging from decreased conduction velocity to conduction blocks and resulting in a variety of symptoms that depend on the location and duration of the lesion.

In the CNS, myelin is formed by the oligodendrocytes, chiefly those lying among the nerve fibers in the white matter. This function is equivalent to that of the Schwann cells in the peripheral nervous system (see Chapter 37). The properties of the myelin sheath—high electrical resistance and low capacitance—permit it to function as an electrical insulator. Small, uninsulated junctures, called the *nodes of Ranvier,* exist between the cells of the myelin sheath. Action potentials jump from node to node (*i.e.*, saltatory conduction), speeding conduction of impulses and reducing the metabolic work required to maintain the ionic gradients necessary for neural conduction.

The process of myelination of the CNS begins early in the fourth month of fetal life. It is incomplete at birth, and some fibers continue to become myelinated during the first year of life.[35] The total amount of myelin increases from birth to maturity. Although myelin is relatively stable, there is continual removal and replacement of individual components. Studies indicate that the myelin formed early in life is the most stable and that newly formed myelin is more easily broken down and replaced.[36] There are two major myelin proteins, proteolipid protein and basic protein, that are incorporated in the myelin sheath and are involved in the replacement process. Myelin enzymes, capable of degrading myelin proteins, may be involved in normal catabolic processes and may have a role in some forms of demyelination.[36]

Multiple sclerosis is characterized by hard, sharp-edged demyelinated patches (*i.e.*, sclerosis) that are macroscopically visible throughout the white matter of the CNS.[37] These lesions, which represent the end result of acute myelin breakdown, are called *plaques*. Oligodendrocytes are decreased in number and may be absent, especially in older lesions. The sequence of myelin breakdown is not well understood, although it is known that the lesions contain small amounts of myelin basic proteins, increased amounts of proteolytic enzymes, macrophages, lymphocytes, and plasma cells. Acute, subacute, and chronic sclerosis is often seen at multiple sites throughout the CNS.

MRI has shown that the lesions of multiple sclerosis may occur in two stages: a first stage that involves the sequential development of small inflammatory lesions and a second stage during which the lesions extend and consolidate and when demyelination and gliosis (*i.e.*, scar tissue development) occur.[38] It is not known whether the inflammatory process, present during the first stage, is directed against the myelin or against the oligodendrocytes that produce myelin. Remyelination of the nervous system was considered to be impossible until a few years ago. Evidence now suggests that remyelination can occur in the CNS if the process that initiated the demyelination is halted before the oligodendrocyte dies.[36]

Etiology

The cause of multiple sclerosis remains unknown. Geographic distribution and migration studies suggest an environmental influence. The disease is more prevalent in the colder northern latitudes; it is more common in the northern Atlantic states, the Great Lakes region, and the Pacific Northwest than in the southern parts of the United States. Other high-incidence areas include northern Europe, Great Britain, southern Australia, and New Zealand. Migration studies have shown that persons who move from a high-risk area tend to retain the risk of their birthplace if they move after age 15 or adopt the risk of their new home if they migrate as children.[5]

Although multiple sclerosis is not directly inherited, there is a familial predisposition in some cases, suggesting a genetic influence on susceptibility. However, studies of monozygotic twins have found that the second twin develops the disease only in 30% of cases, suggesting that an exogenous or environmental trigger such as an infectious agent is required to produce the disease.[39]

There is also a strong association between multiple sclerosis and certain HLA antigens (see Chapter 11).[5]

Many authorities think the disease has an immunologic basis, but this has not been confirmed. The demyelination process in multiple sclerosis is marked by prominent lymphocytic invasion in the lesion. Helper T4 cells and suppressor T8 cells are present. In some persons, a sharp decline in the suppressor T-cell population in the blood accompanies exacerbations of the disease.[5]

Manifestations and Clinical Course

The interruption of neural conduction in the demyelinated nerves is manifested by a variety of symptoms, depending on the location and duration of the lesion. Areas commonly affected by multiple sclerosis are the optic nerve (*i.e.*, visual field), corticobulbar tracts (*i.e.*, speech and swallowing), the corticospinal tracts (*i.e.*, muscle strength), and cerebellar tracts (*i.e.*, gait and coordination), spinocerebellar tracts (*i.e.*, balance), medial longitudinal fasciculus (*i.e.*, conjugate gaze function of the extraocular eye muscles), and posterior cell columns of the spinal cord (*i.e.*, position and vibratory sensation).[40] Typically, an otherwise healthy person suffers an acute or subacute episode of paresthesias, optic neuritis (*i.e.*, visual clouding or loss of vision in part of the visual field with pain on movement of the globe), diplopia, or specific types of gaze paralysis.

Paresthesias are often associated with multiple sclerosis and evidenced as numbness, tingling, burning sensation, or pressure on the face or involved extremities; symptoms can range from annoying to severe. Lhermitte's symptom is an electric-shock–like tingling down the back and onto the legs that is produced by flexion of the neck. Pain from spasticity may also be a factor that can be aided by appropriate stretching exercises. Although pain may not be a prominent symptom, about 80% of persons with multiple sclerosis experience some pain in the course of the disease. Other common symptoms are abnormal gait, bladder and sexual dysfunction, vertigo, nystagmus, fatigue, and speech disturbance. These symptoms are usually painless, last for several days to weeks, and then completely or partially resolve. After a period of normal or relatively normal function, new symptoms appear. Psychologic manifestations, such as mood swings, may represent an emotional reaction to the nature of the disease or, more likely, involvement of the white matter of the cerebral cortex. Depression, euphoria, inattentiveness, apathy, forgetfulness, and loss of memory may occur.

Fatigue is one of the most common problems for persons with multiple sclerosis. Fatigue is often described as a generalized low-energy feeling not related to depression and different from weakness. Fatigue has a harmful impact on activities of daily living and sustained physical activity. Interventions such as spacing activities and setting priorities are often helpful.

Small increases in body temperature can temporarily worsen existing neurologic deficits in persons with multiple sclerosis by blocking impulse conduction in demyelinated nerve fibers. This observation forms the basis for the hot bath test, which is sometimes used to aid in the diagnosis of multiple sclerosis.[41] The test is performed by having the person recline in a whirlpool or hot bath. The water level is adjusted so that both axillae are submerged and the temperature of the water is raised to 110°F while neurologic function is monitored. If new neurologic deficits are observed, the test is terminated, and the water is cooled to reverse the conduction block and its symptoms. Prolonged neurologic sequelae have been observed in persons with multiple sclerosis after unintentional exposure to high environmental temperatures such as those encountered in a hot tub or while sunbathing.[42]

Usually, the course of multiple sclerosis falls into one of four categories, with the progression from one pattern of symptoms to a more serious one (Table 39–2).[43] A small percentage of persons develop an acute form of multiple sclerosis that progresses rapidly and has incomplete remissions of short duration. This form of multiple sclerosis can be fatal within a few months or years. There may also be a subclinical form of the disease, as evidenced by the finding of demyelinated lesions in asymptomatic persons on autopsy.[37] Because of the varied clinical courses of multiple sclerosis, persons in whom the disease is recently diagnosed have some justification for optimism.

Diagnosis

The diagnosis of multiple sclerosis is difficult because there is no specific laboratory test for the disease, manifestations are variable, and there may be lengthy delays between the first appearance of symptoms and recurrence. A definite diagnosis of multiple sclerosis requires evidence of one of the following patterns: two or more episodes of exacerbation separated by 1 month or more and lasting more than 24 hours, with subsequent recovery; a clinical history of clearly defined exacerbations and remissions, with or without complete recovery, followed by progression of symptoms over a period of at least 6 months; or slow and stepwise progression of signs and symptoms over a period of at least 6 months.[40] A person who has not had a relapse or progression of symptoms is described as having stable multiple sclerosis.

MRI can be used as an adjunct to clinical diagnosis. MRI studies can detect the multiplicity of lesions even when CT scans appear normal. A computer-assisted method of MRI can measure lesion size. Many new areas of myelin abnormality are asymptomatic. Serial MRI studies can be done to detect asymptomatic lesions, monitor the progress of existing lesions, and evaluate the effectiveness of treatment. Although MRI can be used to provide evidence of disseminated lesions in persons with the disease, normal findings do not exclude the diagnosis.[40] Electrophysiologic evaluations (*e.g.*, evoked potential studies) and CT scans may assist in the identification and documentation of lesions.

Although no laboratory test can be used to diagnose multiple sclerosis, examination of the cerebrospinal fluid is helpful. A large percentage of patients with mul-

TABLE 39-2

Categories of Symptom Progression in Multiple Sclerosis

Category	Percent of cases	Characteristics
Benign	20	Long symptom-free periods with mild or completely remitting attacks
Relapsing	25	Acute onset of periodic symptoms followed by partial or complete recovery, having plateaus of unchanging impairment
Relapsing-progressive	40	Slow, stepwise deterioration in function highlighted by exacerbations with modest recovery and significant residual impairment
Chronic-progressive	15	Continuous functional deterioration over months or years with risk of life-threatening complications

(National Multiple Sclerosis Society Client and Family Services 1995 Teleconference. Today's symptom control—Tomorrow's new treatments)

tiple sclerosis have elevated IgG levels, and some have oligoclonal patterns (*i.e.*, discrete electrophoretic bands) even with normal IgG levels. Total protein or lymphocyte levels may be mildly elevated in the cerebrospinal fluid. These tests can be altered in a variety of inflammatory neurologic disorders and are not specific for multiple sclerosis.

Treatment

Most treatment measures for multiple sclerosis are directed at modifying the course and managing the primary symptoms of the disease. The variety of symptoms, unpredictable course, and lack of specific diagnostic methods have made the evaluation and treatment of multiple sclerosis difficult. Persons who are minimally affected by the disorder require no specific treatment. The person should be encouraged to maintain as healthy a lifestyle as possible, including good nutrition and adequate rest and relaxation. Physical therapy may help maintain muscle tone. Every effort should be made to avoid excessive fatigue, physical deterioration, emotional stress, and extremes of environmental temperature, which may precipitate an exacerbation of the disease.

The pharmacologic treatment of multiple sclerosis is largely symptomatic and may include the use of dantrolene (Dantrium), baclofen (Lioresal), or diazepam (Valium) for spasticity; cholinergic drugs for bladder problems; and antidepressant drugs for depression. Adrenocorticotrophic hormone (ACTH) and corticosteroids can shorten the duration of an exacerbation. It has been hypothesized that corticosteroids may reduce the inflammation, improve nerve conduction, and have important immunologic effects.[44] Long-term administration does not, however, appear to alter the course of the disease and can have harmful side effects. Several studies have indicated that intensive immunosuppressive therapy with intravenous cyclophosphamide may help arrest the chronic progressive course of active multiple sclerosis. Plasmapheresis has proved beneficial in some cases.

Two substances, copolymer 1 and interferon-β, are undergoing extensive clinical testing. Both agents have shown some benefit in reducing exacerbations in persons with multiple sclerosis that follows a course of relapse, remission, and exacerbations rather than a course of steady progression. Copolymer 1 (COP 1) is a synthetic polypeptide that simulates parts of the myelin basic protein. Its mechanism of action is still uncertain. Interferon-β, a lymphokine that acts as an immune enhancer, has been released for use in treatment of persons with relapsing-progressive multiple sclerosis. The rationale for initial testing of interferons was the hypothesis that the disease might be caused by a persistent or latent CNS viral infection in persons with an altered immune response.[45]

Spinal Cord Injury

Despite the protective mechanisms built in during the development of the CNS, spinal cord injury continues to occur. Estimates of the national population of persons living with spinal cord injuries vary between 180,000 and 200,000. Nationally, there are an additional 8000 to 10,000 new spine injuries that result in paralysis each year.[46] The most frequent cause of spinal cord injury is motor vehicle accidents, followed by falls, violence, sports injuries, and other types of injuries, which include attempted suicide and occupational injuries. Of sports-related injuries, 66% are from diving.[46]

The average age for spinal cord injury is between 16 and 30 years, with 19 years being the most frequent age. As age increases, the cause of injury changes, with falls becoming the most frequent cause. Males sustain spinal cord injuries at a rate four times higher than that of females. Alcohol and drugs have been cited as contributing factors in an increasing number of cases.

Injury to the Vertebral Column

Structure of the Vertebral Column. The spinal column, which is located in the posterior midline of the body, begins at the base of the skull and ends at the coccyx, or "tailbone." There are 32 to 33 individual and fused vertebral bodies, or vertebrae, that make up the spinal column: 7 cervical, 12 thoracic, 5 lumbar, 5 fused sacral, and 3 or 4 fused coccygeal vertebrae. Each vertebra in the vertebral column, with the exception of the first cervical vertebra, shares common characteristics; each consists of an anterior portion, or body, and a posterior portion, called the *vertebral* or *neural arch* (Fig. 39–12). The vertebral arch or posterior elements are composed of two pedicles, two laminae, a spinous process, two transverse processes, and four articular processes known as *facets*. The transverse foramen within the transverse processes of the cervical vertebrae form a passageway for the vertebral artery, vertebral vein, and sympathetic nerves.

The design of the vertebra is to provide bony support and protection for the cord by forming a vertebral foramen or spinal canal. The size and function of the vertebrae are directly related to their specific location in the spinal column. Generally, vertebral bodies increase in size to bear additional weight as they descend along the spinal column. The width of the spinal canal also varies at different levels. The atlas (C1) and the axis (C2) are smaller than the rest of the vertebrae and are formed in a manner that allows flexion, extension, and rotation of the head. The intermediate-sized thoracic vertebrae are heart-shaped and limited in movement, making the thoracic spine, especially the lower levels, more rigid. They also possess tubercles for rib attachment. Each vertebra articulates with the next above and below by means of articular processes called *facets,* which function as sliding synovial joints. The facets provide some support and major limitation of movement. They also can be a frequent source of back pain. The design of the lumbar spine allows for powerful flexion and some extension; these lumbar vertebrae are large and heavy to accommodate the attachment of lower limb muscles and the weight of the thorax, neck, and head.

Fibrocartilaginous disks and strong bands of fibers known as ligaments assist the vertebral column in supporting and protecting the spinal cord. The intervertebral disks contain a firm gelatinous structure called the *nucleus pulposus,* which is surrounded by a layer of fibrocartilage called the *annulus fibrosus*. The intervertebral disks, along with the facet joints, carry all of the compressive loading that the trunk of the body is subjected to.

The vertebrae and intervertebral disks are held in place by the ligaments. There are two major longitudinal ligaments that extend from the axis (C2) to the sacrum on the anterior and posterior surfaces of the vertebral bodies and disks (see Fig. 39–7). These ligaments allow adequate motion and maintenance of alignment between vertebrae; protect the spinal cord by limiting motions within well-defined limits; assist the muscles in providing stability to the spine; and protect the spinal cord in traumatic situations associated with high loads and fast speeds. Other fibrous ligaments that attach at various sites between the parts of neighboring vertebrae also support and limit movement of the spinal column, thereby protecting the spinal cord. Additional stabilizing forces are the rib cage, superficial and deep trunk muscles, and the normal curvature of the spine, which is

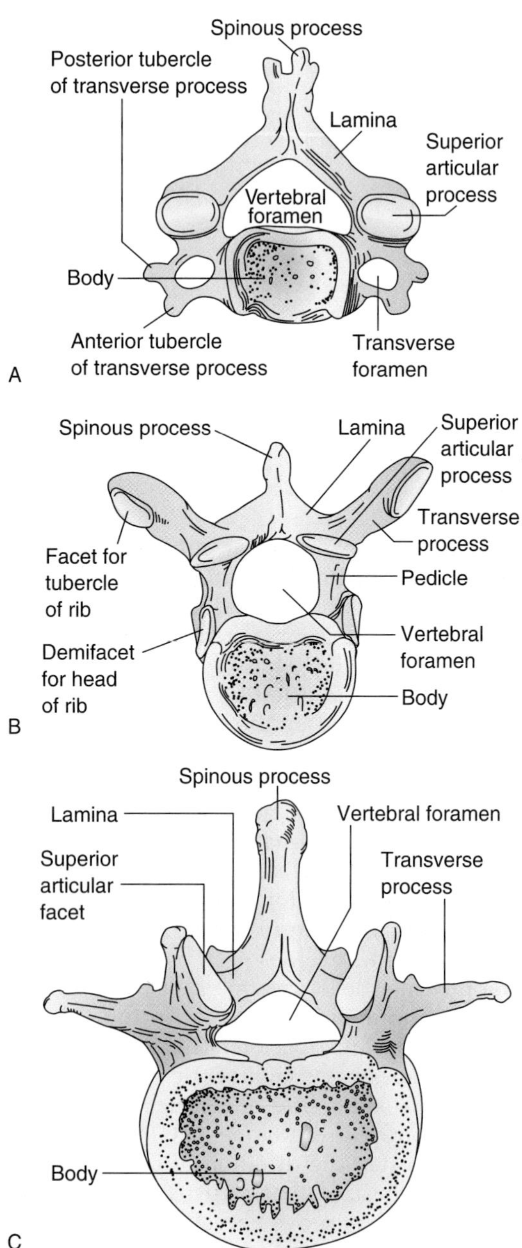

Figure 39–12
Views of three types of vertebrae. (**A**) Fourth cervical vertebra, superior aspect; (**B**) sixth thoracic vertebra, superior aspect; (**C**) third lumbar vertebra, superior aspect.

anteriorly convex at the cervical and lumbar regions and posteriorly convex in the thoracic and sacral levels.

Vertebral Column Injury. Injuries to the vertebral column include fractures, dislocations, and subluxations. A fracture can occur at any part of the bony vertebrae, causing fragmentation of the bone. It most often involves the pedicle, lamina, or processes (*e.g.*, facets). Dislocation or subluxation (*i.e.*, partial dislocation) injury causes the vertebral bodies to become displaced, with one overriding another and preventing correct alignment of the vertebral column. The extent of injury to the vertebral column caused by motion or trauma is related to the amount and direction of motion and the rate of application of force causing the motion. Damage to the ligaments or bony vertebrae may make the spine unstable. In an unstable spine, further unguarded movement of the spinal column can impinge on the spinal canal, causing compression or overstretching of neural tissue.

Most injuries result from some combination of compressive force or bending movement (Fig. 39–13). *Flexion injuries* occur when forward bending of the spinal column exceeds the limits of normal movement. Typical flexion injuries result, for example, when the head is struck from behind, as in a fall with the back of the head as the point of impact. *Extension injuries* occur with excessive forced bending (*i.e.*, hyperextension) of the spine backward. A typical extension injury involves a fall in which the chin or face is the point of impact, causing hyperextension of the neck. Injuries of *flexion and extension* occur more commonly in the cervical spine (C4 to C6) than in any other area. Limitations imposed by the ribs, spinous processes, and joint capsules in the thoracic and lumbar spine make this area less flexible and less susceptible to flexion and extension injuries than the cervical spine. The exact location of increased stiffness and inflexibility can range from T11 to L1. This area is more subject to mechanical failure and accounts for a high number of spine injuries in the thoracolumbar junction.

A *compression injury*, causing the vertebral bones to shatter, squash, or even burst, occurs when there is spinal loading from a high-velocity blow to the top of the head or when landing forcefully on the feet (see Fig. 39–13). This typically occurs at the cervical level (*e.g.*, diving injuries) or in the thoracolumbar area (*e.g.*, falling from a distance and landing on the feet). Compression injuries may occur when the vertebrae are weakened by conditions such as osteoporosis and cancer with bone metastasis. *Axial rotation injuries* can produce highly unstable injuries. Maximal axial rotation occurs in the cervical region, especially between C1 and C2 and at the lumbosacral joint. *Coupling* of vertebral motions is common in injury when two or more individual motions occur (*e.g.*, lateral bending and axial rotation). The motion produced by the external force is called the main motion, and all the accompanying motions are considered coupled motions.

Injury to the Spinal Cord

When the spinal cord becomes injured, maximal physical damage occurs in the gray matter containing the neuronal cell bodies in the center of the spinal cord.[47] Because of their high metabolic rate, the neurons in the gray matter of the spinal cord are more vulnerable to injury than the axons in the surrounding white matter. The white matter tracts have a lower metabolic rate, and their mechanisms for repair are distant from the site of injury; in some cases, axons survive the injury and are

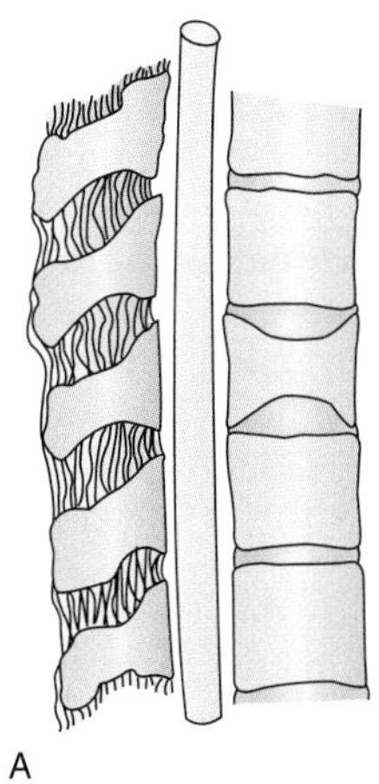

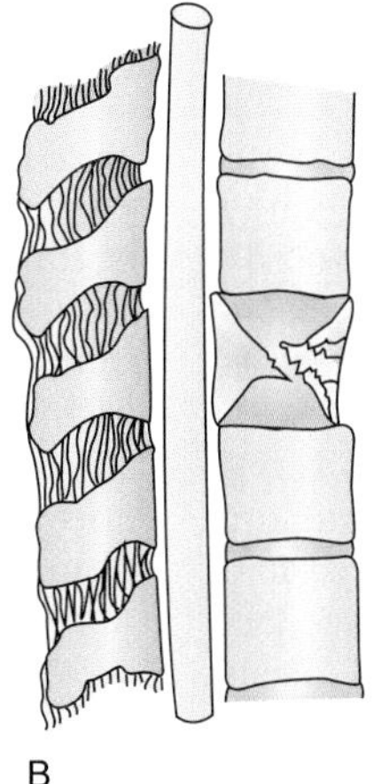

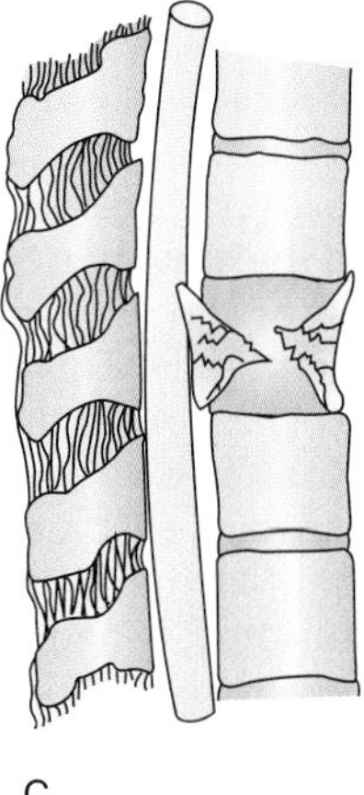

Figure 39–13
Progressive degrees of compression fracture. (**A**) Severe compression fracture showing the biconcave profile produced by the adjacent discs. (**B**) A more severe degree of fracture. A vertical fracture has joined the deformed, concave endplates. The anterior body fragment is comminuted and displaced anteriorly. (**C**) A more severe degree of compression fracture. The posterior body fragment is now comminuted and displaced posteriorly into the spinal canal. Neural damage may occur.

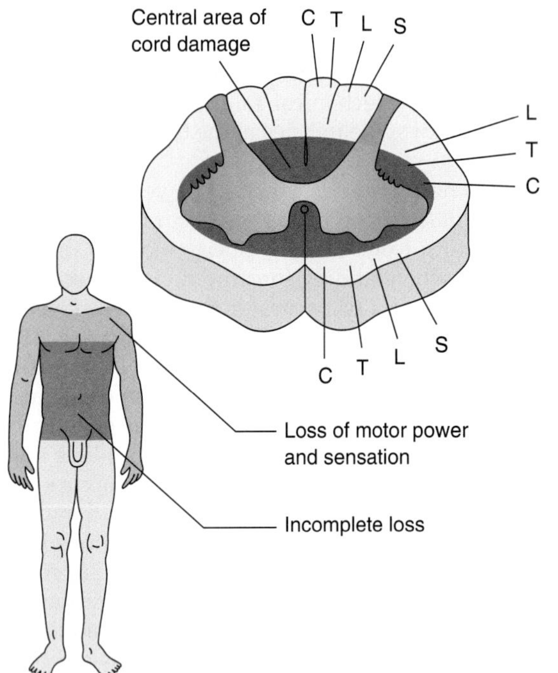

Figure 39–14
Central cord syndrome. A cross section of the cord shows central damage and the associated motor and sensory loss. (C, cervical; T, thoracic; L, lumbar; S, sacral)

salvageable up to 72 hours or more after injury. Three types of pathologic processes occur at the time of spinal cord injury or shortly thereafter: mechanical disruption of neurons at the injury site, injury-related ischemia and hypoxia that contribute to local infarction of neuronal tissue, and development of microhemorrhages or edema at the injury site that result in interruption of neuronal function.[47]

The pathophysiology of spinal cord injury can be divided into two types: primary and secondary. The primary neurologic injury occurs at the time of mechanical injury and is irreversible. It is characterized by small hemorrhages in the gray matter of the cord, followed by edematous changes in the white matter that lead to necrosis of neural tissue. This type of pathology results from the forces of compression, stretch and shear associated with fracture or compression of the spinal vertebrae, dislocation of vertebrae (*e.g.*, flexion, extension, subluxation), and jarring of the cord within the spinal canal (*i.e.*, contusions). Penetrating injuries produce lacerations and direct trauma to the cord and may occur with or without spinal column damage. The most frequent penetrating injuries are caused by gunshot and knife wounds. Lacerations occur when there is cutting or tearing of the spinal cord, which injures nerve tissue and causes bleeding and edema. Even in the presence of complete damage to all neural tissue at the site of injury, the spinal cord frequently remains intact, lending support to the concept that mechanisms secondary to the initial injury play a significant role.

Secondary injuries follow the primary injury and promote the spread of injury.[48] Although there is considerable debate about the pathogenesis of secondary injuries, the tissue destruction that occurs ends in progressive neurologic damage. Following spinal cord injury, several mechanisms of pathology occur, including vascular damage, neuronal injury that leads to loss of reflexes below the level of injury, and release of vasoactive agents and cellular enzymes. Vascular pathology (*i.e.*, vessel trauma and hemorrhage) can lead to ischemia, increased vascular permeability, and edema. Blood flow to the spinal cord may be further compromised by spinal shock that results from a loss of vasomotor tone and neural reflexes below the level of injury. The release of vasoactive substances (*i.e.*, norepinephrine, serotonin, dopamine, and histamine) from the wound tissue causes vasospasm and impedes blood flow in the microcirculation, producing further necrosis of blood vessels and neurons. The release of proteolytic and lipolytic enzymes from injured cells causes delayed swelling, demyelination, and necrosis in the spinal cord.

As in spine trauma, the greater the magnitude of force applied to the spinal cord, the greater is the associated damage. Some areas of hemorrhage and injury may occur rostral and caudal to the site of impact, and the severity of bony injury or radiographic findings may not always correspond with the extent of neurologic damage. Also, the location of bony injury may not coincide with the clinical findings of motor and sensory deficits, such as a C6 compression fracture with motor and sensory level functioning at C7, C4, or C5.

The goal of management of spinal cord injury is to reduce the neurologic deficit and prevent any additional loss of neurologic function. The specific steps in resuscitation and initial evaluation can be carried out at the trauma site or in the emergency room, depending on the urgency of the situation.[48] Most traumatic injuries to the spinal column render it unstable, mandating measures such as immobilization with collars and backboards and limiting the movement of persons at risk or with known spinal cord injury. Every person with multiple trauma or head injury, including victims of traffic and sporting accidents, should be suspected of having sustained an acute spinal cord injury.[49] In-line immobilization without traction is recommended. This includes immobilizing the neck in a neutral position in a rigid cervical collar. The person should be "log rolled" onto a rigid backboard, with the head secured by straps or tape.

The nature of the injury determines further methods of stabilization and treatment. In unstable injuries of the cervical spine, cervical traction improves or restores spinal alignment, decompresses neural structures, and facilitates recovery. Fractures and dislocations of the thoracic and lumbar vertebrae may be initially stabilized by restricting the person to bed rest and turning him or her in log-roll manner to keep the spine rigid. Gunshot or stab wounds of the spinal column may not produce structural instability and require immobilization. The goal of early surgical intervention of an unstable spine is to provide internal skeletal stabilization so that early mobilization and rehabilitation can occur.

The use of high-dose methylprednisone treatment has been shown to improve the outcome from spinal cord injury when given shortly after injury. Methylprednisone is a short-acting corticosteroid that has been used extensively in the treatment of inflammatory and allergic disorders. In acute spinal cord injury, it is thought to stabilize cell membranes, enhance impulse generation, improve blood flow, and inhibit free radical formation.[50] In a prospective, randomized, double-blind controlled study, high-dose methylprednisone treatment, when given within 8 hours of injury, resulted in a significant long-term improvement in maximal motor function.[51] Because methylprednisone has been identified as an effective initial treatment for spinal cord injury in the U.S., it is now considered standard medical treatment to be given within the first 8 hours of injury.

The success of methylprednisolone in improving neurologic functioning after spinal cord injury is expected to lead to the evaluation of other new agents. Other research involves functional electrical stimulation and tissue-bridge implants to reactivate damaged motor systems and promote nerve regeneration. Until a cure is found, prevention of injury through health promotion education, early diagnosis, prompt intervention, and rehabilitation to prevent complications and restore optimal functioning is essential.

Classification and Types of Injury

Alterations in body function that result from spinal cord injury depend on the level of injury and the amount of cord involvement. The American Spinal Injury Association (ASIA) has published *Standards for Neurological and Functional Classification of Spinal Cord Injury.*[52] According to ASIA, *tetraplegia* (a term preferred to quadriplegia), refers to impairment or loss of motor or sensory function (or both) in the cervical segments of the cord after damage of neural elements within the spinal canal. Tetraplegia results in impairment of function in the arms, trunk, legs, and pelvic organs (see Fig. 39–4). It does not include peripheral nerve injuries. *Paraplegia* refers to impairment or loss of motor or sensory function (or both) in the thoracic, lumbar, or sacral segments of the spinal cord from damage of neural elements within the spinal canal. With paraplegia, arm functioning is spared, but depending on the level of injury, functioning of the trunk, leg, and pelvic organs may be involved. Paraplegia also refers to conus medullaris and cauda equina injuries but not injury to peripheral nerves outside the spinal canal.

Further definitions describe the extent of neurologic damage as complete or incomplete injuries. In an *incomplete* spinal cord injury, partial preservation of sensory and motor function is found below the neurologic level of injury and includes the lowest sacral segment (*e.g.*, sparing of S2 to S4 innervation of myocutaneous and deep anal sensation and rectal sphincter control). The necessary test of motor function is the voluntary contraction of the anal sphincter on digital examination. A *complete* injury refers to the absence of sensory and motor function, which includes the lowest sacral segment. The myotome and dermatome charts (see Chapter 40, Fig. 40–1) show skeletal muscle and sensory areas of skin innervated by specific spinal cord segments. The prognosis for return of function is more likely in an incomplete injury because of preservation of axonal function. However, the longer the period since the injury, the less likely it is that improvement will occur.

The level and extent of injury to the spinal cord can be determined by the presenting clinical symptoms, which reflect the predominant area of the cord that is involved. Complete cord injuries can result from severance of the cord, disruption of nerve fibers although they remain intact, or interruption of blood supply to that segment resulting in complete destruction of neural tissue and UMN or LMN paralysis. However, complete severance of the cord is rare. Incomplete injuries may manifest in a variety of patterns but can be organized into certain patterns or "syndromes" that occur more frequently and reflect the predominant area of the cord that is involved.

Central Cord Syndrome. A condition called *central cord syndrome* occurs when injury is predominantly in the central gray or white matter of the cord (see Fig. 39–14).[12] Because the corticospinal tract fibers are organized with those controlling the arms being located more centrally and those controlling the legs located more laterally, some external axonal transmission may remain intact. Motor function of the upper extremities is affected, but the lower extremities may not be affected or may be affected to a lesser degree, with some sparing of sacral sensation. Bowel, bladder, and sexual functions are usually affected to various degrees and may parallel the degree of lower extremity involvement. This syndrome occurs almost exclusively in the cervical cord, rendering the lesion a UMN with spastic paralysis. Central cord damage is more frequent in elderly persons with narrowing or stenotic changes in the spinal canal that are related to arthritis. Damage may also occur in persons with congenital stenosis. As in any incomplete injury, the prognosis for return of function is more likely than in complete injury, and improvement seems to affect the lower extremities to a greater degree than upper extremities because of the nature of the primary injury.

Anterior Cord Syndrome. Anterior artery or *anterior cord syndrome* is usually caused by damage from infarction of the anterior spinal artery resulting in damage to the anterior two thirds of the cord (Fig. 39–15).[12] The deficits result in loss of motor function provided by the corticospinal tracts and the loss of pain and temperature sensation from damage to the lateral spinothalamic tracts. The spinal gray matter largely depends on blood flow from the anterior spinal artery. Loss of the local gray matter can result in reduction in or loss of local reflexes and localized LMNs of the anterior horn. The posterior one third of the cord is relatively unaffected,

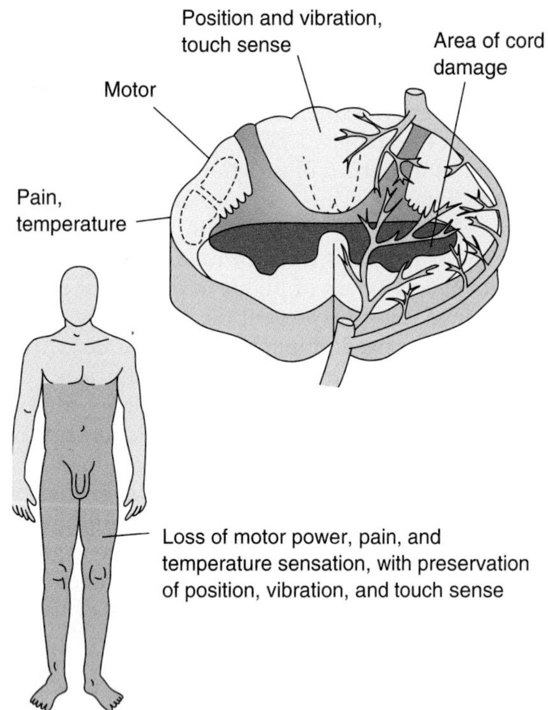

Figure 39–15
Anterior cord syndrome. Cord damage and associated motor and sensory loss are illustrated.

preserving the dorsal column axons conveying position, vibration, and touch sensation.

Brown-Séquard Syndrome. A condition called *Brown-Séquard syndrome* results from damage to a hemisection of the anterior and posterior cord (Fig. 39–16).[12] The effect is a loss of voluntary motor function from the corticospinal tract, proprioception loss from the ipsilateral side of the body, and contralateral loss of pain and temperature sensation from the lateral spinothalamic tracts for all levels below the lesion.

Conus Medullaris Syndrome. *Conus medullaris syndrome* involves damage to the conus medullaris or the sacral cord (*i.e.,* conus) and lumbar nerve roots within the neural canal. Functional deficits resulting from this type of injury usually result in flaccid bowel, bladder, and sexual function. Sacral segments occasionally show preserved reflexes if only the conus is affected. Motor function in the legs and feet may be impaired without significant sensory impairment. Damage to the lumbosacral nerve roots within the canal usually results in LMN and sensory neuron damage known as *cauda equina syndrome.* Functional deficits present as various patterns of asymmetric flaccid paralysis, sensory impairment, and pain.

Because of the variations that occur with incomplete injuries, the discussion in the following sections focuses on complete spinal cord injuries. The physical problems discussed in this chapter are those associated with ventilation and communication, autonomic regulation, sensorimotor integrity, bowel and bladder function, and sexual function.

Alterations in Functional Abilities

Functional abilities after spinal cord injury cover various degrees of sensorimotor loss and altered reflex activity based on the level of cord injury and extent of cord damage. Table 39–3 summarizes the functional abilities by level of injury. Motor function in cervical injuries ranges from complete dependence to independence with or without assistive devices in activities of mobility and self-care. The functional levels of cervical injury are related to C5, C6, C7, or C8 innervation. At the C5 level, deltoid and biceps function is spared, allowing full head, neck, and diaphragm control with good shoulder strength and full elbow flexion. At the C6 level, wrist dorsiflexion by the way of wrist extensors is functional, allowing *tenodesis,* which is the natural bending inward and flexion of the fingers when the wrist is extended and bent backward. Tenodesis is a key movement, because it can be used to pick up objects when finger movement is absent. A functional C7 injury allows full elbow flexion and extension, wrist plantar flexion, and some finger control. At the C8 level, finger flexion is added.

Thoracic cord injuries (T1 to T12) allow full upper extremity control with limited to full control of intercostal and trunk muscles and balance. Injury at the T1 level allows full fine motor control of the fingers. Because of the lack of specific functional indicators at

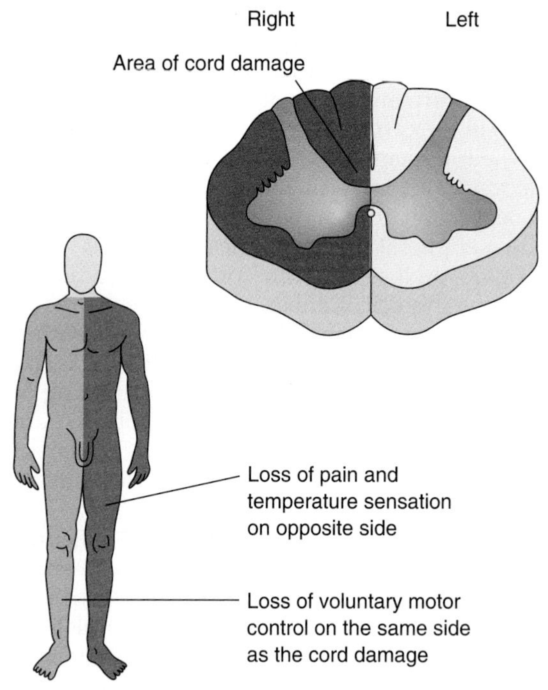

Figure 39–16
Brown-Séquard syndrome. Cord damage and associated motor and sensory loss are illustrated.

TABLE 39-3

Functional Abilities by Level of Cord Injury

Injury Level	Segmental Sensorimotor Function	Dressing, Eating	Elimination	Mobility*
C1	Little or no sensation or control of head and neck; no diaphragm control; requires continuous ventilation	Dependent	Dependent	Limited. Voice or sip-n-puff controlled electric wheelchair
C2 to C3	Head and neck sensation; some neck control. Independent of mechanical ventilation for short periods	Dependent	Dependent	Same as for C1
C4	Good head and neck sensation and motor control; some shoulder elevation; diaphragm movement	Dependent; may be able to eat with adaptive sling	Dependent	Limited to voice, mouth, head, chin, or shoulder-controlled electric chair
C5	Full head and neck control; shoulder strength; elbow flexion	Independent with assistance	Maximal assistance	Electric or modified manual wheel chair, needs transfer assistance
C6	Fully innervated shoulder; wrist extension or dorsiflexion	Independent and/or with minimal assistance	Independent and/or with minimal assistance	Independent in transfers and wheel chair
C7 to C8	Full elbow extension; wrist plantar flexion; some finger control	Independent	Independent	Independent; manual wheelchair
T1 to T5	Full hand and finger control; use of intercostal and thoracic muscles	Independent	Independent	Independent; manual wheelchair
T6 to T10	Abdominal muscle control, partial to good balance with trunk muscles	Independent	Independent	Independent; manual wheelchair
T11 to L5	Hip flexors, hip abductors (L1–3); knee extension (L2–4); knee flexion and ankle dorsiflexion (L4–5)	Independent	Independent	Short distance to full ambulation with assistance
S1 to S5	Full leg, foot and ankle control; innervation of perineal muscles for bowel, bladder, and sexual function (S2–4)	Independent	Normal to impaired bowel and bladder function	Ambulate independently with or without assistance

*Assistance refers to adaptive equipment, set up, or physical assistance.

the thoracic levels, the level of injury is usually determined by sensory level testing.

Functional capacity in the L1 through L5 nerve innervations allows hip flexors, hip abductors (L1 to L3), movement of the knees (L2 to L5), and ankle dorsiflexion (L4 to L5). Sacral (S1 to S5) innervation allows for full leg, foot, and ankle control and innervation of perineal musculature for bowel, bladder, and sexual function.

Alterations in Spinal Reflexes. Altered spinal reflex activity in spinal cord injury is essentially determined by UMN and LMN lesions. UMNs that are fully contained within the CNS are generally affected by any injury at the T12 level or above. This results in spastic paralysis of the affected skeletal muscle groups and muscles that control bowel, bladder, and sexual functions. LMN injuries generally occur with injuries below T12 and result from damage to the peripheral nerves that exit each segment of the spinal cord. The LMN injuries cause flaccid paralysis of involved skeletal muscle groups and muscles that control of bowel, bladder, and sexual function. However, injuries near the T12 level may result in mixed UMN and LMN deficits (*e.g.*, spastic paralysis of the bowel and bladder with flaccid muscle tone).

Spinal shock, or *neurogenic shock,* is the term used to describe the state of areflexia that occurs after cord injury. Spinal shock involves the loss of all or most of the spinal reflexes below the level of injury.[53] It involves the motor pathways, and the manifestations are flaccid paralysis and lack of tendon reflexes and autonomic function, regardless of whether the level of lesion will eventually produce spastic (UMN) or flaccid (LMN) paralysis. The basic mechanisms accounting for the transient spinal shock are unknown. Spinal shock may last for minutes, hours, days, or weeks, after which isolated spinal cord reflex activity returns. Usually, if reflex function returns by the time the person reaches the hospital, the neuromuscular changes are reversible. This kind of reversible spinal shock may occur in football-type injuries, in which jarring of the spinal cord within the canal produces a concussion-like phenomenon that causes a temporary loss of movement and reflexes, followed by full recovery within days. In persons in whom paralysis or weakness persists, hypotension and bradycardia may become critical but manageable problems. Generally, the higher the level of cord injury, the greater is the effect.

Ventilation and Communication Dysfunctions. Ventilation requires movement of the expiratory and inspiratory muscles, all of which receive innervation from the spinal cord. The main muscle of ventilation, the diaphragm, is innervated by segments C3 to C5 through the phrenic nerves. The intercostal muscles, located between the ribs, are innervated by spinal segments T1 through T7. These muscles function in elevating the rib cage and are needed for coughing and deep breathing. The major muscles of expiration are the abdominal muscles, which receive their innervation from levels T6 to T12. By forcing the abdominal viscera against the diaphragm, the muscles exert pressure on the diaphragm and return the thoracic cage to its resting position. Coughing and deep breathing, which are vital to the removal of mucus and foreign particles from the respiratory tract, are facilitated by the elevation of the rib cage and expansion of the anteroposterior and lateral dimensions of the chest wall, followed by strong respiratory and abdominal muscle contraction forcing air out of the lungs.

Although the ability to inhale and exhale may be preserved at various levels of spinal cord injury, functional deficits in ventilation are most apparent in the quality of the breathing cycle and the ability to oxygenate tissues, eliminate carbon dioxide, and mobilize secretions. Cord injuries involving C1 to C3 result in a lack of respiratory effort, and affected patients require assisted ventilation. Although a C3 to C5 injury allows partial or full diaphragmatic function, ventilation is diminished because of the loss of intercostal muscle function, resulting in shallow breaths and a weak cough. Below the C5 level, as less intercostal and abdominal musculature is affected, the ability to take a deep breath and cough is less impaired. Maintenance therapy consists of muscle training to strengthen existing muscles for endurance and mobilization of secretions.

With assisted ventilation, whether continuous or intermittent, ensuring adequate communication of needs is also essential. There are several ways of ensuring communication of needs with the use of verbal or nonverbal communication systems. Verbal approaches may consist of fenestrated tracheal tubes to provide air flow and vibration of the vocal cords, talking tracheostomy tubes, diaphragmatic pacing, electrolarynx-type devices, and mechanical ventilation with an air leak. Nonverbal communication techniques include boards or cards displaying the person's most frequently used words, computerized scanning programs, and mouth-stick control devices.

Autonomic Nervous System Dysfunction. Spinal cord injury not only interrupts the function of the somatic nerves that control skeletal muscle function, it also interrupts visceral afferent input and autonomic outflow from below the site of injury. This affects parasympathetic outflow from the sacral segments of the spinal cord and the sympathetic outflow from the thoracic and lumbar segments. After spinal cord injury, the spinal reflex circuits are largely isolated from the rest of the CNS. Afferent somatic and visceral sensory input that enters the spinal cord through intact segmental nerves is unaffected. Likewise, the efferent outflow from intact reflex centers below the site of injury is largely unaffected. However, the transmission of ascending sensory input to higher centers and descending motor control output from higher centers is blocked at the site of injury. Lacking are the regulation and integration of reflex function from higher autonomic and motor control centers in the brain and brain stem. Interruption of autonomic outflow results in continued function above the level of injury, but the spinal and autonomic reflexes below the level of injury are uncontrolled.

In persons in whom high-level paraplegia or tetraplegia persists beyond the first few hours or days after injury, hypotension and bradycardia may be critical but manageable problems. Circulatory function is impaired by the loss of sympathetic control of heart rate, peripheral vascular resistance, and lack of muscle tone in paralyzed limbs, resulting in sluggish circulating blood flow and venous return. The resulting bradycardia and hypotension can usually be managed with slow fluid resuscitation and body positioning that facilitates venous return. Spinal shock and true hemorrhagic shock (*i.e.,* hypotension and tachycardia) must be differentiated and treated accordingly. Spinal shock is usually self-limited, and the return of reflexes usually occurs in a caudal to rostral direction, with the first returning reflexes being those in the sacral area (*i.e.,* rectal sphincter contraction) followed by those of the lumbar area (*i.e.,* the lower extremities). However, bradycardia and hypotension may persist and become asymptomatic normal parameters. The length of time that it takes to adjust to the altered circulatory status is variable and may be as long as 1 year.

The autonomic regulation of circulatory function and thermoregulation present the most severe problems in spinal cord injury. The higher the level of injury and the greater the body surface area affected, the more profound are the effects on circulation and thermoregulation. Persons with injury at the T6 level or above experience problems in regulating vasomotor tone; those with injuries below the T6 level usually have sufficient sympathetic function to maintain adequate vasomotor function. The level of injury and its corresponding problems may vary among persons and situations, and some dysfunctional effects may be seen at levels below T6. With lower lumbar and sacral injuries, sympathetic function remains essentially unaltered.

Vasovagal Response. The vagus nerve (cranial nerve X) normally exerts a continuous inhibitory effect on heart rate. Vagal stimulation that causes a marked bradycardia by way of the vagus nerve is called the vasovagal response. Visceral afferent input to the vagal centers in the brain stem of persons with tetraplegia or high-level paraplegia can produce marked bradycardia when unchecked by a dysfunctional sympathetic nervous system. Severe bradycardia and even asystole can result when the vasovagal response is elicited by deep endotracheal suctioning or rapid position change. Preventive measures, such as hyperoxygenation before, during, and after suctioning, are advised. Rapid position changes should be avoided or anticipated, and anticholinergic drugs should be immediately available to counteract severe episodes of bradycardia.

Autonomic Dysreflexia. The terms autonomic dysreflexia and autonomic hyperreflexia refer to an acute episode of exaggerated sympathetic reflex responses that occur in persons with spinal cord injury because of a lack of control from higher brain centers. This exaggerated response is usually caused by visceral stimuli that normally cause pain or discomfort in the abdominopelvic region. Autonomic dysreflexia does not occur until spinal shock has resolved and autonomic reflexes return, most often within the first 6 months after injury. It is most unpredictable during the first year after injury but can occur throughout the person's lifetime.

Autonomic dysreflexia is usually characterized by hypertension ranging from mild (20 mm Hg above baseline) to severe hypertension (as high as 300/160 mm Hg), bradycardia, and headache ranging from dull to severe and pounding.[52] The condition is associated with injuries at T6 and above. Usually, persons with injuries at the T6 level or below have sufficient sympathetic outflow to control visceral reflexes. In persons with injuries at T6 or above, sympathetic responses that occur at and below that level of the spinal cord are lost, while baroreceptor function and parasympathetic control of heart rate remain intact. Unregulated sympathetic activity below the level of injury causes vasospasm, hypertension, skin pallor, and gooseflesh associated with the piloerector response. Continued hypertension produces a baroreflex-mediated vagal slowing of heart rate to bradycardic levels. There is an accompanying baroreflex-mediated vasodilatation, flushed skin, and profuse sweating above the level of injury, along with headache, nasal stuffiness, and feelings of anxiety. A person may experience one, several, or all of the symptoms with each episode.

The stimuli initiating the dysreflexic response include visceral distention, such as a full bladder or rectum; stimulation of pain receptors, as occurs with pressure ulcers, ingrown toenails, dressing changes, and diagnostic or operative procedures; and visceral contractions, such as ejaculation, bladder spasms, or uterine contractions. In many cases, the dysreflexic response results from a full bladder.

Autonomic dysreflexia is a clinical emergency, and without prompt and adequate treatment, convulsions, loss of consciousness, and even death can occur. The major components of treatment include monitoring blood pressure while removing or correcting the initiating cause or stimulus. The person should be placed in an upright position, and all support hose or binders should be removed to promote venous pooling of blood and reduce venous return, thereby decreasing blood pressure. If the stimuli have been removed or the stimuli cannot be identified and the upright position established but the blood pressure remains elevated, drugs that block autonomic function are administered. Persons should be monitored for several hours after the dysreflexic event. Prevention of the type of stimuli that trigger the dysreflexic event is advocated.

Postural Hypotension. Postural, or orthostatic, hypotension usually occurs in persons with injuries at T4 to T6 and above and is related to the interruption of descending control of sympathetic outflow to blood vessels in the extremities and abdomen. Pooling of blood, along with gravitational forces, impairs venous return to the heart, and there is a subsequent decrease in cardiac output when the person is placed in an upright position. This usually occurs when the person is placed in the seated position in bed or transferred from the bed to the wheelchair. The signs of orthostatic hypotension include dizziness, pallor, excessive sweating above the level of the lesion, complaints of blurred vision, and possibly fainting. Because of the disruption in autonomic function at the time of injury, the blood pressure and heart rate may already be low but not produce symptoms. Postural hypotension is usually prevented by slow changes in position and measures to promote venous return.

Alterations in Temperature Regulation. The sympathetic nervous system functions in the regulation of body temperature. The central mechanisms for thermoregulation are located in the hypothalamus. In response to cold, the hypothalamus stimulates vasoconstrictor responses in peripheral blood vessels, particularly those of the skin. This results in decreased loss of body heat. Heat production results from increased metabolism, voluntary activity, or shivering. Shivering can almost double the heat production of the body. To reduce heat, hypothalamus-stimulated mechanisms produce vasodilatation of skin blood vessels to dissipate heat and sweating to increase evaporative heat losses.

After spinal cord injury, the communication between the thermoregulatory centers in the hypothalamus and the sympathetic effector responses below the level of injury are disrupted; the ability to control blood vessel responses that conserve or dissipate heat is lost, as are the abilities to sweat and shiver. Higher levels of injury tend to produce greater disturbances in thermoregulation. In tetraplegia and high paraplegia, there are few defenses against changes in the environmental temperature and body temperature tends to assume the temperature of the external environment, a condition known as *poikilothermy*. Persons with lower-level injuries have various degrees of thermoregulation. Disturbances in thermoregulation are chronic and may cause continual loss of body heat. Treatment consists of education in the adjustment of clothing and awareness of how environmental temperatures affect the person's ability to accommodate these changes.

Circulatory System Dysfunction. Edema and deep vein thrombosis are common problems in persons with spinal cord injury. The development of edema is related to decreased peripheral vascular resistance, areflexia or decreased tone in the paralyzed limbs, and immobility that causes increased venous pressure and abnormal pooling of blood in the abdomen, lower limbs, and upper extremities. Orthostatic or dependent edema in the dependent body parts is usually relieved by positioning to minimize gravitational forces or by using compression devices (*e.g.*, support stockings, binders) that encourage venous return.

Deep vein thrombosis occurs as a complication of spinal cord injury in 14% to 100% of affected persons, depending on the method of diagnosis.[54] Although it is seen more frequently in the postacute phase of spinal cord injury, it often has its origin during the events surrounding the initial injury. Impairment of vasomotor tone, initial loss of muscle tone, trauma to the vein wall, hypercoagulability, and immobility predispose to sluggish venous blood flow and the risk of deep vein thrombosis. Prevention includes low-dose heparin, measures to prevent venous pooling of blood, especially in the paralyzed limbs (*e.g.*, range of motion and vascular compression devices), and assessment of risk and presence of deep vein thrombosis beginning immediately after injury.

Sensorimotor Dysfunction. After the period of spinal shock in an UMN injury, isolated spinal reflex activity and muscle tone that is not under the control of higher centers returns. This may result in hypertonia and spasticity of skeletal muscles below the level of injury, where the normal communication pathways to higher centers for voluntary motor control have been interrupted by the spinal cord lesion. These spastic movements are involuntary instead of voluntary, a distinction that needs to be explained to the spinal cord–injured person and his or her family members. Spastic movements in flexor and extensor patterns, which occur below the level of injury, can be tonic (sustained tone) or clonic (intermittent) and are usually heightened initially after injury, reaching a peak and then becoming stable in about 2 years, with further exacerbations caused by other medical conditions.

These movements occur in most spinal injuries above the T12 level in which the stretch reflex arc is preserved. In injuries at T12 or below, the reflex response itself is damaged at the cord or spinal nerve level, preventing spasticity. Spasticity in and of itself is not detrimental to the spinal cord–injured person and may even facilitate maintenance of muscle tone to prevent muscle wasting, improve venous return, and aid in mobility. Spasms become detrimental when they impair safety; the ability to make functional gains in mobility and activities of daily living, such as feeding, dressing, and toileting; and affect vocational and avocational interests. Spasms may also cause trauma to bones and tissues, leading to joint contractures and skin breakdown.

The stimuli for reflex muscle spasm arise from somatic and visceral afferent pathways that enter the cord below the level of injury. The most common of these stimuli are muscle stretching, bladder infections or stones, fistulas, bowel distention or impaction, pressure areas or irritation of the skin, and infections. Because the stimuli that precipitate spasms vary from person to person, careful assessment needs to be done to identify the factors that precipitate spasm in each person. Passive range of motion exercises to stretch spastic muscles should be done twice a day, avoiding stimuli that elicit spasm. Antispasmodic medications (*e.g.*, diazepam, baclofen) may be warranted and need to be carefully monitored for effectiveness. For persons with spasms that do not respond to conventional treatment and oral antispasmodics, alternative invasive methods (*e.g.*, implantable intrathecal infusion pumps) have been approved for use.[55]

Skin. The entire surface of the skin is innervated by cranial or spinal nerves organized into dermatomes showing cutaneous distribution. The central and autonomic nervous systems also play a vital role in skin function. Impulses from the peripheral nervous system carry sensory information to the brain and receive information for motor control and reflex activity at each dermatome.

The sympathetic nervous system, through control of vasomotor and sweat gland activity, influences the health of the skin by providing adequate circulation, excretion of body fluids, and temperature regulation. The lack of sensory warning mechanisms and voluntary motor ability below the level of injury, coupled with circulatory changes, place the spinal cord–injured person at major risk for disruption of skin integrity. Significant factors associated with disruption of skin integrity are pressure, shearing forces, and localized trauma and irritation. Relieving pressure, allowing adequate circulation to the skin, and skin inspection are primary ways of maintaining skin integrity. Of all the complications after spinal cord injury, skin breakdown is the most preventable.

Pain. Pain after spinal cord injury is a diverse and unpredictable experience that, for some persons, can be severe.[56–58] Initially, pain arises from soft tissues such as the skin, muscles, and joint structures and from fractures and dislocations of bony elements. With healing or decompression of neurologic tissue, much of the pain associated with the injury resolves. For many persons, however, chronic pain syndromes develop.[56] About 90% of persons have delayed pain after spinal cord injury; about 40% of these have increasing pain contributing to the disability.[56] Chronic pain is more common among persons with paraplegia than those with tetraplegia.[57]

Four types of pain syndromes occur after spinal cord injury: mechanical, radicular, visceral, and central.[57,58] Mechanical or fracture pain usually occurs at the level of injury related to soft tissue damage, most commonly from damaged facet joints or spinal fracture. It is dull, aching, and often aggravated by movement. Radicular (spinal nerve root) pain presents as an aching or shooting type of pain that radiates into a more or less well-defined nerve root distribution affecting the arm, leg, or trunk. Although the pain occurs in its severest form with incomplete spinal cord lesions, it also occurs with transected cauda equina lesions. The cause of radicular pain in spinal cord injury is obscure but may result from compression or injury of nerve roots by a herniated nucleus pulposus, a fracture fragment, or a dislocated vertebra or neuronal hyperexcitability due to local ischemia. Visceral pain involves a poorly localized, burning discomfort of the abdomen and pelvis. It is often related to some intraabdominal event such as bladder distention or urinary tract infection. It is thought that the cause of visceral pain may be similar to that of central pain. Central pain is a diffuse burning sensation that is experienced in body parts below the level of injury and is aggravated by touch, movement, and visceral distention. The mechanism of central pain is possibly an abnormal firing of deafferented input association or projection neurons. Because this type of pain has resulted from loss of normal sensory input, it is often called *deafferentation pain.*

The management of pain in a person with spinal cord injury begins with assessment measures to determine the type of pain and, if possible, the underlying mechanisms. Transcutaneous electrical nerve stimulation (TENS) and the tricyclic antidepressant drugs (*e.g.*, amitriptyline, doxepin, imipramine) have proved useful in treating central pain. Mechanical pain is often treated with NSAIDs and physical therapy.[58] Anticonvulsant drugs (*e.g.*, carbamazepine, phenytoin) are often effective in relieving radicular pain.[58] The mechanisms of drug action and specifics of chronic pain management are discussed in Chapter 40.

Genitourinary Dysfunction

Among the most devastating consequences of spinal cord injury is the loss of bowel and bladder function. Loss of these functions are apparent immediately after injury and require much time, expense, material, and human energy for management.

Bladder Function. Micturition, or the act of voiding, can be described as the sequence of events involving sensory input that occurs with bladder filling, activation of the spinal reflex voiding center, stimulation and provision of cerebral control, and progression and termination of actual voiding. Although the anatomy and function of the kidneys or production of urine is not greatly altered after spinal cord injury, most affected persons experience some loss of bladder function.

The neural control of bladder function is supplied by sympathetic nerve fibers (T1 to L3) that allow relaxation of the detrusor muscle during bladder filling, sensory signals from bladder stretch receptors that are conducted to the reflex voiding center (S2 to S4) through the pelvic nerves and then reflexly back to the bladder through parasympathetic fibers in these same nerves, and motoneurons from S2 to S4 that travel through the pudendal nerve to supply the voluntary striated muscles of the external sphincter (see Chapter 30). The reflex voiding center coordinates the activity of the detrusor muscle and the external sphincter by way of input from ascending spinal pathways and descending pathways from higher voluntary control centers in the cortex. After resolution of spinal shock, which renders the bladder areflexic, bladder dysfunction is manifested by the disruption of neural pathways between the bladder and the reflex voiding center (*i.e.*, an LMN lesion) or between the reflex voiding center and higher brain centers for communication and coordinated sphincter control (*i.e.*, an UMN lesion). Persons with UMN lesions or spastic bladders lack awareness of bladder filling (*i.e.*, storage) and voluntary control of voiding (*i.e.*, evacuation). In LMN lesions or flaccid bladder dysfunction, lack of awareness of bladder filling and lack of bladder tone render the person unable to void voluntarily or involuntarily. Of specific importance to optimal bladder function is the storage and evacuation of urine under low pressure to prevent damage to the bladder, urethra, and kidneys.

Normally, the low-pressure urine storage mechanism is achieved through sympathetic inhibition of detrusor muscle contractile activity coordinated with increased internal sphincter closing pressure until the reflex voiding threshold is reached. At threshold, the stretched detrusor muscle elicits a parasympathetic response, inducing urethral smooth muscle relaxation along with balanced bladder contraction until complete emptying is achieved. After spinal cord injury, involuntary voiding reflexes (UMN injury) may be elicited during filling along with a higher-level external sphincter response, which may lead to incontinence and prevent complete emptying of the bladder. These reflexes usually occur at high volumes. In LMN injury, there is no bladder function other than storage or external sphincter response, leading to retention with overflow and leakage of urine. This loss of control of bladder emptying influences the quality of life and carries a lifetime threat of severe renal problems.

The principal goals of bladder management are to provide low-pressure drainage to the urinary bladder and prevent complications, with consideration of the person's lifestyle, the potential for cooperation, and support from family and community. Management of neurogenic bladder dysfunction consists of methods of continuous or intermittent drainage, external collection, and manual techniques (*e.g.*, Crede's maneuver, Valsalva's maneuver, bladder tapping).

Bowel Elimination. Bowel elimination is a coordinated function involving the enteric nervous system, the autonomic nervous system, and the CNS. The enteric nervous system consists of a network of nerve fibers within the bowel wall that respond to fecal distention with increased peristalsis. Parasympathetic fibers from the S2 to S4 segments of the spinal cord travel by way of the pelvic nerve to innervate the colon, rectum, and internal anal sphincter. Somatic innervation from the same cord segments travels by way of the pudendal nerve to provide for voluntary control of the striated muscles of the external anal sphincter. Parasympathetic stimulation produces an increase in intestinal motility and a decrease in internal sphincter tone. Sympathetic outflow from the thoracic and lumbar segments (T6 to L3) of the spinal cord has the opposite effect, producing a decrease in intestinal motility and an increase in internal sphincter tone.

Defecation involves a reflex-mediated increase in peristaltic movements of the colon, rectum, and anus, and relaxation of the internal anal sphincter. The defecation reflex, which is integrated in the sacral segments of the spinal cord, proceses incoming signals from the rectum and transmits impulses back to the colon, rectum, and anus by way of parasympathetic fibers in the pelvic nerve. Afferent signals entering the spinal cord also initiate other effects, such as taking a deep breath, closing the glottis, contracting the abdominal muscles, and relaxing the external anal sphincter. Persons with spinal cord injury above the S2 to S4 level develop spastic functioning of the defecation reflex and loss of voluntary control of the external anal sphincter. Damage to the cord at the S2 to S4 level causes flaccid functioning of the defecation reflex and loss of anal sphincter tone. Even though intrinsic contractile responses are intact, without the defecation reflex, peristaltic movements are ineffective in evacuating stool.

The goal of bowel management after spinal cord injury is to establish complete evacuations, which minimize incontinence and complications and afford dignity and independence to the person. The principal methods of bowel management include measures such as a high-fluid and high-fiber diet, mobility at the highest level that is possible, consistent timing of evacuation, privacy, positioning, and chemical (laxatives), mechanical (digital stimulation), and other stimulants (Valsalva's maneuver, peristaltic stimulators).

Sexual Function. Although the physical act of sex itself may change with spinal cord injury, the ability to enjoy a sexual and caring relationship with another person remains and can take on greater importance than before injury.

Spinal cord injury at any level abolishes communication pathways between the genital and higher centers. Erotic and emotional feelings and thoughts, however, may still be experienced in areas above the level of injury, especially when the mouth and neck are stimulated. Extragenital circulatory, musculoskeletal, and respiratory responses such as increased heart rate, breathing, and muscle tone that are mediated by centers above the level of injury may occur.

Sexual function, as in bladder and bowel control, is mediated by the S2 to S4 segments of the spinal cord. The genital sexual response in spinal cord injury, which is manifested by an erection in men and vaginal lubrication in women, may be initiated by mental or touch stimuli, depending on the level of injury. The T11 to L2 cord segments have been identified as the mental-stimuli, or psychogenic, sexual response area, where autonomic nerve pathways in communication with the forebrain leave the cord and innervate the genitalia. The S2 to S4 cord segments have been identified as the sexual-touch, or reflexogenic, reflex center. In a T10 or higher spinal cord injury (UMN lesion), reflex sexual response to genital touch may occur freely. However, a sexual response to mental stimuli (T11 to L2) does not occur because of the spinal lesion blocking the communication pathway. In an injury at T12 or below (LMN lesion), the sexual reflex center may be damaged, and there may be no response to touch. Cord damage below the T12 segment may result in sexual arousal by mental stimuli. For persons with lesions between L2 to S1, sexual response to mental or touch stimuli may occur.

Aids for men with erectile dysfunction include medications, vacuum devices, and penile implants. In women, water-soluble lubricants assist with vaginal lubrication. Orgasm is a cortical experience that arises from the genitalia and is experienced almost simultaneously with contraction of the periurethral and pelvic floor muscles during the sexual response cycle. Without genital sensation, orgasm is absent. However, the severity of injury is not the most important determining factor in the outcome of sexual well-being. Satisfaction is most often the result of good sexual communication and shared intimacy and is independent of orgasm.

In men, the lack of erectile ability or inability to experience penile sensations or orgasm is not a reliable indicator of fertility, which should be evaluated by an expert. In women, fertility is parallel to menses; usually, it is delayed 3 months to 5 months after injury. There are hazards to pregnancy, labor, and birth control devices relative to spinal cord injury that require knowledgeable health care providers but need not be prohibitive.

In summary, multiple sclerosis is an example of a demyelinating disease in which there is a slowly progressive breakdown of myelin and formation of plaques but sparing of the axis cylinder of the neuron. The cause of multiple sclerosis remains unknown. Geographic distributions and migration studies suggest an environmental influence. Interruption of neural conduction in multiple sclerosis is manifested by a variety of disabling signs and symptoms that depend on the neurons that are affected. The most common symptoms are paresthesias, optic neuritis, and motor weakness. The disease is usually characterized by exacerbations and remissions. Initially, near-normal function returns between exacerbations. The variety of symptoms, course of the disease, and lack of specific diagnostic tests make diagnosis and treatment of the disease difficult. Treatment is largely symptomatic.

Spinal cord injury is a disabling neurologic condition most commonly caused by motor vehicle accidents, falls, and sports injuries. It occurs most frequently in males and persons under 30 years of age. Spinal cord injury is caused by abnormal motion or trauma to the spinal column, including injuries caused by excessive forward flexion and lateral bending, rotation, and extension of the spinal column. Dysfunctions of the nervous system after spinal cord injury cover various degrees of sensorimotor loss and altered reflex activity based on the level of injury and extent of cord damage. Depending on the level of injury, the physical problems of spinal cord injury include spinal shock; ventilation and communication problems; autonomic nervous system dysfunction that predisposes to the vasovagal response, autonomic hyperreflexia, impaired body temperature regulation, and postural hypotension; impaired muscle pump and venous innervation leading to edema of dependent areas of the body and risk of deep vein thrombosis; altered sensorimotor integrity that contributes to uncontrolled muscle spasms, altered pain responses, and threat to skin integrity; alterations in bowel and bladder elimination; and impaired sexual function. The treatment of spinal cord injury involves a continuum of care that begins at the moment of injury and continues throughout the person's life.

REFERENCES

1. Berne R.M., Levy M.N. (1988). *Physiology* (2nd ed., pp. 244, 251). St. Louis: C.V. Mosby.
2. Guyton A., Hall J.E. (1996). *Medical physiology* (9th ed., pp. 602–605). Philadelphia: W.B. Saunders.
3. Conn M.P. (1995). *Neuroscience in medicine* (pp. 312–313). Philadelphia: J.B. Lippincott.
4. Penfield W., Rasmussen T. (1950). *The cerebral cortex of man.* New York: Macmillian.
5. Cotran R.S., Kumar V., Robbins S.L. (1994). *Robbins pathologic basis of disease* (5th ed., pp. 1285–1287, 1326–1338). Philadelphia: W.B. Saunders.
6. Smith P.E.M., Calverley P.M.A., Edwards R.H.T., et al. (1987). Practical problems in the respiratory care of patients with muscular dystrophy. *New England Journal of Medicine* 316, 1197.
7. Bartlett R.J., Pericak-Vance M.A., Koh J., et al. (1987). Duchenne muscular dystrophy: High frequency of deletions. *Neurology* 38, 1.
8. Katzung B.G. (1995). *Basic and clinical pharmacology* (6th ed., p. 95). Stamford, CT: Appleton & Lange.
9. Drachman D.B. (1994). Myasthenia gravis. *New England Journal of Medicine* 330 (25), 1797–1810.
10. LaPate G., Pestronk A. (1993). Autoimmune myasthenia gravis. *Hospital Practice* 28 (1A), 109–131.
11. Sellman M.S., Mayer R.F. (1985). Weakness and "tiredness": When to suspect myasthenia gravis. *Geriatrics* 40 (1), 92
12. Hickey J.V. (1997). *Neurological and neurosurgical nursing* (4th ed., pp. 469–480, 431–433). Philadelphia: J.B. Lippincott.
13. Curd J.G., Thorne R.P. (1989). Diagnosis and management of lumbar disk disease. *Hospital Practice* 24 (9), 135–148.
14. Acute Low Back Problems Guideline Panel (1994). *Acute low back problems in adults: Assessment and treatment.* AHCPR publication no. 95–0642. Rockville, MD: Agency for Health Care Policy and Research, Public Health Service, U.S. Department of Health and Human Services.
15. Dawson D.M. (1993). Entrapment neuropathies of the upper extremities. *New England Journal of Medicine* 329 (27), 2013–2018
16. Dawson D.M. (1995). Entrapment neuropathies: Clinical overview. *Hospital Practice* 30 (8), 37–44.
17. Hughes R.A.C. (1992). The management of Guillain-Barré syndrome. *Hospital Practice* 27 (3A), 107–125.
18. Ropper A.H. (1992). The Guillain-Barré syndrome. *New England Journal of Medicine* 326, 1130–1136.
19. Haines D. (Ed.). (1997). *Fundamental neuroscience* (p. 372). New York: Churchill Livingstone.
20. Ng D.C. (1996). Parkinson's disease: Diagnosis and treatment. *Western Journal of Medicine* 165, 234–240.
21. Silverstein P.M. (1996). Moderate Parkinson's disease. *Postgraduate Medicine* 99 (1), 53–68.
22. Youdim M.B.H., Riederer P. (1997). Understanding Parkinson's disease. *Scientific American* 276, 52–59.
23. Rubin E., Farber J.L. *Pathology* (2nd ed., pp. 1429–1431). Philadelphia: J.B. Lippincott.
24. Stacy M., Brownlee H.J. (1996). Treatment options of early Parkinson's disease. *American Family Physician* 53 (4), 1281–1287.
25. Cummings T. (1988). The dementia of Parkinson's disease. *European Neurology* 28 (Suppl. 1), 15–23.
26. Nutt J.G., Woodward W.R., Hammerstad, J.P. (1984). The "on-off" phenomenon in Parkinson's disease. *New England Journal of Medicine* 310, 483–488.
27. The Parkinson Study Group. (1989). Effect of deprenyl on the progression of disability in early Parkinson's disease. *New England Journal of Medicine* 321, 1364–1371.
28. Pascuzzi R.M. (1988). Amyotrophic lateral sclerosis. *Indiana Medicine* 81, 607–612.
29. Beal M.F., Richardson E.P., Martin J.B. (1991). Degenerative disease of the nervous system. In Wilson J., Braunwald E., Isselbacher K.J. (Eds.). *Harrison's principles of internal medicine* (12th ed., pp. 2072–2074). New York: McGraw-Hill.
30. Kassirer J.P. (1994). Riluzole for treatment of amyotrophic lateral sclerosis—Too soon to tell? *New England Journal of Medicine* 330 (9), 636–637
31. Smith R.G., Appel S.H. (1996). Molecular approaches to amyotrophic lateral sclerosis. *Annual Review of Medicine* 46, 133–145.

32. Bensimon G., Lacomblez L., Meininger V., and the ALS/Riluzole Study Group. (1994). A controlled trial of riluzole in amyotrophic lateral sclerosis. *New England Journal of Medicine* 330 (9), 585–591.
33. Anderson D.W., Ellenberg J.H., Leventhal C.M., Reingold S.C., Rodreguez M., Silberberg D.H. (1992). Revised estimate of multiple sclerosis in the United States. *Annuals of Neurology* 31, 333–336.
34. Schapiro R.T., Scheinberg L., Weiner H.L., Wolinsky J.S. (1997). Living with MS: The outlook improves. *Patient Care* 31 (2), 87–113.
35. Cormack D.H. (1987). *Ham's histology* (9th ed., pp. 344–345). Philadelphia: J.B. Lippincott.
36. Norton W.T. (1984). Recent advances in myelin biochemistry. *Annals of the New York Academy of Sciences* 70, 5–10.
37. McFarlin D.E., McFarland H.F. (1982). Multiple sclerosis. *New England Journal of Medicine* 307, 1183–1188.
38. Paty D.W. (1987). Multiple sclerosis: Assessment of disease progression and effects of treatment. *Canadian Journal of Neurology* 14, 518.
39. Gonzalez-Scarano F., Spellman R.S., Nathanson N. (1986). Epidemiology. In McDonald W.E., Silberg D.H. (Eds.). *Multiple sclerosis* (pp. 37–55). Boston: Butterworth.
40. Brod S.A., Lindsey W., Wolinsky J.S. (1996). Multiple sclerosis: Clinical presentation, diagnosis and treatment. *American Family Physician* 54 (4), 1301–1311.
41. Davis F.A. (1984). The hot tub test in multiple sclerosis. In Poser D.W., Scheinber L., McDonald W.I., Ebers G.C. (Eds.). *The diagnosis of multiple sclerosis* (pp. 44–48). New York: Thieme-Stratton.
42. Berger J.R., Sheremata W.A. (1983). Persistent neurological deficit precipitated by hot bath test in multiple sclerosis. *Journal of the American Medical Association* 249, 171.
43. National Multiple Sclerosis Society (1995). Today's symptom control . . . tomorrow's new treatment. *Client and Family Services Teleconference.*
44. Rudick R.A., Goodken D.E., Ransohoff R.M. (1992). Pharmacology of multiple sclerosis. *Cleveland Clinic Journal of Medicine* 59 (3), 267–277.
45. Jacobs L., Johnson K.P. (1994). A brief history of interferons in treatment of multiple sclerosis. *Archives of Neurology* 51 (12), 1245–1251.
46. National SCI Statistics Center. (1994). *Spinal cord injury: Facts and figures at a glance.* Birmingham: University of Alabama.
47. Geisler F.H. (1993). GM-1 ganglioside and motor recovery following human spinal cord injury. *Journal of Emergency Medicine* 11, 49–55.
48. Chiles B.W., Cooper P.R (1996). Acute spinal cord injury. *New England Journal of Medicine* 334 (8), 514–520.
49. Fehling M.G., Louw D. (1996). Initial stabilization and medical management of acute spinal cord injury. *American Family Physician* 42 (1), 155–162.
50. Hilton G., Frei J. (1992). Methylprednisolone for acute spinal cord injury. *Journal of Neuroscience Nursing* 24 (4), 234–237.
51. Bracken M.B. (1993). Pharmacological treatment of acute spinal cord injury: Current status and future projects. *Journal of Emergency Medicine* 11, 43–48.
52. American Spinal Injury Association.(1992). *Standards of neurological and functional classification of spinal cord injury.* Chicago: American Spinal Cord Injury Association.
53. Atkinson P.P., Atkinson J.L.D. (1996). Spinal shock. *Mayo Clinic Proceedings* 71, 384–389.
54. Myllynen P., Kammonen F., Rokkanen P., et al. (1985). Deep venous thrombosis and pulmonary embolism in patients with acute spinal cord injury: A comparison with nonparalyzed patients immobilized due to spinal fractures. *Journal of Trauma* 21, 541–543.
55. Gianino J. (1993). Intrathecal baclofen for spinal spasticity: Implications for nursing practice. *Journal of Neuroscience Nursing* 25, 254–263.
56. Zejdlik C.P. (1992). *Management of spinal cord injury* (2nd ed., pp. 594–601). Boston: Jones & Bartlett.
57. Woolsey R.M. (1986). Chronic pain following spinal cord injury. *Paraplegia* 19 (3 & 4), 27.
58. Farkash A.E., Portenoy R.K. (1986). The pharmacologic management of chronic pain in the paraplegic patient. *Paraplegia* 19 (3 & 4), 41.

ADDITIONAL READINGS

Dituno J.F., Formal C.S. (1994). Chronic spinal cord injury. *The New England Journal of Medicine* 330 (8), 550–556.

Dituno J.F., Young W., Donovan W.H., Creasey G. (1994). The International Standards booklet of neurological and functional classification of spinal cord injury. *Paraplegia* 32, 70–80.

Donovan W.H. (1994). Operative and nonoperative management of spinal cord injury: A review. *Paraplegia* 32, 375–388.

Kernich C.A., Kaminski H.J. (1995). Myasthenia gravis: Pathophysiology, diagnosis, and collaborative care. *Journal of Neuroscience Nursing* 27 (1), 207–215.

Smith R.G., Appel S.H. (1995). Molecular approaches to amyotrophic lateral sclerosis. *Annual Review of Medicine* 46, 133–145.

Wirtz K.M., LaFavor K., Ang R. (1996). Managing chronic spinal cord injury. *Issues in Critical Care, Critical Care Nurse* 16 (4), 24–35.

Wittbrodt E.T. (1996). Drugs and myasthenia gravis. *Archives of Internal Medicine* 157, 399–408.

Young W. (1993). Secondary injury mechanisms in acute spinal cord injury. *Journal of Emergency Medicine* 11, 13–22.

CHAPTER 40

Somatosensory Function and Pain

Sheila Curtis, Camille Kolotylo, and Marion E. Broome

Sensory mechanisms provide a continuous stream of information about the seeming realities of the person, the outside world, and the interactions between the two. The term *somesthesia* (from the Greek words meaning body and sensation) describes a person's awareness of his or her body. The somatosensory component of the nervous system provides an awareness of body sensations such as pain, touch, temperature, and limb position, which are different from the special senses such as vision, hearing, smell, and taste. The sensory receptors for somatosensory function consist of discrete nerve endings in the skin and other body tissues. Between 2 and 3 million sensory neurons deliver a steady stream of encoded information that represent the status of their sensory endings. Only a small proportion of this information reaches awareness; most provides input essential for a myriad of reflex and automatic mechanisms that keep us alive and manage our functioning.

The first part of this chapter describes the organization and control of somatosensory function. The second focuses on pain as a somatosensory modality.

Organization and Control of Somatosensory Function

After you have completed this section of the chapter, you should be able to meet the following objectives:

- Name the three somatosensory modalities
- Define *proprioception* and *kinesthesia*
- Trace the pathway of an impulse that originates in a somatosensory receptor
- State the significance of the dermatomes in a neurologic examination
- Contrast the role of rapid-adapting and slow-adapting afferents in maintaining posture
- Compare the discriminative pathway with the anterolateral pathway, and explain the clinical usefulness of this distinction
- Describe the sensory homunculus in the cerebral cortex

The somatosensory system is designed to provide the central nervous system (CNS) information about the body. Sensory neurons can be divided into three types: general somatic, special somatic, and general visceral afferent neurons. *General somatic afferent neurons* have branches with widespread distribution throughout the body with receptors that result in sensations such as pain, touch, and temperature. *Special somatic afferent* neurons innervate receptors that sense position change and movement of the body. *General visceral afferents* innervate visceral structures and sense fullness and discomfort.

Somesthesia can be subdivided with reference to the location of the sensory nerve endings. Cutaneous modalities include touch and the more complex sensations of itch and tickle; temperature (*i.e.*, warm to hot and cool to cold); and pain, including sharp and dull pain. In deeper structures of the body wall and the limbs, afferent nerve endings supply the deep connective tissues, joint capsules, ligaments, muscles, tendons, periosteum of bone, and blood vessel walls. Some of these sensory endings provide the basis for the coordination of movement and contribute to the experience of body, head, and limb position (*i.e., proprioception*) and movement (*i.e., kinesthesia*). When stimulated at a frequency high enough to be associated with tissue damage, many of these afferents also send a message that is interpreted as pain.

Sensory Systems

Sensory systems are organized as a serial succession of neurons consisting of first-order, or primary, afferent neurons, which transmit sensory information from the periphery; second-order, or secondary, CNS association neurons, which communicate with various reflex networks and sensory pathways that travel directly to the thalamus; and third-order, or tertiary, neurons, which relay information from the thalamus to the cerebral cortex.[1] Many interneurons process and modify the sensory information at the level of the second- and third-order neurons, and myriads more participate before coordinated and appropriate learned-movement responses occur. The number of participating neurons increases exponentially from the primary through the secondary and the secondary through the tertiary levels. By providing multiple parallel projections along with mechanisms for filtering, amplifying, and modulating information, this expansion of the number of participating neurons serves as a safety feature.

The Sensory Unit

A *sensory unit* consists of a dorsal root ganglion neuron; its peripheral branch, which innervates a small region of the periphery; and its central axon, which synapses with a dorsal horn association neuron (see Chapter 37). The many distal endings of the peripheral branch are receptive endings, tuned to specific forms of physical or chemical energy. Less commonly, the peripheral branch terminals innervate specialized receptor cells that are themselves sensitive to specific physical (*e.g.*, baroreceptors) or chemical (*e.g.*, chemoreceptors) stimuli. The peripheral branches of the general somatic afferent neurons divide repeatedly as they supply the skin, fascial sheets, muscles, tendons, joint capsules, periosteum, marrow cavities, and parietal lining of the body cavities. Action potentials that originate from any of the numerous receptive endings of an afferent neuron enter the spinal cord association columns through the dorsal roots of the peripheral nerve. The afferent neuron, in a sense, cannot distinguish among information coming from its various peripheral terminals. If the applied stimulus results in an action potential in any terminal branch, the impulse is transmitted to the dorsal horn association cells in the CNS.

Innervation Patterns

The somesthetic innervation of the body, including the head, retains a basic segmental organizational pattern that was established during embryonic development. Thirty-three paired spinal (*i.e.*, segmental) nerves provide sensory and motor innervation of the body wall, the limbs, and the viscera (see Chapter 37). Sensory input to each spinal cord segment is provided by afferent sensory neurons with cell bodies in the dorsal root ganglia.

The region of the body wall that is supplied by a single pair of dorsal root ganglia is called a *dermatome*. These dorsal root ganglion–innervated strips occur in a regular sequence moving upward from the second coccygeal segment through the cervical segments, reflecting the basic segmental organization of the body and the nervous system (Fig. 40–1). The cranial nerves that innervate the head send their axons to equivalent nuclei in the brain stem. Neighboring dermatomes overlap one another sufficiently so that a loss of one dorsal root or root ganglion results in reduced but not total loss

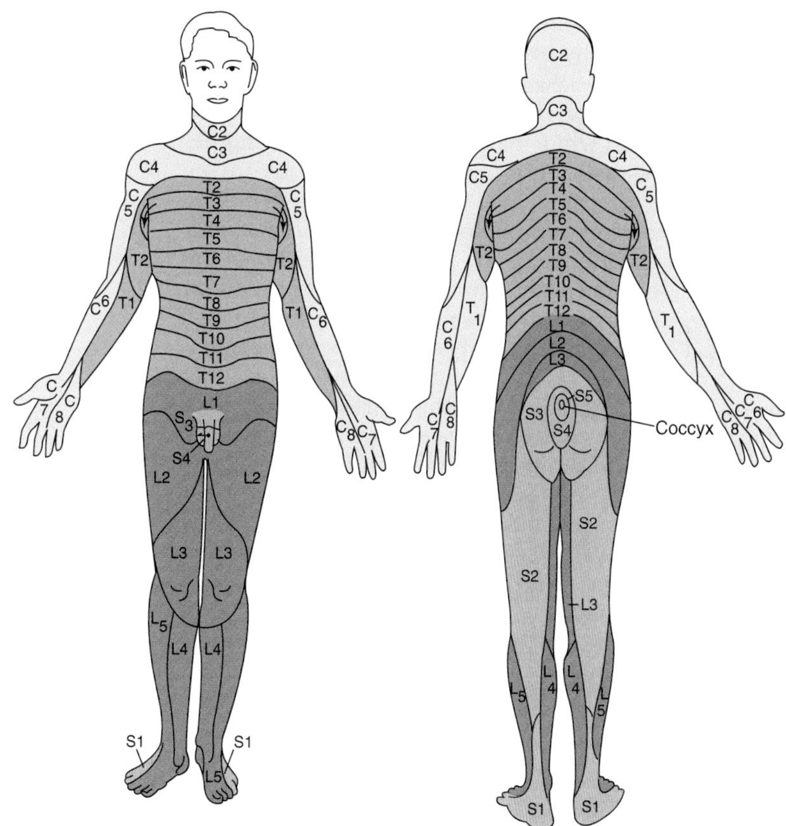

Figure 40–1
Cutaneous distribution of spinal nerves (dermatomes). (Barr, M. [1993]. *The human nervous system.* New York: Harper & Row.)

of sensory innervation of a dermatome (Fig. 40–2). Dermatome maps are helpful in detecting the level and extent of sensory deficits resulting from segmental nerve and spinal cord damage.

Ascending Neural Pathways

Different somesthetic afferents transmit signals related to delicate vibratory or fine tactile stimuli. Other afferents transmit signals from less sensitive pain or temperature receptors. For all classes of somesthetic afferents, the input association cell columns in the dorsal horn of the spinal cord are the source of secondary or association axons that project through spinoreticular tract systems to the reticular activating system of the brain stem. The spinoreticular projections provide the basis for increased wakefulness or awareness after strong somatesthetic stimulation and for the generalized startle reaction that occurs with sudden and intense somesthetic stimuli. The responses of the reticular activating system include postural and autonomic nervous system responses, such as a rise in blood pressure and heart rate, dilation of the pupils, and the pale, moist skin that results from constriction of the cutaneous blood vessels and activation of sweat glands.

The sensory association cell columns relay afferent information to the forebrain, where sensation and perception occur. Two parallel pathways, the *dorsal column discriminative* and the *anterolateral* (*i.e., spinothalamic*) pathways, reach the thalamic level of sensation, each taking a different route through the CNS. These pathways differ in the location of the secondary input association neurons and in the level of the CNS at which the information is projected across the midline to the contralateral thalamus and cortex. Among the advantages of a two-pathway system is that of adding richness to sensation by allowing the same information to be handled in two different ways and providing insurance that if one pathway is damaged the other still provides input.

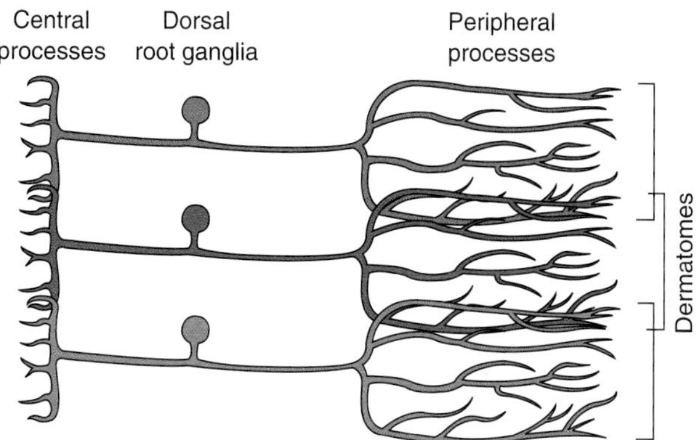

Figure 40–2
The dermatomes formed by the peripheral processes of adjacent spinal nerves overlap on the body surface. The central processes of these fibers also overlap in their spinal distribution.

The Discriminative Pathway. The rapid-transmission discriminative pathway to the thalamus and cerebral cortex involves branches of primary afferent axons that travel up the ipsilateral (i.e., same side) dorsal columns of the spinal cord white matter and synapse with highly evolved somesthetic input association neurons in the medulla. The discriminative pathway uses only three neurons to transmit information from a sensory receptor to the somesthetic strip of parietal cerebral cortex of the opposite side of the brain: the primary sensory neuron that projects its central axon to the dorsal column nuclei; the dorsal column neuron that sends its axon through a rapid conducting tract, the medial lemniscus, that crosses at the base of the medulla and travels to the thalamus on the opposite side of the brain where basic sensation begins; and the thalamic neuron that projects its axons through the somesthetic radiation to the primary sensory cortex, site of discriminative sensation (Fig. 40–3). The medial lemniscus is joined by fibers from the sensory nucleus of the trigeminal nerve (cranial nerve V) that supplies the face. Sensory information arriving at the sensory cortex by this route can be discretely localized and discriminated in terms of intensity grades.

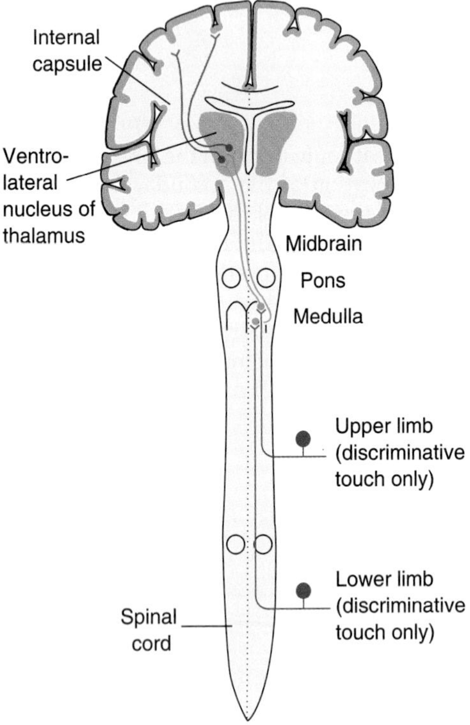

Figure 40–3
Discriminative pathway. This pathway is an ascending system for rapid transmission of sensations that relate joint movement (kinesthesis), body position (proprioception), vibration, and delicate touch. Primary afferents travel up the dorsal columns of the spinal cord white matter and synapse with somesthetic input association neurons in the medulla. Secondary neurons project through the brain stem to the thalamus and synapse with tertiary neurons, which relay the information to the primary somesthetic cortex on the opposite side of the brain.

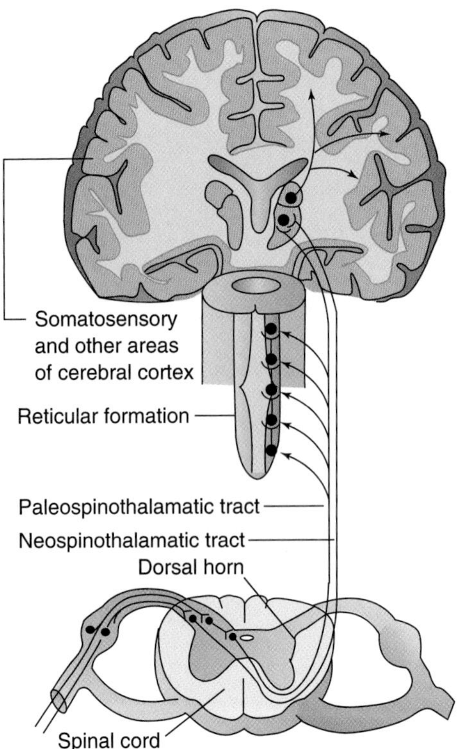

Figure 40–4
Neospinothalamic and paleospinothalamic subdivisions of the anterolateral sensory pathway. The neospinothalamic tract runs to the thalamic nuclei and has fibers that project to the somatosensory cortex. The paleospinothalamic tract sends collaterals to the reticular formation and other structures, from which further fibers project to the thalamus. These fibers influence the hypothalamus and the limbic system as well as the cerebral cortex.

One of the distinct features of this pathway is that it relays precise information regarding spatial orientation. This is the only pathway taken by sensations of joint movement (*i.e.*, kinesthesia), body position (*i.e.*, proprioception), vibration, and delicate, discriminative touch, as is required to differentiate correctly between touching skin at two neighboring points (*i.e.*, two-point discrimination).

The Anterolateral Pathway. In contrast to the three-neuron discriminative pathway, the anterolateral pathway is multisynaptic and therefore slow and crudely graded. It provides for transmission of pain, thermal sensations, crude touch and pressure, and tickle and itch sensations. The anterolateral fibers originate in the dorsal horns at the level of the segmental nerve where the dorsal root afferent neurons enter the spinal cord. They cross in the anterior commissure, within a few segments of origin, to the opposite anterolateral white column where they ascend upward toward the brain.

There are at least two subdivisions in the anterolateral pathway: the neospinothalamic tract and the paleospinothalamic tract (Fig. 40–4). Bright pain travels in the *neospinothalamic tract*, which consists of a sequence of at least three neurons with long axons. It provides for relatively rapid transmission of sensory information to the thalamus. The indirect spinoreticular thalamic pathway consists of bilateral multisynaptic slow-conducting tracts that transmit sensory signals that do not require discrete localization of signal source or discrimination of fine gradations in intensity. This slower-conducting system is also called the *paleospinothalamic tract*, indicating that it is phylogenetically older than the neospinothalamic system.

The anterolateral pathway also projects into the intralaminar nuclei of the thalamus, which have close connections with the limbic cortical systems. This circuitry gives touch its affective or emotional aspects, such as the particular unpleasantness of heavy pressure and the peculiar pleasantness of the tickling and gentle rubbing of the skin.

The Somatosensory Cortex

The somatosensory cortex is located in the parietal lobe, which lies behind the central sulcus and above the lateral sulcus (Fig. 40–5). The strip of parietal cortex that borders the central sulcus is called the *primary sensory cortex* because it receives primary sensory information by way of direct projections from the lateral nuclei of the thalamus. A distorted map of the body and head surface, called the sensory *homunculus*, reflects the density of cortical neurons devoted to sensory input from afferents in corresponding peripheral areas. As depicted in Figure 40–6, much more cortical surface is devoted to areas of the body such as the thumb, forefinger, lips, and tongue, where fine touch and pressure are essential for normal function. The cortical area devoted to body surface area correlates with the density of afferent innervation in that area.

Parallel to and just behind the primary somatosensory cortex (*i.e.*, toward the occipital cortex) lie the somatosensory association areas, which are required to transform the raw material of sensation into meaningful learned perception. Most of the *perceptive* aspects of body sensation, or somesthesia, require the function of

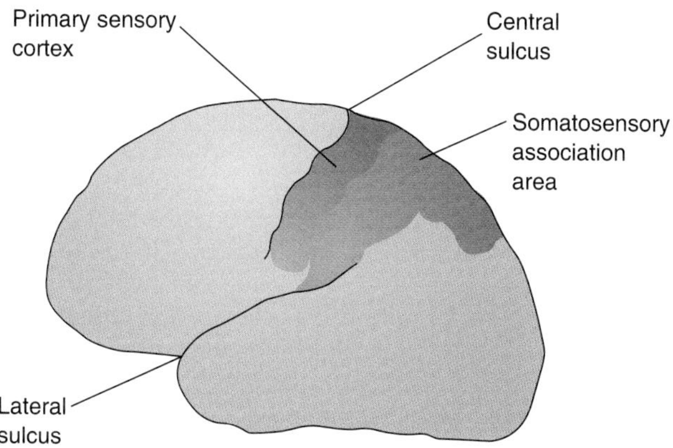

Figure 40–5
Primary somatosensory and association somatosensory cortex.

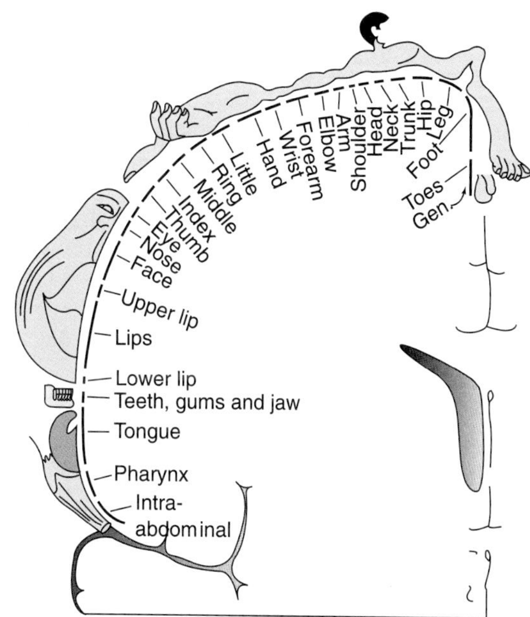

Figure 40–6
Homunculus, as determined by stimulation studies on the human cortex during surgery. (Penfield E., & Rasmussen T. [1955]. *The cerebral cortex of man.* New York: Macmillan. Copyright © by Macmillan Publishing Co., Inc., renewed 1978 by Theodore Rasmussen)

this parietal association cortex. Thalamic association nuclei are also involved. The perceptive aspect, or meaningfulness, of a stimulus pattern involves the integration of present sensation with past learning. For instance, a person's past learning plus present tactile sensation provides the perception of sitting on a soft chair rather than on a hard bicycle seat.

One of the important functions of the discriminative pathway is to integrate the input from multiple receptors. The sense of shape and size of an object in the absence of visualization, called *stereognosis*, is based on precise afferent information from muscle, tendon, and joint receptors. A screwdriver has a different shape from a knife in the texture of its parts (*i.e.*, tactile sensibility) and in its shape based on the relative position of the fingers as they are moved over the object (*i.e.*, proprioception). This complex, interpretive perception requires that the discriminative system must be functioning optimally and that higher-order parietal association cortex processing and prior learning must have occurred.

If the discriminative somesthetic pathway is functional but the parietal associational cortex has become discretely damaged, the person can correctly describe the object but does not recognize that it is a screwdriver. This deficit is called *astereognosis*. If the somesthetic, but not the parietal association cortex, is irritated by a growing tumor or meningeal scar tissue, hallucinations of a "strange tingling sensation" or of "something moving over the skin" are experienced. These usually are unpleasant and without meaning. This abnormal neural firing may cause an *aura* (*i.e.*, sensory seizure), which can then progress to a generalized tonic-clonic seizure. Cortical lesions from strokes or growing tumors usually destroy large areas, affecting the somatosensory and the parietal association cortex. Damage to the somatosensory cortex on the nondominant (usually right) side of the brain can produce a condition called the *hemi-inattention syndrome* in which the entire left side of the body is ignored as if it does not exist as part of the self (see Chapter 38). This syndrome is less evident after lesions of the same region on the dominant side.

Somatosensory Experience

Somatosensory experience can be divided into *modalities*, a term used for qualitative, subjective distinctions between sensations such as touch, heat, and pain. Such experiences require the function of sensory receptors and forebrain structures in the thalamus and cerebral cortex. Sensory experience also involves quantitative sensory discrimination or the ability to distinguish between different levels of sensory stimulation.

Sensory Modality

Receptive endings of different afferent neurons are particularly sensitive to a specific form of physical and chemical energy. They can initiate action potentials to many forms of energy at high energy levels, but they usually are highly tuned to be differentially sensitive to low levels of a particular energy class. For instance, a receptive ending may be particularly sensitive to a small increase in local skin temperature. Stimulating the ending with electric current or strong pressure can also result in action potentials. The amount of energy required, however, is much less for temperature change. Increases in the action potential rate in the *warm* afferent, when the information reaches the thalamus and cerebral cortex, is experienced as the sensation of warmth and at higher rates of action potential generation as hot. Other afferent sensory terminals are most sensitive to slight indentations of the skin, and their signals are subjectively interpreted as *touch*. Cool versus warm, sharp versus dull pain, delicate touch versus deep pressure, and joint movement versus joint position are all based on different populations of afferent neurons or on central integration of simultaneous input from several differently tuned afferents. For example, the sensation of itch results from a combination of high activity in pain- and touch-sensitive afferents, and the sensation of tickle requires a gentle moving tactile stimulus over cool skin.

When this tuned aspect of different primary afferents reaches the forebrain where subjective experience occurs, the qualitative differences between warmth and touch are called *sensory modalities*. These are based on the separate relays of first-order, second-order, and third-order neurons of the receptor-detected information to the thalamus and cortex. But the experience of a modality, such as cold versus warm, is uniquely subjective. The projection pathways for modalities differ considerably in the location of second-order and third-order neurons and the precision with which the sensory information is transmitted to the forebrain.

Stimulus Discrimination

Discrimination of the location of a somesthetic stimulus is called *acuity* and is based on the sensory field within a dermatome innervated by an afferent neuron. High acuity (*i.e.*, the ability to make fine discriminations of location) requires a high density of innervation by afferent neurons. For example, acuity is high on the thumb but lower on the back of the hand. High acuity also requires a projection system through the CNS to the forebrain that preserves distinctions between activity in neighboring sensory fields. Receptors or receptive endings of primary afferent neurons differ as to the intensity at which they begin to fire. This afferent threshold usually is lower than the stimulus threshold required for first brain-level of subjective sensation. For instance, when a single hair on the back of the hand is bent more and more, some bending occurs before action potentials appear in the primary, or tactile, sensory neuron (*i.e.*, afferent threshold). The hair must be bent further and the sensory action potentials must increase in frequency before a person is able to reliably detect the bending of the hair (*i.e.*, subjective sensation threshold). For highly developed discriminative systems, under ideal conditions, these thresholds may correspond closely.

Many factors, such as attention and emotion, can greatly elevate the subjective threshold. After the subjective threshold is reached, the intensity of the experienced sensation is based on the rate of impulse generation in the afferent neuron, such that gradations in stimulus intensity are discriminated proportional to the logarithm of stimulus strength. This means that, after the subjective threshold has been reached, greater changes in stimulus strength are needed for further discrimination. This is known as the *Weber-Fechner principle*. For example, after the subjective threshold has been reached, a person could have difficulty detecting a 1-g increase in weight when holding a 30-g weight or a 10-g increase when holding a 300-g weight. In each case, the ratio of change (*i.e.*, logarithm) remains about 1 to 30.[2] This relation holds true for all sensory systems, including the somesthetic system, and is based on characteristics of the receptor endings.

Some afferent neurons maintain a more or less steady rate of firing to a continuous stimulus. This is true for afferents from muscles, tendons, and joints, where continuous feedback information is necessary for maintaining posture. These slow-adapting afferent neurons contrast with rapid-adapting afferent neurons, which signal only the onset, sudden change, and conclusion of a stimulus. Rapid-adapting afferent neurons are required to signal moving, brief, or vibrating stimuli.

Tactile Sensation

Tactile sensation is important in terms of detecting touch, pressure, and vibration. Touch sensation usually results from stimulation of tactile receptors in the skin and tissues immediately beneath the skin, pressure from deformation of deeper tissues, and vibration from rapidly repetitive sensory signals. Tactile sensation arises from at least six types of specialized receptors in the skin and deeper structures: free nerve ending,[2] Meissner's corpuscles, Merkel's disks, Pacinian corpuscles, hair follicle end-organs, and Ruffini end-organs (Fig. 40–7).[2,3] Free nerve endings are found in skin and many other tissues, including the cornea. They detect touch and pressure.

Meissner's corpuscle is an elongated encapsulated nerve ending that is present in nonhairy parts of the skin. It is particularly abundant in the finger tips, lips, and other areas where the sense of touch is highly developed.

Merkel's disks are dome-shaped receptors found in nonhairy areas and in hairy parts of the skin. In contrast to Meissner's corpuscles, which adapt within a fraction of a second, Merkel's disks transmit an initial strong signal that diminishes in strength but is slow in adapting. For this reason, Meissner's corpuscles are particularly sensitive to the movement of very light objects over the surface of the skin and to low-frequency vibration. Merkel's disks are responsible for giving steady-state signals that allow for continuous determination of touch against the skin.

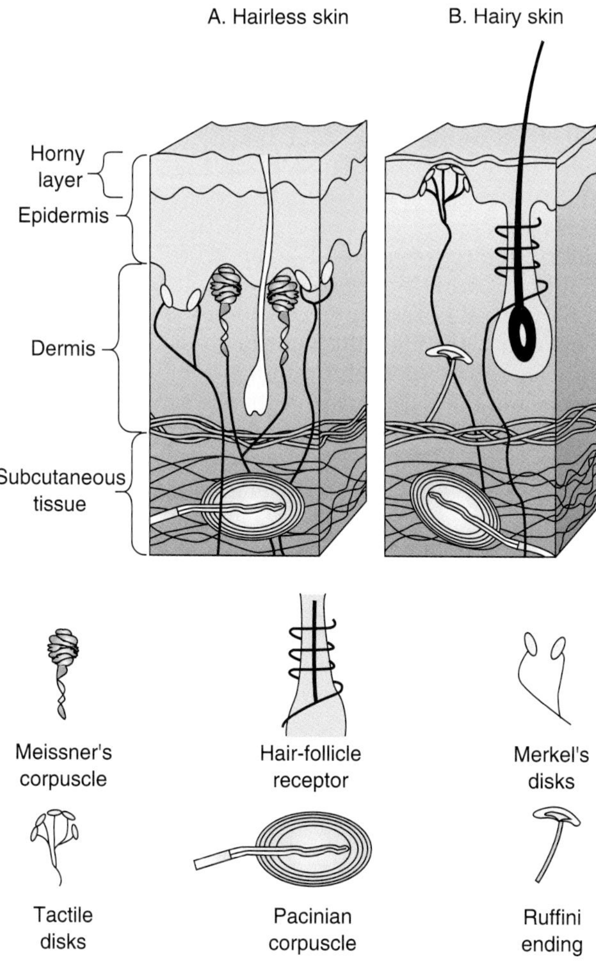

Figure 40–7 Tactile receptors in the skin. (From Rhoades R.A., Tanner G.A. [1996]. *Medical physiology*. Boston: Little, Brown)

The *Pacinian corpuscle* is located immediately beneath the skin and deep in the fascial tissues of the body. This type of receptor, which is stimulated by rapid movements of the tissues and adapts within a few hundredths of a second, is important in detecting tissue vibration. The *hair follicle end-organ* consists of afferent unmyelinated fibers entwined around most of the length of the hair follicle. These receptors, which are rapidly adapting, detect movement on the surface of the body.

The *Ruffini end-organs* are found in the skin and deeper structures, including the joint capsules. These receptors, which have multibranched encapsulated endings, have very little adaptive capacity and are important for signaling continuous states of deformation, such as heavy and continuous touch and pressure.

Almost all the specialized touch receptors, such as Merkel's disks, Meissner's corpuscles, hair follicle receptors, Pacinian corpuscles, and Ruffini's endings, transmit their signals in large myelinated nerve fibers (*i.e.,* type A beta) that have transmission velocities ranging from 25 to 70 m per second. Most free nerve endings transmit signals by way of small myelinated fibers (*i.e.,* type A delta) with conduction velocities of 10 to 30 m per second.[4] Some tactile free nerve endings transmit by way of type C unmyelinated fibers with a velocity of up to 2.5 m per second.[4] The sensory information for tactile sensation enters the spinal cord through the dorsal roots of the spinal nerves. All tactile sensation that requires rapid transmission is transmitted through the discriminative pathway to the thalamus by way of the medial lemniscus. This includes touch sensation requiring a high degree of localization or fine gradations of intensity, vibratory sensation, and sensation that signals movement against the skin.

In addition to the ascending discriminative pathway, tactile sensibility uses a primitive and crude alternative relay to the thalamus. The afferent axons that carry tactile information up the dorsal columns have many branches or collaterals, and some of these synapse in the dorsal horn near the level of dorsal root entry. After several synapses, axons are projected up *both sides* of the anterolateral aspect of the spinal cord to the thalamus. From there, some projections travel to the somesthetic cortex, especially to the side opposite the stimulus. Few fibers travel all the way to the thalamus. Most synapse on reticular formation neurons, which send their axons on toward the thalamus without synapsing. Most synapse on reticular formation neurons that then send their axons on toward the thalamus. Because of these multiple routes, total destruction of the pathway seldom occurs. The lateral nuclei of the thalamus that receive this information are capable of contributing a crude, poorly localized sensation from the opposite side of the body.

The only time this crude alternative system becomes essential is when the discriminative pathway is damaged. Then, despite projection of the anterolateral system information to the somesthetic cortex, only a poorly localized, high-threshold sense of touch remains. Such persons lose all kinesthesia, proprioception, and two-point discrimination. They can detect touch stimuli to one or the other hand, but more force must be delivered to the skin.

Thermal Sensation

Thermal sensation is discriminated by three types of receptors: cold receptors, warmth receptors, and pain receptors. The cold and warmth receptors are located immediately under the skin at discrete but separate points, each serving an area of about 1 mm^2. In some areas there are more cold receptors than warmth receptors. For example, the lips have 15 to 25 cold receptors per square centimeter, compared with 3 to 5 in the same-sized area of the finger.[2] There are correspondingly fewer warmth receptors in these areas. The different gradations of heat and cold result from the relative degrees of stimulation of the different types of nerve endings. The pain receptors are only stimulated by extremes of temperature such as "freezing cold" and "burning hot" sensations. With the exception of pain receptors, thermal receptors tend to adapt rapidly during the first few minutes and then more slowly during the next 30 minutes or so. However, these receptors do not appear to adapt completely, as evidenced by the experience of an intense sense of heat on entering a tub of hot water or the extreme degree of cold initially sensed when going outside on a cold day.

Dorsal root ganglion afferents, with receptive thermal endings in the skin, send their central axons into the segmental dorsal horn of the spinal cord. Cranial nerves that innervate the face and inside of the mouth send their axons to homologous, or equivalent, nuclei of the brain stem. On entering the dorsal horn, thermal signals are processed by second-order input association neurons. These association neurons activate projection neurons whose axons then cross to the opposite side of the cord and ascend in the anterolateral system. Thermal information is projected to the forebrain through the multisynaptic, slow-conducting anterolateral *paleospinothalamic* system to the opposite side of the brain. Thalamic and cortical somesthetic regions for temperature are mixed with those for tactile sensibility. Connections through the medial thalamus into the limbic system provide the potential for the high emotional response to thermal sensation. The ascending information for temperature sensation does not use the discriminative path.

Conduction of thermal information through peripheral nerves is quite slow compared with the rapid tactile afferents. If a person places a foot in a tub of hot water, the tactile sensation of the water on the skin occurs well in advance of the burning sensation. The anterolateral thermal projection system is also quite slow compared with the discriminative tactile pathway. The foot has been removed from the hot water by the local withdrawal reflex well before the excessive heat is perceived by the forebrain. Local anesthetic agents block the small-diameter afferents that carry thermal sensory information before they block the large-diameter axons that carry discriminative touch information. Absence of thermal sensitivity (*i.e.*, athermia) resulting from partial peripheral nerve block or from damage to the anterolateral system is not experienced as a loss of hot and cold sensations. The affected area does not become numb until all tactile information has been blocked from reaching the thalamus and cortex.

Clinical Assessment of Somesthetic Function

Clinically, neurologic assessment of somesthetic function can be done by testing the integrity of spinal segmental nerves. A pinpoint pressed against the skin of the sole of the foot that results in a withdrawal reflex and a complaint of skin pain confirms the functional integrity of the afferent terminals in the skin, the entire pathway through the peripheral nerves of the foot, leg, and thigh to the sacral (S1) dorsal root ganglion, and through the dorsal root into the spinal cord segment. It confirms that the somesthetic input association cells receiving this information are functioning and that the reflex circuitry of the cord segments (L5 to S2) is functioning. In addition, the lower motoneurons of the L4 to S1 ventral horn can be considered operational, and their axons through the ventral roots, the mixed peripheral nerve, and the motoneuron to the muscles producing the withdrawal response can be considered intact and functional. The communication between the lower motoneuron and the muscle cells is functional, and these muscles have normal responsiveness and strength.

Testing is done at each segmental level, or dermatome, moving upward along the body and neck from coccygeal segments through the high cervical levels to test the functional integrity of all the spinal nerves. Similar dermatomes cover the face and scalp, and these, although innervated by cranial segmental nerves, are tested in the same manner.

The observation of a normal withdrawal reflex rules out peripheral nerve disease, disorders of the dorsal root and ganglion, diseases of the myoneural junction, and severe muscle diseases. Normal reflex function also indicates that many major descending CNS tract systems are functioning within normal limits. If the person is able to report the pinprick sensation and accurately identifies its location, many ascending systems through much of the spinal cord and brain are also functioning normally, as are basic intellect and speech mechanisms.

The integrity of the discriminative dorsal column–medial lemniscus pathway compared with the anterolateral tactile pathways is tested with the person's eyes closed by gently brushing the skin with a wisp of cotton, touching an area with two or one sharp point, touching corresponding parts of the body on each side simultaneously or in random sequence, and passively bending the person's finger one way and then another in random order. If only the anterolateral pathway is functional, the tactile threshold is markedly elevated, two-point discrimination and proprioception are missing, and the patient has difficulty discriminating which side of the body received stimulation.

In summary, the somatosensory component of the nervous system provides an awareness of body sensations such as touch, temperature, and pain. Afferent neurons of the dorsal root ganglia innervate a corresponding segment of the body as general soma afferent (*i.e.*, somesthetic) neurons. A sensory unit consists of a single dorsal root ganglion afferent neuron, its terminals in a small region of the periphery, and its central axon that terminates on dorsal horn association neurons. The soma innervated by somesthetic afferent neurons of one set of dorsal root ganglia is called a dermatome. By means of a multisynaptic circuit, any stimuli sufficiently strong to cause tissue damage (*i.e.*, nociceptive stimulus) trigger a highly predictable withdrawal reflex by activating a lower motoneuron–innervated skeletal muscle contraction. Somesthetic afferents transmit the discriminative sensations of vibration and delicate touch, as well as the cruder sensations of pain and temperature.

The tactile system is considered the basic somesthetic system. Loss of temperature or pain sensitivity leaves the person with no awareness of deficiency. However, if the tactile system is lost, total anesthesia (*i.e.*, numbness) of the involved body part results. The tactile system uses two anatomically separate pathways to relay touch information to the opposite side of the forebrain: the dorsal column discriminative pathway and the anterolateral pathway. Both pathways cross to the opposite side of the central nervous system. The discriminative pathway crosses at the base of the medulla, and the anterolateral pathway crosses within the first few segments of entering the cord. Normal delicate touch, vibration, position, and movement sensations use the discriminative, two-neuron pathway to reach the thalamus where tertiary relay occurs to the primary somesthetic strip of parietal cortex. The anterolateral pathway consists of bilateral multisynaptic slow-conducting tracts that preserve crude tactile sensation even when there is considerable damage to the spinal cord. In contrast to the tactile system, temperature sensations of warm-hot and cool-cold result from skin thermal afferents, which project to the thalamus and cortex through the anterolateral system of the opposite side. Testing of the ipsilateral dorsal column (discriminative touch) system or the contralateral temperature projection systems permits diagnostic analysis of the level and extent of damage in spinal cord lesions.

Pain

After you have completed this section of the chapter, you should be able to meet the following objectives:

- Differentiate among the specificity, pattern, and gate-control theories of pain
- Describe the function of nociceptors in response to pain information
- State the difference between the A-delta and C-fiber neurons in the transmission of pain information
- Trace the transmission of pain signals with reference to the neospinothalamic, paleospinothalamic, and reticulospinal pathways
- Compare pain threshold and pain tolerance
- Describe the function of endogenous analgesic mechanisms as they relate to transmission of pain information
- Differentiate acute pain from chronic pain in terms of mechanisms, manifestations, and treatment
- Describe the mechanisms of referred pain, and list the common sites of referral for cardiac and other types of visceral pain
- Describe three methods for assessing pain
- Describe the proposed mechanisms of pain relief associated with the use of heat, cold, transcutaneous electrical nerve stimulation, and acupuncture and acupressure
- State the mechanisms whereby nonnarcotic and narcotic analgesic, tricyclic antidepressant, and anticonvulsive drugs relieve pain

Pain is an "unpleasant sensory and emotional experience associated with actual and potential tissue damage, or described in terms of such damage."[5] It involves anatomic structures, physiologic behaviors, and psychologic, social, cultural, and cognitive factors. Pain can be a prepotent or overwhelming experience, often disruptive to customary behavior, and when severe, it demands and directs all of a person's attention. Pain is the most common symptom that motivates a person to seek professional help. It sends those who suffer to a health care facility more often and with greater speed than any other symptom. Its location, radiation, duration, and severity give important clues to its cause. Despite its unpleasantness, pain can serve a useful purpose because it warns of impending tissue injury, motivating the person to seek relief. For example, an inflamed appendix could progress in severity, rupture, and even cause death were it not for the warning afforded by the pain.

Pain Theories

Traditionally, two theories have been offered to explain the physiologic basis for the pain experience. The first, *specificity theory,* regards pain as a separate sensory modality evoked by the activity of specific receptors that transmit information to pain centers or regions in the forebrain where pain is experienced.[6] The second theory includes a group of theories collectively referred to as *pattern theory.* It proposes that pain receptors share endings or pathways with other sensory modalities, but that different patterns of activity (*i.e.,* spatial or temporal) of the same neurons can be used to signal painful and nonpainful stimuli.[6] For example, light touch applied to the skin would produce the sensation of touch through low-frequency firing of the receptor; intense pressure would produce pain through high-frequency firing of the same receptor.

Both theories focus on the neurophysiologic basis of pain, and both probably apply. Specific nociceptive afferents have been identified and, in addition, almost all afferent stimuli, if driven at a very high frequency, can be experienced as painful. What these theories fail to address are the motivational, cognitive, cultural, and affective components of pain.

Gate control theory, a modification of specificity theory, was proposed by Melzack and Wall in 1965 to meet the challenges presented by the pattern theories. This theory postulated the presence of neural gating mechanisms at the segmental spinal cord level to account for interactions between pain and other sensory modalities.[7] The original gate control theory proposed a spinal cord level network of transmission (*i.e.,* t cells) or projection cells and internuncial neurons that can inhibit the t cells, forming a segmental level gating mechanism that could block projection of pain information to the brain.

According to the gate control theory, the internuncial neurons involved in the gating mechanism are activated by large-diameter, faster-propagating fibers that carry tactile information. The simultaneous firing of the large-diameter touch fibers have the potential for blocking the transmission of impulses from the small-diameter myelinated and unmyelinated pain fibers. Pain therapists have long known that pain intensity can be temporarily reduced during active tactile stimulation. For example, repeated sweeping of a soft-bristled brush on the skin (*i.e.,* brushing) over or near a painful area may result in pain reduction for several minutes to several hours.

Pain modulation is now known to be a much more complex phenomenon than that proposed by the original gate control theory. Tactile information is transmitted by small- and large-diameter fibers. Major interactions between sensory modalities, including the so-called gating phenomenon, occur at several levels of the CNS rostral to the input segment. Perhaps the most puzzling aspect of locally applied stimuli, such as brushing, that can block the experience of pain, is the relatively long-lasting effects (minutes to hours) of such treatments. This prolonged effect has been difficult to explain on the basis of specificity theories, including the gate control theory. Other important factors include the effect of endogenous opioids and their receptors at the segmental and the brain stem level, descending feedback modulation, altered sensitivity, learning, and culture. Despite this complexity, the Melzack and Wall theory has served a useful purpose. It excited interest in pain and stimulated research and clinical activity related to the pain-modulating systems.

Pain Mechanisms and Responses

Scientifically, pain has been viewed within the context of nociception. The term *nociception* is associated with tissue damage (from Latin *nocere,* to injure). Nociceptive stimuli are those that occur at or close to an intensity that causes tissue damage; therefore, they can be objectively defined. Researchers have used the withdrawal reflex (*e.g.,* withdrawal of the hand away from a tissue damaging stimulus) to describe nociceptive stimuli. Such stimuli include pressure from a sharp object, strong electric current to the skin, or application of heat or cold of approximately 10°C above or below skin temperature. This does not imply that pain is experienced whenever noxious stimuli activate nociceptors. Pain occurs when nociceptive stimuli are perceived as painful.

The mechanisms of pain are many and complex. There are first-order neurons and their receptive endings that react to stimuli that threaten the integrity of innervated tissues; second-order neurons, or spinal cord circuitry, that process nociceptive information; third-order tracts or pathways that project pain information to the brain; the thalamus and cortex that integrate and modulate pain; and the person's subjective reaction to the pain experience and associated circumstances.

Pain Receptors and Mediators

Receptors that have pain as their lowest-intensity threshold stimulus are known as nociceptors, or pain receptors. Structurally, the receptive endings of the peripheral pain fibers are free nerve endings. These receptive endings are widely distributed in the skin, dental pulp, some internal organs, periosteum, and meninges. Considerable controversy remains regarding the production of pain by the overstimulation of other receptors, such as those for temperature and pressure. Receptors translate the painful nociceptive stimuli into an electrical impulse that is transmitted to the spinal cord at the dorsal horn. Noxious stimuli evoked by action potentials are transmitted through two afferent nerve types: myelinated fibers called *A-delta fibers* and unmyelinated *C fibers*. The larger A-delta fibers have considerably greater conduction velocities, transmitting impulses at a rate of 5 to 30 m per second. The C fibers are the smallest of all peripheral fibers; they transmit impulses at the rate of 0.5 to 2.0 m per second. C-fiber pain is often described as slow wave pain, because it is slower in onset and longer in duration. The slow postexcitatory potentials generated within C fibers is now believed to be responsible for central sensitization to chronic pain.

Questions remain about how nociceptors are stimulated. In some cases they may be indirectly activated (*e.g.*, mechanical stimulation); at other times, they may be activated by substances released into the tissues by the action of the nociceptive stimuli or as the result of inflammation. The primary afferent neurons release substance P, calcitonin gene-related peptide (CGRP), galanin, and somatostatin. The release of potassium and hydrogen ions, acetylcholine, histamine, and bradykinin occurs as the result of direct tissue injury.[8] Some of these mediators have proinflammatory effects through their action on mast cells, lymphocytes, and other leukocytes. Others such as substance P directly potentiate inflammatory activity. Some of the effects of these peptides may be mediated through sympathetic postganglionic neurons that release prostaglandins, neuropeptide Y, and norepinephrine. These various chemical mediators are effective in producing nociceptive reflexes and the experience of pain by activating peripheral nociceptors, stimulating the release of pain-producing substances, or sensitizing peripheral endings of nociceptors.[9]

Nociceptive stimulation that activates C fibers can cause a characteristic response known as *neurogenic inflammation* that produces vasodilation and increased release of nociceptive mediators. It has been proposed that increasing levels of stimulation can incite pathologic dorsal root reflexes. This may cause neurogenic inflammation to spread to other peripheral tissues by means of antidromic nerve impulses located in the dorsal root ganglia. Retrograde transport and release of inflammatory mediators, such as substance P and CGRP, could cause increasing inflammation and more centrally directed afferent activation. This sets up a vicious cycle, which has implications for persistent pain and hyperalgesia.[8,10,11] Controversy remains as to whether the central events proposed for neurogenic inflammation can be applied to noninflammatory neuropathic pain or causalgia-like problems.[12]

Spinal Cord Circuitry and Pathways

The axons of the A-delta and C fiber neurons travel through the dorsal root to the white matter of the dorsal lateral spinal cord where they bifurcate and ascend or descend one or two segments, projecting collaterals into the dorsal horn association columns of these segments. Activated circuits of the association columns communicate with four categories of circuitry: the segmental level withdrawal reflex, the reticular activating system, the forebrain limbic system, and the thalamus and cortex. The local cord level withdrawal reflex is designed to remove endangered tissue from a damaging stimulus.

From the dorsal horn, axons of association projection neurons cross through the anterior commissure to the opposite side and ascend upward in the previously described *anterolateral sensory pathway*, using the neospinothalamic and paleospinothalamic pathways. Both pathways originate in the periphery, where the A-delta (high-threshold mechanoreceptor) axons are recruited later.

The faster-conducting fibers in the more lateral *neospinothalamic tract* (*i.e.*, discriminate pain pathway) are mainly associated with the sharp, bright, and fast characteristics of acute cutaneous pain. The A-delta afferent fibers synapse with a neuron, which sends axons through the moderately rapid neospinothalamic pathway to the thalamus. Projections of this system to the contralateral parietal somesthetic area provide the precise location of first pain (*i.e.*, bright, sharp, stabbing pain).

The *paleospinothalamic tract* is a slower-conducting multisynaptic tract concerned with the diffuse, dull, aching, and unpleasant sensations that are commonly associated with chronic and visceral pain. This information travels through the small unmyelinated C fibers. This system also projects fibers up the contralateral (*i.e.*, opposite) anterolateral pathway to terminate in several thalamic regions, including the intralateral nuclei, which project to the limbic system. It is associated with the emotional or affective-motivational aspects of pain. *Spinoreticular fibers* from this pathway project bilaterally to the reticular formation of the brain stem. This component of the paleospinothalamic system facilitates avoidance reflexes at all levels. It also contributes to an increase in the electroencephalographic activity associated with alertness and indirectly influences hypothalamic functions associated with sudden alertness, such as increased heart rate and blood pressure. This may explain the tremendous arousal effects of certain pain stimuli. Further projections of these systems send information to the mesencephalic periaqueductal gray and the hypothalamus.

Dorsal horn (second-order) neurons are divided primarily into two types: wide-dynamic-range (WDR) neurons that respond to low intensity stimuli and nociceptive-specific neurons that respond only to noxious or nociceptive stimuli. When stimuli are increased to a noxious level, the WDR neurons respond more intensely. After more severe damage to peripheral sensory afferents, A-delta and C fibers respond more intensely as they are increasingly stimulated. When C fibers are repetitively stimulated at a rate of once per second, each stimulus produces a progressively increasing response from WDR neurons. This phenomenon of amplification of transmitted signals has been called *wind-up* and may explain why pain sensation appears to increase with repeated stimulation. Windup and sensitization of dorsal horn neurons have implications for appropriate and early, or even preemptive, pain therapy to avoid the possibility of spinal cord neurons becoming hypersensitive or subject to firing spontaneously.[8,13]

Brain Centers and Pain Perception

The basic sensation of hurtfulness, or pain, occurs at the level of the thalamus. In the neospinothalamic system, interconnections between the lateral thalamus and the somatosensory cortex are necessary to add precision and discrimination to the pain sensation. Association areas of the parietal cortex are essential to the perception, or learned meaningfulness, of the pain experience. For example, if a mosquito bites a person's index finger on the left hand and only the thalamus is functional, the person complains of pain somewhere on the hand. With the primary sensory cortex functional, the person can localize the pain to the precise area on the index finger. The association cortex is necessary to interpret the buzzing and the sensation that preceded the pain as being related to a mosquito bite. The paleospinothalamic system projects diffusely from the intralaminar nuclei of the thalamus to large areas of the limbic cortex. These connections are probably associated with the hurtfulness and the mood-altering and attention-narrowing effect of pain.

Endogenous Analgesic Mechanisms

The endogenous analgesic system consists of naturally occurring opioids and their receptors. The *opioids* (*e.g.*, endorphins, enkephalins, dynorphin) are morphine-like substances that are synthesized in many regions of the CNS, including the pituitary gland. Endorphins are found primarily in the amygdala, limbic system, hypothalamic-pituitary axis, and other brain stem structures. The enkephalins are found primarily in short interneurons of the *periaqueductal gray* (PAG) of the midbrain, limbic system, basal ganglia, hypothalamus, and the sympathetic nervous system. The discovery of opioid receptors here and in the peripheral nervous system (*e.g.*, cholinergic, enkephalinergic, and serotonergic in the intestinal myenteric plexus) led to a search for natural body substances capable of interacting with these receptors. The natural ligands (*i.e.*, binding molecules) for these opioid receptors are the *endogenous opioid peptides* (*i.e.*, endorphins and enkephalins), which were discovered in 1975. New therapeutic approaches to the treatment of pain were envisioned when it was discovered that these peptides exert inhibitory modulation of pain transmission and that the release of endogenous opioids after CNS stimulation correlated with patient reports of pain relief. These morphine-like substances mimic the peripheral and central effects of morphine and the central effects of other opiate drugs. Since the discovery of the opioids, other neuromodulators for pain have been identified. Norepinephrine and serotonin (5-HT) neurons appear to provide major descending modulation and inhibition for transmission of nociceptive information to the rostral levels of the CNS.[13]

One of the exciting advances in understanding pain is the elucidation of neuroanatomic pathways that arise in the midbrain and brain stem, descend to the spinal cord, and function in the modulation of ascending pain impulses. One such pathway begins in an area of the midbrain called the PAG region. Soon after the introduction of the gate control theory (more appropriately called the gain control theory), it was found that focal stimulation of the midbrain PAG regions produced a state of analgesia. The resultant analgesia lasted for many hours and was sufficient to permit abdominal surgery, although levels of consciousness and reactions to auditory and visual stimuli remained unaffected. A few years later, opioid receptors were found to be highly concentrated in this and other regions of the CNS where electrical stimulation produced analgesia. Because of these findings, the PAG area of the midbrain often is referred to as the *endogenous analgesia center*.

The PAG area receives input from widespread areas of the CNS, including the cerebral cortex, hypothalamus, brain stem reticular formation, and spinal cord by way of the paleospinothalamic and neospinothalamic tracts. This region is intimately connected to the limbic system, which is associated with emotional experience. The neurons of the PAG area have axons that descend into an area called the *nucleus raphe magnus* (NRM) in the rostral medulla. The axons of these NRM neurons project to the dorsal horn of the spinal cord where they terminate in the same layers as the entering primary pain fibers (Fig. 40–8). Stimulation of the medullary nuclei is thought to inhibit pain transmission by dorsal horn projection neurons.[14] There is also evidence of noradrenergic neurons that can inhibit transmission of pain impulses at the level of the spinal cord. Studies indicate that the rostral pons has noradrenergic neurons with axons that project to the medullary nuclei and to the dorsal horn cells of the spinal cord.[15] The discovery that norepinephrine can block pain transmission led to studies directed at the combined administration of opioids and clonidine, a central-acting α-adrenergic agonist for pain relief. Norepinephrine and 5-HT neurons appear to provide the major descending modulation in the dorsal horn.

There are at least two types of cells that affect transmission of nociceptive information to the brain. These cells are called *off-cells* and *on-cells*. The off-cells inhibit, and the on-cells appear to facilitate, the transmission of pain messages.[8,13] 5-HT has been identified as a neuromodulator in the NRM medullary nuclei that project to the spinal cord. It has been shown that tricyclic antidepressant compounds, such as amitriptyline, have analgesic properties independent of their antidepressant effects. These drugs, which enhance the effects of 5-HT by blocking its presynaptic uptake, have been found to be effective in the management of certain types of chronic pain.[16] Neurons that secrete substance P, another neuropeptide, are widely distributed throughout the nervous system. Considerable research data support the role of substance P as a transmitter substance used by unmyelinated C-fiber afferents related to nociception and slow pain.[17] There is evidence that enkephalins and other opioid peptides modulate pain at the spinal level by inhibiting the release of substance P. Other neurotransmitters, such as acetylcholine and neurotensin, may also be involved. Details of the circuitry remain under study.

Pain Threshold, Tolerance, and Reactions

Reactions to pain are affected by pain threshold and tolerance. Although the terms often are used interchange-

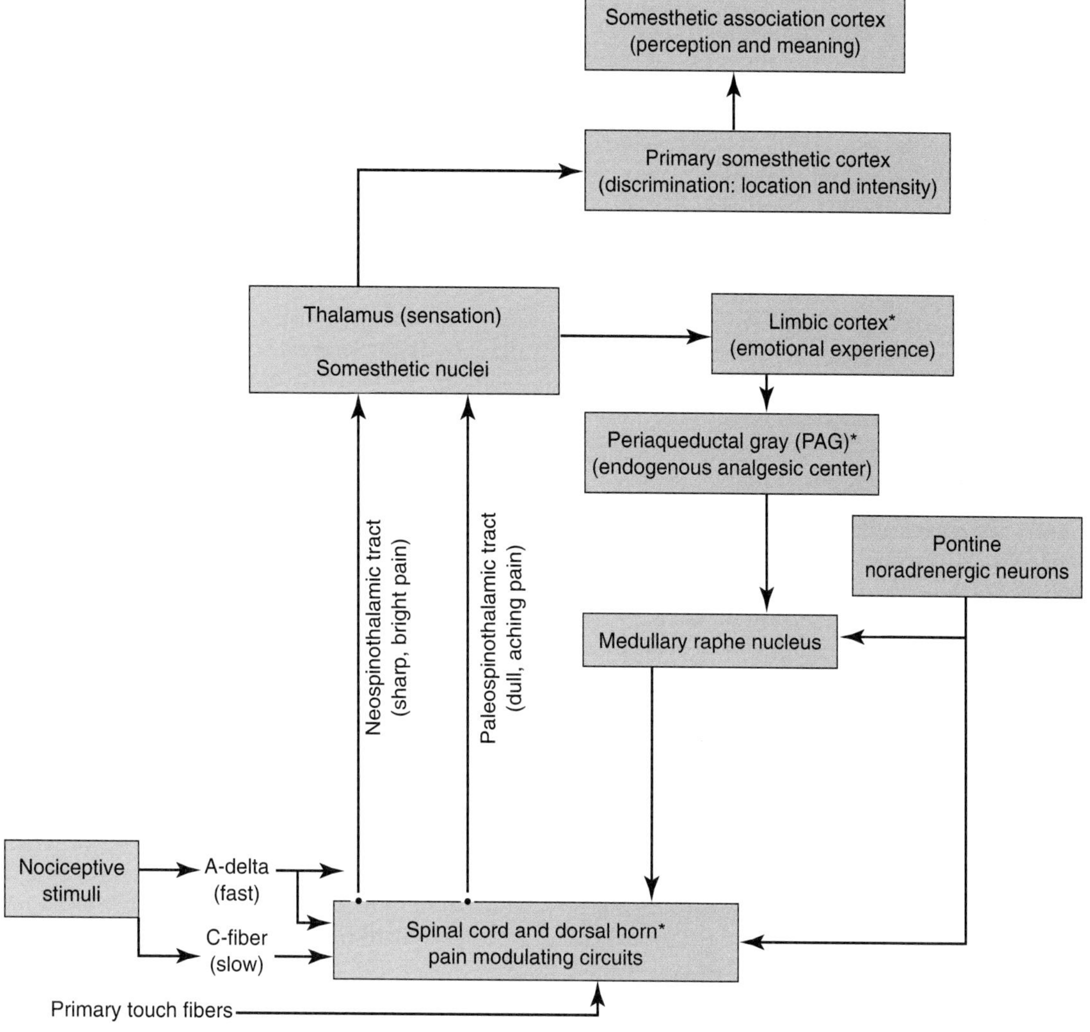

Figure 40–8 ■■■
Primary pain pathways. The transmission of incoming nociceptive impulses is modulated by dorsal horn circuitry that receives input from peripheral touch receptors and from descending pathways that involve the limbic cortical systems (orbital frontal cortex, amygdala, and hypothalamus), periaqueductal endogenous analgesic center in the midbrain, pontine noradrenergic neurons, and the raphe nucleus in the medulla.

ably, pain threshold and pain tolerance are not the same entity. *Pain threshold* is more closely associated with nociceptive (*i.e.,* tissue-damaging) stimuli. *Pain tolerance* relates more to the total pain experience; it is defined as the maximum intensity or duration of pain that a person is willing to endure—the point beyond which the person wants something done about the pain. Tolerance is not necessarily indicative of the severity of pain. Psychologic, familial, cultural, and environmental factors significantly influence the intensity of pain a person is willing to tolerate. Separation and identification of the role of each of these two aspects of pain continue to pose fundamental problems for the pain management team and for pain researchers. The threshold to pain, which is quite uniform from one person to another is more associated with the fast (first) pain pathway. Tolerance to pain, which demonstrates a greater variation from one person to another, is more associated with the slow (second) pain pathway.[8]

Physical reactions to pain may be manifested by facial expressions such as frowning or wrinkling the brows, biting the lips, clenching the teeth, and tensing of limb and body muscles. Protective body movements can be involuntary and voluntary. The previously mentioned withdrawal reaction, which moves the body part away from the pain source, is involuntary. Voluntary movements, such as changes in posture and relaxation exercises, often relieve discomfort.

Responses to Pain

The responses to pain are both physiologic and psychosocial. Pain that persists or is repetitive can result in adaptive responses, with observable decreases in sympathetic activity. Pain receptors show little, if any, adaptation. On the contrary, reactions to long-term pain are centrally mediated. With time, physiologic and psychologic coping mechanisms evolve, but these behavioral responses do not necessarily indicate pain relief. The person may merely be too fatigued to respond.

Physiologic responses to pain involve activation of the sympathetic nervous system, which evokes the fight-or-flight reaction, with catecholamine release from the adrenal medulla. When this occurs, the vessels of the skin and abdominal viscera constrict and those of the heart, brain, lungs, and skeletal muscles dilate as blood is shifted from nonvital to vital parts of the body. The face becomes pallid and the pupils dilate. The respirations become more rapid, the heart rate increases, and the contractions of the heart become more forceful. Muscle tension rises and energy stores are mobilized to supply the body with glucose. A relative decline in parasympathetic activity may result in loss of appetite, nausea, and vomiting. Gastrointestinal motility and digestive gland secretion also diminish. After a period, a parasympathetic rebound response occurs, and the heart rate, blood pressure, and respiratory rate may fall below the prepain level. This is likely when pain is intense but of short duration.

Psychosocial reactions to pain are deeply influenced by the same factors that affect pain tolerance, including past experiences with pain. A verbally competent person may be able to accurately describe the location, duration, and intensity of the pain, as well as his or her ability or willingness to tolerate it. A change in the tone of voice may be as revealing as the words spoken. Previous personal and family experiences with certain diseases, such as cancer, can significantly affect the degree of fear, anxiety, and depression associated with pain and, consequently, the person's reaction to it.

Vocalizations comprise a group of responses such as crying, groaning, grunting, and gasping. Their frequency, loudness, and duration can assume greater significance in situations where the person is too young or too confused to be verbally competent. These manifestations are particularly important in young children and the elderly. Cultural and environmental factors may also play a role in pain perception. For example, a person who values stoicism is unlikely to cry out in public when subjected to painful stimuli, but this may be an acceptable response for someone of another culture.

Types of Pain

The types of pain can be classified into four categories according to source, fast versus slow pain, referral, and duration (acute versus chronic pain).

Source

The sources of pain commonly are divided into four general categories: cutaneous, deep somatic, visceral, and functional or psychogenic.

Cutaneous Pain. Cutaneous pain arises from superficial structures, such as the skin and subcutaneous tissues. A paper cut on the finger is an example of easily localized superficial, or cutaneous, pain. It is a sharp, bright pain with a burning quality and may be abrupt or slow in onset. It can be localized accurately and may be distributed along the dermatomes. Because there is an overlap of nerve fiber distribution between the dermatomes, the boundaries of pain frequently are not as clear-cut as the dermatomal diagrams indicate.

Deep Somatic Pain. Deep somatic pain originates in deep body structures, such as the periosteum, muscles, tendons, joints, and blood vessels. This pain is more diffuse than cutaneous pain. Various stimuli, such as strong pressure exerted on bone, ischemia to a muscle, and tissue damage, can produce deep somatic pain. This is the type of pain one experiences from a sprained ankle. Radiation of pain from the original site of injury can occur. For example, damage to a nerve root can cause a person to experience pain radiating along its fiber distribution.

Visceral Pain. Visceral, or splanchnic, pain has its origin in the visceral organs. Common examples of visceral pain are renal colic, pain caused by cholecystitis, pain associated with acute appendicitis, and ulcer pain. Although the viscera are diffusely and richly innervated, cutting or burning of viscera, as opposed to similar noxious stimuli applied to cutaneous or superficial structures, is unlikely to cause pain. Instead, strong abnormal contractions of the gastrointestinal system, distention, or ischemia affecting the walls of the viscera can induce severe visceral pain. Anyone who has suffered from severe gastrointestinal distress or ureteral colic can readily attest to the misery involved.

Visceral pain is transmitted by small unmyelinated pain fibers that travel with the axons of the autonomic nervous system and project to visceral input association neurons of the cord or brain stem. In addition to sending projections to the forebrain, these input association neurons also project through the paleospinal and spinoreticular pathways into visceral reflex circuits. Visceral pain typically is accompanied by autonomic responses such as nausea, vomiting, sweating, and pallor, and less commonly, shock ensues.

Ascending pathways resulting in the experience of visceral pain have three different overlapping general visceral afferent sources: pharynx through lower esophagus that travel along cranial nerves IX and X, stomach through mid-transverse colon that travel along T1 to L2, and below the mid-transverse colon that travel along S2 to S4. The peripheral general visceral afferent pathways involved travel with the parasympathetic distribution for the upper and lower viscera and with the sympathetic distribution for the intervening viscera. Pain from the viscera may be localized only with difficulty. There are several explanations for this. First, innervation of visceral organs is poorly represented at the forebrain levels (*i.e.*, perception). A second possible explanation is that the brain does not easily learn to localize sensations that originate in organs that are only imprecisely visualized. For example, a cut on the third finger of the right hand can be readily seen, identified, and localized, whereas an inflamed internal organ can be localized only vaguely. A third explanation is that sensory information from thoracic and abdominal viscera can travel by two pathways to the CNS.

Evidence has been mounting for a "new" visceral pain pathway. In the past, pathways carrying nociceptive information were believed to ascend contralaterally, and those carrying discriminative sensory modalities were believed to ascend ipsilaterally. However, animal studies and clinical reports of pain relief after commissural myelotomy (possibly because of unintended dorsal column damage) has led to a case report of intractable pelvic visceral pain relief after a punctate midline myelotomy.[18] The location of this ascending visceral pain pathway, in the ipsilateral posterior (dorsal) columns of the posterior spinal cord, provided accurate neurosurgical access for interruption of only this midline posterior column pathway. Dramatic relief of this severe intractable pelvic pain was immediate and continued up to 10 months postoperatively. The procedure allowed gradual but successful withdrawal of narcotic therapy. No new neurologic deficits were evident postsurgically. More studies are needed to determine the long-term success of midline myelotomy for this and other pain of visceral origin. One exciting aspect of this new finding is that so little of the spinal cord needed to be interrupted to achieve intractable pain relief. It raises the hope that this may open the door to newer more specific and effective means of pain relief in carefully selected patients with severe intractable pain.[18]

Functional or Psychogenic Pain. Pain may have a known or unknown physical source. Whereas organic or somatogenic pain originates in the body, or soma, pain without physical cause (*i.e.*, functional or psychogenic pain) is attributed to the psyche or emotions. In both situations, the physical sensation of pain is the same.

Fast Pain and Slow Pain

Two qualitatively different types of pain can be readily appreciated: fast pain (*i.e.*, first pain) and slow pain (*i.e.*, second pain). Fast pain is a short, well-localized sensation; it starts and stops abruptly when the stimulus is instituted or stopped. Examples are a pinprick or strong pinch. Fast pain has its origin in the free nerve endings of myelinated A-delta axons located in the skin that respond to strong mechanical pressure and high temperature. It is associated with the withdrawal reflex and with the sensation of bright, sharp pain experience. This type of pain can be blocked with local anesthetics. Slow pain is experienced as a throbbing, burning, or aching sensation. It has its origin in the free nerve endings of the very slow conducting unmyelinated C fibers. The slow-pain receptors have chemoreceptor properties and respond to compounds liberated as a result of tissue damage from excessive mechanical, chemical, and cold or hot stimuli. These two fiber-conduction groups of afferents partially explain the two components of pain, the discriminative (*i.e.*, first pain) and the affective-motivational component (*i.e.*, second pain). The farther the stimulus is from the brain, the more time separates the fast and slow components.

Referred Pain

Referred pain is that pain perceived at a site different from its point of origin but innervated by the same spinal segment. It is hypothesized that visceral and somatic afferent neurons converge on the same dorsal horn projection neurons (Fig. 40–9). For this reason, it can be difficult for the brain to correctly identify the original source of pain. Pain that originates in the ab-

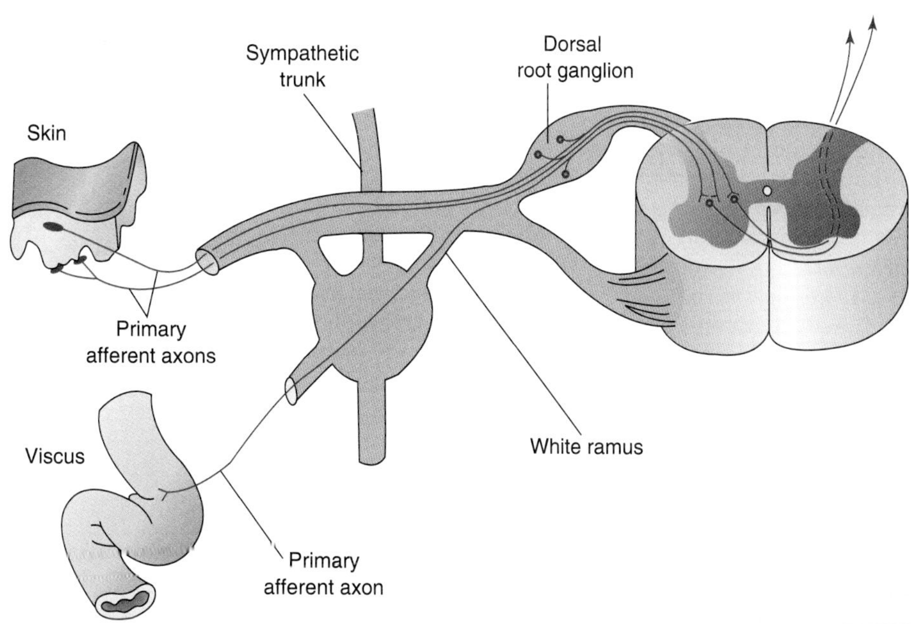

Figure 40–9
Convergence of cutaneous and visceral inputs onto the same second-order projection neuron in the dorsal horn of the spinal cord. Although virtually all visceral inputs converge with cutaneous inputs, most cutaneous inputs do not converge with other sensory inputs.

dominal or thoracic viscera is diffuse and poorly localized and often perceived at a site far removed from the affected area. For example, the pain associated with myocardial infarction commonly is referred to the left arm, neck, and chest.

Referred pain may arise alone or concurrent with pain located at the origin of the noxious stimuli. It may also mask the true origin of nociceptive stimuli. Although the term *referred* usually is applied to pain that originates in the viscera and is experienced as if originating from the body wall, it may also be applied to pain that arises from somatic structures. An example would be pain referred to the chest wall caused by nociceptive stimulation of the peripheral portion of the diaphragm, which receives somatic (somesthetic) innervation from the intercostal nerves. An understanding of pain referral is of great value in diagnosing illness because afferent neurons from visceral or deep somatic tissue enter the spinal cord at the same level as those from the cutaneous areas to which the pain is referred (Fig. 40–10).

The sites of referred pain are determined embryologically as visceral and somatic structure that share the same site for entry of sensory information into the CNS, develop, and move to more distant locations. For example, a person with peritonitis may complain of pain in the shoulder. Internally, there is inflammation of the peritoneum that lines the central part of the diaphragm. In the embryo, the diaphragm originates in the neck, and its central portion is innervated by the phrenic nerve, which enters the cord at the level of the third to fifth segments (C3 to C5). As the fetus develops, the diaphragm descends to its adult position between the thoracic and abdominal cavities, while maintaining its embryonic pattern of innervation. Thus, fibers that enter the spinal cord at the C3 to C5 level carry information from both the neck area and the diaphragm, and the diaphragmatic pain is interpreted by the forebrain as originating in the shoulder or neck area.

Although the *visceral* pleura, pericardium, and peritoneum are said to be relatively free of pain fibers, the *parietal* pleura, pericardium, and peritoneum do react to nociceptive stimuli. Visceral inflammation can involve parietal and somatic structures, and this may give rise to diffuse local or referred pain. For example, irritation of the parietal peritoneum resulting from appendicitis typically gives rise to pain directly over the inflamed area in the lower right quadrant. Such stimuli can evoke pain referred to the umbilical area.

Muscle spasm, or *guarding*, occurs when somatic structures are involved. Guarding is a protective-reflex rigidity; its purpose is to protect the affected body parts (*e.g.*, an abscessed appendix or a sprained muscle). This protective guarding may cause blood vessel compression and give rise to pain of muscle ischemia, causing local and referred pain.

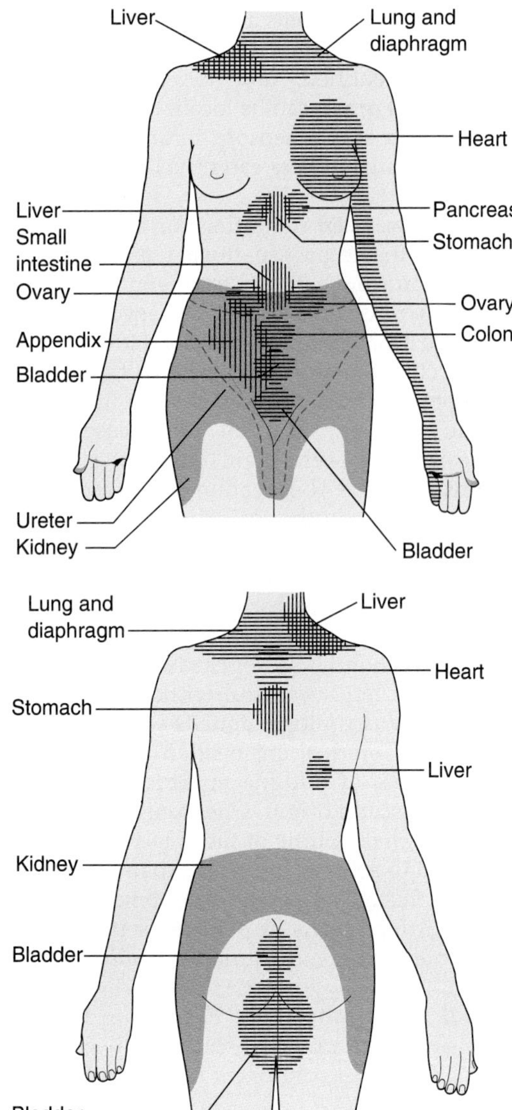

Figure 40–10
Areas of referred pain. (**Top**) Anterior view. (**Bottom**) Posterior view.

Acute and Chronic Pain

Pain can also be classified according to duration and characterized as acute or chronic. The pain research of the past 3 decades has emphasized the importance of differentiating acute pain from chronic pain and dealing with them separately. This is because they differ from each other temporally and in cause, mechanisms, pathophysiology, and function, and the diagnosis of and therapy for each are distinctive (Table 40–1).[16]

Acute Pain. *Acute pain* is defined as pain lasting less than 6 months. It consists of unpleasant sensory, perceptual, and emotional components with associated somatic, autonomic, psychologic, and behavioral responses. Acute pain is caused by noxious, or tissue-damaging events such as trauma or surgery. Acute pain is usually self-limited. It typically subsides when the injury heals. Its purpose is to serve as a protective, or warning, system. Besides alerting the person to the existence of actual or impending tissue damage, it prompts a search for professional help. The pain's location, intensity, duration, and radiation and those factors that aggravate or relieve it are essential diagnostic clues. Unlike chronic pain, it is rare for acute pain to be of unknown origin or to be caused by psychological factors alone. Acute pain commonly is exacerbated by anxiety and secondary reflex musculoskeletal spasms, which usually disappear when the pain is relieved. Inadequately treated pain can provoke physiologic responses that alter circulation and tissue metabolism, and produce physical manifestations such as tachycardia reflective of increased sympathetic activity. Acute pain that is inadequately treated tends to decrease mobility and ambulation and decrease respiratory movements such as deep breathing and coughing to the extent that it may complicate or delay recovery.

Chronic Pain. *Chronic pain* has classically been defined as pain lasting 6 months or longer. In practice, this time frame varies, and the differences between acute and chronic pain are more than temporal. The International Association for the Study of Pain defines chronic pain as that which persists beyond the expected normal time of healing.[19] Chronic pain may be unrelenting as in cancer pain, relatively continuous as in low back pain, or episodic as in pain associated with sickle cell crisis.

Chronic pain is a leading cause of disability in the United States. It has been estimated that 25% to 35% of persons in industrialized nations are afflicted with chronic pain.[20] Unlike acute pain, persistent chronic pain usually serves no useful function. To the contrary, it imposes physiologic, psychologic, family, and economic stresses and may exhaust a person's resources. In contrast to acute pain, psychologic and environmental influences may play an important role in the development of behaviors associated with chronic pain. Chronic pain often is associated with loss of appetite, sleep disturbances, and depression.[21] Amazingly, depression commonly is relieved spontaneously when the pain is removed. The physiology of chronic pain is poorly understood.

Bonica has proposed that chronic pain be divided into syndromes based on mechanisms of origin including peripheral mechanisms, peripheral-central mechanisms, central mechanisms, and psychologic mechanisms.[20] Peripheral mechanisms result from persistent stimulation of nociceptors. Pain emanating from joint and muscle disorders fall into this category. Peripheral-central mechanisms involve abnormal function of the peripheral and central portions of the somatosensory system. These disorders include conditions such as those resulting from partial or complete loss of descending inhibitory influences or spontaneous firing of regenerated nerve fibers. They include conditions such as causalgia, phantom limb pain, and postherpetic neuralgia. Central mechanisms include lesions of the thalamus or other CNS disorders that involve loss of descending inhibitory influences. Psychologic mechanisms can include psychosomatic illness in which emotional stress leads to physiologic reactions, operant mechanisms in which expression of pain produces secondary gain, or psychiatric pain associated with conditions such as schizophrenia.

Persons suffering from chronic pain may not exhibit the somatic, autonomic, or affective behaviors associated with acute pain. As painful conditions become prolonged and continuous, autonomic nervous system responses decrease. Persons with chronic pain are also

TABLE 40-1

Characteristics of Acute and Chronic Pain

Characteristic	Acute Pain	Chronic Pain
Onset	Recent	Continuous or intermittent
Duration	Short duration (less than 6 months)	6 months or more
Autonomic responses	Consistent with sympathetic fight or flight response* Increased heart rate Increased stroke volume Increased blood pressure Increased pupillary dilation Increased muscle tension Decreased gut motility Decreased salivary flow (dry mouth)	Absence of autonomic responses
Psychologic component	Associated anxiety	Increased irritability Associated depression Somatic preoccupation Withdrawal from outside interests Decreased strength of relationships
Other types of response		Decreased sleep Decreased libido Appetite changes

*Responses are approximately proportional to intensity of the stimulus.

thought to have depleted their source of 5-HT and endorphins, leading to decreased pain tolerance. Certain behaviors viewed as acceptable in patients with severe but short-lived pain are not expected or considered appropriate in the chronic situation. With chronic pain, it is important to heed the person's own description of the pain because the expected psychophysiologic responses may or may not be present.

Management of Pain

The therapeutic approaches to acute and chronic pain differ markedly. In acute pain, therapy is directed at providing pain relief while interrupting the nociceptive stimulus. Chronic pain management is more complex and is based on multiple considerations, including life expectancy.

Acute Pain

Acute pain should be aggressively managed and pain medication provided before the pain becomes severe. This allows persons to be more comfortable, more active, and more participant in their care. Part of the reluctance of health care workers to provide adequate relief for acute pain has been fear of addiction. However, addiction to opioid medications is thought to be virtually nonexistent when these drugs are prescribed for acute pain. Usually less medication is needed when the drug is given before the pain becomes severe and the pain pathways become sensitized.

In 1992, the Clinical Practice Guidelines for Acute Pain Management were released.They were developed by a multidisciplinary expert group under the sponsorship of the Agency for Health Care Policy and Research (AHCPR), Public Health Service, U.S. Department of Health and Human Services.[22] The guidelines, which focus on postoperative pain, emphasize the need for a collaborative, interdisciplinary approach to pain control, which includes members of the health care team and input from the patient and the patient's family when appropriate; an individualized proactive pain control plan developed preoperatively by patients and practitioners, because pain is easier to prevent than to bring under control after it has begun; assessment and frequent reassessment of the patient's plan, facilitated by a pain management log or flow sheet; use of drug and nondrug therapies to control or prevent pain; and a formal, institutional approach to management of acute pain, with clear lines of responsibility.

Chronic Pain

Management of chronic pain requires early attempts to prevent pain and adequate therapy for acute bouts of pain. Specific treatment requires an exhaustive search for the cause of the pain. Treatment methods can include neural blockade, electrical modalities, and nonnarcotic and narcotic medications. Nonnarcotic medications such as tricyclic antidepressants, anticonvulsant medications, and nonsteroidal antiinflammatory drugs (NSAIDs) serve as useful adjuncts to opioids for treatment of different types of chronic pain. Cancer is a common cause of chronic pain.

One proposed classification of chronic pain divides affected persons into two broad groups according to life expectancy (brief versus normal). This classification assumes clinical importance primarily if a decision must be reached concerning long-term use of narcotics for pain relief. The goal of chronic malignant pain management should be pain alleviation and prevention. Preemptive therapy tends to reduce sensitization of pain pathways and provides for more effective pain control. In 1994, the AHCPR published Clinical Practice Guidelines for Management of Cancer Pain.[23] This guideline states that there are more than 1 million cases of cancer diagnosed among Americans each year. Unfortunately, pain control remains a significant problem, despite advances in understanding and management of pain. The report emphasizes that pain control merits high priority because it diminishes activity, appetite, and sleep and can further weaken a person already debilitated with cancer. It also emphasizes that pain interferes with productive employment, enjoying recreation, and taking an active part in family life. As with the acute pain guidelines, these guidelines also emphasize the need for a collaborative multidisciplinary approach to management of cancer pain. One of the most important aspects of chronic malignant pain control for the person and their family is access to health care and pain management information. It classifies recommended interventions according to use: analgesics and adjuvant drugs; cognitive or behavioral strategies; physical modalities; palliative radiation and antineoplastic therapies; nerve blocks; and palliative and ablative surgery.[23] Written patient education materials, at an appropriate reading level, should be provided.

Assessment of Pain

The relief and management of pain require careful assessment to consider the cause of the pain, evaluate its severity, location and radiation, and determine the type of pain that is present. As with other disease states, it is preferable to eliminate the cause rather than treat the symptoms. A careful history often provides information about the triggering factors (*i.e.*, injury, infection, or disease) and the site of nociceptive stimuli (*i.e.*, peripheral receptor or visceral organ). Observation of facial expression and posture may provide additional information about the severity and accompanying responses to pain. For example, alterations in normal posture, such as limping, may increase the spread of pain to neighboring myotomes with progressive complaints that worsen with activity and cold. The AHCPR pain guidelines emphasize that the "the single most reliable indicator of the existence and intensity of acute pain—and any resultant affective discomfort or distress—is the patient's self report."[23] This self-report should include pain onset, description, localization, radiation, intensity, quality, pattern, anything that relieves or exacerbates it, and the individual's personal reaction to the pain.

Unlike many other bodily responses, such as temperature and blood pressure, the degree or severity of pain cannot be measured objectively. To overcome this problem, various methods have been developed for quantifying the severity of pain in a given person. Among the methods used for pain measurement are numeric value and visual analog scales, verbal descriptor scales, physiologic and behavioral measures, and multidimensional measures, such as the McGill Pain Questionnaire.[24] Because of the personal nature of pain, most pain instruments are more useful in evaluating individual versus group responses to pain. Pain distress scales, such as *numeric value* and *visual analog* scales, ask a person to give a numeric value to his or her pain, with 0 representing no pain and 10 representing the most intense pain imaginable. The visual analog scale uses a straight line, often 10 cm in length, which represents a continuum of pain intensity. The person is asked to choose a point on the continuum that represents his or her present state of pain intensity. *Verbal descriptor* scales consist of several numerically ranked choices of words such as none, slight, mild, moderate, and severe. The word that is chosen is used to determine the intensity of pain on an ordinal scale.

The *McGill Pain Questionnaire* measures the physiologic and the psychologic dimensions of pain.[25] The instrument is divided into four parts. The first part uses a drawing of the body on which the person indicates the location of pain. The second part uses a list of 20 words to describe the sensory, affective, evaluative, and other qualities of pain, with the selected words being given a numeric score (*e.g.*, words implying the least pain are assigned a value of 1 and next a value of 2, and so on). The third part asks the person to select words such as brief, momentary, and constant to describe the pattern of pain. The fourth part of the instrument evaluates the present pain intensity on a scale of 0 to 5. Another instrument, the *Memorial Pain Assessment Card* can be used to determine the intensity of pain, mood, and effectiveness of analgesia.[23]

Nonpharmacologic Treatment

The treatment of pain may use a number of nonpharmacologic methods, including cognitive-behavioral interventions, physical agents such as heat and cold, and electroanalgesia. These methods are often used as adjunctive therapy.

Cognitive-Behavioral Interventions. Cognitive-behavioral interventions include relaxation, distraction and imagery, and biofeedback. If the person is having surgery, these techniques can be taught preoperatively. *Relaxation* is one of the most evaluated cognitive-behavioral approaches to pain relief. The relaxation methods need not be complex. Relatively simple strategies, such as slow rhythmic breathing and brief jaw relaxation procedures, have been successful in decreasing self-reported pain and analgesic use.

Distraction (*i.e.*, focusing a person's attention on stimuli other than painful stimuli or negative emotions) is used to make pain more tolerable but usually does not eliminate it. It could be considered a type of sensory shielding whereby attention to pain is sacrificed for attention to objective or physical stimuli that are already present or easily obtained. Examples are counting, repeating phrases or poems, engaging in activities that require concentration, such as projects, activities, work, conversation, describing slides or pictures, and rhythmic breathing. Television, adventure movies, music, and humor can also provide diversion. It is a mistake to assume that a person who appears to be able to cope with pain by the use of distraction does not have pain. The person should not be punished for his or her efforts by having appropriate medications withheld.[26]

Imagery consists of using imagination to develop a mental picture—a visual image. In pain management, therapeutic guided imagery (*i.e.*, goal-directed imaging) is used. It can be used in conjunction with relaxation techniques, biofeedback, and other management methods to develop sensory images that can decrease the perceived intensity of pain. It can also be used to lessen anxiety and reduce muscle tension. *Meditation* can also be used, but it requires practice and the ability to concentrate to be effective.

Biofeedback is used to provide feedback to a person concerning the current status of some body function (*e.g.*, finger temperature, temporal artery pulsation, blood pressure, muscle tension). It is a process of learning designed to make the person aware of certain of his or her own body functions for the purpose of modifying these functions at a conscious level. Interest in biofeedback rose with the possibility of using this treatment modality in the management of migraine and tension headaches or for other pain that had a muscle tension component.

Use of Heat and Cold. Physical agents used to provide pain relief include electrical stimulation, heat, and cold. The type of agent that is being used depends on the type of pain being treated and, in many cases, personal preference.

Historically, *heat* (*i.e.*, thermotherapy) has proved to be a useful method for relieving pain. Some of the earliest sources of therapeutic heat were heated stones, sand, oils, and water or simply the radiant heat from the sun or a fire.[27] Currently, application is achieved through a number of methods, such as immersion in hot water, and the use of hot packs, electrically heated pads, infrared rays, and shortwave diathermy, and gel or chemical packs.

Heat dilates blood vessels and increases local blood flow; it can also influence the transmission of pain impulses and it increases collagen extensibility.[28] Overall, an increase in local circulation can reduce the level of nociceptive stimulation by reducing local ischemia caused by muscle spasm or tension, it can increase the removal of metabolites and inflammatory mediators that act as nociceptive stimuli, and it can help to reduce swelling and relieve pressure on local nociceptive endings. Heat information is carried to the posterior horn of the spinal cord and may exert its effect by modulating projection of pain transmission. It may also produce the release of endogenous opioids through placebo-type mechanisms. Limitation in the range of movement often is the result of muscle shortening. Heat alters the viscosity of collagen fibers in ligaments, tendons, and joint structures so that they are more easily extended and can be stretched further before the nociceptive endings are stimulated. Thus, heat often is applied before therapy aimed at stretching joint structures and increasing range of motion. Care must be taken not to use excessive heat. When excessive heat is used, the heat itself becomes a noxious stimulus, which results in the perception of pain. More importantly, this perception of pain should be regarded as a warning signal of impending tissue damage and an indication that removal of the heat source is essential to avoid a burn. In certain circumstances or diseases, use of heat is controversial; and in some conditions where increased blood flow or metabolism (*e.g.*, peripheral vascular disease) would be detrimental, the application of heat is contraindicated. However, because reports at this time do not contraindicate the use of heat on skin, it is still used in control of some pain related to cancer.[23]

Like heat, the application of *cold* may produce a dramatic reduction in the level of pain that some persons perceive. Cold exerts its effect on pain through circulatory and neural mechanisms. The initial response to local application of cold is sudden local vasoconstriction. This initial vasoconstriction is followed by alternating periods of vasodilatation and vasoconstriction during which the body "hunts" for its normal level of blood flow to prevent local tissue damage. This gives rise to the so-called *hunting reflex* whereby the circulation to the cooled area undergoes alternating periods of pallor caused by ischemia and flushing caused by hyperemia.[28] The vasoconstriction is caused by local stimulation of sympathetic fibers and direct cooling of blood vessels; hyperemia, by local autoregulatory mechanisms. In situations of acute injury, cold is used to produce vasoconstriction and prevent extravasation of blood into the tissues; pain relief results from decreased swelling and decreased stimulation of nociceptive endings. The vasodilatation that follows can be useful in removing substances that stimulate nociceptive endings.

Cold can also have a marked and dramatic effect on pain that results from muscle spasm that causes an accumulation of metabolites within the muscle. For example, the severe pain of joint inflammation suffered by persons with rheumatoid arthritis often is appreciably reduced with the application of cold. In terms of pain modulation, cold may reduce afferent activity reaching the posterior horn of the spinal cord by modulating sensory input. The application of cold can be considered a noxious stimulus and may influence the release of endogenous opioids from the PAG area. Cold packs should be flexible to conform to body parts easily; adequately wrapped to protect the skin; and applied no more than 15 minutes at a time. Cold should be used only with great caution in anyone whose whole circulation is compromised.[23]

Stimulus-Induced Analgesia. Stimulation-induced analgesia is one of the oldest known methods of pain relief.[29] Historical references to the use of electricity to decrease or control pain date back to AD 46 when a Roman physician, Scribonius Largus, described how the stimulus from an electric eel was able to provide pain relief for headache and gout.[30] Electrical stimulation methods of pain relief include *transcutaneous electrical nerve stimulation* (TENS) and electrical acupuncture. TENS refers to the transmission of electrical energy across the surface of the skin to the peripheral nerve fibers. TENS units have been developed that are convenient, easily transported, and relatively economical to use. Most are about the size of a transistor radio or cigarette package. These battery-operated units deliver a measurable amount of current to a target site.

The system usually consists of three parts: a pair of electrodes, lead wires, and a stimulator. The electrical stimulation is delivered in a pulsed waveform that can be varied in terms of pulse amplitude, width, and rate. The type of stimulation used varies with the type of pain being treated. Electrode placement is determined by the physiologic pathways and an understanding of the pain mechanisms involved. They may be placed on either side of a painful area, over an affected dermatome, over an affected peripheral nerve where it is most superficial, or over a nerve trunk. For example, the electrodes commonly are placed medial and lateral to the incision when treating postoperative pain.

There is probably no one explanation for the physiologic effects of TENS.[31] Each specific type of stimulator may have different sites of action and may be explained by more than one theory. The gate control theory was proposed as one possible mechanism.[32] According to this theory, pain information is transmitted by small-diameter A-delta and C fibers. Large-diameter afferent A fibers and small-diameter fibers carry tactile information mediating touch, pressure, and kinesthesia. Transcutaneous electrical nerve stimulators were proposed to function on the basis of differentially firing of impulses in the large fibers that carry nonpainful information. Accordingly, increased activity in these larger fibers purportedly modulate transmission of painful information to the forebrain. A second possible explanation is that the high-frequency stimulation (50 to 60 Hz) produced by some units simply acts as a counterirritant.[33] A third possible explanation is that stimulators that produce strong rhythmic contractions may act through the release of endogenous analgesics such as the endorphins and enkephalins that suppress or modulate pain transmission.[34] A fourth, and probably the best, explanation for quick analgesia with brief, intense stimulation, is that it acts as a conduction block.[35] TENS has the advantage that it is noninvasive, easily regulated by the person or health professional, and effective in some forms of acute and chronic pain. Its use can be taught preoperatively, affording a reduction in hospital days and postoperative analgesic medication and, possibly, preventing the development of persistent pain.

Acupuncture and Acupressure. The practice of acupuncture consists of achieving a therapeutic effect by introducing needles into specific points on the surface of the body. Charts are available that describe the points used to relieve pain at certain anatomic sites. Sometimes palpation is used. It typically is useful to stimulate points that are not normally painful but that become so when symptoms are present. The practice of acupuncture dates back thousands of years to ancient China when the stimulation was achieved by using needles made of bone, stone, or bamboo. Interest in acupuncture peaked in the 1970s as communication between the Eastern and Western medical communities became established and reports of complete surgical analgesia by use of acupuncture alone reached the Western world. Later findings indicated that complete analgesia is unlikely. The Chinese are practicing electroacupuncture, in which electrical impulses are passed through the needles. Heat may also be applied to the needles, resulting in heat penetration to the depth of the needle. Various theories of how acupuncture achieves analgesia have been proposed, including the gate control theory and stimulation of endogenous opioid release. Pain relief from acupuncture and electroacupuncture has been shown to be reversible by the morphine antagonist naloxone.

Acupressure is the means of stimulating acupressure points without using needles. It is particularly popular in Japan, where it is called *Shiatsu* (*shi,* meaning finger, and *atsu,* meaning pressure).[32] Pressure may be applied with a finger, thumb, or any blunt instrument. Many techniques are used, including massaging in a circular motion for 3 to 5 minutes, pressing inward toward the center of the body and releasing three times, or vibrating the point with fingertip pressure.

Pharmacologic Treatment

The use of medications to control pain is only one aspect of the overall program for pain relief. These agents have been used for many years to relieve pain of short duration, enabling the person to achieve mobility—for example, after surgery, when exercises such as coughing and deep breathing may be required. Therapy for chronic pain and cancer pain usually requires an interdisciplinary approach to achieve pain management. An analgesic drug is a medication that acts on the nervous system to decrease or eliminate pain without inducing loss of consciousness. Analgesic drugs have no powerful curative effects but may prevent acute pain from progressing to chronic pain. The Management of Cancer Pain Guidelines for Clinical Practice classifies pain medications into three categories: aspirin, NSAIDs, and acetaminophen; opioid analgesics; and adjuvant analgesics.

The ideal analgesic would be potent, nonaddictive, and produce minimal adverse effects. It would be effective without altering the person's state of awareness, would not cause tolerance, and would be inexpensive. Necessary long-term treatment with opioids can result in opioid tolerance (*i.e.,* more drug is needed to achieve the same effect) and physical dependence, but this should not be confused with addiction. Addiction is rare in persons who are treated only during the time that they require pain relief. The unique needs and circumstances presented by each person in pain must be addressed to achieve satisfactory pain management. Elderly persons and those who present with established substance abuse pose special but not insoluble solutions.

Nonnarcotic Analgesics. The nonnarcotic oral analgesic medications include aspirin, the NSAIDs, and acetaminophen. Aspirin, or acetylsalicylic acid, acts centrally and peripherally to block the transmission of pain impulses. It also has antipyretic and antiinflammatory properties, and like steroids, it is known to inhibit prostaglandins, which make the nerves more sensitive to chemicals such as bradykinin. Another group of drugs with aspirin-like properties are the NSAIDs. These drugs act mainly through the inhibition of prostaglandin synthesis. They decrease the sensitivity of blood vessels to bradykinin and histamine, affect lymphokine production from T lymphocytes, reverse vasodilatation, and decrease the release of inflammatory mediators from granulocytes, mast cells, and basophils. Acetaminophen is another alternative to aspirin. Although equivalent to aspirin as an effective analgesic and antipyretic agent, it differs by its lack of antiinflammatory properties.

Opioid Analgesics. The term *opioid* or *narcotic,* is used to refer to a group of medications, natural or synthetic, with morphine-like actions. The older term *opiate* was used to designate drugs derived from opium—morphine, codeine, and many other semisynthetic congeners of morphine. The pain-relieving (*i.e.,* analgesic) and psychopharmacologic properties of morphine have been known for centuries. More recently, it was discovered that the brain contains its own (*i.e.,* endogenous) analgesic, morphine-like chemicals, which comprise a group of peptides known as endorphins. Three distinct families of opioid peptides have been identified: *enkephalins, endorphins,* and *dynorphins.* Each family of opioid peptides is derived from a genetically distinct precursor molecule (*e.g.,* proenkephalin, proendorphin, prodynorphin). Each of these precursors contains a number of biologically active peptides, opioid and nonopioid. The precursor molecules are found in the CNS and in blood and various other tissues.

The opioids exert their action through opioid receptors. There is reasonably firm evidence of four major categories of opioid receptors in the CNS, designated mu (μ), kappa (κ), delta (δ), and sigma (σ); two subtypes of each category have been identified tentatively.[37] Inferences have been drawn from data that attempt to relate pharmacologic effects of opioid drugs to interactions with a particular type of receptor. For example, analgesia is thought to involve mu receptors, largely at supraspinal sites, and kappa receptors, principally within the spinal cord. The function of delta receptors is more speculative. The function of the fourth type, the sigma receptor, is more controversial but may be related to the dysphoria, hallucinogenic, and cardiac stimulant effects of opioids. These receptors are particularly concentrated in areas of the brain where the enkephalins have also been located. Endogenous and exogenous opioids bind to these receptors; some may interact to a variable extent with all four types of receptors and act as an agonist, partial agonist, or antagonist at each.

There is evidence that morphine and other morphine-like opioid agonists produce analgesia primarily through interaction with mu-opioid receptors. Other consequences of mu receptor activation include respiratory depression, miosis, reduced gastrointestinal motility (causing constipation), and feelings of well-being or euphoria. Several types of mu receptors have been identified, based on their affinities for agonists: mu_1 (higher affinity), thought to mediate supraspinal analgesia, and mu_2 (lower affinity), thought to mediate respiratory depression and gastrointestinal actions among others. As more information becomes available regarding the opioids and their receptors, it seems likely that pain medications can be developed that act selectively at certain receptor sites, providing more effective pain control while producing fewer adverse effects and affording less danger of addiction. For example, it might be possible to develop opioid drugs that produce effective analgesia but not undesirable adverse effects, such as respiratory depression and the most common complication, constipation. When used for temporary relief of severe pain, such as that occurring postoperatively, there is much evidence that opioids given routinely before the pain starts or becomes extreme are far more effective than those administered in a sporadic manner; patients seem to require fewer doses and are better able to resume regular activities earlier. Opioids are also used for treatment of pain in persons with limited life expectancy. Too often, because of undue concern about the possibility of addiction, many chronic pain sufferers with a short life expectancy receive inadequate pain relief. Most pain experts agree that it is appropriate to provide the level of opioid necessary to relieve the severe, intractable pain of persons whose life expectancy is limited. Oral medications are preferable to injection; tolerance usually is minimal after a few weeks. Addiction is not considered a problem in cancer patients.[38] In persons with cancer pain, morphine remains the most useful strong opioid. The World Health Organization has recommended that oral morphine be part of the essential medication list and made available throughout the world as the medication of choice.[39] Oral forms of morphine are well absorbed from the gastrointestinal tract and have a half-life of about 2.5 hours and a duration of action of 4 to 6 hours. Liquid forms of the medication usually are given at 4-hour intervals to maintain an adequate blood level for analgesia, while minimizing the potential for toxic side effects.[39]

One approach to opioid administration is the use of continuous infusion pumps. Infusion pumps can be used to deliver opioids by way of the subcutaneous or intravenous route on a continuous or demand basis.[40,41] An alternative approach, patient-controlled analgesia, has proved effective for relieving postoperative pain and for pain management in persons with cancer.[40] This system consists of a microprocessor-controlled infusion pump that delivers the opioid medication through an intravenous cannula. A push button on the system enables patients to deliver their own medication dose as needed. A lockout system, which prevents overdosing, is programmed into the system.

The administration of opioids into the intrathecal or epidural spaces for the relief of acute and chronic pain has gained popularity in clinical practice.[42] The procedure requires the introduction of a catheter into the epidural or intrathecal space by an anesthesiologist or other physician trained in the technique. With this method, every precaution must be taken that no medications or solutions are given that could damage the spinal cord. This method offers the advantage of providing effective analgesia while minimizing the central depressant effects common to systemic opioid administration. This type of pain control is based on the finding of opioid receptors in the cell bodies of the primary afferent neurons in the dorsal root ganglia and in the dorsal horn cells of the spinal cord that are involved in pain transmission.

Adjuvant Analgesics. Adjuvant analgesics include medications such as tricyclic antidepressants, antiseizure medications, and neuroleptic anxiolytic agents. The fact that the pain-suppression system has nonendorphin synapses raises the possibility that potent centrally acting nonopiate medications may be useful in relieving pain. 5-HT has been shown to play an important role in producing analgesia. The tricyclic antidepressant medications (*i.e.*, imipramine, amitriptyline, and doxepin) that block the removal of 5-HT from the synaptic cleft have been shown to produce pain relief in some persons. The medications are particularly useful in some chronic painful conditions, such as postherpetic neuralgia.

Certain antiseizure medications, such as carbamazepine (Tegretol) and phenytoin (Dilantin), have specific analgesic effects that are effective in some pain conditions. These medications, which suppress spontaneous neuronal firing, are particularly useful in the management of pain that occurs after nerve injury. Other agents, such as the corticosteroids, may be used to decrease inflammation and nociceptive stimuli responsible for pain.

Placebo Response. An interesting phenomenon that deserves comment is the placebo response (Latin for "I please"). The definition of a placebo can include the use of any treatment strategy that produces a positive placebo response. This positive reaction occurs because of the person's belief that the treatment will be effective, rather than because of any specific or therapeutic properties of the placebo itself. For example, a *positive placebo reactor* might report pain relief after the administration of a medication believed to be an analgesic, when in fact it was composed of an inert substance. It is believed that the placebo-derived analgesia may be mediated through endogenous opioid pathways.

At one time, placebo reactors were thought to have psychogenic or functional pain that was more imaginary than real. Newer research indicates that most persons are, to a greater or lesser degree, placebo reactors. Numerous studies have shown that 20% to 40% of those with objective physical stimuli for pain consistently report pain relief from a placebo, at least for a short time. Placebos should not be used to distinguish "real" pain from psychogenic pain. Most importantly, placebos should not be used to manage cancer pain.

Surgical Intervention

With rare exception, noninvasive analgesic approaches should precede invasive palliative approaches.[23] Surgery for severe intractable pain of peripheral or central origin has met with some success. It can be used to remove the cause or block the transmission of pain. Persons with phantom limb pain, severe neuralgia, inoperable cancer of certain types, or causalgia sometimes suffer so intensively that they consider suicide as their only means of escape. In these extreme cases, surgery may be the only remaining treatment that seems to offer relief from the agony. Surgical methods to relieve pain usually are considered a last resort because any damage to nerve cell bodies is irreversible. A penalty is paid because of the damage to other systems, predisposing the patient to other problems. Although severed axons may regenerate, full recovery is highly unlikely. After a few weeks or months, the pain often returns and may be more disturbing than the condition for which the surgery was performed. Regenerating nerve fibers may give rise to dysesthesias (*i.e.*, extremely uncomfortable sensations); but if survival time is short, surgery may be warranted. In some cases, such as removal of a tumor pressing on nerve fibers or removal of an inflamed appendix, pain can be completely relieved. Surgery to block the transmission of pain signals along peripheral or central pathways may be successful. Peripherally, nerve section (*i.e.*, neurectomy) or section of a dorsal root ganglion (*i.e.*, rhizotomy) may be considered if neuroaxial opioid infusion or chemical neurolysis are unavailable or unsuccessful. Some success has been reported for this type of surgery, particularly in trigeminal neuralgia.

At the spinal cord level, cordotomy (*i.e.*, severing of the anterolateral quadrant of the cord) and tractotomy (*i.e.*, interruption of the lateral spinothalamic tract) may require deep incisions into the cord to give adequate relief. With such deep incision, bladder function may be affected. The success of these types of surgery depends on the source of pain and the cord level involved. Electrical stimulation or pharmacologic agents, or both, often are used to determine the appropriate surgical site or to eliminate the need for surgery. Hypophysectomy, the removal or chemical interruption of the pituitary gland, has an interesting history. It was done originally in an effort to prevent metastasis in certain hormone-dependent cancers, including some breast cancers. It was found, rather unexpectedly, that the pain often was immediately and totally relieved. It is now most likely to be used to relieve intractable pain caused by disseminated cancer of the prostate or breast that cannot be controlled by morphine or more localized means. The mechanism of pain relief is not yet understood. It is particularly mysterious because the pituitary is a rich source of endogenous opioids. This procedure is not often used, except for such problems as bilateral or diffuse bone pain unrelieved by other measures.

Interdisciplinary Approach

The Clinical Practice Guidelines for acute and cancer pain management emphasize the need for a collaborative, interdisciplinary approach to pain control, including members of the health care team in collaboration with the patient and the patient's family. The interdisciplinary approach to complex chronic pain was introduced more than 30 years ago, and many pain clinics have been established since then. This team approach uses the knowledge and expertise of many health professionals to diagnose and manage complex types of pain. Besides being useful clinically, the team approach is effective in teaching and collaborative research. The acute pain model assumes an objective cause that can be treated and diminished or eliminated within a short time, but the most perplexing difficulties are those relating to chronic pain. Although productive research has improved the outlook for pain modulation and elimination, the interdisciplinary team approach has demonstrated its value in addressing many of the chronic pain problems from the physical, physiologic, and psychosocial aspects simultaneously.

In summary, pain is an elusive and complex phenomenon; it is a symptom common to many illnesses. It is a highly individualized experience that is shaped by a person's culture and previous life experiences, and it is difficult to measure. Traditionally, there have been two principal theories of pain; specificity and pattern theories. Scientifically, pain is viewed within the context of nociception. Nociceptors are receptive nerve endings that respond to noxious stimuli. Neither theory accounts for the motivational, cognitive, cultural, and affective components of pain. Pain can be classified according to source, duration, objective signs, and areas of referral. Reactions to pain, which are affected by pain threshold, pain tolerance, age, gender, and other factors, are manifested through physical reactions, physiologic responses, and psychosocial reactions. Referred pain is pain that is perceived at a site different from its point of origin but innervated by the same spinal segment.

Pain can be acute or chronic; the latter is particularly difficult to manage. Controversy continues as to whether chronic pain should be viewed as a physiologic phenomenon with psychologic correlates or as a psychologic phenomenon with physiologic correlates. A growing body of data suggest that the latter definition may eliminate many of the chronic pain management problems.

Treatment modalities include the use of physiologic, cognitive, and behavioral measures; heat and cold; stimulation-induced analgesic methods; and pharmacologic agents singly or in combination. It is becoming apparent that even with chronic pain, the most effective approach is early treatment or even prevention. After pain is present, the greatest success in the management of problems related to assessment and appropriate, effective treatment is achieved with the use of an interdisciplinary approach.

Alterations in Pain Sensitivity and Special Types of Pain

After you have completed this section of the chapter, you should be able to meet the following objectives:

- Define *hypesthesia, hyperesthesia, hyperalgesia, dysesthesia, paresthesias, anesthesia, hyperpathia, analgesia*, and *hypoalgesia*
- Describe the cause and characteristics and treatment of neuropathic pain, causalgia, trigeminal neuralgia and postherpetic neuralgia
- Cite a possible mechanism of phantom limb pain

Alterations in Pain Sensitivity

Sensitivity and perception of pain varies among persons and in the same person under different conditions and in different parts of the body. Irritation, mild hypoxia, and mild compression of a peripheral nerve often result in hyperexcitability of the sensory nerve fibers or cell bodies. This is experienced as unpleasant hypersensitivity (*i.e., hyperesthesia*) or increased painfulness (*i.e., hyperalgesia*). Possible causes of increased sensitivity to noxious stimuli include a decrease in the threshold of nociceptors, an increase in pain produced by suprathreshold stimuli, and the wind-up phenomenon. Primary hyperalgesia occurs at the site of injury. Secondary hyperalgesia occurs in nearby uninjured tissue.

Hyperpathia is a syndrome in which the sensory threshold is raised, but when it is reached, continued stimulation, especially if repetitive, results in a prolonged and unpleasant experience. This pain can be explosive and radiates through a peripheral nerve distribution. It is associated with pathologic changes in peripheral nerves, such as localized hypoxia. Spontaneous, unpleasant sensations called *paresthesias* occur with more severe irritation (*e.g.*, the pins-and-needles sensation that follows temporary compression of a peripheral nerve). The general term *dysesthesia* is given to distortions (usually unpleasant) of somesthetic sensation that typically accompany partial loss of sensory innervation.

More severe pathology can result in reduced or lost tactile (*e.g., hypesthesia, anesthesia*), temperature (*e.g., hypothermia, athermia*), and pain sensation (*i.e., hypalgesia*). *Analgesia* is the absence of pain on noxious stimulation or the relief of pain without loss of consciousness. The inability to sense pain may result in trauma, infection, and even loss of a body part or parts. Inherited insensitivity to pain may take the form of congenital indifference or congenital insensitivity to pain. In the former, transmission of nerve impulses appears normal but appreciation of painful stimuli at higher levels appears to be absent. In the latter, a peripheral nerve defect apparently exists such that transmission of painful nerve impulses does not result in perception of pain. Whatever the cause, persons who lack the ability to perceive pain are at constant risk of tissue damage because pain is not serving its protective function.

Allodynia (Greek *allo*, other, and *odynia*, painful) is the term used for the puzzling phenomenon of pain that follows a nonnoxious stimulus to apparently normal skin. This term is intended to refer to instances in which otherwise normal tissues may be abnormally innervated or may be referral sites for other loci that give rise to pain with nonnoxious stimuli. It may be that an area is hypersensitive because of inflammation, injury, or another cause, and a normally subthreshold stimulus is sufficient to trigger the sensation of pain. This response is thought to be chemically mediated, possibly the result of tissue damage in the surrounding area. *Trigger points* are highly localized points on the skin or mucous membrane that can produce immediate intense pain at that site or elsewhere when stimulated by light tactile stimulation. *Myofascial trigger points* are foci of exquisite tenderness found in many muscles and can be responsible for pain projected to sites remote from the points of tenderness. Trigger points are widely distributed in the back of the head and neck and in the lumbar and thoracic regions. These trigger points cause reproducible myofascial pain syndromes in specific muscles. These pain syndromes are the major source of pain in clients at chronic pain treatment centers.

Special Types of Pain

Neuropathic Pain

Neuropathic pain is pain that precedes, accompanies, or results from a pathologic change in or dysfunction of a peripheral nerve. It can involve one or several nerves and it may be unilateral or bilateral, depending on its cause. Causes of neuropathic pain include: tumor infiltration of peripheral nerves; compression, constriction, or damage to a peripheral nerve before, during, or after surgery; a side effect of medical treatment, such as radiation (*e.g.*, radiation-induced tumors) or chemotherapy (*e.g.*, nerve damage due to use of neurotoxic agents, such as taxol and vincristine); postherpetic, vasculopathic, and other diseases related to peripheral nerve damage.

Treatment methods include removal of the causative agent if possible and the use of analgesics, local anesthetics, or corticosteroids where appropriate.[23] As a last resort, neurolysis or neurosurgical blockade are sometimes used if less drastic procedures, such as pharmacotherapy, radiation, TENS or other forms of cutaneous stimulation, are not indicated or ineffective.

Causalgia

Causalgia is an extremely painful condition that follows sudden and violent deformation of peripheral nerves of the limbs. This problem often is initiated in combat because of nerve damage by high-velocity missiles (*e.g.*, bullets, metal fragments). The nerve typically is damaged but not severed. The classic syndrome was described by Mitchell in 1864 for men sustaining gunshot wounds to the extremities.[43] The median and sciatica nerves most commonly are affected. The pain is characteristically burning and can be elicited with the slightest movement or touch to the affected area. The pain is excruciating, and even clothing or puffs of air are sufficient to set it off in severe cases. It can be exacerbated by emotional upsets or any increased peripheral sympathetic nerve stimulation. Sympathetic components are part of all variations of causalgia. These are characterized by vascular and trophic (*i.e.*, nutritive) changes to the skin, soft tissue, and bone. Reflex sympathetic dystrophy follows trauma to a portion of an extremity and is a disorder of the sympathetic nervous system characterized by rubor or pallor, sweating or dryness, edema, pain, or skin atrophy.

Treatment by sympathetic blockade usually is successful and may be the reason this condition is considered a dysautonomia (*i.e.*, a dysfunction of the autonomic nervous system). In some cases, prolonged cooling and intravenous administration of guanethidine into the affected limb (with venous outflow blocked for several minutes) has been shown to alleviate the pain for days or longer. Electrical stimulation of the large myelinated fibers that innervate the area from which the pain arises is also effective. Controversy remains regarding the mechanisms involved in these pain-relief measures. The long-term use of opioids is discouraged because of the danger of addiction. Effective treatment is imperative to prevent invalidism and, in severe instances, suicide.

Neuralgia

Neuralgia is characterized by severe, brief, often repetitive attacks of lightning-like or throbbing pain. It occurs along the distribution of a spinal or cranial nerve and usually is precipitated by stimulation of the cutaneous region supplied by that nerve.

Trigeminal Neuralgia. Trigeminal neuralgia, or *tic douloureux*, is one of the most common and severe neuralgias. It is manifested by facial tics or grimaces and characterized by stabbing, paroxysmal attacks of pain that usually are limited to the unilateral sensory distribution of one or more branches of the trigeminal nerve, most often the maxillary or mandibular divisions. Victims describe the pain as excruciating. It may be triggered by light touch, eating, swallowing, shaving, talking, chewing gum, washing the face, or sneezing or have no apparent cause. Stimulation of small-diameter afferent fibers is more likely to provoke attacks than cold, warm, or noxious stimuli. Abnormalities of facial sensation are not likely between attacks. Neurologic deficits are rare, as they are in neuralgias of cranial nerves VII, IX, and X.

Carbamazepine (Tegretol), which is a tricyclic compound, may be used to control the pain of trigeminal neuralgia and may delay or eliminate the need for surgery. Surgical release of vessels, dural structures, or scar tissue surrounding the semilunar ganglion or root in the middle cranial fossa often eliminates the symptoms. If not, destruction or blocking peripheral branches or central root of cranial nerve V produces loss of all sensation, including pain. A more satisfactory treatment is sectioning of the descending spinal tract of nerve V in the brain stem. This may be effective because it removes background inflow of impulses on which spontaneous attacks depend. Dissociation of facial sensation occurs, in that pain and temperature disappear, but there is only a slight decrease in tactile activity. This neurosurgical procedure provides evidence that the nucleus caudalis of the trigeminal complex is necessary for the transmission of facial pain. Considerable controversy remains regarding the pathophysiology of trigeminal neuralgia. Other interventions include avoidance of precipitating factors (*e.g.*, stimulation of trigger spots) and eye injury due to irritation; provision for adequate nutrition; and avoidance of social isolation.

Postherpetic Neuralgia. The pain associated with postherpetic neuralgia (*i.e.*, herpes zoster, or shingles) follows recovery from an infection of the dorsal root ganglia and corresponding areas of innervation by the herpes zoster virus (see Chapter 15). Herpes zoster is caused by the same herpes virus that causes varicella (*i.e.*, chickenpox) and is thought to represent a localized recurrent infection by the varicella virus that has remained latent in the dorsal root ganglia since the initial attack of chickenpox. Reactivation of viral replication is associated with a decline in immunity, such as that which occurs with aging or certain diseases.

During the acute attack of herpes zoster, the reactivated virus travels centrifugally from the ganglia to the skin of the corresponding dermatomes, causing a localized vesicular eruption and hyperpathia (*i.e.*, abnormally exaggerated subjective response to pain). In the acute infection, proportionately more of the large nerve fibers are destroyed. Regenerated fibers appear to have smaller diameters. Older patients have pain, dysesthesia, and hyperesthesia after the acute phase; these are increased by minor stimuli. Because there is a relative loss of large fibers with age, elderly persons are particularly prone to suffering because of the shift in the proportion of large- to small-diameter nerve fibers. Normally, the pain of acute herpes zoster tends to resolve spontaneously with time. Postherpetic neuralgia describes the presence of pain more than one month after the onset of the eruption of herpes zoster. Nearly all patients have acute pain with zoster and 10% to 70% develop postherpetic neuralgia.[44] The risk of postherpetic zoster increases with age.

Postherpetic neuralgia is extremely distressing and most efficaciously treated early (*i.e.*, in the first 3 months), before the condition becomes established. High doses of systemic corticosteroids and an oral antiviral drug such as acyclovir or valacyclovir, a medication that inhibits herpesvirus DNA replication, may reduce the incidence of postherpetic neuralgia when used early in the disease.

A topical anesthetic agent, lidocaine-prilocaine cream or 5% lidocaine gel, is recommended as initial therapy. A tricyclic antidepressant medication, such as amitriptyline or desipramine, may be used for pain relief. Regional nerve blockade (*i.e.*, stellate ganglion, epidural, local infiltration, or peripheral nerve block) has been used with limited success. Topical capsaicin preparations have been used with mixed results because many persons are intolerant of the burning sensation that precedes anesthesia after application.[44]

Phantom Limb Pain

Phantom limb pain, a type of neurologic pain, follows amputation of a limb or part of a limb. As many as 70% of amputees suffer from phantom pain.[45] The pain often begins as sensations of tingling, heat and cold, or heaviness; followed by burning, cramping, or shooting pain. It may disappear spontaneously or persist for many years. One of the troublesome problems of phantom pain is that the person may experience painful sensations that were present before the amputation such as that of a painful ulcer or bunion.[45]

Several theories have been proposed as to the causes of phantom pain.[45] One theory is that the end of a regenerating nerve becomes trapped in the scar tissue of the amputation site. It is known that when a peripheral nerve is cut, the scar tissue that forms becomes a barrier to regenerating outgrowth of the axon. The growing axon often becomes trapped in the scar tissue, forming a tangled growth (*i.e.*, neuroma) of small-diameter axons, including primary nociceptive afferents and sympathetic efferents. It has been proposed that these afferents show increased sensitivity to innocuous mechanical stimuli and to sympathetic activity and circulating catecholamines. A related theory moves the source of phantom limb pain to the spinal cord, suggesting that the pain arises from spontaneous firing of spinal cord neurons that have lost their normal sensory input from the body. In this case a closed self-exciting neuronal loop in the posterior horn of the spinal cord is postulated to send impulses to the brain, resulting in pain. Even the slightest irritation to the amputated limb area can initiate this cycle. The phantom limb pain may arise within the brain itself. In one hypothesis, the pain is caused by changes in the flow of signals through somatosensory areas of the brain. In other words, there appears to be plasticity, even in the adult CNS.

Treatment has been accomplished by the use of sympathetic blocks, transcutaneous electrical nerve stimulation of the large myelinated afferents innervating the area, hypnosis and relaxation training. Controversy continues as to the precise mechanisms responsible for the usefulness of these methods. Many of the complications of limb amputation can be alleviated by immediate fitting of a prosthesis and conscientious stump care. Stump care includes bandaging to support the remaining muscles, protect the soft tissues, and prevent the formation of edematous fluids. Care must be taken to prevent infection. After the amputation wound has healed, the stump must be shrunk and shaped into a conical form to permit the correct fitting of a prosthesis. This is done by the proper application of elastic bandages or devices. The reader is referred to a specialty text for more complete information on stump care.

In summary, pain may occur with or without an adequate stimulus, or it may be absent in the presence of an adequate stimulus—either of which describes a pain disorder. There may be analgesia (*i.e.*, absence of pain), hyperalgesia (*i.e.*, increased sensitivity to pain), hypalgesia (*i.e.*, decreased sensitivity to painful stimuli), hyperpathia (*i.e.*, an unpleasant and prolonged response to pain), or allodynia (*i.e.*, pain produced by stimuli that do not normally cause pain). Causalgia is an extremely painful condition that follows sudden and traumatic deformation of peripheral nerves. Neuralgia is characterized by severe, brief, often repetitiously occurring attacks of lightning-like or throbbing pain that occurs along the distribution of a spinal or cranial nerve and usually is precipitated by stimulation of the cutaneous region supplied by that nerve. Trigeminal neuralgia, or tic douloureux, is one of the most common and severe neuralgias. It is manifested by facial tics or grimaces. Postherpetic neuralgia, or shingles, is caused by an infection of the dorsal root ganglia and corresponding areas of innervation by the herpes zoster virus. Phantom limb pain, a neurologic pain, follows amputation of a limb or part of a limb.

Headache and Associated Pain

After you have completed this section of the chapter, you should be able to meet the following objectives:

- State the importance of distinguishing between primary and secondary type headaches
- Differentiate between the periodicity of occurrence and manifestations of migraine headache, cluster headache, and tension-type headache, and headache due to temporomandibular joint syndrome
- Characterize the nonpharmacologic and pharmacologic methods used in treatment of headache

- Cite the most common cause of temporomandibular joint pain

Headache is one of the major reasons for patient consultation with physicians. Headache is a universally recognized phenomenon that is common, although its cause is unknown. There are many types of headache, including migraine with aura, migraine without aura, tension-type headache, cluster headache, or chronic daily headache (CDH). Classification of headache has been problematic, partly because of the lack of laboratory tests and markers to assist in the diagnosis of headache and also because of frequently seen mixed headache phenomenon. Headache often is interpreted by health care professionals as a nonspecific symptom, making its diagnosis difficult.

Headache can also be a sign of a serious underlying illness such as meningitis, brain tumor, or cerebral aneurysm. Therefore, complaints of head pain should be carefully evaluated to exclude other pathology as a cause of headache. Severe headache, escalating in intensity within a period of minutes to hours should be of particular concern.

Types of Headache

Until 1988, most headache classifications were derived from a 1962 publication of the Ad Hoc Committee on the Classification of Headache.[46] In 1988, the first edition of The Classification and Diagnostic Criteria for Headache Disorders, Cranial Neuralgias, and Facial Pain, prepared by the Headache Classification Committee of the International Headache Society, was published, along with ten general rules considered essential to the correct use of this new system.[47] Although the primary purpose for development of this classification system was research, the operational diagnostic criteria has aided in the diagnosis and treatment of headaches. The chosen criteria for a particular diagnosis represent a compromise between sensitivity and specificity and are expected to help clarify some of the problems of the 1962 classification system. The major classifications of the 1988 classification system are given in Chart 40–1. Subclassifications to the second digit are included for migraine and tension-type headaches because these are the two most commonly encountered types of headaches in clinical practice. Headaches associated with another medical diagnosis are often referred to as *secondary headaches* to distinguish them from headaches such as migraine and cluster headaches in which headache is the *primary* problem.

CHART **40-1**
Classification and Diagnostic Criteria for Headache Disorders, Cranial Neuralgias, and Facial Pain

1. Migraine
   1.1 Migraine without aura
   1.2 Migraine with aura
   1.3 Ophthalmoplegic migraine
   1.4 Retinal migraine
   1.5 Childhood periodic syndromes that may be precursors to or associated with migraine
   1.6 Complications with migraine
   1.7 Migrainous disorder not fulfilling above criteria
2. Tension-type headache
   2.1 Episodic tension-type headache
   2.2 Chronic tension-type headache
   2.3 Headache of the tension-type not fulfilling the above criteria
3. Cluster headache and chronic paroxysmal hemicrania
4. Miscellaneous headaches unassociated with structural lesion
5. Headache associated with head trauma
6. Headache associated with vascular disorders
7. Headache associated with nonvascular intracranial disorders
8. Headache associated with substances or their withdrawal
9. Headache associated with noncephalic infection
10. Headache associated with metabolic disorder
11. Headache or facial pain associated with disorder of cranium, neck, eyes, ears, nose, sinuses, teeth, mouth or other facial or cranial structures
12. Cranial neuralgias, nerve trunk pain, and deafferentation pain
13. Headache not classifiable

(Adapted from Oleson J. [1988]. Classification and diagnostic criteria for headache disorders, cranial neuralgias, and facial pain. *Cephalgia* 8 (Suppl 7), 13–19)

Migraine Headache

There are two categories of migraine headache, those with aura (15%) and those without aura (85%). Migraine headache often presents as a mixed headache with tension-type headache, or may have progressed to CDH, labeled as transformed migraine. These designations make patient classification difficult and it has been suggested that patients be classified as having migraine or tension-type headache if they have both forms.[47] Complicated migraine is a less common form of migraine in which the neurologic symptoms are more disabling, and include migraine with prolonged aura, familial hemiplegic migraine, basilar migraine, ophthalmoplegic migraine, retinal migraine, status migrainosus, and migrainous infarction.[48] Migraine headache without aura is an idiopathic, recurring disorder that lasts for 1 to 3 days, is unilateral in location, of pulsating quality, moderate to severe in intensity, and is aggravated by routine physical activity. These headaches are associated with nausea, photophobia, and phonophobia.[47] Migraine with aura has similar symptoms, with the addition of neurologic symptoms that can unequivocally be localized to the cerebral cortex or brain stem, which develop over 5 to 20 minutes and usually last less than 60 minutes.

The mechanisms of migraine attacks are poorly understood. There are several hypotheses that attempt to explain migraine headache; these include reduction of cerebral regional blood flow, spreading cortical depression (*i.e.,* migraine with aura), and cortical arteriolar vasospasm.[47–49] Other hypotheses include sterile inflammation, biochemical and hormonal changes, the release of substances such as histamine, prostaglandin, and 5-HT, and nitric oxide.[50] It is unclear whether the cause of migraine is neurologic or vascular, but it is clear that it is not psychogenic.[51] The pathophysiology of migraine probably involves cerebrovascular changes as well as changes in 5-HT activity, peripherally and centrally.[48] These effects may be mediated by a central mechanism involving brain stem noradrenergic and serotonergic neurotransmission.

Cluster Headache

Cluster headaches are an infrequent headache disorder affecting more males than females. These headaches tend to occur nightly over weeks or months, followed by a long remission period. Cluster headache is typified by severe, unrelenting, unilateral pain, and most commonly occurs in the orbital, retro-orbital, temporal, supraorbital, and infraorbital region in order of decreasing frequency.[47,52] The headache is rapid in onset and builds to a peak in about 10 to 15 minutes, lasting for 15 to 180 minutes. The pain behind the eye radiates to the ipsilateral trigeminal nerve (*e.g.,* temple, cheek, gum).[48]

Cluster headache can be episodic, chronic, or chronic paroxysmal hemicrania. Episodic cluster headache is characterized by cluster periods of headaches of 7 days to 1 year.[52] Cluster headaches are usually not associated with aura symptoms. They are associated with one or more symptoms such as conjunctival injection, lacrimation, nasal congestion, rhinorrhea, forehead and facial sweating, miosis, ptosis, and eyelid edema. The number of attacks can vary from one to three per day or from one a week to eight or more a day.[47,51] Attacks typically occur in series lasting for weeks or months that are separated by periods of remission, which may last months or years.

The age at onset of cluster headache is usually between 20 and 40 years and men are affected five to six times more often than women.[47] The underlying pathophysiologic mechanisms of cluster headaches are unknown. Hypotheses include the interplay of vascular, neurogenic, metabolic, and humoral factors. Although the trigeminovascular system appears to be involved in the pathogenesis of cluster headache, a theory to explain the symptoms, periodicity, and circadian regularity of cluster headaches does not exist[48] The regularity in the timing of cluster headache may be caused by dysfunction of the hypothalamic biologic clock mechanisms.[52] Ipsilateral lacrimation, nasal stuffiness, and rhinorrhea are thought to result from parasympathetic overactivity. Pain and vasodilation are thought to result from activation of the trigemino-vascular system. Some evidence of neurogenic inflammation has been associated with cluster headache.

Tension-Type Headache

Tension-type headache is the most common headache type with a lifetime prevalence of 88% in women and 69% in men.[53] About 30% of the adult population experiences tension-type headache.[54] Unlike migraine and cluster headaches, tension-type headache is usually not sufficiently severe that it interferes with daily activities but may be bothersome because of its persistence.

Tension-type headaches are described as dull, aching, diffuse, nondescript headaches not associated with nausea or vomiting or worsened by activity and as occurring in a hatband distribution around the head.[48] They can be classified as episodic, chronic, or not fitting these criteria. Episodic tension-type headaches are recurrent and last minutes to days. The pain is pressing or tightening in quality, of mild or moderate intensity, bilateral in location, and does not worsen with physical activity. Although photophobia and phonophobia may be present, nausea is not.[47] Chronic tension-type headache is present for at least 15 days each month for at least 6 months. The quality of the pain is pressing or tightening, mild to moderate in severity, and bilateral. It does not worsen with routine physical activity. Nausea, photophobia, or phonophobia may occur. Chronic tension-type headache may also be associated with disorders of the pericranial or scalp muscles.

The exact mechanisms of tension-type headache are not known and the hypotheses of causation are contradictory. One popular theory is that tension-type headaches result from sustained tension of the muscles of the scalp and neck, while other research indicates no correlation between muscle contraction and tension-type headache.[48] Many authorities now believe that tension-type headaches are forms of migraine headache.[55] The alteration of the platelet 5-HT content in patients with chronic tension-type headaches, which also occurs with migraine headache, suggests that these two types of headaches share some pathophysiologic features.[56] It is thought that migraine headache may be transformed gradually into chronic tension-type headache. With many tension-type headaches there may be no causative factors identifiable, or they may be caused by the overuse of analgesics or caffeine, oromandibular dysfunction, psychogenic stress, anxiety, depression, and muscular stress.[47]

Chronic Daily Headache

Little is known about the prevalence and incidence of CDH. Forty percent of patients seen in headache clinics have chronic daily headache. CDH has not been identified as a separate entity in the International Headache Society headache classification. The cause of CDH is unknown, although there are several hypotheses. These include transformed migraine headache, evolved tension-type headache, new daily persistent headache, and posttraumatic headache. Transformed migraine, a daily or near daily headache, has been found to constitute 77% of CDH in one population.[57] Many of these headaches retain certain characteristics of migraine, while others resemble chronic tension-type headache. CDH may be associated with chronic and episodic tension-type headache. New daily persistent headache may have a fairly rapidly onset, with no history of migraine, tension-type headache, trauma, or psychologic stress. Although overuse of symptomatic medications (*e.g.*, analgesics, ergotamine) have been related to CDH, there is a group of patients where CDH is unrelated to excessive use of medications.

Temporomandibular Joint Pain

Temporomandibular joint (TMJ) syndrome is a common cause of head pain. It is usually caused by an imbalance in joint movement because of poor bite, bruxism (*i.e.*, teeth grinding), or joint problems such as inflammation, trauma, and degenerative changes.[58] The pain is almost always referred and commonly presents as facial muscle pain, headache, neckache, or earache. Referred pain is aggravated by jaw function. Headache associated with this syndrome is common in adults and children and can cause chronic pain problems. The initial therapy for TMJ should be directed toward relief of pain and improvement in function. Treatment of TMJ pain is aimed at correcting the problem, and in some cases this may be difficult.

Diagnosis and Treatment

Diagnosis of headache requires a comprehensive history and physical examination to exclude secondary causes. The history should include factors that precipitate headache such as foods and food additives, missed meals, and association with the menstrual period. A careful medication history is essential because many medications can provoke or aggravate headaches. Alcohol can also cause or aggravate headache. A headache diary in which the person records his or her headaches and concurrent or antecedent events may be helpful in identifying factors that contribute to headache onset.

Nonpharmacologic Treatment

Nonpharmacologic treatment of headaches include a referral to a headache clinic for pharmacologic and nonpharmacologic management of headache. Various nonpharmacologic treatments have been tried with headache sufferers with varying success. Tension-type headaches and CDH are more responsive to nonpharmacologic techniques, such as biofeedback, massage, acupuncture, relaxation, imagery, and physical therapy, than other types of headache.[48,57] Lifestyle changes are important in migraine headache. These interventions are combined with pharmacologic approaches to affect headache relief.

Pharmacologic Treatment

Pharmacologic treatment consists of symptomatic, abortive medications to provide relief during an acute headache and prophylactic medication used to prevent or reduce the frequency and severity of recurrent headaches.[48] Persons with infrequent tension-type headache usually self medicate using over-the-counter analgesics to abort an acute headache episode and do not require prophylactic medication. Patients with migraine and cluster headaches who suffer from frequent and severe headaches, who usually respond poorly to abortive medication, may require prophylactic medication. For patients with CDH, a combination of pharmacologic and behavioral interventions may be necessary.[57]

The medication of choice for acute treatment of tension-type headaches are analgesics, including acetaminophen, acetylsalicylic acid, and NSAIDs.[48] Other medications used concomitantly with analgesics, which are sometimes effective, are sedatives (*e.g.*, butalbital), anxiolytics (*e.g.*, diazepam), and skeletal muscle relaxants (*e.g.*, orphenadrine).[48] Prophylactic treatment for tension-type headache is most effective with antidepressants (*e.g.*, amitriptyline).[48] It has been suggested that because "the dividing line" between migraine and tension-type headache is often vague, the entire range of migraine medications may be tried in refractory cases of tension-type headache or mixed tension-type and migraine headache disorder. Migraine headaches are treated abortively with medications to relieve the acute pain and the associated migraine symptoms. Pharmacologic preparations include 5-HT receptor agonists (*e.g.*, sumatriptan, ergot derivatives), analgesics (*e.g.*, acetaminophen with codeine, morphine, NSAIDs), sedatives, and antiemetic medications (*e.g.*, metoclopramide).[48] Administration of these medications based on the person's specific complaints and rest in a dark, quiet environment are often successful in relieving acute pain and associated symptoms in migraines. For intractable migraine headache, dihydroergotamine given parenterally with an antiemetic, sumatriptan, chlorpromazine, opioid analgesics, or prednisone may be effective.[48] The β-adrenergic blocking medication propranolol is usually the first choice for prophylactic treatment because of empiric support for its effectiveness, its safety, efficacy, and favorable side effect profile.[48] Several other medications that may be effective prophylactically for migraine headache are amitriptyline, verapamil, sodium valproate, methysergide, clonidine, naproxen sodium, lithium carbonate, and phenytoin.

Agents that reach the site of action quickly are the most effective abortive medications to use in cluster headache. The most effective medications are oxygen inhalation and subcutaneous sumatriptan.[48,52] Ergotamine derivatives, analgesics, and opioids are usually ineffective in the treatment of cluster headaches because the attacks are of short duration and self-limited and are almost terminated by the time these medications reach the bloodstream in sufficient levels. Prophylactic medications effective with cluster headaches include ergotamine, verapamil, methysergide, lithium carbonate, corticosteroids, sodium valproate, and indomethacin. CDH, which is thought to be caused by medication rebound, requires discontinuation of the offending medications, attempting to break the cycle of continuous headache. Methods used for headache relief include dihydroergotamine or sumatriptan, initiation of prophylactic medication, and concurrent behavioral intervention (*e.g.*, biofeedback, exercise).[57] Prophylactic treatment includes β-adrenergic blocking agents, antidepressants, calcium channel blockers, and 5-HT antagonists.

In summary, headache is so common that it is experienced by 75% of the population by age 15. There are many types of headache, the most common of which are tension-type (muscle contraction) headache and migraine headache. In 1988, the first edition of The Classification and Diagnostic Criteria for Headache Disorders, Cranial Neuralgias, and Facial Pain, prepared by the Headache Classification Committee of the International Headache Society, was published, along with 10 general rules considered essential to the correct use of this new system.

TMJ syndrome is one of the major causes of headaches. It usually is caused by an imbalance in the joint movement because of poor bite, teeth grinding, or joint problems such as inflammation, trauma, and degenerative changes.

Pain in Children and Adolescents

After you have completed this section of the chapter, you should be able to meet the following objectives:

- State how the pain response may differ in children
- Explain the advantage of intravenously versus intramuscularly administered opioid medications for relief of pain in children

Pain in children was not recognized as a legitimate phenomenon until the late 1970s, when dramatic differences in analgesic administration between children and adults after surgery was described.[59] This inattention to the pain experience in children was related to several factors. The first was the misconception that children do not feel pain, or if they feel it, they do not remember it. A second was the prevalent belief that pain, even if present, exacted only a psychologic cost and there were not physiologic consequences to ignoring pain in children. A third factor was the dearth of reliable and valid pain measurement tools that clinicians and researchers could use to determine if a child was experiencing pain, the intensity of the pain, and where it was located. And finally, exaggerated fears about the effects of analgesia on respiratory status and the potential for addiction in children receiving opioids were prevalent. Research during the past decades has added a great deal to the body of knowledge about pain in children, has provided valuable data to refute previously held misconceptions, and has changed markedly the practices of health professionals.[60–62]

Response to pain occurs early in the human fetus and neonatal period. Although the younger the neonate, the less specific and localized the behavioral reaction, protective and withdrawal reflexes are clearly demonstrated in response to nociceptive stimuli. Pain pathways, cortical and subcortical centers, and neurochemical responses associated with pain transmission are developed and functional by the last trimester of pregnancy. As infants mature and children grow, their responses to pain become more complex and reflective of their maturing cognitive and developmental processes. Children do feel pain and have been shown to reliably and accurately report pain as young as 3 years of age. They also remember pain, as evidenced in studies of children with cancer, whose distress during painful procedures increases over time without intervention and neonates in intensive care units, who demonstrate protective withdrawal responses to heelstick after repeated episodes. The notion that untreated pain exacts a physiologic cost for the human organism has implications for morbidity and mortality as documented in the mid-1980s work of Anand and colleagues.[62,63] These authors documented that nociceptive stimuli produces reverberations throughout the human organism, including cardiovascular, endocrine, and immune systems. The cascade of physiologic responses involving these systems include a depressed immune response, and significant increases in norepinephrine levels and plasma cortisol levels, all of which can have a significant impact on recovery.[62–64]

Pain Assessment

The assessment of pain in children is somewhat complicated, but research during the past 2 decades has resulted in a variety of assessment and measurement tools that health professionals can use. There are a variety of measurement tools that can be used to obtain children's self-reports about pain within a developmental and cultural framework.[65] Faces of actual children are used to elicit young children's reports, while numeric scales (*i.e.*, 1 to 10) and word graphic scales (*i.e.*, none, a little, most I have ever experienced) can be used with older children and adolescents.[66] All of these have been found to be valid and reliable. Another strategy for assessing a child's pain is to use body outlines and ask the child to indicate where the hurt is located.[67] There are some distinct advantages to assessing the intensity and location of a child's pain. Although important, intensity alone does not always determine the type of analgesia used. For instance, the type of pain stimulus (*e.g.*, bladder spasm versus abdominal incision) requires different analgesic approaches to be effective. Children's reports of pain are influenced by a variety of factors, including age, anxiety and fear levels, and parent presence.

Nurses and physicians have reported that they rely most often on the child's physiologic parameters such as heart rate, respiratory rate, and behavior expressions rather than the child's self report of pain.[68] Although there are positive correlations between heart rate, respiratory rate and pain, these parameters are nonspecific for pain and are reflective of an increase in sympathetic nervous system activity that can be related to a variety of factors, such as anxiety and activity. There is no objective physiologic parameter that is specific for pain. Pain experts recommend that health professionals consider the child's report of pain as the gold standard and a primary component of their assessment, in addition to their assessment of the child's behavior and physiologic parameters.

Pain Management

The management of children's pain basically falls into two categories: pharmacologic and nonpharmacologic. In terms of pharmacologic interventions, currently there are a variety of analgesic agents considered safe and effective for use with children and adolescents. As with any person in pain, the type of analgesic used should be matched to the type and intensity of pain. The World Health Organization developed a very useful framework for decision making that suggests that mild pain should be treated with nonopioid agents such as aspirin, acetaminophen, or nonsteroidal anti-inflammatory agents (NSAIDs); moderate pain with weaker opioids such as codeine; and severe pain with stronger opioids, such as morphine.[69] The overriding principle is to treat each child's pain on an individual basis and to match the analgesic agent with the level of pain. A second principle involves maintaining the balance between level of sedation and pain relief such that pain relief is obtained with as little opioid and sedation as possible. One strategy to enable this is to time the administration of analgesia such that pain is prevented, as much as possible, and steady blood level is achieved. This requires that the child receive analgesia on a regular dosing schedule, not "as needed."

The side effects of pain medication vary according to the analgesic agent chosen. Side effects of NSAIDs include bleeding and gastric distress, but these are usually associated with prolonged use and higher doses. These side effects reduce their viability as an option for selected groups of children, such as those with cancer. The most common side effects of opioids include sedation, pruritus, and nausea, while the least common are respiratory depression and addiction. Some of these side effects (*e.g.*, nausea) are more bothersome in children, who often refuse the analgesia while in pain to avoid the side effects. One of the goals of analgesic treatment is to achieve the highest level of analgesia and comfort with the least number of side effects. For some children in severe pain, it is necessary to treat the side effects and the pain to achieve this goal.

The use of nonpharmacologic strategies can be very effective in reducing the amount of overall pain and the overall amount of analgesia used, reducing anxiety, and increasing the child's level of self-control during pain.[70] Children as young as 4 years of age can be taught to use simple distraction and relaxation, and other techniques such as application of heat and cold.[71] Nonpharmacologic techniques based on peripheral stimulation such as heat, TENS, or cryotherapy involve the stimulation of cutaneous afferents that send signals to the central cognitive processing system that compete with pain transmission.[68] In contrast, those techniques that are cognitively based (*i.e.*, relaxation, distraction, imaging), require that an individual's active attention be refocused from pain to another stimulus. This refocusing alters the sensory, evaluative, and affective components of the pain experience. Nonpharmacologic techniques must be taught to children and their parents and the methods used should be developmentally appropriate. If possible, the child and parent should be taught these techniques before the pain experience begins so that they can have an opportunity to practice the technique.[60] Research has provided health professionals with a wide variety of pharmacologic and nonpharmacologic options to treat a child's pain. The application of this research is critical if effective and safe pain care is to be provided.[61]

In summary, the last 2 decades have seen significant changes in the assessment and management of pain in children. Research has led to the recognition that pain is a legitimate phenomenon in children, and it has physiologic and psychologic consequences that can significantly affect recovery. Children experience and remember pain, and even young children are able to accurately and reliably report their pain.

As previous misconceptions have been dispelled regarding the ability of the fetus, neonate, and young child to experience pain, more research has been stimulated. This has changed the clinical practice of health professionals involved in the assessment of children's pain. Pain management in children is improving as exaggerated fears and misconceptions concerning the risks of addiction and respiratory depression in children treated with opioids are also dispelled.

Pharmacologic (including the use of opioids) and nonpharmacologic pain management interventions have been shown to be effective in children. Nonpharmacologic techniques must be based on the developmental level of the child and should be taught to both children and parents.

REFERENCES

1. Martin J.H., Jessell T.M. (1991). Anatomic substrates for somatic sensation. In Kandel E.R., Schwartz J.H. (Eds.). *Principles of neuroscience* (3rd ed., pp. 353–366). New York: Elsevier.
2. Guyton A., Hall J.E. (1996). *Textbook of medical physiology* (9th ed., pp. 595–607). Philadelphia: W.B. Saunders.
3. Rhoades R.A., Tanner G.A. (1996). *Medical Physiology*. (pp. 60–70). Boston: Little, Brown.

4. Gebhart GE. (1995). Somatovisceral sensation. In Conn P.M. (Ed.). *Neuroscience in Medicine* (pp. 433–455), Philadelphia, J.B. Lippincott.
5. Ready L.B. (Chair) (1992). *International Association for the Study of Pain Task Force on Chronic Pain.* Seattle: IASP Publications.
6. Bonica J.J. (1991). History of pain concepts and pain theory. *Mount Sinai Journal of Medicine* 58 (3), 191–202.
7. Melzack R., Wall P.D. (1965). Pain mechanisms: A new theory. *Science* 150, 971.
8. Cross S.A. (1994). Pathophysiology of pain. *Mayo Clinic Proceedings* 69, 375–383.
9. Kelley D.D., Jessell T.M. (1991). Pain and analgesia. In Kandel E.R., Schwartz J.H. (Eds.). *Principles of neuroscience* (3rd ed., pp. 385–399). New York: Elsevier.
10. Lisney S.J.W. (1995). The development of peripheral inflammation: Is a centrally generated neuromechanism involved? *Pain Forum* 4:153–154.
11. Sluka K.A., Willis W.D., Westlund K.N. (1995). The role of dorsal root reflexes in neurogenic inflammation. *Pain Forum* 4:141–149.
12. Ochoa J., Serra J. (1995). Dorsal root reflexes: Do they play a role in chronic "neuropathic" pain? *Pain Forum* 4:155–157.
13. Markenson J.A. (1996). Mechanisms of chronic pain. *American Journal of Medicine* 101 (Suppl. 1A), 6S–18S.
14. Cooper J.R., Bloom F.E., Roth R.H. (1991). *The biochemical basis of neuropharmacology* (6th ed., p. 263). New York: Oxford University Press.
15. Basabaum A.I. (1987). Cytochemical studies of the neural circuitry underlying pain and pain control. *Acta Neurochirurgica (Wien)* 38 (Suppl.), 5.
16. Fields H.L., Heinricher M.M., Mason P. (1991). Neurotransmitters in nociceptive modulatory circuits. *Review of Neuroscience* 14, 219.
17. Saria A. (1987). The role of substance P and other neuropeptides in transmission of pain. *Acta Neurochirurgica (Wien)* 38 (Suppl.), 33.
18. Nauta H.J.W., Hewitt E., Westlund K.N., Willis W.D. (1997). Surgical interruption of a midline dorsal column visceral pain pathway. *Journal of Neurosurgery* 80:538–542.
19. Grichnick K., Ferrante F.M. (1991). The difference between acute and chronic pain. *Mount Sinai Journal of Medicine* 58, 217–220.
20. Bonica J.J. (1990). *The management of pain* (2nd ed., pp. 159–197). Philadelphia: Lea & Febiger.
21. Ruoff G.E. (1996). Depression in the patient with chronic pain. *Journal of Family Practice* 43 (6 Suppl.), S25–S33.
22. Acute Pain Management Guideline Panel. (1992). *Acute pain management: Operative or medical procedures and trauma.* AHCPR Pub. No. 92-0032. Rockville, MD: Agency for Health Care Policy and Research, Public Health Service U.S. Department of Health and Human Services.
23. Jacox A., Carr D.B., Payne R., et al. (1994). *Management of Cancer Pain. Clinical Practice Guideline No. 9.* AHCPR Pub. No. 94-0592. Rockville, MD: Agency for Health Care Policy and Research, Public Health Service U.S. Department of Health and Human Services.
24. Chapman C.R., Syrjala K.L. (1990). Measurement of pain. In Bonica J.J. *Management of Pain* (2nd ed., pp 580–594) Philadelphia: Lea & Febiger.
25. Melzack R. (1975). The McGill Pain Questionnaire: Major properties and scoring methods. *Pain* 22, 1.
26. Licht S. (1984). History of therapeutic heat and cold. In Lehman J.F. (Ed.). *Therapeutic heat and cold* (3rd ed.). Baltimore: Williams & Wilkins.
27. Nigel P.P. (1988). Heat and cold. In Wells P.E., Frampton V., Bowsher D. (Eds.). *Pain management in physical therapy* (pp. 169–180). East Norwalk, CT: Appleton & Lange.
28. Keating W. (1961). Cold vasodilatation after adrenaline. *Journal of Physiology* 159, 101.
29. Chapman C.R. (1979). Contribution of research on acupuncture and transcutaneous electrical stimulation to the understanding of pain mechanisms and pain relief. In Roland F., Beers J., Bassett E.G. (Eds.). *Mechanisms of pain and analgesic compounds* (pp. 7–183). New York: Raven Press.
30. Hymes A. (1984). A review of the historical area of electricity. In Mannheimer J.S., Lampe G.N. (Eds.). *Clinical transcutaneous electrical stimulation* (p. 1). Philadelphia: F.A. Davis.
31. Michel T.H. (Ed.). (1985). *International perspectives in physical therapy* (pp. 96–97, 129–130). Edinburgh: Churchill Livingstone.
32. Wolf S.L. (1984). Neurophysiologic mechanisms of pain modulation: Relevance to TENS. In Mannheimer J.S., Lampe G.N. (Eds.). *Clinical transcutaneous electrical stimulation* (p. 41). Philadelphia: F.A. Davis.
33. Anderson S.A. (1979). Pain control by sensory stimulation. In Bonica J.J. (Ed.). *Advances in pain research and therapy* (p. 569). New York: Raven Press.
34. Sjolund B.H., Terenius L., Erickson M.B.E. (1977). Increased cerebrospinal fluid levels of endorphin after electroacupuncture. *Acta Physiologica Scandinavica* 100, 382.
35. Ignelzi R.J., Nyquist J.K. (1979). Excitability changes in peripheral nerve fibers after repetitive electrical stimulation: Implications for pain modulation. *Journal of Neurosurgery* 51, 824.
36. Sherman J.E., Liebeskind J.C. (1980). An endorphinergic centrifugal substrate of pain modulation: Recent findings, current concepts and complexities. In Bonica J.J. (Ed.). *Pain.* New York: Raven Press.
37. Way W.L., Way L., Field H. (1995). Opioid analgesics and antagonists. In Katzung H. (Ed.). *Basic & clinical pharmacology* (6th ed., 460–477). East Norwalk, CT: Appleton & Lange.
38. Melzak R. (1990). The tragedy of needless pain. *Scientific American* 262 (2), 2–8.
39. Swerdlow M., Stjerward J. (1982). Cancer pain relief—An urgent problem. *World Health Forum* 3, 325–330.
40. Fields H.L., Levine J.D. (1984). Pain—mechanisms and management. *Western Journal of Medicine* 141, 347.
41. Dennis E.M.P. (1984). An ambulatory infusion pump for pain control: A nursing approach to home care. *Cancer Nursing* 7, 309.
42. Lieb R.A., Hurtig J.B. (1985). Epidural and intrathecal narcotics for pain management. *Heart and Lung* 14, 164.
43. Jaffe J.H., Martin W.R. (1990). Opioid analgesics and antagonists. In A.G. Gilman, L.S. Goodman, T.W. Rall, et al. (Eds.). *Goodman and Gilman's The pharmacological basis of therapeutics* (8th ed., pp. 485–497). New York: Macmillan.
44. Kost R.G., Straus S.E. (1996). Postherpetic neuralgia—Pathogenesis, treatment and prevention. *New England Journal of Medicine* 335 (1), 32–42.
45. Melzak R. (1992). Phantom pain. *Scientific American* 120–123.
46. Friedman A.P. (Chair). (1962). Ad Hoc Committee on the Classification of Headache: Classification of headache. *Archives of Neurology* 6, 173–176.
47. Olesen J. (Chair). (1988). Headache Classification Committee of the International Headache Society. The classifica-

tion and diagnostic criteria for headache disorders, cranial neuralgias, and facial pain. *Cephalalgia* 8 (Suppl. 7), 1–96.

48. Alldredge B.K. (1996). Headache. In Young L.Y., Koda-Kimble M.A. (Eds.). *Applied therapeutics: The clinical use of drugs* (6th ed., pp. 50–1–50–19). Vancouver, WA: Applied Therapeutics.
49. Lauritzen M. (1994). Review article. Pathophysiology of the migraine aura: The spreading depression theory. *Brain* 117, 199–210.
50. Thomsen L.L., Olesen J. (1996). The role of nitric oxide in migraine pain. In Campbell J.N. (Ed.). *Pain 1996—An updated review: Refresher course syllabus* (pp. 129–134). Seattle: IASP Press.
51. Olesen J. (1996). Headache. Presented at the meeting of the International Association for the Study of Pain, 8th World Congress on Pain, Vancouver, Canada.
52. Mathew N.T. (1996). Cluster headache. In Campbell J.N. (Ed.). *Pain 1996—An updated review: Refresher course syllabus* (pp. 135–142). Seattle: IASP Press.
53. Rasmussen B.J., Jensen R., Schroll M., Olesen J. (1991). Epidemiology of headache in a general population: A prevalence study. *Journal of Clinical Epidemiology* 44 (11), 1147–1157.
54. Edmeads J. G. (1996). Tension-type: The "other" headache. *Headache: Newsletter of the American Council for Headache Education,* 7 (3), 1–2.
55. Berman G.D., Saper J.R., Solomon G.D. (1996). Chronic headache: Management strategies that make sense. *Patient Care* Jan 30, 54–66.
56. Silberstein S.D. (1993). Advances in understanding the pathophysiology of headache. *Neurology* 42 (Suppl. 2), 6.
57. Mathew N.T. (1996). Chronic daily headache. In Campbell J.N. (Ed.). *Pain 1996—An updated review: Refresher course syllabus* (pp. 143–153). Seattle: IASP Press.
58. Okeson J.P. (1996). Temporomandibular disorders in the medical practice. *Journal of Family Practice* 43 (4), 347–356.
59. Eland J., Anderson J. (1977). The experience of pain in children. In Jacox A. (Ed). *Pain: A sourcebook for nurses and other professionals.* Boston: Little, Brown.
60. Broome M., Foley M.K., Rehwaldt M. (1995). The utilization of cognitive-behavioral pain interventions by children and parents. In *Key aspects of caring for the acutely ill: Technical aspects, patient education and quality of life.* New York: Springer Publishing.
61. Broome M., Richtsmeier A., Maikler V., Alexander M. (1996). Pediatric pain practices: A survey of health professionals. *Journal of Pain and Symptom Management* 4, 315–319.
62. Anand K.J.S., Hickey P.R. (1987). Pain and its effects in the human neonate and fetus. *New England Journal of Medicine* 317 (21), 1321.
63. Anand K., Sippell W., Aynsley-Green A. (1987). Randomized trial of fentanyl anesthesia in preterm babies undergoing surgery: Effects on the response. *Lancet* 1, 243–1248.
64. Fitzgerald M., Anand K. (1993). Developmental neuroanatomy and neurophysiology of pain. In Schechter N., Berde C., Yaster M. (Eds.). *Pain in infants, children and adolescents* (pp. 11–32). Baltimore: Williams & Wilkins.
65. Acute Pain Management Guideline Panel. (1992). *Acute pain management: Operative or medical procedures and trauma.* AHCPR Pub. No. 92–0032. Rockville, MD: Agency for Health Care Policy and Research, Public Health Service U.S. Department of Health and Human Services.
66. Beyer J. (In Press). Establishing construct validity for a pain assessment tool for African-American and Hispanic children. *Journal of Pediatric Nursing.*
67. Savedra M., Tesler M., Holzemer W., Brokaw P. (1995). A strategy to assess the temporal dimension of pain in children and adolescents. *Nursing Research* 44 (5), 272–275.
68. Watt-Watson J., Donovan M. (1992). *Nursing management of the patient in pain.* Philadelphia J.B. Lippincott.
69. World Health Organization. (1990). *Cancer pain relief and palliative care.* Report of the WHO Expert Committee (Technical Report Series. 804). Geneva Switzerland: WHO.
70. Slifer K., Babbit R.L., Cataldo M. (1995). Stimulation and counterconditioning as adjuncts to pharmacotherapy for invasive pediatric procedures. *Journal of Developmental and Behavioral Pediatrics* 36, 133–141.
71. Vessey J., Carlson K., McGill J. (1995). Use of distraction with children during an acute pain experience. *Nursing Research* 43, 369–372.

ADDITIONAL READINGS

Adams R.D., Victor M. (1993). *Principles of neurology* (5th ed.). New York: McGraw-Hill.

Al-Chaer E.D., Lawand N.B., Westlund K.N., et al. (1955). The dorsal column (DC) is more important for visceral pain than the spinothalamic tract? [abstract] *Society for Neuroscience* 21, 644.

Al-Chaer E.D., Lawand N.B., Westlund K.N., et al. (1996). Visceral nociceptive input into the ventral posterolateral nucleus of the thalamus: a new function for the dorsal column pathway. *Journal of Neurophysics* 76, 2661–2674.

Bonica J.J. (1990). The management of pain (vol. I & II, 2nd. ed.). Philadelphia: Lea and Febiger.

Casey K.L. (1996). Match and mismatch: Identifying the neuronal determinants of pain. *Annals of Internal Medicine* 124 (11), 995–998.

Cassidy J.T. (1994). Progress in diagnosing and understanding chronic pain syndromes in children. *Current Opinion in Rheumatology* 6, 544–546.

Cleary J., Carbone P.F. (1995). Pharmacologic management of cancer pain. *Hospital Practice* 30 (11), 41–49.

Gloth F.M. III. (1996). Concerns of chronic analgesic therapy in elderly patients. *American Journal of Medicine* 101 (Suppl. 1A): 20S–23S.

Hickey J.V., Brown R.P. (1997). Management of chronic pain: A neuroscience perspective, pp. 361–372. In Hickey J.V. (Ed.). *Neurological and neurosurgical nursing* (4th ed.). Philadelphia: J.B. Lippincott.

Kitahata L.M. (1994). Pain pathways and transmission. *Yale Journal of Biology and Medicine* 66, 437–442.

Kost R.G., Strauss S.E. (1996). Postherpetic neuralgia—Pathogenesis, treatment, and prevention. *New England Journal of Medicine* 335, 32–42.

Kryst S., Scherl E. (1994). A population-based survey of the social and personal impact of headache. *Headache* 19 (1), 18–24.

Lister B.J. (1996). Dilemmas in the treatment of chronic pain. *American Journal of Medicine* 101 (Suppl. 1A), 2S–4S.

MacEvilly M., Buggy D. (1996). Back pain and pregnancy: A review. *Pain* 64:405–414.

McGuire D.B., Yarbro C.H., Ferrell B.R. (1995). Cancer pain management (2nd ed.). Boston: Jones and Bartlett Publishers.

Ochoa J.L. (1993). The human sensory unit and pain. New concepts, syndromes, and tests. *Muscle and Nerve* 16, 1009–1016.

Saper J.R. (1997). Diagnosis and treatment of migraine. *Headache* 37 (Suppl 1), S1–S14.

Schott G.D. (1994). Visceral afferents: Their contribution to "sympathetic dependent" pain. *Brain* 17, 397–413.

Sorkin L.S. (1991). Nociceptive transmission within the spinal cord. *The Mount Sinai Journal of Medicine* 58 (3), 208–215.

Stein C. (1995). The control of pain in peripheral tissues by opioids. *New England Journal of Medicine* 332 (25), 1685–1690.

Tyring S.K. (1996). Early treatment of herpes zoster. *Hospital Practice* 31 (7), 137–144.

Walco G.A., Cassidy R.C., Schrechter N.L. (1994). The ethics of pain control in infants and children. *New England Journal of Medicine* 331 (8), 541–543.

Wall P.D. (1992). The placebo effect: An unpopular topic. *Brain* 51, 1–3.

Warren S., Capra N.F., Yezierski R.P. (1997). The somatosensory system II: Touch, temperature, and nociception. In Haynes D.E. (Ed.). *Fundamental neuroscience* (pp. 238–240). New York: Churchill Livingstone.

Wiener S.L. (1993). *Differential diagnosis of acute pain by body region*. New York: McGraw-Hill.

UNIT XI

Alterations in Special Senses

Of all the ancient civilizations, it was the Greeks who led the way in understanding the body and its workings. One of the earliest Greek anatomists was Alcmaeon of Croton (c. 500 BC). Through his animal dissections, Alcmaeon came to recognize many structures and was the first to mention the eye in his writings. He described the optic nerve and decided that three things were necessary for vision—external light, the "fire" in the eye (he assumed there must be fire in the eye because a blow to the eye produces sparks, or stars), and the liquid in the eyeball.

The Greeks also developed early surgical procedures, among them techniques for the removal of cataracts. However, it was the Roman encyclopedist Aulus Cornelius Celsus (1st century AD), whose most important surviving works are concerned with medicine, who provided a vivid description of the procedure:

> *The needle is to be sharp enough to penetrate, yet not too fine; and this to be inserted straight through...at a spot between the pupil of the eye and the angle adjacent to the temple, away from the middle of the cataract, in such a way that no vein is wounded. The needle, however, should not be inserted timidly. When the spot is reached, the needle is to be sloped against the colored area [lens] itself and rotated gently, guiding it little by little below the pupil; when the cataract has passed below the pupil, it is pressed upon more firmly in order that it may settle below.*

CHAPTER 41

Control of Special Senses

Sheila M. Curtis, Edward W. Carroll, and Robin L. Curtis

The Eye and Visual Function

After you have completed this section of the chapter, you should be able to meet the following objectives:

- Describe the structures and functions of the eyelids and lacrimal apparatus
- Name the layers of the eyeball and relate their structure to the overall function of the eye
- Compare the location and contents of the anterior and posterior chambers of the eye
- Discuss the function of the lens and distinguish between refraction and accommodation
- Explain the difference between myopia and hyperopia
- Characterize the structure of the retina, differentiating the three layers of neurons and the functions of rods and cones
- Trace a visual image from the time it reaches the retina to its perception in the visual and association cortices

The optic globe, or eyeball, is a remarkably mobile, nearly spherical structure contained within a pyramid-shaped cavity of the skull called the *orbit* (Fig. 41–1). The eyeball consists of three layers: an outer supporting fibrous layer, the sclera; a vascular layer, the uveal tract; and a neural layer, the retina. The interior is filled with transparent media, the aqueous and vitreous humors, which allow the penetration and transmission of light to photoreceptors in the retina. The exposed surface of the eye is protected by the eyelid, a mucous membrane–lined skin flap that provides a means for shutting out most light. Tears bathe the anterior surface of the eye; they prevent friction between it and the lid, maintain hydration of the cornea, and protect the eye from irritation by foreign objects. The two eyes with their associated extraocular muscles permit directional rotation of the eyeball to provide slightly different images of the same object. This results in binocular vision with depth perception.

Orbit

The eyeball is located within the bony orbit of the skull. The orbit is a pyramid-shaped cavity with walls formed

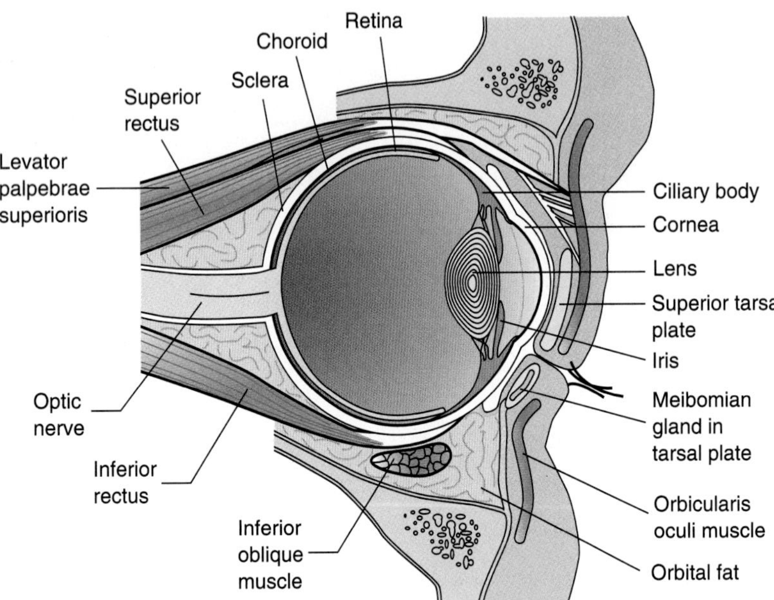

Figure 41–1
The eye and its appendages, lateral view.

by the union of seven cranial and facial bones: the frontal, maxillary, zygomatic, lacrimal, sphenoid, ethmoid, and palatine bones (Fig. 41–2). The superior surface of the maxillary bone forms the main floor of the orbit. The maxillary, lacrimal, and ethmoid bones form the medial wall of the orbit. The shape of the lateral wall of the orbit is triangular; it is formed anteriorly by the zygomatic bone and posteriorly by the sphenoid bone. It forms the thickest part of the orbit, particularly at the orbital margin, where the wall is most likely to be exposed to trauma.

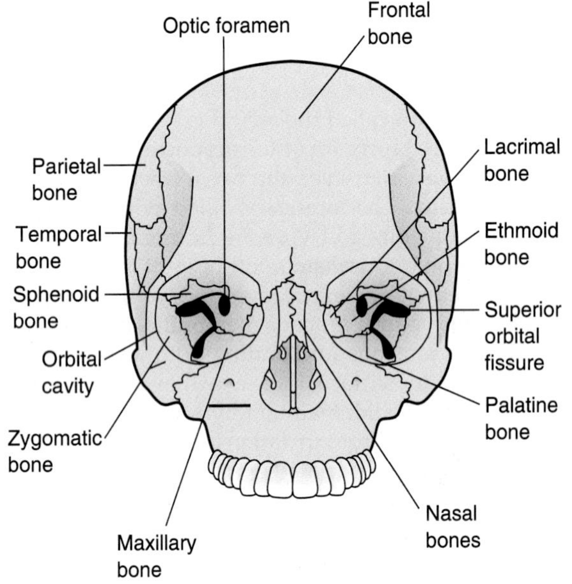

Figure 41–2
Anterior view of the skull shows the orbital cavity and optic foramen that form an opening for the optic nerve, blood vessels (*e.g.*, ophthalmic artery), and sympathetic nerves that supply the eye.

The apex of the orbital pyramid, at the posterior medial part of the orbit, is pierced by an opening called the *optic foramen*. The optic nerve, ophthalmic artery, and sympathetic nerves from the carotid plexus pass through this foramen. Among other functions, these sympathetic nerve fibers innervate the pupillary dilator muscle. A larger opening, the superior orbital fissure, permits passage of branches of cranial nerves (CN) III, IV, V_1 (*i.e.*, ophthalmic division of the trigeminal nerve), and VI. These cranial nerves provide motor innervation of the extrinsic (CN III, IV, and V_1) and intrinsic eye muscles (CN III) and sensory innervation of the orbit and its contents.

The eyeball occupies only the anterior one fifth of the orbit; the remainder is filled with muscles, nerves, the lacrimal gland, and adipose tissue that supports the normal position of the optic globe. A layer of fascia known as Tenon's capsule surrounds the globe of the eye from the cornea to the posterior segment and separates the eye from the orbital fat.

Eyelid

The upper and lower eyelids, the *palpebrae*, are modified folds of skin that protect the eyeball. The palpebral fissure is the oval opening between the upper and lower eyelids. The angle where the upper and lower lids meet is referred to as the *canthus*; the lateral canthus is the outer, or temporal, angle, and the medial canthus is the inner, or nasal, angle (Fig. 41–3). A line through the lateral and medial canthi defines the angle of the palpebral

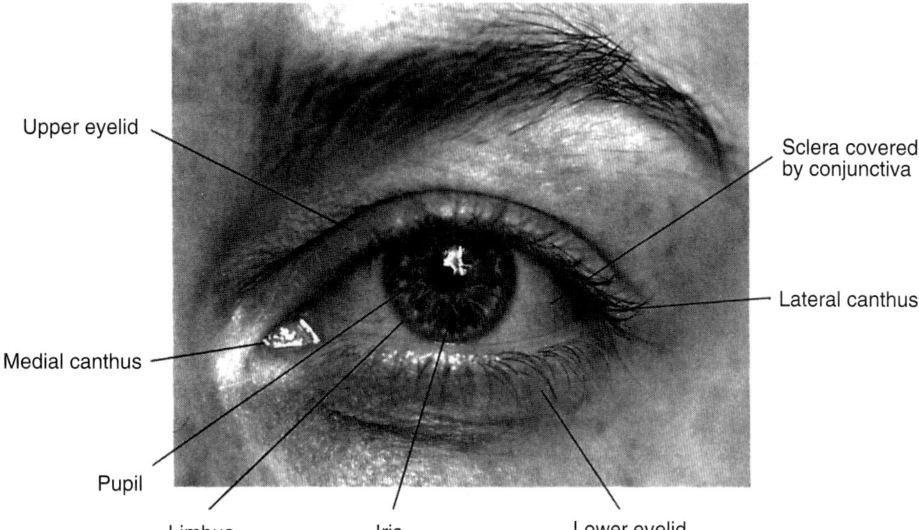

Figure 41–3
Left eye.

fissure and is usually horizontal. In children with Down syndrome (trisomy 21), this line has an upward and outward slant (see Chapter 4). A fold of skin, the *epicanthic fold,* covers the medial canthus and is characteristic of members of the Asian race and of persons with certain chromosomal abnormalities.

In each lid, a tarsus, or plate of dense connective tissue, gives the lid its shape (Fig. 41–4). Each tarsus contains modified sebaceous glands, called meibomian glands, the ducts of which open onto the eyelid margins. The sebaceous secretions of the meibomian glands enable airtight closure of the lids and prevent rapid evaporation of tears. Sympathetic axons, through the sympathetic plexus, innervate the superior tarsal muscle that assists the levator palpebrae (CN III) to adjust the height of the palpebral opening.

The lacrimal gland is the source of serous secretions called *tears.* This gland lies in the orbit, superior and lateral to the eyeball (Fig. 41–5). Approximately 12 small ducts connect the lacrimal gland to the superior conjunctival fornix. Tears, which contain about 98% water, 1.5% sodium chloride, and the antibacterial enzyme lysozyme, are essential to vision because of their lubricant and possibly antibacterial properties. Lubrication between the layers of conjunctiva permits comfortable eye and lid movement. Tears drain from the eye through a reddish elevation, the lacrimal caruncle, located in the medial canthus into the nasolacrimal duct, which opens into the nasal cavity.

Conjunctiva

The conjunctiva is a thin mucous membrane that lines the inner surface of both eyelids and covers the anterior surface of the optic globe to the *limbus,* or corneal-scleral junction (Fig. 41–6). The portion of the conjunctiva that lines the eyelids is called the *palpebral conjunctiva,* and the

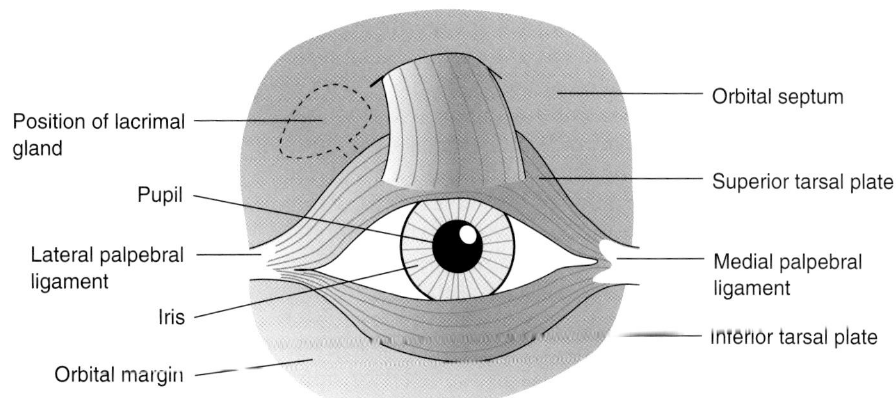

Figure 41–4
Anterior view of the right orbit shows the superficial structures.

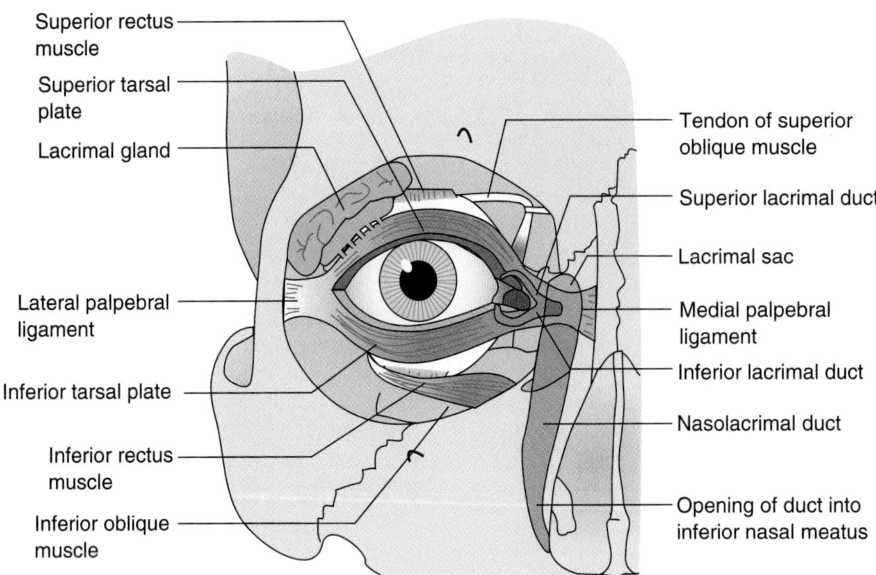

Figure 41–5 The eye and its appendages: anterior view.

part that covers the eyeball is called the *bulbar (ocular) conjunctiva.* When the eyes are closed, the conjunctiva lines the closed conjunctival sac. The conjunctiva is extremely sensitive to irritation and inflammation. The lining of the upper lid is innervated by the ophthalmic division (V_1) of the trigeminal cranial nerve and that of the lower lid, by the maxillary division (V_2) of the same nerve.

Eyeball

The wall of the eyeball is composed of three layers: the sclera or outer supporting layer, the choroid or middle vascular layer, and the retina, which is composed of the neuronal retinal layer and outer pigmented layer (Fig. 41–6). The optic globe is separated into two cavities, an anterior, fluid-filled cavity and a posterior cavity, the vitreous body, which is filled with a gel-like material. The anterior cavity is separated into an anterior and posterior chamber by the lens and by the ciliary body and its processes.

Sclera and Cornea

The outer layer of the eyeball consists of a tough, opaque, white fibrous layer called the *sclera.* Its strong yet elastic properties maintain the shape of the globe. The sclera is continuous with the cornea anteriorly and with the cranial dural sheath that surrounds and protects the optic nerve posteriorly. This sheath is continuous except for the lamina cribrosa, a number of tiny holes at the optic disk, through which the optic nerve axons exit the retina. In an inherited collagen disease known as *osteogenesis imperfecta* (see Chapter 46), the sclera is thin, and the pigmented choroid shows through, providing a bluish cast to the sclera. Subconjunctival hemorrhage frequently is associated with even mild trauma to the head or optic globe. In jaundice, the sclera appears yellow because of staining from excessive levels of circulating bilirubin.

At the anterior part of the eyeball, the sclera is continuous and connects to the transparent cornea at the limbus. The major part of refraction (*i.e.,* bending) of light rays and focusing of vision occurs at this point. The cornea has three layers: an extremely thin outer epithelial layer, which is continuous with the bulbar (ocular) conjunctiva; a middle layer called the *substantia propria or stroma;* and an inner endothelial layer, which lies adjacent to the aqueous humor of the anterior chamber. The thick substantia propria constitutes 90% of the cornea; its anterior condensation, called Bowman's membrane, is attached to the basement membrane of the epithelial layer. Descemet's membrane, the basement membrane of the endothelium, separates the endothelium from the substantia propria. The substantia propria is composed of regularly arranged collagen bundles embedded in a mucopolysaccharide matrix. The regular organization of the collagen fibers, which makes the substantia propria transparent, is necessary for light transmission. Hydration within a limited range is necessary to maintain the spacing of the collagen fibers and transparency.

Uveal Tract

The middle vascular layer, or uveal tract, of the eye includes the choroid, the ciliary body, and the iris. The uveal tract is an incomplete ball with gaps at the pupil and at the optic disk, where it is continuous with the arachnoid and pial layers surrounding the optic nerve. The choroid is rich in dispersed melanocytes, which prevent the diffusion of light through the wall of the optic globe. The pigment of these cells absorbs light within the eyeball and light that penetrates the retina. The light-absorptive function prevents the scattering of light and is important for visual acuity, particularly with high background illumination levels.

The ciliary body is an anterior continuation of the choroid layer. It has smooth muscle and secretory functions. Its smooth muscle function contributes to alteration in lens shape; its secretory function contributes to the production of aqueous humor.

The iris is an adjustable diaphragm that permits alteration in pupil size and therefore in the amount of light entering the eye. The pupillary diameter can be varied from approximately 2 to 8 mm. The posterior surface of the iris is formed by a two-layer epithelium continuous with those layers covering the ciliary body. The anterior layer contains the dilator, or radial, muscles of the iris (Fig. 41–7). Just anterior to these muscles is the loose, highly vascular connective tissue stroma. Embedded in this layer are concentric rings of smooth muscle cells that compose the sphincter muscle of the pupil. The anteriormost layer of the iris forms a highly irregular anterior surface and contains many fibroblasts and melanocytes. Eye color differences result from the density of the pigment. The amount of pigment decreases from dark brown eyes through shades of brown and gray to blue.

Several mutations affect the pigment of the uveal tract, including albinism. Albinism is a genetic (autosomal recessive trait) deficiency of tyrosinase, the enzyme needed for the synthesis of melanin by the melanocytes. Tyrosinase-negative albinism, also called *classic albinism*, is characterized by an absence of tyrosinase; affected persons have white hair, pink skin, and light blue eyes. In these persons, excessive light penetrates the unpigmented iris and, to some extent, the anterior sclera and unpigmented choroid. Their photoreceptors are flooded with excess light, and visual acuity is markedly reduced. Excess stimulation of the photoreceptors at normal or high illumination levels is experienced as painful photophobia. Tyrosinase-positive albinism results from a genetic defect in which a reduced but variable amount of tyrosinase is synthesized by the pigment cells. Hair and skin color vary among affected persons. Reduced choroid and iris pigment results in variable acuity and photophobic abnormalities. A third type of hereditary defect involves the absence of pigment in the choroid and iris with normal pigmentation elsewhere. This *ocular albinism* results from a genetic abnormality located on the X chromosome. Other hereditary syndromes include reduced or absent pigment in the choroid and iris pigment, as in phenylketonuria. Persons with classic albinism and those with ocular albinism usually have continuous back-and-forth excursion eye movements (*i.e.*, physiologic nystagmus), which makes reading difficult.

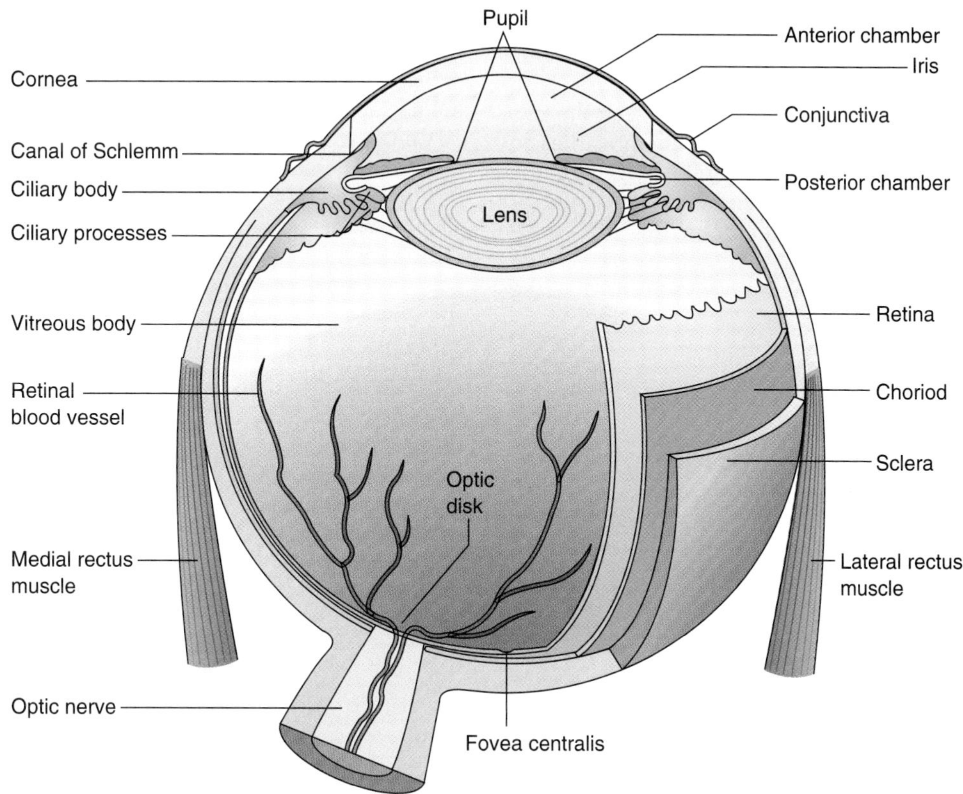

Figure 41–6 ■■■
Transverse section of the eyeball.

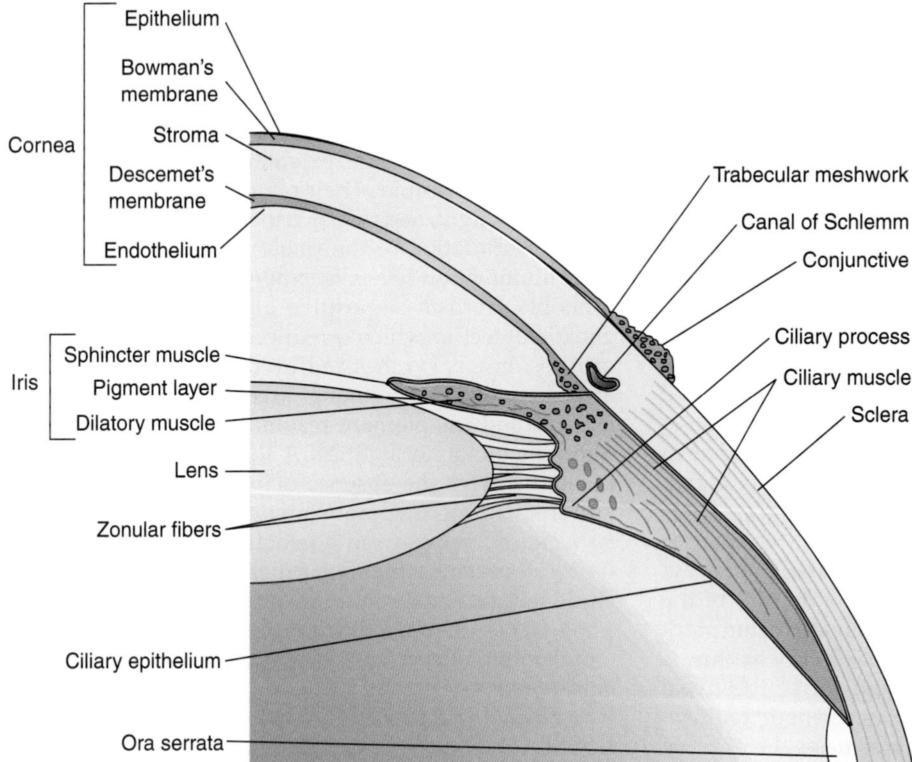

Figure 41–7 Anterior chamber angle and surrounding structures.

Anterior and Posterior Chambers

The fluid-filled anterior cavity of the eye is divided by the iris into the anterior and posterior chambers, with the pupil forming the only passageway between the two chambers (see Fig. 41–6). The anterior chamber lies in front of the iris and the posterior chamber, which is the smaller of the two, lies posterior to the iris and anterior to the lens. The gel-like vitreous humor fills the posterior cavity of the globe.

The transparent aqueous humor, which fills the space between the cornea and lens, is secreted by the ciliary epithelium in the posterior chamber. The secreted aqueous humor flows slowly through the thin passageway between the lens and the iris and is reabsorbed by a specialized region at the iridocorneal angle. At the iridocorneal angle, the aqueous humor normally passes through a porous trabeculated region of the sclera (see Fig. 41–7) that permits entry into a circular venous ring called the *canal of Schlemm* and from there into the anterior ciliary veins.

Lens

The function of the eye is to transform light energy into nerve signals that can be transmitted to the cerebral cortex for interpretation. Optically, the eye is similar to a camera. It contains a lens system that inverts an image, an aperture (*i.e.,* pupil) for controlling light exposure, and a retina that corresponds to the film and records the image (Fig. 41–8).

The lens is an avascular transparent biconvex body, whose posterior side is more convex than the anterior side. It measures about 9 to 10 mm in the transverse diameter and about 4 mm in the anteroposterior diameter. A thin, homogeneous, and highly elastic carbohydrate-containing lens capsule is attached to the surrounding ciliary body by delicate suspensory radial ligaments called *zonules*, which hold the lens in place (see Fig. 41–7). In providing for a change in lens shape, the tough elastic sclera acts as a bow, and the zonule and lens capsule act as the bow string. The lens capsule is normally under tension, and the lens is flattened. Some of the smooth muscle fibers of the ciliary body are oriented parallel to the scleral surface and insert more anteriorly at the scleral-corneal junction. Many of the fibers are oriented radially as a sphincter around the eyeball. Contraction of the muscle fibers of the ciliary body results in a bending-in of the anterior sclera, relieving the tension on the zonules and the lens capsule. Under these conditions, the rather elastic lens assumes a nearly spherical shape. Altering the normally flat lens shape to a more spherical shape increases the focusing power of the lens, bringing the focused image of a near object forward to the retinal surface.

Refraction

When light passes from one medium to another, its velocity is decreased or increased, and the direction of light transmission is changed. The bending of light at an angulated surface is called *refraction*. When light rays pass through the center of a lens, their direction is not changed; however, other rays passing peripherally through a lens are bent (Fig. 41–9). Usually, the refractive power of a lens is described as the distance (in meters) from its surface to the point at which the rays come into focus (*i.e.*, focal length) or as the reciprocal of this distance (*i.e.*, diopters). For example, a lens that brings an object into focus at 0.5 m has a refractive power of 2 diopters (1.0/0.5 = 2.0). With a fixed power lens, the closer an object is to the lens, the further behind the lens the focus point is. The closer the object, the stronger and more precise the focusing system must be.

In the eye, the major refraction of light begins at the convex corneal surface. Further refraction occurs as light moves from the posterior corneal surface to the aqueous humor, from the aqueous humor to the anterior lens surface, and from the posterior lens surface to the vitreous humor. The focusing surface of the eye, the retina, is at a fixed distance from the lens; adjustability in the refractive power of the lens is needed to keep the image of close objects in sharp focus on the retina. This is called *accommodation*. The adjustable lens shape and the adjustable pupillary opening must be under the control of a feedback system that makes these adjustments while evaluating image sharpness. All of this is accomplished by accommodation and pupillary reflexes under the control of the visual acuity centers in the primary visual and association cortices. These areas provide feedback control for modifying lens shape and therefore visual acuity.

Disorders of Refraction. A perfectly shaped optic globe and cornea result in optimal visual acuity (*i.e.*, emmetropia), producing a sharp image in focus at all points on the retinal surface in the posterior part, or fundus, of the eye (see Fig. 41–9). Unfortunately, individual differences in formation and growth of the eyeball and cornea frequently result in inappropriate image focal formation. If the eyeball is too short from front to back, the image is focused posterior to (in back of) the retina. This is called *hyperopia* or *farsightedness*. In such cases, the accommodative changes of the lens can bring distant images into focus, but near images become blurred. This type of defect is corrected by appropriate biconvex lenses. If the eyeball is too long from front to back, an infinitely distant target is focused anterior to (in front of) the retina. This condition is called *myopia* or *nearsightedness* (see Fig. 41–9). Persons with myopia can see close objects without problems because the accommodative changes in their lens brings near objects into focus, but distant objects are blurred. Myopia can be corrected with an appropriate biconcave lens. Radial keratotomy, a form of refractive corneal surgery, can be performed to correct the defect. This surgical procedure involves the use of radial incisions to alter the corneal curvature.

Refractive defects of the corneal surface do not permit the formation of a sharp image. However, the accommodative reflex continues its unsuccessful attempts to alter the shape of the lens by ciliary muscle contraction to alter the lens shape. The discomfort or pain

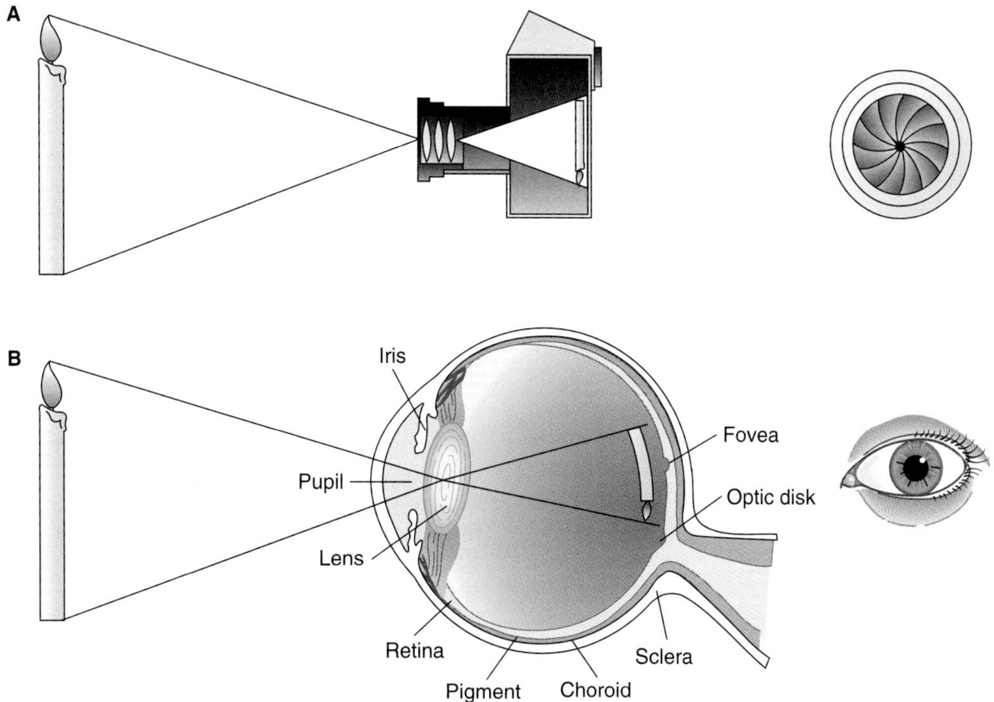

Figure 41–8
Comparison of lens of the eye and camera. (Kandel E.R., Schwartz J.H., Jessel T.M. [1991]. *Principles of neural science* [3rd ed.]. New York: Elsevier.)

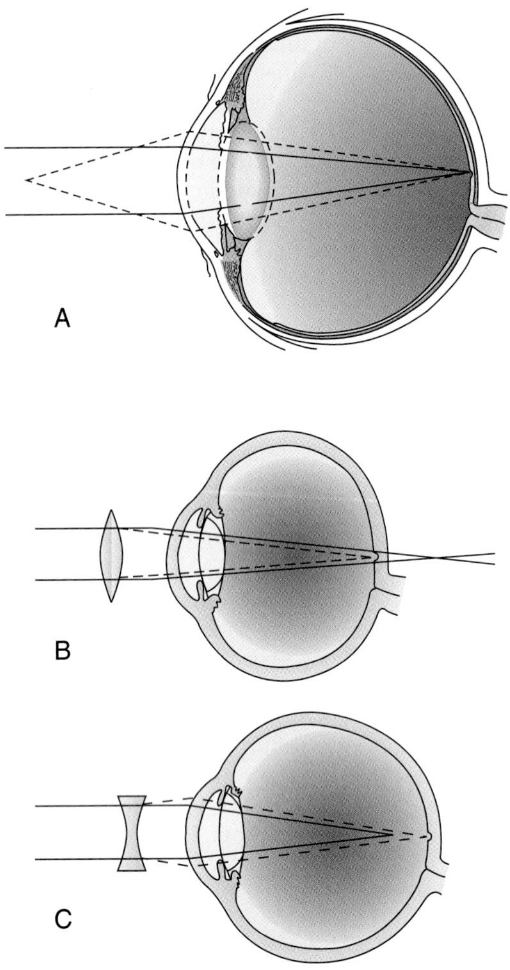

Figure 41–9
(**A**) Accommodation. The *solid lines* represent rays of light from a distant object, and the *dotted lines* represent rays from a near object. The lens is flatter for the former and more convex for the latter. In each case the rays of light are brought to a focus on the retina. (**B**) Hyperopia corrected by a biconvex lens, as shown by the *dotted lines.* (**C**) Myopia corrected by a biconcave lens, shown by the *dotted lines.*

associated with continuous muscle contraction is experienced as eyestrain. Nonuniform curvature of the refractive medium (*e.g.*, horizontal plane vs vertical plane) is called *astigmatism*. Astigmatism usually is the result of a defect in the cornea, but it can result from defects in the lens or the retina. Spherical aberration, another refractive error, involves a cornea with nonspherical surfaces. Lens correction is available for both these refractive errors.

Accommodation

Accommodation is the process whereby a clear image is maintained as gaze is shifted from a far to a near object. It requires convergence of the eyes, pupillary constriction, and thickening of the lens through contraction of the ciliary muscle. Accommodation is under the control of the parasympathetic portion of the oculomotor (III) cranial nerve. The cell bodies of this nerve are contained in the oculomotor nuclear complex located in the midbrain, and its preganglionic axons synapse with postganglionic neurons of the ciliary ganglion in the orbit. The postganglionic axons enter the back of the eye and travel in the choroid layer to the ciliary muscle fibers.

Visual function must be present to evaluate and adjust the clarity of the image. Accommodation depends on the functional integrity of the entire visual system, including the forebrain and midbrain circuitry. Accommodation does not occur during sleep. An absolutely blind person cannot accommodate, nor can a person in a coma.

Disorders of Accommodation. Paralysis of the ciliary muscle and thereby of accommodation is called *cycloplegia.* Pharmacologic cycloplegia is sometimes necessary to facilitate ophthalmoscopic examination of the fundus of the eye, especially in small children who are unable to hold a steady fixation during the examination. The lens shape is totally under the control of the pretectal region and parasympathetic pathways by way of the oculomotor nerve to the ciliary muscle. Accommodation is lost with destruction of this pathway.

Presbyopia is a change in the lens that occurs as a result of aging. The lens consists of transparent fibers arranged in concentric layers, of which the external layers are the newest and softest. There is no loss of lens fibers with aging. Instead, additional fibers are added to the outermost portion of the lens. As the lens ages, it thickens, and its fibers become less elastic, so that the range of focus or accommodation is diminished to the point where reading glasses become necessary for near vision.

Retina

Function and Organization

The function of the retina is to receive visual images, partially analyze them, and transmit this modified information to the brain. It is composed of two layers: the outer melanin-containing layer and the inner neural layer. The light-sensitive neural retina covers the inner aspect of the eyeball. A non–light-sensitive portion of the retina, along with the retinal pigment epithelium, continues anteriorly to form the posterior surface of the iris. The wavy border where the light sensitive and the non–light-sensitive retina meet is called the *ora serrata.* The single pigment layer is separated from the vascular portion of the choroid by a thin layer of elastic tissue, Bruch's membrane, which contains collagen fibrils in its superficial and deep portions. The cells of the pigmented layer receive their nourishment by diffusion from the choroid vessels. The tight junctions that join the endothelial cells of the retinal blood vessels form a blood–retina barrier.

The neural retina is composed of three layers of neurons: a posterior layer of photoreceptors, a middle layer of bipolar cells, and an inner layer of ganglion cells that communicate with the photoreceptors. A superficial marginal layer contains the axons of the ganglion cells as they collect and leave the eye by way of the optic nerve (Fig. 41–10). These fibers lie adjacent to the vitreous humor. The interneurons, composed of horizontal and amacrine cells, have cell bodies in the bipolar layer, and they play an important role in modulating retinal function. Light must pass through the transparent inner layers of the sensory retina before it reaches the photoreceptors.

Photoreceptors

There are two types of photoreceptors: rods, capable of black-white discrimination, and cones, capable of color discrimination. Both types of photoreceptors are thin, elongated, mitochondria-filled cells with a single, highly modified cilium (see Fig. 41–10). The cilium has a short base, or inner segment, and a highly modified outer segment. The plasma membrane of the outer segment is highly folded to form membranous disks (rods) or conical shapes (cones) containing visual pigment. These disks are continuously synthesized at the base of the outer segment and shed at the distal end. The discarded membranes are phagocytized by the retinal pigment cells. If this phagocytosis is disrupted, as in retinitis pigmentosa (see Chapter 42), the sensory retina degenerates.

Rods. Photoreception involves the transduction of light energy into an altered ionic membrane potential of the rod cell. Light passing through the eye penetrates the nearly transparent neural elements to produce decomposition of the photochemical substance (*i.e.*, visual pigment) called *rhodopsin* in the outer segment of the rod. Light that is not trapped by a rhodopsin molecule is absorbed by the retinal pigment melanin or the more superficial choroid melanin. Rhodopsin consists of a protein called opsin and a vitamin A–derived pigment called *retinal*. During light stimulation, rhodopsin is broken down into its component parts, opsin and retinal; retinal is subsequently converted into vitamin A. The reconstitution of rhodopsin occurs during total darkness; vitamin A is transformed into retinal, and then opsin and retinal combine to form rhodopsin. Because there are considerable stores of vitamin A in the retinal pigment cells and in the liver, a vitamin A deficiency must exist for weeks or months to have an impact on the photoreceptive process. Reduced sensitivity to light, a symptom of vitamin A deficiency, first affects night vision and is quickly reversed by injection or ingestion of the vitamin.

A pattern of light on the retina falls on a massive array of photoreceptors. These photoreceptors communicate with bipolar and other interneurons before action potentials in ganglion cells relay the message to specific regions of the brain and the brain stem associated with vision. For rods, this microcircuitry involves the convergence of signals from many rods on a single ganglion cell. This arrangement maximizes spatial summation and the detection of stimulated (light versus dark) receptors. Rod-based vision is particularly sensitive to detecting light, especially moving light stimuli, at the expense of clear pattern discrimination. Rod vision is particularly adapted for night and low-level illumination.

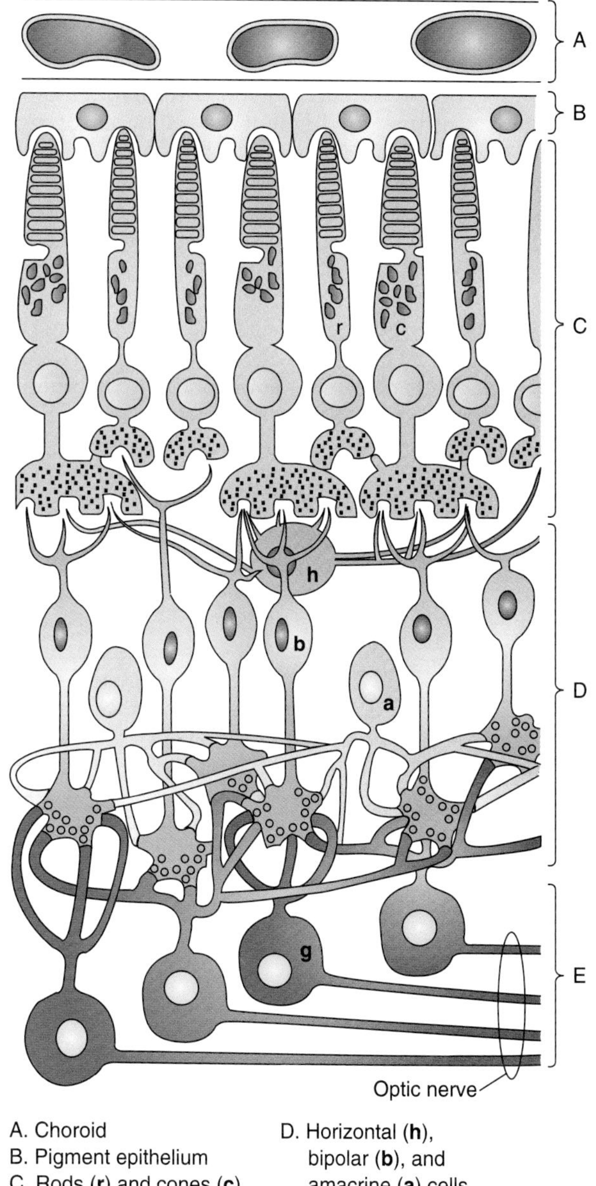

Figure 41–10
Organization of the human retina. The various layers are described in the text. (Modified from Dowling J.F., Boycott B.B. [1966]. Organization of the primate retina: Electron microscopy. *Proceedings of the Royal Society of London* 166, 80–111.)

Dark adaptation is the process by which rod sensitivity increases to the optimum level. This requires approximately 4 hours in total or near-total darkness and involves only rod receptor (black and white) vision. During daylight or high-intensity bombardment the concentration of vitamin A increases, and the concentration of the photopigment retinal decreases. During dark adaptation, increased synthesis of retinal from vitamin A results in a higher concentration of rhodopsin available to capture light energy.

Cones and Color Sensitivity. Cone receptors that are selectively sensitive to different wavelengths of light provide the basis for color vision. Three types of cones, or cone-color systems, respond to the blue, green, and red portions of the visible electromagnetic spectrum. This selectivity reflects the presence of one of three color-sensitive molecules to which the photochemical substance (*i.e.,* visual pigment) is bound. The decomposition and reconstitution of the cone visual pigments are believed to be similar to that of the rods. The color a person perceives depends on which set of cones or combination of sets of cones is stimulated in a given image.

Cones do not have the dark adaptation of rods. Consequently, the dark-adapted eye is a rod receptor eye with only black-gray-white experience (*i.e., scotopic vision*). The light-adapted eye (*i.e., photopic vision*) adds the capacity for color discrimination. Rhodopsin has its maximum sensitivity in the blue-green region of the electromagnetic spectrum. If red lenses are worn in daylight, the red cones (and green cones to some extent) are in use; the rods and blue cones are essentially in the dark, and therefore the dark adaptation proceeds. This method is used by military and night-duty airport control tower personnel to allow adaptation to take place before they go on duty in the dark.

Macula and Fovea. An area approximately 1.5 mm in diameter near the center of the retina, called the *macula lutea* (*i.e.,* yellow spot), is especially capable of acute and detailed vision. This area is composed entirely of cones. In the central portion of the macula, the *fovea centralis* (*i.e.,* foveola), the blood vessels and innermost layers are displaced to one side instead of resting on top of the cones (Fig. 41–11). This allows light to pass unimpeded to the cones without passing through several layers of retina. The density of cones drops off rapidly away from the fovea. There are no rods in the fovea, but their numbers increase as the cones decrease in density toward the periphery of the retina. Many cones are connected on a one-to-one basis with ganglion cells. Retinal microcircuitry for cones emphasizes the detection of edges. This type of circuitry favors high acuity. A concentration of acuity-favoring cones at the fovea supports the use of this part of the retina for fine analysis of focused central vision.

Color Blindness. Color blindness is a misnomer for a condition in which persons appear to confuse, mismatch, or experience reduced acuity for color discrimination. Such persons are often unaware of their defect until they attempt to discriminate between red and green traffic lights or demonstrate difficulty matching colors. Most often the result of genetic factors, the deficit can result from the defective function of one or more of the three

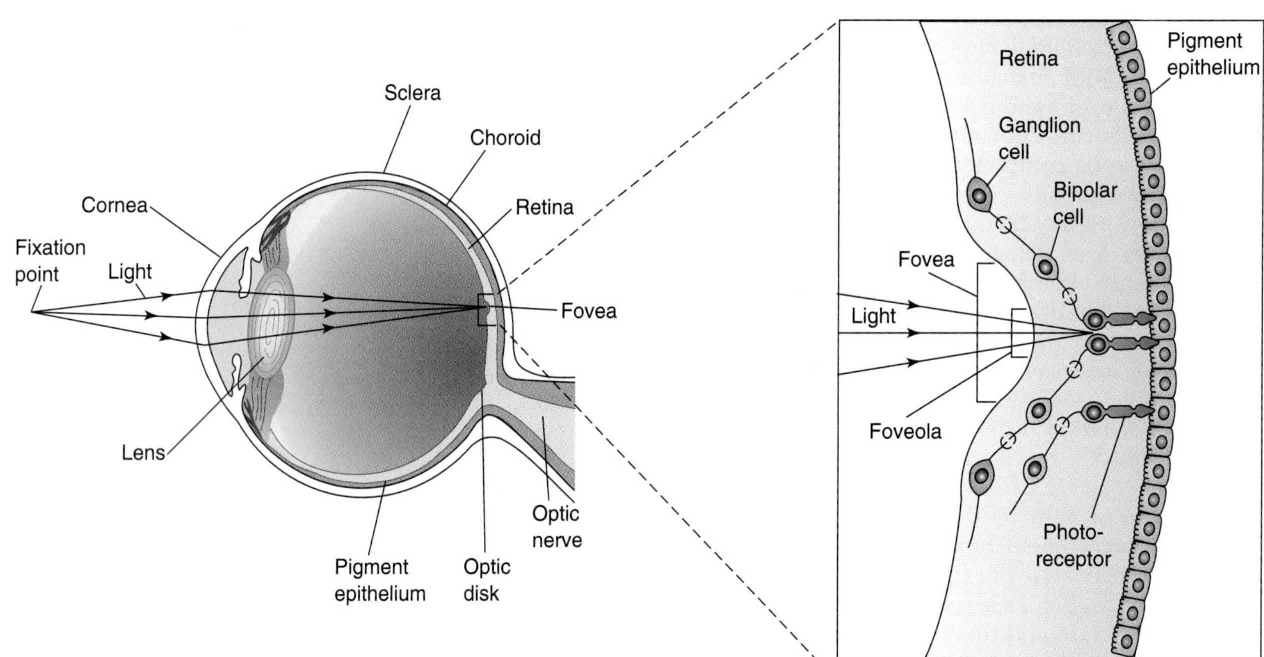

Figure 41–11
Location of fovea in the retina. (Kandel E.R., Schwartz J.H., Jessel T.M. [1991]. *Principles of neural science* [3rd ed.]. New York: Elsevier.)

color-cone mechanisms. The deficiency is usually partial but can be complete. Rarely are two of the color mechanisms missing. When this does occur, usually red and green are missing. Persons with no color mechanisms are rare. For them, the world is experienced entirely as black, gray, and white.

The genetically color-blind person has never experienced the full range of normal color vision and is unaware of what he or she is missing. Color discrimination is necessary for everyday living, and color-blind persons, knowingly or unknowingly, make color discriminations based on other criteria, such as brightness or position. For example, the red light of a traffic signal is always the upper light, and the green is the lower light. The color-blind person gets into trouble when brightness differences are minimal and discrimination must be based on hue and saturation qualities.

The genes responsible for color blindness affect receptor mechanisms rather than central acuity. The gene for red and green mechanisms is sex linked (*i.e.,* on the X chromosomes), resulting in a much higher incidence among males of red, green, or red-green color blindness. The gene affecting the blue mechanism is autosomal. Acquired color defects are more complex but tend to follow a general rule: disease of the more peripheral retina affects blue discrimination, and disease of the more central retina affects red and green discrimination. This is because there are no blue cones in the central fovea.

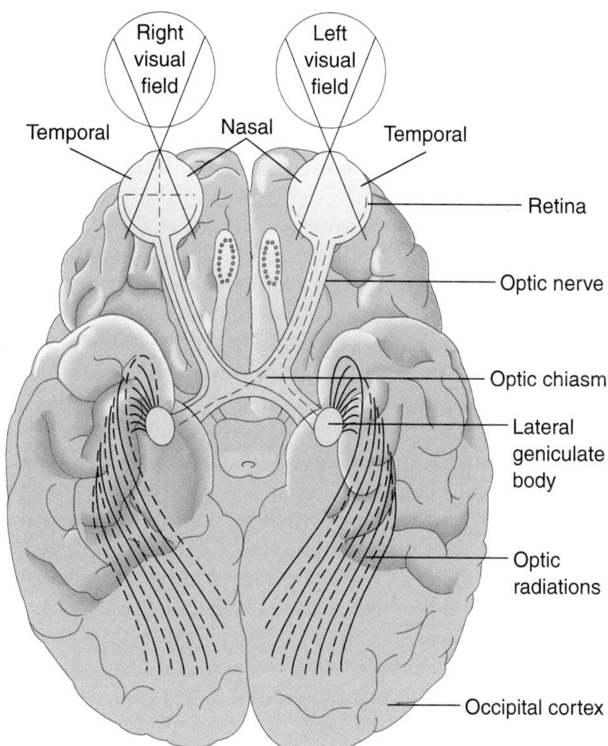

Figure 41–12
Diagram of optic pathways. Note the crossing of fibers from the medial half of each retina.

Neural Pathways and Cortical Centers

Full visual function requires the normally developed brain-related functions of photoreception and pupillary reflex. These functions depend on the integrity of all visual pathways, including retinal circuitry and the pathway from the optic nerve to the visual cortex and other visual regions of the brain and brain stem.

Visual information is carried to the brain by axons of the retinal ganglion cells, which form the optic nerve. Surrounded by pia mater, cerebrospinal fluid, arachnoid, and dura mater, the optic nerve represents an outgrowth of the brain rather than a peripheral nerve. The optic nerve extends from the back of the optic globe through the orbit and the optic foramen, into the middle fossa, and on to the optic chiasm at the base of the brain—a distance of 40 to 50 mm in the adult (Fig. 41–12). Axons from the nasal half of the retina remain medial, and those from the temporal retina remain lateral in the optic nerve.

The two optic nerves meet and fuse at the optic chiasm, located on the ventral and most rostral end of the brain stem, just in front of the infundibular stalk of the pituitary gland. In the optic chiasm, axons from the nasal retina of each eye cross to the contralateral side and travel with the axons of the temporal retina of the contralateral eye to form the optic tracts. One optic tract contains fibers from both eyes that transmit information from the same visual field.

The fibers of the optic tracts move laterally around the cerebral peduncles to synapse in the dorsal lateral geniculate nucleus (LGN) of the thalamus. Axons from these neurons in the LGN form the optic radiations to the primary visual cortex in the calcarine area of the occipital lobe. The LGN receives input from the visual cortex, the oculomotor centers in the brain stem, and the brain stem reticular formation; this input is thought to modify the pattern and strength of the retinal input.

The pattern of information transmission that was established in the optic tract is retained in the optic radiations. For example, the axons from the right visual field, represented by the nasal retina of the right eye and the temporal retina of the left eye, are united at the chiasm and continue through the left optic tract and left optic radiation to the left visual cortex, where visual experience is first perceived. The left primary visual cortex receives two representations of the right visual field. Because the left LGN and the left primary visual cortex retain physical separation of information from the left and right visual fields, interaction between these slightly disparate representations occurs and provides the basis for the sensation of depth in the near visual field.

Visual Cortex

The primary visual cortex (area 17 or V1) surrounds the calcarine fissure, which lies within the occipital lobe. It is at this level that visual sensation is first experienced (Fig. 41–13). Immediately surrounding area 17 (V1) are the visual association cortices (areas 18 [V2, V3, V4] and 19 [V5]) and several other association cortices. These association cortices, together with their thalamic nuclei, must be functional for added meaningfulness of visual perception. This higher-order aspect of the visual experience depends on previous learning.

Approximately 1 million retinal ganglion cell axons pass through the optic nerve and tract to reach the LGN in the thalamus, and more than 100 million axons arising from geniculate neurons provide the input to the billions of neurons in the visual cortex. Here, the spatial representation of the visual field is retained in a distorted retinal map. The proportion of cells of the LGN and of the primary visual area devoted to analysis of the central visual field is greatly expanded compared with that of the peripheral retina. From 80% to 90% of the cellular mass and area of the primary visual cortex is concerned with central vision. This intense level of neural representation supports the high degree of visual activity characteristic of central vision; it exists at the retina and all levels of the visual pathway.

Circuitry in the primary visual cortex and the visual association areas is extremely discrete with respect to the location of retinal stimulation. For example, specific neurons respond to the moving edge of a particular inclination, specific colors, or familiar shapes. This fine-grained organization of the visual cortex, with functionally separate and multiple representations of the same visual field, provides the major basis for visual sensation and perception. Because of this discrete circuitry, lesions of the visual cortex must be large to be detected clinically.

A flash of light delivered to the retina evokes potentials that can be measured and recorded by placing electrodes on the scalp over the occipital lobes. The waves of the evoked potentials, called pattern-reversed-evoked potentials or visual-evoked potentials, have proven to be a useful tool for clinical evaluation of the functional integrity of successive levels of the visual pathway.

Pupillary Reflex

The pupillary reflex, which controls the size of the pupillary opening, is controlled by the autonomic nervous system. The sphincter muscle that produces pupillary constriction is innervated by postganglionic parasympathetic neurons of the ciliary ganglion and other scattered ganglion cells between the scleral and choroid layers (Fig. 41–14). The autonomic portion of the oculomotor (CN III) cranial nerve nucleus (*i.e.*, Edinger-Westphal nucleus), located in the midbrain, provides the preganglionic innervation for these parasympathetic axons. Innervation for the dilator muscle is derived from thoracic sympathetic preganglionic neurons that send axons along the sympathetic chain to innervate the postganglionic neurons in the superior cervical ganglion. The postganglionic neurons send axons along the internal carotid and ophthalmic arteries to the posterior surface of the optic globe. These axons travel between the scleral and choroid layers to reach the dilator muscles of the iris.

The pupillary reflex is controlled by a region in the midbrain called the *pretectum*. The pretectal areas on each side of the brain are connected, accounting for the binocular aspect of the light reflex. These areas project axons to the Edinger-Westphal nuclei of the midbrain, which contain the parasympathetic preganglionic neurons that innervate the ciliary ganglion and control the sphincters of the iris. Midbrain-level evaluation with feedback control provides an automatic brightness control mechanism. The functional importance of this reflex

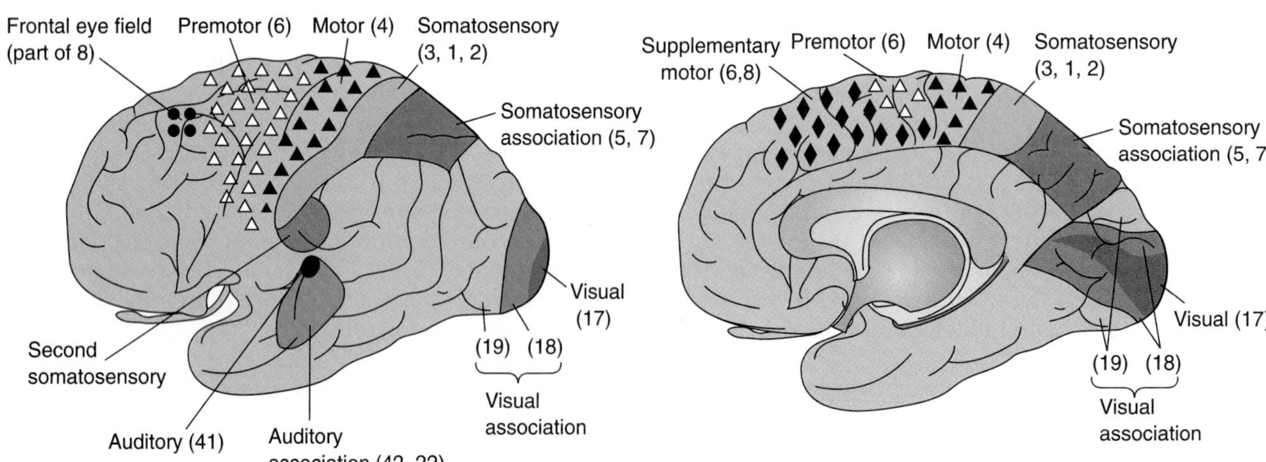

Figure 41–13
Lateral view of the cortex with the lateral sulcus pried open to expose the insula (**left**) and medial view of the cortex (**right**), illustrating the location of the visual, visual association, auditory, and auditory association areas. (Nolte J. [1981]. *The human brain* [p. 271]. St. Louis: C.V. Mosby. Reproduced with permission)

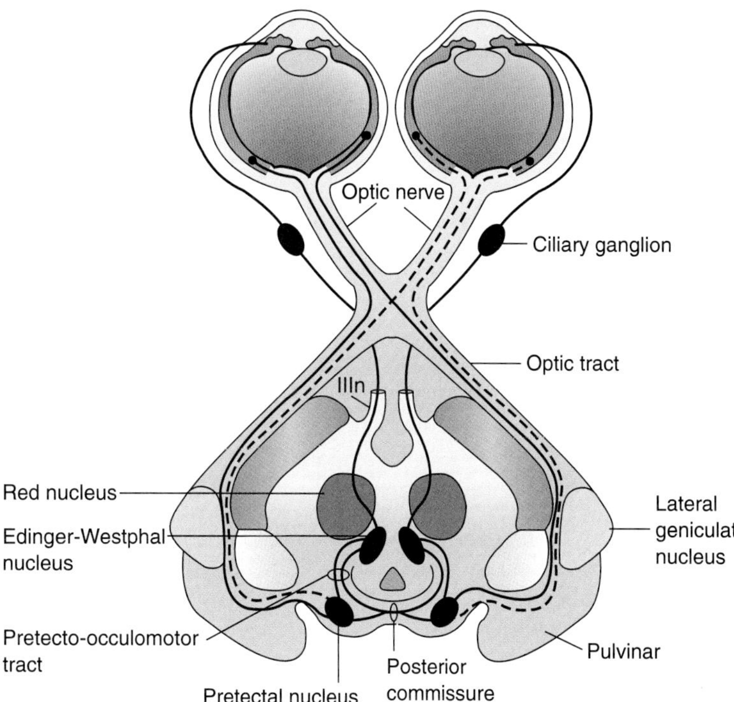

Figure 41–14
Diagram of the path of the pupillary light reflex. (Reproduced with permission from Walsh F.B., Hoyt W.F. [1969]. *Clinical neuro-opthalmology* [3rd ed., vol. 1]. Baltimore: Williams & Wilkins)

mechanism is its rapidity, compared with the slow light and dark-adaptive retinal mechanism.

Visual Fields

The visual field refers to the area that is visible during fixation of vision in one direction. Because visual system deficits are often expressed with reference to the visual field rather than to direct measures of neural function, the terminology for normal and abnormal visual characteristics is usually based on visual field orientation.

Most of the visual field is binocular, or seen by both eyes. This binocular field is subdivided into central and peripheral portions. The central portion of the retina provides high visual acuity and corresponds to the field focused on the central fovea; the peripheral and surrounding portion provides the capacity to detect objects, particularly moving objects. Beyond the visual field shared by both eyes, the left lateral periphery of the visual field is seen exclusively by the left nasal retina, and the right peripheral field is seen by the right nasal retina.

As with a camera, the simple lens system of the eye inverts the image of the external world on each retina. The right and left sides of the visual field are also reversed. The right binocular visual field is seen by the left retinal halves of each eye: the nasal half of the right eye and the temporal half of the left eye.

Once the level of the retina is reached, the nervous system plays a consistent role. The upper half of the visual field is received by the lower half of the retinas of both eyes, and the representations of this upper half of the field are carried in the lower half of each optic nerve to synapse in the lower half of the LGN of each side of the brain. Neurons in this part of the LGN send their axons through the inferior half of the optic radiation, which loops into the temporal lobe to the lower half of the primary visual cortex on each side of the brain. Because of the lateral separation of the two eyes, the visual field as viewed by the two eyes results in a slightly different image of the world by each eye, called *binocular disparity*. Disparity between the laterally displaced images seen by the two eyes provides a powerful source of three-dimensional depth perception for objects within a distance of 30 m. Beyond that distance, the binocular disparity becomes insignificant, and depth perception is based on other cues, such as the superimposition of the image of near objects over that of far objects or the relatively faster movement of near objects than of far objects.

In summary, the optic globe, or eyeball, is a nearly spherical structure protected posteriorly by the bony structures of the orbit and anteriorly by the eyelids. The eye is continuously bathed by a protective layer of tears. The conjunctiva lines the inner surface of the eyelids and covers the optic globe to the junction of the cornea and sclera. The wall of the eye is made up of three layers: an outer fibrous coat that has a white opaque region called the sclera and a transparent window known as the cornea; a highly pigmented middle vascular layer known as the choroid; and an inner neural layer, the retina. The interior of the eye is divided into a smaller fluid-filled anterior cavity and a larger vitreous-filled posterior segment. The anterior segment of the eye is divided into an anterior and posterior chamber, separated by the pupil and closely adjacent lens. Aqueous humor, secreted by the ciliary epithelium, flows through a thin passageway between the lens and iris and then moves through a porous trabeculated region of the sclera into the canal of Schlemm for entry into the venous system.

The function of the eye is similar to a camera; it contains a lens, an aperture for controlling light exposure (*i.e.*, pupil), and the retina, which corresponds to the film and records the image. The lens is a biconvex, avascular, colorless, and almost transparent structure that is suspended behind the iris. It is enclosed within a thin, homogeneous, highly elastic, and carbohydrate-containing lens capsule that is held in place by suspensory ligaments called zonules. The shape of the lens is controlled by the ciliary muscle that contracts and relaxes the zonule fibers to change the tension on the lens capsule, thereby altering the focus of the lens.

Refraction refers to the ability to focus an object on the retina. The refractive properties of the eye depend on the size and shape of the eyeball and the cornea and on the focusing ability of the lens. Errors in refraction occur when the visual image is not focused on the retina because of individual differences in the size or shape of the eyeball or cornea. In hyperopia, or farsightedness, the image falls in back of the retina. In myopia, or nearsightedness, the image falls in front of the retina.

Accommodation is the process whereby a clear image is maintained as the gaze is shifted from a far to a near object. It requires convergence of the eyes, pupillary constriction, and thickening of the lens through contraction of the ciliary muscle. Paralysis of the ciliary muscle and thereby of accommodation is called cycloplegia. The lens shape is totally under the control of the pretectal region and the parasympathetic pathway by way of the oculomotor nerve to the ciliary muscle. Accommodation is lost with the destruction of this pathway. Presbyopia is a change in the lens that occurs as a result of aging such that the lens becomes thicker and less able to change shape and accommodate for near vision.

The retina covers the inner aspect of the posterior two thirds of the eyeball and is continuous with the optic nerve. It contains the photoreceptors for vision: the rods, which are capable of black and white discrimination, and the cones, which are capable of color vision. Visual information is carried to the brain by axons of the retinal ganglion cells forming the optic nerve. The two optic nerves meet and fuse in the optic chiasm. The axons of each nasal retina cross in the chiasm and join the uncrossed fibers from the temporal retina of the opposite eye in the optic tract. From the optic chiasm, the crossed fibers of the nasal retina of one eye and the uncrossed temporal fibers of the eye pass to the LGN and then to the primary visual cortex, which is located in the calcarine fissure of the occipital lobe.

The Ear and Auditory and Vestibular Function

After you have completed this section of the chapter, you should be able to meet the following objectives:

- List the structures of the external, middle, and inner ear and cite their function
- Explain how the frequency and intensity of a tone is transformed into the experience of pitch at a particular loudness
- Explain the function of the vestibular system in terms postural reflexes and maintaining a stable visual field despite marked changes in head position

The ears are paired organs that are responsible for hearing and the maintenance of equilibrium and effective posture. The ear consists of an external ear, a middle ear, and an inner ear. The external and middle ear functions capture, transmit, and amplify sound. The inner ear contains the receptive organs that are selectively stimulated by sound waves (*i.e.*, hearing) or head position and motion (*i.e.*, vestibular function).

The Auditory System

Hearing is a specialized sense that provides the ability to perceive vibration of sound waves. The compression waves that produce sound have frequency and intensity. *Frequency* indicates the rate of change with time (reported in cycles per second [cps] or Hertz [Hz]). Most persons cannot hear compression waves that have a frequency higher than 20,000 Hz. Waves of higher frequency are called ultrasonic waves, meaning that they are above the audible range. In the audible frequency range, the subjective experience correlated with sonic frequency is the pitch of a sound. Waves below 20 to 30 Hz are experienced as a rattle or drum beat rather than a tone. The human ear is most sensitive to waves in the frequency range of 1000 to 3000 Hz.

Wave intensity is represented by amplitude or units of sound pressure. By convention, the *intensity* (in power units, or ergs per square centimeter) of a sound is expressed as the ratio of intensities between the sound and a reference value. A 10-fold increase in sound pressure is called a *bel*, after Alexander Graham Bell. This representation often is too crude to be of use; the most often used unit is the decibel (db), or one tenth of a bel. In the normal sonic environment, about 1 db of increased intensity (loudness) can be detected. The region of audible speech sounds falls between 42 and 70 db.

The ear receives sound waves, distinguishes their frequency, translates this information into nerve impulses, and transmits them to the central nervous system (CNS). The auditory system can be divided into five parts: the external ear, the middle ear, the inner ear, auditory brain stem pathways, and the primary and auditory association cortices of the brain's temporal lobe.

External Ear

The external ear is called the *pinna,* or *auricle.* It is supported by elastic cartilage and shaped like a funnel. The funnel shape concentrates high-frequency sound entering from the lateral-forward direction into the *external acoustic meatus,* or *ear canal* (Fig. 41–15). The shape also helps to prevent front-back confusion of sound sources. The anterior portion of the pinna and the external ear canal are innervated by branches of the mandibular division of the trigeminal (CN V) cranial nerve. The posterior portions, including the back of the external ear and the posterior wall of the ear canal, are innervated by auricular branches of the facial (CN VII), glossopharyngeal (CN IX), and vagus (CN X) cranial nerves. Because of the vagal innervation, the insertion of a speculum or an otoscope into the external ear canal can stimulate coughing or vomiting reflexes, particularly in young children.

The external ear canal extends from the auricle to the tympanic membrane, or eardrum. Its outer two thirds is supported by elastic cartilage, and its inner one third is supported by the tympanic bone. It is somewhat S shaped and acts as a resonator, amplifying frequencies around 3500 Hz. A thin layer of skin containing fine hairs, sebaceous glands, and ceruminous glands lines the ear canal. The ceruminous glands secrete cerumen, or earwax, which has certain antimicrobial properties and is thought to serve a protective function.

Middle Ear

The middle ear is a tiny cavity, roughly the shape of a red blood cell set on edge, located in the petrous (stony) temporal bone. Its lateral wall is formed by the tympanic membrane, and its medial wall is formed by the bone dividing the middle and inner ear. Two tissue-covered openings in the medial wall, the oval and the round windows, provide for the transmission of sound waves between the air-filled middle ear and the fluid-filled inner ear. Posteriorly, the middle ear is continuous with small air pockets in the temporal bone called *mastoid air spaces* or *cells* (see Fig. 41–15). In early life, these air spaces are filled with hematopoietic tissue. Replacement of hematopoietic tissue with air sacs begins during the third year of life and is completed at puberty. The *eustachian tube,* or *auditory tube,* connects the middle ear with the nasopharynx. The middle ear is filled with the air that reaches it from the nasopharynx by way of the auditory tube; it is lined with a mucous membrane that is continuous with the pharynx and mastoid air cells.

Three tiny bones, the *auditory ossicles,* are suspended from the roof of the middle ear cavity and connect the tympanic membrane with the oval window (see Fig. 41–15). They are connected by synovial joints and are covered with the epithelial lining of the cavity. The *malleus* (hammer) has its handle firmly fixed to the upper half of the tympanic membrane. The head of the malleus articulates with the *incus* (anvil), which articulates with

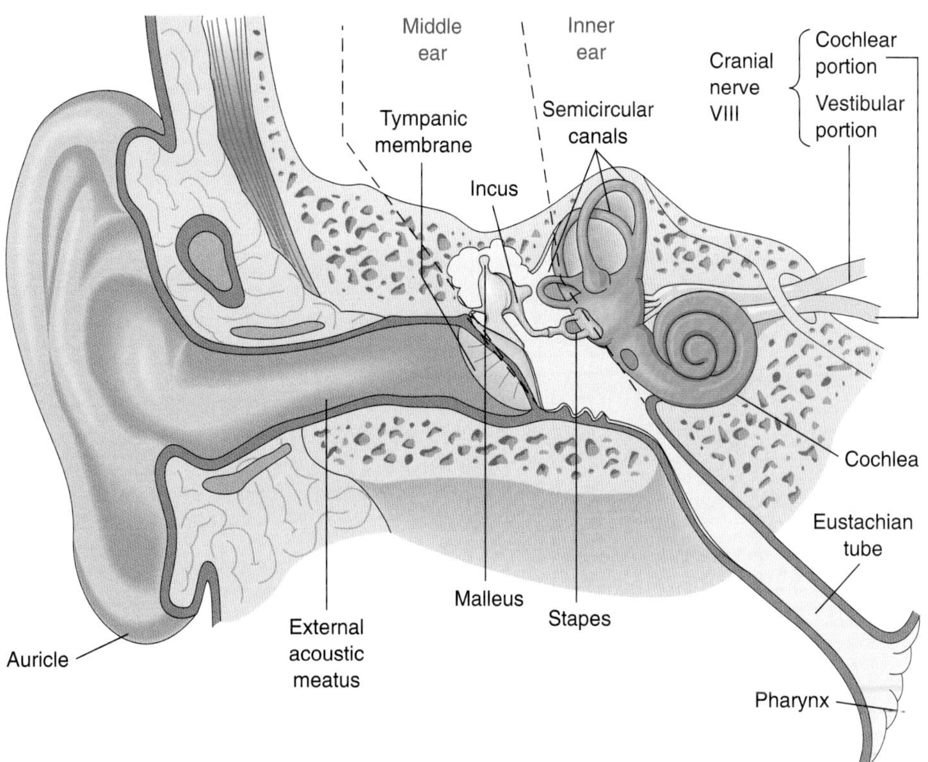

Figure 41–15
External, middle, and internal subdivisions of the ear.

the *stapes* (stirrup), which is inserted and sealed into the oval window by an annular ligament. The ossicles are arranged so that their lever movements transmit vibrations from the tympanic membrane to the oval window and from there to the fluid in the inner ear. It is the pistonlike action of the stapes footplate that sets up compression waves in the inner ear fluid.

Air and liquid offer different degrees of impedance (resistance) to the transmission of sound waves. The bones of the middle ear serve as impedance-matching devices between the low impedance of the air and the high impedance of the cochlear fluid. This matching is accomplished by concentrating the pressure from the large area of the tympanic membrane (43 to 55 mm^2) to the small area of the oval window (about 3 mm^2) and by amplifying the air-transmitted sound waves into the force required to set up compression waves in the fluid of the inner ear. The latter is accomplished by the ossicular lever system, which increases the pressures from the tympanic membrane to the oval window.

Two tiny skeletal muscles, the *tensor tympani* and the *stapedius*, insert into the ossicles. The tensor tympani, which is innervated by the CNV, is positioned in the roof of the auditory tube and inserts on the base of the malleus handle. The functional role of this muscle is in dispute. The stapedius muscle alters the movement of the stapes, reducing the displacement of fluid in the inner ear. Reflex contraction of this muscle by means of the facial nerve, the stapedial reflex, provides a protective mechanism for the delicate inner ear structures when high-intensity sound occurs.

Inner Ear

The inner ear contains a labyrinth, or system of intercommunicating channels, and the receptors for hearing and position sense. The outer bony wall of the inner ear, the bony labyrinth, encloses a thin-walled, membranous duct system, the membranous labyrinth (Fig. 41–16). Two separate fluids are found in the inner ear. A fluid called the *periotic fluid* (*i.e.*, perilymph) separates the bony labyrinth from the membranous labyrinth, and one called the *otic fluid* (*i.e.*, endolymph) fills the membranous labyrinth. The composition of periotic fluid is similar to that of the cerebrospinal fluid (CSF), and a tubular perilymphatic duct connects the periotic fluid with the CSF in the arachnoid space of the posterior fossa. The otic fluid has a potassium content that is similar to intracellular fluid. A small-diameter tubular extension, the endolymphatic sac, connects this system with the subdural space near the jugular foramen, providing an exit for the slowly circulating otic fluid.

The bony labyrinth is divided into a series of perilymph-filled interconnected cavities: the cochlea, the semicircular ducts, the utricle, and the saccule (Fig. 41–17). The membranous labyrinth floats within the bony labyrinth. It is embryologically derived from a delicate ectodermal sac and is made up of a single layer of cuboidal cells. Localized dilations of the membranous labyrinth develop specialized sensory regions of columnar epithelium: the ciliated hair cells of an ampulla of each semicircular canal, the maculae of the utricle and sacculus, and the organ of Corti of the cochlear duct. The cochlea, which contains the auditory receptors, is enclosed in a bony tube shaped like a snail shell that winds around a central bone column called the *modiolus.* The semicircular ducts, the utricle, and the saccule contain the receptors for head position sense. The entire bony labyrinth occupies a volume with a diameter that is less than the size of a dime.

The membranous cochlear duct is a triangular structure that stretches across the cochlea, separating it into two parallel tubes, each containing periotic fluid: the scala vestibuli and the scala tympani. One side of the cochlear duct, the basilar membrane, stretches under ten-

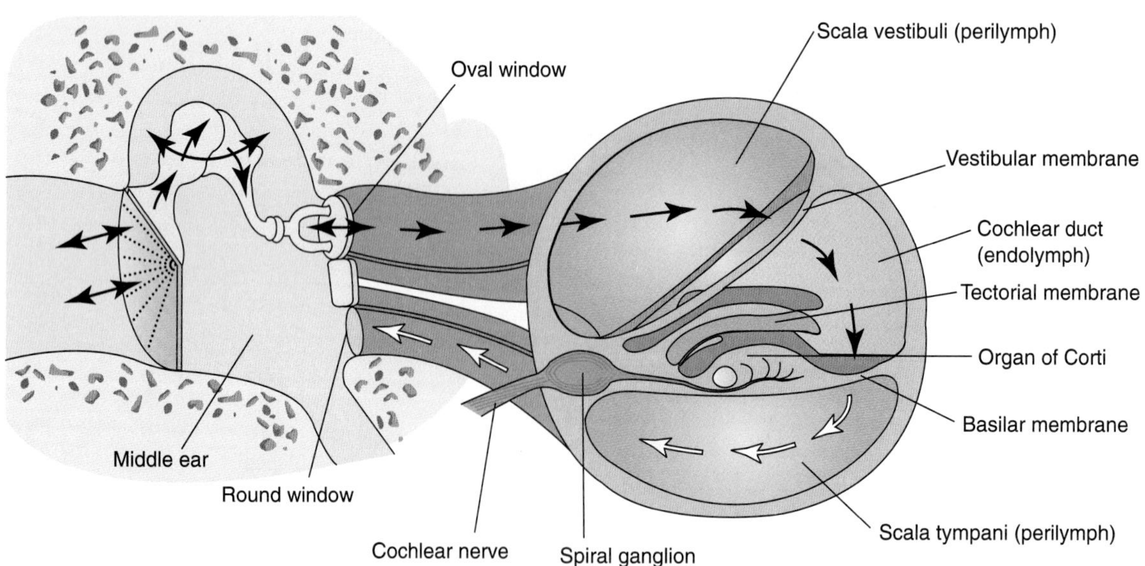

Figure 41–16
Path taken by sound waves reaching the inner ear.

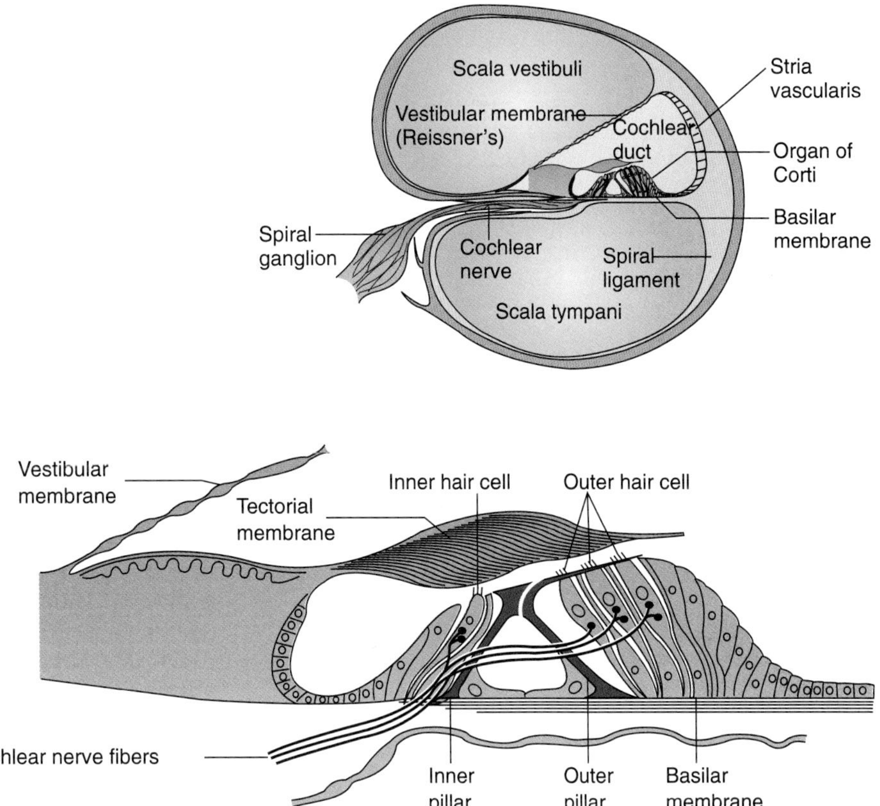

Figure 41–17
(**Top**) Portion of cochlea. Notice the relation of the cochlear duct to the scalae, vestibuli, and tympani. (**Bottom**) Spiral organ of Corti has been removed from the cochlear duct and greatly enlarged.

sion laterally from the modiolus to an elastic spiral ligament. The second side, the vestibular membrane (*i.e.*, Reissner's membrane), is a delicate double layer of squamous epithelial cells. The third side consists of a well-vascularized epithelium, the stria vascularis, which is the source of otic fluid. The cochlear duct separates the scala vestibuli and the scala tympani from the base of the cochlea throughout its two and one-half spiral turns to its apex. An opening at the apex, called the helicotrema, permits fluid waves to move between the two scalae. Sound waves, delivered by the stapes footplate to the periotic fluid, travel throughout the fluid of the inner ear, including up the scala vestibuli, to the apex of the cochlea. The fluid pressure wave results in compensatory displacements of the round window, compressing the air of the middle ear cavity and auditory canal.

The basilar membrane becomes progressively more massive from base to distal apex and resonates to higher frequencies near the base and to lower frequencies toward the apex as the fluid pressure wave travels up the cochlear spiral. This "tuned" aspect of the basilar membrane results in increased amplitude of displacement at the resonant locations, responding to a particular sound frequency and greater firing of cochlear neurons innervating this region. This mechanism provides the major basis for the discrimination of sound frequency.

Perched on the basilar membrane and extending along its entire length is the organ of Corti, an elaborate arrangement of columnar epithelium. Continuous rows of hair cells separated into inner and outer rows can be found within the cell arrangement. The cells have hairlike cilia that protrude through openings in an overlying supporting reticular membrane into the endolymph of the cochlear duct. A gelatinous mass, the tectorial membrane, extends from the medial side of the duct to enclose the cilia of the outer hair cells. The traveling compression waves moving from base to apex through the periotic fluid distort the organ of Corti, causing the hairs to be bent against the less flexible tectorial membrane. Each inner hair cell is innervated by several nerve fibers and the outer hair cells by many cochlear afferent neuron terminals.

Several theories exist about the mechanism for transduction of mechanical sound into afferent nerve signals. The bending of the hair cells in the organ of Corti due to the vibrational effects of sound waves and the effects of two fluids of slightly different ionic content, the periotic fluid and the otic fluid, on nerve impuse generation, probably contribute. It is generally agreed that the inner rows of hair cells, transducing different frequencies, are arranged sequentially with those transducing the higher tones located on the lower (basal) end of the cochlear duct and those transducing lower tones located near its apex (Fig. 41–18). Selective destruction of hair cells in a

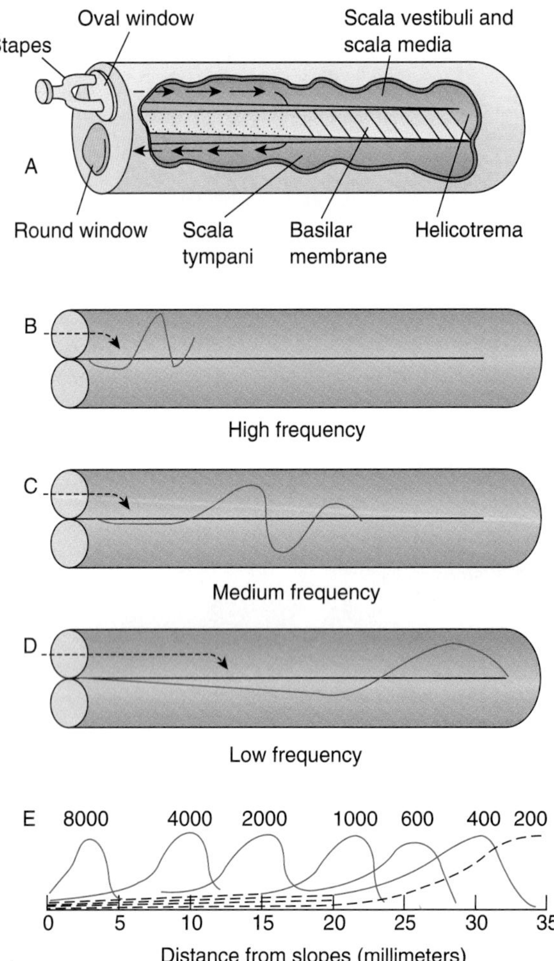

Figure 41–18
(**Top**) Movement of fluid in the cochlea after forward thrust of the stapes. (**A,B,C**) "Traveling waves" along the basilar membrane for high-, medium-, and low-frequency sounds. (**D**) Amplitude pattern of vibration of the basilar membrane for a medium-frequency sound. Amplitude patterns for sounds of all frequencies between 200 and 8000 per second, showing the points of maximum amplitude (the resonance points) on the basilar membrane for the different frequencies. (Modified from Guyton A.C., Hall J.E. [1996]. *Textbook of medical physiology* [9th ed., pp. 665–666]. Philadelphia: W.B. Saunders)

particular segment of the cochlea can lead to hearing loss of particular tones. The outer rows of hair cells appear to provide the signals on which the experience of sound loudness, a correlate of sound physical intensity, is based.

Neural Pathways

Afferent fibers from the organ of Corti have their cell bodies in the spiral ganglion in the central portion of the cochlea. Nerve fibers from the spiral ganglion (*i.e.*, vestibulocochlear, or auditory, nerve [VIII]) travel to the cochlear nuclei located in the caudal pons (Fig. 41–19). Many of the secondary nerve fibers from the cochlear nuclei pass to the opposite side of the pons. These secondary fibers may project to cell groups called the trapezoid, the superior olivary nucleus, or rostrally toward the inferior colliculus of the midbrain. Ipsilateral projections and interconnections between the nuclei of the two sides occur throughout the central auditory system. Consequently, impulses from either ear are transmitted through the auditory pathways to both sides of the brain stem.

A number of reflexes, initiated by sound stimuli, involve the central auditory pathways in the brain stem. Very-high-intensity sound results in a protective stapedial reflex by which the movement of the middle ear ossicular chain is dampened, and this involves the trapezoid nuclei. Analysis of the direction of the sound based on comparison of the timing and intensity of the stimuli reaching the two ears initially occurs in the superior olivary nuclei. Sudden, intense sounds result in the auditory startle reflex in which the eyes, head, and body are suddenly turned toward the source, the ipsilateral shoulder is flexed, the elbow is extended, and body support is shifted to the contralateral leg. The heart rate rapidly increases, the skin blanches, the pupils dilate, and respiration stops momentarily. This startle response pattern involves the inferior colliculi, where the directional responses are organized. The trapezoid nuclei have extensive connections with the brain stem respiratory and cardiovascular centers, providing the linkage to the alarm aspects of the startle reflex.

From the inferior colliculus, the auditory pathway passes to the medial geniculate nucleus of the thalamus, where all the fibers synapse. Considerable evidence supports the capability of this level of organization to provide crude auditory experience, including crude tone and intensity discrimination and the directionality of a sound source. From the medial geniculate nucleus, the auditory tract spreads by way of the auditory radiation to the primary auditory cortex (area 41) located mainly in the superior temporal gyrus and insula (see Fig. 41–13). This area and its corresponding higher-order thalamic nucleus are required for high-acuity loudness discrimination and for precise discrimination of pitch. The auditory association cortex (areas 42 and 22) borders the primary cortex on the superior temporal gyrus. This area and its associated high-order thalamic nuclei are necessary for auditory gnosis, or the meaningfulness of sound, to occur. Experience and the precise analysis of momentary auditory information are integrated during this process.

The Vestibular System

The vestibular receptive organs, which are located in the inner ear, and their CNS connections contribute to the reflex activity necessary for effective posture and movement in a physical world governed by momentum and a gravitational field. Because the vestibular apparatus is part of the inner ear and located in the head, it is head motion and acceleration that are sensed. The vestibular system serves two general and related functions. It maintains and assists recovery of stable body and head position through control of postural reflexes, and it maintains a stable visual field despite marked changes in head position.

Peripheral Vestibular Structures

The peripheral apparatus of the vestibular system is contained within the bony labyrinth of the inner ear adjacent to and continuous with the cochlea of the auditory system. The vestibular apparatus is divided into five prominent structures: three semicircular ducts, a utricle, and a saccule (Fig. 41–20). The receptors of these structures are differentiated into the angular acceleration-deceleration receptors of the semicircular ducts and the linear acceleration-deceleration and static gravitational receptors of the utricle and saccule. The utricle and saccule are two widened membranous sacs within the bony vestibule. The utricle connects the ends of each semicircular duct. The saccule communicates with the utricle through a small duct and with the cochlear duct of the auditory apparatus through the ductus reuniens.

Small patches of hair cells are located in the floor of the utricle (*i.e.,* utricular macula), in the side wall of the saccule (*i.e.,* saccular macula), at the base of each semicircular duct (*i.e.,* cristae), and along the floor of the cochlear duct (*i.e.,* organ of Corti; Fig. 41–21). Each hair cell has several microvilli and one true cilium called a *kinocilium.* At the apical end of each inner hair cell is a projecting bundle of rodlike structures called *stereocilia.* Ganglion cells, homologous with dorsal root ganglion cells, form three afferent ganglia: the superior vestibular ganglion, which innervates the hair cells of the utricular macula and the cristae of the superior and horizontal semicircular ducts; the inferior vestibular ganglion, which innervates the saccular macula and the cristae of the inferior semicircular duct; and the spiral, or acoustic, ganglion, which innervates the cochlear duct. The central axons of these ganglion cells become the superior and inferior vestibular nerves and the cochlear auditory nerve. They often are collectively called the *eighth cranial nerve,* and they enter the side of the nearby medullary-pontine junction of the brain stem. The axons of the vestibular nerves terminate in the four vestibular nuclei (*i.e.,* superior, lateral, medial, and inferior vestibular nuclei).

Semicircular Ducts

The three semicircular ducts, each about two thirds of a circle, are arranged at right angles to one another, with the horizontal duct tilted at about 12 degrees above the normal horizontal plane of the head (see Fig.41–20). The horizontal ducts on the two sides of the head are in the same plane and the superior (anterior) duct of one side is parallel with the inferior (posterior) duct on the other side, and the two function as a pair. Near its junction with the utricle, each semicircular duct has an en-

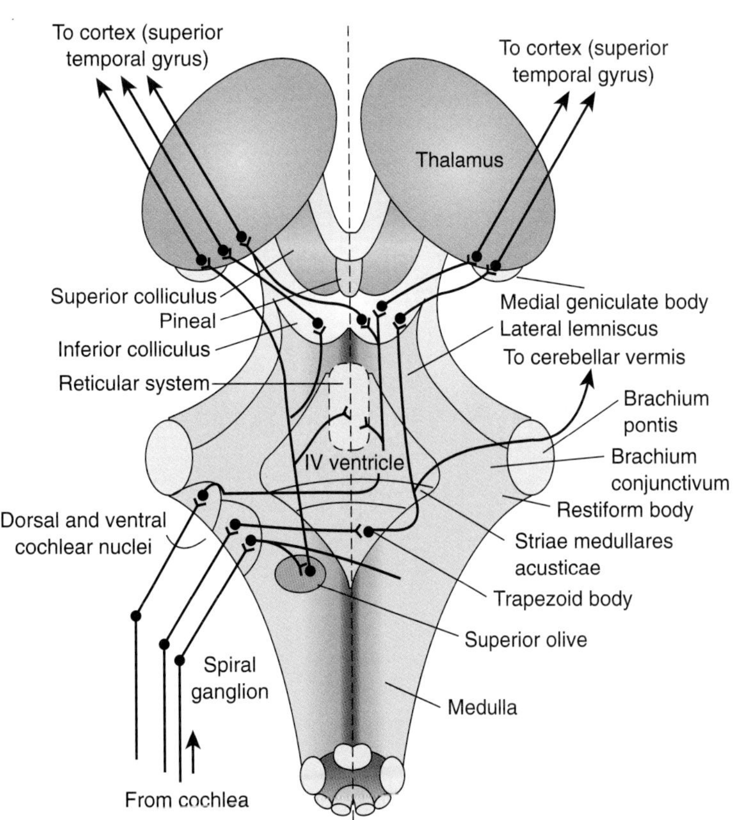

Figure 41–19
Simplified diagram of the main auditory pathways superimposed on a dorsal view of the brain stem. The cerebellum and cerebral cortex were removed. (Reproduced with permission from Ganong W. [1975]. *Review of medical physiology* [7th ed.]. Los Altos, CA: Lange)

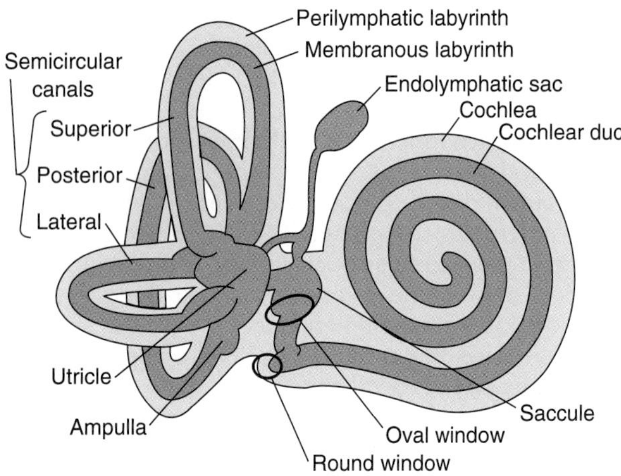

Figure 41–20
The labyrinth of the inner ear, showing the semicircular canals and the utricle and saccule, organs devoted to the sensation of rotary motion and static position. (Rhoades R.A., Tanner G.A. [1996]. *Medical physiology* [p. 83]. Boston: Little, Brown)

largement, called the *ampulla*. Each ampulla contains a hair cell sensory surface raised into a crest, or crista, at right angles to the duct. The stereocilia of each hair cell extend into a flexible gelatinous mass, called the *cupula*, which essentially closes off fluid flow through the semicircular ducts.

When the head begins to rotate around the axis of a semicircular duct (*i.e.*, undergoes angular acceleration), the momentum of the otic fluid causes an increase in pressure to be applied to one side of the cupula. This is similar to the lagging behind of the water in a glass that is suddenly rotated, except that the otic fluid cannot flow past the cupula and instead applies a differential pressure to its two sides, bending it and the stereocilia of the hair cells. All of the hair cells face in the same direction; when the stereocilia are bent toward the kinocilium, the frequency of action potentials in the primary afferent vestibular neuron leaving the ampulla is increased. Bending in the other direction decreases the action potential frequency. Action potentials in the vestibular afferents are transmitted past the vestibular ganglia through the vestibular cranial nerve (CN VIII) to the vestibular nuclei of the caudal pons.

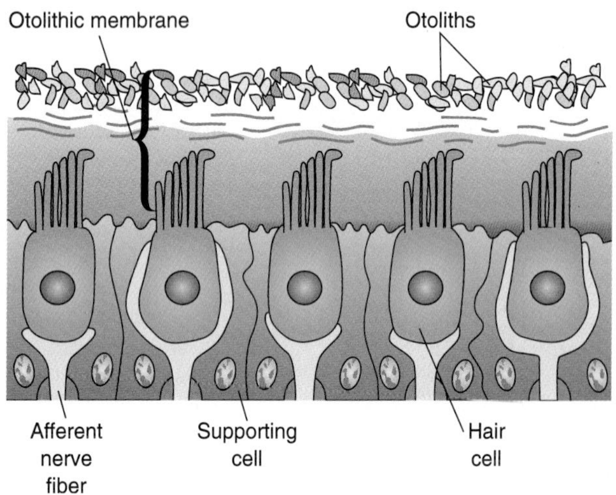

Figure 41–21
The relation of the otoliths to the sensory cells in the macula of the utricle and saccule. (Adapted from Selkurt F.D. [Ed.] [1982]. *Basic physiology for the health sciences* [2nd ed.]. Boston: Little, Brown)

Maximal stimulation of the afferents of a semicircular duct results when rotation of the head occurs exactly in the plane of the membranous duct. Because of the orientation of the three semicircular ducts, angular accelerations of the head result in action potentials in at least one and usually more than one of the vestibular nerve branches to the three cristae. If the angular acceleration reduces to a steady angular velocity, friction between the otic fluid and the duct wall gradually results in a reduction of pressure and then in a loss of differential pressure on the two sides of the cupula—a form of sensory adaptation. On sudden reduction or cessation of head rotation, the momentum of the otic fluid applies pressure on the cupula from the opposite direction. The semicircular duct system provides a mechanism for signaling the direction and rate of accelerations and decelerations in head rotation to the CNS.

Utricle and Saccule

The hair cell surface (*i.e.*, macula) of the utricle is oriented approximately in the horizontal plane. The macula of the saccule is oriented in the vertical plane. In both instances, the stereocilia of the hair cells extend into a gelatinous mass within the otic fluid. Myriad microscopic crystals of calcium carbonate and calcium phosphate, called *otoliths*, are embedded in this gelatinous material, adding considerably to its total mass. The gelatinous mass with its otoliths is called the *otolithic membrane*. When the head is tilted, the gelatinous mass shifts its position because of the pull of the gravitational field, bending the stereocilia of the macular hair cells. Although each hair cell becomes hyperpolarized (*i.e.*, less excitable) or hypopolarized (*i.e.*, more excitable) depending on the direction in which the cilia are bending, the hair cells are oriented in all directions, making these sense organs sensitive to static or changing head position in relation to the gravitational field. The central connections from the maculae provide the mechanism by which head, body, and eye postural adjustments occur in response to tilting the head and by which a stable visual fixation point of the optic field, as well as postural support of a stable head position, is maintained. Projections to the forebrain provide the basis for sensations of head tilt away from the horizontal plane.

In addition to this rather static tilt reception function, the utricle and saccule provide linear acceleration and deceleration reception. When the head is accelerated in a linear manner, such as the initial or terminal phase of an elevator ride or during automobile acceleration or deceleration, differential movement between the head and the otolithic membranes provides the basis for reflex compensatory bracing of neck, trunk, and limbs. The utricle and saccule also provide the input data on which the air-righting reflexes are based. A cat dropped from an upside-down position lands on its feet and does so even if blindfolded. Most vestibular reflexes, including air-righting, are functional at birth. If a neonate is supported in the prone position and the support is momentarily (and with great care) removed, the trunk is extended and all four limbs are extended as falling begins. In the supine position, the trunk is flexed and the limbs are flexed as the fall progresses. However, the head-on-body vestibular reflexes of the infant are not sufficiently operational during the first 6 weeks or so after birth to maintain head posture. This is why the neonate's head must be supported when the neonate is lifted in the supine position.

Neural Pathways

The nerve fibers from the vestibular receptors travel in the vestibular portion of the vestibulocochlear nerve (CN VIII) to the superior, medial, lateral, and inferior vestibular nuclei located at the junction of the medulla and pons (Fig. 41–22). Primary vestibular afferent axons project to two areas of the cerebellar cortex: the midline, or vermis, and the flocculus. The vermis projection contributes to head, body, and limb coordination by providing constant information on head position with reference to gravity and of linear or angular head velocity or acceleration. The floccular projection is part of the network that provides adaptability to the system, such as compensation for asymmetric function of unilateral damage.

Medial Longitudinal Fasciculus. A fiber tract called the *medial longitudinal fasciculus* (MLF) extends from the midbrain to the upper part of the spinal cord; it lies close to the medial plane and connects the vestibular nuclei with motor nuclei, particularly those of cranial nerves III, IV, VI, and XI. In addition to complex internal circuitry, neurons from the vestibular nuclei project into the nearby reticular formation and provide powerful control on postural reflexes of the eyes, head, body, and limbs. Projections extend into the pons lateral gaze control center, to the vertical and torsional gaze control regions, to the sixth cranial nerve nuclei, to the MLF, to the fourth and third nerve nuclei, and to cervical-level lower motoneurons (LMNs) innervating the sternocleidomastoid and other neck muscles that control head turning and posture. The MLF projections primarily control horizontal or lateral turning and conjugate gaze. Extensive projections into and through the reticular formation follow the central tegmental fasciculus pathway that controls the vertical and rotatory (torsion) gaze reflexes.

The term *nystagmus* is used to describe the involuntary rhythmic and oscillatory eye movements that preserve eye fixation on stable objects in the visual field during angular and rotational movements of the head. These vestibular-controlled eye movements are initiated by impulses generated by the movement of the otic fluid

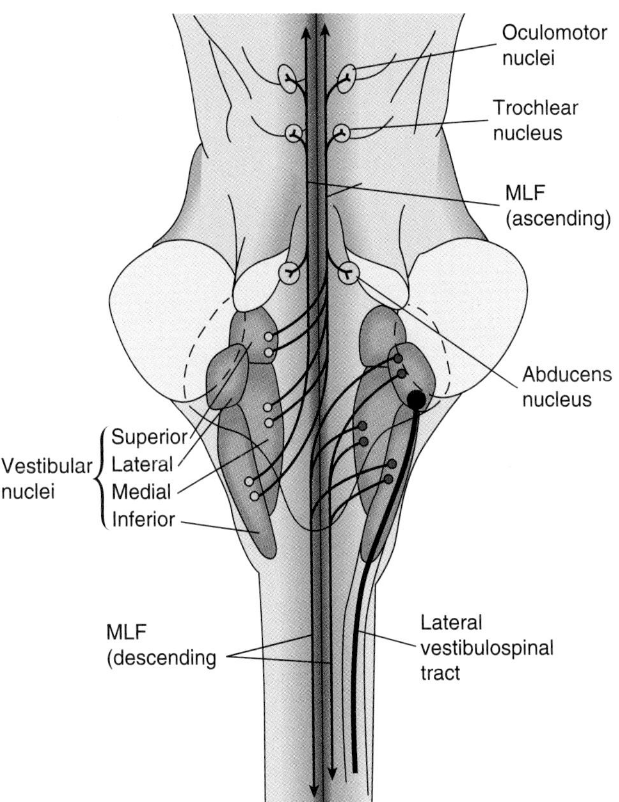

Figure 41–22 ■■■
The ascending (*left*) and descending (*right*) vestibular pathways. Ipsilateral inhibitory and contralateral excitatory ascending projections from the vestibular nuclei course through the medial longitudinal fasciculus (MLF) and target motor neurons in the abducens, trochlear, and oculomotor nuclei. The ascending connections mediate the vestibulo-ocular reflex. Bilateral descending fibers in the MLF project primarily to motor neurons in the cervical spinal cord that innervate the dorsal neck muscles, forming the basis for the vestibulocollic reflex. The lateral vestibulospinal tract arises from the lateral vestibular nuclei and descends ipsilaterally in the spinal cord, targeting primarily motor neurons that innervate axial extensor muscles that maintain posture.

within the semicircular ducts, transmitted to the vestibular nuclei, and relayed through the MLF to the appropriate motor nuclei for the extraocular muscles controlling conjugate eye movement. As the body and head begin rotation, the eyes in a conjugate manner move in exactly the opposite direction, maintaining the previous fixation point (Fig. 41–23). This is called the slow phase of nystagmus. If the rotation continues beyond the range of lateral eye movement, a quick (*i.e.*, rapid phase of nystagmus) conjugate eye correction (*i.e.*, saccadic return) occurs as if to obtain a new stable fixation point, and then the slow phase continues again. This nystagmus pattern continues as long as angular acceleration continues. When a steady rotational velocity is reached, compensatory nystagmus movements gradually wane as the disparity between the movement of endolymph and the semicircular duct wall is lost and the pressure on the two sides of the cupula is

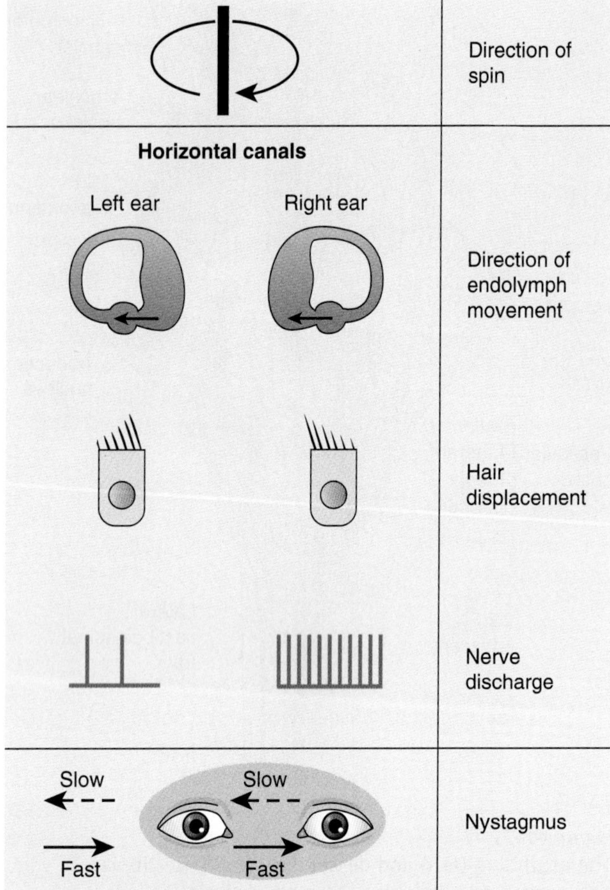

Figure 41–23
Effect of spinning a subject clockwise. (Sekurt F.E. [1982]. *Basic physiology for the health professions* [2nd ed., p. 140]. Boston: Little, Brown)

equalized. Clinically, the direction of nystagmus is named for the fast, or saccadic phase. The reflex circuitry is in precise control of motor units in the nuclei that innervate the extrinsic eye muscles by way of cranial nerves III, IV, and VI. The precision of nystagmus movements is as great in persons whose eyes are closed and in the congenitally blind as normal-sighted persons. If the eyes are not allowed to move, or if stimulation is strong, the head also moves in a nystagmoid manner as a result of vestibular control of the sternocleidomastoid muscles by cranial nerve XI.

Nystagmus can be classified in terms of the direction of eye movement: horizontal, vertical, rotary (torsional), or mixed. If head rotation is continued, friction between otic fluid and semicircular duct walls results in otic fluid rotating at the same velocity as the head, and nystagmus adapts to a stable eye posture. If rotation is suddenly stopped, vestibular nystagmus reappears in precisely the direction opposite to angular accelerating nystagmus. This results because the inertia of the otic fluid is again bending ampullar hair cells of a now stationary ampulla. Because the observer does not have to rotate the subject, demonstration of postrotary nystagmus is often used to evaluate the function of vestibular reflexes. Nystagmus is always abnormal if it occurs spontaneously or is sustained. Nystagmus eye movements can be tested by rotation or caloric stimulation (see Chapter 43).

Thalamic and Cortical Projections. Some of the neurons of the vestibular nuclei project their axons rostrally to the ventrolateral nuclei of the thalamus. In addition to the intrathalamic circuitry, thalamic projections go to the primary vestibular cortex near the somesthetic area of the parietal lobe. These thalamic and cortical projections provide the basis for the subjective experiences of position in space, rotation, and vertigo that accompany the onset or sudden cessation of head rotation. During such episodes, nystagmus is observed.

Postural Reflexes

Sudden changes in balance or orientation, such as falling to the right or left or backward or forward, result in powerful reflexes needed to maintain equilibrium and posture. The descending portion of the MLF, essentially a medial vestibulospinal tract, continues at least into thoracic cord levels and provides vestibular control of the muscle tone of axial muscles, including the dorsal back muscles. A rapidly conducting lateral vestibulospinal tract descends the spinal cord to provide powerful vestibular control of the LMNs of the upper and lower limbs. As the head begins to tip (*i.e.,* rotate) on the neck or moves as part of general body tipping, the vestibular system activates the appropriate extensor muscles of the neck, trunk, and limbs, opposing the direction of the tilt. These powerful reflex adjustments in muscle tone assist in maintaining stable head and therefore body postural support during static posture and during passive or active movement.

All the vestibular nuclei receive input from the cerebellum and the vestibular nerve. The cerebellar connections of the vestibular system are necessary for adjustments of temporally smooth, coordinated movements to ongoing head movement, tilt, or angular acceleration. For instance, accurate grasping can occur during a fall, indicating cerebellar adjustments based on vestibular information during the performance of a smooth, accurate movement.

Vestibular reflexes are quite powerful, and considerable learning is required to inhibit or greatly modify them, as is necessary for acrobatic pilots, divers, and gymnasts. Dancers and skaters who engage in rapid spinning movements also learn to use or at least partially inhibit these reflexes.

In summary, hearing is a specialized sense whose external stimulus is the vibration of sound waves. The ear receives the sound waves, distinguishes their frequencies, translates this information into nerve impulses, and transmits these to the CNS. The auditory system consists of the outer ear, middle ear, and inner ear, auditory pathways, and auditory cortex. The middle ear is a tiny air-filled cavity located in the temporal

Doll's-Head Eye Response

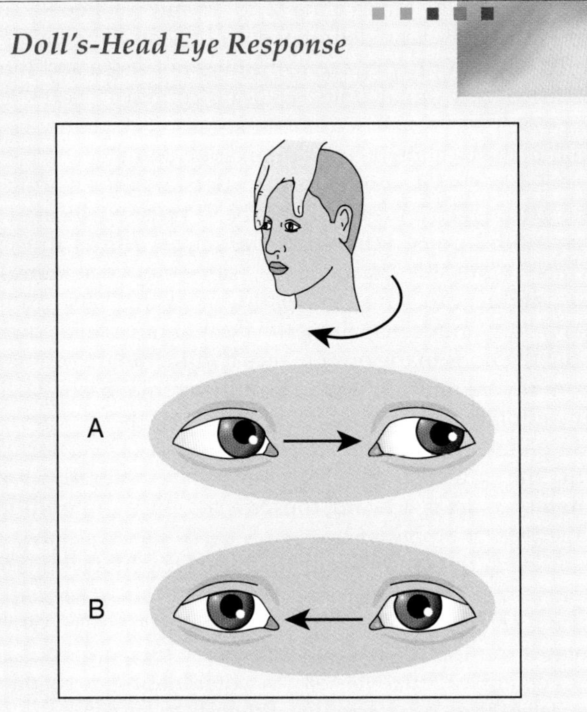

The *doll's-head eye response* demonstrates the always-present vestibular static reflexes without forebrain interference or suppression. Severe damage to the forebrain or to the brain stem rostral to the pons often results in loss of rostral control of these static vestibular reflexes. If the person's head is moved from side to side or up and down, the eyes will move in conjugate gaze to the opposite side (A), much like that those of a doll with counterweighted eyes. If doll's-head phenomenon is observed, brain stem function at the level of the pons is considered intact (in a comatose person). In the unconscious person without intact brain stem function and vestibular static reflexes, the eyes stay in midposition (fixed) or turn in the same direction (B) as the head is turned.

bone. The auditory tube connects the middle ear to the nasopharynx and allows equalization of pressure between the middle ear and the atmosphere. The inner ear contains the receptors for hearing.

The vestibular system plays an essential role in the equilibrium sense, which is closely integrated with the visual and proprioceptive (position) senses. The receptors for the vestibular system, which are located in the semicircular ducts of the inner ear, respond to changes in linear and angular acceleration of the head. The vestibular nerve fibers travel in the vestibulocochlear (CN VIII) nerve to the vestibular nuclei located at the junction of the medulla and pons. Some of the fibers pass through the nuclei to the cerebellum. The cerebellar connections are necessary for temporally smooth, coordinated movements during ongoing head movements, tilt, and angular acceleration. The vestibular nuclei also connect with the nuclei of the oculomotor (CN III), trochlear (CN IV), and abducens (CN VI) nerves. Vestibular control of conjugate eye movements preserves eye fixation on stable objects in the visual field during head movement. The term nystagmus is used to describe vestibular-controlled eye movements that occur in response to angular and rotational movements of the head. Neurons of the vestibular nuclei also project to the thalamus, to the temporal cortex, and to the somatesthetic area of the parietal cortex. The thalamic and cortical projections provide the basis for the subjective experiences of position in space and of rotation and vertigo.

Eye Movements and Conjugate Gaze Reflex Mechanisms

After you have completed this section of the chapter, you should be able to meet the following objectives:

- Name the six extraocular muscles and relate their function to the movements of the optic globe during conjugate, vergent, and gaze movements of the eye
- Characterize conjugate gaze, slow pursuit, saccadic, and optokinetic eye movements
- Describe normal nystagmus eye movements

To make full use of the visual function of the eyes, it is necessary that the two eyes point toward the same fixation point and that the retinal and CNS visual acuity mechanisms are functioning. Despite the somewhat different view of the external world for each eye (*i.e.*, binocular disparity), it is important that these two images become fused (*i.e.*, binocular fusion), which is a forebrain function. Binocular fusion is controlled by ocular reflex mechanisms that adjust the orientation of each eye to produce a single image. If these reflexes fail, double vision (*i.e.*, diplopia) occurs. To be effective, these reflexes must adjust eye movements for viewing objects at various distances. During distance vision, reflex mechanisms are required to maintain parallel orientation of the two eyes, called *conjugate gaze reflexes*. In contrast to parallel or conjugate eye movements, at distances closer than approximately 30 feet, reflexes must alter eye orientation away from parallel if a common fixation point is to be obtained. These constitute a second category of reflexes, called *vergence reflexes*, which turn the eyes toward each other (*i.e.*, convergence), as when a target is approaching the observer, or away from each other (*i.e.*, divergence), as when the target is receding (Table 41–1).

The concept of "optical grasp" has been used to characterize the reflexes that enable the eyes to grasp and "hang onto" a visual target. Bilaterally linked or *yoked* rotation of the two eyes in response to visual, auditory, vestibular, or somesthetic stimuli use a basic repertoire of eye movement reflexes built into the circuitry of the central nervous system. These reflexes are normally operative at or within a few weeks of birth.

Conjugate and vergence movements are further subdivided into relatively slow and very rapid, or *saccadic*, movements. In general, the slow movements permit continuous fixation on a visual target during movements of the target or rotations of the head. The rapid or saccadic movements permit a resetting of the fixation point to a new location. This section of the chapter is discusses the extrinsic muscles and their innervation, conjugate gaze movements, and vergence movements.

Extrinsic Eye Muscles and Their Innervation

Binocular vision depends on three pairs of extraocular muscles—the medial and lateral recti, the superior and inferior recti, and the superior and inferior obliques (Fig. 41–24). Each of the three sets of muscles in each eye is reciprocally innervated so that one muscle relaxes when the other contracts. The medial and lateral recti contract reciprocally to move the eye from side to side (*i.e.*, adduct and abduct); the superior and inferior recti contract to move the eye up and down (*i.e.*, elevate and depress). The oblique muscles rotate (*i.e.*, intort and extort) the eye around its optic axis. A seventh muscle, the *levator palpebrae superioris*, elevates the upper lid.

The extraocular muscles are innervated by three cranial nerves. The trochlear cranial nerve (CN IV) innervates the superior oblique, the abducens cranial nerve (CN VI) innervates the lateral rectus, and the oculomotor cranial nerve (CN III) innervates the remaining four muscles. The motor units in the extraocular muscles are quite small, with one LMN innervating 2 to 10 muscle fibers. This gives the CNS very delicate control of muscle generated force through progressive recruitment of more and more of these very small units. Delicate control is necessary, because a very small eye movement results in a very large shift in the location of a distant fixation point.

Table 41–1 describes the function and innervation of the extraocular muscles. The CN VI nucleus, located in the caudal pons, innervates the lateral rectus muscle, which rotates the *ipsilateral* (*i.e.*, same side) eye laterally (*i.e.*, abduction). The long pathway of the VIth cranial nerve (*i.e.*, abducens) along the floor of the cranial cavity from the pons to the orbit makes it vulnerable to damage from severe injury or fracture of the cranial base. Partial or complete damage to this nerve results in weakness or complete paralysis of the muscle. Medial gaze is normal, but the affected eye fails to rotate laterally with attempted gaze toward the affected side, a condition called *medial strabismus*.

The IVth cranial nerve nucleus, located at the junction of the pons and midbrain, innervates the *contralateral* or *opposite side* superior oblique muscle, which rotates the top of the globe inward toward the nose, a movement called *intorsion*. In combination with other muscles, it also contributes strength to moving the innervated eye downward and inward. The superior oblique muscle neurons cross over the roof of the midbrain, drop vertically through the roof of the cavernous sinus, and then enter the orbit. This short pathway is rarely damaged, and signs of dysfunction are usually the result of a small brain stem stroke affecting the IVth cranial nerve nucleus or from damage to the midbrain level vertical gaze networks.

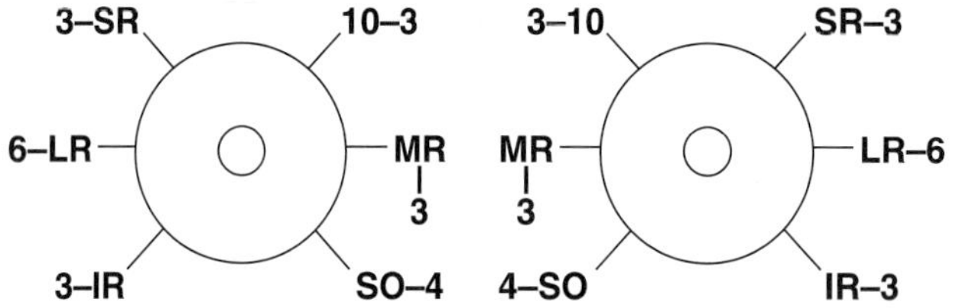

3–SR 10–3 3–10 SR–3
6–LR MR–3 MR–3 LR–6
3–IR SO–4 4–SO IR–3

TABLE 41–1

Eye in Primary Position: Extrinsic Ocular Muscle Actions

Muscle*	Innervation	Primary	Secondary	Tertiary
MR: medial rectus	III	Adduction		
LR: lateral rectus	VI	Abduction		
SR: superior rectus	III	Elevation	Intorsion	Adduction
IR: inferior rectus	III	Depression	Extorsion	Adduction
SO: superior oblique	IV	Intorsion	Depression	Abduction
IR: inferior oblique	III	Extorsion	Elevation	Abduction

*In the schema of the functional roles of the six extraocular muscles, the major directional force applied by each muscle is indicated by arrows. These muscles are arranged in functionally opposing pairs per eye and in parallel opposing pairs for conjugate movements of the two eyes. The numbers associated with each muscle indicate the cranial nerve innervation: 3, oculomotor (III) cranial nerve; 4, trochlear (IV) cranial nerve; 6, abducens (VI) cranial nerve.

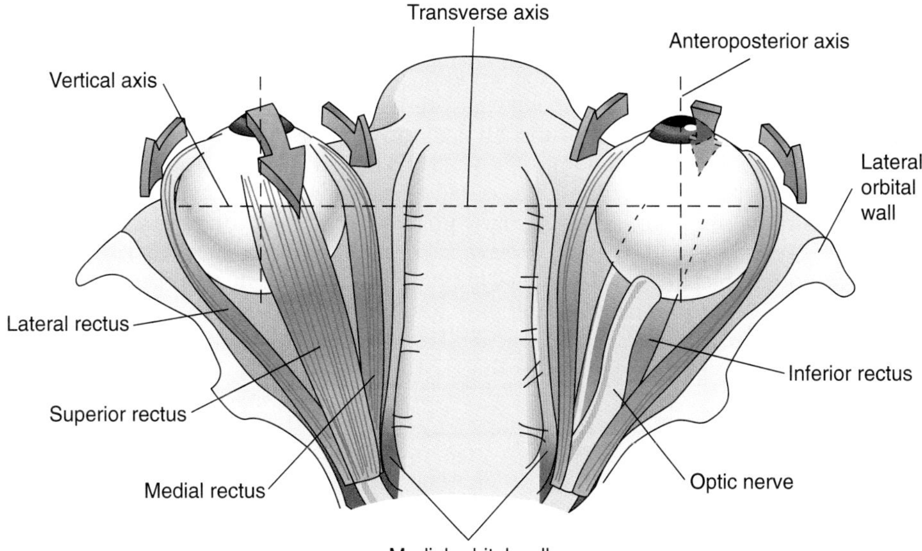

Figure 41–24
Extraocular eye muscles. (Williams & Warwick. [1975]. *Functional neuroanatomy of man* [p. 1126]. Philadelphia: W.B. Saunders)

The IIIrd cranial nucleus, which extends through a considerable part of the midbrain, contains clusters of LMNs for each of the five eye muscles it innervates: the ipsilateral superior rectus, inferior rectus, inferior oblique, and medial rectus. The fifth muscle, the levator palpebrae superioris, elevates the upper lid and is only involved in vertical gaze eye movements. As the eyes rotate upward, the upper lid is reflexively retracted, and in the downward gaze, the upper lid becomes slightly lowered, restricting the exposure of the conjunctiva to air and reducing the effects of drying. The medial rectus, superior rectus, and inferior rectus rotate the eyes in the directions indicated in Table 41–1. The inferior rectus works in opposition to the superior rectus. Because of its plane of attachment to the globe, the internal oblique rotates the eye in the frontal plane (*i.e.*, torsion), pulling the top of eye laterally (*i.e.*, extorsion).

Tremor refers to involuntary rhythmic oscillatory eye movements, occurring approximately 10 times per second. As a result of this quivering motion, there is constant movement of a stable optical image over the retinal photoreceptors. Small-range optical tremor is a normal and useful independent function of each eye. Tremor results from inequality in the number of motor units active in opposing extraocular muscles at any moment. The central mechanism that prevents the experience of blurring is not understood. One function of the fine optic tremor is to constantly move a bright image onto a new bank of cones, permitting previously stimulated receptors to quickly recover from adaptation. A role in the improvement in contrast has also been suggested.

Conjugate Eye Movements

The term *conjugate gaze* refers to the use of both eyes to look steadily in one direction. During conjugate eye movements, the optical axes of the two eyes are maintained parallel with each other as the eyes rotate in their sockets. Although the conjugate reflexes are essential to efficient visual function during head movement or target movement, their circuitry is so deeply embedded in central nervous system function that they are present and can be elicited when the eyes are closed, during sleep, and in deep coma, and they function normally and accurately in congenitally blind persons.

Conjugate gaze movements include lateral gaze, vertical gaze, oblique gaze, and torsional gaze. Lateral gaze movements are in the horizontal plane and are controlled by a *lateral gaze center* of interneurons within the VIth cranial nerve nucleus on the side of abduction (see Fig. 41–22). Vertical gaze upward or downward is controlled by a *vertical gaze center* of interneurons within and near the IIIrd cranial nerve nucleus. Oblique gaze involves a combination of lateral and vertical gaze controls. Torsional gaze movements involve ocular rotation around the optical axis of the eyes, and although they occur frequently, they are more difficult to observe. The *torsional gaze center* involves interneurons within the IVth cranial nerve nucleus on both sides. Each of these control centers maintains a moderate level of tonic activity (*i.e.*, low level of "spontaneous" action potentials) in each opposing pair of muscles. This has the effect of maintaining a neutral position of eye posture. More and more motor units are automatically recruited when an eye deviates from this neutral position. When released from a directional signal, the eyes automatically return to the neutral position.

Communication between the eye muscle nuclei of each side occurs primarily through the posterior commissure at the rostral end of the midbrain. Longitudinal communication between the three nuclei occurs in or near the previous described MLF (see Fig. 41–22). Each pair of eye muscles is reciprocally innervated, by way of the MLF or other associated pathways, so that as one muscle contracts the other relaxes. For example, at the same time that the LMNs of cranial nerve VI produce lateral rotation (*i.e.,* abduction) of the left eye, interneurons of the left cranial nerve VI communicate with the right cranial nerve III by way of the MLF to move the right eye medially (adduction). These MLF-linked communication paths are vulnerable to damage in the caudal midbrain and pons. Damage to the pontine MLF on one side results in a loss of this linkage such that lateral deviation in the ipsilateral eye is no longer linked to adduction on the contralateral side (*i.e.,* internuclear ophthalmoplegia). If the MLF is damaged bilaterally, the linkage is lost for lateral gaze in either direction.

Slow Conjugate Eye Movements

Slow conjugate gaze reflexes, which are integrated by the vestibular and visual systems, hold a steady visual fixation point on the fovea during brief head movements. The vestibular nuclei send controlling signals to the appropriate gaze centers, moving the eyes in the *opposite direction* to that of the head and at precisely the same rate as the head movement, thereby allowing the eyes to maintain a constant distant fixation point, whatever the direction of movement.

A specialized part of the conjugate gaze network, a nucleus in the floor of the fourth ventricle, called the *nucleus prepositus hypoglossi,* converts the vestibular afferent signals into the appropriate velocity and range of gaze movements. This mechanism can adapt to alterations in vestibular input. Destruction of the vestibular nerve of one side results in a severe sensation of falling, reduced muscle tone, and nystagmus toward the damaged side. Adaptive recovery is rapid, with only minor signs remaining within a few weeks after damage. The adaptive mechanism involves vestibular afferent collaterals that project to the flocculus of the archicerebellum, which projects to nucleus prepositus hypoglossi and to the vestibular nuclei. Destruction of this region of cerebellar cortex prevents any further adaptive changes to occur.

The vestibulo-ocular reflexes, although powerful, can be avoided or altered to some extent by learned forebrain mechanisms. For instance, spinning skaters and dancers learn to minimize the reflex by rotating their head in the direction opposite to the spin, reducing vestibular input and the conjugate movements. Fixing attention on a visual stimulus can also override the reflex.

The optokinetic slow gaze reflexes result in conjugate eye movements that follow a moving visual stimulus. These vestibulo-ocular reflexes hold the moving visual fixation point on the fovea while the head position remains stationary. They can be superseded by visual stimuli, if the stimulus has high contrast and relatively high intensity. This reflex mechanism requires high-definition directional signals that move in consort as if the opposite were true (*i.e.,* as if the head were moving through a visual environment). Probably everyone has had the experience of moving through space, even though the head is stationary, when a nearby bus or train moves in the opposite direction. If a rotating visual environment has less contrast, if the cortical visual system is functional, and if the subject "attends" to a particular visual target in the moving visual field, optokinetic slow following of the target also occurs.

Conjugate following of a rotating visual environment can occur at a subcortical level or at a visual cortical level. Although the optokinetic conjugate eye movement reflexes provide a powerful experience of movement through space, they also operate in persons with damage to their visual cortex (*i.e.,* cortical blindness) but with functional subcortical visual reflex mechanisms. In this instance, there is no visual perception of movement during the optokinetic conjugate movements.

A third class of slow conjugate gaze mechanisms involves smooth visual pursuit or tracking movements that maintain an object at a fixed point in the center of the visual fields of both eyes. The object may be moving and the eyes following it, or the object may be stationary and the head of the observer moving. In smooth pursuit, the visual cortical areas dominate and use the vestibular system's slow eye reflex systems through direct projections on the vestibular nuclei. The superior colliculus apparatus provides specific directional motor controls required to move the conjugate focal point to the moving target. The superior colliculus also operates through tectobulbar projection on the vestibular nuclei. Temporal and spatial smoothing adjustments are provided by visual cortical projections of the cerebellar vermis. Unlike the optokinetic reflexes, smooth visual pursuit reflexes depend on the perception of and attention to a clear, localized visual target. It does not occur with clouded vision or with cortical blindness. Testing for smooth pursuit requires the tester to move his finger or some other small but distinct target, such as a small flashlight, in an irregular fashion in the plane of focus in front of the subject and observe whether the target-following conjugate gaze is a continuous (smooth) following of the target location.

Fast Saccadic Eye Movements

When slow conjugate deviation reaches the limit to which the optic globes can rotate in the orbits, a reflex mechanism called *saccadic movement* occurs. It is an extremely rapid corrective conjugate rotation that has the function of finding a new point at the edge of the visual field onto which fixation is shifted, jumping from one point to another at a rate of two to three jumps per second. The jumps are called *saccades.* During the saccade, a person does not experience the blur of the rapidly moving visual field. The mechanism by which visual experience is momentarily shut off is not understood. Saccades are a component of vestibular, optokinetic, startle, and motor-driven scanning movements. It is an automatic reflex that, in most situations, operates at the brain stem level. It also is the sole mechanism by which changes in a fixation point are accomplished through learned motor control.

The saccade involves a very rapid conjugate rotation of the eyes. The central networks must overcome optic globe inertia, rotate the eyes rapidly, and then stop the motion and hold a new position, retaining a bilaterally parallel orientation throughout. The neurons involved in saccadic eye movements are mostly concentrated in three locations, depending on the plane of rotation. In the horizontal plane, the cells controlling the saccade are located in the medial pontine reticular formation at and slightly rostral to the VIth cranial nerve nucleus. Interneurons controlling saccades in the vertical plane are clustered in a nucleus next to and within the MLF in the rostral midbrain. Saccades in the oblique plane involve interaction between both of the these areas. These saccade-producing areas control the interocular nucleus network. They are under the control of vestibular, retinal, startle, and motor system input. Saccades also occur for torsional eye rotation, but the location in the midbrain reticular formation of the controlling interneurons has not been thoroughly investigated.

The saccade mechanism is integrated into the vestibulo-ocular reflexes. During head rotation, the compensatory conjugate rotation in the opposite direction reaches its orbital limit, and a saccade occurs, rapidly shifting the conjugate gaze ahead to a new environmental fixation point, and then the slow-phase compensatory rotation begins again. The vestibular nuclei control the direction of the saccade through projections onto the directional saccade centers. The fast ocular rotation is in the plane of head rotation and in the same direction as the head rotation. The saccade is immediately followed by a new vestibulo-ocular slow rotation in the direction opposite to that of head rotation. With momentary lapses during the saccade, a stable visual image is available most of the time during rotational acceleration. As with the vestibulo-ocular reflex slow phase, the visual experience is not required for this automatic reflex sequence to occur, and the sequence of slow, fast, slow, fast movement components continues with the eyes closed or even in the congenitally blind.

Optokinetic Nystagmus. The sequence of alternating slow ocular rotation and fast saccadic phase eye movements is called *nystagmus.* Optokinetic-induced slow conjugate eye reflexes alternate with fast-phase (saccadic) reflexes, a condition called *optokinetic nystagmus.* If the moving visual stimulus situation continues until slow ocular rotation reaches its limit within the orbit, the saccade moves the conjugate gaze to a new fixation point on the moving visual environment behind the previous one, at the opposite side of the available visual field. It is followed by a new slow-phase optokinetic movement that matches the direction and rate of movement of the visual environment. As with the slow phase of optokinetic reflexes, the fast or saccadic phase does not require a functional visual cortex. The subcortical, retinal projection to the superior colliculus map of the visual field interacts with a tectobulbar projection onto the saccade centers and continues the inhibition of vestibular system control of eye movements.

Optically induced nystagmus has been used to test visual acuity in infants and persons in whom verbal communication is ineffective. If the reflex can be induced by surrounding the infant with a set of rotating vertical black and white stripes, this indicates that retinal and brain stem components are functional. The width of the stripes can then be systematically reduced until the reflex is lost, providing an objective, nonverbal method of testing retinal level of visual acuity.

The Startle Reflex. A saccadic shift of gaze toward the source of a sudden, unexpected visual, auditory, tactile, or painful stimulation is a component of the startle pattern. This is functionally a *visual grasping reflex,* redirecting conjugate gaze in the direction of the startle stimulus. The startle saccade involves superior collicular domination of the conjugate gaze mechanism. Rapid head turning, turning of the body, and extension of the ipsilateral upper limb also occur. Learned shifting of conjugate gaze from one visual target to another involves the frontal eye fields under the domination of the motor, premotor, and prefrontal cortex. Visual input to the visual cortex and to the superior colliculus provides the required directional information. The frontal eye fields dominate the superior colliculus–saccadic gaze mechanism. Motor-driven shifts to a new visual target can only occur as saccades; therefore, blur is not experienced.

The saccadic conjugate eye movement component of the startle reflex pattern involves reception of an adequate input pattern by the superior colliculus superimposed on visual, auditory, and somesthetic maps of the external environment. Directional high-contrast retinal input reaches the superior colliculus through retinal ganglion cell collaterals that leave the optic tracts just before entry into the thalamus. The vision-related thalamic nucleus, the lateral geniculate nucleus, also projects to the superior colliculus. Coded signals for a high-intensity auditory stimulus reach the inferior colliculus through the ascending auditory pathway through the lateral lemniscus. The directionality aspect of an auditory signal is analyzed in the superior olivary nuclei, and codes for this aspect of the stimulus are also projected to subnuclei of the inferior colliculus. A collateral pathway interconnects the inferior colliculus with the superior colliculus auditory map of the surrounding environment. A tactile or nociceptive (*i.e.,* pain or temperature) code reaches the superior colliculus through collaterals of the ascending somesthetic pathways, the medial lemniscus, and especially the anterior lateral spinothalamic system. Superior colliculus output through tectobulbar fibers reach and dominate the directional saccadic or rapid eye movement networks. Vestibular input control of eye and head rotation is superseded by the startle reaction pattern, although vestibular reflex control of postural support continues during the startle behavioral pattern.

Learned Motor Control of Saccadic Conjugate Eye Movements. Rapid, or saccadic, conjugate eye movements are not limited to vestibular, startle, or visual reflexes. A person learns to control the direction of visual fixation and to change from fixation point to fixation point during visual searching of the environment, as when reading a map or searching the woods for game. A specialized area of the lateral premotor cortex on the middle frontal gyrus, called the frontal eye fields, has direct control of saccadic eye movements. The frontal eye fields receive input from the visual cortex, motion-sensitive parietal cortex (*i.e.*, parietal eye fields), higher-order premotor cortex, and lateral prefrontal cortex. Projections from frontal eye fields are a part of the corticobulbar system, and they impinge on the directional motor fields of the superior colliculus and directly on the saccadic gaze centers. The frontal eye fields of one hemisphere controls saccades toward the contralateral side and has subareas dedicated to the various directional dimensions of saccadic movement.

Frontal cortical control of saccadic eye movements becomes an integrated component of planned, learned motor patterns. A person cannot move her or his conjugate gaze smoothly from fixation point to fixation point. The eyes always move between the fixation points in one or in a series of jerky saccades. This learned skill is an important but not often recognized aspect of the acquired motor skills necessary for daily survival. Motor control of saccadic eye movements supersedes vestibular system control, except during very rapidly accelerating head rotation. As with visual control of eye movements, vestibular reflex control of head and body postural support continues to function normally.

Motor control of saccadic conjugate eye movements can only occur when attention is directed at a specific visual target. Ordinarily, a functional cortical visual system also is necessary. However, with the eyes closed, these movements occur during a search for an imaginary target (based on learning), and they occur in sleep during vivid visual dreams that take place during rapid eye movement (REM) sleep.

Vergence Eye Movements

Vergence (disconjugate) movements are those that move the eyes in opposite directions to keep the image of an object precisely positioned on the fovea of each eye. The vergence system is driven by retinal disparity (*i.e.*, differential placement of an object's image on each retina).

When a target within about 30 feet of the eyes moves in the longitudinal dimension of the optical axis, toward or away from the eyes, a reflex mechanism provides redirection of the optical axes of each eye away from parallel (*i.e.*, in opposite directions) in the horizontal plane (*i.e.*, vergence gaze), which permits continued binocular focus on the near target. Convergence and divergence, which assist in maintaining a binocularly fixed image in near vision, have a major role in accurate depth perception. Perception of depth is a higher-order function of the cortical visual system and is based on one or more of several classes of stimuli, such as superimposition and relative movement. Retinal disparity, or differences in the retinal image of a visual target, is a major contributor to depth perception in near vision. Accurate depth perception is important for precise manipulation of tools or other objects with which humans are especially skilled.

The stimulus for vergence reflexes is the same as that for accommodation: blur of the retinal image. The accommodation mechanism searches for a sharp image by varying the shape and therefore the focal point of the lens. The vergence mechanism searches for the sharpest binocular image by varying the degree of convergence or divergence of the two eyes. Vergence movements may involve the following of a receding target (*i.e.*, slow divergence), and the rate of change of divergence must be matched to the movement of the target. At a fixation distance of approximately 30 feet, the retinal images become essentially identical and binocular orientation becomes parallel. Following an incoming target (*i.e.*, slow convergence) conforms to the same principles but in the opposite direction. Functional vision and attention to the visual target are necessary for vergence movements to occur.

Slow Vergence Eye Movements

Slow vergence movements (*i.e.*, convergence, divergence) result from projections from the primary and secondary visual cortex bilaterally on nuclei in the pretectum region of the midbrain. These nuclei control a vergence gaze center adjacent to the IIIrd cranial nerve nucleus. This projects bilaterally on the medial rectus LMNs of the IIIrd cranial nerve and through the MLF bilaterally on VIth nerve nucleus of lateral rectus LMNs. Simultaneous bilateral facilitation of the medial rectus motor units of each side with bilateral inhibition of the lateral rectus muscles results in convergence. Simultaneous bilateral facilitation of the lateral rectus motor units combined with bilateral inhibition of medial rectus motor units results in divergence. Coordination between the two sides involves axons crossing in the posterior commissure.

The fact that convergence and divergence reflexes depend on a functional cortical visual system and on the capability for at least momentarily maintained attention should be emphasized. These reflexes do not occur in a blind person, in a comatose person, or in a person who is highly distractible and unable to concentrate on obtaining a clear image of a near target.

Fast Convergence and Divergence Eye Movements

Rapid changes in vergence occur when focus is redirected from a near to a far target, or vice versa. A saccadic-like mechanism provides such rapid changes in the vergence system. The person experiences no blur during fast changes in vergence. However, vision must be intact, and attention must be directed to the change of fixation point.

Other Reflexes Associated With Vergence Eye Movements

When a visual image becomes blurred, an automatic reflex mechanism alters the curvature of the lens in a search for a clearer image. This *accommodation reflex* only occurs if the primary visual cortex is functioning and then only if the subject is "attending" a particular fixation point. Several occipital association areas apparently also are involved. The network for accommodation involves occipital cortical projections on the Edinger-Westphal part of the IIIrd cranial nerve nucleus complex. Parasympathetic preganglionic neurons project axons through cranial nerve III to postganglionic neurons of the ciliary ganglion, which innervate the ciliary muscle. Contraction of this muscle results in rounding-up of the lens (*i.e.,* moving the focal point forward), which has the effect of bringing the external focal point closer to the eye. Bilateral coordination between accommodation in the two eyes involves communication through the posterior commissure in the rostral midbrain. Accommodative changes are required to maintain a sharp focus (*i.e.,* minimize blur) of a target moving toward the eye if the distance is less than about 30 feet.

Three other reflex mechanisms are intimately correlated with the accommodative mechanism: convergence-divergence, pupillary constriction-dilation, and widening-narrowing of the palpebral opening. *Convergence* of the two eyes is an automatic component of the accommodation reflex complex. Visual cortical projections to pretectal nuclei control both processes in both eyes. If the target is moving away, focal length and divergence must be smoothly adjusted to maintain a clear image.

In near vision, a narrow pupillary opening (*i.e.,* miosis) facilitates the clarity of the retinal image. This must be balanced against the resultant decrease in light intensity reaching the retina. The *pupillary reflex* component of accommodation also involves visual cortical projection on the pretectum and pretectal control of the part of the Edinger-Westphal nucleus that controls the sphincter of the pupil. During changes from near to far vision, pupillary dilation partially compensates for the reduced size of the retinal image by increasing the amount of light entering the pupil. Opening the pupil involves pretectal (pretectospinal) projections on sympathetic preganglionic neurons at high thoracic cord levels. Axons of these pass through the T1 through T3 white rami and rostrally in the sympathetic trunk to innervate postganglionic cells of the superior cervical ganglion. The latter cells send axons forward through the internal carotid plexus to eventually reach the radial (dilator) smooth muscle of the pupil.

A third component of accommodation involves the reflex *narrowing of the palpebral opening* during near vision and widening during far vision. Narrowing involves inhibition of the IIIrd cranial nerve–innervated levator palpebrae superioris and facilitation of the VIIth cranial nerve–innervated orbicularis oculi. Widening involves the opposite muscle actions. The width of the palpebral opening is under the same visual cortex to pretectal nuclei control as are the other components of accommodation.

Accommodation and its correlated reflexes, convergence-divergence, pupillary constriction-dilation, and changes in the diameter of the palpebral opening, require a functional visual cortical system and attention directed at a particular visual target. These reflex adjustments can be slow and smooth, or they can involve sudden, saccade-like jumps from near to distance vision and vice versa.

In summary, ocular reflexes, whether controlling a parallel orientation of the two eyes (i.e., conjugate gaze) in distance vision or converging or diverging the two optical axes in near vision, have a common function: the search for and the maintenance of a maximally clear binocular foveal image of the visual target. Reflex linkage mechanisms are required that continuously maintain the parallel orientation of the two eyes during head movements, movement of the visual surroundings, movement of a specific visual target within a stable visual field, and rapid shifting of attention from one visual target to another. The concept of optical grasp has been used to characterize the reflex mechanisms that hang onto a visual target, freeing the organism to concentrate on other aspects of the constant struggle to survive.

The conjugate gaze mechanism involves the interocular nuclear network, which coordinates the actions of the extraocular muscles of the two sides through connections between the IIIrd, IVth, and VIth cranial nerve nuclei. Conjugate gaze is controlled by interneurons in the VIth nucleus (i.e., lateral gaze center), in the IIIrd nerve nucleus (i.e., vertical gaze center), and in the IVth nerve nucleus (i.e., torsional gaze center). The MLF is particularly important in linking the IIIrd and VIth nerve nuclei during lateral gaze, and unilateral damage to this pathway disconnects the abduction of the ipsilateral eye with the medial rotation of the other (i.e., internuclear ophthalmoplegia). Slow conjugate gaze occurs in the direction and a rate precisely opposite to head rotation. Optokinetic slow conjugate gaze occurs automatically if a high-contrast visual environment is rotated. This involves retinal and thalamic projection to the superior colliculus, a network that controls slow conjugate gaze by dominating the vestibular conjugate control system. If the visual environment is stable but a moving target passes across the visual field, a slow, smooth conjugate following of the target can occur. This smooth pursuit conjugate gaze requires a functional cortical visual system and attention directed toward the moving target. Visual cortical control of the superior colliculus–conjugate gaze mechanism is involved. Modulation of this function involves the cerebellar vermis and flocculus.

Saccadic eye movement consist of small jumping movements that represent rapid shifts in conjugate gaze orientation. Separate specialized networks exist for controlling horizontal, vertical, and torsional saccadic movements. Because of an unknown mechanism, no visual sense of blurring occurs during a saccade. Saccades occur on continued head rotation when eye rotation reaches its orbital limit, rapidly moving the eyes forward in the direction of rotation to a new fixation point, and then the slow vestibulo-ocular reflex occurs again.

The sequence of slow ocular rotation, a saccade, slow rotation, and so on is called nystagmus. Nystagmus can be induced by the rotation of a high-contrast visual environment (i.e., optokinetic nystagmus). If the visual environment includes high-contrast lines or bars, subcortical visual system domination of the saccadic mechanism occurs, and the function of the superior colliculus is critically important. If the cortical visual system is functional and the person attends a particular target in the moving visual environment, optokinetic nystagmus also occurs. Cortical visual projection on the same saccade control system is involved.

A saccadic shift of gaze toward the source of a sudden, unexpected visual, auditory, tactile, or painful stimulation is a component of the startle pattern. This is functionally a visual grasping reflex, redirecting conjugate gaze in the direction of the startle stimulus. Within approximately 30 feet of the retinas, when a visual target moves in the longitudinal dimension of the optical axis, a reflex mechanism provides changes in the optical axes of the two eyes away from parallel (*i.e.*, vergence gaze), which permits continued binocular focus on the target. Maintaining a foveal focal point of a visual target in each eye provides disparate retinal images, and retinal disparity contributes to the perception of depth.

Convergence or divergence can be slow and smooth, much like smooth pursuit, or can be sudden and rapid, much like a saccade. Attending the target and a functional visual cortical system are required. Visual cortical projection on pretectal nuclei control the divergence and convergence networks associated with the IIIrd cranial nerve nuclei. Vergence eye movements are one component of several reflexes associated with accommodation. These include reflex control of pupillary diameter and of palpebral diameter.

BIBLIOGRAPHY

Bear M.F., Connors B.W., Paradiso M.A. (1996). *Neuroscience.* Baltimore: Williams & Wilkins.

Conn P.M. (Ed.) (1995). *Neuroscience in medicine.* Philadelphia: J.B. Lippincott.

Evans N.M. (1995). *Ophthalmology* (2nd ed.). New York: Oxford University Press.

Forrester J., Dick A., McMenamin P., Lee W. (1996). *The eye: Basic sciences in practice* (p. 208). Philadelphia: W.B. Saunders.

Goldberg M., Eggers H.M., Gouras P. (1991). The ocular motor system. In Kandel E.R., Schwartz J.H., Jessel T.M. (Eds.). *Principles of neural science* (3rd ed., pp. 660–678). New York: Elsevier.

Guyton A.C., Hall J.E. (1996). *Textbook of medical physiology* (9th ed., pp. 663–673,707–713). Philadelphia: W.B. Saunders.

Kelly J.P. (1991). The sense of balance. In Kandel E.R., Schwartz J.H., Jessel T.M. (Eds.). *Principles of neural science* (3rd. ed., pp. 500–511). New York: Elsevier.

Kingsley R.E. (1996). *Concise text of neurosciences.* Baltimore: Williams & Wilkins.

Kline L.B., Bajandas F.J. (1996). *Neuro-ophthalmology review manual* (4th ed.). Thorofare, NJ: Slack.

Marieb E.N. (1995). *Human anatomy and physiology* (3rd ed.). Redwood City, CA: Benjamin Cummings Publishing Company.

Martini F.H. (1995). *Fundamentals of anatomy and physiology* (3rd ed.). Englewood Cliffs, NJ: Prentice Hall.

Parent A. (1996). *Carpenter's neuroanatomy.* Baltimore: Williams & Wilkins.

Ross M.H., Romrell L.J., Kaye G.I. (1995). *Histology: A text and atlas* (pp. 740–767). Baltimore: Williams & Wilkins.

Spencer R.F. (1996). The oculomotor system. In Conn P.M. *Neuroscience in medicine* (pp. 249–260). Philadelphia: J.B. Lippincott.

Zolton B. (1996). *Vision, perception, and cognition* (3rd ed.). Thorofare, NJ: Slack.

CHAPTER 42

Alterations in Vision

Sheila M. Curtis and Edward W. Carroll

Almost 11.5 million persons in the United States suffer from some degree of visual impairment. Of these, 12% are unable to see well enough to read ordinary newsprint even with the aid of glasses, and another 4% are classified as legally blind.[1] Of the more than 95.2 million persons older than 40 years, 3 million are visually impaired (*i.e.*, vision <20/40 in the better eye with glasses). More than 900,000 persons older than 40 years of age are considered legally blind (*i.e.*, vision of 20/200 or worse in the better eye with glasses).[2] The rates of blindness and visual impairment increase with age, with the elderly most affected. At the other end of the age spectrum are visual disorders that originate in utero, infancy, or early childhood.

Alterations in vision can result from disorders of the orbit and surrounding structures, intraocular pressure (glaucoma), lens (cataract), vitreous and retina, visual pathways and visual cortex, and extraocular muscles and eye movement. Visual impairment due to common types of eye disorders is illustrated in Figure 42–1.

Disorders of the Orbit and Surrounding Structures

After you have completed this section of the chapter, you should be able to meet the following objectives:

- Differentiate exophthalmos from proptosis
- Define entropion and ectropium
- Explain the differences in marginal blepharitis, a hordeolum, and a chalazion in terms of causes and manifestations
- State the causes and treatment of dry eye

Because the walls of the orbit are rigid, any space-occupying lesion results in protrusion of the eyeball, a condition called *exophthalmos*. Exophthalmos may be caused by swelling or trauma of orbital tissues, tumors of the orbit, or forward displacement of the eye because of endocrine disorders of pituitary or hypothalamic origin. It is commonly seen in persons with a form of hyperthyroidism called *Graves' disease* (see Chapter 35). When the eyelid also protrudes, the condition is known as *proptosis*. This condition causes a delay in lid closure (*i.e.*, lid lag) and, in severe cases, prevents the lids from closing completely, which results in constant exposure and subsequent drying of the cornea. Because the optic nerve has sufficient length within the orbit, protrusion greater than 5 mm is required before nerve damage occurs.

Enophthalmos, or deeply sunken eyes, may be an individual characteristic, but the condition also occurs with severe loss of orbital fat during malnutrition and starvation. Severe developmental defects during the first month of fetal life can result in the absence of one or both optic globes, called *anophthalmos*, and growth defects during the last 3 months of gestation can result in abnormally small eyes, called *microphthalmos*.

Disorders of the Eyelid

Normally, the edges of the eyelids, or palpebrae, are in such a position that the palpebral conjunctiva that lines the eyelids is not exposed and the eyelashes do not rub against the cornea. Turning in of the lid is called *entropion*. It is usually caused by scarring of the palpebral conjunctiva or degeneration of the fascial attachments to the lower lid that occurs with aging. Turning inward of the eyelashes causes corneal irritation. *Ectropion* refers to eversion of the lower lid. The condition is usually bilateral and caused by relaxation of the orbicularis oculi muscle because of seventh nerve weakness or the aging process. Ectropion causes tearing and ocular irritation and may lead to inflammation of the cornea.

Entropion and ectropion can be treated surgically. Electrocautery penetration of the lid conjunctiva can also be used to treat mild forms of ectropion. Contraction of the scar tissue that follows tends to draw the lid up to its normal position.

Eyelid Inflammation

Blepharitis, or inflammation of the eyelid margins, is a common disorder of the eyelid margins. There are two main types: seborrheic and staphylococcal. The seborrheic form is usually associated with seborrhea (*i.e.*, dandruff) of the scalp or brows. Staphylococcal blepharitis may be caused by *Staphylococcus aureus*, in which case it is often ulcerative.[3] The chief symptoms are irritation, burning, redness, and itching of the eyelid margins. Treatment includes careful cleaning with a wet applicator or clean washcloth to remove the scales. A nonirritating baby shampoo can be used. When the disorder is associated with a microbial infection, an antibiotic ointment is prescribed.

A *hordeolum*, or *sty*, is caused by infection of the sebaceous glands of the eyelid and can be internal or external (Fig. 42–2). The main symptoms are pain, redness, and swelling. The treatment is similar to that for abscesses in other parts of the body. Heat in the form of warm compresses is applied, and antibiotic ointment may be used. Incision or expression of the infectious contents of the abscess may be necessary.

A *chalazion* is a small nodule that is formed by fatty degeneration of a hordeolum (Fig. 42–3). It is treated by surgical excision.

Eyelid Weakness

The two striated muscles that provide movement of the eyelids are the levator palpebrae superioris and the orbicularis oculi, which is a circular ring of muscle that surrounds the eye (see Chapter 41). The levator palpebrae, which is innervated by the oculomotor cranial nerve (CN III), raises the upper lid. The orbicularis oculi, which is supplied by the facial nerve (CN VII), closes the lid. The palpebral portion of this muscle is used for gentle closure, and the orbital portion is used for forcible closure of the lids.

Drooping of the eyelid is called *ptosis*. It can result from weakness of the levator muscle (innervated by CN III) that elevates the upper lid in conjunction with the unopposed action of the orbicularis oculi that forcefully closes the palpebral fissure. Weakness of the orbicularis oculi causes an open eyelid, but not ptosis. Neurologic causes of eyelid weakness include damage to the innervating cranial nerves or to the nerves' central nuclei in the midbrain and the caudal pons. Interruption of the sympathetic innervation from the superior cervical ganglion to smooth muscle in the upper eyelid can cause a mild form of ptosis, called *pseudoptosis*.

The facial nerve (CN VII) reaches the orbicularis oculi after exiting the skull under the parotid gland and traveling deep to the skin across the face. Trauma to the zygomatic and buccal branches of the facial nerve with resultant weakness of the orbicularis oculi muscle is relatively common. Weakness of the orbicularis oculi is tested by placement of the examiner's fingers on the muscular

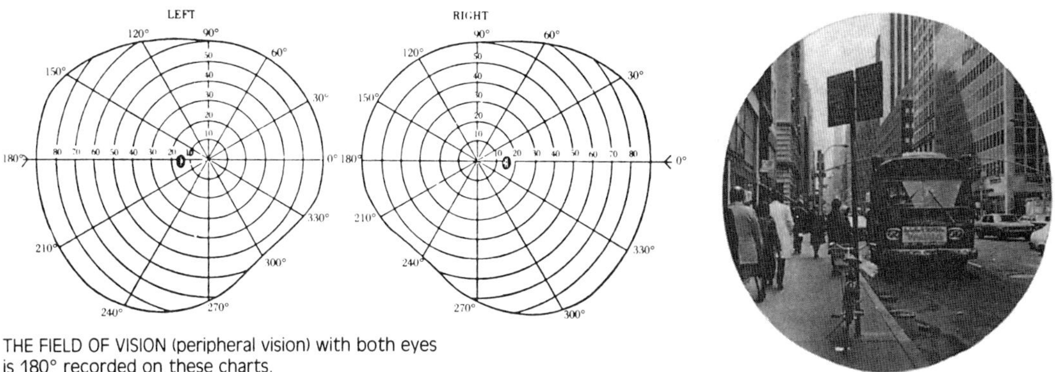

THE FIELD OF VISION (peripheral vision) with both eyes is 180° recorded on these charts.

NORMAL VISION A person with normal or 20/20 vision sees this street scene.

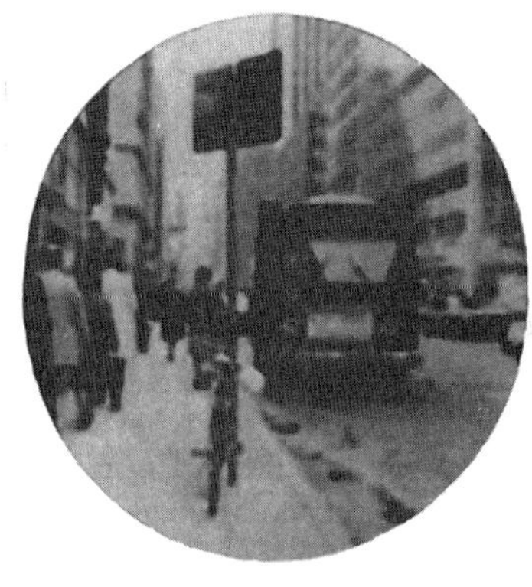

CATARACT Diminished acuity from an opacity of the lens. The field of vision is unaffected. There is no scotoma, but the person has an overall haziness of the view, particularly in glaring light conditions.

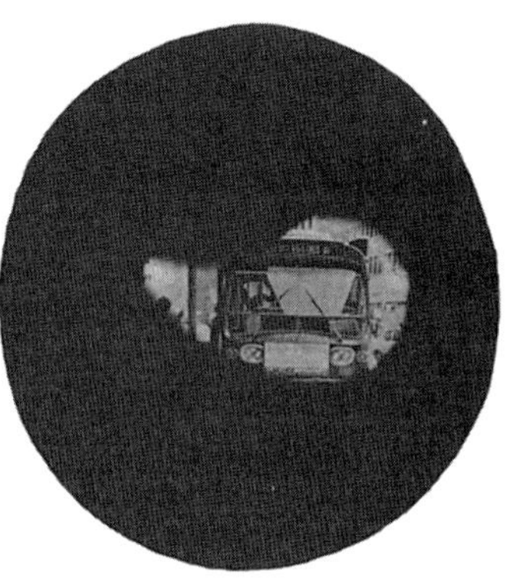

GLAUCOMA Advanced glaucoma involves loss of peripheral vision but the individual still retains most of his central vision.

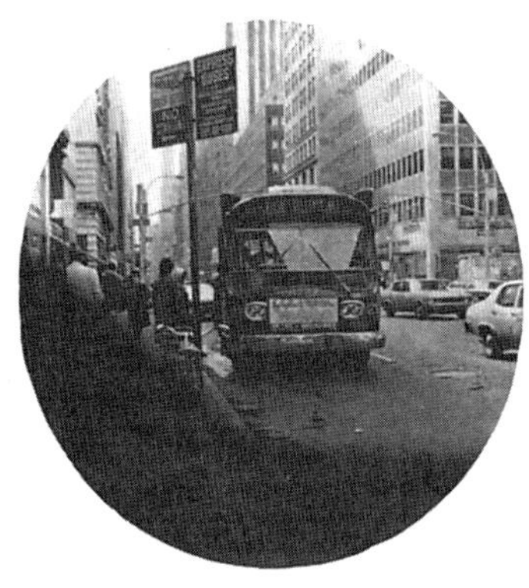

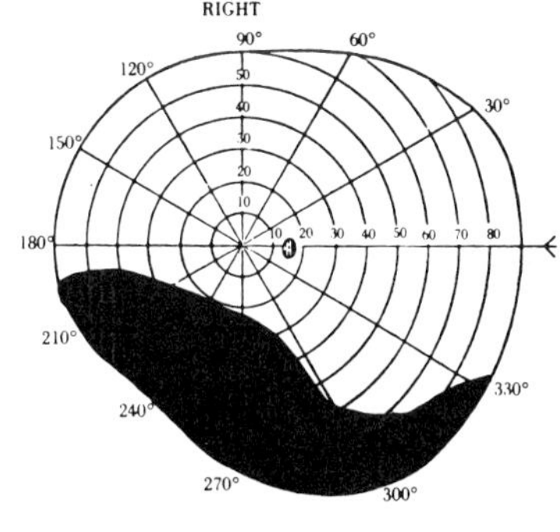

RETINAL DETACHMENT shown here in the active stage. There are many causes for detachment, but the hole or tear allows fluid to lift the retina from its normal position. This elevated retina causes a field or vision defect, seen as a dark shadow in the peripheral field. It may be above, or below as illustrated.

Figure 42–1 ■ ■ ■
Photographs representing the eye diseases, done as if the camera were the right eye. The accompanying visual field chart showing the area of visual loss also represents the right eye. (Photo courtesy The Lighthouse, The New York Association for the Blind)

sphincter ring while the eye is open and then asking the person to close the eye. *Bell's palsy*, which involves paralysis of muscles on one side of the face due to a lesion of the facial nerve or its nucleus in the caudal pons, may result in eyelid weakness, hyperacusis (*i.e.*, acute sense of hearing or painful sensitivity to sound), and disorders of lacrimation and salivation from involvement of the lacrimal, submandibular, and sublingual glands.

Damage to the oculomotor nerve is much less common than damage to the facial nerve, because the oculo-

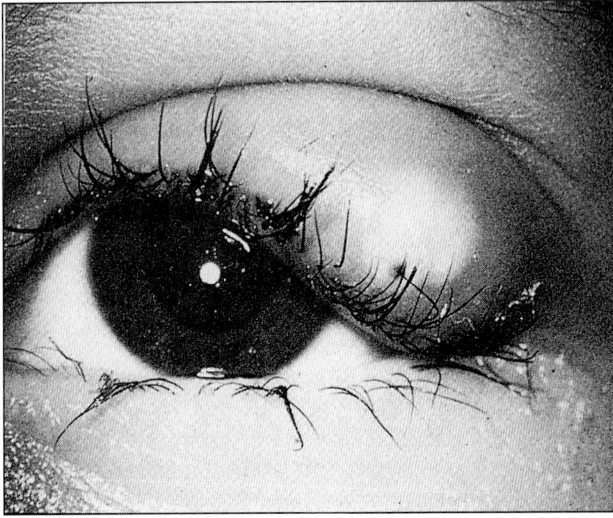

Figure 42–2
Internal hordeolum, left upper eyelid pointing on skin side. (Courtesy of A. Rosenburg. From Vaughn D.G., Asbury T., Riordan-Eva P. [1995]. *General ophthalmology.* Stamford, CT: Appleton-Lange.)

motor nerve is protected by the skull throughout its path. However, ptosis resulting from cranial nerve III injury can occur in cases of midbrain stroke and basal skull fractures and from tumors located deep in the orbit or in the cavernous sinus.

Disorders of the Lacrimal Apparatus

The lacrimal gland is the source of the serous secretions called tears. This gland lies in the orbit, superior and lateral to the eyeball (Chapter 41, Fig. 41–5). Approximately 12 small ducts connect the tear gland to the superior conjunctival fornix. Tears, which contain about 98% water, 1.5% sodium chloride, and the antibacterial enzyme lysozyme, are essential to the maintenance of vision because of their lubricant and antibacterial properties. Lubrication between the two layers of conjunctiva permits comfortable eye and lid movement.

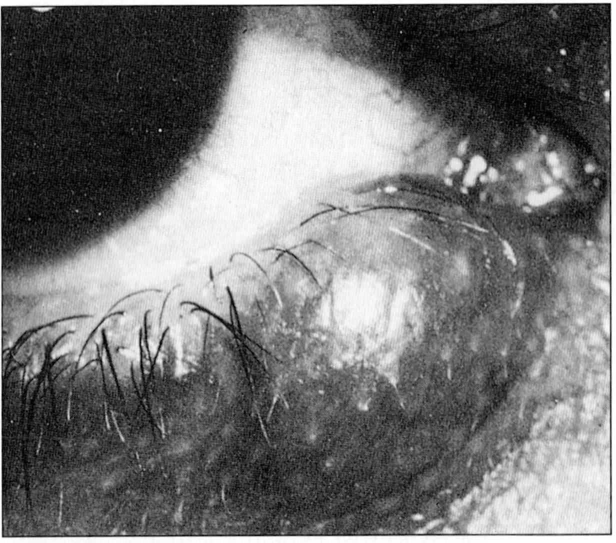

Figure 42–3
Chalazion, right lower eyelid. (Courtesy of K. Tabbara. From Vaughn D.G., Asbury T., Riordan-Eva P. [1995]. *General ophthalmology.* Stamford, CT: Appleton-Lange.)

Dry Eyes

The thin film of tears that covers the cornea is essential in preventing drying and damage of the outer layer of the cornea. The tear film is composed of three layers: the superficial lipid layer, derived from the meibomian glands and thought to retard evaporation; the aqueous layer, secreted by the lacrimal glands; and the mucinous layer that overlies the cornea and epithelial cells.[3] Because the epithelial cell membranes are relatively hydrophobic and cannot be wetted by aqueous solutions alone, the mucinous layer plays an essential role in wetting these surfaces. Periodic blinking of the eyes is needed to maintain a continuous tear film over the ocular surface. Disruption of any of the tear film components or of the blinking action of the eyelids can lead to the interruption of the tear film and result in dry spots on the cornea.

Several conditions reduce the functioning of the lacrimal glands. With aging, the lacrimal glands tend to diminish their secretion, and as a result, many older persons awaken from a night's sleep with highly irritated eyes. Dry eyes also result from loss of reflex lacrimal gland secretion because of congenital defects, infection, irradiation, damage to the parasympathetic innervation of the gland, and medications such as antihistamines and drugs with an anticholinergic action. Wearing contact lenses tends to contribute to eye dryness through decreased blinking.

Sjögren's syndrome is a systemic disorder in which lymphocytes and plasma cells infiltrate the lacrimal and parotid glands. The disorder is associated with diminished salivary and lacrimal secretions, resulting in keratoconjunctivitis sicca (dry eye syndrome) and xerostomia (*i.e.,* dry mouth). The syndrome occurs mainly in women near menopause and is often asssociated with connective tissue disorders such as rheumatoid arthritis. Persons with dry eyes complain of a dry or gritty sensation in the eye, burning, itching, inability to produce tears, photosensitivity, redness, pain, and difficulty in moving the eyelids. Dry eyes and the absence of tears can cause keratinization of the cornea and conjunctival epithelium. In severe cases, corneal ulcerations can occur. Consequent corneal scarring can cause blindness.

The treatment of dry eyes includes frequent instillation of artificial tear solutions into the conjunctival sac. More prolonged duration of action can be obtained from topical preparations containing methylcellulose or polyvinyl alcohol. An ointment is useful for prolonged lubrication. These artificial tear preparations are generally safe and without side effects. However, the preservatives necessary to maintain their sterility are potentially damaging to the cornea.

Dacryocystitis

Dacryocystitis is an infection of the lacrimal sac. It occurs most often in infants or in persons older than 40 years of age. It is usually unilateral and most often occurs secondary to obstruction of the nasolacrimal duct. Often the cause of the obstruction is unknown, although there may be a history of severe trauma to the midface. The symptoms include tearing and discharge, pain, swelling, and tenderness. The treatment includes application of heat (*e.g.*, warm compresses) and antibiotic therapy. In chronic forms of the disorder, surgical repair of the tear duct may be necessary.

In infants, dacryocystitis usually is caused by failure of the nasolacrimal ducts to open spontaneously before birth. When one of the ducts fails to open, a secondary dacryocystitis may develop. These infants are usually treated with gentle massage of the tear sac, instillation of antibiotic drops into the conjunctival sac, and if that fails, probing of the tear duct.

In summary, the optic globe, or eyeball, is protected posteriorly by the bony structures of the orbit and anteriorly by the eyelids. It is continuously bathed by a protective film of tears. Protrusion of the eyes is called exophthalmos, and the condition of deeply sunken eyes is called enophthalmos.

The eyelids serve to protect the eye. Entropion, which refers to turning in the upper eyelid and eyelashes, is discomforting and causes corneal irritation. Extropion, or eversion of the lower eyelid, causes tearing and the potential for corneal inflammation. Marginal blepharitis is the most common disorder of the eyelids. It is commonly caused by a staphylococcal infection or seborrhea (i.e., dandruff). Ptosis refers to drooping of the upper lid, which is caused by injury to CN III. A milder form, pseudoptosis, can be caused by interruption of sympathetic innervation to portions of the principal elevator muscle of the upper eyelid (i.e., levator palpebrae superioris).

Tears protect the cornea from drying and irritation. Impaired tear production or conditions that prevent blinking and the spread of tears produce drying of the eyes and predispose them to corneal irritation and injury.

Disorders of the Conjunctiva, Cornea, and Uveal Tract

After you have completed this section of the chapter, you should be able to meet the following objectives:

- Compare symptoms associated with the red eye caused by conjunctivitis, corneal irritation, and acute glaucoma
- List at least four causes of red eye
- Describe the appearance of corneal edema
- Characterize the manifestations, treatment, and possible complications of bacterial, *Acanthamoeba*, and herpes keratitis

The outer wall of the eyeball (optic globe) is composed of the sclera, which is modified anteriorly to form the cornea, through which light rays enter the eye. The middle vascular layer, or uveal tract, of the eye includes the choroid, the ciliary body, and the iris. The choroid layer contains many of the blood vessels that nourish the structures of the eyeball.

Conjunctivitis

The conjunctiva is a thin layer of mucous membrane that lines the inner surface of the eyelid and covers the optic globe to the junction of the cornea and sclera. Conjunctivitis, or inflammation of the conjunctiva (*i.e.*, red eye or pink eye), is one of the most common forms of eye disease. It varies from mild hyperemia with tearing (*i.e.*, hay fever conjunctivitis) to a severe necrotizing process (*i.e.*, membranous conjunctivitis). Conjunctivitis may result from bacterial or viral infection, allergens, chemical agents, physical irritants, or radiant energy. Infections may extend from areas adjacent to the conjunctiva or may be bloodborne, such as in measles or chickenpox. Newborns can contract conjunctivitis during the birth process.

The main symptoms of conjunctivitis are redness of the eye, which is most obvious peripherally; ocular discomfort or foreign body sensation; a gritty or burning sensation; and tearing. Severe pain suggests corneal rather than conjunctival disease. Itching is common in allergic conditions. A discharge, or exudate, may be present with all types of conjunctivitis and may cause transient blurring of vision. It is usually watery when the conjunctivitis is caused by allergy, a foreign body, or viral infection and mucopurulent in the presence of bacterial or fungal infection. A characteristic of many forms of conjunctivitis is papillary hypertrophy. This occurs because the palpebral conjunctiva is bound to the tarsus by fine fibrils. As a result, inflammation that develops between the fibrils causes the conjunctiva to be elevated in mounds called *papillae*. When the papillae are small, the conjunctiva has a smooth, velvety appearance. A red papillary conjunctivitis suggests bacterial or chlamydial conjunctivitis. In allergic conjunctivitis, the papillae often become flat-topped, polygonal, and milky in color and have a cobblestone appearance. Excessive edema of the bulbar or ocular conjunctiva is called *chemosis*.

Allergic Conjunctivitis

Allergic conjunctivitis (*e.g.*, hay fever) is a common disorder associated with exposure to allergens such as pollen. It causes bilateral tearing, itching, and redness of the eyes. The treatment includes the use of cold compresses, antihistamines, and vasoconstrictor eye drops. Topical lodoxamide (Alomide), a mast cell stabilizer, is available for treatment of mild to moderate manifestations.[4] Levocabastine (Livostin) is currently the only histamine H_1 antagonist available. Ketorolac (Acular) is a nonsteroidal antiinflammatory agent that has been shown to be useful for treatment of allergic conjunctivitis.[4] Topical vasoconstrictor and antihistamine combinations are available as over-the-counter preparations. These preparations are useful but often produce rebound hyperemia.[4] The local application of corticosteroids may be used on a short-term basis.

Bacterial Conjunctivitis

Common agents of bacterial conjunctivitis are *Streptococcus pneumoniae, Staphylococcus aureus, Haemophilus influenzae,* and several members of the genus *Moraxella*.[5] All of these organisms produce a copious, purulent discharge. The eyelids are sticky, and there may be excoriation of the lid margins. Treatment may include local application of antibiotics. The disorder is usually self-limited, lasting about 10 to 14 days if untreated. Scrupulous personal hygiene and prompt adequate treatment of infected persons and their contacts are effective.

Infection may also be caused by *Neisseria gonorrhoeae*. In persons with gonococcal conjunctivitis, corneal disease may lead to perforation. If the cornea is not involved, the infection may be treated with an appropriate antibiotic administered intramuscularly. Topical antibiotics may be used concurrently.[4]

Viral Conjunctivitis

Etiologic agents of viral conjunctivitis include adenoviruses, herpesviruses, and enteroviruses.[6] Adenovirus type 3 infection is usually associated with pharyngitis, fever, and malaise. It causes generalized hyperemia, copious tearing, and minimal exudate. Children are affected more often than adults. Swimming pools contaminated because of inadequate chlorination are common sources of infection. Infections due to adenoviruses types 4 and 7 are often associated with acute respiratory disease. These viruses are rapidly disseminated when large groups mingle with infected individuals (*e.g.*, military recruits). Adenovirus type 8 epidemics are associated with inadequate sterilization of ophthalmic equipment. There is no specific treatment for this type of viral conjunctivitis; it usually lasts 7 to 14 days. Preventive measures include scrupulous personal hygiene such as avoiding shared use of eyedroppers, eye makeup, goggles, and towels.[6,7]

Herpes simplex virus conjunctivitis is characterized by unilateral infection, irritation, mucoid discharge, pain, and mild photophobia. Herpetic vesicles may develop on the eyelids and lid margins. Although the infection is usually caused by the type 1 herpesvirus, it can also be caused by the type 2 virus. It is often associated with herpes simplex virus keratitis, in which the cornea shows discrete epithelial lesions.

Treatment involves the use of systemic or local antiviral agents. Topical antiviral agents such as vidarabine, trifluridine, or idoxuridine usually provide prompt relief.[8] Local corticosteroid preparations increase the activity of the herpes simplex virus, apparently by enhancing the destructive effect of collagenase on the collagen of the cornea. The use of these medications should be avoided in those suspected of having herpes simplex conjunctivitis or keratitis. Local application of interferon has been reported to decrease the spread of herpes simplex keratitis, but the lesions produced by these viruses are not cured. Interferon has a potentiating effect when used with trifluridine.[9]

Chlamydial Conjunctivitis

Inclusion conjunctivitis is usually a benign suppurative conjunctivitis transmitted by the type of *Chlamydia trachomatis* that causes venereal infections (see Chapter 52). It is spread by contaminated genital secretions and occurs in newborns of mothers having *C. trachomatis* infections of the birth canal. It can also be contracted through swimming in unchlorinated pools. The incubation period varies from 5 to 12 days, and the disease may last for several months if untreated. The infection is usually treated with systemic erythromycin and topical tetracycline ointment.

A more serious form of infection is caused by a different strain of *C. trachomatis*. This form of chlamydial infection affects the conjunctiva and causes ulceration and scarring of the cornea. It is the leading cause of preventable blindness in the world. Although the agent is widespread, it is seen mostly in dry and sandy regions and among poor people and nomads.[10] In the United States, the infection is largely confined to Native Americans living in the Southwest. It is transmitted by direct human contact, contaminated objects (fomites), and flies. Of particular concern is pervasive spread of chlamydial infection if this form of conjunctivitis is untreated.

Ophthalmia Neonatorum

Ophthalmia neonatorum is a form of conjunctivitis that occurs in newborns younger than 1 month of age. It is seen most commonly in the newborn and is usually contracted during or soon after vaginal delivery. There are many causes, including *N. gonorrhoeae, Pseudomonas,* and *C. trachomatis*.[11] Epidemiologically, these infections reflect those sexually transmitted diseases most common in a particular area. Once the most common form of conjunctivitis in the newborn, gonococcal ophthalmia neonatorum has an incidence of 0.3% of live births in the United States; *C. trachomatis* has an incidence of 8.2% of live births.[11] Drops of 0.5% erythromycin or 1% silver nitrate are applied immediately after birth to prevent gonococcal ophthalmia. Silver nitrate instillation may cause mild, self-limited conjunctivitis.

Signs of ophthalmia neonatorum include redness and swelling of the conjunctiva, swelling of the eyelids, and discharge, which may be purulent. The conjunctivitis caused by silver nitrate occurs within 6 to 12 hours of birth and clears within 24 to 48 hours.[11] The incubation period for *N. gonorrhoeae* is 2 to 5 days and for *C. trachomatis,* 5 to 14 days. Infection should be suspected when conjunctivitis develops 48 hours after birth.[11] Ophthalmia neonatorum is a potentially blinding condition, and it can cause serious and potentially systemic manifestations. It requires immediate diagnosis and treatment.

Diagnosis

The diagnosis of conjunctivitis is based on history, physical examination, and microscopic and culture studies to identify the cause. Because a red eye may be the sign of several eye conditions, it is important to differentiate between redness caused by conjunctivitis and that caused by more serious eye disorders, such as corneal lesions and acute glaucoma. In contrast to corneal lesions and acute glaucoma, conjunctivitis produces injection (*i.e.*, enlargement and redness) of the peripheral conjunctival blood vessels rather than those radiating around the corneal limbus, and it causes mild discomfort rather than moderate to severe discomfort associated with corneal lesions or the severe and deep pain associated with acute glaucoma. Conjunctivitis does not affect vision, nor does it cause pupillary dilation, as does acute glaucoma. It does not produce changes in the appearance of the cornea. The clarity of the cornea may be changed in corneal injury, depending on the cause, and is steamy or cloudy in acute glaucoma. Infectious forms of conjunctivitis are often bilateral and may involve other family members and close associates. Unilateral disease suggests sources of irritation such as foreign bodies or chemical irritation.

Disorders of the Cornea

The cornea is avascular and derives its nutrient and oxygen supply by diffusion from blood vessels of the adjacent sclera, from the aqueous humor at its deep surface, and from tears. The corneal epithelium is heavily innervated by sensory neurons (trigeminal cranial nerve [V], ophthalmic division [V_1]). Epithelial damage causes discomfort that ranges from a foreign body sensation and burning of the eyes to severe stabbing or knifelike incapacitating pain. Reflex lacrimation is common. Disorders of the cornea include trauma and infections, abnormal corneal deposits, and arcus senilis.

Corneal Trauma

Trauma that causes abrasions of the cornea can be extremely painful, but if minor, the abrasions usually heal in a few days. The epithelial layer is capable of regeneration, and small defects heal without scarring. If the stroma is damaged, healing occurs more slowly, and the danger of infection is increased. Injuries to Bowman's membrane and the stromal layer heal with scar formation and permanent opacification. Opacities of the cornea impair the transmission of light. A minor scar can severely distort vision, because it disturbs the refractive surface.

The integrity of the epithelium and the endothelium is necessary to maintain the hydration of the cornea within a limited range. Damage to either structure leads to edema and loss of transparency. Among the causes of corneal edema are prolonged and uninterrupted wearing of hard contact lenses, which can deprive the epithelium of oxygen, disrupting its integrity. The edema disappears spontaneously when the cornea comes in contact with the atmosphere. Corneal edema also occurs when there is a sudden rise in intraocular pressure. If intraocular pressure rises rapidly above 50 mm Hg, as in acute glaucoma, subendothelial edema develops. With corneal edema, the cornea appears dull, uneven, and hazy. Visual acuity decreases, and iridescent vision (*i.e.*, rainbows around lights) occurs. Iridescent vision results from epithelial and subepithelial edema, which splits white light into its component parts with blue in the center and red on the outside.

Keratitis

Keratitis refers to inflammation of the cornea. It can be caused by infections, hypersensitivity reactions, ischemia, defects in tearing, trauma, and interruption in sensory innervation, as occurs with local anesthesia. Scar tissue formation due to keratitis is the leading cause of blindness and impaired vision throughout the world. Most of this vision loss is preventable if the condition is diagnosed early and appropriate treatment is instituted.

Keratitis can be divided into two types: ulcerative, in which part of the epithelium, stroma, or both are destroyed, and nonulcerative, in which all the layers of the epithelium are affected by the inflammation but the epithelium remains intact. Causes of ulcerative keratitis include infectious agents such as those causing conjunctivitis (*e.g.*, *Staphylococcus*, *Streptococcus pneumoniae*, *Chlamydia*), exposure trauma, and use of extended-wear contact lens. Bacterial keratitis tends to be aggressive and demands immediate care. Exposure trauma may result from deformities of the lid, paralysis of the lid muscles, or severe exophthalmos. Mooren's ulcer is a chronic, painful, indolent ulcer that occurs in the absence of infection. It is usually seen in older persons and may affect both eyes. Nonulcerative keratitis is associated with a number of diseases, including syphilis, tuberculosis, and lupus erythematosus. It may also result from a viral infection entering through a small defect in the cornea.

Generally, peripheral involvement of the cornea is related to the same disorders that affect the conjunctiva. *Acanthamoeba* is a free-living protozoa that thrives in contaminated water. It is an increasingly serious and sight-threatening complication of wearing soft contact lens, particularly when homemade saline solutions are used for cleaning.[12] It is characterized by pain that is disproportionate to the clinical manifestations, redness of the eye, and photophobia. The disorder is commonly misdiagnosed as herpes keratitis. Diagnosis is confirmed by scrapings and culture with specially prepared medium. In the early stages of infection, epithelial debridement may be beneficial. Treatment includes intensive use of topical antibiotics. However, the organism may encyst within the corneal stroma, making treatment more difficult. Keratoplasty may be necessary in advanced disease to arrest the progression of the infection.

Symptoms of keratitis include photophobia, discomfort, and lacrimation. The discomfort may range from foreign body sensation to severe pain. Defective vision results from the changes in transparency and curvature of the cornea that occur. An ulcerated area stains green when a drop of fluorescein dye is instilled.

Herpes Simplex Keratitis

Herpes simplex virus keratitis is the most common cause of corneal ulceration in the United States. Most cases are caused by herpes simplex virus type 1 infections. However, in neonatal infections acquired during passage through the birth canal, about 80% are caused by herpes simplex virus type 2.[13] The disease can occur as a primary or recurrent infection. Primary infections cause follicular conjunctivitis and blepharitis, characterized by a rounded cobblestone pattern of avascular lesions. Epithelial keratitis may develop. After the initial primary infection, the virus may persist in a quiescent or latent state that remains in the trigeminal ganglion and possibly in the cornea without causing signs of infection. During childhood, mild primary herpes simplex virus infection may go unnoticed.[13]

Recurrent infection may be precipitated by various poorly understood, stress-related factors that reactivate the virus. Involvement is usually unilateral. The first symptoms are irritation, photophobia, and tearing. There may be some reduction in vision when the lesion affects the central part of the cornea. Because corneal anesthesia occurs early in the disease, the symptoms may be minimal, and the person may delay seeking medical care. There is often a history of fever blisters or other herpetic infection, but corneal lesions may be the only sign of recurrent herpes infection. Most typically, the corneal lesion involves the epithelium and has a typical branching pattern (Fig. 42–4). These epithelial lesions heal without scarring. Topical antiviral agents such as trifluridine (Viroptic) drops, idoxuridine (IDU) drops, or vidarabine (Vira-A) ointment are used to promote healing. Corticosteroid drugs are contraindicated because they increase viral replication.

Lesions that involve the stromal layer of the cornea produce increasingly severe corneal opacities. They are thought to have an immune rather than an infectious cause. Stromal keratitis may be treated with topically applied corticosteroids to suppress the immune response. The most common cause of corneal blindness in the Western world is stromal scarring from herpes simplex keratitis.[13]

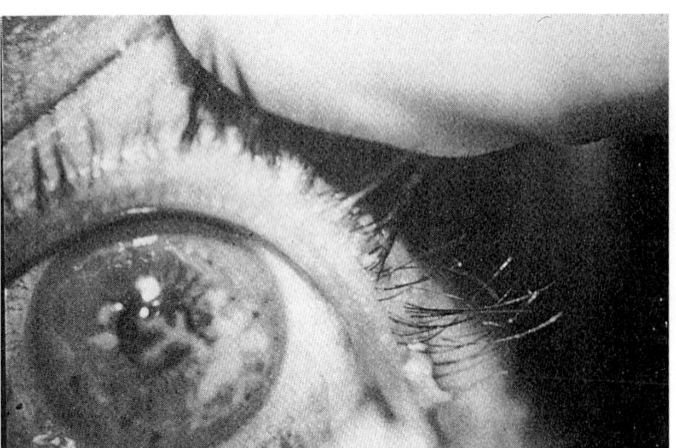

Figure 42–4
Dendritic figures seen in herpes simplex keratitis. (From Vaughn D.G., Asbury T., Riordan-Eva P. [1995]. *General ophthalmology.* Stamford, CT: Appleton-Lange.)

Abnormal Corneal Deposits

The cornea is frequently the site of deposition of abnormal metabolic products. In hypercalcemia, calcium salts can precipitate within the cornea, producing a cloudy band keratopathy. Cystine crystals are deposited in cystinosis, cholesterol esters in hypercholesterolemia, and a golden ring of copper (*i.e.,* Kayser-Fleischer ring) in hepatolenticular degeneration due to Wilson's disease. Pharmacologic agents, such as chloroquine, can result in crystal deposits in the cornea.

Arcus Senilis

Arcus senilis is an extremely common, bilateral, benign corneal degeneration that may occur at any age, but it is more common in the elderly. It consists of a grayish white infiltrate, about 2 mm wide, that occurs at the periphery of the cornea. It represents an extracellular lipid infiltration and is commonly associated with hyperlipidemia. Arcus senilis does not produce visual symptoms, and there is no treatment for the disorder.

Corneal Transplantation

Advances in ophthalmologic surgery permit corneal transplantation using a cadaver cornea. Unlike kidney or heart transplantation procedures, which are associated with considerable risk of rejection of the transplanted organ, the use of cadaver corneas entails minimal danger of rejection, because this tissue is not exposed to the vascular and therefore the immunologic defense system. Instead, the success of this type of transplantation operation depends on the prevention of scar tissue formation, which would limit the transparency of the transplanted cornea.

Uveitis

Inflammation of the entire uveal tract, which supports the lens and neural components of the eye, is called *uveitis.* It is one of several inflammatory disorders of ocular tissue with clinical features in common and an immunologically based cause.[13] One of the serious consequences of uveitis can be the involvement of the underlying retina. Parasitic invasion of the choroid can result in local atrophic changes that usually involve the retina; examples include toxoplasmosis and histoplasmosis. Sarcoid deposition in the form of small nodules results in irregularities of the underlying retinal surface.

In summary, the conjunctiva lines the inner surface of the eyelids and covers the optic globe to the junction of the cornea and sclera. Conjunctivitis, also called red eye or pink eye, may result from bacterial or viral infection, allergens, chemical agents, physical agents, or radiant energy. It is important to differentiate between redness caused by conjunctivitis and that caused by more serious eye disorders, such as acute glaucoma or corneal lesions.

Keratitis, or inflammation of the cornea, can be caused by infections, hypersensitivity reactions, ischemia, trauma, defects in tearing, or trauma. Trauma or disease that involves the stromal layer of the cornea heals with scar formation and permanent opacification. These opacities interfere with the transmission of light and may impair vision.

The uveal tract is the middle vascular layer of the eye. It contains melanocytes that prevent diffusion of light through the wall of the optic globe. Inflammation of the uveal tract (uveitis) can affect visual acuity.

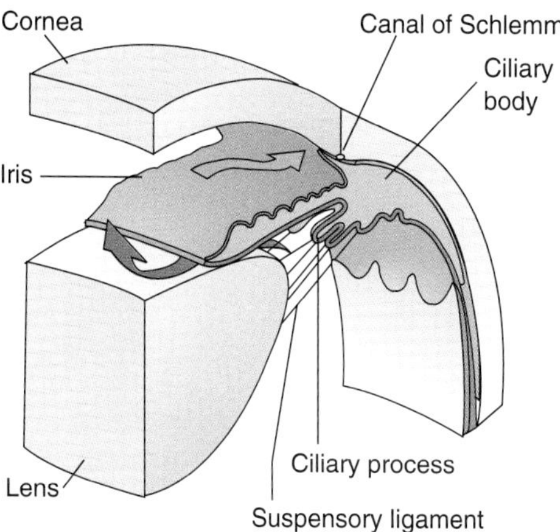

Figure 42–5
Enlarged view of the anterior portion of the eyeball. *Arrows* indicate the flow of aqueous humor.

Glaucoma

After you have completed this section of the chapter, you should be able to meet the following objectives:

- Describe the formation and outflow of aqueous humor from the eye and relate to the development of glaucoma
- Compare closed-angle and open-angle glaucoma
- Explain why glaucoma leads to blindness

Glaucoma includes a group of conditions that produce an elevation in intraocular pressure. If left untreated, the pressure may increase sufficiently to cause ischemia and degeneration of the optic nerve, leading to progressive blindness. Glaucoma is a major contributor to the incidence of more than 80,000 to 150,000 legally blind persons in the United States.[14] It is the second leading cause of irreversible blindness in the United States and the most common cause among African Americans. Although the latter have been reported to have an incidence six times that of whites, they are only twice as likely to receive appropriate health care.[15] The condition is often asymptomatic, and a significant loss of peripheral vision may occur before medical attention is sought, emphasizing the need for routine screening for early diagnosis and treatment of increased intraocular pressure in persons older than 40.

Control of Intraocular Pressure

The aqueous humor helps maintain intraocular pressure and serves a nutritive function, facilitating metabolism of the lens and posterior cornea. It contains a low protein concentration and a high concentration of ascorbic acid, glucose, and amino acids. It also mediates the exchange of respiratory gases.

The aqueous humor is formed by the ciliary epithelium in the posterior chamber and flows through the pupil to the angle formed by the cornea and the iris. Here it filters through the trabecular meshwork and enters the canal of Schlemm for return to the venous circulation (Fig. 42–5). The secretion of aqueous humor is an active process that continues regardless of the pressure exerted by the secreted fluid. The secretory activity of the ciliary epithelium requires the enzyme carbonic anhydrase.

The interior pressure of the eye must exceed atmospheric pressure to prevent the eyeball from collapsing. The hydrostatic pressure of the aqueous humor results from a balance of several factors, including the rate of secretion, resistance to flow through the narrow opening between the lens and iris at the entrance into the anterior chamber, and resistance to resorption at the trabeculated region of the sclera at the iridocorneal angle. Normally, the rate of aqueous production is equal to the rate of aqueous outflow, and the intraocular pressure is maintained within a normal range of 9 to 21 mm Hg. However, data suggest that the value is closer to 12 ± 1 mm Hg in young, healthy adults during daylight hours. The mean value increases by approximately 1 mm Hg per decade after 40 years of age.[16]

Abnormalities in the balance between aqueous production and outflow lead to increased intraocular pressure, a disease complex called *glaucoma.* Rarely is intraocular pressure increased by overproduction of aqueous humor; it usually results from interference with aqueous outflow from the anterior chamber. As intraocular pressure rises because of impaired outflow, the canal of Schlemm is compressed, causing a further reduction in aqueous outflow. The sustained increase in intraocular pressure that occurs with glaucoma leads to a gradual loss of peripheral vision (see Fig. 42–1), followed by loss of central vision.

Types of Glaucoma

Glaucoma is commonly classified as closed-angle (*i.e.,* narrow-angle) or open-angle (*i.e.,* wide-angle) glaucoma, depending on the location of the compromised aqueous humor circulation and resorption. Glaucoma may occur as a congenital or an acquired condition, and

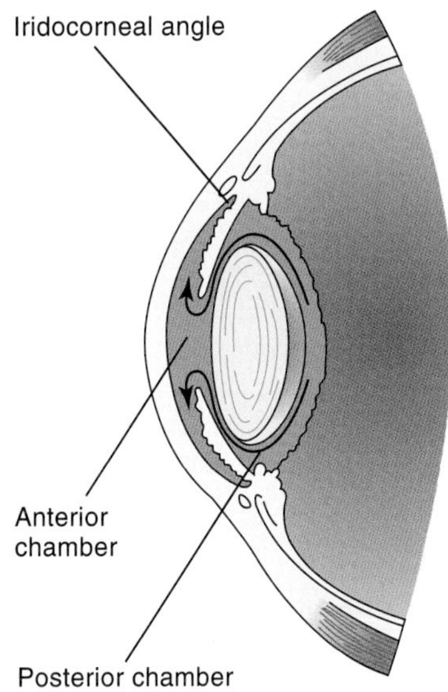

Figure 42–6
Narrow anterior chamber and iridocorneal angle in closed-angle (narrow-angle) glaucoma.

it may manifest as a primary or secondary disorder. Primary glaucoma occurs without evidence of preexisting ocular or systemic disease. Secondary glaucoma can result from inflammatory processes that affect the eye, from tumors, or from the blood cells of trauma-produced hemorrhage that obstruct the outflow of aqueous humor. Obstruction of the anterior chamber angle can accompany a number of pathologic processes, such as adhesions of the iris to the cornea or lens.[13]

Closed-Angle Glaucoma

In closed-angle glaucoma, the anterior chamber is narrow, and outflow becomes impaired when the iris thickens as the result of pupil dilation (Fig. 42–6). As the iris thickens, it restricts the circulation between the base of the iris and the sclera (*i.e.*, pupillary-block mechanism), reducing or restricting the circulation between the posterior and anterior chambers and reducing or eliminating access to the angle where aqueous reabsorption occurs.[14] Approximately 5% to 10% of all cases of glaucoma fall into this category. Closed-angle glaucoma usually occurs as the result of an inherited anatomic defect that causes a shallow anterior chamber. This defect is exaggerated by the anterior displacement of the peripheral iris that occurs in older persons because of the increase in lens size that occurs with aging.

The symptoms of closed-angle glaucoma are related to sudden, intermittent increases in intraocular pressure. These occur after prolonged periods in the dark, emotional upset, and other conditions that cause extensive and prolonged pupil dilation. Administration of pharmacologic agents such as atropine that cause pupillary dilation (mydriasis) can also precipitate an acute episode of increased intraocular pressure in persons with the potential for closed-angle glaucoma. Attacks of increased intraocular pressure are manifested by ocular pain and blurred or iridescent vision caused by corneal edema. The pupil may be enlarged and fixed. The symptoms are often spontaneously relieved by sleep and conditions that promote pupillary constriction. With repeated or prolonged attacks, the eye becomes reddened, and edema of the cornea may develop, giving the eye a hazy appearance. A unilateral, often excruciating, headache is common. Nausea and vomiting may occur, causing the headache to be confused with migraine.

Some persons with congenitally narrow anterior chambers never develop symptoms, and others develop symptoms only when they are elderly. Because of the dangers of vision loss, those with narrow anterior chambers should be warned about the significance of blurred vision, halos, and ocular pain. Sometimes, decreased visual acuity and an unreactive pupil may be the only clue to closed angle glaucoma in the elderly.

Primary Open-Angle Glaucoma

Primary open-angle glaucoma is the most common form of glaucoma. It tends to manifest after age 35, with an incidence of 0.5% to 2% among persons 40 years of age and older.[13] The condition is characterized by an abnormal increase in intraocular pressure that occurs in the absence of an obstruction between the trabecular meshwork and the anterior chamber. Instead, it usually occurs because of an abnormality of the trabecular meshwork that impairs the flow of aqueous humor between the anterior chamber and the canal of Schlemm. Risk factors for this disorder include an age of 40 years and older, family history of the disorder, diabetes mellitus, and myopia. In some persons, the use of moderate amounts of topical corticosteroid medications can cause an increase in intraocular pressure. Sensitive persons may also sustain an increase in intraocular pressure with the use of systemic corticosteroid drugs. Primary open-angle glaucoma is usually asymptomatic and chronic, causing progressive loss of visual field unless it is appropriately treated. Because it is usually asymptomatic, routine screening using applanation tonometry is the best means of detecting the disorder.

Diagnosis. Intraocular pressure can be estimated by direct palpation or measured indirectly by means of a tonometer. Direct palpation, by gentle use of the examiner's index fingers on each upper tarsal plate, is not quantitative but can indicate whether the eye is soft or hard. Two types of tonometers are used for measuring intraocular pressure: contact tonometers such as the Goldmann applanation tonometer that is placed on the anesthetized eye, and the noncontact tonometer, which uses an air pulse. Applanation tonometry is the most accurate clinically applicable method to measure the intraocular pressure. It functions by flattening the curvature of the cornea to a degree dependent on the pressure applied and the resistance of the cornea to deformation. As long as the cornea is structurally intact, its resistance to deformation varies directly with intraocular pressure. Although the noncontact tonometer is not as accurate as the contact applanation tonometer, it does not require eye drops, because no instrument touches the eye. Another familiar method, Schiotz tonometry, requires only a hand-held instrument—the Schiotz contact tonometer. It is less accurate than the Goldman applanation tonometer but may be used when an irregular corneal surface precludes use of other devices.

Increased intraocular pressure causes damage to optic nerve axons in the region of the optic nerve that can be recognized on ophthalmoscopic examination. The normal optic disk has a centrally placed depression called the *optic cup*. With progressive atrophy of axons caused by increased intraocular pressure, pallor of the optic disk develops, and the size and depth of the optic cup increase. Because changes in the optic cup precede the visual field loss, regular ophthalmoscopic examination is important for detecting eye changes that occur with increased intraocular pressure. Stereoscopic viewing during slit-lamp examination improves the accuracy of evaluation.[17]

The depth of the anterior chamber can be evaluated by transillumination or by a technique called *gonioscopy*. Gonioscopy uses a special contact lens and mirrors or prisms so that the angle of the anterior chamber can be seen and measured. The transillumination method requires only a penlight. The light source is held at the temporal side of the eye and directed horizontally across the iris. In persons with a normal-sized anterior chamber, the light passes through the chamber to illuminate both halves of the iris. In persons with a narrow anterior chamber, only the half of the iris adjacent to the light source is illuminated (Fig. 42–7).

Advances in computer technology allow detection and quantification of visual changes due to glaucoma. These tests of vision include color vision analysis, blue-on-yellow visual field testing and testing of contrast sensitivity, dark adaptation, and other tests of retinal function. In the future, these tests are likely to be used in detecting visual field defects not currently detected by standard means.[14]

Treatment. The treatment of closed-angle glaucoma is primarily surgical. It involves creating an opening between the anterior and posterior chambers with laser or incisional iridectomy to allow aqueous humor to bypass the pupillary block. The anatomic abnormalities responsible for closed-angle glaucoma are usually bilateral, but progression may not be symmetric. In contrast to closed-angle glaucoma, which can be treated surgically, open-angle glaucoma is usually treated medically.

Most glaucoma drugs exert their effect by acting on the parasympathetic (cholinergic) or sympathetic (adrenergic) branches of the autonomic nervous system within the eye. These drugs are applied topically as eye drops and exert their major effects locally, rather than systemically. The α- and β-adrenergic receptors interact in a complex way to control aqueous humor production and outflow. The β-adrenergic blockers are usually the drugs of first choice for lowering intraocular pressure. In general, β-adrenergic activation tends to increase aqueous outflow, and inhibition tends to reduce aqueous production. Nonselective and selective β_1 and β_2 blockers are available; the selection of an agent may be based on cardiac or pulmonary side effects. Nonselective adrenergic agents such as epinephrine stimulate both α and β receptors and tend to cause more systemic side effects such as tachycardia. Dipivefrin is a prodrug that is converted to epinephrine within the eye and seldom causes side effects. Apraclonidine, an α-$_2$ agonist reduces intraocular pressure by decreasing aqueous humor formation.

Acetylcholine is the postganglionic neuromediator for the parasympathetic system; it increases aqueous outflow through contraction of the ciliary muscle and pupillary constriction (miosis). Acetylcholine is broken down by the enzyme acetylcholinesterase. The most commonly used miotic drug is pilocarpine, which functions as a direct cholinergic agonist. Echothiophate, another miotic agent, acts indirectly by inhibiting the breakdown of acetylcholine by acetylcholinesterase.

Carbonic anhydrase inhibitors reduce the secretion of aqueous humor by the ciliary epithelium. Until recently,

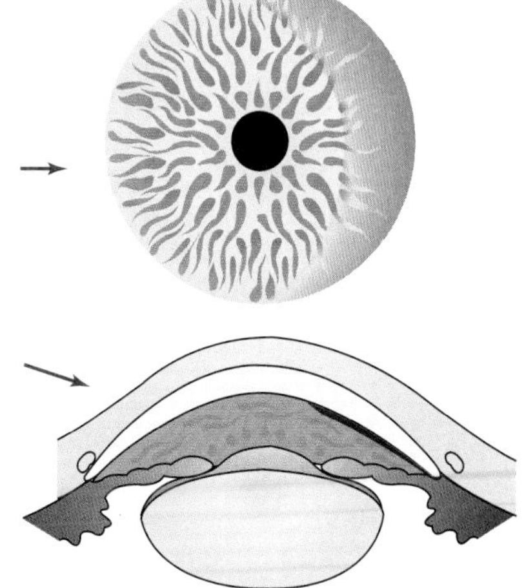

Figure 42–7
Transillumination of the iris. In the eye with a normal anterior chamber, the iris is evenly illuminated by light shining obliquely into the anterior chamber. In the eye with a narrow anterior chamber, the iris is unevenly illuminated and shadowed.

these drugs (*i.e.*, methazolamide and acetazolamide) had to be taken orally, and systemic side effects were common. A topical carbonic anhydrase inhibitor, dorzolamide, acts locally, eliminating the side effects associated with the oral forms of the drug.[14]

When a reduction in intraocular pressure cannot be maintained through pharmacologic methods, surgical treatment may become necessary. Until recently, the main surgical treatment for open-angle glaucoma was a filtering procedure in which an opening is created between the anterior chamber and the subconjunctival space. An argon or neodymium-aluminum-garnet (Nd:YAG) laser technique, in which multiple spots are applied 360 degrees around the trabecular meshwork, has been developed.[3] The microburns resulting from the laser treatment scar rather than penetrate the trabecular meshwork, a process that is thought to enlarge the outflow channels by increasing the tension exerted on the trabecular meshwork. Cryotherapy, diathermy, and high-frequency ultrasound may be used in some cases to destroy the ciliary epithelium and reduce aqueous humor production.

Congenital or Infantile Glaucoma

Congenital glaucoma is caused by a disorder in which the anterior chamber retains its fetal configuration, with aberrant trabecular meshwork extending to the root of the iris, or is covered by a membrane. The incidence of congenital glaucoma is 1 case per 5000 to 10,000 live births. An X-linked recessive mode of inheritance is common, producing a high incidence among males.[18] The earliest symptoms are excessive lacrimation and photophobia. Affected infants tend to be fussy, have poor eating habits, and rub their eyes frequently. Diffuse edema of the cornea usually occurs, giving the eye a grayish white appearance. Chronic elevation of the intraocular pressure before the age of 3 years causes enlargement of the entire globe (*i.e.*, buphthalmos). Early surgical treatment is necessary to prevent blindness.

In summary, glaucoma is one of the leading causes of blindness in the United States. It is characterized by conditions that cause an increase in intraocular pressure and that, if untreated, can lead to atrophy of the optic disk and progressive blindness. The aqueous humor is formed by the ciliary epithelium in the posterior chamber and flows through the pupil to the angle formed by the cornea and the iris. Here it filters through the trabecular meshwork and enters canal of Schlemm for return to the venous circulation. Glaucoma results from overproduction or the impeded outflow of aqueous humor from the anterior chamber of the eye.

There are two major forms of glaucoma: closed-angle and open-angle. Closed-angle glaucoma is caused by a narrow anterior chamber and blockage of the outflow channels at the angle formed by the iris and the cornea. This occurs when the iris becomes thickened during pupillary dilation. Open-angle glaucoma is caused by microscopic obstruction of the trabecular meshwork. Open-angle glaucoma is usually asymptomatic, and considerable loss of the visual field often occurs before medical treatment is sought. Routine screening by applanation tonometry provides one of the best means for early detection of glaucoma before vision loss has occurred.

Cataracts

After you have completed this section of the chapter, you should be able to meet the following objectives:

- Describe the changes in eye structure that occur with cataract
- Cite risk factors associated with cataract
- Characterize the visual changes that occur with cataract
- Describe the treatment of persons with cataracts

A cataract is a lens opacity that interferes with the transmission of light to the retina. It has been estimated that 5 to 10 million persons in the United States are visually disabled because of cataracts.[1] Cataracts are the most common cause of age-related visual loss in the world; they are found in about 50% of those between 65 and 74 years of age and in 70% of those older than 75. In most cases of cataract, vision can be restored or improved by surgical intervention. An estimated 1.35 million procedures are performed each year in the United States.[19]

Causes and Types of Cataracts

The cause of cataract development is thought to be multifactorial, with different factors being associated with different types of opacities. Several risk factors have been proposed, including the effect of aging, genetic influences, environmental and metabolic influences, and injury.[19] Long-term exposure to sunlight (UVB radiation) and heavy smoking have been associated with increased risk of cataract formation.[19] In some cases, cataracts occur as a developmental defect (*i.e.*, congenital cataracts) or secondary to trauma or diseases.

Disorders of carbohydrate metabolism are the most common metabolic causes of cataract. Normally, glucose enters lens cells by diffusion and is reduced to sorbitol (an alcohol) by the intracellular enzyme aldose reductase. Sorbitol diffuses out of the lens fibers slowly, creating an osmotic gradient for the entry of water. In uncontrolled diabetes mellitus, the entry of water into the lens fibers accelerates, with increased production of osmotically active sorbitol. The lens fibers swell and change their refractive properties, causing myopic changes and blurring of vision. The condition is slowly reversible unless it is longstanding, in which case lens fiber destruction and permanent cataracts occur. The sugar galactose exerts the same effect in persons with galactosemia.

Cataracts can result from a number of drugs. Dinitrophenol, a drug widely used for weight reduction during the 1930s; triparanol; chlorpromazine; and the corticosteroid drugs have all been implicated as causative agents in cataract formation. Busulfan, a cancer treatment drug, has been clearly linked to cataract formation. Frequent examination of lens transparency should accompany the use of these and any other substances with cataract-forming effects.

Traumatic Cataract

Traumatic cataracts are most often caused by foreign body injury to the lens or blunt trauma to the eye. Foreign body injury that interrupts the lens capsule allows aqueous and vitreous humor to enter the lens and initiate cataract formation. Other causes of traumatic cataract are overexposure to heat (*e.g.*, glassblower's cataract) or to ionizing radiation. The radiation dose necessary to cause a cataract varies with the amount and type of energy; younger lenses are most vulnerable.

Congenital Cataract

A congenital cataract is one that is present at birth. Among the causes of congenital cataracts are genetic defects, toxic environmental agents, and viruses such as rubella. A maternal rubella infection during the first trimester can cause congenital cataract. Exposure of the embryo to ionizing radiation levels as low as 50 centigray (cGy), such as occurs during a barium enema or fluoroscopy, can also induce congenital cataract. Cataracts and other developmental defects of the ocular apparatus depend on the total dose and the embryonic stage at the time of exposure. During the last trimester of fetal life, genetically or environmentally influenced malformation of the superficial lens fibers can occur. Most congenital cataracts are not progressive and are not dense enough to cause significant visual impairment. However, if the cataracts are bilateral and the opacity is significant, lens extraction should be done on one eye by the age of 2 months to permit the development of vision and prevent nystagmus. If the surgery is successful, the other eye should be done soon after.

Senile Cataract

Cataract is the most common cause of age-related vision loss in the world. With normal aging, the nucleus and the cortex of the lens enlarge as new fibers are formed in the cortical zones of the lens. In the nucleus, the old fibers become more compressed and dehydrated. Metabolic changes occur. Lens proteins become more insoluble, and concentrations of calcium, sodium, potassium, and phosphate increase. During the early stages of cataract formation, a yellow pigment and vacuoles accumulate in the lens fibers. The unfolding of protein molecules, cross-linking of sulfhydryl groups, and conversion of soluble to insoluble proteins lead to the loss of lens transparency. The onset is gradual, and the only symptoms are increasingly blurred vision and visual distortion.

Manifestations

The manifestations of cataract depend on the extent of opacity and whether the defect is bilateral or unilateral. With the exception of traumatic or congenital cataract, most cataracts are bilateral. Age-related cataracts, which are the most common type, are characterized by increasingly blurred vision and visual distortion (see Fig. 42–1). Vision for far and near objects decreases. Dilation of the pupil in dim light improves vision. With nuclear cataracts (those involving the lens nucleus), the refractive power of the anterior segment often increases to produce an acquired myopia. Persons with hyperopia may experience a "second sight" or improved reading acuity until increasing opacity reduces acuity. Central lens opacities may divide the visual axis and cause an optical defect in which two or more blurred images are seen. In addition to decreased visual acuity, cataracts tend to cause light entering the eye to be scattered, thereby producing glare or the abnormal presence of light in the visual field. On ophthalmoscopic examination, cataracts may appear as a gross opacity filling the pupillary aperture or as an opacity silhouetted against the red background of the fundus.

Diagnosis and Treatment

Diagnosis of cataract is based on the Snellen vision test and on the degree of visual impairment. A Snellen acuity of 20/50 is a common requirement for drivers of motor vehicles. Visual impairment is based on the person's assessment of visual function and disability due to glare. Other tests of potential vision (*e.g.*, the ability to see well after surgery), such as electrophysiologic testing in which the response to visual stimuli is measured electronically, may be done.

There is no effective medical treatment for cataract. Use of strong bifocals, magnification, appropriate lighting, and visual aids may be used as the cataract progresses. Surgery is the only treatment for correcting cataract-related vision loss. Surgery usually involves lens extraction and intraocular lens implantation. One of the greatest advances in cataract surgery has been the development of reliable lens implants. The use of extracapsular surgery, which leaves the posterior capsule of the lens intact, has further improved the outcomes of cataract surgery. One of the advances in extracapsular surgery is phacoemulsification, or breaking up of the lens using sound waves. In the future, it is anticipated that lasers may be used for this purpose. Another advance in cataract surgery has been the use of a Nd:YAG laser to remove capsular opacities that develop in about 25% of persons who have extracapsular surgery.

The American Academy of Ophthalmology standard for when cataract surgery should be performed is when "best corrected" visual acuity is 20/50 or worse in the affected eye.[20] However, surgery may still be indicated when a person's best corrected acuity is 20/40 or better, if there is disabling glare or work-related disability or if the cataract threatens to cause other eye problems, such as secondary glaucoma or uveitis. Surgery is commonly performed on an outpatient basis and with the use of local anesthesia.

In summary, a cataract is a lens opacity. It can occur as the result of congenital influences, metabolic disturbances, infection, injury, and aging. The most common type of cataract is the senile cataract that occurs with aging. The treatment for a totally opaque or mature cataract is surgical extraction. An intraocular lens implant may be inserted during the surgical procedure to replace the lens that has been removed; otherwise, thick convex lenses or contact lenses are used to compensate for the loss of lens function.

Disorders of the Vitreous and Retina

After you have completed this section of the chapter, you should be able to meet the following objectives:

- Relate the phagocytic function of the retinal pigment epithelium to the development of retinitis pigmentosa
- Cite the manifestations and long-term visual effects of papilledema, central artery and central venous occlusions
- Describe the pathogenesis of background and proliferative diabetic retinopathies and their mechanisms of visual impairment
- Explain how prematurity and oxygen administration interact in producing retinopathy of prematurity
- Discuss the cause of retinal detachment
- Explain the pathology and visual changes associated with macular degeneration

The posterior segment, which constitutes five sixths of the eyeball, contains the transparent vitreous humor and the neural retina. The innermost layer of the eyeball, the fundus, is is visualized through the pupil with an ophthalmoscope.

Disorders of the Vitreous

The vitreous humor (*i.e.*, vitreous body) is a colorless, amorphous, biologic gel that fills the posterior cavity of the eye. It consists of about 99% water, some salts, glycoproteins, proteoglycans, and dispersed collagen fibrils. The vitreous is attached to the ciliary body and the peripheral retina in the region of the ora serrata and to the periphery of the optic disk.

Disease, aging, and injury can disturb the factors that maintain the water of the vitreous humor in suspension, causing liquefaction of the gel to occur. With the loss of gel structure, fine fibers, membranes, and cellular debris develop. When this occurs, floaters (images) can often be noticed as these substances move within the vitreous cavity during head movement. In disease, blood vessels may grow from the surface of the retina or optic disk onto the posterior surface of the vitreous, and blood may fill the vitreous cavity.

During development, the distal portion of the hyaloid artery within the vitreous body normally degenerates; the proximal portion remains as the central artery of the optic nerve. If the distal portion persists, cysts or a cord of tissue may remain within the vitreous body. In addition, failure of the distal portion to degenerate may result in colobomas (*i.e.*, fissures or pits) within the iris, retina, or optic nerve.[21]

In a procedure called a *vitrectomy*, the removal and replacement of the vitreous with a balanced saline solution can restore sight in some persons with vitreous opacities resulting from hemorrhage or vitreoretinal membrane formations that cause legal blindness. In this procedure, a small probe with a cutting tip is used to remove the opaque vitreous and membranes. The procedure is difficult and requires complex instrumentation. It is of no value if the retina is not functional.

Disorders of the Retina

The function of the retina is to receive visual images, partially analyze them, and transmit this modified information to the brain. Disorders of the retina and its function include derangements of the pigment epithelium (*e.g.*, retinitis pigmentosa); ischemic conditions caused by disorders of the retinal blood supply; disorders of the retinal vessels such as retinopathies that cause hemorrhage and the development of opacities; separation of the pigment and sensory layers of the retina (*i.e.*, retinal detachment); retinopathy of prematurity; and abnormalities of Bruch's membrane and choroid (*e.g.*, macular degeneration). Because the retina has no pain fibers, most diseases of the retina are painless and do not cause redness of the eye.

Retinitis Pigmentosa

Retinitis pigmentosa is a group of hereditary diseases that causes slow degenerative changes in the retinal receptors. There are several modes of inheritance, including dominant, recessive, sex-linked, or sporadic.[13] In the United States, the incidence for all types of retinitis pigmentosa is 1 case in 3500 persons; the incidence of the carrier state may be 1 in 80. Slow destruction of the rods occurs, progressing from the peripheral to the central regions of the retina. Based on research with animal models, one probable mechanism of the disorder is a defect in phagocytic mechanisms of the pigment cells that cause membrane debris to accumulate and destroy the photoreceptors. The destruction results in dark lines and areas in which the pigment of the retinal pigment layer is unmasked by receptor loss. Night blindness, the first symptom of the disorder, often begins in early youth, with gross visual handicap occurring in the middle or advanced years. Some initial data suggest treat-

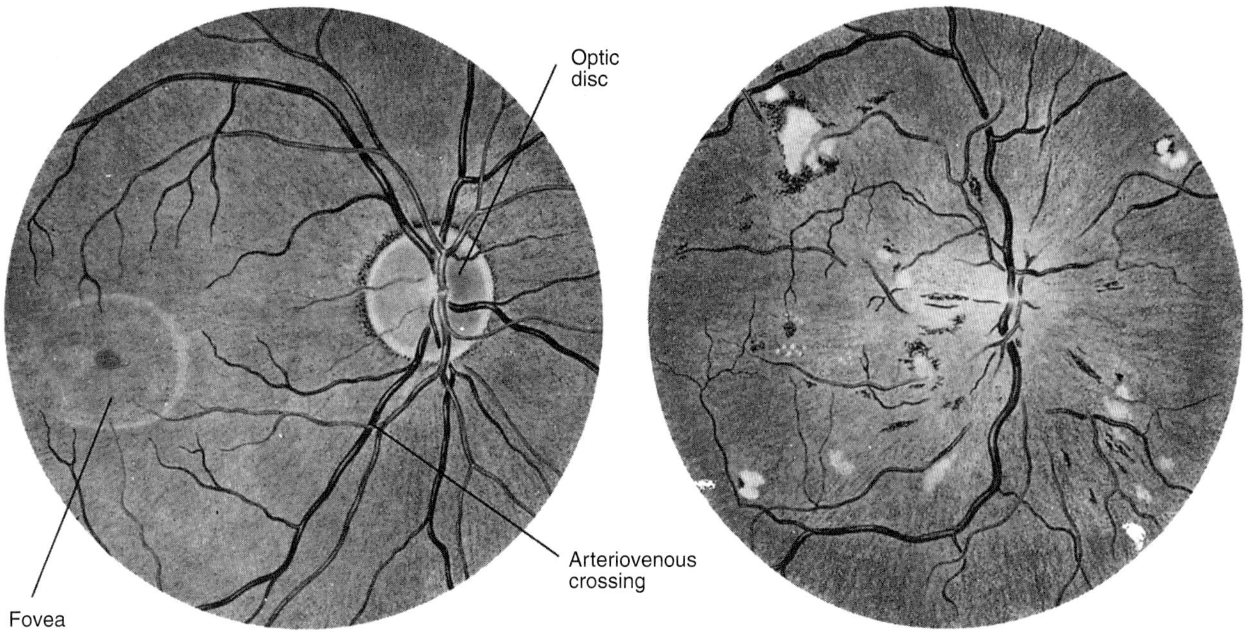

Figure 42–8
Fundus of the eye as seen in retinal examination with an ophthalmoscope: (**left**) normal fundus; (**right**) pathologic fundus. The macula fovea is not evident, but one can see flame-shaped hemorrhages and interrupted arteriovenous crossings.

ment with 11-*cis*-vitamin A over a 2-year period may at least delay the progress of retinitis pigmentosa.[9]

Disorders of Retinal Blood Supply

The blood supply for the retina is derived from two sources: the choriocapillaries of the choroid and the branches of the central retinal artery. The nutritional needs of the retina, including oxygen and the supply to the pigment cells and rods and cones, involve diffusion from blood vessels in the choroid. Because the choriocapillaries provide the only blood supply for the fovea centralis (*i.e.*, foveola), detachment of this part of the sensory retina from the pigment epithelium causes irreparable visual loss.

The bipolar, horizontal, amacrine, and ganglion cells, as well as the ganglion cell axons that gather at the optic disk, are supplied by branches of the retinal artery. The central artery of the retina is a branch of the ophthalmic artery. It enters the globe through the optic disk. Branches of this artery radiate over the entire retina, except for the central fovea, which is surrounded by, but is not crossed by, arterial branches. The retinal veins follow a distribution parallel to the arterial branches and carry venous blood to the central vein of the retina, which exits the back of the eye through the optic disk.

Funduscopic examination of the eye with an ophthalmoscope provides an opportunity to examine the retinal blood vessels and other aspects of the retina (Fig. 42–8). Because the retina is an embryonic outgrowth of the brain and the blood vessels are to a considerable extent representative of brain blood vessels, the ophthalmoscopic examination of the fundus of the eye provides an opportunity for the study and diagnosis of metabolic and vascular diseases of the brain and of pathologic processes that are specific to the retina.

The functioning of the retina, like that of other cellular portions of the central nervous system (CNS), depends on an oxygen supply from the vascular system. One of the earliest signs of decreased perfusion pressure in the head region is a graying-out or blackout of vision, which usually precedes loss of consciousness. This can occur during large increases in intrathoracic pressure, which interferes with the return of venous blood to the heart, as occurs with Valsalva's maneuver, with systemic hypotension, and during sudden postural movements under conditions of decreased vascular adaptability.

Ischemia of the retina occurs during general circulatory collapse. If a person survives cardiopulmonary arrest, for instance, permanently decreased visual acuity can occur as a result of edema and the ischemic death of retinal neurons. This is followed by primary optic nerve atrophy proportional to the extent of ganglionic cell death. The ophthalmic artery, the source of the central artery of the retina, takes its origin from the internal carotid artery. Intermittent retinal ischemia can accompany internal carotid or common carotid stenosis. In addition to ipsilateral intermittent blindness, contralateral hemiplegia or sensory deficits may accompany the episodes, depending on the competency of the circle of Willis in providing the brain with alternative arterial support. Treatment with anticoagulants or surgical endarterectomy may provide relief. Arteritis of the ophthalmic and central artery occurs more frequently in older persons, and if severe, it can result in occlusive disease and permanent visual deficits.

Papilledema. The central retinal artery enters the eye through the optic *papilla* in the center of the optic nerve. The central vein of the retina exits the eye along the same path. The entrance and exit of the central artery and veins of the retina through the tough scleral tissue at the optic papilla can be compromised by any condition causing persistent increased intracranial pressure. The most common of these conditions are cerebral tumors, subdural hematomas, hydrocephalus, and malignant hypertension.

The thin-walled, low-pressure veins are the first to collapse, with the consequent backup and slowing of arterial blood flow. Under these conditions, capillary permeability increases, and leakage of fluid results in edema of the optic papilla, called *papilledema.* The interior surface of the papilla is normally cup-shaped and can be evaluated through an ophthalmoscope. With papilledema, sometimes called *choked disk,* the optic cup is distorted by protrusion into the interior of the eye. Because this sign does not occur until the intracranial pressure is significantly elevated, compression damage to the optic nerve fibers passing through the lamina cribrosa may have begun. As a warning sign, papilledema occurs quite late. Unresolved papilledema results in the destruction of the optic nerve axons and blindness.

Central Retinal Artery Occlusion. Complete occlusion of the central artery of the retina results in sudden unilateral blindness (*i.e.,* anopsia). This is an uncommon disorder of older persons and most often is caused by embolism or atherosclerosis. Because the retina has a dual blood supply, the survival of retinal structures is possible if blood flow can be reestablished within approximately 90 minutes.[3] If blood flow is not restored, the infarcted retina swells and opacities. Because the receptors of the central fovea are supplied with blood from the choroid, they survive (*i.e.,* macular sparing). A cherry-red spot, indicating a healthy fovea, is surrounded by the pale white, opacified retina. Although the nerve fibers of the optic disks are adequately supplied by the choroid, the disk becomes pale after death of the ganglion cells and their axonal processes (*i.e.,* optic nerve fibers), resulting in optic nerve atrophy.

Occlusions of branches of the central artery, called branch arterial occlusions, are essentially retinal strokes. These occur mainly as a result of emboli and local infarction in the neural retina. The opacification that follows is often slowly resolved, and retinal transparency is restored. Local blind spots or *scotomas* may occur after destruction of local elements of the retina. Loss of the axons of destroyed ganglion cells results in some optic nerve atrophy.

Central Retinal Vein Occlusion. Occlusion of the central retinal vein results in venous dilation, stasis, and reduced flow through the retinal veins. It is usually monocular and causes rapid deterioration of visual acuity because of an accompanying increase in capillary wall fragility and a lack of arterial inflow. Superficial and deep hemorrhages may occur throughout the retina.

Among the causes of central retinal vein obstruction are hypertension, diabetes mellitus, and conditions such as sickle cell anemia that slow venous blood flow. The reduction in blood flow results in neovascularization with fibrovascular invasion of the space between the retina and the vitreous humor. In addition to obstructing normal visual function, the new vessels are fragile and prone to hemorrhage. Escaped blood may fill the space between the retina and vitreous, producing the appearance of a sudden veil over the visual field. The blood can find its way into the aqueous humor (*i.e.,* hemorrhagic glaucoma). Photocoagulation of the spreading new blood vessels with high-intensity light or laser beam is used to prevent blindness and eye pain. As the hemorrhage is resolved, degenerating blood products can produce contraction of the vitreous and formation of fibrous tissue within it, causing tears and detachment of the retina.

Much more common are local vein occlusions with regional and focal capillary microhemorrhages that produce the same but more restricted pathologic effects. These microhemorrhages result in the formation of rings of yellow exudate composed of lipid and lipoprotein blood-breakdown products. Microhemorrhages deep in the neural retina are somewhat restricted by the vertical organization of the neural elements and result in dot hemorrhages. Microhemorrhages in the layer of ganglionic cell axon bundles result in the appearance of cotton-wool spots on the fundus.

Retinopathies

Disorders of the retinal vessels result in microaneurysms, neovascularization, hemorrhage, and formation of retinal opacities. *Microaneurysms* are outpouchings of the retinal vasculature. On ophthalmoscopic examination, they appear as minute, unchanging red dots associated with blood vessels. These microaneurysms tend to leak plasma, resulting in localized edema that gives the retina a hazy appearance. Microaneurysms can be identified with certainty using fluorescein angiography; the fluorescein dye is injected intravenously, and the retinal vessels are subsequently photographed using a special ophthalmoscope and fundus camera. The microaneurysms may bleed, but areas of hemorrhage and edema tend to clear spontaneously. However, they reduce visual acuity if they encroach on the macula and cause degeneration before they are absorbed.

Neovascularization involves the formation of new blood vessels. They can develop from the choriocapillaries, extending between the pigment layer and the sensory layer, or from the retinal veins, extending between the sensory retina and the vitreous cavity and sometimes into the vitreous. These new blood vessels are fragile, leak protein, and tend to bleed. Neovascularization occurs in a number of conditions that impair retinal circulation, including stasis because of hyperviscosity of blood or decreased flow, vascular occlusion, sickle cell disease, sarcoidosis, diabetes mellitus, and retinopathy of prematurity. Research links the formation of new blood vessels with a vascular endothelial growth factor (VEGF) produced by the lining of blood vessels.[22] The cause of new blood vessel formation is uncertain. The vitreous humor is thought to contain a substance that normally inhibits neovascularization, and this factor is apparently suppressed under conditions in which the new blood vessels invade the vitreous cavity.

Hemorrhage can be preretinal, intraretinal, or subretinal. Preretinal hemorrhages occur between the retina and the vitreous. These hemorrhages tend to be large because the blood vessels are only loosely restricted; they may be associated with a subarachnoid or subdural hemorrhage and are usually regarded as a serious manifestation of the disorder. They usually reabsorb without complications unless they penetrate into the vitreous. Intraretinal hemorrhages occur because of abnormalities of the retinal vessels, diseases of the blood, increased pressure within the retinal vessels, or vitreous traction on the vessels. Systemic causes include diabetes mellitus, hypertension, and blood dyscrasias. Subretinal hemorrhages are those that develop between the choroid and pigment layer of the retina. A common cause of subretinal hemorrhage is neovascularization. Photocoagulation may be used to treat microaneurysms and neovascularization.

Light normally passes through the transparent inner portions of the sensory retina before reaching the photoreceptors. *Opacities* such as hemorrhages, exudate, cotton-wool patches, edema, and tissue proliferation can produce a localized loss of transparency observable with an ophthalmoscope. *Exudates* are opacities resulting from inflammatory processes. The development of exudates often results in the destruction of the underlying retinal pigment and choroid layer. *Deposits* are localized opacities consisting of lipid-laden macrophages or accumulated cellular debris. *Cotton-wool patches* are retinal opacities with hazy, irregular outlines. They occur in the nerve fiber layer and contain cell organelles. Cotton-wool patches are associated with retinal trauma, severe anemia, papilledema, and diabetic retinopathy.

Diabetic Retinopathy. Diabetic retinopathy is the third leading cause of blindness for all ages in the United States. It ranks first as the cause of newly reported cases of blindness in persons between the ages of 20 and 74 years, with 12% of all cases caused by diabetes.[23] In the United States, approximately 125,000 cases of diabetic retinopathy are diagnosed each year.[22] The risk of blindness for the nation's 12 million diabetics is 25 times that of the general population. Ocular symptoms occur in 20% to 40% of persons with diabetes mellitus.[19]

Diabetic retinopathy can be divided into two types: nonproliferative (*i.e.,* background) and proliferative. Background or nonproliferative retinopathy is confined to the retina. It involves thickening of the retinal capillary walls and microaneurysm formation. Ruptured capillaries cause small intraretinal hemorrhages, and microinfarcts may cause cotton-wool exudates. A sensation of glare (because of the scattering of light) is a common complaint. The most common cause of decreased vision in persons with background retinopathy is macular edema.[24] It represents fluid accumulation within the retina stemming from a breakdown in the blood-retina barrier.

Proliferative diabetic retinopathy represents a more severe retinal change than background retinopathy. It is characterized by formation of fragile blood vessels (*i.e.,* neovascularization) at the disk and elsewhere in the retina. These vessels grow in front of the retina along the posterior surface of the vitreous or into the vitreous. They threaten vision in two ways. First, because they are abnormal, they tend to bleed easily, leaking blood into the vitreous cavity and decreasing visual acuity. Second, the blood vessels attach firmly to the retinal surface and posterior surface of the vitreous, such that normal movement of the vitreous may exert a pull on the retina, causing retinal detachment and progressive blindness. Because early proliferative diabetic retinopathy is likely to be asymptomatic, it must be identified early, before bleeding occurs and obscures the view of the fundus or leads to fibrosis and retinal attachment.

The American Diabetes Association, American College of Physicians, and American Academy of Ophthalmology have developed screening guidelines for diabetic retinopathy.[25] These guidelines recommend that persons with type I diabetes be screened annually for retinopathy beginning 5 years after the onset of diabetes. In general, screening is not indicated before the start of puberty. Persons with type II diabetes should have an initial examination for retinopathy shortly after diagnosis. After the initial eye examination, every person with diabetes should have regular ocular follow-up visits, at least once each year and more frequently if warranted by the severity of the retinopathy. The ocular examination by the ophthalmologist should include acuity measurements, slit-lamp biomicroscopy, and direct and indirect ophthalmoscopy of the retina through fully dilated pupils. When indicated, color fundus photographs and fluorescein angiograms should be done. When planning pregnancy, women with preexisting diabetes should be counseled about the risk of developing retinopathy or progression of existing retinopathy. Women who become pregnant should have a comprehensive eye examination during the first trimester and close follow-up throughout pregnancy.

Growing evidence suggests that careful control of blood sugar levels in persons with diabetes mellitus may retard the onset and progression of retinopathy. The Diabetes Control and Complication Trial Research Group demonstrated that intensive management of persons with type I diabetes to maintain blood glucose levels at near-normal levels reduced the risk of retinopathy by 76% in persons with no retinopathy and slowed the progress by 54% in persons with early disease.[26]

Laser photocoagulation provides the major direct treatment modality for diabetic retinopathy. Treatment strategies include laser photocoagulation applied directly to leaking microaneurysms and grid photocoagulation with a checkerboard pattern of laser burns applied to diffuse areas of leakage and thickening.[24] Because laser photocoagulation destroys the proliferating vessels and the ischemic retina, it reduces the stimulus for further neovascularization. Laser phototherapy also decreases macular edema and increases the chance of visual improvement in persons with nonproliferative retinopathy.[27] Vitrectomy has proved effective in removing vitreous hemorrhage and severing vitreoretinal membranes that develop.

Hypertensive Retinopathy. Long-standing systemic hypertension results in the compensatory thickening of arteriolar walls, which effectively reduces capillary perfusion pressure. Ordinarily, a retinal blood vessel is transparent and seen as a red line; in venules, the red cells resemble a string of boxcars. On ophthalmoscopy, arteries in persons with long-standing hypertension appear paler than veins because they have thicker walls. The thickened arterioles in chronic hypertension become opaque and have a copper-wiring appearance. Edema, microaneurysms, intraretinal hemorrhages, exudates, and cotton-wool spots are all observed.[18] Malignant hypertension involves swelling of the optic disk as a result of the local edema produced by escaped fluid. If the condition is permitted to progress long enough, serious visual deficits result.

Protective thickening of arteriolar walls cannot occur with sudden increases in blood pressure. Therefore, hemorrhage is likely to occur. Trauma to the optic globe or the head, sudden high blood pressure in eclampsia, and some types of renal disease are characteristically accompanied by edema of the retina and optic disk and by an increased likelihood of hemorrhage.

Atherosclerosis of Retinal Vessels. In atherosclerosis, the lumen of the arterioles becomes narrowed. As a result, the retinal arteries become tortuous and narrowed. At sites where the arteries cross and compress veins, the red cell column of the vein appears distended. Exudate accumulates on arteriolar walls as plaque or cytoid bodies. Deep and superficial hemorrhages are common. Atheromatous plaques of the central artery are associated with increased danger of stasis, thrombi of the central veins, and occlusion.

Retinopathy of Prematurity. Retinopathy of prematurity, previously called *retrolental fibroplasia*, is a potentially blinding abnormal proliferation of retinal blood vessels that is unique to the preterm infant. The improved survival rates of low-weight premature infants during the past several decades has resulted in an increased incidence of retinopathy of prematurity.[28] The survival rate for infants weighing 500 to 750 g at birth approaches 60%, and for those weighing 751 to 1000 g, it approaches 90%.[29]

The immature retina has two blood supplies, the choroidal and the inner retinal vessels. The choroidal blood vessels, which lie on the outside of the retina, develop early and are the sole supplier of nourishment for the immature retina. Vascularization of the inner retina begins during the 16th week of gestation as the retinal vessels grow and advance outward in a 360-degree circle from the optic nerve; they reach the *ora serrata,* the anterior serrated edge of the neural retina, at the nasal periphery by 32 weeks and reach the temporal periphery by about the 40th week of gestation.[30] Retinopathy of prematurity develops at the site of these newly forming retinal vessels. Normally, these vessels develop under hypoxic conditions that exist in utero. Unfortunately, most premature babies require some supplemental oxygen to sustain extrauterine life. When confronted with the hyperoxic conditions that occur when a baby is born prematurely, these immature vessels constrict and are obliterated.

After cessation of oxygen therapy, the blood vessels that were not obliterated begin to proliferate and grow rapidly in an attempt to reestablish and complete the vascularization of the inner retina. This area of rapid vascular growth usually forms an abrupt, rather than a gradual, junction between the vascular and avascular retina; the vessels are often abnormal and weak and can grow into the vitreous body, where they may cause leakage of fluid or hemorrhage with resultant formation of scar tissue. As the scar tissue shrinks, it can exert traction on the retina, causing retinal detachment and permanent loss of vision.

The more premature the infant, the greater is the risk of retinopathy developing. The incidence of retinopathy of prematurity in infants weighing 500 to 750 g is almost 100%, with severe disease developing in about 30% of these infants; the incidence of retinopathy in those weighing 751 to 1000 g is almost 80%, with severe disease occurring in about 10% of the infants.[29]

In 1984, the Committee for the Classification of Retinopathy of Prematurity developed an international system for classification that divides the visual retina into three concentric zones (*i.e.,* 360-degree circles spaced between the optic nerve and the ora serrata) and characterizes the extent of involvement by the number of clock hours (*i.e.,* retinal segments) involved.[31] The system includes four stages of retinopathy. In *stage I disease,* a flat, white line of demarcation has developed, separating the vascularized retina from the undeveloped avascular retina. In *stage II disease,* the line of demarcation has height and width; it extends out of the plane of the retina into the vitreous. In *stage III disease,* extraretinal proliferation of vascular tissue is present along the ridge of the demarcation line and may extend into the vitreous. A plus (+) is added to the stage (*e.g.,* III+ retinopathy of prematurity) when the retinal vasculature posterior to the ridge becomes enlarged, dilated, and tortuous. *Stage IV* disease is characterized by detachment of the retina. Retinal detachment results in blindness. Treatment should be initiated before stage IV disease.

It has been recommended that all infants with a birth weight of less than 1600 g and who have received extended oxygen therapy should undergo repeated ophthalmic screening for retinopathy of prematurity.[3] If no disease or stage I or II disease is detected, repeat ophthalmic examinations should be scheduled according to the infant's level of risk until the retina is completely vascularized.[32] In many cases of stage I and II disease, partial or complete regression may occur in one or both eyes. Infants having stage III+ disease in zones I or II in five contiguous or eight cumulative clock hours (threshold retinopathy of prematurity) should be treated promptly because rapid progression to stage IV disease is possible.

Treatment consists of cryotherapy to the vascular portion of the retina. During cryotherapy, the trained ophthalmologist or ocular surgeon places the cryoprobe on the outside of the eye to produce transscleral freezing and destruction of the abnormal vessels. Cryotherapy can reduce the risk of an unfavorable outcome of retinopathy of prematurity by 50%.[32] Because the incidence of myopia and astigmatism is greater among children treated with cryotherapy, infants requiring treatment should be closely followed by an ophthalmologist.

Retinal Detachment

Retinal detachment involves the separation of the sensory retina from the pigment epithelium (Fig. 42–9). It occurs when traction on the inner sensory layer or a tear in this layer allows fluid, usually vitreous, to accumulate between the two layers. Retinal detachment that results from breaks in the sensory layer of the retina is called *rhegmatogenous detachment* (*rhegma* in Greek, meaning rent or hole). The vitreous is normally adherent to the retina at the optic disk, macula, and periphery of the retina. When the vitreous shrinks, it separates from the retina at the posterior pole of the eye (posterior vitreous detachment), but at the periphery, the vitreous pulls on the attached retina, which can lead to tearing of the retina. Vitreous fluid can enter the tear and contribute to further separation of the retina from its overlying pigment layer.

Persons with high grades of myopia may have abnormalities in the peripheral retina that predispose to sudden detachment. Intraocular surgery such as cataract extraction may produce traction on the peripheral retina that causes eventual detachment months or even years after surgery.[24] Detachment may result from exudates that separate the two retinal layers. Exudative detachment may be caused by intraocular inflammations, intraocular tumors, or certain systemic diseases. Inflammatory processes include posterior scleritis, uveitis, or parasitic invasion. Retinal detachment can also follow trauma immediately or at some later time.

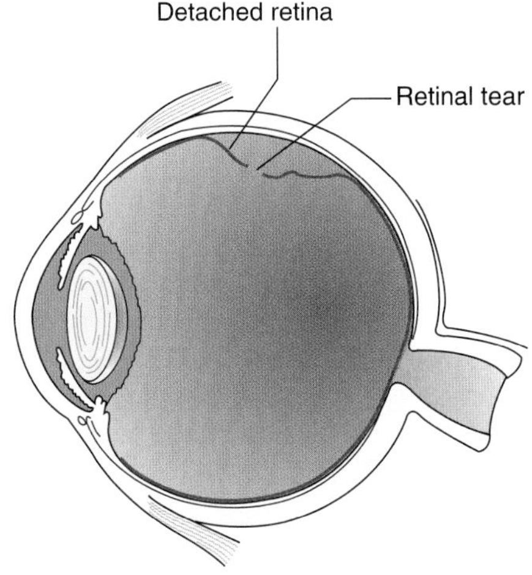

Figure 42–9 Detached retina.

Detachment of the neural retina from the retinal pigment layer separates the receptors from their major blood supply, the choroid. If retinal detachment continues for some time, permanent destruction and blindness of that part of the retina occur. The bipolar and ganglion cells survive because their blood supply, by way of the retinal arteries, remains intact. Without receptors, however, there is no visual function. The primary symptom of retinal detachment is loss of vision. Sometimes, flashing lights or sparks, followed by small floaters or spots in the field of vision, occur as the retina pulls away from the posterior pole of the eye.[24] There is no pain. As detachment progresses, the person perceives a dark curtain progressing across the visual field (see Fig. 42–1). Because the process begins in the periphery and spreads circumferentially and posteriorly, initial visual disturbances may involve only one quadrant of the visual field. Large peripheral detachments may occur without involvement of the macula, so that visual acuity remains unaffected. The tendency, however, is for detachments to enlarge until all of the retina is detached.

Diagnosis is based on the ophthalmoscopic appearance of the retina. Treatment is aimed at closing retinal tears and reattaching the retina. Rhegmatogenous detachment usually requires surgical treatment. Scleral buckling or pneumatic retinopexy are the most commonly used surgical techniques. Scleral buckling is the primary surgical procedure performed to reattach the retina. The procedure requires careful location of the retinal break and treatment with diathermy, cryotherapy, or laser to produce chorioretinal adhesions that seal the retinal tears so that the vitreous can no longer leak into the subretinal space. With scleral buckling, a piece of silicone (*i.e.*, the buckle) is sutured and infolded into the sclera, physically indenting the sclera so it comes in contact with the separated pigment and retinal layers. Pneumatic retinopexy involves the intraocular injection of an expandable gas instead of a piece of silicone to form the indentation. An overall reattachment rate of 90% is reported, but the visual results depend on the preoperative status of the macula.[3] The most common cause of failure after surgical treatment for detached retina is the development of membranes on the retina. Intraocular instruments have been refined for microsurgical removal of membranes from the retinal surface and reattaching the retina.[24]

Macular Degeneration

Macular degeneration is characterized by destructive changes of the yellow-pigmented area surrounding the central fovea resulting from vascular disorders. Age-related macular degeneration is the most common cause of reduced vision in the United States. It is the leading cause of blindness among persons older than 75 and of newly reported cases of blindness among those older than 65 years.[24] The cause of macular degeneration is unknown, although nutritional, hemodynamic, degenerative, and phototoxic factors are under investigation. Although rare, macular degeneration can occur as a hereditary condition in young persons and sometimes in adults.

Macular degeneration is characterized by the loss of central vision, usually in both eyes. The person may find it difficult to see at long distances (*e.g.*, in driving), do close work (*e.g.*, reading), see faces clearly, or distinguish colors. However, the person may not be severely incapacitated because the peripheral retinal function usually remains intact. With the help of low-vision aids, patients can usually continue their normal activities.

There are two types of age-related macular degeneration: an atrophic nonexudative or "dry" form and an exudative or "wet" form.[33] The atrophic form is characterized by a gradual, progressive bilateral vision loss from atrophy and degeneration of the rod and cone photoreceptors. The exudative form is characterized by the formation of a neovascular membrane that separates the pigmented epithelium from the neuroretina. These new blood vessels have weaker walls than normal and are prone to leakage. This combination allows the leakage of serous or hemorrhagic fluid into the subretinal space, causing separation of the pigmented epithelium from the neurosensory retina. Over time, the subretinal hemorrhages organize to form scar tissue. When this happens, retinal tissue death and loss of all visual function in the corresponding macular area occurs. Between 80% and 85% of those with age-related macular degeneration have the atrophic form, but 80% to 85% of severe vision loss can be ascribed to the exudative form.[34]

Although there is no treatment for the dry form of macular degeneration, argon laser photocoagulation may be useful in treating the wet form.[33,35] Persons with macular degeneration should be reassured that loss of central vision does not progress to loss of peripheral vision; most persons can maintain their independence assisted by low-vision aids. Pale yellow spots that may occur individually or in groups throughout the macula are called *drusen*. They are the most common indication of age-related macular degeneration.

Tests of Retinal Function

The diagnosis of retinal disease is based on history, tests of visual acuity, refraction, visual field tests, color vision tests, and often fluorescein angiography. Electroretinography (ERG) can be used to measure the electrical activity of the retina in response to a flash of light. Recorded ERG represents the difference in electrical potential between an electrode placed in a corneal contact lens and one placed on the forehead. The test can be used to evaluate retinal function in persons with an opaque lens or vitreous body. The electro-oculogram (EOG) records the electrical potentials between the front of the eye and the retina in the back of the eye. It is recorded from two electrodes, one placed above and the other lateral to the eye. The EOG measures eye movement and is frequently used in sleep studies.

In summary, the retina covers the inner aspect of the posterior two thirds of the eyeball and is continuous with the optic nerve. It contains the neural receptors for vision, and it is here that light energy of different frequencies and intensities is converted to graded local potentials, which are then converted to action potentials and transmitted to visual centers in the brain. The photoreceptors normally shed portions of their outer segments. These segments are phagocytized by cells in the pigment epithelium. Failure of phagocytosis, as occurs in one form of retinitis pigmentosa, results in degeneration of the pigment layer and blindness.

The retina receives its blood from two sources: the choriocapillaries, which supply the pigment layer and the outer portion of the sensory retina adjacent to the choroid, and the branches of the retinal artery, which supply the inner half of the retina. The retinal blood vessels are normally apparent through the ophthalmoscope. Disorders of retinal vessels can result from a number of local and systemic disorders, including diabetes mellitus, and hypertension. They cause vision loss through changes that result in hemorrhage, the production of opacities, and the separation of the pigment epithelium and sensory retina. Retinopathy of prematurity is a potentially blinding disorder of preterm infants who require oxygen therapy. The disorder involves the formation of new fragile blood vessels that may cause leakage of fluid and hemorrhage with scar formation. Retinal detachment involves separation of the sensory receptors from their blood supply; it causes blindness unless reattachment is promptly accomplished.

Disorders of Neural Pathways and Cortical Centers

After you have completed this section of the chapter, you should be able to meet the following objectives:

- Characterize what is meant by a visual field defect
- Explain the use of perimetry in the diagnosis of a visual field defect
- Define the terms hemianopia, quadrantanopia, heteronymous hemianopia, and homonymous hemianopia and relate to disorders of the optic pathways
- Describe visual defects associated with disorders of the visual cortex and visual association areas
- Describe tests used in assessing the pupillary reflex and cite the possible causes of abnormal pupillary reflexes

Full visual function requires the normally developed brain-related functions of photoreception, visual sensation and perception, and the pupillary reflex. These functions depend on the integrity of all visual pathways, including the retinal circuitry and the pathway from the optic nerve.

Visual Field Defects

Visual field defects result from damage to the visual pathways or the visual cortex. Perimetry or visual field testing, in which the visual field of each eye is measured and plotted in an arc, is used to identify defects and determine the location of lesions. The periphery of the opposite visual field is represented on the medial surface and in the depths of a deep medial calcarine sulcus of the occipital cortex (area 17). The central, high acuity part of the visual half-field extends somewhat over the occipital pole. The visual association cortex surrounds the primary cortex on the superior, lateral, and inferior occipital lobe. This area is required for complex analysis and learned meaningfulness of visual stimuli.

All of us possess a hole, or *scotoma*, in our visual field, of which we are unaware. Because the optic disk, where the optic nerve fibers exit the retina, does not contain photoreceptors, a corresponding location in the visual field constitutes a blind spot (Fig. 42–10). Local retinal damage caused by small vascular lesions (*i.e.*, retinal stroke) and other localized pathology can produce additional blind spots. As with the normal blind spot, persons are not usually aware of the existence of scotomata in their visual fields unless they encounter problems seeing objects in certain restricted parts of the visual field.

Absences near or in the center of the bilateral visual field can be annoying and even disastrous. Although the hole is not recognized as such, the person finds that a part of a printed page appears or disappears, depending on where the fixation point is held. Most persons learn to position their eyes so as to use the remaining central foveal vision for high-acuity tasks. Defects in the peripheral visual field, including the monocular peripheral fields, are less annoying but potentially more dangerous. The person who is unaware of the defect, when walking or driving an automobile, does not see cars or bicyclists until their image reaches the functional visual field—sometimes too late to avert an accident. With careful education, a person can learn to shift the gaze constantly to obtain visual coverage of important parts of the visual field. If the damage is at the retinal or optic nerve level, only the monocular field of the damaged eye becomes a problem. A lesion affecting the central foveal vision of one eye can result in complaints of eye strain during reading and other close work, because only one eye is really being used. Localized damage to the optic tracts, lateral geniculate nucleus (LGN), optic radiation, or primary visual cortex affects corresponding parts of the visual fields of both eyes.

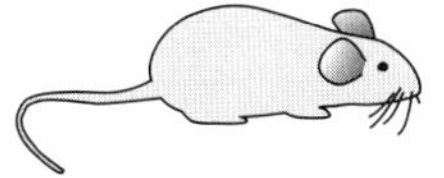

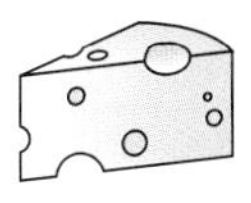

Figure 42–10.
Hold figure approximately 1 foot in front of your face. Close left eye and concentrate on the mouse with your right eye. Slowly move the figure toward you. The cheese will "disappear" when its image comes into focus on the optic disc or "blind spot" of the retina.

Disorders of the Optic Pathways

The visual pathway extends from the front to the back of the head. It is much like a telephone line between distant points in that damage at any point along the pathway results in functional defects (Fig. 42–11). Among the disorders that can interrupt the visual pathway are vascular lesions, trauma, and tumors. For example, normal visual system function depends on vascular adequacy in the ophthalmic artery and its branches; the central artery of the retina; the anterior and middle cerebral arteries, which supply the intracranial optic nerve, chiasm, and optic tracts; and the posterior cerebral artery, which supplies the LGN, optic radiation, and visual cortex. The adequacy of the posterior cerebral artery function depends on that of the vertebral and basilar arteries that supply the brain stem. Vascular insufficiency in any one of these arterial systems can seriously affect vision.

Examination of visual system function is of particular diagnostic use, because lesions at various points along the pathway have characteristic symptoms that assist in the localization of pathology. Visual field defects of each eye and of the two eyes together are useful in localizing lesions affecting the system. Blindness in one eye is called *anopia*. If half of the visual field for one eye is lost, the defect is called *hemianopia;* loss of a quarter field is called *quadrantanopia*. Enlarging pituitary tumors can produce longitudinal damage through the optic chiasm with loss of the medial fibers of the optic nerve representing both nasal retinas and both temporal visual half-fields. Loss of the temporal or peripheral visual fields on both sides results in a narrow binocular field, commonly called *tunnel vision*. The loss of different half-fields in the two eyes is called a *heteronymous* loss, and the abnormality is called *heteronymous hemianopia*. Destruction of one or both lateral halves of the chiasm is common with multiple aneurysms of the circle of Willis. Here, the function of the left or both temporal retinas occurs, and the nasal fields of the left or of both eyes are lost. The loss of the nasal fields of both eyes is called *bitemporal heteronymous anopia*. With both eyes open, the person with bilateral defects still has the full binocular visual field.

Loss of the optic tract, LGN, full optic radiation, or complete visual cortex on one side results in loss of the corresponding visual half-fields in each eye. *Homonymous* means the same for both eyes. In left-side lesions, the right visual field is lost for each eye and is called *complete right homonymous hemianopia*. Partial injury to

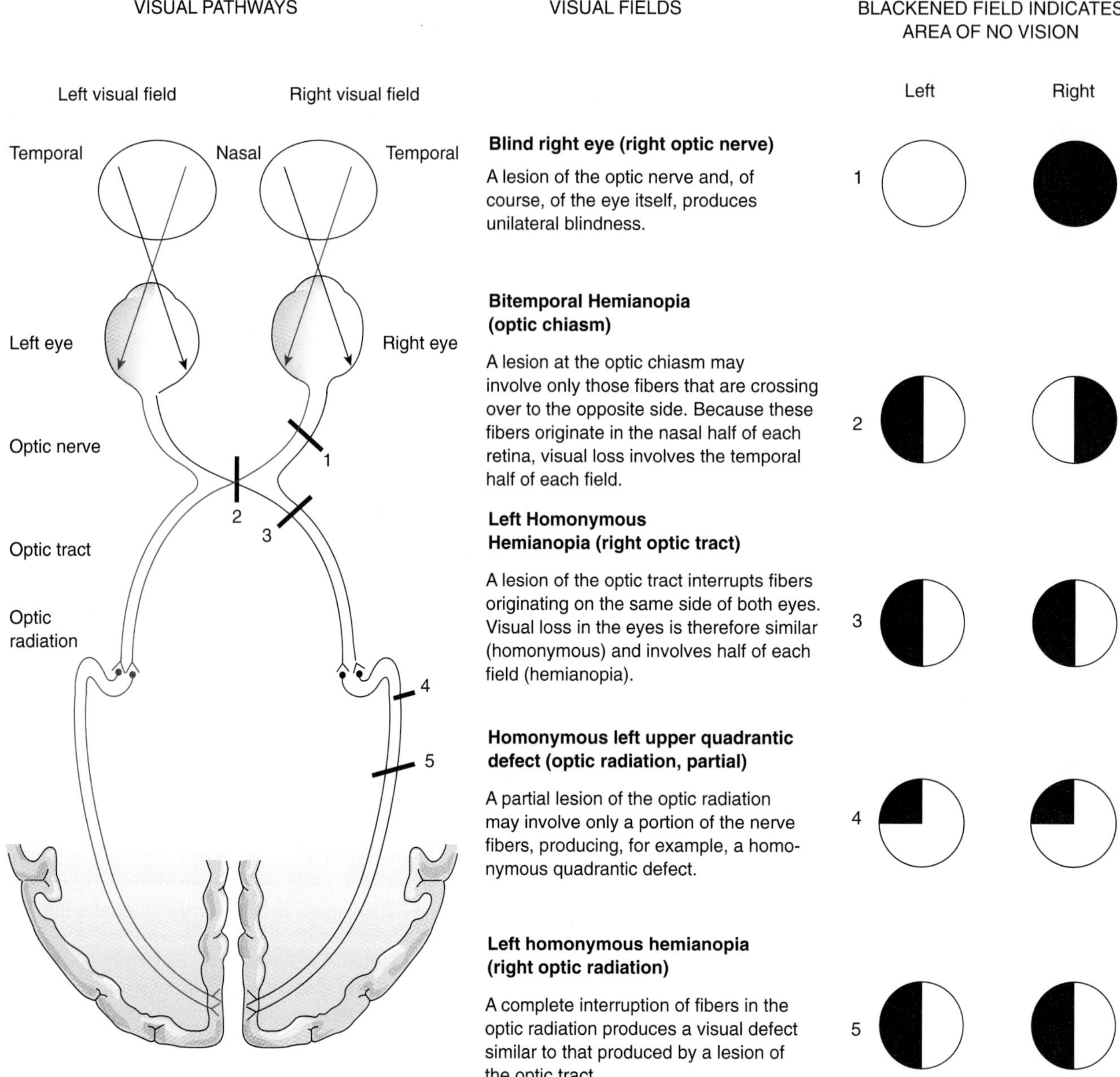

VISUAL PATHWAYS
VISUAL FIELDS
BLACKENED FIELD INDICATES AREA OF NO VISION
Left visual field
Right visual field
Left
Right
Temporal
Nasal
Temporal
Left eye
Right eye
Optic nerve
Optic tract
Optic radiation
1
2
3
4
5
Blind right eye (right optic nerve)
A lesion of the optic nerve and, of course, of the eye itself, produces unilateral blindness.
Bitemporal Hemianopia (optic chiasm)
A lesion at the optic chiasm may involve only those fibers that are crossing over to the opposite side. Because these fibers originate in the nasal half of each retina, visual loss involves the temporal half of each field.
Left Homonymous Hemianopia (right optic tract)
A lesion of the optic tract interrupts fibers originating on the same side of both eyes. Visual loss in the eyes is therefore similar (homonymous) and involves half of each field (hemianopia).
Homonymous left upper quadrantic defect (optic radiation, partial)
A partial lesion of the optic radiation may involve only a portion of the nerve fibers, producing, for example, a homonymous quadrantic defect.
Left homonymous hemianopia (right optic radiation)
A complete interruption of fibers in the optic radiation produces a visual defect similar to that produced by a lesion of the optic tract.

Figure 42–11
Visual field defects produced by selected lesions in the visual pathways.

the left optic tract, LGN, or optic radiation can result in the loss of a quarter of the visual field in both eyes. This is called *homonymous quadrantanopia*, and depending on the lesion, it can involve the upper (superior) or lower (inferior) fields. Because the optic radiation fibers for the superior quarter of the visual field traverse the temporal lobe, superior quadrantanopia is more common. The LGN, optic radiation, and visual cortex all receive their major blood supply from the posterior cerebral artery; unilateral occlusion of this artery results in complete loss of the opposite field (*i.e.*, homonymous hemianopia). Bilateral occlusion of these arteries results in total cortical blindness.

Disorders of the Visual Cortex

Discrete damage in the binocular portion of the primary visual cortex can also result in scotomata in the corresponding visual fields. If the visual loss is in the central high-acuity part of the field, severe loss of visual acuity and pattern discrimination occurs. The central, high-acuity portion of the visual field is located at the occipital pole. This region can be momentarily compressed against the occipital bone (*i.e.*, contrecoup) after severe trauma to the frontal part of the cranium. Mechanical trauma to the cortex results in firing of neurons, experienced as flashes of light or "seeing stars." Destruction of the polar visual cortex causes severe loss of visual acuity and pattern discrimination. Such damage is permanent and cannot be corrected with lenses.

The bilateral loss of the entire primary visual cortex, called *cortical blindness*, eliminates all visual experience. Crude analysis of visual stimulation at reflex levels, such as eye-orienting and head-orienting responses to bright moving lights, pupillary reflexes, and blinking at sudden bright lights, may be retained even though vision has been lost. Extensive damage to the visual association cortex (areas 18 and 19) that surrounds an intact primary visual cortex results in a loss of the learned meaningfulness of visual images (*i.e.*, visual agnosia). The patient can see the patterns of color, shapes, and movement, but can no longer recognize formerly meaningful stimuli. Familiar objects can be described but not named or reacted to meaningfully. However, if other sensory modalities, such as hearing and touch, can be applied, full recognition occurs. This disorder represents a problem of recognition rather than intellect.

Testing of Visual Fields

Crude testing of the binocular visual field and the visual field of each individual eye (*i.e.*, monocular vision) can be accomplished without specialized equipment. In the confrontation method, the examiner stands or sits 2 to 3 feet in front of the person to be tested and instructs the person to focus on an object such as a penlight with one eye closed. The object is moved from the center toward the periphery of the person's visual field and from the periphery toward the center, and the person is instructed to report the presence or absence of the object. By moving the object through the vertical, horizontal, and oblique aspects of the visual field, a crude estimate can be made of the visual field. If the test object is kept midway between the examiner and the person being tested, the examiner can close the corresponding eye and compare the person's monocular vision with his or her own. This test is based on the assumption that the examiner's peripheral field of vision is within normal limits. Large field defects can be estimated by the confrontation method, and it may be the only way for testing young children and uncooperative adults. Rapidly presenting the examiner's fingers toward the eyes and observing for a reflex blink to the threat is sometimes the only way to detect a visual field deficit in someone with decreased consciousness.

Accurate determination of the presence, size, and shape of smaller holes, or scotomata, in the visual field of a particular eye can be demonstrated by the ophthalmologist only through the use of perimetry. This is done by having the person look with one eye toward a central spot directly in front of the eye while the head is stabilized by a chin rest or bite board. A small dot of light or a colored object is moved back and forth in all areas of the visual field. The person reports whether the stimulus is visible and, if a colored stimulus is used, what the perceived color is. A hemispheric support is used to control and standardize the movement of the test object, and a plot of radial coordinates of the visual field is made. Perimetry provides a means of determining alterations from normal and, with repeated testing, a way of following the progress of the disease or treatment.

Disorders of the Pupillary Reflex

The pupillary reflex, which controls the size of the pupillary opening, is controlled by the autonomic nervous system. Normal function of the pupillary reflex mechanism is tested by shining a penlight into one eye of the person being tested. To avoid accommodation, the person is asked to stare into the distance. A rapid constriction of the pupil exposed to light should occur; this is called the direct light reflex or direct pupillary reflex. Because the reflex is normally bilateral, the contralateral pupil should also constrict, a reaction called the consensual light reflex or consensual pupillary reflex. Reflex pupillary dilation occurs more quickly in lightly pigmented eyes than in more darkly pigmented eyes. By shining the light first into one eye and then into the other eye and noting the response of both pupils, considerable information can be gathered about the function of the CNS circuitry.

The circuitry of the light reflex is partially separated from the main visual pathway. This is illustrated by the fact that the pupillary reflex remains unaffected when lesions to the optic radiations or the visual cortex occur. The cortically blind person retains direct and consensual light reflexes. The light reflex also functions under light anesthetic levels and is used to evaluate the depth of anesthesia. When the reflex is lost, the anesthesia is approaching a level that depresses the respiratory reflexes.

Careful attention to inappropriate or unequal pupil diameters is diagnostically important. The integrity of the dual control of pupillary diameter is somewhat vulnerable to trauma, tumor enlargement, or vascular disease. Damage to the oculomotor nucleus or nerve eliminates innervation of four of the six extraocular muscles and the levator muscle of the upper lid, and it results in permanent pupillary dilation, called *mydriasis*, in the affected eye. Persons with mydriasis experience discomfort in normal or brightly lit environments because of loss of pupillary constriction in the affected eye.

Lesions affecting descending brain control of sympathetic outflow that passes through the cervical spinal cord, ascending sympathetic preganglionic axons of the sympathetic ganglia, or sympathetic postganglionic axonal plexus in the wall of the carotid artery can interrupt the sympathetic control of the iris dilator muscle, resulting in permanent pupillary constriction, called *miosis*. Tumors of the orbit that compress structures behind the eye can eliminate all pupillary reflexes, usually before destroying the optic nerve.

The function of the sympathetic and parasympathetic control of the iris (and pupillary size) is differentially affected by many pharmacologic agents. Bilateral pupillary constriction is characteristic of opiate usage. Pupillary dilation results when topical parasympathetic blocking agents such as atropine or homatropine are applied and sympathetic pupillodilatory function is left unopposed. These medications are used by ophthalmologists to facilitate the examination of the transparent media and fundus of the eye. Miotic drugs such as pilocarpine have the opposite effect, facilitating aqueous humor circulation.

In summary, visual information is carried to the brain by axons of the retinal ganglion cells that form the optic nerve. The two optic nerves meet and fuse in the optic chiasm. The axons of each nasal retina cross in the chiasm and join the uncrossed fibers of the temporal retina of the opposite eye in the optic tract. From the optic chiasm, the crossed fibers of the nasal retina of one eye and the uncrossed temporal fibers of the other eye pass to the LGN and then to the primary visual cortex, which is located in the calcarine fissure of the occipital lobe. Damage to the visual pathways or visual cortex leads to visual field defects that can be identified through visual field testing or perimetry and used to determine the lesion's location. Damage to the visual association cortex can result in seeing an object, although with loss of learned recognition (*i.e.*, visual agnosia).

The pupillary reflex, which controls the size of the pupil, is controlled by the autonomic nervous system. The parasympathetic nervous system controls pupillary constriction, and the sympathetic nervous system controls pupillary dilation.

Disorders of Eye Movement

After you have completed this section of the chapter, you should be able to meet the following objectives:

- Explain the difference between paralytic and nonparalytic strabismus
- Define *amblyopia* and explain its pathogenesis
- Explain the need for early diagnosis and treatment of eye movement disorders in children

Normal vision depends on the coordinated action of the entire visual system and a number of central control systems. It is through these mechanisms that an object is simultaneously imaged on the fovea of both eyes and perceived as a single image. Strabismus and amblyopia are two disorders that affect this highly integrated system. Although strabismus may develop in later life, it is seen most commonly in children, among whom its incidence is approximately 2%.

Strabismus

Strabismus, or *squint*, refers to any abnormality of eye coordination or alignment that results in loss of binocular vision (Fig. 42–12). When images from the same spots in visual space do not fall on corresponding points of the two retinas, diplopia, or double vision, occurs.

In standard terminology, the disorders of eye movement are described according to the direction of movement. *Esotropia* refers to medial deviation, *exotropia* refers to lateral deviation, *hypertropia* refers to upward deviation, *hypotropia* refers to downward deviation, and *cyclotropia* refers to torsional deviation. The term *concomitance* refers to equal deviation in all directions of gaze. A *nonconcomitant strabismus* is one that varies with the direction of gaze. Strabismus may be divided into paralytic (nonconcomitant) forms, in which there is weakness or paralysis of one or more of the extraocular muscles, and nonparalytic (concomitant) forms, in which there is no primary muscle impairment. Strabismus is called *intermittent*, or *periodic*, when there are periods in which the eyes are parallel. It is *monocular* when the same eye always deviates and the fellow eye fixates. Figure 42–13 illustrates abnormalities in eye movement associated with esotropia and exotropia.

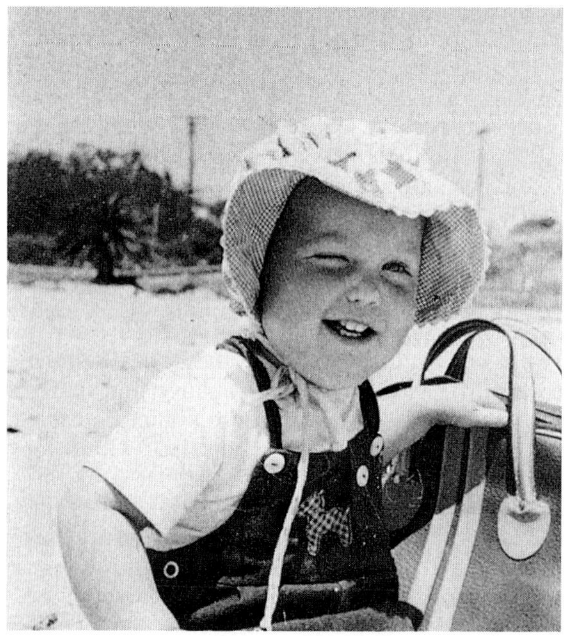

Figure 42–12
Photograph of a child with intermittent exotropia squinting in the sunlight. (Vaughn D.G., Asbury T., Riordon-Eva P. [1995]. *General ophthalmology* [p. 239]. Stamford, CT: Appleton & Lange.)

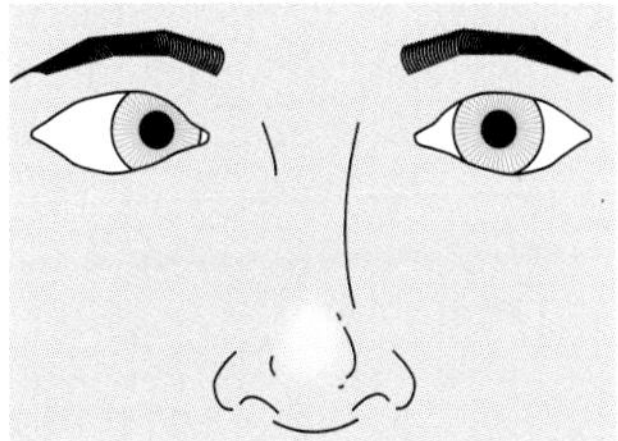

A Primary position: right esotropia

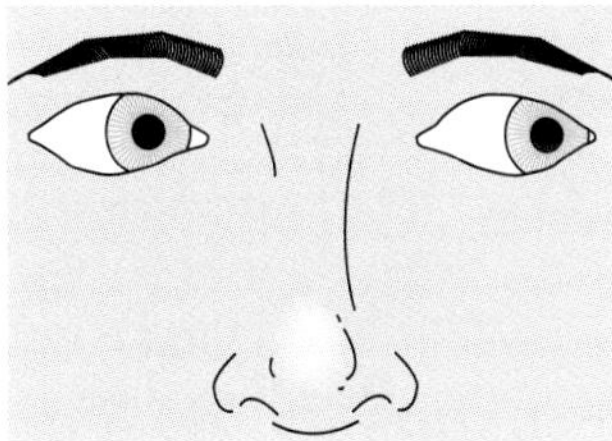

B Left gaze: no deviation

C Right gaze: left esotropia

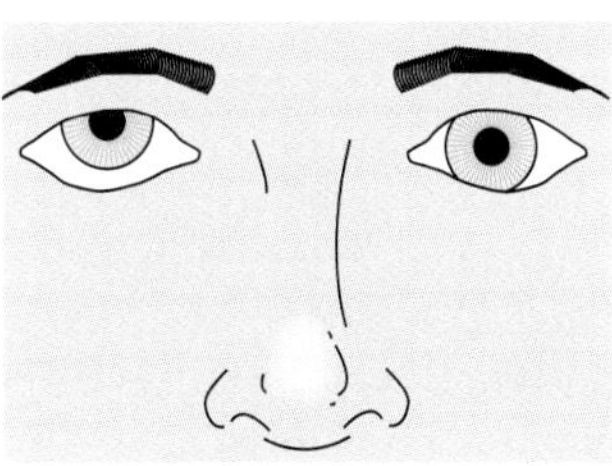

D Right hypertropia

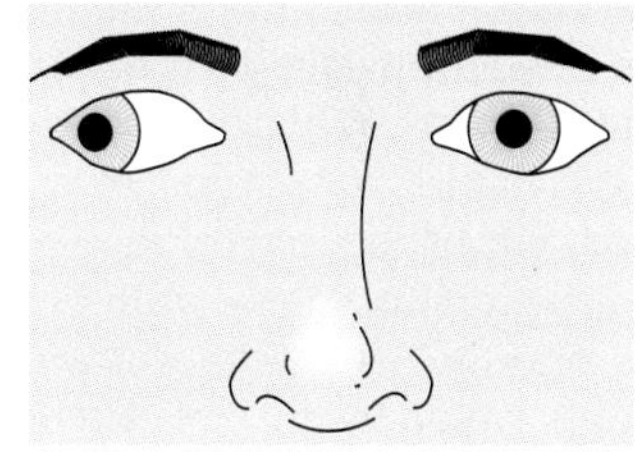

E Right exotropia

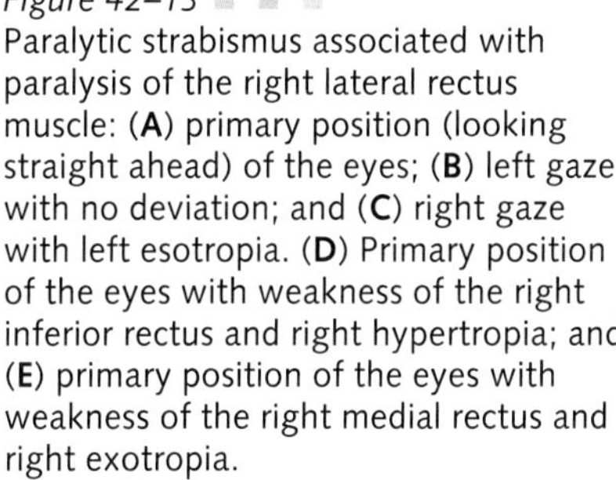

Figure 42–13
Paralytic strabismus associated with paralysis of the right lateral rectus muscle: (**A**) primary position (looking straight ahead) of the eyes; (**B**) left gaze with no deviation; and (**C**) right gaze with left esotropia. (**D**) Primary position of the eyes with weakness of the right inferior rectus and right hypertropia; and (**E**) primary position of the eyes with weakness of the right medial rectus and right exotropia.

Strabismus affects approximately 4% of children younger than 6 years of age. Because 30% to 50% of children suffer permanent secondary loss of vision, or amblyopia, early diagnosis and treatment are essential.[36]

Paralytic Strabismus

Paralytic strabismus results from paresis (*i.e.,* weakness) or plegia (*i.e.,* paralysis) of one or more of the extraocular muscles. When the normal eye fixates, the affected eye is in the position of primary deviation. In the case of esotropia, there is weakness of one of the lateral rectus muscles, usually the result of weakness of the abducens (VI) cranial nerve. When the affected eye fixates, the unaffected eye is in a position of secondary deviation. The secondary deviation of the unaffected eye is greater than the primary deviation of the affected eye. This is because the affected eye requires an excess of innervational impulse to maintain fixation; the excess impulses also are distributed to the unaffected eye (*i.e.,* Hering's law of equal innervation), causing overaction of its muscles.[3]

Paralytic strabismus is uncommon in children but accounts for nearly all cases of adult strabismus; it can be caused by a number of conditions. Paralytic strabismus is most commonly seen in adults who have had cerebral vascular accidents and may also occur as the first sign of a tumor or inflammatory condition involving the CNS. One type of muscular dystrophy exerts its effects on the extraocular muscles. Initially eye movements in all directions are weak, with later progression to bilateral optic immobility. Weakness of eye movement and lid elevation is often the first evidence of myasthenia gravis. The pathway of the oculomotor (III), trochlear (IV), and abducens (VI) cranial nerves through the cavernous sinus and the back of the orbit make them vulnerable to basal skull fracture and tumors of the cavernous sinus (*e.g.,* cavernous sinus syndrome) or orbit (*e.g.,* orbital syndrome).[37] In infants, paralytic strabismus can be caused by birth injuries affecting the extraocular muscles or the cranial nerves supplying these muscles. It can also result from congenital anomalies of the muscles. In general, paralytic strabismus in an adult with previously normal binocular vision causes diplopia. This does not occur in persons who have never developed binocular vision.

Nonparalytic Strabismus

In nonparalytic strabismus, there is no extraocular muscle weakness or paralysis, and the angle of deviation is always the same in all fields of gaze. With persistent deviation, secondary abnormalities may develop because of overaction or underaction of the muscles in some fields of gaze. Nonparalytic esotropia is the most common type of strabismus. The disorder may be accommodative, nonaccommodative, or a combination of the two. Accommodative strabismus is caused by disorders such as uncorrected hyperopia, in which the esotropia occurs with accommodation. The onset of this type of esotropia characteristically occurs between 18 months and 4 years of age, because accommodation is not well developed until that time. The disorder is most often monocular but may be alternating. About 50% of the cases of esotropia are accommodative in nature. The causes of nonaccommodative strabismus are obscure. The disorder may be related to faulty muscle insertion, fascial abnormalities, or faulty innervation. There is evidence that idiopathic strabismus may have a genetic basis; siblings may have similar disorders.

Diagnosis and Treatment

Examination by a qualified practitioner is indicated in any infant whose eyes are not aligned at all times during waking hours after 3 months of age.[3,39] Diagnostic measures emphasize two major areas: ocular deviation due to altered extrinsic muscle function and visual acuity.

Rapid assessment of extraocular muscle function is accomplished by three methods. First, in a somewhat darkened room and with the child staring straight ahead, a penlight is pointed at the midpoint between the two eyes, and a bright dot of reflected light can be seen on the cornea of each eye. With normal eye alignment, the reflected light should appear at the same spot on the cornea of each eye. Nonparallelism of the two eyes indicates muscle imbalance because of weakness or paralysis of the deviant eye. In a second method, the child is asked to follow the movement of a small object (*e.g.*, a pencil point, lighted penlight) as it is moved through the extremes of what are called the six cardinal positions of gaze. In extreme lateral gaze, normal subjects can show a few quick beats of a jerky or nystagmoid movement. Nystagmoid movement is abnormal if it is prolonged or present in any other eye posture. The third method, called the cover-uncover test, eliminates binocular fusion as a factor in maintaining parallelism between the eyes and is used to determine which eye is used for fixation. The child's attention is directed toward a fixed object such as a small picture or tongue blade. A light should not be used, because it may not stimulate accommodation. If a mild weakness is present, the eye with blocked vision drifts into a resting position, the extent of which depends on the relative strength of the muscles. The eye should snap back when the card is removed. The test is always done for near and far fixation. Visual acuity is evaluated to obtain a comparison of the two eyes. A tumbling E chart (or similar test chart) can be used for young children.[38]

Treatment of strabismus is directed toward the development of normal visual acuity, correction of the deviation, and superimposition of the retinal images to provide binocular vision. Nonsurgical and surgical methods can be used. In children, early treatment is important; the ideal age to begin is 6 months. Nonsurgical treatment includes occlusive patching, pleoptics (*i.e.*, eye exercises), and prism glasses. Because prolonged occlusive patching leads to loss of useful vision in the covered eye, patching is alternated between the affected and unaffected eye. This improves the vision in the affected eye without sacrificing vision in the unaffected eye. Prism glasses compensate for an abnormal alignment of an optic globe. Long-acting miotics in weak strengths (*e.g.*, echothiophate iodide solution [Phospholine Iodide], demecarium bromide [Humorsol]) may be used in treating accommodative esotropia. In young children, these drugs can be used instead of glasses. They act by altering the accommodative convergence relation in a favorable manner so that fusion is maintained despite accommodation. Miosis also allows for clearer vision with less accommodation in near and far vision. Surgical procedures may be used to strengthen a muscle or weaken a muscle by altering its length or attachment site.

Amblyopia

Amblyopia describes a condition of diminished vision (uncorrectable by lenses) in which no detectable organic lesion of the eye is present. This condition is sometimes referred to as *lazy eye*. Types of amblyopia include deprivation occlusion, strabismus, refractive, and organic amblyopia. It is caused by visual deprivation (*e.g.*, cataracts, severe ptosis) or abnormal binocular interactions (*e.g.*, strabismus, anisometropia) during visual immaturity. Normal development of the thalamic and cortical circuitry necessary for binocular visual perception requires simultaneous binocular use of each fovea during a critical period early in life (0 to 5 years). In infants with unilateral cataracts that are dense, central, and larger than 2 mm in diameter, this time is before 2 months of age.[3] In conditions causing abnormal binocular interactions, one image is suppressed to provide clearer vision. In esotropia, vision of the deviated eye is suppressed to prevent diplopia. A similar situation exists in anisometropia, in which the refractive indexes of the two eyes are different. Although the eyes are correctly aligned, they are unable to focus together, and the image of one eye is suppressed. In animal experiments, monocular deprivation results in reduced synaptic density in the LGN and the primary visual cortical areas that process input from the affected eye or eyes.[34]

The reversibility of amblyopia depends on the maturity of the visual system at the time of onset and the duration of the abnormal experience. If esotropia is involved, some persons alternate eyes and do not experience diplopia. With late-adolescent or adult onset, this habit pattern must be unlearned after correction.

Peripheral vision is less affected than central foveal vision in amblyopia. Suppression becomes more evident with high illumination and high contrast. It is as if the affected eye did not possess central vision and the person learns to fixate with the nonfoveal retina. If bilateral congenital blindness or near blindness (*e.g.*, from cataracts) occurs and remains uncorrected during infancy and early childhood, the person remains without pattern vision and has only overall field brightness and color discrimination. This is essentially bilateral amblyopia.

The treatment of children with the potential for developing amblyopia must be instituted well before the age of 6 to avoid the suppression phenomenon. Surgery for congenital cataracts and ptosis should be done early. Severe refractive errors should be corrected. In strabismus, alternately blocking vision in one eye and then the other forces the child to use both eyes for form discrimination. The duration of occlusion of vision in the good eye must be short (2 to 5 hours per day) and closely monitored, or deprivation amblyopia can develop in the good eye as well.[40] Although amblyopia is not likely to occur after the age of 8 or 9, some plasticity in central circuitry is evident even in adulthood.[41] For example, after refractive correction for longstanding astigmatism in adults, visual acuity improves slowly, requiring several months to reach normal levels.

In summary, disorders of eye movement include strabismus and amblyopia. Strabismus refers to abnormalities in the coordination of eye movements with loss of binocular eye alignment. This inability to focus a visual image on corresponding parts of the two retinas results in diplopia. Esotropia refers to medial deviation, exotropia refers to lateral deviation, hypertropia refers to upward deviation, hypotropia refers to downward deviation, and cyclotropia refers to torsional deviation. Paralytic strabismus is caused by weakness or paralysis of the extraocular muscles. Nonparalytic strabismus results from the inappropriate length or insertion of the extraocular muscles or from accommodation disorders. Amblyopia (*i.e.*, lazy eye) is a condition of diminished vision that cannot be corrected by lenses and one in which no detectable organic lesion in the eye can be observed. It results from inadequately developed CNS circuitry because of visual deprivation (*e.g.*, cataracts) or abnormal binocular interactions (*e.g.*, strabismus, anisometropia) during the period of visual immaturity.

REFERENCES

1. National Society to Prevent Blindness. (1980). *Vision problems in the U.S.* New York: Prevent Blindness of America.
2. Tielsch J.M., Sommers A., Witt K., Katz J., Royall RM., and the Baltimore Eye Survey Research Group. (1990). Blindness and visual impairment in an American Urban Population. *Archives of Ophthalmology* 108, 286–290.
3. Vaughan D.G., Ashbury T., Riordan-Eva P. (1995). *General ophthalmology* (14th ed., pp. 79, 90–91, 169–170, 200–203, 225, 233). Norwalk, CT: Appleton Lange.
4. Hara J.H. (1996). The red eye: Diagnosis and treatment. *American Family Physician* 54 (8), 2423–2430.
5. Black J.G. (1996). *Microbiology: Principles and applications* (p. 253). Upper Saddle River, NJ: Prentice Hall.
6. Benenson A.S. (Ed.). (1990). *Control of communicable disease in man* (15th ed., pp. 103–104, 442). Washington, DC: APHA.
7. McLean D.M., Smith J.A. (1991). *Medical microbiology synopsis* (p. 164). Philadelphia: Lea & Febiger.
8. Abel S.R. (1996). Eye disorders. In Young L.Y., Koda-Kimble M.A. (Eds.). *Applied therapeutics: The clinical use of drugs* (6th ed., pp. 49–1—49–11). Vancouver, WA: Applied Therapeutics.
9. Mauger T.F., Craig E.L. (1994). *Havener's ocular pharmacology*. (6th ed., pp. 2–3, 307–313, 397–398, 484) St. Louis: C.V. Mosby Co.
10. Cotran R.S., Kumar V., Robbins S.L. (1994). *Robbins' pathologic basis of disease* (5th ed., pp. 327, 1466). Philadelphia: W.B. Saunders.
11. Nelson L. (1996). Disorders of the conjunctiva. In Behrman R.E., Kliegman R.M., Arvin A.M. (Eds.). *Nelson textbook of pediatrics* (15th ed., pp. 1779–1781). Philadelphia: W.B. Saunders.
12. Bacon A.S., Dart J.K., Ficker L.A., et al. (1993). Acanthamoeba keratitis. *Ophthalmology* 100 (8), 238–243.
13. Evans N.M. (1995). *Ophthalmology* (2nd ed., pp. 43–44, 68–69, 113–116, 205). New York: Oxford Press.
14. Rosenberg L.F. (1995). Glaucoma: Early detection and therapy for prevention of vision loss. *American Family Physician* 52 (8), 2289–2298.
15. Javitt J.C., McBean A.M., Nicholson G.A., et al. (1991). Underestimation of glaucoma among Black Americans. *New England Journal of Medicine* 325, 1418–1422.
16. Martin X.D. (1992). Normal intraocular pressure in man. *Ophthalmologicia* 205, 57–63.
17. Quigley H.A. (1993). Open-angle glaucoma. *New England Journal of Medicine* 328 (15), 1097–1106.
18. Rubin E., Farber J.L. (*1994*). Pathology (2nd ed., pp. 1466–1479). Philadelphia: J.B. Lippincott.
19. Agency for Health Care Policy and Research, Cataract Management Guideline Panel. (1993). *Cataract in adults: Management of functional impairment*. Bethesda: U.S. Department of Health and Human Services.
20. Quality of Care Committee—Anterior Segment Panel. (1989). *Cataract in the otherwise healthy eye*. San Francisco: American Academy of Ophthalmology.
21. Sadler T.W. (1995). *Langman's medical embryology* (7th ed., pp. 424–425, 360, 363). Baltimore; Williams & Wilkins.
22. Aiello LP., Avery R.L., Aerig P.G., et al (1994). *New England Journal of Medicine* 331, 1480–1487.
23. Al E. (1992). Current management of diabetic retinopathy. *Western Journal of Medicine* 157, 67–70.
24. D'Amico D.J. (1994). Diseases of the retina. *New England Journal of Medicine* 331 (2), 95–106.
25. Writing Committee American College of Physicians, American Diabetes Association, American Academy of Ophthalmology. (1992). Screening guidelines for diabetic retinopathy. *Annals of Internal Medicine* 116 (8), 686–685.
26. Diabetes Control and Complications Trial Research Group. (1993). The effect of intensive treatment of diabetes on the development and progression of long-term complications in insulin-dependent diabetes mellitus. *New England Journal of Medicine* 329 (14), 977–986.
27. Murphy R.P. (1995). Management of diabetic retinopathy. *American Family Physician* 51 (4), 785–796.
28. Valenine R.H., Jackson J.C., Kalina R.E., et al. (1989). Increased survival of low birth weight infants: Impact on the incidence of retinopathy of prematurity. *Pediatrics* 84, 442–445.

29. Kretzer F.L., Hittner H.M. (1988). Retinopathy of prematurity: Clinical implications of retinal development. *Archives of Disease in Childhood* 63, 1151–1167.
30. Shapiro C. (1986). Retrolental fibroplasia: What we know and what we don't know. *Neonatal Network* 4 (6), 33–45.
31. The Committee for the Classification of Retinopathy of Prematurity. (1984). An international classification of retinopathy of prematurity. *Archives of Ophthalmology* 102, 1130–1134.
32. Cryotherapy for Retinopathy of Prematurity Cooperative Group. (1988). Multicenter trial of cryotherapy for retinopathy of prematurity: Preliminary results. *Pediatrics* 81, 697–706.
33. Capino D.G., Leibowitz H.M. (1988). Age-related macular degeneration. *Hospital Practice* 22 (3A), 23–42.
34. Woods S. (1992). Macular degeneration. *Nursing Clinics of North America* 27, 755–761.
35. Macular Photocoagulation Study Group. (1991). Argon laser photocoagulation for neovascular maculopathy. *Archives of Ophthalmology* 109, 1109–1114.
36. Lavrich J.B., Nelson L.B. (1993). Diagnosis and management of strabismus disorders. *Pediatric Clinics of North America* 40 (4), 737–751.
37. Kline L.B., Bajandas F.J. (1996). *Neuro-ophthalmology review manual* (chap. 4–7). Thorofare, NJ: Slack.
38. Scheiman M. (1997). *Understanding and managing vision defects* (pp. 26–27). Thorofare, NJ: Slack.
39. Rubein S.E., Nelson S.B. (1993). Amblyopia: Diagnosis and management. *Pediatric Clinics of North America* 40 (4), 727–735.
40. Wong-Riley M.T.T., Carroll E.W. (1984). The effect of impulse blockage on cytochrome oxidative activity in the monkey visual system. *Nature* 307, 262–264.
41. Carroll E.W., Wong-Riley M.T.T. (1987). Recovery of cytochrome oxidase activity in the adult macaque visual system after termination of impulse blockage due to tetrodotoxin [abstract 13]. Society for Neuroscience. New Orleans, LA, 1987.

BIBLIOGRAPHY

Ciner E.B., Macks B., Shanel-Klatsch E. (1991). A cooperative early demonstration project for early intervention service. *Occupational Therapy Practice* 3, 42–56.

Chandrasoma P., Taylor C.R. (1995). *Concise pathology* (2nd ed., pp. 482–493). Norwalk, CT: Appleton & Lange.

Clark C.M., Lee D.A. (1995). Prevention and treatment of complications of diabetes mellitus. *New England Journal of Medicine* 332 (18), 1210–1216.

Frank K.J., Dieckert J.P. (1996). Diabetic eye disease: A primary care perspective. *Southern Medical Journal* 89 (5), 463–470.

O'Hara M. (1993). Ophthalmia neonatorium. *Pediatric Clinics of North American* 40 (4), 715–724.

Javitt C., Wang F., West S. (1996). Blindness to cataract: Epidemiology and prevention. *Annual Review of Public Health* 17, 159–177.

Ramachandran V.S. (1992). Blind spots. *Scientific American* 266 (5), 86–91.

Roberts D.K., Terry J.E. (1996). *Ocular disease: Diagnosis and Treatment* (2nd ed., pp. 41–43). Boston: Butterworth-Heinemann.

Sher N.A., Trobe J.D., Weingeist T.A. (1995). New options for vision loss. *Patient Care* 29 (1A), 55–76.

Tielsch J.M. (1995). The epidemiology and control of open angle glaucoma: A population-based perspective. *Annual Review of Public Health* 17, 121–136.

CHAPTER 43

Alterations in Hearing and Vestibular Function

Carol Mattson Porth and Robin L. Curtis

The ears are paired organs consisting of an external and middle ear, which function in capturing, transmitting, and amplifying sound, and an inner ear that contains the receptive organs that are stimulated by sound waves (*i.e.*, hearing) or head position and movement (*i.e.*, vestibular function). Hearing loss may be the most common physical disability suffered by persons in the United States. More than 13 million persons in the United States have some hearing impairment. Of these, 6 million are seriously handicapped, and more than 1.7 million are deaf. Although not as debilitating, otitis media is a common disease of childhood. Vertigo is another common cause of disability, particularly among the elderly. This chapter is divided into two parts: the first focuses on disorders of the ear and auditory function and the second on disorders of the inner ear and vestibular function.

Alterations in Auditory Function

After you have completed this section of the chapter, you should be able to meet the following objectives:

- Describe two common disorders of the outer ear
- Relate the functions of the auditory or eustachian tube to the development of middle ear problems, including otitis media
- Explain why infants and young children are prone to develop otitis media
- List three common symptoms of otitis media
- Describe the disease process that occurs with otosclerosis and relate it to the hearing loss that occurs
- Characterize tinnitus
- Differentiate between conductive and sensorineural hearing loss and cite the more common causes of each
- List at least three drug groups that have potential ototoxicity
- Cite the impact of damage to Wernicke's area in the brain

Disorders of the External Ear

The external ear is a funnel-shaped structure that conducts sound waves to the tympanic membrane. The function of the external ear is disturbed when sound transmission is obstructed by impacted cerumen or inflammation of the external ear (*i.e.*, otitis externa).

Impacted Cerumen

Cerumen, or earwax, is a protective secretion produced by the outer portion of the ear canal. Although the ear is normally self-cleaning, the cerumen can accumulate and narrow the canal. Repeated unskilled attempts to remove the wax may pack it more deeply into the ear canal. Impacted cerumen usually produces no symptoms until the canal becomes completely occluded, at which point a feeling of fullness, loss of hearing, tinnitus (*i.e.*, ringing in the ears), or coughing because of vagal stimulation develops.

In most cases, the accumulated cerumen can be removed with detergent ear drops. A few drops of dilute hydrogen peroxide solution (6.5% carbamide peroxide in glycerol) can be instilled into the ear to soften the wax. A number of commercial products are available for this purpose. When necessary, the ear may be irrigated with warm water. Warm water is used to avoid a vestibular caloric response. The ear canal should be dried thoroughly after irrigation to avoid introducing an infection. Cerumen may also be removed using an otoscope and a wire loop or blunt cerumen curette.

Otitis Externa

Otitis externa is an inflammation of the external ear that may vary in severity from a mild eczematoid dermatitis to severe cellulitis. It can be caused by infectious agents, irritation (*e.g.*, wearing earphones), or allergic reactions. Predisposing factors include moisture in the ear canal after swimming (*i.e.*, swimmer's ear) or bathing and trauma resulting from scratching or attempts to clean the ear. Most infections are caused by gram-negative bacteria (*e.g.*, *Pseudomonas, Proteus*) or fungi that grow in the presence of excess moisture. Otitis externa commonly is manifested by itching, redness, tenderness, and narrowing of the ear canal because of swelling. Inflammation of the pinna or canal makes movement of the ear painful. There may be watery or purulent drainage and intermittent deafness.

Treatment usually includes the use of ear drops containing an appropriate antibiotic in combination with a topical corticosteroid to reduce inflammation. Protection of the ear from additional moisture and avoidance of trauma from scratching is important. Preventing recurrences is important, particularly in persons who swim frequently. Instillation of a dilute alcohol, acetic acid, or Burow's solution (available in over-the-counter ear drops) immediately after swimming is usually an effective prophylaxis.

Dermatoses (*i.e.*, seborrheic, contact, and atopic dermatitis) are common causes of inflammation of the external ear canal and can be precursors of acute inflammation caused by scratching and introduction of infectious organisms.

Pruritus

Pruritus of the external ear and ear canal is a common problem. It is most commonly self-induced by overzealous cleaning with soap and water or use of cotton swabs to remove protective cerumen from the ear canal.

Treatment includes application of mineral oil to reduce dryness and avoidance of scratching, irritation, and removal of cerumen. Corticosteroid ear drops may be used when inflammation is present. Severe pruritus may also be caused by allergy in persons with hay fever. Medications used for treatment of the allergy and corticosteroid ear drops are usually effective in relieving the pruritus.

Disorders of the Middle Ear

The middle ear consists of the tympanic membrane, or eardrum, which separates the outer ear from the inner ear; the auditory tube, which connects the middle ear with the nasopharynx; and the bony ossicles, which connect the tympanic membrane with the oval window (see Chapter 41, Fig. 41–15). It is located in an air-filled space within the petrous portion of the temporal bone.

The tympanic membrane, which separates the external ear from the middle ear, has three layers: an outer layer of thin skin continuous with the lining of the external ear canal, a middle layer of tough collagenous fibers mixed with fibrocytes and some elastic fibers, and an inner epithelial layer continuous with the lining of the middle ear. It is attached in a manner that allows it to vibrate freely when audible sound waves enter the external auditory canal. When viewed through an otoscope, the tympanic membrane appears as a shallow, almost circular cone pointing inward toward its apex, the umbo (Fig. 43–1). The landmarks include the lightened stripe over the handle of the malleus; the umbo at the end of the handle; the pars tensa, which constitutes most of the drum; and the pars flaccida, the small area above the malleus attachment. Light usually is reflected from the pars tensa at about the 4-o'clock position. The tympanic membrane is semitransparent, and a small whitish cord, which traverses the middle ear from back to front, can be seen just under its upper edge. This is the chorda tympani, a branch of the intermedius component of the facial cranial nerve (CN VII).

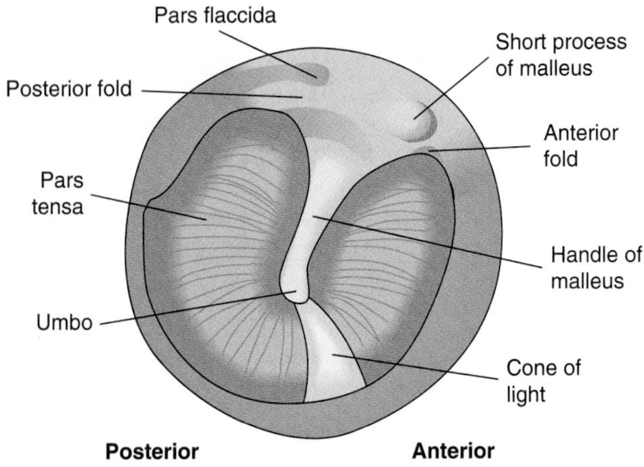

Figure 43–1
Right eardrum.

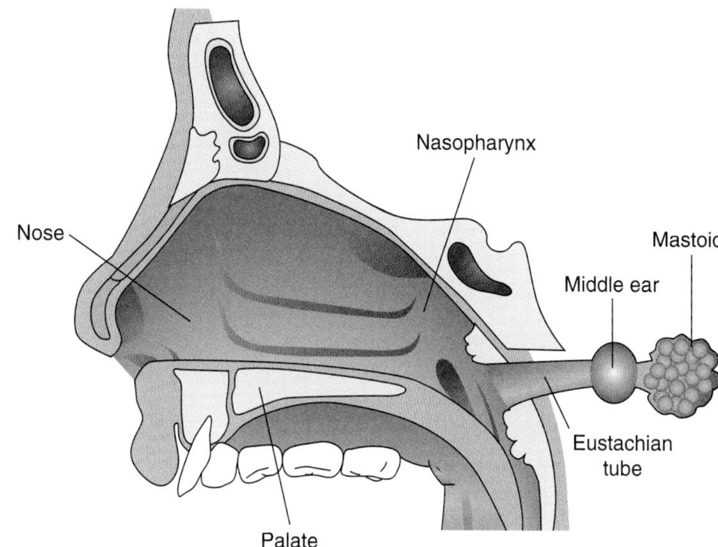

Figure 43–2
Nasopharynx–eustachian tube–mastoid air cell system. (Bluestone C.D. [1981]. Recent advances in pathogenesis, diagnosis, and management of otitis media. *Pediatric Clinics of North America* 28 [4], 36. Reproduced with permission)

Auditory Tube Dysfunction

There is a gap in the bone between the anterior and medial walls of the middle ear for a canal, called the *eustachian tube*, or *auditory tube*, which connects with the nasopharynx (Fig. 43–2). The middle ear is filled with the air that reaches it from the nasopharynx by way of the auditory tube. The auditory tube is lined with a mucous membrane that is continuous with the pharynx and mastoid air cells. Infections from the nasopharynx can travel from the nasopharynx along the mucous membrane of the auditory tube to the middle ear, causing otitis media. Near the opening of the auditory tube, the columnar epithelial lining changes to the pseudostratified ciliated-columnar surface of the pharynx, which contains occasional mucus-secreting cells. Hypertrophy of the mucus-secreting cells contributes to the mucoid secretions that develop during certain types of otitis media.

The auditory tube, which connects the middle ear with the nasopharynx, serves three basic functions: ventilation of the middle ear, along with equalization of middle ear and ambient pressures; protection of the middle ear from unwanted nasopharyngeal sound waves and secretions; and drainage of middle ear secretions into the nasopharynx.[1] The nasopharyngeal entrance to the auditory tube, which usually is closed, is opened by the action of the CN V–innervated tensor veli palatini muscles (Fig. 43–3). Opening of the auditory tube, which normally occurs with swallowing and yawning reflexes, provides the mechanism for equalizing the pressure of the middle ear with that of the atmosphere. This equalization ensures that the pressures on both sides of the tympanic membrane are the same, so that sound transmission is not reduced and rupture does not result from sudden changes in external pressure, as occurs during plane travel.

Abnormalities in auditory tube function are important factors in the pathogenesis of middle ear infections. There are two important types of auditory tube dysfunction: abnormal patency and obstruction (Fig. 43–3). The abnormally patent tube does not close or does not close completely. In infants and children with an abnormally patent tube, air and secretions are often pumped into the auditory tube during crying and nose blowing. Obstruction can be functional or mechanical. Functional obstruction results from the persistent collapse of the auditory tube because of a lack of tubal stiffness or poor function of the tensor veli palatini muscle that controls opening of auditory tube. It is

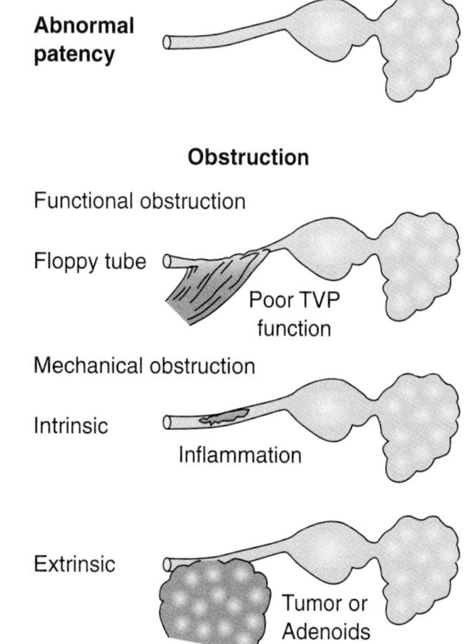

Figure 43–3
Pathophysiology of the eustachian tube. TVP, tensor veli palatini. (Bluestone C.D. [1981]. Recent advances in the pathogenesis, diagnosis, and management of otitis media. *Pediatric Clinics of North America* 28 [4], 737. Reproduced with permission)

common in infants and young children, because the amount and stiffness of the cartilage supporting the auditory tube are less than in older children and adults. Age-related changes in the craniofacial base also render the muscle responsible for opening the auditory tube less efficient in this age group. Mechanical obstruction can be intrinsic or extrinsic; the most common obstruction is caused by intrinsic swelling resulting from upper respiratory tract infection or allergy.[2] Extrinsic obstruction can result from the enlargement of adenoid tissue or a tumor. With obstruction, air in the middle ear is absorbed, causing a negative pressure and the transudation of serous fluid into the middle ear. This can result in sterile otitis media with effusion.

Barotrauma

Barotrauma represents injury resulting from the inability to equalize the barometric stress on the middle ear imposed by air travel or less commonly by underwater diving. It occurs most often during air travel when there is a sudden change in atmospheric pressure. The pressure in the middle ear parallels that of atmospheric pressure; it decreases at high altitudes and increases at lower altitudes. The problem occurs during rapid airplane descent, when the negative pressure in the middle ear tends to cause the auditory tube to collapse. If air cannot pass back through the auditory tube, hearing loss and discomfort develop. This most often occurs in persons who travel while suffering from an upper respiratory tract infection. Autoinflation measures such as yawning, swallowing, and chewing gum seem to facilitate opening of the auditory tube, which equalizes air pressure in the middle ear. Systemic decongestants (*e.g.*, pseudoephedrine) may be used to prevent symptoms. Acute negative pressure that persists on the ground is treated with decongestants and attempts at autoinflation. Myringotomy (*i.e.*, surgical incision in the tympanic membrane) provides immediate relief and may be used in cases of acute otalgia and hearing loss. Repeated episodes of barotrauma in persons who must use frequent air travel may be treated with insertion of ventilating tubes.

Otitis Media

Otitis media represents a spectrum of diseases in which fluid is present in the middle ear. Otitis media can be acute, subacute, or chronic. It may or may not be infectious in origin. In acute otitis media, signs and symptoms of inflammation accompany the accumulation of fluid or effusion. Otitis media may occur in any age group, although children are most commonly affected; it is the most common diagnosis made by physicians who care for children. Infants and young children are at highest risk for otitis media; the peak prevalence is between 6 and 36 months of age.[3]

Acute Otitis Media. Acute otitis media is characterized by a suppurative (purulent or pus-containing) or serous (serum-type) exudate. Most cases of otitis media follow an upper respiratory tract infection that has been present for several days. *Streptococcus pneumoniae, Haemophilus influenzae,* and *Moraxella catarrhalis* are the most frequently isolated organisms.[3–6] The mucosal lining of the middle ear is continuous with the auditory tube and nasopharynx; most middle ear infections enter by way of the auditory tube (see Fig. 43–2). There are two reasons for the increased risk in infants and young children: the auditory tube is shorter, more horizontal, and wider in this age group than in older children and adults; and infection can spread more easily through the canal of the infant who spends most of the day lying in bed. Bottle-fed babies have a higher incidence of otitis media than breast-fed babies, probably because bottle-fed babies are held in a more horizontal position during feeding, and swallowing while in the horizontal position facilitates the reflux of milk into the middle ear. Breast-feeding also provides for the transfer of protective maternal antibodies to the infant.

The incidence of otitis media is higher among children with craniofacial anomalies (*e.g.*, cleft palate, Down syndrome) and among Alaskan natives (Inuits [Eskimos]) and Native Americans.[7] Other risk factors include male gender, sibling with history of otitis media, group day care attendance, and exposure to tobacco smoke.

Acute suppurative otitis media is characterized by otalgia (*i.e.*, earache), fever (up to 104°F), and hearing loss. The patient may have rhinorrhea, vomiting, and diarrhea. Pain usually increases as purulent exudate accumulates behind the tympanic membrane. An infant may cry and rub the infected ear, and an older child may complain of sharp or severe pain in the ear. If the tympanic membrane ruptures because of excessive pressure, the pain is relieved, and purulent drainage is observed in the external ear canal.

Diagnosis and Treatment. Diagnosis of acute otitis media often is made by otoscopic examination of the tympanic membrane. A bulging, lusterless membrane with subsequent obliteration of the bony landmarks and cone of light are observed. Gentle movement of the pinna can help to differentiate otitis media from otitis externa. This maneuver does not produce pain in purulent otitis media but causes severe discomfort in otitis externa. A culture of middle ear effusion fluid may be used for verifying the presence of a microorganism and identifying its type. A needle can be inserted through the inferior part of the tympanic membrane to obtain a specimen of effusion fluid, or a culture can be made of the drainage in the external ear canal when the tympanic membrane has perforated.

The use of the pneumatic otoscope permits the introduction of air into the canal for the purpose of determining tympanic membrane flexibility. The movement of this membrane is decreased in some cases of acute otitis media and absent in chronic middle ear infection. Tympanometry is an important advance in the identification of middle ear disease. A tympanogram is obtained by inserting a small probe into the external auditory canal; a tone of fixed characteristics is then presented through the probe, and the mobility of the tympanic membrane is measured electronically while the external canal pressure is artificially varied.

The treatment of acute otitis media includes the use of appropriate antibiotic therapy. Additional supportive therapy, including analgesics, antipyretics, and local heat, may be indicated. Myringotomy may be done to relieve pressure on the tympanic membrane, reduce pain and hearing loss, and prevent the ragged opening that can follow spontaneous rupture of the tympanic membrane. A middle ear effusion may persist after the course of antibiotic therapy. The effusion often clears spontaneously and does not require further treatment. If there is evidence of continued infection, treatment with another antimicrobial agent may be indicated.

Recurrent Otitis Media. Recurrent otitis media is characterized by repeated episodes of otitis media that occur with almost every respiratory tract infection. Most children with recurrent otitis media respond well to treatment and have fewer recurrences with advancing age. Some children have persistent middle ear effusion with superimposed recurrent episodes of acute otitis media.

Pressure-equalization (ventilating) tubes may be used in the treatment of children with recurrent or chronic otitis media. Insertion of the tubes is one of the most commonly performed surgical procedures in the United States; the long-term benefits are controversial. Indications for tube insertion include the persistence of middle ear fluid for 3 or more months per episode, the presence of speech-language delay, and conductive hearing loss of 20 decibels (db) or more. The tubes are usually placed under general anesthesia. The ears of children with the tubes must be kept out of water. Spontaneous extrusion of the tubes usually occurs after 5.5 to 7 months.[8] The adverse effects include recurrent otorrhea; persistent perforation, scarring, and atrophy of the tympanic membrane; and cholesteatoma.

Otitis Media With Effusion. Otitis media with effusion is a condition in which serous fluid accumulates in the middle ear. The condition may be acute, as in a viral infection, or it may follow successfully treated otitis media. Signs of otitis media with effusion include conductive hearing loss, eardrum retraction, and a fluid level or air bubbles visible through the tympanic membrane. A persistent middle ear effusion is one that persists after the initial 10 to 14 days of treatment for acute otitis. One possible explanation for the persistent effusion is that inflammatory mediators associated with an acute episode of otitis media damages the mucus-secreting cells of the middle ear, leading to a persistent hypersecretory state.[7] Persistent middle ear effusion is usually asymptomatic, although some children may complain of feeling of fullness of the ears.

Persistent middle ear effusions often resolve spontaneously. The treatment is often one of "watch and wait." Topical and systemic decongestants are usually of little value in clearing middle ear effusion. If the effusion persists for 3 months or longer, treatment with antibiotics is recommended.[9] Corticosteroids may be used in conjunction with the antibiotics, although this practice is controversial. Tympanostomy tube placement may be considered in children with hearing loss and in whom effusion has lasted longer than 3 months.[7]

Complications. Complications of otitis media are uncommon, but they can follow inadequate treatment. The most common are those associated with the aural (ear) cavity, tympanic membrane, and surrounding temporal bone. Intracranial complications are rare but are the most serious. One of the most common complications of otitis media is persistent conductive hearing loss. Fluid may be present in the middle ear for weeks or months after an acute bout of otitis media. This may impair hearing and affect the child's learning of language skills. Hearing loss that is associated with fluid collection usually resolves when the effusion clears. Permanent hearing loss may occur as the result of damage to the tympanic membrane or other middle ear structures.

Perforation of the tympanic membrane occurs most often after acute otitis media; although it usually heals spontaneously, tympanoplasty may be necessary. Adhesive otitis media involves an abnormal healing reaction to an inflamed middle ear. It produces irreversible thickening of the mucous membranes and may cause impaired movement of the ossicles and possibly conductive hearing loss. Tympanosclerosis involves the formation of whitish plaques and nodular deposits on the submucosal surface of the tympanic membrane, with possible adherence of the ossicles and conductive hearing loss.

A cholesteatoma is a saclike mass containing silvery white debris of keratin, which is shed by the squamous epithelial lining of the tympanic membrane. As the lining of the epithelium sheds and desquamates, the lesion expands and erodes the surrounding tissues. The lesion, which is associated with chronic middle ear infection, is insidiously progressive, and erosion may involve the temporal bone, causing intracranial complications. The treatment involves microsurgical techniques to remove the cholesteatomatous material.

The mastoid antrum and air cells constitute a portion of the temporal bone and may become inflamed as an extension of an acute or chronic otitis media. Because of the use of antibiotics, acute mastoiditis, a complication of acute otitis media, is unusual. If it does occur, there is necrosis of the mastoid process and destruction of the bony intercellular matrix, which are visible by radiologic examination. Mastoid tenderness and drainage of exudate through a perforated tympanic membrane can occur. Chronic mastoiditis can develop as the result of chronic middle ear infection. The usefulness of antibiotics for this condition is limited. Mastoid or middle ear surgery, along with other medical treatment, may be indicated.

Intracranial complications, although rare, can develop if the infection spreads through vascular channels, by direct extension, or through preformed pathways such as the round window. These complications are seen more often with chronic suppurative otitis media and mastoiditis. They include meningitis, focal encephalitis, brain abscess, lateral sinus thrombophlebitis or thrombosis, labyrinthitis, and facial nerve paralysis. Any child who develops persistent headache, tinnitus, stiff neck, or visual or other neurologic symptoms should be investigated for possible intracranial complications.

Otosclerosis

Otosclerosis is a familial, autosomal dominant disorder that causes conductive deafness, sensorineural hearing loss, and tinnitus. It is a disorder of the otic capsule (*i.e.*, bone surrounding the inner ear) and the stapes. Otosclerosis may begin at any time in life but usually does not appear until after puberty, most frequently between the ages of 20 and 30. The disease process accelerates during pregnancy.

Otosclerosis begins with resorption of bone in one or more foci. During active bone resorption, the bone structure appears spongy and softer than normal (*i.e.*, osteospongiosis). The resorbed bone is replaced by an overgrowth of new, hard sclerotic bone. The process is slowly progressive, involving more areas of the temporal bone, especially in front of and posterior to the stapes footplate. As it invades the footplate, the pathologic bone increasingly immobilizes the stapes, reducing the transmission of sound. Pressure of otosclerotic bone on inner ear structures or the vestibulocochlear nerve (CN VIII) may contribute to the development of tinnitus, sensorineural hearing loss, and vertigo.

The symptoms of otosclerosis involve an insidious hearing loss. Initially, the affected person is unable to hear a whisper or someone speaking at a distance. In the earliest stages, the bone conduction by which the person's own voice is heard remains relatively unaffected. Then the person's own voice sounds unusually loud, and the sound of chewing becomes intensified. Because of bone conduction, most of these persons can hear fairly well on the telephone, which provides an amplified signal. Many are able to hear better in a noisy environment, probably because the masking effect of background noise causes other persons to speak louder.

The treatment of otosclerosis can be medical or surgical. A carefully selected, well-fitting hearing aid may allow a person with conductive deafness to lead a normal life. Sodium fluoride has been used in the medical treatment of osteospongiosis. Because much of the conductive hearing loss associated with otosclerosis is caused by stapedial fixation, the surgical treatment involves stapedectomy with stapedial reconstruction using the patient's own stapes or a stapedial prosthesis. The argon laser beam may be used in the surgical procedure.

Disorders of the Inner Ear

Tinnitus

Tinnitus (from the Latin *tinniere*, meaning to ring) is the perception of abnormal ear or head noises, not produced by an external stimulus. Although it is often described as "ringing of the ears," it may also assume a hissing, roaring, or whooshing sound. Tinnitus may be constant, pulsed, or intermittent.

Intermittent periods of mild, high-pitched tinnitus lasting for several minutes are common in normal-hearing persons. Impacted cerumen is a benign cause of tinnitus, which resolves after the ear wax is removed. Medications such as aspirin and stimulants such as nicotine and caffeine can cause transient tinnitus. The physiologic mechanism underlying tinnitus is unknown. It seems likely that there are several mechanisms, including abnormal firing of auditory receptors, transmission of signals, and alterations in central processing of the signal. Tinnitus is a symptom, and the diagnosis relies heavily on the person's description of the problem, including onset, frequency, description, and location of the tinnitus; perceived cause; and extent to which the person is bothered by the problem. A history of medication or stimulant use and dietary factors that may cause tinnitus should obtained. Tinnitus often accompanies hearing disorders, and tests of auditory function are usually done.

Treatment methods include elimination of drugs or other substances such as caffeine, some cheeses, red wine, and foods containing monosodium glutamate (MSG) that are suspected of causing tinnitus. The use of an externally produced sound may be used to mask or inhibit the tinnitus. Medications, including antihistamines, anticonvulsant drugs, calcium-channel blockers, benzodiazepines, and antidepressants, have been used for tinnitus alleviation, but none produce lasting relief without side effects. For persistent tinnitus, psychologic interventions may be needed to help the person deal with the stress and distraction associated with the condition.

Hearing Loss

There are many causes of hearing loss or deafness. Most fit into the categories of conductive, sensorineural, or mixed deficiencies that involve a combination of conductive and sensorineural function deficiencies of the same ear. Chart 43–1 summarizes common causes of conductive and sensorineural hearing loss. Hearing loss may be congenital or acquired, sudden or progressive, unilateral or bilateral, partial or complete.

Conductive Hearing Loss

Conductive hearing loss can occur when auditory stimuli are not adequately transmitted through the auditory canal, tympanic membrane, middle ear, or ossicle chain to the inner ear. Temporary hearing loss can occur as the result of impacted cerumen in the outer ear or fluid in the middle ear. More permanent causes of hearing loss are thickening or damage of the tympanic membrane or otosclerosis.

Sensorineural Hearing Loss

Sensorineural, or perceptive, hearing loss occurs with disorders that affect the inner ear, auditory nerve, or auditory pathways of the brain. With this type of deafness, sound waves are conducted to the inner ear, but abnormalities of the cochlear apparatus or auditory nerve

CHART 43-1
Common Causes of Conductive and Sensorineural Hearing Loss

Conductive Hearing Loss

External Ear Conditions
- Impacted ear wax or foreign body
- Otitis externa

Middle Ear Conditions
- Trauma
- Otitis Media
- Otosclerosis

Sensorineural Hearing Loss

Trauma
- Head injury
- Noise

Inflammation
- Infection (viral, bacterial, meningitis)

Autoimmune

Endocrine
- Diabetes
- Hypothyroidism

Degenerative
- Presbycusis

Vascular
- Atherosclerosis
- Sudden deafness

Ototoxicity
- Aminoglycosides
- Salicylates
- Diuretics

Tumors
- Vestibular schwannoma (acoustic neuroma)
- Meningioma
- Metastatic

Idiopathic
- Ménière's disease

decrease or distort the transfer of information to the brain. Tinnitus accompanies cochlear nerve irritation. Abnormal function resulting from damage or malformation of the central auditory pathways and circuitry is included in this category.

Sensorineural hearing loss may have a genetic cause, result from intrauterine infections such as maternal rubella, or developmental malformations of the inner ear. It has been estimated that 50% of profound deafness in children has a genetic basis.[10] Trauma to the inner ear, tumors that encroach on the inner ear or sensory neurons, vascular disorders with hemorrhage, or thrombosis of vessels that supply the inner ear are causes of sensorineural deafness. Other causes of sensorineural deafness are infections and drugs. Sudden sensorineural hearing loss represents an abrupt loss of hearing that occurs instantaneously or on awakening. It is most commonly caused by viral infections, circulatory disorders, or rupture of the labyrinth membrane that can occur during tympanotomy.[11]

Environmentally induced deafness can occur through direct exposure to excessively intense sound, as in the workplace or at a concert. This type of deafness was once called "boilermaker's deafness" because of the intense reverberating sound to which riveters were exposed when putting together boiler tanks. Sustained or repeated exposure to noise pollution at sound intensities greater than 100 to 120 db can cause corresponding mechanical damage to the organ of Corti on the "tuned" basilar membrane. If damage is severe, permanent sensorineural deafness to the offending sound frequencies results. Wearing earplugs or ear protection is important under many industrial conditions and for musicians and music listeners exposed to high sound amplification. Noise pollution often is characterized by high-intensity sounds of a specific frequency that cause corresponding damage to the organ of Corti.

A number of infections can cause hearing loss. Deafness or some degree of hearing impairment is the most common serious complication of bacterial meningitis in infants and children, reportedly resulting in sensorineural hearing loss in 5% to 35% of persons who survive the disease.[10] The mechanism causing hearing impairment seems to be suppurative labrynthitis or neuritis resulting in the loss of hair cells and damage to the auditory nerve. Untreated suppurative otitis media can also cause sensorineural hearing loss through the same mechanisms. Congenital and acquired syphilis can cause unilateral or bilateral sensorineural hearing loss.

Among the neoplasms that impair hearing are acoustic neuromas. Acoustic neuromas are benign Schwann cell tumors affecting CN VIII. These tumors are usually unilateral and cause hearing loss by compressing the cochlear nerve or interfering with blood supply to the nerve and cochlea. Other neoplasms that can affect hearing include meningiomas and metastatic brain tumors.

Drugs that damage inner ear structures are labeled ototoxic. Vestibular symptoms of ototoxicity include lightheadedness, giddiness, and dizziness; if severe, cochlear symptoms that consist of tinnitus or hearing loss occur. Hearing loss is sensorineural and may be bilateral or unilateral, transient or permanent. Several classes of drugs have been identified as having ototoxic potentials: aminoglycoside antibiotics and other basic antibiotics with similar ototoxic potential, antimalarial drugs, loop diuretics, and salicylates. Many other drug groups have been implicated in causing ototoxicity. The risk of ototoxicity depends on the total dose of the drug and its concentration in the bloodstream. It is increased in persons with impaired kidney functioning and in those previously or currently treated with another potentially ototoxic drug. Table 43–1 lists drugs with the potential for producing ototoxicity.

Presbycusis

The term *presbycusis* is used to describe degenerative hearing loss that occurs with advancing age. About 23% of persons between ages 65 and 75 years and 40% of the population older than 75 years are affected.[12] The degenerative changes that impair hearing may begin in the fifth decade of life and not be clinically apparent until later.[13] Onset may

TABLE 43-1
Major Ototoxic Drugs

Drug	Affects Auditory Function	Affects Vestibular Function
Aminoglycoside Antibiotics		
Amikacin	+	0
Gentamicin	+	+
Kanamycin	+	+
Neomycin	+	+
Streptomycin	+	+
Tobramycin	+	+
Others	+	+
Other Antibiotics		
Colistin (topical middle ear)	0	+
Erythromycin (intravenous)	+*	0
Minocycline	0	+
Polymyxin B (topical middle ear)	0	+
VAncomycin	+	0
Antimalarial Drugs		
Chloroquine and quinine	+*	0
Loop Diuretics		
Ethacrynic acid	+	+
Furosemide	+*	0
Bumetanide	+*	0
Others	+*	0
Salicylates	+*	0
Cisplatin	+	0

+, yes; 0, no.
*Effects are rarely permanent.

be associated with chronic noise exposure or vascular disorders.[13] The disorder involves loss of neuroepithelial (hair) cells, neurons, and the stria vascularis.[10] High-frequency sounds are affected more than low-frequency sounds, because high and low frequencies distort the base of the basilar membrane, but only low frequencies affect the distal (apical) region. Through the years, permanent mechanical damage to the organ of Corti is more likely to occur near the base of the cochlea, where the high sonic frequencies are discriminated. Men are affected earlier and experience a greater loss than women.

Diagnosis

Hearing loss may be estimated by having the person report soft whispered, normal spoken, or shouted words. A ticking watch may also be used, but this only tests the higher frequencies.

The *audiogram* is an important method of analyzing a person's hearing. It is done by an audiologist and requires highly specialized sound production and control equipment. Pure tones of controlled intensity are delivered, usually to one ear at a time, and the minimum intensity needed for hearing to be experienced is plotted as a function of frequency.

Tuning forks are used to differentiate conductive and sensorineural hearing loss. A 512-Hz or higher frequency tuning fork is used, because frequencies below this level elicit a tactile response. The *Weber test* evaluates conductive hearing loss by lateralization of sound. It is done by placing the lightly vibrating tuning fork on the forehead or vertex of the head. In persons with conductive losses, the sound is louder on the side with the hearing loss, but in persons with sensorineural loss, it radiates to the side with the better hearing. The *Rinne test* compares air and bone conduction. The test is done by alternately placing the tuning fork on the mastoid bone and in front of the ear canal. In conductive losses, bone conduction exceeds air conduction; in sensorineural losses, the opposite occurs.

The *brain stem–evoked response* (BSER) is a noninvasive method that permits functional evaluation of certain defined parts of the central auditory pathways. Scalp electrodes and high-gain amplifiers are required to produce a record of the electrical wave activity elicited during repeated acoustic stimulations of either or both ears. With this method, certain of the early waves that come from discrete portions of the pons and midbrain auditory pathways can be correlated with specific sensorineural abnormalities. *Imaging studies* such as computed tomography scans and magnetic resonance imaging can be done to determine the site of a lesion and the extent of damage.[1]

Treatment

Conduction deafness can be corrected through the use of electrical amplification methods, such as hearing aids. Hearing aids deliver sound stimuli directly to the skull bones with sufficient added power to directly vibrate the inner ear apparatus. This method bypasses the middle ear conduction apparatus. Amplification is of no assistance with sensorineural hearing loss. With sensorineural deficit, a hearing aid serves only to increase the intensity of a signal experienced as distorted. In mixed hearing loss, amplification can provide improvement only for the conduction problems that are part of the syndrome. Although most standard tests for auditory acuity use pure tone stimuli, intelligibility of sound stimuli is not necessarily correlated with pure tone loss. Damage to the important communicative function of auditory language produces a social isolation that is potentially damaging to a person's mental attitude and motivation for rehabilitation.

Surgically implantable cochlear prostheses for the profoundly deaf have been developed. These prostheses are inserted into the scala tympani of the cochlea and work by providing direct stimulation to the auditory nerve, bypassing the stimulation that typically is provided by transducer cells but that is absent or nonfunctional in a deaf cochlea. For the implant to work, the auditory nerve must be functional. Early implants used a single electrode. Later implants use multielectrode placement, enhancing speech perception. Much of the progress in implant performance has been achieved through improvements in the speech processors that convert sound into electrical stimuli.

Advances in the development of the multichannel implant has improved performance such that cochlear implants have been established as an effective option for adults and children with profound hearing impairment. Most persons who are deafened after learning speech derive substantial benefit when cochlear implants are used in conjunction with lip reading; some are able to understand some speech without lip-reading; and some are able to communicate by telephone. A National Institutes of Health Consensus Panel on Cochlear Implants in Adults and Children concluded that cochlear implantation improves the communication ability in most adults with severe to profound deafness and frequently leads to positive psychologic and social benefits. The Consensus Panel recommended that children at least 2 years of age and adults with profound deafness should be considered as candidates for implantation.[14] The Panel also concluded that optimal educational and rehabilitation services are important for adults and critical for children to maximize the benefits available from the implant. One limitation is that the earliest age for implantation in children is no earlier than 2 years of age, which is beyond the critical period of auditory input for the acquisition of oral language.

Disorders of the Central Auditory Pathways

The auditory pathways in the brain involve communication between the two sides of the brain at many levels. As a result, strokes, tumors, abscesses, and other focal abnormalities seldom produce more than a mild reduction in auditory acuity on the side opposite the lesion. For intelligibility of auditory language, lateral dominance becomes important. On the dominant side, usually the left side, the more medial and dorsal portion of the associational auditory cortex is of crucial importance. This area is called *Wernicke's area,* and damage to it is associated with auditory receptive aphasia (and agnosia of speech). Persons with damage to this area of the brain can speak intelligibly and read normally but are unable to understand the meaning of major aspects of audible speech.

Irritative foci that affect the auditory radiation or the primary auditory cortex can produce roaring or clicking sounds, which appear to come from the auditory environment of the opposite side (*i.e.,* auditory hallucinations). Focal seizures that originate in or near the auditory cortex often are immediately preceded by the perception of ringing or other sounds preceded by a prodrome (*i.e.,* aura). Damage to the auditory association cortex, especially if bilateral, results in deficiencies of sound recognition and memory (*i.e.,* auditory agnosia). If the damage is in the dominant hemisphere, speech recognition can be affected (*i.e.,* sensory or receptive aphasia).

In summary, disorders of the auditory system include infections of the external and middle ear, otosclerosis, and conduction and sensorineural deafness. Otitis externa is an inflammatory process of the external ear. The middle ear is a tiny air-filled cavity located in the temporal bone. The auditory tube connects the middle ear to the nasopharynx and allows for equalization of pressure between the middle ear and the atmosphere. Infections can travel from the nasopharynx to the middle ear along the auditory tube, causing otitis media, or inflammation of the middle ear. The auditory tube is shorter and more horizontal in infants and young children, and infections of the middle ear are a common problem in these age groups.

Otitis media can be acute, subacute, or chronic. Acute suppurative otitis media, usually follows an upper respiratory tract infection and is characterized by otalgia, fever, and hearing loss. The effusion that accompanies otitis media can persist for weeks or months, interfering with hearing and impairing speech development.

Otosclerosis is a familial disorder of the otic capsule. It causes bone resorption followed by excessive replacement with sclerotic bone. The disorder eventually causes immobilization of the stapes and conduction deafness.

Deafness, or hearing loss, can develop as the result of a number of auditory disorders. It can be conductive, sensorineural, or mixed. Conduction deafness occurs when transmission of sound waves from the external to the inner ear is impaired. Sensorineural deafness can involve cochlear structures of the inner ear or the neural pathways that transmit auditory stimuli. Sensorineural hearing loss can result from genetic or congenital disorders, trauma, infections, vascular disorders, tumors, or ototoxic drugs. Treatment of hearing loss includes the use of hearing aids and, in some cases of profound deafness, implantation of a cochlear prosthesis.

Disorders of Vestibular Function

After you have completed this section of the chapter, you should be able to meet the following objectives:

- Relate the function of the vestibular system to nystagmus and vertigo
- Differentiate the structures of peripheral and central vestibular function
- Characterize the physiologic cause of motion sickness
- Compare the manifestations and pathology associated with benign positional vertigo and Ménière's disease
- Differentiate the manifestations of peripheral and central vestibular disorders

The vestibular receptive organs, which are located in the inner ear, and their CNS connections contribute to the reflex activity necessary for effective posture and movement in a physical world governed by momentum and a gravitational field. Because the vestibular apparatus is part of the inner ear and located in the head, it is head motion and acceleration that are sensed. The vestibular system serves two general and related functions. It maintains and assists recovery of stable body and head position through control of postural reflexes, and it maintains a stable visual field despite marked changes in head position.

Vestibular Function

The vestibular system plays an essential role in the equilibrium sense, which is closely integrated with the visual and proprioceptive (position) senses. The receptors for the vestibular system, which are located in the semicircular ducts of the inner ear, respond to changes in linear and angular acceleration of the head. The vestibular nerve fibers travel in the vestibulocochlear (VIII) cranial nerve to the vestibular nuclei located at the junction of the medulla and pons. Some of the fibers pass through the nuclei to the cerebellum. The cerebellar connections are necessary for temporally smooth, coordinated movements during ongoing head movements, tilt, and angular acceleration. The vestibular nuclei also connect with the nuclei of the oculomotor (III), trochlear (IV), and abducens (VI) cranial nerves. Vestibular control of conjugate eye movements serves to preserve eye fixation on stable objects in the visual field during head movement. Neurons of the vestibular nuclei also project to the thalamus, to the temporal cortex, and to the somatesthetic area of the parietal cortex. The thalamic and cortical projections provide the basis for the subjective experiences of position in space and of rotation. The vestibular system also connects with a chemoreceptor trigger zone, which stimulates the vomiting center in the brain. This accounts for the nausea and vomiting that is often associated with vestibular disorders.

Disorders of vestibular function can be peripheral, involving the labyrinth, or central, involving the vestibular connections. Abnormal nystagmus, tinnitus, and hearing loss are other common manifestations of vestibular dysfunction, as are autonomic manifestations such as perspiration, nausea, and vomiting.

Vertigo

Disorders of vestibular function are characterized by a condition called *vertigo,* in which a hallucination of motion occurs. The person is stationary and the environment is in motion (*i.e.,* objective vertigo), or the person is in motion and the environment is stationary (*i.e.,* subjective vertigo).

Vertigo should be differentiated from dizziness, which is accompanied by lightheadedness, fainting, or unsteadiness (Table 43–2). Dizziness, which is characterized by a feeling of lightheadedness or "blacking out," is commonly caused by postural hypotension (see Chapter 18). Dizziness and unsteadiness when walking may be caused by disorders of sensory input (*e.g.,* proprioception) rather than vestibular function and are usually corrected by touching a stationary object such as the wall or a table.

Depending on the cause, vertigo may be treated pharmacologically. There are two types of drugs used in the treatment of vertigo.[15] The first are drugs that are used to suppress the hallucination of motion. These include drugs such as antihistamines and anticholinergic drugs that suppress the vestibular system. The second type are drugs used to relieve the nausea and vomiting that commonly accompany the condition. Antidopinergic drugs are commonly used for this purpose.

Vestibulo-ocular Reflexes and Nystagmus

The term *nystagmus* is used to describe the vestibulo-ocular reflexes that occur in response to ongoing head rotation (see Chapter 41). The vestibulo-ocular reflexes produce slow compensatory conjugate eye rotations that occur in precisely the direction opposite to ongoing head rotation and provide for continuous, ongoing reflex stabilization of the binocular fixation point. This reflex can be demonstrated by holding a pencil vertically in front of the eyes and moving it from side to side through a 10-degree arch at a rate of about five times per second. At this rate of motion, the pencil appears blurred, because a different and more complex reflex, smooth pursuit, cannot compensate quickly enough.[16] However, if the pencil is maintained in a stable position and the head is moved back and forth at the same rate, the image of the pencil is clearly defined. The eye movements are the same in both cases. The reason that the

TABLE 43-2

Differences in Pathology and Manifestations of Dizziness Associated with Benign Positional Vertigo, Presyncopy, and Disequilibrium State

Type of disorder	Pathology	Symptoms
Benign positional vertigo	Disorder of otoliths	Vertigo initiated by a change in head position, usually lasts less than a minute
Presyncope	Orthostatic hypotension	Lightheadedness and feeling faint on assumption of standing position
Disequilibrium	Sensory (*e.g.,* vision, proprioception) deficits	Dizziness and unsteadiness when walking, especially when turning; Relieved by additional proprioceptive stimulation such as touching wall or table

pencil image remains clear in the second situation is because the vestibulo-ocular reflexes keeps the image of the pencil on the retinal fovea. The vestibulo-ocular reflexes are "hard wired" in the CNS and occur almost with the same precision with the eyes closed or in the congenitally blind. They can be modified, however, by visual control and by motor system intervention.

When compensatory vestibulo-ocular reflexes carry the conjugate eye rotations to their physical limit, a very rapid conjugate movement (*i.e.*, saccade) moves the eyes in the direction of head rotation to a new fixation point, followed by a slow vestibulo-ocular reflex as the head continues to rotate past the new fixation point. This pattern of slow-fast-slow movements is called nystagmus.

Spontaneous nystagmus that occurs without head movement or visual stimuli is always pathologic. It seems to appear more readily and more severely with fatigue and to some extent can be influenced by psychologic factors. Nystagmus derived from the CNS, in contrast to peripheral end-organ or CN VIII sources, seldom is accompanied by vertigo. If present, the vertigo is of mild intensity.

Motion Sickness

Motion sickness is a form of normal physiologic vertigo. It is caused by repeated rhythmic stimulation of the vestibular system, such as is encountered in car, air, or boat travel. Vertigo, malaise, nausea, and vomiting are the principal symptoms. Autonomic signs, including lowered blood pressure, tachycardia, and excessive sweating, may occur. Hyperventilation, which commonly accompanies motion sickness, produces changes in blood volume and pooling of blood in the lower extremities leading to postural hypotension and sometimes to syncope. Some persons experience a variant of motion sickness, complaining of sensing the rocking motion of the boat after returning to ground. This usually resolves after the vestibular system becomes accustomed to the stationary influence of being back on land.

Motion sickness can usually be suppressed by supplying visual signals that more closely match the motion signals being supplied to the vestibular system. For example, looking out the window and watching the environment move when suffering from motion sickness associated with car travel provides the vestibular system with the visual sensation of motion, but reading a book provides the vestibular system the miscue that the environment is stable. Motion sickness usually decreases in severity with repeated exposure. Anti–motion sickness drugs may be also used to reduce or ameliorate the symptoms. These drugs work by suppressing the activity of the vestibular system.

Disorders of Peripheral Vestibular Function

The peripheral vestibular system consists of a set of paired inner ear sensory organs, each sending messages to a set of single central brain centers that interpret signals relating to the body's position in space and control eye movement. Disorders of peripheral vestibular function occur when these signals are distorted, as in benign positional vertigo, or are *unbalanced* by unilateral involvement of one of the vestibular organs, as in Ménière's disease. The inner ear is vulnerable to injury caused by fracture of the petrous portion of the temporal bones; infection of nearby structures, including the middle ear and meninges; and by bloodborne toxins and infections. Damage to the vestibular system can occur as an adverse effect of certain drugs or from allergic reactions to foods. The aminoglycosides (*e.g.*, streptomycin, gentamicin) have a specific toxic affinity for the vestibular portion of the inner ear. Alcohol can cause transient episodes of vertigo.

Severe irritation or damage of the vestibular end-organs or nerves results in severe balance disorders reflected by instability of posture, dystaxia, and falling accompanied by vertigo. With irritation, falling is away from the affected side; with destruction, it is toward the affected side. Adaptation to asymmetric stimulation occurs within a few days, after which the signs and symptoms diminish and eventually are lost. After recovery, there usually is a slightly reduced acuity for tilt, and the person walks with a somewhat broadened base to improve postural stability. The neurologic basis for this adaptation to unilateral loss of vestibular input is not understood. After adaptation to the loss of vestibular input from one side, the loss of function of the opposite vestibular apparatus produces signs and symptoms identical to those resulting from unilateral rather than bilateral loss. Within weeks, adaptation is again sufficient for locomotion and even for driving a car. Such a person relies heavily on visual and proprioceptive input and has severe orientation difficulty in the dark, particularly when traversing uneven terrain.

Benign Positional Vertigo

Benign positional vertigo (BPV) is the most common cause of pathologic vertigo. It is characterized by brief periods of vertigo, usually lasting less than 1 minute, that are precipitated by a change in head position.[16–18] It typically occurs when turning over in bed, getting in and out of bed, bending over and straightening up, or extending the head to look up. The condition may result from head injury, viral infection, vascular occlusion, or as an isolated symptom of unknown cause. The latter is more common in the elderly. BPV is thought to result from damage to the delicate sensory organs of the inner ear, the semicircular ducts, and otoliths. In persons with BPV, the otoliths from the utricle become dislodged and settle into the posterior semicircular duct, which is the most dependent part of the inner ear. The shift in otoliths causes the posterior duct to become more sensitive, such that any movement of the head in the plane parallel to the posterior duct may cause vertigo and nystagmus. There is usually a several-second delay between head movement and onset of vertigo, representing the time that it takes to generate the exaggerated otic fluid activity. Symptoms usually subside with continued movement, probably because the movement causes the otoliths to be redistributed throughout the endolymph system and away from the posterior duct.

Diagnosis is based on tests that involve the use of change in head position to elicit vertigo and nystagmus.[17,18] BPV is often successfully treated using habituation exercises.

Acute Vestibular Neuronitis

Acute vestibular neuronitis, sometimes called labyrinthitis, is characterized by an acute onset of vertigo, nausea, and vomiting lasting several days and not associated with auditory or other neurologic manifestations. Most persons gradually improve over 1 to 2 weeks, but some develop recurrent episodes. A large percentage report an upper respiratory tract illness 1 to 2 weeks before onset of symptoms, suggesting a viral origin. The condition can also occur in persons with herpes zoster oticus. In some persons, attacks of acute vestibulopathy recur over months or years. There is no way to determine whether a person who suffers a first attack will have repeated attacks.

Ménière's Disease

Ménière's disease is a disorder of inner ear involvement, auditory and vestibular, caused by an overaccumulation of endolymph. Unlike BPV, Ménière's disease is associated with vertigo that lasts for hours, and unlike other peripheral vestibular disorders, affected persons have cochlear symptoms—sensorineural hearing loss, tinnitus, and a sensation of ear fullness. The disorder is usually unilateral, resulting in rotary nystagmus caused by an imbalance in vestibular control of eye movements.

The disorder is caused by fluid distention of the endolymph system, sometimes referred to as *endolymphatic hydrops*. Herniation and rupture of the endolymphatic membrane may occur when there is massive distention of the endolymph.[19] The condition is thought be caused by impaired reabsorption of endolymph in the endolymph duct or sac. A number of conditions, such as trauma, infection, allergy, adrenal-pituitary insufficiency, and hypothyroidism, are associated with Ménière's disease. The most common form of the disease is an idiopathic form thought to be caused by a single viral injury to the fluid transport system of the inner ear. One area of investigation has been the relation between immune disorders and Ménière's disease.

Ménière's disease is characterized by fluctuating episodes of tinnitus, feelings of ear fullness, and violent rotary vertigo that often renders the person unable to sit or walk. There is a need to lie quietly with the head fixed in a comfortable position, avoiding all head movements that aggravate the vertigo. Symptoms referable to the autonomic nervous system, including pallor, sweating, nausea, and vomiting, usually are present. The more severe the attack, the more prominent are the autonomic manifestations. A fluctuating hearing loss occurs, and initially, there is a return to normal after the episode subsides. As the disease progresses, it becomes more severe and permanent. Because the disorder is unilateral and because the sense of hearing is bilateral, many persons with the disorder are not aware of the full extent of their hearing loss.

Methods used in the diagnosis of Ménière's disease include audiograms, vestibular testing by electronystagmography, and petrous pyramid radiographs. The administration of hyperosmolar substances, such as glycerin and urea, often produces acute temporary hearing improvement in persons with Ménière's disease and sometimes is used as a diagnostic measure of endolymphatic hydrops. The diuretic furosemide may also be used for this purpose.

The management of Ménière's disease focuses on attempts to reduce the distention of the endolymphatic space and can be medical or surgical. Pharmacologic management consists of suppressant drugs (*e.g.*, prochlorperazine, promethazine, diazepam), which act centrally to decrease the activity of the vestibular system. Diuretics are used to reduce endolymph fluid volume. Histamine analogues, which directly reduce inner ear fluid mainly by decreasing cochlear blood flow, are being studied.[20] A low-sodium diet is recommended in addition to these medications. The steroid hormone prednisone may be used to maintain satisfactory hearing and resolve dizziness. Streptomycin therapy has been used for ablation of the vestibular system.[21] Surgical methods include the creation of an endolymphatic shunt in which excess endolymph from the inner ear is diverted into the subarachnoid space or the mastoid and vestibular nerve section. Advances in vestibular nerve section have facilitated the monitoring of CN VII and CN VIII potentials. These methods are used to prevent hearing damage.[21]

Disorders of Central Vestibular Function

Abnormal nystagmus and vertigo can occur as a result of CNS pathology. Compression of the vestibular nuclei by cerebellar tumors invading the fourth ventricle results in progressively severe signs and symptoms. In addition to abnormal nystagmus and vertigo, vomiting and a broad-base and dystaxic gait become progressively more evident. Some drugs (*e.g.*, anticonvulsants) can also cause abnormal nystagmus. Centrally derived nystagmus usually has equal excursion in both directions (*i.e.*, pendular). In contrast to peripherally generated nystagmus, CNS-derived nystagmus is relatively constant rather than episodic, can occur in any direction rather than being primarily in the horizontal or torsional (rotatory) dimensions, often changes direction through time, and cannot be suppressed by visual fixation. Repeated induction of nystagmus results in rapid diminution or "fatigue" of the reflex with peripheral abnormalities, but fatigue is not characteristic of central lesions. Congenital and lifelong nystagmus abnormalities are not uncommon and occur as part of a number of hereditary syndromes. Nystagmus can also accompany other motor defects in cerebral palsy and degenerative syndromes such as multiple sclerosis. Abnormal nystagmus can make reading and other tasks that require precise eye positional control difficult.

Diagnostic Tests of Vestibular Function

Diagnosis of vestibular disorders is based on a description of the symptoms, a history of trauma or exposure to agents that are destructive to vestibular structures, and physical examination. Tests of eye movements (*i.e.*, nystagmus) and muscle control of balance and equilibrium often are used. The tests of vestibular function focus on the horizontal semicircular reflex, because it is the easiest reflex to stimulate rotationally and calorically and to record using electronystagmography.

Electronystagmography

Electronystagmography (ENG) is a precise and objective diagnostic method of evaluating nystagmus eye movements. Electrodes are placed lateral to the outer canthus of each eye and above and below each eye. A ground electrode is placed on the forehead. With ENG, the velocity, frequency, and amplitude of spontaneous or induced nystagmus and the changes in these measurements brought by a loss of fixation, with the eyes open or closed, can be quantified. The advantages of ENG are that it is easily administered, is noninvasive, does not interfere with vision, and does not require head restraint.[22]

Caloric Stimulation

Caloric testing involves elevating the head 30 degrees and irrigating each external auditory canal separately with 30 to 50 ml of ice water. The resulting changes in temperature, as conducted through the petrous portion of the temporal bone, set up convection currents in the otic fluid that mimic the effects of angular acceleration. In an unconscious person with a functional brain stem and intact oculovestibular reflexes, the eyes exhibit a jerk nystagmus lasting 2 to 3 minutes, with the slow component toward the irrigated ear followed by rapid movement away from the ear. With impairment of brain stem function, the response becomes perverted and eventually disappears. An advantage of the caloric stimulation method is the ability to test the vestibular apparatus on one side at a time. The test is never done on a person who does not have an intact eardrum or who has blood or fluid collected behind the eardrum.

Rotational Tests

Rotational testing involves rotation using a rotatable chair or motor-driven platform. Unlike caloric testing, rotational testing depends only on the inner ear and is unrelated to conditions of the external ear or temporal bone. A major disadvantage of the method is that both ears are tested simultaneously.

Motor-driven platforms can be precisely controlled, and multiple graded stimuli can be delivered in a relatively short period. For rotational testing, the person is seated in a chair mounted on the motor-driven platform. Testing is usually performed in the dark without visual influence and with selected light stimuli. Eye movements are monitored using ENG. A rotatable chair, the Bárány chair that is much like a barber's chair, can be used for assessing postrotational vestibular reflexes. The person is strapped into the chair with the head positioned so that the plane of one pair of semicircular ducts is in the horizontal plane (*i.e.*, plane of rotation); each of the three primary planes of the ducts is tested in turn. The person is rotated until a steady rate of rotation is achieved. The chair is suddenly stopped, and the ensuing postrotational reflex nystagmus and the compensatory movements of the body and limbs are observed. Vestibular reflexes are very powerful. The examiner should use extreme caution whenever testing the vestibular reflexes of a person on a motor-driven platform or with a Bárány chair.

Romberg Test

The Romberg test is used to demonstrate disorders of static vestibular function. The person being tested is requested to stand with feet together and arms extended forward so that the degree of sway and arm stability can be observed. The person is then asked to close his or her eyes. When visual clues are removed, postural stability is based on proprioceptive sensation from the joints, muscles, and tendons and from static vestibular reception. Deficiency in vestibular static input is indicated by greatly increased sway and a tendency for the arms to drift toward the side of deficiency.

If vestibular input is severely deficient, the subject falls toward the deficient side. Care must be taken, because defects of proprioceptive projection to the forebrain also result in some arm drift and postural instability toward the deficient side. Only if two-point discrimination and vibratory sensation from the lower and upper limbs are bilaterally normal can the deficiency be attributed to the vestibular system.

Treatment of Vestibular Disorders

Pharmacologic Methods

Among the methods used to treat vertigo are the antivertigo or anti–motion sickness drugs. Drugs used in the treatment of vertigo include anticholinergic drugs (*e.g.*, scopolamine, atropine), monoaminergic drugs (*e.g.*, amphetamine, ephedrine), and antihistamines (*e.g.*, meclizine [Antivert], cyclizine [Marezine], dimenhydrinate [Dramamine], and promethazine [Phenergan]). Animal studies have documented that drugs with anticholinergic or monoaminergic activity diminish the excitability of neurons in the vestibular nuclei. Although the antihistamines have long been used in treating vertigo, little is known about their mechanism of action. Most of these drugs have some anticholinergic activity, and some enhance sympathetic activity by blocking the reuptake of monoamines at the synaptic nerve terminals.

Vestibular Rehabilitation

Vestibular rehabilitation, a relatively new treatment modality for peripheral vestibular disorders, has met with considerable success.[23,24] It commonly is done by physical therapists and uses a home exercise program that incorporates habituation exercises, balance retraining exercises, and a general conditioning program.[24] The habituation exercises take advantage of physiologic fatigue of the neurovegetative response to repetitive movement or positional stimulation and are done to decrease motion-provoked vertigo, lightheadedness, and unsteadiness. The exercises are selected to provoke the vestibular symptoms. The person moves quickly into the position that causes symptoms, holds the position until the symptoms subside (*i.e.*, fatigue of the neurovegetative response), relaxes, and then repeats the exercise for a prescribed number of times. The exercises usually are repeated twice daily. The habituation effect is characterized by decreased sensitivity and duration of symptoms. It may occur in as quickly as 2 weeks or take as long as 6 months.[24]

Balance-retraining exercises consist of activities directed toward improving individual components of balance that may be abnormal. General conditioning exercises, a vital part of the rehabilitation process, are individualized to the person's preferences and lifestyle. They should consist of motion-oriented activity that the person is interested in and should be done on a regular basis, usually four to five times per week.[24]

In summary, disorders of the vestibular system include motion sickness and Ménière's disease. Ménière's disease, which is caused by an overaccumulation of endolymph, is characterized by severe disabling episodes of tinnitus, feelings of ear fullness, and violent rotary vertigo. The diagnosis of vestibular disorders is based on a description of the symptoms, a history of trauma or exposure to agents destructive to vestibular structures, and tests of eye movements (*i.e.*, nystagmus) and muscle control of balance and equilibrium. Among the methods used in the treatment of vertigo that accompanies vestibular disorders are the antivertigo or anti–motion sickness drugs. These drugs act by diminishing the excitability of neurons in the vestibular nucleus.

REFERENCES

1. Weissman J.L. (1996). Hearing loss. *Radiation* 199, 593–611.
2. Bluestone C.D., Klein J. (1995). *Otitis media in infants and children*. Philadelphia: W.B. Saunders.
3. Eden A.N., Fireman P., Stool S.E. (1995). The rise in acute otitis media. *Patient Care* 29 (19), 22–56.
4. Swanson J.A., Hoecker J.L. (1996). Otitis media in young children. *Mayo Clinic Proceedings* 71, 179–183.
5. Berman S. (1995). Otitis media in children. *New England Journal of Medicine* 332 (23), 1560–1565.
6. Shapiro A.M., Bluestone C.D. (1995). Otitis media reassessed. *Postgraduate Medicine* 97 (5), 73–82.
7. Klein J.O. (1994). Otitis Media. *Clinical Infectious Diseases* 19, 823–833.
8. Heald M.M., Matkin N.D., Merideth K.E. (1990). Pressure-equalization (PE) tubes in treatment of otitis media: National survey of otolaryngologists. *Laryngology—Head and Neck Surgery* 102, 334–338.
9. Stool S.E., Berg A.O., Carney C.J., et al. (1994). Otitis media with effusion in young children. In *Clinical practice guideline no. 12*. AHCPR Publication No. 95–0622. Rockville, MD: Department of Health and Human Services, Agency for Health Care Policy and Research.
10. Nadol J.G. (1993). Hearing loss. *New England Journal of Medicine*. 329 (15) 1092–1101.
11. Yamasoba T., Kikuchi S., O'uchi T., Higo R., Tokumaru A. (1993). Sudden sensorineural hearing loss associated with slow blood flow of the vertibrobasilar system. *Annals of Otorhinolaryngology* 102 (11), 873–877.
12. Gates G.A. (Chairperson). (1989). Invitational Geriatric Otorhinolaryngology Workshop: Presbycusis. *Otolaryngology—Head and Neck Surgery* 100, 266–271.
13. Saeed S., Ramsden R. (1994). Hearing loss. *The Practitioner* 238, 454–460.
14. NIH Consensus Development Panel on Cochlear Implants in Adults and Children. (1995). Cochlear implants in adults and children. *Journal of the American Medical Association* 274 (24), 1955–1961.
15. Rascol O., Hain T.C., Brefel C., Benazet M., Clanet M., Montastruc J. (1995). Antivertigo drugs and drug-induced vertigo. *Drugs* 50 (5), 777–789.
16. McGee S.R. (1995). Dizzy patients. *Western Journal of Medicine* 162, 37–42.
17. Mohr D.N. (1986). The syndrome of paroxysmal positional vertigo. *Western Journal of Medicine* 145, 645–650.
18. Lempert T., Gresty M.A., Bronstein A.M. (1995). Benign positional vertigo: Recognition and treatment. *British Medical Journal* 311, 489–491.
19. Paparella M.M (1991). Pathogenesis and pathophysiology of Meniere's disease. *Acta Otolaryngology (Stockholm)* (Suppl 484), 26–35.
20. Brooks C.B. (1996). The pharmacological treatment of Meniere's disease. *Clinical Otolaryngology* 21, 3–11.
21. Dickens J.R.E., Graham S.S. (1990). Meniere's disease—1983–1989. *American Journal of Otology* 11 (1), 51–65.
22. Baloh R.W. (1989). Modern vestibular function testing. *Western Journal of Medicine* 150, 59–67.
23. Horak F.B., Jones-Rycewicz C., Black F.W., et al. (1992). Effects of vestibular rehabilitation on dizziness and imbalance. *Otolaryngology—Head and Neck Surgery* 106, 175–180.
24. Smith-Whellock M., Shepard N.T., Telian S.A. (1991). Physical therapy program for vestibular rehabilitation. *American Journal of Otolology* 12, 218–225.

ADDITIONAL READINGS

Bluestone C.D. (1989). Modern management of otitis media. *Pediatric Clinics of North America* 36, 1371–1387.

Brackemann D.E. (1990). Surgical treatment of vertigo. *Journal of Laryngology and Otology* 164, 849–859.

Clark M.R. (1994) Chronic dizziness: An integrated approach. *Hospital Practice* 29 (12), 57–64.

Froehling D.A., Silverstein M.D., Mohr D.N., Beatty C.W. (1994). Does this dizzy patient have a serious form of vertigo. *Journal of the American Medical Association* 271 (5), 385–388.

Gantz B.J., Schindler R.A., Snow J.B. (1995). Adult hearing loss: Some tips or pearls. *Patient Care* 29 (17), 77–89.

Langman A.W., Jackler R.K., Sooy F.A. (1991). Stapedectomy: Long-term hearing results. *Laryngoscope* 101, 810–814.

Lempert T., Gresty M.A., Bronstein A.M. (1995). Benign positional vertigo: Recognition and treatment. *British Medical Journal* 311, 489–491.

Mulrow C.D. (1991). Screening for hearing impairment in the elderly. *Hospital Practice* 26, 79–86.

Paradise J.L. (1992). Antimicrobial prophylaxis for recurrent otitis media. *Annals of Otolaryngology* 101, 33–36.

Sade J., Luntz M. (1991). Adenoidectomy in otitis media. *Annals of Otology, Rhinology, and Laryngology* 100, 226–231.

Swan I.R. (1989). The Rinne tuning fork test. *Hospital Practice* 24, 99–102.

Skeletal and Musculotendinous Function

Some of the most significant investigations of the skeleton and muscles took place during the Renaissance—a time that celebrated the human body and lifted the knowledge of the body and its workings out of medieval murkiness.

The first comprehensive description of musculature was presented by Andreas Vesalius (1514–1564), a professor of anatomy and surgery at Padua. The product of his scrupulous dissections was the masterwork De Humani Corporis Fabrica *(On the Structure of the Human Body), the second volume of which dealt with muscles and their structure. The work was beautifully illustrated with elegantly poised cadavers set against backgrounds of medieval Italy. Vesalius' effort successfully challenged many of the long-held pronouncements of Galen. The studies of artist Leonardo da Vinci (1452–1519) sought not to dispute or confirm previous teachings but to learn of the "divine form" so that it could be better rendered. A physician of the time wrote that "in order that he might be able to paint the various joints and muscles as they bend and extend according to the laws of nature, he [Leonardo] dissected in medical schools the corpses of criminals, indifferent to this inhuman and nauseating work." Although da Vinci was primarily a painter studying anatomy for the sake of art, there is little doubt that had his anatomic drawings been published during his lifetime or shortly after, science would have been advanced by years.*

UNIT XII

CHAPTER 44

Structure and Function of the Skeletal System

Without the skeletal system, movement in the external environment would not be possible. The bones of the skeletal system serve as a framework for the attachment of muscles, tendons, and ligaments. The skeletal system protects and maintains soft tissues in their proper position, provides stability for the body, and maintains the body's shape. The bones act as a storage reservoir for calcium, and the central cavity of some bones contains the hematopoietic connective tissue in which blood cells are formed.

The skeletal system consists of the axial and appendicular skeleton. The axial skeleton, which is composed of the bones of the skull, thorax, and vertebral column, forms the axis of the body. The appendicular skeleton consists of the bones of the upper and lower extremities, including the shoulder and hip. For our purposes, the skeletal system is considered to include the bones and cartilage of the axial and appendicular skeleton, as well as the connective tissue structures (*i.e.*, ligaments and tendons) that connect the bones and join muscles to bone.

Characteristics of Skeletal Tissue

After you have completed this section of the chapter, you should be able to meet the following objectives:

- Cite the common components of cartilage and bone
- Compare the properties of the intercellular collagen and elastic fibers of skeletal tissue
- Cite the characteristics and name at least one location of elastic cartilage, hyaline cartilage, and fibrocartilage
- Name and characterize the function of the four types of bone cells
- State the function of parathyroid hormone, calcitonin, and vitamin D in terms of bone formation and metabolism
- State the location and function of the periosteum and the endosteum

Two types of connective tissue are found in the skeletal system: cartilage and bone. Each of these connective tissue types consists of living cells, nonliving intercellular protein fibers, and an amorphous, or shapeless, ground substance. The tissue cells are responsible for secreting and maintaining the intercellular substances in which they are housed. These substances provide the structural characteristics of the tissue. For example, the intercellular matrix of bone is impregnated with calcium salts, providing the hardness that is characteristic of this tissue.

Two main types of intercellular fibers are found in skeletal tissue: collagenous and elastic. Collagen is an inelastic and insoluble fibrous protein. Because of its molecular configuration, collagen has great tensile strength; the breaking point of collagenous fibers found in human tendons is reached with a force of several hundred kilograms per square centimeter. Fresh collagen is colorless, and tissues that contain large numbers of collagenous fibers generally appear white. The collagen fibers in tendons and ligaments give these structures their white color. Elastin is the major component of elastic fibers that allows them to stretch several times their length and rapidly return to their original shape when the tension is released. Ligaments and structures that must undergo repeated stretching contain a high proportion of elastic fibers.

Cartilage

Cartilage is a firm but flexible type of connective tissue consisting of cells and intercellular fibers embedded in an amorphous, gel-like material. It has a smooth and resilient surface and a weight-bearing capacity exceeded only by that of bone.

Cartilage is essential for growth before and after birth. It is able to undergo rapid growth while maintaining a considerable degree of stiffness. In the embryo, most of the axial and appendicular skeleton is formed first as a cartilage model and is replaced by bone. In postnatal life, cartilage continues to play an essential role in the growth of long bones and persists as articular cartilage in the adult.

There are three types of cartilage: elastic cartilage, hyaline cartilage, and fibrocartilage. *Elastic cartilage* contains some elastin in its intercellular substance. It is found in areas, such as the ear, where some flexibility is important. Pure cartilage is called *hyaline cartilage* (from a Greek word meaning glass) and is pearly white. It is the type of cartilage seen on the articulating ends of fresh soup bones found in the supermarket. *Fibrocartilage* has characteristics that are intermediate between dense connective tissue and hyaline cartilage. It is found in the intervertebral disks, in areas where tendons are connected to bone, and in the symphysis pubis.

Hyaline cartilage is the most abundant type of cartilage. It forms much of the cartilage of the fetal skeleton. In the adult, hyaline cartilage forms the costal cartilages that join the ribs to the sternum and vertebrae, many of the cartilages of the respiratory tract, the articular cartilages, and the epiphyseal plates.

Cartilage cells, which are called *chondrocytes*, are located in lacunae. These lacunae are surrounded by an uncalcified, gel-like intercellular matrix of collagen fibers and ground substance. Cartilage is devoid of blood vessels and nerves. The free surfaces of most hyaline cartilage, with the exception of articular cartilage, is covered by a layer of fibrous connective tissue called the *perichondrium*.

It has been estimated that about 65% to 80% of the wet weight of cartilage is water held in its gel structure. Because cartilage has no blood vessels, this tissue fluid allows the diffusion of gases, nutrients, and wastes between the chondrocytes and blood vessels outside the cartilage. Diffusion cannot take place if the cartilage matrix becomes impregnated with calcium salts, and cartilage dies if it becomes calcified.

Bone

Bone is connective tissue in which the intercellular matrix has been impregnated with inorganic calcium salts so that it has great tensile and compressible strength but is light enough to be moved by coordinated muscle contractions. The intercellular matrix is composed of two types of substances—organic matter and inorganic salts. The organic matter, including bone cells, blood vessels, and nerves, constitutes about one third of the dry weight of bone; the inorganic salts make up the other two thirds.

The organic matter consists primarily of collagen fibers embedded in an amorphous ground substance. The inorganic matter consists of hydroxyapatite, an insoluble macrocrystalline structure of calcium phosphate salts, and small amounts of calcium carbonate and calcium fluoride. Bone may also take up lead and other heavy metals, thereby removing these toxic substances from the circulation. This can be viewed as a protective mechanism. The antibiotic tetracycline is readily bound to calcium deposited in newly formed bones and teeth. When tetracycline is given during pregnancy, it can be deposited in the teeth of the fetus, causing discoloration and deformity. Similar changes can occur if the drug is given for long periods to children younger than 6 years of age.

Types of Bone

There are two types of mature bones, cancellous and compact bone (Fig. 44–1). Both types are formed in lay-

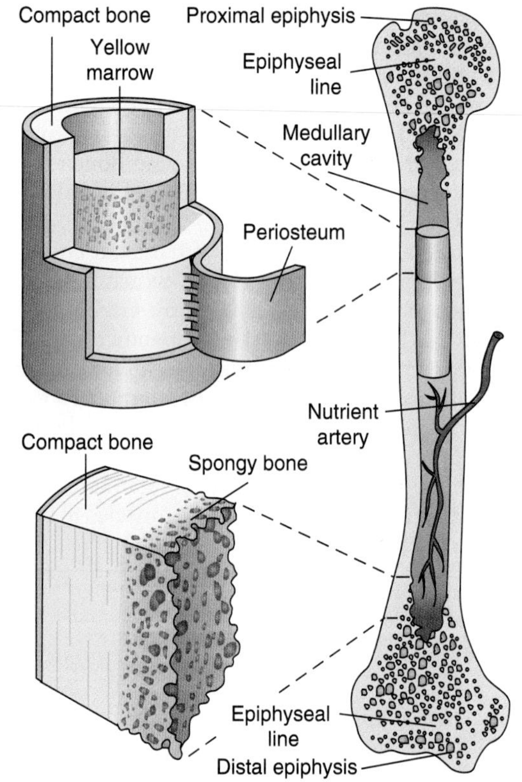

Figure 44–1
A long bone shown in longitudinal section.

ers and are therefore called lamellar bone. Cancellous, or spongy, bone is found in the interior of bones and is composed of trabeculae, or spicules, of bone, which form a latticelike pattern. These latticelike structures are lined with osteogenic cells and filled with red or yellow bone marrow. Cancellous bone is relatively light, but its structure is such that it has considerable tensile strength and weight-bearing properties. Compact, or cortical, bone has a densely packed calcified intercellular matrix that makes it more rigid than cancellous bone. The relative quantity of compact and cancellous bone varies in different types of bones throughout the body and in different parts of the same bone, depending on the need for strength and lightness. Compact bone is the major component of tubular bones. It is also found along the lines of stress on long bones and forms an outer protective shell on other bones.

Bone Cells

Four types of bone cells participate in the formation and maintenance of bone tissue: osteogenic cells, osteoblasts, osteocytes, and osteoclasts (Table 44–1).

Osteogenic Cells. The undifferentiated osteogenic cells are found in the periosteum, endosteum, and epiphyseal plate of growing bone. These cells differentiate into osteoblasts and are active during normal growth; they may also be activated in adult life during healing of fractures and other injuries. Osteogenic cells also participate in the continual replacement of worn-out bone tissue.

Osteoblasts. The osteoblasts, or bone-building cells, are responsible for the formation of the bone matrix. Bone formation occurs in two stages: ossification and calcification. Ossification involves the formation of osteoid, or prebone. Calcification of bone involves the deposition of calcium salts in the osteoid tissue. The osteoblasts synthesize collagen and other proteins that make up osteoid tissue. They also participate in the calcification process of the osteoid tissue, probably by controlling the availability of calcium and phosphate. Osteoblasts secrete the enzyme alkaline phosphatase, which is thought to act locally in bone tissue to raise calcium and phosphate levels to the point at which precipitation occurs. The activity of the osteoblasts undoubtedly contributes to the rise in serum levels of alkaline phosphatase that follows bone injury and fractures.

Osteocytes. The osteocytes are mature bone cells that are actively involved in maintaining the bony matrix. Death of the osteocytes results in the resorption of this matrix. The osteocytes lie in a small lake filled with extracellular fluid, called a *lacuna*, and are surrounded by a calcified intercellular matrix. Extracellular fluid-filled passageways permeate the calcified matrix and connect with the lacunae of adjacent osteocytes. These passageways are called *canaliculi*. Because diffusion does not occur through the calcified matrix of bone, the canaliculi serve as communicating channels for the exchange of nutrients and metabolites between the osteocytes and the blood vessels on the surface of the bone layer.

The osteocytes, together with their intercellular matrix, are arranged in layers, or lamellae. In compact bone, 4 to 20 lamellae are arranged concentrically around a central haversian canal, which runs essentially parallel to the long axis of the bone. Each of these units is called a *haversian system*, or *osteon*. The haversian canals contain blood vessels that carry nutrients and wastes to and from the canaliculi (Fig. 44–2). The blood vessels from the periosteum enter the bone through tiny openings called *Volkmann's canals* and connect with the haversian systems. Cancellous bone is also composed of lamellae, but its trabeculae are usually not penetrated by blood vessels. Instead, the bone cells of cancellous bone are nourished by diffusion from the endosteal surface through canaliculi, which interconnect their lacunae and extend to the bone surface.

Osteoclasts. Osteoclasts are bone cells that function in the resorption of bone, removing the mineral content and the organic matrix. Unlike the osteoblasts, which originate in osteogenic cells, the osteoclasts are formed by the fusion of blood-derived monocytes. Although the mechanism of osteoclast formation and activation remains elusive, it is known that parathyroid hormone (PTH) increases the number and resorptive function of the osteoclasts. Calcitonin is thought to reduce the number and resorptive function of the osteoclasts. The mechanism whereby osteoclasts exert their resorptive effect on bone is unclear. These cells may secrete an acid that

TABLE 44–1

Function of Bone Cells

Type of Bone Cell	Function
Osteogenic cells	Undifferentiated cells that differentiate into osteoblasts. They are found in the periosteum, endosteum, and epiphyseal growth plate of growing bones.
Osteoblasts	Bone-building cells that synthesize and secrete the organic matrix of bone. Osteoblasts also participate in the calcification of the organic matrix.
Osteocytes	Mature bone cells that function in the maintenance of bone matrix. Osteocytes also play an active role in releasing calcium into the blood.
Osteoclasts	Bone cells responsible for the resorption of bone matrix and the release of calcium and phosphate from bone.

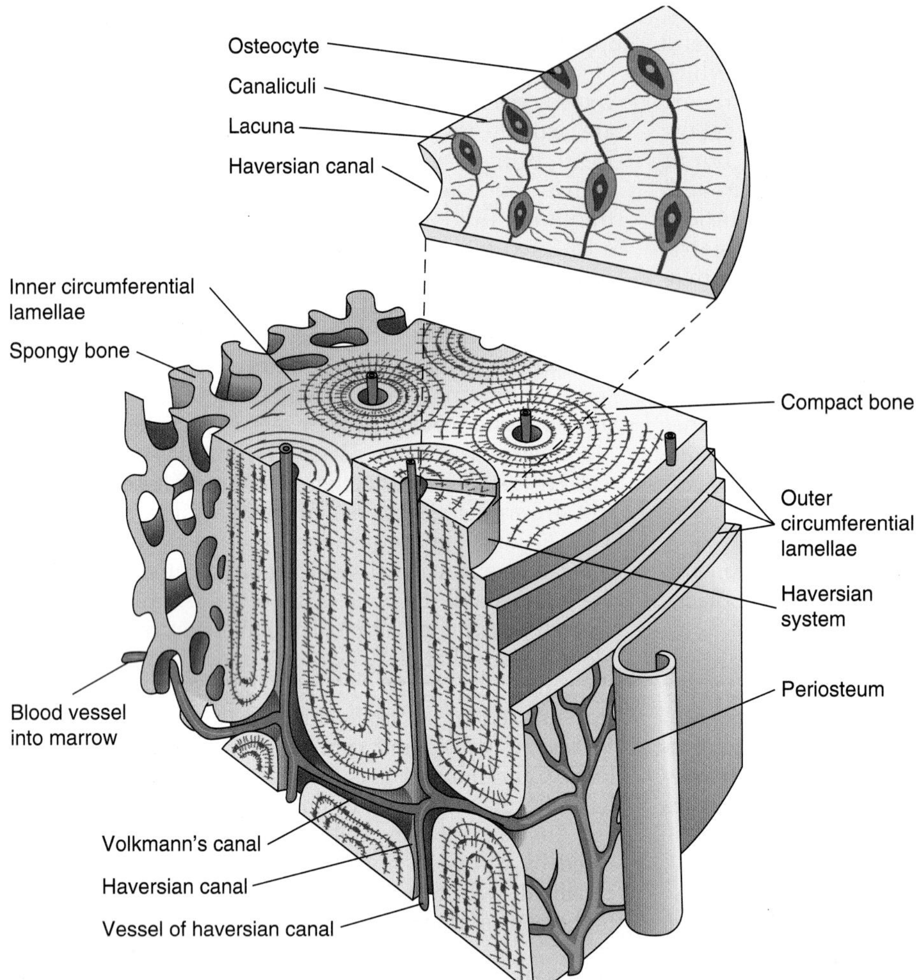

Figure 44–2 Haversian systems as seen in a wedge of compact bone tissue. The periosteum has been peeled back to show a blood vessel entering one of Volkmann's canals. (**Upper right**) Osteocytes lying within lacunae; canaliculi permit interstitial fluid to reach each lacuna.

removes calcium from the bone matrix, releasing the collagenic fibers for digestion by osteoclasts or mononuclear cells.

Periosteum and Endosteum

Bones are covered, except at their articular ends, by a membrane called the periosteum (see Fig. 44–1). The periosteum has an outer fibrous layer and an inner layer that contains the osteogenic cells needed for bone growth and development. The periosteum contains blood vessels and acts as an anchorage point for vessels as they enter and leave the bone. The endosteum is the membrane that lines the spaces of spongy bone, the marrow cavities, and the haversian canals of compact bone. It is composed mainly of osteogenic cells. These osteogenic cells contribute to the growth and remodeling of bone and are necessary for bone repair.

Hormonal Control of Bone Formation and Metabolism

The process of bone formation and mineral metabolism is complex. It involves the interplay between the action of PTH, calcitonin, and vitamin D. Other hormones, such as cortisol, growth hormone, thyroid hormone, and the sex hormones, also influence bone formation directly or indirectly. The actions of PTH, calcitonin, and vitamin D are summarized in Table 44–2.

Parathyroid Hormone

PTH is one of the important regulators of calcium and phosphate levels in the blood. The hormone is secreted by the parathyroid glands. There are two pairs of parathyroid glands located on the dorsal surface of right and left lobes of the thyroid gland.

PTH prevents serum calcium levels from falling below and serum phosphate levels from rising above normal physiologic concentrations. The secretion of PTH is regulated by negative feedback according to serum levels of ionized calcium (see Chapter 26). PTH, which is released from the parathyroid gland in response to a decrease in plasma calcium, restores the concentration of the calcium ion to just above the normal set point. This inhibits further secretion of the hormone. Other factors, such as serum phosphate and arterial blood pH, indirectly influence parathyroid secretion by altering the

TABLE 44-2

Actions of Parathyroid Hormone, Calcitonin, and Vitamin D

Actions	Parathyroid Hormone	Calcitonin	Vitamin D
Intestinal absorption of calcium	Increases indirectly through increased activation of vitamin D	Probably not affected	Increases
Intestinal absorption of phosphate	Increases	Probably not affected	Increases
Renal excretion of calcium	Decreases	Increases	Probably increases but less effect than PTH
Renal excretion of phosphate	Increases	Increases	Increases
Bone resorption	Increases	Decreases	1,25-$(OH)_2D_3$ increases
Bone formation	Decreases	Uncertain	24,25-$(OH)_2D_3$ increases (?)
Serum calcium levels	Produces a prompt increase	Decreases with pharmacologic doses	No effect
Serum phosphate levels	Prevents an increase	Decreases with pharmacologic doses	No effect

amount of calcium that is complexed to phosphate or bound to albumin.

PTH maintains serum calcium levels by initiating release of calcium from bone, by conservation of calcium by the kidney, by enhanced intestinal absorption of calcium through activation of vitamin D, and by reduction of serum phosphate levels (Fig. 44–3). PTH also increases the movement of calcium and phosphate from bone into the extracellular fluid. Calcium is immediately released from the canaliculi and bone cells; a more prolonged release of calcium and phosphate is mediated by increased osteoclast activity. In the kidney, PTH stimulates tubular reabsorption of calcium while reducing the reabsorption of phosphate. The latter effect ensures that increased release of phosphate from bone during mobilization of calcium does not produce an elevation in serum phosphate levels. This is important because an increase in calcium and phosphate levels could lead to crystallization within soft tissues. PTH increases intestinal absorption of calcium because of its ability to stimulate activation of vitamin D by the kidney.

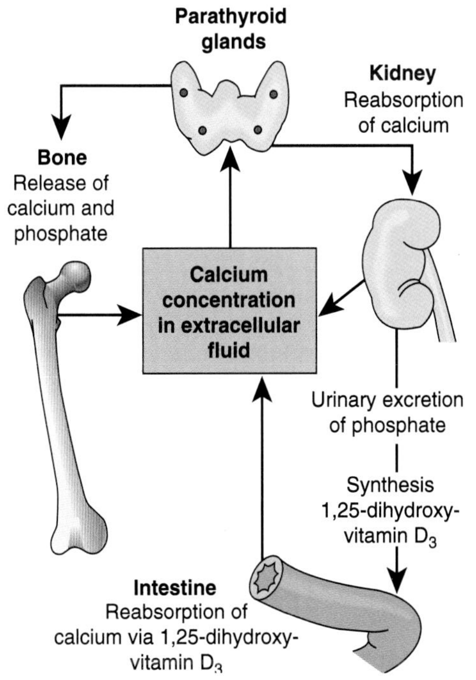

Figure 44–3
Regulation and actions of parathyroid hormone.

Calcitonin

Whereas PTH increases blood calcium levels, the hormone calcitonin lowers blood calcium levels. Calcitonin, sometimes called thyrocalcitonin, is secreted by the parafollicular, or C, cells of the thyroid gland.

Calcitonin inhibits the release of calcium from bone into the extracellular fluid. It is thought to act by causing calcium to become sequestered in bone cells and by inhibiting osteoclast activity. Calcitonin also reduces the renal tubular reabsorption of calcium and phosphate; the decrease in serum calcium level that follows administration of pharmacologic doses of calcitonin may be related to this action.

The major stimulus for calcitonin synthesis and release is a rise in serum calcium. The role of calcitonin in overall mineral homeostasis is uncertain. There are no clearly definable syndromes of calcitonin deficiency or excess, which suggests that calcitonin does not directly alter calcium metabolism. It has been suggested that the physiologic actions of calcitonin are related to the postprandial handling and processing of dietary calcium. This theory proposes that after meals calcitonin maintains parathyroid secretion at a time when it normally would be reduced by calcium entering the blood from the digestive tract. Although excess or deficiency states associated with alterations in physiologic levels of calcitonin have not been observed, it has been shown that pharmacologic doses of the hormone reduce osteoclastic activity. Because of this action, calcitonin has proved effective in the treatment of Paget's disease (see Chapter 46). The hormone is also used to reduce serum calcium levels during hypercalcemic crises.

Salmon calcitonin, which differs from human calcitonin in 9 of 32 amino acids, is 100 times more potent than human calcitonin. The higher potency may be related to higher affinity for receptor sites and slower degradation by peripheral tissues. Calcitonin used clinically is often a synthetic preparation containing the amino acid sequence of salmon calcitonin.

Vitamin D

Vitamin D and its metabolites are not vitamins but steroid hormones. There are two forms of vitamin D: vitamin D_2 (ergocalciferol) and vitamin D_3 (cholecalciferol). The two forms differ by the presence of a double bond, but they have identical biologic activity. The term *vitamin D* is used to indicate both forms.

Vitamin D has little or no activity until it has been metabolized to compounds that mediate its activity. Figure 44–4 depicts sources of vitamin D and pathways for activation. The first step of the activation process occurs in the liver, where vitamin D is hydroxylated to form the metabolite 25-hydroxyvitamin D_3 (25-OH D_3). From the liver, 25-OH D_3 is transported to the kidneys, where it undergoes conversion to 1,25-dihydroxyvitamin D_3 [1,25-$(OH)_2D_3$] or 24,25-dihydroxyvitamin D_3 [24,25-$(OH)_2D_3$]. Other metabolites of vitamin D have been and are still being discovered.

There are two sources of vitamin D: intestinal absorption and skin production. Intestinal absorption occurs mainly in the jejunum and includes vitamin D_2 and vitamin D_3. The most important dietary sources of vitamin D are fish, liver, and irradiated milk. Because vitamin D is fat soluble, its absorption is mediated by bile salts and occurs by means of the lymphatic vessels. In the skin, ultraviolet radiation from sunlight spontaneously converts 7-dehydrocholesterol provitamin D_3 to vitamin D_3. A circulating vitamin D–binding protein provides a mechanism to remove vitamin D from the skin and makes it available to the rest of the body.

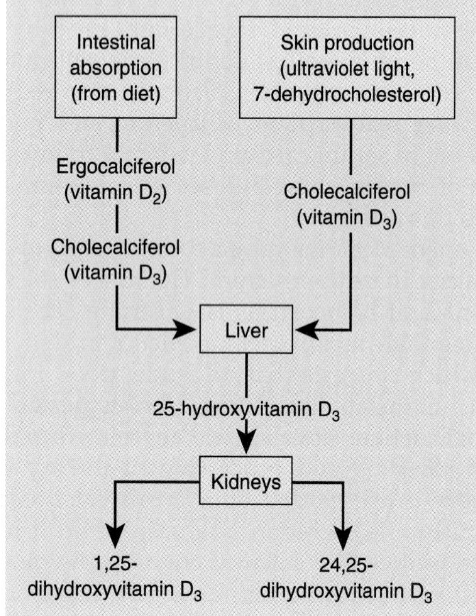

Figure 44–4
Sources and pathway for activation of vitamin D.

With adequate exposure to sunlight, the amount of vitamin D that can be produced by the skin is usually sufficient to meet physiologic requirements. The importance of sunlight exposure is evidenced by population studies that report lower vitamin D levels in countries, such as England, that have less sunlight than the United States. Elderly persons who are housebound or institutionalized frequently have low vitamin D levels. The deficiency often goes undetected until there are problems such as pseudofractures or electrolyte imbalances. Seasonal variations in vitamin D levels probably reflect changes in sunlight exposure.

The most potent of the vitamin D metabolites is 1,25-$(OH)_2D_3$. This metabolite increases intestinal absorption of calcium and promotes the actions of PTH on resorption of calcium and phosphate from bone. Bone resorption by the osteoclasts is increased and bone formation by the osteoblasts is decreased; there is also an increase in acid phosphatase and a decrease in alkaline phosphatase. Intestinal absorption and bone resorption increase the amount of calcium and phosphorus available to the mineralizing surface of the bone. The role of 24,25-$(OH)_2D_3$ is less clear. There is evidence that 24,25-$(OH)_2D_3$, in conjunction with 1,25-$(OH)_2D_3$, may be involved in normal bone mineralization.

The regulation of vitamin D activity is influenced by several hormones. PTH and prolactin stimulate 1,25-$(OH)_2D_3$ production by the kidney. States of hyperparathyroidism are associated with increased levels of 1,25-$(OH)_2D_3$, and hypoparathyroidism leads to lowered levels of this metabolite. Prolactin may have an ancillary role in regulating vitamin D metabolism during pregnancy and lactation. Calcitonin inhibits 1,25-$(OH)_2D_3$ production by the kidney. In addition to hormonal influences, changes in the concentration of ions such as calcium, phosphate, hydrogen, and potassium exert an effect on 1,25-$(OH)_2D_3$ and 24,25-$(OH)_2D_3$ production. Under conditions of deprivation of phosphate and calcium, 1,25-$(OH)_2D_3$ levels are increased, whereas hyperphosphatemia and hypercalcemia decrease the levels of metabolite.

In summary, skeletal tissue is composed two type of connective tissue: cartilage and bone. These skeletal structures are composed of similar tissue types; each has living cells and nonliving intercellular fibers and ground substance that is secreted by the cells. Cartilage is a firm, flexible type of skeletal tissue that is essential for growth before and after birth. There are three types of cartilage: elastic, hyaline, and fibrocartilage. Hyaline cartilage, which is the most abundant type, forms the costal cartilages that join the ribs to the sternum and vertebrae, many of the cartilages of the respiratory tract, and the articular cartilages.

The characteristics of the various skeletal tissue types are determined by the intercellular matrix. In bone, this matrix is impregnated with calcium salts to provide hardness and strength. There are four types of bone cells: osteocytes, or mature bone cells; osteoblasts, or bone-building cells; osteoclasts, which function in bone resorption; and osteogenic cells, which differentiate into osteoblasts; and osteogenic cells, which differentiate into osteoblasts. A typical long bone has a shaft, or diaphysis, and two ends, called epiphyses. Densely packed compact bone forms the outer shell of a bone, and latticelike cancellous bone forms the interior. Bones are covered by a membrane called the periosteum, which contains blood vessels and acts as an anchorage point for vessels as they enter and leave the bone. The endosteum is the membrane that lines the spaces of spongy bone, the marrow cavities, and the haversian canals of compact bone.

The process of bone formation and mineral metabolism involves the interplay among the actions of PTH, calcitonin, and vitamin D. PTH acts to maintain serum levels of ionized calcium; it increases the release of calcium and phosphate from bone, increases the conservation of calcium and elimination of phosphate by the kidney, and increases intestinal reabsorption of calcium through vitamin D. Calcitonin inhibits the release of calcium from bone and increases renal elimination of calcium and phosphate, thereby serving to lower serum calcium levels. Vitamin D functions as a hormone in regulating body calcium. It increases absorption of calcium from the intestine and promotes the actions of PTH on bone.

Skeletal Structures

After you have completed this section of the chapter, you should be able to meet the following objectives:

- Characterize the structure of bones based on their shape and list the structures of long bones
- State the characteristics of tendons and ligaments
- State the difference between synarthrodial and diarthrodial joints
- Describe the source of blood supply to a diarthrodial joint
- Explain why pain is often experienced in all the joints of an extremity when only a single joint is affected by a disease process
- Describe the structure and function of a bursa
- Explain the pathology associated with a torn meniscus of the knee

Classification of Bones

Bones are classified by shape as long, short, flat, and irregular. Long bones are found in the upper and lower extremities. Short bones are irregularly shaped bones located in the ankle and the wrist. Except for their surface, which is compact bone, these bones are spongy throughout. Flat bones are composed of a layer of spongy bone between two layers of compact bone. They are found in areas such as the skull and rib cage, where extensive protection of underlying structures is needed or, as in the scapula, where a broad surface for muscle attachment must be provided. Irregular bones, because of their shapes, cannot be classified in any of the previous groups. This group includes bones such as the vertebrae and the bones of the jaw.

A typical long bone has a shaft, or *diaphysis,* and two ends, called *epiphyses.* Long bones are usually narrow in the midportion and broad at the ends so that the weight they bear can be distributed over a wider surface. The shaft of a long bone is formed mainly of compact bone roughly hollowed out to form a marrow-filled medullary canal. The ends of long bones are covered with articular cartilage that rests on a bony plate, the subchondral bone.

In growing bones, the part of the bone shaft that funnels out as it approaches the epiphysis is called the *metaphysis* (Fig. 44–5). It is composed of bony trabeculae that have cores of cartilage. In the child, the epiphysis is separated from the metaphysis by the cartilaginous growth plate. After puberty, the metaphysis and epiphysis merge, and the growth plate is obliterated.

Bone marrow occupies the medullary cavities of the long bones throughout the skeleton and the cavities of cancellous bone in the vertebrae, ribs, sternum, and flat

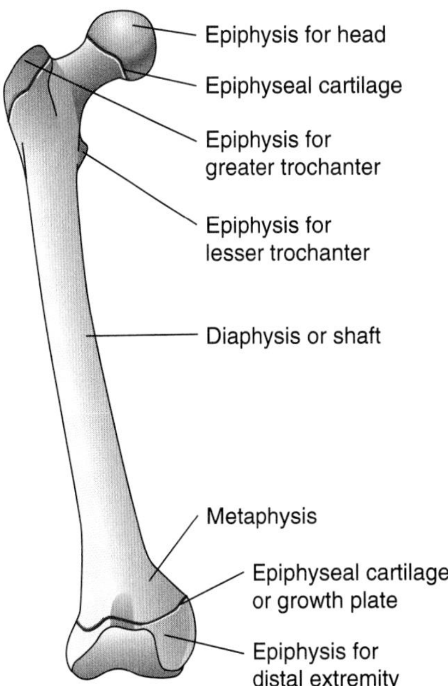

Figure 44–5
A femur, showing epiphyseal cartilages for the head, metaphysis, trochanters, and distal end of the bone.

bones of the pelvis. The cellular composition of the bone marrow varies with age and skeletal location. Red bone marrow contains developing red blood cells and is the site of blood cell formation. Yellow bone marrow is composed largely of adipose cells. At birth, nearly all of the marrow is red and hematopoietically active. As the need for red blood cell production decreases during postnatal growth, red marrow is gradually replaced with yellow bone marrow in most of the bones. In the adult, red marrow persists in the vertebrae, ribs, sternum, and ilia.

Tendons and Ligaments

In the skeletal system, tendons and ligaments are dense connective tissue structures that connect muscles and bones. Tendons connect muscles to bone, and ligaments connect the movable bones of joints. Tendons can appear as cordlike structures or as flattened sheets, called aponeuroses, such as in the abdominal muscles.

The dense connective tissue found in tendons and ligaments has a limited blood supply and is composed largely of intercellular bundles of collagen fibers arranged in the same direction and plane. This type of connective tissue provides great tensile strength and can withstand tremendous pull in the direction of fiber alignment. At the sites where tendons or ligaments are inserted into cartilage or bone, a gradual transition from pure dense connective tissue to bone or cartilage occurs. In cartilage this transitional tissue is called *fibrocartilage.*

Tendons that may rub against bone or other friction-generating surfaces are enclosed in double-layered sheaths. An outer connective tissue tube is attached to the structures surrounding the tendon, and an inner sheath encloses the tendon and is attached to it. The space between the inner and outer sheath is filled with a fluid similar to synovial fluid.

Joints and Articulations

Articulations, or joints, are areas where two or more bones meet. The term *arthro* is the prefix used to designate a joint. For example, *arthrology* is the study of joints, and *arthroplasty* is the repair of a joint. There are two classes of joints, based on movement and the presence of a joint cavity: synarthroses and diarthroses.

Synarthroses

Synarthroses are joints that lack a joint cavity and move little or not at all. There are three types of synarthroses: synostoses, synchondroses, and syndesmoses. *Synostoses* are nonmovable joints in which the surfaces of the bones are joined by dense connective tissue or bone. The bones of the skull are joined by synostoses; they are joined by dense connective tissue in children and young adults and by bone in older persons. *Synchondroses* are joints in which bones are connected by hyaline cartilage and have limited motion. The ribs are attached to the sternum by this type of joint. *Syndesmoses* permit a certain amount of movement; they are separated by a fibrous disk and joined by interosseous ligaments. The symphysis pubis of the pelvis and the bodies of the vertebrae that are joined by intervertebral disks are examples of syndesmoses.

Diarthroses

Diarthrodial joints (*i.e.*, synovial joints) are freely movable joints. Most joints in the body are of this type. Although they are classified as freely movable, their movement ranges from almost none (*e.g.*, sacroiliac joint) to simple hinge movement (*e.g.*, interphalangeal joint) to movement in many planes (*e.g.*, shoulder or hip joint). The bony surfaces of these joints are covered with thin layers of articular cartilage, and the cartilaginous surfaces of these joints slide past each other during movement. As discussed in Chapter 47, diarthrodial joints are the joints most frequently affected by rheumatic disorders.

In a diarthrodial joint, the articulating ends of the bones are not connected directly but are indirectly linked by a strong fibrous capsule (*i.e.*, joint capsule) that surrounds the joint and is continuous with the periosteum (Fig. 44–6). This capsule supports the joint and helps to hold the bones in place. Additional support may be provided by ligaments that extend between the bones of the joint.

The joint capsule consists of two layers: an outer fibrous layer and an inner membrane, the synovium. The synovium surrounds the tendons that pass through the joints and the free margins of other intraarticular structures such as ligaments and menisci. The synovium forms folds that surround the margins of articulations but do not cover the weight-bearing articular cartilage. These folds permit stretching of the synovium so that movement can occur without tissue damage.

The synovium secretes a slippery synovial fluid with the consistency of egg white. This fluid acts as a

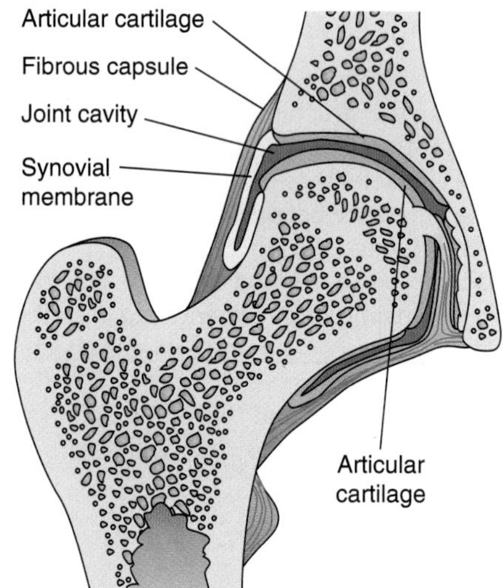

Figure 44–6
Diarthrodial joint, showing the articular cartilage, fibrous joint capsule, joint cavity, and synovial membrane.

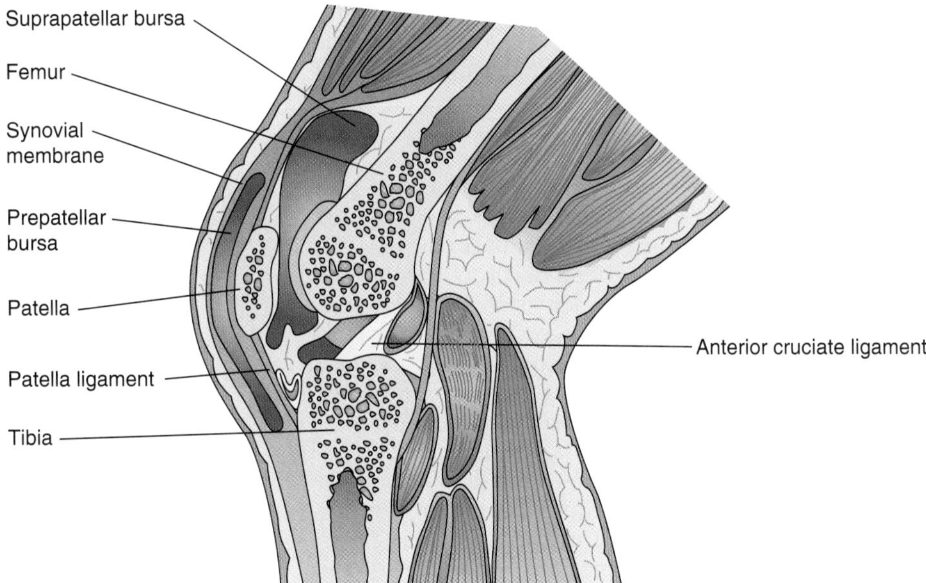

Figure 44–7
Sagittal section of knee joint, showing prepatellar and suprapatellar bursae.

lubricant and facilitates the movement of the articulating surfaces of the joint. Normal synovial fluid is clear or pale yellow, does not clot, and contains fewer than 100 cells/mm^3. The cells are predominantly mononuclear cells derived from the synovium. The composition of the synovial fluid is altered in many inflammatory and pathologic joint disorders. Aspiration and examination of the synovial fluid play an important role in the diagnosis of joint diseases.

The articular cartilage is an example of hyaline cartilage and is unique in that its free surface is not covered with perichondrium. It has only a peripheral rim of perichondrium, and calcification of the portion of cartilage abutting the bone may limit or preclude diffusion from blood vessels supplying the subchondral bone. Articular cartilage is apparently nourished by the diffusion of substances contained in the synovial fluid bathing the cartilage. Regeneration of most cartilage is slow; it is accomplished primarily by growth that requires the activity of perichondrium cells. In articular cartilage, which has no perichondrium, superficial injuries heal slowly.

Blood Supply and Innervation

The blood supply to a joint arises from blood vessels that enter the subchondral bone at or near the attachment of the joint capsule and form an arterial circle around the joint. The synovial membrane has a rich blood supply, and constituents of plasma diffuse rapidly between these vessels and the joint cavity. Because many of the capillaries are near the surface of the synovium, blood may escape into the synovial fluid after relatively minor injuries. Healing and repair of the synovial membrane are usually rapid and complete. This is important because synovial tissue is injured in many surgical procedures that involve the joint.

The nerve supply to joints is provided by the same nerve trunks that supply the muscles that move the joints. These nerve trunks also supply the skin over the joints. As a rule, each joint of an extremity is innervated by all the peripheral nerves that cross the articulation; this accounts for the referral of pain from one joint to another. For example, hip pain may be perceived as pain in the knee.

The tendons and ligaments of the joint capsule are sensitive to position and movement, particularly stretching and twisting. These structures are supplied by the large sensory nerve fibers that form proprioceptor endings (see Chapter 37). The proprioceptors function reflexively to adjust the tension of the muscles that support the joint and are particularly important in maintaining muscular support for the joint. For example, when a weight is lifted, there is a proprioceptor-mediated reflex contraction and relaxation of appropriate muscle groups to support the joint and protect the joint capsule and other joint structures. Loss of proprioception and reflex control of muscular support leads to destructive changes in the joint.

The synovial membrane is innervated only by autonomic fibers that control blood flow. It is relatively free of pain fibers, as evidenced by the fact that surgical procedures on the joint are often done under local anesthesia. The joint capsule and the ligaments have pain receptors; these receptors are more easily stimulated by stretching and twisting than other joint structures. Pain arising from the capsule tends to be diffuse and poorly localized.

Bursae

In some diarthrotic joints, the synovial membrane forms closed sacs that are not part of the joint. These sacs, called *bursae*, contain synovial fluid. Their purpose is to prevent friction on a tendon. Bursae occur in areas where pressure is exerted because of close approximation of joint structures (Fig. 44–7). Such conditions occur when tendons are deflected over bone or where skin must move freely over bony tissue. Bursae may become injured or inflamed, causing discomfort, swelling, and limitation in movement of the involved area. A bunion is an inflamed bursa of the metatarsophalangeal joint of the great toe.

Intraarticular Menisci

Intraarticular menisci are fibrocartilage structures that develop from portions of the articular disk that occupied the space between articular cartilage surfaces during fetal development. Menisci may extend part way through the joint and have a free inner border, as at the lateral and medial articular surfaces of the knee, or they may extend through the joint, separating it into two separate cavities, as in the sternoclavicular joint. The menisci of the knee joint may be torn as the result of an injury. The detached portion may interfere with joint motion and cause recurring pain and locking or giving way of the joint. When this happens, the injured structure is often removed surgically. After removal, a new structure sometimes grows in from the fibrous capsule of the joint. The new meniscus is almost a complete duplicate of the old, except that it is made up of dense connective tissue rather than the fibrocartilage of the original structure.

In summary, bones are classified on the basis of their shape as long, short, flat, or irregular. Long bones are found in the upper and lower extremities; short bones in the ankle and wrist; flat bone in the skull and rib cage; and irregular bones in the vertebrae and jaw. Tendons and ligaments are dense connective skeletal tissue that connect muscles and bones. Tendons connect muscles to bones, and ligaments connect the movable bones of joints.

Articulations, or joints, are areas where two or more bones meet. Synarthroses are joints in which bones are joined together by fibrous tissue, cartilage, or bone; they lack a joint cavity and move little or no movement. Diarthrodial or synovial joints are freely movable. The surfaces of the articulating ends of bones in diarthrodial joints are covered with a thin layer of articular cartilage, and they are enclosed in a fibrous joint capsule. The joint capsule consists of two layers: an outer fibrous layer and an inner membrane, the synovium. A slippery fluid called the synovial fluid, which is secreted by the synovium into the joint capsule, acts as a lubricant and facilitates movement of the joint's articulating surfaces. Bursae, which are closed sacs containing synovial fluid, prevent friction in areas where tendons are deflected over bone or where skin must move freely over bony tissue.

Menisci are fibrocartilaginous structures that develop from portions of the articular disk that occupied the space between the articular cartilage during fetal development. The menisci may have a free inner border, or they may extend through the joint, separating it into two cavities. The menisci in the knee joint may be torn as a result of injury.

BIBLIOGRAPHY

Cormack D.H. (1987). *Ham's histology* (9th ed., pp. 234–338). Philadelphia: J.B. Lippincott.

DeLuca H.F. (1988). The vitamin D story: A collaborative effort of basic science and clinical medicine. *FASEB Journal* 2:244–236.

Hall A. C., Guyton J.F. (1996). *Textbook of medical physiology* (9th ed., pp. 989–998). Philadelphia: W.B. Saunders.

Junqueira L.C., Carneiro J., Kelly O. (1995). *Basic histology* (8th ed., pp. 124–151). Los Altos, CA: Lange Medical Publications.

Rhoades R.A., Tanner G.A. (1996). *Medical physiology* (pp. 725–735). Boston: Little, Brown.

CHAPTER 45

Alterations in Skeletal Function: Trauma and Infection

Kathleen E. Gunta

The musculoskeletal system includes the bones, joints, and muscles of the body together with associated structures such as ligaments and tendons. This system, which constitutes more than 70% of the body, is subject to a large number of disorders. These disorders affect persons in all age groups and walks of life and cause pain, disability, and deformity. The discussion in this chapter focuses on the effects of trauma, infections, and ischemia on musculoskeletal structures such as bones, muscles, tendons, and ligaments.

Injury and Trauma of Musculoskeletal Structures

After you have completed this section of the chapter, you should be able to meet the following objectives:

- Describe the physical agents responsible for soft tissue trauma
- Name the three types of soft tissue injuries
- Compare muscle strains and ligamentous sprains
- Describe the healing process of soft tissue injuries
- Differentiate open from closed fractures
- List the signs and symptoms of a fracture
- Describe the fracture healing process
- Relate individual and local factors to the healing process in bone
- Explain the importance of immobilization for fracture healing
- Explain why muscle and joint function should be maintained during fracture healing
- Differentiate the early complications of fractures from later complications of fracture healing

Trauma, which commonly includes injury to musculoskeletal structures, is the third leading cause of death in the United States. A broad spectrum of injuries result from numerous physical forces. Injuries to the musculoskeletal system include blunt tissue trauma, disruption of tendons and ligaments, and fractures of bony structures.

Many of the external physical agents that cause injury to the musculoskeletal system are typical for a particular environmental setting, an activity, or an age group. Trauma resulting from high-speed motor accidents is ranked as the number one killer of adults younger than 35 years of age. Motorcycle accidents are especially common in young men, with fractures of the distal tibia, midshaft femur, and radius occurring most often.

Trauma in children is usually the result of an accident. Bicycle-related injuries account for more than 50,000 emergency room visits annually, with most involving the 5- to 14-year-old age group.[1] Accidents caused by all-terrain or off-road vehicles are becoming increasingly common.

Elderly persons are at particular risk for injuries caused by falls. Impaired hearing and sight, dizziness, and unsteadiness of gait contribute to falls in the older person. These falls are often compounded by osteoporosis, or bone atrophy, which makes fractures more likely. Fractures of the vertebrae, proximal humerus, and hip are particularly common in this age group.

Soft Tissue Injury

Most skeletal injuries are accompanied by soft tissue injuries. These injuries include contusions, hematomas, and lacerations. They are discussed here because of their association with musculoskeletal injuries.

A *contusion* is an injury to soft tissue that results from direct trauma and is usually caused by striking a body part against a hard object. With a contusion, the skin overlying the injury remains intact. Initially, the area becomes ecchymotic (*i.e.*, black and blue) because of local hemorrhage; later, the discoloration gradually changes to brown and then to yellow as the blood is reabsorbed.

A large area of local hemorrhage is called a *hematoma* (*i.e.*, blood tumor). Hematomas cause pain as blood accumulates and exerts pressure on nerve endings. The pain increases with movement or when pressure is applied to the area. The pain and swelling of a hematoma take longer to subside than that accompanying a contusion. A hematoma may become infected because of bacterial growth. Unlike a contusion, which does not drain, a hematoma may eventually split the skin because of increased pressures and produce drainage.

The treatment for a contusion and a hematoma consists of elevating the affected part and applying cold for the first 24 hours to reduce the bleeding into the area. A hematoma may need to be aspirated. After the first 24 hours, heat or cold should be applied intermittently for 20 minutes at a time.

A *laceration* is an injury in which the skin is torn or its continuity is disrupted. The seriousness of a laceration depends on the size and depth of the wound and on whether there is contamination from the object that caused the injury. Puncture wounds from nails or rusted material may result in the growth of toxic bacteria, leading to gas gangrene or tetanus.

Lacerations are usually treated by wound closure, which is done after the area is sufficiently cleaned; the closed wound is covered with a sterile dressing. It is important to minimize contamination of the wound and to control bleeding. Contaminated wounds and open fractures are copiously irrigated and debrided, and the skin is usually left open to heal to prevent the development of an anaerobic infection or a sinus tract.

Strains and Sprains

Tendons and ligaments, which connect bones and muscles, can be severed by cutting injuries or damaged by forcible twisting or stretching. A *strain* is a stretching injury to a muscle or a musculotendinous unit caused by mechanical overloading. This type of injury may result from an unusual muscle contraction or an excessive forcible stretch. Although there is usually no external evidence of a specific injury, pain, stiffness, and swelling exist. The most common sites for muscle strains are the lower back and the cervical region of the spine. The elbow and the shoulder are also supported by musculotendinous units that are subject to strains. Foot strain is associated with the weight-bearing stresses of the feet; it may be caused by inadequate muscular and ligamentous support, overweight, or excessive exercise such as standing, walking, or running.

A *sprain*, which involves the ligamentous structures surrounding the joint, resembles a strain, but the pain and swelling subside more slowly (Fig. 45–1). It is usually caused by abnormal or excessive movement of the joint. With a sprain, the ligaments may be incompletely torn or, as in a severe sprain, completely torn or ruptured. The signs of sprain are pain, rapid swelling, heat, disability, discoloration, and limitation of function. Any joint may be sprained, but the ankle joint is most commonly involved. Most ankle sprains occur when the foot is turned inward under a person, forcing the ankle into inversion beyond the structural limits. Other common sites of sprain are the knee (*i.e.*, the collateral ligament and anterior cruciate ligament) and elbow (*i.e.*, the ulnar side). As with a strain, the soft tissue injury that occurs with a sprain is not evident on the radiograph (x-ray). Occasionally, however, a chip of bone is evident when the entire ligament, including part of its bony attachment, has been ruptured or torn from the bone.

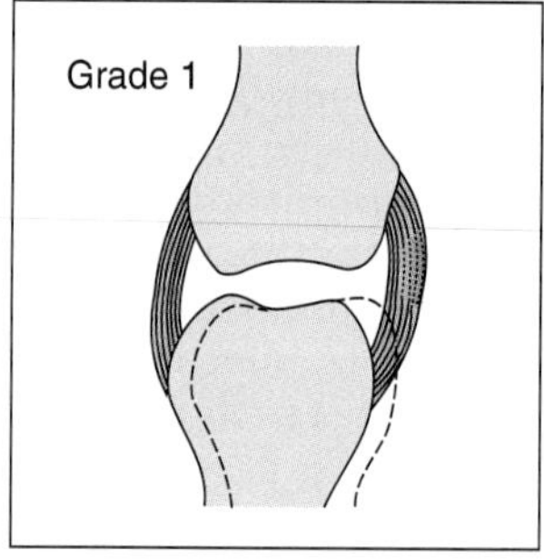

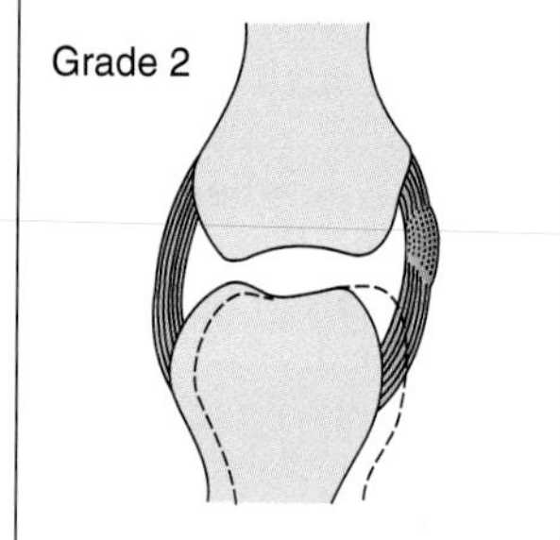

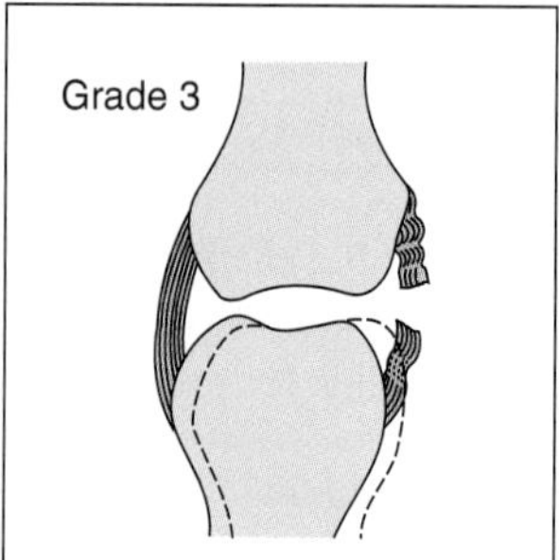

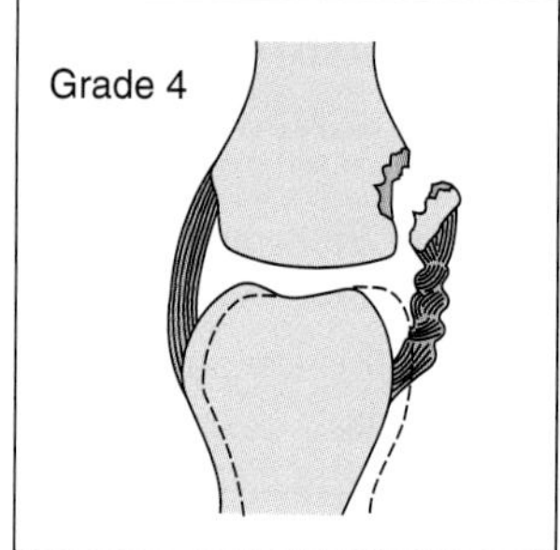

Figure 45–1
Degrees of sprain on the medial side of the right knee: grade 1, mild sprain of the medial collateral ligament; grade 2, moderate sprain with hematoma formation; grade 3, severe sprain with total disruption of the ligament; and grade 4, severe sprain with avulsion of the medial femoral condyle at the insertion of the medial collateral ligament. (Adapted from Spickler L.L. [1983]. Knee injuries of the athlete. *Orthopedic Nursing* 2 [5], 12–13)

A tear of the meniscus can be associated with a sprained knee. Meniscus tears can be described by their appearance (*e.g.*, parrot-beak, bucket handle) or their location (*e.g.*, posterior horn, anterior horn). Meniscus injury commonly occurs as the result of a rotational injury from a sudden or sharp pivot or a direct blow to the knee as in hockey, basketball, or football. The injured knee is edematous and painful, especially with hyperflexion and hyperextension. A loose fragment may cause knee instability and locking. Diagnosis is made by examination and confirmed by arthroscopy.

Healing of the dense connective tissues in tendons and ligaments is similar to that of other soft tissues. If properly treated, injuries usually heal with the restoration of the original tensile strength. Repair is accomplished by fibroblasts from the inner tendon sheath or, if the tendon has no sheath, from the loose connective tissue that surrounds the tendon. Capillaries infiltrate the injured area during the initial healing process and supply the fibroblasts with the materials they need to produce large amounts of collagen. Formation of the long collagen bundles begins within 4 to 5 days, and although tensile strength increases steadily thereafter, it is not sufficient to permit strong tendon pulls for 4 to 5 weeks.[2] During the first 3 weeks, there is a danger that muscle contraction will pull the injured ends apart, causing the tendon to heal in the lengthened position. There is also a danger that adhesions will develop in areas where tendons pass through fibrous channels, such as in the distal palm of the hands, rendering the tendon useless.

The treatment of muscle strains and ligamentous sprains is similar in several ways. For an injured extremity, elevation of the part followed by local application of cold may be sufficient. Compression, accomplished through the use of adhesive wraps or a removable splint, helps reduce swelling and provides support. A cast is applied for severe sprains, especially those severe enough to warrant surgical repair. Immobilization for a muscle strain is continued until the pain and swelling have subsided. In a sprain, the affected joint is immobilized for several weeks. Immobilization may be followed by graded active exercises. Early diagnosis, treatment, and rehabilitation are essential in preventing chronic ligamentous instability.

In the lumbar and cervical spine regions, muscle strains are more common than sprains. For these strains, treatment usually consists of bed rest, traction, application of heat, and massage. Cold should be used during the first 24 hours to reduce pain and swelling of the affected area. Exercises, correct posture, and good body mechanics help to reduce the risk of reinjury. Mechanical low back pain is becoming increasingly common in the adolescent athlete. Overuse, especially hyperextension of the lumbar spine in such sports as track, wrestling, gymnastics, and diving, can tear the muscles, fascia, and ligaments. Chronic low back pain may indicate a stress fracture. Fractures near the top and bottom surface of the vertebrae can occur when the growing lumbar spine is overstressed, causing the disks to push into the bone. Early detection and treatment are important to prevent complications and prevent disability.

Rotator cuff injury occurs in one or more of the four muscles that lie deep in the shoulder bridging the glenohumeral joint. It is caused by excessive usage, a direct blow or stretch injury usually involving throwing or swinging, as with baseball pitchers or tennis players. Complete tears of the rotator cuff usually occur in young persons after severe trauma. Overuse syndrome has a slower onset and is seen in older persons with minor or no trauma. Rotator cuff tendinitis, also known as *shoulder impingement syndrome,* is also common, especially in swimmers.

Many physical examination maneuvers are used to define shoulder pathology. The history and mechanism of injury are important. In addition to standard radiographs, an arthrogram, computed tomography (CT) scan, or magnetic resonance imaging (MRI) scan may be obtained. Arthroscopic examination under anesthesia is done for diagnostic purposes and operative arthroscopy to repair severe tears. Conservative treatment with anti-inflammatory agents, steroid injections, and physical therapy is often done. A period of rest is followed by a customized exercise and rehabilitation program to improve strength, flexibility, and endurance. The rotator cuff is not unlike other muscle groups of the body in that its risk of injury increases when asked to perform a high-stress function in an unconditioned state.

Dislocations

Dislocation of a joint is the loss of articulation of the bone ends within the joint capsule caused by displacement or separation of the bone end from its position in the joint. It usually follows a severe trauma that disrupts the holding ligaments. Dislocations are seen most often in the shoulder and acromioclavicular joints. A *subluxation* is a partial dislocation in which the bone ends within the joint are still in partial contact with each other.

Dislocations can be congenital, traumatic, or pathologic. Congenital dislocations occur in the hip and knee. Traumatic dislocations occur after falls, blows, or rotational injuries. For example, car accidents often cause dislocations of the hip and accompanying acetabular fractures because the direction of impact. This is true of persons wearing seat belts and those who are unrestrained. In the shoulder and patella, dislocations may become recurrent, especially in athletes. They recur with the same motion but require less and less force each time. Pathologic dislocation in the hip is a late complication of infection, rheumatoid arthritis, paralysis, and neuromuscular diseases. Dislocations of the phalangeal joints are not serious and are usually reduced by manipulation. Less common sites of dislocation, seen mainly in young adults, are the wrist and midtarsal region. They are usually the result of direct force, such as a fall on an outstretched hand.

Diagnosis of a dislocation is made by physical examination and confirmed by radiographs. The symptoms are pain, deformity, and limited movement. With recurrent dislocations, the person often senses the impending dislocation and may have a look of apprehension when range of joint motion is tested.

The treatment depends on the site, mechanism of injury, and associated injuries such as fractures. Dislocations that do not reduce spontaneously usually require manipulation or surgical repair. Various surgical procedures can also be used to prevent redislocation of the patella, shoulder, or acromioclavicular joints. Immobilization is necessary for several weeks after reduction of a dislocation to allow healing of the joint structures. In dislocations affecting the knee, alternatives to surgery are isometric quadriceps-strengthening exercises and a temporary brace. Surgical procedures, such as joint replacement, may be necessary in certain pathologic dislocations.

Recurrent subluxation and dislocation of the patella (*i.e.*, knee cap) are common injuries in young adults. They account for about 10% of all athletic injuries and are more common in females. Sports such as skiing or tennis may cause stress on the patella. These sports involve external rotation of the foot and lower leg with knee flexion, a position that exerts rotational stresses on the knee. There is often a sensation of the patella "popping out" when the dislocation occurs. Other complaints include the knee giving out, swelling, crepitus, stiffness, and loss of range of motion. Congenital knee variations are predisposing factors. Treatment can be difficult, but nonsurgical methods are used first. They include immobilization with the knee extended, bracing, administration of salicylates, and isometric quadriceps-strengthening exercises. Surgical intervention is often necessary.

Chondromalacia

Chondromalacia, or softening of the articular cartilage, is seen most commonly on the undersurface of the patella and occurs most frequently in young adults. It can be the result of recurrent subluxation of the patella or overuse in strenuous athletic activities. Persons with this disorder typically complain of pain, particularly when climbing stairs or sitting with the knees bent. Occasionally, the person experiences weakness of the knee.

The treatment consists of rest, isometric exercises, and application of ice after exercise. Part of the patella may be surgically removed in severe cases. In less severe cases, the soft portion is shaved, using a saw inserted through an arthroscope.

Loose Bodies

Loose bodies are small pieces of bone or cartilage inside the joint. These can be the result of trauma to the joint or may occur when cartilage has worn away from the articular surface, causing a part of the surface bone to die. When this happens, a piece of bone separates and becomes free floating. The symptoms are painful catching and locking of the joint. Loose bodies are commonly seen in the knee, elbow, hip, and ankle. The loose body repeatedly gets caught in the crevice of a joint, pinching the underlying healthy cartilage; unless the loose body is removed, it may cause osteoarthritis and restricted movement. The treatment consists of removal using operative arthroscopy.

Fractures

Normal bone can withstand considerable compression and shearing forces and, to a lesser extent, tension forces. A fracture is any break in the continuity of bone that occurs when more stress is placed on the bone than it is able to absorb. Grouped according to cause, fractures can be divided into three major categories: fractures caused by sudden injury, fatigue or stress fractures, and pathologic fractures. The most common fractures are those resulting from sudden injury. The force causing the fracture may be direct, such as a fall or blow, or indirect, such as a massive muscle contraction or trauma transmitted along the bone. For example, the head of the radius or clavicle can be fractured by the indirect forces that result from falling on an outstretched hand. A fatigue fracture results from repeated wear on a bone. Pain associated with overuse injuries of the lower extremities, especially posterior medial tibial pain, is one of the most common symptoms that physically active persons such as runners experience. Stress fractures in the tibia may be confused with "shin splints," a nonspecific term for pain in the lower leg from overuse in walking and running, because they frequently do not appear on x-ray films until 2 weeks after the onset of symptoms.

A pathologic fracture occurs in bones that are already weakened by disease or tumors. Fractures of this type may occur spontaneously with little or no stress. The underlying disease state can be local, as with infections, cysts, or tumors, or it can be generalized, as in osteoporosis, Paget's disease, or disseminated tumors.

Classification

Fractures are usually classified according to location, type, and direction or pattern of the fracture line (Fig. 45–2).

Location. A long bone is divided into three parts: proximal, midshaft, and distal (see Fig. 45–2). A fracture of the long bone is described in relation to its position in the bone. Other descriptions are used when the fracture affects the head or neck of a bone, involves a joint, or is near a prominence such as a condyle or malleolus.

Types. The type of fracture is determined by its communication with the external environment, the degree of break in continuity of the bone, and the character of the fracture pieces. A fracture can be classified as open or closed. When the bone fragments have broken through

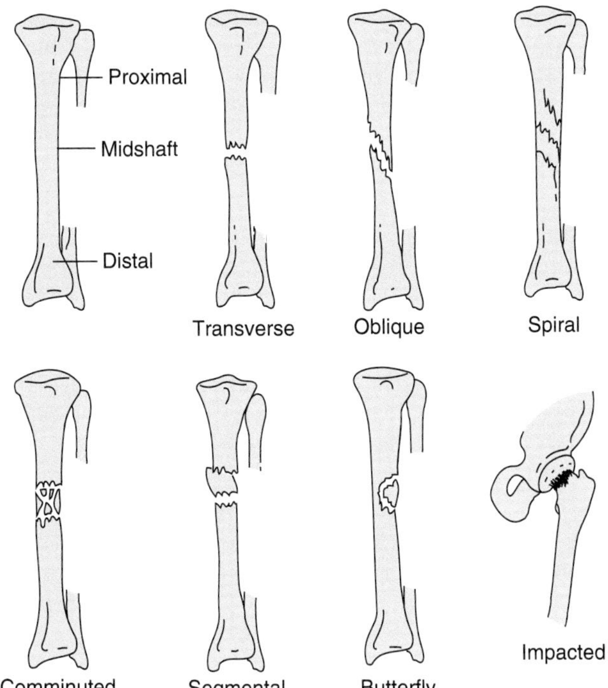

Figure 45–2
Classification of fractures. Fractures are classified according to location (proximal, midshaft, or distal), the direction of fracture line (transverse, oblique, spiral), and type (comminuted, segmental, butterfly, or impacted).

the skin, the fracture is called an *open* or *compound fracture.* Open fractures are often complicated by infection, osteomyelitis, delayed union, or nonunion. In a *closed fracture,* there is no communication with the outside skin.

The degree of a fracture is described in terms of a partial or complete break in the continuity of bone. A *greenstick fracture,* which is seen in children, is an example of a partial break in bone continuity and resembles the kind seen when a young sapling is broken. This kind of break occurs because children's bones, especially until about age 10, are more resilient than the bones of adults.

A fracture is also described by the character of the fracture pieces. A *comminuted fracture* has more than two pieces. A *compression fracture,* as occurs in the vertebral body, involves two bones that are crushed or squeezed together. A fracture is called *impacted* when the fracture fragments are wedged together. This type usually occurs in the humerus and is often less serious and generally treated without surgery.

Patterns. The direction of the trauma or mechanism of injury produces a certain configuration or pattern of fracture. *Reduction* is the restoration of a fractured bone to its normal anatomic position. The pattern of a fracture indicates the nature of the trauma and provides information about the easiest method for reduction. Transverse fractures are caused by simple angulatory forces. A spiral fracture results from a twisting motion, or torque. A transverse fracture is not likely to become displaced or lose its position after it is reduced. On the other hand, spiral, oblique, and comminuted fractures are often unstable and may change position after reduction.

Manifestations

The signs and symptoms of a fracture include pain, tenderness at the site of bone disruption, swelling, loss of function, deformity of the affected part, and abnormal mobility. The deformity varies according to the type of force applied, the area of the bone involved, the type of fracture produced, and the strength and balance of the surrounding muscles.

In long bones, three types of deformities—angulation, shortening, and rotation—are seen. Severely angulated fracture fragments may be felt at the fracture site and often push up against the soft tissue to cause a tenting effect on the skin. Bending forces and unequal muscle pulls cause angulation. Shortening of the extremity occurs as the bone fragments slide and override each other because of the pull of the muscles on the long axis of the extremity (Fig. 45–3). Rotational deformity occurs when the fracture fragments rotate out of their normal longitudinal axis; this can result from rotational strain produced by the fracture or unequal pull by the muscles that are attached to the fracture fragments. A crepitus or grating sound may be heard as the bone fragments rub against each other. In the case of an open fracture, there is bleeding from the wound where the bone protrudes. Blood loss from a pelvic fracture or multiple long bone fractures can cause hypovolemic shock in a trauma victim.

Shortly after the fracture has occurred, nerve function at the fracture site may be temporarily lost. The area may become numb, and the surrounding muscles may become flaccid. This condition has been called *local shock.* During this period, which may last for a few minutes to a half-hour, fractured bones may be reduced with little or no pain. After this brief period, pain sensation returns and, with it, muscle spasms and contractions of the surrounding muscles.

Healing

Bone healing occurs in a manner similar to soft tissue healing. It is, however, a more complex process and takes longer. Although the exact mechanisms of bone healing are open to controversy, five stages of the healing process have been identified: hematoma formation, cellular proliferation, callus formation, ossification, and

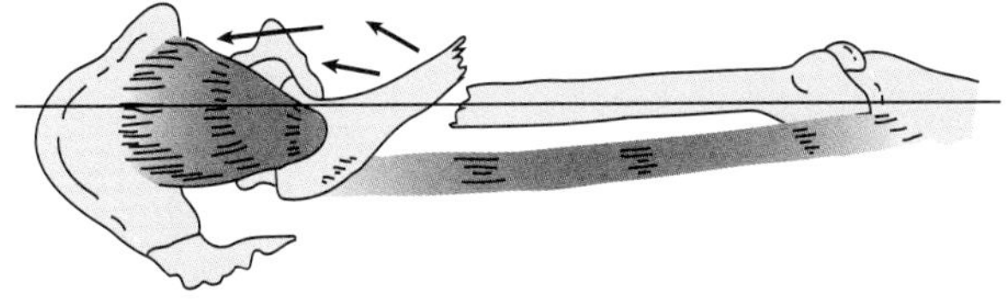

Figure 45–3
Displacement and overriding of fracture fragments of a long bone (femur) caused by severe muscle spasm.

remodeling (Fig. 45–4). The degree of response during each of these stages is in direct proportion to the extent of trauma.

Hematoma Formation. Hematoma formation occurs during the first 48 to 72 hours after fracture. It develops as blood from torn vessels in the bone fragments and surrounding soft tissue leaks between and around the fragments of the fractured bone. As a result of hematoma formation, clotting factors remain in the injured area to initiate the formation of a fibrin meshwork, which serves as a framework for the ingrowth of fibroblasts and new capillary buds. Granulation tissue, the result of fibroblasts and new capillaries, gradually invades and replaces the clot. When a large hematoma develops, healing is delayed because macrophages, platelets, oxygen, and nutrients for callus formation are prevented from entering the area.

Cellular Proliferation. Three layers of bone structure are involved in the cellular proliferation that occurs during bone healing: the periosteum, or outer covering of the bone; the endosteum, or inner covering; and the medullary canal, which contains the bone marrow. During this process, the osteoblasts, or bone-forming cells, multiply and differentiate into a fibrocartilaginous callus. The fibrocartilaginous callus is softer and more flexible than callus. Cellular proliferation begins distal to the fracture, where there is a greater supply of blood. After a few days, a fibrocartilage "collar" becomes evident around the fracture site. The collar edges on either side of the fracture eventually unite to form a bridge, which connects the bone fragments.

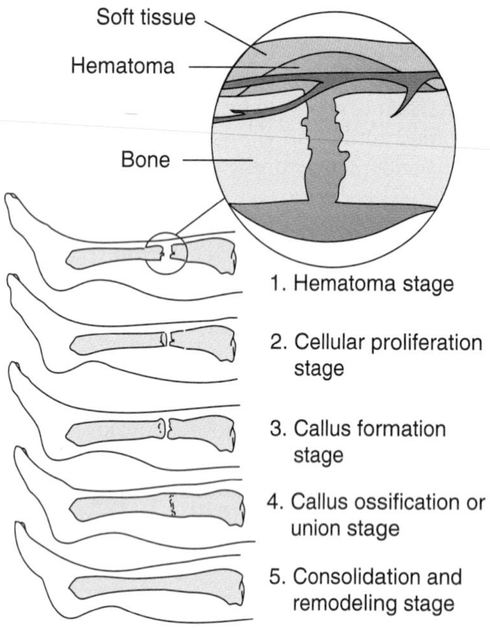

Figure 45–4
Healing of a fracture. During hematoma formation (1), a locally formed clot serves as a fibrin meshwork for subsequent cellular invasion. Cellular proliferation (2) involves the invasion of the hematoma area by fibroblastic and endothelial cells. During callus formation (3), osteoblasts enter the area and produce the osteoid matrix. Callus formation is followed by union (4). The remodeling of the healed fracture is the last stage of the healing process (5).

Callus Formation. During the early stage of callus formation, the fracture becomes "sticky" as osteoblasts continue to move in and through the fibrin bridge to help keep it firm. Cartilage forms at the level of the fracture, where there is less circulation. In areas of the bone with muscle insertion, periosteal circulation is better, bringing in the nutrients necessary to bridge the callus. The bone calcifies as mineral salts are deposited. This stage occurs in 3 to 4 weeks.

Ossification. Ossification involves the final laying down of bone. This is the stage at which the fracture has been bridged and the fracture fragments are firmly united. Mature bone replaces the callus, and the excess callus is gradually resorbed by the osteoclasts (*i.e.,* cells that resorb bone). The fracture site feels firm and immovable and appears united on the radiograph. At this point, it is safe to remove the cast.

Remodeling. Remodeling involves resorption of the excess bony callus that develops within the marrow space and encircling the external aspect of the fracture site. The remodeling process is directed by mechanical stress and direction of weight bearing. It continues according to Wolff's law—bone responds to mechanical stress by becoming thicker and stronger in relation to its function.

Healing Time. Healing time depends on the site of the fracture, the condition of the fracture fragments, hematoma formation, and other local and host factors. In general, fractures of long bones, displaced fractures, and fractures with less surface area heal slower. Function usually returns within 6 months after union is complete. However, return to complete function may take longer.

Factors Affecting Healing. Factors that influence bone healing are those specific to the patient and the following local factors:

* Nature of the injury or the severity of the trauma, including fracture displacement, edema and arterial occlusion with crushing injuries
* Degree of bridge formation that develops during bone healing
* Amount of bone loss (*e.g.,* it may be too great for the healing to bridge the gap)
* Type of bone that is injured (*e.g.,* cancellous bone heals faster than cortical bone)
* Degree of immobilization that is achieved (*e.g.,* movement disrupts the fibrin bridge and cartilage forms instead of bone)

- Local infection, which retards or prevents healing
- Local malignancy, which must be treated before healing can proceed
- Bone necrosis, which prevents blood flow into the fracture site
- Intraarticular fractures (those through a joint), which may heal more slowly and may eventually produce arthritis

Individual factors that may delay bone healing are the patient's age; current medications; debilitating diseases, such as diabetes and rheumatoid arthritis; local stress around the fracture site; circulatory problems, coagulation disorders; and poor nutrition.

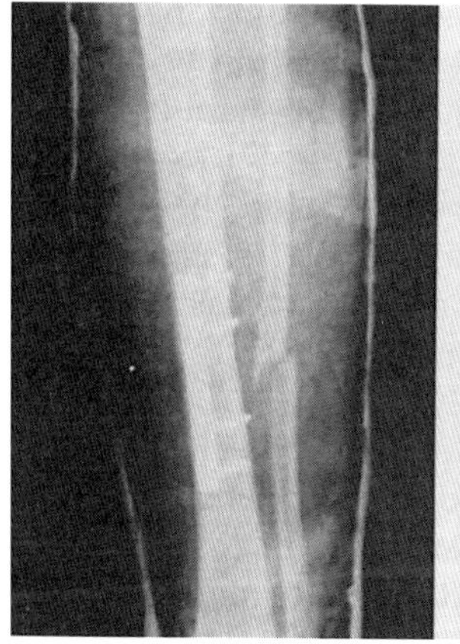
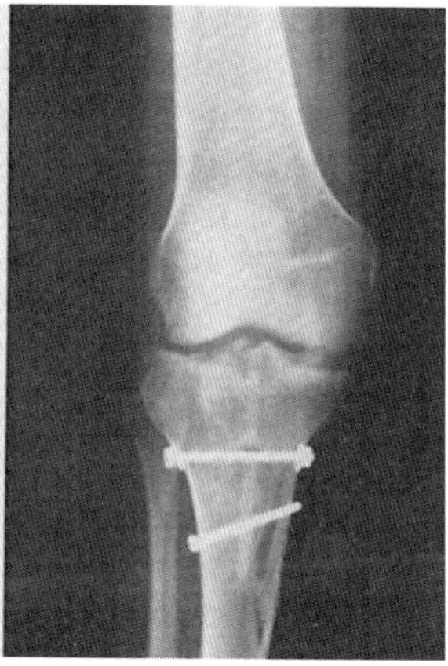

Figure 45–5
(Left) Internal fixation of the tibia with compression plate. **(Right)** Internal fixation of an intraarticular fracture of the upper tibia with a screw and bolt.

Diagnosis and Treatment

A *splint* is a device for immobilizing the movable fragments of a fracture. When a fracture is suspected, the injured part should always be splinted before it is moved. This is essential for preventing further injury.

Diagnosis is the first step in the care of fractures and is based on history and physical manifestations. X-ray examination is used to confirm the diagnosis and direct the treatment. The ease of diagnosis varies with the location and severity of the fracture. In the trauma patient, the presence of other more serious injuries may make diagnosis more difficult. A thorough history includes the mechanism, time, and place of the injury; first recognition of symptoms; and any treatment initiated. A complete history is important, because a delay in seeking treatment or weight bearing on a fracture may have caused further injury or displacement of the fracture.

Treatment of fractures depends on the general condition of the patient, the presence of associated injuries, the location of the fracture, its displacement, and whether the fracture is open or closed. There are three objectives for treatment of fractures: reduction of the fracture, immobilization, and preservation and restoration of the function of the injured part.

Reduction. Reduction of a fracture is directed toward replacing the bone fragments to as near to a normal anatomic position as possible. This can be accomplished by closed manipulation or surgical (open) reduction. Closed manipulation uses methods such as manual pressure and traction. Fractures are held in reduction by external or internal fixation devices. Surgical reduction involves the use of various types of hardware to accomplish internal fixation of the fracture fragments (Fig. 45–5). Primary closure of crush injuries in the extremities is delayed until tissue viability is determined. The wound is first debrided and immobilized with an external fixation device. Reconstruction is done later using cancellous bone grafts, using microvascular composite tissue grafts, or by means of tissue regeneration with distraction devices.[3]

Immobilization. Immobilization prevents movement of the injured parts and is the single most important element in obtaining union of the fracture fragments. Immobilization can be accomplished through the use of external devices, such as splints, casts, external fixation devices, or traction, or by means of internal fixation devices inserted during surgical reduction of the fracture.

Splints are made from many different materials. Metal splints or air splints may be used during transport to a health care facility as a temporary measure until the fracture has been reduced and another form of immobilization instituted. Plaster of Paris splints, which are molded to fit the extremity, work well. Splinting should be done if there is any suspicion of a fracture, because motion of the fracture site can cause pain, bleeding, more soft tissue damage, and nerve or blood vessel compression. If the fracture has sharp fragments, movement can cause perforation of the skin and conversion of a closed fracture into an open one. When a splint is applied to an extremity, it should extend from the joint above the fracture site to the joint below it.

Casts, which are made of plaster or synthetic material, are commonly used to immobilize fractures of the extremities. They are often applied with a joint in partial flexion to prevent rotation of the fracture fragments. Without this flexion, the extremity, which is essentially a cylinder, tends to rotate within the cylindrical structure of the cast.

The application of a cast brings the risk of impaired circulation to the extremity because of blood vessel compression. A cast applied shortly after a fracture may not be large enough to accommodate the swelling that inevitably occurs in the hours that follow. After a cast is applied, the peripheral circulation must be observed carefully until this danger has passed. If the circulation becomes inadequate, the parts that are exposed at the distal end of the cast (*i.e.,* the toes with a leg cast and the fingers with an arm cast) usually become cold and cyanotic or pale. An increase in pain may occur initially, followed by paresthesia (*i.e.,* tingling or abnormal sensation) or anesthesia as the sensory neurons that supply the area are affected. There is a decrease in the amplitude or absence of the pulse in areas where the arteries can be palpated. Capillary refill time, which is assessed by applying pressure to the fingernail and observing the rate of blood return, is prolonged to longer than 3 seconds. This condition demands immediate measures, such as splitting the cast, to restore the circulation and prevent permanent damage to the extremity. A casted extremity should always be elevated above the level of the heart for the first 24 hours to minimize swelling.

A brace may be used after a cast is removed or instead of a cast, as with a tibial stress fracture.

With *external fixation devices,* pins or screws are inserted directly into the bone above and below the fracture site. They are secured to a metal frame and adjusted to align the fracture. This method of treatment is used primarily for open fractures, infections such as osteomyelitis and septic joints, unstable closed fractures, and limb lengthening.

Limb-lengthening devices are used for traumatic losses of bone and soft tissue. Limb-lengthening systems, such as the Ilizarov external fixator (Fig. 45–6), are used to lengthen or widen bones, correct angular or rotational defects, or immobilize fractures.[4] The apparatus is applied with a surgical technique called a corticotomy, which is a percutaneous osteotomy that preserves the periosteal and endosteal tissues. A circular external apparatus is attached to bone by tensioned Kirschner wires. The corticotomy site is gradually distracted or pulled apart by about 1 mm per day until the desired length is achieved. The continuous distraction activates regeneration of bone, soft tissue, nerves, and blood vessels. New bone forms (*i.e.,* osteogenesis) in the distraction gap. This newly formed bone can fill posttraumatic defects or those formed after resection for osteomyelitis, consolidate nonunions, regenerate bone in limb lengthening, correct deformities, and eliminate the need for bone grafting. The apparatus is left on until the desired length is achieved and consolidation is complete.

Another method for achieving immobility and maintaining reduction is *traction.* Traction is a pulling force applied to an extremity or part of the body while a counterforce, or countertraction, pulls in the opposite direction. Countertraction is usually exerted by the body's weight on the bed. Traction is used to maintain alignment of the fracture fragments and reduce muscle spasm.

Effective traction prevents movement of the fracture site. Fractures caused by trauma are associated with muscle injury and spasm. These muscle contractions cause overriding and displacement of the bone fragments, particularly when the fractures affect long bones. The five goals of traction therapy are to correct and maintain the skeletal alignment of entire bones or joints; to reduce pressure on a joint surface; to correct, lessen, or prevent deformities such as contractures and dislocations; to decrease muscle spasm; and to immobilize a part to promote healing. Traction may be used as a temporary measure before surgery or as a primary treatment method.

There are three types of traction: manual traction, skin traction, and skeletal traction. *Manual traction* con-

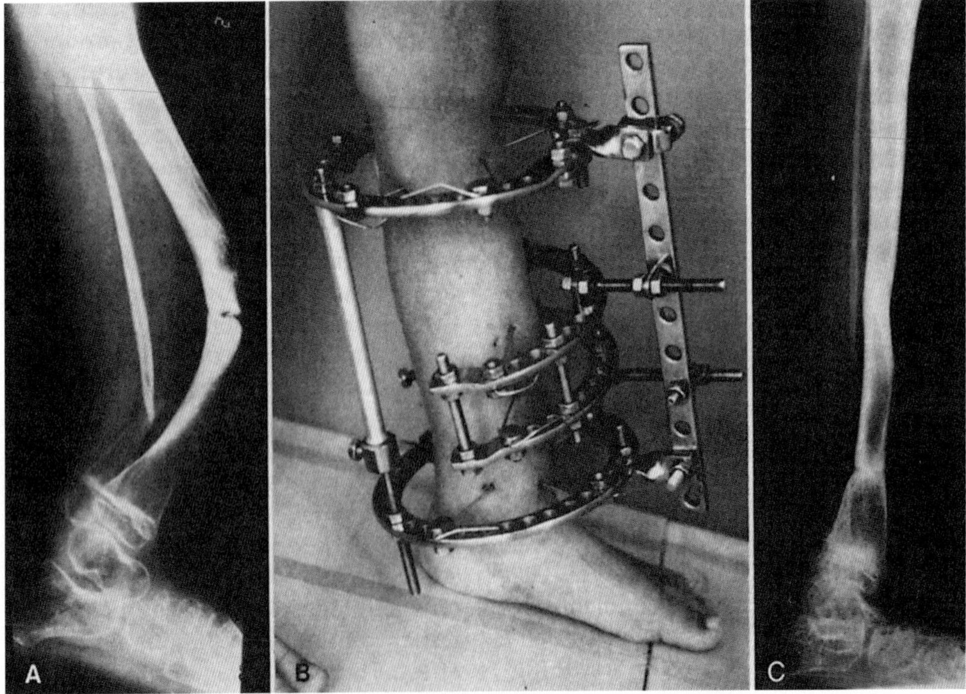

Figure 45–6
Ilizarov device used to treat a tibial fracture with anterolateral bow and medullary sclerosis: before (**A**), with Ilizarov device in place (**B**), and three-year follow-up lateral roentgenograph (**C**). (Paley D., Catagni M, Argnani F. et al. [1992]. Treatment of congenital pseudoarthrosis of the tibia using Ilizarov technique. *Clinical Orthopedics and Related Research, 280,* 84)

sists of a steady, firm pull that is exerted by the hands. It is a temporary measure used to manipulate a fracture during closed reduction, for support of a neck injury during transport when a cervical spine fracture is suspected, or for reduction of a dislocated joint. *Skin traction* is a pulling force applied to the skin and soft tissue. It is accomplished by strips of adhesive, flannel, or foam secured to the injured part.

Skeletal traction is a pulling force applied directly to the bone. Pins, wires, or tongs are inserted through the skin and subcutaneous tissue into the bone distal to the fracture site. Skeletal traction provides an excellent pull and can be used for long periods with large amounts of weight. It is commonly used for fractures of the femur, the humerus, and the cervical spine (*e.g.*, Crutchfield tongs applied to the skull). Skeletal traction is also used in maintaining alignment of fractures that are casted and in certain types of reconstructive foot surgery. Pin tract infection is a complication of skeletal traction. Larger pins are associated with a greater risk for infection.

Preservation and Restoration of Function. During the period of immobilization required for fracture healing, the preservation and restoration of the function of muscles and joints are an ongoing process in the unaffected and the affected extremities. Exercises designed to preserve function, maintain muscle strength, and reduce joint stiffness should be started early. Active range of motion, in which the person moves the extremity, is done on unaffected extremities, and isometric, or muscle-tensing, exercises are done on the affected extremities. In some instances, an electrical muscle stimulator is applied directly to the skin to stimulate isometric muscle contraction as a means of preventing disuse atrophy. After the fracture has healed, a program of physical therapy may be necessary. However, the most important factor in restoring function is the person's own active exercises.

Muscles tend to atrophy during immobilization because of lack of use. Joints stiffen as muscles and tendons contract and shorten. The degree of muscle atrophy and joint stiffness depends on several factors. In adults, the degree of atrophy and muscle stiffness are directly related to the length of immobilization, with longer periods of immobility resulting in greater stiffness. Children have a natural tendency to move on their own, and this movement maintains muscle and joint function. They usually have less atrophy and recover sooner after the source of immobilization has been removed. Associated soft tissue injury, infection, and preexisting joint disease increase the risk of stiffness. Although limbs are immobilized in a functional position, casts are removed as soon as fracture healing has taken place so that joint stiffness does not occur.

Complications

The complications of fractures can be divided into two groups: the early complications associated with loss of skeletal continuity, injury from bone fragments, pressure from swelling and hemorrhage, or development of fat emboli and the complications associated with fracture healing. The early complications of fractures depend on the severity of the fracture and the area of the body that is involved. For example, bone fragments from a skull fracture may cause injury to brain tissue, or multiple rib fractures may lead to a flail chest and respiratory insufficiency. With flail chest, the chest wall on the fractured side becomes so unstable that it may move in the opposite direction as the person breathes (*i.e.*, in during inspiration and out during expiration).

Compartment Syndrome. Compartment syndrome is the result of increased pressure within a limited anatomic space that compromises circulation and threatens the viability and function of the nerves and muscles within a closed compartment (see Chapter 17). It can be acute or chronic. Acute compartment syndrome can occur after a fracture or crushing injury when excessive swelling around the site of injury results in increased pressure (30 mm Hg or more) within a closed compartment. This increase in pressure occurs because fascia, which covers and separates muscles, is inelastic and unable to compensate for the extreme swelling.

The condition causes severe pain because of passive stretching of soft tissue and skin. Nerve compression may cause changes in sensation (*e.g.*, paresthesias such as burning or tingling or loss of sensation), diminished reflexes, and eventually the loss of motor function. Compression of blood vessels may cause muscle ischemia and loss of function. Muscles and nerves may be permanently damaged if the pressure is not relieved. In contrast to the diminished or absent pulses that occur when ischemia is caused by a tight bandage or cast, the arterial pulses are typically normal in compartment syndrome.[5] The compartment syndrome is more common with crushing injuries, in closed fractures, and when external compression of a limb produces a tourniquet effect. The most common sites are the four compartments of the lower leg (*i.e.*, deep posterior, superficial posterior, lateral, and anterior compartments) and the dorsal and volar compartments of the forearm.

Treatment is directed at reducing the compression of blood vessels and nerves. Constrictive dressings and casts are loosened. Intracompartmental pressure can be measured by means of a catheter or needle inserted into the compartment. A fasciotomy, or transection of the fascia that is restricting the muscle compartment, may be required when the pressure in the area rises above 30 mm Hg, which is roughly equal to the perfusion pressure in the capillary beds. Delay in diagnoses and treatment of compartment syndrome can lead to irreversible nerve and muscle damage.[6]

Chronic compartment syndrome occurs most often in young adults after activity that involves repetitive strain on lower extremities, such as long-distance running or marching. Although the exact mechanism is unclear, exercise causes an increase in compartment size.[6] The compartment is stretched and becomes inflamed. The fascia is scarred, less elastic, and unable to compensate for further compartment volume. Pain is experienced during activity. Tissue pressure measurements are usually done. Conservative measures, such as shoe orthotics, stretching exercises, and activity modification are attempted. A fasciotomy is done for persistent symptoms.

Fat Emboli. Fat emboli result from intracellular fat globules in the lung parenchyma and peripheral circulation after a long-bone fracture or other major trauma. There are two theories about the origin of fat emboli: mechanical and biochemical. The mechanical theory is that fat globules are released from the bone marrow or subcutaneous tissue at the fracture site into the venous system through torn veins and are lodged in the lungs, brain, or other organs (*i.e.*, mechanical theory).[7] The biochemical theory postulates that the fat emboli develop intravascularly secondary to an alteration in lipid stability caused by increased release of tissue lipases, catecholamines, glucagon, or other steroid hormones in response to the stress of injury.[8] The circulating free fatty acids affect the pneumonocytes, producing abnormalities in gas exchange (*i.e.*, biochemical theory). The mechanical and biochemical theories are not mutually exclusive. There is support for the mechanical theory in studies that have correlated the severity of pulmonary failure with the quantity of fat embolization.[9] Fat emboli may also be caused by exogenous sources of fat, such as blood transfusions, intravenous fat emulsions, or bone marrow transplantation.

Fat embolism syndrome (FES) describes a respiratory deficiency state caused by decreased alveolar diffusion of oxygen because of fat embolism. Three degrees of severity are seen: subclinical, overt clinical, and fulminating. Although the subclinical and overt clinical forms of FES respond well to treatment, the fulminating form is often fatal. There are three possible outcomes when fat emboli enter the pulmonary circulation: (1) small emboli can mold to vessel caliber, pass through the lung, and enter the systemic circulation, where they are trapped in the tissues or eliminated through the kidney; (2) the fat particles can be broken down by alveolar cells and eliminated through sputum; or (3) local lipolysis can occur with the release of free fatty acids.[10] Free fatty acids cause direct injury to the alveolar capillary membrane, which leads to hemorrhagic interstitial pneumonitis with disruption of surfactant production and development of the adult respiratory distress syndrome. The fat globules also become coated with platelets, causing thrombocytopenia. Serotonin released by the sequestered platelets causes bronchospasm and vasodilatation.

Clinically, the incidence of fat embolization is related to fractures of bones containing the most marrow (*i.e.*, long bones and the bones of the pelvis). Although fat embolization occurs with fractures or operative fixation of fractures, FES only occurs in a small percentage of cases. Initial symptoms begin to develop within a few hours to 3 to 4 days after injury and do not appear beyond 1 week after the injury. The first symptoms include a subtle change in behavior and signs of disorientation resulting from emboli in the cerebral circulation combined with respiratory depression. There may be complaints of substernal chest pain and dyspnea accompanied by tachycardia and a low-grade fever. Diaphoresis, pallor, and cyanosis become evident as respiratory function deteriorates. A petechial rash that does not blanch with pressure often occurs 2 to 3 days after the injury. This rash is usually found on the anterior chest, axillae, neck, and shoulders. It may also appear on the soft palate and conjunctiva. The rash is thought to be related to embolization of the skin capillaries or thrombocytopenia.

An important part of the treatment of fat emboli is early diagnosis. Arterial blood gases should be assayed immediately after recognition of clinical manifestations. In a person suspected of having FES, a sustained arterial oxygen tension (PO_2) of less than 60 mm Hg, an arterial carbon dioxide tension (PCO_2) of more than 55 mm Hg, or a blood pH of less than 7.3 is diagnostic.[11] Urinary fat bodies are so common after injury that they are of no diagnostic value. Treatment is directed toward correcting hypoxemia and maintaining adequate fluid balance. Mechanical ventilation may be required. Corticosteroid drugs are administered to decrease the inflammatory response of lung tissues, decrease the edema, stabilize the lipid membranes to reduce lipolysis, and combat the bronchospasm. Corticosteroids are also given prophylactically to high-risk persons. The only preventive approach to FES is early stabilization of the fracture.

Impaired Healing. *Union* of a fracture has occurred when the fracture is solid enough to withstand normal stresses and it is clinically and radiologically safe to remove the external fixation. In children, fractures generally heal within 4 to 6 weeks; in adolescents, they heal within 6 to 8 weeks; and in adults, they heal within 10 to 18 weeks.

Delayed union is the failure of a fracture to unite within the normal period (*e.g.*, 20 weeks for a fracture of the tibia or femur in an adult). The treatment for delayed union consists in determining and correcting the cause of the delay. *Malunion* is healing with deformity, angulation, or rotation that is visible on x-ray films. It is usually treated by surgery. Early aggressive treatment, especially of the hand, can prevent malunion and result in earlier alignment and return of function. *Nonunion* is failure to produce union and cessation of the processes of bone repair. It is seen most often in the tibia, especially with open fractures or crushing injuries. It is characterized by mobility of the fracture site and pain on weight bearing. Muscle atrophy and loss of range of motion may also occur. Nonunion is usually established 6 to 12 months after the time of the fracture. The complications of fracture healing are summarized in Table 45–1.

Treatment methods for impaired bone healing encompass surgical interventions, including bone grafts, bracing, external fixation, or electrical stimulation of the bone ends. Electrical stimulation is thought to stimulate the osteoblasts to lay down a network of bone. Three types of commercial bone growth stimulators are available: a noninvasive model, which is placed outside the cast; a semi-noninvasive model, in which pins are inserted around the fracture site; and a totally implantable

TABLE 45-1
Complications of Fracture Healing

Complication	Manifestations	Contributing Factors
Delayed union	Failure of fracture to heal within predicted time as determined by x-ray	Large displaced fracture Inadequate immobilization Large hematoma Infection at fracture site Excessive loss of bone Inadequate circulation
Malunion	Deformity at fracture site Deformity or angulation on x-ray	Inadequate reduction Malalignment of fracture at time of immobilization
Nonunion	Failure of bone to heal before the process of bone repair stops Evidence on x-ray Motion at fracture site Pain on weight bearing	Inadequate reduction Mobility at fracture site Severe trauma Bone fragment separation Soft tissue between bone fragments Infection Extensive loss of bone Inadequate circulation Malignancy Bone necrosis Noncompliance with restrictions

type, in which a cathode coil is wound around the bone at the fracture site and is operated by a battery pack implanted under the skin. The Ilizarov method of circular external fixation is being used with increasing frequency to treat nonunions, especially those that are infected.

In summary, many external physical agents can cause trauma to the musculoskeletal system. Particular factors, such as environments, activity, or age, can place a person at greater risk for injury. Some soft tissue injuries such as contusions, hematomas, and lacerations are relatively minor and easily treated. Muscle strains and ligamentous sprains are caused by mechanical overload on the connective tissue. They heal more slowly than the minor soft tissue injuries and require some degree of immobilization. Healing of soft tissue begins within 4 to 5 days of the injury and is primarily the function of fibroblasts, which produce collagen. Joint dislocation is caused by trauma to the supporting structures. Repeated trauma to the joint can cause articular softening (*i.e.*, chondromalacia) or the separation of small pieces of bone or cartilage, called loose bodies, within the joint.

Fractures occur when more stress is placed on a bone than the bone can absorb. The nature of the stress determines the type of fracture and the character of the resulting bone fragments. Healing of fractures is a complex process that takes place in five stages: hematoma formation, cellular proliferation, callus formation, ossification, and remodeling. For satisfactory healing to take place, the affected bone has to be reduced and immobilized. This is accomplished by a surgically implanted internal fixation device or devices such as splints, casts, or traction or external fixation apparatus. The complications associated with fractures can occur early when soft tissue, blood vessels, and nerves are damaged or later when the healing process is interrupted. Local factors related to the healing environment and the person's general physical condition affect the healing process.

Bone Infections

After you have completed this section of the chapter, you should be able to meet the following objectives:

- Explain the implications of bone infection
- Describe how an acute form of osteomyelitis becomes chronic

Bone infections are difficult to treat and eradicate. Their effects can be devastating; they can cause pain, disability, and deformity. Chronic bone infections may drain for years because of a sinus tract. This occurs when a passageway develops from an abscess or cavity within the bone to an opening through the skin.

Iatrogenic Bone Infections

Iatrogenic bone infections are those inadvertently brought about by surgery or other treatment. These infections include complications of pin tract infection in skeletal traction, septic (infected) joints in joint replacement surgery, and wound infection after any surgery. Measures to prevent these infections include

(1) preparation of the skin to reduce bacterial growth before surgery or insertion of traction devices or wires; (2) strict operating room protocols, including disinfection of the operative site and a wide surrounding field with draping to prevent egress of the patient's and operating room personnel's flora into the area, presence of laminar air flow systems, use of hoods for operating room personnel, and limiting the number of personnel in the room; (3) prophylactic use of antibiotics, including topical wound irrigation; and (4) maintenance of sterile technique after surgery when working with drainage tubes and dressing changes. Because of the danger of infection, orthopedic wounds are kept covered with a sterile dressing until they are closed.

Osteomyelitis

Osteomyelitis represents an acute or chronic pyogenic infection of the bone. The term *osteo* refers to bone, and *myelo* refers to the marrow cavity, both of which are involved in this disease. Osteomyelitis can be caused by hematogenous (through the bloodstream) seeding, direct extension, or direct contamination of an open fracture or wound. In most cases, *Staphylococcus aureus* is the infecting organism.[12] *S. aureus* possess the ability to adhere to the connective tissue elements of bone through the elaboration of extracellular polysaccharides.

The most common cause of osteomyelitis is the direct contamination of bone from an open wound. It may be the result of an open fracture, a gunshot wound, or a puncture wound. Inadequate irrigation or debridement, introduction of foreign material into the wound, and extensive tissue injury increase the bone's susceptibility to infection. If the infection is not sufficiently treated, the acute infection may become chronic. Osteomyelitis may also occur as a complication of surgery, such as in the sternum after open heart surgery or in extremities after bone allograft or total joint replacement.

Acute Hematogenous Osteomyelitis

Acute hematogenous osteomyelitis occurs as the result of localization of a bloodborne infection in the bone. It is seen most commonly in children younger than 10 years of age.[13]

In children, it commonly begins in the metaphyseal region of long bones and is usually preceded by staphylococcal or streptococcal infections of the skin, sinuses, teeth, or middle ear. Thrombosis occurring as the result of local trauma may predispose to localization of the infection consequent to bacteremia.[13]

In the adult, hematogenous osteomyelitis usually affects the axial skeleton and the irregular bones in the wrist and ankle. It is most common in debilitated patients and in those with a history of chronic skin infections, chronic urinary tract infections, and intravenous drug use and in those who are immunologically suppressed. Intravenous drug users are at risk for infections with *Streptococcus* and *Pseudomonas*.

The condition usually manifests as an acute febrile systemic illness lasting 48 hours or less and accompanied by the signs of local bone involvement. Although the incidence of the acute form of osteomyelitis has declined, there is an apparent increase in the subacute form.[13b] Subacute osteomyelitis has an insidious onset in which symptoms are typically present for 2 weeks or more before diagnosis. The infection generally begins in the metaphysis of the bone where the nutrient artery channels terminate and the blood flow is sluggish. Because of the bone's rigid structure, there is little room for swelling, and the purulent exudate that forms finds its way to the surface of the bone to form a subperiosteal abscess. The blood supply to the bone may become obstructed by septic thrombi, in which case the ischemic bone becomes necrotic. It separates from the viable surrounding bone to form a fragment of bone known as a sequestrum (Fig. 45–7).

The signs and symptoms of acute hematogenous osteomyelitis are those of bacteremia accompanied by symptoms referable to the site of the bone lesion. There is often pain on movement of the affected extremity, loss of movement, and local tenderness followed by redness and swelling. X-ray studies may appear normal initially, but they show evidence of periosteal elevation and increased osteoclastic activity after an abscess has formed. Changes are evident on a bone scan 10 to 14 days before any changes are seen on x-ray films.

The treatment of acute osteomyelitis begins with identification of the causative organism through blood cultures, aspiration cultures, and Gram's stain. Antibiotics are first given intravenously and then orally. The amount of time that the affected limb needs to be rested and pain control measures used are based on the person's symptoms. Debridement and surgical drainage may also be necessary.

Chronic Osteomyelitis

Chronic osteomyelitis has long been recognized as a disease. The incidence, however, has decreased in the last century because of improvements in surgical techniques and antibiotic therapy. Chronic osteomyelitis includes all inflammatory processes of bone, excluding those in rheumatic diseases, that are caused by microorganisms. It may be the result of delayed or inadequate treatment of acute hematogenous osteomyelitis or osteomyelitis caused by direct contamination of bone. Acute osteomyelitis is considered to have become chronic when the infection persists beyond 6 to 8 weeks or when the acute process has been adequately treated and is expected to resolve but does not. Chronic osteomyelitis can persist for years; it may appear spontaneously, after a minor trauma, or when resistance is lowered.

The hallmark feature of chronic osteomyelitis is the presence of infected dead bone, a sequestrum, that has separated from the living bone. A sheath of new bone, called the involucrum, forms around the dead bone. Radiologic techniques such as x-ray films, bone scans, and sinograms are used to identify the infected site.

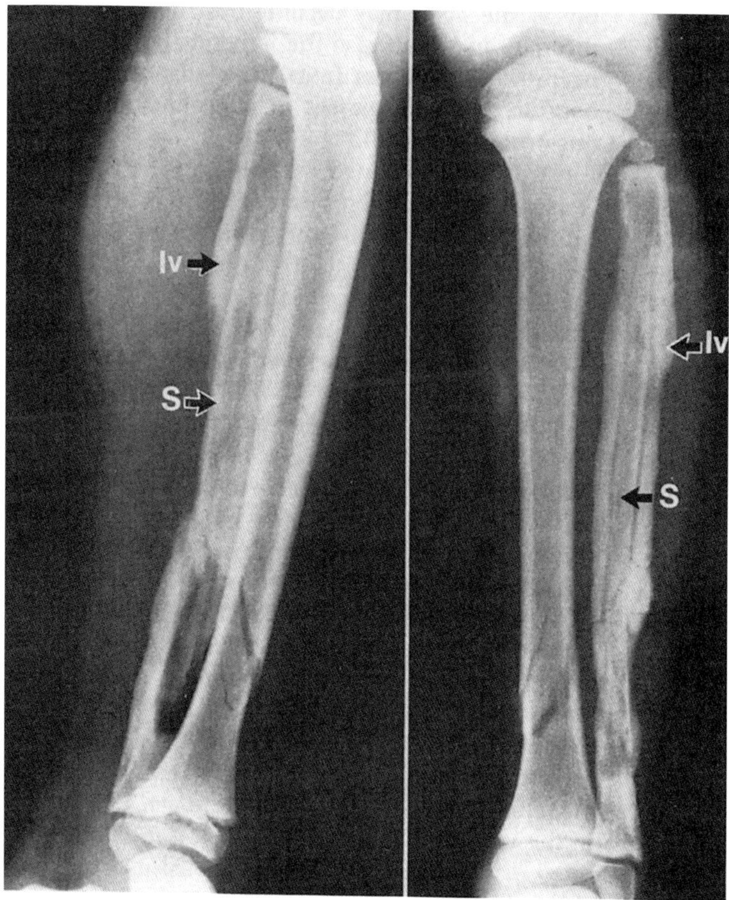

Figure 45–7
Hematogenous osteomyelitis of the fibula of 3 months' duration. The entire shaft has been deprived of its blood supply and has become a sequestrum (S) surrounded by new immature bone, involucrum (Iv). Pathologic fractures are present in the lower tibia and fibula.

Chronic osteomyelitis or infection around a total joint prosthesis can be difficult to diagnose, because the classic signs of infection are not apparent and the blood leukocyte count may not be elevated. A subclinical infection may exist for years. Bone scans are used in conjunction with bone biopsy for a definitive diagnosis.

The treatment of chronic bone infections begins with wound cultures to identify the microorganism and its sensitivity to antibiotic therapy. Although intravenous antibiotic therapy is still the primary treatment, antibiotic-laden beads, implanted at the site are an effective measure, especially for open fractures. The goal in selecting antimicrobial treatment for osteomyelitis is to use the drug with the highest bactericidal activity and least toxicity and at the lowest cost.[14] Methicillin-resistant *S. aureus* has become increasingly common, especially in persons with total joint replacements, those treated in intensive care units or trauma centers, residents of long-term care facilities, and patients with indwelling catheters and intravascular devices.[15]

Initial antibiotic therapy is followed by surgery to remove foreign bodies (*e.g.*, metal plates, screws) or sequestra and by long-term antibiotic therapy. Immobilization of the affected part is usually necessary, with restriction of weight bearing on a lower extremity. External fixation devices are used. The Ilizarov method has been used in Russia for osteomyelitis since 1951.[16] With this method, chronic refractory osteomyelitis can frequently be cured because the mass regeneration of new bone within the focus of infection serves as a highly vascularized bone graft.[17]

Tuberculosis of the Bone or Joint

Tuberculosis can spread from one part of the body, such as the lungs or the lymph nodes, to the bones and joints. When this happens, it is called extrapulmonary or miliary tuberculosis. It is caused by *Mycobacterium tuberculosis*. The disease is localized and progressively destructive but not as contagious as primary pulmonary tuberculosis. In about 50% of cases, it affects the vertebrae, but it is also frequently seen in the hip and knee.[18] Tuberculosis can also affect the joints and soft tissues. The disease is characterized by bone destruction and abscess formation. Local symptoms include pain, immobility, and muscle atrophy; joint swelling, mild fever, and leukocytosis may also occur. Diagnosis is confirmed by a positive culture. The most important part of the treatment is antituberculosis drug therapy.

Because of improved methods to prevent and treat tuberculosis, its incidence had diminished in recent decades. However, the incidence is on the rise again: in 1986, there was an increase of 2.5%, the first substantial rise since 1952.[19] Tuberculosis has increased because of the spread of disease in communal settings (*e.g.*, jails, shelters, nursing homes), the human immunodeficiency virus epidemic, and the influx of immigrants who have come to the United States from countries where the disease is endemic.[20] Unfortunately, the diagnosis of tuberculosis in the bones and joints may still be missed.

In summary, bone infections occur because of the direct or indirect invasion of the skeletal circulation by microorganisms, most commonly the bacterium *S. aureus*. Tuberculosis of the bone, which is characterized by bone destruction and abscess formation, is caused by spread of the infection from the lungs or lymph nodes. Osteomyelitis, or infection of the bone and marrow, can be an acute or chronic disease. Acute osteomyelitis is seen most often as a result of the direct contamination of bone by a foreign object. Chronic osteomyelitis is a long-term process that can recur spontaneously at any time throughout a person's life. The incidence of all types of bone infection has been dramatically reduced since the advent of antibiotic therapy. Iatrogenic infections are those inadvertently brought about by surgery or other treatments.

Osteonecrosis

After you have completed this section of the chapter, you should be able to meet the following objectives:

- Define *osteonecrosis*
- Cite four major causes of osteonecrosis
- Characterize the blood supply of bone and relate to the pathologic features of the condition
- Describe the methods used in diagnosis and treatment of the condition

Osteonecrosis, or death of a segment of bone, is a condition caused by the interruption of blood supply to the marrow, medullary bone, or cortex. It is a relatively common disorder and can occur in the medullary cavity of the metaphysis and the subchondral region of the epiphysis, especially in the proximal femur, distal femur, and proximal humerus.[12] It is a common complicating disorder of Legg-Calvé-Perthes disease, sickle cell disease, steroid therapy, and hip surgery. The rates of osteonecrosis among persons treated with corticosteroids range from 5% to 25%. More than 10% of 500,000 joint replacements performed annually in the United States are for treatment of osteonecrosis.

Although bone necrosis results from ischemia, the mechanisms producing the ischemia are varied and include mechanical vascular interruption such as occurs with a fracture; thrombosis and embolism (*e.g.*, sickle cell disease, nitrogen bubbles caused by inadequate decompression during deep sea diving); vessel injury (*e.g.*, vasculitis, radiation therapy); and increased intraosseous pressure with vascular compression (*e.g.*, steroid-induced osteonecrosis). In many cases, the cause of the necrosis is uncertain. Other than fracture, the most common causes of bone necrosis are idiopathic (*i.e.*, those of unknown cause) and prior steroid therapy. Chart 45–1 lists disorders associated with osteonecrosis.

Bone has a rich blood supply that varies from site to site. The flow in the medullary portion of bone originates in nutrient vessels from an interconnecting plexus that supplies the marrow, trabecular bone, and endosteal half of the cortex. The outer cortex receives its blood supply from periosteal, muscular, metaphyseal, and epiphyseal vessels that surround the bone. Some bony sites such as the head of the femur have only limited collateral circulation so that interruption of the flow, such as with a hip fracture, can cause necrosis of a substantial portion of medullary and cortical bone and irreversible damage.

The pathologic features of bone necrosis are the same, regardless of cause. The site of the lesion is related to the vessels involved. There is necrosis of cancellous bone and marrow. The cortex is usually not involved because of collateral blood flow. In subchondral infarcts (*i.e.*, ischemia below the cartilage), a triangular or wedge-shaped segment of tissue that has the subchondral bone plate as its base and the center of the epiphysis as its apex undergo necrosis. When medullary infarcts occur in fatty marrow, death of bone results in calcium release and necrosis of fat cells with the formation of free fatty acids. Released calcium forms an insoluble "soap" with free fatty acids. Because bone lacks mechanisms for resolving the infarct, the lesions remain for life.

One of the most frequent causes of osteonecrosis is that associated with administration of corticosteroids.[21,22] Despite numerous studies, the mechanism of steroid-induced osteonecrosis remains unclear. The con-

CHART **45-1**
Causes of Osteonecrosis

Mechanical disruption of blood vessels
- Fractures
- Legg-Calvé-Perthes disease
- Blount's disease

Thrombosis and embolism
- Sickle cell disease
- Nitrogen bubbles in decompression sickness

Vessel injury
- Vasculitis
- Connective tissue disease
    - Systemic lupus erythematosus
    - Rheumatoid arthritis
- Radiation therapy
- Gaucher's disease

Increased introsseous pressure
- Steroid-induced osteonecrosis

dition may develop following the administration of very high, short-term doses; during long-term treatment; or even from intraarticular injection. Although the risk increases with the dose and duration of treatment, it is difficult to predict who will be affected. The interval between corticosteroid administration and onset of symptoms is rarely less than 6 months and may be more than 3 years. There is no satisfactory method for preventing progression of the disease.

The symptoms associated with bone necrosis are varied and depend on the extent of infarction. Typically, subchondral infarcts cause chronic pain that is initially associated with activity but that gradually becomes more progressive until it is experienced at rest. Subchondral infarcts often collapse and predispose the patient to severe secondary osteoarthritis.

Diagnosis of osteonecrosis is based on history, physical findings, radiographic findings, and the results of special imaging studies, including CT scans and technetium-99m bone scans. MRI is particularly effective in the diagnosis of osteonecrosis. Plain radiographs are used to define and classify the course of the disease, particularly of the hip.

Treatment of osteonecrosis depends on the underlying pathology. In some cases, only short-term immobilization, nonsteroidal antiinflammatory drugs, exercises, and limitation in weight bearing are used. Osteonecrosis of the hip is particularly difficult to treat. In persons with early disease, limitation of weight bearing through the use of crutches may allow the condition to stabilize. Although several surgical approaches have been used, the most definitive treatment of advanced osteonecrosis of the knee or hip is prosthetic replacement.

In summary, osteonecrosis is a common condition that has long been recognized but is not fully understood. Death of bone is caused by disruption in the blood supply from intravascular or extravascular processes. Sites with poor collateral circulation, such as the femoral head are most seriously affected. Causative factors include corticosteroids. Symptoms include pain that varies in severity, depending on the extent of infarction. Total joint replacement is the most frequently used treatment for advanced osteonecrosis.

REFERENCES

1. Centers for Disease Control. (1987). Bicycle-related injuries: Data from the National Electronic Injury Surveillance System. *Morbidity and Mortality Weekly Report* 36, 269.
2. Wright P.H., Brashear H.R. (1980). The local response to trauma. In Wilson F.C. (Ed.). *The musculoskeletal system: Basic processes and disorders* (2nd ed., p. 264). Philadelphia: J.B. Lippincott.
3. Martini Z., Castaman E. (1987). Tissue regeneration in the reconstruction of lost bone and soft tissue in the limbs: A preliminary report. *British Journal of Plastic Surgery* 40, 142.
4. Paley D., Catagni M., Argnani F., et al. (1992). Treatment of congenital pseudoarthrosis of the tibia using Ilizarov technique. *Clinical Orthopaedics and Related Research* 280, 81.
5. Ross D. (1996). Chronic compartment syndrome. *Orthopedic Nursing* 15 (3), 23.
6. Rorabeck C.H. (1984). The treatment of compartment syndromes of the leg. *Journal of Bone and Joint Surgery, British* 66, 93.
7. Fabian T.C. (1993). Unraveling the fat embolism syndrome. *New England Journal of Medicine* 329 (13), 961.
8. Maylan J.A., Evenson M.A. (1979). Diagnosis and treatment of fat embolism. *Annual Review of Medicine* 28, 885.
9. Pell A.C.H., Hughes D., Keating J., Christie J., Buscittil A., Sutherland G.R. (1993). Fulminating fat embolism syndrome caused by paradoxical embolism through patent foramen ovale. *New England Journal of Medicine* 329 (13), 926.
10. Oldman G.L., Weise W. (1979). Fat embolism. *Arizona Medicine* 36, 885.
11. Lindeque B.G.P., Schoeman H.S., Dommisse G.F., et al. (1987). Fat embolism and the fat embolism syndrome. *Journal of Bone and Joint Surgery* 1, 128.
12. Cotran R.S., Kumar V., Robbins S.L.(1994). *Robbins pathologic basis of disease* (5th ed., pp. 1230–1232, 1229–1230). Philadelphia: W.B. Saunders.
13. Narashimhan N., Marks M. (1996) Osteomyelitis and septic arthritis. In Behrman R.F., Kliegman R.M., Arvin A.M (Eds.). *Nelson textbook of pediatrics* (15th ed., pp. 724–728). Philadelphia: W.B. Saunders.

13b.Jones N.S., Anderson D.J., Stiles P.J. (1987). Osteomyelitis in a general hospital. *Journal of Bone and Joint Surgery, British* 69, 779.

14. Mader J.T., Landon G.C., Calhoun J. (1993). Antimicrobial treatment of osteomyelitis. *Clinical Orthopaedics* 195, 87.
15. Bitar C.M., Mayahll C.G., Lamb V.A., et al. (1987). Outbreak due to methicillin-and-rifampin resistant *Staphylococcus aureus*: Epidemiology and eradication of the resistant strain from the hospital. *Infection Control* 8 (1), 15.
16. Ilizarov G.A., Ledyaev V.I. (1992). The replacement of long tubular bone defects by lengthening distraction osteotomy of one of the fragments. *Clinical Orthopaedics and Related Research* 280, 7.
17. Green S.A. (1991). Osteomyelitis: The Ilizarov perspective. *Orthopedic Clinics of North America* 22 (3), 515.
18. Childs S.G. (1996). Osteoarticular *Mycobacterium tuberculosis*. *Orthopedic Nursing* 15 (3), 28.
19. Tuberculosis, final data—United States, 1986. (1988). *Morbidity and Mortality Weekly Report* 36, 817.
20. Alland D., Kalkut G., Moss A., et al. (1994). Transmission of tuberculosis in New York City: An analysis of DNA fingerprinting and epidemiologic methods. *New England Journal of Medicine* 330 (24), 1710.
21. Mankin H.J. (1992). Nontraumatic necrosis of bone (Osteonecrosis). *New England Journal of Medicine* 326 (22), 1473–1479.
22. Simkin P.S., Gardner G.C. (1994). Osteonecrosis: Pathogenesis and practicalities. *Hospital Practice* 29 (3), 73–84.

ADDITIONAL READINGS

Anderson P.A., Rivara F.P., Maier R.V., et al. (1991). The epidemiology of seat belt—associated injuries. *Journal of Trauma* 31 (1), 60.

Barden R.M., Sinkora G.L. (1991). Bone stimulators for fusions and fractures. *Nursing Clinics of North America* 26 (3), 89.

Cattaneo R., Catagni M., Johnson E.E. (1992). The treatment of infected nonunions and segmental defects of the tibia by means of Ilizarov. *Clinical Orthopaedics* 280, 143.

Dirschl D.R., Wilson F.C. (1991). Topical antibiotic irrigation in prophylaxis of operative wound infections in orthopedic surgery. *Orthopedic Clinics of North America* 22, 419.

Folcik M.A. (1991). Meniscal injuries. *Nursing Clinics of North America* 26 (1), 181.

Lester B., Mallik A. (1996). Impending malunions of the hand. *Clinical Orthopaedics* 327, 55.

Long J.S. (1996). Shoulder arthroscopy. *Orthopedic Nursing* 15 (2), 21.

Merritt K. (1988). Factors increasing the risk of infection in patients with open fracture. *Journal of Trauma* 28, 823.

Ross D. (1991). Acute compartment syndrome. *Orthopedic Nursing* 10 (2), 33.

Sly D.A. (1991). Orthopedic complication: Compartment syndrome, fat embolization syndrome, and venous thromboembolism. *Nursing Clinics of North America* 26 (1), 113.

Whitelaw G.P., Wetzler M.J., Levy A.S., et al. (1991). A pneumatic leg brace for the treatment of tibial stress fracture. *Clinical Orthopaedics and Related Research* 270, 301.

CHAPTER 46

Alterations in Skeletal Function: Congenital Disorders, Metabolic Bone Disease, and Neoplasms

Kathleen E. Gunta

During childhood, skeletal structures grow in length and diameter and sustain a large increase in bone mass. The term *modeling* refers to the formation of the macroscopic skeleton, which ceases at maturity, usually between 18 and 20 years of age. Bone remodeling replaces existing bone and occurs in children and adults. It involves resorption and formation of bone. With aging, bone resorption and formation are no longer perfectly coupled, and there is loss of bone. Alterations in musculoskeletal structure and function may develop as a result of normal growth and developmental processes or as a result of impairment of skeletal development due to hereditary or congenital influences. Other skeletal disorders can occur later in life as a result of metabolic disorders or neoplastic growth.

Alterations in Skeletal Growth and Development

After you have completed this section of the chapter, you should be able to meet the following objectives:

- Describe the function of the epiphysis in skeletal growth
- Differentiate between toeing-in and toeing-out
- Describe common torsional deformities that occur in infants and small children, proposed mechanisms of development, diagnostic methods, and treatment
- Define *genu varum* and *genu valgum*
- List the problems that occur because of defective tissue synthesis in osteogenesis imperfecta
- Characterize the abnormalities associated with developmental dysplasia of the hip and methods of diagnosis
- Describe the treatment for a newborn with clubfoot
- Define the term osteochondroses and describe the pathology and symptomatology of Legg-Calvé-Perthes disease and Osgood-Schlatter disease
- Describe the pathology associated with a slipped capital femoral epiphyseal and explain why early treatment is important
- Differentiate between infantile, idiopathic, and neuromuscular scoliosis
- Discuss the diagnosis and treatment of idiopathic scoliosis

Bone Growth and Remodeling

Embryonic Development

The skeletal system develops from the mesoderm, the thin middle layer of embryonic tissue. Development of the vertebrae of the axial skeleton begins at about the fourth week in the embryo; during the ninth week, ossification begins with the appearance of ossification centers in the lower thoracic and upper lumbar vertebrae. The paddle-shaped limb buds of the lower extremities make their appearance late in the fourth week. The hand pads are developed by day 33 to 36, and the finger rays are evident on day 41 to 43 of embryonic development.[1]

Bone Growth in Childhood

During the first two decades of life, the skeleton undergoes general overall growth. The long bones of the skeleton, which grow at a relatively rapid rate, are provided with a specialized structure called the *epiphyseal growth plate*. As long bones grow in length, the deeper layers of cartilage cells in the growth plate multiply and enlarge, pushing the articular cartilage farther away from the metaphysis and diaphysis of the bone.[2] As this happens, the mature and enlarged cartilage cells at the metaphyseal end of the plate become metabolically inactive and are replaced by bone cells (Fig. 46–1). This process allows bone growth to proceed without changing the shape of the bone or causing disruption of the articular cartilage. The cells in the growth plate stop dividing at puberty, at which time the epiphysis and metaphysis fuse.

Several factors can influence the growth of cells in the epiphyseal growth plate. Epiphyseal separation can occur in children as the result of trauma. The separation usually occurs in the zone of the mature enlarged cartilage cells, which is the weakest part of the growth plate. The blood vessels that nourish the epiphysis, which pass through the growth plate, are ruptured when the growth plate separates. This can cause cessation of growth and a shortened extremity.

The growth plate is also sensitive to nutritional and metabolic changes. Scurvy (*i.e.*, vitamin C deficiency) impairs the formation of the organic matrix of bone, causing slowing of growth at the epiphyseal plate and cessation of diaphyseal growth. In rickets (*i.e.*, vitamin D deficiency), calcification of the newly developed bone on the metaphyseal side of the growth plate is impaired. Thyroid and growth hormones are required for normal growth. Alterations in these and other hormones can affect growth (see Chapter 35).

Growth in the diameter of bones occurs as new bone is added to the outer surface of existing bone along with an accompanying resorption of bone on the endosteal or inner surface. Such oppositional growth allows for widening of the marrow cavity while preventing the

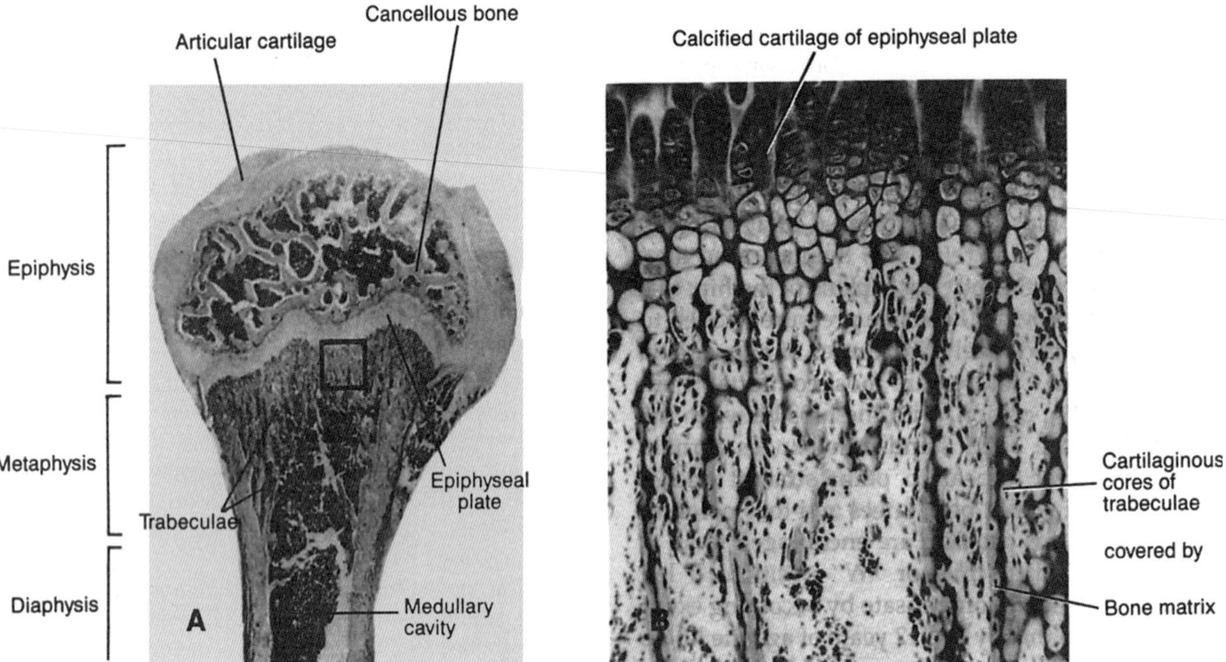

Figure 46–1
(**A**) Low-power photomicrograph of one end of a growing long bone (rat). Osteogenesis has spread from the epiphyseal center of ossification so that only the articular cartilage above and the epiphyseal disk below remain cartilaginous. On the diaphyseal side of the epiphyseal plate (disk), metaphyseal trabeculae extend down into the diaphysis. (**B**) Medium-power photomicrograph of the area indicated in **A,** showing trabeculae on the diaphyseal side of the epiphyseal plate (disk). These have cores of calcified cartilage on which bone has been deposited. The cartilaginous cores of the trabeculae were formerly partitions between columns of chondrocytes in the epiphyseal plate (disk).

cortex from becoming too thick and heavy. In this way, the shape of the bone is maintained. As a bone grows in diameter, concentric rings are added to the bone surface, much as rings are added to a tree trunk; these rings form the lamellar structure of mature bone. Osteocytes, which develop from osteoblasts, become buried in the rings. Haversian channels form as periosteal vessels running along the long axis become surrounded by bone.

Alterations During Normal Growth Periods

Infants and children undergo changes in muscle tone and joint motion during growth and development. Toeing-in, toeing-out, bowlegs, and knock-knees occur frequently in infancy and childhood.[3] These changes usually cause few problems and are corrected during normal growth processes. The normal folded position of the fetus in utero causes physiologic flexion contractures of the hips and a froglike appearance of the lower extremities (Fig. 46–2). The hips are externally rotated, and the patellae point outward, whereas the feet appear to point forward because of the internal pulling force of the tibiae. During the first year of life, the lower extremities begin to straighten out in preparation for walking. Internal and external rotation become equal, and the hips extend. Flexion contractures of the shoulders, elbows, and knees are also commonly seen in newborns, but they should disappear by 3 months of age.[4]

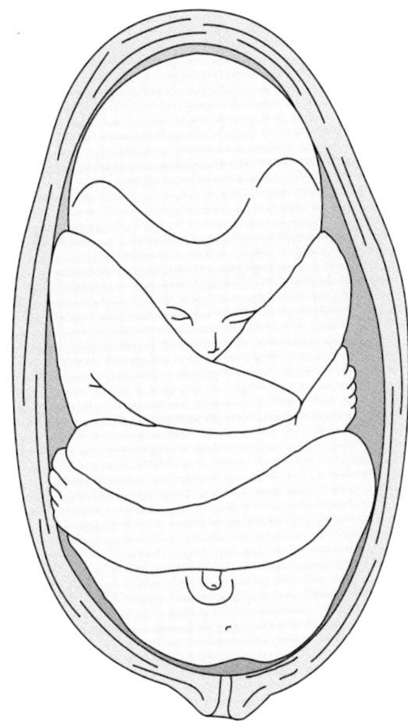

Figure 46–2
Position of fetus in utero, with tibial bowing and legs folded. (Dunne K.B., Clarren S.K. [1986]. The origin of prenatal and postnatal deformities. *Pediatric Clinics of North America* 33[6], 1282)

Torsional Deformities

All infants and toddlers have lax ligaments that become tighter with age and assumption of the weight-bearing posture. The hypermobility that accompanies joint laxity along with torsional, or twisting, forces exerted on the limbs during growth are responsible for a number of variants seen in young children. Torsional forces caused by intrauterine positions or sleeping and sitting patterns twist the growing bones and can produce the deformities as a child grows and develops.

In infants, the femur is normally rotated to an anteverted position with the femoral head and neck rotated anteriorly with respect to the femoral condyles. Femoral anteversion (*i.e.*, medial rotation) decreases from an average 40 degrees at birth to about 15 degrees at maturity. The normal tibia is externally rotated about 5 degrees at birth and 15 degrees at maturity. Torsional abnormalities frequently demonstrate a familial tendency.

Toeing-in and Toeing-out. The foot progression angle describes the angle between the axis of the foot and the line of progression. It is determined by watching the child walking and running. Figure 46–3 illustrates the position of the foot in toeing-in and toeing-out.

Toeing-in (*i.e.*, metatarsus adductus) is the most common congenital foot deformity, affecting boys and girls equally. It can be caused by torsion in the foot, lower leg, or entire leg. Toeing-in due to adduction of the forefoot (*i.e.*, congenital metatarsus adductus) is usually the result of the fetal position maintained in utero. It may occur in one foot or both feet. A supple deformity can be passively manipulated into a straight position and requires no treatment. Treatment consisting of serial long leg casting or a brace that pushes the metatarsals (not the hindfoot) into abduction is usually required in a fixed deformity (*i.e.*, one in which the forefoot cannot be passively manipulated into a straight position).

Toeing-out is a common problem in children and is caused by external femoral torsion. This occurs when the femur can be externally rotated to about 90 degrees but internally rotated only to a neutral position or slightly beyond. When a child habitually sleeps in the prone position, the femoral torsion persists, and an external tibial torsion may also develop. If external tibial torsion is present, the feet point lateral to the midline of the medial plane. External tibial torsion rarely causes toeing-out; it only intensifies the condition. Toeing-out usually corrects itself as the child becomes proficient in walking. Occa-

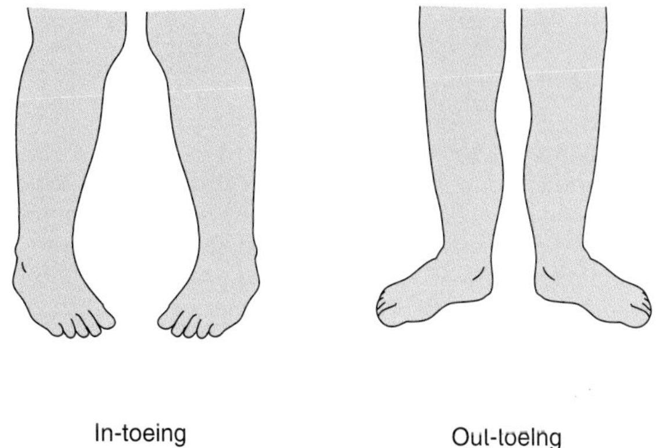

Figure 46–3
Position of feet in in-toeing and out-toeing

sionally, a night splint is used. Toeing-in and toeing-out are less noticeable when the child is running or barefoot. Overcorrection of a supple foot deformity can cause flatfoot deformity, but a rigid deformity that is untreated can cause pain and improper fitting of footwear.

Tibial Torsion. Tibial torsion is determined by measuring the thigh-foot angle, which is done with the ankle and knee positioned at 90 degrees (Fig. 46–4*A*). In this position, the foot normally rotates outward. *Internal tibial torsion* (*i.e.*, bowing of the tibia) is a rotation of the tibia that makes the feet appear to turn inward. It is the most common cause of toeing-in in children younger than 2 years of age. It is present at birth and may fail to correct itself if children sleep on their knees with the feet turned in or sit on in-turned feet. It is thought to be caused by genetic factors and intrauterine compression, such as an unstretched uterus during a first pregnancy or intrauterine crowding with twins or multiple fetuses. Tibial torsion improves naturally with growth, but this may take years.[5] The Denis Browne splint, a bar to which shoes are attached, may be used to put the feet into mild external rotation while the child is sleeping.

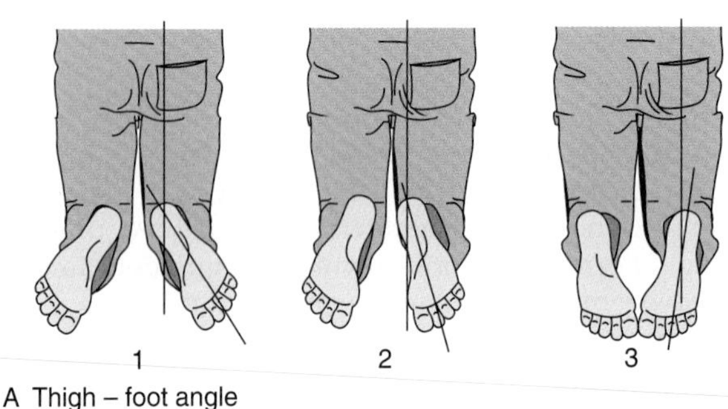

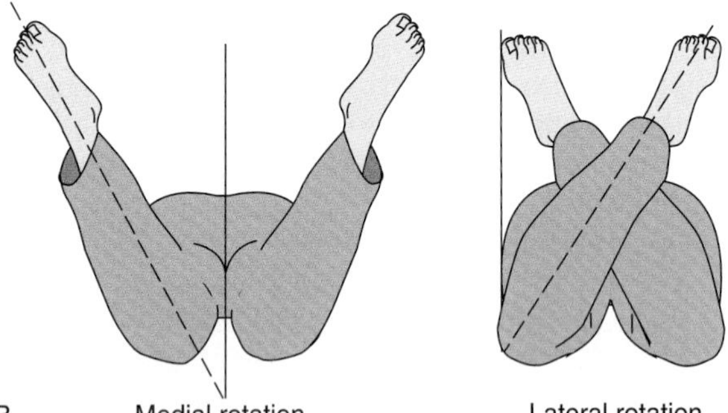

Figure 46–4
(**A**) Assessment for tibial torsion using thigh–foot angle. When child is in the prone position with the knee flexed, with normal alignment there is slight external rotation (2); internal tibial torsion produces inward rotation (3), and external tibial torsion; outward rotation (1). (**B**) Hip rotation is measured with child prone and knees flexed at 90° angle. On outward rotation the leg produces internal (medial) hip and femoral rotation; on inward rotation the leg produces external hip and femoral rotation. (Adapted from Stahelli L.T. [1986]. Torsional deformity. *Pediatric Clinics of North America*. 33[6],p. 1378, and Kliegman R.M., Neider M.I., Super S.M. [eds]. *Practical strategies in pediatric diagnosis and therapy.* Philadelphia: W.B. Saunders.)

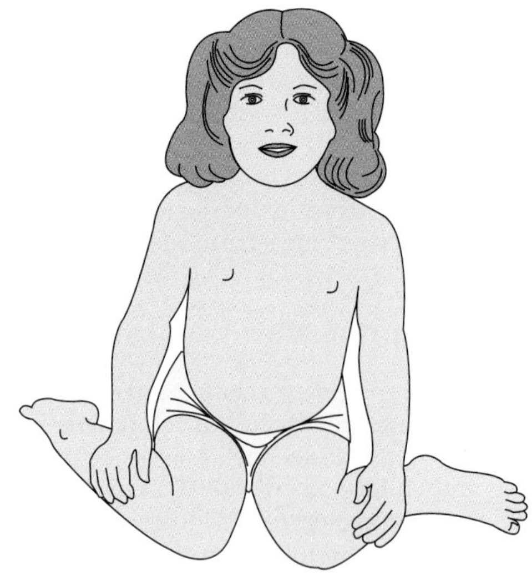

Figure 46–5
Typical sitting position of child with femoral anteversion. (Staheli L.T. [1986]. Torsional deformities. *Pediatric Clinics of North America 33*[6], 1382)

External tibial torsion, a much less common disorder, is associated with calcaneovalgus foot and is caused by a normal variation of in utero positioning or a neuromuscular disorder. It is characterized by an abnormally positive thigh-foot angle of 30 to 50 degrees. The condition corrects itself naturally, and treatment is observational. Significant improvement begins during the first year with the onset of ambulation and is usually complete by 2 to 3 years of age.[6] The normal adult exhibits 20 degrees tibial torsion.

Femoral Torsion. Femoral torsion refers to abnormal variations in hip rotation. Hip rotation is measured at the pelvic level with the child in the prone position and the knees flexed at a 90-degree angle. In this position, the hip is in a neutral position. Rotating the lower leg outward produces internal or medial femoral rotation; rotating it inward produces external or lateral rotation (Fig. 46–4*B*). During measurement of hip rotation, the legs are allowed to fall to full internal rotation by gravity alone; lateral rotation is measured by allowing the legs to fall inward and cross. Hip rotation in flexion and extension can also be measured with computed tomography (CT). By 1 year of age, there is normally about 45 degrees of internal and 45 degrees of external rotation.[6]

Internal femoral torsion (*i.e.*, femoral anteversion) is a normal variant commonly seen during the first 6 years of life, especially in 3- and 4-year-old girls.[3,7] Characteristically, internal rotation exceeds external rotation by 30 degrees or more. The condition is thought to be related to increased laxity of the anterior capsule of the hip such that it does not provide the stable pressure needed to correct the anteversion that is present at birth. Children are most comfortable sitting in the "W" position with their hips between their knees (Fig. 46–5). It is believed that this position allows the lower leg to act as a lever, producing torsional changes in the femur. When the child stands, the knees turn in, and the feet appear to point straight ahead; when the child walks, knees and toes point in. Children with this problem are encouraged to sit cross-legged or in the so-called tailor position. If left untreated, the tibiae compensate by becoming externally rotated so that by 8 to 12 years of age the knees may turn in but the feet no longer do. This can result in patellofemoral malalignment with patella subluxation or dislocation and pain. A derotational osteotomy may be done in severe cases or if there is functional disability.

External femoral torsion is an uncommon disorder. It is usually associated with slipped capital femoral epiphysis (discussed later). It is characterized by excessive external rotation of the hip. Idiopathic external femoral torsion is usually a bilateral disorder. When the disorder is unilateral, slipped capital femoral epiphysis should be excluded. External femoral torsion is usually benign and treatment is observational.

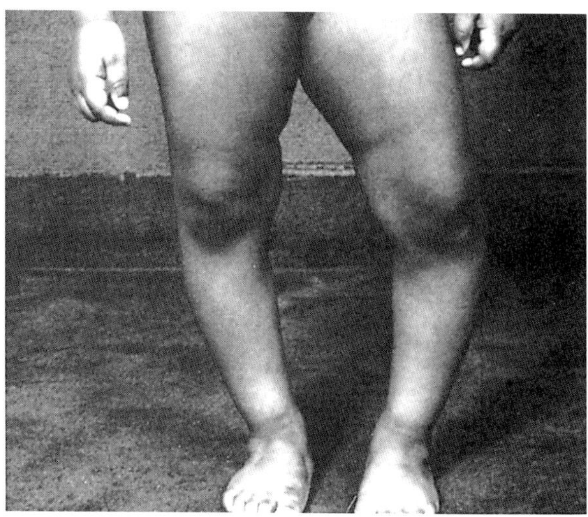

Figure 46–7
Rotational deformity of the proximal tibia, especially when unilateral, suggests tibia vera (Blount's disease).

Genu Varum and Genu Valgum

Genu varum (*i.e.*, bowlegs) is an outward bowing of the knees greater than 1 inch when the medial malleoli of the ankles are touching (Fig. 46–6). Most infants and toddlers have some bowing of their legs up to age 2. If there is a large separation between the knees (>15 degrees) after age 2, the child may require bracing. The child should also be evaluated for diseases such as rickets or tibia vara (*i.e.*, Blount's disease).

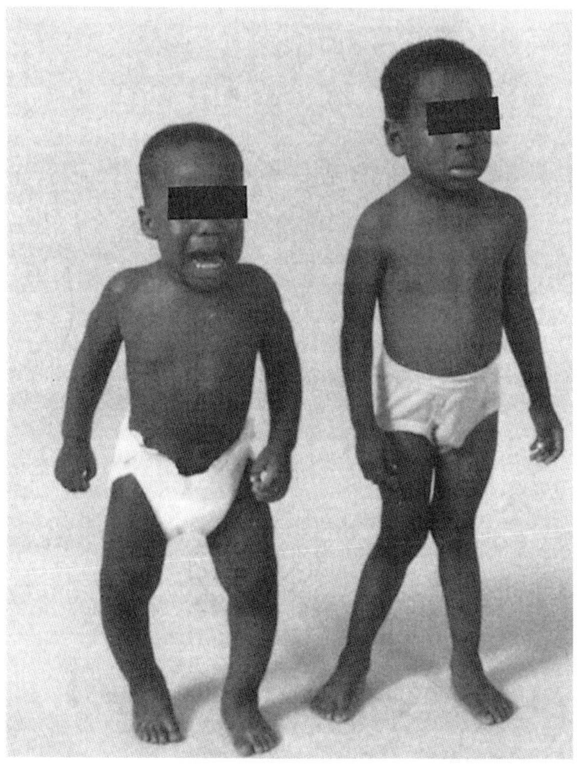

Figure 46–6
Normal genu varum (bowlegs) in a toddler (*left*) and genu valgum (knock-knees) in a toddler (*right*), which is often seen in children between 2 and 6 years of age.

Genu valgum (*i.e.*, knock-knees) is a deformity in which there is decreased space between the knees (see Fig. 46–6). The medial malleoli in the ankles cannot be brought in contact with each other when the knees are touching. It is seen most frequently in children between the ages of 2 and 6 years and should resolve by 7 to 10 years of age. The condition is usually the result of lax medial collateral ligaments of the knee and may be exacerbated by sitting in the "M position." Genu valgum can be ignored up to age 7, unless it is more than 15 degrees, unilateral, or associated with short stature. It usually resolves spontaneously and rarely requires treatment. If genu varum or genu valgum persists and is uncorrected, osteoarthritis may develop in adulthood as a result of abnormal intraarticular stress. Genu varum can cause gait awkwardness and increased risk of sprains and fractures. Uncorrected genu valgum may cause subluxation and recurrent dislocation of the patella, with a predisposition to chondromalacia and joint pain and fatigue.

Blount's disease, or idiopathic tibia vara, is a developmental deformity of the medial half of proximal tibial epiphysis that results in a progressive varus angulation below the knee (Fig. 46–7). It is the most common cause of pathologic genu varum and seen most often in black children, females, obese children, and early walkers.[8] Onset can occur early as in infancy or later as during adolescence. Adolescent Blount's disease occurs in the second decade of life, is seen in persons who are above the 95th percentile in height and weight, and is usually unilateral.[9] Long leg braces are used for treatment in early onset disease. If progression occurs, or onset is late, surgery is done to correct the angulation and prevent further progression.

Flatfoot

Flatfoot (*i.e.*, pes planus) is a deformity characterized by the absence of the longitudinal arch of the foot. Infants normally have a wider and fatter foot than adults. The fat pads that are normally accentuated by pliable muscles create an illusion of fullness often mistaken for flatfeet. Until the longitudinal arch develops at 2 to 3 years of age, all children have flatfeet. The true criterion for flatfoot is that the head of the talus points medially and downward, so that the heel is everted and the forefoot must be inverted (toed-in) for the metatarsal heads to be planted equally on the ground. Weight bearing may cause pain in the longitudinal arch and up the leg.

There are two types of flatfeet—flexible and rigid. Most children with flexible (or supple) flatfeet have loose ligaments, allowing the feet to sag when they gain weight.[10] In supple flatfeet, the arch disappears only with weight bearing. No special treatment is needed for flexible flatfeet, and it is usually recommended that children with the disorder wear regular shoes. The rigid flatfoot is fixed with no apparent arch in any position. It is seen in conjunction with congenitally tight heel cords, neuromuscular diseases such as cerebral palsy, or juvenile rheumatoid arthritis.

In the adult, treatment of flatfeet is conservative and aimed at relieving fatigue, pain, and tenderness. Supportive well-fitting shoes with arch supports may be helpful and prevent ligaments from becoming overstretched. Women may complain of pain in the forefoot when wearing poorly fitting high heels. Surgery may be done in cases of severe and persistent symptoms.

Hereditary and Congenital Deformities

Congenital deformities are abnormalities that are present at birth. They range in severity from mild limb deformities, which are relatively common, to major limb malformations, which are relatively rare. There may be a simple webbing of the fingers or toes (*i.e.*, syndactyly) or the presence of an extra digit (*i.e.*, polydactyly). Joint contractures and dislocations produce more severe deformity, as does the absence of entire bones, joints, or limbs. An epidemic of limb deformities occurred from 1957 to 1962 as a result of maternal ingestion of thalidomide. This drug was withdrawn from the market in 1961.

Congenital deformities are caused by many factors, some as yet unknown. These factors include genetic influences, external agents that injure the fetus (*e.g.*, radiation, alcohol, medications, viruses), and in utero environmental factors. As discussed in Chapter 4, the fourth through the seventh week of gestation is the most vulnerable period for the development of limb deformities.

Osteogenesis Imperfecta

Osteogenesis imperfecta is a hereditary disease characterized by defective synthesis of connective tissue, including bone matrix. It is one of the most common hereditary bone diseases, with an occurrence rate of approximately 1 case in 20,000 births.[11] Although it is usually transmitted as an autosomal dominant trait, a distinct form of the disorder with multiple lethal defects is thought to be inherited as an autosomal recessive trait.[12]

The disorder is characterized by thin and poorly developed bones that are prone to multiple fractures (Fig. 46–8). These children have short limbs and a soft, thin cranium with bifrontal prominences that give a triangular appearance to the face. Other problems associated with defective connective tissue synthesis include short stature, thin skin, blue or gray sclera, abnormal tooth development, hypotonic muscles, loose-jointedness, scoliosis, and a tendency for hernia formation. Hearing loss is common in adults with this disorder because of otosclerosis of the middle and inner ear.

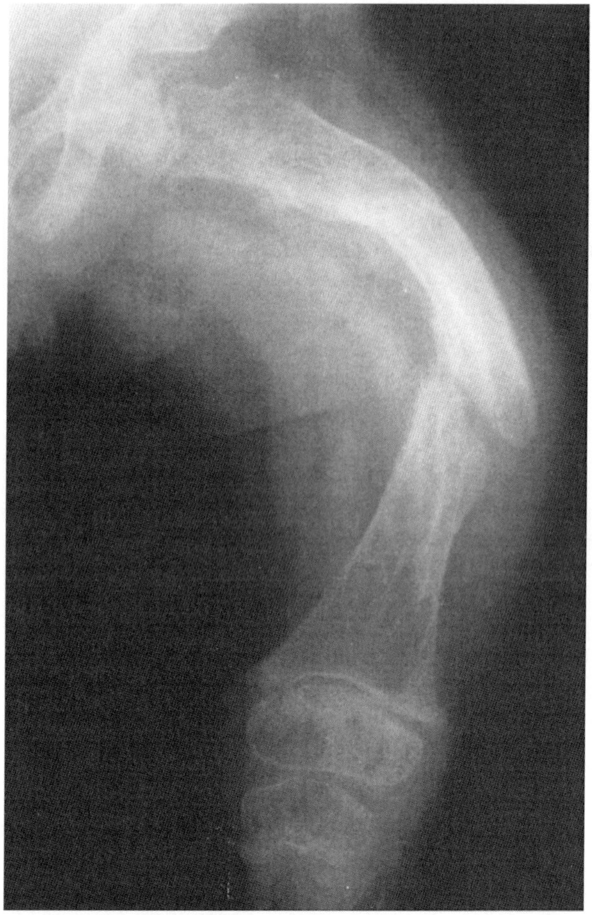

Figure 46–8
Osteogenesis imperfecta in a 1-year-old child. Recurrent fractures typically develop through the diaphyses of long bones.

The most serious defects occur when the disorder is inherited as a recessive trait. Severely affected fetuses have multiple intrauterine fractures and bowing and shortening of the extremities. Many of these babies are stillborn or die during infancy. Less severe affliction occurs when the disorder is inherited as a dominant trait. The skeletal system is not so weakened, and fractures often do not appear until the child becomes active and starts to walk or even later in childhood. These fractures heal rapidly, although with a poor-quality callus. In some cases, parents may be suspected of child abuse when the child is admitted to the health care facility with multiple fractures.

There is no known medical treatment for correction of the defective collagen synthesis that is characteristic

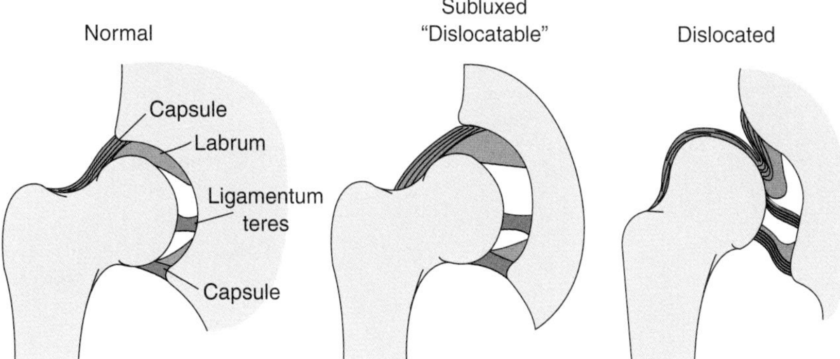

Figure 46–9
Normal and abnormal relationships of hip joint structure. (Adapted from Dunn P.M. [1969]. Congenital dislocation of the hip. *Proceedings of the Royal Society of Medicine* 62,1035–1037.)

of osteogenesis imperfecta. Instead, treatment modalities focus on preventing and treating fractures. Precise alignment is necessary to prevent deformities. Nonunion is common, especially with repeated fractures at a progressively deforming site. Surgical intervention is often needed to correct deformities (*e.g.*, internal fixation of long bones may be done with an intramedullary rod that "grows" with the child), stabilize fractures, remove hardware devices after a nonunion, and, occasionally, amputate the site of a failed bone graft.

Developmental Dysplasia of the Hip

Developmental dysplasia of the hip, formerly known as *congenital dislocation of the hip,* is an abnormality in hip development that leads to a wide spectrum of hip problems seen in infants and children, including hips that are unstable, malformed, subluxated, or dislocated.[13–15] In less severe cases, the hip joint may be unstable with excessive laxity of the joint capsule or subluxed, so that the joint surfaces are separated and there is a partial dislocation (Fig. 46–9). With dislocated hips, the head of the femur is located outside of the acetabulum.

The results of newborn screening programs have shown that 1 of 100 infants have some evidence of hip instability; however, dislocation of the hip is seen in 1.5 of every 1000 live births.[14] Of infants found to have hip instability at birth, 58% were stable when reexamined at 1 week, and by 2 months, 90% were stable.[13] In white infants, developmental dysplasia of the hips occurs most frequently in first-born children and is six times more common in female than in male infants.[16] It is thought that the instability of the hip is a consequence of laxity of the ligaments, which is genetically determined, and dislocation is the result of environmental factors such as fetal position, breech delivery, or when the uterus is tight and prevents fetal movement.

Normal development of the hip requires that a normal positional relation exist between the femoral head and the acetabulum. If this relation is not maintained, there may be a delay in the maturation, size, and development of the femoral head and the acetabulum. Early diagnosis of a dislocatable hip is important, because treatment is easiest and most effective if begun during the first 6 months of life. Repeated dislocation causes damage to the femoral head and the acetabulum.

Clinical examinations to detect dislocation of the hip should be done at birth and every several months during the first year of life. Several examination techniques are used to screen for a dislocatable hip. In infants, signs of dislocation include asymmetry of the hip or gluteal folds, shortening of the thigh so that one knee (on the affected side) is higher than the other, and limited abduction of the affected hip (Fig. 46–10). The asymmetry of gluteal folds is not definitive but indicates the need for further evaluation. A specific examination method involves an attempt to manually dislocate and reduce the abnormal hip while the infant is in the supine position with both knees flexed (*i.e.*, Barlow's maneuver). With gentle downward pressure being applied to the knees, the knee and thigh are manually abducted as an upward and medial pressure is applied to the proximal thigh (Fig. 46–11). In infants with the disorder, the initial downward pressure on the knee produces a dislocation of the hip, a positive Barlow's sign. This is followed by a palpable or audible click (*i.e.*, Ortolani's sign) as the hip is reduced and moves back into the acetabulum. In an older child, instability of the hip may produce a delay in standing or walking and eventually cause a characteristic waddling gait. When the thumbs are placed over the anterior iliac crest and the hands are

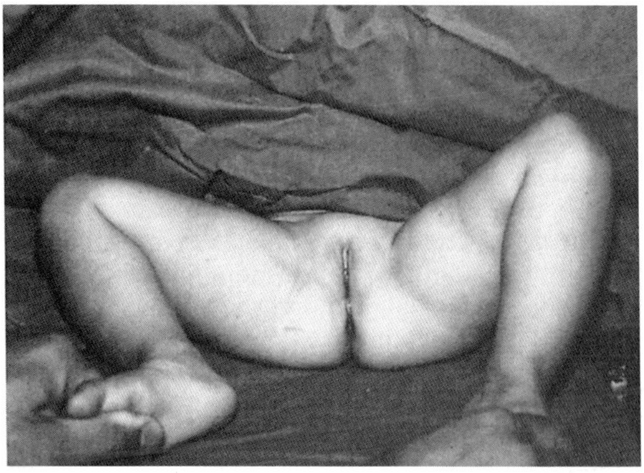

Figure 46–10
An 18-month-old girl has congenital dysplasia of the left hip.

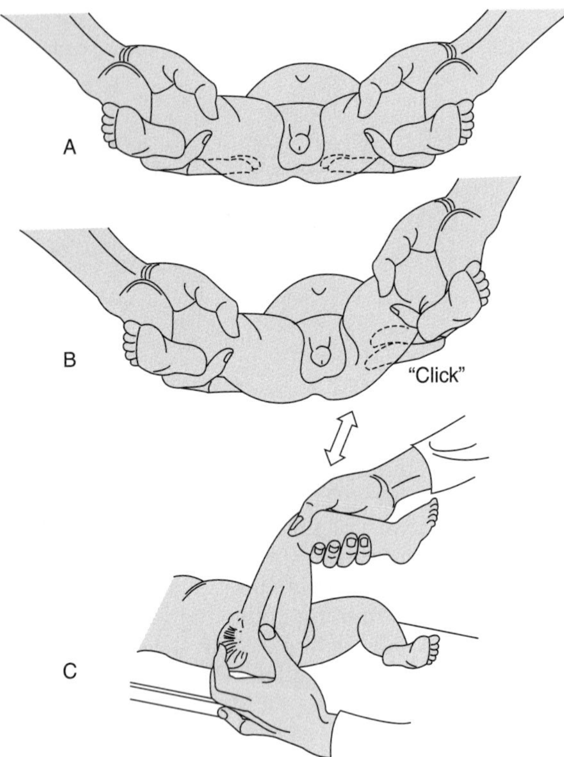

Figure 46–11
Congenital dislocation of the hip. (**A**) in the newborn, both hips can be equally flexed, abducted, and externally rotated without producing a "click." (**B**) A diagnosis of a congenital dislocation of the hip may be confirmed by Ortolani's "click" test. The involved hip cannot be abducted as far as the opposite one, and there is a "click" as the hip reduces. (**C**) Telescoping of the femur to aid in the diagnosis of a congenitally dislocated hip. (*Hoppenfeld's physical examination of the spine and extremities.* [1976]. New York: Appleton-Century-Crofts)

placed over the lateral pelvis in examination, the levels of the thumbs are not even; the child is unable to elevate the opposite side of the pelvis (positive Trendelenburg's test). Diagnosis is confirmed by radiography. Ultrasound is proving to be a useful diagnostic method in newborns and infants from birth to 4 months of age.[13]

The treatment of a dislocated hip is begun as soon as the diagnosis has been made. The best results are obtained if the treatment is begun before changes in the hip structure (*e.g.,* 2 to 3 months) prevent it from being reduced by gentle manipulation or abduction devices. The Pavlik harness is used on newborns (up to 6 months) to maintain the femoral head in the acetabulum. The harness allows the child more mobility as the leg is slowly and gently brought into abduction. Infants with dislocated hips caused by anatomic changes and toddlers who may lack development of the acetabular socket require more aggressive treatment, such as open reduction and joint reconstruction.

Treatment at any age includes reduction of the dislocation and immobilization of the legs in an abducted position. The most serious complication of any treatment is avascular necrosis of the femoral head as a result of the forced abduction. With children younger than years of age, gentle traction is used when reduction cannot be easily obtained. This treatment is followed by several months of immobilization in a hip spica cast, plaster splints, or an abduction splint such as a Ilfeld splint. Older children or adults with a unreduced dislocatable hip may require hip surgery because of damage to the articulating surface of the joint. These persons have considerable problems after surgery because of soft tissue contractures.

Congenital Clubfoot

Clubfoot, or talipes, is a congenital deformity of the foot that can affect one or both feet. Like congenital dislocation of the hip, its occurrence follows a multifactorial inheritance pattern. The condition has an incidence of 1 case per 1000 live births and occurs twice as often in males as in females.[17] Clubfoot is associated with chromosomal abnormalities and may be associated with other congenital syndromes that are transmitted by mendelian inheritance patterns (see Chapter 4). However, it is most commonly idiopathic and found in normal infants in whom no genetic or chromosomal abnormality or other extrinsic cause can be found.

In forefoot adduction, which accounts for about 95% of idiopathic cases, the foot is plantar flexed and inverted. This is the so-called equinovarus type in which the foot resembles a horse's hoof (Fig. 46–12). The other 5% of cases are of the calcaneovalgus type, or reverse clubfoot, in which the foot is dorsiflexed and everted. The reverse clubfoot can occur as an isolated condition or in association with multiple congenital defects. At birth, the feet of many infants assume one of these two positions, but they can be passively overcorrected or brought back into the opposite position. If the foot cannot be overcorrected, some type of correction may be necessary. Although the exact cause of clubfoot is unknown, three theories are generally accepted: an anomalous development occurs during the first trimester of pregnancy, the leg fails to rotate inward and move from the equinovarus position at about the third month, or the soft tissues in the foot do not mature and lengthen.

Clubfoot varies in severity from a mild deformity to one in which the foot is completely inverted. Treatment is begun as soon as the diagnosis is made. When treatment is initiated during the first few weeks of life, a nonoperative procedure is effective within a short period. Serial manipulations and casting are used to gently correct each component in the forefoot varus, the hindfoot varus, and the equinus. The treatment is continued until the foot is in a normal position with full correction evident clinically and on radiographic studies. Surgery may be required for severe deformities or when nonoperative treatment methods are unsuccessful. About 30% to 50% of idiopathic deformities are corrected with casts; the others require surgery.[18] An external distractor such as the Ilizarov external fixator may be used to correct the deformity of a relapsed or neglected clubfoot.

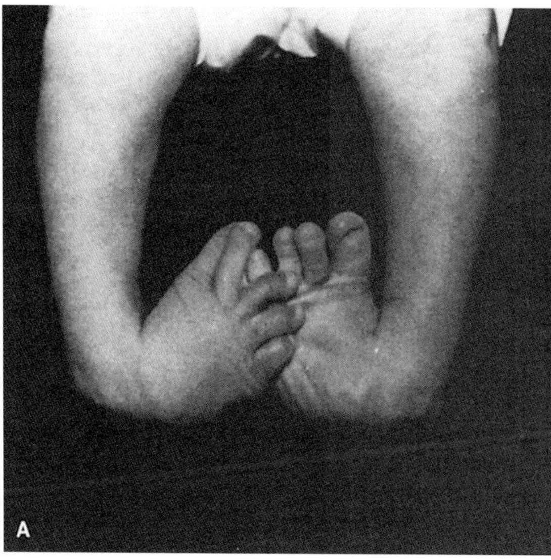

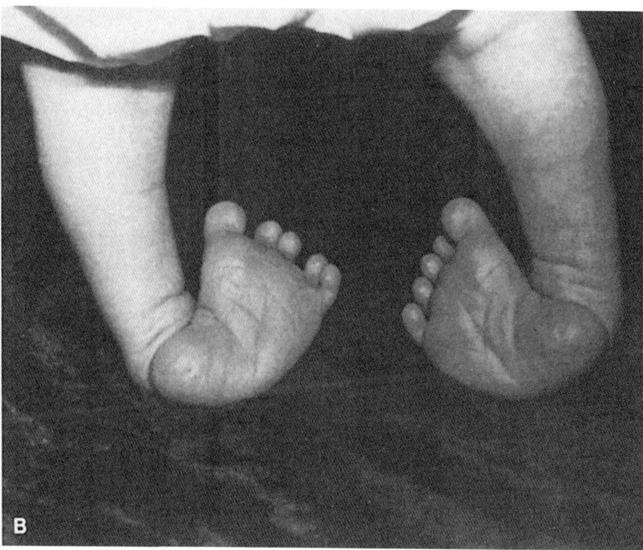

Figure 46–12 ■ ■ ■
Severe clubfoot deformity. The heel is in severe varus, and the forefoot is adducted and inverted. The cavus deformity results from the slightly pronated position of the forefoot in relation to the hindfoot.

Juvenile Osteochondroses

The term *juvenile osteochondroses* is used to describe a group of children's diseases in which one or more growth ossification centers undergo a period of degeneration, necrosis, or inactivity that is followed by regeneration and usually deformity. The osteochondroses are separated into two groups according to their causes. The first group consists of the true osteonecrotic osteochondroses, so called because the diseases are caused by localized osteonecrosis of an apophyseal or epiphyseal center (*e.g.*, Legg-Calvé-Perthes disease, Freiberg's infraction, Panner's disease, Kienböck's disease). The second group of juvenile osteochondroses are caused by abnormalities in ossification of cartilaginous tissue resulting from a genetically determined normal variation or from trauma (*e.g.*, Osgood-Schlatter disease, Blount's disease, Sever's disease, Scheuermann's disease). The discussion in this section focuses on Legg-Calvé-Perthes disease from the first group and Osgood-Schlatter disease from the second group.

Legg-Calvé-Perthes Disease

Legg-Calvé-Perthes disease, or coxa plana, is an osteonecrotic disease of the proximal femoral (capital) epiphysis, which is the growth center for the head of the femur. It occurs in 1 of 1200 children, affecting primarily those between ages 2 and 13 years, with a peak incidence between 4 and 9 years.[19] It occurs primarily in boys and is much more common in whites than African Americans. Although no definite genetic pattern has been established, it occasionally affects more than one family member.

The cause of Legg-Calvé-Perthes disease is unknown. The disorder is usually insidious in onset and occurs in otherwise healthy children. It may, however, be associated with acute trauma. The children usually affected have a shorter stature. Undernutrition has been suggested as a causative factor. When girls are affected, they usually have a poorer prognosis than boys because they are skeletally more mature. This means that they would have a shorter period for growth and remodeling than boys of the same age. Although both legs can be affected, in 85% of cases, only one leg is involved.[5]

The primary pathologic feature of Legg-Calvé-Perthes disease is an avascular necrosis of the bone and marrow involving the epiphyseal growth center in the femoral head. The disorder may be confined to part of the epiphysis, or it may involve the entire epiphysis. In severe cases, there is a disturbance in the growth pattern that leads to a broad, short femoral neck. The necrosis is followed by slow absorption of the dead bone over 2 to 3 years. Although the necrotic trabeculae are eventually replaced by healthy new bone, the epiphysis rarely regains its normal shape. The process occurs in four predictable stages, each with its distinctive radiologic characteristics.[14,19,20]

1. The incipient or synovitis stage is characterized by synovial inflammation and increased joint fluid. This stage usually lasts 1 to 3 weeks.
2. During the aseptic or avascular stage, the ossification center becomes necrotic. This stage may last from several months to a year. Damage to the femoral head is determined by the degree of necrosis that occurs during this stage.
3. The regenerative or revascularization stage involves the resorption of the necrotic bone. This stage lasts 1 to 3 years, during which the necrotic bone is gradually replaced by new immature bone cells and the contour of the bone is remodeled.

4. The healed or residual stage is characterized by the formation and replacement of immature bone cells by normal bone cells. Remodeling of the femoral head continues throughout the growing years but is ultimately determined by the amount of collapse that has occurred during the avascular stage.

Legg-Calvé-Perthes disease has an insidious onset with a prolonged course. The main symptoms are pain in the groin, thigh, or knee and difficulty in walking. The child may have a painless limp with limited abduction and internal rotation and a flexion contracture of the affected hip. The age of onset is important because young children have a greater capability for remodeling of the femoral head and acetabulum, and thus less flattening of the femoral head occurs. Early diagnosis is important and is based on correlating physical symptoms with radiographic findings that are related to the stage of the disease.

The goal of treatment is to reduce deformity and preserve the integrity of the femoral head. Conservative and surgical interventions are used in the treatment of Legg-Calvé-Perthes disease. Children younger than 4 years of age with little or no involvement of the femoral head may require only periodic observation. In all other children, some intervention is needed to relieve the force of weight bearing, muscular tension, and subluxation of the femoral head. It is important to maintain the femur in a well-seated position in the concave acetabulum to prevent deformity. This is done by keeping the hip in abduction and mild internal rotation.

The initial treatment usually involves bed rest with Russell's or Buck's traction (see Chapter 45) or with a device to keep the legs separated in abduction with mild internal rotation (*e.g.*, hip spica cast, abduction brace). After the inflammatory stage (usually several weeks in length) has subsided, the child is allowed up but is not permitted to bear weight on the femoral head. The child walks with crutches and may be required to wear a brace, splint, or walking cast. Surgery may be done to contain the femoral head within the acetabulum. This treatment is usually reserved for children older than 6 years who at the time of diagnosis have more serious involvement of the femoral head. The best surgical results are obtained when surgery is done early, before the epiphysis becomes necrotic.

Osgood-Schlatter Disease

Osgood-Schlatter disease is a partial separation of the tonguelike epiphysis of the tibial tuberosity caused by sudden or continued strain from the patellar tendon during growth. It occurs most frequently in boys between the ages of 11 and 15 years and in girls between 8 and 13 years.[20] The disorder is characterized by pain in the front of the knee that is associated with inflammation and thickening of the patellar tendon. An ossification center of growing cartilage forms within the tibial tubercle, making it susceptible to the pull of the quadriceps muscle. A partial avulsion or tearing of the tubercle is the result of extraordinary stress placed on the knee during a critical growth period. Follow-up studies have indicated that the disorder may be a mechanical tendonitis with partial avulsion of the tibial tubercle.

With Osgood-Schlatter disease, pain is usually associated with specific activities such as kneeling, running, bicycle riding, or stair climbing. The symptoms are self-limiting; although they may recur during growth periods, they usually resolve after closure of the tibial growth plate. In some cases, limitations on activity, braces to immobilize the knee, antiinflammatory agents, and application of cold are necessary to relieve the pain. The objective of treatment is to release tension on the quadriceps to permit revascularization and reossification of the tibial tubercle. Surgery may be indicated to excise painful bony fragments from the patellar tendon. Occasionally, minor symptoms or an increased prominence of the tibial tubercle may continue into adulthood. In some cases, a high riding patella can cause dislocation with chondromalacia of the patella and result in degenerative arthritis.

Slipped Capital Femoral Epiphysis

Normally, the proximal femoral epiphysis unites with the neck of the femur between ages 16 and 19 years. Before this time (10 to 14 years in girls and 10 to 16 years in boys), the femoral head may slip from its normal position directly at the head of the femur and become displaced medially and posteriorly.[19] The head is held in the acetabulum by the ligamentum teres, and the neck of the femur is pulled upward and outward (Fig. 46–13). This produces an anterolateral and superior adduction with extension deformity. About 2 of 100,000 children suffer a slipped capital femoral epiphysis.[19] It is the most common disorder of the hip in adolescents.

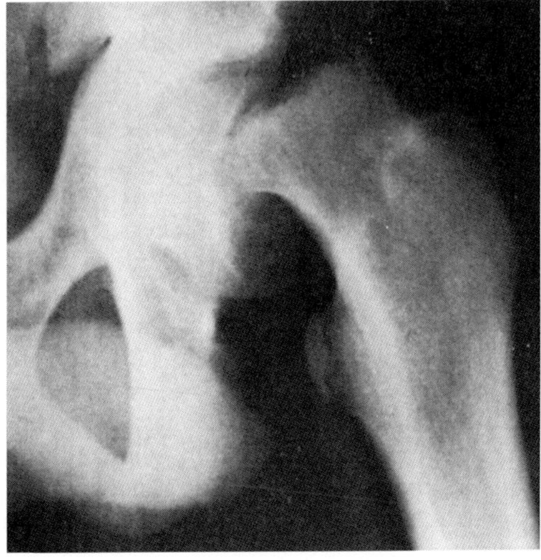

Figure 46–13
Completely slipped upper femoral epiphysis.

The cause of slipped capital femoral epiphysis is obscure, but it may be related to the child's susceptibility to stress on the femoral neck as a result of genetics or abnormal structure. Boys are affected twice as often as girls, and in about one half of cases, the condition is bilateral.[8] Affected children are often overweight with poorly developed secondary sex characteristics or, in some instances, are extremely tall and thin. In many cases, there is a history of rapid skeletal growth preceding displacement of the epiphysis. The condition may also be affected by nutritional deficiencies or endocrine disorders such a hypothyroidism, hypopituitarism, and hypogonadism. Rapid growth after administration of growth hormone has been associated with displacement of the epiphysis.

Children with the condition often complain of referred knee pain accompanied by difficulty in walking, fatigue, and stiffness. The diagnosis is confirmed by radiographic studies in which the degree of slipping is determined and graded according to severity. Early treatment is imperative to prevent lifelong crippling. Avoidance of weight bearing on the femur and bed rest are essential parts of the treatment. Traction or gentle manipulation under anesthesia is used to reduce the slip. Surgical insertion of pins to keep the femoral neck and head of the femur aligned is a common method of treatment for children with moderate or severe slips. Crutches are used for several months after surgical correction to prevent full weight bearing until the growth plate is sealed by the bony union.

Children with the disorder must be followed closely until the epiphyseal plate closes. Long-term prognosis depends on the amount of displacement that occurs. Complications include avascular necrosis, leg shortening, malunion, and problems with the internal fixation. Degenerative arthritis may develop, requiring joint replacement later in life.

Scoliosis

Scoliosis is a lateral deviation of the spinal column that may or may not include rotation or deformity of the vertebrae. It has been estimated that more than 500,000 adults in the United States have scoliosis.[21] It is most commonly seen during adolescence and is eight times more common among girls than boys. Scoliosis can develop as the result of another disease condition, or it can occur without known cause. Idiopathic scoliosis accounts for 75% to 80% of cases of the disorder. The other 20% to 25% of cases result from more than 50 different causes, including poliomyelitis, congenital hemivertebrae, neurofibromatosis, and cerebral palsy. Although minor curves are relatively common (affecting approximately 2% of the population), it has been estimated that fewer than 0.1% of U.S. school children have severe idiopathic scoliosis. Earlier studies that indicated a more widespread problem were probably based on inclusion of children with serious systemic diseases such as poliomyelitis.

Types of Scoliosis

Scoliosis is classified as postural or structural. With postural scoliosis, there is a small curve that corrects with bending. It can be corrected with passive and active exercises. Structural scoliosis does not correct with bending. It is a fixed deformity classified according to the cause: congenital, neuromuscular, and idiopathic.

Congenital Scoliosis. Congenital scoliosis is caused by disturbances in vertebral development during the sixth to eighth week of embryologic development. There are structural anomalies in the vertebrae that can cause a severe curvature. The child may have other anomalies and neurologic complications if the spine is involved. Early diagnosis and treatment of progressive curves are essential for children with congenital scoliosis.

Neuromuscular Scoliosis. Neuromuscular scoliosis develops from neuropathic or myopathic diseases. Neuropathic scoliosis is seen with cerebral palsy, myelodysplasia, and poliomyelitis. There is often a long C-shaped curve from the cervical to the sacral region. In children with cerebral palsy, severe deformity may make treatment difficult. Myopathic neuromuscular scoliosis develops with Duchenne's muscular dystrophy and is usually not severe.

Idiopathic Scoliosis. Idiopathic scoliosis is a structural spinal curvature for which no cause has been established. It seems likely that genetics is involved, and mother-daughter pairings are common. Growth and mechanical factors also seem to play a role.

Idiopathic scoliosis can be divided into three groups on the basis of age at onset: infantile (birth to 3 years), juvenile (4 to 10 years), and adolescent (11 years and older).[22] The infantile form is rare in the United States. It is seen primarily in the United Kingdom and Europe. It affects males more often than females, and most curves are convex and to the left rather than to the right, as in other forms of scoliosis. Although most forms of juvenile scoliosis regress spontaneously, some progress and are difficult to treat effectively. Juvenile idiopathic scoliosis is uncommon. However, in many children with the diagnosis of adolescent scoliosis, the onset may have occurred when they were juveniles but was not diagnosed until later. Adolescent scoliosis is the most common type and accounts for about 80% of all cases of idiopathic scoliosis. Adolescent scoliosis is seen most commonly in females. An increase in joint laxity, which causes excessive joint motion and is commonly found in girls, has been associated with development of idiopathic scoliosis.[23]

Although the curve may be present in any area of the spine, the most common curve is a right thoracic curve, which produces a rib prominence on the convex side and hypokyphosis from rotation of the vertebral column around its long axis as the spine begins to curve. A spinal curvature of less than 10 degrees is considered a normal variant, not scoliosis.[24,25] Curves greater than 40 degrees are usually considered severe.

Manifestations

Scoliosis is usually first noticed because of the deformity it causes. A high shoulder, prominent hip, or projecting scapula may be noticed by a parent or in a school screening program. In girls, difficulty in hemming or fitting a dress may call attention to the deformity. Idiopathic scoliosis is usually a painless process, although pain may be present in severe cases, usually in the lumbar region. The pain may be caused by pressure on the ribs or on the crest of the ilium. There may be shortness of breath as a result of diminished chest expansion and gastrointestinal disturbances from crowding of the abdominal organs. Adults with less severe deformity may experience mild backache. If scoliosis is left untreated, the curve may progress to an extent that compromises cardiopulmonary function and creates a risk for neurologic complications.

Diagnosis and Treatment

Early diagnosis of scoliosis can be important in the prevention of severe spinal deformity. The cardinal signs of scoliosis are uneven shoulders or iliac crest, prominent scapula on the convex side of the curve, malalignment of spinous processes, asymmetry of the flanks, asymmetry of the thoracic cage, and rib hump or paraspinal muscle prominence when bending forward (Fig. 46–14). A complete physical examination is necessary for children with scoliosis, because the defect may be indicative of other underlying pathology.

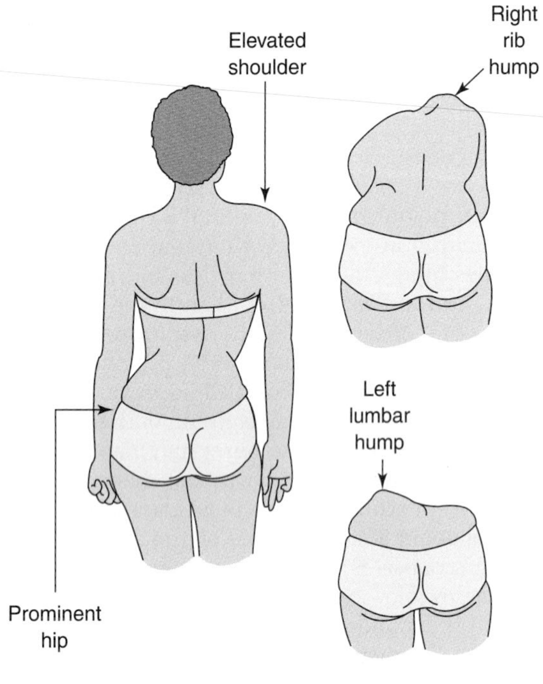

Figure 46–14
Scoliosis. Abnormalities to be determined at initial screening examination. (Gore D.R., Passhel R., Sepic S., & Dalton A. [1981]. Scoliosis screening: Results of a community project. *Pediatrics* 67[2]. Copyright 1981 by the American Academy of Pediatrics)

School screening programs were instituted with the assumption that early detection and treatment of spinal curves would halt progression of the defect. The Scoliosis Research Society has recommended annual screening for all children between 10 and 14 years of age. The American Academy of Pediatrics has recommended screening during routine health supervision visits at the ages of 10, 12, 14, and 16 years. Scoliosis screening is required by law in some states.[21] The U.S. Preventative Task Force examined evidence regarding the effectiveness of routine screening for adolescent idiopathic scoliosis. After reviewing studies regarding the natural history of curve projection, accuracy of screening tests, effectiveness of treatment, potential adverse effects, costs, and burden of suffering, the Task Force issued a statement that "there is insufficient evidence to recommend for or against routine screening of asymptomatic adolescents for idiopathic scoliosis."[21] The Task Force also indicated that there is a great need for clinical research to demonstrate the effectiveness or ineffectiveness of routine screening. Studies that will provide these data are underway, and recommendations regarding screening must be updated when this information becomes available.[26]

Diagnosis of scoliosis is made by physical examination and confirmed by radiographs. A scoliometer should be used at the apex of the curvature to quantify a prominence; a scoliometer reading of greater than 10 degrees requires referral to a physician. The curve is measured by determining the amount of lateral deviation present on x-ray films and is labeled right or left for the convex portion of the curve. Other radiographic procedures may be done, including CT, magnetic resonance imaging (MRI), and myelography.

The treatment of scoliosis depends on the severity of the deformity and the likelihood of progression. Larger curves are more likely to progress. Age of presentation is also important. Curves that are detected before menarche are more likely to progress than those detected after menarche. For persons with lesser degrees of curvature (10 to 20 degrees), the trend has been away from aggressive treatment and toward a "wait and see" approach, taking advantage of the more sophisticated diagnostic methods that are now available. Treatment is considered for physiologically immature patients with curves between 20 and 30 degrees. Curves between 30 and 40 degrees are usually considered for bracing, and those greater than 40 to 45 degrees are considered for surgery.

A brace may be used to control the progression of the curvature during growth and can provide some correction. The most commonly used brace is the Milwaukee brace, which was developed by Blount and Schmitt in the 1940s (Fig. 46–15). This was the first brace to provide some degree of active correction. It involves a pelvic mold, various pads, and two metal upright supports around the throat. It is cumbersome, and compliance with wearing the brace has been shown to be lacking. Studies across the United States found that fewer than 50% of patients consistently wore their braces. In an effort

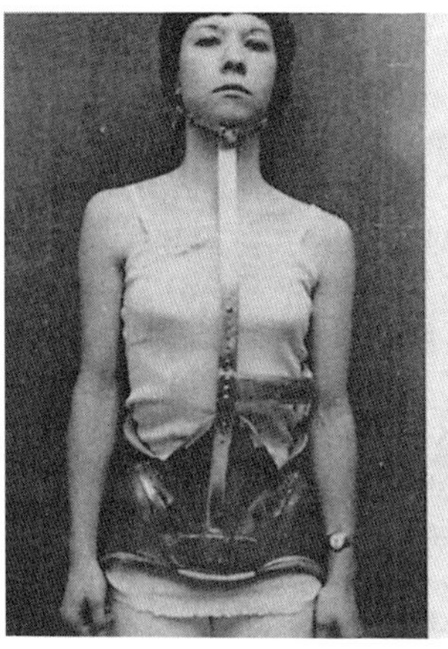
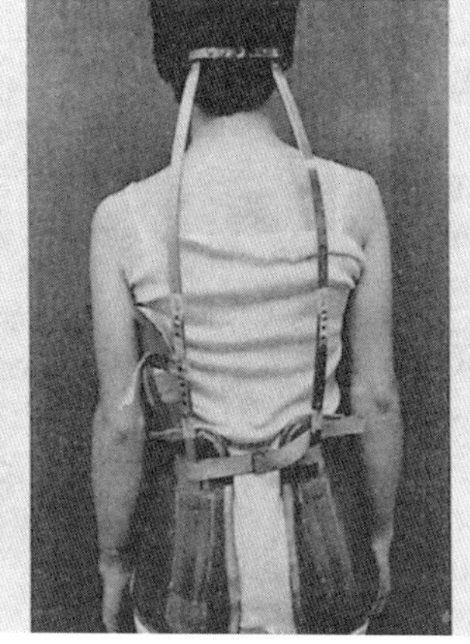
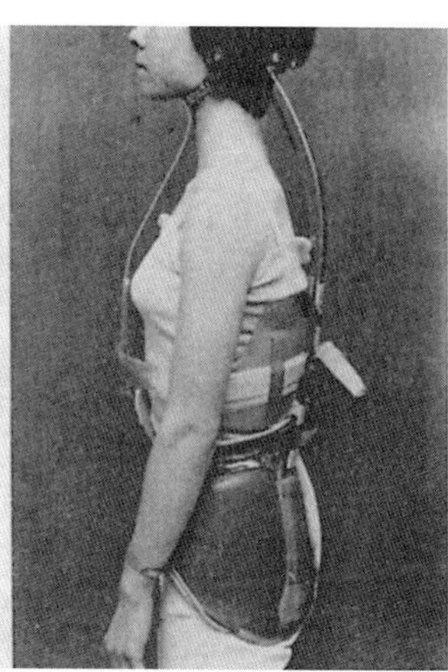

Figure 46–15 ■■■
The Milwaukee brace as seen from front, back, and side.

to improve compliance, a number of new bracing techniques were developed. They include underarm or thoracolumbosacral orthoses (TLSO). These orthoses consist of easily concealed, prefabricated forms that are modified to suit the patient. Although probably less effective than the Milwaukee brace, they are more cosmetically acceptable. Another alternative is the Charleston brace, which provides more dramatic correction but is only worn at night. Although the TLSO and Charleston braces are probably more acceptable to the patient, long-term data related to their effectiveness are not available.

Surgical intervention with instrumentation and spinal fusion is done in severe cases—when the curvature has progressed to 40 degrees or beyond at the time of diagnosis or when curves of a lesser degree are compounded with imbalance or rotation of the vertebrae. Unlike bracing, which is intended to halt progression of the curvature, surgical intervention is used to decrease the curve (Fig. 46–16). Instrumentation helps correct the curve and balance, and spinal fusion maintains the spine in the corrected position. Several methods of instrumentation (*i.e.*, rods that attach to the vertebral column) are used, including Harrington rod instrumentation and posterior spinal fusion, Dwyer (or Zielke) instrumentation and anterior spinal fusion, segmental (Luque) spinal instrumentation and posterior spinal fusion, or Cotrel-Dubousset bilateral segmental fixation. An anterior approach is usually used as the first stage of a two-stage procedure. Combined

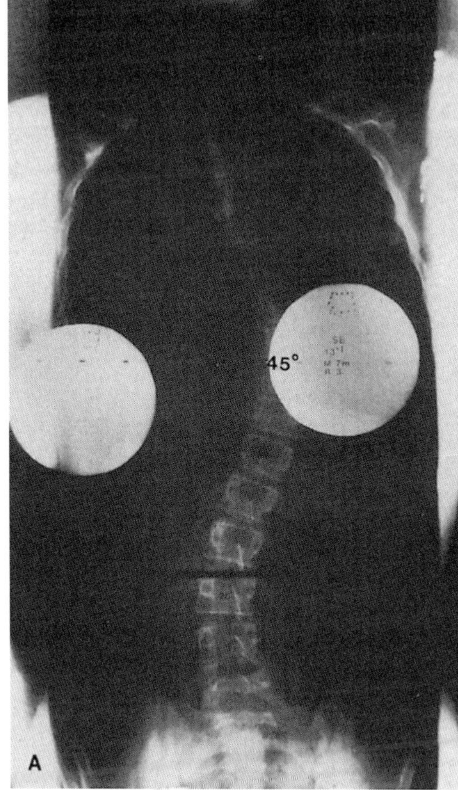

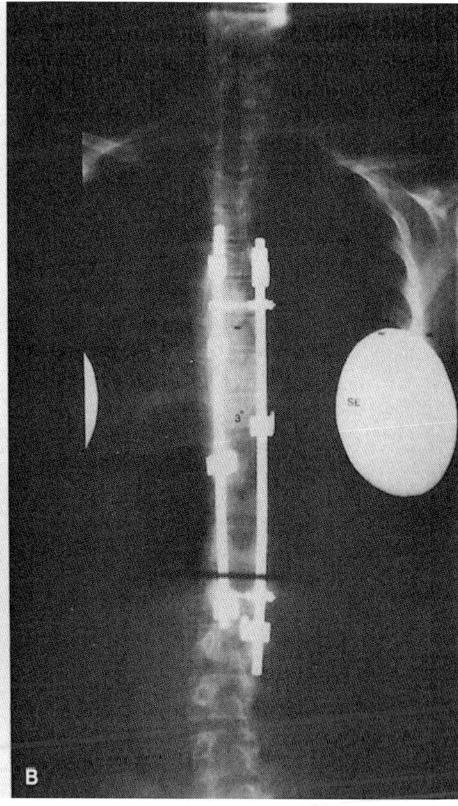

Figure 46–16 ■■■
(**A**) A 13-year-old girl has a curved spine that progressed from 23 to 45 degrees despite bracing. (**B**) After spinal fusion and Cotrel-Dubousset instrumentation, the curvature is 3 degrees.

anterior and posterior surgery is used for more severe curvatures. Despite great advances in spinal surgery, no one method seems to be the best for all cases.

In summary, skeletal disorders can result from congenital or hereditary influences or from factors that occur during normal periods of skeletal growth and development. Newborn infants undergo normal changes in muscle tone and joint motion, causing torsional conditions of the femur or tibia. Many of these conditions are corrected as skeletal growth and development take place. Osteogenesis imperfecta is a rare autosomal hereditary disorder characterized by defective synthesis of connective tissue, including bone matrix. It results in poorly developed bones that fracture easily. Developmental dysplasia of the hip includes a range of structural abnormalities. Dislocated hips are always treated to prevent changes in the anatomic structure. Other childhood skeletal disorders, such as the osteochondroses, slipped capital femoral epiphysis, and scoliosis, are not corrected by the growth process. These disorders are progressive, can cause permanent disability, and require treatment. Disorders such as congenital dislocation of the hip and congenital clubfoot are present at birth. Both of these disorders are best treated during infancy. Regular examinations during the first year of life are recommended as a means of achieving early diagnosis of such disorders.

Metabolic Bone Disease

After you have completed this section of the chapter, you should be able to meet the following objectives:

- Name the three factors responsible for maintaining the equilibrium of bone tissue
- Cite the functions of osteoclasts and osteoblasts in bone remodeling and relate them to the actions of parathyroid hormone, vitamin D, and estrogen
- Describe risk factors that contribute to the development of osteoporosis and relate them to the prevention of the disorder
- Describe the primary features of osteoporotic bone
- Describe the action of estrogen, calcitonin, fluorides, and biphosphonates in the treatment of osteoporosis
- Describe the pathogenesis and manifestations of osteomalacia and rickets
- Characterize the cause and manifestations of Paget's disease

The process of bone resorption and formation is continuous throughout life. This process is called *bone remodeling*. There are two types of bone remodeling: structural and internal remodeling. Structural remodeling involves deposition of new bone on the outer aspect of the shaft at the same time that bone is resorbed from the inner aspect of the shaft. It occurs during growth and results in a bone having adult form and shape. Internal remodeling largely involves the replacement of trabecular bone and is continuous during adulthood.

In the adult, about 25% of trabecular bone is replaced each year, compared with 3% of compact bone.[27] In the adult skeleton, bone remodeling proceeds in cycles that involve resorption of old bone by osteoclasts and subsequent formation of new bone by osteoblasts (Fig. 46–17). After the bone formation has ceased, the bone is covered by a distinct type of terminally differentiated osteoblasts.

The sequence of bone resorption and bone formation is activated by one of many stimuli, including the actions of parathyroid hormone and calcitonin. It begins with osteoclastic resorption of existing bone, during which the organic (protein matrix) and the inorganic (mineral) components are removed. The sequence proceeds to the formation of new bone by osteoblasts. In the adult, the length of one sequence (*i.e.*, bone resorption and formation) is about 4 months. Ideally, the replaced bone should equal the absorbed bone. If it does not, there is a net loss of bone. In the elderly, for example, bone resorption and formation are no longer perfectly coupled, and bone mass is lost.

The three major influences on the equilibrium of bone tissue are mechanical stress; calcium and phosphate levels in the extracellular fluid; and hormones and local growth factors and cytokines, which influence bone resorption and formation. Mechanical stress stimulates osteoblastic activity and formation of the organic matrix. It is important in preventing bone atrophy and in healing fractures. Bone serves as a storage site for extracellular calcium and phosphate ions. Consequently, alterations in the extracellular levels of these ions affect

Quiescent bone surface covered by lining cells

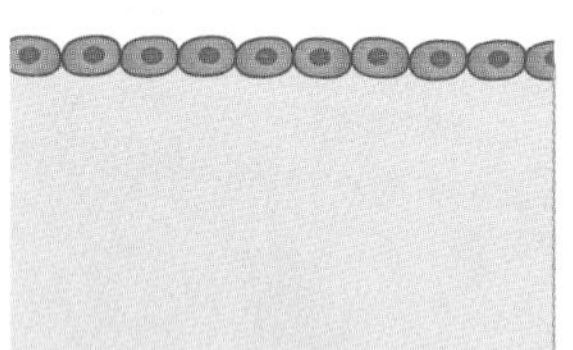

Osteoclasts on the bone surface resorbing old bone

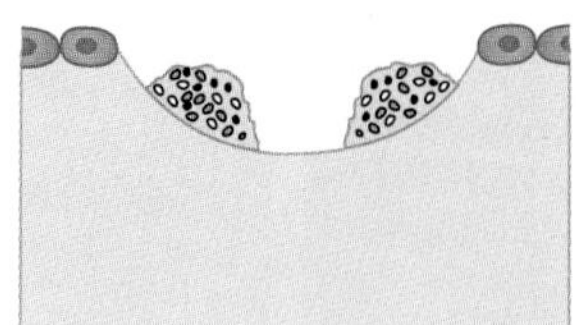

Osteoblasts filling the resorption cavity with osteoid

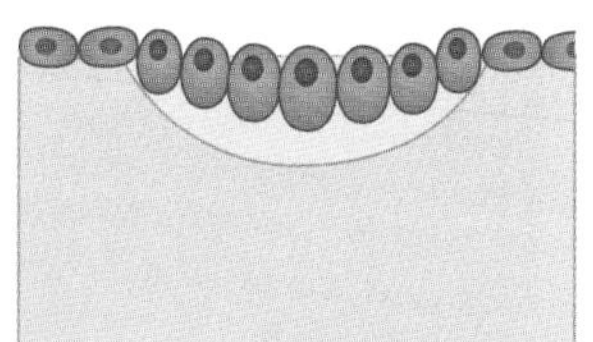

Osteoid becoming mineralized

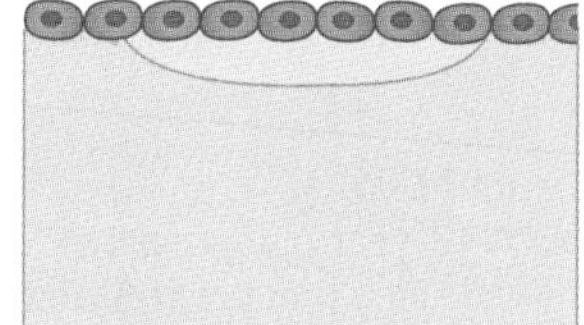

Figure 46–17
The process of bone resorption by the osteoclasts and subsequent bone formation by the osteoblasts.

their deposition in bone (see Chapter 26). Vitamin C is required for proper collagen formation. A deficiency of vitamin C can result in a disease called *scurvy*. In the absence of vitamin C, the epiphyseal plates and bony shaft of growing bone are so thin and fragile that they are predisposed to fractures. In the adult, vitamin C deficiency affects bone maintenance rather than growth. Vitamin D is needed for intestinal absorption of calcium and phosphate. Blood levels of calcium and phosphate are regulated by parathyroid hormone and calcitonin. Parathyroid hormone promotes bone resorption, and calcitonin inhibits bone resorption.

Osteoclasts and osteoblasts are derived from progenitor cells in the bone marrow.[27] The osteoclasts originate from hematopoietic precursors and osteoblasts from stromal (supporting) cells in the bone marrow. However, the development of osteoclasts from hematopoietic precursors cannot take place unless stromal-osteoblastic cells are present. The effects of systemic hormones and local influences on osteoclast development are mediated by stromal-osteoblastic cells. The differentiation and function of osteoclasts and osteoblasts are regulated by chemical messengers, including colony-stimulating factors and other cytokines (see Chapter 11). Interleukin-6, which is produced in response to systemic hormones such as parathyroid hormone and vitamin D, stimulates the early stages of osteoclast development. Interleukin-6 is thought to be involved in the abnormal bone resorption associated with Paget's disease. The inhibitory effects of estrogen on bone resorption are thought to be mediated through the inhibition of interleukin-6. With aging, the ability of the bone marrow to produce osteoblastic precursors is decreased.

Osteopenia

Osteopenia is a condition that is common to all metabolic bone diseases. It is characterized by a reduction in bone mass greater than expected for age, race, or sex, and it occurs because of a decrease in bone formation, inadequate bone mineralization, or excessive bone deossification. Osteopenia is not a diagnosis but a term used to describe an apparent lack of bone seen on x-ray studies. The major causes of osteopenia are osteoporosis, osteomalacia, malignancies such as multiple myeloma, and endocrine disorders such as hyperparathyroidism and hyperthyroidism.

Osteoporosis

Osteoporosis refers to increased porosity of bone due to loss of bone mass. Although osteoporosis can occur as the result of an endocrine disorder or malignancy, it is most often associated with the aging process. After attaining maximal bone mass at age 30, the rate of bone loss for both sexes is approximately 0.5% per year, and it increases to about 1% per year or more in menopausal women.[28] An estimated 25 million Americans are affected with osteoporosis, and more than 1.5 million suffer from fractures related to osteoporosis each year.[29] Bone mass positively correlates with the amount of skin pigmentation; whites have the least amount of bone mass, and African Americans have the most.[30] Although osteoporosis is uncommon among African-American women, many cases are seen among postmenopausal women with brown and yellow skin. One of the reasons for the increased risk in postmenopausal women of white or Asian descent may be that their original bone mass is less and that the losses associated with aging therefore affect them sooner. Osteoporosis is rare in children. When it does occur, it is related to such causes as the excess corticosteroid levels associated with Cushing's syndrome, colon disease, prolonged immobility, or osteogenesis imperfecta.

The development of osteoporosis involves many factors. It is related to hormone levels, physical fitness, and general nutrition. It is thought that an indirect action of estrogen is the suppression of bone resorption. This action is reduced after menopause. Exercise helps to prevent involutional bone loss and may serve to prevent or delay the progression of osteoporosis. Poor nutrition or an age-related decrease in intestinal absorption of calcium because of deficient activation of vitamin D may contribute to osteoporosis, particularly in the elderly.[31] Persons with endocrine disorders such as hyperthyroidism, hyperparathyroidism, Cushing's syndrome, or diabetes mellitus are at high risk for developing osteoporosis. The prolonged use of medications that increase calcium excretion, such as aluminum-containing antacids, corticosteroids, and anticonvulsants, is also associated with bone loss.[32] Other risk factors found to be associated with osteoporosis are a diet high in protein, cigarette smoking, alcohol ingestion, and a family history of osteoporosis.

Pathogenesis

The pathogenesis of osteoporosis is unclear, but most data suggest an imbalance between bone resorption and formation such that bone resorption exceeds bone formation. There appears to be a decrease in the number and activity of osteoblasts or bone-building cells and an increase in activity of osteoclasts or bone-resorbing cells.[12,33] Decreases in sex hormone levels, which seem to act as intermediates to prevent bone loss, in men and women are somehow important in the pathogenesis of osteoporosis. During early menopause, there is osteoclast-mediated rapid bone loss. This is caused by increased remodeling activation and increased rate and depth of osteoclastic bone reabsorption. There are structural changes in the cancellous and cortical bone structure. In postmenopausal women, these changes can be reversed by estrogen therapy. Bone loss is slower after early menopause because of a decrease in remodeling by the osteoclasts. There is some evidence that osteoporosis is caused, at least in part, by abnormalities in local factors, such as prostaglandins, interleukins, and growth factors, that influence bone cell function.[34] Further study is needed, particularly because local factors cannot be measured directly but must be identified with in vitro organ-culture methods and tissues from laboratory animals.

Osteoporotic changes occur in the diaphysis and the metaphysis of bone. The diameter of the bone enlarges with age, causing the outer supporting cortex to become thinner. In severe osteoporosis, the bones begin to resemble the fragile structure of a fine porcelain vase. There is loss of trabeculae from cancellous bone and thinning of the cortex to such an extent that minimal stress causes fractures (Fig. 46–18). The changes that occur with osteoporosis have been explained by two distinct disease processes affecting women early and late in life.[34] Type I is caused by early postmenopausal estrogen deficiency and is manifested by loss of trabecular bone, with a predisposition to fractures of the vertebrae and distal radius. Type II (*i.e.*, senile osteoporosis) is caused by a calcium deficiency and is a slower process in which cortical and trabecular bone are lost. Hip fractures, which are seen later in life, result from the second type. The different pathogenic mechanisms and presentations make it difficult to generalize about osteoporosis.

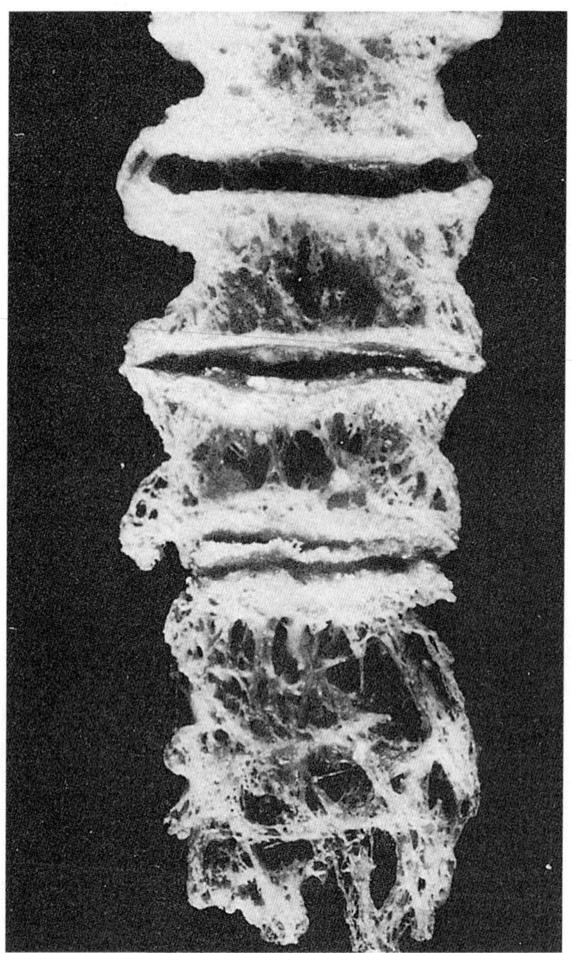

Figure 46–18
Vertebral osteoporosis in a speciman cleared of soft tissue, leaving only the residual bone structure. (From Cotra R.S., Kumar, V. and Robbins S. *Robbins pathologic basis of disease* [5th ed.]. Philadelphia: WB Saunders)

Manifestations

The first clinical manifestations of osteoporosis are pain accompanied by skeletal fractures—a vertebral compression fracture or fractures of the hip, pelvis, humerus, or any other bone. Unfortunately, fractures represent an end stage of the disease. Women who present with fractures are much more likely to suffer another fracture than are women of the same age without osteoporosis. Wedging and collapse of vertebrae causes a loss of height in the vertebral column and kyphosis, a condition commonly referred to as dowager's hump. Usually, there is no generalized bone tenderness. When pain occurs, it is related to fractures. Systemic symptoms such as weakness and weight loss suggest that the osteoporosis may be caused by underlying disease.

Diagnosis and Treatment

An important advance in diagnostic methods used for the identification of osteoporosis has been the use of bone-density assessment. The clinical method of choice for bone density studies is dual energy x-ray absorptiometry (DEXA) of the spine and hip. Simpler single or dual photon beams to assess density of the calcaneous (and the wrists, hips, or spine) can also be used. In the United States, the National Osteoporosis Foundation sets the diagnostic criteria at 2.0 standard deviations below peak value. According to these standards, most women would be candidates for treatment by age 60.[28] Measurement of bone density has become increasingly common for early detection and fracture prevention. Excessive loss of height indicates some probability of low bone mass.[35] Measurement of serial heights in older adults is another simple way to screen for osteoporosis. A further advance in the diagnosis of osteoporosis is the refinement of risk factors, permitting better analysis of risk pertaining to particular persons.[36]

Prevention and early detection of osteoporosis is essential to the prevention of the associated deformities and fractures. It is important to identify persons in high-risk groups so treatment can be begun early. Postmenopausal women of small stature or lean body mass, those with sedentary lifestyles, those whose calcium intake is poor, and those suffering from diseases that demineralize bone are at greatest risk. Other risk factors include an age of 80 or greater, maternal history of hip fracture, caffeine intake exceeding two cups of coffee each day, previous hyperthyroidism, current anticonvulsant therapy, and current use of long-acting benzodiazepines. Risk factors for osteoporosis are listed in Chart 46–1.

Regular exercise and adequate calcium intake are important factors in preventing osteoporosis. Weight-bearing exercises such as walking, jogging, rowing, and weight lifting are important in the maintenance of bone mass. Studies have indicated that premenopausal women need more than 1000 mg and postmenopausal women need 1500 mg of calcium daily.[28,29] This means that adults should drink three to four glasses of milk daily or substitute other foods that are high in calcium. Because most older American women do not consume a sufficient

CHART **46-1**
Risk Factors Associated with Osteoporosis

Personal Characteristics

Advanced age
Female
Caucasian (fair, thin skin)
Small bone structure
Postmenopausal
Family history

Lifestyle

Sedentary
Calcium deficiency (long-term)
High-protein diet
Excessive alcohol intake
Excessive caffeine intake
Smoking

Drug and Disease Related

Aluminum-containing antacids
Anticonvulsants
Heparin
Corticosteroids or Cushing's disease
Gastrectomy
Diabetes mellitus
Chronic obstructive lung disease
Malignancy
Hyperthyroidism
Hyperparathyroidism
Rheumatoid arthritis

quantity of dairy products to meet their calcium needs, calcium supplementation is recommended. Calcium tablets vary in content of elemental calcium, with calcium carbonate tablets providing the greatest amount. The popular 500-mg tablet provides 200 mg of elemental calcium and 20% of the recommended daily requirement. The usual dose is 500 mg taken three times a day with meals to avoid gastric upset.

There is still conflicting data on recommendations for vitamin D supplementation. Deficient activation of vitamin D may be an important factor in the impaired intestinal absorption of calcium in the elderly.[36] On the basis of this evidence, 1,25-dihydroxyvitamin D_3 is being studied as a treatment for osteoporosis. A daily intake of 400 to 800 IU of vitamin D is recommended, because vitamin D optimizes calcium absorption and inhibits increased parathyroid secretion, which stimulates calcium resorption from bone.

Estrogen therapy in postmenopausal women in the United States is relatively common and is becoming less controversial. If begun soon after menopause, estrogen prevents early-stage bone loss.[29] Studies have indicated that the beneficial effects from administering estrogen to women continue into their seventies.[32] Although the incidence of endometrial cancer is increased by administration of estrogen, this risk is reduced by concurrent administration of progestin.[29] Whether estrogen increases the risk of breast cancer remains to be determined.

Active treatment of osteoporosis uses four types of agents: gonadal hormones (estrogen), calcitonin, fluorides, and bisphosphonates. Calcitonin can be used to decrease osteoclastic activity. It has some effect on bone pain, but until recently, it was only available as an injectable drug. A nasal-spray formulation is now available. Fluoride appears to combat osteoporosis by directly inducing bone formation. In early studies, the quality of the bone was questionable. Because the new bone is laid down on existing bone, the treatment must be started while there is still adequate bone onto which the fluoride-induced bone can be built. The use of cyclic, intermittent, slow-release sodium fluoride has shown some promise.[29]

The biphosphonates are analogues of endogenous inorganic pyrophosphate that the body cannot break down. In bone, they bind to hydroxyapatite and prevent bone resorption through the inhibition of osteoclast activity. Etidronate (Didronel), the prototypical agent, also inhibits osteoblastic activity and bone formation. It is given in a 2-week cycle for osteoporosis. The cycle is repeated every 10 to 12 weeks to permit the body to achieve excess formation of bone in relation to resorption.[37] Alendronate (Fosamax) is a newer form of biphosphonate that is taken once per day. It is reported to have little or no deleterious effect on osteoblastic activity and bone formation. Another biphosphate, residronate, is in the advanced stages of clinical trials. Further research is needed to determine if the increases in bone density seen with biphosphonates can be maintained and if they are quality bone deposits.

Persons with osteoporosis have many special needs. In treating fractures, it is important to minimize immobility. Surgical intervention is done for stable fracture fixation that allows early restoration of mobility and function. This means early weight bearing on the lower extremities. Walking and swimming are encouraged. Unsafe conditions that predispose persons to falls and fractures should be corrected or avoided.

Osteomalacia and Rickets

In contrast to osteoporosis, which causes a loss of total bone mass and results in brittle bones, osteomalacia and rickets produce a softening of the bones and do not involve the loss of bone matrix. About 60% of bone is mineral content, about 30% is organic matrix, and the remainder is living bone cells. The organic matrix and the inorganic mineral salts are needed for normal bone consistency. If the inorganic mineral salts are removed from fresh bone (by dilute nitric acid), the organic matrix that remains still resembles a bone, but it is so flexible that it can be tied in a knot. When a bone is placed over a hot flame, the organic material is destroyed, and the bone becomes brittle.

Osteomalacia

Osteomalacia is a generalized bone condition in which inadequate mineralization of bone matrix results from a calcium or phosphate deficiency, or both. It is sometimes referred to as the adult form of rickets

There are two main causes of osteomalacia: insufficient calcium absorption from the intestine because of a lack of calcium or resistance to the action of vitamin D and phosphate deficiency due to increased renal losses or decreased intestinal absorption. Vitamin D is a fat-soluble vitamin that is absorbed intact through the intestine or produced in the skin as a result of ultraviolet irradiation. Vitamin D that is absorbed from the intestine or synthesized in the skin is inactive. Vitamin D is activated in a two-step process that begins in the liver and is completed in the kidney. Vitamin D deficiency is most commonly caused by reduced vitamin D absorption as a result of biliary tract or intestinal diseases that impair fat and fat-soluble vitamin absorption. Lack of vitamin D in the diet is rare in the United States because many foods are fortified with the vitamin. Anticonvulsant medications, such as phenobarbital and phenytoin, induce hepatic hydroxylases that accelerate breakdown of the active forms of vitamin D.

A form of osteomalacia called *renal rickets* occurs in persons with chronic renal failure. It is caused by the inability of the kidney to activate vitamin D and excrete phosphate and is accompanied by hyperparathyroidism, increased bone turnover, and increased bone resorption. Another form of osteomalacia results from renal tubular defects that cause excessive phosphate losses. This form of osteomalacia is commonly referred to as *vitamin D–resistant rickets* and is often a familial disorder. It is inherited as an X-linked dominant gene passed by mothers to one half of their children and by fathers to their daughters only. This form of osteomalacia affects boys more severely than girls. Longstanding primary hyperparathyroidism causes increased calcium resorption from bone and hypophosphatemia, which can lead to rickets in children and osteomalacia in adults. Another cause of phosphate deficiency is the long-term use of antacids, such as aluminum hydroxide, that bind dietary forms of phosphate and prevent their absorption.

The incidence of osteomalacia is high among the elderly because of diets deficient in calcium and vitamin D and is often compounded by the intestinal malabsorption problems that accompany aging. Osteomalacia is often seen in cultures in which the diet is deficient in vitamin D, such as in northern China, Japan, and northern India. Women in these areas have a higher incidence of the disorder than men because of the combined effects of pregnancy, lactation, and more indoor confinement. Osteomalacia is occasionally seen in strict vegetarians; persons who have had a gastrectomy; and those on long-term anticonvulsant, tranquilizer, sedative, muscle relaxant, or diuretic drugs. There is also a greater incidence of osteomalacia in the colder regions of the world, particularly during the winter months, probably because of lessened exposure to sunlight.

The clinical manifestations of osteomalacia are bone pain, tenderness, and fractures as the disease progresses. In severe cases, muscle weakness is often an early sign. The cause of muscle weakness is unclear. The combined effects of gravity, muscle weakness, and bone softening contribute to the development of deformities. There may be a dorsal kyphosis in the spine, rib deformities, a heart-shaped pelvis, and marked bowing of the tibiae and femurs. Osteomalacia predisposes a person to pathologic fractures in the weakened areas, especially in the distal radius and proximal femur. In contrast to osteoporosis, it is not a significant cause of hip fractures. There may be delayed healing and poor retention of internal fixation devices. Osteomalacia is usually accompanied by a compensatory or secondary hyperparathyroidism stimulated by low serum calcium levels. Parathyroid hormone reduces renal absorption of phosphate and removes calcium from the bone. Serum calcium levels are only slightly reduced in osteomalacia.

Diagnosis and Treatment

Diagnostic measures are directed toward identifying osteomalacia and establishing its cause. Diagnostic methods include x-ray studies, laboratory workup, bone scan, and bone biopsy. X-ray findings typical of osteomalacia are the development of transverse lines or pseudofractures called Looser's zones or milkman's fractures. These are apparently caused by stress fractures that are inadequately healed or by the mechanical inadequacy of penetrating nutrient vessels.[12] A bone biopsy may be done to confirm the diagnosis of osteomalacia in a person with nonspecific osteopenia who shows no improvement after treatment with exercise, vitamin D, and calcium.

The treatment of osteomalacia is directed at the underlying cause. If the problem is nutritional, restoring adequate amounts of calcium and vitamin D to the diet may be sufficient. The elderly with intestinal malabsorption may also benefit from vitamin D. The least expensive and most effective long-term treatment is a diet rich in vitamin D (*i.e.*, fish, dairy products, and margarine) along with careful exposure to the midday sun. Vitamin D is specific for adult osteomalacia and vitamin D–resistant rickets, but large doses are usually needed to overcome the resistance to its calcium absorption action and to prevent renal loss of phosphate. The biologically active form of vitamin D, 25-OH vitamin D (calciferol) or 1,25-$(OH)_2$ vitamin D (calcitriol), is available for use in the treatment of osteomalacia resistant to vitamin D (*i.e.*, osteomalacia resulting from chronic liver disease and kidney failure). If osteomalacia is caused by malabsorption, the treatment is directed toward correcting the primary disease condition. For example, adequate replacement of pancreatic enzymes is of paramount importance in pancreatic insufficiency. In renal tubular disorders, the treatment is directed at the altered renal physiology.

Rickets

The vitamin D–deficiency rickets seen in children is called *infantile* or *nutritional rickets.* It is a disturbance in the formation of bone in the growing skeleton and affects the epiphyseal plate and the bones of the immature child. It is characterized by softened and deformed bones caused by failure of the organic matrix of bone to calcify normally. Rickets occurs primarily in underdeveloped areas of the world and in urban areas where pigmented ethnic groups have migrated from sunny to cloudy climates. It is seen most often in infants 6 to 24 months of age.

Nutritional rickets is caused by a lack of vitamin D in the diet or malabsorption diseases. Inadequate amounts of calcium and phosphorus in the diet also play a part in the development of rickets. The bony changes are a result of inadequate absorption of calcium. The pathology of rickets is the same as that of osteomalacia seen in adults. Because rickets affects children during periods of active growth, the structural changes seen in the bone are somewhat different. Bones become deformed; ossification at epiphyseal plates is delayed and disordered. This results in widening of the epiphyseal cartilage plate. Any new bone that does grow is unmineralized.

The symptoms of rickets are usually noticed between 6 months and 3 years of age. The child usually has stunted growth, with a height sometimes far below the normal range. Weight is often not affected so that the children, many of whom present with a protruding abdomen (*i.e.*, rachitic potbelly), have been described as presuming a Buddha-like appearance when sitting. Early symptoms are lethargy and muscle weakness, which may be accompanied by convulsions or tetany related to hypocalcemia. Irritability is common. In severe cases, children lose their skin pigment, develop flabby subcutaneous tissue, and have poorly developed musculature. The ends of long bones and ribs are enlarged. The thorax may be abnormally shaped, with prominent rib cartilage (*i.e.*, rachitic rosary). The legs exhibit bowlegged or knock-kneed deformities. The skull is enlarged and soft, and closure of the fontanels is delayed. The child is slow to develop teeth and may have difficulty standing. Rickets is treated with a balanced diet sufficient in calcium, phosphorus, and vitamin D. Exposure to sunshine is also important, especially for premature infants and those on artificial milk feedings. Supplemental vitamin D in excess of normal requirements is given for several months. Maintaining good posture, positioning, and bracing in older children are used to prevent deformities. After the disease is controlled, deformities may have to be surgically corrected as the child grows.

Paget's Disease

Paget's disease (*i.e.*, osteitis deformans) is discussed separately because it is not a true metabolic disease. It is a progressive skeletal disorder that involves excessive bone destruction and repair and is characterized by increasing structural changes of the long bones, spine, pelvis, and cranium. The disease usually begins during the fifth decade and has a slight male dominance.[12] In children, hyperostosis corticalis deformans juvenilis (a rare inherited disorder), hyperphosphatemia, and diseases that cause diaphyseal stenosis may mimic Paget's disease and are sometimes referred to as juvenile Paget's disease.

The cause of Paget's disease is unknown. One theory proposes that it may be caused by a virus capable of inciting osteoclastic activity.[38] It has been suggested a virus or viruses induce secretion of interferon-6, which is a potent inducer of osteoclastic proliferation, by infected macrophages and fibroblasts.[12] The disease usually begins insidiously and progresses slowly over many years. An initial osteolytic phase is followed by an osteoblastic sclerotic phase. During the initial osteolytic phase, abnormal osteoclasts proliferate. Bone resorption occurs so rapidly that new bone formation cannot keep up, and the bone is replaced by fibrous tissue. The two processes of destruction and rebuilding occur simultaneously. The bones increase in size and thickness because of accelerated bone resorption followed by abnormal regeneration. Irregular bone formation results in sclerotic and osteoblastic lesions. The result is a thick layer of coarse bone with a rough and pitted outer surface that has the appearance of pumice. Histologically, the Paget's lesions show increased vascularity and bone marrow fibrosis with intense cellular activity. The bone has a somewhat mosaic pattern caused by areas of density outlined by heavy blue lines, called *cement lines*.

The disease varies in severity from a simple lesion to involvement of many bones. It may be present long before it is clinically detected. The clinical manifestations of Paget's disease depend on the specific area involved. About 20% of persons with the disorder are totally asymptomatic, and the disease is discovered accidentally.[39] Involvement of the skull causes headaches, intermittent tinnitus, vertigo, and eventual hearing loss. In the spine, collapse of the anterior vertebrae causes kyphosis of the thoracic spine. The femur and tibia become bowed. Softening of the femoral neck can cause coxa vara (*i.e.*, reduced angle of the femoral neck). Coxa vara, in combination with softening of the sacral and iliac bones, causes a waddling gait. When the lesion affects only one bone, it may cause only mild pain and stiffness. Progressive deossification weakens and distorts the bone structure. The deossification process begins along the inner cortical surfaces and continues until the substance of the bone disappears. Pathologic fractures may occur, especially in the bones subjected to the greatest stress (*e.g.*, upper femur, lower spine, pelvic bones). These fractures often heal poorly, with excessive and poorly distributed callus.

Other manifestations of Paget's disease include nerve palsy syndromes from lesions in the upper extremities, mental deterioration, and cardiovascular disease. Cardiovascular disease is the most serious complication and is listed as the most common cause of death of those with advanced generalized Paget's disease. It is caused by vasodilation of the vessels in the skin and subcutaneous tissues overlying the affected bones. When one third to one half of the skeleton is affected, the increased blood flow may lead to high-output cardiac failure. Ventilatory capacity may be limited by rib and spine involvement.

Osteogenic sarcomas, most commonly osteosarcomas, occur in 5% to 10% of persons with Paget's disease, with a slight predominance in men. One fifth of all osteogenic sarcomas in persons 50 years or older originate in persons with Paget's disease.[40] The bones most often affected, in order of frequency, are the femur, pelvis, humerus, and tibia. There appears to be a close histopathogenic relationship between Paget's disease and the associated sarcoma.[40]

Diagnosis of Paget's disease is based on characteristic bone deformities and x-ray changes. Elevated levels of serum alkaline phosphatase and urinary hydroxyproline support the diagnosis, and continued surveillance of these levels may be used to monitor the effectiveness of treatment. Bone scans are used to detect the rapid bone turnover indicative of active disease and to monitor the response to treatment. The scan cannot identify bone activity resulting from malignant lesions. Bone biopsy may be done to differentiate the lesion from osteomyelitis or a primary or metastatic bone tumor.

The treatment of Paget's disease is based on the degree of pain and the extent of the disease. Pain can be reduced with nonsteroidal or other antiinflammatory agents. Suppressive agents such as calcitonin, mithramycin, and diphosphate compounds are used to manage pain and prevent further spread of the disease and neurologic defects. Calcitonin and etidronate, a biphosphonate agent, inhibits osteoclast-mediated bone resorption. Nasal calcitonin is becoming available as a replacement for parenterally administered forms. Mithramycin is a cytotoxic agent that causes osteoclasts to reduce their resorption of bone. Because this drug is toxic, it is reserved for resistant cases. Decreases in serum alkaline phosphatase and urinary hydroxyproline levels and radiologically evident improvement indicate a response to treatment. However, symptomatic improvement is usually considered the best measure of success.

In summary, in addition to its structural function, the skeleton is a homeostatic organ. Metabolic bone diseases such as osteoporosis, osteomalacia, rickets, and Paget's disease are the result of a disruption in the equilibrium of bone formation and resorption. Osteoporosis, which is the most common of the metabolic bone diseases, occurs when the rate of bone resorption is greater than that of bone formation. It is seen frequently in postmenopausal women and is the major cause of fractures in persons older than 45 years of age. Osteomalacia and rickets are caused by inadequate mineralization of bone matrix, primarily because of a deficiency of vitamin D. Paget's disease results from excessive osteoclastic activity and is characterized by the formation of poor-quality bone. The success rate of the various drugs and hormones that are used to treat metabolic bone diseases varies. Further research is needed to clarify the cause, pathology, and treatment of these diseases.

Neoplasms

After you have completed this section of the chapter, you should be able to meet the following objectives:

- Differentiate between the properties of benign and malignant bone tumors
- Name the three major symptoms of bone cancer
- Contrast osteogenic sarcoma and chondrosarcoma
- List the primary sites of tumors that frequently metastasize to the bone
- State the three primary goals for treatment of metastatic bone disease

Neoplasms in the skeletal system are usually referred to as bone tumors. Primary malignant tumors of the bone are uncommon, constituting about 1% of all adult cancers and 15% of pediatric malignancies.[41] Metastatic disease of the bone, however, is relatively common. Primary bone tumors may arise from any of the skeletal components, including osseous bone tissue, cartilage, and bone marrow. The discussion in this section focuses on primary benign and malignant bone tumors of osseous or cartilaginous origin and metastatic bone disease. Tumors of bone marrow origin (*i.e.*, leukemia and multiple myeloma) are discussed in Chapter 9.

Like other types of neoplasms, bone tumors may be benign or malignant. The benign types, such as osteochondromas and giant cell tumors, tend to grow rather slowly and usually do not destroy the supporting or surrounding tissue or spread to other parts of the body. Malignant tumors, such as osteosarcoma and Ewing's sarcoma, grow rapidly and can spread to other parts of the body through the bloodstream or lymphatics. Specific types of bone tumors affect different age groups. They are virtually unknown in infancy, rare in children younger than 10 years of age, and peak during the teen years. Adolescents have the highest incidence, with a rate of 3 cases per 100,000.[41] The two major forms of bone cancer in children and young adults are osteosarcoma and Ewing's sarcoma. It is unusual for either condition to be seen after age 25.[40] Primary lymphoma of bone is seen after 25 years, with a peak incidence at 40 years of age. Chondrosarcoma is most common in those 50 years of age and older.[40] The classification of benign and malignant bone tumors is described in Table 46–1.

Characteristics of Bone Tumors

There are three major symptoms of bone tumors: pain, presence of a mass, and impairment of function (Chart 46–2).[42] Pain is a feature common to almost all malignant tumors but may or may not occur with benign tumors. For example, a benign bone cyst is usually asymptomatic until a fracture occurs. Pain that persists at night and is not relieved by rest suggests malignancy. A mass or hard lump may be the first sign of a bone tumor. A malignant tumor is suspected when a painful mass exists that is enlarging or eroding the cortex of the bone. The ease of discovery of a mass depends on the location of the tumor; a small lump arising on the surface of the tibia is easy to detect, whereas a tumor that is deep in the medial portion of the thigh may grow to a considerable size before it is noticed. Benign and malignant tumors may cause the bone to erode to the point where it cannot withstand the strain of ordinary use. In such cases, even a small amount of bone stress or trauma pre-

TABLE 46-1.
Classification of Primary Bone Neoplasms

Tissue Type	Benign Neoplasm	Malignant Neoplasm
Bone	Osteoid osteoma Benign osteoblastoma	Osteosarcoma Parosteal osteogenic sarcoma
Cartilage	Osteochondroma Chondroma Chrondroblastoma Chondromyxoid fibroma	Chondrosarcoma
Lipid	Lipoma	Liposarcoma
Fibrous and fibroosseous tissue	Fibrous dysplasia	Fibrosarcoma Malignant fibrous histiocytoma
Miscellaneous	Giant cell tumor	Malignant giant cell Ewing's sarcoma
Bone marrow		Multiple myeloma Reticulum cell sarcoma

cipitates a pathologic fracture. A tumor may produce pressure on a peripheral nerve, causing decreased sensation, numbness, a limp, or limitation of movement.

Benign Neoplasms

Benign bone tumors usually are limited to the confines of the bone, have well-demarcated edges, and are surrounded by a thin rim of sclerotic bone. The four most common types of benign bone tumors are osteoma, chondroma, osteochondroma, and giant cell tumor.

An *osteoma* is a small bony tumor found on the surface of a long bone, flat bone, or the skull. It is usually composed of hard, compact (ivory osteoma) or spongy (cancellous) bone. It may be excised or left alone.

A *chondroma* is a tumor composed of cartilage. It grows outward from the bone (*i.e.*, ecchondroma) or within the bone (*i.e.*, enchondroma). These tumors may become large and are especially common in the hands and feet. A chondroma may persist for many years and then take on the attributes of a malignant chondrosarcoma. A chondroma is usually not treated unless it becomes unsightly or uncomfortable.

An *osteochondroma* is the most common form of benign tumor in the skeletal system. It grows only during periods of skeletal growth, originating in the epiphyseal cartilage plate and growing out of the bone like a mushroom. An osteochondroma is composed of cartilage and bone and usually occurs singly but may affect several bones in a condition called multiple exostoses. Malignant changes are rare, and excision of the tumor is done only when necessary.

A *giant cell tumor*, or osteoclastoma, is an aggressive tumor of multinucleated cells that often behaves like a malignant tumor, metastasizing through the bloodstream and recurring locally after excision. It occurs most often in young adults, predominantly female, and is most commonly found in the knee, wrist, or shoulder. The tumor begins in the metaphyseal region, grows into the epiphysis, and may extend into the joint surface. Pathologic fractures are common, because the tumor destroys the bone substance. Clinically, pain may occur at the tumor site, with gradually increasing swelling. X-ray films show destruction of the bone with expansion of the cortex.

The treatment of giant cell tumors depends on their location. If the affected bone can be eliminated without loss of function, such as the clavicle or fibula, the entire bone or part of it may be removed. When the tumor is near a major joint, such as the knee or shoulder, a local excision is done. Irradiation may be used to prevent recurrence of the tumor.

CHART 46-2
Symptoms of Bone Cancer

- Bone pain in an adult or child that comes on slowly but lasts for as long as a week, is constant or intermittent, and may be worse at night.
- Unexplained swelling or lump on the bones of the arms, legs, thigh, or other parts of the body that is firm and slightly tender and may be felt through the skin. It may interfere with normal movement and can cause the bone to break.

These symptoms are not sure signs of cancer. They may also be caused by other, less serious problems. Only a physician can tell for sure.

(Adapted from U.S. Department of Health and Human Services [1993]. *What you need to know about cancers of the bone.* NIH publication no. 93–1571. Bethesda: U.S. Government Printing Office)

Malignant Bone Tumors

In contrast to benign tumors, malignant tumors tend to be ill defined, lack sharp borders, and extend beyond the confines of the bone, showing that it has destroyed the cortex. Malignant bone tumors are rare before age 10, have their peak incidence in the teen years, and have a high mortality rate. There is much morbidity and trauma from the often mutilating surgical excision.

The diagnosis of bone tumors includes radiologic staging and biopsy. Radiographs give the most general diagnostic information, such as malignant versus benign and primary versus metastatic status. The radiograph demonstrates the region of bone involvement, extent of destruction, and amount of reactive bone formed. Radioisotope scans are used to estimate the local intramedullary extent of the tumor and screen for other skeletal areas of involvement. CT scans further aid diagnosis and anatomic localization and can identify small pulmonary metastases not seen by conventional radiographs. MRI is the most accurate method of evaluating the intramedullary extent of bone tumor and can demarcate the soft structures in relation to neurovascular structures without the use of a contrast media. It is best used in conjunction with a CT scan.[43] A biopsy is also done because the definitive treatment of most bone tumors is based on pathologic interpretation of the biopsy specimen. A bone biopsy can be performed by means of a large needle or open surgical methods.

The treatment of malignant bone tumors primarily involves surgical removal of the tumor, with amputation of the limb or wide resection of the tumor and surrounding tissue. Preoperative, intraoperative, or postoperative irradiation; chemotherapy; or chemotherapy plus irradiation are used. Radiation therapy is used as a definitive and adjuvant treatment to slow the progression of the cancer, decrease bone pain, and prevent pathologic fractures. A pathologic fracture spreads the tumor cells through formation of a hematoma. Because high-grade bone and soft tissue sarcomas produce clinically undetectable metastases called micrometastases, immunotherapy, irradiation, and chemotherapy are often used in combination as adjuvant therapy. Chemotherapy is the most effective modality for controlling metastases. Extremely aggressive drug combinations have been developed, particularly for the pediatric and young adult age groups.

Many advances have been made in the limb-salvage and reconstructive surgical procedures being used as an alternative to limb amputation. The tumor must have minimal soft tissue involvement and no involvement of major blood vessels. A prosthetic metal implant or allograft (*i.e.*, cadaveric bone transplant) is used to fill the bony defect resulting from surgery.

Osteosarcoma

Osteosarcoma represents 60% of all bone tumors occurring in children and adolescents. The peak incidence is between the ages of 15 and 25 years. The male to female ratio increases to about 1.6 to 1 during late adolescence and adulthood.[41] It it most commonly seen during periods of maximal growth. The primary tumor is most often located at the anatomic sites associated with maximum growth velocity—the distal femur, proximal tibia, and proximal humerus. Persons affected with osteosarcoma are usually tall and are found to have a high plasma level of somatomedin. Bone tumors in the elderly, often with Paget's disease, are more common in the humerus, pelvis, and proximal femur.

Osteosarcoma is a malignant tumor of mesenchymal cells, characterized by the direct formation of osteoid or immature bone by malignant osteoblasts. These cells synthesize thin, wispy, and purposeless fragments of bone. Osteogenic sarcomas are aggressive tumors that grow rapidly; they are often eccentrically placed in the bone and move from the metaphysis of the bone out to the periosteum, with subsequent spread to adjacent soft tissues.

The causes of osteosarcoma are unknown. The correlation of age and location of most of the tumors with the period of maximum growth suggests some relation to increased osteoblastic activity. Paget's disease, which is linked to osteosarcoma in adults, is also associated with increased osteoblastic activity. Irradiation from an internal source, such as the radioactive pharmaceutical technetium used in bone scans, or an external source, such as x-ray films, has also been associated with osteosarcoma.

The primary clinical feature of osteosarcoma is localized pain and swelling in the affected bone, usually of sudden onset. Patients and their families often associate the symptoms with recent trauma.[43] The skin overlying the tumor may be warm, shiny, and stretched, with prominent superficial veins. The range of motion of the adjacent joint may be restricted. Osteosarcoma usually begins as a firm white or reddish mass and later becomes softer with a viscous interior (Fig. 46–19). The tumor infrequently metastasizes to the lymph nodes, because the cells are unable to grow within the node. Nodal metastases usually occur only in the late course of disseminated disease. Most often, the tumor cells exit the primary tumor through the venous end of the capillary, and early metastasis to the lung is common. Lung metastases, even if massive, are usually relatively asymptomatic. The prognosis for a patient with osteosarcoma depends on the aggressiveness of the disease, radiologic features, presence or absence of pathologic fracture, size of the tumor, rapidity of tumor growth, and sex of the person.

Chemotherapy, using various drug combinations, is the most effective treatment for metastatic osteosarcoma. The treatment for sarcomas is surgery in combination with chemotherapy and radiation therapy used both preoperatively and postoperatively. In the past, treatment usually entailed amputation above the level of the tumor. Limb-salvage surgical procedures, using a metal prosthesis or cadaver allografts, are becoming a standard alternative. Studies have shown that limb-salvage surgery has no adverse effects on the long-term survival of persons with osteosarcoma. The success of limb salvage appears to depend on the use of a wide surgical margin, improved radiographic imaging studies, multiagent chemotherapy, and more refined surgical reconstructive techniques.[44,45] Advanced imaging techniques and the use of angiography assist the surgeon in determining the best type of definitive surgery. Successful limb conservation has been achieved in a limited

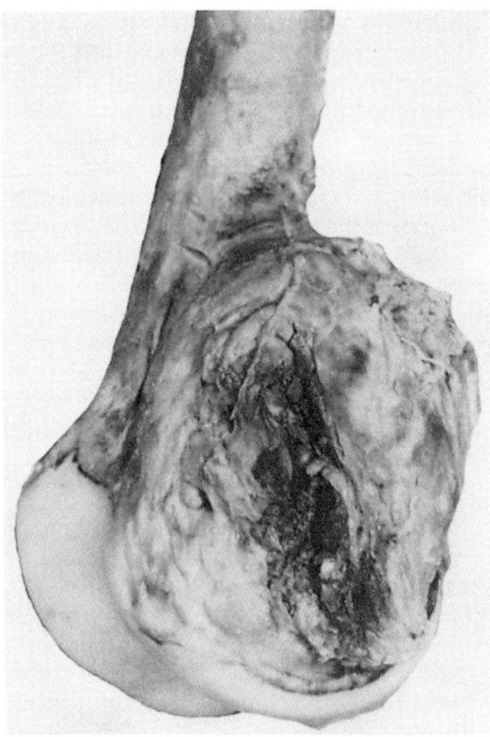

Figure 46–19
Photograph of an osteosarcoma of the distal femur. The neoplasm has broken through the bone and formed a large soft tissue mass.

population with a technique involving en bloc resection (*i.e.*, removal of the tumor and a portion of uninvolved soft tissue as a whole), extracorporeal irradiation, and reimplantation of the irradiated bone.[46]

Irradiation is used for inoperable tumor, such as in the mandible, maxilla, or pelvis. Interstitial implantation of iridium-192 seeds or iodine-125 performed 5 to 6 days after surgery is another treatment under investigation. The use of immunotherapy, including interferon, is still in the experimental stage, as it is with other types of cancers.

Chondrosarcoma

Chondrosarcoma, a malignant tumor of cartilage that can develop within the medullary cavity or peripherally, is the second most common form of malignant bone tumor. It occurs primarily in middle or later life and slightly more often in males. A genetic defect in fetal cartilage can increase the likelihood of developing a chondrosarcoma. The tumor arises from points of muscle attachment to bone, particularly the knee, shoulder, hip, and pelvis. Chondrosarcomas can arise from underlying benign lesions.[41]

Chondrosarcomas are slow growing, metastasize late, and are often painless. They can remain hidden in an area such as the pelvis for a long time. This type of tumor, like many primary malignancies, tends to destroy bone and extend into the soft tissues beyond the confines of the bone of origin. Chondrosarcomas mainly affect the bones of the trunk, pelvis, or proximal femur and rarely develop in the distal portion of a bone. Irregular flecks and ringlets of calcification often are prominent radiographic findings. Early diagnosis is important, because chondrosarcoma responds well to early radical surgical excision. It is generally resistant to radiation therapy and available chemotherapeutic agents.

Ewing's Sarcoma

Ewing's sarcoma is the third most common type of primary bone tumor, and it is highly malignant. It commonly occurs in males younger than 25 years of age, with the incidence highest among teenagers.[40] Ewing's tumor arises from immature bone marrow cells and causes bone destruction from within. It usually occurs in the shaft of long bones or any portion of the pelvis.

Manifestations of Ewing's tumor include pain, tenderness, fever, and leukocytosis. Pathologic fractures are common because of bone destruction. Immediate combination chemotherapy is the first-line treatment of Ewing's sarcoma.[40] Wide resection of the tumor is done if the nerves and blood vessels are free of disease. Most protocols use several courses of intensive chemotherapy before surgery and continue it for a year after surgery. Ewing's sarcoma is more radiosensitive than most bone tumors, but there is risk of a secondary radiation-induced osteosarcoma.

Metastatic Bone Disease

Skeletal metastases are the most common malignancy of osseous tissue, accounting for about one half of the million cancers diagnosed each year in the United States.[47] Metastatic lesions are seen most often in the ribs, spine, and pelvis and are less common in anatomic sites that are further removed from the trunk of the body. Tumors that frequently spread to the skeletal system are those of the breast, lung, prostate, kidney, and thyroid, although any cancer can ultimately involve the skeleton. More than 80% of bone metastases result from primary lesions in the breast, lung, or prostate.[48] The incidence of metastatic bone disease is highest in persons older than 40 years of age. There are typically several bony metastases, with or without metastatic spread to other organs. Solitary lesions are most commonly seen with cancers of the kidney and thyroid. Because of the effectiveness of current cancer treatment modalities, cancer patients are living longer, and the incidence of clinically apparent skeletal involvement appears to be increasing in the long run. These skeletal metastases cause great pain, increase the risk of fractures, and increase the disability of the cancer patient.

Metastasis to the bone frequently occurs without involving other organs, because the blood flow in the veins of the skeletal system is sluggish. These are thin-walled, valveless veins, and there are many storage sites along the way. The pattern of metastasis is often related to the specific vascular pathway involved (*e.g.*, metastases to the shoulder girdle and pelvis occur when prostatic cancers invade the vertebral vein system). If metastasis is limited to the skeletal system, without other major organ involvement, a person can live for many years. Death is usually a consequence of metastasis to vital organs rather than a consequence of the primary tumor.

The major symptom of bone metastasis is pain with evidence of an impending pathologic fracture. Pain is caused by stretching of the periosteum of the involved bone or by nerve entrapment, as in the nerve roots of the spinal cord by the vertebral body. X-ray examinations are used along with CT or bone scans to detect, diagnose, and localize metastatic bone lesions. About one third of persons with skeletal metastases have positive bone scans without radiologic findings. This is because 50% of the trabecular bone must be destroyed before a lesion is visible on plain radiographs.[49] Arteriography using radiopaque contrast media may be helpful in outlining the tumor margins. A bone biopsy usually is done when there is a question regarding the diagnosis or treatment. A closed needle biopsy with CT localization is particularly useful with spine lesions. Serum levels of alkaline phosphatase and calcium are often elevated in persons with metastatic bone disease. Hypercalcemia occurs in 10% to 20% of persons with metastatic bone disease because of bone lysis.[49]

The primary goals in treatment of metastatic bone disease are to prevent pathologic fractures and to promote survival with maximum functioning, allowing the person to maintain as much mobility and pain control as possible. Treatment methods include chemotherapy, irradiation, and surgical stabilization. The discovery of new and more effective drugs along with the use of combination protocols has increased the effectiveness of chemotherapy in treating metastatic bone disease. Local irradiation can effect rapid pain relief within 1 to 2 weeks in more than 50% of patients.[50] Radiation therapy is primarily used as a palliative treatment to alleviate pain and prevent pathologic fractures. Bracing may be ordered for an unstable spine. It is difficult to find a comfortable fit when there is metastasis to the ribs or pelvis. Steroid drugs may also be helpful. The biphosphonates inhibit osteoclastic activity and subsequent bone-induced osteolysis. Biphosphonates are used in metastatic bone disease to relieve the symptoms, enable bone healing to occur, and delay complications.

Hypercalcemia occurs in 10% to 20% of persons with metastatic bone disease because of bone lysis.[50] Symptoms include dulling of consciousness, stupor, weakness, muscle flaccidity, and decreased neural excitability. A total serum calcium level greater than 12 mg/dl requires treatment with diuretics and intravenous sodium chloride (see Chapter 26).

Pathologic fractures occur in about 10% to 15% of persons with metastatic bone disease. The affected bone appears to be eaten away on x-ray images and, in severe cases, crumbles on impact, much like dried toast. Many pathologic fractures occur in the femur, humerus, and vertebrae. In the femur, fractures occur because the proximal aspect of the bone is under great mechanical stress. Lesions may be treated prophylactically with surgery and radiation therapy to prevent pathologic fractures. Flexible intramedullary rods may be used to stabilize long bones. After a pathologic fracture has occurred, bracing, intramedullary nailing of the femur and spine stabilization may be done. Because adequate fixation is often difficult in diseased bone, cement (*i.e.*, methylmethacrylate) is often used with internal fixation devices to stabilize the bone. The selection of a treatment modality for prevention or treatment of pathologic fractures depends on the severity of the lesion, the degree of pain, and the life expectancy of the patient. The goal is to provide flexibility, mobility, and pain relief. Surgeons employ a certain degree of aggressiveness in treating metastatic lesions so that patients can function as normally as possible, even if life expectancy is as short as 3 months.[50]

In summary, bone tumors, like any other type of neoplasm, may be benign or malignant. Benign bone tumors grow slowly and usually do not destroy the surrounding tissues. Malignant tumors can be primary or metastatic. Primary bone tumors are rare, grow rapidly, metastasize to the lungs and other parts of the body through the bloodstream, and have a high mortality rate. Metastatic bone tumors are usually multiple, originating primarily from cancers of the breast, lung, and prostate. The incidence of metastatic bone disease is probably increasing because the improved treatment methods enable persons with cancer to live longer. Advances in chemotherapy, radiation therapy, and surgical procedures have substantially increased the survival and cure rates for many types of bone cancers. A primary goal in metastatic bone disease is the prevention of pathologic fractures.

REFERENCES

1. Moore K.L. (1988). *The developing human* (pp. 72–81, 334–349). Philadelphia: W.B. Saunders.
2. Cormack D.H. (1993). *Essential histology* (pp. 174–178). Philadelphia: J.B. Lippincott.
3. Bruce R.W. (1996). Torsional and angular deformities. *Pediatric Clinics of North America* 43 (4), 867–881.
4. Kunin K.B., Clarren S.K. (1986). The origin of prenatal and postnatal deformities. *Pediatric Clinics of North America* 33 (6), 1277–1297.
5. Sponseller P.D. (1994). Bone, joint, and muscle problems. In Oski F.S. (Ed.). *Principles and practices of pediatrics* (2nd ed., pp. 1016–1048). Philadelphia: J.B. Lippincott.
6. Thompson G.H., Scoles P.V. (1996). Bone and joint disorders. In Behrman R.E., Kliegman R.M., Arvin A.M. *Nelson textbook of pediatrics* (15th ed., pp. 1915–1949). Philadelphia: W.B. Saunders.
7. Staheli L.T. (1986). Torsional deformity. *Pediatric Clinics of North America* 33 (6), 1373–1383.
8. Schoppee K. (1995). Blount disease. *Orthopedic Nursing* 14 (5), 31.
9. Pizzutillo P.D. (1994). The pediatric leg and knee. In Weinstein S.L., Buckwalter J.A. (Eds.). *Turek's orthopaedics: Principles and their application* (5th ed., pp. 573–584). Philadelphia: J.B. Lippincott.

10. Wenger D.R., Leach J. (1986). Foot deformities in infants and children. *Pediatric Clinics of North America* 33 (6), 1411–1429.
11. Tachdjian M.O. (1990). *Pediatric orthopedics.* Philadelphia: W.B. Saunders.
12. Cotran R.S., Kumar V., Robbins S.L. (1994). *Pathologic basis of disease* (5th ed., pp. 441, 1213–1271). Philadelphia: W.B. Saunders.
13. Aronsson D.D., Goldberg M.J., Kling T.F., Roy D.R. (1994). Developmental dysplasia of the hip. *Pediatrics* 94 (2), 201–208.
14. Weinstein S.L. (1994) The pediatric hip. In Weinstein S.L, Buckwalter J.A. (Eds.). *Turek's orthopaedics: Principles and their application* (5th ed., pp. 487–519). Philadelphia J.B. Lippincott.
15. Novacheck T.F. (1996). Developmental dysplasia of the hip. *Pediatrics* 43 (4), 829–848.
16. Shoppee K. (1992). Developmental dysplasia of the hip. *Orthopedic Nursing* 11 (5), 30.
17. Weinstein S.L. (1994). The pediatric foot. In Weinstein S.L, Buckwalter J.A. (Eds.). *Turek's orthopaedics: Principles and their application* (5th ed., pp. 615–653). Philadelphia: J.B. Lippincott.
18. Hoffinger S.A. (1996). Evaluation and management of pediatric foot deformities. *Pediatric Clinics of North America* 43 (5), 1091–1101.
19. Koops S., Quanbeck D. (1996). Three common causes of childhood hip pain. *Pediatric Clinics of North America* 43 (5), 1056–1065.
20. Salmon S.W., Mooney N.E. Verdisco L.A. (1991) *Core curriculum in orthopedic nursing* (pp 344–351, 359–361, 326–330). Pitman, NJ: National Association of Orthopedic Nurses.
21. U.S. Preventative Services Task Force. (1993). Screening for adolescent idiopathic scoliosis [review]. *Journal American Medical Association* 269 (20), 2667–2672.
22. Weinstein S. (1994). The thoracolumbar spine. In Weinstein S.L, Buckwalter J.A. (Eds.). *Turek's orthopaedics: Principles and their application* (5th ed., pp. 447–483), Philadelphia: J.B. Lippincott.
23. Binns M. (1988). Joint laxity in idiopathic adolescent scoliosis. *Journal of Bone and Joint Surgery, British* 70, 420.
24. Rinsky L.A. (1992) Advances in treatment of idiopathic scoliosis. *Hospital Practice* 27 (4), 49–55.
25. Skaggs D.L., Bassett G.S. (1996). Adolescent idiopathic scoliosis: An Update. *American Family Physician* 53 (7), 2327–2334.
26. U.S. Preventative Services Task Force. (1993). Screening for adolescent idiopathic scoliosis: Policy statement. *Journal of the American Medical Association* 269, 2664–2666.
27. Manolagas S.C., Jilka R.L. (1995). Bone marrow, cytokines, and bone remodeling. *New England Journal of Medicine* 332 (5), 305–310.
28. Barzel U.S. (1996). Osteoporosis: Taking a fresh look. *Hospital Practice* 30 (5), 59–68.
29. Riggs B.L., Melton L.J. (1992). The prevention and treatment of osteoporosis. *New England Journal of Medicine* 327 (9), 620–627.
30. Gordon G.S., Vaughn C. (1980). Osteoporosis: Early detection, prevention, and treatment. *Consultant* 25, 64.
31. Liscum B. (1992). Osteoporosis: The silent disease. *Orthopedic Nursing* 11 (4), 21.
32. Gambert S.R., Schulz B.M., Hamdy B.C. (1995). Osteoporosis: Clinical features, prevention, and treatment. *Endocrinology and Metabolic Clinics of North America* 24, 317–371.
33. Bellantoni M.F. (1996). Osteoporosis prevention and treatment. *American Family Physician* 54 (3), 986–992.
34. Riggs B.L. (1987). Pathogenesis of osteoporosis. *American Journal of Obstetrics and Gynecology* 156, 1342.
35. Hunt A.H. (1996). The relationship between height change and bone mineral density. *Orthopedic Nursing* 15 (3), 57.
36. Fraser D.R. (1995). Vitamin D. *Lancet* 345, 104.
37. Gray M.A. (1994). Osteoporosis medications: What's your source of information. *Orthopedic Nursing* 13 (5), 55.
38. Wallach S. (1982). Treatment of Paget's disease. *Advances in Internal Medicine* 27, 1.
39. Hamdy R.C. (1990). Paget's disease of bone. *Hospital Practice* 25 (10), 33–41.
40. Mankin H.J., Willett C.G., Harmon D.C. (1991). Malignant tumors of the bone. In Holleb A.I., Fink D.J., Murphy G.P. (Eds.). *American Cancer Society textbook of clinical oncology* (pp. 355–358). Atlanta: American Cancer Society.
41. American Cancer Society (1996). Cancer statistics 1996. *CA: A Cancer Journal for Clinicians* 46 (11), 8.
42. U.S. Department of Health and Human Services. (1990). *What you need to know about cancers of the bone.* NIH Publication No 90–1571. Bethesda: U.S. Government Printing Office.
43. Meyer W. (1996). Neoplasms of bone. In Behrman R.E., Kliegman R.M., Arvin A.M. (Eds.). *Nelson textbook of pediatrics* (15th ed., pp. 1467–1470). Philadelphia: W.B. Saunders.
44. Bridge J.A., Schwartz H.S., Neff J.R. (1995). Bone sarcoma. In Abeloff M.D., Armitage J.O., Lichter A.S., Niederhuber J.E. (Eds.). *Clinical oncology* (pp. 1715–1797) New York: Churchill Livingstone.
45. Dmroh T.A., Pritchard D.J. (1995). Current combined treatment of high grade osteosarcoma. *Oncology* 9 (4), 327.
46. Uyttendaele D., DeSchyver A., Claessen H. (1988). Limb conservations in primary bone tumors by resection, extracorporeal irradiation and re-implantation. *Journal of Bone and Joint Surgery, British* 70, 348.
47. Boring C.C., Squires T., Tong T. (1991). Cancer statistics, 1991. *Cancer* (4), 19.
48. Mauch P.M., Drew M.A. (1985). Treatment of metastatic cancer to bone. In DeVita V.T., Hellman S., Rosenberg S.A. (Eds.). *Cancer: Principles of practice of oncology* (2nd ed., pp. 2132, 2133, 2135). Philadelphia: J.B. Lippincott.
49. Piasecki P.A. (1996). Nursing care of the patient with metastatic bone disease. *Orthopedic Nursing* 15, 25.
50. Rubens R.D., Coleman R.E. (1995). Bone metastases. In Abeloff M.D., Armitage J.O., Lichter A.S., Niederhuber J.E. (Eds.). *Clinical oncology* (pp. 643–666). New York: Churchill Livingstone.

ADDITIONAL READINGS

Birch J.C., Herrig J.H., Roach J.W., et al. (1988). Cotrel-Dubousset instrumentation in idiopathic scoliosis. *Clinical Orthopaedics and Related Research* 228, 25.

Christodouloy A.G., Prince H.G., Webb J.K., et al. (1987). Adolescent idiopathic thoracic scoliosis: A prospective trial with and without bracing during postoperative care. *Journal of Bone and Joint Surgery* 69 (1), 13.

Consensus Development Conference. (1991). Prophylaxis and treatment of osteoporosis. *American Journal of Medicine* 90, 107–110,.

Corbett D. (1988). Information needs of parents of a child with Pavlik harness. *Orthopedic Nursing* 7 (2), 20.

Cornell C.N. (1990). Management of fractures in patients with osteoporosis. *Orthopedic Clinics of North America* 21 (11), 125.

Cummings S.R., et al. (1995) Risk factors in hip fracture in white women. *New England Journal of Medicine* 332, 767.

Einhorn T.A., Levine B. (1990). Nutrition and bone. *Orthopedic Clinics of North America* 21 (1), 43.

Gelberman R.H., Cohen M.S., Desai S.S., et al. (1987). Femoral anteversion: A clinical assessment of idiopathic intoeing gait in children. *Journal of Bone and Joint Surgery, British* 69, 75.

Gerther J.M., Root L. (1990). Osteogenesis imperfecta. *Orthopedic Clinics of North America* 21 (1), 151.

Goldberg C.J., Dowling F.E., Fogary E.E., Moore D.P. (1995). School scoliosis screening and the United States Preventive Services Task Force: An examination of long-term results. *Spine* 20, 1368–1374.

Habermann E.T., Lopez R.A. (1989). Metastatic disease of bone and treatment of pathologic fractures. *Orthopedic Clinics of North America* 20 (3), 469.

Jaffe N. (1989). Chemotherapy for malignant bone tumors. *Orthopedic Clinics of North America* 20 (3), 487.

Kaplan F.S., Soffer S.R., Fallon M.D., et al. (1988). Osteomalacia as a very late manifestation of primary hyperparathyroidism. *Clinical Orthopaedics and Related Research* 228, 26.

Klein M.J., Kehan S., Lewis M.M. (1989). Osteosarcoma: Clinical and pathological considerations. *Orthopedic Clinics of North America* 30 (3), 327.

Mankin H.J. (1990). Rickets, osteomalacia, and renal dystrophy: An update. *Orthopedic Clinics of North America* 21 (1), 81.

McKibbin B., Freedman L., Howard C., et al. (1988). The management of congenital dislocation of the hip in the newborn. *Journal of Bone and Joint Surgery, British* 70, 423.

O'Connor M.I., Pritchard D.J. (1991). Ewing's sarcoma: Prognostic factors, disease control, and the re-emerging role of surgical treatment. *Clinical Orthopaedics and Related Research* 262, 78.

Renshaw T.S. (1988). Screening school children for scoliosis. *Clinical Orthopaedics and Related Research* 229, 26.

Rodts M.F. (1987). Surgical intervention for adult scoliosis. *Orthopedic Nursing* 6 (6), 11.

Shane E. (1988). Osteoporosis. *Contemporary Issues in Endocrinology and Metabolism* 5, 151.

Sambrook P.N. (1995). The treatment of postmenopausal osteoporosis. *New England Journal of Medicine* 333 (22), 1495–1496.

Thomas I.H., Cole W.G., Waters K.D. (1987). Function after partial pelvic resection of Ewing's sarcoma. *Journal of Bone and Joint Surgery, British* 69, 271.

Winter R.B. (1986). Adolescent idiopathic scoliosis. *New England Journal of Medicine* 314, 1379.

CHAPTER 47

Alterations in Skeletal Function: Rheumatic Disorders

Debra Ann Bancroft and Janice Smith Pigg

Arthritis is a descriptive term applied to more than 100 rheumatic diseases, ranging from localized, self-limiting conditions to those that are systemic, autoimmune processes. Arthritis affects persons in all age groups and is the second leading cause of disability in the United States.[1,2] The common use of the term *arthritis* oversimplifies the nature of the varied disease processes, the difficulty in differentiating one form of arthritis or rheumatic disease from another, and the complexity of treatment of these usually chronic conditions. These diverse conditions share inflammation of the joint as a prominent or accompanying symptom. In the systemic rheumatic diseases—those affecting body systems in addition to the musculoskeletal system—the inflammation is primary, resulting from an immune response, probably autoimmune in origin. In rheumatic conditions limited to a single or few diarthrodial joints, the inflammation is secondary, resulting from the degenerative process and joint irregularities as the bone attempts to remodel itself.

Not yet included in the classification of rheumatic diseases, but being reported in the literature, are the frequent joint complaints in persons who are positive for human immunodeficiency virus (HIV) infection. The HIV epidemic, through its selective immunosuppression, is providing new insights into the pathogenic immunologic processes that occur in rheumatic diseases.[3]

The disabling effects of arthritis may be manifested in an individual's personal, social, and employment activities. To effectively help persons with arthritis, health care providers must have a working knowledge of the specific disease and an understanding of the underlying pathologic processes. Basic education is fundamental in rectifying misconceptions.

Although arthritis cannot be cured, much can be done to control its progress. Fear of being crippled is a major concern that should be addressed so the disease can be perceived realistically. All aspects of treatment require that the person with arthritis accept responsibility for the health care program. Family members should be included in education programs; their support in integrating prescribed treatment regimens is important. Because many unproven remedies for arthritis are offered, patients need information on how to assess the validity of the available treatments. The Arthritis Foundation provides information and community services to persons with arthritis and their families.

This chapter focuses on systemic autoimmune rheumatic diseases, arthritis associated with spondylitis, osteoarthritis syndromes, metabolic diseases associated with arthritis, and rheumatic disease in children and the elderly. A review of normal joint structures is presented in Chapter 44.

Systemic Autoimmune Rheumatic Diseases

After you have completed this section of the chapter, you should be able to meet the following objectives:

- Describe the difficulty in defining the term *arthritis*
- Describe the pathologic changes that may be found in the joint of a person with rheumatoid arthritis
- List the extraarticular manifestations of rheumatoid arthritis
- Describe the immunologic process that occurs in systemic lupus erythematosus
- List four major organ systems that may be involved in systemic lupus erythematosus

Systemic autoimmune rheumatic diseases are a group of chronic disorders that are characterized by diffuse inflammatory vascular lesions and degenerative changes in connective tissue. These disorders share similar clinical features and may affect many of the same organs. Rheumatoid arthritis, systemic lupus erythematosus, polymyalgia rheumatica, temporal arteritis, and juvenile arthritis and dermatomyositis, which share an autoimmune systemic pathogenesis, are discussed in this chapter.

Rheumatoid Arthritis

Rheumatoid arthritis is a systemic inflammatory disease that affects 0.3% to 1.5% of the population, with women affected two to three times more frequently than men.[1] Although the disease occurs in all age groups, its prevalence increases with age. The peak incidence among women is between the ages of 40 and 60, with the onset at 30 to 50 years.

Etiology and Pathogenesis

Although the cause of rheumatoid arthritis remains somewhat mysterious, evidence points to the importance of immunologic events (see Chapters 11 and 12). About 70% to 80% of those with the disease have a substance called the *rheumatoid factor*, which is an antibody that reacts with a fragment of immunoglobulin G (IgG), an autologous (self-produced) antibody, to form immune complexes.[4]

Why the body would begin to produce antibodies against its own IgG remains unclear. An infectious agent, such as a virus, may alter the immunoglobulin so that it is recognized as foreign. Another possibility is that genetic predisposition plays a role in the development of the response. Sixty percent of persons with rheumatoid arthritis have the major histocompatibility complex (MHC) antigen, human lymphocyte antigen (HLA) DR4.[1] HLA-DR4 may play a role in identifying susceptibility to rheumatoid arthritis and be related to the severity of the disease.

Rheumatoid factor has been found in the blood, synovial fluid, and synovial membrane of affected individuals. Much of the rheumatoid factor is produced by lymphocytes in the inflammatory infiltrate of the synovial tissue.[5] The role of the autoimmune process in joint destruction remains obscure. At the cellular level, polymorphonuclear leukocytes, macrophages, and lymphocytes are attracted to the area. The polymorphonuclear leukocytes and macrophages phagocytize the immune complexes and, in the process, release lysosomal enzymes capable of causing destructive changes in the joint cartilage (Fig. 47–1). The inflammatory response that follows attracts additional lymphocytes and plasma cells, setting into motion a chain of events that perpetuates the condition. As the inflammatory process advances, the synovial cells and the subsynovial tissue undergo reactive hyperplasia. Vasodilation and increased blood flow cause warmth and redness. Swelling results from the increased capillary permeability that accompanies the inflammatory process.

Characteristic of rheumatoid arthritis is the development of an extensive network of new blood vessels in the synovial membrane, which contributes to the advancement of the rheumatoid synovitis. This destructive vascular granulation tissue, which is called *pannus*, extends from the synovium to involve the "bare area," a region of unprotected bone at the junction between cartilage and subchondral bone. Pannus is a feature of rheumatoid arthritis that differentiates it from other forms of inflammatory arthritis (Fig. 47–2).[6] The inflammatory cells found in the pannus have a destructive effect on the adjacent cartilage and bone. Eventually, pannus develops between the joint margins, leading to reduced joint motion and the possibility of eventual ankylosis. With progression of the disease, joint inflammation and the resulting structural changes can lead to

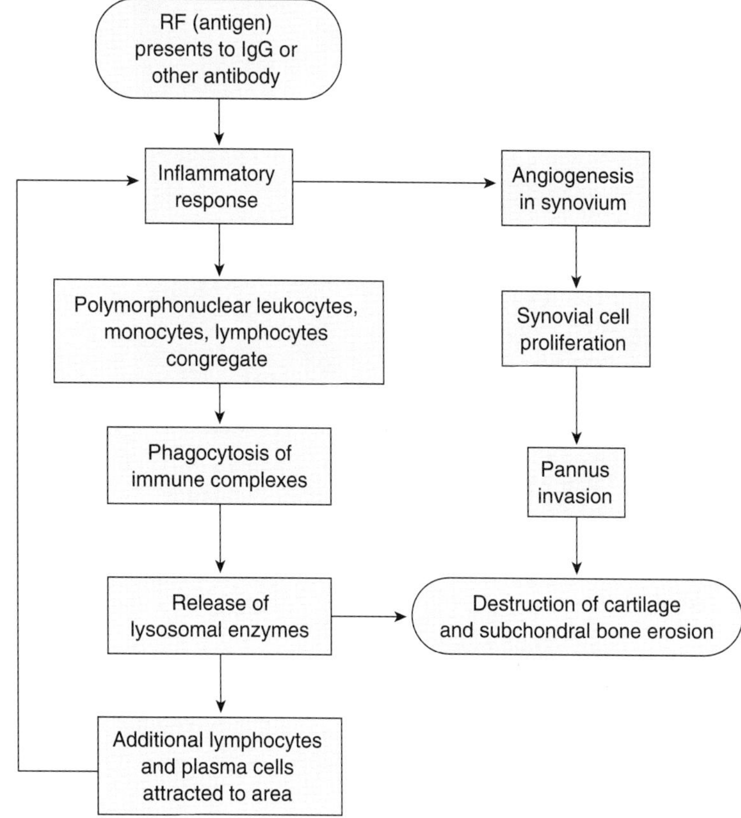

Figure 47–1
Disease process in rheumatoid arthritis.

joint instability, muscle atrophy from disuse, stretching of the ligaments, and involvement of the tendons and muscles. The effect of the pathologic changes on joint structure and function is related to the degree of disease activity, which can change at any time. Unfortunately, the destructive changes are irreversible.

Clinical Manifestations

Rheumatoid arthritis is often associated with extraarticular as well as articular manifestations. It usually has an insidious onset marked by systemic manifestations such as fatigue, anorexia, weight loss, and generalized aching and stiffness. The disease, which is characterized by

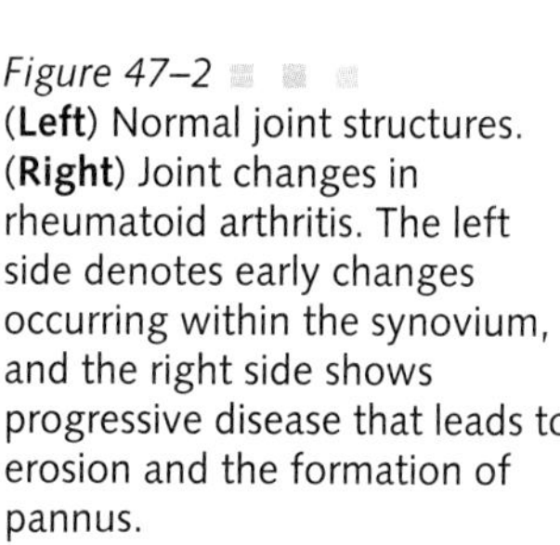

Figure 47–2
(**Left**) Normal joint structures. (**Right**) Joint changes in rheumatoid arthritis. The left side denotes early changes occurring within the synovium, and the right side shows progressive disease that leads to erosion and the formation of pannus.

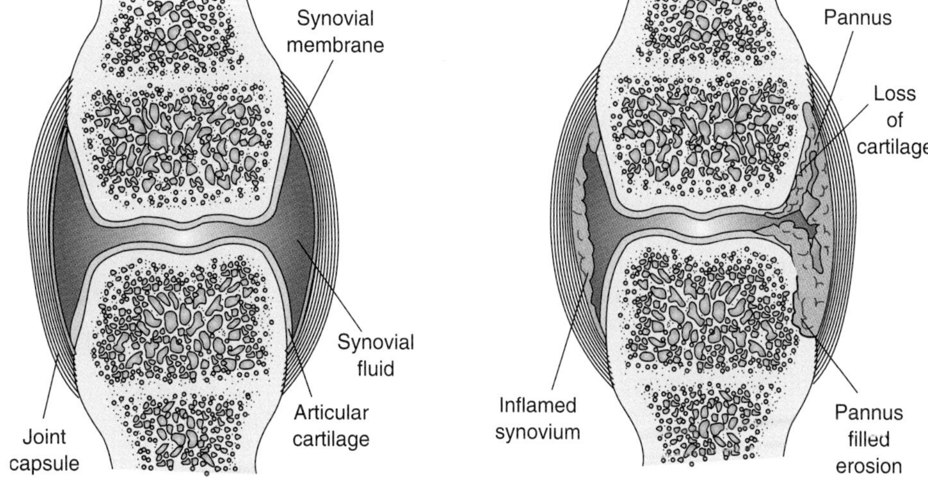

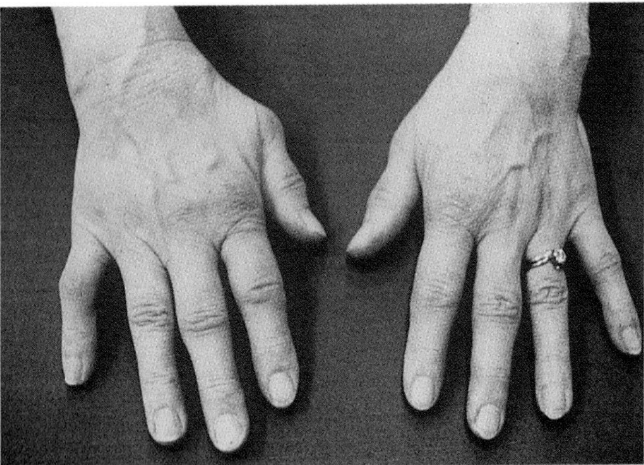

Figure 47–3
Inflammation of finger proximal interphalangeal joints in early stages of rheumatoid arthritis, giving the fingers a spindle-shaped appearance. (Reprinted from the ARHP Arthritis Teaching Slide Collection. Used with permission of the American College of Rheumatology.)

exacerbations and remissions, may involve only a few joints for brief durations, or it may be relentlessly progressive and debilitating. About 3% of those with the disease have a progressive, unremitting form that does not respond to aggressive therapy.[2]

Joint Manifestations. Joint involvement is usually symmetric and polyarticular. Any diarthrodial joint can be involved. The person may complain of joint pain and stiffness that lasts 30 minutes and frequently for several hours. The limitation of joint motion that occurs early in the disease is usually because of pain; later, it is because of fibrosis. The most frequently affected joints initially are the fingers, hands, wrists, knees, and feet. Later, other diarthrodial joints may become involved. Spinal involvement is usually limited to the cervical region. In the hands, there is usually bilateral and symmetric involvement of the proximal interphalangeal (PIP) and metacarpophalangeal (MCP) joints in the early stages of rheumatoid arthritis; the distal interphalangeal (DIP) joints are rarely affected. The fingers often take on a spindle-shaped appearance because of inflammation of the PIP joints (Fig. 47–3).

Progressive joint destruction may lead to subluxation (*i.e.*, dislocation of the joint resulting in misalignment of the bone ends) and instability of the joint and in limitation of movement. Swelling and thickening of the synovium can result in stretching of the joint capsule and ligaments. When this occurs, muscle and tendon imbalance develop, and mechanical forces applied to the joints through daily activities produce joint deformities. In the MCP joints, the extensor tendons can slip to the ulnar side of the metacarpal head, causing ulnar deviation of the finger (Fig. 47–4). Subluxation of the MCP joints may develop when this deformity is present. Hyperextension of the PIP joint and partial flexion of the DIP joint is called a *swan neck deformity*. After this condition becomes fixed, severe loss of function occurs, because the person can no longer make a fist. Flexion of the PIP joint with hyperextension of the DIP joint is called a *boutonnière deformity*.

The knee is one of the most commonly affected joints and is responsible for much of the disability associated with the disease.[1] Active synovitis may be apparent as visible swelling that obliterates the normal contour over the medial and lateral aspects of the patella. The bulge sign, which involves milking fluid from the lateral to the medial side of the patella, may be used to determine the presence of excess fluid when it is not visible. Joint contractures, instability, and genu valgus (knock-knee) deformity are other possible manifestations. Severe quadriceps atrophy can contribute to the disability. A *Baker's cyst* may occur in the popliteal area behind the knee. This is caused by enlargement of the bursa and usually does not cause symptoms unless the cyst ruptures, in which case symptoms mimicking thrombophlebitis appear.

Disease activity can limit flexion and extension of the ankle, which can create difficulty in walking. Involvement of the metatarsophalangeal joints can cause subluxation, hallux valgus, and hammer toe deformities.

Neck discomfort is common. In rare cases, long-standing disease can lead to neurologic complications such as occipital headaches, muscle weakness, and numbness and tingling in the upper extremities. More severe neurologic complications, but less common, are dislocation of the first cervical vertebra and subluxation of the odontoid process of the second vertebra into the foramen magnum, which can lead to paralysis and is potentially fatal.

Extraarticular Manifestations. Although characteristically a joint disease, rheumatoid arthritis can affect a number of other tissues. Extraarticular manifestations probably occur with a fair degree of frequency but are

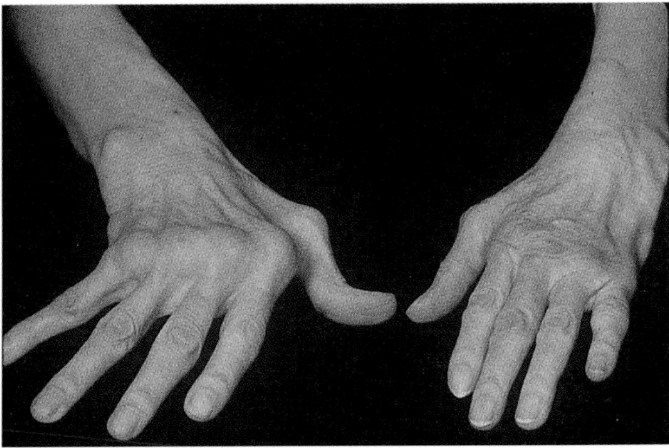

Figure 47–4
Subluxation of the metacarpophalangeal joints of the fingers in rheumatoid arthritis (swan neck deformity). (Reprinted from the ARHP Arthritis Teaching Slide Collection. Used with permission of the American College of Rheumatology.)

usually mild enough to cause few problems. They are most likely to occur in persons with rheumatoid factor .

Because rheumatoid arthritis is a systemic disease, it may be accompanied by complaints of fatigue, weakness, anorexia, weight loss, and low-grade fever when the disease is active. The erythrocyte sedimentation rate (ESR), which is commonly elevated during inflammatory processes, has been found to correlate with the amount of disease activity.[7] Anemia associated with a low serum iron level or low iron-binding capacity is common.[1] This anemia is generally resistant to iron therapy.

Rheumatoid nodules are granulomatous lesions that develop around small blood vessels. The nodules may be tender or nontender, movable or immovable, and small or large. Typically, they are found over pressure points such as the extensor surfaces of the ulna. The nodules may remain unless surgically removed, or they may resolve spontaneously.

Vasculitis is an uncommon manifestation of rheumatoid arthritis in persons with a long history of active arthritis and high titers of rheumatoid factor. It is possible that some persons have vasculitis that remains silent. Vasculitis is caused by the inflammatory process affecting the small and medium-sized arterioles. Manifestations include ischemic areas in the nail fold and digital pulp that appear as brown spots. Ulcerations may occur in the lower extremities, particularly around the malleolar areas. In some cases, neuropathy may be the only symptom of vasculitis. The visceral organs, such as the heart, lungs, and gastrointestinal tract, may also be affected.

Other extraarticular manifestations include eye lesions such as episcleritis and scleritis, hematologic abnormalities, pulmonary disease, cardiac complications, infection, and Felty's syndrome (*i.e.,* leukopenia with or without splenomegaly).

Diagnosis and Treatment

The diagnosis of rheumatoid arthritis is based on findings of the history, physical examination, and laboratory tests. Information should be elicited regarding the duration of symptoms, systemic manifestations, stiffness, and family history. The criteria for rheumatoid arthritis developed by the American Rheumatism Association are useful in establishing the diagnosis (Chart 47–1). At least four of the criteria must be present to make a diagnosis of rheumatoid arthritis. Practitioners must realize that these criteria were developed for use in epidemiologic studies and are designated for classification purposes and *not* as diagnostic criteria, but they can be used as guidelines for diagnosing the illness in individual patients.

In the early stages, the disease is often difficult to diagnose. On physical examination, the affected joints show signs of inflammation, swelling, tenderness, and possibly warmth and reduced motion. The joints have a soft, spongy feeling because of the synovial thickening and inflammation. Body movements may be guarded to prevent pain. Changes in joint structure are usually not visible early in the disease.

Rheumatoid factor test results are not diagnostic for rheumatoid arthritis, but they can be of value in differentiating rheumatoid arthritis from other forms of arthritis. Between 1% and 5% of healthy persons have rheumatoid factor, and its presence seems to be more common with advancing age.[1] A person can have rheumatoid arthritis without having rheumatoid factor. Radiologic findings also are not diagnostic in rheumatoid arthritis, because joint erosions are often not seen on radiographic images in the early stages of the disorder. Synovial fluid analysis can be helpful in the diagnostic process. The fluid has a cloudy appearance, because the white blood cell count is elevated as a result of inflammation, whereas the complement components of the synovial fluid are depressed.

The treatment goals for a person with rheumatoid arthritis are to reduce pain, minimize stiffness and swelling, maintain mobility, and become an informed health care consumer. The treatment plan includes education about the disease and its treatment, rest, therapeutic exercises, and medications. Because of the chronicity of the disease and the need for continuous, long-term adherence to the prescribed treatment modalities, it is important that the treatment be integrated with the person's lifestyle.

Strategies to aid in symptom control also involve regulating activity by pacing, establishing priorities, and setting realistic goals. Support groups and group education experiences benefit some persons. The home and work environments should be assessed, and interventions should be incorporated as the situation warrants.

CHART 47-1
Proposed 1987 Revised American Rheumatism Association Criteria for Rheumatoid Arthritis

Four or more of the following conditions must be present to establish a diagnosis of rheumatoid arthritis:

1. Morning stiffness for at least 1 hour and present for at least 6 weeks
2. Swelling of three or more joints for at least 6 weeks
3. Swelling of wrist, metacarpophalangeal or proximal interphalangeal joints for 6 or more weeks
4. Symmetric joint swelling
5. Hand roentgenogram changes typical of rheumatoid arthritis that must include erosions or unequivocal bony decalcification
6. Rheumatoid nodules
7. Serum rheumatoid factor identified by a method that is positive in less than 5% of normals

(*Primer on the rheumatic diseases* [10th ed.]. [1993]. Atlanta: Arthritis Foundation. Used with the permission of the Arthritis Foundation)

Both physical and emotional rest are important aspects of care. Physical rest reduces joint stress. Rest of specific joints is recommended to relieve pain. For example, sitting reduces the weight on an inflamed knee, and the use of lightweight splints reduces undue movement of the hand or wrist. Some persons find that discomfort increases with emotional stress; with emotional rest, muscles relax, and discomfort is reduced. Although rest is essential, therapeutic exercises also are important in maintaining joint motion and muscle strength. Range of motion exercises involve the active and passive movement of joints. Isometric (muscle tensing) exercises may be used to strengthen muscles. These exercises are frequently taught by a physical therapist and performed daily at home. The difference between normal activity and therapeutic exercise should be emphasized. Aerobic exercise can be an important component of the treatment regimen of selected patients. Studies have shown that, although persons with rheumatoid arthritis have generally low levels of physical fitness, they can benefit from individualized exercise programs without experiencing joint damage or flares of the disease.[8]

Instruction in the safe use of heat and cold modalities to relieve discomfort and in the use of relaxation techniques is also important. Proper posture, positioning, body mechanics, and the use of supportive shoes can provide further comfort. There is often a need for information about the principles of joint protection and work simplification. Some persons need assistive devices to reduce pain and improve their ability to perform activities of daily living. The goals of pharmacologic therapy for rheumatoid arthritis are to reduce pain, decrease inflammation, maintain or restore joint function, and prevent bone and cartilage destruction. Medications used to achieve these goals are classified as those that provide relief of arthritis symptoms and those that have the potential for modifying the course of the disease.[9]

The trend in management of rheumatoid arthritis is toward a more aggressive pharmacologic approach earlier in the disease. A window of opportunity for improved disease management occurs within 2 years of disease onset. Early treatment is based on the theory that T-cell–dependent pathways, which manifest early in the inflammatory process, are more responsive to treatment than later in the process, when disease progression may be controlled by activated fibroblasts and macrophages and the disease may be more resistant to treatment.[4]

Nonsteroidal antiinflammatory drugs (NSAIDs) are generally the first choice in the treatment of rheumatoid arthritis. The NSAIDs inhibit the production of prostaglandins, which have a damaging effect on joint structures. NSAIDs, including salicylates (*e.g.*, aspirin), provide analgesic and antiinflammatory effects. Effectiveness, side effects, cost, and dosing schedules are considered when selecting an NSAID. There is a wide range of responses to the various NSAIDs, and the particular NSAID that works best for any one individual is not always predictable. The incidence of adverse reactions to the NSAIDs increases with age and long-term use and may include gastric irritation, renal failure, hepatic changes, anemia, rashes, headaches, and confusion.

Second-line drug therapy is initiated early in disease if joint symptoms persist despite use of NSAIDs. Disease-modifying antirheumatic drugs (DMARDs) include gold salts, hydroxychloroquine, sulfasalazine, methotrexate, and azathioprine. Methotrexate has become the drug of choice because of its potency, and it is relatively fast acting (*i.e.*, improvement is seen in 1 month) compared with the slower-acting DMARDs, which can take 3 to 4 months to work. Methotrexate is thought to interfere with purine metabolism leading to the release of adenosine, a potent antiinflammatory compound. All of the DMARDs can be toxic and require close monitoring for adverse effects, especially those related to bone marrow suppression.[9]

Corticosteroid drugs may be used to reduce discomfort. To avoid long-term side effects, they are only used in specific situations for short-term therapy at a low dose level. They may be used for unremitting disease with extraarticular manifestations. Corticosteroids may interrupt the inflammatory and immune cascade at several levels, such as by interfering with inflammatory cell adhesion and migration, by impairing prostaglandin synthesis, and by inhibiting neutrophil superoxide production.[9] This medication does not modify the disease and is unable to prevent joint destruction. Intraarticular corticosteroid injections can provide rapid relief of acute or subacute inflammatory synovitis (after infection is excluded) in a few joints. They should not be repeated more than a few times each year.

A newer approach to rheumatoid arthritis treatment is combination therapy. This approach is still considered experimental, but it has been shown to be effective in early studies. Individual drugs with different mechanisms of action are given simultaneously to control the disease.[7] A typical drug combination may include hydroxychloroquine, azathioprine, and methotrexate or gold plus methotrexate. This combination is given in addition to an NSAID. Drugs are then tapered as symptoms subside and clinical remission is achieved.[10]

Plasmapheresis, leukapheresis, lymphapheresis, thoracic duct drainage, chemical or local radiation synovectomy, and total body irradiation are procedures considered experimental. These therapies modulate immune function and have been effective, but they are not practical for routine use. Some research and experimental treatments have focused on immunobiologics. The new treatments delete the destructive cells in the immune system rather than suppressing all of the immune system cells, which occurs with such drugs as methotrexate and azathioprine. Monoclonal antibodies, antitumor necrosis factor antibodies, and T-cell receptor peptide therapy are being tested as alternatives to traditional rheumatoid arthritis treatment.[11] These new treatments may hold promise for the future.

Surgery may be a part of the treatment of rheumatoid arthritis. Synovectomy may be indicated to reduce pain and joint damage when synovitis does not respond to medical treatment. The most common soft tissue surgery is tenosynovectomy (*i.e.*, repair of damaged tendons) of the hand to release nerve entrapments. Total joint replacements (*i.e.*, arthroplasty) may be indicated to reduce pain and increase motion. Arthrodesis (*i.e.*, joint fusion) is indicated in only extreme cases when there is so much soft tissue damage and scarring or infection that a replacement is impossible.

Although the course of rheumatoid arthritis is unpredictable, the past 25 years have brought more effective treatment for the disease. Patients with arthritis symptoms are being diagnosed and treated earlier. Criteria have been developed for remission in rheumatoid arthritis (Chart 47–2).

Systemic Lupus Erythematosus

Systemic lupus erythematosus (SLE) is a chronic inflammatory disease that can affect virtually any organ system, including the musculoskeletal system. It is a major rheumatic disease, with a prevalence of about 1 case per 2000 persons. Approximately 500,000 persons in the United States are afflicted with this disease. There is a female predominance of 9 to 1 over men, and this ratio is closer to 30 to 1 during the childbearing years. SLE is more common in African Americans, Hispanics, and Asians than whites, and the incidence in some families is higher than others.

Etiology and Pathogenesis

The cause of SLE is unknown. It is characterized by the formation of autoantibodies and immune complexes. Persons with SLE appear to have B-cell hyperreactivity and increased production of antibodies against self (*i.e.*, autoantibodies) and nonself antigens. These B cells are polyclonal, meaning that there are multiple B cell clones, each producing a different type of antibody. Antibodies have been identified against an array of nuclear and cytoplasmic cell components. B-cell hyperreactivity could result from several mechanisms. In theory, excessive functioning of helper T cells or defective functioning of suppressor T cells could alter the B-cell response (see Chapter 11).

The development of autoantibodies can result from a combination of factors, including genetic, hormonal, immunologic, and environmental factors.[12] Genetic predisposition is evidenced by the occurrence of familial cases of SLE, especially among identical twins. The increased incidence among African Americans compared with whites also suggests genetic factors. As many as four genes may be involved in the expression of SLE in humans. Genes linked to the HLA-DR and DQ loci in the MHC class II molecules show strong support for a genetic link in the development of SLE.[13]

Studies also suggest that an imbalance in sex hormone levels may play a role in the development of the disease, especially because the disease is so prevalent among women. Androgens appear to protect and estrogens seem to favor the development of SLE. It has been suggested that an imbalance in sex hormone levels may lead to a heightened helper T-cell and weakened suppressor T-cell immune response that could lead to the development of autoantibodies.[1]

Possible environmental triggers include ultraviolet light, chemicals (*e.g.*, hydralazine, procainamide, hair dyes), some foods, and possibly infectious agents.[13] Ultraviolet (UV) light, specifically UVB associated with exposure to the sun or unshielded fluorescent bulbs, may trigger exacerbations. Photosensitivity occurs in approximately one third of SLE patients.

The pathologic process probably begins with the activation of polyclonal B cells, causing exaggerated production of autoantibodies. The autoantibodies combine with corresponding antigens to form immune complexes. These immune complexes are deposited in vascular and tissue surfaces, triggering an inflammatory response and ultimately causing local tissue injury. Some autoantibodies that have been identified in SLE are antinuclear antibodies (ANA), including anti-DNA. Other antibodies may be produced against various cells, including red blood cell surface antigens, platelets, coagulation factors, and other antibodies. Autoantibodies against red blood cells can lead to anemia and those against platelets to thrombocytopenia. Certain drugs may provoke a lupuslike disorder in susceptible persons, particularly in elderly persons. The most common of these drugs are hydralazine and procainamide. Other drugs, such as quinidine, chlorpromazine, methyldopa, isoniazid, and phenytoin, have also been known to produce this syndrome. The disease usually recedes when the drug is discontinued.

Clinical Manifestations

SLE can manifest in a variety of ways. The disease has been called the *great imitator* because it has the capacity for affecting many different body systems, including the

CHART **47-2**

Proposed Criteria for Clinical Remission in Rheumatoid Arthritis

Five or more of the following requirements must be fulfilled for at least 2 consecutive months:

1. Duration of morning stiffness not exceeding 15 minutes
2. No fatigue
3. No joint pain (by history)
4. No joint tenderness or pain on motion
5. No soft tissue swelling in joints or tendon sheaths
6. Erythrocyte sedimentation rate (Westergren method) less than 30 mm/h for a female or 20 mm/h for a male

(*Primer on rheumatic diseases* [10th ed.]. [1993]. Atlanta: Arthritis foundation. Used with permission of the Arthritis Foundation)

musculoskeletal system, the skin, the cardiovascular system, the lungs, the kidneys, the central nervous system (CNS), and the red blood cells and platelets. The onset may be acute or insidious, and the course of the disease is characterized by exacerbations and remissions. Rare cases result in death with weeks or months.

Arthralgias and arthritis are among the most commonly occurring early symptoms of SLE; approximately 90% of all persons with the disease complain of joint pain at some point during the course of their disease.[13] The polyarthritis of SLE initially can be confused with other forms of arthritis, especially rheumatoid arthritis, because of the symmetric arthropathy. However, on radiologic examination, articular destruction is rarely found. Ligaments, tendons, and the joint capsule may be involved, causing varied deformities in approximately 30% of persons with the disease. Flexion contractures, hyperextension of the interphalangeal joint, and subluxation of the carpometacarpal joint contribute to the deformity and subsequent loss of function in the hands. Other musculoskeletal manifestations of SLE include tenosynovitis, rupture of the intrapatellar and Achilles tendons, and avascular necrosis, frequently of the femoral head.

Skin manifestations can vary greatly and may be classified as acute, subacute, or chronic. The acute skin lesions comprise the classic malar or "butterfly" rash on the nose and cheeks (Fig. 47–5). This rash is seen in SLE but may be associated with other skin lesions, such as hives or livedo reticularis (i.e., reticular cyanotic discoloration of the skin, often precipitated by cold) and fingertip lesions, such as periungual erythema, nail fold infarcts, and splinter hemorrhages. Hair loss is common. Mucous membrane lesions tend to occur during periods of exacerbation. Sun sensitivity may occur in SLE even after mild sun exposure.

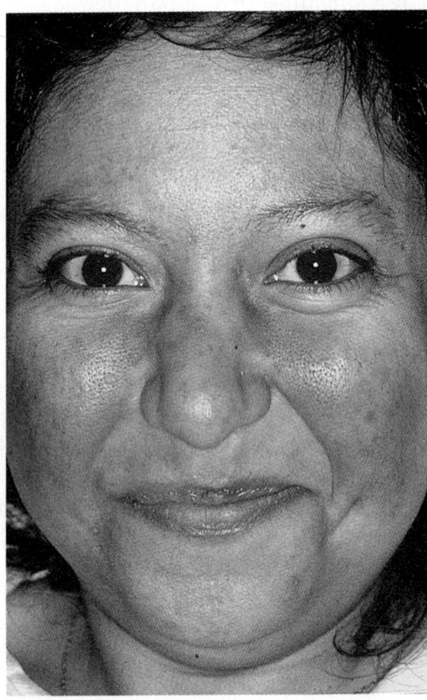

Figure 47–5
The butterfly (malar) rash of systemic lupus erythematosus. (Reprinted from the ARHP Arthritis Teaching Slide Collection. Used with permission of the American College of Rheumatology.)

Renal involvement occurs in about 50% of persons with SLE. Several forms of glomerulonephritis may occur, including mesangial, focal proliferative, diffuse proliferative, and membranous (see Chapter 28). Interstitial nephritis may also occur. Nephrotic syndrome causes proteinuria with resultant edema in the legs, abdomen, and around the eyes. Renal failure may or may not be preceded by the nephrotic syndrome. Kidney biopsy is the best determinant of renal damage and the extent of treatment needed.

Pulmonary involvement in SLE occurs in 40% to 50% of patients and is manifested primarily by pleural effusions or pleuritis. Less frequently occurring pulmonary problems include acute pneumonitis, pulmonary hemorrhage, chronic interstitial lung disease, and pulmonary embolism.

Pericarditis is the most common of the cardiac manifestation, occurring in up to 30% to 40% of persons with SLE and often accompanied by pleural effusions. Myocarditis affects as many as 25% of those with SLE. Congenital heart block can occur in infants of mothers with lupus who have a specific type of ANA (anti-Ro) in their serum. Secondary heart disease is also a problem in those with lupus. Hypertension may be associated with lupus nephritis and long-term corticosteroid use. Ischemic heart disease can occur in older patients with longer-duration lupus. Infective carditis is rare but can occur with valvular lesions.[12]

The CNS is involved in 30% to 75% of persons with SLE. The pathologic basis for the CNS symptoms is not entirely clear. It has been ascribed to an acute vasculitis that impede blood flow, causing strokes or hemorrhage; an immune response involving antineuronal antibodies that attack nerve cells; or production of antiphospholipids that damage blood vessels and cause blood clots in the brain. Seizures can occur and are more frequent when renal failure is present. Psychotic symptoms, including depression and unnatural euphoria as well as decreased cognitive functioning, confusion, and altered levels of consciousness may develop. More research is being done on the role of psychologic factors triggering the onset of lupus.

Hematologic disorders may manifest as hemolytic anemia, leukopenia, lymphopenia, or thrombocytopenia. Lymphadenopathy may also occur in 50% of all lupus patients.[12] Discoid SLE (i.e., chronic cutaneous lupus) involves plaquelike lesions on the head, scalp, and neck. These lesions first appear as red, swollen patches of skin, and later there can be scarring, depigmentation, and plugging of hair follicles. Ninety percent of patients with discoid lupus have disease that only involves the skin.

Subacute cutaneous lupus erythematosus (SCLE) is a less severe form of lupus. The skin lesions in this condition may resemble psoriasis. These lesions are found in sun-exposed areas such as the face, chest, upper back, and arms. Patients with SCLE may have mild systemic problems, which are usually limited to joint and muscle pains. There is a low incidence of lupus nephritis among those with SCLE.

Diagnosis and Treatment

The diagnosis of SLE can be complicated and difficult. The American College of Rheumatology has defined 11 criteria to be considered in the diagnosis of the disease, but these are intended for use in clinical trials rather than for individual diagnosis.[14] Diagnosis is based on a complete history, physical examination, and analysis of the blood work. No single test can diagnose lupus in all persons.

The most common laboratory test performed is the immunofluorescence test for ANA. Ninety-five percent of persons with untreated SLE have high ANA levels. The ANA test is not specific for lupus, and positive ANA results may be found in healthy persons or may be associated with other disorders. The anti-DNA antibody test is more specific for the diagnosis of lupus.[13] Other serum testing may reveal moderate to severe anemia, thrombocytopenia, and leukocytosis or leukopenia. Additional immunologic tests may be done to give support to the diagnosis or to differentiate SLE from other connective tissue diseases.

Treatment of lupus focuses on managing the acute and chronic symptoms of the disease. Communication and trust between health care providers and the person with SLE are the basis for long-term disease management. The person with SLE is the best source of information about the pattern of his or her disease activity. Teamwork can reduce the need for unnecessary hospitalization, testing, expense, and anxiety. The goals of treatment include preventing progressive loss of organ function, reducing the possibility of exacerbations, minimizing disability from the disease process, and preventing complications from medication therapy.[15] Treatment with medications may be as simple as a drug to reduce inflammation, such as an NSAID. NSAIDs can control fever, arthritis, and mild pleuritis. An antimalarial drug may be the next medication considered to treat cutaneous and musculoskeletal manifestations of lupus. Adrenal corticosteroids are used to treat more significant symptoms of SLE, such as renal and CNS disorders. High-dose corticosteroid treatment is used for acute symptoms, and the drug is tapered to the lowest therapeutic dose as soon as possible to minimize the adverse effects. Immunosuppressive drugs are used in cases of severe disease. Cyclophosphamide, under closely monitored circumstances, has been found to be beneficial in the treatment of lupus nephritis.[16]

Systemic Sclerosis

Systemic sclerosis, often prefixed by the term progressive, is sometimes called *scleroderma*. The condition is systemic and may involve the lungs, esophagus, heart, duodenum, and kidneys. In this disorder, the skin is thickened through fibrosis with an accompanying fixation to the subdermal structures, including the sheaths or fascia covering tendons and muscles. African Americans and women are more susceptible to this disease than white men. Clinical manifestations include muscular atrophy, pain, edema, calcification, and arthrodesis. Studies have indicated that if heart, lung, or kidney involvement is to become severe, it tends to do so early in disease and is a predictor of shortened survival.[17] The cause of this rare disorder, although characterized by proliferative vascular changes, is not well understood.

A variant of systemic sclerosis is the *CREST* syndrome. This acronym represents the manifestations of *calcinosis, Raynaud's phenomenon, esophageal dysmotility, sclerodactyly* (localized scleroderma of the fingers), and *telangiectasia*.

Polymyositis and Dermatomyositis

Polymyositis and dermatomyositis are chronic inflammatory myopathies. The pathogenesis is multifactorial and includes cellular and humoral immune mechanisms. Systemic manifestations are common, and cardiac and pulmonary complications often adversely affect the outcome. These conditions are characterized by symmetric proximal muscle weakness and occasional muscle pain and tenderness.

In summary, rheumatoid arthritis is a systemic inflammatory disorder that affects 0.3% to 1.5% of the population. Women are affected more frequently than men. This form of arthritis, the cause of which is unknown, has a chronic course and is usually characterized by remissions and exacerbations. Joint involvement is symmetric and begins with inflammatory changes in the synovial membrane. As joint inflammation progresses, structural changes can occur, leading to joint instability and eventual deformity. Systemic manifestations include weakness, anorexia, weight loss, and low-grade fever. Some extraarticular features include rheumatoid nodules, and vasculitis. The treatment goals include reducing pain, stiffness, and swelling, maintaining mobility, and assisting the person to become an informed health care consumer.

SLE is a chronic autoimmune disorder that affects multiple body systems. There is no known cause of lupus, but the disease may result from an immunoregulatory disturbance brought about by a combination of genetic, hormonal, and environmental factors. Some drugs have been shown to induce lupus, especially in the elderly. There is an exaggerated production of autoantibodies, which interact with antigens to produce an immune complex. These immune complexes produce an inflammatory response in affected tissues. Treatment focuses on preventing loss of organ function, controlling inflammation, and minimizing complications of medication therapy.

Systemic sclerosis, often prefixed by the term progressive, is sometimes called scleroderma. In this disorder, the skin is thickened through fibrosis with an accompanying fixation to the subdermal structures, including the sheaths or fascia covering tendons and muscles. Polymyositis and dermatomyositis are chronic inflammatory myopathies. The pathogenesis is multifactorial and includes cellular and humoral immune mechanisms.

Arthritis Associated With Spondylitis

After you have completed this section of the chapter, you should be able to meet the following objectives:

- Cite a definition of the seronegative spondlyoarthropathies
- Cite the primary features of ankylosing spondylitis
- Describe how the site of inflammation differs in spondyloarthropathies from that in rheumatoid arthritis
- Contrast and compare ankylosing spondylitis, reactive arthritis, and psoriatic arthritis in terms of cause, pathogenesis, and clinical manifestations

The spondlyoarthropathies are an interrelated group of multisystem inflammatory disorders that primarily affect the axial skeleton, particularly the spine. Inflammation develops at sites where ligament inserts into bone rather than in the synovium. Sacroiliitis is the pathologic hallmark. The person with spondyloarthropathy sometimes also has inflammation and involvement of the peripheral joints, in which case the signs and symptoms overlap with other inflammatory types of arthritis. However, the spondyloarthropathies differ from rheumatoid arthritis in that there is an absence of the rheumatoid factor factor; these disorders are often referred to as *seronegative spondyloarthropathies* (Table 47–1).

The seronegative spondyloarthropathies include ankylosing spondylitis, juvenile ankylosing spondylitis, reactive arthritis, enteropathic arthritis (i.e., inflammatory bowel disease), and psoriatic arthritis. There is clinical evidence of overlap between the various seronegative spondyloarthropathies. In none of these disorders is the cause or pathogenesis well understood. There is a striking association with the HLA-B27 antigen, but the presence of the HLA-B27 antigen by itself is neither necessary nor sufficient for the development of any of the diseases.

Ankylosing Spondylitis

Ankylosing spondylitis is a chronic, systemic inflammatory disease of the axial skeleton, including the sacroiliac joints, intervertebral disk spaces, and the apophyseal and costovertebral articulations. Bilateral sacroiliitis is a primary feature of the disease. Occasionally, large synovial joints (i.e., hips, knees, and shoulders) may be involved. The small peripheral joints are usually not affected. The sites of ligament insertion into bone are eroded by inflammatory cells, with subsequent formation of woven bone. Ankylosing spondylitis may cause fibrosis, calcification, and ossification of joints, with progression to ankylosis. The joint becomes ankylosed when bone replaces ligament throughout its length.

The disease generally brings to mind an image of a person bent over looking at the floor and unable to straighten up. X-ray films show a rigid, bamboolike spine. Fortunately, few persons develop a progressive disease pattern that leads to this outcome. The disease spectrum ranges from an asymptomatic sacroiliitis to a progressive disease that can affect many body systems. The progressive disease pattern usually affects men.

Etiology and Pathogenesis

This disorder is more common than was once believed; it probably affects about 2% to 8% of the HLA-B27–posi-

TABLE **47-1**

Comparison of the Spondyloarthropathies

Characteristic	Ankylosing Spondylitis	Reiter's disease	Psoriatic Arthritis	Inflammatory Bowel Disease
Age at onset	Young adult	Young to middle age	Any age	Any age
Type of onset	Gradual	Sudden	Variable	Gradual
Sacroillitis	>95%	20%	20%	10%
Peripheral joint involvement	25%	90%	All (about 5% to 7% of those patients with psoriasis)	Occasional
HLA-B27 (in whites)	>90%	75%	<50%	<50%
Eye involvement	25% to 30%	Common	Occasional	Occasional

(Adapted from Arnett F.C., Khan M.A., Willikens R.F. [1989]. A new look at ankylosing spondylitis. *Patient Care*, 23 [19], 82–101)

tive white population.[18] Epidemiologic findings indicate that genetic and environmental factors play a role in the pathogenesis of the disease. Clinical manifestations usually begin in late adolescence or early adulthood and are slightly more common in men that in women. The disease evolves more slowly and is less severe in women.

The pathogenesis of ankylosing spondylitis is not well understood. The presence of mononuclear cells in acutely involved tissue suggests an immune response. The HLA-B27 antigen remains one of the best-known examples of an association between a disease and a hereditary marker. Although about 90% of those with ankylosing spondylitis possess the HLA-B27 antigen and nearly 100% of those who also have uveitis or aortitis have the marker, the HLA-B27 antigen is also present in about 8% of the normal population. Several theories have been advanced to account for the association between the HLA-B27 antigen and ankylosing spondylitis. One possibility is that the gene that determines the HLA-B27 antigen may be linked to other genes that determine pathologic autoimmune phenomena or that lead to increased susceptibility to infections or environmental agents. A second theory postulates molecular mimicry; an autoimmune reaction to an antigenic determinant site in the host's tissues may occur as a consequence of an immunologic response to an identical or closely related antigen of a foreign agent, usually an infectious agent.

Clinical Manifestations

The person with ankylosing spondylitis typically complains of low-back pain, which may be persistent or intermittent. The pain, which becomes worse when resting, particularly when lying in bed, may initially be blamed on muscle strain or spasm from physical activity. Lumbosacral pain may also be present, with discomfort in the buttocks and hip areas. Sometimes, pain can radiate to the thigh in a manner similar to that of sciatic pain. Prolonged stiffness is present in the morning and after periods of rest. Mild physical activity or a hot shower helps reduce pain and stiffness. Sleep patterns are frequently interrupted because of these manifestations. Walking or exercise may be needed to provide the comfort needed to return to sleep. Muscle spasm may also contribute to discomfort.

Loss of motion in the spinal column is characteristic of the disease. The severity and duration of disease activity influence the degree of mobility. Loss of lumbar lordosis occurs as the disease progresses, and this is followed by kyphosis of the thoracic spine and extension of the neck. A spine fused in the flexed position is the end result in severe ankylosing spondylitis. A kyphotic spine makes it difficult for the patient to look ahead and to maintain balance while walking. The heart and lungs are constricted in the chest cavity. Abnormal weight bearing can lead to degeneration and destruction of hips, necessitating joint replacement procedures. Peripheral arthritis is more common in hips and shoulders. The incidence of hip joint involvement varies from 17% to 36% and potentially is more crippling than involvement in any other joint.[1] A lower age at onset and a presenting manifestation of hip joint involvement indicate a greater likelihood of progression to needing total hip replacement. The most common extraskeletal involvement is acute anterior uveitis, which occurs in 25% to 30% of patients sometime in the course of their disease.[1] Systemic features of weight loss, fever, and fatigue may be apparent. Sometimes, the fatigue is a greater problem than pain or stiffness. Osteoporosis can occur, especially in the spine, which contributes to the risk of spinal fracture. Fusion of the costovertebral joints can lead to reduced lung volume.

The disease process varies considerably among individuals. Exacerbations and remissions are common; their unpredictability can create uncertainty in planning daily activities and in setting goals. Fortunately, most of those affected are able to lead productive lives. The prognosis for ankylosing spondylitis is generally good. The first decade of disease predicts the remainder. Severe disease usually occurs early and is marked by peripheral arthritis, especially of the hip. Mortality is low (6%), and significant disability occurs in fewer than 20% of persons with the disorder.

Diagnosis and Treatment

The early and precise diagnosis of ankylosing spondylitis is closely related to a favorable prognosis. Early recognition allows for implementation of a conservative and usually effective treatment program on a lifelong basis. The diagnosis of ankylosing spondylitis is based on history, physical examination, and x-ray examination. Several methods are available to assess mobility and detect sacroiliitis. These methods include pressure on the sacroiliac joints with the person in a forward-bending position to elicit pain and muscle spasm, measurement of the distance between the tips of fingers and the floor in a bent-over position with straight knees, and a modified Schöber's test in which contralateral flexion of the back is measured. Although these measures alone do not provide a diagnosis of ankylosing spondylitis or other spondyloarthropathies, they can provide useful measurements for monitoring the disease status. Chest expansion may be used as an indirect indicator of thoracic involvement, which usually occurs late in the disease course. Measurements are taken at the fourth intercostal space. Normally, the chest expands by 4 to 5 cm with inspiration. This measurement is more difficult to obtain in women and less specific in older persons with normally decreased expansion, in smokers, or in those with emphysema.

Laboratory findings frequently include an elevated ESR. The patient may also have a mild normocytic normochromic anemia. HLA typing is not diagnostic of the disease and should not be used as a routine screening procedure. Radiologic evaluations help differentiate sacroiliitis from other diseases. In early disease, x-ray images may be normal. Vertebrae are normally concave on the anterior border. In ankylosing spondylitis, the vertebrae take on a squared appearance (Fig. 47–6). Progressive spinal changes usually follow an ascending pattern up the spine.

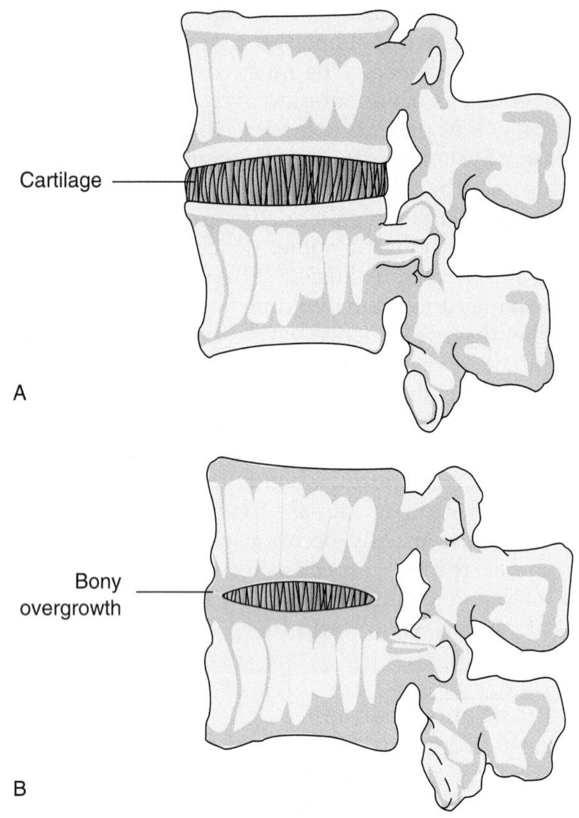

Figure 47–6
The bony overgrowth (**B**) of the vertebra characteristic of ankylosing spondylitis is evident when compared with normal vertebra (**A**).

Treatment is directed at controlling pain and maintaining mobility by suppressing inflammation. The patient should be instructed in proper posture and positioning. This includes sleeping in a supine position on a firm mattress and using one small pillow or no pillow. Sleeping in extension may reduce the possibility of flexion contractures. A bed board may be used to supply additional firmness. Therapeutic exercises are important to assist in maintaining motion in peripheral joints and in the spine. Muscle-strengthening exercises for extensor muscle groups are also prescribed. Heat applications or a shower or bath may be beneficial before exercise to improve ease of movement. These strategies can also be used in the morning or at bedtime to reduce stiffness and pain. Immobilizing joints is *not* recommended. Maintaining ideal weight reduces the stress on weight-bearing joints. Smoking should be discouraged, because it can exacerbate respiratory problems. Swimming is an excellent general conditioning exercise that avoids joint stress and enhances muscle tone. Occupational counseling or job evaluation may be warranted because of postural abnormalities. NSAIDs are used to reduce inflammation, which helps to control pain and reduce muscle spasm. Phenylbutazone is highly effective, but its use should be limited to persons with severe disease in whom other agents have failed because of potential bone marrow suppression with long-term usage.

Most peripheral joint pain and limitations of motion occur in the hip. Total hip replacement surgery helps reduce pain and increase mobility. Anesthesia can be problematic for persons with cervical rigidity or with reduced chest expansion. These factors must be weighed before surgery is considered.

Reactive Arthritis

The reactive arthropathies may be defined as sterile inflammatory joint disorders that are distant in time and place from the initial inciting infective process. A reactive arthritis is a seronegative arthritis in which an infective trigger mechanism is suspected. The list of triggering agents is continuously increasing and may be divided into urogenic, enterogenic, and respiratory tract associated and the idiopathic arthritides. In some cases, the identity of the causative agent is unknown.

Rheumatic fever is a classic form of reactive arthritis. Recognition of newer forms of reactive arthritis include reactions to *Chlamydia pneumoniae* infection and hepatitis B vaccination. Reactive arthritis has been observed in persons with acquired immunodeficiency syndrome (AIDS). Spondyloarthropathies such as Reiter's syndrome and psoriatic arthritis are more severe and frequent in HIV-infected patients than in the general population. It is thought the immune system response to HIV infection is selective and largely spares the natural killer cells, and these residual functioning components of the immune response may be critical in the pathogenesis of these conditions. In contrast, rheumatoid arthritis and SLE dramatically improve as immunodeficiency develops.[3] Reactive arthritis may result from the presence of a foreign substance within the joint tissue, as in silicone implants in the small joints of the hand or feet or after exposure to industrial gases and oils. However, there is no evidence of antigenicity of the causative substance. In the strictest sense, the definition of reactive arthritis includes a possibility of immunologic sensitization before arthritic development.[18] Having the HLA-B27 marker is not a prerequisite for development of reactive arthritis.

Similarities exist between reactive arthritis and bacterial arthritis. Several bacteria cause both diseases. When cultured bacteria are isolated from the synovial fluid, the diagnosis is bacterial arthritis. When they cannot be isolated, even though there has been a preceding infection, the diagnosis of reactive arthritis is made.

Reactive arthritis may follow a self-limited course; it may involve recurrent episodes of arthritis, or in a small number of cases, it may follow a continuous unremitting course. The treatment is largely symptomatic. NSAIDs are used in treating the arthritic symptoms. Vigorous treatment of possible triggering infections is thought to prevent relapses of reactive arthritis, but in many cases, the triggering infection passes unnoticed or is mild, and the patient only contacts a physician at the time of definite arthritis. Short antibiotic courses at this time are not effective.

Reiter's Syndrome

Reiter's syndrome is considered to be a clinical manifestation of reactive arthritis that may be accompanied by extraarticular symptoms such as uveitis, bowel inflammation, and carditis. Reiter's syndrome develops in a genetically susceptible host after an infection by bacteria, *Chlamydia trachomatis* in the genitourinary tract or *Salmonella, Shigella, Yersinia,* or *Campylobacter* in the gastrointestinal tract.

The term *Reiter's syndrome* may soon be relegated to history as the pathogenesis becomes better understood. Alternative designations include sexually reactive arthritis (SARA) and BASE syndrome (*i.e.,* HLA-B27, arthritis, sacroiliitis, and extraarticular inflammation).[1] Reiter's syndrome was the first rheumatic disease to be recognized in association with HIV infection. Symptoms of arthritis may precede any overt signs of HIV disease. Treatment with agents such as methotrexate and azathioprine may further suppress the immune response and provoke a full expression of AIDS.

Enteropathic Arthritis

Arthritis that is associated with an inflammatory bowel disease is generally considered an enteropathic arthritis because the intestinal disease is directly involved in the pathogenesis. Most cases of enteropathic arthritis are classified among the spondyloarthropathies. These include cases in which the arthritis is associated with inflammatory bowel disease (*i.e.,* ulcerative colitis and Crohn's disease), the reactive arthritides triggered by enterogenic bacteria, some of the undifferentiated spondyloarthropathies, Whipple's disease, and reactions after intestinal bypass surgery.[1] There is no direct relation between the activity of the bowel disease and the degree of arthritis activity.

Psoriatic Arthritis

Psoriatic arthritis is a seronegative inflammatory arthropathy. There seems to be a clinical similarity between reactive arthritis and psoriatic arthritis, suggesting a bacterial or other infectious trigger. Genetic susceptibility factors play an important role in expression of the psoriatic skin disease and the arthritis. The pathologic state of the synovium is similar to that in rheumatoid arthritis, with a few exceptions.

Although the arthritis can antedate detectable skin rash, the definite diagnosis of psoriatic arthritis cannot be made without evidence of skin or nail changes typical of psoriasis. Psoriatic arthritis falls into five subgroups: oligoarticular, or asymmetric (48%); spondyloarthropathy (24%); polyarticular, or symmetric (18%); distal interphalangeal (8%); and mutilans (2%).[19] This heterogeneous clinical presentation suggests more than one disease is associated with psoriasis or various clinical responses to a common cause. At least 20% of those with psoriatic arthritis have an elevated serum level of uric acid. The abnormally elevated serum uric acid level is caused by the rapid skin turnover of psoriasis, the breakdown of nucleic acid, and the metabolism to uric acid. This finding may lead to a misdiagnosis of gout. Psoriatic arthritis tends to be slowly progressive but has a more favorable prognosis than rheumatoid arthritis.

Basic management is similar to the treatment of rheumatoid arthritis. Suppression of the skin disease may be important in helping control the arthritis. Often, affected joints are surprisingly functional and only minimally symptomatic.

In summary, spondyloarthropathies affect the axial skeleton, particularly the spine. Inflammation develops at sites where ligaments insert into bone. They include ankylosing spondylitis, reactive arthritis, enteropathic arthritis, and psoriatic arthritis. Because they lack the rheumatoid factor factor, they are referred to as seronegative spondyloarthropathies. Ankylosing spondylitis is considered a prototype of this classification category. Bilateral sacroiliitis is the primary feature of ankylosing spondylitis. The disease spectrum ranges from asymptomatic sacroiliitis to a progressive disorder affecting many body systems. The cause remains unknown; however, a strong association between the HLA-B27 antigen and ankylosing spondylitis has been identified. Loss of motion in the spinal column is characteristic of the disease. Peripheral arthritis may occur in some persons. Other forms of spondyloarthritis include reactive arthritis, enteropathic arthritis, and psoriatic arthritis. Although there are overlapping features for each of the spondyloarthropathies, identifying etiologic differences and clinical manifestations is important for determining treatment.

Osteoarthritis Syndromes

After you have completed this section of the chapter, you should be able to meet the following objectives:

- Compare rheumatoid arthritis and osteoarthritis in terms of joint involvement, level of inflammation, and local and systemic manifestations
- Describe the pathologic joint changes associated with osteoarthritis
- Characterize the treatment of osteoarthritis

Osteoarthritis, formerly called *degenerative joint disease,* is the most prevalent form of arthritis. It is second only to cardiovascular disease as the cause of chronic disability in adults.[20] Osteoarthritis is more of a disease process than a specific entity. The term encompasses a heterogeneous collection of syndromes. Clinical subsets include osteoarthri-

CHART 47–3
Causes of Osteoarthritis

Postinflammatory disorders
- Rheumatoid arthritis
- Septic joint

Posttraumatic disorders
- Acute fracture
- Ligament or meniscal injury
- Cumulative occupational or recreational trauma

Anatomic or bony disorders
- Hip dysplasia
- Avascular necrosis
- Paget's disease
- Slipped capital femoral epiphysis
- Legg-Perthes disease

Metabolic disorders
- Calcium crystal deposition
- Hemachromatosus
- Acromegaly
- Wilson's disease
- Ochronosis

Neuropathic arthritis
- Charcot joint

Hereditary disorders of collagen
Idiopathic or primary variants

tis of the hand, of the knee, of the hip, of the foot, and of the spine. It can lead to loss of mobility and chronic pain, often causing significant disability, especially when the involved joints are critical to carrying out daily activities. Fortunately, changes in the traditional conservative management of this underemphasized condition are occurring. Attitudes regarding the inevitability of the limitations imposed by this condition are changing on the part of health care providers and persons with the disease.

One third of all adults in the United States have x-ray evidence of osteoarthritis of the hand, foot, knee, or hip. Although radiographic incidence of knee osteoarthritis increases with advancing age, the incidence of symptomatic osteoarthritis of the knee decreases.[21] The joint changes associated with osteoarthritis are progressive loss of articular cartilage and synovitis resulting from the inflammation caused by the attempts of the bone to remold itself, creating osteophytes or spurs. These changes are accompanied by joint pain, stiffness, limitation of motion, and possibly by joint instability and deformity. Although there may be periods of mild inflammation, it is not the severe destructive type seen in the inflammatory forms of rheumatic diseases such as rheumatoid arthritis.

Osteoarthritis can occur as a primary idiopathic or a secondary disorder, although this distinction is not always clear. Idiopathic or primary variants of osteoarthritis occur as localized or generalized (*i.e.*, more than three joints) syndromes. Chart 47–3 lists examples of the posttraumatic disorders, anatomic and bony disorders, metabolic disorders, neuropathic arthritis, and hereditary disorders of collagen.

Gender and age interact to influence the time of onset and, with race, the pattern of joint involvement. Men are more commonly affected at a younger age than women, but the rate of women affected exceeds that of men by middle age. Hand osteoarthritis is more likely to affect white women, whereas knee osteoarthritis is more common in black women. The incidence of hip osteoarthritis is less among the Chinese than Europeans, perhaps representing the influence of other factors such as occupation, obesity, or heredity. Obesity is a risk factor for osteoarthritis of the knee in women and a contributory biomechanical factor in the pathogenesis of the disease. Weight loss reduces the risk of developing symptomatic osteoarthritis of the knee.[22] Excess fat may have a direct metabolic effect on cartilage beyond the effects of excess joint stress. Heredity influences the occurrence of hand osteoarthritis in the distal interphalangeal joint. Bone mass may influence the risk of developing osteoarthritis. Theoretically, thinner subchondral bone mass may provide a greater shock-absorbing function than denser bone, allowing less direct trauma to the cartilage. Studies also implicate immunologic factors in the perpetuation and acceleration of osteoarthritic changes.[23]

Pathogenesis

Osteoarthritis is not a simple consequence of aging; it is an active metabolic disorder of the articular cartilage and subchondral bone (*i.e.*, bony plate that supports the

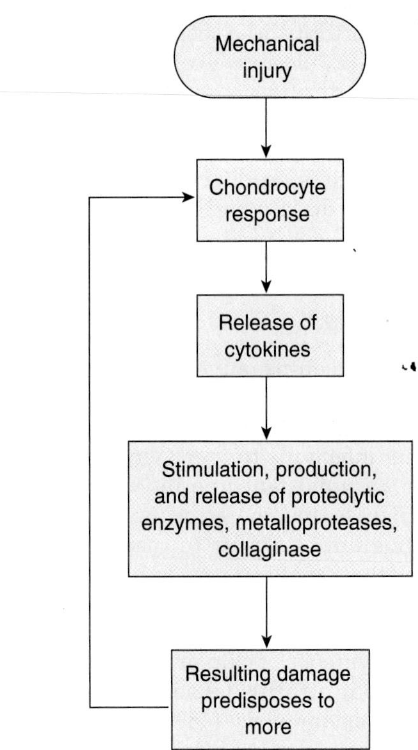

Figure 47–7
Disease process in osteoarthritis.

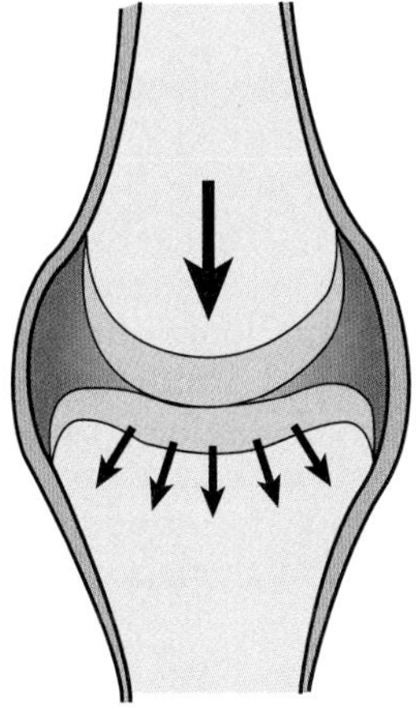

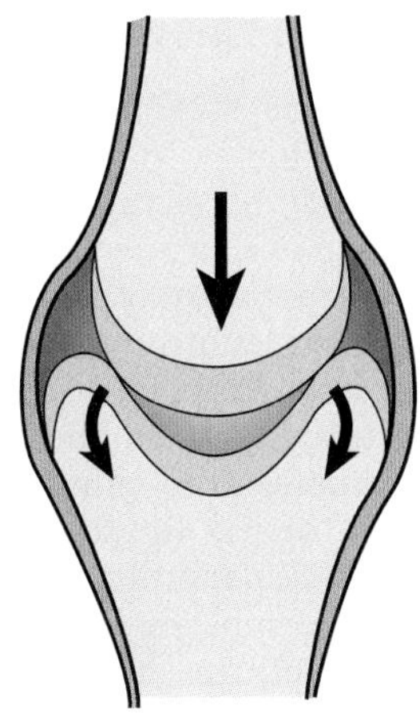

Figure 47–8
(**Left**) A joint normally undergoes deformation of the articular cartilage and the subchondral bone when carrying a load. This maximizes the contact area and spreads the force of the load. (**Right**) If the joint does not deform with a load, the stresses are concentrated and the joint breaks down. (Redrawn from Brandt K.D., & Radin E. [1987]. The physiology of articular stress: Osteoarthroses. *Hospital Practice* [January 15], 111)

articular cartilage) of diarthrodial joints (Fig. 47–7). Popularly known as "wear and tear" arthritis, the changes that occur in osteoarthritis are much more complex.

A balance between mechanical stress and the ability of the joint tissues to resist that stress exists in the diarthrodial joints. Osteoarthritis represents deterioration of the articular cartilage caused by a physiologic imbalance between the stress applied to the joint tissues and the ability of the joint tissues to withstand the stress. Either the articular cartilage underlying bone is normal, but excessive loads applied to the joints cause the tissues to fail, or a physiologic reasonable load is applied to the joint, but the articular cartilage or bone is defective.

Articular cartilage plays two essential mechanical roles in joint physiology. First, the articular cartilage serves as a remarkably smooth weight-bearing surface. In combination with synovial fluid, the articular cartilage provides extremely low friction during movement of the joint. Second, the cartilage transmits the load down to the bone, dissipating the mechanical stress. The subchondral bone protects the overlying articular cartilage, providing it with a pliable bed and absorbing the energy of the force (Fig. 47–8).

Cartilage is a specialized type of connective tissue. As with other types of tissue, it consists of cells (*i.e.*, chondrocytes) nested in an extracellular matrix. In articular cartilage, the extracellular matrix is composed of water, proteoglycans, collagen, and ground substance. The proteoglycans, which are large macromolecules made up of disaccharides and amino acids, afford elasticity and stiffness, permitting articular cartilage to resist compression. The ground substance constitutes a highly hydrated semisolid gel. Collagen molecules consist of polypeptide chains that form long fibrous strands. They provide form and tensile strength. The primary function of the collagen fibers is to provide a rigid scaffold to support the chondrocytes and ground substance of cartilage. The hydrated proteoglycan molecules, because of their macromolecular size and charge, are trapped within the collagen meshwork of the extracellular matrix. Because of the inextensibility of the collagen fibers, the proteoglycans are prevented from expanding to their maximum size. This confers a high osmotic pressure within the tissue.

Mechanical injury results in a chondrocyte response that leads to eventual degradation in the upper layers of cartilage. It is thought that injury leads to the release of cytokines such as interleukin-1. These chemical messengers stimulate production and release of extracellular proteolytic enzymes, metalloproteases, and collagenase. The resulting damage predisposes the chondrocytes to more injury. Inadequate repair mechanisms and imbalances between the proteases and their inhibitors may further contribute to disease progression (Fig. 47–9).

Under physiologic conditions of impact loading, the joint is protected with passive and active mechanisms. Passive mechanisms include microfractures and deformation of the subchondral bone. Deformation is essential for maximizing the contact area and for minimizing the stress (see Fig. 47–8). A progressive increase in the number of microfractures in subchondral bone may be detrimental to normal joint function, because the remodeled trabeculae may be stiffer than normal and less effective as shock absorbers. Under such circumstances, the subchondral bone cannot deform normally with a load. The increased incongruity of joint surfaces that occurs normally with loading is dimin-

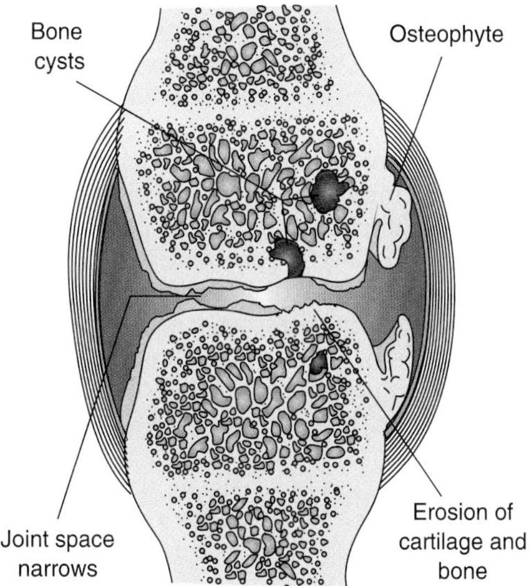

Figure 47–9
Joint changes in osteoarthritis. The left side denotes early changes and joint space narrowing with cartilage breakdown. The right side shows more severe disease progression with lost cartilage and osteophyte formation.

ished, and stress is concentrated at contact areas on the articular cartilage.

Under conditions of repeated movement, articular cartilage is highly resistant to wear. However, repetitive impact loading rapidly leads to joint failure, accounting for the high prevalence of osteoarthritis specific to vocational or avocational sites, such as the shoulders and elbows of baseball pitchers, ankles of ballet dancers, and knees of basketball players. Although this process is occurring in the cartilage, changes are also taking place in the underlying subchondral bone. The subchondral bone plate thickens and can become eburnated (*i.e.*, an ivorylike mass). Sclerosis, or formation of new bone and cysts, usually occurs in the juxtaarticular bone (*i.e.*, bone near the joint). New bone that forms at the joint margins is called an *osteophyte*, or spur.

To further understand the pathology of osteoarthritis, the lubrication of the joint must be considered. Under high loads such as weight bearing, lubrication depends on a film of interstitial fluid squeezed out of the cartilage with compression of the opposing surfaces of the joint. The greater the load is, the better the lubrication. With depletion of proteoglycans from the cartilage matrix in osteoarthritis, the mechanisms that normally operate under high loads to produce a pressurized lubricating film may be impaired. Attempts to devise artificial lubricants have been unsuccessful, because they impede the flow of interstitial fluid into and out of the cartilage surface.

Immobilization also can produce degenerative changes in articular cartilage. Cartilage degeneration due to immobility may result from loss of the pumping action of lubrication that occurs with joint movement. These changes are more marked and appear earlier in areas of contact but occur also in areas not subject to mechanical compression. By 3 weeks after remobilization, all biochemical, metabolic, and morphologic abnormalities in the cartilage that result from immobilization are reversed. Although cartilage atrophy is rapidly reversible with activity after a period of immobilization, impact exercise during the period of remobilization can prevent reversal of the atrophy. Slow, gradual remobilization may be important in preventing cartilage injury and has clinical implications with respect to instructions to patients concerning the recommended level of physical activity after removal of a cast. This balance between enough activity to lubricate and nourish cartilage and overloaded activity that further damages cartilage reasonably confuses patients who have difficulty in understanding whether they should use an affected joint or rest it.

Mild synovitis may occur in osteoarthritis. This inflammation represents a reactive process and is more likely to be seen in advanced disease. The synovitis may be related to the release of free cartilage proteoglycans from the deteriorating articular cartilage. Immunologic factors may also be involved. Calcium pyrophosphate and apatite crystals are common in osteoarthritic knee effusions.[1]

Clinical Manifestations

The manifestations of osteoarthritis may occur suddenly or insidiously. Initially, pain may be described as aching and may be somewhat difficult to localize. It worsens with use or activity and is relieved by rest. In later stages of disease activity, night pain may be experienced during rest. Pain can occur at rest, several hours after the use of the involved joints. Crepitus and grinding may be evident when the joint is moved. As the disease advances, even minimal activity may cause pain because of the limited range of motion resulting from intraarticular and periarticular structural damage.

The most frequently affected joints are the hips, knees, lumbar and cervical vertebrae, proximal and distal joints of the hand, the first carpometacarpal joint, and the first metatarsophalangeal joints of the feet. Table 47–2 identifies the joints that are commonly affected by osteoarthritis and the common clinical features correlated with the disease activity of each particular joint. A single joint or several may be affected. Although a single weight-bearing joint may be involved initially, other joints often become affected because of the additional stress placed on them while trying to protect the original joint. It is not unusual for a person having a knee replacement to discover soon after the surgery is done that the second knee also needs to be replaced. Other clinical features are limitations of joint motion and joint instability. Joint enlargement usually results from new bone formation; the joint feels hard, in contrast with the soft, spongy feeling characteristic of the joint in rheumatoid arthritis. Sometimes, mild synovitis or increased synovial fluid can cause joint enlargement.

Diagnosis and Treatment

The diagnosis of osteoarthritis is usually determined by history and physical examination, x-ray studies, and laboratory findings that exclude other diseases. Although osteoarthritis is often contrasted with rheumatoid arthritis for diagnostic purposes, the differences are not always readily apparent. Other rheumatic diseases may be superimposed on osteoarthritis. Psychologic factors, severity of joint disease, and educational level affect the expression of symptoms.[24]

Characteristic radiologic changes initially include medial joint space narrowing, followed by subchondral bony sclerosis, formation of spikes on the tibial eminence, and osteophytes. The results of laboratory studies are usually normal because the disorder is not a systemic disease. The ESR may be slightly elevated in generalized osteoarthritis or erosive inflammatory variations of the disease. If inflammation is present, there may be a slight increase in the blood cell count. The synovial fluid is usually normal.

Because there is no cure, the treatment of osteoarthritis is symptomatic and includes physical rehabilitative, pharmacologic, and surgery measures. Physical

TABLE 47-2 Clinical Features of Osteoarthritis

Joint	Clinical Features
Cervical spine	Localized stiffness; radicular or nonradicular pain; posterior osteophyte formation may cause vascular compression
Lumbar spine	Low back pain and stiffness; muscle spasm; decreased back motion; nerve root compression causing radicular pain; spinal stenosis
Hip	Most common in older male adults; characterized by insidious onset of pain, localized to groin region or inner aspect of the thigh; may be referred to buttocks, sciatic region, or knee; reduced hip motion; leg may be held in external rotation with hip flexed and adducted; limp or shuffling gait; difficulty getting in and out of chairs
First carpometacarpal joint (CMC)	Tenderness at base of thumb; squared appearance to joint
Proximal interphalangeal joint (PIP) Bouchard's nodes	Same as for distal interphalangeal joint disease
Distal interphalangeal joint (DIP) Heberden's nodes	Occurs more frequently in women; usually involves multiple DIPs, lateral flexor deviation of joint, spur formation at joint margins, pain and discomfort following joint use
Knee	Localized discomfort with pain on motion; limitation of motion; crepitus; quadriceps atrophy due to lack of use; joint instability; genu varus or valgus; joint effusion
First metatarsal phalangeal joint (MTP)	Insidious onset; irregular joint contour; pain and swelling aggravated by tight shoes

measures are aimed at improving the supporting structures of the joint and strengthening opposing muscle groups involved in cushioning weight-bearing forces. This includes a balance of rest and exercise, use of splints to protect and rest the joint, use of heat and cold to relieve pain and muscle spasm, and adjusting the activities of daily living. Weight reduction is helpful when the knee is involved. The involved joint should not be further abused, and steps should be taken to protect and rest it. This includes weight reduction (when weight-bearing surfaces are involved) and the use of a cane or walker if the hips and knees are involved. Muscle-strengthening exercises may help protect the joint and decrease pain.[25]

Oral medications are aimed at reducing inflammation or providing analgesia. The most popular medications used in the treatment of osteoarthritis are the NSAIDs, many of which are available without a prescription. Ongoing research may confirm that some NSAIDs impede the repair mechanisms in early cartilage lesions. There is growing concern about the side effects of NSAIDs. Studies have shown the pain of osteoarthritis may arise from causes other than an inflamed synovium, such as stretching of the joint capsule, ligaments, or nerve endings in the periosteum over osteophytes to nontrabecular microfractures; intraosseous hypertension; bursitis or tendinitis; or muscle spasm. In such cases, the pain may be relieved by an NSAID because of the analgesic action of the drug rather than an antiinflammatory effect.[26] For many persons, acetaminophen in doses as high as 4000 mg/day may be as effective and less toxic than NSAIDs.

If the patient becomes more limited or the regimen is unsuccessful in adequately relieving symptoms, corticosteroid injections may be helpful, especially for those who have an effusion of the joint. Injections are usually limited to a total of four and not more than three within 1 year, because their use is thought to accelerate joint destruction.

Viscosupplementation is a new concept in treatment and is based on the hypothesis that joint lubrication is abnormal in osteoarthritis. Hyaluronate is injected into the joint weekly for 3 to 5 weeks. Controlled studies have shown this approach to be equally efficacious as

NSAIDs. Speculation that other agents may be chondroprotective has initiated other studies, but these results have not been confirmed in humans.

Surgery is considered when the person is having severe pain and joint function is severely reduced. Procedures include arthroscopic lavage and debridement, bunion resections, osteotomies to change alignment of the knee and hip joints, and decompression of the spinal roots in osteoarthritic vertebral stenosis. Total hip replacements have provided effective relief of symptoms and improved range of motion for many persons, as have total knee replacements, although the latter procedure has produced less consistent results. Joint replacement is available for the first carpometacarpal joint. Arthrodesis is used in advanced disease to reduce pain; however, this results in loss of motion.

Investigations are underway that use animal models of abrasion of the subchondral bone to permit vascular invasion to stimulate cartilage resorption and replacement with fibrocartilage and that place chondral grafts and progenitor cells under the periosteum.[27] Future management of osteoarthritis lies in the development of techniques to identify and monitor cartilage lesions at an earlier stage. Potential approaches include bone scanning, magnetic resonance imaging, and arthroscopy.

In summary, osteoarthritis, the most common form of arthritis, is a localized condition affecting primarily the weight-bearing joints. Risk factors for osteoarthritis progression include older age, osteoarthritis in multiple joints, neuropathy, and for knees, obesity. The disorder is characterized by degeneration of the articular cartilage and subchondral bone. It has been suggested that the cellular events responsible for the development of osteoarthritis begin with some type of abnormal mechanical insult or stimuli, including hormones and growth factors, drugs, mechanical stresses, and the extracellular environment. Studies also implicate immunologic factors in the perpetuation and acceleration of the osteoarthritic change. As cartilage ages, biochemical events such as collagen fatigue and fracture occur with less stress. Attempts at repair by increased matrix synthesis and cellular proliferation maintain the integrity of the cartilage until failure of reparative processes allows the degenerative changes to progress. Joint enlargement usually results from new bone formation, which causes the joint to feel hard. Pain and stiffness are primary features of the disease. Inflammatory mediators (e.g., prostaglandins) may increase the inflammatory and degenerative response.

Treatment is directed toward the relief of pain and maintenance of mobility while preserving the articular cartilage. Although there is no known cure for osteoarthritis, appropriate treatment can reduce pain, maintain or improve joint mobility, and limit functional disability.

Metabolic Diseases Associated With Rheumatic States

After you have completed this section of the chapter, you should be able to meet the following objectives:

- Relate the metabolism and elimination of uric acid to the pathogenesis of crystal-induced arthropathy
- State why asymptomatic hyperuricemia is a laboratory finding and not a disease
- Describe the clinical manifestations, diagnostic measures, and methods used in treatment of gouty arthritis

Metabolic bone and joint disorders result from biochemical and metabolic disorders that affect the joints. Metabolic and endocrine diseases associated with joint symptoms include amyloidosis, osteogenesis imperfecta, diabetes mellitus, hyperparathyroidism, thyroid disease, AIDS, and hypermobility syndromes. The discussion in this chapter is limited to the crystal-induced arthropathy, monosodium urate, or gout.

Crystal-Induced Arthropathies

Crystal deposition within joints produces arthritis. In gout, monosodium urate or uric acid crystals are found in the joint cavity. Another condition where calcium pyrophosphate dihydrate (CPPD) crystals are found in the joints is sometimes referred to as pseudogout or chondrocalcinosis. A brief discussion of pseudogout is found later in this chapter in the section about rheumatic diseases and the elderly.

Gout

The manifestations of the heterogeneous group of diseases known as the gout syndrome include acute gouty arthritis with recurrent attacks of severe articular and periarticular inflammation; tophi or the accumulation of crystalline deposits in articular surfaces, bones, soft tissue, and cartilage; gouty nephropathy or renal impairment; and uric acid kidney stones. Primary gout is predominantly a disease of men, with peak incidence in the fourth or sixth decade. Only 3% to 7% of cases occur in women, and most of these are in postmenopausal women.[28]

Uric Acid Metabolism and Elimination

Uric acid is a metabolite of the purines, adenine and guanine. Normally, about two thirds of the uric acid produced each day is excreted through the kidneys; the rest is eliminated through the gastrointestinal tract. Normal renal handling of uric acid involves three steps: filtration, reabsorption, and secretion. Uric acid is freely filtered in the glomerulus, completely reabsorbed in the proximal tubule, and is secreted back into the tubular fluid by another mechanism in the distal end of the proximal tubule or distal tubule (see Chapter 25). The tubular secretion and postsecretory reabsorption determine the final concentration of uric acid in the urine.

Most persons with gout have reduced urate clearance. For them, the serum urate level becomes elevated so that a normal amount of urate can be excreted and urate homeostasis can be achieved. Most persons with increased production of urate have increased excretion of uric acid. However, with kidney damage, an increased amount of uric acid is eliminated by the gastrointestinal tract.

Small doses of uricosuric agents may preferentially reduce secretion and increase uric acid retention, but therapeutic doses block reabsorption and increase uric acid elimination. The salicylates reduce secretion and cause retention of uric acid when given at doses used for pain relief; very large doses are needed to block reabsorption and secretion. Consequently, aspirin and other salicylates are not recommended for use as an analgesic in persons with gout. Some of the diuretics, including the thiazides, which are weak acids, are secreted by the proximal tubular cells and can also interfere with the excretion of uric acid.

Etiology and Pathogenesis

Hyperuricemia reflects a metabolic derangement in extracellular fluids. Hyperuricemia is defined as a serum urate concentration greater than 7.0 mg/dl as measured by the specific uricase method.[29] Monosodium urate crystal deposition develops when hyperuricemia exists. Asymptomatic hyperuricemia is a laboratory finding and not a disease. Most persons with hyperuricemia do not develop gout. Hyperuricemia may occur because of overproduction of uric acid, underexcretion of uric acid, or a combination of the two. Primary and secondary forms of hyperuricemia exist. Primary forms result from genetic defects in purine metabolism. Secondary forms of hyperuricemia are related to certain disease conditions and medications.

An attack of gout occurs when the monosodium urate crystals precipitate within the joint and initiate an inflammatory response. This may follow a sudden rise in the serum urate levels. The excess urate is not soluble and therefore precipitates. An attack can also occur with a sudden drop in the urate level. In either situation, crystals are released into the synovial fluid, and an inflammatory response is initiated.

Phagocytosis of urate crystals by the polymorphonuclear leukocytes occurs and leads to polymorphonuclear cell death with the release of lysosomal enzymes. As this process continues, the inflammation causes destruction of the cartilage and subchondral bone. Tophi are large, hard nodules that have irregular surfaces and contain crystalline deposits of monosodium urate that incite an inflammatory response. They are most commonly found in the synovium, olecranon bursa, Achilles tendon, subchondral bone, and extensor surface of the forearm and may be mistaken for rheumatoid nodules. Tophi usually do not appear until 10 years or more after the first gout attack. This stage of gout, called *chronic tophaceous gout,* is characterized by more frequent and prolonged attacks, which are often polyarticular.

Crystal deposition usually occurs in peripheral areas of the body, such as the great toe and the pinnae of the ear. Sodium urate is less soluble at temperatures below 37°C. The peripheral tissues are cooler than other parts of the body, and this may at least partially explain why gout occurs most frequently in peripheral joints.

Clinical Manifestations

The typical acute attack of gout is monarticular and usually affects the first metatarsophalangeal joint. The tarsal joints, insteps, ankles, heels, knees, wrists, fingers, and elbows may also be initial sites of involvement. Acute gout often begins at night and may be precipitated by excessive exercise, certain medications, foods, alcohol, or dieting. The onset of pain is typically abrupt, and redness and swelling are observed. The attack may last for days or weeks. Pain may be severe enough to be aggravated even by the weight of a bed sheet covering the affected area.

In the early stages of gout after the initial attack has subsided, the person is asymptomatic, and joint abnormalities are not evident. This is referred to as intercritical gout. After the first attack, it may be months or years before another attack. As attacks recur with increased frequency, joint changes occur and become permanent.

Diagnosis and Treatment

Although hyperuricemia is the biochemical hallmark of gout, the presence of hyperuricemia cannot be equated with gout, because many persons with this condition never develop gout. A definitive diagnosis of gout can be made only when monosodium urate crystals are in the synovial fluid or in tissue sections of tophaceous deposits. Synovial fluid analysis is useful in excluding other conditions, such as septic arthritis, pseudogout, and rheumatoid arthritis. The next step is to determine if the disorder is related to overproduction or to underexcretion of uric acid. The uric acid level is determined, and a 24-hour urine sample is collected. Ideally, the person should be on a purine-free diet during the time the urine specimen is being collected. Urate urine values above the normal range of 264 to 588 mg/day indicate an overproduction of uric acid.[13] The normal serum urate concentration is 5.0 to 5.7 mg/dl in men and 3.7 to 5.0 mg/dl in women.[30]

The objectives in the treatment of gout are the termination and prevention of the acute attacks of gouty arthritis and the correction of hyperuricemia, with consequent inhibition of further precipitation of sodium urate and absorption of urate crystal deposits already in the tissues. Management of acute gout is directed toward reducing joint inflammation. Hyperuricemia and related problems of tophi, joint destruction, and renal problems are treated after the acute inflammatory process has subsided. NSAIDs, particularly indomethacin and ibuprofen, are used for treating acute gouty arthritis. Alternative therapies include colchicine and intraarticular deposition of corticosteroids. Treatment with colchicine is used early in the acute stage. Although the drug is usually given orally, a more rapid response is obtained when colchicine is given intravenously. The nausea and diarrhea that may occur with large oral doses are avoided when the drug is given intravenously. The acute symptoms of gout usually subside within 48 hours after treatment with oral colchicine has been instituted and within 12 hours after intravenous administration of the drug.

NSAIDs are effective during the acute stage when used at their maximum dosage and are sometimes preferred to colchicine because they have fewer toxic side effects. Phenylbutazone is usually effective but is used only on a short-term basis because long-term use can cause bone marrow suppression. The corticosteroid drugs are not recommended for treatment of gout unless all other medications have proved unsuccessful. Intraarticular injections of corticosteroid agents may be used when only one joint is involved and the person is unable to take colchicine or nonsteroidal drugs.

With the exception of phenylbutazone, the drugs used to treat acute gout have no effect on the serum urate level and are valueless in tophaceous gout and the control of hyperuricemia. After the acute attack has been relieved, the hyperuricemia is treated. One method is to reduce hyperuricemia through the use of allopurinol or a uricosuric agent (*i.e.*, probenecid or sulfinpyrazone, a phenylbutazone derivative). These compounds are not used in the treatment of acute gouty arthritis and, if given, only tend to exacerbate and prolong the inflammation. These uricosuric medications prevent the tubular reabsorption of urate. The serum urate concentrations are monitored to determine efficacy and dosage. These drugs are usually started in small doses and gradually increased over 7 to 10 days. Aspirin should not be used with these medications, because it decreases the urinary excretion of uric acid. Allopurinol is the preferred antihyperuricemic therapy for patients with frequent attacks of gout, significant hyperuricemia (>9 to 11 mg/dl), significant hyperuricosuria (>800 to 1000 mg/day), tophi, uric acid urolithiasis, or urate nephropathy. Allopurinol inhibits xanthine oxidase, an enzyme needed for the conversion of hypoxanthine to xanthine and xanthine to uric acid. There is a slight possibility that xanthine kidney stones can develop if allopurinol is used for many years. It is usually reserved for the person who does not have an adequate response or is unable to tolerate other forms of treatment. Treatment of hyperuricemia is aimed at maintaining normal uric acid levels and requires lifelong treatment. Prophylactic colchicine or NSAIDs may be used between gout attacks. If the uric acid level is normal and the person has not had recurrent attacks of gout, these medications may be discontinued.

Gout can be effectively controlled by medical management; often it is not, because many persons with gout have a limited understanding of the disease and therefore a low compliance with treatment. Education about the disease and its management is fundamental to the treatment and management of gout. The sufferer should be made aware that the prognosis is very good and that the disease, although chronic, can be controlled in almost all cases. Some changes in lifestyle may be needed, such as maintenance of ideal weight, moderation in alcohol consumption, and avoiding purine-rich foods, such as liver, kidney, sardines, anchovies, and sweetbreads, particularly by patients with excessive tophaceous deposits. Adherence to the lifelong use of medications may be the only major lifestyle change necessary for many persons.

In summary, crystal-induced arthropathy is characterized by crystal deposition within the joint. However, hyperuricemia is a laboratory finding and not a disease. Gout is the prototype of this group. Acute attacks of arthritis occur with gout and are characterized by the presence of monosodium urate crystals in the joint. The disorder is accompanied by hyperuricemia, which results from overproduction of uric acid or from the reduced ability of the kidney to rid the body of excess uric acid. Management of acute gout is first directed toward the reduction of joint inflammation; then the hyperuricemia is treated. Hyperuricemia is treated with uricosuric agents, which prevent the tubular reabsorption of urate, or with medication that inhibits the production of uric acid. Although gout is chronic, it can be controlled with appropriate lifestyle changes by most patients.

Rheumatic Diseases in Children and the Elderly

After you have completed this section of the chapter, you should be able to meet the following objectives:

- List three types of juvenile rheumatoid arthritis and differentiate among their major characteristics
- Name one rheumatic disease that affects only the elderly population

Rheumatic Diseases in Children

Children can be affected with almost all of the rheumatic diseases. In addition to disease-specific differences, these conditions affect not only the child but the family. Growth and development require special attention. Adherence to the treatment program requires intervention with the child and parents. School issues also must be addressed.

Juvenile Rheumatoid Arthritis

Juvenile rheumatoid arthritis (JRA) is a chronic disease that affects approximately 60,000 to 200,000 children in the United States.[1] It is characterized by synovitis and can influence epiphyseal growth by stimulating growth of the affected side. Generalized stunted growth may also occur.

Systemic onset (*i.e.*, Still's disease) affects about 20% of children with JRA.[1] The symptoms of Still's disease include a daily intermittent high fever, which is usually accompanied by a rash, generalized lymphadenopathy, hepatosplenomegaly, leukocytosis, and anemia. Most of these children also have joint involvement by the disease. Systemic symptoms usually subside in 6 to 12 months. This form of JRA can also make an initial appearance in adulthood. Infections, heart disease, and adrenal insufficiency may cause death.

A second subgroup of JRA, pauciarticular arthritis, affects no more than four joints.[10] This disease affects 55% to 75% of children with JRA. Pauciarticular arthritis affects two distinct groups. The first group generally consists of girls younger than 6 years of age with chronic uveitis. The results of ANA testing in this group are usually positive. The second group, who have late-onset arthritis, is most commonly made up of males. The HLA-B27 test results are positive in more than one half of this group. They are affected by sacroiliitis, and the arthritis usually occurs in the lower extremities.

The third subgroup of JRA, accounting for about 20% of the total, is polyarticular onset disease. It affects more than four joints during the first 6 months of the disease. This form of arthritis more closely resembles the adult form of the disease than the other two subgroups. Rheumatoid factor is sometimes present and may indicate a more active disease process. Systemic features include a low-grade fever, weight loss, malaise, anemia, stunted growth, slight organomegaly (*e.g.*, hepatosplenomegaly), and adenopathy.[1]

The prognosis for most children with rheumatoid arthritis is good. NSAIDs are the first-line drugs used in treating JRA. Salicylates have been replaced by agents such as naproxen, ibuprofen, and ketoprofen. The second-line agent is low-dose methotrexate or, less often, sulfasalazine. Gold salts, hydroxychloroquine, and D-penicillamine are rarely used.[31] Other aspects of treatment of children with JRA are similar to those used for the adult with rheumatoid arthritis. Children are encouraged to lead as normal a life as possible.

Systemic Lupus Erythematosus

The features of SLE in children are similar to the disease in adults. The incidence in children is 10 times lower, estimated to occur in 0.6 of 100,000 children. The occurrence in the sexes is almost equal until pubescence, and it then approaches the sex ratio seen in adults. The clinical manifestations of SLE in children reflect the extent and severity of systemic involvement. The best prognostic indicator in children is the extent of renal involvement, which is more common and more severe in children than in adults with SLE. Infectious complications are the most common cause of death (40%) in children with SLE.

Children with SLE may present with constitutional symptoms, including fever, malaise, anorexia, and weight loss. Symptoms of the skin, musculoskeletal, central nervous, cardiac, pulmonary, and hematopoietic systems are similar to those of adults. Endocrine abnormalities include Cushing's syndrome from long-term corticosteroid use and autoimmune thyroiditis. Adolescents often experience menstrual disturbances, which tend to resolve with disease remission.[32]

Treatment of SLE in children is similar to that of adults. The use of NSAIDs, corticosteroids, antimalarials, and immunosuppressive agents depends on the symptoms. Corticosteroids may cause stunting of growth and necrosis of femoral heads and other joints. Immunization schedules should be maintained using attenuated rather than live vaccines. Rest periods should be balanced with exercise; children should be encouraged to maintain as normal a schedule as possible.[33] The diversity of the clinical manifestations of SLE in the young requires the establishment of a comprehensive program.[34]

Juvenile Dermatomyositis

Juvenile dermatomyositis (JDMS) is an inflammatory myopathy primarily involving skin and muscle and associated with a characteristic rash. JDMS can affect children of all ages, with a mean age at onset of 8 years. There is an increased incidence among females. The cause is unknown.

Symmetric proximal muscle weakness, elevated muscle enzymes, evidence of vasculitis, and electromyographic changes confirming an inflammatory myopathy are diagnostic for JDMS. Generalized vasculitis is not seen in the adult form of the disease. The rash may precede or follow the onset of proximal muscle weakness. Periorbital edema, erythema, and eyelid telangiectasia are common.

Calcifications can occur in 30% to 50% of children with JDMS and are by far the most debilitating symptom. The calcifications appear at pressure points or sites of previous trauma. JDMS is treated primarily with corticosteroids to reduce inflammation. Occasionally, immunosuppressives are used in cases of refractory disease.[1]

Juvenile Spondyloarthropathies

Ankylosing spondylitis, reactive arthritis, psoriatic arthritis, and spondylarthropathies associated with ulcerative colitis and regional enteritis can affect children and adults. In children, spondyloarthritis manifests in peripheral joints first, mimicking pauciarticular JRA, with no evidence of sacroiliac or spine involvement for months to years after onset. The spondylarthropathies are more common in boys and commonly occur in children who have a positive family history. HLA-B27 typing is helpful in diagnosing children because of the unusual presentation of the disease.

Management of the disease involves physical therapy, education, attention to school and growth and development issues. Medication includes the use of salicylates or other NSAIDs such as tolmetin or indomethacin. More severe disease or symptoms may require systemic corticosteroids.[1]

Rheumatic Diseases in the Elderly

Arthritis is the most common complaint of elderly persons. The pain, stiffness, and muscle weakness impact daily life, often threatening independence and quality of life. Symptoms of the rheumatic diseases also can have an indirect effect and even threaten the duration of life for the elderly. The weakness and gait disturbance that are often a part of the rheumatic diseases can contribute to the likelihood of falls and fracture, causing suffering, increased health care costs, further loss of independence, and the potential for a decreased life span.

The elderly cope less well with mild to moderately severe disease that in younger persons is less likely to lead to serious disability for the same degree of impairment. Unfortunately, the elderly and often their health care providers think the problems associated with arthritis are an inevitable consequence of aging and fail to benefit from measures that can improve the quality of life.

Because arthritis is the leading cause of change in the functional status of older adults, a functional approach to the problems of the elderly is appropriate. Inactivity is a societal expectation of the elderly. What activity there is tends to be of the nature of leisurely walking, and deconditioning occurs.

Older patients often have multiple problems complicating diagnosis and management. The diagnosis of an elderly patient with a musculoskeletal problem must consider a wide variety of disorders that are usually regarded as outside the range of typical rheumatic disease. Among these are metastatic malignancy, multiple myeloma, musculoskeletal disorders accompanying endocrine or metabolic disorders, orthopedic conditions, and neurologic disease. The diagnosis may be missed if the assumption is that musculoskeletal problems in the older person are caused by osteoarthritis.

An increased incidence of false-positive tests for rheumatoid factor and ANAs occurs for the elderly population with or without rheumatic disease, because older persons are better producers of autoantibodies than younger persons. There are differences in the manifestations, diagnosis, and treatment of some of the rheumatic diseases in the elderly. The usual presentation of these conditions was discussed earlier in this chapter. One form of rheumatic disease that has a predilection for the elderly is polymyalgia rheumatica.

Rheumatoid Arthritis

The prevalence of rheumatoid arthritis increases with advancing age, at least until age 75.[25] Seropositive patients are more likely to have had an acute onset with systemic features and higher disease activity. Patients with seronegative, elderly-onset rheumatoid arthritis have a disease that generally follows a mild course. The close resemblance of the manifestations of seronegative rheumatoid arthritis in the elderly to those of polymyalgia rheumatica has led to speculation concerning the relation of these syndromes.[35] It may be that rheumatoid arthritis in the elderly is a broad disorder that includes a number of distinct subsets with characteristic manifestations, courses, and outcomes.

Systemic Lupus Erythematosus

SLE is another condition with different manifestations in the elderly.[36] The disease is less frequently accompanied by renal involvement. However, pleurisy, pericarditis, arthritis, and symptoms closely resembling polymyalgia rheumatica are more common tan in younger patients. The characteristics of lupus in the elderly closely resemble those of drug-induced lupus, leading to speculation that the syndrome may result from one of the multiple drugs that are taken by many elderly patients.

Osteoarthritis

Osteoarthritis is by far the most common form of arthritis among the elderly. It is the greatest cause of disability and limitation of activity in older populations. It has been suggested that osteoarthritis begins at a very young age, expressing itself in the elderly only after a long period of latency. Too often, it is accepted by the patient or expected by the physician. Osteoarthritis presents a major management problem, but there is much that can be done. Self-control by maintaining a positive attitude and sense of self-esteem is a frequent coping strategy.[37]

Crystal-Induced Arthropathies

The incidence of clinical gout increases with advancing age, in part because of the increased involvement of joints after years of continued hyperuricemia.[38] High serum urate levels rarely occur in women before menopause; initial attacks of clinical gout occur around the age of 70, or 20 years after menopause.[39] Gouty attacks in elderly women may be precipitated by the use of diuretics.

The treatment of gout is more difficult in the elderly. Although colchicine may be effective in controlling the symptoms of chronic gout, it may cause diarrhea in some patients, limiting its effectiveness in maintenance therapy.

As part of the tissue-aging process, osteoarthritis develops with associated cartilage degeneration. Calcium pyrophosphate crystals are shed into the joint cavity. These crystals may produce a low-grade chronic inflammation—the chronic pseudogout syndrome. The accumulation of calcium pyrophosphate and related crystalline deposits in articular cartilage is common in the elderly. There are no medications that can remove the crystals from the joints. Although it may be asymptomatic, presence of the crystals may contribute to more rapid cartilage deterioration. This condition may coexist with severe osteoarthritis.

Polymyalgia Rheumatica

Of the forms of arthritis affecting the elderly, polymyalgia rheumatica is one of the more difficult to diagnose and one of the most important to identify. Elderly women are especially at risk. Polymyalgia rheumatica is a common syndrome of older patients, rarely occurring before age 50 and usually after age 60. The onset can be abrupt, with the patient going to bed feeling well and awakening with pain and stiffness in the neck, shoulders, and hips.

Diagnosis is based on the pain and stiffness persisting for at least 1 month and an elevated ESR. The diagnosis is confirmed when the symptoms respond dramatically to a small dose of prednisone, a corticosteroid. Biopsies have shown that the muscles are normal, despite the name, but that a nonspecific inflammation affecting the synovial tissue is present. It is possible that a number of patients are erroneously diagnosed as having rheumatoid arthritis or osteoarthritis. For patients with an elevated Westergren ESR (>50 mm), the diagnosis is usually based on a 3-day trial of prednisone treatment.[40] Patients with polymyalgia rheumatica typically exhibit striking clinical improvement about the second day. Patients with rheumatoid arthritis also show improvement, although usually days later.

Treatment with NSAIDs provides relief for some patients, but most require continuing therapy with prednisone, with gradual reduction of the dose over the course of 1.5 to 2 years, using the patient's symptoms as the primary guide. Patients need close monitoring during the maintenance phase with prednisone. Because their symptoms are relieved, they often quit taking the prednisone and their symptoms recur, or doses are missed and the decreased dosage leads to an increase in symptoms. Unless careful assessment reveals the frequency of missed doses, the physician may be misled into increasing the dosage when it is not needed. Because of the side effect of the corticosteroids, the goal is to use the lowest dose of the drug necessary to control the symptoms. Weaning patients off low-dose prednisone therapy after this length of time can be difficult and extended over some time. Health care providers must work closely with the elderly patient to make sure the correct dosage is taken as the amount is slowly decreased. Even a small error in dosage can set the tapering program back by weeks or months.

A certain percentage of patients with polymyalgia rheumatica also have giant cell arteritis (*i.e.*, temporal arteritis), frequently with involvement of the ophthalmic arteries. The two conditions are considered to represent different manifestations of the same disease. Giant cell arteritis, a form of systemic vasculitis, is a systemic inflammatory disease of large and medium-sized arteries (see Chapter 17). The inflammatory response seems to be a T-cell response to an antigen.

Clinical manifestations of giant cell arteritis usually begin insidiously and may exist for some time before being recognized (Chart 47–4).[41] It is potentially dangerous if missed or mistreated, especially if the temporal artery or other vessels supplying the eye are involved, in which case blindness can quickly ensue without treatment. The condition is responsive to appropriate therapy. For those patients at risk, adherence to the medication program is critical, with preservation of sight being the goal. Because this complication can occur so quickly and is relatively asymptomatic, it is vital that the patient understands the importance of taking the correct dose regularly as prescribed. Treatment consists of large doses of prednisone. The usual side effects occur, some of which (osteoporosis) are more common than that normally expected. This dosage is continued for 4 to 6 weeks and then decreased gradually.

CHART **47-4**
Signs and Symptoms of Giant Cell Arteritis

- Constitutional symptoms
  - Malaise
  - Fatigue
  - Fever (usually low grade)
  - Weight loss
  - Cough
  - Sore throat
- Polymyalgia rheumatica syndrome
  - Limb girdle pain and stiffness
- Manifestations related to vascular involvement
  - New type of headache
  - Scalp tenderness, especially over temporal area
  - Visual loss
  - Diplopia
  - Aortic arch syndrome
- Ischemic optic neuropathy
  - Atrophy
- Claudication of jaw or arm

Localized Musculoskeletal Disorders

The elderly are also prone to localized musculoskeletal syndromes. Years of wear frequently lead to a range of inflammatory disorders, including bursitis and tendinitis. These are known collectively as *impingement syndromes.* An example is a disorder in the shoulder where the rotator cuff rides against the acromion. Tennis elbow (only 5% of those with this problem actually play tennis), or humeral epicondylitis, is also frequently seen among the elderly. Other localized inflammatory conditions of the musculoskeletal system affecting the elderly are fibrositis or fibromyalgia and Dupuytren's contracture.

Management of Rheumatic Disease in the Elderly

In addition to diagnosis-specific treatment, the elderly require special considerations. Management techniques that rely on modalities other than drugs are particularly important for the elderly. These include splints, walking aids, muscle-building exercise, and local heat. Muscle-strengthening and stretching exercises are particularly effective in the elderly person with age-related losses in muscle function and should be instituted early. Rest, the cornerstone of conservative therapy, is hazardous in the elderly, who can rapidly lose muscle strength.

The NSAIDs may be less well tolerated by the elderly, and the side effects are more likely to be serious. In addition to bleeding from the gastrointestinal tract and renal insufficiency, there may be cognitive dysfunction, manifested by forgetfulness, inability to concentrate, sleeplessness, paranoid ideation, and depression. Misoprostol should be considered in conjunction with treatment with NSAIDs to prevent ulcer formation, and the patient should be monitored for renal insufficiency.[42]

Even such tasks as the frequent visits to the physician's office for the laboratory monitoring that is necessary with drugs such as gold can be difficult or impossible for elderly patients who live in a cold climate during the winter. For the patient who no longer drives or does not want to, transportation can be a barrier. Elderly patients often hesitate to ask family or friends to take them to the doctor every week.

The elderly are more likely to conceal symptoms than to elaborate on them, because they feel they are a part of the aging process or that "nothing can be done." One of the ways to enhance a person's ability to combat the symptoms of arthritis is by enforcing a greater sense of control. The elderly patient should be involved in the management and treatment program.

Joint arthroplasty is used for pain relief and increased function. Chronologic age is not a contraindication for surgical treatment of arthritis. In appropriately selected elderly candidates, survival and functional outcome after surgery are equivalent to those in younger age groups. The more sedentary activity level of the elderly makes them even better candidates for joint replacement, because they put less stress and demand on the new joint.

In summary, rheumatic diseases that affect children can be similar to the adult disease, but there are also manifestations unique to the younger population. In addition to disease-specific differences, children with chronic diseases have to be approached with different priorities than adults. Managing rheumatic diseases in children requires a team approach to address issues of the family, school, growth and development, and coping strategies and requires a comprehensive disease management program.

Arthritis is the most common complaint of elderly population. The pain, stiffness, and muscle weakness impact daily life, often threatening independence and quality of life. There is a difference in the manifestations, diagnosis, and treatment of some of the rheumatic diseases in the elderly. Osteoarthritis is the most common form of arthritis among the elderly. The prevalence of rheumatoid arthritis and gout increases with advancing age. One form of rheumatic disease that has a predilection for the elderly is polymyalgia rheumatica. A certain percentage of patients with polymyalgia rheumatica also have giant cell arthritis, frequently with involvement of the ophthalmic arteries. If this condition is untreated, it carries a serious threat of blindness.

REFERENCES

1. Schumacher H.R. (Ed.). (1993). *Primer on the rheumatic diseases* (10th ed.). Atlanta: Arthritis Foundation.
2. Harris E.D. (1989). The clinical features of rheumatoid arthritis. In Kelly W.N., Harris E.D., Ruddy S., Sledge C.B. (Eds.). *Textbook of rheumatology* (3rd ed., pp. 943–981). Philadelphia: W.B. Saunders.
3. Winchester R. (1994). HIV and rheumatic diseases. *Bulletin on the Rheumatic Diseases* 43 (2), 5–8.
4. Pope R.M. (1996). Rheumatoid arthritis: Pathogenesis and early recognition. *American Journal of Medicine* 100 (2A), 3s–9s.
5. Harris E.D. (1992). Excitement in synovium: The rapid evolution of understanding of rheumatoid arthritis and expectations for therapy. *Journal of Rheumatology Supplement* 32 (19), 3–5.
6. Klippel J.H., Dieppe P.A. (1994). *Rheumatology.* St. Louis: Mosby.
7. Semble E.L. (1995). Rheumatoid arthritis: New approaches for its evaluation and management. *Archives of Physical Medicine and Rehabilitation* 76, 190–201.
8. Minor M.A., et al. (1989). Efficacy of physical conditioning exercise in patients with rheumatoid arthritis and osteoarthritis. *Arthritis and Rheumatism* 32, 1396–1405.
9. Moncur C., Williams H.J. (1993). Rheumatoid arthritis: Status of drug therapies. *Physical Therapy* 75 (6), 511–525.
10. Chan K.A., et al. (1994). The lag time between onset of symptoms and diagnosis of rheumatoid arthritis. *Arthritis and Rheumatism* 37 (6), 814–820.
11. McGuire C., Ridgway H.J. (1993). Aggressive drug therapy for rheumatoid arthritis. *Hospital Practice* 28 (9), 45–52.
12. Boumpas D.T., et al. (1995). Systemic lupus erythematosus: Emerging concepts. *Annals of Internal Medicine* 122 (12), 940–950.
13. Mills J.A. (1994). Medical progress: Systemic lupus erythematosus. *New England Journal of Medicine* 330 (26), 1871–1878.
14. Tan E.M., Cohen A.S., Fries J.F., et al. (1982). The 1982 revised criteria for the classification of systemic lupus erythematosus. *Arthritis and Rheumatism* 25 (11), 1271–1277.
15. Pigg J.S., Bancroft D.A. (1996). Management of patients with rheumatic diseases. In Smeltzer S.C., Bare B.C. (Eds.). *Brunner and Suddarth's textbook of medical-surgical nursing* (8th ed., pp. 1443–1472). Philadelphia: J.B. Lippincott.
16. Van Vollenhoven R.F. (1996) Systemic lupus erythematosus: Managing early, mild disease. *Journal of Musculoskeletal Medicine* 13 (8), 24–39.
17. Clements P.J. (1994). Systemic sclerosis: Natural history and management strategies. *Journal of Musculoskeletal Medicine* 11 (11), 43–50.
18. Toivanen A, Toivanen P. 1994. Epidemiologic aspects, clinical features, and management of ankylosing spondylitis and reactive arthritis. *Current Opinion Rheumatology* 6 (4): 354–359.

19. Smiley J.D. (1995). Psoriatic arthritis. *Bulletin on the Rheumatic Diseases* 44 (4), 1–2.
20. Arnold W.J. (1995). Case management study: Osteoarthritis of the knee. *Bulletin on the Rheumatic Diseases* 44 (6), 1–2.
21. Felson D.T., Zhang Y., Anthony J.M., Naimark A., Anderson J.J. (1992). Weight loss reduces the risk for symptomatic knee osteoarthritis in women: The Framingham Study. *Annals of Internal Medicine* 116, 535–539.
22. Howell D.S., Altman R.D. (1993). Cartilage repair and conservation in osteoarthritis. A brief review of some experimental approaches to chondroprotection. *Rheumatic Diseases Clinics of North America* 19 (3):713–724.
23. Hochberg M.C., et al. for the American College of Rheumatology. (1995). Guidelines for the medical management of osteoarthritis. Part II: Osteoarthritis of the knee. *Arthritis and Rheumatism* 38 (11), 1541–1546.
24. Lawrence R.C., Hochberg M.D., Kelsey J.L., et al. (1989). Estimates of the prevalence of selected arthritic and musculoskeletal diseases in the United States. *Journal of Rheumatology* 16, 427–441.
25. Schilke J.M., Johnson G.O., Housh T.J., O'Dell J.R. (1996). Effects of muscle-strength training on the functional status of patients with osteoarthritis of the knee joint. *Nursing Research* 45 (2), 68–72.
26. Brandt K.D. (1993). Should osteoarthritis be treated with nonsteroidal anti-inflammatory drugs? *Rheumatic Disease Clinics of North America* 19 (3):697–712.
27. Howell D.S., Altman R.D. (1993). Cartilage repair and conservation in osteoarthritis. *Rheumatic Disease Clinics of North America* 19 (3), 713–724.
28. Levinson D.J., Becker M.A. (1993). Clinical gout and the pathogenesis of hyperuricemia. In McCarty D.J., Koopman W.J. (Eds.). *Arthritis and allied conditions* (12th ed., pp. 1733–1805). Philadelphia: Lea & Febiger.
29. Wortman R.L. (1993). Management of hyperuricemia. In McCarty D.J., Koopman W.J. (Eds.), *Arthritis and allied conditions* (12th ed., pp. 1807--1818). Philadelphia: Lea & Febiger.
30. Yeomans A.C. (1991). Assessment and management of gouty arthritis. *Nurse Practitioner* 16 (4), 20, 21, 25, 26.
31. Giannini E.H., Cawkwell G.D. (1995). Drug treatment in children with juvenile rheumatoid arthritis. *Pediatric Clinics of North America* 42 (5), 1099–1125.
32. Alsaeid K., Ayoub E.M. (1992). Systemic lupus erythematosus in children: Part one: Diagnosis complicated by a lengthy differential list. *Journal of Musculoskeletal Medicine* 9 (9), 29–39.
33. Fuller C., Hartley B. (1991). Systemic lupus erythematosus in adolescents. *Journal of Pediatric Nursing* 6 (4), 252–257.
34. Alsaeid K., Ayoub E.M. (1992). Systemic lupus erythematosus in children: Part two: Management team acts to control symptoms. *Journal of Musculoskeletal Medicine* 10 (10), 30–39.
35. Van Schaardenburg D, Breedveld FC. (1994). Elderly-onset rheumatoid arthritis. *Seminars in Arthritis and Rheumatology* 23 (6), 367–378.
36. Maddison P.J. (1987). Systemic lupus erythematosus in the elderly. *Journal of Rheumatology* 14 (S13), 182–187.
37. Burke M, Flaherty MJ. (1993). Coping strategies and health status of elderly arthritic women. *Journal Advanced Nursing* 18 (1), 7–13.
38. Calkins E. (1991). Arthritis in the elderly. *Bulletin on the Rheumatic Diseases* 40 (3), 3.
39. Campbell S.M. (1988). Gout: How presentation, diagnosis, and treatment differ in the elderly. *Geriatrics* 43, 71–77.
40. Powell M.A. (1991). Polymyalgia rheumatica. *Journal of the American Academy of Nurse Practitioners* 3 (4), 188–189.
41. Kachroo A, Tello C, Bais R, Panush RS. (1996). Giant cell arteritis: Diagnosis and management. *Bulletin on the Rheumatic Diseases* 45 (5), 2–5.
42. American College of Rheumatology Ad Hoc Committee on Clinical Guidelines. (1996). Guidelines for monitoring drug therapy in rheumatoid arthritis. *Arthritis and Rheumatism* 30 (5), 723–731.

ADDITIONAL READINGS

Arnett F.C. (1990). Revised criteria for the classification of rheumatoid arthritis. *Orthopedic Nursing* 9 (2), 58–64.

Arnett F.C. (1991). Pathogenesis of the spondyloarthropathies. *Bulletin on the Rheumatic Diseases* 40 (6), 1–3.

Arnett F.C. (1992). Genetic aspects of human lupus. *Clinical Immunology* 63 (1), 4–6.

Bunning R.D., Materson R.S. (1991). A rational program of exercise for patients with osteoarthritis. *Seminars in Arthritis and Rheumatism 21* (S), 3343.

Campbell S.M. (1991). Rheumatoid arthritis. *Hospital Medicine* 27 (1), 55–62.

Collo M.C.B., Johnson J.L., Finch W.R., Felicetta J.V. (1991). Evaluating arthritic complaints. *Nurse Practitioner* 16 (2), 9–20.

Ellman M.H. (1992). Treating acute gouty arthritis. *Journal of Musculoskeletal Medicine* 3 (3), 71–77.

Hamerman D. (1989). The biology of osteoarthritis. *New England Journal of Medicine* 320 (20), 1322–1330.

Harris E.D. (1992). Excitement in synovium: The rapid evolution of understanding of rheumatoid arthritis and expectations for therapy. *Journal of Rheumatology* 19 (S32), 18–20.

Hess E.V. (1991). Drug-related lupus. *Bulletin on the Rheumatic Diseases* 40 (4), 1–8.

Kale S.A., Raymond M.K. (1990). Osteoarthritis: The patient-centered approach: Part 1—Evaluation. *Consultant* Aug, 24–26.

Kovar P.A., Allegrante J.P., MacKenzier R., Peterson M.G.E., Gutin B., Charlson M.E. (1992). Supervised fitness walking in patients with osteoarthritis of the knee. *Annals of Internal Medicine* 116 (7), 529–534.

Lorig K., Fries J.F. (1990) *The arthritis helpbook.* Reading, MA: Addison-Wesley.

Minor M.A. (1994). Exercise in the management of osteoarthritis of the knee and hip. *Arthritis Care Research* 7 (4):198– 204.

Morrey B.F. (1992). Primary osteoarthritis of the knee: A stepwise management plan. *Journal of Musculoskeletal Medicine* 9 (9), 79–94.

Pincus T., Callahan L.F. (1992). Early mortality in RA predicted by poor clinical status. *Bulletin on the Rheumatic Diseases* 41 (4), 1–5.

Ramanujam R., Schumacher H.R. (1992). Ankylosing spondylitis: Early recognition and management. *Journal of Musculoskeletal Medicine* 1 (1), 75--91.

Smith C.A., Arnett F.C. (1991). Epidemiologic aspects of rheumatoid arthritis. *Clinical Orthopedic Research* 265, 23–35.

Watts R.A., Isaacs J.D. (1992). Immunotherapy of rheumatoid arthritis. *Annals of the Rheumatic Diseases* 51 (5), 577–579.

Wegner S.T., Belza B., Gall E.P. (1996). *Clinical care in the rheumatic diseases.* Atlanta: American College of Rheumatology.

Reproductive System

There is a long history of misunderstanding and myths about human reproduction, especially the female reproductive system. Early on, the uterus was deemed the most important structure of the female reproductive anatomy. One of the first representations of the uterus appears in ancient Egyptian hieroglyphs (c. 2900 BC). Its importance was a direct result of the understanding that it was from the uterus that a child was born. That a woman was the carrier of the next generation was enough to establish her importance to society. However, society also imposed harsh restrictions on women that made it difficult, if not impossible, for further understanding. Until the Renaissance, custom and manners dictated that a woman's body could not be represented unless it was fully clothed.

To a regrettable extent, the associations made in ancient times that surmised a destiny for women based on the anatomy peculiar to their sex still affect how woman are viewed today. The Greek philosopher Plato (427?–347? BC) postulated that the unused womb became "indignant" and wandered around the body, inhibiting the body's "spirits," or life force, and causing disease. The reasonings of Aristotle (384–332 BC) were equally fanciful. It was he, believing as others of the time did that women were irrational and prone to emotional outbursts, who provided the nomenclature for the womb, naming it hystera *(ustera). Their concept that emotional excitability or instability was the domain of women is confirmed by another word that was coined by the Greeks: hysteria.*

UNIT XIII

CHAPTER 48

Structure and Function of the Male Reproductive System

Stephanie M. Stewart

The male genitourinary system is composed of the paired gonads, or testes, genital ducts, accessory organs, and penis. The dual function of the testes is to produce male sex androgens (*i.e.,* male sex hormones), mainly testosterone, and spermatozoa (*i.e.,* male germ cells). The internal accessory organs produce the fluid constituents of semen, and the ductile system aids in the storage and transport of spermatozoa. The penis functions in urine elimination and sexual function. This chapter focuses on the structure of the male reproductive system, spermatogenesis and control of male reproductive function, neural control of sexual function, and changes in function that occur at puberty and as a result of the aging process.

Structure of the Male Reproductive System

After you have completed this section of the chapter, you should be able to meet the following objectives:

- Characterize the embryonic development of the male reproductive organs and genitalia
- Describe the structure and function of the testes and scrotum, the genital ducts, accessory organs, and penis

Embryonic Development

The sex of a person is determined at the time of fertilization by the sex chromosomes. In the early stages of embryonic development, the tissues from which the male and female reproductive organs develop are undifferentiated. Until approximately the seventh week of gestation, it is impossible to determine whether the embryo is male or female unless the chromosomes are studied. Until this time, the genital tracts of the male and the female consist of two wolffian ducts, from which the male genitalia develop, and two müllerian ducts, from which the female genital structures develop. During this period of gestation, the gonads (*i.e.,* ovaries and testes) are also undifferentiated.

Between the sixth and eighth weeks of gestation, the testes begin development under the influence of the Y chromosome. During this time, the testicular cells of the male embryo begin producing an antimüllerian hormone and testosterone. The antimüllerian hormone inhibits development of the female genital organ from the müllerian ducts. Testosterone stimulates the wolffian ducts to develop into the epididymis, vas deferens, and seminal vesicles. Testosterone is also the precursor of a third hormone, dihydrotestosterone, which functions in the formation of the male urethra, prostate, and external genitalia. In the absence of testosterone, a male embryo with an XY chromosomal pattern develops female genitalia.

Testicular development and the embryonic production of testosterone requires a Y chromosome. Gonadal sex determination is determined by a testis-determining gene (or genes) located on the short arm of the Y chromosome. In the presence of the testis-determining gene, the embryonic gonads develop into testes, and in its absence, the gonads develop into ovaries.

Testes and Scrotum

The testes, or male gonads, are two egg-shaped structures located outside the abdominal cavity in the scrotum. Embryologically, the testes develop in the abdominal cavity and then descend through the inguinal canal into a pouch of peritoneum (which becomes the tunica vaginalis) in the scrotum during the seventh to the ninth month of fetal life. As they descend, the testes pull their arteries, veins, lymphatics, nerves, and conducting excretory ducts with them. These structures are encased by the cremaster muscle and layers of fascia that constitute the spermatic cord. The descent of the testes is thought to be mediated by testosterone, which is active during this stage of development. After descent of the testes, the inguinal canal closes almost completely. Failure of this canal to close predisposes to the development of an inguinal hernia later in life.

The testes are enclosed in a double-layered membrane, the *tunica vaginalis*, which is derived embryologically from the abdominal peritoneum (Fig. 48–1). An outer covering, the *tunica albuginea*, is a tough, white, fibrous sheath that resembles the sclera of the eye. The tunica albuginea protects the testes and gives them their ovoid shape. The cremaster muscles, which are bands of skeletal muscle arising from the internal oblique muscles of the trunk, elevate the testes. The testes receive their arterial blood supply from the long testicular arteries, which branch from the aortic artery. The testicular veins, which drain the testes, arise from a venous network called the *pampiniform plexus* that surrounds the testicular artery. The testes are innervated by fibers from both divisions of the autonomic nervous system. Associated sensory nerves transmit pain impulses, resulting in excruciating pain, especially when the testes are hit forcibly.

The scrotum, which houses the testes, is made up of a thin outer layer of skin that forms rugae, or folds, and is continuous with the perineum and outer skin of the groin. Under the outer skin lies a thin layer of fascia and smooth muscle (*i.e.*, dartos muscle). This layer contains a septum that separates the two testes. The dartos muscle responds to changes in temperature. When it is cold, the muscle contracts, bringing the testes closer to the body, and the scrotum becomes shorter and heavily wrinkled. When it is warmer, the muscle relaxes, allowing the scrotum to fall away from the body.

The location of the testes in the scrotum is important for sperm production, which is optimal at 2°C to 3°C below body temperature. Two systems maintain the temperature of the testes at a level consistent with sperm production. One is the pampiniform plexus of testicular veins that surround the testicular artery. This plexus absorbs heat from the arterial blood, cooling it as it enters the testes. The other is the cremaster muscles, which respond to decreases in testicular temperature by moving the testes closer to the body. Prolonged exposure to elevated temperatures, as a result of prolonged fever or the dysfunction of thermoregulatory mechanisms, can impair spermatogenesis. Some tight-fitting undergarments hold the testes against the body and are thought to contribute to a decrease in sperm counts and infertility by interfering with the thermoregulatory function of the scrotum. Cryptorchidism, the failure of the testes to descend into the scrotum, also exposes the testes to the higher temperature of the body.

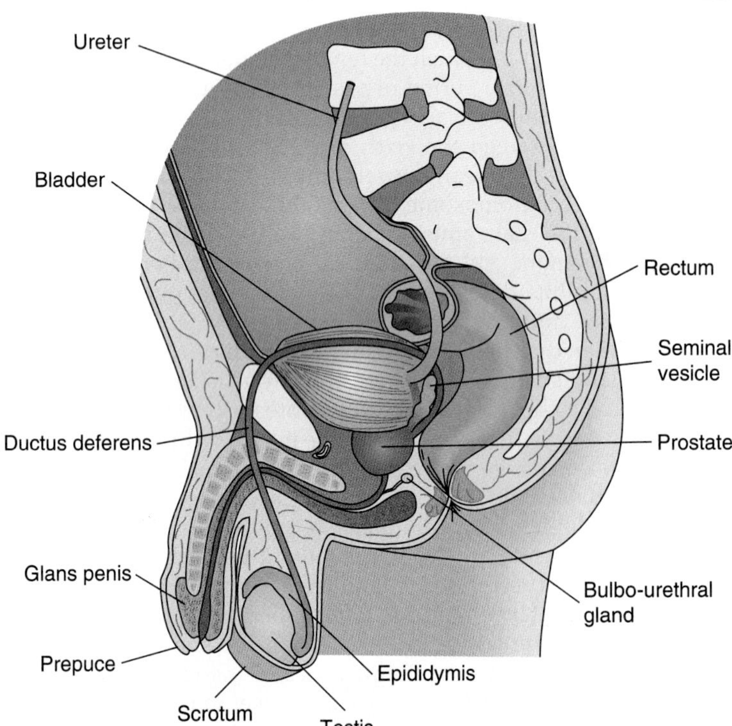

Figure 48–1 The structures of the male reproductive system, including the testes, the scrotum, and the excretory ducts.

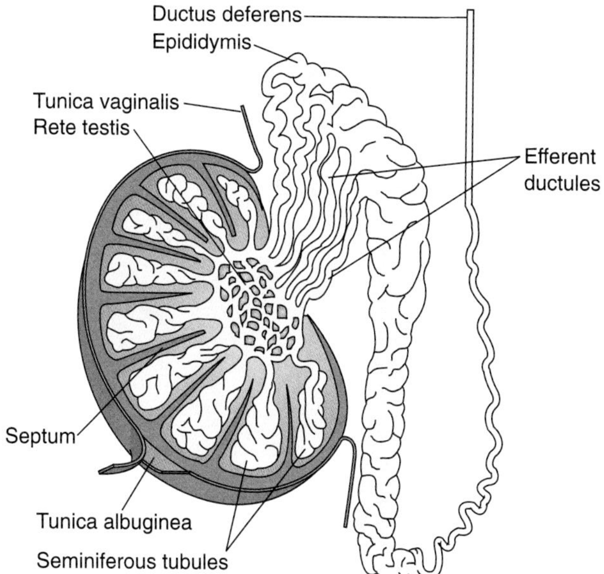

Figure 48–2
The parts of the testes and epididymis.

Genital Duct System

Internally, the testes are composed of several hundred compartments or lobules (Fig. 48–2). Each lobule contains one or more coiled *seminiferous tubules.* These tubules are the site of sperm production. As the tubules lead into the *efferent ducts,* the seminiferous tubules become the *rete testis.* From the rete testis, 10,000 to 20,000 efferent ducts emerge to join the *epididymis,* which is the final site for sperm maturation. Because the spermatozoa are not motile at this stage of development, peristaltic movements of the ductal walls of the epididymis aid in their movement. The spermatozoa continue their migration through the ductus deferens, also called the *vas deferens.* The *ampulla* of the vas deferens serves as a storage reservoir for sperm. Sperm are stored in the ampulla until they are released through the penis during ejaculation (Fig. 48–3). Spermatozoa can be stored in the genital ducts for as long as 42 days and still maintain their fertility. Surgical disconnection of the vas deferens in the scrotal area (*e.g.,* vasectomy) serves as an effective method of male contraception. Because sperm are stored in the ampulla, men can remain fertile for 4 to 5 weeks after performance of a vasectomy.

Accessory Organs

The male accessory organs consist of the seminal vesicles, the prostate gland, and the bulbourethral glands. Spermatozoa are transported through the reproductive structures by movement of the seminal fluid, which is combined with secretions from the genital ducts and accessory organs. The spermatozoa plus the secretions from the genital ducts and accessory organs make up the *semen* (from the Latin word meaning seed).

The *seminal vesicles* consist of two highly tortuous tubes that secrete fluid for the semen. Each of the paired seminal vesicles is lined with secretory epithelium containing an abundance of fructose, prostaglandins, and several other proteins. The fructose secreted by the seminal vesicles provides the energy for sperm motility. The prostaglandins are thought to assist in fertilization by making the cervical mucus more receptive to sperm and by causing reverse peristaltic contractions in the uterus and fallopian tubes to move the sperm toward the ovaries.

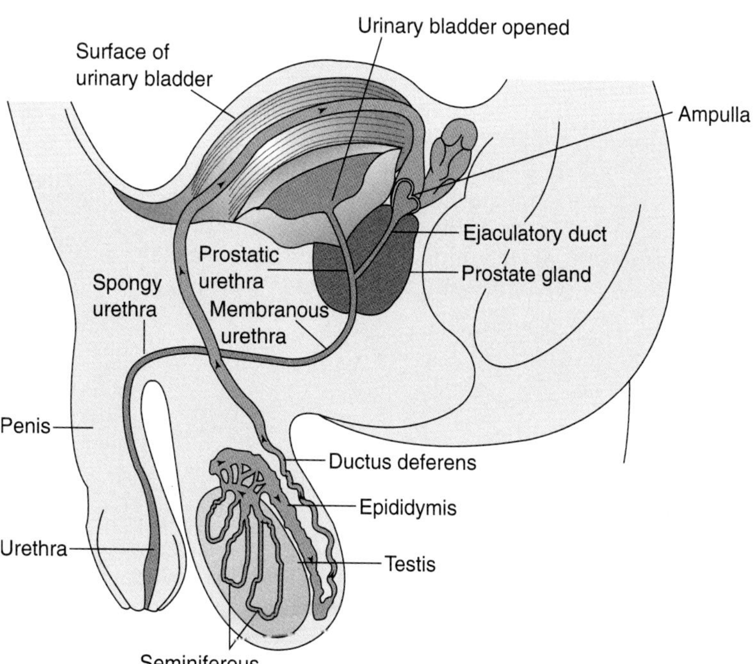

Figure 48–3
The excretory ducts of the male reproductive system and the path that sperm follows as it leaves the testis and travels to the urethra.

Each seminal vesicle joins its corresponding vas deferens to form the ejaculatory duct, which enters the posterior part of the prostate and continues through until it ends in the prostatic portion of the urethra. During the emission phase of coitus, each vesicle empties fluid into the ejaculatory duct, adding bulk to the semen. About 70% of the ejaculate originates in the seminal vesicles.

The prostate is a fibromuscular and glandular organ lying just inferior to the bladder. The prostate gland secretes a thin, milky, alkaline fluid containing citric acid, calcium, acid phosphate, a clotting enzyme, and a profibrinolysin. During ejaculation, the capsule of the prostate contracts, and the added fluid increases the bulk of the semen. Both vaginal secretions and the fluid from the vas deferens are strongly acidic. Because sperm mobilization occurs at a pH of 6.0 to 6.5, the alkaline nature of the prostatic secretions is essential for successful fertilization of the ovum. The bulbourethral or Cowper's glands lie on either side of the membranous urethra and secrete an alkaline mucus, which further aids in neutralizing acids from the urine that remain in the urethra.

The prostate gland also functions in the elimination of urine and consists of a thin, fibrous capsule that encloses the circularly oriented smooth muscle fibers and collagenous tissue that surround the urethra where it joins the bladder. The segment of urethra that traverses the prostate gland is called the *prostatic urethra*. It is lined by a thin, longitudinal layer of smooth muscle that is continuous with the bladder wall. The smooth muscle incorporated with the prostate gland is derived primarily from the longitudinal bladder musculature. This smooth muscle represents the true involuntary sphincter of the posterior urethra in the male. Because the prostate surrounds the urethra, enlargement of the gland can produce urinary obstruction.

The prostate gland is made up of many secretory glands arranged in three concentric areas surrounding the prostatic urethra into which they open. The component glands of the prostate include the small mucosal glands associated with the urethral mucosa, the intermediate submucosal glands that lie peripheral to the mucosal glands, and the large main prostatic glands that are situated toward the outside of the gland. It is the overgrowth of the mucosal glands that causes benign prostatic hypertrophy in older men (see Chapter 49).

Penis

The penis is the external genital organ through which the urethra passes. Anatomically, the external penis consists of a shaft that ends in a tip called the *glans* (Fig. 48–4). The loose skin of the penis shaft folds to cover the glans, forming the *prepuce*, or *foreskin*. The glans of the penis contains many sensory nerves, making this the most sensitive portion of the penile shaft. It is the foreskin that is removed during circumcision.

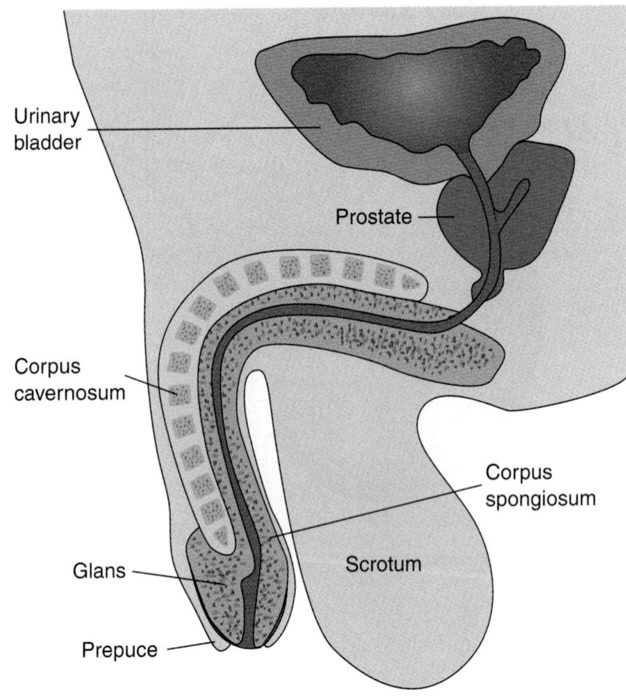

Figure 48–4
Sagittal section of the penis, showing the prepuce, glans, corpus cavernosum, and corpus spongiosum.

The cylindrical body or shaft of the penis is composed of three masses of erectile tissue held together by fibrous strands and covered with a thin layer of skin. The two lateral masses of tissue are called the *corpora cavernosa*. The third ventral mass is called the *corpus spongiosum*. The corpora cavernosa and corpus spongiosum are cavernous sinuses that are normally relatively empty but become engorged with blood during penile erection.

In summary, the male reproductive system consists of a pair of gonads (*i.e.*, testes), a system of excretory ducts (*i.e.*, seminiferous tubules and efferent ducts), the accessory organs (*i.e.*, epididymis, seminal vesicles, prostate, and Cowper's glands), and the penis. The sex of a person is determined by the sex chromosomes at the time of fertilization. During the seventh week of gestation, the XY chromosome pattern in the male is responsible for the development of the testes, with the subsequent production of testosterone and testosterone-stimulated development of the internal and external male genital structures. Before this period of embryonic development, the tissues from which the reproductive structures of the male and female develop are undifferentiated. In the absence of testosterone production, the male embryo with an XY chromosomal pattern develops female genitalia.

Spermatogenesis and Hormonal Control of Male Reproductive Function

After you have completed this section of the chapter, you should be able to meet the following objectives:

- Describe the process of spermatogenesis
- State the functions of testosterone
- Draw a diagram illustrating the secretion, site of action, and feedback control of gonadotropin-releasing hormone, luteinizing hormone, and follicle-stimulating hormone
- Describe the function of follicle-stimulating hormone in terms of spermatogenesis

During childhood, the gonads remain essentially quiescent. At puberty, the male gonads and testes begin to mature and to carry out spermatogenesis and hormone production. Around the age of 10 or 11 years, the adenohypophysis, or anterior pituitary, under the control of the hypothalamus begins to secrete the gonadotropins that stimulate testicular function and cause the interstitial cells of Leydig to begin producing testosterone. About the same time, hormonal stimulation induces mitotic activity of the germ cells that develop in sperm. After cell maturation has begun, the testes begin to enlarge rapidly as the individual tubules grow. Full maturity and spermatogenesis are usually attained by age 15 or 16.

Spermatogenesis

Spermatogenesis refers to the generation of spermatozoa or sperm. It begins at an average age of 13 and continues throughout the reproductive years of a man's life. Spermatogenesis occurs in the seminiferous tubules of the testes. These tubules, if placed end to end, would measure about 750 feet. The outer layer of the seminiferous tubules are made up of connective tissue and smooth muscle; the inner lining is composed of Sertoli's cells, which are embedded with sperm in various stages of development. Sertoli's cells secrete a special fluid that contains nutrients to bathe and nourish the immature germ cells; they provide digestive enzymes that play a role in spermiation (*i.e.*, converting the spermatocytes to sperm); and they are thought to play a role in shaping the head and tail of the sperm. Sertoli's cells also secrete several hormones, including müllerian inhibitory factor, which is secreted by the testes during fetal life to inhibit development of fallopian tubes; estradiol, the principal feminizing sex hormone, which seems to be required in the male for spermatogenesis; and inhibin, which controls the function of Sertoli's cells through feedback inhibition of FSH from the anterior pituitary gland.

In the first stage of spermatogenesis, small and unspecialized diploid germinal cells located immediately adjacent to the tubular wall, called the *spermatogonia*, undergo rapid mitotic division and provide a continuous source of new germinal cells. As these cells multiply, the more mature spermatogonia divide into two daughter cells, which grow in size and become the *primary spermatocytes*—the precursors of sperm. Over several weeks, large primary spermatocytes divide by a process called *meiosis* to form two smaller secondary spermatocytes. Each of the secondary spermatocytes divides to form two *spermatids*, each containing 23 chromosomes. Meiosis is a unique form of cell division that occurs only in the gonads. It consists of two consecutive nuclear divisions with formation of four daughter cells, each containing a single set of 23 chromosomes rather than a pair of 46 chromosomes, as occurs during mitotic cell division in other body cells (see Chapter 3).

The spermatid elongates into a *spermatozoon*, or mature *sperm* cell, with a head and tail (Fig. 48–5). The outside of the anterior two thirds of the head, called the *acrosome*, contains enzymes necessary for penetration and fertilization of the ovum. The to-and-fro flagellar motion of the tail provides movement for the sperm. The energy for this process is supplied by the mitochondria in the tail. Normal sperm move in a straight line at a velocity of 1 mm to 4 mm per minute. This allows them

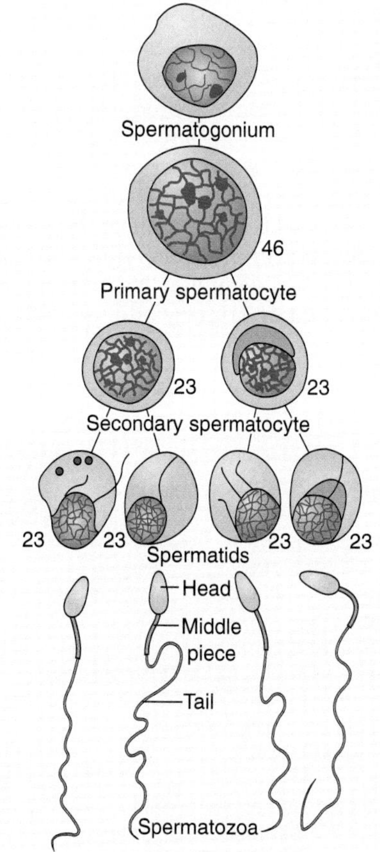

Figure 48–5
The various stages of spermatogenesis.

to move through the female genital tract. When the sperm grow to full size, they move to the epididymis to further mature and gain mobility. A small quantity of sperm can be stored in the epididymis, but most are stored in the vas deferens or the ampulla of the vas deferens. With excessive sexual activity, storage may be no longer than a few days. The sperm can live for many weeks in the male genital tract; however, in the female genital tract, their life expectancy is 1 or 2 days. Frozen sperm have been preserved for years.

The entire process of spermatogenesis takes about 60 to 70 days. The sperm count in a normal ejaculate is about 100 million to 400 million. Infertility may occur when insufficient numbers of motile, healthy sperm are present.

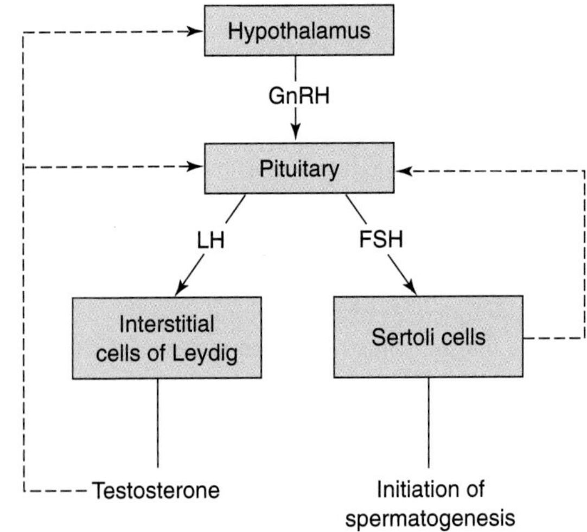

Figure 48–6
Hypothalamic-pituitary feedback control of spermatogenesis and testosterone levels in the male.

Hormonal Control of Male Reproductive Function

The male sex hormones are called androgens. Testosterone is the main androgen produced in the testes. The adrenal cortex also produces androgens, although in much smaller quantities than in the testes. More than 95% of the testosterone is secreted by the testes; the remainder is secreted by the adrenals.

Testosterone is secreted by the interstitial Leydig's cells in the testes. It is metabolized in the liver and excreted by the kidneys. In the bloodstream, testosterone exists in a free or a bound form. The bound form is attached to plasma proteins, including albumin and the sex-hormone–binding protein produced by the liver. Only about 2% of circulating testosterone is unbound and therefore able to enter the cell and exert its metabolic effects.

Testosterone exerts a variety of biologic effects in the male (Chart 48–1). In the male embryo, testosterone is essential for the appropriate differentiation of the internal and external genitalia. Testosterone is essential to the development of primary and secondary male sex characteristics during puberty and for the maintenance of these characteristics during adult life. Androgens function as anabolic agents in males and females to promote metabolism and musculoskeletal growth.

The hypothalamus and the anterior pituitary gland play an essential role in promoting spermatogenic activity in the testes and maintaining the endocrine function of the testes by means of the gonadotropic hormones. The synthesis and release of the gonadotropic hormones from the pituitary gland are regulated by the gonadotropin-releasing factor, which is synthesized by the hypothalamus and secreted into the hypothalamo-hypophysial portal circulation (Fig. 48–6).

Two gonadotropic hormones are secreted by the pituitary gland: follicle-stimulating hormone (FSH) and luteinizing hormone (LH). In the male, LH is also called interstitial cell-stimulating hormone (ICSH). The production of testosterone by the interstitial cells of Leydig is regulated by LH (see Fig. 48–6).

FSH binds selectively to the Sertoli's cells surrounding the seminiferous tubules, where it functions in the initiation of spermatogenesis. Under the influence of FSH, the Sertoli's cells produce androgen-binding protein, plasminogen activator, and inhibin. Androgen-binding protein binds testosterone and serves as a carrier of testosterone in the Sertoli's cells and as a storage site for testosterone. Although FSH is necessary for the initiation of spermatogenesis, full maturation of the spermatozoa requires testosterone. Androgen-binding protein also serves as a carrier of testosterone from the testes to the epididymis. Plasminogen activator, which converts plasminogen to plasmin, functions in the final detachment of mature spermatozoa from the Sertoli's cells.

CHART **48-1**
Main Actions of Testosterone

Induces differentiation of the male genital tract during fetal development
Induces development of primary and secondary sex characteristics
- Gonadal function
- External genitalia and accessory organs
- Male voice timbre
- Male skin characteristics
- Male hair distribution

Anabolic effects
- Promotes protein metabolism
- Promotes musculoskeletal growth
- Influences subcutaneous fat distribution

Promotes spermatogenesis (in FSH-primed tubules) and maturation of sperm

Circulating levels of the gonadotropic hormones are regulated in a negative feedback manner by testosterone. High levels of testosterone suppress LH secretion through a direct action on the pituitary and an inhibitory effect on the hypothalamus. FSH is thought to be inhibited by a substance called *inhibin*, produced by Sertoli's cells. Inhibin suppresses FSH release from the pituitary gland. The pituitary gonadotrophic hormones and the Sertoli's cells in the testes form a classic negative feedback loop in which FSH stimulates inhibin and inhibin suppresses FSH. Unlike the cyclic hormonal pattern in the female, in the male, FSH, LH, and testosterone secretion and spermatogenesis occur at relatively unchanging rates during adulthood.

In summary, the function of the male reproductive system is under the negative feedback control of the hypothalamus and the anterior pituitary gonadotropic hormones FSH and LH. Spermatogenesis is initiated by FSH, and the production of testosterone is regulated by LH. Testosterone, the major sex hormone in the male, is produced by the interstitial Leydig's cells in the testes. In addition to the differentiation of the internal and external genitalia in the male embryo, testosterone is essential for the development of secondary male characteristics during puberty, the maintenance of these characteristics during adult life, and spermatozoa maturation.

Neural Control of Sexual Function and Aging Changes

After you have completed this section of the chapter, you should be able to meet the following objectives:

- Describe the autonomic nervous system control of erection, emission, and ejaculation
- Describe changes in the male reproductive system that occur with aging

In the male, the stages of the sexual act involve erection, emission, ejaculation, and detumescence. The physiology of the sexual act involves a complex interaction between spinal cord reflexes, higher neural centers, the vascular system, and the endocrine system.

Neural Control

The most important source of impulse stimulation for initiating the male sexual act is the glans penis, which contains a highly organized sensory system. Afferent impulses from sensory receptors in the glans penis pass through the pudendal nerve to ascending fibers in the spinal cord by way of the sacral plexus. Stimulation of other perineal areas, such as the anal epithelium, the scrotum, and the testes, can transmit signals to higher brain centers, such as the limbic system and cerebral cortex, through the cord, adding to sexual satisfaction.

The psychic element to sexual stimulation, such as thinking sexual thoughts, can cause erection and ejaculation. Although psychic involvement and higher-center functions contribute to the sex act, they are not necessary for sexual performance. Genital stimulation can produce erection and ejaculation in some men with complete transection of the spinal cord (see Chapter 39).

Erection involves the shunting of blood into the corpus cavernosum. It is controlled by the sympathetic, parasympathetic, and nonsympathetic-nonparasympathetic systems. Nitric oxide is the locally released nonsympathetic-nonparasympathetic mediator that produces relaxation of vascular smooth muscle. In the flaccid or detumescent state, sympathetic discharge through α-adrenergic receptors maintains contraction of the arteries that supply the penis and vascular sinuses of the corpus cavernosa and corpus spongiosum (Fig. 48–7). Parasympathetic stimulation produces erection by inhibiting sympathetic neurons that cause detumescence and by stimulating the release of nitric oxide to effect a rapid relaxation of the penile blood vessels. During sexual stimulation, parasympathetic impulses also cause the urethral and bulbourethral glands to secrete mucous to aid in lubrication. Parasympathetic innervation is effected through the pelvic nerve and sacral segments of the spinal cord. Sympathetic innervation exits the spinal cord at the L1 and L2 levels.

Erectile dysfunction can be caused by disease or dysfunction of the brain, spinal cord, cavernous or pudendal nerves, terminal nerve endings or receptors. Table 48–1 lists the levels of neural dysfunction and the effects on erectile function. Intracavernous injection of papaverine (a vasodilator), phentolamine (an α-adrenergic blocking drug), or alprostadil (a prostaglandin E_1) can be used to achieve erection in men who are impotent.

Emission and ejaculation, which constitute the culmination of the male sexual act, are a function of the sympathetic nervous system. As with erection,

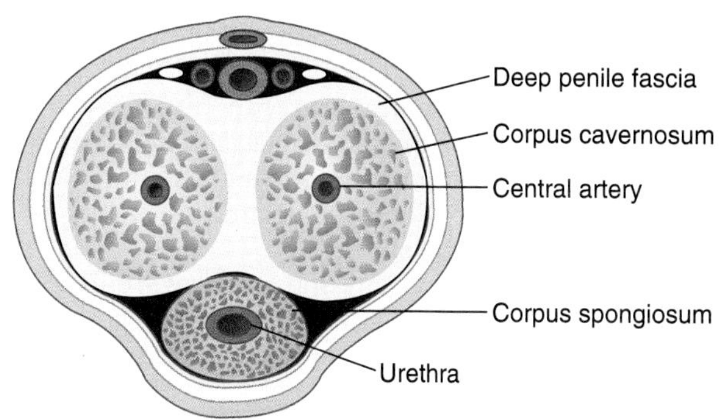

Figure 48–7
Erectile tissue of the penis.

TABLE 48-1

Neurologic Causes of Erectile Dysfunction

Level of Neurologic Disorder	Erectile Dysfunction
Brain disorders (*e.g.*, brain tumor, stroke, Parkinson's disease, Alzheimer's disease)	Increased central inhibition; disinterest
Spinal cord injury	
Upper motoneuron lesion	Often retain ability for reflexogenic erectile function if sacral cord segments are preserved
Lower motoneuron lesion	Often results in loss of cord reflexes that control erection
Pudendal nerve (*e.g.*, trauma, radical prostatic or rectal surgery)	Loss of erectile function due to nerve damage
Peripheral neuropathies (*e.g.*, diabetes, chronic alcoholism)	Affects peripheral nerves and nerve endings and results in deficiency of transmitter release

emission and ejaculation are mediated through spinal cord reflexes. With increasing intensity of the sexual stimulus, reflex centers of the spinal cord begin to emit sympathetic impulses that leave the cord at the L1 and L2 level and pass through the hypogastric plexus to the genital organs to initiate emission, which is the forerunner of ejaculation. Emission causes the sperm to move from the epididymis to the urethra. Efferent impulses from the spinal cord produce contraction of smooth muscle in the vas deferens and ampulla that move sperm forward and close the internal urethral sphincter to prevent retrograde ejaculation into the bladder.

Ejaculation represents the expulsion of the sperm from the urethra. It involves contraction of the seminal vesicles and prostate gland, which add fluid to the ejaculate and propel it forward. Ejaculation is accompanied by contraction of the ischiocavernous and bulbocavernous muscles at the base of the penis. The filling of the internal urethra elicits signals that are transmitted through the pudendal nerves from the spinal cord, giving the sudden feeling of fullness of genital organs. Rhythmic increases in pressure in the urethra cause the semen to be propelled to the exterior, resulting in ejaculation. At the same time, rhythmic contractions of the pelvic and trunk muscles produce thrusting movements of the pelvis and penis, which help propel the ejaculate into the vagina.

The period of emission and ejaculation is called *male orgasm*. After ejaculation, erection ceases within 1 to 2 minutes. A man usually ejaculates about 2 to 5 ml of semen. The ejaculate may vary with frequency of intercourse. It is less with frequent ejaculation and may increase two to four times its normal amount during periods of abstinence. The semen that is ejaculated is 98% fluid and about 2% sperm.

The role of circulating androgens in regard to sexual function remains unclear. It is apparent that sexual desire and performance depend on some threshold level of testosterone; however, this level varies from man to man. Studies of hypogonadal and castrated males show a variety of sexual behavior ranging from complete loss of libido to normal sexual activity. It may be that the role of testosterone in male sexuality is in the area of sexual interest and motivation, with individual intrapsychic factors playing a significant role.

Aging Changes

Like other body systems, the male reproductive system undergoes degenerative changes as a result of the aging process; it becomes less efficient with age. The declining physiologic efficiency of male reproductive function occurs gradually and involves the endocrine, circulatory, and neuromuscular systems. Compared with the marked physiologic change in aging females, the changes in the aging male are more gradual and less drastic. Gonadal and reproductive failure are not generally related directly to age, because a male remains fertile into advanced age; 80- and 90-year-old men have been known to father children. Contrary to popular belief, many investigators consider that there is no physiologic basis for what has been called the male climacteric; instead, they attribute it to psychologic mechanisms. An aging man may experience midlife crisis with concomitant psychosomatic manifestations that mimic the symptomatology of menopause. Most experts agree that decline in male sexual desire parallels decline in physical vigor and represents the aging of all the body tissues and neural structures.

As the male ages, his reproductive system differs measurably in structure and function from that of the younger male. Male sex hormone levels, particularly of testosterone, decrease with age, with the decline starting later on the average than in women. The sex hormones play a part in the structure and function of the reproductive system and other body systems from conception to old age; they affect protein synthesis, salt and water balance, bone growth, and cardiovascular function. Decreasing levels of testosterone affect sexual energy, muscle strength, and the genital tissues. The testes become smaller and lose their firmness. The seminiferous tubules, which produce spermatozoa, thicken and begin a degenerative process that finally inhibits sperm production, resulting in a decrease of viable spermatozoa.[9] The prostate gland enlarges, and its contractions become weaker. The force of ejaculation decreases because of a reduction in the volume and viscosity of the seminal fluid. The seminal vesicle changes little from childhood to puberty. The pubertal increases in the fluid capacity of the gland remain throughout adulthood and decline after age 60. After age 60, the walls of the seminal vesicles thin, the epithelium decreases in height, and the muscle layer is replaced by connective tissue. Age-related changes in the penis consist of fibrotic changes in the trabeculae in the corpus spongiosum, with progressive sclerotic changes in arteries and veins. Sclerotic changes also follow in the corpora cavernosa, with the condition becoming generalized in 55- to 60-year-old men.

As a sexual partner, the aging male exhibits some differences in responsiveness and activity from his younger counterpart. Masters and Johnson studied the significant aging changes in the physiology of the sex act.[11] They observed that frequency of intercourse, intensity of sensation, speed of attaining erection, and force of ejaculation are all reduced.

Many social and cultural practices do not support or encourage sexual activity in the elderly. Research, however, indicates that sexual thought and feeling continue into old age and that sexual activity continues for most healthy older persons. Most gerontologists agree that continued sexual interest and activity can be therapeutic for the elderly.

Sexual dysfunction in the elderly male is often directly related to the general physical condition of the person. Diseases that accompany aging can have direct bearing on male reproductive organs. Various cardiovascular, respiratory, hormonal, neurologic, and hematologic disorders can be responsible for secondary impotence. For example, vascular disease affects male potency because it may impair blood flow to the pudendal arteries or their tributaries, resulting in loss of blood volume with subsequent poor distention of the vascular spaces of erectile tissue. Other diseases affecting potency include hypertension, diabetes, cardiac disease, and malignancies of the reproductive organs.

One of the greatest inhibitors of sexual functioning in older men is the loss of self-esteem and the development of a negative self-image. The emphasis on youth pervades much of our society. The image of success for a man often involves qualities of masculinity and sexual attractiveness. When queried about success, men often mention such things as work, managing money well, participating in sports or other activities, discussing politics or world events, advising younger persons, and being attractive to women. When a man feels good about himself and expresses self-confidence, sexual attractiveness is communicated regardless of age. Many older men live in environments that are not sensitive to the importance of helping them maintain a positive self-image. Premature cessation of the aforementioned esteem-building activities can contribute to loss of libido and zest for life in the elderly man.

In summary, the sex act involves erection, emission, ejaculation, and detumescence. The physiology of these functions involves a complex interaction between autonomic-mediated spinal cord reflexes, higher neural centers, and the vascular system. Erection is mediated by the parasympathetic nervous system and emission and ejaculation by the sympathetic nervous system. Like other body systems, the male reproductive system undergoes changes as a result of the aging process. The changes occur gradually and involve parallel changes in endocrine, circulatory, and neuromuscular function. Testosterone levels decrease, the size and firmness of the testes decrease, sperm production declines, and the prostate gland enlarges. There is usually a decrease in frequency of intercourse, intensity of sensation, speed of attaining erection, and force of ejaculation. However, sexual thought, interest, and activity usually continue into old age.

BIBLIOGRAPHY

Aboseif S.R. (1988). Hemodynamics of penile erection. *Urologic Clinics of North America* 15, 1.

Blackmore C. (1988). The impact of orchiectomy on the sexuality of the man with testicular cancer. *Cancer Nursing* 11, 33.

Breitiung J.C. (1987). *Caring for the older adult* (pp. 100–111). Philadelphia: W.B. Saunders.

Carnevali D.L., Patrick M. (1986). *Nursing management of the elderly* (pp. 60–61). Philadelphia: J.B. Lippincott.

Croft L.H. (1982). *Physiology of aging* (pp. 47–65). Boston: John Wright.

Fergusson D.M., Lawton J.M., Shannon J.T. (1988). Neonatal circumcision and penile problems: An 8-year longitudinal study. *Pediatrics* 81, 537.

George F.C. (1992). Sexual differentiation. In Griffin J.E., Ojeda S.R. (Eds.). *Textbook of endocrine physiology* (2nd ed., pp. 118–133). New York: Oxford University Press.

Greenspan F.S., Baxter J.D. (1994). *Basic and clinical endocrinology* (pp. 401–403). Norwalk, CT: Appleton & Lange.

Guyton A.C. (1991). *Textbook of medical physiology* (8th ed., pp. 885–893). Philadelphia: W.B. Saunders.

Guyton A.C., Hall J. (1996). *Textbook of medical physiology* (9th ed., pp. 1003–1016). Philadelphia: W.B. Saunders.

Herzog L.W., Alvarez S.R. (1986). The frequency of foreskin problems in uncircumcised children. *American Journal of Diseases of Children* 140, 254.

Lue T.F. (1992). Male sexual dysfunction. In Smith D.R. (Ed.). *General urology* (13th ed., pp. 696–711). Norwalk, CT: Appleton & Lange.

Lue T.F. (1995). Male sexual dysfunction. In Tanagho E.A., McAnnich J.W. (Eds.). *Smith's general urology* (14th ed., pp. 273–292). Norwalk, CT: Appleton & Lange.

Masters W.H., Johnson V. (1970). *Human sexual inadequacy* (pp. 337–338). Boston: Little, Brown.

Merry B.J., Holehan A.M. (1994). Aging of the male reproductive system. In Timinas P.S. (Ed.). *Physiological basis of aging and geriatrics* (2nd ed., 171–178). Boca Raton: CRC Press.

Rhoades R.A., Tanner G.A. (1996). *Medical Physiology* (pp. 737–756). Boston: Little, Brown.

Steinke E.E., Bergen M.B. (1986). Sexuality and aging: A review of the literature from a nursing perspective. *Journal of Gerontological Nursing* 12, 6.

CHAPTER 49

Alterations in Structure and Function of the Male Genitourinary System

Stephanie M. Stewart

The male genitourinary system is subject to structural defects, inflammation, and neoplasms, all of which can affect urine elimination, sexual function, and fertility. This chapter discusses disorders of the penis, the scrotum and testes, and the prostate.

Disorders of the Penis

After you have completed this section of the chapter, you should be able to meet the following objectives:

- State the difference between hypospadias and epispadias
- Cite the significance of phimosis
- Describe the pathology of priapism
- Describe the anatomic changes that occur with Peyronie's disease
- Describe the appearance of balanitis xerotica obliterans
- List the signs of penile cancer

The penis is the external male genitalia through which the urethra passes to the exterior of the body. It is involved in urinary and sexual function. Disorders of the penis include congenital and acquired defects, inflammatory conditions, and neoplasms.

Hypospadias and Epispadias

Hypospadias and epispadias are congenital disorders of the penis resulting from embryologic defects in the development of the urethral groove and penile urethra (Fig. 49–1). In hypospadias, which affects about 1 of 500 male infants, the termination of the urethra is on the ventral surface of the penis.[1] Epispadias, in which the opening of the urethra is on the dorsal surface of the penis, is a less common defect. Both of these abnormalities are often accompanied by other congenital urogenital defects. Testes are undescended in 10% of boys born with hypospadias, and the incidence of chordee (*i.e.*, ventral bowing of the penis) and inguinal hernia is also common. In the newborn with severe hypospadias and undescended testes, the differential diagnosis should consider ambiguous genitalia and masculinization that is seen in females with congenital adrenal hyperplasia. Because many chromosomal aberrations result in ambiguity of the external genitalia, chromosomal studies are often recommended for male infants with hypospadias and cryptorchidism.[1]

Surgery is the treatment of choice for hypospadias and epispadias. Circumcision is avoided because the foreskin is used for surgical repair. Factors that influence the timing of surgical repair include anesthetic risk, penile size, and the psychologic effect of the surgery on the child. In mild cases, the surgery is done for cosmetic

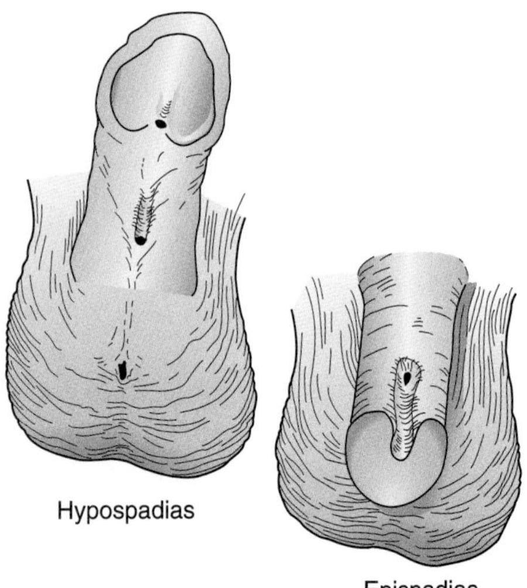

Figure 49–1
Hypospadias and epispadias.

reasons only. In more severe cases, repair becomes essential for normal sexual functioning and to prevent the psychologic sequelae of having malformed genitalia. In contrast to the practices of several decades ago, when surgical repair was often delayed until the child was 2 to 6 years of age, surgical repair is now done between the ages of 6 to 12 months. Some studies of male psychologic adjustment favor repair before the age of 1 year. With advances in surgical techniques, the use of fine suture materials, and advances in anesthesia and pain control, the repair of these conditions results in safe and reliable outcomes. The procedure is usually done on an outpatient basis or during a 24-hour hospital stay.[2]

Phimosis and Paraphimosis

Phimosis refers to a tightening of the penile foreskin that prevents its retraction over the glans. Embryologically, the foreskin begins to develop during the eighth week of gestation as a fold of skin at the distal edge of the penis that eventually grows forward over the base of the glans. By the 16th week of gestation, the prepuce and the glans are adherent. Only a small percentage of newborns have a fully retractable foreskin. With growth, a space develops between the glans and foreskin, and by 3 years of age, about 90% of male children have retractable foreskins.

Because the foreskin of many males cannot be fully retracted in early childhood, it is important that the area be cleaned thoroughly. There is no need to retract the foreskin forcibly, because this could lead to infection, scarring, or paraphimosis. As the child grows, the foreskin becomes retractable, and the glans and foreskin should be cleaned routinely. If symptomatic phimosis occurs after childhood, it can cause difficulty with voiding or sexual activity. Circumcision is then the treatment of choice.[3]

In a related condition called *paraphimosis*, the foreskin is so tight and constricted that it cannot cover the glans. A tight foreskin can constrict the blood supply to the glans and lead to ischemia and necrosis. Many cases of paraphimosis result from the foreskin being retracted for an extended period, as in the case of catheterized uncircumcised males.

Priapism

Priapism is an involuntary prolonged abnormal and painful erection that is not associated with sexual excitement. Priapism is a true urologic emergency, because the presence of priapism for 24 to 48 hours can result in fibrosis of the erectile tissue with significant risk of subsequent impotence. Many men regard priapism with embarrassment rather than alarm and often delay medical treatment.

Priapism is caused by impaired blood flow in the corpora cavernosa of the penis. Two mechanisms for priapism have been proposed: low-flow (ischemic) priapism, in which there is stasis of blood flow in the corpora cavernosa with a resultant failure of detumescence, and high-flow (nonischemic) priapism, which involves persistent arterial flow into the corpora cavernosa. In high-flow priapism, there is no hypoxia of local tissue, the penis is less rigid, and the pain is less than in stasis priapism.

Priapism is classified as primary (idiopathic) or secondary to a disease or drug effect. Primary priapism is the result of conditions such as trauma, infection, and neoplasms. Secondary causes include hematologic conditions such as leukemia, sickle cell disease, and thrombocytopenia; neurologic conditions such as stroke, spinal cord injury, and other central nervous system lesions; and renal failure. Various medications, such as antihypertensive drugs, anticoagulant drugs, antidepressant drugs, alcohol, and marijuana, can contribute to the development of priapism. Currently, intracavernous injection therapy for impotence is one of the more common causes of priapism.

Priapism can occur at any age. It can occur in the newborn and in two other age groups. The first peak is in children between the ages of 5 and 10 years. In this age group, the disorder is most frequently associated with sickle cell disease or neoplasms. The second peak occurs in men between the ages of 20 and 50 years.

The diagnosis of priapism is usually based on clinical findings. Blood gas studies using intracaveranal aspirate may be helpful in differentiating ischemic low-flow priapism from nonischemic high-flow priapism. Corporeal caversonagraphy, Doppler studies of penile blood flow, penile ultrasound, and computed tomography (CT) scans may be used to determine intrapelvic pathology.

Initial treatment measures include analgesics, sedation, and hydration. Urinary retention may necessitate catheterization. Local measures include ice packs and cold saline enemas, aspiration and irrigation of the corpus cavernosum with plain or heparinized saline, or instillation of α-adrenergic drugs. If less aggressive treatment does not produce detumescence, a temporary surgical shunt may be established between the corpus cavernosum and the corpus spongiosum.

The prognosis for whether fibrosis or erectile failure will occur is determined by the severity and duration of blood stasis. In high-flow priapism, the damaging effects of decreased oxygen tension and intracavernal blood pressure are less pronounced than in stasis priapism. Normal erectile potency can be restored even after a long duration of high-flow priapism. Persistent stasis priapism, in contrast, is known to result in impaired erectile function and tissue fibrosis unless resolved within 24 hours of onset.[4]

Peyronie's Disease

Peyronie's disease involves a localized and progressive fibrosis of unknown origin that affects the tunica albuginea (*i.e.*, the tough fibrous sheath that surrounds the corpora cavernosa) of the penis. It is characterized initially by an inflammatory process that results in dense fibrous plaque formation. The plaque is usually on the dorsal midline of the shaft (Fig. 49–2). This plaque may become calcified and bony. The fibrous tissue prevents lengthening of the involved area during erection, making intercourse difficult and painful. There is no pain when the penis is in the nonerect state. The disease usually occurs in middle-aged or elderly men. Although the cause of the disorder is unknown, the dense microscopic plaques are consistent with findings of severe vasculitis.[5]

The erectile dysfunction associated with Peyronie's disease may be caused by the disease or impaired erection. It is often difficult to determine whether it is of arterial, venous, or functional origin. Doppler ultrasound may be used to assess causation of the disorder. Although surgical interventions can be used to correct the disorder, it is often delayed, because in many cases the disorder is self-limiting.[6] Less invasive treatments include injecting hydrocortisone into the fibrous area, administering vitamin E, using ultrasound wave therapy, or administering fibrolytic agents such as potassium para-aminobenzoate.

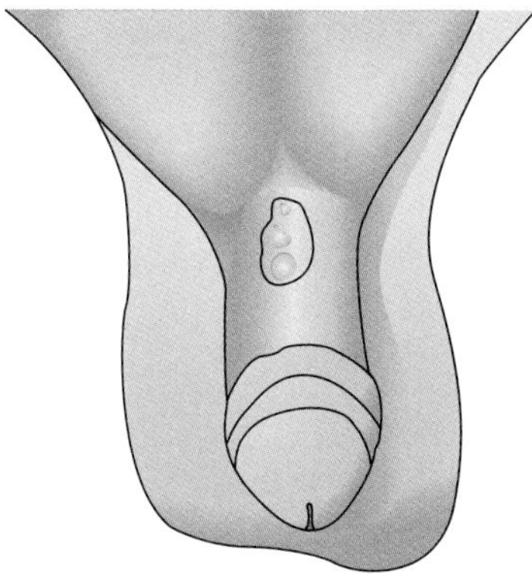

Figure 49–2
In Peyronie's disease, there are palpable, nontender, hard plaques just beneath the skin, usually along the dorsum of the penis.

Balanitis and Balanoposthitis

Balanitis is an acute or chronic inflammation of the glans penis. *Balanoposthitis* refers to inflammation of the glans and prepuce. It is usually encountered in males with phimosis or a large, redundant prepuce that interferes with cleanliness and predisposes to bacterial growth within the accumulated secretions and smegma (*i.e.*, debris from the desquamated epithelia). If left untreated, the condition may cause ulcerations of the mucosal surface of the glans; these ulcerations may lead to inflammatory scarring of the phimosis and further aggravate the condition.

Acute superficial balanoposthitis is characterized by erythema of the glans and prepuce. An exudate in the form of malodorous discharge may be present. Extension of the erythema and edema may result in phimosis. The condition may result from infection, trauma, or irritation. Infective balanoposthitis may be caused by a wide variety of organisms. *Chlamydia* and *Mycoplasma* have been identified as causative organisms in this disease. The inflammatory reaction is nonspecific, and correct identification of the specific agent requires bacterial smears and cultures.

Balanitis xerotica obliterans is a chronic, sclerosing, atrophic process of the glans penis that occurs in uncircumcised males. It is clinically and histologically similar to the lichen sclerosus that is seen in females. Typically, the lesions consist of whitish plaques on the surface of the glans penis and the prepuce. The foreskin is thickened and fibrous and is not retractable. Treatment measures include circumcision and topical or intralesional injections of corticosteroids.[7]

Cancer of the Penis

Squamous cell cancer of the penis is most common in men between 45 and 60 years of age. In the United States, it accounts for less than 1% of male genital tumors; however, in other countries of the world, it accounts for 10% to 20% of male cancers.[8]

The cause of penile cancer is unknown. There is an association between penile cancer and poor genital hygiene and phimosis. This type of cancer is rare in Jewish and Muslim men, who are circumcised routinely. Phimosis is found in about 75% of the males with squamous cell carcinoma of the penis and is the most common abnormality associated with the tumor.[9] Although studies have yielded conflicting results, it has been hypothesized that smegma may serve as a carcinogenic agent. However, there is increasing evidence of a viral role in the development of cancer of the penis; studies have shown that certain types of papillomavirus may be implicated. Ultraviolet radiation may also have a carcinogenic effect on the penis. Males who were treated for psoriasis with ultraviolet A or B therapies (*i.e.*, PUVA or PUVB) have had a reported increased incidence of genital squamous cell carcinomas. Because of this observation, it is suggested that men should shield their genital area when using tanning salons.[9]

The tumor begins as a small lump or ulcer on the penis. If phimosis is present, there may be painful swelling, purulent drainage, or difficulty in urinating. Palpable lymph nodes may be present in the inguinal region. Cavernsonagraphy, CT scans, and magnetic resonance imaging (MRI) may be used in the diagnostic workup.

Penile cancer tends to be slow growing. When it is diagnosed early, it is highly curable. The greatest hindrance to early diagnosis is a delay in seeking medical attention. Treatment options vary according to stage, size, location, and invasiveness of the tumor. Surgery remains the mainstay of treatment. Superficial primary lesions that are freely movable, do not invade the corpora, and show no evidence of metastatic disease can be treated with sleeve resection. Partial or total penectomy is indicated for invasive lesions. About 65% of invasive penile cancers are stage III tumors with lymph node involvement.[9] For these men, bilateral lymph node dissection is indicated.

Cumulative data reveal that males with penile cancer have an overall 5-year survival rate of 65% to 90%. The most important prognostic indicator is the lymph node status. For men with tumor-positive inguinal lymph nodes, the 5-year survival rate is 30% to 50%, and with positive iliac nodes, it is 20%.[10]

In summary, disorders of the penis can be congenital or acquired. Hypospadias and epispadias are congenital defects in which there is malpositioning of the urethral opening: it is located on the ventral surface in hypospadias and on the dorsal surface in epispadias. Phimosis is the condition in which the opening of the foreskin is too tight to permit retraction over the glans. Prolonged, painful, and nonsexual erection that can lead to thrombosis with ischemia and necrosis is called priapism. Peyronie's disease is characterized by the growth of a band of fibrous tissue on top of the penile shaft. Balanitis is an acute or chronic inflammation of the glans penis, and balanoposthitis is an inflammation of the glans and prepuce. Cancer of the penis accounts for less than 1% of male genital cancers in the United States. Although the tumor is slow growing and highly curable when diagnosed early, the greatest hindrance to successful treatment is a delay in seeking medical attention.

Disorders of the Scrotum and Testes

After you have completed this section of the chapter, you should be able to meet the following objectives:

- State the physical manifestations of cryptorchidism
- Describe the potential risks associated with cryptorchidism
- Compare the cause, appearance, and significance of hydrocele, hematocele, spermatocele, and varicocele
- State the difference between extravaginal and intravaginal testicular torsion
- Describe the symptoms of epididymitis
- State the manifestations and possible complications of mumps orchitis
- Relate environmental factors to development of scrotal cancer
- State the cell types involved in seminoma, embryonal carcinoma, teratoma, and choriocarcinoma tumors of the testes

The scrotum is a skin-covered pouch that contains the testes and their accessory organs. Defects of the scrotum and testes include cryptorchidism, disorders of the scrotal sac, vascular disorders, inflammation of the scrotum and testes, and neoplasms.

Cryptorchidism

The testes develop intraabdominally in the fetus and usually descend into the scrotum through the inguinal canal during the seventh to ninth months of gestation. Cryptorchidism, or undescended testes, occurs when one or both of the testicles fail to move down into the scrotal sac. The undescended testes may remain within the lower abdomen or at a point of descent within the inguinal canal (Fig. 49–3). The cause of cryptorchidism is poorly understood. Most cases are idiopathic, but some may result from genetic or hormonal factors.[11] The incidence of cryptorchidism is directly related to birth weight and gestational age; infants who are born prematurely or are small for gestational age have the highest incidence of the disorder. In 75% of term infants and 95% of premature infants born with cryptorchidism, spontaneous testicular descent occurs within the first year of life. Spontaneous descent rarely occurs after the age of 1 year.[1]

In children with cryptorchidism, histologic abnormalities of the testes reflect intrinsic defects in the testi-

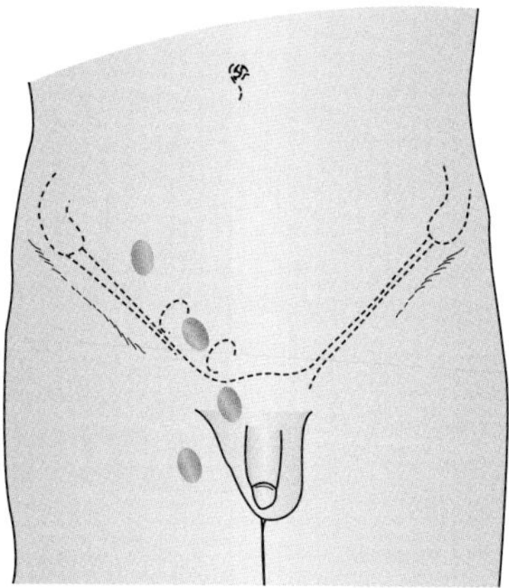

Figure 49–3
Possible locations of undescended testicles.

cle or adverse effects of the extrascrotal environment. These changes begin as early as 2 years of age. There is an arrest of germ cell development and changes in the spermatic tubules. The Leydig cells are not affected. Temperatures in the inguinal canal are 1 to 2 degrees higher than in the scrotum. This increased temperature may damage the undescended testicle. When the disorder is unilateral, it may also produce morphologic changes in the descended testis, possibly reflecting autosensitization through the production of antibodies against spermatozoa, germinal epithelium, or Sertoli's cells. These testicular changes may cause infertility and increase the risk of testicular cancer in later life.

Males with unilateral or bilateral cryptorchidism usually have decreased sperm counts in the undescended testis and the contralateral testis. Spermatogonia counts in males with cryptorchidism never reach the normal counts that are found in males whose testes have descended in the usual manner. Studies have shown abnormalities in the sperm density and hormonal levels of men who underwent orchiopexy (*i.e.*, surgical fixation of the testes in the scrotum) between the ages of 4 and 12 years. The increased risk of testicular cancer is not significantly affected by orchiopexy, hormonal therapy, or late spontaneous descent after the age of 2 years.[12]

The major manifestation of cryptorchidism is the absence of one or more of the testes from the scrotum. The testis is either not palpable or can be felt external to the inguinal ring. The testes are not palpable in 15% to 20% of males with cryptorchidism. Improved techniques for testicular localization include ultrasonography (*i.e.*, visualization of the testes by recording the pulses of ultrasonic waves directed into the tissues), gonadal venography and arteriography (*i.e.*, radiography of the veins and arteries of the testes after the injection of a contrast medium), and laparoscopy (*i.e.*, examination of the interior of the abdomen using a visualization instrument).

Undescended testes due to cryptorchidism should be differentiated from retractable testes that retract into the inguinal canal in response to an exaggerated cremaster muscle reflex. Retractable testes are usually palpable at birth but become nonpapable later. They can be brought down with careful palpation in a warm room. Retractable testes usually assume a scrotal position during puberty. They have none of the complications associated with undescended testicles due to cryptorchidism.[1]

The treatment goals for the male with cryptorchidism include measures to enhance fertility, place the gonad in a favorable place for cancer detection, and improve cosmetic appearance. Regardless of the type of treatment that is employed, it should be carried out before the child is 2 years of age.[1] Treatment modalities for children with unilateral or bilateral cryptorchidism include initial hormone therapy with human chorionic gonadotropin (hCG) or luteinizing hormone–releasing hormone (LHRH), a hypothalamic hormone that stimulates production of the gonadotropic hormones by the anterior pituitary gland. For children who do not respond to hormonal treatment, surgical placement and fixation of the testes in the scrotum (*i.e.*, orchiopexy) have proved effective.

Treatment of males with undescended testis should include lifelong follow-up considering the sequelae of testicular cancer and infertility. Children should be reevaluated 1 year after surgery for testes location and mobility. Parents need to be aware of the potential issues of infertility and increased risk of testicular cancer. On reaching puberty, boys should be instructed in the necessity of testicular self-examination.[13] Some practitioners recommend a postpubertal testicular biopsy for males with a history of cryptorchidism.

Hydrocele

The testes and epididymis are completely surrounded by the tunica vaginalis, a serous pouch derived from the peritoneum during the fetal descent of the testes from the abdomen into the scrotum. The tunica vaginalis has an outer parietal layer and a deeper visceral layer that adheres to the dense fibrous covering of the testes, the tunica albuginea. A space exists between these two layers that typically contains a few milliliters of clear fluid. A hydrocele forms when excess fluid collects within the layers of the tunica vaginalis (Fig. 49–4). It may be unilateral or bilateral and can develop as a primary congenital defect or as a secondary condition. Acute hydrocele may develop after local injury, epididymitis or orchitis, gonorrhea, lymph obstruction, germ cell testicular tumor, or as a side effect of radiation therapy. Chronic hydrocele is more common. Fluid collects about the testis, and the mass grows gradually. Its cause is unknown, and it usually develops in men older than 40 years.

Most cases of hydrocele in male infants and children are caused by a patent processus vaginalis, which is continuous with the peritoneal cavity. It is also a form of indirect inguinal hernia. Most hydroceles of infancy close spontaneously; therefore, they are not repaired before the age of 1 year. If the hydrocele persists

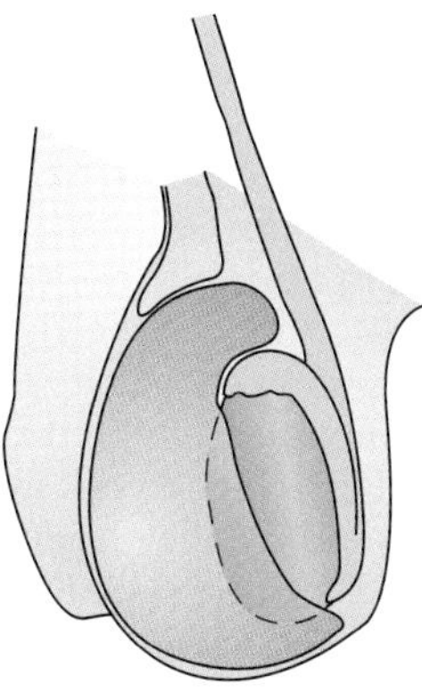

Figure 49–4
Hydrocele.

beyond 18 months of age, surgical treatment is usually indicated.

Hydroceles are palpated as cystic masses that may attain massive proportions. If there is enough fluid, the mass may be mistaken for a solid tumor. Transillumination of the scrotum (*i.e.*, shining a light through the scrotum for the purposes of visualizing its internal structures) or ultrasonography can help to determine whether the mass is solid or cystic and whether the testicle is normal. A dense hydrocele that does not illuminate should be differentiated from a testicular tumor. If a hydrocele develops in a young man without apparent cause, careful evaluation is needed to exclude cancer or infection.

In an adult male, a hydrocele is a relatively benign condition. The condition is often asymptomatic, and no treatment is necessary. When symptoms do occur, the feeling may be that of heaviness in the scrotum or pain in the lower back. In cases of secondary hydrocele, the primary condition is treated. If the hydrocele is painful or cosmetically undesirable, surgical correction is indicated. Surgical repair may be done inguinally or transcrotally.[14]

Hematocele

A hematocele is an accumulation of blood in the tunica vaginalis, which causes the scrotal skin to become dark red or purple. It may develop as a result of an abdominal surgical procedure, scrotal trauma, a bleeding disorder, or a testicular tumor.

Spermatocele

A spermatocele is a painless, sperm-containing cyst that forms at the end of the epididymis. It is located above and posterior to the testis, is attached to the epididymis, and is separate from the testes. Spermatoceles may be solitary or occur in groups and are usually less than 1 cm in diameter. They are freely movable and should transilluminate. Spermatoceles rarely cause problems, but a large one may become painful and require excision.

Varicocele

Varicocele is characterized by varicosities of the pampiniform plexus, a network of veins supplying the testes. The left side is more commonly affected, because the left internal spermatic vein inserts into the left renal vein at a right angle, whereas the right spermatic vein usually enters the inferior vena cava. Incompetent valves are more common in the left internal spermatic veins, causing a reflux of blood back into the veins of the pampiniform plexus. The force of gravity resulting from the upright position also contributes to venous dilatation. If the condition persists, there may be damage to the elastic fibers and hypertrophy of the vein walls, as occurs in formation of varicose veins in the leg.

The presence of a varicocele may be associated with male infertility. The exact mechanism whereby varicocele produces infertility is not understood. One theory suggests that, because a varicocele may be caused by a retrograde flow of blood down the internal spermatic vein, metabolites may be refluxed down the vein, producing adverse effects on sperm production. A second theoretical mechanism involves the effect of heat on the testes. This theory proposes that a varicocele can cause an increase in scrotal temperature, a factor that is thought to impair spermatogenesis. A third theory links epididymal conditions within the epididymis with infertility. Several factors in the epididymis determine motility and maturation of the spermatozoa, including blood supply, tissue androgens, and electrolyte composition. The retrograde flow of blood in the pampiniform plexus could adversely affect environmental conditions in the epididymis and thereby impair the maturation of the spermatozoa, leading to disturbances in motility. There is also the possibility that occult epididymal obstruction accounts for impaired spermatogenesis and infertility. Several of these factors may interact and impair fertility in the presence of varicocele.

Varicoceles are rarely found before puberty, and the incidence is highest in men between 15 and 35 years of age. Symptoms of varicocele include an abnormal feeling of heaviness in the left scrotum, although many varicoceles are asymptomatic. Usually, the varicocele is readily diagnosed on physical examination with the patient in the standing and recumbent positions. Typically, the varicocele disappears in the lying position because of venous decompression into the renal vein. Scrotal palpation of a varicocele has been compared with feeling a "bag of worms." Small varicoceles are sometimes difficult to identify. Valsalva's maneuver (*i.e.*, forced expiration against a closed glottis) may be used to accentuate small varicosities. A hand-held Doppler stethoscope is used while the patient performs Valsalva's maneuver. If the varicocele is present, a distinct venous rush is heard because of the sudden occurrence of retrograde blood flow. Other diagnostic aids include real-time ultrasound, radioisotope scanning, spermatic venography,[15] and scrotopenogram.[16]

Treatment options include surgical ligation or embolization or sclerosing by way of a percutaneous transvenous catheter under fluoroscopic guidance. Both can be performed as outpatient procedures. The benefits of the percutaneous technique include a slightly lower recurrence rate and more rapid return to full physical activity.[15] It has been shown that 40% of men with abnormalities in their semen and a varicocele show some degree of improvement in fertility after obliteration of the dilated veins. Aside from improving fertility, other reasons for surgery include the relief of the sensation of "heaviness" and cosmetic improvement.

Testicular Torsion

Testicular torsion is a twisting of the spermatic cord that suspends the testis (Fig. 49–5). It is the most common acute scrotal disorder in the pediatric and young-adult

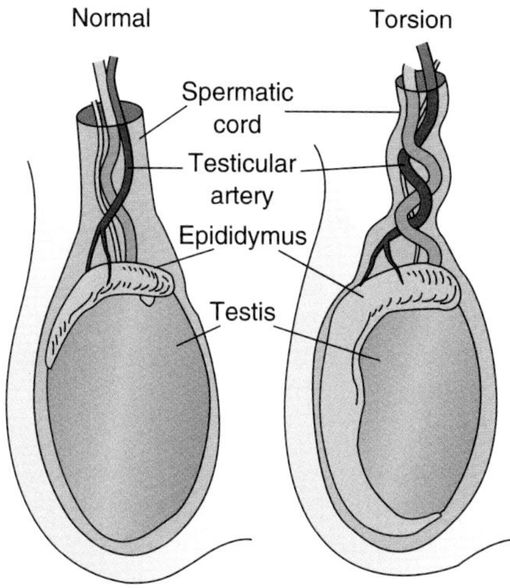

Figure 49–5
Testicular torsion.

population. Testicular torsion can be divided into two distinct clinical entities, depending on the level of spermatic cord involvement: extravaginal and intravaginal torsion.

In *extravaginal torsion,* the less common form of testicular torsion, the testicle and the fascial tunicae that surround it rotate around the spermatic cord at a level well above the tunica vaginalis. Extravaginal torsion occurs almost exclusively in neonates. The torsion probably occurs during fetal or neonatal descent of the testes before the tunica adheres to the scrotal wall. At birth or shortly thereafter, a firm, smooth, painless scrotal mass is identified. The scrotal skin appears red, and some edema is present. Differential diagnosis is relatively easy because testicular tumors, epididymitis, and orchitis are exceedingly rare in neonates; a hydrocele is softer and can be transilluminated, and physical examination can exclude the presence of hernia. Treatment includes elective unilateral surgical exploration and orchiectomy (*i.e.*, removal of the testis).[17]

Intravaginal torsion is considerably more common than extravaginal torsion. It occurs when the testis rotates on the long axis within the tunica vaginalis. In most cases, congenital abnormalities of the tunica vaginalis or spermatic cord exist. The tunica vaginalis normally surrounds the testes and epididymis, allowing the testicle to rotate freely within the tunica. Although anomalies of suspension vary, the epididymal attachment may be loose enough to permit torsion between the testis and the epididymis. More commonly, the testis rotates about the distal spermatic cord. Because this abnormality is developmental, bilateral anomalies are common.

Intravaginal torsion occurs most frequently in males between the ages of 8 and 18 years and is rarely seen after age 30. Males usually present in severe distress within hours of onset and often have nausea, vomiting, and tachycardia. The affected testis is large and tender, with pain radiating to the inguinal area. Extensive cremaster muscle contraction causes a thickening of the spermatic cord.

Testicular torsion must be differentiated from epididymitis, orchitis, and trauma to the testis. On physical examination, the testicle is often high in the scrotum and in an abnormal orientation. These changes are caused by the twisting and shortening of the spermatic cord. The degree of scrotal swelling and redness depends on the duration of symptoms. The testis are firm and tender. The cremasteric reflex, normally elicited by stroking the medial aspect of the thigh and observing testicular retraction, is frequently absent. Urinalysis should be performed, because pyuria indicates an infectious process rather than torsion. A Doppler ultrasound and testicular radionuclide scanning aid in the diagnosis.[18]

Testicular torsion is a true surgical emergency, and early recognition and treatment are necessary if the testicle is to be saved. Treatment includes surgical detorsion and orchiectomy. Orchiectomy is carried out when the testis is deemed nonviable after surgical detorsion. Testicular salvage rates are directly related to the duration of torsion. Studies have shown a more than 80% testicular salvage rate if detorsion is performed in less than 3 hours and a 20% testicular salvage rate if more than 12 hours have elapsed before detorsioning.[17] Because the opposite testicle usually is affected by the same abnormal attachments, prophylactic fixation of that testis should be performed.

Epididymitis

Epididymitis is an inflammation of the epididymis, the elongated cordlike structure that lies along the posterior border of the testis, whose function is the storage, transport, and maturation of spermatozoa. There are two major types of epididymitis: sexually transmitted infections associated with urethritis and primary nonsexually transmitted infections associated with urinary tract infections and prostatitis. Most cases of epididymitis are caused by bacterial pathogens.

In primary nonsexual infections, the pressure associated with voiding or physical strain may force urine containing pathogens from the urethra or prostate up the ejaculatory duct and through the vas deferens and into the epididymis. Infections may also reach the epididymis through the lymphatics of the spermatic cord. In rare cases, organisms from other foci of infection reach the epididymis through the bloodstream. In children, the disorder is usually associated with congenital urinary tract abnormalities and infection with gram-negative rods. Sexually transmitted acute epididymitis occurs mainly in young men without underlying genitourinary disease and is most commonly caused by *Chlamydia trachomatis* and *Neisseria gonorrhoeae* (singly or in combination). In men older than 35 years of age, epididymitis is often associated with pathogens such as *Escherichia coli*, *Pseudomonas*, and gram-positive cocci.

Epididymitis is characterized by unilateral pain and swelling, accompanied by erythema and edema of the overlying scrotal skin that develops over a period of 24 to 48 hours. Initially, the swelling and induration are limited to the epididymis. However, the distinction between the testis and epididymis becomes less evident as the inflammation progresses, and the testis and epididymis become one mass. There may be tenderness over the groin (spermatic cord) or in the lower abdomen. Fever and complaints of dysuria occur in about one half of cases. Whether urethral discharge is present or not depends on the organism causing the infection; it usually accompanies gonorrheal infections, is common in chlamydial infections, and is less common in infections by gram-negative organisms.

Laboratory findings usually reveal an elevated white blood cell count. Urinalysis and urine culture are important in the diagnosis of epididymitis, with bacteriuria and pyuria suggestive of the disorder. The cause of epididymitis can be differentiated by Gram's stain examination or culture of a midstream urine specimen or a urethral specimen.

Treatment during the acute phase (which usually lasts for 3 to 4 days) includes bed rest, scrotal elevation and support, and antibiotics. Bed rest with scrotal support improves lymphatic drainage. The choice of antibiotics is determined by age, physical findings, urinalysis, Gram's stain results, cultures, and sexual history. Oral analgesics and antipyretics are usually indicated. Sexual activity or physical strain may exacerbate the infection and worsen the symptoms and should be avoided.

Orchitis

Orchitis, an infection of the testes, can be precipitated by a primary infection in the genitourinary tract, such as urethritis, cystitis, or seminal vesiculitis. Many infections from other parts of the body spread to the testes through the bloodstream or the lymphatics. Orchitis can develop as a complication of a systemic infection, such as parotitis (*i.e.*, mumps), scarlet fever, or pneumonia. Probably the best known of these complications is orchitis caused by the mumps virus. Mumps orchitis does not occur in prepubertal males. However, about 20% to 35% of adolescent boys and young men with mumps develop this form of orchitis.[19]

The onset of mumps orchitis is sudden; it usually occurs about 3 to 4 days after the onset of the parotitis and is characterized by fever, painful enlargement of the testes, and small hemorrhages into the tunica albuginea. Unlike epididymitis, the urinary symptoms are absent. The symptoms usually run their course in 7 to 10 days. Microscopically, an acute inflammatory response is seen in the seminiferous tubules, with proliferation of neutrophils, lymphocytes, and histiocytes causing distention of the tubules. The residual effects that are seen after the acute phase include hyalinization of the seminiferous tubules and atrophy of the testes. Spermatogenesis is irreversibly damaged in about 30% of testes damaged by mumps orchitis.[19] If both testes are involved, permanent sterility results, but androgenic hormone function is usually maintained.[19]

Neoplasms

Tumors can develop in the scrotum or the testes. Benign scrotal tumors are common and often do not require treatment. Carcinoma of the scrotum is rare and is usually associated with exposure to carcinogenic agents. Almost all solid tumors of the testes are malignant.

Scrotal Cancer

Cancer of the scrotum was the first cancer directly linked to a specific occupation when, in the 1800s, it was associated with chimney sweeps.[20] Studies have linked this cancer to exposure to tar, soot, and oils. Most squamous cell cancers of the scrotum are linked to poor hygiene and chronic inflammation. Exposure to ultraviolet A radiation (*e.g.*, PUVA) or human papillomavirus has also been associated with the disease. Malignant tumors of the scrotum are rare in the United States but are 20 times more common in the United Kingdom. The mean age of presentation with the disease is 60 years; often preceded by 20 to 30 years of chronic irritation.

In the early stages, cancer of the scrotum may appear as a small tumor or wartlike growth that eventually ulcerates. The thin scrotal wall lacks the tissue reactivity needed to block the malignant process; more than one half of the cases seen involve metastasis to the lymph nodes. Because this tumor does not respond well to chemotherapy or irradiation, the treatment includes wide local excision of the tumor with inguinal and femoral node dissection.[21] The prognosis correlates with lymph node involvement.

Testicular Cancer

Approximately 5000 men are diagnosed with testicular cancer each year. This accounts for 1% of all male cancers and 3% of male urogenital cancers. Although relatively rare, it is the most common cause of cancer in the 15- to 35-year-old age group. In the past, testicular cancer was a leading cause of death among males entering their most productive years. However, during the past 20 years, advances in therapy have transformed an almost invariably fatal disease into one that is highly curable. With the exception of men with advanced metastatic disease at the time of presentation or those who relapse after primary chemotherapy, most men with these tumors are cured with available therapy.

Although the cause of testicular cancer is unknown, congenital and acquired factors have been implicated as contributing factors. The strongest association has been with cryptorchid testis. The incidence of testicular cancer is 35 times higher in males with cryptorchid testes.[22] Administration of exogenous estrogen to the mother during pregnancy has been associated with an increased relative risk of testicular tumors of 2.8% to 5.3% over the expected incidence.[10] Other acquired factors such as trauma and infection have also been implicated, although a causal relation has not been established.

Often the first sign of testicular cancer is a slight enlargement of the testicle that may be accompanied by some degree of discomfort. This may be an ache in the abdomen or groin or a sensation of dragging or heaviness in the scrotum. Frank pain may be experienced in the later stages, when the tumor is growing rapidly and hemorrhaging occurs. Testicular cancer can spread when the tumor may be barely palpable.

The prognosis and extent of treatment required for testicular cancer are related to the stage of the disease at the time of presentation. A delay in seeking medical attention is related to increased stage of the disease and decreased treatment effectiveness. Recognition of the importance of prompt diagnosis and treatment has resulted in the development of a procedure for testicular self-examination and an emphasis on public education programs about this type of cancer. The American Cancer Society strongly advocates that every young adult male examines his testes at least once each month as a means of early detection of testicular cancer. The examination should be done after a warm bath or shower, when the scrotal skin is relaxed. To do this self-examination, each testicle is examined with the fingers of both hands by rolling the testicle between the thumb and fingers to check for the presence of any lumps. If any lump, nodule, or enlargement is noted, it should be brought immediately to the attention of a physician.

The diagnosis of testicular cancer requires a thorough urologic history and physical examination. A painless testicular mass may be cancer. Conditions that produce an intrascrotal mass similar to testicular cancer include epididymitis, orchitis, hydrocele, or hematocele. The examination for masses should include palpation of the testes and surrounding structures, transillumination of the scrotum, and abdominal palpation. Testicular ultrasound can be used to differentiate testicular masses. The intravenous pyelogram may be used to evaluate kidney structure. CT scans and MRI are used in assessing metastatic spread.

There are several systems for classification of testicular cancer. The Armed Forces Institute of Pathology (AFIP) classification system divides testicular cancer into germinal (germ cell) tumors arising from the spermatozoa and their derivatives and nongerminal cell tumors arising from other cellular components of the testes.

Germ cell tumors, which constitute about 95% of all testicular tumors, can be divided into two groups: seminomas and nonseminomas.[11] The peak incidence of seminoma occurs in men between 30 and 40 years of age and that of nonseminoma in men between ages 20 and 30 years. Seminomas are thought to arise from the seminiferous epithelium of the testes. They are the most common type of testicular cancer, accounting for approximately 30% of all germ cell tumors.[11]

Nonseminoma germ cell tumors are classified into three histologic types: embryonal carcinoma, teratoma, and choriocarcinoma. Embryonal carcinomas represent about 20% of all germ cell tumors. They are less differentiated and more aggressive than seminomas. Teratomas are derived from totipotential germ cells that have the capacity to differentiate into tissues representing any of the three germ layers of the embryo—ectoderm, mesoderm, or endoderm. They constitute less than 5% of germ cell tumors and can occur at any age from infancy to old age. They usually behave as benign tumors in children; in adults, they often contain minute foci of cancer cells. Choriocarcinoma, a highly malignant form of cancer that is identical to tumors that arise in the placental tissue, accounts for 1% of testicular cancers. Each of these basic histologic types can occur as a pure form or as a combination of cell types. Forty percent of testicular cancers are of mixed tissue types.[10] The most common mixture is teratocarcinoma, which contains embryonal carcinoma and teratoma elements.

The clinical staging (TNM classification) for testicular cancer is as follows: stage I, tumor confined to testes; stage II, tumor spread to retroperitoneal lymph nodes; stage III, distant metastases (see Chapter 5). Staging procedures include CT scans of the chest, abdomen, and pelvis; ultrasonography for detection of bulky inferior nodal metastases; venacavography; and lymphangiography. Radiographic methods are used to detect metastatic spread.

Tumor markers, assayed by radioimmunoassay methods that measure protein antigens produced by malignant cells, provide information about the existence of a tumor and the type of tumor present, and these studies may detect tumors that are too small to be found on physical examination or radiographs. Three tumor markers are useful in evaluating the tumor response: *α-fetoprotein* (AFP), a glycoprotein that is normally present in fetal serum in large amounts; *hCG*, a hormone that is normally produced by the placenta in pregnant women; and *lactate dehydrogenase* (LDH), a cellular enzyme normally found in muscle, liver, kidney, and brain.[10] During embryonic development, the totipotential germ cells of the testes travel down normal differentiation pathways and produce different protein products. The reappearance of these protein markers in the adult suggests activity of the undifferentiated cells in a testicular germ cell tumor.

The basic treatment of all testicular cancers includes orchiectomy, which is done at the time of diagnostic exploration. The widely used surgical procedure is the unilateral radical orchiectomy by way of an inguinal incision. Surgical therapy is advantageous because it enables precise staging of the disease. Recommendations for further therapy (*e.g.*, retroperitoneal dissection, chemotherapy, radiation therapy) are based on the pathologic findings from the surgical procedure.

Seminomas are radiosensitive; the treatment of stage I or II seminoma is irradiation of the retroperitoneal and homolateral lymph nodes to the level of the diaphragm. Patients with bulky retroperitoneal or distant metastases are often treated with multiagent chemotherapy. Seminoma is probably the most curable of all solid tumors. Retroperitoneal lymph node dissection is widely used after orchiectomy to treat stage II and nonseminomatous germ cell tumors. Patients who have extensive retroperitoneal or chest metastasis are best treated with multiagent chemotherapy after orchiectomy.

With appropriate treatment, the prognosis for men with testicular cancer is excellent. The 5-year survival rate for patients with stage I and II disease exceeds 90%. Patients with stage III tumors have an overall survival rate of approximately 70%, with prognosis related to the degree of distant metastases. Even patients with mild or moderate lung metastases have excellent chances for long-term survival.

Therapy for testicular cancer can have potentially adverse effects on sexual functioning. It has been reported that up to 50% of men who had been treated for testicular cancer had some type of sexual dysfunction. Men who have retroperitoneal lymph node dissection may experience retrograde ejaculation or failure to ejaculate because of severing of the sympathetic plexus. A nerve-sparing technique can be used in cases without extensive disease and can preserve seminal emission and fertility in 90% of these men.

In summary, disorders of the scrotum and testes include cryptorchidism (*i.e.*, undescended testicles), hydrocele, hematocele, spermatocele, varicocele, and testicular torsion. Inflammatory conditions can involve the scrotal sac, epididymis, or testes. Tumors can arise in the scrotum or the testes. Scrotal cancers are usually associated with exposure to petroleum products such as tar, pitch, and soot. Testicular cancer accounts for 3% of cancers of the male genitourinary system. With present treatment methods, a large percentage of men with these tumors can be cured. Testicular self-examination is recommended as a means of early detection of this form of cancer.

Disorders of the Prostate

After you have completed this section of the chapter, you should be able to meet the following objectives:

- Compare the pathology and symptoms of acute bacterial prostatitis, chronic bacterial prostatitis, nonbacterial prostatitis, and prostatodynia
- Describe the urologic manifestations of benign prostatic hyperplasia
- List the methods used in the diagnosis and treatment of prostatic cancer

The prostate is a firm glandular structure that surrounds the urethra. It produces a thin, milky, alkaline secretion that aids sperm motility by helping to maintain an optimum pH. The contraction of the smooth muscle in the gland promotes semen expulsion during ejaculation.

Prostatitis

Prostatitis refers to a variety of inflammatory disorders of the prostate gland, some bacterial in nature and some not. It may occur spontaneously, as a result of catheterization or instrumentation, or secondary to other diseases of the male genitourinary system. There are four types of prostatitis: acute bacterial, chronic bacterial, nonbacterial, and prostatodynia.

Acute Bacterial Prostatitis

Acute bacterial prostatitis is relatively rare but dramatic in its presentation. Symptoms include high fever, chills, malaise, myalgia, arthralgia, frequent and urgent urination, dysuria, and urethral discharge. Dull aching pain is present in the perineum, rectum, or sacrococcygeal region. Rectal examination reveals a swollen, tender, warm prostate with scattered soft areas. Prostatic massage produces a thick discharge with white blood cells that grows large numbers of pathogens on culture. These pathogens often include gram-negative enteric bacteria such as *Pseudomonas* and gram-positive staphylococci and streptococci.

Treatment of acute bacterial prostatitis depends on the severity of symptoms. It usually includes bed rest, adequate hydration, antipyretics, analgesics (often narcotics) or spasmolytic drugs to alleviate pain, and stool softeners. Hospitalization may be necessary. A suprapubic catheter may be indicated if voiding is difficult or painful.

Acute prostatitis usually responds to appropriate antimicrobial therapy chosen in accordance with the sensitivity of the causative agents in the urethral discharge. Depending on the urine culture results, antibiotic therapy is usually continued for at least 4 weeks. Because acute prostatitis is often associated with anatomic abnormalities, a thorough urologic examination is usually performed after treatment is completed.

A persistent fever indicates the need for further investigation for an additional site of infection or a prostatic abscess. CT scans and transrectal ultrasound of the prostate are useful in the diagnosis of prostatic abscesses. Prostatic abscesses, which are relatively uncommon since the advent of effective antibiotic therapy, are found more commonly in males with diabetes mellitus. Prostatic abscesses are usually associated with bacteremia; prompt drainage by transperitoneal or transurethral incision followed by appropriate antimicrobial therapy is usually indicated.[19]

Chronic Bacterial Prostatitis

In contrast to acute bacterial prostatitis, chronic bacterial prostatitis is a subtle disorder that is difficult to treat. The symptoms of chronic prostatitis are variable and include frequent and urgent urination, dysuria, perineal discomfort, and low-back pain. Occasionally, myalgia and arthralgia accompany the other symptoms. Secondary epididymitis is sometimes associated with the disorder. Many men suffer relapsing lower or upper urinary tract infections because of recurrent invasion of the bladder by the prostatic bacteria. Bacteria may exist in the prostate gland even when the prostatic fluid is sterile. Organisms responsible for chronic bacterial prostatitis are usually the gram-negative enterobacteria (*E. coli, Proteus mirabilis*, or *Klebsiella pneumoniae*) or *Pseudomonas aeruginosa*. Occasionally, a gram-positive organism such as *Streptococcus faecalis* is the causative organism. Infected prostatic calculi may develop and contribute to the chronic infection.

The most accurate method of establishing a diagnosis is by localizing cultures. It is based on sequential collections of the first part of the voided urine (urethral specimen), midstream specimen (bladder specimen), the expressed prostatic secretion (obtained by prostatic massage), and the urine voided after prostatic massage. The last two specimens are considered prostatic urine. A positive expressed prostatic specimen establishes the diagnosis of bacterial prostatitis, excluding nonbacterial prostatitis and prostatodynia.

Even after an accurate diagnosis has been established, treatment for chronic prostatitis is often difficult and frustrating. Unlike their action in the acutely inflamed prostate, antibacterial drugs penetrate poorly into the chronically inflamed prostate. Long-term therapy (4 to 6 months) with an appropriate low-dose oral antimicrobial agent such as trimethoprim-sulfamethoxazole, carbenicillin indanyl sodium, minocycline, or erythromycin is often used to treat the infection. Transurethral prostatectomy may be indicated when the infection is not cured or adequately controlled by medical therapy, particularly when prostate stones are present.

Nonbacterial Prostatitis

A large group of men with prostatitis suffer from pains along the penis, testicles, and scrotum; painful ejaculation, low-back pain; rectal pain along the inner thighs; urinary symptoms; decreased libido; and impotence, but they have no bacteria in the urinary system. Men with nonbacterial prostatitis often have inflammation of the prostate with an elevated white blood cell count and abnormal inflammatory cells in their prostatic secretions. The cause of the disorder is unknown, and efforts to prove the presence of unusual pathogens (*e.g.*, mycoplasmas, chlamydiae, trichomonads, viruses) have been largely unsuccessful. It is also thought that nonbacterial prostatitis may be an autoimmune disorder. Those affected may be treated with tetracycline, with erythromycin, or if mycosis is present, with an antifungal treatment. Because nonbacterial prostatitis does not usually respond to antibiotic therapy, treatment is often directed toward symptom control. Antiinflammatory agents such as ibuprofen may be used to provide symptom relief.

Prostatodynia

Men with prostatodynia have symptoms resembling those of nonbacterial prostatitis but have negative urine culture results and no evidence of prostatic inflammation (*i.e.*, negative leukocyte count results). The cause of prostatodynia is unknown, but because of the absence of inflammation, the search for the cause of symptoms associated with prostatodynia has been directed toward extraprostatic sources. In some cases, there is an apparent functional obstruction of the bladder neck near the external urethral sphincter; during voiding, this results in higher than normal pressures within the prostatic urethra that cause intraprostatic urine reflux and chemical irritation of the prostate by urine. In other cases, there is an apparent myalgia (*i.e.*, muscle pain) associated with prolonged tension of the pelvic floor muscles. Emotional stress has been implicated in other cases.

Benign Prostatic Hyperplasia

Benign prostatic hyperplasia is an age-related, nonmalignant enlargement of the prostate gland. It is one of the most common diseases of aging men. It has been reported that 51% of men between the ages of 60 and 69 years have clinical evidence of benign prostatic hyperplasia.[23] Benign prostatic hyperplasia is characterized by the formation of large discrete lesions in the periurethral region of the prostate. Although the condition has traditionally been referred to as benign prostatic hypertrophy (BPH), the basic process is one of hyperplasia rather than hypertrophy.

The exact cause of the hyperplasia is unknown. The fact that the condition occurs largely in older men suggests a relation to changes in the hormonal balance associated with aging. Both androgens (testosterone) and estrogens appear to contribute to the process. Dihydrotestosterone, believed to be the biologically active metabolite of testosterone, is thought to be the ultimate mediator of hyperplasia, with estrogen serving to sensitize the prostatic tissue to the growth-producing effects of dihydrotestosterone. Although the exact source is uncertain, small amounts of estrogen are produced in the male. It has been postulated that a relative increase in estrogen levels that occurs with aging may facilitate the action of androgens within the prostate despite a decline in testicular output of testosterone.

The symptoms of benign prostatic hyperplasia are related to the compression of the urethra, with accompanying bladder distention and hypertrophy, urinary tract infection, and renal disease. The typical picture includes outflow obstruction with a decreased caliber and force of the urinary stream. As the obstruction increases, acute retention may occur with overdistention of the bladder. The residual urine in the bladder causes increased frequency of urination and a constant desire to empty the bladder, which becomes worse at night. With marked bladder distention, overflow incontinence may occur with the slightest increase in intraabdominal pressure.

It is now thought that the single most important factor in the evaluation and treatment of BPH is the man's own experiences related to the disorder.[23] The American Urological Society Symptom Index consists of seven questions, each with a score of 0 (mild) to 7 (severe). A maximum score of 35 indicates severe symptoms. Total scores below 7 are considered mild; those between 8 and 20, moderate; and scores over 20, severe.[24]

The clinical significance of benign prostatic hyperplasia resides in its tendency to compress the urethra and cause partial or complete obstruction of urinary outflow. The resulting obstruction to urinary flow can give rise to urinary tract infection, destructive changes of the bladder wall, hydroureter, and hydronephrosis. Hypertrophy and changes in bladder wall structure develop in stages. Initially, the hypertrophied fibers form trabeculations and then herniations, or sacculations; finally, diverticula develop as the herniations extend through the bladder wall (see Fig. 30–4). Because urine is seldom completely emptied from them, these diverticula are readily infected. Back pressure on the ureters and collecting system of the kidneys promotes hydroureter, hydronephrosis, and danger of eventual renal failure.

In 1994, the Agency for Health Care Policy and Research published clinical practice guidelines for management of BPH.[25] These guidelines suggest that the initial evaluation of men for a diagnosis of BPH includes history, physical examination, digital rectal examination, urinalysis, blood tests for serum creatinine and prostate-specific antigen (PSA), and urine flow rate. Blood and urine analyses are used as adjuncts to determine benign prostatic hyperplasia complications. Urinalysis is done to detect bacteria, white blood cells, or microscopic hematuria in the presence of infection and inflammation. The serum creatinine test is used as an estimate of the glomerular filtration rate and renal function. The PSA test is used to screen for prostatic cancer. These evaluation measures along with the symptom index are used to describe the extent of obstruction, determine if other diagnostic tests are needed, and establish the need for treatment.

The digital rectal examination is used to examine the external surface of the prostate. Enlargement of the prostate due to BPH usually produces a large, palpable prostate with smooth rubbery surface. Hardened areas of the prostate gland suggest cancer and should be biopsied. An enlarged prostate found during a rectal examination does not always correlate with the degree of urinary obstruction. Some men can have greatly enlarged prostate glands with no urinary obstruction, but others may have severe symptoms without a palpable enlargement of the prostate. The reason for this variation in symptoms is related to different characteristics of the enlarged prostate. For example, a man may have an enlarged gland that protrudes into the soft surrounding tissue without compressing the urethra, producing no symptoms.

Among the objective signs of benign prostatic hyperplasia are a large residual volume and reduced urine flow rate. The bladder may be seen and palpated as retention of urine increases. Residual urine measurement may be made by ultrasonography or postvoiding catheterization for residual urine volume. Residual urines greater than 100 ml are considered high. Uroflowometry provides an objective measure of urine flow rate. The patient is asked to void with a relatively full bladder (at least 150 ml) into a device that electronically measures the force of the stream and urine flow rate. A urinary flow rate of greater than 14 ml per second is considered normal, and less than 10 ml per second is indicative of obstruction.

In the past, intravenous urography was used extensively for visualization of the urinary tract; however, with new imaging techniques, routine urography is seldom considered necessary. Transabdominal or transrectal diagnostic ultrasound can be used to evaluate the kidneys, ureters, and bladder. Abdominal radiographs may be used to reveal the size of the gland. Urethrocystoscopy is indicated in men with a history of hematuria, stricture disease, urethral injury, or prior lower urinary tract surgery. It is used to evaluate the length and diameter of the urethra, the size and configuration of the prostate, and bladder capacity. It also detects the presence of trabeculations, bladder stones, and small bladder cancers. CT scans, MRI studies, and radionuclide scans are reserved for rare instances of tumor detection.

Treatment of BPH is determined by the degree of symptoms that the condition produces and complications due to obstruction. When a man develops mild symptoms related to BPH, a "watch and wait" stance is often taken by the physician. The condition does not always run a predictable course. It may remain stable or even improve. However, when more severe signs of obstruction develop, treatment is indicated to provide comfort and to avoid serious renal damage.

Until the 1980s, surgery was the mainstay of treatment to alleviate urinary obstruction due to BPH. Currently, there is an emphasis on less invasive methods of treatment, including use of pharmacologic agents, hyperthermia, laser prostatectomy, and prostatic stents.

Pharmacologic management includes use of α-adrenergic blocking drugs and hormonal manipulation. The presence of α-adrenergic receptors in prostatic smooth muscle has prompted the use of α-adrenergic blocking drugs to relieve prostatic obstruction and increase urine flow. Hormonal manipulation involves the use of drugs that block the action of androgens at the prostate cellular level. The prostate normally requires enzymatic conversion of testosterone to dihydrotestosterone. Several drugs can be used for hormonal treatment of BPH. Finasteride is an an antiandrogen that exerts its effect by blocking the enzyme that converts testosterone to dihydrotestosterone. Side effects of the drug, including impotence and decreased libido, are minimal. Flutamide, another antiandrogen drug, blocks action of androgens at the prostate cellular level by binding to nuclear androgen receptors.

The surgical removal of an enlarged prostate can be accomplished by several approaches: transurethral, suprapubic, or perineal. The transurethral prostatectomy (TURP) is the most commonly used technique in the United States. With this approach, an instrument is introduced through the urethra, and prostate tissue removed using a resectoscope and electrocautery. Immediate complications of TURP include the inability to urinate, postoperative hemorrhage or clot retention, and urinary tract infection. Late complications of TURP include impotence, incontinence, and bladder neck contractures. Retrograde ejaculation is another problem that may occur because of resection of bladder neck tissue.

Several alternative procedures for treatment of benign prostatic hyperplasia have been developed. A new surgical approach is the transurethral incision of the prostate (TUIP). This procedure involves making one or two incisions in the bundle of smooth muscle where the prostate gland is attached to the bladder. The gland is split to reduce pressure on the urethra. TUIP is helpful for smaller prostate glands that cause obstruction.

Another alternative to TURP is laser prostatectomy or transurethral ultrasound-guided laser-induced prostatectomy (TULIP). With this procedure, an instrument with a laser source is inserted into the urethra. The laser beam destroys the prostate gland while sparing the surrounding tissue. Laser surgery involves a one-night hospital stay and a less traumatic recovery with fewer side effects than traditional surgery.

A balloon dilation approach for removing the obstruction is another new technique. This procedure may be performed on an outpatient basis, with recovery in 2 to 10 days compared with 6 to 12 weeks after surgical procedures. The procedure is not done if the postvoiding residual urine exceeds 500 ml, if prostate cancer is suspected, if the prostatic urethra is longer than 8 cm, or if the prostate is larger than 40 g.[26] Transrectal ultrasound is used to monitor balloon dilation of the prostate. Because this procedure is still relatively new, studies are needed to evaluate long-term results.

Other new and experimental forms of treatment for BPH include microwave hyperthermia, high-intensity focused ultrasound, and transurethral needle ablation. Microwave hyperthermia, delivered to the prostate through a transrectal or transurethral approach, produces heat-induced tissue damage. The procedure is limited to medium-sized enlargements of the prostate. The procedure is still experimental in the United States.[23] High-intensity focused ultrasound uses ultrasonic energy with resultant heat and tissue damage to destroy discrete areas of the prostate gland. This method reduces the volume of prostate tissue and improves symptoms. Controlled trials are being conducted to determine its usefulness. Transurethral needle ablation involves the use of high-frequency radio waves to cause thermal damage to prostate tissue. The energy is usually delivered by transurethral needles and controlled by thermocoupled measurements.[23]

For men who have heart or lung disease or a condition that precludes major surgery, a stent may be used to widen and maintain the patency of the urethra. A stent is a device made of tubular mesh. The insertion of a stent is done under local or regional anesthesia. Within several months, the lining of the urethra grows to cover the inside of the stent.

Prostatic Cancer

Prostatic cancer is the most common male cancer in the United States and is second to lung cancer as a cause of cancer-related deaths in men. An estimated 318,000 new cases were diagnosed in the United States in 1996, compared with an estimated 165,000 new cases diagnosed in 1993. The increase in diagnosed cases is thought to reflect earlier diagnosis because of widespread use of PSA testing, which was approved by the Food and Drug Administration in 1994.[27]

The incidence of prostate cancer varies markedly from country to country and varies among races in the same country.[28] African-American males have the highest reported incidence for prostate cancer at all ages. Prostate cancer also tends to be diagnosed at a later stage in African-American men, and the 5-year survival rate for African-American compared with white men is lower (62 % versus 72%). Japanese-American men have the lowest incidence of prostate cancer. Prostate cancer is also a disease of aging. It rarely occurs before age 40, and its incidence increases progressively, reaching a peak among men in their eighties.

The precise cause of prostatic cancer is unclear. As with other cancers, it appears that the development of prostate cancer requires multiple steps involving genes that control cell replication and growth, including those that initiate the transformation and those that promote the transformation process.

Hereditary and environmental factors may be involved in the development of prostate cancer.[28] The incidence of prostate cancer appears to be higher in male relatives of men with prostate cancer. It has been estimated that men who have an affected first-degree relative (*e.g.*, father, brother) and an affected second-degree relative (*e.g.*, grandfather, uncle) have an eightfold increase in risk.[29] Although there appears to be an increased risk for the development of prostate cancer in men with affected relatives, no genetic markers have been described. Suspected environmental factors include dietary fat and occupational exposure. Male hormone levels may also play a role. There is insufficient evidence linking socioeconomic status, infectious agents, smoking, vasectomy, sexual behavior, or BPH to the pathogenesis of prostate cancer.

Epidemiologic research that has associated diet with prostate cancers may help to explain the higher incidence of prostate cancer in Western society. It has been observed that immigrants to the United States from low-risk countries such as Japan have incidence rates that are somewhere between that of their original country and that of the United States, suggesting that environmental factors may play a role in promoting the transformation process. It has been suggested that dietary patterns, including increased dietary fats, may alter the production of sex hormones and affect the risk of prostate cancer. In support of the role of dietary fats as a risk factor for prostate cancer has been the observation that the diet of Japanese men, who have a low rate of prostate cancer, is much lower in fat content than that of U.S. men, who have a much higher incidence.[28]

Workers in certain industries have excess mortality rates due to prostatic cancer, suggesting an environmental influence. A higher incidence of prostate cancer has been observed among men who have had prolonged occupational exposure to cadmium through welding, alkaline battery production, or electroplating. Other work-related exposures include farmers, typesetters, shipfitters, and those involved in horticulture.

In terms of hormonal influence, higher serum levels of testosterone have been proposed as a major risk determinant of prostatic cancer. Evidence favoring a hormonal influence include the presence of steroid receptors in the prostate, the requirement of sex hormones for normal growth and development of the prostate, and the fact that prostate cancer almost never develops in men who have been castrated. The response of prostatic cancer to estrogen administration or androgen deprivation further supports a correlation between the disease and testosterone levels.

Screening

Most prostate cancers are asymptomatic, indicating the need for screening tests that can detect the disease in its early stage. The screening tests currently available are digital rectal examination, PSA testing, and transrectal ultrasound. PSA is a glycoprotein secreted into the cytoplasm of benign and malignant prostatic cells and is not found in other normal tissues or tumors. However, a positive PSA test can only indicate the possible presence of prostate cancer. It can also be positive in cases of benign prostatic hyperplasia and prostatitis. It has been reported that one third of men with elevated PSA levels have prostate cancer determined by biopsy, and two thirds do not.[30] Measures to increase the specificity of PSA testing in terms of predicting prostate cancer are being developed and evaluated. For example, because PSA levels increase with age, age-specific ranges have been established. PSA density (*i.e.*, PSA level/prostate volume as measured by rectal ultrasound) is being evaluated as a method of predicting the presence of prostate cancer in men with a postive PSA test.

The American Cancer Society and the American Urological Association recommend that men 50 years of age or older should undergo annual measurement of PSA and rectal examination for early detection of prostate cancer. Men at high risk for prostate cancer such as blacks and those with a strong family history should undergo annual screening beginning at age 40 years.[31]

A new approach, transrectal ultrasonography, may detect cancers that are too small to be detected by physical examination. This method is not used for first line detection because of its expense, but it may benefit men who are at high risk for development of prostate cancer.

Diagnosis

The diagnosis of prostate cancer is confirmed through biopsy methods. Two new biopsy techniques, fine-needle aspiration and automated core biopsy, are available for this purpose. Both of these methods can be done without anesthesia, cause little discomfort, and can be done on an outpatient basis. The fine-needle aspiration technique is done transrectally or transperitoneally and uses a flexible aspiration needle guide and aspiration syringe. The aspirated material is placed on slides, dried, and stained for microscopic study. The automated core biopsy method is done transrectally; it uses a spring-powered device that on activation allows an inner trocar needle to cut through the tissue in a fraction of a second. This method has the advantage of obtaining tissue samples for histologic examination.

Transrectal ultrasonography, a continuously improving method of imaging, is a proven method for detecting prostatic cancers as small as 5 mm in diameter. It is credited with detecting lesions that are out of the range of the examining finger in digital examinations. It is also used to guide a biopsy needle and document the exact location of the biopsied tissue. Newly developed small probes for transrectal MRI have been shown to be sensitive indicators of the presence of cancer within the prostate. This method may prevent unnecessary biopsies and can be expected to be used increasingly in the early diagnosis of prostatic cancer. Radiologic examination of the bones of the skull, ribs, spine, and pelvis can be used to reveal metastases, although radionuclide bone scans are more sensitive. Excretory urograms are used to delineate changes due to urinary tract obstruction and renal involvement. Lymphangiography is often done to determine pelvic node metastases.

Depending on the size and location of prostatic cancer at the time of diagnosis, there may be changes associated with the voiding pattern similar to those found in benign prostatic hyperplasia. These include urgency, frequency, nocturia, hesitancy, dysuria, hematuria, or blood in the ejaculate. On physical examination, the prostate is nodular and fixed. Bone metastasis is often characterized by low-back pain. Pathologic fractures can occur at the site of metastasis. Men with metastatic disease may have experienced weight loss, anemia, or shortness of breath.

Treatment

Treatment of prostate cancer is based on determining the extent of the disease. Cancer of the prostate, like other forms of cancer, is graded and staged (see Chapter 5). Well-differentiated tumors are assigned a grade of 1, and poorly differentiated tumors are assigned a grade of 5. In 1992, the American Joint Commission for Cancer and the International Union Against Cancer adopted the TNM system for staging prostate cancer. Stage A cancers are asymptomatic and discovered on histologic examination of prostatectomy specimens.[31] The incidence of stage A tumors increases with age and approaches 60% in men older than 80.[11] Between 75% and 95% of men with stage A1 cancers do not show evidence of progressive disease when followed for 10 years or longer. Those with progressive stage A1 cancers are usually younger men (<60 years) with a longer life expectancy. Approximately 30% to 50% of stage 2B can be expected to progress, with a mortality rate of 20% if left untreated.[11] Stage B cancers are palpable on digital examination but are confined to the prostate gland. About 5% to 10% of men with prostate cancer are detected at this stage by rectal examination.[11] Stage C tumors have extended beyond the prostate but have not produced clinically evident metastases. Stage D cancers are those with distant metastasis. More than 75% of men with prostate cancer present with stage C or D disease.[11]

Two tumor markers, PSA and serum acid phosphatase, are important in the staging and management of prostatic cancer. In untreated cases, the level of PSA correlates with the volume and stage of disease. A rising PSA after treatment is consistent with progressive disease whether it is locally recurring or metastatic. Measurement of PSA is used to detect recurrence after total prostatectomy. Because the prostate is the source of PSA, levels of the antigen should drop to zero after the surgery; a rising PSA indicates recurring disease. Serum acid phosphatase is less sensitive than PSA and is used less frequently. However, it is more predictive of metastatic disease and may be used for that purpose.

Cancer of the prostate is treated by surgery, radiotherapy, and hormonal manipulations. Men with stage A1 disease are usually treated with watchful waiting unless they are relatively young. Radical prostatectomy and radiation therapy are used as curative methods of treatment in early disease that is limited to the prostate (*i.e.*, stages A2 and B). The use of nerve-sparing methods of radical prostatectomy has improved the outcomes of surgical intervention. Radiation therapy is being used increasingly in the treatment of stage C disease. Systemic chemotherapy has not proven beneficial in this disease.

Metastatic disease (stage D) is usually treated with androgen-deprivation therapy.[32] Orchiectomy or estrogen therapy is often effective in reducing symptoms and extending survival. The LHRH analogs (*e.g.*, leuprolide, buserelin, nafarelin) are a new class of drugs that block luteinizing hormone release from the pituitary and reduce testosterone levels without orchiectomy or estrogen therapy. When given continuously and in therapeutic doses, these drugs desensitize LHRH receptors in the pituitary, thereby preventing the release of the luteinizing hormone. The antiandrogens (*i.e.*, flutamide and bicalutamide) block the uptake and actions of androgens in the target tissues. Complete androgen blockade can be achieved by combining an antiandrogen with an LHRH agent or orchiectomy. In men with metastatic prostate cancer, treatment with a combination of an LHRH agonist and flutamide seems to increase survival, particularly in those with minimal disease. Although testosterone is the main circulating androgen, the adrenal gland also secrets androgens. Inhibitors of adrenal androgen synthesis (*i.e.*, ketoconazole, aminoglutethimide, and glucocorticosteroids) may be used for treating men with advanced prostatic cancer who present with spinal cord compression, bilateral ureteral obstruction, or disseminated intravascular clotting.

In summary, the prostate is a firm glandular structure that surrounds the urethra. Inflammation of the prostate occurs as an acute or a chronic process. Chronic prostatitis is probably the most common cause of relapsing urinary tract infections in men. Benign prostatic hyperplasia is a common disorder in men older than 50 years of age. Because the prostate encircles the urethra, benign prostatic hyperplasia exerts its effect through obstruction of urinary outflow from the bladder. Advances in the treatment of benign prostatic hyperplasia include laser surgery, balloon dilation, prostatic stents, and pharmacologic treatment using α-adrenergic receptor blockers and agents that block the effects of androgens on the prostate.

Prostatic cancer is the most common male cancer in the United States and is second to lung cancer as a cause of cancer-related deaths of men. An estimated 318,000 new cases were diagnosed in the United States in 1996, almost twice as many as diagnosed in 1993. The increase is thought to reflect earlier diagnosis because of widespread use of PSA testing, which was approved by the Food and Drug Administration in 1994. The incidence increases with age; more than 80% of all prostate cancers are diagnosed in men older than 65. Most prostate cancers are asymptomatic and are incidentally discovered on rectal examination. Screening for prostate cancer has become recognized as a method for early identification of prostate cancer. The American Cancer Society suggests that every man 50 years of age or older should have a rectal examination and PSA test done as part of his annual physical examination. Cancer of the prostate, like other forms of cancer, is graded and staged. Treatment, which is based on the extent of the disease, includes surgery, radiotherapy, and hormonal manipulation.

REFERENCES

1. Behrman R., Kleigman R.M., Nelson W. (1996). *Nelson's textbook of pediatrics* (15th ed., p. 1546–1549). Philadelphia: W.B. Saunders.
2. Downie L.L., Lucarotti C.L. (1996). My child has hypospadias. *Plastic Surgical Nursing* 16 (1), 23–26.
3. Duckett J.W., Snow B.W. (1986). Disorders of the urethra and penis. In Walsh P.C., Gittes R.F, Permutter A.D. (Eds.). *Campbell's urology* (5th ed., pp. 200–239). Philadelphia: W.B. Saunders.
4. Bakht F.R. (1989). Genitourinary emergencies in the male patient. *Primary Care* 16 (4), 905–923.
5. McAninch J.W. (1995). Disorders of the penis and male urethra. In Tanagho E.A., McAninch J.W. (Eds.). *Smith's general urology* (14th ed., pp. 662–669). Norwalk, CT: Appleton & Lange.
6. Ralph D.J., Hughes T., Lees W.R., et al. (1992). Preoperative assessment of Peyronie's disease using colour Doppler sonography. *British Journal of Urology* 69, 629–631.
7. Vohra S., Badlani G. (1992). Balanitis and balanoposthitis. *Urological Clinics of North America* 19, 143–147.
8. Burgers J.K., Badalament R.A., Drago J.R. (1992). Penile cancer, clinical presentation, diagnosis and staging. *Urologic Clinics of North America* 79 (2), 247–255.
9. Grossman H.B. (1992). Premalignant and early carcinomas of the penis and scrotum. *Urologic Clinics of North America* 19 (2), 221–225.
10. Presti J.C., Herr H.W. (1995). Genital tumors. In Tanagho E.A., McAninch J.W. (Eds.). *Smith's general urology* (14th ed., pp. 442–445). Norwalk, CT: Appleton & Lange.

11. Cotran R.S., Kumar V., Robbins S.L. (1994). *Pathologic basis of disease* (5th ed., pp. 1011, 1029–1030). Philadelphia: W.B. Saunders.
12. Gillenwater J.Y., Grayhoch J.T., Howards S.S., et al. (1991). *Adult and pediatric urology* (2nd ed.). St. Louis: C.V. Mosby.
13. Rozanski T.A., Bloom D.A. (1995). The undescended testis, theory and management. *Urologic Clinics of North America* 22 (1), 107–115.
14. Derkson D.J., Smith A.Y. (1989). Genitourinary problems in the male patient. *Primary Care* 16 (4), 981–995.
15. Thomas A.J., Geisinger M.A. (1990). Current management of varicoceles. *Urologic Clinics of North America* 17 (4), 893–895.
16. Kim Y.C., Choi H.K. (1992). Clinical value of scrotopenogram for evaluating varicocele and erectile dysfunction. *Urology* 29 (2), 150–156.
17. Fontanarosa P.M., Hellman M.G. (1991). The acute scrotum. *Topics in Emergency Medicine* 3 (1), 84—92.
18. Tonetti J.A., Tonetti F.W. (1990). Testicular torsion or acute epididymitis: Diagnosis and treatment. *Journal of Emergency Nursing* 16 (2), 96–98.
19. Meares E.M. (1995). Nonspecific infections of the genitourinary tract. In Tanagho E.A., McAninch J.W. (Eds.). *Smith's general urology* (14th ed., pp. 237–238). Norwalk, CT: Appleton & Lange.
20. Mebcow M.M. (1975). Percivall Pott (1713–1788): 200th anniversary of first report of occupation-induced cancer of the scrotum in chimney sweepers (1745). *Urology* 6, 745.
21. Lowe F.C. (1992). Squamous cell carcinoma of the scrotum. *Urologic Clinics of North America* 19 (2), 297–405.
22. Lasater S.J. (1990). Testicular cancer: A perioperative challenge. *AORN Journal* 51 (2), 513–523.
23. Narayan P. (1995). Neoplasms of the prostate gland. In Tanagho E.A., McAninch J.W. (Eds.). *Smith's general urology* (14th ed., pp. 392–433). Norwalk, CT: Appleton & Lange.
24. Barry M.J., et al. (1992). The American Urological Association Index of Benign Prostatic Hypertrophy. *Journal of Urology* 148, 1549.
25. Agency of Health Care Policy and Research. (1994). *Clinical practice guidelines for benign prostatic hyperplasis.* AHCPR publication no. 94-0582. Rockville: U.S. Department of Health and Human Services.
26. Osterling J.E. (1995). Benign prostatic hyperplasia. *New England Journal of Medicine* 332 (2), 99–109.
27. Garnick M.B., Fair W.R. (1996). Prostate cancer: Emerging concepts, part I. *Annals of Internal Medicine* 125, 118–125.
28. Pienta K.J., Esper P.S. (1993). Risk factors for prostate cancer. *Annals of Internal Medicine* 118, 793–803.
29. Steinber G.D., Carter B.S., Beaty T.L., et al. (1990). The familial aggregation of prostate cancer: A case control study [abstract]. *Journal of Urology 143,* 131A.
30. Woolf S.H. (1995). Screening for prostate cancer with prostate specific antigen: An examination of the evidence. *New England of Medicine* 333 (21), 1401–1405.
31. Catalona W.J. (1987). Diagnosis, staging, and surgical treatment of prostatic cancer. *Archives of Internal Medicine* 147, 361.
32. Catona W.J. (1994). Management of cancer of the prostate. *New England of Medicine* 331 (15), 996–1004.

ADDITIONAL READINGS

Baren J.M. (1996). Acute scrotum: Serious or benign. *Emergency Medicine* 8, 24–45.

Davenport M. (1996). Acute problems of the scrotum. *British Medical Journal* 312 (7028), 435–438.

Damjanov I. (1995). Testicular cancer. *Scientific American Science and Medicine* 1 (1), 48–57.

Garnick M.B., Fair W.R. (1996). Prostate cancer: Emerging concepts, part II. *Annals of Internal Medicine* 125, 205–12.

Garin M. (1994). The dilemmas of prostate cancer. *Scientific American* 270 (4), 72–81.

Jacobson S.J., Bergstralh E.J., Guess H.A., Oesterling J.E., et. al. (1996). Predictive properties of serum prostate-specific antigen testing in a community based setting. *Archives of Internal Medicine* 156, 2462–2468.

Lepar H., Ossterling J.E., Wasson J.H. (1996). BPH management minimal to maximal. *Patient Care* 30 (4), 8–30.

Rosanski T.A. Bloom D.A. (1995). The undescended testis: Theory and good management. *Urologic Clinics of North America* 22 (1), 107–115.

Weldon V.E. (1996). Should we and can we cure prostate cancer? *Western Journal of Medicine* 164 (4), 341–342.

CHAPTER 50

Structure and Function of the Female Reproductive System

Patricia McCowen Mehring

The female genitourinary system consists of internal paired ovaries, uterine tubes, uterus, vagina, external mons pubis, labia majora, labia minora, clitoris, urethra, and perineal body. Although the female urinary structures are anatomically separate from the genital structures, their anatomic proximity provides a means for cross-contamination and shared symptomatology between the two systems (Fig. 50–1). This chapter focuses on the internal and external genitalia. It includes a discussion of hormonal and physical changes that occur throughout the life cycle in response to the gonadotropic hormones. The reader is referred to a specialty text for a discussion of pregnancy.

Reproductive Structures

After you have completed this section of the chapter, you should be able to meet the following objectives:

- Describe the anatomic relation of the structures of the external genitalia
- Name the three layers of the uterus and describe their function
- Cite the location of the ovaries in relation to the uterus, fallopian tubes, broad ligaments, and ovarian ligaments
- Explain the function of the fallopian tubes
- State the function of endocervical secretions

External Genitalia

The external genitalia are located at the base of the pelvis in the perineal area and include the mons pubis, labia majora, labia minora, clitoris, and perineal body. The urethra and anus, although not genital structures, usually are considered in a discussion of the external genitalia. The external genitalia, also known collectively as the vulva, are diagrammed in Figure 50–2.

The *mons pubis* is a rounded, skin-covered fat pad located anterior to the symphysis pubis. Puberty stimulates an increase in the amount of fat and the development of darker and coarser hair over the mons. Normal pubic hair distribution in the female follows an inverted triangle with the base centered over the mons. Hair color and texture varies from person to person and among racial groups. There is an abundance of sebaceous glands in the skin that can become infected owing to normal variations in glandular secretions or poor hygiene. The mons pubis is the most common site of pubic lice infestation in the female.

The *labia majora* (singular, labium majus) are analogous to the male scrotum. These structures are the outermost lips of the vulva, beginning anteriorly at the base of the mons pubis and ending posteriorly at the anus. The labia majora are composed of folds of skin and fat and become covered with hair at the onset of puberty. Before puberty, the labia majora have a skin covering

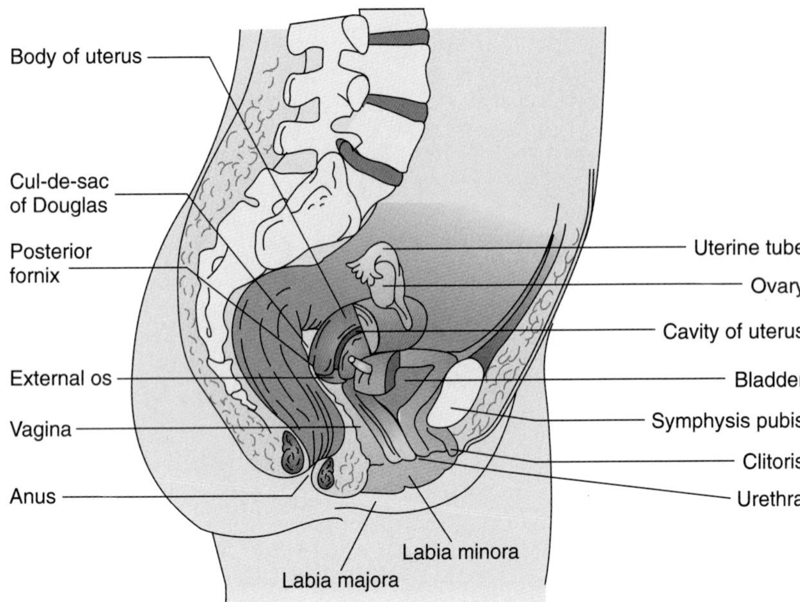

Figure 50–1
Female reproductive system as seen in sagittal section.

similar to that covering the abdomen. With sufficient hormonal stimulation, the labia of a mature woman close over the urethral and vaginal openings; this can change after childbirth or surgery.

The *labia minora* (singular, labium minus) are located between the labia majora. These delicate cutaneous structures are smaller than the labia majora and are composed of skin, fat, and some erectile tissue. Unlike the skin of the labia majora, that of the labia minora is hairless and usually light pink. The labia minora begin anteriorly at the hood of the clitoris and end posteriorly at the base of the vagina. The area between them is called the vestibule. Within the vestibule are located the urethral and vaginal openings and the *Bartholin's lubricating glands*. During sexual arousal, the labia minora become distended with blood; with resolution, the labia throb and then return to normal size. The sebaceous glands secrete odoriferous fluid in the presence or absence of sexual arousal.

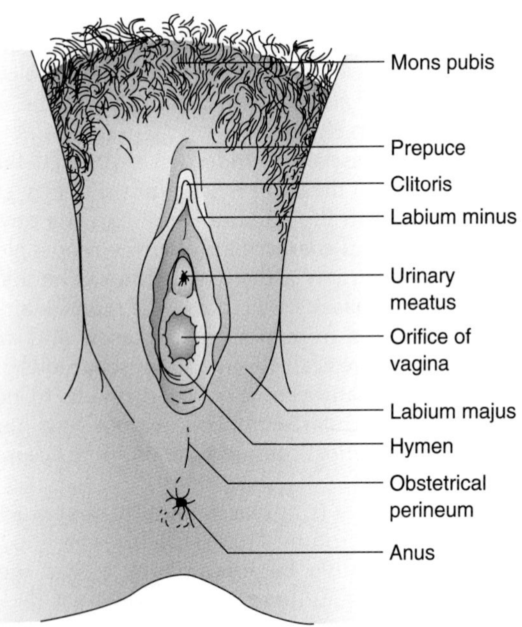

Figure 50–2
External genitalia of the female.

The *clitoris* is located below the clitoral hood, or prepuce, which is formed by the joining of the two labia minora. The female clitoris is an erectile organ, rich in blood and nerve supply. Analogous to the male penis, it is a highly sensitive organ that becomes distended during sexual stimulation.

The *urethra*, or urinary meatus, is the external opening of the internal urinary bladder. The urethra is posterior to the clitoris and usually is closer to the vaginal opening than to the clitoris. The urethra, vaginal opening, and Bartholin's glands lie within the vestibule. The urethral opening is the site of the Skene's glands, which have a lubricating function.

The vaginal orifice, commonly known as the *introitus*, is the opening between the external and internal genitalia. The size and shape of the opening are determined by a connective tissue membrane called the hymen that surrounds the introitus. The opening may be oval, circular, or sievelike and may be partially or completely occluded. Occlusion may occur because of the presence of an intact or partially intact hymen. Contrary to popular notion, an intact hymen does not indicate virginity, because this tissue can be stretched without tearing. At puberty, an intact hymen may require surgical intervention to permit discharge of menstrual fluids.

The *perineal body* is that tissue located posterior to the vaginal opening and anterior to the anus. It is composed of fibrous connective tissue and is the site of insertion of several perineal muscles.

Internal Genitalia

Vagina

Connecting the internal and external genitalia is a fibromuscular tube called the *vagina*. The vagina, which is essentially free of sensory nerve fibers, is located behind the urinary bladder and urethra and anterior to the rectum. The uterine cervix projects into the vagina at its upper end, forming recesses called *fornices*. The vagina functions as a route for discharge of menses and other secretions. It also serves as an organ of sexual fulfillment and reproduction.

The membranous vaginal wall forms two longitudinal folds and several transverse folds, or rugae. The vagina is lined with mucus-secreting stratified squamous epithelial cells. Vaginal tissue usually is moist, with a pH maintained within the bacteriostatic range of 3.8 to 4.2.

The epithelial cells of the vagina, like other tissues of the reproductive system, respond to changing levels of the ovarian sex hormones. Estrogen stimulates the proliferation and maturation of the vaginal mucosa; this results in a thickening of the vaginal mucosa and an increased glycogen content of the epithelial cells. The glycogen is fermented to lactic acid by the lactobacilli (*i.e.*, Döderlein's bacilli) that are part of the normal vaginal flora, accounting for the mildly acid pH of vaginal fluid. The vaginal ecology can be disrupted at many levels, rendering it susceptible to infection. Pregnancy and the use of oral contraceptive agents increase the amount of estrogen within the system. Diabetes or a prediabetic state may increase the glycogen content of the cells. The use of systemic antibiotics may decrease the number of lactobacilli within the vagina.

Decreased estrogen stimulation after menopause causes the vaginal mucosa to become thin and dry, often resulting in dyspareunia (*i.e.*, painful intercourse), atrophic vaginitis, and occasionally in vaginal bleeding. During a routine pelvic examination, the estrogen level can be estimated by examining the cellular structure and configuration of the vaginal epithelial cells. This test is known as the *maturation index*. The maturation index is a cytologic evaluation of vaginal scrapings that determines the ratio of parabasal (least mature), intermediate, and superficial (most mature) cells. Typically, this index is 0–40–60 during the reproductive years. With diminished estrogen levels, there is a shift to the left, producing an index of 30–40–30 during the perimenopausal period and an index of 75–25–0 during the postmenopausal period.

Uterus and Cervix

The uterus is a thick-walled muscular organ. This pear-shaped hollow structure is located between the bladder and the rectum. The uterus can be divided into three parts: the portion above the insertion of the fallopian tubes, called the *fundus;* the lower constricted part, called the *cervix;* and the portion between the fundus and the cervix, called the *body of the uterus* (Fig. 50–3). The uterus is supported on both sides by four sets of ligaments: the broad ligaments, which run laterally from the body of the uterus to the pelvic side walls; the round ligaments, which run from the fundus laterally into each labium majus; the uterosacral ligaments, which run from the uterocervical junction to the sacrum; and the cardinal or transverse cervical ligaments.

The wall of the uterus is composed of three layers: the perimetrium, the myometrium, and the endometrium. The *perimetrium* is the outer serous covering that is derived from the abdominal peritoneum. This outer layer merges with the peritoneum that covers the broad ligaments. Anteriorly, the perimetrium is reflected over the bladder wall, forming the vesicouterine pouch; posteriorly, it extends to form the *cul-de-sac*, or *pouch of Douglas*. Because of the proximity of the perimetrium to the urinary bladder, infection of this organ often causes uterine symptoms, particularly during pregnancy.

The middle muscle layer, the *myometrium*, forms the major portion of the uterine wall. It is continuous with

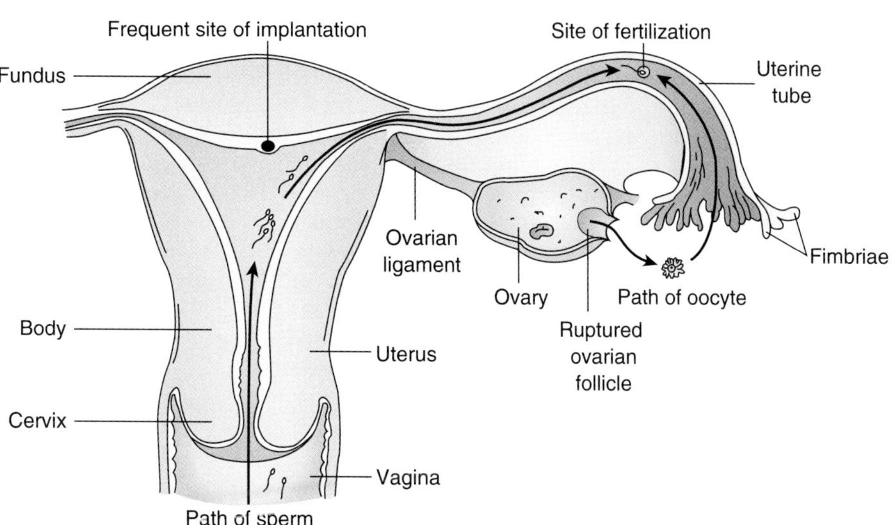

Figure 50–3 Schematic drawing of female reproductive organs, showing the path of the oocyte as it moves from the ovary into the fallopian (uterine) tube; the path of sperm is also shown, as is the usual site of fertilization.

the myometrium of the fallopian tubes and the vagina and extends into all the supporting ligaments with the exception of the broad ligaments. The inner fibers of the myometrium run in various directions, giving it an interwoven appearance. Contractions of these muscle fibers help to expel menstrual flow and the products of conception during miscarriage or childbirth. When pain accompanies the contractions associated with menses, it is called *dysmenorrhea*. The myometrium has an amazing ability to change length during pregnancy and labor, increasing the uterine capacity more than 4000 times.

The *endometrium*, the inner layer of the uterus, is continuous with the lining of the fallopian tubes and vagina. The endometrium is made up of a basal and a superficial layer. The superficial layer is shed during menstruation and regenerated by cells of the basal layer. Ciliated cells promote the movement of tubal-uterine secretions out of the uterine cavity into the vagina.

The round cervix is the neck of the uterus that projects into the vagina. The cervix is a firm structure, composed of a connective tissue matrix of glands and muscular tissue elements, that becomes soft and pliable under the influence of hormones produced during pregnancy. Glandular tissue provides a rich supply of protective mucus that changes in character and quantity during the menstrual cycle and during pregnancy. The cervix is richly supplied with blood from the uterine artery and can be a site of significant blood loss during delivery.

The opening of the cervix, the *os*, forms a pathway between the uterus and the vagina. The vaginal opening is called the external os and the uterine opening, the internal os. The space between these two openings is the endocervical canal. Secretions from the columnar epithelium of the endocervix protect the uterus from infection, alter receptivity to sperm, and form a mucoid "plug" during pregnancy. The endocervical canal provides a route for menstrual discharge and sperm entrance.

Fallopian Tubes

The fallopian, or uterine, tubes are slender, cylindrical structures attached bilaterally to the uterus and supported by the upper folds of the broad ligament. The end of the fallopian tube nearest the ovary forms a funnel-like opening with fringed fingerlike projections, called *fimbriae*, that pick up the ovum after its release into the peritoneal cavity following ovulation (see Fig. 50–3). The fallopian tubes are formed of smooth muscle and lined with a ciliated, mucus-producing epithelial layer. The beating of the cilia, along with contractile movements of the smooth muscle, propels the nonmobile ovum toward the uterus. If coitus has occurred recently, fertilization normally occurs in the middle to outer portion of the fallopian tube. Besides providing a passageway for ova and sperm, the fallopian tubes provide for drainage of tubal secretions into the uterus.

Ovaries

By the third month of fetal life, the ovaries of the female have fully developed and descended to their permanent pelvic position. Remnants of the primitive genital system provide lateral supporting attachments to the uterus; in the mature female, these supporting structures evolve into the round and suspensory ligaments. Remnants that do not evolve may form cysts, which may become symptomatic later in life.

Oogenesis is the process of generation of ova by mitotic division that begins at the sixth week of fetal life. These primitive germ cells ultimately provide the 1 to 2 million oocytes that are present in the ovaries at birth. At puberty, this number is reduced through cell death to about 300,000.

The neonate's ovaries are smooth, pale, and elongated. They become shorter, thicker, and heavier before the onset of menarche, which is initiated by pituitary influence. The initial hormonal stimulus for this development is believed to come from ovarian rather than systemic estrogen.

In the adult, the ovaries are flat, almond-shaped structures that are 3 to 5 cm long and weigh 2 to 3 g. They are located on either side of the uterus below the fimbriated ends of the two oviducts, or fallopian tubes. The ovaries are attached to the posterior surface of the broad ligament and to the uterus by the ovarian ligament. They are covered with a thin layer of surface epithelium that is continuous with the lining of the peritoneum. The integrity of this covering is periodically broken at the time of ovulation.

The ovaries, like the male testes, have a dual function: they store the female germ cells, or ova, and produce the female sex hormones, estrogen and progesterone. Unlike the male gonads, which produce sperm throughout a man's reproductive life, the female gonads contain a fixed number of ova at birth that diminishes throughout a woman's life.

Structurally, the mature ovary is divided into a highly vascular inner medulla, which contains supporting connective tissue, and an outer cortex of stroma and epithelial follicles (*i.e.*, vesicles), which contain the primary oocytes, or germ cells. After puberty, the pituitary gonadotropic hormones—follicle stimulating hormone (FSH) and luteinizing hormone (LH)—stimulate primordial follicles to develop into mature graafian follicles. The graafian follicle produces estrogen, which begins to stimulate the development of the endometrium in the uterus. Although several follicles begin to develop during each ovulatory cycle, only one or two complete the entire developmental process and rupture to release a mature ovum. After ovulation, the follicle becomes luteinized; as the corpus luteum, it produces estrogen and progesterone to support the endometrium until conception occurs or the cycle begins again.

In summary, the female reproductive system consists of internal paired ovaries, uterine tubes, uterus, vagina, external mons pubis, labia majora, labia minora, clitoris, urethra, and perineal body. The genitourinary system as a whole serves sexual and reproductive functions throughout the life cycle. The uterus is a thick-walled muscular organ. The wall of the uterus is composed of three layers: the outer perimetrium; the myometrium or muscle layer, which is continuous with the myometrium of the fallopian tubes and the vagina; and the inner lining or endometrium, which is continuous with the lining of the fallopian tubes and vagina. The gonads, or ovaries, which are internal in the female (unlike the testes in the male) have the dual function of storing the female germ cells, or ova, and producing the female sex hormones. Through the regulation and release of sex hormones, the ovaries influence the development of secondary sexual characteristics, regulation of menstrual cycles, maintenance of pregnancy, and advent of menopause.

Menstrual Cycle

After you have completed this section of the chapter, you should be able to meet the following objectives:

- Describe the feedback control of estrogen and progesterone levels by means of gonadotropin-releasing hormone, LH, FSH, and ovarian follicle function
- List the actions of estrogen and progesterone
- Describe the four functional compartments of the ovary
- Relate FSH and LH levels to the stages of follicle development and to estrogen and progesterone production
- Describe the endometrial changes that occur during the menstrual cycle
- Describe the composition of normal cervical mucus and the changes that occur during the menstrual cycle
- Describe the physiology of normal menopause

Between menarche (*i.e.*, first menstrual bleeding) and menopause (*i.e.*, last menstrual bleeding), the female reproductive system undergoes cyclic changes called the *menstrual cycle.* This includes the maturation and release of oocytes from the ovary during ovulation and periodic vaginal bleeding resulting from the shedding of the endometrial lining. It is not necessary for a woman to ovulate to menstruate; anovulatory cycles do occur. The menstrual cycle produces changes in the breasts, uterus, skin, ovaries, and perhaps other unidentified tissues. The maintenance of the cycle affects biologic and sociologic aspects of a woman's life, including fertility, reproduction, sexuality, and femaleness.

Hormonal Control

Normal menstrual function results from interactions among the central nervous system, hypothalamus, anterior pituitary, ovaries, and associated target tissues. Although each part of the system is essential to normal function, the ovaries are primarily responsible for controlling the cyclic changes and the length of the menstrual cycle. In most women in the middle reproductive years, menstrual bleeding occurs every 25 to 35 days, with a median length of 28 days.

The hormonal control of the menstrual cycle is complex. For example, the biosynthesis of estrogens that occurs in adipose tissue may be a significant source of the hormone. There is evidence that a certain minimum body weight (48 kg) and fat content (16% to 24%) are necessary for menarche to occur and for the menstrual cycle to be maintained. Although menarche is variable, this is supported by the observation of amenorrhea in women with anorexia nervosa, chronic disease, and malnutrition and in those who are long-distance runners. In women with anorexia nervosa, gonadotropin and estradiol secretion, including LH release and responsiveness to gonadotropin-releasing hormone (GnRH), can revert to prepubertal levels. With resumption of weight gain and attainment of sufficient body mass, the normal hormonal pattern usually is reinstated. Obesity or significant weight gain is also associated with oligomenorrhea or amenorrhea and infertility, although the mechanism is not well understood.

Hypothalamic and Pituitary Hormones

Growth, prepubertal maturation, reproductive cycle, and sex hormone secretion in males and females are regulated by FSH and LH from the anterior pituitary gland (Fig. 50–4). Because these hormones promote the growth of cells in the ovaries and testes as a means of stimulating the production of sex hormones, they are called the gonadotropic hormones. The secretion of LH and FSH is stimulated by GnRH from the hypothalamus.

In addition to LH and FSH, the anterior pituitary secretes a third hormone—prolactin. Its primary function is the stimulation of lactation in the postpartum period. During pregnancy, prolactin, along with other

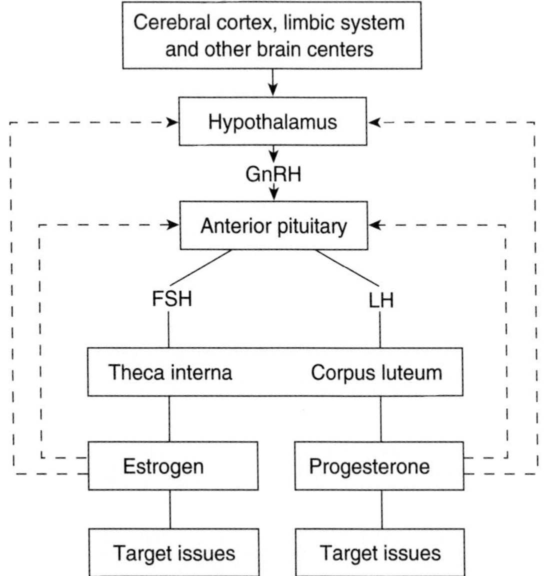

Figure 50–4
Hypothalamic-pituitary feedback control of estrogen and progesterone levels in the female.

hormones such as estrogen, progesterone, insulin, and cortisol, contributes to breast development in preparation for lactation. Although prolactin does not appear to play a physiologic role in ovarian function, hyperprolactinemia leads to hypogonadism. This may include an initial shortening of the luteal phase with subsequent anovulation, oligomenorrhea or amenorrhea, and infertility. Prolactin production by the pituitary normally is inhibited by a hypothalamic inhibiting factor. Hyperprolactinemia may occur as an adverse effect of drug treatment using phenothiazine derivatives (*i.e.,* antipsychotic drugs). These drugs are thought to act at the level of the hypothalamus to increase prolactin release by the pituitary.

Ovarian Hormones

The ovaries produce estrogens, progesterone, and androgens. Ovarian hormones are secreted in a cyclic pattern as a result of the interaction between the hypothalamic-releasing factors and the pituitary gonadotropic hormones.

The steroid sex hormones enter cells by passive diffusion, bind to specific receptor proteins in the cytoplasm, and then move to the nucleus, where they bind to specific sites on the chromosomes. These hormones exert their effects through gene-hormone interactions, which stimulate the synthesis of specific messenger ribonucleic acid (see Chapter 3). The number of hormonal receptor sites on a cell is not fixed; evidence suggests that they are constantly being removed and replaced. An increase or a decrease in the number of receptors can serve as a mechanism for regulating hormonal activity. For example, estrogen may induce the development of an increased number of estrogen receptors in some tissues and may stimulate the synthesis of progesterone receptors. In contrast, progesterone may cause a reduction in the number of estrogen and progesterone receptors.

Estrogens. Estrogens are a family of structurally related female sex hormones synthesized and secreted by cells in the ovaries and, in small amounts, by cells in the adrenal cortex. Androgens can be converted to estrogens peripherally, especially in fat tissue. Three estrogens occur naturally in humans: estrone (E_1), estradiol (E_2), and estriol (E_3). Of these, estradiol is the most biologically potent and the most abundantly secreted product of the ovary. Estrogens are secreted throughout the menstrual cycle. Two peaks occur: one before ovulation and one in the middle of the luteal phase. Estrogens are transported in the blood bound to specific plasma globulins (which can also bind testosterone), inactivated and conjugated in the liver, and then excreted in the bile.

Estrogens are necessary for the normal physical maturation of the female. In concert with other hormones, estrogens provide for the reproductive processes of ovulation, implantation, pregnancy, parturition, and lactation by stimulating the development and maintaining the growth of the accessory organs. In the absence of androgens, estrogens stimulate the intrauterine development of the vagina, uterus, and uterine tubes from the embryonic müllerian system. They also stimulate the stromal development and ductal growth of the breasts at puberty; are responsible for the accelerated pubertal skeletal growth phase and for closure of the epiphyses of the long bones; contribute to the growth of axillary and pubic hair; and alter the distribution of body fat to produce the typical female body contours, including the accumulation of body fat around the hips and breasts. Larger quantities stimulate pigmentation of the skin in the nipple, areolar, and genital regions.

In addition to their effects on the growth of uterine muscle, estrogens play an important role in the development of the endometrial lining. During anovulatory cycles, continued exposure to estrogens for prolonged periods leads to abnormal hyperplasia of the endometrium and abnormal bleeding patterns. When estrogen production is poorly coordinated during the normal menstrual period, inappropriate bleeding and shedding of the endometrium can also occur (see Chapter 51).

Estrogens have a number of important extragenital metabolic effects. They are responsible for maintaining the normal structure of skin and blood vessels in women. Estrogens decrease the rate of bone resorption by antagonizing the effects of parathyroid hormone on bone; for this reason, osteoporosis is a common problem in estrogen-deficient postmenopausal women. In the liver, estrogens increase the synthesis of transport proteins for thyroxine, estrogen, testosterone, and other hormones. Estrogens also affect the composition of the plasma lipoproteins; they produce an increase in high-density lipoproteins (HDLs), a slight reduction in low-density lipoproteins (LDLs), and a reduction in cholesterol levels (see Chapter 17). Estrogens have additional cardioprotective actions, including direct antiatherosclerotic effects on the arterial wall (*i.e.,* vasodilation and antiplatelet function), improved peripheral glucose metabolism with subsequent decreased circulating insulin levels, and direct effects on cardiac function (*i.e.,* increased left ventricular diastolic filling and stroke volume output). Estrogens increase plasma triglyceride levels and they enhance the coagulability of blood by effecting increased circulating levels of plasminogen and factors II, VII, IX, and X.

The estrogens cause moderate retention of sodium and water. Most women retain sodium and water and gain weight just before menstruation. This occurs because the estrogens facilitate the loss of intravascular fluids into the extracellular spaces, producing edema and increased sodium and water retention by the kidneys because of the decreased plasma volume. The actions of estrogens are summarized in Table 50–1.

Progesterone. Although the word *progesterone* refers to a substance that maintains pregnancy, progesterone is secreted as part of the normal menstrual cycle. The corpus luteum of the ovary secretes large amounts of progesterone after ovulation, and the adrenal cortex secretes small amounts. The hormone circulates in the blood attached to a specific plasma protein. It is metabolized in the liver and conjugated for excretion in the bile.

TABLE 50-1

Actions of Estrogens

General Function	Specific Actions
Growth and development	
Reproductive organs	Stimulate development of vagina, uterus, and fallopian tubes in utero and of secondary sex characteristics during puberty
Skeleton	Accelerate growth of long bones and closure of epiphyses at puberty
Reproductive processes	
Ovulation	Promote growth of ovarian follicles
Fertilization	Alter the cervical secretions to favor survival and transport of sperm
	Promote motility of sperm within the fallopian tubes by decreasing mucus viscosity
Implantation	Promote development of endometrial lining in the event of pregnancy
Vagina	Proliferate and cornify vaginal mucosa
Cervix	Increase mucus consistency
Breasts	Stimulate stromal development and ductal growth
General metabolic effects	
Bone resorption	Decrease rate of bone resorption
Plasma proteins	Increase production of thyroid and other binding globulins
Lipoproteins	Increase high-density and slightly decrease low-density lipoproteins

The local effects of progesterone on reproductive organs include the glandular development of the lobular and alveolar tissue of the breasts and the cyclic glandular development of the endometrium. Progesterone can also compete with aldosterone at the level of the renal tubule, causing a decrease in sodium reabsorption, with a resultant increase in secretion of aldosterone by the adrenal cortex, as occurs in pregnancy. Although the mechanism is uncertain, progesterone increases basal body temperature and is responsible for the increase in body temperature that occurs with ovulation.

Smooth muscle relaxation under the influence of progesterone plays an important role in maintaining pregnancy by decreasing uterine contractions and is responsible for many of the common discomforts of pregnancy, such as edema, nausea, constipation, flatulence, and headaches. The increased progesterone present during pregnancy and the luteal phase of the menstrual cycle enhances the ventilatory response to carbon dioxide, leading to a measurable change in arterial and alveolar carbon dioxide (PCO_2) levels.

Androgens. The normal female produces androgens, estrogens, and progesterone. About 25% of these androgens are secreted from the ovaries, 25% from the adrenal cortex, and 50% from ovarian or adrenal precursors. In the female, androgens contribute to normal hair growth at puberty and may have other important metabolic effects.

Ovarian Follicle Development and Ovulation

The tissues of the adult ovary can be conveniently divided into four compartments, or units: the stroma, or supporting tissue; the interstitial cells; the follicles; and the corpus luteum. The stroma is the connective tissue substance of the ovary in which the follicles are distributed. The interstitial cells are estrogen-secreting cells that resemble the Leydig's cells, or interstitial cells, of the testes.

Beginning at puberty, a cyclic rise in the anterior pituitary gonadotropic hormones FSH and LH stimulates the development of several graafian, or mature, follicles. Follicles at all stages of development can be found in both ovaries, except in menopausal women (Fig. 50–5). Most follicles exist as primary follicles, each of which consists of a round oocyte surrounded by a single layer of flattened epithelium-derived granulosa cells and a basement membrane. The primary follicles constitute an inactive pool of follicles from which all the ovulating follicles develop. Under the influence of endocrine stimulation, 6 to 12 primary follicles develop into secondary follicles once every ovulatory cycle. During the development of the secondary follicle, the primary oocyte increases in size, and the granulosa cells proliferate to form a multilayered wall around it. During this time, a membrane called the zona pellucida develops and surrounds the oocyte and small pockets of fluid begin to appear between the granulosa cells. Blood vessels, however, do not penetrate the basement membrane; the granulosa cell layer remains avascular until after ovulation has occurred.

As the follicles mature, FSH stimulates the development of the cell layers. Cells from the surrounding stromal tissue align themselves to form a cellular wall called the theca. The cells of the theca become differentiated into two layers: an inner theca interna, which lies adjacent to the follicular cells, and an outer theca externa. As the follicle enlarges, a single large cavity, or antrum, is formed, and a portion of the granulosa cells and the oocytes are displaced to one side of the follicle by the fluid that accumulates. The secondary oocyte remains surrounded by a crown of granulosa cells, the corona radiata. As the follicle ripens, ovarian estrogen is produced by the granulosa cells. Selection of a dominant follicle occurs with the con

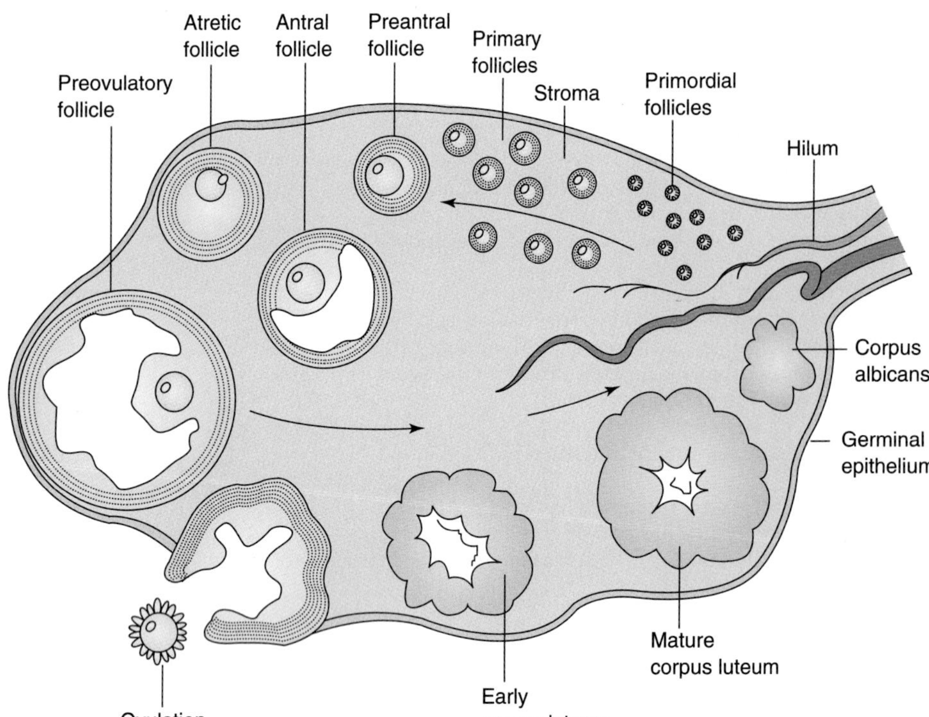

Figure 50–5 Schematic diagram of an ovary, showing the sequence of events in the origin, growth, and rupture of an ovarian follicle and the formation and retrogression of a corpus luteum. The atretic follicles are those that show signs of degeneration and death.

version to an estrogen microenvironment; the lesser follicles, although continuing to produce some estrogen, atrophy or become atretic. The dominant follicle accumulates a greater mass of granulosa cells, and the theca becomes richly vascular, giving the follicle a hyperemic appearance. High levels of estrogen exert a negative feedback effect on FSH, inhibiting multiple follicular development and causing an increase in LH levels. This represents the follicular stage of the menstrual cycle. As estrogen suppresses FSH, the actions of LH predominate, and the mature follicle (measuring about 20 mm) bursts; the oocyte, along with the corona radiata, is ejected from the follicle. The ovum normally is then picked up and transported through the fallopian tube toward the uterus.

After ovulation, the follicle collapses, and the luteal stage of the menstrual cycle begins. The granulosa cells are invaded by blood vessels and yellow lipochrome-bearing cells from the theca layer. A rapid accumulation of blood and fluid forms a mass called the *corpus luteum*. Leakage of this blood onto the peritoneal surface that surrounds the ovary is thought to contribute to the *mittelschmerz* (middle, or intermenstrual, pain) of ovulation. During the luteal stage, progesterone is secreted from the corpus luteum. If fertilization does not take place, the corpus luteum atrophies and is replaced by white scar tissue (*i.e.*, corpus albicans); the hormonal support of the endometrium is withdrawn and menstruation occurs. In the event of fertilization, human chorionic gonadotropin is produced by the trophoblastic cells within the blastocyst and prevents luteal regression. The corpus luteum remains functional for 3 months and provides hormonal support for pregnancy until the placenta is fully functional. Figure 50–6 shows the hormonal changes that occur during the development of the ovarian follicle and ovulation.

Endometrial Changes

The endometrium consists of two distinct layers, or zones, that are responsive to hormonal stimulation: a basal layer and a functional layer. The basal layer lies adjacent to the myometrium and is not sloughed during menstruation. The functional layer arises from the basal layer and undergoes proliferative changes and menstrual sloughing. It can be subdivided into two components: a thin, superficial, compact layer and a deeper spongiosa layer that makes up most of the secretory and fully developed endometrium. The endometrial cycle can be divided into three phases: the proliferative, or preovulatory, phase, during which the glands and stroma of the superficial layer grow rapidly under the influence of estrogen; the secretory, or postovulatory, phase, during which progesterone produces glandular dilation and active mucus secretion and the endometrium becomes highly vascular and edematous; and the menstrual phase, during which the superficial layer degenerates and sloughs off.

Cervical Mucus

Cervical mucus is a complex heterogeneous secretion produced by the glands of the endocervix. It is composed of 92% to 98% water and 1% inorganic salts, mainly sodium chloride. The mucus also contains simple sugars, polysaccharides, proteins, and glycoproteins. Its pH usually is alkaline, ranging from 6.5 to 9.0. Its characteristics are strongly influenced by serum levels of estrogen and progesterone. Estrogen stimulates the production of large amounts of clear, watery mucus through which sperm can penetrate most easily. Progesterone, even in the presence of estrogen, reduces the secretion of mucus. During the luteal phase of the menstrual cycle, mucus is scant, viscous, and cellular (see Fig. 50–6).

Two methods are used to examine the properties of cervical mucus and correlate them with hormonal activity. *Spinnbarkeit* is the property that allows cervical mucus to be stretched or drawn into a thread. Spinnbarkeit can be estimated by stretching a sample of cervical mucus between two glass slides and measuring the maximum length of the thread before it breaks. At midcycle, spinnbarkeit usually exceeds 10 cm. A second method of estimating hormonal levels is ferning, or arborization. *Ferning* refers to the characteristic microscopic pattern that results from the crystallization of the inorganic salts in the cervical mucus when it is dried. As the estrogen levels increase, the composition of the cervical mucus changes, so that dried mucus begins to demonstrate ferning in the latter part of the follicular phase. The absence of ferning can indicate inadequate estrogen stimulation of the endocervical glands or inhibition of the endocervical glands by increased secretion of progesterone. Persistent ferning throughout the menstrual cycle suggests anovulatory cycles or insufficient progesterone secretion.

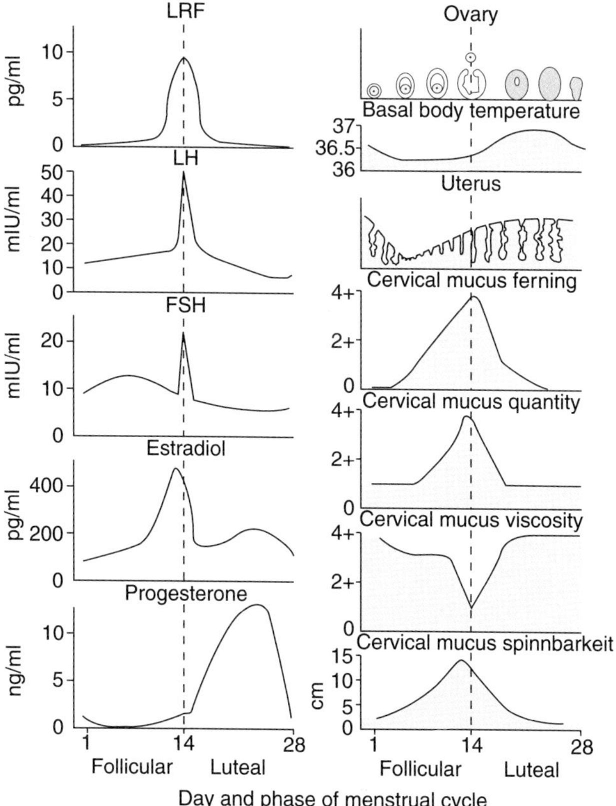

Figure 50–6
Hormonal and morphologic changes during the normal menstrual cycle. (Hershman J.M. [1982]. *Endocrine pathophysiology* [2nd ed.]. Philadelphia: Lea & Febiger)

Menopause

Menopause is the cessation of menstrual cycles. Like menarche, it is more of a process than a single event. Most women stop menstruating between 48 and 55 years of age. Perimenopause (the years immediately surrounding menopause) precedes menopause by approximately 4 years and is characterized by menstrual irregularity and other menopausal symptoms. *Climacteric* is a more encompassing term that refers to the entire transition to the nonreproductive period of life. Premature ovarian failure describes the approximately 1% of women who experience menopause before the age of 40. A woman who has not menstruated for a full year or has an FSH level greater than 30 mIU is considered menopausal.

Menopause results from the gradual cessation of ovarian function and the resultant diminished levels of estrogen. Although estrogens derived from the adrenal cortex continue to circulate in a woman's body, they are insufficient to maintain the secondary sexual characteristics in the same manner as ovarian estrogens. As a result, breast tissue, body hair, skin elasticity, and subcutaneous fat decrease; the ovaries and uterus diminish in size; and the cervix and vagina become pale and friable. The woman may find intercourse painful and traumatic, although some type of vaginal lubrication may be helpful.

Systemically, a woman may experience significant vasomotor instability secondary to the decrease in estrogens and the relative increase in pituitary FSH. This instability may give rise to "hot flashes," palpitations, dizziness, and headaches as the blood vessels dilate. A woman may feel anxious or depressed about these uncontrollable and unpredictable events.

Societal mores influence behaviors. A society that emphasizes youthfulness, fitness, and vigor may not look on aging as a positive process, and menopause is regarded as a hallmark of advancing age. A woman who focuses her energy on beauty and youth may feel frustrated or depressed by the natural aging process. A woman who values her other, nonphysical attributes may welcome advancing age as a time when she may more fully develop as a person.

In summary, between the menarche and menopause, the female reproductive system undergoes cyclic changes called the menstrual cycle. The normal menstrual function results from complex interactions among the hypothalamus, which produces GnRH; the anterior pituitary gland, which synthesizes and releases FSH, LH, and prolactin; the ovaries, which synthesize and release estrogens, progesterone, and androgens; and associated target tissues, such as the endometrium and the vaginal mucosa. Although each component of the system is essential for normal functioning, the ovarian hormones are largely responsible for controlling the cyclic changes and length of the menstrual cycle. Estrogens are necessary for the normal physical maturation of the female, for growth of ovarian follicles, for generation of a climate that is favorable to fertilization and implantation of the ovum, and for promoting the development of the endometrium in the event of pregnancy. Estrogens also have a number of extragenital effects, including prevention of bone resorption and regulation of the composition of cholesterol-carrying lipoproteins (HDL and LDL) in the blood. The functions of progesterone include the glandular development of the lobular and alveolar tissue of the breasts and the cyclic glandular development of the endometrium, and maintenance of pregnancy. Androgens contribute to hair distribution in the female and may have important metabolic effects.

Breasts

After you have completed this section of the chapter, you should be able to meet the following objectives:

- Describe the anatomy of the female breast
- Describe the influence of hormones on breast development
- Characterize the changes in breast structure that occur with pregnancy, lactation, and menopause

Although anatomically separate, the breasts are functionally related to the female genitourinary system in that they respond to the cyclic changes in sex hormones and produce milk for infant nourishment. The breasts are also important for their sexual function and for cosmetic appearance. Breast cancer represents the most common malignancy among females in the United States. The high rate of breast cancer has drawn even greater attention to the importance of the breasts throughout the life span.

Structure

The breasts, or mammary tissues, are located between the third and seventh ribs of the anterior chest wall and are supported by the pectoral muscles and superficial fascia. They are specialized glandular structures that have an abundant shared nerve, vascular, and lymphatic supply (Fig. 50–7). What are commonly called breasts are two parts of a single anatomic breast. This contiguous nature of breast tissue is important in health and illness. Men and women alike are born with rudimentary breast tissue, with the ducts lined with epithelium. In women, the pituitary release of FSH, LH, and prolactin at puberty stimulates the ovary to produce and release estrogen. This estrogen stimulates the growth and proliferation of the ductile system. With the onset of ovulatory cycles, progesterone release stimulates the growth and development of ductile and alveolar secretory epithelium. By adolescence, the breasts have developed characteristic fat deposition patterns and contours.

Structurally, the breast consists of fat, fibrous connective tissue, and glandular tissue. The superficial fibrous connective tissue is attached to the skin, a fact that is important in the visual observation of skin movement over the breast during breast self-examination. The breast mass is supported by the fascia of the pectoralis major and minor muscles and by the fibrous connective tissue of the breast. Fibrous tissue ligaments, called *Cooper's ligaments*, extend from the outer boundaries of the breast to the nipple area in a radial manner, like the

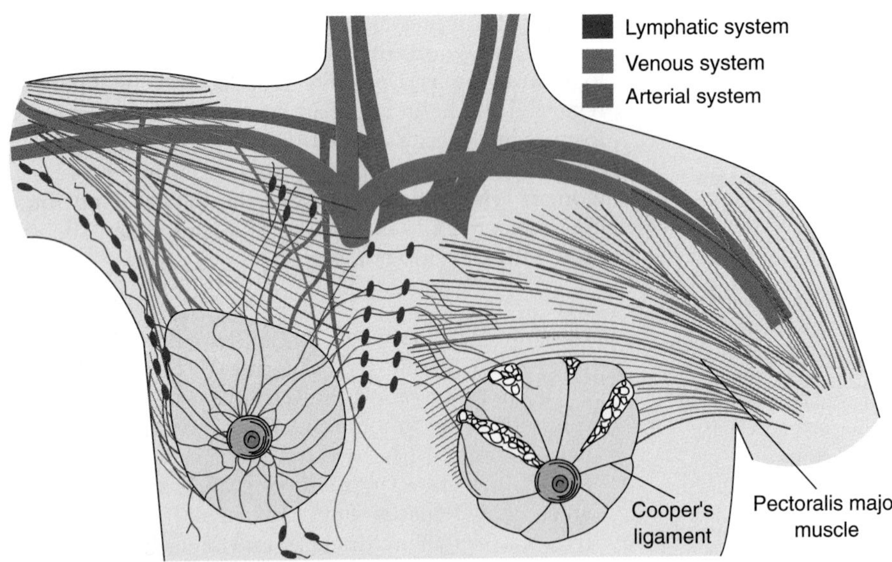

Figure 50–7 The breasts, showing the shared vascular and lymphatic supply as well as the pectoral muscles.

spokes on a wheel (see Fig. 50–7). These ligaments further support the breast and form septa that divide the breast into 15 to 25 lobes. Each lobe consists of grapelike clusters, alveoli or glands, which are interconnected by ducts. The alveoli are lined with secretory cells capable of producing milk or fluid under the proper hormonal conditions (Fig. 50–8). The route of descent of milk and other breast secretions is from alveoli to duct, to intralobar duct, to lactiferous duct and reservoir, to nipple. Breast milk is produced secondary to complex hormonal changes associated with pregnancy. Fluid is produced and reabsorbed during the menstrual cycle. The breasts respond to the cyclic changes in the menstrual cycle with fullness and discomfort.

The nipple is made up of epithelial, glandular, erectile, and nervous tissue. Areolar tissue surrounds the nipple and is recognized as the darker smooth skin between the nipple and the breast. The small bumps or projections on the areolar surface are Montgomery's tubercles, sebaceous glands that keep the nipple area soft and elastic. At puberty and during pregnancy, increased levels of estrogen and progesterone cause the areola and nipple to become darker and more prominent and Montgomery's glands to become more active. The erectile tissue of the nipple is responsive to psychologic and tactile stimuli, which contributes to the sexual function of the breasts.

There are many individual variations in breast size and shape. The shape and texture vary with hormonal, genetic, nutritional, and endocrine factors and with muscle tone, age, and pregnancy. A well-developed set of pectoralis muscles supports the breast mass higher on the chest wall. Poor posture, significant weight loss, and lack of support may cause the breasts to droop.

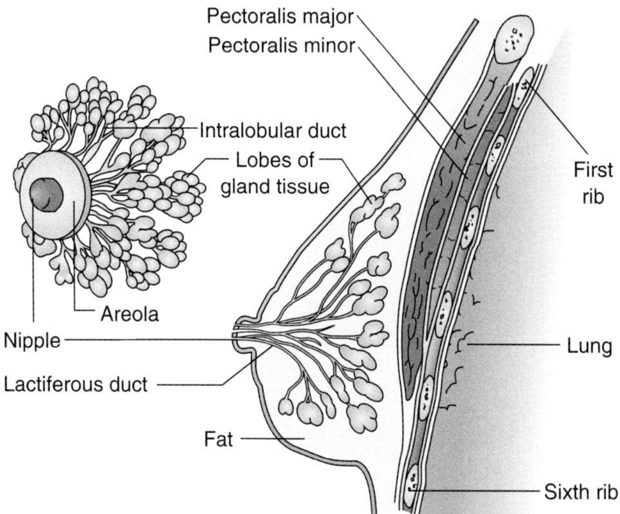

Figure 50–8
The breast, showing the glandular tissue and ducts of the mammary glands.

Pregnancy

During pregnancy, the breasts are significantly altered by increased levels of estrogen and progesterone. Estrogen stimulates increased vascularity of the breasts and the growth and extension of the ductile structures, causing "heaviness" of the breasts. Progesterone causes marked budding and growth of the alveolar structures. The alveolar epithelium assumes a secretory state in preparation for lactation. The progesterone-induced changes that occur during pregnancy may confer some protection against cancer. Cellular changes that occur within the alveolar lining are thought to change the susceptibility of these cells to estrogen-mediated changes later in life.

Lactation

During lactation, milk is secreted by alveolar cells, which are under the influence of the anterior pituitary hormone prolactin. Milk ejection from the ductile system occurs in response to the release of oxytocin from the posterior pituitary. The suckling of the infant provides the stimulus for milk ejection. Suckling produces feedback to the hypothalamus, stimulating the release of oxytocin from the posterior pituitary. Oxytocin causes contraction of the myoepithelial cells lining the alveoli and ejection of milk into the ductal system. A woman may have breast leakage for 3 months to 1 year after the termination of breast-feeding as breast tissue and hormones regress to the nonlactating state. Overzealous breast stimulation with or without pregnancy can likewise cause breast leakage.

Changes with Menopause

At the onset of menopause, the levels of estrogen and progesterone are gradually reduced, and the breasts regress because of loss of glandular tissue. The lobular-alveolar structures atrophy, leaving fat, connective tissue, and ducts. The breasts become pendulous with the decrease in tissue mass.

In summary, the breast is a complex structure of variable size, consistency, and composition. Although anatomically distinct, the breasts are functionally related to the female genitourinary system in that they respond to cyclic changes in sex hormones and produce milk for infant nourishment. Breast tissue is not static but changes throughout the life cycle with development of the alveolar structures in preparation for lactation during pregnancy, milk production during pregnancy, and replacement of glandular tissue with adipose tissue during menopause.

BIBLIOGRAPHY

Benson R.C. (1983). *Handbook of obstetrics and gynecology* (8th ed., p. 20). Los Altos, CA: Lange Medical Publications.

Speroff L., Glass R.H., Kase N.G. (1994). *Clinical gynecologic endocrinology and infertility* (5th ed). Baltimore: Williams & Wilkins.

Greenspan F.S., Baxter J.D. (1994). *Basic and clinical endocrinology* (4th ed). Norwalk, CT: Appleton & Lange.

Guyton A., Hall J.E. (1996). *Textbook of medical physiology* (9th ed., pp. 1017–1032). Philadelphia: W.B. Saunders.

Rhoades R.A., Tanner G.A. (1996). *Medical physiology* (pp. 757–776). Boston, Little Brown.

CHAPTER 51

Alterations in Structure and Function of the Female Reproductive System

Patricia McCowen Mehring

Disorders of the female genitourinary system have widespread effects on physical and psychological function, affecting sexuality and reproductive function. The reproductive structures are located close to other pelvic structures, particularly those of the urinary system, and disorders of the reproductive system may affect urinary function. This chapter focuses on infection and inflammation, benign conditions, and neoplasms of the female reproductive structures; disorders of pelvic support and uterine position; and alterations in menstruation. An overview of infertility is also included.

Disorders of the External Genitalia and Vagina

After you have completed this section of the chapter, you should be able to meet the following objectives:

- Compare the extragenital abnormalities associated with vulvitis, Bartholin's cyst, epidermal cysts, nevi, vulvar dystrophy, vulvodynia, and cancer of the vulva

- Characterize the symptoms and frequency of recurrence of vulvar vestibulitis, cyclic vulvovaginitis, vulvar dysesthesia, and vulvar dermatoses
- State the role of Döderlein's bacilli in maintaining the normal ecology of the vagina
- Describe the conditions that predispose to vaginal infections and the methods used to prevent and treat these infections
- Cite the association between diethylstilbestrol and adenocarcinoma of the vagina

Disorders of the External Genitalia

Vulvitis and Folliculitis

Vulvitis is characterized by inflammation and pruritus (*i.e.,* itching) of the vulva. It is not considered a specific disease but typically accompanies other local and systemic disorders. The cause often is an irritating vaginal discharge. *Candida albicans,* a yeast, is the most common cause of chronic vulvar pruritus, particularly in women with diabetes mellitus. Vulvitis may also be a component of sexually transmitted diseases such as herpes genitalis and human papillomavirus (HPV) infection (*i.e.,* condyloma). Local dermatologic reactions to chemical irritants, such as laundry products, perfumed soaps or sprays, and spermicides, or to allergens, such as poison ivy, can also cause inflammation. Vulvar itching may be caused by atrophy that is part of the normal aging process.

Management of vulvitis focuses on appropriate treatment of underlying causes and comfort measures to relieve the irritation. These include keeping the area clean and dry; using warm sitz baths with baking soda, wet dressings, or Burow's solution soaks (a mild astringent); or applying a mild hydrocortisone cream for the immediate relief of symptoms.

Folliculitis is an infection that involves the hair follicles of the mons or labia majora. The infection, characterized by small red papules or pustules surrounding the hair shaft, is relatively common because of the density of bacteria in this area and the occlusive nature of clothing covering the genitalia. Treatment includes thorough cleaning of the area with germicidal soap, followed by the application of a mild bacterial ointment, such as Neosporin or Polysporin.

Bartholin's Cyst and Bartholin Abscess

Bartholin's cyst is a fluid-filled sac. Bartholin's cyst results from the occlusion of the duct system within Bartholin's gland. When the cyst becomes infected, the contents become purulent; if the infection goes untreated, a bartholinian abscess can result. The obstruction that causes cyst and abscess formation most commonly follows a bacterial, chlamydial, or gonococcal infection. Cysts can attain the size of an orange and frequently recur (Fig. 51–1). Abscesses can be extremely tender and painful. Asymptomatic cysts require no treatment. The treatment of symptomatic cysts consists of the administration of appropriate antibiotics, local application of moist heat, and incision and drainage. Cysts that frequently are abscessed or are large enough to cause blockage of the introitus may require surgical intervention (*i.e.,* marsupialization).

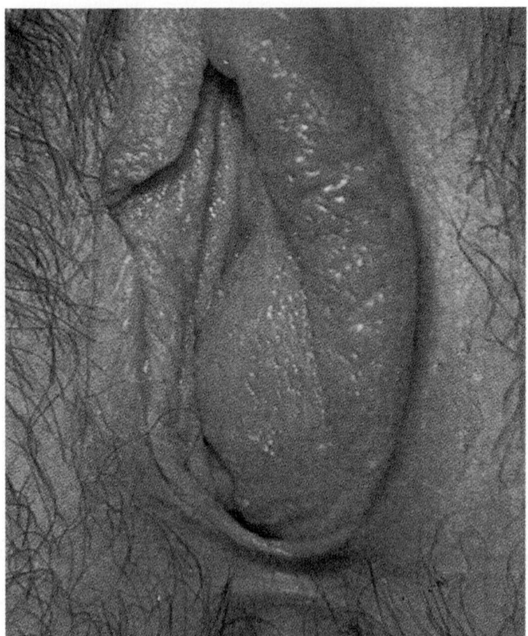

Figure 51–1
Bartholin's gland cyst. The 4-cm lesion is located to the right of and posterior to the vaginal introitus.

Epidermal Cysts

Epidermal cysts (*i.e.,* sebaceous or inclusion cysts) are common semisolid tumors of the vulva. These small nodules are lined with keratinizing squamous epithelium and contain cellular debris with a sebaceous appearance and odor. Epidermal cysts may be solitary or multiple and have a yellow appearance when stretched or compressed. They usually resolve spontaneously, and treatment is unnecessary unless they become infected or significantly enlarged.

Nevi

Nevi (*i.e.,* moles) occur on the vulva as elsewhere on the body. They can be singular or multiple, flat or raised, and may vary in degree of pigmentation from flesh-colored to dark brown or black. Nevi are asymptomatic but should be observed for changes that could indicate cancer. Nevi may resemble melanomas or basal cell carcinomas, and excisional biopsy is recommended when doubt exists (see Chapter 15).

Vulvar Dystrophy

Vulvar dystrophy, characterized by white lesions of the vulva, is a common condition that was once considered to be precancerous. The lesions may be categorized as lichen sclerosus, squamous cell hyperplasia, or other dermatoses, depending on clinical and histologic characteristics. Lichen sclerosus patches are hypopigmented, parchment-thin, and atrophic (Fig. 51–2). Hyperplastic lesions are thick, gray-white plaques. Both can be pruritic. Lichen sclerosus responds best to topical application of testosterone propionate in petroleum jelly. It is often necessary to initially treat the severe pruritus with an intermediate to potent topical corticosteroid. Hyperplastic areas respond well to a combination steroid (*e.g.*, betamethasone valerate) and antipruritic cream (*e.g.*, crotamiton [Eurax]) and to the removal of any irritants (*e.g.*, detergents, perfumes). Lichen sclerosus frequently recurs, and lifetime maintenance therapy is suggested. Hyperplastic areas that occur within the field of lichen sclerosis may be sites of malignant change and warrant close follow-up and possible biopsy.[1]

Vulvodynia

Vulvodynia, also referred to as vulvar pain syndrome or burning vulva syndrome, is a chronic vulvar discomfort characterized by burning, stinging, irritation, and rawness. It includes several disorders. Pain at onset of intercourse (*i.e.*, insertional dyspareunia), localized point tenderness near the vaginal opening, and sensitivity to tampon placement, tight-fitting pants, bicycling, or prolonged sitting are characteristic of *vulvar vestibulitis*. When the condition demonstrates episodic flares that only occur before menses or after coitus, it is referred to as *cyclic vulvovaginitis*. Symptoms that are generally noncyclic and pruritic and develop progressively during the perimenopausal or postmenopausal years are characteristic of *vulvar dermatoses*.

Vulvar dysesthesia, also known as idiopathic or essential vulvodynia, involves severe, constant, widespread burning that interferes with daily activities.[2] Although the cause is unknown, the quality of pain with vulvar dysesthesia resembles reflex sympathetic dystrophy or pudendal neuralgia and is possibly the result of myofascial restrictions affecting sacral and pelvic floor enervation.

Possible causes for other classifications include candidal hypersensitivity with chronic recurrent yeast infections, chemical or drug irritations, especially to prolonged use of topical steroid creams, elevated urinary levels of calcium oxalate, immunoglobulin A deficiency and dermatoses such as lichen sclerosus, lichen planus, or squamous cell hyperplasia. Previous links to HPV infection have not been supported by studies, and the finding of subclinical HPV in women with vulvodynia is now thought to be a secondary or unrelated phenomenon. Herpes simplex virus (HSV) may be related to episodic vulvodynia and long-term viral suppressive therapy may be of benefit to women with known HSV who experience multiple outbreaks each year.[3]

Treatment for this chronic, often debilitating problem is aimed at symptom relief and elimination of suspected underlying problems. Careful history taking and physical assessment is essential for differential diagnosis and treatment. Regimens can include long-term vaginal or oral antifungal therapy, avoidance of potential irritants, cleaning with water only or a gentle soap, sitz baths with baking soda, emollients such as vitamin E or vegetable oil for lubrication, low-oxalate diet plus calcium citrate supplements (calcium binds oxalate in the bowel and citrate inhibits the formation of oxalate crystals), topical anesthetic or steroid ointments, antidepressants, physical therapy, and surgery. Psychosocial support is often needed because this condition can cause strain in sexual, family, and work relationships.

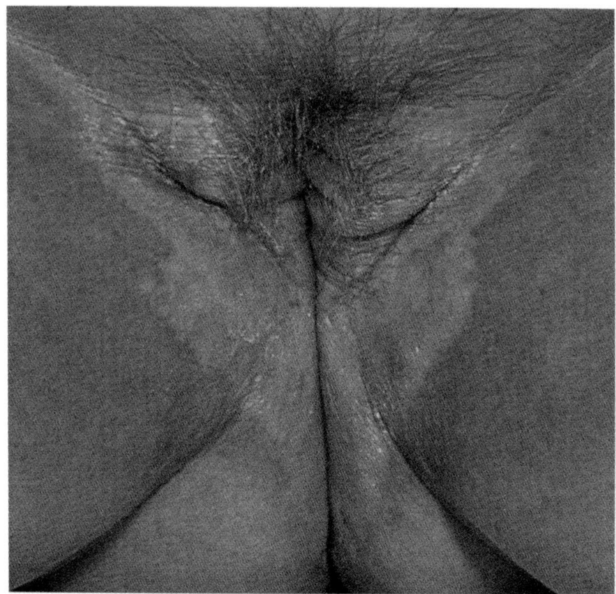

Figure 51–2
Lichen sclerosus of vulva. The sharply demarcated white lesion affects the vulva and perineum.

Cancer of the Vulva

Carcinoma of the vulva accounts for about 5% of all cancers of the female genitourinary system. Invasive carcinoma most frequently is seen in women who are age 60 or older; almost one half are older than 70. The mean age for carcinoma in situ is 10 years younger than for invasive carcinoma.[4]

A significant rise in the incidence of vulvar intraepithelial neoplasia (VIN) among women in their twenties and thirties appears to be caused by the oncogenic (cancer-promoting) potential of certain strains of HPV that are sexually transmitted. VIN is a proliferative intraepithelial squamous process characterized by abnormal epithelial maturation, nuclear enlargement, and nuclear atypia. The extent of replacement of epithelial cells by abnormal cells determines the grade of VIN: I, II, or III.[1] Full-thickness replacement, VIN III, is synonymous with carcinoma in situ (CIS). Histologic staging for VIN uses the same differentiation as cervical cancer (Table 51–1). VIN lesions may take many forms that are presumed to progress to invasive carcinoma if not treated.

About 85% to 90% of invasive cancers of the vulva are epidermoid carcinomas that originate in the epidermal layer of the vulva. The initial lesion may appear as an inconspicuous thickening of the skin, a small raised area or lump, or an ulceration that fails to heal. A lesion may be single or multiple and vary in color from white

TABLE 51-1

Cervical Intraepithelial Neoplasia Grading System

Grade	Extent of Involvement	Differentiation of Lesion
CIN I (mild dysplasia)	Initial one third of epithelial layer	Well differentiated
CIN II (moderate dysplasia)	Initial two thirds of epithelial layer	Less well differentiated
Cin III (severe dysplasia or cancer in situ [CIS])	Full-thickness involvement	Undifferentiated

(Data from Rubin E., Farber J.L. [1994]. *Pathology* [pp. 928–929]. Philadelphia: J.B. Lippincott)

to velvety red or black. The lesions may resemble eczema or dermatitis and may produce few symptoms, other than pruritus, local discomfort, and exudation. A recurrent, persistent, pruritic vulvitis may be the only complaint. The symptoms frequently are treated with various home remedies before medical treatment is sought. The lesion often becomes secondarily infected, and this causes pain and discomfort. The malignant lesion gradually spreads superficially or as a deep furrow involving all of one labial side. Because there are many lymph channels around the vulva, the cancer metastasizes freely to the regional lymph nodes. The most common extension is to the superficial inguinal, deep femoral, and external iliac lymph nodes.

Less common types of cancer found on the vulva include extramammary Paget's disease (intraepithelial or invasive), carcinoma of Bartholin's gland (1% of vulvar cancers), basal cell carcinoma (1% to 2% of vulvar cancers), malignant melanoma (5% of vulvar cancers), and sarcoma (<2% of vulvar cancers).[4]

Early diagnosis is important in the treatment of vulvar carcinoma. Because malignant lesions can vary in appearance and commonly are mistaken for other conditions, biopsy and treatment often are delayed. Treatment is primarily wide surgical excision of the lesion for noninvasive cancer and vulvectomy with node resection for invasive cancer. Local chemotherapeutic agents (*e.g.*, fluorouracil) and colposcopically guided laser therapy are used to treat focal areas of cancer in cases where surgery is contraindicated. The 5-year survival rate for women with lesions less than 3 cm in diameter and minimal node involvement is about 65% after surgical treatment. Follow-up visits every 3 months for the first 2 years after surgery and every 6 months thereafter are important to detect recurrent disease or a second primary cancer. The 5-year survival rate for patients who have larger lesions in conjunction with three or more positive nodes is about 75% after surgical treatment.[4] After pelvic lymphadenopathy is established, the prognosis is poor.

Disorders of the Vagina

The normal vaginal ecology depends on the delicate balance of hormones and bacterial flora. Normal estrogen levels maintain a thick, protective squamous epithelium that contains glycogen. Döderlein's bacilli, part of the normal vaginal flora, metabolize glycogen, and in the process, produce the lactic acid that normally maintains the vaginal pH below 4.5. Disruptions in these normal environmental conditions predispose to infection.

Vaginitis

Vaginitis is inflammation of the vagina; it is characterized by vaginal discharge and burning, itching, redness, and swelling of vaginal tissues. Pain often occurs with urination and with sexual intercourse. Vaginitis may be caused by chemical irritants, foreign bodies, and infectious agents. The causes of vaginitis differ in various age groups. In premenarchal girls, most vaginal infections have nonspecific causes, such as poor hygiene, intestinal parasites, or the presence of foreign bodies. *C. albicans, Trichomonas vaginalis,* and bacterial vaginosis are the most common causes of vaginal discharge in the childbearing years and can be transmitted sexually (see Chapter 52). In postmenopausal women, atrophic vaginitis is the most common form.

Atrophic vaginitis is an inflammation of the vagina that occurs after menopause or removal of the ovaries and their estrogen supply. Estrogen deficiency results in a lack of regenerative growth of the vaginal epithelium, rendering these tissues more susceptible to infection and irritation. Döderlein's bacilli disappear, and the vaginal secretions become less acidic. The symptoms of atrophic vaginitis include itching, burning, and painful intercourse. These symptoms usually can be reversed by local application of estrogen creams or by vaginal suppositories.

Every woman has a normal vaginal discharge during the menstrual cycle, but it should not cause burning or itching or have an unpleasant odor. These symptoms suggest inflammation or infection. Because these symptoms are common to the different types of vaginitis, precise identification of the organism is essential for proper treatment. A careful history should include information about systemic disease conditions, the use of drugs such as antibiotics that foster the growth of yeast, dietary habits, stress, and other factors that alter the resistance of vaginal tissue to infections. A physical examination usually is done to evaluate the nature of the discharge and its effects on the genital structures.

Microscopic examination of a saline wet-mount smear (prepared by placing a sample of vaginal mucus in one to two drops of normal saline) is the primary means of identifying the organism responsible for the infection. A small amount of 10% to 20% potassium hydroxide (KOH) is added to a second specimen on the slide to aid in the identification of *C. albicans*. KOH destroys the cellular material making the epithelial cells become increasingly transparent so that the hyphae and buds that are characteristic of *Candida* become much easier to see. Culture methods may be needed when the organism is not apparent on the wet-mount preparation.

The prevention and treatment of vaginal infections depend on proper health habits and accurate diagnosis and treatment of ongoing infections. Measures to prevent infection include development of daily hygiene habits that keep the genital area clean and dry, maintenance of normal vaginal flora and healthy vaginal mucosa, and avoidance of contact with organisms known to cause vaginal infections. Perfumed products, such as feminine deodorant sprays, douches, bath powders, soaps, and even toilet paper, can be irritating and may alter the normal vaginal flora. Tight clothing prevents the dissipation of body heat and evaporation of skin moisture and promotes favorable conditions for the growth of pathogens and irritation. Nylon and other synthetic undergarments, pantyhose, and swimsuits hold body moisture next to the skin and harbor infectious organisms, even after they have been washed. Cotton undergarments that withstand hot water and bleach (*i.e.*, a fungicide) may be preferable for women to prevent such infections. Swimsuits and other garments that cannot withstand hot water or bleaching should be hung in the sunlight to dry. Women should be taught to wipe the perineal area from front to back to avoid bringing rectal contamination into the vagina. Avoiding sexual contact whenever an infection is known to exist or suspected should limit that route of transmission.

Cancer of the Vagina

Primary cancers of the vagina are extremely rare. They account for about 1% to 2% of all cancers of the female reproductive system. Like vulvar carcinoma, carcinoma of the vagina is largely a disease of older women, with a mean age of 55 years for invasive cancer. The exception to that is the clear cell adenocarcinoma associated with diethylstilbestrol (DES) exposure in utero, which is associated with an age range of 7 to 42 years.[5] Vaginal cancers may result from local extension of cervical cancer, from local irritation such as occurs with prolonged use of a pessary, or from exposure to sexually transmitted herpesvirus or HPV.

About 85% of vaginal cancers are epidermoid carcinomas, with other common types being adenocarcinomas, sarcomas, and melanomas.[4] Maternal ingestion of DES in early pregnancy has been associated with the development of clear cell adenocarcinoma in female offspring who were exposed in utero. Between 1940 and 1975, DES, a nonsteroidal synthetic estrogen, commonly was prescribed to prevent miscarriage. Its association with adenocarcinoma of the vagina was not discovered until the late 1960s. A tumor registry of clear cell adenocarcinoma of the genital tract in young women was established in 1971, and more than 600 cases have now been reported. The incidence of clear cell adenocarcinoma of the vagina is low, about 0.1% in young women who were exposed in utero to synthetic estrogen. This is fortunate, because at the time of the banning of DES, an estimated 4 million American women had taken the drug. Although only a small percentage of girls exposed to estrogen actually develop clear cell adenocarcinoma, 75% to 90% of them develop benign adenosis (*i.e.*, ectopic extension of cervical columnar epithelium into the vagina, which normally is stratified squamous epithelium), which may predispose to cancer. Any girl exposed to DES should be encouraged to have semiannual gynecologic examinations beginning at age 14 or menarche with an initial examination that includes careful colposcopic inspection of the cervix and vagina. Because the upper age limit for this type of cancer is unknown, there is no age at which a DES daughter can be considered risk free.[5]

The most common symptom of vaginal carcinoma is abnormal bleeding. Twenty percent of women are asymptomatic, with the cancer being discovered during a routine pelvic examination. The anatomic proximity of the vagina to other pelvic structures (*e.g.*, urethra, bladder, rectum) permits early spread to these areas. Pelvic pain, dysuria, constipation, and vaginal discharge can be associated symptoms. Vaginal epidermoid carcinoma most often is detected in the upper posterior one third of the vagina, with adenocarcinoma more often found on the lower anterior and lateral vaginal vault. Cancer can develop anywhere within the vagina, and visualization during physical examination should always cover the entire vault. Women should continue to have vaginal cytology studies (Papanicolaou's test [Pap smear]) at least every 3 years after hysterectomy to exclude development of vaginal cancer. Diagnosis requires a biopsy of suspicious lesions or areas.

Treatment of vaginal cancer must take into consideration the size, location, and spread of the lesion and the woman's age. Radical surgery and radiation therapy are both curative. When there is upper vaginal involvement, radical surgery includes a total hysterectomy, pelvic lymph node dissection, partial vaginectomy, and placement of a graft from the buttock to the area from which the vagina was excised. Vaginal reconstruction is often possible to allow for sexual intercourse. The ovaries usually are preserved unless they are diseased. Extensive lesions and those located in the middle or lower vaginal area usually are treated by radiation therapy. The prognosis depends on the stage of the disease, the involvement of lymph nodes, and the degree of mitotic activity of the tumor. With appropriate treatment and follow-up, the 5-year survival rate for stage I or II disease is 70% to 75%. This drops to 30% to 40% for stage III disease. Few survive stage IV disease.[4] For DES-related cancers, the 5-year survival rate is about 93% for stage I disease.[5]

In summary, the surface of the vulva is affected by disorders that affect skin on other parts of the body. These disorders include inflammation (*i.e.*, vulvitis and folliculitis), epidermal cysts, and nevi. Although these disorders are not serious, they can be distressing because they produce severe discomfort and itching. Bartholin's cysts are the result of occluded ducts within the Bartholin's glands. They often are painful and can become infected. Vulvar dystrophies are characterized by thinning and hyperplastic thickening of vulvar tissues. Vulvodynia is a chronic vulvar pain syndrome with several classifications and variable treatment results. Cancer of the vulva, which accounts for 3% to 5% of all female genitourinary cancers, is associated with genital herpesvirus and HPV infections.

The normal vaginal ecology depends on the delicate balance of hormones and bacterial flora. Normal estrogen levels maintain a thick protective squamous epithelium that contains glycogen. Döderlein's bacilli, which are part of the normal vaginal flora, metabolize glycogen and, in the process, produce the lactic acid that normally maintains the vaginal pH below 4.5. Disruptions in these normal environmental conditions predispose to vaginal infections. Vaginitis or inflammation of the vagina is characterized by vaginal discharge and burning, itching, redness, and swelling of vaginal tissues. It may be caused by chemical irritants, foreign bodies, and infectious agents. Primary cancers of the vagina are extremely rare, accounting for 1% to 2% of all cancers of the female reproductive system. Daughters of women treated with DES to prevent miscarriage are at increased risk of developing adenocarcinoma of the vagina.

Disorders of the Cervix and Uterus

After you have completed this section of the chapter, you should be able to meet the following objectives:

- Describe the importance of the cervical transformation zone in the development of cervical cancer
- Compare the lesions associated with nabothian cysts and cervical polyps
- List the complications of untreated cervicitis
- Compare the age distribution and risk factors for cervical and endometrial cancer
- Characterize the development of cervical cancer from the appearance of atypical cells to the development of invasive cervical cancer
- Relate the importance of Papanicolaou's test in early detection and decreased incidence of deaths from cervical cancer
- Describe the methods used in the treatment of cervical cancer
- Compare the pathology and manifestations of endometriosis and adenomyosis
- Cite the major early symptom of endometrial cancer
- Compare intramural and subserosal leiomyomas

Disorders of the Uterine Cervix

The cervix is composed of two distinct types of tissue. The exocervix, or visible portion, is covered with stratified squamous epithelium, which also lines the vagina. The endocervical canal is lined with columnar epithelium. The junction of these two tissue types (*i.e.*, squamocolumnar junction) appears at various locations on the cervix at different points in a woman's life (Fig. 51–3). During periods of high estrogen production, particularly fetal existence, menarche, and the first pregnancy, the cervix everts or turns outward, exposing the columnar epithelium to the vaginal environment. The combination of estrogen and low vaginal pH leads to a gradual transformation from columnar to squamous epithelium—a process called *metaplasia* (see Chapter 2). The dynamic area of change where metaplasia takes place is called the *transformation zone*.[6]

The transformation zone is a critical area for the development of cervical cancer. During metaplasia, the newly developed squamous epithelial cells are vulnerable to genetic change if exposed to carcinogenic agents (*i.e.*, cancer-producing substances). *Dysplasia* means disordered growth or development. Although initially a reversible cell change, untreated dysplasia can develop into carcinoma.

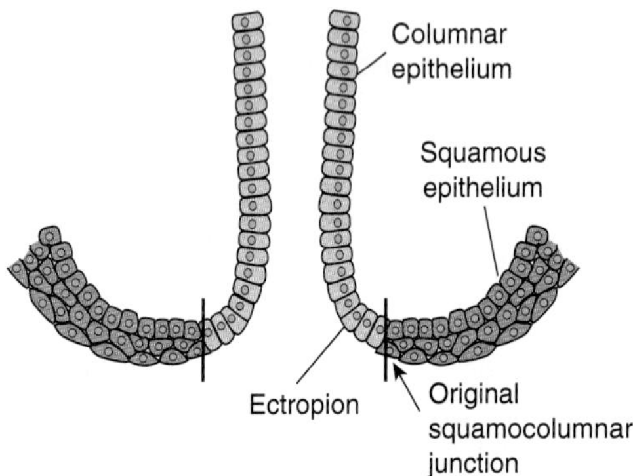

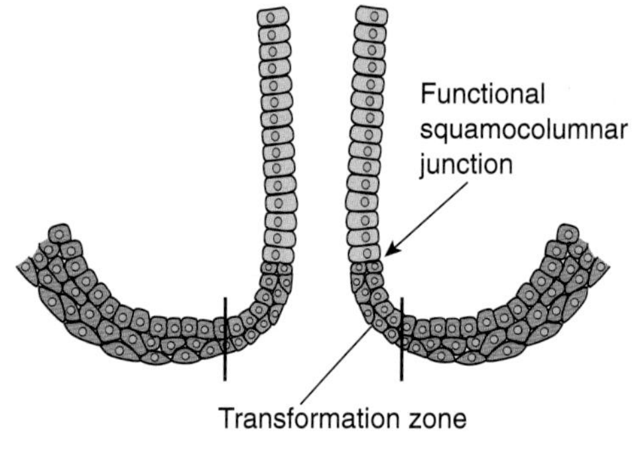

Figure 51–3
The transformation zone of the cervix.

Metaplasia can result in retention cysts, called *nabothian cysts*, that develop when mucus becomes trapped within the deeper clefts of the columnar epithelial cells. These are benign cysts that require no treatment unless they become so numerous that they cause cervical enlargement. The nabothian cyst farthest away from the external cervical os indicates the outer aspect of the transformation zone. The transformation zone is the area of the cervix that must be sampled to have an adequate Pap smear and the area most carefully examined during colposcopy.

Cervicitis and Cervical Polyps

Cervicitis is an acute or chronic inflammation of the cervix. Acute cervicitis may result from the direct infection of the cervix or may be secondary to a vaginal or uterine infection. It may be caused by a variety of infective agents, including *C. albicans, T. vaginalis, Neisseria gonorrhoeae, Gardnerella vaginalis, Chlamydia trachomatis, Ureaplasma urealyticum*, and herpes simplex virus. *Chlamydia* is the organism most commonly associated with mucopurulent cervicitis.[4] Chronic cervicitis represents a low-grade inflammatory process. It is common in parous women and may be a sequela to minute lacerations that occur during childbirth, instrumentation, or other trauma. The organisms usually are of a nonspecific type, often staphylococcal, streptococcal, or coliform bacteria.

With acute cervicitis, the cervix becomes reddened and edematous. Irritation from the infection results in copious mucopurulent drainage and leukorrhea. The symptoms of chronic cervicitis are less well defined: the cervix may be ulcerated or normal in appearance; it may contain nabothian cysts; the cervical os may be distorted by old lacerations or everted to expose areas of columnar epithelium; and a mucopurulent drainage may be present.

Untreated cervicitis may extend to include the development of pelvic cellulitis, low back pain, painful intercourse, cervical stenosis, dysmenorrhea, and further infection of the uterus or fallopian tubes. Depending on the causative agent, acute cervicitis is treated with appropriate antibiotic therapy. Diagnosis of chronic cervicitis is based on vaginal examination, colposcopy, cytologic smears, and occasionally on biopsy to exclude malignant changes. The treatment usually involves cryosurgery or cauterization, which causes the tissues to slough and leads to eradication of the infection. Colposcopically guided laser vaporization of abnormal epithelium is the newest but most expensive treatment for cervicitis.

Polyps are the most common lesions of the cervix. They can be found in women of all ages, but their incidence is higher during the reproductive years. Polyps are soft, velvety-red lesions; they usually are pedunculated and often are found protruding through the cervical os. They usually develop as a result of inflammatory hyperplasia of the endocervical mucosa. Polyps typically are asymptomatic but may have associated postcoital bleeding. Most are benign, but they should be removed and examined by a pathologist to exclude malignant change.

Cancer of the Cervix

Cervical cancer is readily detected and, if detected early, it is the most easily cured of all the cancers of the female reproductive system. According to the American Cancer Society, an estimated 15,700 cases of invasive cervical cancer were diagnosed in 1996, with approximately 4900 deaths from cervical cancer during the same period. By comparison there were 65,000 new cases of cervical carcinoma in situ (*i.e.*, precancerous lesion) diagnosed, indicating that a large number of potentially invasive cancers are cured by early detection and effective treatment. The death rate has steadily declined over the past 50 years with the introduction of more sensitive and readily available screening methods (*e.g.*, Pap smear, colposcopy, cervicography), consistent use of a standardized grading system that guides treatment, and more effective treatment methods. However, the mortality rate is more than twice as high for black women than for white women. The 5-year survival rate for all cervical cancer patients is 68%. For women with localized disease, the 5-year survival rate is 91%, but only 51% of cancers are discovered that early.[7]

Carcinoma of the cervix is considered a sexually transmitted disease. It is rare among celibate women. Risk factors include early age at first intercourse, multiple sexual partners, a promiscuous male partner, smoking, and a history of sexually transmitted diseases.[8] Certain strains of HPV have been identified in invasive carcinoma of the cervix, whereas others are more often associated with dysplasia or cancer in situ. Because these viruses are spread by sexual contact, their association with cervical cancer provides a tempting hypothesis to explain the relation between sexual practices and cervical cancer. HPV is discussed further in Chapter 52.

One of the most important advances in the early diagnosis and treatment of cancer of the cervix was made possible by the observation that this cancer arises from precursor lesions, which begin with the development of atypical cervical cells.[9] These gradually progress to cancer in situ and to invasive cancer of the cervix. Atypical cells differ from normal cervical squamous epithelium. There are changes in the nuclear and cytoplasmic parts of the cell and more variation in cell size and shape (*i.e.*, dysplasia). Cancer in situ is localized to the epithelial layer, whereas invasive cancer of the cervix spreads to deeper layers.

A system of grading devised to describe the dysplastic changes of cancer precursors uses the term *cervical intraepithelial neoplasia* (CIN). The CIN system grades according to extent of involvement of the epithelial thickness of the cervix (see Table 51–1). After cancer has been diagnosed, the general preference is to use the International Federation of Gynecology and Obstetrics (FIGO) classification system to describe the histologic and clinical stage of the disease (Table 51–2). The development of an internationally accepted grading system

TABLE 51–2

Stages of Gynecologic Cancer

Stage	Description*
0	Rarely used; refers to preinvasive lesions
I	Cancer is confined to organ in which it originated
II	Cancer involves some of the structures surrounding the organ of origin
III	Regional spread of cancer with lymph node involvement
IV	Distant spread of cancer with metastasis

*This table represents a generic staging system used for most gynecologic cancers. The International Federation of Gynecology and Obstetrics (FIGO) system is a defined staging system used for each specific site and can be found in most cancer textbooks.

has significantly increased the database for cervical cancer and the consistency of that database.

The atypical cellular changes that precede frank neoplastic changes consistent with cancer of the cervix can be recognized by a number of direct and microscopic techniques, including the Pap smear, colposcopy, and cervicography. The precursor lesions can exist in a reversible form, which may regress spontaneously, or may progress and undergo malignant change. Cancers of the cervix have a long latent period; untreated dysplasia gradually progresses to carcinoma in situ, which may remain static for 7 to 10 years before it becomes invasive. After the preinvasive period, growth is rapid, and if the cancer is untreated, death follows within 2 to 5 years of the onset of symptoms.[4]

The purpose of the Pap smear (see Chapter 5) is to detect the presence of abnormal cells on the surface of the cervix or within the endocervix. This test detects precancerous and cancerous lesions. Although the American Cancer Society has suggested that the Pap smear need not be done annually if there have been three normal tests in succession, many clinicians maintain that performing an annual test is the safest course to follow. If the woman has risk factors, such as previous HPV infection, DES exposure in utero, or a strong family history of cervical cancer, more frequent Pap smears may be recommended.

Pap smears are only about 80% to 90% accurate in diagnosing CIN even under optimal circumstances. Care must be taken to obtain an adequate smear from the transformation zone that includes endocervical cells and to ensure that the cytologic examination is done by a competent laboratory. New techniques of specimen collection, slide preparation and processing, and computer-assisted evaluation of Pap smears are in the early stages of marketing and offer hope of improved accuracy in diagnosis of precancerous cervical changes.

The accepted format for reporting cervical and vaginal cytologic diagnoses, called *The Bethesda System* (TBS), was developed during a National Cancer Institute Workshop in 1989 and updated in 1991. TBS includes three components: a statement of specimen adequacy (*i.e.*, satisfactory, satisfactory but limited by . . ., unsatisfactory); general categorization (*i.e.*, within normal limits or other); and a descriptive diagnosis of findings (infection, reactive and reparative changes, hormonal balance, and epithelial cell abnormalities). Table 51–3 presents terms used to describe epithelial cell abnormalities.

In June 1992, the National Cancer Institute convened a workshop of experts to develop guidelines for management of abnormal cervical cytology based on the classifications in TBS. The minimally abnormal Pap smear (*i.e.*, atypical squamous cells of undetermined significance [ASCUS], low-grade squamous intraepithelial lesion [LSIL]) presents the greatest challenge to clinicians. The uncertain significance of ASCUS is often related to inflammation, atrophy, or other temporary or reversible processes. Even squamous intraepithelial lesions (SIL) regress spontaneously in about 60% of patients, and costly evaluation or aggressive treatment may not be warranted. Follow-up with repeat Pap smears at 3- to 6-month intervals is usually appropriate. If compliance with follow-up observation is uncertain, colposcopy, endocervical curettage, or directed biopsy may be used to confirm the presence of a lesion so treatment can be selected.[10]

The presence of normal endometrial cells in a cervical cytologic sample during the luteal phase of the menstrual cycle or during the postmenopausal period has been associated with endometrial disease and warrants further evaluation with endometrial biopsy. This demonstrates that shedding of even normal cells at an inappropriate time may indicate disease. Because adenocarcinoma of the cervix is being detected more frequently, especially in women younger than 35 years of age, an AGCUS Pap result warrants further evaluation by endocervical or endometrial curettage, hysteroscopy or ultimately a cone biopsy if the abnormality cannot be located or identified through other means.

Diagnosis of cervical cancer requires pathologic confirmation. Pap smear results demonstrating SIL often require further evaluation by colposcopy. This is a vaginal examination that is done using a colposcope, an instrument that affords a well-lighted and magnified stereoscopic view of the cervix. During colposcopy, the cervical tissue may be stained with an iodine solution (*i.e.*, Schiller's test) or acetic acid solution to accentuate topographic or vascular changes that can differentiate normal from abnormal tissue. A biopsy sample may be obtained from suspicious areas and examined microscopically.

A final diagnostic tool in areas where colposcopy is not readily available is cervicography, a noninvasive photographic technique that provides permanent objective documentation of normal and abnormal cervical patterns. Acetic acid (5%) is applied to the cervix, a cervicography camera is used to take photos, and the projected cervicogram (*i.e.*, slide after film developing) can be sent for expert evaluation. In one study, the cervicogram was found to give a greater yield of CIN than Pap smear alone.[11]

Before the availability of colposcopy, many women with abnormal Pap smears required surgical cone biopsy for further evaluation. Cone biopsy involves the removal of a cone-shaped wedge of cervix, including the entire transformation zone and at least 50% of the endocervical canal. Postoperative hemorrhage, infection, cervical stenosis, infertility, and incompetent cervix are possible sequelae that warrant avoidance of this procedure unless it is truly necessary. Diagnostic conization is still indicated when a lesion is partly or completely beyond colposcopic view or colposcopically directed biopsy fails to explain the cytology.

The *loop electrode excision procedure* (LEEP), a refinement of loop diathermy techniques dating back to the 1940s, is quickly becoming the first-line management for SIL. This outpatient procedure allows for the simultaneous diagnosis and treatment of dysplastic lesions found on colposcopy. It uses a thin, rigid, wire loop electrode attached to a generator that blends high-frequency, low-voltage current for cutting and a modulated higher voltage for coagulation. In skilled hands, this wire can remove the entire transformation zone, providing adequate treatment for the lesion while providing a specimen for further histologic evaluation. The width and depth of the tissue excised are controlled by the size and shape of the loop and the speed and pressure that is applied during the procedure. This can help avoid the problems that can occur after surgical cone biopsy (*e.g.*, stenosis, incompetent cervix). Bleeding can be minimized by fulguration of the base with electrocoagulation or by applying a thin layer of Monsel's gel (*i.e.*, chemical cautery). Although long-term results are not available, this procedure, which requires only local anesthesia, appears to provide a lower-cost, office-based alternative to cone biopsy.

Early treatment of cervical cancer involves removal of the lesion by one of various techniques. Biopsy or local cautery may be therapeutic in and of itself. Electrocautery, cryosurgery, or carbon dioxide laser therapy may be used to treat moderate to severe dysplasia that is limited to the exocervix (*i.e.*, squamocolumnar junction clearly visible). Therapeutic conization becomes necessary if the lesion extends into the endocervical canal and can be done surgically or with LEEP in the physician's office.[12]

Depending on the stage of involvement of the cervix, invasive cancer is treated with radiation therapy, surgery, or both. External beam irradiation and intracavitary cesium irradiation (*i.e.*, insertion of a closed metal cylinder containing cesium) can be used in the treatment of cervical cancer. Intracavitary radiation provides direct access to the central lesion and increases the tolerance of the cervix and surrounding tissues, permitting curative levels of radiation to be used. External beam radiation sterilizes metastatic disease in pelvic lymph nodes and other structures, as well as shrinking the cervical lesion to optimize the intracavitary radiation. Surgery can include extended hysterectomy (*i.e.*, removal of

TABLE 51-3

Epithelial Cell Abnormalities

Squamous Cell

ASCUS: atypical squamous cells of undetermined significance
- Favor reactive (probably benign)
- Favor dysplasia (consider same as SIL)

LSIL: low-grade squamous intraepithelial lesion
- Includes HPV effect and mild dysplasia (CIN I)

HSIL: high-grade squamous intraepithelial lesion
- Includes moderate and severe dysplasia of cancer in situ (CIN II and III)

SCC: squamous cell carcinoma

Glandular Cell

Presence of endometrial cells
- Out of phase in a menstruating woman
- In a postmenopausal woman
- No menstrual history available

AGCUS: atypical glandular cells of undetermined significance
- Endometrial
- Endocervical
- Not otherwise specified

Adenocarcinoma
- Specify site: endometrial, endocervical, extrauterine, not specified

the uterus, fallopian tubes, ovaries, and upper portion of the vagina) without pelvic lymph node dissection, radical hysterectomy with pelvic lymph node dissection, or pelvic exenteration (*i.e.*, removal of all pelvic organs, including the bladder, rectum, vulva, and vagina). The choice of treatment usually is influenced by the woman's age and health.[4]

Disorders of the Uterus

Endometritis

Inflammation or infection of the endometrium is an ill-defined entity that produces variable symptoms. The presence of plasma cells is required for diagnosis. Endometritis can occur as a postpartum or postabortal infection, with gonococcal or chlamydial salpingitis, after instrumentation or surgery, or can be associated with an intrauterine device or tuberculosis.[13] Causative organisms, in addition to *N. gonorrhoeae, Chlamydia*, and *Mycobacterium tuberculosis*, include *Escherichia coli, Proteus, Pseudomonas, Klebsiella, Bacteroides*, and *Mycoplasma* species. Abnormal vaginal bleeding, mild to severe uterine tenderness, fever, malaise, and foul-smelling discharge have been associated with endometritis, but the clinical picture is variable. Treatment involves oral or intravenous antibiotic therapy, depending on the severity of the condition.

Endometriosis

Endometriosis is the condition in which functional endometrial tissue is found in ectopic sites outside the uterus. The site may be the ovaries, broad ligaments, pouch of Douglas (cul-de-sac), pelvis, vagina, vulva, perineum, or intestines. Rarely, endometrial implants have been found in the nostrils, umbilicus, lungs, and limbs.

The cause of endometriosis is unknown. There appears to have been an increase in its incidence in the developing Western countries during the past four to five decades. About 10% to 15% of premenopausal women have some degree of endometriosis. The incidence may be higher in women with infertility (23% to 40%) or women younger than 20 years of age with chronic pelvic pain (50%).[14] It is more common in women who have postponed childbearing. Risk factors for endometriosis may include early menarche; regular periods with shorter cycles (≤27 days), longer duration (>7 days), or heavier flow; increased menstrual pain; and other first-degree relatives with the condition.

Several theories attempt to account for endometriosis. One theory suggests that menstrual blood containing fragments of endometrium is forced upward through the fallopian tubes into the peritoneal cavity. Retrograde menstruation is not an uncommon phenomenon, and it is unknown why endometrial cells implant and grow in some women but not in others. Another proposal is that dormant, immature cellular elements spread over a wide area during embryonic development persist into adult life and that the ensuing metaplasia accounts for the development of ectopic endometrial tissue. Another theory suggests that the endometrial tissue may metastasize through the lymphatics or vascular system.

The gross pathologic changes that occur in endometriosis differ with location and duration. In the ovary, the endometrial tissue may form cysts (*i.e.*, endometriomas filled with old blood that resembles chocolate syrup [*chocolate cysts*]). Rupture of these cysts can cause peritonitis and adhesions. Elsewhere in the pelvis, the tissue may take the form of small hemorrhagic lesions that may be black, bluish, or red and clear or opaque. Some may be surrounded by scar tissue. These ectopic implants respond to hormonal stimulation in the same way normal endometrium does, becoming proliferative, then secretory, and finally undergoing menstrual breakdown. Bleeding into the surrounding structures can cause pain and the development of significant pelvic adhesions. Extensive fibrotic tissue can develop and cause bowel obstruction.

Endometriosis may be difficult to diagnose because its symptoms mimic those of other pelvic disorders. The severity of the symptoms does not always reflect the extent of the disease. The classic triad of dysmenorrhea, dyspareunia, and infertility strongly suggests endometriosis. Accurate diagnosis can be accomplished only through laparoscopy. This minimally invasive surgery allows direct visualization of pelvic organs to determine the presence and extent of endometrial lesions.

The treatment modalities for endometriosis fall into three categories: pain relief, endometrial suppression, and surgery. In young, unmarried women, simple observation and antiprostaglandin analgesics (*i.e.*, nonsteroidal antiinflammatory drugs [NSAIDs]) may be sufficient treatment. The use of hormones to induce physiologic amenorrhea is based on the observation that pregnancy affords temporary relief by inducing atrophy of the endometrial tissue. This can be accomplished through administration of progesterone, oral contraceptive pills, danazol (a synthetic androgen), or long-acting gonadotropin-releasing hormone analogues that inhibit the pituitary gonadotropins and suppress ovulation.[15]

Surgery is the most definitive therapy for many women with endometriosis. In the past, laparoscopic use of cautery was limited to mild endometriosis without extensive adhesions. With the advent of carbon dioxide or potassium-titanyl-phosphate (KTP) lasers, in-depth treatment of endometriosis or pelvic adhesions can be accomplished by means of laparoscopy. Advantages of laser surgery include better hemostasis, more precision in vaporizing lesions with less damage to surrounding tissue, and better access to areas that are not well visualized or would be difficult to reach with cautery. The KTP laser is particularly useful for endometriosis because of its flexible fiberoptic delivery system, which allows tissue incision and vaporization in addition to photocoagulation, and its green beam, which makes visualization and fine focusing easier.[16] Radical treatment involves total hysterectomy and bilateral salpingo-oophorectomy (*i.e.*, removal of the fallopian tubes and ovaries) when the symptoms are unbearable or the woman's childbearing is completed.

Treatment offers relief but not cure. Recurrence of endometriosis is not uncommon, regardless of the treatment (except for radical surgery). According to one source, recurrence rates confirmed by surgery were 10% after 3 years and 35% after 5 years.[4] Pregnancy may delay but does not preclude recurrence.

Adenomyosis

Adenomyosis is the condition in which endometrial glands and stroma are found within the myometrium, interspersed between the smooth muscle fibers. In contrast to endometriosis, which usually is a problem of young, infertile women, adenomyosis typically is found in multiparous women in their late 30s or 40s. It is thought that events associated with repeated pregnancies, deliveries, and uterine involution may cause the endometrium to be displaced throughout the myometrium. Adenomyosis frequently coexists with uterine myomas or endometrial hyperplasia. The diagnosis of adenomyosis often occurs as an incidental finding in a uterus removed for symptoms suggestive of myoma or hyperplasia. Adenomyosis resolves with menopause. Hysterectomy (with preservation of the ovaries in premenopausal women) is the treatment of choice. Efforts to control this condition with pelvic irradiation or medication to suppress ovarian stimulation have been largely unsuccessful.[17]

Endometrial Cancer

Endometrial cancer is the most common cancer found within the female pelvis; it occurs more than twice as often as cervical cancer. In 1996, the American Cancer Society estimated that there would be 34,000 cases diagnosed and 6000 deaths from endometrial cancer.[7] Endometrial cancer occurs more frequently in older women (peak ages of 55 to 65), with only a 2% to 5% incidence among women younger than 40 years of age.

Prolonged estrogen stimulation with excessive growth (*i.e.*, hyperplasia) of endometrium has been identified as a major risk factor for endometrial cancer. Estrogens are synthesized in body fats from adrenal and ovarian androgen precursors. Endometrial hyperplasia and endometrial cancer appear to be related to obesity and anovulatory cycles. Anovulatory dysfunction that causes infertility at any age or occurs with declining ovarian function in perimenopausal women can also result in unopposed estrogen and increase the risk of endometrial cancer. Diabetes mellitus, hypertension, polycystic ovary syndrome (previously called Stein-Leventhal syndrome) are conditions that alter estrogen metabolism and elevate estrogen levels. Women with estrogen-secreting ovarian tumors are also at increased risk for endometrial cancer, as are women receiving unopposed estrogen therapy (*i.e.*, estrogen therapy without progesterone).

A sharp rise in endometrial cancer was seen in the 1970s among middle-aged women who had received estrogen therapy for menopausal symptoms. It was later determined that it was not the estrogen exposure that increased the risk of cancer, but that the hormone was administered without progesterone. It is the presence of progesterone in the second half of the menstrual cycle that matures the endometrium and the withdrawal of progesterone that ultimately results in endometrial sloughing. Long-term unopposed estrogen exposure without periodic addition of progesterone allows for continued endometrial growth. Hyperplasia may develop, with or without the presence of atypical cells, and can progress to carcinoma if left untreated. Hyperplasia usually regresses after treatment with cyclic progesterone. Sequential oral contraceptives (estrogen alone or 15 days followed by 7 days of combined estrogen and progestin) were withdrawn from the market in the 1970s because of increased risk of endometrial hyperplasia. In contrast, combination oral contraceptives (estrogen and progestin in each pill) effectively prevent hyperplasia and decrease the risk of cancer by 50%.[18] Tamoxifen, a drug that blocks estrogen receptor sites and is used in treatment of breast cancer, exerts a weak estrogenic effect on the endometrium and represents another exogenous risk factor for endometrial cancer.

A small subset of women who develop endometrial cancer do not exhibit increased estrogen levels or preexisting hyperplasia. These women usually acquire the disease at an older age. These tumors arise from clones of cancer-initiated mutant cells and are more poorly differentiated. This type of endometrial cancer generally has a poorer prognosis than that associated with prolonged estrogen stimulation and endometrial hyperplasia.[18]

The major symptom of endometrial hyperplasia or overt endometrial cancer is abnormal, painless bleeding. In menstruating women, this takes the form of bleeding between periods or excessive prolonged menstrual flow. In postmenopausal women, any bleeding is abnormal and warrants investigation. Abnormal bleeding is an early warning sign of the disease, and because endometrial cancer tends to be slow growing in its early stages, the chances of cure are good if prompt medical care is sought. Later signs of uterine cancer may include cramping, pelvic discomfort, postcoital bleeding, lower abdominal pressure, and enlarged lymph nodes. Although the Pap smear can identify a small percentage of endometrial cancers, it is not a good screening test for this gynecologic cancer. Endometrial biopsy (*i.e.*, tissue sampling obtained in an office procedure by direct aspiration of the endometrial cavity) is far more accurate; 80% to 90% of endometrial cancers are identified if adequate tissue is obtained. Dilatation and curettage (D&C), which consists of dilating the cervix and scraping the uterine cavity, is the definitive procedure for diagnosis, because it provides a more thorough evaluation. Transvaginal ultrasound used to measure the endometrial thickness is being evaluated as an initial test for postmenopausal bleeding, because it is less invasive than endometrial biopsy and less costly than D&C when biopsy is not possible.

Surgery and radiation therapy are the most successful methods of treatment for endometrial cancer. When used alone, radiation therapy has a 20% lower cure rate than surgery for stage I disease. It may be the best option, however, in women who are not good surgical candidates. Total abdominal hysterectomy with bilateral salpingo-oophorectomy plus sampling of regional lymph nodes and peritoneal washings for cytologic evaluation of occult disease is the treatment of choice whenever possible. Postoperative radiation therapy is added in cases of advanced disease for more complete treatment and to prevent recurrence or metastasis. Preoperative radiation is rarely used today. With early diagnosis and treatment, the 5-year survival rate ranges from 83% to 95%. This decreases to 18.7% for stage IV disease.[4]

Leiomyomas

Leiomyomas are benign neoplasms of smooth muscle origin. They are also known as *myomas* and sometimes called *fibroids*. These are the most common form of pelvic tumor and are believed to occur in one of every four or five women older than 35 years of age. They are

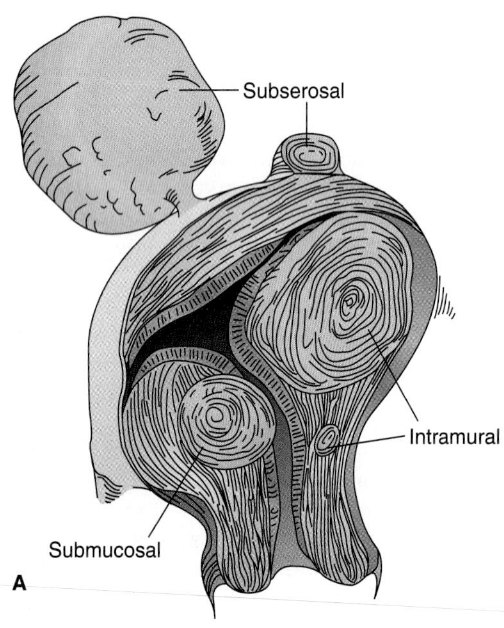

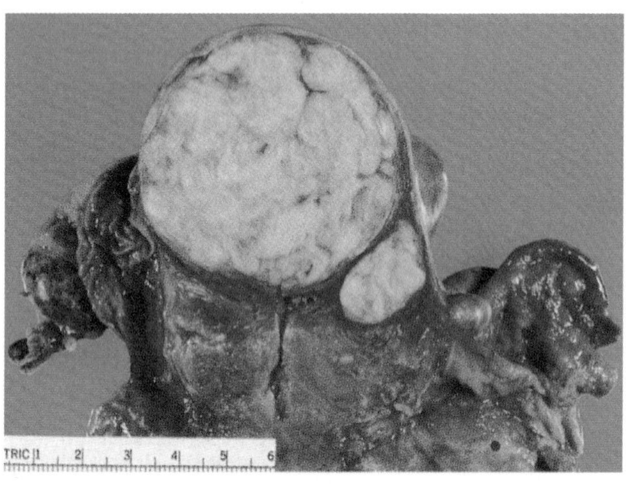

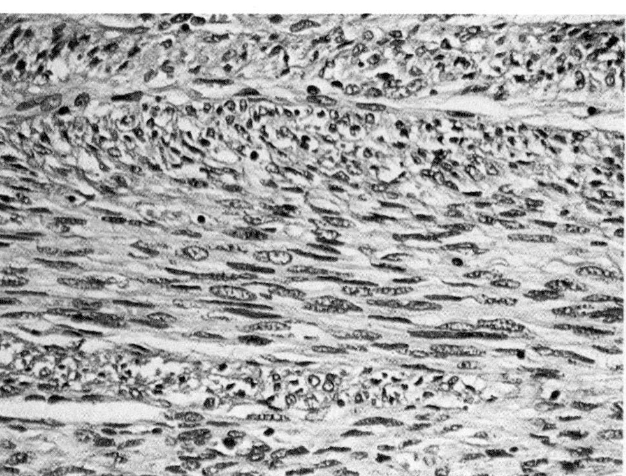

Figure 51–4
(**A**) Submucosal, intramural, and subserosal leiomyomas. (**B,C**) Leiomyoma of the uterus: (**B**) a bisected uterus displays a prominent, sharply circumscribed, fleshy tumor; (**C**) microscopically, smooth muscle cells intertwine in bundles, some of which are cut longitudinally (elongated nuclei) and others transversely. (**A** redrawn from Green T.H. [1977]. *Gynecology: Essentials of clinical practice* [3rd ed.] Boston: Little, Brown.)

seen more often and their rate of growth is more rapid in black women than in white women. Leiomyomas usually develop in the corpus of the uterus; they may be submucosal, subserosal, or intramural (Fig. 51–4). Intramural fibroids are embedded within the myometrium. They are the most common type of fibroids, taking the form of a symmetric enlargement of the nonpregnant uterus. *Subserosal* tumors are located beneath the perimetrium of the uterus. These tumors are recognized as irregular projections on the uterine surface; they may become pedunculated, displacing or impinging on other genitourinary structures and causing hydroureter or bladder problems. *Submucosal* fibroids displace endometrial tissue and are more likely to cause bleeding, necrosis, and infection than either of the other types.

Leiomyomas may be asymptomatic and be discovered during a routine pelvic examination, or they may cause bleeding, particularly at the time of the menstrual period. Their rate of growth is variable, but they may increase in size during pregnancy or with exogenous estrogen stimulation (*i.e.*, oral contraceptives or menopausal estrogen replacement therapy). Interference with pregnancy is rare unless the tumor is submucosal and interferes with implantation or obstructs the cervical outlet. These tumors may outgrow their blood supply, become infarcted, and undergo degenerative changes. Most leiomyomas regress with menopause, but if bleeding, pressure on the bladder, pain, or other problems persist, hysterectomy may be required. Myomectomy (*i.e.*, removal of just the tumors) can be done to preserve the uterus for future childbearing. Caesarean section may be recommended if the uterine cavity is entered during myomectomy. Gonadotropin-releasing hormone antagonists (*e.g.*, leuprolide [Lupron]) may be used to suppress leiomyoma growth before surgery.

In summary, disorders of the cervix and uterus include inflammatory conditions (*i.e.*, cervicitis and endometritis), cancer (*i.e.*, cervical and endometrial cancer), endometriosis, and leiomyomas. Cervicitis is an acute or chronic inflammation of the cervix. Acute cervicitis may result from the direct infection of the cervix or may be secondary to a vaginal or uterine infection. It may be caused by a variety of infective agents. Chronic cervicitis represents a low-grade inflammatory process resulting from trauma or nonspecific infectious agents. Cervical cancer is readily detected, and if detected early, it is the most easily cured of all the cancers of the female reproductive system. It arises from precursor lesions that can be detected on a Pap smear; the condition can be cured if detected and treated early.

Endometritis represents an ill-defined inflammation or infection of the endometrium that produces variable symptoms. Endometriosis is the condition in which functional endometrial tissue is found in ectopic sites outside the uterus such as the ovaries, broad ligaments, pouch of Douglas (cul-de-sac), pelvis, vagina, vulva, perineum, or intestines. It causes dysmenorrhea, dyspareunia, and infertility. Adenomyosis is the condition in which endometrial glands and stroma are found within the myometrium, interspersed between the smooth muscle fibers. Endometrial cancer is the most common cancer found within the female pelvis; it occurs more than twice as often as cervical cancer. Prolonged estrogen stimulation with hyperplasia of the endometrium has been identified as a major risk factor for endometrial cancer.

Leiomyomas are benign uterine wall neoplasms of smooth muscle origin. They can develop in the corpus of the uterus, and can be submucosal, subserosal, or intramural. Submucosal fibroids displace endometrial tissue and are more likely to cause bleeding, necrosis, and infection than either of the other types.

Disorders of the Fallopian Tubes and Ovaries

After you have completed this section of the chapter, you should be able to meet the following objectives:

- List the common causes and symptoms of pelvic inflammatory disease
- State the causative factors associated with tubal pregnancy
- Describe the symptoms of a tubal pregnancy
- State the underlying cause of ovarian cysts
- Differentiate benign ovarian cyst from polycystic ovary syndrome (previously called Stein-Leventhal syndrome)
- List the hormones produced by the three types of functioning ovarian tumors
- State the reason that ovarian cancer may be difficult to detect in an early stage

Pelvic Inflammatory Disease

Pelvic inflammatory disease (PID) is an inflammation of the upper reproductive tract that involves the uterus (*i.e.*, endometritis), fallopian tubes (*i.e.*, salpingitis), or ovaries (*i.e.*, oophoritis). About 80% of women with acute salpingitis have *N. gonorrhoeae* or *C. trachomatis* identified within the reproductive tract.[19] PID is a polymicrobial infection and the cause varies by geographic location and population.[20] In addition to the primary causative agents already mentioned *Mycoplasma hominis*, *Ureaplasma urealcyticum*, *Bacteroides*, *Peptostreptococcus*, *E. coli*, *Haemophilus influenzae*, and *Streptococcus agalactiae* may be involved. The organisms ascend through the endocervical canal to the endometrial cavity and then to the tubes and ovaries. The endocervical canal is slightly dilated during menstruation; bacteria can gain entrance to the uterus and other pelvic structures. After entering the upper reproductive tract, the organisms multiply rapidly in the favorable environment of the sloughing endometrium and ascend to the fallopian tube.

Factors that predispose women to the development of PID include ages 16 to 24, unmarried status, nulliparity, history of multiple sexual partners, and previous history of PID. Although the use of an intrauterine contraceptive device (IUD) has been associated with a threefold to fivefold increased risk of developing PID, studies have shown that women with only one sexual partner who are at low risk of acquiring sexually transmitted diseases (STD) have no significant risk of developing PID from using an IUD.

The symptoms of PID include lower abdominal pain, which may start just after a menstrual period; purulent cervical discharge; adnexal tenderness; and an exquisitely painful cervix. Fever (greater than 100.4°F [41°C]), increased erythrocyte sedimentation rate, and an elevated white blood cell count (>10,000 cells/μl) commonly are seen, even though the woman may not appear acutely ill. A newer test involves measurement of C reactive protein (CRP) in the blood. Elevated CRP levels equate with inflammation.

Treatment may involve hospitalization with intravenous administration of antibiotics. If the condition is diagnosed early, outpatient antibiotic therapy may be sufficient. Antibiotic regimens should be selected according to STD treatment guidelines, which are published every 4 years by the Centers for Disease Control. Treatment is aimed at preventing complications, which can include pelvic adhesions, infertility, ectopic pregnancy, chronic abdominal pain, and tubo-ovarian abscesses. Accurate diagnosis and appropriate antibiotic therapy may decrease the severity and frequency of PID sequelae.

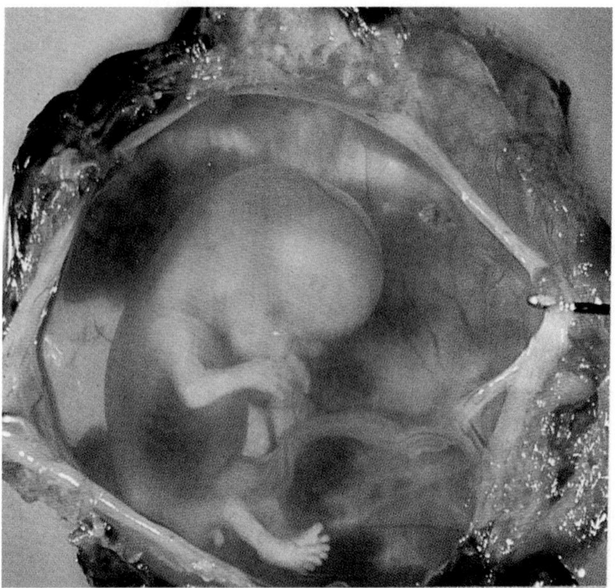

Figure 51–5
Ectopic pregnancy. An enlarged fallopian tube has been opened to disclose a minute fetus.

Ectopic Pregnancy

Although pregnancy is not discussed in detail in this text, it is reasonable to mention ectopic pregnancy, because it represents a true gynecologic emergency and should be considered when a woman of reproductive age presents with the complaint of pelvic pain.[21] Ectopic pregnancy occurs when a fertilized ovum implants outside the uterine cavity. The most common site for ectopic pregnancy is the fallopian tube (Fig. 51–5). According to the Centers for Disease Control, between 1970 and 1987, the number of ectopic pregnancies increased from 17,800 to 88,000; the rate of occurrence among females between the ages of 15 to 44 rose from 4.5 to 16.8 per 1000 reported pregnancies (*i.e.*, live births, abortions, and ectopics). Although complications from ectopic pregnancy are one of two leading causes of maternal death in the United States, the death rate has steadily declined to its current rate of 3.4 per 10,000 ectopic pregnancies.[22]

The cause of ectopic pregnancy is delayed ovum transport, which may result from decreased tubal motility or distorted tubal anatomy (*i.e.*, narrowed lumen, convolutions, or diverticula). Factors that may predispose to the development of an ectopic pregnancy include PID, therapeutic abortion, tubal ligation or tubal reversal, previous ectopic pregnancy, intrauterine exposure to DES, infertility, and the use of fertility drugs to induce ovulation. Contraceptive failure with progestin-only birth control pills or the "morning-after pill" has also been associated with ectopic pregnancy.[4]

The site of implantation within the tube (*e.g.*, isthmus, ampulla) may determine the onset of symptoms and the timing of diagnosis. As the tubal pregnancy progresses, the surrounding tissue is stretched. The pregnancy eventually outgrows its blood supply, at which point the pregnancy terminates or the tube itself ruptures because it can no longer contain the growing pregnancy. Symptoms can include lower abdominal discomfort—diffuse or localized to one side—which progresses to severe pain caused by rupture, spotting, syncope, referred shoulder pain from bleeding into the abdominal cavity, and amenorrhea. Physical examination usually reveals adnexal tenderness; an adnexal mass is found in only 50% of cases. Culdocentesis (*i.e.*, needle aspiration from the cul-de-sac) may reveal blood if rupture has occurred. Quantitative β-human chorionic gonadotropin (hCG) pregnancy tests may detect lower than normal hCG production. Pelvic ultrasound studies after 5 weeks' gestation may demonstrate an empty uterine cavity or presence of the gestational sac outside the uterus. Definitive diagnosis may require laparoscopy. Differential diagnosis for this type of pelvic pain includes ruptured ovarian cyst, threatened or incomplete abortion, PID, acute appendicitis, and degenerating fibroid.

Treatment is generally surgical: a laparoscopic salpingostomy to remove the ectopic pregnancy if the fallopian tube has not ruptured or salpingectomy to remove the tube if it has. In salpingostomy, a linear incision is made in the tube and allowed to heal closed without suturing to decrease scar tissue formation; this procedure preserves fertility but requires careful surgical technique to minimize the risk of recurrent ectopic pregnancies. Laparoscopic treatment of ectopic pregnancy is well tolerated and more cost effective than laparotomy because of shorter convalescence and the reduced need for postoperative analgesia. When possible, it is the preferred method of treatment. In laparotomy, an open incision is made into the abdominopelvic cavity; this procedure becomes necessary when there is uncontrolled internal bleeding, when the ectopic site cannot be visualized through the laparoscope, or when the surgeon is not trained in operative laparoscopy.[2]

Methotrexate, a chemotherapeutic agent, has been successfully used to eliminate residual ectopic pregnancy tissue after laparoscopy or in cases where the pregnancy is unruptured and surgery is contraindicated. The drug is given for 1 to 8 days and is better tolerated when given orally. Adverse effects can include oral lesions, transient elevation of liver enzyme levels, and anemia. Close follow-up with weekly monitoring of hCG levels is necessary until the pregnancy is completely resolved.

Cancer of the Fallopian Tube

Cancer of the fallopian tube is rare, accounting for less than 1% of all female genital tract cancers. Fewer than 3000 cases have been reported. Diagnosis of this cancer is extremely difficult, and the disease may be well advanced when found. Most primary tubal cancers are papillary adenocarcinomas, and these tumors develop bilaterally in 40% to 50% of patients.[4]

Symptoms are uncommon, but intermittent serosanguineous vaginal discharge, abnormal vaginal bleeding, and colicky low abdominal pain have been reported. An adnexal mass may be present; however, the preoperative diagnosis in most cases is leiomyoma or ovarian tumor. Treatment is total hysterectomy, bilateral salpingo-oophorectomy, and pelvic lymph node dissection. More extensive procedures may be warranted, depending on the stage of the disease. The 5-year survival rates vary from 0% to 44%; if metastasis has occurred, the prognosis is poor.

Benign Ovarian Cysts and Tumors

The ovaries have a dual function: they produce germ cells, or ova, and they synthesize the female sex hormones. Disorders of the ovaries frequently cause menstrual and fertility problems. Benign conditions of the ovaries can present as primary lesions of the ovarian structures or as secondary disorders related to hypothalamic, pituitary, or adrenal dysfunction.

Ovarian Cysts

Cysts are the most common form of ovarian tumor. Many are benign. A follicular cyst is one that results from occlusion of the duct of the follicle. Each month, several follicles begin to develop and are blighted at various stages of development. These follicles form cavities that fill with fluid, producing a cyst. The dominant follicle normally ruptures to release the egg (*i.e.*, ovulation) but occasionally persists and continues growing. Likewise, a luteal cyst is a persistent cystic enlargement of the corpus luteum that is formed after ovulation and does not regress in the absence of pregnancy. Functional cysts are asymptomatic unless there is substantial enlargement or bleeding into the cyst. This can cause considerable discomfort or a dull, aching sensation on the affected side. The cyst may become twisted or may rupture into the intraabdominal cavity. These cysts usually regress spontaneously.

Ovarian dysfunction associated with infrequent or absent menses in obese, infertile women was first reported in the 1930s by Stein and Leventhal, for whom the syndrome was originally named. *Polycystic ovary disease* is characterized by numerous cystic follicles or follicle cysts. Once thought to be relatively rare, it appears that this clinical entity is one of the most common endocrinologic disorders among women in the reproductive years. The syndrome is characterized by various degrees of hirsutism, obesity, and infertility. Anovulation, causing amenorrhea or irregular menses, commonly accompanies the finding of bilaterally enlarged polycystic ovaries. Whether this condition is a primary ovarian defect or a result of hypothalamic-pituitary dysfunction is still being debated.

Most women with polycystic ovary disease have elevated luteinizing hormone (LH) levels with normal estrogen and follicle-stimulating hormone (FSH) production. Elevated levels of testosterone, dehydroepiandrosterone sulfate (DHAS), or androstenedione are not uncommon, and these women occasionally have hyperprolactinemia or hypothyroidism. The diagnosis can be suspected from the clinical picture and confirmed with ultrasound or laparoscopic visualization of the ovaries. When fertility is desired, the condition usually is treated by the administration of the hypothalamic-pituitary–stimulating drug clomiphene citrate to induce ovulation. This drug is used carefully because it can induce extreme enlargement of the ovaries. When medication is ineffective, laser surgery to puncture the multiple follicles can be helpful to restore normal ovulatory function. If fertility is not desired, oral contraceptives can induce regular menses and prevent the development of endometrial hyperplasia caused by unopposed estrogen. Chronic anovulation can increase a woman's risk of endometrial cancer, cardiovascular disease, and hyperinsulinemia leading to diabetes mellitus. Treatment is essential for anyone with this condition.[23]

Benign and Functioning Ovarian Tumors

Serous cystadenoma and mucinous cystadenoma are the most common benign ovarian neoplasms. Some of these adenomas, however, are considered to have low malignant potential. They are asymptomatic unless the size is sufficient to cause abdominal enlargement. *Endometriomas* are the chocolate cysts that develop secondarily to ovarian endometriosis (see the endometriosis section earlier in this chapter). *Ovarian fibromas* are connective tissue tumors composed of fibrocytes and collagen.

They range in size from 6 to 20 cm. *Cystic teratomas,* or *dermoid cysts,* are derived from primordial germ cells and are composed of various combinations of well-differentiated ectodermal, mesodermal, and endodermal elements. Not uncommonly, they contain sebaceous material, hair, or teeth. Treatment for all ovarian tumors is surgical excision. Ovarian tissue that is not affected by the tumor can be left intact if frozen-section analysis does not reveal malignancy. When ovarian tumors are very large, as is frequently the case with serous or mucinous cystadenomas, the entire ovary must be removed.

The three types of *functioning ovarian tumors* are estrogen secreting, androgen secreting, and mixed estrogen-androgen secreting. These tumors may be benign or cancerous. One such tumor, the granulosa cell tumor, is associated with excess estrogen production. When it develops during the reproductive period, the persistent and uncontrolled production of estrogen interferes with the normal menstrual cycle, causing irregular and excessive bleeding, endometrial hyperplasia, or amenorrhea and fertility problems. When it develops after menopause, it causes postmenopausal bleeding, stimulation of the glandular tissues of the breast, and other signs of renewed estrogen production. Androgen-secreting tumors (*i.e.,* Sertoli-Leydig cell tumor or androblastoma) inhibit ovulation and estrogen production. They tend to cause hirsutism and development of masculine characteristics, such as baldness, acne, oily skin, breast atrophy, and deepening of the voice. The treatment is surgical removal of the tumor.

Ovarian Cancer

Ovarian cancer is the second most common female genitourinary cancer and the most lethal. In 1996, 26,700 new cases of ovarian cancer were reported in the United States, two thirds of which were in advanced stages of the disease. Most of these women die of the disease (14,800 women in 1996).[7] The incidence of ovarian cancer increases with age, being greatest between the ages of 65 and 84. Ovarian cancer is difficult to diagnose, and 60% to 70% of women have metastatic disease before the time of discovery. The most significant risk factor for ovarian cancer appears to be ovulatory age—the length of time during a woman's life when her ovarian cycle is not suppressed by pregnancy, lactation, or oral contraceptive use. The incidence of ovarian cancer is much lower in countries where women bear numerous children than in the United States.

Cancer of the ovary is complex because of the diversity of tissue types that originate in the ovary. As a result of this diversity, there are several types of ovarian cancers. Malignant neoplasms of the ovary can be divided into three categories: epithelial tumors, germ cell tumors, and gonadal stromal tumors. Epithelial tumors account for about 80% of cases. These different cancers display various degrees of virulence, depending on the type of tumor and degree of differentiation involved. A well-differentiated cancer of the ovary may have produced symptoms for many months and still be found operable at the time of surgery. A poorly differentiated tumor may have been clinically evident for only a few days but found to be widespread and inoperable. Often no correlation exists between the duration of symptoms and the extent of the disease.

Most cancers of the ovary produce no symptoms, or the symptoms are so vague that the woman seldom seeks medical care until the disease is far advanced. These vague discomforts include abdominal distress, flatulence, and bloating, especially after ingesting food. These gastrointestinal manifestations may precede other symptoms by months. Many women take antacids or bicarbonate of soda for a time before consulting a physician. The physician may also dismiss the woman's complaints as being caused by other conditions, further delaying diagnosis and treatment. It is not fully understood why the initial symptoms of ovarian cancer are manifested as gastrointestinal disturbances. It is thought that biochemical changes in the peritoneal fluids may irritate the bowel or that pain originating in the ovary may be referred to the abdomen and be interpreted as a gastrointestinal disturbance. Clinically evident ascites (*i.e.,* fluid in the peritoneal cavity) is seen in about one fourth of women with malignant ovarian tumors and is associated with a worse prognosis.

No good screening tests or other early methods of detection exist for ovarian cancer. The serum tumor marker CA 125 is a cell surface antigen; its level is elevated in 80% to 90% of women with stage II nonmucinous ovarian epithelial cancers. The result is negative, however, for as many as 50% of women with stage I disease. In a postmenopausal woman with a pelvic mass, an elevated CA 125 has a positive predictive value of greater than 70% for cancer. It can also be used in monitoring therapy and recurrences when preoperative levels have been elevated. Despite its role in diagnostic evaluation and follow-up, CA 125 is not cancer or tissue specific for ovarian cancer. Levels are also elevated in the presence of endometriosis, uterine fibroids, pregnancy, liver disease, and other benign conditions and with cancer of the endometrium, cervix, fallopian tube, and pancreas. Because it lacks sensitivity and specificity, CA 125 has limited value as a single screening test, but combining CA 125 with other serum tumor markers (*e.g.,* CA 15–3, TAG 72.3) may improve specificity.[24]

Transvaginal ultrasonography (TVS) has been used to evaluate ovarian masses for malignant potential. As a screening test, it has demonstrated 80% to 90% sensitivity and 83% to 95% specificity. Because the lifetime risk of developing ovarian cancer is 1 in 70 women with no family history of the disease, the cost of universal screening for ovarian cancer using the available technology has been estimated at $1 million to save one woman. The combined use of sonography and CA 125 to screen all women older than age 45 would cost about $14 billion annually.[25] The National Institutes of Health Consensus Panel convened in 1995 recommended no widespread screening of women for ovarian cancer. CA 125 with TVS is suggested only for women who are part of a family with hereditary ovarian cancer syndrome (*i.e.*, two or more affected first-degree relatives), which is fewer than 1% of women.[26] Molecular biologic studies have identified tumor suppressor genes that may play a role in the cause of ovarian cancer. Overexpression, mutation, or deletion of various genes of chromosome 17 may explain the increased risk for these women. Further evaluation in this area is ongoing and may eventually lead to identification of appropriate screening techniques for ovarian cancer.

When ovarian cancer is suspected, surgical evaluation is required for diagnosis, complete and accurate staging, and cytoreduction and debulking procedures to reduce the size of the tumor. At the time of surgery, the uterus, fallopian tubes, ovaries, and omentum are removed; the liver, diaphragm, retroperitoneal and aortic lymph nodes, and peritoneal surface are examined and biopsies are taken as needed. Cytologic washings are done to test for cancerous cells in the peritoneal fluid. Recommendations regarding treatment beyond surgery and prognosis depend on the stage of the disease. Women with limited disease (*i.e.*, stage Ia or Ib that is well differentiated) generally do not require adjuvant treatment; women with intermediate disease (*i.e.*, stage Ib or II) or advanced disease (*i.e.*, stage III or IV) can benefit from chemotherapy with cisplatin and cyclophosphamide. When this combination therapy fails, salvage chemotherapy with newer drugs such as paclitaxel (Taxol) may prolong survival. Irradiation no longer plays a major role in treatment of ovarian cancer because of the difficulty in irradiating the entire abdomen without causing life-threatening damage to vital organs.

The lack of accurate screening tools and the resistant nature of ovarian cancers significantly affects success of treatment and survival. Five-year survival is 91% for women whose ovarian cancer is detected and treated early; however, only 23% of all cases are detected at the localized stage. Overall, the 5-year survival rate is 44%.[7]

In summary, PID is an inflammation of the upper reproductive tract that involves the uterus (*i.e.*, endometritis), fallopian tubes (*i.e.*, salpingitis), or ovaries (*i.e.*, oophoritis). It is most commonly caused by *N. gonorrhoeae* or *C. trachomatis*. Accurate diagnosis and appropriate antibiotic therapy are aimed at preventing complications such as pelvic adhesions, infertility, ectopic pregnancy, chronic abdominal pain, and tubo-ovarian abscesses.

Ectopic pregnancy occurs when a fertilized ovum implants outside the uterine cavity; the common site is the fallopian tube. Causes of ectopic pregnancy are delayed ovum transport resulting from complications of PID, therapeutic abortion, tubal ligation or tubal reversal, previous ectopic pregnancy, or other conditions such use of fertility drugs to induce ovulation. It represents a true gynecologic emergency, often necessitating surgical intervention. Cancer of the fallopian tube is rare; the diagnosis is difficult, and the condition usually is well advanced when diagnosed.

Disorders of the ovaries include benign cysts, functioning ovarian tumors, and cancer of the ovary; they are usually asymptomatic unless there is substantial enlargement or bleeding into the cyst or the cyst becomes twisted or ruptures. Polycystic ovarian disease (formerly known as Stein-Leventhal syndrome) is characterized by numerous cystic follicles or follicle cysts; it causes various degrees of hirsutism, obesity, and infertility. Benign ovarian tumors consist of endometriomas, which are chocolate cysts that develop secondarily to ovarian endometriosis; ovarian fibromas, which are connective tissue tumors composed of fibrocytes and collagen; and cystic teratomas or dermoid cysts, which are derived from primordial germ cells and are composed of various combinations of well-differentiated ectodermal, mesodermal, and endodermal elements. Functioning ovarian tumors are of three types: estrogen secreting, androgen secreting, and mixed estrogen-androgen secreting and may be benign or cancerous. Cancer of the ovary is the second most common female genitourinary cancer and the most lethal. It can be divided into three categories: epithelial tumors, germ cell tumors, and gonadal stromal tumors. There are no effective screening methods for ovarian cancer, and often the disease is well advanced at the time of diagnosis.

Disorders of Pelvic Support and Uterine Position

After you have completed this section of the chapter, you should be able to meet the following objectives:

- Characterize the function of the supporting ligaments and pelvic floor muscles in maintaining the position of the pelvic organs, including the uterus, bladder, and rectum
- Describe the manifestations of cystocele, rectocele, and enterocele
- Explain how uterine anteflexion, retroflexion, and retroversion differ from normal uterine position
- Describe the cause and manifestations of uterine prolapse

The uterus and the pelvic structures are maintained in proper position by the uterosacral ligaments, round ligaments, broad ligament, and cardinal ligaments. The two cardinal ligaments maintain the cervix in its normal position. The uterosacral ligaments normally hold the uterus in a forward position (Fig. 51–6). The broad ligament suspends the uterus, fallopian tubes, and ovaries within the pelvis. The vagina is encased in the semirigid structure of the strong supporting fascia. The muscular floor of the pelvis is a strong, slinglike structure that supports the uterus, vagina, urinary bladder, and rectum (Fig. 51–7).

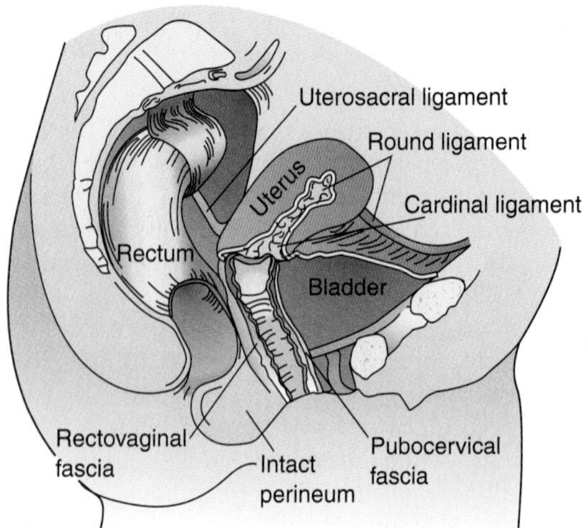

Figure 51–6
Normal support of the uterus and vagina.

In the female anatomy, nature is faced with the problems of supporting the pelvic viscera against the force of gravity and increases in intraabdominal pressure associated with coughing, sneezing, defecation, and laughing while at the same time allowing for urination, defecation, and normal reproductive tract function, especially the delivery of a baby. Three supporting structures are provided for the abdominal pelvic diaphragm. The bony pelvis provides support and protection for parts of the digestive tract and genitourinary structures, and the peritoneum holds the pelvic viscera in place. The main support for the viscera, however, is the pelvic diaphragm, made up of muscles and connective tissue that stretch across the bones of the pelvic outlet. The openings that must exist for the urethra, rectum, and vagina cause an inherent weakness in the pelvic diaphragm. Congenital or acquired weakness of the pelvic diaphragm results in widening of these openings, particularly the vagina, with the possible herniation of pelvic viscera through the pelvic floor (*i.e.*, prolapse).

Relaxation of the pelvic outlet usually comes about because of overstretching of the perineal supporting tissues during pregnancy and childbirth. Although the tissues are stretched only during these times, there may be no difficulty until later in life, such as the fifth or sixth decade, when further loss of elasticity and muscle tone occurs. Even in a woman who has not borne children, the combination of aging and postmenopausal changes may give rise to problems related to relaxation of the pelvic support structures. The three most common conditions associated with this relaxation are cystocele, rectocele, and uterine prolapse. These may occur separately or together.

Cystocele

Cystocele is a herniation of the bladder into the vagina. It occurs when the normal muscle support for the bladder is weakened, and the bladder sags below the uterus. The vaginal wall stretches and bulges downward

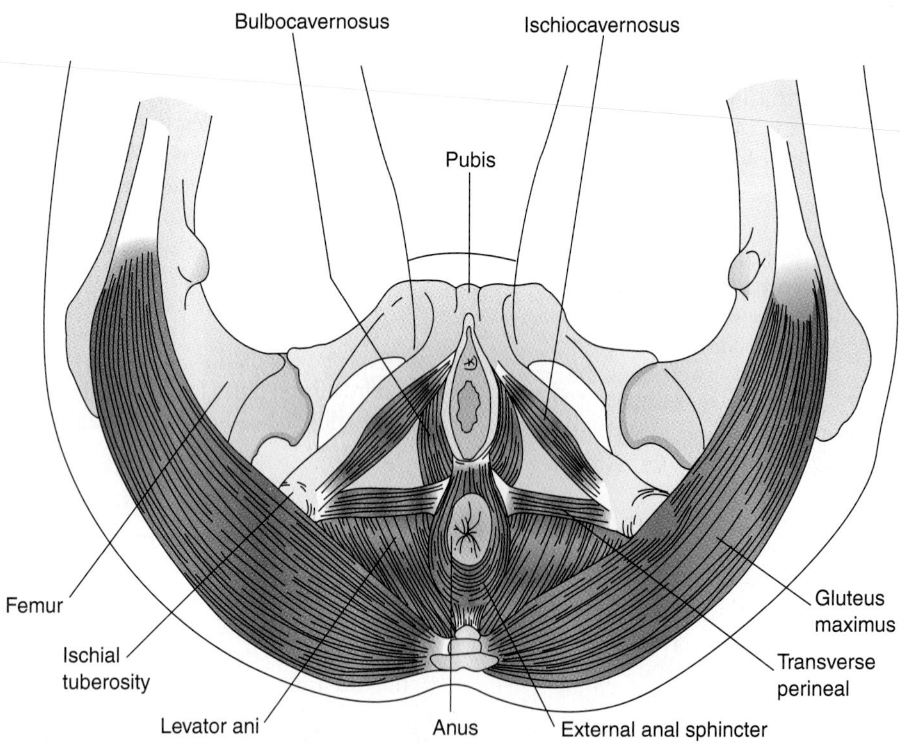

Figure 51–7
Muscles of the pelvic floor (female perineum).

because of the force of gravity and the pressure from coughing, lifting, or straining at stool. The bladder herniates through the anterior vaginal wall, and a cystocele forms (Fig. 51–8).

The symptoms include an annoying bearing-down sensation, difficulty in emptying the bladder, frequency and urgency of urination, and cystitis. Stress incontinence may occur at times of increased abdominal pressure, such as during squatting, straining, coughing, sneezing, laughing, or lifting.

Rectocele and Enterocele

Rectocele is the herniation of the rectum into the vagina. It occurs when the posterior vaginal wall and underlying rectum bulge forward, ultimately protruding through the introitus as the pelvic floor and perineal muscles are weakened. The symptoms include discomfort because of the protrusion of the rectum and difficulty in defecation (see Fig. 51–8). Digital pressure (*i.e.*, splinting) on the bulging posterior wall of the vagina may become necessary for defecation.

The area between the uterosacral ligaments just posterior to the cervix may weaken and form a hernial sac into which the small bowel protrudes when the woman is standing. This defect, called an *enterocele*, may extend into the rectovaginal septum. It may be congenital or acquired through birth trauma. Enterocele can be asymptomatic or cause a dull, dragging sensation and occasionally cause low backache.

Uterine Prolapse

Uterine prolapse is the bulging of the uterus into the vagina that occurs when the primary supportive ligaments (*i.e.*, cardinal ligaments) are stretched. Prolapse is ranked as first, second, or third degree, depending on how far the uterus protrudes through the introitus. First-degree prolapse shows some descent, but the cervix has not reached the introitus. In second-degree prolapse, the cervix or part of the uterus has passed through the introitus. The entire uterus protrudes through the vaginal opening in third-degree prolapse (*i.e.*, procidentia).

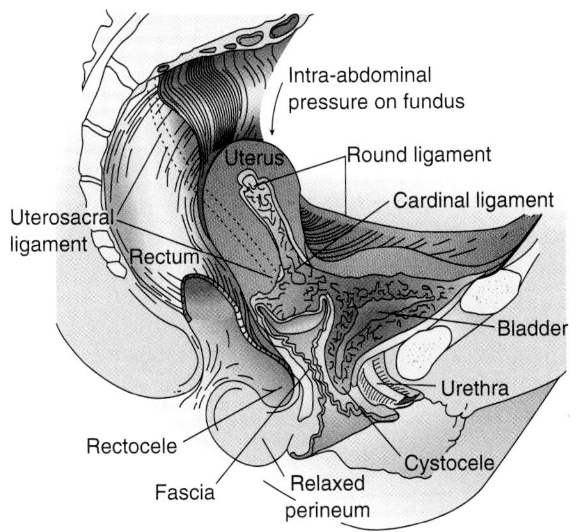

Figure 51–8
Relaxation of pelvic support structures with descent of the uterus as well as formation of cystocele and rectocele.

The symptoms associated with uterine prolapse result from irritation of the exposed mucous membranes of the cervix and vagina and the discomfort of the protruding mass. Prolapse often is accompanied by perineal relaxation, cystocele, or rectocele. Like cystocele, rectocele, and enterocele, it most commonly occurs in multiparous women, because childbearing is accompanied by injuries to pelvic structures and uterine ligaments. It may also result from pelvic tumors and neurologic conditions, such as spina bifida and diabetic neuropathy, that interrupt the innervation of pelvic muscles. A pessary may be inserted to hold the uterus in place and may stave off surgical intervention in women who want to have children or in older women for whom the surgery may pose a significant health risk.

Treatment of Pelvic Support Disorders

Most of the disorders of pelvic relaxation require surgical correction. These are elective surgeries and usually are deferred until after the childbearing years. The symptoms associated with the disorders often are not severe enough to warrant surgical correction. In other cases, the stress of surgery is contraindicated because of other physical disorders; this is particularly true of older women, in whom many of these disorders occur.

There are a number of surgical procedures for the conditions that result from relaxation of pelvic support structures. Removal of the uterus through the vagina (*i.e.*, vaginal hysterectomy) with appropriate repair of the vaginal wall (*i.e.*, colporrhaphy) often is done when uterine prolapse is accompanied by cystocele or rectocele. A vesicourethral suspension may be done to alleviate the symptoms of stress incontinence. Repair may involve abdominal hysterectomy along with anteroposterior repair. Kegel exercises, which strengthen the pubococcygeus muscle, may be helpful in cases of mild cystocele or rectocele or after surgical repair to help maintain the improved function.

Variations in Uterine Position

Variations in the position of the uterus are common. Some variations are innocuous; others, which may be the result of weakness and relaxation of the perineum, give rise to various problems that compromise the structural integrity of the pelvic floor, particularly after childbirth.

The uterus usually is flexed about 45 degrees anteriorly, with the cervix positioned posteriorly and downward in the anteverted position. When the female is standing, the angle of the uterus is such that it lies

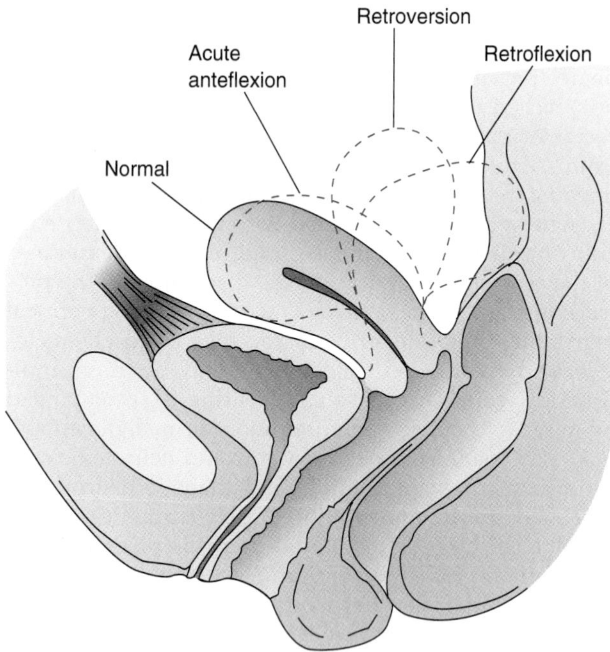

Figure 51–9
Variations in uterine position.

practically horizontal, resting lightly on the bladder. Asymptomatic, normal variations in the axis of the uterus in relation to the cervix (*i.e.*, flexion) and physiologic displacements that arise after pregnancy or with cul-de-sac pathology include anteflexion, retroflexion, and retroversion (Fig. 51–9). An anteflexed uterus is flexed forward on itself. Retroflexion is flexion backward at the isthmus. Retroversion describes the condition in which the uterus inclines posteriorly while the cervix remains tilted forward. Simple retroversion of the uterus is the most common displacement, found in 30% of normal women. It usually is a congenital condition caused by a short anterior vaginal wall and relaxed uterosacral ligaments; together these force the uterus to fall back into the cul-de-sac of Douglas. Retroversion can also follow certain diseases, such as endometriosis and PID, which produce fibrous tissue adherence with retraction of the fundus posteriorly. Large leiomyomas may also cause the uterus to move into a posterior position. Dyspareunia with deep penetration or low back pain with menses can be associated with retroversion. Most symptoms in these women are caused by the associated condition (*e.g.*, adhesions, fibroids) rather than congenital retroversion.

In summary, alterations in pelvic support frequently occur because of weaknesses and relaxation of the pelvic floor and perineum. Cystocele and rectocele involve herniation of the bladder or rectum into the vagina. Uterine prolapse occurs when the uterus bulges into the vagina. Pelvic relaxation disorders typically result from overstretching of the perineal supporting muscles during pregnancy and childbirth. The loss of elasticity in these structures that is a normal accompaniment of aging contributes to these problems. Variations in uterine position are common; they include anteflexion, retroflexion, and retroversion. These disorders, which often are innocuous, can be the result of a congenital shortness of the vaginal wall, development of fibrous adhesions secondary to endometriosis or PID, or displacement caused by large uterine leiomyomas.

Menstrual Disorders

After you have completed this section of the chapter, you should be able to meet the following objectives:

- Define the terms *amenorrhea, hypomenorrhea, oligomenorrhea, menorrhagia, metrorrhagia,* and *menometrorrhagia*
- State the function of alterations in estrogen and progesterone levels as a cause of dysfunctional menstrual cycles
- Compare the symptoms of primary dysmenorrhea with those of secondary dysmenorrhea
- Characterize the manifestation of the premenstrual syndrome, its possible causes, and the methods of treatment

Dysfunctional Menstrual Cycles

Although unexplained uterine bleeding can occur for many reasons, such as pregnancy, abortion, blood dyscrasias, and neoplasms, the most frequent cause in the nonpregnant female is what are commonly called dysfunctional menstrual cycles or bleeding. Dysfunctional cycles may take the form of *amenorrhea* (*i.e.*, absence of menstruation), *hypomenorrhea* (*i.e.*, scanty menstruation), *oligomenorrhea* (*i.e.*, infrequent menstruation, periods more than 35 days apart), *menorrhagia* (*i.e.*, excessive menstruation), or *metrorrhagia* (*i.e.*, bleeding between periods). *Menometrorrhagia* is heavy bleeding during and between menstrual periods.

Dysfunctional menstrual cycles are related to alterations in the hormones that support normal cyclic endometrial changes. Estrogen deprivation causes retrogression of a previously built-up endometrium and bleeding. Such bleeding often is irregular in amount and duration, with the flow varying with the time and degree of estrogen stimulation and with the degree of estrogen withdrawal. A lack of progesterone can cause abnormal menstrual bleeding; in its absence, estrogen induces development of a much thicker endometrial layer with a richer blood supply. The absence of progesterone results from the failure of any of the developing ovarian follicles to mature to the point of ovulation, with the subsequent formation of the corpus luteum and production and secretion of progesterone.

Periodic bleeding episodes alternating with amenorrhea are caused by variations in the number of functioning ovarian follicles present. If a number are present and active and if new follicles assume functional capacity, high levels of estrogen develop, causing the endometrium to proliferate for weeks or even months. In time, estrogen withdrawal and bleeding develop. This can occur for two reasons: an absolute estrogen deficiency may develop when several follicles simultaneously degenerate, or a relative deficiency may develop as the needs of the enlarged endometrial tissue mass exceed the capabilities of the existing follicles, even though estrogen levels remain constant. Estrogen and progesterone deficiency are associated with the absence of ovulation, hence the term *anovulatory bleeding*. Because the vasoconstriction and myometrial contractions that normally accompany menstruation are caused by progesterone, anovulatory bleeding seldom is accompanied by cramps, and the flow frequently is heavy. Anovulatory cycles are common among adolescents during the first several years after menarche, when ovarian function is becoming established, and among perimenopausal women, whose ovarian function is beginning to decline.

Dysfunctional menstrual cycles can originate as a primary disorder of the ovaries or as a secondary defect in ovarian function related to hypothalamic-pituitary stimulation. The latter can be initiated by emotional stress, marked variation in weight (*i.e.,* sudden gain or loss), or nonspecific endocrine or metabolic disturbances. Organic causes of irregular menstrual bleeding include endometrial polyps, submucosal myoma (*i.e.,* fibroid), blood dyscrasia, infection, endometrial cancer, polycystic ovarian disease, and pregnancy.

The treatment of dysfunctional bleeding depends on what is identified as the probable cause. A detailed history with emphasis on bleeding pattern and a physical examination should be the minimum evaluation that is done. Endocrine studies (FSH-LH ratio, prolactin, testosterone, DHAS), β-hCG pregnancy test, endometrial biopsy, D&C with or without hysteroscopy, and progesterone withdrawal tests may be needed for diagnosis. If organic problems are excluded and alterations in hormone levels are the primary cause, treatment may include the use of oral contraceptives, cyclic progesterone therapy, or long-acting progesterone injections.[27]

Amenorrhea

There are two types of amenorrhea: primary and secondary. Primary amenorrhea is the failure to menstruate by age 16 or by age 14 if failure to menstruate is accompanied by absence of secondary sex characteristics. Secondary amenorrhea is the cessation of menses for at least 6 months in a woman who has established normal menstrual cycles. Primary amenorrhea usually is caused by gonadal dysgenesis, congenital müllerian agenesis, testicular feminization, or a hypothalamic-pituitary-ovarian axis disorder. Causes of secondary amenorrhea include ovarian, pituitary, or hypothalamic dysfunction; intrauterine adhesions (*i.e.,* Asherman's syndrome); infections (*e.g.,* tuberculosis, schistosomiasis); pituitary tumor; anorexia nervosa; or strenuous physical exercise, which can alter the critical body fat-muscle ratio needed for menses to occur.[27]

Diagnostic evaluation resembles that for dysfunctional uterine bleeding, with the possible addition of a computed tomographic (CT) scan to exclude a pituitary tumor. Treatment is based on correcting the underlying cause and inducing menstruation with cyclic progesterone or combined estrogen-progesterone regimens.

Dysmenorrhea

Dysmenorrhea is pain or discomfort with menstruation. Although not usually a serious medical problem, it causes some degree of monthly disability for a significant number of women. There are two forms of dysmenorrhea: primary and secondary. Primary dysmenorrhea is menstrual pain that is not associated with a physical abnormality or pathology. It usually occurs with ovulatory menstruation beginning 6 months to 2 years after menarche. Symptoms may begin 1 to 2 days before menses, peak on the first day of flow, and subside within several hours to several days. Severe dysmenorrhea may be associated with systemic symptoms such as headache, nausea, vomiting, diarrhea, fatigue, irritability, dizziness, and syncope. The pain typically is described as dull, lower abdominal aching or cramping, spasmodic or colicky in nature, often radiating to the lower back, labia majora, or upper thighs.

Secondary dysmenorrhea is menstrual pain caused by specific organic conditions, such as endometriosis, uterine fibroids, adenomyosis, pelvic adhesions, IUDs, or PID. Laparoscopy often is required for diagnosis of secondary dysmenorrhea if medication for primary dysmenorrhea is ineffective.

Treatment for primary dysmenorrhea is directed at symptom control. Although analgesic agents such as aspirin and acetaminophen may relieve minor uterine cramping or low back pain, prostaglandin synthetase inhibitors, such as ibuprofen, naproxen, mefenamic acid, and indomethacin, are more specific for dysmenorrhea and the treatment of choice if contraception is not a concern. Ovulation suppression and symptomatic relief of dysmenorrhea can be instituted simultaneously with the use of oral contraceptives. Relief of secondary dysmenorrhea depends on identifying the cause of the problem. Medical or surgical intervention may be needed to eliminate the problem.

Premenstrual Syndrome

The premenstrual syndrome (PMS) is a distinct clinical entity characterized by a cluster of physical and psychologic symptoms limited to 3 to 14 days preceding menstruation that are relieved by onset of the menses. According to surveys, 25% to 40% of the adult female population in the United States experience mild to moderate monthly symptoms that they attribute to PMS; 2% to 8% report extreme or severe symptoms.[28] How many of these women have symptoms that are severe enough to warrant treatment is unknown. The incidence of PMS seems to increase with age. It is less common in women in their teens and twenties, and the highest number of women seeking help for the problem are in their mid-thirties. There is some dispute about whether PMS occurs more frequently in women who have not had children or in those who have had children. The disorder is not culturally distinct; it affects non-Westerners and Westerners.

The physical symptoms of PMS include painful and swollen breasts, bloating, abdominal pain, headache, and backache. Psychologically, there may be depression, anxiety, irritability, and behavioral changes. In some cases, there are puzzling alterations in motor function, such as clumsiness and altered handwriting. Women with PMS may report one or several symptoms, with symptoms varying from woman to woman and from month to month in the same patient. Signs and symptoms associated with this disorder are summarized in Table 51–4. PMS can significantly affect a woman's ability to perform at normal levels. She may lose time from or function ineffectively at work. Family responsibilities and relationships may suffer. Students have had lower grades during the premenstrual period. More crimes are committed by females during the premenstrual phase of the cycle, and more lives are lost to suicide during this period.

Although the causes of PMS are poorly documented, they are probably multifactorial. Like dysmenorrhea, only recently has PMS become recognized as a bona fide disorder rather than merely a psychosomatic illness.

There has been a tendency to link the disorder with endocrine imbalances such as hyperprolactinemia, estrogen excess, and alteration in the estrogen-progesterone ratio. Prolactin concentration affects sodium and water retention, is higher in the luteal phase than in the follicular phase, and can be increased by estrogens, stress, hypoglycemia, pregnancy, and oral contraceptives.[28] Estrogens stimulate anxiety and nervous tension, and increased progesterone levels may produce depression. The role of hormonal factors in the cause of PMS is supported by two well-established phenomena. First, women who have undergone a hysterectomy but not an oophorectomy may have cyclic symptoms that resemble PMS. Second, PMS symptoms are rare in postmenopausal women. Research has failed to confirm these theories.

Other hypotheses suggest that increased aldosterone may contribute to symptoms associated with fluid retention (*e.g.*, headache, bloating, breast tenderness, weight gain); that pyridoxine (vitamin B_6) deficiency may lead to estrogen excess or decrease production of the neurotransmitters dopamine and serotonin, which may contribute to PMS symptoms; or that decreased prostaglandin E_1 (PGE_1) concentrations can lead to abnormal sensitivity to prolactin, with associated fluid retention, irritability, and depression. In addition, increased appetite, binge eating, fatigue, and depression have been associated with altered endorphin activity and subclinical hypoglycemia.[28–30] There is also evidence that learned beliefs about menstruation can contribute to the production of PMS or at least affect the woman's response to the symptoms.

Diagnosis focuses on identification of the symptom clusters by means of prospective charting for at least 3 months. A complete history and physical examination are necessary to exclude other physical causes of the symptoms. Depending on the symptom pattern, blood studies, including thyroid hormones, glucose, and prolactin assays, may be done. Psychosocial evaluation is helpful to exclude emotional illness that is merely exacerbated premenstrually.

In the past, the treatment of PMS has been largely symptomatic. Attempts have been made to effect weight loss and reduce fluid retention through the use of diuretics. Tranquilizer drugs were used to treat mood changes, and pain was treated with mild analgesics. Treatment is to some extent still directed toward somatic complaints. Relief of somatic pain does not, however, totally resolve PMS suffering. The latest approach is to recommend an integrated program of personal assessment by diary, regular exercise, avoidance of caffeine, and a diet low in simple sugars and high in lean proteins. Additional therapeutic regimens include vitamin or mineral supplements (particularly pyridoxine, vitamin E, and magnesium), natural progesterone supplements, low-dose monophasic oral contraceptives, gonadotropin-releasing hormone agonists, bromocriptine for prolactin suppression, danazol (a synthetic androgen), spironolactone (an aldosterone antagonist and steroidogenesis inhibitor),

TABLE 51–4

Symptoms of Premenstrual Syndrome (PMS) by System

Body System	Symptoms
Cerebral	Irritability, anxiety, nervousness, fatigue, and exhaustion; increased physical and mental activity; lability; crying spells; depressions; inability to concentrate
Gastrointestinal	Craving for sweets or salts, lower abdominal pain, bloating, nausea, vomiting, diarrhea, constipation
Vascular	Headache, edema, weakness, or fainting
Reproductive	Swelling and tenderness of the breasts, pelvic congestion, ovarian pain, altered libido
Neuromuscular	Trembling of the extremities, changes in coordination, clumsiness, backache, leg aches
General	Weight gain, insomnia, dizziness, acne

evening primrose oil (which contains linoleic acid, a precursor of prostaglandin PGE_1), and lithium for marked functional impairment from affective symptoms.[29,30]

The daily use of prescribed relaxation techniques during the premenstrual period can improve physical and emotional symptoms.[28] Management includes education and support directed toward lifestyle changes. Drug therapy should be used cautiously until well-controlled studies establish criteria for use and effective treatment results. The placebo effect may account for symptom relief in a significant number of women. It is unlikely that a single cause or treatment for PMS will ever be found. Evaluation and management should focus on identifying and controlling the individual symptom clusters when possible.

In summary, menstrual disorders include dysfunctional menstrual cycles, dysmenorrhea, and premenstrual syndrome. Dysfunctional menstrual cycles occur when the hormonal support of the endometrium is altered. Estrogen deprivation causes retrogression of a previously built-up endometrium and bleeding. A lack of progesterone can cause abnormal menstrual bleeding; in its absence, estrogen induces development of a much thicker endometrial layer with a richer blood supply. The absence of progesterone results from the failure of any of the developing ovarian follicles to mature to the point of ovulation, with the subsequent formation of the corpus luteum and production and secretion of progesterone. Dysfunctional menstrual cycles produce amenorrhea, oligomenorrhea, metrorrhagia, or menorrhagia. Dysmenorrhea is characterized by pain or discomfort during menses. It can occur as a primary or secondary disorder. Primary dysmenorrhea is not associated with other disorders and begins soon after menarche. Secondary dysmenorrhea is caused by a specific organic condition, such as endometriosis or pelvic adhesions. It occurs in women with previously painless menses. PMS represents a cluster of physical and psychologic symptoms that precede menstruation by 1 to 2 weeks. The true incidence and nature of PMS has only recently been recognized, and its cause and methods for treatment are still under study.

Disorders of the Breast

After you have completed this section of the chapter, you should be able to meet the following objectives:

- Describe changes in breast function that occur with galactorrhea, mastitis, and ductal ectasia
- Describe the manifestations of fibrocystic disease and state why it is often referred to as a catchall for breast irregularities
- Cite the risk factors for breast cancer, the importance of breast self-examination, and recommendations for mammography
- Describe the methods used in the diagnosis and treatment of breast cancer

Most breast disease may be described as benign or cancerous. Breast tissue is never static; the breast is constantly responding to changes in hormonal, nutritional, psychologic, and environmental stimuli that cause continual cellular changes. Benign breast conditions are nonprogressive; some forms of benign disease, however, increase the risk of malignant disease. In light of this, strict adherence to a dichotomy of benign versus malignant disease may not always be appropriate. This dichotomy is, however, useful for the sake of simplicity and clarity.

Galactorrhea

Galactorrhea is the secretion of breast milk in a nonlactating breast. Galactorrhea may result from vigorous nipple stimulation during lovemaking, exogenous hormones, internal hormonal imbalance, or local chest infection or trauma. A pituitary tumor may produce large amounts of prolactin and cause galactorrhea. Galactorrhea occurs in men and women and usually is benign. Observation may be continued for several months before diagnostic hormonal screening.

Mastitis

Mastitis is inflammation of the breast. It most frequently occurs during lactation but may also result from other conditions.

In the lactating woman, inflammation results from an ascending infection that travels from the nipple to the ductile structures. The offending organisms originate from the suckling infant's nasopharynx or the mother's hands. During the early weeks of nursing, the breast is particularly vulnerable to bacterial invasion because of minor cracks and fissures that occur with vigorous suckling. Infection and inflammation cause obstruction of the ductile system. The breast area becomes hard, inflamed, and tender if not treated early. Without treatment, the area becomes walled off and may abscess, requiring incision and drainage. It is advisable for the mother to continue breast-feeding during antibiotic therapy to prevent this.

Mastitis is not confined to the postpartum period; it can occur as a result of hormonal fluctuations, tumors, trauma, or skin infection. Cyclic inflammation of the breast occurs most frequently in adolescents, who commonly have fluctuating hormone levels. Tumors may cause mastitis secondary to skin involvement or lymphatic obstruction. Local trauma or infection may develop into mastitis because of ductal blockage of trapped blood, cellular debris, or the extension of superficial inflammation.

The treatment for mastitis symptoms may include application of heat or cold, excision, aspiration, mild analgesics, antibiotics, and a supportive brassiere or breast binder.

Ductal Disorders

Ductal ectasia manifests in older women as a spontaneous, intermittent, usually unilateral, grayish green nipple discharge. Palpation of the breast increases the discharge. Ectasia occurs during or after menopause and is symptomatically associated with burning, itching, pain, and a pulling sensation of the nipple and areola. The disease results in inflammation of the ducts and subsequent thickening. The treatment requires removal of the involved ductal mass.

Intraductal papillomas are benign epithelial tissue tumors that range in size from 2 mm to 5 cm. Papillomas usually manifest with a bloody nipple discharge. The tumor may be palpated in the areolar area. The papilloma is probed through the nipple, and the involved duct is removed.

Fibroadenoma and Fibrocystic Disease

Fibroadenoma is seen in premenopausal women, most commonly in the third and fourth decade. The clinical findings include a firm, rubbery, sharply defined round mass. On palpation, the mass "slides" between the fingers and is easily movable. These masses usually are singular; only 15% are multiple or bilateral. Fibroadenoma is asymptomatic and usually found by accident. It is not thought to be precancerous. Treatment involves simple excision.

Fibrocystic breast disease (mammary dysplasia) is a condition typified by the development of fibrosis and cystic tissue formation. It is the single most common disorder of the breast and accounts for 50% to 75% of the surgical procedures on the female breast. The term *fibrocystic disease* has become a catchall for breast irregularities that occur bilaterally, change cyclically, and in younger women, are accompanied by dull, aching pain and heaviness. Some clinicians think that the term is overused and that the breast changes associated with this process are a result of hormonally modulated proliferative activity with incomplete resolution. This incomplete resolution may be a result of excess hormonal stimulation or hypersensitive breast epithelium.[31] Some investigators think fibrocystic disease may be part of a continuum of breast pathology related to cancer, particularly when the fibrocystic disease includes epithelial hyperplasia or demonstrable calcifications.

Fibrocystic disease usually presents as nodular (*i.e.*, "shotty"), granular breast masses that are more prominent and painful during the luteal or progesterone-dominant portion of the menstrual cycle. Discomfort ranges from heaviness to exquisite tenderness, depending on the degree of vascular engorgement and cystic distention. Diagnosis is made by physical examination, biopsy (*i.e.*, aspiration or tissue sample), and mammography. The use of mammography for diagnosis in high-risk groups younger than age 35 on a routine basis is still controversial. Mammography may be helpful in establishing the diagnosis, but increased breast tissue density in women with fibrocystic disease may make an abnormal or cancerous mass difficult to discern among the other structures. Hand-held ultrasonography can be useful in clarifying inconclusive mammographic densities.

Treatment for fibrocystic breast disease usually is symptomatic. Aspirin, mild analgesics, and local application of heat or cold may be recommended. Some physicians attempt to aspirate prominent or persistent cysts and send any fluid obtained to the laboratory for cytologic analysis. Women are advised to avoid foods that contain xanthines (*e.g.*, coffee, cola, chocolate, and tea) in their daily diets, particularly premenstrually. Vitamin E may be helpful in reducing mastalgia (*i.e.*, breast pain), and women should be encouraged to wear a good supporting brassiere. Danazol can be used for women with severe pain, although the potential for adverse effects warrants trying other methods first.

There is controversy regarding the relation between fibrocystic disease and cancer of the breast. It appears that the catchall term "fibrocystic disease" encompasses several disorders, some of which may undergo malignant changes. Nonproliferative lesions (70%) do not demonstrate an added risk for cancer; proliferative lesions without atypia (26%) may have a slightly increased risk for cancer. The remaining 4% of women with fibrocystic disease show proliferative lesions with atypia on biopsy and have a four times increased risk of cancer.[31] Any discrete mass or lump on the breast should be viewed as possible carcinoma, and cancer should be excluded before the conservative measures used to treat fibrocystic disease are used.

Breast Cancer

Cancer of the breast is the most common female cancer. One in eight women in the United States will have breast cancer in her lifetime. In 1996, breast cancer affected 184,000 American women and killed almost 44,000 women. Although breast cancer mortality has shown a slight decline, it is second only to lung cancer as a cause of cancer-related deaths in women. An additional 260 deaths occurred from breast cancer in males.

Risk factors for breast cancer include gender (*i.e.*, <1% incidence and mortality rates for men); increasing age (*i.e.*, 77% of new diagnoses each year occur in women older than 50 years of age); personal or family history of breast cancer (*i.e.*, at highest risk are those with multiple first-order relatives); history of benign breast disease (*i.e.*, primary "atypical" hyperplasia); and hormonal influences that promote breast maturation and may increase chance of cell mutation (*i.e.*, early menarche, late menopause, and no term pregnancies or first child after age 30). Two breast cancer susceptibility genes—*BRCA1* on chromosome 17 and *BRCA2* on chromosome 13—may account for most inherited breast cancers (see Chapter 5). However, most family history of breast cancer does not represent a direct genetic link, but rather it indicates inherited hormonal risk factors or lifestyle similarities that increase risk.[32] Seventy percent of women older than 50 years of age diagnosed with breast cancer have no identifiable risk factors other than age and gender.[33]

Detection

Cancer of the breast may manifest clinically as a mass, a puckering, nipple retraction, or unusual discharge. Many cancers are found by women themselves through breast self-examination (BSE)—sometimes when only a thickening or subtle change in breast contour is noticed. The variety of symptoms and potential for self-discovery underscore the need for regular, systematic self-examination. BSE should be done routinely by women older than 20 years. Premenopausal women should conduct the examination right after menses. This time is most appropriate in relation to cyclic breast changes that occur in response to fluctuations in hormone levels. Postmenopausal women and women who have had a hysterectomy should perform the examination on the same day of every month. Examination should be done in the shower or bath or at bedtime. The most important aspect of BSE is to devise a regular, systematic, convenient, and consistent method of examination. As an adjunct to BSE, women should have a clinical examination by a trained health professional at least every 3 years between ages 20 and 40, and annually after age 40.

X-ray mammography is the only effective screening technique for the early detection of clinically inapparent lesions. A generally slow-growing form of cancer, breast cancer may have been present for 2 to 9 years before it reaches 1 cm, the smallest size mass normally detected by palpation. Mammography can disclose lesions as small as 1 mm and clustering of calcifications that may warrant biopsy to exclude cancer. The American Cancer Society recommends a baseline mammogram between ages 35 and 40, studies every 1 to 2 years between 40 and 49 years, and annual evaluation for women after age 50. About 40% of breast cancers can be detected only by palpation and another 40% only by mammography.[4] The most comprehensive approach to screening is a combination of BSE, clinical evaluation by a health professional, and mammography.

Diagnosis and Classification

Procedures used in the diagnosis of breast cancer include physical examination, mammography, ultrasonography, percutaneous needle aspiration, stereotactic needle biopsy (*i.e.,* core biopsy), and excisional biopsy. Figure 51–10 illustrates the appearance of breast cancer on mammography. Breast cancer often manifests as a solitary, painless, firm, fixed lesion with poorly defined borders. It can be found anywhere in the breast but is most

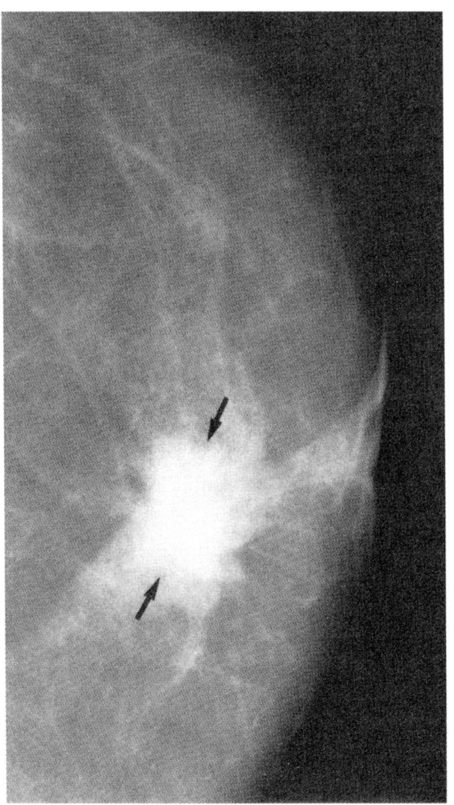

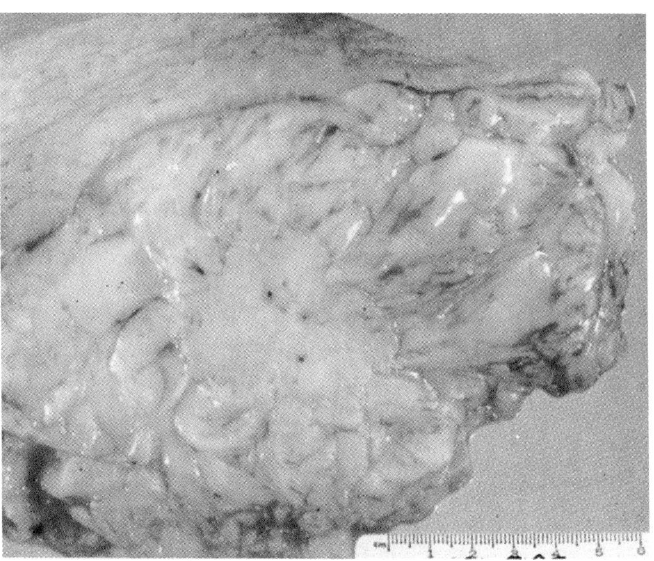

Figure 51–10
Carcinoma of the breast. (**A**) Mammogram. An irregularly shaped, dense mass (*arrows*) is seen in this otherwise fatty breast. (**B**) Mastectomy specimen. The irregular white, firm mass in the center is surrounded by fatty tissue.

common in the upper outer quadrant. Because of the variability in presentation, any suspicious change in breast tissue warrants further investigation. The diagnostic use of mammography enables additional definition of the clinically suspicious area (*e.g.*, appearance, character, calcification). Placement of a wire marker under radiographic guidance can ensure accurate surgical biopsy of nonpalpable suspicious areas. Ultrasonography is useful as a diagnostic adjunct to differentiate cystic from solid tissue in women with nonspecific thickening.

Fine-needle aspiration is a simple in-office procedure that can be performed repeatedly in multiple sites and with minimal discomfort. It can be accomplished by stabilizing a palpable mass between two fingers or in conjunction with hand-held sonography to define cystic masses or fibrocystic changes and to provide specimens for cytologic examination. Fine-needle aspiration can identify the presence of malignant cells, but it cannot differentiate in situ from infiltrating cancers. Stereotactic needle biopsy is an outpatient procedure done with the guidance of a mammography machine. After the lesion is localized radiologically, a large-bore needle is mechanically thrust quickly into the area, removing a core of tissue. Discomfort is similar to ear piercing, and even when multiple cores are obtained, healing occurs quite rapidly. Cells are available for histologic evaluation with a 96% accuracy in detecting cancer. This procedure is less costly than excisional biopsy.[34] Excisional biopsy to remove the entire lump provides the only definitive diagnosis of breast cancer, and often is therapeutic without additional surgery. Magnetic resonance imaging techniques, positron emission tomography, and computer-based or digital mammography are being evaluated as additional diagnostic modalities for breast cancer.

Tumors are classified histologically according to tissue characteristics and staged clinically according to tumor size, nodal involvement, and presence of metastasis. It is recommended that estrogen and progesterone receptor analysis be performed on surgical specimens. Information about the presence or absence of estrogen and progesterone receptors can be used in predicting tumor responsiveness to hormonal manipulation. High levels of both receptors improve the prognosis and increase the likelihood of remission.

Treatment

The treatment methods for breast cancer are controversial. They may include surgery, chemotherapy, radiation therapy, and hormonal manipulation. Radical mastectomy (*i.e.*, removal of the entire breast, underlying muscles, and all axillary nodes) is rarely used today as a primary surgical therapy unless breast cancer is advanced at the time of diagnosis. Modified surgical techniques (*i.e.*, mastectomy plus axillary dissection or lumpectomy for breast conservation) accompanied by chemotherapy or radiation therapy have achieved outcomes comparable to radical surgical methods and constitute the preferred treatment methods.

The prognosis is related more to the extent of nodal involvement than to the extent of breast involvement. Greater nodal involvement requires more aggressive postsurgical treatment, and many cancer specialists believe that a diagnosis of breast cancer is not complete until dissection and testing of the axillary lymph nodes has been accomplished. Adjuvant systemic therapy refers to the administration of chemotherapy or hormonal therapy to women without detectable metastatic disease. The goal of this therapy depends on nodal involvement, menopausal status, and hormone receptor status.[33] Tamoxifen is a nonsteroidal antiestrogen that binds to estrogen receptors and blocks the effects of estrogens on the growth of malignant cells in the breast. Studies have shown decreased cancer recurrence, decreased mortality rates, and increased 5-year survival rates in women with estrogen-receptor–positive tissue samples. The 5-year survival rate for localized cancer is 96%; with nodal involvement, it is about 75%, and it is about 20% with distant metastasis.

Paget's Disease

Paget's disease accounts for 1% of all breast cancers. The disease presents as an eczemoid lesion of the nipple and areola (Fig. 51–11). Paget's disease is usually associated with an infiltrating, intraductal carcinoma. When the lesion is limited to the nipple only, axillary metastasis is about 5%. Complete examination is required and includes a mammogram and biopsy. Treatment depends on the extent of spread.

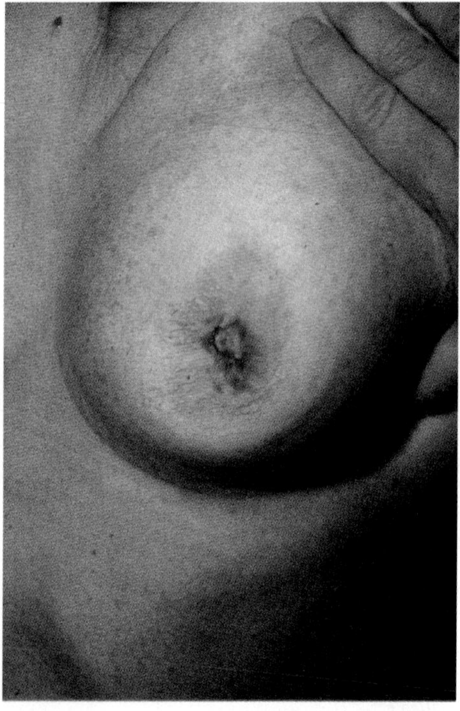

Figure 51–11
Paget disease of the nipple. An erythematous, scaly, and weeping "eczema" involves the nipple.

In summary, the breasts are subject to benign and malignant disease. Mastitis is inflammation of the breast, occurring most frequently during lactation. Galactorrhea is an abnormal secretion of milk that may occur as a symptom of increased prolactin secretion. Ductal ectasia and intraductal papilloma cause abnormal drainage from the nipple. Fibroadenoma and fibrocystic disease are characterized by abnormal masses in the breast that are benign. By far the most important disease of the breast is breast cancer, which is a significant cause of death of women. BSE and mammography afford a woman the best protection against breast cancer. They provide the means for early detection of breast cancer and, in many cases, allow early treatment and cure.

Infertility

After you have completed this section of the chapter, you should be able to meet the following objectives:

- Provide a definition of infertility
- List male and female factors that contribute to infertility
- Briefly describe methods used in the treatment of infertility

Infertility is the inability to conceive a child after 1 year of unprotected intercourse. It affects about 15% of couples in the United States. *Primary infertility* refers to situations in which there has been no prior conception. *Secondary infertility* is infertility that occurs after one or more previous pregnancies. *Sterility* is the inability to father a child or to become pregnant because of congenital anomalies, disease, or surgical intervention. About 1% to 2% of U.S. couples are affected by sterility.

The complexity of the process that must occur to achieve a pregnancy is taken for granted by most couples. For some couples, pregnancy occurs far too easily, whereas for others, no amount of money, hard work, love, patience, or medical resources seems to be able to bring about this amazing, desired event. Although a full discussion of the diagnosis and treatment of infertility is beyond the scope of this book, an overview of the areas in which problems can occur is presented.

The causes of infertility are almost equally divided between male factors (30% to 40%), female factors (30% to 40%), and combined factors (30% to 40%). In about 10% to 15% of infertile couples, the cause remains unknown even after a full workup.

Male Factors

For pregnancy to occur, the male must be able to provide sperm in sufficient quantity, delivered to the upper end of the vagina, with adequate motility to traverse the female reproductive tract. The male contribution to this process is assessed by means of a semen analysis, which evaluates volume of semen (normally 2 to 5 ml), sperm density (>20 million/ml), motility (>50% good progressive), viability (>50%), morphology (>60% normal), and viscosity (full liquefaction within 20 minutes). The specimen is best collected by masturbation into a sterile container after 3 days of abstinence. Because of variability in specimens, abnormal results should lead to a repeat test before the need for treatment is presumed.

Azoospermia is the absence of sperm; *oligospermia* refers to decreased numbers of sperm; and *asthenospermia* refers to poor motility of sperm. Tests of sperm function include cervical mucus penetration tests (*e.g.*, postcoital test, Penetrak), sperm penetration assay (*i.e.*, Hamster Zona Free Ovum test), and sperm antibody testing.

The causes of male infertility include varicocele, ejaculatory dysfunction, hyperprolactinemia, hypogonadotropic hypogonadism, infection, immunologic problems (*i.e.*, sperm antibodies), obstruction, and congenital anomalies. Risk factors for sperm problems include a history of mumps orchitis, cryptorchidism (*i.e.*, undescended testes), testicular torsion, hypospadias, previous urologic surgery, infection, and exposure to known gonadotoxins.[35] Treatment depends on the cause and may include surgery, medication, or the use of artificial insemination to deliver a more concentrated specimen directly to the cervical canal or uterine fundus. Artificial insemination with donor sperm can be offered if the male is sterile and this is an acceptable alternative to husband and wife.

Female Factors

The female contribution to pregnancy is more complex, requiring production and release of a mature ovum capable of being fertilized; production of cervical mucus that assists in sperm transport and maintains sperm viability within the female reproductive tract; patent fallopian tubes with the motility potential to pick up and transfer the ovum to the uterine cavity; development of an endometrium that is suitable for the implantation and nourishment of a fertilized ovum; and a uterine cavity that allows for growth and development of a fetus. Each of these factors is discussed briefly, along with an overview of diagnostic tests and treatment.

Ovulatory Dysfunction

In a normally menstruating female, ovulatory cycles begin several months to a year after menarche. Release of FSH from the pituitary causes the development of several primordial follicles within the ovary. At some point, a dominant follicle is selected and the remaining follicles undergo atresia. When the dominant follicle has become large enough to contain a mature ovum (16 to 20 mm in diameter) and is producing sufficient estradiol to ensure adequate proliferation of the endometrium, production of LH increases (*i.e.*, the LH surge), and the increased LH level induces release of the ovum from within the follicle (*i.e.*, ovulation).

After ovulation, under the influence of LH, the former follicle luteinizes and begins producing progesterone in addition to estradiol. The progesterone stimulates the development of secretory endometrium, which has the capability to nourish a fertilized ovum if one should implant.

The presence of progesterone after ovulation causes a rise in the woman's basal body temperature (BBT). This thermogenic property of progesterone provides the basis for the simplest, most inexpensive beginning test of ovulatory function—the measurement of BBT. Women should be able to detect at least a 0.4°F rise in their BBT (at rest) after ovulation that should be maintained throughout the luteal phase. This biphasic temperature pattern demonstrates that ovulation has taken place, where in the cycle it occurred, and the length of the luteal phase. BBT can be influenced by many other factors, including restless sleep, alcohol intake, drug use, fever due to illness, and change in usual rising time. However, as an initial step in the infertility investigation, it can provide useful information to direct other forms of testing.

Endometrial biopsy, the removal of a sample of the endometrium during an office procedure, provides histologic evidence of secretory endometrium and the level of maturation of the lining. In a normal cycle, the luteal phase should be 14 days long. Without pregnancy and the subsequent secretion of hCG, the corpus luteum begins to degenerate 7 to 10 days after the LH surge. The luteal phase of the cycle is so consistent that a pathologist can tell by evaluating a section of endometrium that it is representative of a particular day of the luteal phase. The pathologist's assessment of maturation is compared with the arrival of the next menses. If a discrepancy of more than 2 days exists, the woman is said to have a luteal phase defect (LPD). This diagnosis indicates that, although ovulation is occurring, endometrial development is insufficient and implantation may not be possible. Pregnancy requires fertilization and implantation. LPD can also be suggested by an abnormal serum progesterone level 7 days after ovulation. It can be treated directly with supplemental progesterone after ovulation or with the use of clomiphene citrate to stimulate increased pituitary production of FSH and LH.

Anovulation (*i.e.*, no ovulation) and oligo-ovulation (*i.e.*, irregular ovulation) are other forms of ovulatory dysfunction. These problems can be identified by the tests for LPD previously described. Ovulatory problems can be primary problems of the ovary or secondary problems related to endocrine dysfunction. When disturbances in ovulation are confirmed, it is reasonable to evaluate other endocrine functions before initiating treatment. If the results of tests for pituitary hormones (*e.g.*, FSH, LH, prolactin), thyroid studies, and tests of adrenal function (*e.g.*, DHAS, androstenedione) are normal, ovulatory dysfunction is primary and should respond to treatment. Abnormalities in any of the other endocrine areas should be further evaluated as needed and treated appropriately. Hyperprolactinemia responds well to bromocriptine, but pituitary microadenoma may need to be excluded first. Hypothyroidism requires thyroid replacement, and hyperthyroidism requires suppressive therapy and, sometimes, surgical intervention with thyroid replacement later. Adrenal suppression can be instituted with dexamethasone, a glucocorticoid analogue. Normal ovulatory function may resume without further intervention; if not, treatment can be concurrent with management of other endocrine problems.

Cervical Mucus Problems

High preovulatory levels of estradiol stimulate the production of large amounts of clear, stretchy cervical mucus that aids the transport of sperm into the uterine cavity and helps to maintain an environment that keeps the sperm viable for up to 72 hours. Insufficient estrogen production (*i.e.*, inherent or secondary to treatment with clomiphene citrate, an antiestrogen), cervical abnormalities from disease or invasive procedures (*e.g.*, DES exposure, stenosis, conization), and cervical infection (*e.g.*, chlamydial infection, mycoplasmal infection, gonorrhea) can adversely affect the production of healthy cervical mucus.

A postcoital test (Sims-Huhner) involves evaluation of the cervical mucus 1 to 8 hours after intercourse within the 48 hours before ovulation. A sample of cervical mucus is obtained using a special syringe and evaluated grossly for amount, clarity, and stretch (*i.e.*, spinnbarkeit) and microscopically for cellularity, for number and quality of motile sperm, and for the presence of ferning after the sample has air-dried on the slide. To obtain good-quality mucus, it is essential to obtain the sample within the 48 hours before ovulation. Tests may have to be repeated within the same cycle or in subsequent cycles to ensure appropriate timing.

If inadequate estrogen effect is seen (poor-quality mucus), supplemental oral estrogen can be given in the first 9 days of the next cycle, and the test can be repeated. Administration of mucolytic expectorants (1 teaspoon four times daily, starting on day 10 and continuing until ovulation is confirmed) may also improve the quality of the mucus. If mucus is good but sperm are inadequate in number or motility, further evaluation of the male may be needed. The man and woman should be tested for sperm antibodies when repeated postcoital tests reveal that the sperm are all dead or agglutinated. Artificial insemination with the husband's sperm can bypass the cervical mucus.

Cervical cultures for gonorrhea, chlamydial infection, and mycoplasmal infection should be obtained with the postcoital test if they have not already been acquired. If the cultures give positive results, treatment should be instituted as needed.

Uterine Cavity Abnormalities

Alterations within the uterine cavity can occur because of DES exposure, submucosal fibroids, cervical polyps, bands of scar tissue, or congenital anomalies (*e.g.*, bicornuate septum, single horn). These defects may be suspected from the patient's history or pelvic examination but require hysterosalpingography (*i.e.*, x-ray study in which dye is placed through the cervix to outline the uterine cavity and demonstrate tubal patency) or hysteroscopy (*i.e.*, study in which a lighted fiberoptic scope placed through the cervix under general anesthesia allows direct visualization of the uterine cavity) for confirmation. Treatment is surgical when possible.

Tubal Factors

Tubal patency is required for fertilization and can be disrupted secondary to PID, ectopic pregnancy (*i.e.*, after salpingectomy or salpingostomy), large myomas, endometriosis, pelvic adhesions, and previous tubal ligation. Hysterosalpingography can reveal the location and type of any blockage, such as fimbrial, cornual, or hydrosalpinx. Sometimes, microsurgical repair is possible.

Even when tubal patency is demonstrated, it is possible for tubal disease to make ovum pick up impossible. Contrary to popular belief, the ovum is not extruded directly into the fallopian tube. The tube must be free to move to engulf the ovum after release. Pelvic adhesions from previous infection, surgery, or endometriosis can interfere with the tube's mobility. Laparoscopic evaluation of the pelvis is needed for diagnosis. Laser ablation or cautery can be used to lyse adhesions and to remove endometriosis through the laparoscope or, if severe, by means of laparotomy.

New Technologies

In vitro fertilization (IVF) was developed in 1978 for women with significantly damaged or absent tubes to provide them with an opportunity for pregnancy where none normally exists. The ovaries are superstimulated to produce multiple follicles using clomiphene citrate, human menopausal menotropins (*e.g.*, Pergonal, Humegon), pure FSH (*e.g.*, Metrodin, Fertinex), or a combination of these drugs.

Follicular maturation is monitored by means of ultrasonography and assay of serum estradiol levels. When preovulatory criteria are met, an injection of hCG is given to simulate an LH surge; 35 hours later, the follicles are aspirated laparoscopically or, more often, by the ultrasound-guided transvaginal route. The follicular fluid is evaluated microscopically for the presence of ova. When found, they are removed and placed into culture media in an incubator.

The eggs are inseminated with semen from the husband that has been prepared by a washing technique that removes the semen, begins the capacitation process, and allows the strongest sperm to be used for fertilization. When very low numbers of normal motile sperm are available, microsurgical techniques can be used to assist with fertilization. A procedure called *partial zona dissection* involves the creation of a small opening in the protective layer (*i.e.*, zona pellucida) that surrounds the egg. With *subzonal insertion*, several sperm are inserted into the space just beneath the protective layer. The most definitive form of micromanipulation is a procedure called *intracytoplamsic sperm injection*, where a single spermatozoa is injected directly into the cytoplasm of the egg.

Between 12 and 24 hours after insemination, the ova are evaluated for signs of fertilization. If signs are present, the ova are returned to the incubator, and 48 to 72 hours after egg retrieval, the fertilized eggs are placed back into the woman's uterus by means of a transcervical catheter. A procedure similar to partial zona dissection can be performed just before embryo transfer to help the fertilized egg escape from within the zona pellucida. This "assisted hatching" improves the chances of implantation.

Hormonal supplementation of the luteal phase often is used to increase the possibility of implantation. The overall live delivery rate for 1994, as reported by the National In Vitro Fertilization and Embryo Transplantation registry, was 20.7% per egg retrieval.[35] Indications for IVF have been expanded to include male factors (*i.e.*, severe oligospermia or asthenospermia), immunologic infertility, severe endometriosis, and idiopathic or unknown infertility. The substantial risk of multiple births with IVF procedures has been reduced with the availability of cryopreservation, which allows freezing of excess embryos and limits the number of fresh embryos transferred. The live delivery rate in 1994 after frozen embryo transfer was 15.4%.

An outgrowth of IVF technology is gamete intrafallopian transfer (GIFT), which uses similar ovarian stimulation protocols and laparoscopic egg retrieval and involves placing ovum and sperm directly into the fallopian tube during the same laparoscopy procedure. This procedure requires at least one patent fallopian tube and was developed primarily to try to increase the pregnancy rate in women with idiopathic infertility. The basic premises are that, if a transportation problem is interfering with ovum pick up, GIFT could solve that problem and that implantation may result more often if fertilization occurs within the body. The live delivery rate for 1994 was 28.4%.[36] The multiple birth rate with GIFT is similar to that with IVF.

Newer reproductive technologies include zygote intrafallopian transfer (ZIFT) and tubal embryo transplant (TET). With ZIFT, the zygote is placed laparosopically into the fallopian tube after the traditional IVF procedure. With TET, the embryos are transferred into the fallopian tubes transcervically using ultrasound guidance or by means of hysteroscopy. The theoretic advantages of these procedures involve tubal factors that may facilitate implantation. Live delivery rate for ZIFT-related procedures in 1994 was 29.1%.

By mid-1992, more than 30,000 babies had been born worldwide using some type of assisted reproductive technology, and an additional 6000 births per year have occurred since then. Future research will focus on understanding and improving the implantation process.

In summary, infertility is the inability to conceive a child after 1 year of unprotected intercourse. Male factors are related to number, motility, and ability of sperm to penetrate the cervical mucus and the ovum. Causes of male infertility include varicocele, ejaculatory dysfunction, hyperprolactinemia, hypogonadotropic hypogonadism, infection, immunologic problems (*i.e.*, sperm antibodies), obstruction, and congenital anomalies. Risk factors for sperm problems include a history of mumps orchitis, cryptorchidism (*i.e.*, undescended testes), testicular torsion, hypospadias, previous urologic surgery, infection, and exposure to known gonadotoxins.

The female contribution to pregnancy is more complex, requiring production and release of a mature ovum capable of being fertilized; production of cervical mucus that assists in sperm transport and maintains sperm viability within the female reproductive tract; patent fallopian tubes with the mobility potential to pick up and transfer the ovum to the uterine cavity; development of an endometrium that is suitable for the implantation and nourishment of a fertilized ovum; and a uterine cavity that allows for growth and development of a fetus.

Evaluation and treatment of infertility can be lengthy and highly stressful for the couple. Options for therapy continue to expand, but newer treatment modalities, such as IVF, GIFT, ZIFT, and TET are expensive, and financial resources can be strained while couples seek their sometimes elusive dream of having a child.

REFERENCES

1. Wilkinson E.J., Stone I.K. (1995). *Atlas of vulvar disease* (pp. 16, 33–35, 101). Baltimore: Williams & Wilkins.
2. Spadt S.K. (1995). Suffering in silence: Managing vulvar pain patients. *Contemporary Nurse Practitioner* 11 (12), 32.
3. Jones J.D., Lehr S.T. (1994). Vulvodynia: Diagnostic techniques and treatment modalities. *Nurse Practitioner* 19 (4), 40.
4. DeCherney A.H., Pernooll M.L. (1994). *Current obstetric and gynecologic diagnosis and treatment* (pp. 315, 909–919, 931–945, 717, 807, 945, 966, 1125). Norwalk, CT: Appleton & Lange.
5. National Cancer Institute, National Child Health & Human Development, National Institutes of Health. (1995). *Clear cell carcinoma; Resource guide for DES-exposed daughters and their families* (pp. 3, 5, 24). Rockville, MD: National Institutes of Health.
6. Glass R.H. (1993). *Office gynecology* (pp. 135). Baltimore: Williams & Wilkins.
7. American Cancer Society. (1996). *Cancer facts and figures 1996* (pp. 13–15). New York: American Cancer Society.
8. Gries-Griffin J. (1995). Abnormal Pap test results: meaning and management. *ADVANCE for Nurse Practitioners* 7, 17–18.
9. Huff B.C. (1996). Prevention, screening and early detection of gynecologic cancers. *VOICE-AWHONN* 4 (5), 11.
10. Kurman R.J., et al. (1996). Interim guidelines for management of abnormal cytology. *Journal of the American Medical Association* 271 (23), 1868.
11. Tawa K., Forsythe A., et al. (1988). A comparison of Papanicolaou smear and the cervicogram: Sensitivity, specificity, and cost analysis. *Obstetrics and Gynecology* 71, 242.
12. Ferenczy A., Wright T.C. Jr. (1993). Managing abnormal Papanicolaou findings: Large loop excision of the transformation zone. *Female Patient* 18 (3), 18.
13. Danforth D.N., Scott J.R. (1986). *Obstetrics and gynecology* (5th ed., pp. 918, 1080). Philadelphia: J.B. Lippincott.
14. Keitz M.D., Olive D.L. (1993). Diagnostic and therapeutic options in endometriosis. *Hospital Practice* 28(10), 16.
15. Zivnuska J. (1995). Endometriosis: An overview of diagnosis and treatment. *ADVANCE for Nurse Practitioners* 1, 16.
16. Daniell J.F., Miller W., Tosh R. (1986). Initial evaluation of the use of the potassium-titanyl-phosphate (KTP/532) laser in gynecology laparoscopy. *Fertility and Sterility* 46 (3), 373.
17. Pavlik R.M. (1996). For an operational definition of endometrial hyperplasia. *Contemporary Obstetrics and Gynecology* 10, 117.
18. Ferenczy A. (1996). For an operational definition of endometrial hyperplasia. *Contemporary Obstetrics and Gynecology* 10, 17.
19. Centers for Disease Control. (1993). STD treatment guidelines 1993. *Morbidity and Mortality Weekly Report* 39 (24).
20. Kottmann L.M. (1995). Pelvic inflammatory disease: An overview. *Journal of Obestetric, Gynecologic, and Neonatal Nurses* 24 (8), 761.
21. Centers for Disease Control. (1990). Ectopic pregnancy mortality 1970–1987. *Morbidity and Mortality Weekly Report* 39 (24).
22. Centers for Disease Control. (1993). STD treatment guidelines 1993. *Morbidity and Mortality Weekly Report* 39 (24), 75.
23. Speroff L., Glass R.H., Kase N.G. (1994). *Clinical Gynecology: Endocrinology and infertility* (pp. 473). Baltimore: Williams & Wilkins.
24. Bast R., Fenoglia-Preiser CM., Ozer H., Sidransky D. (1993). Clinical application of tumor markers. *Contemporary Obstetrics and Gynecology* 11, 66.
25. Orange L.M. (1994). Cost prohibits large-scale ovarian cancer screen. *OB-GYN News* 29 (17), 2.
26. National Institutes of Health Consensus Development Panel on Ovarian Cancer. (1995). Ovarian cancer: screening and follow-up. *Journal of the American Medical Association* 273, 491–497.
27. Murata J.M. (1991). Abnormal genital bleeding and secondary amenorrhea. *Journal of Obstetric, Gynecologic, and Neonatal Nursing* 19 (1), 31, 33.
28. Stair W.L., Lrmmel L.L., Shannon MT. (1995). *Women's primary health care: Protocols for practice* (pp. 12–141, 12–153). Washington, DC: American Nurses Publishing.
29. Mastranelo R. (1994). Taming the beast known as PMS. *ADVANCE for Nurse Practitioners* 10, 11–14.
30. Chuong C.J., Pearsall-Otey L.R., Rosenfeld B.L. (1995). A practical guide for relieving PMS. *Contemporary Nurse Practitioner* 5 (6), 34–37.
31. Kuhrik N.S., Bohner D.G., Moore S., Kuhric M. (1994). Evaluating women for fibrocystic breast condition. *American Journal of Nursing* 7, 16A.
32. American Cancer Society. (1995). *Breast cancer facts and figures 1996* (pp. 1–10). Atlanta: American Cancer Society.
33. Goldman S. (1994). Evaluating breast masses. *Contemporary Obstetrics and Gynecology* 6 (7), 17.
34. Shapiro T.J., Clark P.M. (1995). Breast cancer: What the primary provider needs to know. *Nurse Practitioner* 20 (3), 36–38.
35. Jarow J.P., Lipschultz L.I. (1987). Urologic evaluation of male infertility. *Contemporary Obstetrics and Gynecology* (Special Issue), 85.
36. Society for Assisted Reproductive Technology. (1996). Assisted reproductive technology in the United States & Canada: 1994 results generated from the American

Society for Reproductive Medicine/Society for Assisted Reproductive Technology Registry. *Fertility and Sterility* 66 (5), 697.

ADDITIONAL READINGS

Bayer S.R., DeCherney A.H. (1993). Clinical manifestations & treatment of dysfunctional uterine bleeding. *Journal of the American Medical Association* 269 (14), 1823–1828.

Brucks J.A. (1997). A practical approach to ovarian cancer. *Clinical Excellence for Nurse Practitioners* 1 (1), 35–45.

Guist R.M., Iwamotoa K., Hatch E.E. (1995). Diethylstilbestrol revisited: A review of long-term health effects. *Annals of Internal Medicine* 122, 778–788.

Hillard P.A. (1995). Abnormal uterine bleeding in adolescents. *Contemporary Nurse Practitioner* 9 (10), 21–28.

Hillis S.D. (1994). PID prevention: Clinical and societal stakes. *Hospital Practice* 29 (4), 121–130.

Klemm P.R., Guarnieri C. (1996). Cervical cancer: A developmental perspective. *Journal of Obstetric, Gynecologic, and Neonatal Nurses* 25 (7), 629–634.

Mallon W.K. (1996). When is vaginal bleeding an emergency? *Emergency Medicine* 5, 29–39.

Mandelblatt J.S., Phillips R.N. (1996). Cervical cancer: How often—and why—to screen older women. *Geriatrics* 51 (6), 45–48.

Olive D.L., Schwartz L.B. (1993). Endometriosis. *New England Journal of Medicine* 328 (24), 1759–1769.

Palerma G.D., Cohen J., Rosenwaks Z. (1996). Intracytoplasmic sperm injection: A powerful tool to overcome fertilization failure. *Fertility and Sterility* 65 (5), 899–908.

Sale P.G. (1995). Genitourinary infection in older women. *Journal of Obstetric, Gynecologic, and Neonatal Nurses* 24 (8), 769–775.

CHAPTER 52

Sexually Transmitted Diseases

Patricia McCowen Mehring

The incidence and types of sexually transmitted diseases (STDs), as reported in the professional literature and public health statistics, are increasing. It must be recognized, however, that the incidence of disease is based on clinical reports, and many STDs are not reportable or not reported. The agents of transmission include bacteria, chlamydiae, viruses, fungi, protozoa, parasites, and unidentified microorganisms (see Chapter 10). Portals of entry include the mouth, genitalia, urinary meatus, rectum, and skin. All STDs are more common in persons who have more than one sexual partner, and it is not uncommon for a person to be concurrently infected with more than one type of STD. This chapter discusses the manifestations of STDs in men and women in terms of infections of the external genitalia, vaginal infections, and infections that have systemic effects and genitourinary manifestations. Human immunodeficiency virus (HIV) infection is presented in Chapter 13.

Infections of the External Genitalia

After you have completed this section of the chapter, you should be able to meet the following objectives:

- Define what is meant by a *sexually transmitted disease* (STD)
- Give a reason why the reported incidence of STDs may not accurately reflect the true incidence
- List common portals of entry for STDs
- Name the organisms responsible for condylomata acuminata, genital herpes, molluscum contagiosum, chancroid, granuloma inguinale, and lymphogranuloma venereum
- State the significance of condyloma acuminata
- Explain the recurrent infections in genital herpes

Some STDs primarily affect the mucocutaneous tissues of the external genitalia. These include human papillomavirus infection, genital herpes, molluscum contagiosum, chancroid, granuloma inguinale, and lymphogranuloma venereum.

Human Papillomavirus

Condylomata acuminata, or genital warts, are the most common manifestation of the human papillomavirus (HPV). Although recognized for centuries, HPV-induced genital warts have become one of the fastest rising STDs of the past decade. The Centers for Disease Control and Prevention (CDC) estimate that 20 million Americans carry the virus and that up to 1 million new cases are diagnosed each year.[1] The current prevalence of HPV is difficult to determine, because it is not a reportable disease and estimates are based only on visible HPV lesions.

The incubation period for HPV ranges from 6 weeks to 8 months; subclinical infection may be present for months to years before the disease manifests itself clinically. Although HPV infections often are asymptomatic, they can be detected by the presence of characteristic warty lesions.

Structurally, there are four types of condylomas or warts: papillous, flat, spiked, and exophytic.[2] Papillous condylomas are soft, pink, fleshy growths of external genitalia. They often are difficult to differentiate from normal genital tissue and may require biopsy for definitive diagnosis. Until recently, papillous condylomas were the only type of condyloma recognized. The flat condyloma, discovered in 1977, is the most virulent type. The flat condyloma, which is a macular, flat, granular lesion, typically is found on the cervix or introitus in women and on the frenulum or upper shaft of the penis in men. The lesions, which frequently are invisible to the naked eye, become readily apparent when the affected area is soaked with a 5% acetic acid solution. Biopsy may be required to differentiate these lesions from other hyperkeratotic or precancerous lesions. Spiked condylomas, which are less common, are small, pointed projections found primarily in the vagina. Exophytic or inverted condylomas grow only within the glands of the cervix and can mimic carcinoma in situ.

A relation between HPV and genital neoplasms has become increasingly apparent over the past 20 years. HPV DNA has been identified in more than 90% of cervical cancers.[3] Seventy types of HPV have been identified. Twenty of these affect the anogenital area. Type 16 (50%) and type 18 (20%) appear to be the most virulent. Types 31, 33, 35, 39, 45, 51, 52, 56, and 58 are less common but have also demonstrated malignant potential. These high-risk HPV types account for 10% of condylomas, but are present in 40% of low-grade dysplasias and 85% of high-grade lesions.[3,4] In contrast, types 6, 11, 42, 43, and 44 account for 70% to 90% of genital warts but are generally benign, with only a low potential for dysplasia (15% to 35%). Numerous studies have demonstrated that HPV infection is common and that its presence alone is not sufficient to induce neoplasia. Cofactors that may increase the risk for cancer include smoking, immunosuppression, other STDs—particularly herpes—and exposure to hormonal alteration (*e.g.*, pregnancy, oral contraceptives).[3,4] This association with premalignant and malignant changes has increased the concern about diagnosis and treatment of this viral infection.

Genital condylomas should be considered in any woman who presents with the primary complaint of vulvar pruritus or who has had an abnormal Papanicolaou test (Pap smear). Microscopic examination of a wet-mount slide preparation and cultures are used to exclude associated vaginitis. Acetic acid soaks are used before inspecting the vulva under magnification, and specimens for biopsy are taken from questionable areas. Colposcopic examination of the cervix and vagina may be advised as a follow-up measure when there is an abnormal Pap smear or when HPV lesions are identified on the vulva. Evaluation and treatment of sexual partners may be suggested.

Treatment is aimed at prevention of cancer and control of symptomatic infections, because systemic eradication of the virus is not possible with available therapies. The CDC identifies several acceptable treatment alternatives. Podophyllin (10% to 25%) has long been used for visible external growths. Multiple applications of this cytotoxic agent may be required for resolution of lesions. The amount of drug used and the surface area treated should be limited with each treatment session to avoid systematic absorption and toxicity. This treatment is contraindicated in pregnancy for the same reason. Purified podophyllotoxin is less toxic and is applied by the individual at home. An alternative first-line therapy for vulvar, vaginal, or penile condylomas is the topical application of a 50% to 80% solution of trichloroacetic acid. This weak destructive agent produces an initial burning in the affected area, followed in several days by a sloughing of the superficial tissue. Several applications 1 to 2 weeks apart may be necessary to eradicate the virus. Vulvar, vaginal, and penile condylomas may also be treated with electrocautery. Topical 5-fluorouracil (Efudex) and laser therapy have been used successfully in the treatment of vaginal condylomas.[5]

Because it can penetrate deeper than other forms of therapy, cryotherapy (*i.e.*, freezing therapy) is often the treatment of choice for cervical HPV lesions. Laser surgery can be used to remove large or widespread lesions of the cervix, vagina, vulva, or lesions that have failed to respond to other first-line methods of treatment. Interferon, in the form of a topical application or as an intralesional injection has not shown any advantage over other available forms of treatment. Sexual abstinence is suggested during any type of treatment.[1–3,5–6]

The recurrence rate for HPV infection is high, sometimes occurring as early as 3 to 6 weeks after treatment. Originally, it was assumed that reinfection from sexual partners was the primary cause, but recurrences result from a persistent HPV infection existing in a latent state in the apparently normal tissue near the treated lesions.[2] Stress and trauma appear to be two possible factors in the reactivation of the latent virus. Extending the area of treatment 5 mm beyond the lesion border is recommended and may decrease the likelihood of recurrences. Research eventually may lead to the prevention or eradication of this form of what appears to be a sexually transmitted precursor to neoplasia.

Genital Herpes

Genital herpes is caused by the herpes simplex virus (HSV). Because herpesvirus infection is not reportable in all states, reliable data on its true incidence and prevalence are lacking. In 1996, it was reported that the number of infected persons in the United States increased from 25 million in 1980 to 44 million by 1990, with an estimated 2 million new cases occurring each year.[7]

There are five types of herpesviruses that cause infections in humans: HSV-1, which causes cold sores, and HSV-2, which causes genital herpes; varicella-zoster virus, which causes chickenpox and shingles; Epstein-Barr virus, which causes infectious mononucleosis and

Burkitt's lymphoma; and cytomegalovirus, which causes cytomegalic inclusion disease.

The herpesviruses are neurotropic; they grow within neurons and share the biologic property of latency. *Latency* refers to the ability to maintain disease potential in the absence of clinical signs and symptoms. In genital herpes, the virus ascends through the peripheral nerves to the sacral dorsal root ganglia (Fig. 52–1). The virus can remain dormant in the dorsal root ganglia, or it can reactivate, in which case the viral particles are transported back down the nerve root to the skin, where they multiply and cause a lesion to develop. During the dormant or latent period, the virus replicates in a different manner so that the immune system or available treatments have no effect on it. It is not known what reactivates the virus. It may be that the body's defense mechanisms are altered. Numerous studies have shown that host responses to infection influence initial development of the disease, severity of infection, development and maintenance of latency, and frequency of HSV recurrences.[8]

HSV-1 and HSV-2 can cause genital lesions. HSV is shed from active lesions and usually is transmitted by contact with infectious lesions or genital secretions. HSV-1 often is transmitted by kissing. When a person has a cold sore on the mouth, HSV-1 may be spread to the genital area by autoinoculation after poor handwashing or through oral intercourse. HSV-2 usually is transmitted by sexual contact but can be passed to an infant during childbirth if the virus is actively being shed from the genital tract.

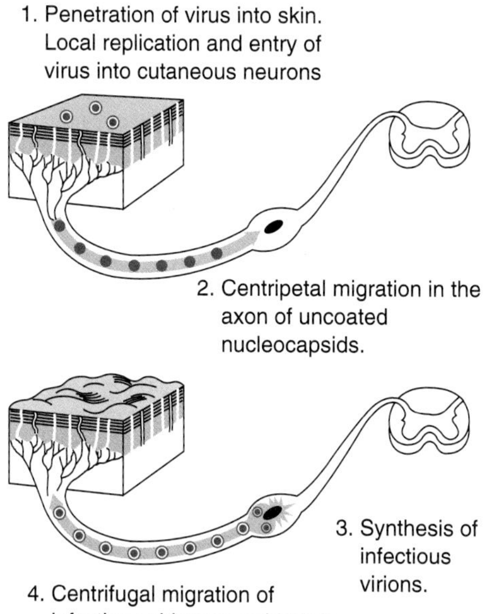
1. Penetration of virus into skin. Local replication and entry of virus into cutaneous neurons
2. Centripetal migration in the axon of uncoated nucleocapsids.
3. Synthesis of infectious virions.
4. Centrifugal migration of infectious virions to epidermis

Figure 52–1
Pathogenesis of primary mucocutaneous herpes simplex virus infection. (Corey L., & Spear P.G. [1986]. Infections with herpes simplex viruses. Pt. 1. *New England Journal of Medicine, 314*, 686)

The incubation period for HSV is 2 to 10 days. Genital HSV infection may manifest as a primary or a nonprimary form of infection. Primary infections are infections that occur in a person who is seronegative for antibody to HSV-1 or HSV-2. Nonprimary infections refer to the clinical appearance of genital herpes in a person who is seropositive for antibodies to HSV-1 or HSV-2, implying a previous asymptomatic exposure.

The initial symptoms of primary genital herpes infections include tingling, itching, and pain in the genital area followed by eruption of small pustules and vesicles. These lesions rupture on about the fifth day to form wet ulcers that are excruciatingly painful to touch and can be associated with dysuria, dyspareunia, and urine retention. Involvement of the cervix and urethra is seen in more than 80% of women with primary infections.[9] In men, the infection can cause urethritis and lesions of the penis and scrotum. Rectal and perianal infections are possible with anal contact. Systemic symptoms associated with primary infections include fever, headache, malaise, muscle ache, and lymphadenopathy. Primary infections may be debilitating enough to require hospitalization, particularly in women.

Untreated primary infections typically are self-limited and last for about 2 to 4 weeks. The symptoms usually worsen for the first 10 to 12 days. This period is followed by a 10- to 12-day interval during which the lesions crust over and gradually heal. Nonprimary episodes of genital herpes manifest with less severe symptoms that usually are of shorter duration and have fewer systemic manifestations. Except for the greater tendency of HSV-2 to recur, the clinical manifestations of HSV-2 and genital HSV-1 are similar. Genital HSV-2 infections are twice as likely to be reactivated and recur 8 to 12 times more often than genital HSV-1 infections.[8]

Recurrent HSV infections result from reactivation of the virus stored in the dorsal root ganglia of the infected dermatomes. An outbreak may be preceded by a prodrome of itching, burning, or tingling at the site of future lesions. Because patients have already developed immune lymphocytes from the primary infection, recurrent episodes have fewer lesions, fewer systemic symptoms, less pain, and a shorter duration (7 to 10 days). Frequency and severity of recurrences vary from person to person. Numerous factors, including emotional stress, lack of sleep, overexertion, other infections, vigorous or prolonged coitus, and premenstrual or menstrual distress, have been identified as triggering mechanisms.

Asymptomatic disease is significant. In the United States, only 20% to 25% of the estimated 55 million individuals with genital herpes in 1996 were aware of their condition.[9] Some persons possess antibodies to HSV-1 or HSV-2 without any history of clinical disease. Asymptomatic shedding of the virus can occur from these persons and from those whose recurrences result in viral excretion into saliva or cervical secretions without development of overt lesions. Although transmission of the disease was thought to occur primarily during symptomatic periods of viral excretion (*i.e.*, prodrome or actual outbreak), it has been estimated that up to 70% of transmission occurs through exposure during periods of asymptomatic shedding.[7]

Diagnosis of genital herpes is based on the symptoms, appearance of the lesions, and identification of the virus from a Tzanck smear or cultures taken from the lesions. Depending on the laboratory, a preliminary report on cultures takes from 2 to 5 days, and a final negative report takes from 10 to 12 days to establish. The stability of the virus in transport media is good for 48 to 72 hours, making mail transport possible. The likelihood of obtaining a positive culture decreases with each day that has elapsed after a lesion develops. The chance of obtaining a positive culture from a crusted lesion is slight, and patients suspected of having genital herpes should be instructed to have a culture within 24 hours of developing new lesions.

A Tzanck smear is done by scraping a debrided lesion with a cytology spatula and smearing the exudate on a slide, allowing the slide to dry, and sending it to a laboratory for microscopic identification of multinucleated giant cells. About 50% of Tzanck smear results are falsely negative. They are, however, available in 24 to 48 hours, compared with the 2 to 5 days required for culture tests. Newer tests for HSV-1 and HSV-2 include immunofluorescence assays that use monoclonal antibodies, DNA-hybridization procedures, and combined tissue culture and immunologic detection (*i.e.*, modified viral culture). These methods provide faster, cheaper diagnosis but require special equipment and training to perform and are less specific than viral culture techniques.[3,6] These types of testing are continually being improved and should be in wider use in the near future.

There is no known cure for genital herpes, and the methods of treatment are largely symptomatic. The antiviral drugs acyclovir, valacyclovir, and famciclovir have become the cornerstone for management of genital herpes. By interfering with viral DNA replication, these drugs decrease the frequency of recurrences, shorten the duration of active lesions, reduce the number of new lesions formed, and decrease viral shedding with primary infections. Valacyclovir, the active component of acyclovir, and famciclovir have greater bioavailability, which enables improved dosing schedules and increased compliance. Episodic intervention reduces the duration of viral shedding and the healing time for recurrent lesions.[10] Continuous antiviral suppressive therapy may be advised when more than six outbreaks occur within 1 year. These drugs are well tolerated, with few adverse effects. This long-term suppressive therapy does not limit latency, and reactivation of the disease frequently occurs after the drug is discontinued.[3] Topical treatment with antibacterial soaps, lotions, dyes, ultrasonography, and ultraviolet light has been tried with little success. Sometimes symptomatic relief can be obtained with cool compresses (*i.e.*, Burow's soaks), sitz baths, topical anesthetic agents, and oral analgesic drugs.

Good hygiene is essential to prevent secondary infection with HSV infections. Fastidious handwashing is recommended to avoid hand-to-eye spread of the infection. HSV infection of the eye is the most frequent cause of corneal blindness in the United States.[9] To prevent spread of the disease, intimate contact should be avoided until lesions are completely healed.

Because up to 65% of infected neonates die if they contract herpes infections during vaginal delivery, active infection during labor may necessitate cesarean delivery. Recommendations from the American College of Obstetrics and Gynecologists direct care providers to obtain cultures when a pregnant woman has active lesions, but vaginal delivery is acceptable if visible lesions are not present at the onset of labor. Weekly surveillance cultures from women with a history of HSV are no longer suggested. Because women with HSV-2 may be at increased risk for developing cervical cancer, it is recommended that they obtain annual Pap smears and be alert to the development of suspicious vulvar lesions that may warrant biopsy.

Molluscum Contagiosum

Molluscum contagiosum is a common viral disease of the skin that gives rise to multiple umbilicated papules. The disease is mildly contagious; it is transmitted by skin-to-skin contact, fomites, and autoinoculation. Lesions are domelike and have a dimpled appearance. A curdlike material can be expressed from the center of the lesion. Necrosis and secondary infection are possible. Diagnosis is based on the appearance of the lesion and microscopic identification of intracytoplasmic molluscum bodies. Molluscum is a benign and self-limited disease.

The goal of treatment is to prevent its spread for cosmetic reasons.[3] When indicated, treatment consists of removing the top of the papule with a sterile needle or scalpel, expressing the contents of each lesion, and applying alcohol or silver nitrate to the base. Electrodesiccation, cryosurgery, laser, and surgical biopsy are alternative treatments but seldom are needed unless lesions are large or extend over a wide area.

Chancroid

Chancroid (*i.e.*, soft chancre) is a disease of the external genitalia and lymph nodes. The causative organism is the gram-negative bacterium *Haemophilus ducreyi*, which causes acute ulcerative lesions with profuse discharge. This disease had become somewhat uncommon in the United States, but it is increasing in frequency and may be a leading cause of genital ulcers in many parts of the country.[11] It is more prevalent in Southeast Asia, the West Indies, and North Africa. A highly infectious disease, chancroid usually is transmitted by sexual intercourse or through skin and mucous membrane abrasions. Autoinoculation may lead to multiple chancres.

Lesions begin as macules, progress to pustules, and then rupture. This painful ulcer has a necrotic base and jagged edges. In contrast, the syphilitic chancre is nontender and indurated. Subsequent discharge can lead to further infection of self or others. On physical examination, lesions and regional lymphadenopathy (*i.e.*, buboes) may be found. Secondary infection may cause significant tissue destruction. Diagnosis is confirmed through the use of Gram stain and culture. The organism has shown resistance to treatment with sulfamethoxazole alone and to tetracycline. The CDC recommends treatment with azithromycin, erythromycin, or ceftriaxone.[5]

Granuloma Inguinale

Granuloma inguinale (*i.e.*, granuloma venereum) is caused by a gram-negative bacillus, *Calymmatobacterium donovani*, which is a tiny, encapsulated, intracellular parasite. This disease is almost nonexistent in the United States. It most frequently is found in India, Brazil, the West Indies, and parts of China, Australia, and Africa.

Granuloma inguinale causes ulceration of the genitalia, beginning with an innocuous papule. The papule progresses through nodular or vesicular stages until it begins to break down as pink, granulomatous tissue. At this final stage, the tissue becomes thin and friable and bleeds easily. There are complaints of swelling, pain, and itching. Extensive inflammatory scarring may cause late sequelae, such as lymphatic obstruction with the development of enlarged and elephantoid external genitalia. The liver, bladder, bone, joint, lung, and bowel tissue may become involved. Genital complications include tubo-ovarian abscess, fistula, vaginal stenosis, and occlusion of vaginal or anal orifices. Lesions may become neoplastic.

Diagnosis is made through the identification of Donovan bodies (*i.e.*, large mononuclear cells filled with intracytoplasmic gram-negative rods) in tissue smears, biopsy samples, or culture. A 3-week period of treatment with doxycycline, tetracycline, erythromycin, or gentamicin is used in treating the disorder.[5]

Lymphogranuloma Venereum

Lymphogranuloma venereum is an acute and chronic venereal disease caused by *Chlamydia trachomatis* types L1, L2, and P3. The disease, although found worldwide, has a low incidence outside the tropics. Most cases reported in the United States are in men.

The lesions of lymphogranuloma can incubate for a few days to several weeks and thereafter cause small painless papules or vesicles that may go undetected. An important characteristic of the disease is the early (1 to 4 weeks later) development of large, tender, and sometimes fluctuant inguinal lymph nodes called buboes. There may be flulike symptoms with joint pain, rash, weight loss, pneumonitis, tachycardia, splenomegaly, and proctitis. In later stages of the disease, a small percentage of affected persons develop elephantiasis of the external genitalia, caused by lymphatic obstruction or fibrous strictures of the rectum or urethra from inflammation and scarring. Urethral involvement may cause pyuria and dysuria. Anorectal structures may be compromised to the point of incontinence. Complications of lymphogranuloma infection may be minor or extensive, involving compromise of whole systems or progression to a cancerous state.

Diagnosis usually is accomplished by means of a complement fixation test for *Chlamydia* group antibody. High titers for this antibody differentiate this group from other chlamydial subgroups. Treatment involves 3 weeks of doxycycline, tetracycline, or erythromycin.[11] Surgery may be required to correct sequelae such as strictures or fistulas.

In summary, STDs that primarily affect the external genitalia include HPV (condyloma acuminata), genital herpes (HSV-2), molluscum contagiosum, chancroid, granuloma inguinale, and lymphogranuloma venereum. The lesions of these infections occur on the external genitalia of male and female sexual partners. Of concern is the relation between HPV and genital neoplasms. Genital herpes is caused by a neurotropic virus (HSV-2) that ascends through the peripheral nerves to reside in the sacral dorsal root ganglia. The herpes virus can be reactivated and produce recurrent lesions in genital structures that are supplied by the peripheral nerves of the affected ganglia. There is no permanent cure for herpes infections. Molluscum contagiosum is a benign and self-limited infection that is only mildly contagious. Chancroid, granuloma inguinale, and lymphogranuloma venereum produce external genital lesions with various degrees of inguinal lymph node involvement. These diseases are uncommon in the United States.

Vaginal Infections

After you have completed this section of the chapter, you should be able to meet the following objectives:

- State the difference between wet-mount slide and culture methods of diagnosis of STDs
- Compare the signs and symptoms of infections caused by *Candida albicans*, *Trichomonas vaginalis*, and bacterial vaginosis

Candidiasis, trichomoniasis, and bacterial vaginosis are vaginal infections that can be sexually transmitted. Although these infections can be transmitted sexually, the male partner usually is asymptomatic.

Candidiasis

Also called yeast infection, thrush, and moniliasis, candidiasis is the second leading cause of vulvovaginitis in the United States. Approximately 75% of reproductive-age women in the United States experience one episode in their lifetime; 40% to 45% experience two or more infections.[12]

The causative organism is *Candida*, a genus of yeast-like fungi. The species most commonly identified is *Candida albicans* (Fig. 52–2), but other candidal species, such as *C. glabrata* and *C. tropicalis*, have caused symptoms. Another 18 separate strains of *C. albicans* with various levels of virulence have been identified.[13] These organisms are present in 25% of healthy women without causing symptoms,[12] and the decision of the CDC to classify candidiasis as an STD is controversial. The possibility of sexual transmission has been recognized for many years; however, candidiasis requires a favorable environment for its growth. The gastrointestinal tract also serves as a reservoir for this organism, and candidiasis can develop through autoinoculation in women who are not sexually active. Although studies have documented the presence of *Candida* on the penis of male partners of women with vulvovaginal candidiasis, few men develop balanoposthitis that requires treatment.[12]

Causes for the overgrowth of *C. albicans* include antibiotic therapy, which suppresses the normal protective bacterial flora; high hormone levels owing to pregnancy or the use of oral contraceptives, which cause an increase in vaginal glycogen stores; and diabetes mellitus or HIV infection, because they compromise the immune system. Food allergies, hypothyroidism, endocrine disorders, dietary influences, tight-fitting clothing, and douching have also been suggested as possible contributors to the development of vulvovaginal candidiasis.[3,12]

In obese persons, *Candida* may grow in skin folds underneath the breast tissue, the abdominal flap, and the inguinal folds. Vulvar pruritus accompanied by irritation, dysuria, dyspareunia, erythema, and an odorless, thick, cheesy vaginal discharge are the predominant symptoms of the infection. Accurate diagnosis is made by identification of budding yeast filaments (*i.e.*, hyphae) or spores on a wet-mount slide using 20% potassium hydroxide (see Fig. 52–2). The pH of the discharge, which is checked with litmus paper, typically is less than 4.5. When the wet-mount technique is negative but the clinical manifestations are suggestive of candidiasis, a culture may be necessary.

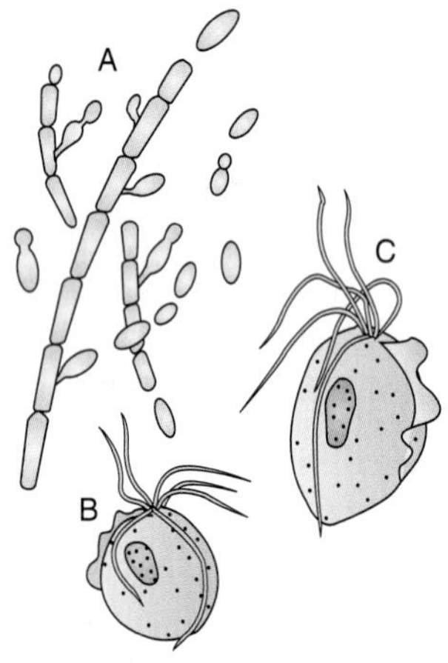

Figure 52–2
Organisms that cause vaginal infections. **(A)** *Candida albicans* (blastospores and pseudohyphae). **(B,C)** *Trichomonas vaginalis.*

Antifungals such as clotrimazole, miconazole, butaconazole, and terconazole, in various forms, are effective in treating candidiasis.[5] These drugs, with the exception of terconazole, are available without prescription for use by women who have had a previously confirmed diagnosis of candidiasis. Oral fluconazole has been shown to be as safe and effective as the standard intravaginal regimens.[14] Gentian violet solution (1%) applied to the vagina by swabs or tampon, potassium sorbate douches, or boric acid soaks to the vulva are treatment adjuncts. Tepid sodium bicarbonate baths, clothing that allows adequate ventilation, and the application of cornstarch to dry the area may increase comfort during treatment. Chronic vulvovaginal candidiasis, defined as three or more mycologically confirmed episodes within 1 year, affects approximately 5% of women and is difficult to manage and presents a challenge to researchers to find a means of eradicating this nonserious but aggravating affliction.

Candidiasis can be confused with Döderlein cytolysis—an excess of lactobacilli—which can present with a similar clinical picture. In the case of Döderlein cytolysis, wet-mount and culture techniques show only excessive lactobacilli but no yeast. Treatment for Döderlein cytolysis involves use of a sodium bicarbonate douche two to three times each week to raise the vaginal pH and decrease the symptoms.

Trichomoniasis

An anaerobic protozoan that can be transmitted sexually, *Trichomonas vaginalis* is shaped like a turnip and has three or four anterior flagella (see Fig. 52–2). Trichomonads can reside in the paraurethral glands of both sexes. Males harbor the organism in the urethra and prostate and are asymptomatic. Although 10% to 25% of women are asymptomatic, trichomoniasis is a common cause of vaginitis when some imbalance allows the protozoan to proliferate. This extracellular parasite feeds on the vaginal mucosa and ingests bacteria and leukocytes. The infection causes a copious, frothy, malodorous, green or yellow discharge. There commonly is erythema and edema of the affected mucosa, with occasional itching and irritation. Sometimes, small hemorrhagic areas, called strawberry spots, appear on the cervix.

Diagnosis is made microscopically by identification of the protozoan on a wet-mount slide preparation. The pH of the discharge usually is greater than 6.0. Special culture media are available for diagnosis but are costly and not needed for diagnosis.

Because the organism resides in other urogenital structures besides the vagina, systemic treatment is recommended. The treatment of choice is oral metronidazole (Flagyl), a medication that is effective against anaerobic protozoans.[5] Metronidazole is chemically similar to disulfiram (Antabuse), a drug used in the treatment of alcohol addiction that causes nausea, vomiting, flushing of the skin, headache, palpitations, and lowering of the blood pressure when alcohol is ingested. Alcohol should be avoided during and for 24 to 48 hours after treatment. Gastrointestinal disturbances and a metallic taste in the mouth are potential adverse effects of the drug. Metronidazole has not been proven safe for use during pregnancy and is used only after the first trimester for fear of potential teratogenic effects. Sexual partners should be treated to avoid reinfection, and abstinence is recommended until the full course of therapy is completed.

Bacterial Vaginosis (Nonspecific Vaginitis)

Considerable controversy exists regarding the organisms responsible for a vaginal infection that produces a characteristic fishy or ammonia-smelling discharge yet fails to produce an inflammatory response that is characteristic of most infections. A number of terms have been used to describe the nonspecific vaginitis that cannot be attributed to one of the accepted pathogenic organisms, such as *T. vaginalis* or *C. albicans*.

In 1955, Gardner and Dukes isolated an organism from women with this type of vaginitis and proposed the name *Haemophilus vaginalis*, apparently because the gram-negative organism required blood for growth.[15] In 1963, gram-positive isolates were found, and the organism was renamed *Corynebacterium vaginale*. Because the organism did not meet all the criteria of corynebacteria, it was renamed *Gardnerella vaginalis* in 1980, after its original discoverer, and admitted to a taxonomic genus of its own.[16] The development of a special agar on which *G. vaginalis* could be cultured led to the discovery that 40% to 70% of women harbor this organism as part of their normal vaginal flora. Further study revealed that abnormal discharge frequently contained highly motile, crescent-shaped rods called *Mobiluncus* and many more anaerobic than aerobic bacteria.[17] It has been suggested that the presence of anaerobes, which produce ammonia or amines from amino acids, favors the growth of *G. vaginalis* by raising vaginal pH. Because of the presence of anaerobic bacteria and the lack of an inflammatory response, a new term, *bacterial vaginosis*, was proposed.[18]

Bacterial vaginosis is the most prevalent form of vaginal infection seen by health care professionals. Its relation to sexual activity is not clear. Sexual activity is believed to be a catalyst rather than a primary mode of transmission, and endogenous factors play a role in the development of symptoms. The predominant symptom of bacterial vaginosis is a thin, grayish white discharge that has a foul, fishy odor. Burning, itching, and erythema usually are absent because the bacteria has only minimal inflammatory potential. Bacterial vaginosis may be carried asymptomatically by men and women.

The diagnosis is made when at least three of the following characteristics are present: homogeneous discharge, production of a fishy, amine odor when a 10% potassium hydroxide solution is dropped onto the secretions, vaginal pH above 4.5 (usually 5.0 to 6.0), and appearance of characteristic "clue cells" on wet-mount microscopic studies. Clue cells are squamous epithelial cells covered with masses of coccobacilli, often with large clumps of organisms floating free from the cell. Because *G. vaginalis* can be a normal vaginal flora, cultures should not be done routinely. They are of limited clinical value, because it is believed that the condition is caused by a combination of *G. vaginalis* and anaerobic bacteria.

The mere presence of *G. vaginalis* in an asymptomatic woman is not an indication for treatment. When indicated, treatment is aimed at eradicating the anaerobic component of bacterial vaginosis to reestablish the normal balance of the vaginal flora. The CDC recommends oral metronidazole, although failure rates may range from 30% to 70%. Alternative therapies include metronidazole vaginal gel, clindamycin vaginal cream, or oral clindamycin. Treatment of sexual partners is not recommended.[11]

Preterm labor, premature rupture of membranes, chorioamnionitis, and postpartum endometritis have been linked to the organisms associated with bacterial vaginosis. Oral or cream clindamycin formulations can be used for treatment during the first trimester of pregnancy; oral or vaginal metronidazole can be used after the first trimester for treatment failures. Routine screening for bacterial vaginosis is not being advocated, but symptomatic women should be treated.[19]

In summary, candidiasis, trichomoniasis, and bacterial vaginosis are common vaginal infections that become symptomatic because of changes within the vaginal ecosystem. Only trichomoniasis is spread through sexual contact. Trichomoniasis is caused by an anaerobic protozoan. The infection incites the production of a copious, frothy, yellow or green, malodorous discharge. Candidiasis, also called a yeast infection, is the form of vulvovaginitis that women are most familiar with. Candida can be present without producing symptoms; usually some host factor, such as altered immune status, contributes to the development of vulvovaginitis. It can be treated with over-the-counter medications. Bacterial vaginosis is the most common cause of vaginal discharge. It is a nonspecific type of infection that produces a characteristic fishy-smelling discharge. The infection is thought to be caused by the combined presence of *G. vaginalis* and anaerobic bacteria. The anaerobe raises the vaginal pH, thereby favoring the growth of *G. vaginalis*.

Vaginal-Urogenital-Systemic Infections

After you have completed this section of the chapter, you should be able to meet the following objectives:

- Compare the signs and symptoms of gonorrhea in the male and female
- Describe the three stages of syphilis
- State the genital and nongenital complications that can occur with chlamydial infections, gonorrhea, nonspecific urogenital infection, and syphilis
- State the treatment for chlamydial urogenital infections, gonorrhea, nonspecific urogenital infections, and syphilis

Some STDs infect genital and extragenital structures. Among the infections of this type are chlamydial infections, gonorrhea, nonspecific urogenital infection, and syphilis. Many of these infections also pose a risk to babies born to infected mothers. Some infections, such as syphilis, may be spread to the infant while in utero; others, such as chlamydial and gonorrheal infections, can be spread to the infant during the birth process.

Chlamydial Infections

C. trachomatis is an obligate intracellular bacterial pathogen that is closely related to gram-negative bacteria. It resembles a virus in that it requires tissue culture for isolation, but like a bacteria, it has RNA and DNA and is susceptible to some antibiotics.

C. trachomatis can be serologically subdivided into types A, B, and C, which are associated with trachoma; types L1, L2, and L3, which are associated with lymphogranuloma venereum; and types D through K, which are associated with genital infections and their complications. The organism causes a wide variety of genitourinary infections, including nongonococcal urethritis in men and pelvic inflammatory disease in women. *Chlamydia* can cause significant ocular disease in neonates; it is a leading cause of blindness in underdeveloped countries. In these countries, the organism is spread primarily by flies, fomites, and nonsexual personal contact. In industrial countries, the organism is spread almost exclusively by sexual contact and, therefore, affects primarily the genitourinary structures.

Although chlamydial infections are not reportable in all states, their incidence is estimated to be more than twice that of gonorrhea. The most prevalent STD in the United States, chlamydial infections occur at a rate of 3 to 10 million new cases each year according to CDC estimates, predominantly among individuals younger than 25 years of age.[20]

The chlamydial organism exists in two forms: the elementary body, which is the infectious particle capable of entering uninfected cells, and the initiator or reticulate body, which multiplies by binary fission to produce the inclusions identified in stained cells. The 48-hour growth cycle starts with attachment of the elementary body to the susceptible host cell, following which it is ingested by a process that resembles phagocytosis (Fig. 52–3). Once within the cell, the elementary body is organized into the reticulate body, the metabolically active form of the organism that is capable of reproduction. The reticulate body is not infectious and cannot survive outside the body. The reticulate bodies divide within the cell for up to 36 hours and then condense to form new elementary bodies, which are released when the infected cell bursts.

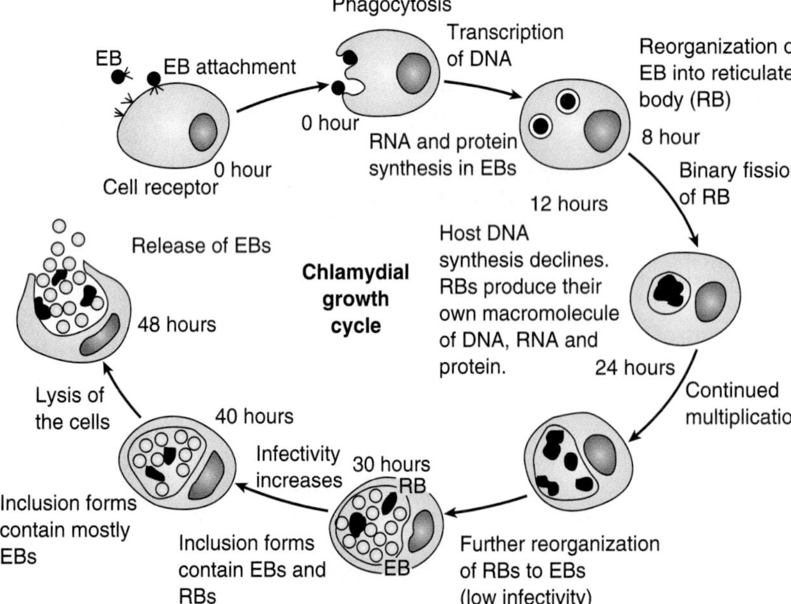

Figure 52–3 Chlamydial growth cycle. EB, elementary body; RB, reticulate body. (Thompson S.E., & Washington A.E. [1983]. Epidemiology of sexually transmitted *Chlamydia trachomatis* infections. *Epidemiologic Reviews, 5,* 96–123)

The signs and symptoms of chlamydial infections resemble those produced by gonorrhea. In women, chlamydial infections may cause urinary frequency, dysuria, and vaginal discharge. The most common symptom is a mucopurulent cervical discharge. The cervix itself frequently hypertrophies and becomes erythematous, edematous, and extremely friable. The organism may cause pelvic inflammatory disease, which leads to infertility or ectopic pregnancy. These complications result in an estimated 2.5 million outpatient visits each year and an annual cost exceeding $5 billion.[21] The most significant difference between chlamydial and gonococcal salpingitis is that chlamydial infections may be asymptomatic or subclinically nonspecific. This can lead to greater fallopian tube damage and increase the reservoir for further chlamydial infections.

Routine screening for sexually active adolescents and young adults has been suggested by the CDC in an effort to minimize these serious sequelae of asymptomatic infection. Between 25% and 50% of infants born to mothers with cervical chlamydial infections develop ocular disease (*i.e.*, inclusion conjunctivitis), and 10% to 20% develop chlamydial pneumonitis.

In men, chlamydial infections cause urethritis, including meatal erythema and tenderness, urethral discharge, dysuria, and urethral itching. Prostatitis and epididymitis with subsequent infertility may develop. The most serious complication that can develop with nongonococcal urethritis is Reiter's syndrome, a systemic condition characterized by urethritis, conjunctivitis, arthritis, and mucocutaneous lesions (see Chapter 47).

Diagnosis of chlamydial infections takes several forms. The identification of polymorphonuclear leukocytes on Gram stain of male discharge or cervical discharge is presumptive evidence. The two available serologic tests can be misleading. Complement fixation tests are the most useful in diagnosing lymphogranuloma venereum. The microimmunofluorescent test is more sensitive for *C. trachomatis* types D through K, but it does not distinguish among acute, chronic, or carrier states. The high rates of antichlamydial antibodies in sexually active populations render serodiagnosis inconclusive.[3] Tissue cultures are definitive but slow (requiring at least 3 days), costly, and not always available. Nonculture methods, such as direct fluorescent antibody test (DFA) and an enzyme-linked immunosorbent assay (ELISA), which use antibodies against an antigen in the *Chlamydia* cell wall, have been developed. These are less expensive, rapid tests that require less sophisticated laboratory techniques but have a lower sensitivity than culture (sensitivity ranges from 70% to 100% and specificity from 94% to 100% for either type of test). The positive predictive value of these tests is excellent among high-risk groups, but false-positive results occur more often in populations with lower risks.

Amplified DNA probe assays, such as the polymerase chain reaction (PCR) or ligase chain reaction (LCR) have demonstrated specificity of near 100% (same as culture) and sensitivity of 94%. Sensitivity of cell culture has been estimated at 70% to 85% for endocervical specimens and 50% to 75% for male urethral specimens. Amplified DNA testing can be performed on urine and swab specimens from the distal vagina and the traditional endocervical and urethral specimens, making it an easy, convenient means of accurate detection.[20–23] Cost may be a factor in determining which type of testing to use.

The CDC recommends the use of azithromycin or doxycycline in the treatment of chlamydial infection; penicillin is ineffective.[5] Antibiotic treatment of both sexual partners simultaneously is recommended. Abstinence from sexual activity is encouraged to facilitate cure.

Gonorrhea

Gonorrhea is a reportable disease caused by the bacterium *Neisseria gonorrhoeae*. In 1995, there were 395,493 reported cases of gonorrhea in the United States. Of these reported cases, more than 90% involved persons between 15 and 44 years of age, with the heaviest concentration among young adults (15 to 24 years). Although the incidence of gonorrhea has continued to decline since its peak in 1975, there has been an increase in infections caused by antibiotic-resistant strains during that period.[24]

The gonococcus is a pyogenic (*i.e.*, pus-forming), gram-negative diplococcus that evokes inflammatory reactions characterized by purulent exudates. Humans are the only natural host for *N. gonorrhoeae*. The organism grows best in warm, mucus-secreting epithelia. The portal of entry can be the genitourinary tract, eyes, oropharynx, anorectum, or skin.

Transmission usually is by heterosexual or homosexual intercourse. Autoinoculation of the organism to the conjunctiva is possible. Neonates born to infected mothers can acquire the infection during passage through the birth canal and are in danger of developing gonorrheal conjunctivitis, with resultant blindness, unless treated promptly. An amniotic infection syndrome characterized by premature rupture of the membranes, premature delivery, and increased risk of infant morbidity and mortality has been identified as an additional complication of gonococcal infections in pregnancy.[19] Genital gonorrhea in young children should raise the possibility of sexual abuse.

The infection commonly manifests 2 to 7 days after exposure. It typically begins in the anterior urethra, accessory urethral glands, Bartholin's or Skene's glands, and the cervix. If untreated, gonorrhea spreads from its initial sites upward into the genital tract. In males, it spreads to the prostate and epididymis; in females, it commonly moves to the fallopian tubes. Pharyngitis may follow oral-genital contact. The organism can also invade the bloodstream (*i.e.*, disseminated gonococcal infection), causing serious sequelae such as bacteremic involvement of joint spaces, heart valves, meninges, and other body organs and tissues.[19]

Persons with gonorrhea may be asymptomatic and may unwittingly spread the disease to their sexual partners. Men are more likely to be symptomatic than women. In men, the initial symptoms include urethral pain and a creamy, yellow, sometimes bloody discharge. The disorder may become chronic and affect the prostate, epididymis, and periurethral glands. Rectal infections are common in homosexual men. In women, recognizable symptoms include unusual genital or urinary discharge, dysuria, dyspareunia, pelvic pain or tenderness, unusual vaginal bleeding (including bleeding after intercourse), fever, and proctitis. Symptoms may occur or increase during or immediately after menses, because the bacterium is an intracellular diplococcus that thrives in menstrual blood but cannot survive long outside the human body. There may be infections of the uterus and development of acute or chronic infection of the fallopian tubes (*i.e.*, salpingitis), with ultimate scarring and sterility.

Diagnosis is based on the history of sexual exposure and symptoms. It is confirmed by identification of the organism on Gram stain or culture. A Gram stain usually is an effective means of diagnosis in symptomatic males (*i.e.*, those with discharge). In women and asymptomatic men, a culture usually is preferred because the Gram stains often are unreliable. A specimen should be collected from the appropriate site (*i.e.*, endocervix, urethra, anal canal, or oropharynx), plated onto selective Thayer-Martin media, and placed in a carbon dioxide environment. *N. gonorrhoeae* is a fastidious organism with specific nutrient and environmental needs. Optimal growth requires a pH of 7.4, temperature of 35.5°C, and an atmosphere that contains 2% to 10% carbon dioxide.[25] The accuracy of culture results is affected if transport is delayed or growth requirements are not available. The search for methods to provide rapid and accurate diagnosis of *N. gonorrhoeae* continues. An enzyme immunoassay for detecting gonococcal antigens (Gonozyme) is available but has several requirements that limit its usefulness. Detection by means of amplified DNA probes is possible using urine and urethral swab specimens and may be cost effective in high risk populations.

Testing for other STDs, particularly syphilis and chlamydial infections, is suggested at the time of examination. Pregnant women are routinely screened at the time of their first prenatal visit; high-risk populations should have repeat cultures during the third trimester. Neonates are routinely treated with various antibacterial agents applied to the conjunctiva within 1 hour of birth to protect against undiagnosed gonorrhea and other diseases.

The standard treatment of gonorrhea has been with the use of injectable penicillin and oral probenecid, a drug that delays the renal excretion of penicillin. Patients who were allergic to penicillin were treated with oral tetracycline for 7 days instead. The current treatment recommendation to combat tetracycline- and penicillin-resistant strains of *N. gonorrhea* is ceftriaxone in a single injection. For a symptomatic patient, particularly the male partner, it is common practice to treat both partners before culture results are available because of the potential loss of reproductive capacity. Persons with the disease, particularly pregnant women, should be followed with repeated cultures to determine the effectiveness of treatment. Patients are instructed to refrain from intercourse or to use condoms until cultures show negative results.

Because of the high rate of concomitant chlamydial infections (30% to 50%) in women with gonococcal pelvic inflammatory disease, the CDC now recommends a treatment regimen for gonorrhea that treats both infections. The combination regimen supplements the single-dose ceftriaxone treatment with a 7-day treatment of oral doxycycline. Another alternative is a single injection of spectinomycin and a 7-day treatment with doxycycline. In pregnant women, erythromycin can be substituted for tetracycline.[11]

Nonspecific Urogenital Infection

Nonspecific urogenital infection is chiefly a disease of the male urethra but may involve the cervix, urethra, Bartholin's glands, vagina, and fallopian tubes in the female. In about 50% of cases, the disease is secondary to chlamydial infection. *Chlamydia* is a formidable pathogen because of its long-term effects and its ability to affect the neonate. This disease entity, like nonspecific vaginitis, will probably be named more specifically as the causative agents are identified.

Diagnosis is made through the use of cultures. Treatment consists of various antibiotic regimens, dictated by the organism and antibiotic sensitivity.

Syphilis

Syphilis is a reportable disease caused by a spirochete, *Treponema pallidum*. During 1995, 16,501 new cases of primary and secondary syphilis were reported in the United States.[24] This represents a steady decline from the 50,000 cases reached in 1990 following an epidemic resurgence of this problem between 1985 and 1990. The populations that have experienced the largest rise in the incidence of syphilis are blacks and Hispanics in urban areas and women of all racial and ethnic backgrounds. The reasons for the reversal in the trend of decreasing incidence that characterized the years before 1985 are unknown. Budget reductions in syphilis control programs, the practice of trading sex with multiple partners for illegal drugs, and the increased use of cocaine among women of childbearing age have been contributing factors. Likewise, no data exist to identify which STD control programs may be responsible for the actual decline of syphilis among all racial groups and in both sexes.[26]

T. pallidum is spread by direct contact with an infectious, moist lesion, usually through sexual intercourse. Bacteria-laden secretions may transfer the organism during kissing or intimate contact. Skin abrasions provide another possible portal of entry. There is rapid transplacental transmission of the organism from the mother to the fetus after 16 weeks' gestation, so that active disease in the mother during pregnancy can produce congenital syphilis in the fetus. Untreated syphilis can cause prematurity, stillbirth, and congenital defects and active infection in the infant. Once treated for syphilis, a pregnant woman usually is followed throughout pregnancy by repeat testing of serum titers.

The clinical disease is divided into three stages: primary, secondary, and tertiary. Primary syphilis is characterized by the appearance of a chancre at the site of exposure. Chancres typically appear within 3 weeks of exposure but may incubate for 1 week to 3 months. The primary chancre begins as a single, indurated, buttonlike papule up to several centimeters in diameter that erodes to create a clean-based ulcerated lesion on an elevated base. These lesions usually are painless and located at the site of sexual contact. Primary syphilis is readily apparent in the male, where the lesion is on the penis or scrotum. Although chancres can develop on the external genitalia in females, they are more common on the vagina or cervix, and primary syphilis may therefore go untreated. There usually is an accompanying regional lymphadenopathy. The disease is highly contagious at this stage, but because the symptoms are mild, it frequently goes unnoticed. The chancre usually heals within 3 to 12 weeks, with or without treatment.

The timing of the second stage of syphilis varies even more than that of the first, lasting from 1 week to 6 months. The symptoms of a rash (especially on the palms and soles), fever, sore throat, stomatitis, nausea, loss of appetite, and inflamed eyes may come and go for a year but usually last for 3 to 6 months. Secondary manifestations may include alopecia and genital condylomata lata. Condylomata lata are elevated, red-brown lesions that may ulcerate and produce a foul discharge. They are 2 to 3 cm in diameter, contain many spirochetes, and are highly contagious.

After the second stage, syphilis frequently enters a latent phase that may last the lifetime of the person or progress to tertiary syphilis at some point. Persons can be infective during the first 1 to 2 years of latency.

Tertiary syphilis is a delayed response of the untreated disease. It can occur as long as 20 years after the initial infection. Only about one third of those with untreated syphilis progress to the tertiary stage of the disease, and about one half of these develop symptoms. About one third undergo spontaneous cure, and the remaining one third continue to have positive serologic tests but do not develop structural lesions.[25] When syphilis does progress to the symptomatic tertiary stage, it commonly takes one of three forms: development of localized destructive lesions called gummas, development of cardiovascular lesions, or development of central nervous system lesions. The syphilitic gumma is a peculiar rubbery, necrotic lesion that is caused by noninflammatory tissue necrosis. Gummas can occur singly or multiply and vary in size from microscopic lesions to large, tumorous masses. They most commonly are found in the liver, testes, and bone. Central nervous system lesions can produce dementia, blindness, or injury to the spinal cord, with ataxia and sensory loss (*i.e.*, tabes dorsalis). Cardiovascular manifestations usually result from scarring of the medial layer of the thoracic aorta with aneurysm formation (see Chapter 17). These aneurysms produce enlargement of the aortic valve ring with aortic valve insufficiency.

T. pallidum does not produce endotoxins or exotoxins but evokes a humoral immune response that provides the basis for serologic tests. Two types of antibodies—nonspecific and specific—are produced. The nonspecific antibodies can be detected by flocculation tests such as the Venereal Disease Research Laboratory (VDRL) test.[2] Because these tests are nonspecific, positive results can occur with diseases other than syphilis. The tests are easy to perform, rapid, and inexpensive and frequently are used as a screening test for syphilis. Results become positive 4 to 6 weeks after infection or 1 to 3 weeks after the appearance of the primary lesion. Because these tests are quantitative, they can be used to measure the degree of disease activity or treatment effectiveness. The VDRL titer usually is high during the secondary stage of the disease and becomes less so during the tertiary stage. A falling titer during treatment suggests a favorable response. The fluorescent treponemal antibody absorption (FTA-ABS) or microhemagglutinin test is used to detect specific antibodies to *T. pallidum*. These qualitative tests are used to determine whether a positive result on a nonspecific test such as the VDRL is attributable to syphilis. The test results remain positive for life.

T. pallidum cannot be cultured. The diagnosis of syphilis is based on serologic tests or dark-field microscopic examination with identification of the spirochete in specimens collected from lesions. Because the disease's incubation period may delay test sensitivity, serologic tests usually are repeated after 6 weeks if the initial test results were negative.

The treatment of choice for syphilis is penicillin. Because of the spirochetes' long generation time, effective tissue levels of penicillin must be maintained for several weeks. Long-acting injectable forms of penicillin are used. Tetracycline or doxycycline is used for treatment in persons who are sensitive to penicillin. Erythromycin is the treatment of choice in pregnancy or in case of penicillin allergy. Sexual partners should be evaluated and treated prophylactically even though they may show no sign of infection. All treated individuals should be reexamined clinically and serologically at 3 and 36 months after completing therapy.[11]

In summary, the vaginal-urogenital-systemic STDs—chlamydial infections, gonorrhea, nonspecific urogenital infection, and syphilis—can severely involve the genital structures and manifest as systemic infections. Gonorrheal and chlamydial infections can cause a wide variety of genitourinary complications in men and women, and both can cause ocular disease and blindness in neonates born to infected mothers. Nonspecific urogenital infection is primarily a disease of the male urethra but may involve the cervix, urethra, Bartholin's glands, vagina, and fallopian tubes in the female. Syphilis is caused by a spirochete, *T. pallidum*. It can produce widespread systemic effects and is transferred to the fetus of infected mothers by way of the placenta.

REFERENCES

1. Garchustsky M. (1996). Human papillomavirus. *ADVANCE for Nurse Practioners* 5, 22.
2. DeCherney A.H., Pernoll M.L. (1994). *Current Obstetric and Gynecologic Diagnosis and Treatment* (pp. 692, 758). Norwalk, CT: Appleton & Lange.
3. Glass R.H. (1993). *Office gynecology* (4th ed., pp. 3, 9, 15, 59). Baltimore: Williams & Wilkins.
4. Schiffman M.H. (1993). Latest HPV findings: Some clinical implications. *Contemporary OB-GYN* 10, 28.
5. Centers for Disease Control. (1993). STD treatment guidelines 1993. *MMWR Morbidity and Mortality Weekly Report* 42, (RR-14).
6. Youngkin E.Q. (1995). Sexually transmitted diseases. Current and emerging concerns. *Journal of Obstetric, Gynecologic, and Neonatal Nursing* 24 (8), 754, 745.
7. Orange L.M. (1996). Herpes virus clarified by diagnostic techniques. *OB-GYN News* Jan 15, 14.
8. Corey L., Spear P.G. (1986). Infections with herpes simplex viruses—Part 1. *New England Journal of Medicine* 314, 686.
9. Corey L., Spear P.G. (1986). Infections with herpes simplex viruses—Part 2. *New England Journal of Medicine* 314, 749.
10. Sacks S.L., Aoki F.Y., Diaz-Mitoma F., et al. (1996). Patient-initiated twice daily oral famcyclovir for early recurrent genital herpes. *JAMA* 276 (1), 44.
11. Tucker ME. (1996). Chancroid on the rise causing genital ulcers. *OB-GYN News* Oct 15, 9.
12. Freeman SB. (1995). Common genitourinary infections. *JOGNN* 24 (8), 736, 737.
13. Robertson W.H. (1988). Mycology of vulvovaginitis. *American Journal of Obstetrics and Gynecology* 158, 989.
14. Sobel J.D., Brooker D., Stein G.E., et al. (1995). Single oral dose fluconazole compared with conventional clotrimazole topical therapy of *Candida* vaginitis. *American Journal of Obstetrics and Gynecology* 69, 962.
15. Gardner H.L., Dukes C.D. (1955). *Haemophilus vaginalis* vaginitis. *American Journal of Obstetrics and Gynecology* 69, 62.
16. Jones B.M. (1983). *Gardnerella* vaginitis. *Medical Laboratory Sciences* 40, 53.
17. Thomason J.L., Schreckenberger P.C., Spellacy W.N., et al. (1984). Clinical and microbiological characterization of patients with nonspecific vaginosis associated with motile, curved anaerobic rods. *Journal of Infectious Diseases* 149, 814.
18. Eschenback D.A. (1984). Diagnosis of bacterial vaginosis (nonspecific vaginitis): Role of the laboratory. *Clinical Microbiology Newsletter* 6, 18.
19. Ament L.A., Whalen E. (1996). Sexually transmitted diseases in pregnancy: Diagnosis, impact, and intervention. *Journal of Obstetric, Gynecologic and Neonatal Nursing* 15 (8), 663, 668.
20. Centers for Disease Control. (1993). Recommendations for the prevention and management of Chlamydia trachomatis infections. *MMWR* Morbidity and Mortality Weekly Report 42 (RR-12), 3, 14–19.
21. Quinn T.C., Gaydos C., Shepard M., et al. (1996). Epidemiologic and microbiolgic correlates of *Chlamydia trachomatis* infection in sexual partners. *Journal of the American Medical Association* 276 (21), 1737.
22. Lee H.H., Chenesky M.A., Schachter J., et al. (1995). Diagnosis of *Chlamydia trachomatis* genitourinary infections in women by ligase chain reaction assay of urine. *Lancet* 345, 213–216.
23. Zoler M.L. (1995). Kits supplant STD speculum examination. *OB-GYN News* 30 (22), 3.
24. Centers for Disease Control. (1996). Summary of notifiable diseases—United States, 1995. *MMWR Morbidity and Mortality Weekly Report* 44 (53), 10.
25. Sweet R.L., Gibbs R.S. (1985). *Infectious disease of the female genital tract* (pp. 39–40, 103–122). Baltimore: Williams & Wilkins.
26. Centers for Disease Control. (1993). Surveillance of primary and secondary syphilis—United States, 1991. *MMWR* Morbidity and Mortality Weekly Report 42 (SS-3), 13.

ADDITIONAL READINGS

Buckley H.B. (1992). Syphilis–A review and update of the "new" infection of the 90s. *Nurse Practioner* 17 (8), 25.

Erickson M.J. (1994). Chlamydial infections: Combating the silent threat. *American Journal of Nursing—NP* 6, 16B-F.

Holmes K., March P., Sparling P.F., et al. (1990). *Sexually transmitted diseases*. New York: McGraw-Hill.

MCourty M.K. (1995). Vaginal infections: Keys to treatment. *Contemporary Nurse Practioner* 5 (6), 18–23.

Sharts-Hopko N.C. (1997). STDs in women: What you need to know. *AJN* 97 (4), 46–54.

Webb T. (1994). Sexually transmitted diseases: Barrier methods key to protection. *ADVANCE for Nurse Practioners*, 5, 17–20.

US Public Health Service. (1995). Sexually transmitted diseases and HIV infection. *Nurse Practioner* 20 (2), 66–71.

Integrated Body Function

French physiologist Claude Bernard (1813–1878) was the first to theorize that, in a closely orchestrated process, the body strives to achieve and maintain a steady state. In the middle of the 19th century, Bernard proposed his concept of the milieu intèrieur, *or the stable internal environment, regulated by a multitude of interacting control mechanisms geared to maintain the body's chemical and physical status. He proposed that internal secretions functioned as a part of the body's regulatory mechanism, maintaining a balance in response to a range of changing conditions imposed by the external environment.*

Through his experiments, Bernard discovered a number of mechanisms that were dedicated to maintaining homeostasis. One of his discoveries was the process by which internal temperature is kept constant. He was able to show that the nervous system responds to internal cold by sending chemical messages to the blood vessels to constrict in order to conserve body heat. The product of his considerable work is the classic Introduction to the Study of Experimental Medicine *(1865).*

UNIT XIV

CHAPTER 53

Stress and Adaptation

Health is a dynamic state in which energy must be expended continuously to adapt to life stresses. Much of this energy is used to recruit physiologic and psychologic behaviors that oppose or compensate for perceived threats to the integrity of the internal environment. In this respect, the human body is truly an amazing structure—able to withstand exposure to environmental stresses while maintaining its internal environment within the confines of what is called *normal*.

From astronauts who have traveled to the moon and from explorers of the ocean's depths, we have learned that vital physiologic functions such as heart rate, blood pH, and body temperature remain remarkably similar to those observed under normal environmental conditions. Even in advanced disease states, the body retains much of its adaptive capacity and is able to maintain the internal environment within relatively normal limits.

Health and Adaptation

After you have completed this section of the chapter, you should be able to meet the following objectives:

- Explain the purpose of adaptation
- Describe the components of a control system including the function of a negative feedback system
- Cite Cannon's four features of homeostasis

Adaptation implies the ability to respond and maintain stability, physiologically and psychologically, during rapidly changing conditions in the internal and external environments. Adaptation and homeostasis are idealized concepts. In practice, the body has available to it a wide variety and range of responses for adjusting to the external and internal environments, and conditions do not always return to their original state.

Adaptation affects the whole person. When adapting to stress, the body uses behaviors that are most efficient and effective; it does not use long-term mechanisms when short-term adaptation mechanisms are sufficient. The increase in heart rate that accompanies a febrile illness is a temporary response designed to deliver additional oxygen to the tissues during the short period when the elevated temperature increases the metabolic needs of the tissues; the increase in heart rate also expedites delivery of heat-carrying blood to the skin surface, where the heat can be lost to the external environment. On the other hand, adaptive responses such as hypertrophy of the left ventricle in persons with systemic hypertension are long-term responses.

Of particular interest are the differences in the body's response to stressors that threaten the integrity of the body's physiologic environment and those that threaten the integrity of the person's psychosocial environment. Many of the body's responses to physiologic stressors are controlled on a moment-by-moment basis by feedback mechanisms that limit their application and duration of action. For example, the baroreflex-mediated rise in heart rate that occurs when a person moves from the recumbent to the standing position is almost instantaneous and subsides within seconds. Furthermore, the response to physiologic stressors that threaten the integrity of the internal environment is specific to the stress; the body does not usually raise the body temperature when a rise in heart rate is needed. In contrast, the response to psychologic stressors is not regulated with the same degree of specificity and feedback control; instead, the effect may be inappropriate and sustained.

Constancy of the Internal Environment

The environment in which body cells live is not the external environment that surrounds the organism, but a local fluid environment that surrounds each cell. It is from this internal environment that body cells receive their nourishment, and it is into this fluid that they secrete their wastes. Even the contents of the gastrointestinal tract and lungs do not become part of the internal environment until they have been absorbed into the extracellular fluid. A multicellular organism is able to survive only as long as the composition of the internal environment is compatible with the survival needs of the individual cells. Even a small change in the pH of the body fluids can disrupt the metabolic processes of individual cells.

Claude Bernard, a 19th century physiologist, was the first to describe clearly the central importance of a stable internal environment (*milieu intèrieur*). Bernard recognized that body fluids that surround the cells and the various organ systems provide the means for exchange between the external and the internal environments.

1. Constancy in an open system, such as our bodies represent, requires mechanisms that act to maintain this constancy. Cannon based this proposition on insights into the ways by which steady states such as glucose concentrations, body temperature, and acid-base balance were regulated.
2. Steady-state conditions require that any tendency toward change automatically met with factors that resist change. An increase in blood sugar results in thirst as the body attempts to dilute the concentration of sugar in the extracellular fluid.
3. The regulating system that determines the homeostatic state consists of a number of cooperating mechanisms acting simultaneously or successively. Blood sugar is regulated by insulin, glucagon, and other hormones that control its release from the liver or its uptake by the tissues.
4. Homeostasis does not occur by chance, but is the result of organized self-government.

(Cannon W.B. [1932]. *The wisdom of the body* (pp. 299–300). New York: W.W. Norton)

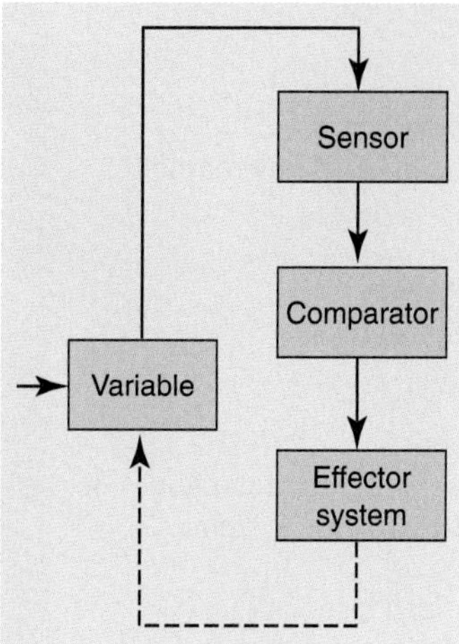

Figure 53–1
A simple control system consisting of a sensor that monitors a physiologic variable, a comparator that compares the actual value of the monitored variable with the setpoint of the system, and an effector system that functions to correct the disturbance (*solid line*). The *broken line* represents feedback control.

Homeostasis

The concept of a stable internal environment was supported by Walter B. Cannon, who proposed that this kind of stability, which he called *homeostasis*, was achieved through a system of carefully coordinated physiologic processes that oppose change.[1] He pointed out that these processes were largely automatic.

Cannon emphasized that homeostasis involves resistance to external disturbances and resistance to disturbances from within. In his book *Wisdom of the Body*, published in 1939, Cannon presented four tentative propositions to describe the general features of homeostasis.[1] These propositions are described in the box. With this set of propositions, Cannon emphasized that when a factor is known to shift homeostasis in one direction, it is reasonable to expect the existence of mechanisms that have the opposite effect. In the homeostatic regulation of blood sugar, for example, mechanisms that both raise and lower blood sugar would be expected to play a part. As long as the responding mechanism to the stress can recover homeostasis, the integrity of the body and the status of normality are retained.

Control Systems

A homeostatic control system is a collection of interconnected components that function to keep a physical or chemical parameter of the body relatively constant. At least three essential components exist in a control system: a *sensor*, which detects changes in product or function; a *comparator*, which compares the sensed value with an acceptable range; and an *effector system*, which returns the function or product to the acceptable range (Fig. 53–1).

The ability of the body to function under conditions of change in the internal and external environment depends on the thousands of control systems that regulate body function. The body's control systems regulate cellular function, control the life processes, and integrate functions of the different organ systems. The most intricate of these control systems are the genetic control systems that regulate cellular function, including cell structure and replication. Other control systems regulate function within organs and systems, and still others operate throughout the body to integrate the functions of the different organ systems. The concentration of carbon dioxide in the extracellular spaces is regulated by the respiratory and nervous systems, and the blood sugar concentration is controlled mainly by the liver and hormones from the endocrine pancreas.

Of recent interest has been the neuroendocrine control systems that influence behavior. Biochemical messengers that exist in our brain control nerve activity, information flow, and ultimately behavior.[3] These control systems function in producing the normal emotional reactions to stress. In persons with mental health disorders, they can interact in the production of symptoms associated with the disorder. The field of neuropharmacology has focused on the modulation of the endogenous messengers and signaling systems that control behavior in treatment of mental disorders such as anxiety disorders, depression, and schizophrenia.

System Efficiency

The effectiveness of a system is determined by the amount of change—amplification or gain—that occurs within the system in response to changes in external chemical or physical parameters. In his textbook of physiology, Arthur Guyton uses the example of a 1°F change in body temperature (from 98°F to 99°F) that occurs when the ambient temperature is increased from 60°F to 110°F.[2] As body temperature rises because of the change in external temperature, sensors in the system detect the error, and sufficient compensation, in terms of radiation and evaporative heat losses from the skin, returns the temperature to within 1°F of the setpoint of the system. Were it not for the efficiency of the control system, the body temperature would have risen 50°F instead of 1°F (Fig. 53–2).[2]

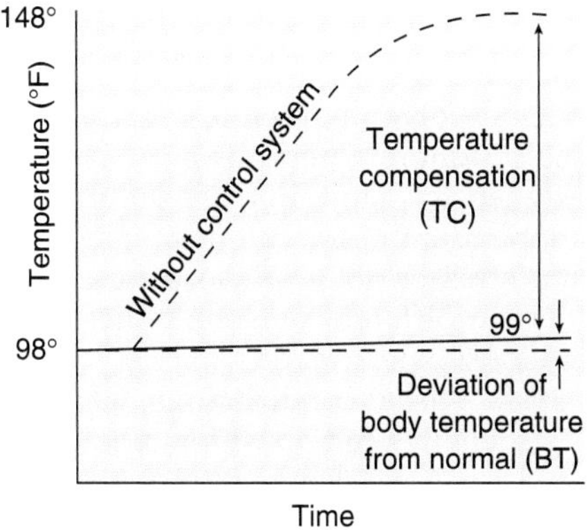

Figure 53–2
Effects on body temperature of suddenly increasing the air temperature 50°F, showing the hypothetical effect without a control system and the actual effect with a normal control system. (Guyton A. [1986]. *Textbook of medical physiology* [7th ed.]. Philadelphia: W.B. Saunders)

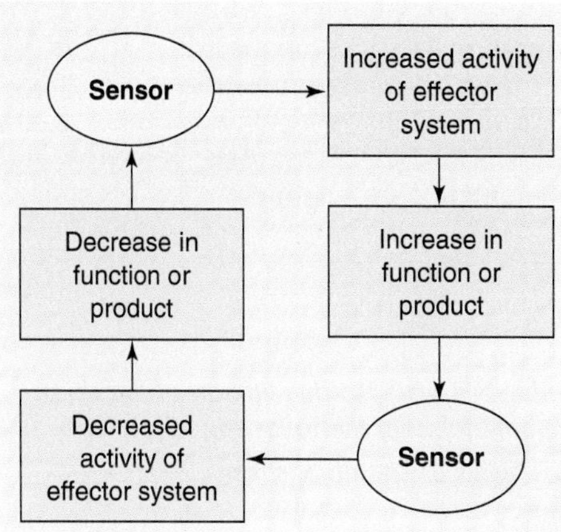

Figure 53–3
Negative feedback control of a body function, hormone level, or biochemical product.

Feedback Systems

Most control systems in the body operate by *negative feedback mechanisms*, which function in a manner similar to the thermostat on a heating system. When the monitored function decreases below the setpoint of the system, the feedback mechanism causes the function to increase, and when the function is increased above the setpoint, the feedback mechanism causes it to decrease (Fig. 53–3). For example, in the negative feedback mechanism that controls blood glucose levels, an increase in blood glucose stimulates an increase in insulin, which enhances the removal of glucose from the blood. When sufficient glucose has left the bloodstream to cause blood glucose levels to fall, the release of glucose from the liver and the recruitment of other counterregulatory mechanisms cause the blood glucose to return to normal.

The reason most physiologic control systems function under negative rather than *positive feedback mechanisms* is that a positive feedback mechanism interjects instability rather than stability into a system. It produces a cycle in which the initiating stimulus produces more of the same. In a positive feedback system, exposure to an increase in environmental temperature would invoke compensatory mechanisms designed to increase rather than decrease body temperature.

In summary, physiologic and psychologic adaptation involves the ability to maintain the constancy of the internal environment and behavior in the face of a wide range of changes in the internal and external environments. It involves positive and negative feedback control systems that regulate cellular function, control life's processes, regulate behavior, and integrate the function of the different body systems.

Stress

After you have completed this section of the chapter, you should be able to meet the following objectives:

- State Selye's definition of *stress*
- Define *stressor*
- Cite two factors that influence the nature of the stress response
- Compare specific and nonspecific stress responses
- Explain the interactions of the nervous system in mediating the stress response
- Describe the stress responses of the autonomic nervous system, the endocrine system, the immune system, and the musculoskeletal system

The increased focus on health promotion has hightened interest in the roles that stress and altered adaptive processes play in the development of disease.[4] Hypertension, heart disease, and peptic ulcer are but a few of the diseases associated with stress. Stress may contribute directly to the production of disease, or it may contribute to the development of behaviors such as smoking, overeating, and drug abuse, which increase the risk of disease.

For the most part, the stress response is meant to be acute and of a time-limited nature. The time-limited nature of the process renders the accompanying catabolic and immunosuppressive effects advantageous. It is the chronicity of the stress response that is thought to be disruptive of physical and mental health.

The Stress Response

Hans Selye, the world-renowned endocrinologist and pioneer in the field of stress research, described *stress* as the nonspecific response of the body to any demand made on it.[5] As a young medical student, Selye noticed that patients suffering from diverse disease conditions had many signs and symptoms in common. He observed that "whether a man suffers from a loss of blood, an infectious disease, or advanced cancer, he loses his appetite, his muscular strength, and his ambition to accomplish anything; usually the patient also loses weight and even his facial expression betrays that he is ill."[5] Selye referred to this as the "syndrome of just being sick."

Selye observed a triad of adrenal enlargement, thymus atrophy, and gastric ulcers in rats used in his original studies and assumed that the hypothalmic-pituitary-adrenal axis (HPA) played a pivotal role in the stress response. To Selye, the response to stress was a process that enabled the body to resist the stressor in the best possible way by enhancing the function of the system best able to respond to it. He called this response the *general adaptation syndrome* (GAS). The GAS involves three stages: the alarm stage, the stage of resistance, and the stage of exhaustion.

The alarm stage is characterized by a diffuse response, and no body organ or system is predominantly active. During the resistance stage, the body selects the most effective and economic channels of defense. During this stage, the increased cortisol levels that were present during the first stage drop, because they are no longer needed. During the third stage—the stage of exhaustion—the reaction spreads because of "wear and tear" on the most appropriate channel of adaptation.[6]

Selye contended that many ailments, such as various emotional disturbances, mildly annoying headaches, insomnia, upset stomach, gastric and duodenal ulcers, and certain types of rheumatic disorders, and cardiovascular and kidney diseases, appear to be initiated or encouraged by the "body itself because of its faulty adaptive reactions to potentially injurious agents."[5]

The events or environmental agents responsible for initiating the stress response are called *stressors*. According to Selye, stressors may be endogenous, arising from within the body, or exogenous, arising from outside the body.[5] In explaining the stress response, Selye proposed that two factors determine the nature of the stress response: the properties of the stressor and the conditioning of the person being stressed.[5] Selye indicated that not all stress was detrimental; hence, he coined the terms *eustress* and *distress*.[6] For example, the joy of becoming a new parent and the sorrow of losing a parent are completely different experiences, yet their stressor effect—the nonspecific demand for adjustment to a new situation—can be similar. The specific stress responses alert a person to the presence of the stressor, whereas the nonspecific effects, which involve neuroendocrine responses such as increased autonomic nervous system (ANS) activity, are designed to maintain or reestablish normality and are independent of specific responses. The ability of the same stressor to produce different responses and disorders in different persons indicates the adaptive capacity of the person, or what Selye called *conditioning factors*. These conditioning factors may be internal (*e.g.*, genetic predisposition, age, sex) or external (*e.g.*, exposure to environmental agents, life experiences, dietary factors).[5]

Selye also indicated that mild, brief, and controllable periods of stress could be perceived as positive stimuli to emotional and intellectual growth and development. It is the severe, protracted, and uncontrolled situations of psychologic and physical distress that are disruptive of health.

Neuroendocrine-Immune Interactions

A normally functioning stress system integrates large numbers of incoming signals and provides appropriate output. The central stress system, which is located in a pivotal position in the brain, receives inputs from the environment and body through various sensory systems, from circulating mediators that are carried in the blood stream, and from various parts of the brain such as the cerebral cortex and the limbic system. In addition, immune cells such as monocytes and lymphocytes can penetrate the blood–brain barrier and take up residence in the brain, where they secrete cytokines and other inflammatory mediators that influence the stress response.[7] In responding to the various inputs, the stress system sends output to the HPA axis, the ANS, and the immune system.[7–8]

The manifestations of the stress response—a pounding headache, cold moist hands, a stiff neck, and increased incidence of infections—reflect for the most part the nonspecific aspects of the stress response. The integration of these responses, which occurs at the level of the central nervous system (CNS), is elusive and complex. It relies on communication among the cerebral cortex, the limbic system, the thalamus, the hypothalamus, the pituitary gland, and the reticular activating system (RAS) (Fig. 53–4). The cerebral cortex is involved with vigilance, cognition, and focused attention, and the limbic system with the emotional components (*e.g.*, fear, excitement, rage, and anger) of the stress response. The thalamus functions as the relay center and is important in receiving, sorting out, and distributing sensory input. The hypothalamus functions in coordinating the endocrine and ANS responses. The RAS modulates mental alertness, ANS activity, and skeletal muscle tone, but it does this using input and output from other neural structures. The musculoskeletal tension that occurs during the stress response reflects the increased activity of the RAS and its influence on the muscle spindles and the gamma loop (*i.e.*, descending neural pathways, gamma motor neurons, spindle muscle fibers, afferent neurons, and alpha motor neurons), which control muscle tone (see Chapter 37). Muscle tension can remain as a prolonged manifestation of the stress response and can cause stiffness of the neck, backache, headaches, and other complaints.

Central to the neuroendocrine component of the stress response are corticotropin-releasing factor (CRF), which functions in the control of endocrine response to stress, and the locus ceruleus–norepinephrine pathway, which functions in the regulation of the sympathetic nervous system component of the ANS. The CRF and ANS responses seem to participate in a positive feedback loop so that activation of one system tends to activate the other as well.

The CRF system is widespread throughout the nervous system but is best characterized by its concentration in the hypothalamus and its role in the functioning of the HPA axis. CRF sets into motion a coordinated series of physiologic and behavioral responses that are adaptive during stressful situations. Each of the anterior pituitary hormones is under the direct influence

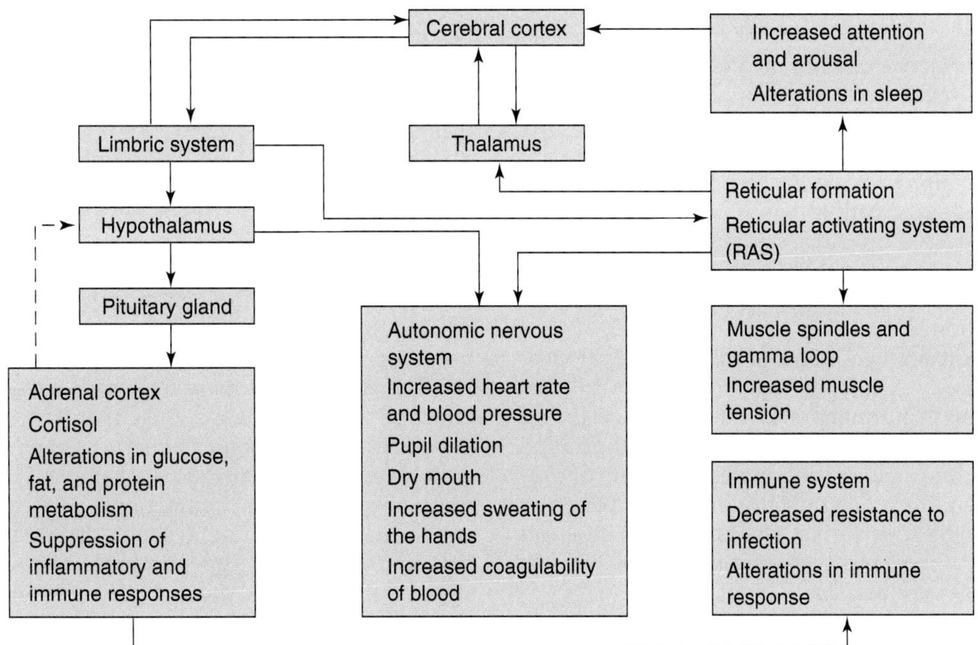

Figure 53–4
Stress pathways. The *broken line* represents negative feedback.

of the hypothalamus, and their secretion can be influenced by suprahypothalamic stimuli such as environmental signals, sleep rhythms, and physical and emotional stress. CRF has also been found outside the HPA axis, and its presence during increased emotionality suggests that the CRF has a role in coordinating behavioral and autonomic responses to stress. Moderate levels of CRF appear to enhance arousal and promote cautious restraint, but large amounts produce anxiety, hyperresponsiveness to stress, and sensory stimuli.

Sympathetic Nervous System Responses

The sympathetic division of the ANS confers an adaptive advantage during a stressful situation. The sympathetic nervous system manifestation of the stress reaction has been called the *fight-or-flight response.* This is the most rapid of the stress responses and represents the basic survival response of our primitive ancestors when confronted with the perils of the wilderness and its inhabitants. In the presence of danger, the alternatives were clear—run away or stand up and fight. The heart and respiratory rates increase, the hands and feet become moist, the pupils dilate, the mouth becomes dry, and the activity of the gastrointestinal tract decreases. The ANS is also involved in less-threatening situations.

Endocrine Responses

A wide variety of hormones are highly responsive to stressful situations. Systems responsible for reproduction, growth, and immunity are directly linked to the stress system, and each is profoundly influenced by the effectors of the stress response.

The most widely studied hormonal mechanisms have been those associated with the HPA axis that regulates body levels of adrenocortical hormones (mainly cortisol). The influence of emotion and stress on cortisol production is largely mediated through the CNS by way of the hypothalamus and CRF-regulated control of the adrenocorticotrophic hormone (ACTH). Cortisol is involved in maintaining blood glucose levels, facilitating fat metabolism, supporting vascular responsiveness, and modulating CNS function. Cortisol also affects mineral turnover in bone, hematopoiesis, gastric acid secretion, protein and collagen synthesis, immune responses, and renal function.

Although growth hormone is initially elevated at the onset of stress, prolonged activation leads to suppression of growth hormone and somatomedin C and other growth factors. The decrease in growth hormone and somatomedin C, along with increased levels of glucocorticoids, can exert a chronically inhibitory effect on growth. Although speculative, the effects of stress on growth hormone may provide one of the vital links in failure to thrive in children (see Chapter 35).

A corollary to the influence on growth hormone is the effect of stress on thyroid hormone. Stress is associated with decreased levels of thyroid-stimulating hormone and inhibition of conversion of thyroxine to the more biologically active triiodothyronine in peripheral tissues. Although the exact mechanisms are unknown, both responses are related to increased levels of glucocorticoids and may conserve energy during stress.

Other hormones, such as the antidiuretic hormone (ADH) and the sex hormones, are involved in the stress response. ADH, also known as vasopressin, increases water retention by the kidneys, produces vasoconstriction of blood vessels, and appears to synergize CRF's capacity to increase the release of ACTH. The reproductive hormones and growth hormone are inhibited by various components of the HPA axis.[5] Sepsis and severe trauma can induce anovulation and amenorrhea in women and decreased spermatogenesis and decreased levels of testosterone in men.

Immune Responses

The hallmark of the stress response, as first described by Selye, is the endocrine–immune interactions (*i.e.,* increased corticosteroid production and atrophy of the thymus) that are known to suppress the immune response. Much of the literature regarding stress and the immune response focuses on the causal role of stress in immune-related diseases. It has been suggested that the reverse may occur; emotional and psychologic stress may be a manifestation of alterations in the CNS resulting from the immune response. In the case of cancer, this could mean that the subjective feelings of helplessness and hopelessness that have been repeatedly related to the onset and progression of cancers may arise secondary to the CNS effects of products released by immune cells during the early stage of the disease.[10]

Occurrence of the oral disease acute necrotizing gingivitis, in which the normal bacterial flora of the mouth become invasive, is known by dentists to be associated with acute stress, such as final examinations.[11] Similarly, herpes simplex type 1 (*i.e.,* cold sores) infection often develops during periods of inadequate rest, fever, ultraviolet radiation, and emotional upset. The resident herpes virus is kept in check by body defenses, probably T lymphocytes, until a stressful event occurs and causes suppression of the immune system. Psychologic stress is associated in a dose-response manner with an increased risk of developing the common cold, and this risk is attributable to increased rates of infection rather than frequency of symptoms after infection.[12]

The exact mechanism by which stress produces its effect on the immune response is unknown and probably varies from person to person, depending on genetic endowment and environmental factors. The most significant arguments for interactions between the neuroendocrine and immune systems derive from evidence that immune and neuroendocrine cells share common signal pathways (*i.e.,* messenger molecules and receptors), that hormones and neuropeptides can alter the function of immune cells, and that immune system and its products (*e.g.,* cytokines) can modulate neuroendocrine function.[13] Receptors for a number of CNS-controlled hormones and neuromediators reportedly have been found on lymphocytes. Among these are receptors for glucocorticoids, insulin, testosterone, prolactin, catecholamines, estrogens, acetylcholine, and growth hormone, suggesting that these hormones influence lymphocyte function. For example, cortisol is known to suppress immune function, and pharmacologic doses of cortisol are used clinically to suppress the immune response. There is evidence that the immune system, in turn, influences neuroendocrine function. It has been observed that the HPA system is activated by cytokines such as interleukin-1, interleukin-2, interleukin-3, and tumor necrosis factor that are released from immune cells.

A second possible route of neuroendocrine regulation of immune function is through the sympathetic nervous system and release of catecholamines. The lymph nodes, thymus, and spleen are supplied with ANS nerve fibers. Centrally acting CRF activates the ANS through multisynaptic, descending pathways, and circulating epinephrine acts synergistically with CRF and cortisol to inhibit the function of the immune system.

In summary, stress is defined in many ways. Hans Selye, the world-renowned endocrinologist and pioneer in the field of stress research, defined stress as the nonspecific response of the body to any demands made on it. The event or environmental agent that produces the stress is called a stressor. Stressors may be physical, psychologic, or social. They include mental and physical effort and extremes of temperature, hunger, thirst, fatigue, and other everyday experiences. Most stressors produce specific and nonspecific responses. The specific responses alert the person to the nature of the stressor and assist in establishing definitive measures to deal with it. The nonspecific responses are designed to maintain or reestablish normality.

Factors Affecting Adaptation to Stress

After you have completed this section of the chapter, you should be able to meet the following objectives:

- List at least six factors that influence a person's adaptive capacity
- Relate experience and previous learning to the process of adaptation
- Contrast anatomic and physiologic reserve
- Propose a way by which social support may serve to buffer stress

Adaptation is affected by previous experience and learning, physiologic reserve, time, genetic endowment and age, health status, nutrition, sleep-wake cycles, and psychosocial factors (Fig. 53–5).

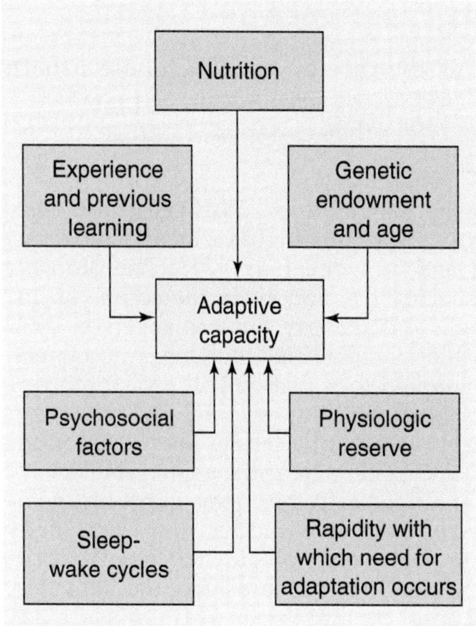

Figure 53–5
Factors affecting adaptation.

Adaptive Capacity

The ability to adapt to a wide range of environments and stressors is not peculiar to humans. According to René Dubos, a microbiologist known for his study of human response to the total environment, "adaptability is found throughout life and is perhaps the one attribute that distinguishes most clearly the world of life from the world of inanimate matter."[11] Living organisms, no matter how primitive, do not submit passively to the impact of environmental forces. They attempt to respond adaptively, each in its own unique and most suitable manner. The higher the organism is on the evolutionary scale, the larger its repertoire of adaptive mechanisms and its ability to select and limit aspects of the environment to which it responds. The most fully evolved mechanisms are the social responses through which individuals or groups modify their environments, their habits, or both to achieve a way of life that is suited to their needs.[14]

Human beings, because of their highly developed nervous system and intellect, usually have alternative mechanisms for adapting and have the ability to control many aspects of their environment. Air conditioning and central heating limit the need to adapt to extreme changes in environmental temperature. The control of microbial growth, immunization, and the availability of antibiotics eliminate the need to respond to common infectious agents. On the other hand, modern technology creates new challenges for adaptation and provides new sources of stress, such as increased noise, air pollution, changes in the pathogenicity of microbial agents from exposure to chemicals and drugs in the environment, and alterations in biologic rhythms imposed by shift work and transcontinental flights.

Previous Experience and Learning

Dubos cites the case of an old Chinese fisherman (the type depicted on the scrolls of the Sung era) as an example of the effect that experience and learning have on adaptation:[14]

> The fisherman appears fully at ease and relaxed in his primitive boat, floating on a misty lake, or even a polluted and crowded harbor. He has probably experienced many tribulations in the course of his years of struggle and poverty but has survived by becoming almost totally identified with his environment. He is so well adapted to it that he will probably live for many more years, without modern comfort, sanitation, or medical care, just by letting his existence be ruled by what he considers to be the unalterable laws of the seasons and nature. In the course of his life, he developed different protective mechanisms that increased his immunologic, physiologic, and psychic resistance to the physicochemical hardships, the parasites, and the social conflicts that threatened him every day. He has elected to spend the rest of his life in the environment in which he has evolved and to which he has become adapted. Robust though he appears and really is, he probably would soon become sick if he moved into an area where the parasites, physiologic stresses, and social customs differ from the ones among which he has spent his early life.

Physiologic Reserve

The trained athlete is able to increase cardiac output sixfold to sevenfold during exercise. The safety margin for adaptation of most body systems is considerably greater than that needed for normal activities. The red blood cells carry more oxygen than the tissues can use, the liver and fat cells store excess nutrients, and bone tissue stores calcium in excess of that needed for normal neuromuscular function. The ability of body systems to increase their function given the need to adapt is known as the *physiologic reserve*. Many of the body organs, such as the lungs, kidneys, and adrenals, are paired to provide *anatomic reserve* as well. Both organs are not needed to ensure the continued existence and maintenance of the internal environment. Many persons function normally with only one lung or one kidney. In kidney disease, for example, signs of renal failure do not occur until about 90% of the functioning nephrons have been destroyed.

Time

Adaptation is most efficient when changes occur gradually rather than suddenly. It is possible, for instance, to lose a liter or more of blood through chronic gastrointestinal bleeding over a week without developing signs of shock. However, a sudden hemorrhage that causes loss of an equal amount of blood is likely to cause hypotension and shock.

Genetic Endowment

Adaptation is further affected by the availability of adaptive responses and flexibility in selecting the most appropriate and economical response. The greater the number of available responses, the more effective is the capacity to adapt.

Genetic endowment can ensure that the systems that are essential to adaptation function adequately. Even a gene that has deleterious effects may prove adaptive in some environments. In Africa, the gene for sickle cell anemia persists in some populations because it provides some resistance to infection with the parasite that causes malaria.

Age

The capacity to adapt is decreased at the extremes of age. The ability to adapt is impaired by the immaturity of an infant much as it is by the decline in functional reserve that occurs with age. For example, the infant has difficulty concentrating urine because of immature renal structures and is therefore less able than an adult to cope with decreased water intake or exaggerated water losses. A similar situation exists in the elderly from age-related changes in renal function.

Health Status

Physical and mental health status determines physiologic and psychologic reserves and is a strong determinant of the ability to adapt. For example, persons with heart disease are less able to adjust to stresses that require the recruitment of cardiovascular responses. Severe emotional stress often produces disruption of physiologic function and limits the ability to make appropriate choices related to long-term adaptive needs. Those who have worked with acutely ill persons know that the will to live often has a profound influence on survival during life-threatening illnesses.

Nutrition

There are 50 to 60 essential nutrients, including minerals, lipids, certain fatty acids, vitamins, and specific amino acids. Deficiencies or excesses of any of these nutrients can alter a person's health status and impair the ability to adapt. The importance of nutrition to enzyme function, immune response, and wound healing is well known. On a worldwide basis, malnutrition may be one of the most common causes of immunodeficiency.

Among the problems associated with dietary excess are obesity and alcohol abuse. Obesity is a common problem. It predisposes to a number of health problems, including atherosclerosis and hypertension. Alcohol commonly is used in excess. It acutely affects the brain function and, with long-term use, can seriously impair the function of the liver, brain, and other vital structures.

Sleep-Wake Cycles

Sleep is considered to be a restorative function in which energy is restored and tissues are regenerated.[15] Sleep occurs in a cyclic manner, alternating with periods of wakefulness and increased energy use. Biologic rhythms play an important role in adaptation to stress, the development of illness, and response to medical treatment. Many rhythms such as rest and activity, work and leisure, and eating and drinking oscillate with a frequency similar to that of the 24-hour light-dark solar day. The term *circadian*, from the Latin *circa* (about) and *dies* (day), is used to describe these 24-hour diurnal rhythms.

The stress of sleep disorders and alterations in the sleep-wake cycle has been shown to alter immune function, the normal circadian pattern of hormone secretion, and physical and psychologic functioning.[16] The two most common manifestations of an alteration in the sleep-wake cycle are insomnia and sleep deprivation or increased somnolence. In some persons, stress may produce sleep disorders, and in others, sleep disorders may lead to stress. Acute stress and environmental disturbances, loss of a loved one, recovery from surgery, and pain are common causes of transient and short-term insomnia. Air travel and jet lag constitute additional causes of altered sleep-wake cycles, as does shift work. In persons with chronic insomnia, the bed often acquires many unpleasant secondary associations and becomes a place of stress and worry rather than a place of rest.[17]

Psychosocial Factors

Several studies have related social factors and life events to illness. Scientific interest in the social environment as a cause of stress has gradually broadened to include the social environment as a resource that modulates the relation between stress and health. Presumably, persons who can mobilize strong supportive resources from within their social relationships are better able to withstand the negative effects of stress on their health. Studies suggest that social support has direct and indirect positive effects on health status and serves as a buffer or modifier of the physical and psychosocial effects of stress.[18]

Social networks contribute in a number of ways to a person's psychosocial and physical integrity. The configuration of significant others that constitutes this network functions to mobilize the resources of the person; these friends, colleagues, and family members share the person's tasks and provide monetary support, materials and tools, and guidance in improving problem-solving capabilities.[18] Persons with ample social networks are not as likely to experience many types of stress such as being homeless or being lonely.[19] There is also evidence that persons who have social supports or social assets may live longer and have a lower incidence of somatic illness.[20]

Social support has been viewed in terms of the number of relationships a person has and the person's perception of these relationships.[21] Close relationships with others can involve positive effects and the potential for conflict and may, in some situations, leave the person less able to cope with life stressors.

In summary, adaptation is affected by a number of factors, including experience and previous learning, the rapidity with which the need to adapt occurs, genetic endowment and age, health status, nutrition, sleep-wake cycles, and psychosocial factors.

REFERENCES

1. Cannon W.B. (1932). *The wisdom of the body* (pp. 299–300). New York: W.W. Norton.
2. Guyton A.C. (1986). *Textbook of medical physiology* (7th ed., p. 8). Philadelphia: WB Saunders.
3. Wilcox R.E., Gonzales R,A. (1995). Introduction to neurotransmitters, receptors, signal transduction, and second messengers. In Schatzberg A.F., Nemeroff C.B. (Eds.). *Textbook of psychopharmacology* (pp. 3–29). Washington, DC: American Psychiatric Press.
4. Chrousos G.P. (1992). The concepts of stress and stress system disorders. *Journal of the American Medical Association* 267 (9), 1244–1252.
5. Selye H. (1973). The evolution of the stress concept. *American Scientist* 61, 692.
6. Selye H. (1974). *Stress without distress* (p. 6). New York: New American Library.
7. Reichlin S. (1993). Neuroendocrine-immune interactions. *New England Journal of Medicine* 329 (17), 1246–1253.
8. Black P.H. (1995). Psychoneuroimmunology: Brain and immunity. *Scientific American Science and Medicine* Nov/Dec, 16–25.
9. Heinrichs S.C., Menzaghi F., Pich E.M., et al. (1995). The role of CRF in behavioral aspects of stress. *Annals of New York Academy of Science* 771, 92–101.
10. Dantzer R., Kelley K.W. (1989). Stress and immunity: An integrated view of relationships between the brain and immune system. *Life Sciences* 44, 1995–2008.
11. Dworkin S.F. (1969). Psychosomatic concepts and dentistry: Some perspectives. *Journal of Peridontology* 40, 647.
12. Cohen S., Tyrrell D.A.J., Smith A.P. (1991). Psychological stress and susceptibility to the common cold. *New England Journal of Medicine* 325, 606–612.
13. Falaschi P., Martocchia A., Proietti A., Pastore R., D'urso R. (1994). Immune system and the hypothalamus-pituitary-adrenal axis. *Annals New York Academy of Science* 741, 223–231.
14. Dubos R. (1965). *Man adapting* (pp. 256, 258, 261, 264). New Haven: Yale University Press.
15. Adams K., Oswold I. (1983). Protein synthesis, bodily renewal and sleep-wake cycle. *Clinical Science* 65, 561–567.

16. Gillin J.C., Byerley W.F. (1990). The diagnosis and management of insomnia. *New England Journal of Medicine* 322, 239–248.
17. Moldofsky H., Lue F.A., Davidson J.R., et al. (1989). Effects of sleep deprivation on human immune functions. *FASEB Journal* 3, 1972–1977.
18. Broadhead W.E., Kaplan B.H., James S.A., et al. (1983). The epidemiologic evidence for a relationship between social support and health. *American Journal of Epidemiology* 117, 521–537.
19. Greenblatt M., Becerra R.M., Serafetinides E.A. (1982). Social networks and mental health: An overview. *American Journal of Psychiatry* 139 (8), 977.
20. House J.S., Robbins C., Metzner H.L. (1982). The association of social relationships and activities with mortality: Prospective evidence from the Tecumseh Community Health Study. *American Journal of Epidemiology* 16, 123.
21. Tilden V.P., Weinert C. (1987). Social support and the chronically ill individual. *Nursing Clinics of North America* 33, 613–620.

CHAPTER 54

Alterations in Nutritional Status

Joan Pleuss

"You are what you eat" is a familiar maxim. To a great extent, nutrition determines how a person looks, feels, and acts. The need for adequate nutrition begins at the time of conception and continues throughout life. Nutrition provided by food or supplements in the proper proportions enables the body to maintain life, to grow physically and intellectually, to heal and repair tissue, and to maintain the stamina necessary for well-being. This chapter addresses nutritional status, overnutrition and obesity, and undernutrition.

Nutritional Status

After you have completed this section of the chapter, you should be able to meet the following objectives:

- Define *nutritional status*
- Define *calorie* and state the number of calories derived from the oxidation of 1 g of protein, fat, or carbohydrate
- Explain the difference between anabolism and catabolism
- Relate the processes of glycogenolysis and gluconeogenesis to the regulation of blood glucose by the liver
- Define *basal metabolic rate* and cite factors that affect it
- State the purpose of the recommended daily allowance of calories, proteins, fats, carbohydrates, vitamins, and minerals
- Describe methods used for a nutritional assessment
- State the factors used in determining body mass index and explain its use in evaluating body weight in terms of undernutrition and overnutrition

Nutritional status describes the condition of the body related to the availability and use of nutrients. Nutrients provide the energy and materials necessary for performing the activities of daily living; for maintaining healthy skin, muscles, and other body tissues; for replacing and healing tissues; and for the effective functioning of all body systems, including the immune and respiratory systems. Poor nutritional status can cause illness and prevent recuperation from illness.

Nutrients are derived from the digestive tract through the ingestion of foods or, in some cases, through liquid feedings that are delivered directly into the gastrointestinal tract by a synthetic tube (*i.e.,* tube feedings). The exception occurs in persons with certain illnesses in which the digestive tract is bypassed and the nutrients are infused directly into the circulatory system. Once inside the body, nutrients are used for energy or as the building blocks for tissue growth and repair. When excess nutrients are available, they frequently are stored for future use. If the required nutrients are unavailable, the body adapts by conserving and using its nutrient stores.

Energy Metabolism

Energy is measured in heat units called *calories*. A calorie, spelled with a small *c* and also called a *gram calorie,* is the amount of heat or energy required to raise the temperature of 1 g of water by 1°C. A *kilocalorie* (kcal), or *large calorie,* is the amount of energy needed to raise the temperature of 1 kg of water by 1°C. Because a calorie is so small, kilocalories are often used in nutritional and physiologic studies. The oxidation of proteins provides 4 kcal/g; fats, 9 kcal/g; carbohydrates, 4 kcal/g, and alcohol, 7 kcal/g.

All body activities require energy, whether they involve an individual cell, a single organ, or the entire body. *Metabolism* is the organized process through which nutrients such as carbohydrates, fats, and proteins are broken down, transformed, or otherwise converted into cellular energy. The process of metabolism is unique in that it enables the continual release of energy, and it couples this energy with physiologic functioning. For example, the energy used for muscle contraction is derived largely from energy sources that are stored in muscle cells and then released as the muscle contracts. Because most of our energy sources come from the nutrients in the food that is eaten, the ability to store energy and control its release is important.

Adipose Tissue

More than 90% of body energy is stored in the adipose tissues of the body. Adipocytes, or fat cells, occur singly or in small groups in loose connective tissue. In many parts of the body, they cushion body organs such as the kidneys. In addition to isolated groups of fat cells, entire regions of fat tissue are committed to fat storage. Collectively, fat cells constitute a large body organ that is metabolically active in the uptake, synthesis, storage, and mobilization of lipids, which are the main source of fuel storage for the body. Some tissues, such as liver cells, are able to store small amounts of lipids, but when these lipids accumulate, they begin to interfere with cell function. Adipose tissue not only serves as a storage site for body fuels, but also provides insulation for the body, fills body crevices, and protects body organs.

Studies of adipocytes in the laboratory have shown that fully differentiated cells do not divide. However, such cells have a long life span, and anyone born with large numbers of adipocytes runs the risk of becoming obese. Some immature adipocytes capable of division are present in postnatal life; these cells respond to estrogen stimulation and are the potential source of additional fat cells during postnatal life.[1] Fat deposition results from proliferation of these existing immature adipocytes and can occur as a consequence of excessive caloric intake when a woman is breast-feeding or during estrogen stimulation around the time of puberty. An increase in fat cells may also occur during late adolescence and in middle-aged persons who are already overweight.

There are two types of adipose tissue: white fat and brown fat. White fat, which despite its name is cream colored or yellow, is the prevalent form of adipose tissue in postnatal life. It constitutes 10% to 20% of body weight in adult males and 15% to 25% in adult females. At body temperature, the lipid content of fat cells exists as oil. It consists of *triglycerides,* which are three molecules of fatty acids esterified to a glycerol molecule. Triglycerides, which contain no water, have the highest caloric content of all nutrients and are an efficient form of energy storage. Fat cells synthesize triglycerides, the major fat storage form, from dietary fats and carbohydrates. Insulin is required for transport of glucose into fat cells. When calorie intake is restricted for any reason, fat cell triglycerides are broken down, and the resultant fatty acids and glycerol are released as energy sources.

Brown fat differs from white fat in terms of its thermogenic capacity or ability to produce heat. Brown fat, the site of diet-induced thermogenesis and nonshivering thermogenesis, is found primarily in early neonatal life in humans and in animals that hibernate. In humans, brown fat decreases with age but is still detectable in the sixth decade. This small amount of brown fat has a minimal effect on energy expenditure.

Anabolism and Catabolism

There are two phases of metabolism: anabolism and catabolism. *Anabolism* is the phase of metabolic storage and synthesis of cell constituents. Anabolism does not provide energy for the body; it requires energy. *Catabolism* involves the breakdown of complex molecules into substances that can be used in the production of energy. The chemical intermediates for anabolism and catabolism are called *metabolites* (*e.g.,* lactic acid is a metabolite formed when glucose is broken down in the absence of oxygen). Both anabolism and catabolism are catalyzed by *enzyme systems* located within body cells. A *substrate* is a substance on which an enzyme acts. Enzyme systems selectively transform fuel substrates into cellular energy and facilitate the use of energy in the process of assembling molecules to form energy substrates and storage forms of energy.

Because body energy cannot be stored as heat, the cellular oxidative processes that release energy are low-temperature reactions that convert food components to chemical energy that can be stored. The body transforms carbohydrates, fats, and proteins into the intermediary compound, adenosine triphosphate (ATP). ATP is called the energy currency of the cell, because almost all body cells store and use ATP as their energy source (see Chapter 1). The metabolic events involved in ATP formation allow cellular energy to be stored, used, and replenished.

Glucose Metabolism

Glucose is a six-carbon molecule; it is an efficient fuel that, when metabolized in the presence of oxygen, breaks down to form carbon dioxide and water (Fig. 54–1). Although many tissues and organ systems are able to use other forms of fuel, such as fatty acids and ketones, the brain and nervous system rely almost exclusively on glucose as a fuel source. The nervous system can neither store nor synthesize glucose; instead it relies on the minute-by-minute extraction of glucose from the blood to meet its energy needs. In the fed and early fasting state, the nervous system requires about 100 to 115 g of glucose per day to meet its metabolic needs.

The liver regulates the entry of glucose into the blood. Glucose ingested in the diet is transported from the gastrointestinal tract, through the portal vein, and to the liver before it gains access to the circulatory system (Fig. 54–2). The liver stores and synthesizes glucose. When blood sugar is increased, the liver removes glucose from the blood and stores it for future use. Conversely, the liver releases its glucose stores when blood sugar drops. In this way, the liver acts as a buffer system to regulate blood sugar levels. Blood sugar levels usually reflect the difference between the amount of glucose released into the circulation by the liver and the amount of glucose removed from the blood by body cells.

Excess glucose is stored in two forms. It can be converted to fatty acids and stored in fat cells as triglycerides, or it can be stored in the liver and skeletal muscle as glycogen. Small amounts of glycogen are also stored in the skin and in some of the glandular tissues.

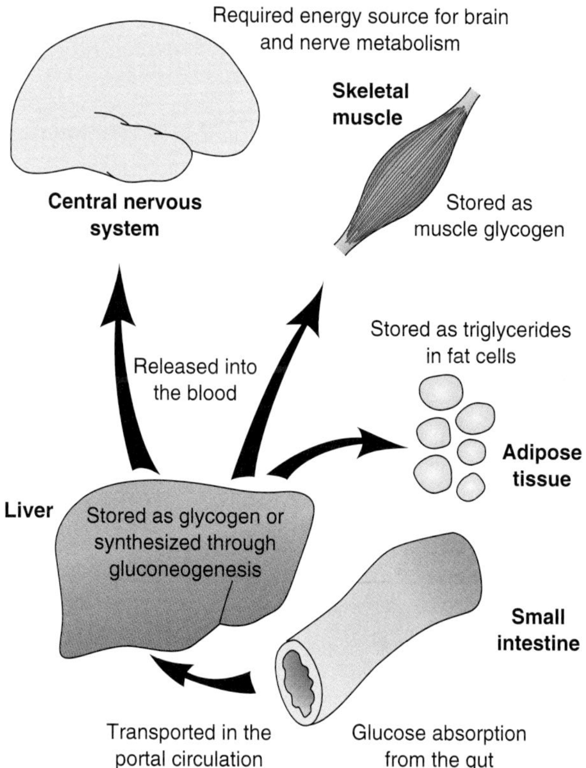

Figure 54–2 ■■■
Regulation of blood glucose by the liver.

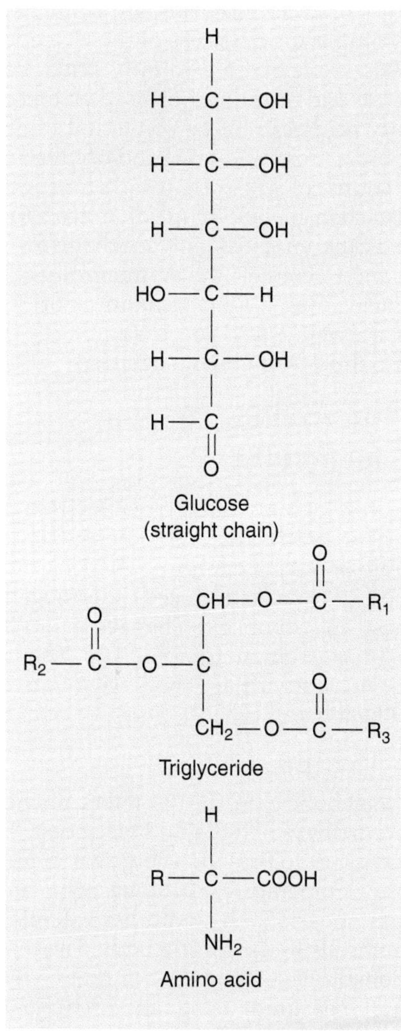

Figure 54–1 ■■■
Glucose, triglyceride, and amino acid structure.

Glycogenolysis. Glycogenolysis, or the breakdown of glycogen, is controlled by the action of two hormones: glucagon and epinephrine. Epinephrine is more effective in stimulating glycogen breakdown in muscle, whereas the liver is more responsive to glucagon. The synthesis and degradation of glycogen are important because they help maintain blood sugar levels during periods of fasting and strenuous exercise. Only the liver is able to release its glucose stores into the blood for use by other tissues, such as the brain and nervous system. Glycogen breaks down to form a phosphorylated glucose molecule, and in this form, it is too large to pass through the cell membrane. The liver, but not skeletal muscle, has the enzyme glucose-6-phosphatase, which is needed to remove the phosphate group and to allow the glucose molecule to enter the bloodstream.

Although rare, there are several genetic disorders that impair glycogen breakdown, causing an excessive accumulation of glycogen. *Von Gierke's disease* involves a genetic deficiency of glucose-6-phosphatase. Children with this disease have stunted growth, liver enlargement, hypoglycemia, and hyperlipidemia resulting from mobilization of fatty acids. McArdle's disease is characterized by a deficiency in the muscle enzyme phosphorylase. The disorder, which is limited to skeletal muscle, causes muscle cramps during strenuous exercise.

Gluconeogenesis. The synthesis of glucose is referred to as *gluconeogenesis*, or the building of glucose from new sources. The process of gluconeogenesis, most of which occurs in the liver, converts amino acids, lactate, and glycerol into glucose. Although fatty acids can be used as fuel by many body cells, they cannot be converted to glucose.

Glucose produced through the process of gluconeogenesis is either stored in the liver as glycogen or released into the general circulation. During periods of food deprivation or when the diet is low in carbohydrates, gluconeogenesis provides the glucose that is needed to meet the metabolic needs of the brain and other glucose-dependent tissues. Several hormones stimulate gluconeogenesis, including glucagon, glucocorticoid hormones from the adrenal cortex, and thyroid hormone.

Fat Metabolism

The average American diet provides about 33% of calories in the form of fats. In contrast to glucose, which yields only 4 kcal/g, each gram of fat yields 9 kcal. Another 30% to 50% of the carbohydrates consumed in the diet are converted to triglycerides for storage.

A triglyceride contains three fatty acids linked by a glycerol molecule (see Fig. 54–1). Fatty acids and triglycerides can be derived from dietary sources, they can be synthesized in the body, or they can be mobilized from fat depots. Excess carbohydrate is converted to triglyceride and is transported by lipoproteins in the blood to adipose cells for storage. One gram of anhydrous (water-free) fat stores more than six times as much energy as one hydrated gram of glycogen. One reason weight loss is greatest at the beginning of a fast or weight-loss program is that this is when the body uses its water-containing glycogen stores. Later, when the body begins to use energy stored as triglycerides, water losses are decreased and weight loss tends to plateau.

The mobilization of fat for use in energy production is facilitated by the action of lipases (*i.e.*, enzymes) that break the triglycerides into three fatty acids and a glycerol molecule. The activation of lipases and the subsequent mobilization of fatty acids are stimulated by epinephrine, glucocorticoid hormones, growth hormones, and glucagon. After triglyceride breakdown, the fatty acids and the glycerol molecule leave the fat cell and enter the circulation. In the circulation, many of the fatty acids are transported to the liver, where they are removed from the blood and are used by liver cells as a source of energy or converted to ketones.

The efficient burning of fatty acids requires a balance between carbohydrate and fat metabolism. The ratio of fatty acid and carbohydrate use is altered in situations that favor fat breakdown, such as diabetes mellitus and fasting. In these situations, the liver produces more ketones than it can use; this excess is released into the bloodstream. Ketones can be an important source of energy, because even the brain adapts to the use of ketones during prolonged periods of starvation. A problem arises, however, when fat breakdown is accelerated and the production of ketones exceeds tissue use. Because ketone bodies are organic acids, they cause *ketoacidosis* when they are present in excessive amounts.

Protein Metabolism

About three-fourths of body solids are proteins. Proteins are essential for the formation of all body structures, including genes, enzymes, contractile proteins in muscle, matrix of bone, and hemoglobin of red blood cells.

Amino acids are the building blocks of proteins. Twenty amino acids are present in body proteins in significant quantities. Each amino acid has an acidic group (COOH) and an amino group (NH_2) (see Fig. 54–1). Unlike glucose and fatty acids, there is only a limited facility for the storage of excess amino acids in the body. Most of the stored amino acids are contained in body proteins. Amino acids in excess of those needed for protein synthesis are converted to fatty acids, ketone bodies, or glucose and are stored or used as metabolic fuel. Because fatty acids cannot be converted to glucose, the body must break down proteins and use the amino acids as a major source of substrate for gluconeogenesis during periods when metabolic needs exceed food intake. The liver has the enzymes and mechanisms needed to deaminate and to convert the amino groups (NH_2) from the amino acid to urea. The breakdown or degradation of proteins and amino acids occurs primarily in the liver, which is also the site of gluconeogenesis.

Energy Expenditure

The expenditure of body energy results from four mechanisms of heat production (*i.e.*, thermogenesis): basal metabolic rate or resting energy equivalent, diet-induced thermogenesis, exercise-induced thermogenesis, and thermogenesis in response to changes in environmental conditions (discussed in Chapter 56). The amount of energy used varies with age, body size, rate of growth, and state of health.

Basal Metabolic Rate

The basal metabolic rate (BMR) refers to the chemical reactions occurring when the body is at rest. These reactions are necessary to provide energy for maintenance of normal body temperature, cardiovascular and respiratory function, muscle tone, and other essential activities of tissues and cells in the resting body. The resting metabolic rate constitutes 65% to 70% of body energy needs. The BMR is measured using an instrument called a *metabolator* that measures the rate of oxygen use by a person. Oxygen consumption is measured under basal conditions: after a full night's sleep, after at least 12 hours

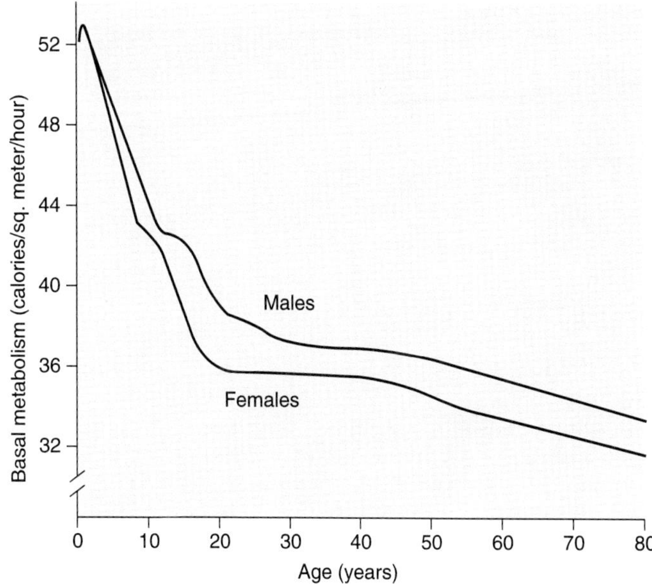

Figure 54–3
Normal basal metabolic rates at different ages for each sex. (Guyton A.C., Hall J.E. [1996]. *Medical physiology* [9th ed., p. 909]. Philadelphia: W.B. Saunders)

without food, and while the person is awake and at rest in a warm and comfortable room. The BMR is then calculated in terms of calories per hour and normally averages about 60 calories per hour in young men and 53 calories per hour in young women. Women generally have a 5% to 10% lower BMR than men because of their higher percentage of adipose tissue. Factors that affect the BMR are age, sex, physical state, and pregnancy. A progressive decline in the normal BMR occurs with aging (Fig. 54–3).[1] The BMR can be used to predict the calorie needs for maintenance of nutrition.

The resting energy equivalent (REE) is used for predicting energy expenditure. Several equations that determine REE have been published. Although the Harris-Benedict equation has been the most widely used, research indicates that the World Health Organization equation has better predicting value (Table 54–1).[2] Multiplying the REE by a factor of 1.2 usually adequately predicts the caloric needs for maintenance of nutrition during health. A factor of 1.5 usually provides the needed nutrients during repletion and during illnesses such as pneumonia, long-bone fractures, cancer, peritonitis, and recovery from most types of surgery.

Diet- and Exercise-induced Thermogenesis

The diet-induced thermogenesis, or thermic effect of food, describes the energy used by the body for the digestion, absorption, and assimilation of food after its ingestion. It is energy expended over and above the caloric value of the food and accounts for about 10% of the total calories expended. When food is eaten, the metabolic rate rises and then returns to normal within a few hours.

The amount of energy expended for physical activity is determined by the type of activity performed, the length of participation, and the person's weight and physical fitness. Table 54–2 gives the energy expenditures for various activities.

Dietary Reference Intakes

The Dietary Reference Intakes include the Recommended Dietary Allowances, Adequate Intake, Estimated Average Requirement, and Tolerable Upper Intake Level. The *Recommended Dietary Allowances* (RDA) is an intake that meets the nutrient need of almost all healthy persons in a specific age and gender group (Table 54–3). The RDA should be used in advis-

TABLE **54–1**

Equations for Predicting Resting Energy Expenditure (REE) from Body Weight Alone

Sex and Age Range (Yr)	Equation to Derive REE in kcal/day*	SD†
Males		
0–3	(60.9 × wt) − 54	53
3–10	(22.7 × wt) + 495	62
10–18	(17.5 × wt) + 651	100
18–30	(15.3 × wt) + 679	151
30–60	(11.6 × wt) + 879	164
>60	(13.5 × wt) + 487	148
Females		
0–3	(61.0 × wt) − 51	61
3–10	(22.5 × wt) + 499	63
10–18	(12.2 × wt) + 746	117
18–30	(14.7 × wt) + 496	121
30–60	(8.7 × wt) + 829	108
>60	(10.5 × wt) + 596	108

*Weight (wt) of person in kilograms.
†Standard deviation (SD) of the differences between actual and computed values.
(Adapted from Food and Nutrition Board, National Research Council, NAS: *Recommended dietary allowances* [10th ed.]. Washington, DC: National Academy Press, 1989)

TABLE 54–2

Energy Expenditure per Hour During Different Types of Activity for a 70-kg Man

Form of Activity	Calories per Hour
Sleeping	65
Awake lying still	77
Sitting at rest	100
Standing relaxed	105
Dressing and undressing	118
Tailoring	135
Typewriting rapidly	140
"Light" exercise	170
Walking slowly (2.6 mph)	200
Carpentry, metal working, industrial painting	240
"Active" exercise	290
"Severe" exercise	450
Sawing wood	480
Swimming	500
Running (5.3 mph)	570
"Very severe" exercise	600
Walking very fast (5.3 mph)	650
Walking up stairs	1100

(Extracted from data compiled by Professor M.S. Rose. Guyton, A. [1986]. *Medical physiology* [7th ed.]. Philadelphia: W.B. Saunders)

ing persons about the level of nutrient intake they need to decrease the risk of chronic disease.

An *Adequate Intake* (AI) is set when there is not enough scientific evidence to estimate an average requirement. The AI is derived from experimental or observational data that show a mean intake that appears to sustain a desired indicator of health. An *Estimated Average Requirement* is the intake that meets the estimated nutrient need of half of the persons in a specific group. This figure is used as the basis for developing the RDA and is expected to be used by nutrition policy makers in the evaluation of the adequacy of a nutrient for a specific group and for planning how much of the nutrient the group should consume.

The *Tolerable Upper Intake Level* is the maximum intake that is judged unlikely to pose a health risk in almost all healthy persons in a specified group. It refers to the total intakes from food, fortified food, and nutrient supplements. This value is not intended to be a recommended level of intake, and there is no established benefit for persons who consume nutrients at the RDA or AI levels.

The Dietary Reference Intakes are regularly reviewed and updated by the Food and Nutrition Board of the Institute of Medicine, National Academy of Science. Calcium, phosphorus, magnesium, and vitamin D were the first nutrients to be reviewed and given new recommendations since 1989. The recommendations include a higher AI for calcium for almost all age groups (1300 mg/day for ages 9–18 years; 1000 mg/day for ages 19–50 years; and 1200 mg/day for persons 51 years of age and older). The Panel on Folate and Other B Vitamins is expected to complete its work in 1998. It is expected that these recommendations will replace some of the current RDA values.

The United States RDA (USRDA) was established for the purpose of labeling foods. It takes the highest value of each nutrient for children older than 4 years of age and for adults (excluding pregnancy and lactation); therefore, the USRDA sometimes provides a margin of nutritional safety higher than the RDA.

Proteins, fats, carbohydrates, vitamins, and minerals each have their own function in providing the body with what it needs to maintain life and health. Recommended allowances have not been established for every nutrient; some are given as a safe and adequate intake, but others, such as carbohydrates and fats, are expressed as a percentage of the calorie intake.

Nutritional Needs

Calories

Energy requirements are greater during growth periods. Infants require approximately 115 kcal/kg at birth, 105 kcal/kg at 1 year, and 80 kcal/kg of body weight between 1 to 10 years of age. During adolescence, boys require 45 kcal/kg of body weight and girls require 38 kcal/kg of body weight. During pregnancy, a woman needs an extra 300 kcal per day above her usual requirement, and during the first 3 months of breast-feeding, she requires an additional 500 kcal.[3] Table 54–4 can be used to predict the caloric requirements of healthy adults.

Proteins

Proteins are required for growth and maintenance of body tissues, enzymes and antibody formation, fluid and electrolyte balance, and nutrient transport. Proteins are composed of amino acids, nine of which are essential to the body. These are leucine, isoleucine, methionine, phenylalanine, threonine, tryptophan, valine, lysine, and histidine. The foods that provide these essential amino acids in adequate amounts are milk, eggs, meat, fish, and poultry. Dried peas and beans, nuts, seeds, and grains contain all the essential amino acids but in less than adequate proportions. These proteins need to be combined with each other or with complete proteins to meet the amino acid requirements for protein synthesis. Diets that are inadequate in protein can result in kwashiorkor. If calories and protein are inadequate, protein-calorie malnutrition occurs.

Unlike carbohydrates and fats, which are composed of hydrogen, carbon, and oxygen, proteins contain 16% nitrogen; therefore, nitrogen excretion is an indicator of protein intake. If the amount of nitrogen taken in by way of protein is equivalent to the nitrogen excreted, the person is said to be in *nitrogen balance*. A person is in positive nitrogen balance when the nitrogen consumed by way of protein is greater than the amount excreted. This occurs during growth, pregnancy, or healing after surgery or injury. A negative nitrogen balance often occurs during fever, illness, infection, trauma, or burns when more nitrogen is excreted than is consumed. Tissue wasting ensues.

Fats

Dietary fats are composed primarily of triglycerides (*i.e.,* a mixture of fatty acids and glycerol). The fatty acids are saturated (*i.e.,* no double bonds), monounsaturated (*i.e.,* one double bond), or polyunsaturated (*i.e.,* two or more double bonds). The saturated fatty acids elevate blood cholesterol, whereas the monounsaturated and polyunsaturated fats lower blood cholesterol. Saturated fats are generally from animal sources and remain solid at room temperature. With the exception of coconut and palm oils (which are saturated), unsaturated fats are found in plant oils and are usually liquid at room temperature.

Dietary fats provide energy, serve as carriers for the fat-soluble vitamins, are precursors of prostaglandins, and are a source of fatty acids. The polyunsaturated fatty acid linoleic acid is the only fatty acid that is required. A deficiency of linoleic acid results in dermatitis. The daily requirement is 5 g or 1% to 2% of the total daily calories. Because vegetable oils are rich sources of linoleic acid, this level can be met by including two teaspoons of oil.

Other than the requirement for linoleic acid, there is no specific requirement for dietary fat, provided there is adequate nutrition available for energy. Fat is the most concentrated source of energy. It is recommended that 30% or less of the calories in the diet should come from fats.[4]

Cholesterol is the major constituent of cell membranes and is synthesized by the body. Cholesterol metabolism and transport are discussed in Chapter 16. The daily dietary recommendation for cholesterol is less than 300 mg.

Carbohydrates

Dietary carbohydrates are composed of simple sugars, complex carbohydrates, and undigested carbohydrates (*i.e.,* fiber). Because of their vitamin, mineral, and fiber content, it is recommended that the bulk of the carbohydrate content in the diet be in the complex form rather than as simple sugars that contain few nutrients. Sucrose (*i.e.,* table sugar) is implicated in the development of dental caries.

There is no specific dietary requirement for carbohydrates. All of the energy requirements can be met by dietary fats and proteins. Although some tissues, such as the nervous system, require glucose as an energy source, this need can be met through the conversion of amino acids and the glycerol part of the triglyceride molecule to glucose. The fatty acids from triglycerides are converted to ketones and used for energy by other body tissues. A carbohydrate-deficient diet usually results in the loss of tissue proteins and the development of ketosis. Because protein and fat metabolism increases the production of osmotically active metabolic wastes that must be eliminated through the kidneys, there is danger of dehydration and electrolyte imbalances. The amount of carbohydrate needed to prevent tissue wasting and ketosis is 50 to 100 g/day. In practice, most of the daily energy requirement should be from carbohydrate. This is because protein is an expensive source of calories and because it is recommended that no more than 30% of the calories in the diet be derived from fat. The current recommendation is that the diet should provide 50% to 60% of the calories as carbohydrates.

Vitamins

Vitamins are a group of organic compounds that act as catalysts in various chemical reactions. A compound cannot be classified as a vitamin unless it is shown that a deficiency of it causes disease. Contrary to popular belief, vitamins do not provide energy directly. As catalysts, they are part of the enzyme systems required for the release of energy from protein, fat, and carbohydrates. Vitamins are also necessary for the formation of red blood cells, hormones, genetic materials, and the nervous system. They are essential for normal growth and development.

There are two types of vitamins: fat-soluble and water-soluble. The four fat-soluble vitamins are vitamins A, D, E, and K. The nine required water-soluble vitamins are thiamine, riboflavin, niacin, pyridoxine, pantothenic acid, B_{12}, folic acid, biotin, and vitamin C. Because the water-soluble vitamins are excreted in the urine, it is less likely that they may become toxic to the body, but the fat-soluble vitamins are stored in the body, and they may reach toxic levels. Table 54–5 lists sources and functions of vitamins.

Minerals

Minerals serve many functions. They are involved in acid-base balance and in the maintenance of osmotic pressure within body compartments. Minerals are components of vitamins, hormones, and enzymes. They maintain normal hemoglobin levels, have functions within the nervous system, and are involved in muscle contraction and skeletal development and maintenance. Minerals that are present in relatively large amounts in the body are called *macrominerals*. These include calcium, phosphorus, sodium, chloride, potassium, magnesium, and sulfur. The remainder are classified as *trace minerals*; they include iron, manganese, copper, iodine, zinc, cobalt, fluorine, and selenium. Table 54–6 lists mineral sources and functions.

Fiber

Fiber, the portion of food that cannot be digested by the human intestinal tract, increases stool bulk and facilitates bowel movements. Fiber decreases the incidence of digestive diseases and colorectal cancer and lowers blood sugar and cholesterol.[5] The amount of fiber believed beneficial is a daily intake of 20 to 30 g.

Nutritional Assessment

The nutritional status can be assessed by evaluating the person's dietary intake, taking anthropometric measurements, performing a physical examination, and con-

TABLE 54-3

Food and Nutrition Board, National Academy of Sciences–National Research Council Recommended Dietary Allowances,* Revised 1989 Designed for the Maintenance of Good Nutrition of Practically all Healthy People in the United States

Category	Age (Years) or Condition	Weight (kg)	Weight (lb)	Height (cm)	Height (in)	Protein (G)	Fat-Soluble Vitamins: Vitamin A (μg RE)‡	Vitamin D (μg)§	Vitamin E (mg α-TE)‖	Vitamin K (μg)
Infants	0.0–0.5	6	13	60	24	13	375	7.5	3	5
	0.5–1.0	9	20	71	28	14	375	10	4	10
Children	1–3	13	29	90	35	16	400	10	6	15
	4–6	20	44	112	44	24	500	10	7	20
	7–10	28	62	132	52	28	700	10	7	30
Males	11–14	45	99	157	62	45	1000	10	10	45
	15–18	66	145	176	69	59	1000	10	10	65
	19–24	72	160	177	70	58	1000	10	10	70
	25–50	79	174	176	70	63	1000	5	10	80
	51+	77	170	173	68	63	1000	5	10	80
Females	11–14	46	101	157	62	46	800	10	8	45
	15–18	55	120	163	64	44	800	10	8	55
	19–24	58	128	164	65	46	800	10	8	60
	25–50	63	138	163	64	50	800	5	8	65
	51+	65	143	160	63	50	800	5	8	65
Pregnant						60	800	10	10	65
Lactating	1st 6 mo					65				
	2nd 6 mo					62	1200	10	11	65

*The allowances, expressed as average daily intakes over time, are intended to provide for individual variations among most normal persons as they live in the United States under usual environmental stresses. Diets should be based on a variety of common foods to provide other nutrients for which human requirements have been less well defined.

†Weights and heights of Reference Adults are actual medians for the U.S. population of the designated age, as reported by NHANES II. The median weights and heights of those younger than 19 years of age were taken from Hamill et al. (1979) (see pages 16–17). The use of these figures does not imply that the height-to-weight ratios are ideal.

ducting laboratory tests. The nutritional assessment can provide information regarding the adequacy of the diet, the person's body size compared with normal ranges, and the possibility of overnutrition or undernutrition.

Nutritional assessment remains more of an art than a science. A global assessment obtains information about many facets of nutrition, including current physical symptoms, any functional impairment, acute and chronic illnesses, a detailed physical examination, and history of dietary intake. Clinical assessment is probably one of the most valid methods of making a nutritional diagnosis and planning nutritional care.[6]

Diet Assessment

A nutritional assessment begins with an evaluation of the person's diet. This can be accomplished by recording the food consumed by actual observation or by 24-hour recall and through the administration of a questionnaire or diet history. Each technique has its own shortcomings, such as the tendency to alter behavior when it is known that the behavior is being observed or reported.

TABLE 54-4

Caloric Requirements Based on Body Weight and Activity Level

	Sedentary	Moderate	Active
Overweight	20–25 kcal/kg	30 kcal/kg	35 kcal/kg
Normal	30 kcal/kg	35 kcal/kg	40 kcal/kg
Underweight	30 kcal/kg	40 kcal/kg	45–50 kcal/kg

(Adapted from Goodhart R.S., Shils M.E. [1980]. *Modern nutrition in health and disease* [6th ed.]. Philadelphia: Lea and Febiger.)

Water-Soluble Vitamins							Minerals						
Vitamin C (mg)	*Thiamin (mg)*	*Riboflavin (mg)*	*Niacin (mg NE)*	*Vitamin B_6 (mg)*	*Folate (μg)*	*Vitamin B_{12} (μg)*	*Calcium (mg)*	*Phosphorus (mg)*	*Magnesium (mg)*	*Iron (mg)*	*Zinc (mg)*	*Iodine (μg)*	*Selenium (μg)*
30	0.3	0.4	5	0.3	25	0.3	400	300	40	6	5	40	10
35	0.4	0.5	6	0.8	35	0.5	600	500	60	10	5	50	15
40	0.7	0.8	9	1.0	50	0.7	800	800	80	10	10	70	20
45	0.9	1.1	12	1.1	75	1.0	800	800	120	10	10	90	20
45	1.0	1.2	13	1.4	100	1.4	800	800	170	10	10	120	30
50	1.3	1.5	17	1.7	150	2.0	1200	1200	270	12	15	150	40
60	1.5	1.8	20	2.0	200	2.0	1200	1200	400	12	15	150	50
60	1.5	1.7	19	2.0	200	2.0	1200	1200	350	10	15	150	70
60	1.5	1.7	19	2.0	200	2.0	800	800	350	10	15	150	70
60	1.2	1.4	15	2.0	200	2.0	800	800	350	10	15	150	70
50	1.1	1.3	15	1.4	150	2.0	1200	1200	280	15	12	150	45
60	1.1	1.3	15	1.5	180	2.0	1200	1200	300	15	12	150	50
60	1.1	1.3	15	1.6	180	2.0	1200	1200	280	15	12	150	55
60	1.1	1.3	15	1.6	180	2.0	800	800	280	15	12	150	55
60	1.0	1.2	13	1.6	180	2.0	800	800	280	10	12	150	55
70	1.5	1.6	17	2.2	400	2.2	1200	1200	320	30	15	175	65
95	1.6	1.8	20	2.1	280	2.6	1200	1200	355	15	19	200	75
90	1.6	1.7	20	2.1	260	2.6	1200	1200	340	15	16	200	75

‡Retinol equivalents. 1 retinol equivalent = 1 μg retinol or 6 μg β-carotene. See text for calculation of vitamin A activity of diets as retinol equivalents.

§As cholecalciferol. 10 μg cholecalciferol = 400 IU of vitamin D.

‖α-Tocopherol equivalents. 1 mg D-αtocopherol = 1 α-TE. See text for variation in allowances and calculation of vitamin E activity of the diet as α-tocopherol equivalents.

¶1 NE (niacin equivalent) is equal to 1 mg of niacin or 60 mg of dietary tryptophan.

Health Assessment

Health assessment, including a health history and physical examination, reveals weight changes, muscle wasting, fat stores, functional status, and nutritional status. Comparison of the person's current weight with previous weights identifies whether the person's weight is stable, changed drastically, or tends to fluctuate. For example, recent rapid weight loss can be a sign of cancer, a malfunctioning thyroid gland, or self-imposed starvation. A history of fluctuating weight could be associated with bulimia. Degradation of muscle, or muscle wasting, is a serious sign of malnutrition. Decreased ability to initiate or complete activities of daily living could result from a decrease in energy caused by a poor diet, a neurologic malfunction such as multiple sclerosis, or symptoms related to chronic obstructive pulmonary disease. Quality of the hair, absence of body hair, condition of gums, and skin lesions could signal poor nutritional status.

Anthropometric Measurements

Anthropometric measurements provide a means for assessing body composition, particularly fat stores and skeletal muscle; it is done by measuring height, weight, circumferences, and thickness of various skinfolds. These measurements are used to determine growth patterns in children and appropriateness of current weight in adults. Body weight is the most frequently used method of assessing nutritional status; it should be used in combination with measurements of body height to establish whether a person is underweight or overweight.

Relative weight is the actual weight divided by the desirable weight and multiplied by 100. A relative weight greater than 120% is indicative of obesity. Recent changes in weight are probably a better indication of undernutrition than a low relative weight. A loss of 10% of body weight or more within the past 6 month period is usually considered predictive of a poor clinical outcome, especially if weight loss is continuing.[7]

The body mass index (BMI) uses height and weight to determine healthy weight. It is calculated by dividing the weight in kilograms by the height in meters squared (BMI = weight [kg]/height [m^2]). A BMI between 19 and 25 has the lowest statistical health risk.[8] A BMI of 25 to 30 is considered overweight; greater than 30 as obese; and greater than 45 as very or morbidly obese.

Body weight reflects lean body mass and adipose tissue and cannot be used as a method for describing

TABLE 54-5
Sources and Functions of Vitamins

Vitamin	Major Food Sources	Functions
Fat-Soluble Vitamins		
Vitamin A (retinol, provitamin, carotenoids)	Retinol: liver, butter, whole milk, cheese, egg yolks; provitamin A: carrots, leafy green vegetables, sweet potatoes, pumpkin, winter squash, apricots, cantaloupe, fortified margarine	Essential for normal retinal function; plays an essential role in cell growth and differentiation, particularly epithelial cells. Epidemiologic evidence suggests a role in preventing certain cancers
Vitamin D (calciferol)	Vitamin D—fortified dairy products, fortified margarine, fish oils, egg yolk	Increases intestinal absorption of calcium and promotes ossification of bones and teeth
Vitamin E (tocopherol)	Vegetable oil, margarine, shortening, green and leafy vegetables, wheat germ, whole-grain products, egg yolk, butter, liver	Functions as an antioxidant protecting vitamins A and C and fatty acids; prevents cell membrane injury
Water-Soluble Vitamins		
Vitamin C (ascorbic acid)	Broccoli, sweet and hot peppers, collards, brussel sprouts, kale, potatoes, spinach, tomatoes, citrus fruits, strawberries	Potent antioxidant involved in many oxidation-reduction reactions; required for synthesis of collagen; increases absorption of nonheme iron; is involved in wound healing and drug metabolism
Thiamin (vitamin B_1)	Pork, liver, meat, whole grains, fortified grain products, legumes, nuts	Coenzyme required for several important biochemical reactions in carbohydrate metabolism. Thought to have an independent role in nerve conduction
Riboflavin (vitamin B_2)	Liver, milk, yogurt, cottage cheese, meat, fortified grain products	Coenzyme that participates in a variety of important oxidation-reduction reactions and important component of a number of enzymes
Niacin (nicotinamide, nicotinic acid)	Liver, meat, poultry, fish, peanuts, fortified grain products	Essential component of the coenzymes nicotinamide adenine dinucleotide (NAD) and nicotinamide dinucleotide diphosphate (NADP), which are involved in many oxidative reduction reactions
Folacin (folic acid)	Liver, legumes, green leafy vegetables	Coenzyme in amino acid and nucleoprotein metabolism; promotes red cell formation
Vitamin B_6 (pyridoxine)	Meat, poultry, fish, shellfish, green and leafy vegetables, whole-grain products, legumes	A major coenzyme involved in the metabolism of amino acids. Required for synthesis of heme
Vitamin B_{12}	Meat, poultry, fish, shellfish, eggs, dairy products	Coenzyme involved in nucleic acid synthesis; assists in development of red cells and maintenance of nerve function
Biotin	Kidney, liver, milk, egg yolks, most fresh vegetables	Coenzyme in fat synthesis, amino acid metabolism, and glycogen formation
Pantothenic acid	Liver, kidney, meats, milk, egg yolk, whole-grain products, legumes	Coenzyme involved in energy metabolism

(Data from *Vitamin facts*, National Dairy Council, and other sources.)

body composition or the percentage of fat tissue present. Statistically, the best percentage of body fat for men is between 12% and 20%, and for women, it is between 20% and 30%.[9] During physical training, body fat usually decreases, and lean body mass increases.

Several types of anthropometric measurements can be used to estimate body fat. Skinfold measurement, although difficult to perform and subject to error when used on obese persons, can be used together with equations and tables to estimate the percentage of lean body mass and fat tissue.[10] Body circumferences are usually a more objective measurement and provide the information needed to calculate waist and hip ratio.

Densitometry by underwater weighing is more accurate than skinfold thickness or body circumference measurements in determining the percentage of body fat, although there are limitations. It requires access to special equipment; assumes a constant density of lean

TABLE 54-6
Sources and Functions of Minerals

Mineral	Major Sources	Functions
Calcium	Milk and milk products, fish with bones, greens	Bone formation and maintenance; tooth formation, vitamin B absorption, blood clotting, nerve and muscle function
Chloride	Table salt, meats, milk, eggs	Regulates pH of stomach, acid-base balance, osmotic pressure of extracellular fluids
Cobalt	Organ meats, meats	Aids in maturation of red blood cells (as part of B_{12} molecule)
Copper	Cereals, nuts, legumes, liver, shellfish, grapes, meats	Catalyst for hemoglobin formation, formation of elastin and collagen, energy release (cytochrome oxidase and catalase), formation of melanin, formation of phospholipids for myelin sheath of nerves
Fluoride	Fluorinated water	Strengthens bones and teeth
Iodine	Iodized salt, fish (saltwater and anadromous)	Thyroid hormone synthesis and its function in maintenance of metabolic rate
Iron	Meats, heart, liver, clams, oysters, lima beans, spinach, dates, dried nuts, enriched and whole-grain cereals	Hemoglobin synthesis, cellular energy release (cytochrome pathway), killing bacteria (myeloperoxidase)
Magnesium	Milk, green vegetables, nuts, bread, and cereals	Catalyst of many intracellular nerve impulses, retention of reactions, particularly those related to intracellular enzyme reactions; low magnesium levels produce an increase in irritability of the nervous system, vasodilatation, and cardiac dysrhythmias
Phosphorus	Meats, poultry, fish, milk and cheese, cereals, legumes, nuts	Bone formation and maintenance; essential component of nucleic acids and energy exchange forms such as adenosine triphosphate (ATP)
Potassium	Oranges, dried fruits, bananas, meats, potatoes, peanut butter, coffee	Maintenance of intracellular osmolality, acid-base balance, transmission of nerve impulses, catalyst in energy metabolism, formation of proteins, formation of glycogen
Sodium	Table salt, cured meats, meats, milk, olives	Maintenance of osmotic pressure of extracellular fluids, acid-base balance, neuromuscular function; absorption of glucose
Zinc	Whole-wheat cereals, eggs, legumes	Integral part of many enzymes including carbonic anhydrase, which facilitates combination of carbon dioxide with water in red blood cells; component of lactate dehydrogenase, which is important in cellular metabolism; component of many peptidases; important in digestion of proteins in gastrointestinal tract

body mass, which is subject to error; and necessitates an estimation of residual gas volumes in the lungs, which is often difficult.

Another method of estimating body fat is bioelectrical impedance. This method is performed by attaching electrodes at the wrist and ankle that send a harmless current through the body. The flow of the current is affected by the amount of water within the body. Because fat-free tissue contains virtually all the water and the conducting electrolytes, measurements of the resistance (*i.e.*, impedance) to current flow can be used to estimate the percentage of body fat present. Bioelectrical impedance is one of the most widely available techniques for assessing body fat. The method is relatively inexpensive, easy to use, and portable.

Dual photon absorptiometry also determines body fat. However, it is expensive, requires exposure to a small amount of radiation, and is difficult to use in the very obese. Its advantages are that it requires minimal cooperation on the part of the person being tested and that it provides a bone mineral estimate.

Computed tomography (CT) and magnetic resonance imaging (MRI) can be used to provide quantitative pictures from which the thickness of fat can be determined. CT scans can also be used to provide quantitative estimates of regional fat and give a ratio of intraabdominal to extraabdominal fat.

Laboratory Studies

Various laboratory tests on blood can aid in evaluating nutritional status. Some of the most commonly performed tests are serum albumin to assess the protein status, total lymphocyte count and delayed hypersensitivity reaction to assess cellular immunity, and creatinine-height index to assess skeletal protein. Vitamin and mineral deficiencies can be determined by measurements of their levels in blood, saliva, and other body tissues or by measuring nutrient-specific chemical reactions. All of these tests are limited by confounding factors and therefore need to be evaluated along with other clinical data.

In summary, nutritional status describes the condition of the body related to the availability and use of nutrients. Nutrients provide the energy and materials necessary for performing the activities of daily living and for the growth and repair of body tissues. Metabolism is the organized process whereby nutrients such as carbohydrates, fats, and proteins are broken down, transformed, or otherwise converted to cellular energy. Glucose, fats, and amino acids from proteins serve as fuel sources for cellular metabolism. These fuel sources are ingested during meals and stored for future use. Glucose is stored as glycogen or converted to triglycerides in fat cells for storage. Fats are stored in adipose tissue as triglycerides. Amino acids are the building blocks of proteins, and most of the stored amino acids are contained in body proteins and as fuel sources for cellular metabolism. Energy is measured in heat units called kilocalories.

The expenditure of body energy results from heat production (*i.e.*, thermogenesis) associated with the basal metabolic rate or basal energy equivalent, diet-induced thermogenesis, exercise-induced thermogenesis, and thermogenesis in response to changes in environmental conditions.

The body requires more than 40 nutrients on a daily basis. Nutritional status reflects the continued daily intake of nutrients over time and the deposition and use of these nutrients within the body. The RDA is the recommended daily intake of essential nutrients considered to be adequate to meet the known nutritional needs of healthy persons. The RDA has 17 age and sex classifications and includes recommendations for calories, protein, fat, carbohydrates, vitamins, and minerals. The nutritional status of a person can be assessed by evaluation of dietary intake, anthropometric measurements, health assessment, and laboratory tests. Health assessment includes a health history and physical examination to determine weight changes, muscle wasting, fat stores, functional status, and nutritional status. Anthropometric measurements are used for assessing body composition; they include height and weight measurements and measurements to determine the composition of the body in relation to lean body mass and fat tissue (*e.g.*, skinfold thickness, body circumferences, densitometry, bioelectrical impedance, and CT scans).

Overnutrition and Obesity

After you have completed this section of the chapter, you should be able to meet the following objectives:

- Define and discuss the causes of obesity and health risks associated with obesity
- Differentiate upper and lower body obesity and their implications in terms of health risk
- Discuss the treatment of obesity in terms of diet, behavior modification, exercise, social support, and surgical methods

"Nicotine in the lungs is invisible, alcoholism may be hidden, but the results of addiction to food . . . cannot be concealed. Fat on the hips is irrevocably public."[11] Obesity is a major health problem in affluent countries. Many believe obesity should be considered a chronic disease.[12] This would decrease the stigma associated with obesity and recognize it as a heterogenous disorder that should be treated individually. Hopefully, this would also result in more health care professionals and patients developing realistic treatment goals. One third of the U.S. population is estimated to be overweight (BMI >27.8 for males and >27.3 for females). This represents an 8% increase from previous surveys.[13]

Because body weight measures muscle mass and body fat, overweight does not necessarily indicate obesity. Obesity is defined strictly as an excess of adipose tissue.[14]

Causes of Obesity

The excess body fat of obesity often significantly impairs health. This excess body fat is generated when the calories consumed exceed those expended through exercise and activity. The physiologic mechanisms that lead to this imbalance still are not understood.[15] The discovery of a hormone called *leptin* has added some knowledge. Leptin informs the brain of the amount of adipose tissue in the body.[16] The brain may then make adjustments in energy intake or output. Leptin is the product of the *OB* gene, and increased linkage to the gene has been found in the massively obese.[17] Research indicates that obesity may be the result of leptin resistance.[18]

Other factors contributing to this imbalance are numerous and probably exist in different combinations among obese persons. Heredity; socioeconomic, cultural, and environmental factors; psychologic influences; and activity levels have all been implicated as causative or contributing factors in the development of obesity. Contrary to popular belief, endocrine disorders rarely cause obesity.

Epidemiologic surveys indicate that the prevalence of overweight is related to social and economic conditions. The second (1976 through 1980) National Health and Nutrition Examination Survey has shown that, if American women were divided into two groups according to economic status, the prevalence of obesity is much higher among those in the poverty group.[19] In contrast, men above the poverty level had a higher prevalence of overweight than men below the poverty level.

Obesity is known to run in families, suggesting a hereditary component. The question that surrounds this observation is whether the disorder arises because of genetic endowment or environmental influences. Studies of twin and adopted children have provided evidence that heredity contributes to the disorder. It is now believed that the heritability of the BMI is about 33%.[20]

Although genetic factors may explain some of the individual variations in terms of excess weight, environmental influences also must be taken into account. These influences include family dietary patterns, decreased level of activity because of labor-saving devices, reliance on the automobile for transportation, and easy access to food. The obese may be greatly influenced by the availability of food, its flavor, time of day, and other cues. The composition of the diet may also be a causal factor, and the percentage of dietary fat independent of total calorie intake may play a part in the development of obesity.[21] Others feel this evidence is weak, because the data is based on food reports.[22] Obesity is associated with increased food intake.[23] These studies used double-labeled water for measuring energy expenditure, and intake proved that food records underestimated the energy intake in the obese. Psychologic factors include using food as a reward, comfort, or means of getting attention. Eating may be a way to cope with tension, anxiety, and mental fatigue. Some persons may overeat and use obesity as a means of avoiding emotionally threatening situations.

It has been suggested that the increased prevalence of obesity in the United States has resulted from increased caloric intake together with a sedentary lifestyle and energy-saving conveniences.[24] A review of the literature reveals that the obese are consistently more sedentary compared with their normal-weight counterparts. They float more when swimming, play less tennis, and walk less per day. Even when a reasonable number of calories are consumed, fewer are expended because of inactivity. A low rate of energy expenditure may contribute to the prevalence of obesity in some families.[25] Infants who become overweight by 3 months of age have a lower energy expenditure than normal-weight infants.[26]

Types of Obesity

Two types of obesity based on distribution of fat have been described: upper body obesity, also referred to as *central, abdominal, android,* or *male obesity,* and lower body obesity, also known as *peripheral, gluteal-femoral, gynoid,* or *female obesity.* The obesity type is determined by dividing the waist by the hip circumference. A waist-hip ratio greater than 1.0 in men and 0.8 in women indicates upper body obesity (Fig. 54–4). Research suggests that fat distribution may be a more important factor for morbidity and mortality than overweight or obesity.

Central obesity can be further differentiated into intraabdominal, or visceral, fat and subcutaneous fat by the use of CT or MRI scans. However, intraabdominal fat is usually synonymous with central fat distribution. Generally, men have more intraabdominal fat and women more subcutaneous fat. As men age, the proportion of intraabdominal fat to subcutaneous fat increases. After menopause, women tend to acquire more central fat distribution. Increasing weight gain, alcohol, and low levels of activity are associated with central obesity. These changes place persons with upper body obesity at greater risk for ischemic heart disease, stroke, and death independent of total body fat. They also tend to exhibit hypertension, elevated levels of triglycerides and decreased levels of high-density lipoproteins, hyperinsulinemia and diabetes mellitus, breast and endometrial cancer, gallbladder disease, menstrual irregularities, and infertility. Visceral fat is also associated with abnormalities of metabolic and sex hormone levels.[27] Weight loss causes a loss of visceral fat and has resulted in improvements in metabolic and hormonal abnormalities.[29,30] Although peripheral obesity is associated with varicose veins in the legs and mechanical problems, it does protect against heart disease.[28]

In terms of weight reduction, some studies have shown that persons with upper body obesity are easier to treat than those with lower body obesity. Other studies have shown no difference in terms of success with weight-reduction programs between the two types of obesity.

Health Risks Associated With Obesity

Social ostracism and isolation are not the only complications of obesity. Obese persons are more likely to develop high blood pressure, hyperlipidemia, cardiovascular disease, glucose intolerance, insulin resistance,

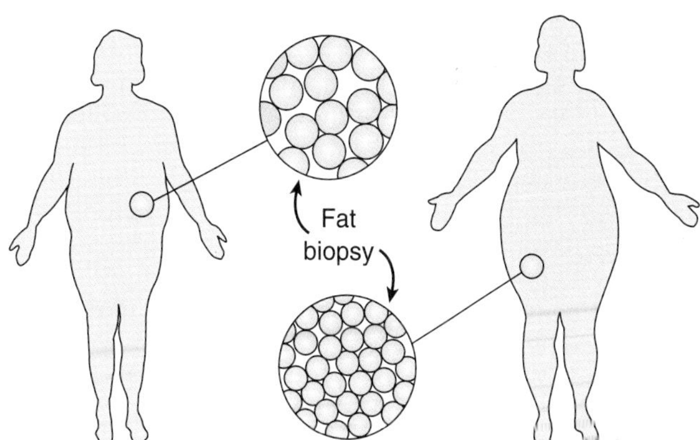

Figure 54–4
Distribution of body fat and size of fat cells in persons with upper and lower body obesity. (Courtesy of Ahmed Kissebah, M.D., Ph.D., Medical College of Wisconsin, Milwaukee)

diabetes, gallbladder disease, infertility, and cancer of the endometrium, breast, prostate, and colon.[31]

The increased weight associated with obesity stresses the bones and joints, increasing the likelihood of arthritis. Because some drugs are lipophilic and exhibit increased distribution in fat tissue, the administration of these drugs, including some anesthetic agents, can be more dangerous in obese persons. If surgery is required, the obese person heals slower than the same-age nonobese person.

It is only with morbid obesity that respiratory function is usually impaired. Sleep apnea and respiratory impairment are prevalent in the morbidly obese population (see Chapter 28). Other respiratory derangements include increased oxygen need to supply the increased body mass, increased respiratory rate to compensate for the resistance offered by chest and body fat, and decreased ventilation to the lower lungs. Obesity increases the risk of various diseases and health problems and heightens the medical risk of other coexisting disorders.

Massive obesity, because of its close association with so many health problems, can be regarded as a disease in its own right.[32] In men who have never smoked, the risk of mortality increases from 1.06 at a BMI of 24.5 to 1.67 at a BMI higher than 26.[33] The waist-hip ratio was a less reliable predictor of mortality in women than BMI.

Treatment of Obesity

Studies have shown that weight reduction in obese persons is beneficial to health. Weight losses in the modest range of 5 to 10 pounds have been shown to lower blood pressure and blood lipids and improve insulin resistance and glucose tolerance [34–36] Weight loss greater than this does not appear to result in greater risk reduction. Recommendations were made for healthy and healthier weights for adults younger than 60 years.[37] Because disease risk occurs at a BMI greater than 25, a healthy weight is defined as one that is at a BMI less than 25. The target should be stabilized by age 21 years and maintained. However, because one third of the population exceeds the healthy weight target, a healthier weight target is defined for those individuals. This goal is achieved by a weight loss of 10 to 16 pounds by those who have not been diagnosed with a weight-related disease. No further weight loss should be attempted until the new weight is stabilized for 6 months and becomes the usual weight. For those individuals who have not been successful at maintaining a weight loss or do not wish to pursue a further decrease in weight, it is suggested that they sustain a stable current weight. Individuals who have a chronic health problem should consult their physician for advice.

Treatment should be actively pursued in individuals with upper body obesity, even if no complications exist.[28] Individuals with peripheral obesity who are at low risk do not require such pursuit. However, because this type of obesity is associated with risks, treatment should be offered.[38] Treatment goals should be broadened for all individuals from weight loss to achieving the best possible weight for overall health.[39] The goals may include stable weight, small weight losses, or prevention of weight gain. There is no single effective treatment for obesity. Treatment methods should include nutritionally adequate and healthful diets, behavior modification, exercise, social support, and in situations of morbid obesity, surgical methods.[40] Ideally, to ensure successful weight maintenance, the individual should be in a program for a minimum of 6 months to possibly 2 years. The team involved should include a physician, nurse, dietitian, psychologist, and exercise physiologist.[41] Appetite suppressant medications are being added to the treatment plan.

Treatment results are discouraging. By 5 years after initially successful weight loss, the result is a net loss of 0 pounds.[15] Some factors have been shown to be a good predictor of positive outcomes. These include social support, willingness to increase physical activity, ability to develop self-control, cognitive coping ability, reasonable expectations, ownership and responsibility, self-efficacy, and self-acceptance.[41] Treatment matching is also possible if the clients are screened for health risk, motivation, previous attempts at weight loss, and eating disorders.[42] Because 25% to 50% of persons who seek treatment for obesity are binge eaters, it is imperative that they receive treatment designed to help them with this problem.[43] This decreases frustration for the caregiver and the client and increases the likelihood of success. There is general agreement that a weight loss of 1 to 2 pounds per week is the most effective and safest.[44] Weight loss in the first 2 to 3 weeks is an unreliable indicator of future weight loss, because this loss includes substantial amounts of water. The macronutrient content of the diet while attempting weight loss does not appear to be a factor in the amount of weight lost.[45] A low-fat diet, however, is believed to correlate with weight maintenance.[45a]

For individuals who have experienced dieting failure, the motivational technique should be to help them develop regular exercise habits and reduce the amount of fat eaten. The technique should be implemented in the following order: development of therapist and peer support, cessation of dieting and normalization of eating patterns, gradual increases in exercise, gradual reduction in dietary fat, and acceptance of what weight loss is achieved through prudent eating and exercise habits.[46]

There is also division within the health care community about the benefit and risks of dieting. Several challenges must be addressed: identify individuals who will be helped or harmed by dieting, reduce the severity and frequency of dieting for those where the cost exceeds the benefits, understand the physical and psychologic reasons why some persons can lose and others cannot, develop safe and effective means for weight loss and its maintenance, and target weight loss methods to individuals who stand to benefit.[47]

Behavior modification focuses on new behaviors. These are achieved through record keeping, stimulus control, cognitive restructuring, and use of support systems. It has proven successful for achieving and maintaining weight loss and has also reported the lowest attrition rates. However, the average loss of any behavioral program reported in the literature is 1 pound per week, with 16 pounds being the average total achieved.

Very-low-calorie diets may be used for severely obese persons in conjunction with behavior modification techniques. The very-low-calorie diets usually contain 400 to 800 calories of a liquid protein fortified with electrolytes and vitamins. Weight loss averages 2 to 4 pounds (0.9 to 1.8 kg) per week. Because of risks from severe calorie restriction, these diets require medical supervision and frequent laboratory testing. Side effects include fatigue, gout, gallstones, cardiac complications, orthostatic hypotension, and fluid and electrolyte disorders. Because severe calorie restriction is undesirable for pregnant and lactating women, these diets are contraindicated for that group, as well as for children, who still require protein for growth. Because of the cost and lack of long-term maintenance, very-low-calorie diets have lost their popularity.

Exercise is an important part of a weight-loss program. Research suggests exercise alone is not effective and must be combined with an energy-deficient diet.[48] It increases energy expenditure and helps preserve lean body tissue during weight loss. Continued exercise after weight loss predicts a greater chance of long-term success.[49] The exercise used was low-intensity aerobic exercise with an emphasis on increasing frequency and duration rather than intensity. Exercise may also help to prevent the compensatory decrease in metabolic rate occurring with a reduction in calories that often makes weight loss difficult.[50] However, there is a high dropout rate from exercise programs. Many overweight persons feel self-conscious, and some types of activities may prove to be uncomfortable or painful. For this reason, many weight-loss programs encourage walking for 10 to 15 minutes three to four times each week. The effect of this simple prescription may have long-lasting effects and may encourage other forms of exercise. Recommendations such as using the stairs instead of the elevator and walking instead of using the car for short distances are encouraged. More strenuous types of exercise may require cardiovascular screening for establishing risk and developing an individualized exercise program.

The surgical treatment for obesity is usually reserved for persons who have a BMI greater than 40 and have resisted other methods of treatment. Two types of gastric surgeries, gastric bypass and vertical-banded gastroplasty, are used for treating obesity.[51] Gastric bypass procedures establish a direct connection between the stomach and the small intestine. In one procedure, the stomach immediately adjacent to the esophagus is connected by way of a loop of intestine to the jejunum closing the larger portion of the stomach so that the stomach contents bypass part of the upper intestine. The smaller upper portion of the stomach is designed to hold 50 to 60 ml of food, causing a feeling of fullness with a small amount of food. Gastroplasty procedures are designed to reduce the size of the stomach to a 15 to 30 ml capacity pouch with a narrow stoma into the remainder of the stomach. This greatly reduces the amount of food which can be eaten at one time. Weight loss averages between 40 and 70 kg.[52] Mortality rates are less than 1%, and morbidity rates are less than 10% in centers that specialize in this treatment. There is a decrease in all complications and risk factors of obesity, together with increased life expectancy and improved psychosocial measures.[53]

The use of medications to effect weight loss is returning to the treatment of obesity. This treatment modality should be limited to persons who have a BMI greater than 27, possess other risk factors, and have been unsuccessful with other weight-loss interventions.[54] The medications should be used as an adjunct to a diet and exercise program and should be continued if there is at least a 4-pound weight loss in the first month. There is little data on the safety and benefits of therapy lasting longer than 1 year.

Weight cycling has no effect on metabolic variables, central obesity, or cardiovascular risk factors or future amount of weight loss.[55] More research is needed to determine its effect on dietary preference for fat, psychologic adjustment, disordered eating, and mortality.[56,57] It is postulated that perhaps it is the underlying obesity and not the weight fluctuation that affects life expectancy.[58]

Emphasis is being placed on the prevention of obesity.[59]. It has been theorized that it is preventable because the effect of heredity factors is no more than moderate. A more active lifestyle together with a low-fat diet (<30% calories) is seen as the strategy for prevention. The target audience should be young children, adolescents, and young adults.[60] Tools needed to achieve this goal include promotion of regular meals, avoidance of snacking, substituting water for calorie-containing beverages, decreased television viewing time, low-fat diet, and increased activity. Other experts target the high-risk period from 25 to 35 years, menopause,[61] and the year after successful weight loss.

Childhood Obesity

Obesity is the most prevalent nutritional disorder affecting the pediatric population in the United States. The findings from the National Health and Nutrition Study (NHANES) III, conducted between 1988 and 1994, showed that 14% of children and 12% of adolescents were overweight. The definition for overweight for the the NHANES III study was a BMI at or above the sex- and age-specific 95th percentile.[62] A diagnosis of obesity is made when the triceps skinfold is greater than the 85th percentile and the weight for height is greater than 120% of ideal when controlled for age and sex.[63] Children who are 120% of weight expected for their height are overweight, but they are overfat only when the triceps skinfold result is greater than the 85th percentile. This distinction is important in preventing misdiagnosis of obesity and creating anxiety for the parents and child.

Childhood obesity is determined by a combination of hereditary and environmental factors. It is associated with obese parents, higher socioeconomic status, increased parental education, small family size, and sedentary lifestyle.[60] Children with overweight parents are at highest risk; for those with two overweight parents there is a 70% risk of becoming obese. Television viewing is associated with consumption of calorie-dense snacks and decreased physical activity; time spent watching television has been directly related to obesity. Obese children appear to have a deficit in recognizing hunger sensations, stemming perhaps from parents who use food as gratification. These children may also have been exposed to an overprotective and perhaps rigid environment.

Because adolescent obesity is predictive of adult obesity, treatment of childhood obesity is desirable.[63b] Weight loss without adverse health effects and maintenance of that loss are the goals.[62] In young children who have mild to moderate weight problems, weight maintenance or a reduced rate of weight gain is sufficient. When weight loss is required, a loss of 1 pound per month is reasonable together with permanent changes in food consumption and activity. Each child should be assessed and treated individually. Group treatment should only be used for those with less serious problems. The focus, however, should be on normalizing food intake, particularly fat intake, and increasing physical activity. If weight gain can be slowed or maintained during growth, lean body mass increases and some of the abnormal metabolic effects of obesity may be reversed. Family members need to be involved so they can learn to provide appropriate support and assist the child in taking responsibility for his or her own actions. Highly restrictive diets should be limited to the rare child or adolescent who has morbid complications. They should not be used for children or adolescents with renal, liver, or cardiac disease. These diets should contain a minimum of 2 g protein/kg body weight.[62] There should be close monitoring for sustained nitrogen losses, cardiac dysrhythmias, and cholelithiasis. Commercial diets are not recommended.

In summary, obesity is defined as excess body fat resulting from consumption of calories in excess of those expended for exercise and activities. Heredity; socioeconomic, cultural, environmental factors; psychologic influences; and activity levels have been implicated as causative factors in the development of obesity. The health risks associated with obesity include hyperlipidemia and cardiovascular disease, including hypertension; insulin resistance, glucose intolerance, and diabetes mellitus; menstrual irregularities and infertility; cancer of the endometrium, breast, prostate, and colon; and gallbladder disease. There are two types of obesity—upper body and lower body obesity. Upper body obesity is associated with a higher incidence of complications. The treatment of obesity focuses on nutritionally adequate weight-loss diets; behavior modification; exercise; social support; and, in situations of marked obesity, surgical methods. Obesity is the most prevalent nutritional disorder affecting the pediatric population in the United States.

Undernutrition

After you have completed this section of the chapter, you should be able to meet the following objectives:

- List the major causes of malnutrition and starvation
- State the difference between protein-calorie starvation (*i.e.*, marasmus) and protein malnutrition (*i.e.*, kwashiorkor)
- Explain the effect of malnutrition on muscle mass, respiratory function, acid-base balance, wound healing, immune function, bone mineralization, the menstrual cycle, and testicular function
- State the causes of malnutrition in the hospitalized patient
- Compare the eating disorders and complications associated with anorexia nervosa and the binge-purge syndrome

Undernutrition ranges from the selective deficiency of a single nutrient to starvation in which there is deprivation of all ingested nutrients. Undernutrition can result from willful eating behaviors as in anorexia nervosa and the binge-purge syndrome, lack of food availability, or health problems that impair food intake and decrease its absorption and use. There is general agreement that malnutrition is the most widespread cause of morbidity and mortality throughout the world. In the United States, poverty, homelessness, and hunger promote malnutrition among all age groups. Weight loss and malnutrition are common during illness, recovery from trauma, and hospitalization.

Malnutrition and Starvation

Malnutrition and starvation are conditions in which a person does not receive or is unable to use an adequate amount of calories and nutrients for body function. Among the many causes of starvation, some are willful, such as the person with anorexia nervosa who does not consume enough food to maintain weight and health, and some are medical, such as persons with Crohn's disease who are unable to absorb their food. Most cases of food deprivation result in semistarvation. Malnutrition can occur in persons with chronic obstructive lung disease when their air hunger interferes with their ability to eat; eventually, the resultant malnutrition further complicates their respiratory status and food consumption.

Protein and Calorie Malnutrition

In malnutrition and starvation, the amount of food consumed and absorbed is drastically reduced. Most of the literature on malnutrition and starvation has dealt with infants and children in underdeveloped countries. The classic approach to the study of this population commonly divides cases into marasmus and kwashiorkor, with intermediate cases of marasmic kwashiorkor combining certain features of each condition.

Protein-calorie malnutrition, also referred to as *marasmus* is characterized by loss of muscle and fat stores. Marasmus is characterized by progressive wasting from inadequate food intake that is equally deficient in calories and protein. The person appears emaciated having sparse, dry, and dull hair and depressed heart rate, blood pressure, and body temperature. The child with marasmus has a wasted appearance, with stunted growth and loss of subcutaneous fat, but with relatively normal skin, hair, liver function, and affect.

Kwashiorkor is caused by protein deficiency. The term *kwashiorkor* comes from the African word meaning *the disease suffered by the displaced child*, because the condition develops soon after a child is displaced from the breast after the arrival of a new baby and placed on a starchy gruel feeding. The child with kwashiorkor is characterized by edema, desquamating skin, discolored hair, enlarged abdomen, anorexia, and extreme apathy. The serum albumin level is less that 3.0 g/dl, and there is pitting edema of the extremities. There is less weight loss and wasting of skeletal muscles than in marasmus. Other manifestations include skin lesions, easily pluckable hair, enlarged liver and distended abdomen, cold extremities, and decreased cardiac output and tachycardia.

Marasmus-kwashiorkor is an advanced protein and calorie deficit together with increased protein requirement or loss. This results in a rapid decrease in anthropometric measurements with obvious edema and wasting and loss of organ mass.

Starvation

Starvation implies the lack of food intake. Depending on the prestarvation state, the metabolic events of starvation permit life to continue for months without caloric intake. In healthy, normally fed persons, there is fuel enough to last for more than 80 days, assuming previous use of 2000 kcal/day; about 85% of these calories are stored in fat tissue, 14% in body proteins, and 1% in stored carbohydrate sources.[64] Despite the limited carbohydrate stores, which are depleted within 12 to 24 hours without food, a continuing supply of glucose is essential for survival. The central nervous system uses about 115 g of glucose a day, and red blood cells, bone marrow, kidneys, and peripheral nervous system use another 36 g of glucose.[64] One of the critical adaptive mechanisms in starvation is the production of new glucose (*i.e.*, gluconeogenesis). The liver uses glycerol, lactate, and amino acids in the synthesis of glucose. The glycerol skeleton, obtained from triglycerides released from fat cells, plays a significant role in glucose synthesis. The predominant fuel for other tissues is fatty acids and ketones. For this reason, a state of ketosis is common during starvation.

Proteins have vital enzymatic and structural functions, and the body avoids using them as a fuel source until the late stages of starvation. Eventually, protein wasting ensues, with substantial weight loss, the most well-known and easily recognized sign of starvation. This weight loss is caused by loss of lean body tissue and fat along with diuresis. The importance of protein conservation to survival has been demonstrated in animal studies, in which a premorbid increase in nitrogen excretion due to protein use heralded the final stages of starvation.[64] Death from starvation rather than from hypoglycemia occurs when one third to one half of the body's protein is lost.[64]

Daily weight loss can range from 1 pound to several pounds, depending on the stage of starvation. Wound healing is poor, and the body is unable to fight off infection because of multiple immunologic malfunctions throughout the body. The muscles used for breathing become weakened, and respiratory function becomes compromised as muscle proteins are used as a fuel source. A reduction in respiratory function has many implications, especially for persons with burns, trauma, infection, or chronic respiratory disease and for persons who are being mechanically ventilated because of respiratory failure.

Although intellectual functioning remains intact despite the ketosis that occurs during starvation, depression and emotional lability are common. There is a diminished appetite and decreased desire for fluids because of the altered hypothalamic function that occurs with ketosis. A marked decrease in libido is observed with starvation. The female experiences anovulation and amenorrhea, and the male experiences decreased testicular function. The kidney does not go untouched by starvation. Calcium and phosphate are excreted as bone is dissolved, and uric acid is retained, which can cause gout.

Malnutrition in Hospitalized Patients

Malnutrition increases morbidity, mortality, incidence of complications, and length of hospital stay. Persons may enter the hospital in a malnourished state. This malnutrition may be caused by poverty, inadequate food storage and preparation facilities, addiction to drugs or alcohol, adherence to fad diets, or even poorly fitting dentures. The malnutrition may result from a disease or disability that alters nutrient requirement, use, or excretion. The hospitalized patient often finds eating a healthful diet difficult and commonly has restrictions on food and water intake in preparation for tests and surgery. Pain, medications, special diets, and stress can decrease appetite. Even when the patient is well enough to eat, eating alone in a room where unpleasant treatments may be given is not conducive to eating. Protein-calorie malnutrition usually develops in the hospitalized patient secondary to physiologic stress or injury. After protein-calorie malnutrition develops, it alters nutritional requirements and intake and use of nutrients. Severe body protein depletion can occur rapidly.

Although hospitalized patients may appear to need fewer calories because they are on bed rest, their actual need for caloric intake may be higher because of other energy expenditures. For example, more calories are expended during fever, when the metabolic rate is increased. There may also be an increased need for protein to support tissue repair after trauma or surgery. Hospitals have nutrition support teams who assess patients' needs for nutrition intervention, select the appropriate nutrition therapy, and monitor the effectiveness and tolerance of the intervention.

Eating Disorders

An eating disorder is a complex disorder involving issues and behaviors relating to food and weight and involving relationships with others.[65] It results in gross disturbance in eating behavior that jeopardizes a person's physical and psychologic health. Eating disorders develop despite a normally functioning gastrointestinal tract and appetite. Anorexia nervosa, bulimia, and the binge-eating syndrome are chronic problems in which there is a preoccupation with food, eating, and weight loss.

Anorexia Nervosa

Anorexia nervosa was first described in the scientific literature over 100 years ago by Sir William Gull.[66] Anorexia nervosa is a self-starvation syndrome in which a person willingly loses an excessive amount of weight (15% or more of original body weight), exhibits muscle wasting, suffers from disturbances in body image, has a preoccupation with food, and experiences unreasonable fears about gaining weight. The term *anorexia*, meaning loss of appetite, is a misnomer because hunger is actually felt, but in this case, it is denied.

Anorexia nervosa is more prevalent among young women than men. The disorder typically begins in teenage girls who are obese or perceive themselves as being obese. An interest in weight reduction becomes an obsession, with severely restricted caloric intake and frequently with excessive physical exercise.

Many organ systems are affected by the malnutrition that occurs in persons with anorexia nervosa. The severity of the abnormalities tends to be related to the degree of malnutrition and is reversed by refeeding. The most frequent complication of anorexia is amenorrhea and loss of secondary sex characteristics with decreased levels of estrogen, which can eventually lead to osteoporosis. Constipation, cold intolerance and failure to shiver in cold, bradycardia, hypotension, decreased heart size, electrocardiographic changes, blood abnormalities, and skin with lanugo (*i.e.*, increased amounts of fine hair) are common. Unexpected sudden deaths have been reported; the risk appears to increase as weight drops to less than 35% to 40% of ideal weight. It is believed that these deaths are caused by myocardial degeneration and heart failure rather than dysrhythmias.

The most exasperating aspect of the treatment of anorexia is the inability of the person with anorexia to recognize there is a problem. Because anorexia is a form of starvation, it can lead to death if left untreated. A multidisciplinary approach appears to be the most effective method of treating persons with the disorder.[65] The goals of treatment are eating and weight gain, resolution of issues with the family, healing of pain from the past, and efforts to work on psychologic, relationship, and emotional issues.

Bulimia Nervosa and Binge Eating

Bulimia nervosa and binge eating are eating disorders that encompass an array of distinctive behaviors, feelings, and thoughts. *Bulimia nervosa* is characterized by secretive episodes or binges of eating large quantities of easily consumed high-caloric foods, such as doughnuts and ice cream. The periods of overeating are followed by compensatory behaviors such as fasting, self-induced vomiting, or abuse of laxatives or diuretics. These individuals also have a sense of a lack of control over eating during episodes of binge eating. The binge-eating disorder is not associated with inappropriate compensatory behaviors.

Persons who experience bulimia nervosa or binge-eating disorders are usually women in their late teens through mid-thirties. Their weight may fluctuate, although not to the dangerously low levels seen in anorexia nervosa. The thoughts and feelings of persons with binge-eating disorders range from fear of not being able to stop eating to a concern about gaining too much weight. They also experience feelings of sadness, anger, guilt, shame, and low self-esteem.

The complications of bulimia nervosa include those resulting from overeating, self-induced vomiting, and cathartic and diuretic abuse. Among the complications of self-induced vomiting are dental disorders, parotitis, and fluid and electrolyte disorders. Dental abnormalities, such as sensitive teeth, increased dental caries, and periodontal disease, occur with frequent vomiting because the high-acid content of the vomitus causes tooth enamel to dissolve. Esophagitis, dysphagia, and esophageal stricture are common. With frequent vomiting, there is often reflux of gastric contents into the lower esophagus because of relaxation of the lower esophageal sphincter. Vomiting may lead to aspiration pneumonia, especially in intoxicated or debilitated persons. Potassium, chloride, and hydrogen are lost in the vomitus, and frequent vomiting also predisposes to metabolic acidosis with hypokalemia (see Chapter 27). An unexplained physical response to vomiting is the development of benign, painless parotid gland enlargement.

The primary goal of therapy for binge-eating disorders is to establish a regular, healthful eating pattern. Unlike those who suffer from anorexia nervosa, persons with bulimia nervosa or binge eating are upset by the behaviors practiced and the thoughts and feelings experienced, and they are more willing to accept help. Persons with binge-eating disorders who have been successfully treated for their eating disorder have reported that making meal plans, eating a balanced diet at three regular meals a day, avoiding high-sugar foods and other binge foods, recording food intake and binge-eating episodes, exercising regularly, finding alternative activities, and avoiding alcohol and drugs are helpful in maintaining their more healthful eating behaviors after treatment. Antidepressant medications have been used effectively in the treatment of bulimia nervosa.[67]

In summary, undernutrition can range from a selective deficiency of a single nutrient to starvation in which there is deprivation of all ingested nutrients. Malnutrition and starvation are among the most widespread causes of morbidity and mortality in the world. The body adapts to starvation through the use of fat stores and glucose synthesis to supply the energy needs of the central nervous system. Malnutrition is common during illness, recovery from trauma, and hospitalization. The effects of malnutrition and starvation on body function are widespread. They include loss of muscle mass, impaired wound healing, impaired immunologic function, decreased appetite, loss of calcium and phosphate from bone, anovulation and amenorrhea in women, and decreased testicular function in men.

Anorexia and binge eating are eating disorders that result in malnutrition. In anorexia nervosa, distorted attitudes about eating lead to serious weight loss and malnutrition. Bulimia nervosa is characterized by secretive episodes or binges of eating large quantities of easily consumed high-caloric foods, followed by compensatory behaviors such as fasting, self-induced vomiting, or abuse of laxatives or diuretics. Binge-eating disorder is characterized by eating large quantities of food but not associated with inappropriate compensatory behaviors.

REFERENCES

1. Guyton A.C., Hall J.E. (1996). *Textbook of medical physiology* (9th ed., p. 909). Philadelphia: W.B. Saunders.
2. Garrell D.R., Bobin N., DeFonge L.H.M. (1996). Should we still use the Harris and Benedict equations? *Nutrition in Clinical Practice* 11, 99.
3. Subcommittee on the Tenth Edition of The RDAS. (1989). *Recommended dietary allowances* (10th ed). Commission on Life Sciences–National Council. Washington DC: National Academic Press.
4. Summary of the second report of the National Cholesterol Education Program (NCEP) Expert Panel on Detection, Evaluation, and Treatment of High Blood Cholesterol in Adults. (1993). *Journal of the American Medical Association* 269, 3015.
5. Bennett W.G., Cerda J.J. (1996). Benefit of dietary fiber: Myth or medicine? *Postgraduate Medicine* 99, 153.
6. Hill G.L., Windsor J.A. (1995). Nutritional assessment in clinical practice. *Nutrition* 11 (2 suppl), 198.
7. Detsky A.S., Smalley P.S., Chang J. (1994). Is this patient malnourished? Journal of the American Medical Association 271, 54.
8. World Health Organization. (1989). *Measuring obesity: Classification and description of anthropometric data.* Copenhagen: World Health Organization.
9. Abernathy R.P., Black D.R. (1996). Healthy body weight: An alternative perspective. *American Journal of Clinical Nutrition* 63 (Suppl.), 448S.
10. Womersley J., Durnin J.V.G.A. (1977). A comparison of skinfold method with extent of "overweight" and various weight-height relationships in assessment of obesity. *British Journal of Nutrition* 38, 271.
11. Epstein L.G., Wing R.R., Voloski A. (1985). Childhood obesity. *Pediatric Clinics of North America* 32, 2.
12. Yanovski S.Z. (1993). A practical approach to treatment of the obese patient. *Archives of Family Medicine* 2, 309.
13. Kuczmarski R.J., Flegal K.M., Campbell S.M., et al. (1994). Increasing prevalence of overweight among U.S. adults: The National Health and Nutrition Examination Surveys, 1960 to 1991. Journal of the American Medical Association 272, 205.
14. Gray D.S. (1989) Diagnosis and prevalence of obesity. *Medical Clinics of North America* 73, 1.
15. NIH Technology Assessment Conference Panel. (1992). Methods for voluntary weight loss and control. *Annals of Internal Medicine* 116, 942.
16. Editorial. (1996). Leptin in humans: Current progress and future directions. *Clinical Chemistry* 42, 843.
17. Bray G. A. (1996). Leptin and leptinomania. *Lancet* 348, 140.
18. Tartaglia L.A., Dembski M., Weng X., et al. (1995). Identification and expression cloning of a leptin receptor, OB-R. *Cell* 83, 1263.
19. *Plan and operation of the National Health and Nutrition Examination Survey, 1976–1980.* DDHS Publication (PHS) 81–1317, Vital and Health Statistics, Series 1, No. 15. Hyattsville, MD: National Center for Health Statistics.
20. Bouchard C. (1994). *The genetics of obesity.* Boca Raton: CRC Press.
21. Schutz Y., Flatt J.P., Jequier E. (1989). Failure of dietary fat intake to promote fat oxidation: A factor favoring the development of obesity. *American Journal of Clinical Nutrition* 50, 307.
22. Gibney M.J. (1995). Epidemiology of obesity in relation to nutrient intake. *International Journal of Obesity* 19 (Suppl. 5), 51.
23. Lichtman S.W., Pisarski K., Berman E.R. (1992). Discrepancy bet self-reported and actual calorie intake and exercise in obese subjects. *New England Journal of Medicine* 327, 1893.
24. McGinnis J.M. (1992). The public health burden of a sedentary lifestyle. *Medical Science Sports Exercise* 24, 51–96.
25. Bogardus C., Lillioja S., Ravussin E., et al. (1987). Familial dependence of the resting metabolic rate. *New England Journal of Medicine* 315, 96.
26. Roberts S.B., Savage J., Coward W., et. al. (1988). Energy expenditure and intake in infants born to lean and overweight mothers. *New England Journal of Medicine* 318, 461.
27. Kissebah A.H., Krakower G.R. (1994). Regional adiposity and morbidity. *Physiological Reviews* 74, 761.
28. Ashwell M. (1994). Obesity in men and women. *International Journal of Obesity* 18 (Suppl. 1), S1.
29. Fujoka S., Matsuzawa Y., Tounaja K., et al. (1991). Improvement of glucose and lipid metabolism associated with selective reduction of intra-abdominal fat in premenstrual women with visceral fat obesity. *International Journal of Obesity* 15, 853.
30. Pleuss J.A., Hoffman R.C., Sonnenberg C.E., et al. (1993). Effects of abdominal fat on insulin and androgen levels. *Obesity Research* 1 (Suppl. 1), 25F.

31. Pi-Sunyer F.X. (1993). Medical hazards of obesity. *Annals of Internal Medicine* 119, 655.
32. Dwyer J. (1996). Policy and healthy weight. *Preventive Medicine* 25, 30.
33. Lee I., Manson J.E., Hennekens C.H., et al. (1993). Body weight and mortality: A 27-year follow-up of middle-aged men. Journal of the American Medical Association 270 (23), 2823.
34. Kannel W.B., D'Agostino R.B., Cobb J.L. (1996). Effect of weight on cardiovascular disease. *American Journal of Clinical Nutrition* 63 (Suppl), 419S.
35. Pi-Sunyer F.X. (1996). Weight and non-insulin-dependent diabetes mellitus. *American Journal of Clinical Nutrition* 63 (Suppl.), 426S.
36. McCarron D.A., Reusser M.E. (1996). Body weight and blood pressure regulation. *American Journal of Clinical Nutrition* 63 (Suppl.), 423S.
37. Meisler J.G., St. Jeor S. (1996). Summary and recommendations from the American Health Foundation's Expert Panel on Healthy Weight. *American Journal of Clinical Nutrition* 63 (Suppl.), 474S.
38. Young T.K., Gelskey D.E. (1995). Is noncentral obesity metabolically benign? Journal of the American Medical Association 274, 1939.
39. Food and Nutrition Board, Institute of Medicine. (1995). *Weighing the options.* Washington, D.C.: National Academy Press.
40. Position of the American Dietetic Association. (1997). Weight management. *Journal of the American Dietetic Association* 97, 71.
41. Turner L.W., Wang M.Q., Westerfield R.C. (1995). Preventing relapse in weight control: A discussion of cognitive and behavioral strategies. *Psychological Reports* 77, 651.
42. Brownell K.D., Kramer F.M. (1989). Behavioral management of obesity. *Medical Clinics of North America* 73, 185.
43. Robinson J.I., Hoerr S.L., Petersmarck K., et al. (1995). Redefining success in obesity intervention: The new paradigm. *Journal of the American Dietetic Association* 95, 422.
44. Technology Assessment Conference Panel. (1993). Methods for voluntary weight loss and control: Technology assessment conference statement. *Annals of Internal Medicine* 119 (7 Pt 2), 764.
45. Golay A., Allaz A., Morel Y., et al. (1996). Similar weight loss with low- or high-carbohydrate diets. *American Journal of Clinical Nutrition* 63, 174.
45a. Hill J.O., Drougas, H., Peters J.C. (1993). Obesity treatment: Can diet composition play a role? *Annals of Internal Medicine* 119 (7 Pt 2), 694.
46. Foreyt J.P., Goodrick G.K. (1993). Weight management without dieting. *Nutrition Today* March / April, 4.
47. Brownell K.D., Rodin J. (1994). The dieting maelstrom. *American Psychologist* 49, 781.
48. Wood P.D. (1996). Clinical applications of diet and physical activity in weight loss. *Nutrition Review* 54, 5131.
49. Pronk N.P., Wing R.R. (1994). Physical activity and long-term maintenance of weight loss. *Obesity Research* 2, 587.
50. Leibel R.L., Rosenbaum M., Hirsch J. (1995). Changes in energy expenditure resulting from altered body weight. *New England Journal of Medicine* 332, 621.
51. Stunkard A.J. (1996). Current views on obesity. *American Journal of Medicine* 100, 230.
52. Kral J.G. (1992). Review of surgical techniques for treating obesity. *American Journal of Clinical Nutrition* 55, 552S.
53. Pories W.J., MacDonald K.G. Jr., Morgan E.J., et al. (1992). Surgical treatment of obesity and its effect on diabetes: 10-year follow-up. *American Journal of Nutrition*, 55, 582S.
54. Task Force on Prevention and Treatment of Obesity. (1996). Long-term pharmacotherapy in the management of obesity. Journal of the American Medical Association 276, 1907.
55. Jeffery R.W. (1996). Does weight cycling present a health risk? *American Journal of Clinical Nutrition* 63 (Suppl.), 452S.
56. Muls E., Kempen K., Vansant G., et al. (1995). Is weight cycling detrimental to health? A review of the literature in humans. *International Journal of Obesity & Related Metabolic Disorders* 19 (Suppl. 3), S46.
57. Williamson D.F. (1996). "Weight cycling" and mortality: How do the epidemiologists explain the role of intentional weight loss? *Journal American College of Nutrition* 15, 6.
58. Garn S.M. (1996). Fractionating healthy weight. *American Journal of Clinical Nutrition* 63 (Suppl.), 412S.
59. Task Force on Prevention and Treatment of Obesity. (1994). Towards prevention of obesity: Research directives. *Obesity Research* 2, 571.
60. Klish W.J. (1995). Childhood obesity: Pathophysiology and treatment. *Acta Paediatricia Japonica* 37, 1.
61. Wing R.R. (1995). Changing diet and exercise behaviors in individuals at risk for weight gain. *Obesity Research* 3 (Suppl. 2), 277s.
62. Update: Prevalence of overweight among children, adolescents, and adults—United States, 1988–1994, *Mortality and Morbidity Weekly Report* 46, 199.
63a. Dietz W.H., Robinson T.N. (1993). Assessment and Treatment of childhood obesity. *Pediatrics in Review* 14, 337.
63b. Eck L.H., Klesge R.C., Hanson C.L. et al. (1992). Children at familial risk for obesity: An examination of dietary intake, physical activity and weight status. *International Journal of Obesity* 16, 71.
64. Sauded K., Felig P. (1976). The metabolic events of starvation. *American Journal of Medicine* 60, 117.
65. Position of The American Dietetic Association. (1994). Nutrition intervention in the treatment of anorexia nervosa, bulimia nervosa, and binge eating. *Journal of the American Dietetic Association* 94, 902.
66. Gull W.W. (1974). Anorexia nervosa. *Transactions of the Clinical Society of London* 7, 22.
67. Advokat C., Kutlesic V. (1994). Pharmacology of the eating disorders. *Neuroscience and Biobehavioral Reviews* 19, 59.

ADDITIONAL READINGS

Alford B.B., Blankenship A.C., Hagen R.D. (1990). The effects of variations in carbohydrate, protein, and fat content of the diet upon weight loss, blood values, and nutrient intake of adult obese women. *Journal of the American Dietetic Association* 90, 534.

Ballard-Barbash R., Swanson C.A. (1996). Body weight: Estimation of risk for breast and endometrial cancers. *American Journal of Clinical Nutrition* 63 (Suppl.), 437S.

Bandini L.J., Schoeller D.A., Cyr H.Y.N., et al. (1990). Validity of reported energy intake in obese and nonobese adolescents. *American Journal of Clinical Nutrition* 52, 421.

Blackburn G. (1995). Effect of degree of weight loss on health benefits. *Obesity Research* 3 (Suppl. 2), 211S.

Bray G.A. (1992). Pathophysiology of obesity. *American Journal of Clinical Nutrition* 55 (Suppl.), 488S.

Elks M.L. (1996). Appetite suppressants as adjuncts in the treatment of obesity. *Journal of Family Practice* 42, 287.

Felson D. (1996). Weight and osteoarthritis. *American Journal of Clinical Nutrition* 63 (Suppl.), 430S.

Manson J.E., Faich G.A. (1996). Pharmacotherapy for obesity: Do the benefits outweigh the risks? *New England Journal of Medicine* 335, 659.

Wilmore J.H. (1996). Increasing physical activity: Alterations in body mass and composition. *American Journal of Clinical Nutrition* 63 (Suppl.), 456S.

Wood P.D. (1996). Clinical applications of diet and physical activity in weight loss. *Nutrition Review* 54, S131.

Zerbe K. (1996). Anorexia nervosa and bulimia nervosa. *Postgraduate Medicine* 99 (1), 161.

CHAPTER 55

Alterations in Activity Tolerance

Mary Kay Jiricka

Health includes physical and psychological components; it involves the ability to work, exercise, participate in leisure activities, and perform activities of daily living. To be able to perform these activities requires that the body have sufficient physiologic and psychological energy and stamina. When the body can no longer meet these energy demands, fatigue occurs. Fatigue may be acute, as in that resulting from increased physical activity, or it may be chronic. Conditions that impair health can affect a person's activity reserve and impose certain restrictions, such as bed rest and immobility, on the ability to perform work and other activities. This chapter focuses on activity tolerance, the ability to do work, and the body's response to exercise; activity intolerance and fatigue; and activity intolerance as it relates to the physiologic and psychosocial responses to immobility and bed rest.

Activity Tolerance

After you have completed this section of the chapter, you should be able to meet the following objectives:

- Describe the body's physiologic and psychological responses to exercise and work
- Define the term *maximal oxygen consumption* and state how it is measured
- Identify one physical method and two paper and pencil tools to assess work performance
- Differentiate acute from chronic fatigue
- List at least four health problems that are associated with chronic fatigue
- Define *chronic fatigue syndrome* and describe assessment findings, presenting symptoms, and laboratory values associated with the disorder
- Discuss treatment modalities for chronic fatigue syndrome

Activity is defined as the process of exerting energy for the purpose of accomplishing an effect. Human beings interact with their environment in a pattern of activity cycles. These cycles include periods of rest and periods of activity, and they have both physical and psychological elements. Rest is characterized by inactivity and requires minimal energy expenditure. Activity denotes the process of movement and requires the expenditure of energy. One form of activity is *exercise*. Like activity, exercise is characterized by movement and energy expenditure, but exercise differs from activity in that it results in an overall conditioning of the body when performed on a regular basis. This section of the chapter focuses on the physiologic and psychosocial responses to activity, specifically the effects of exercise and increased workload on the body.

There is increasing interest in the preventative and therapeutic effects of exercise. A regular program of exercise is recommended as a means of maintaining weight control and cardiovascular fitness. The athletically fit person has more reserves to call on when he or she becomes ill. Exercise is becoming recognized as an integral part of the treatment regimen for many diseases. It is recommended as a means of lowering low-density lipoproteins and increasing high-density lipoproteins in persons with hyperlipidemia, in improving the regulation of blood glucose in persons with diabetes, and in improving activity tolerance in persons with cardiac and respiratory diseases. Regular exercise also has psychological benefits. Exercise training can improve self-esteem, remedy depressive moods, and enhance the quality of life.

Activity Tolerance and Work Performance

There are two main types of exercise: aerobic and isometric. Aerobic exercise involves the use of oxygen for transforming substrates such as glucose, fatty acids, and amino acids into energy. Aerobic exercise training results in muscles that use oxygen more efficiently such that the body can do more work with less cardiac and respiratory effort. Isometric exercise involves activities such as weight lifting or movement against resistance. It is used to improve overall muscle strength and tone. Whereas aerobic activities involve a change in muscle length such as occurs with walking and running, with isometric exercise, the muscle fibers exert work while remaining the same length. Most exercise programs use a combination of aerobic and isometric activities.

Physiologic Responses

Physical activity or exercise involves four major components: cardiopulmonary fitness; muscle strength, flexibility, and endurance; availability of energy substrates to meet the increased energy demands imposed by increased physical activity; and motivation and mental endurance.

Cardiopulmonary Responses. The cardiopulmonary responses, which include the circulatory functions of the heart and blood vessels and the gas exchange functions of the respiratory system, work to supply oxygen and energy substrates to the working muscle groups and exchange oxygen and carbon dioxide with the atmosphere. Aerobic or cardiopulmonary exercise involves repetitive and rhythmic movements; it uses large muscle groups and results in the body's ability to perform vigorous exercise for an extended period. Exercise places a major stress on the cardiovascular system and causes various physiologic responses.[1,2]

The principal factor that determines how long and effectively a person is able to exercise is determined by the capacity of the heart, lungs, and circulation to deliver oxygen to the working muscles. The term *maximal oxygen consumption* ($\dot{V}O_2max$) represents this principle. $\dot{V}O_2max$ is determined by the rate at which oxygen is delivered to the working muscles, the oxygen-carrying capacity of the blood, and the amount of oxygen extracted from the blood by the working muscles. It is measured as the volume of oxygen consumed, usually measured in liters or milliliters per unit time (*i.e.*, liters/minute). The $\dot{V}O_2max$ is an important determinant of the person's capacity to perform work and can increase up to 22-fold with strenuous exercise.[3]

As the cardiovascular system responds to increased activity and exercise, the heart rate, the amount of blood that the heart pumps with each beat (*i.e.*, stroke volume), and arterial blood pressure increase. The increase in heart rate is mediated through neural, hormonal, and intrinsic cardiovascular mechanisms. With anticipation of exercise, the vasomotor center of the brain is stimulated to initiate a mass discharge of sympathetic activity along with a concomitant inhibition of parasympathetic mechanisms. Stimulation of the sympathetic nervous system causes the release of the sympathetic neurotransmitters, norepinephrine and epinephrine. These transmitters produce an increase in heart rate and contractility. At the start of exercise, the heart rate rises immediately and continues to increase until a plateau is reached. This plateau, or steady-state heart rate, is maintained until the exercise or activity is terminated. Also contributing to the increased heart rate are intrinsic mechanisms in the heart. During exercise, increased blood return to the heart stimulates right atrial stretch receptors that serve to increase the heart rate. Release of epinephrine and norepinephrine from the adrenal glands helps to sustain the increased heart rate.[1,2,4]

During exercise, the cardiac output may increase from a resting level of 4 to 8 L/minute to as high as 15 L/minute for women and as high as 22 L/minute for men. The increase in cardiac output results from an increase in heart rate and stroke volume. One factor that is thought to contribute to the cardiac output is the stimulation of the heart muscle by norepinephrine and epinephrine. These neurotransmitters cause the heart to beat faster and more forcefully. Another factor that contributes to the increased cardiac output is the stretching of the myocardial fibers by increased venous return. The increased stretch of the myocardial fibers results in a more forceful contraction and a more complete emptying of the ventricles with each beat, a response called the *Frank-Starling mechanisms* (see Chapter 16).[2,4]

With the onset of exercise, the systolic blood pressure rises, reflecting the increased cardiac output and larger stroke volume being ejected from the heart. The diastolic blood pressure changes little during exercise. This is believed to be related to the peripheral vasodilatation that occurs because of the metabolic waste products that accumulate during exercise. The increased systolic pressure and the fact that the diastolic blood pressure does not change results in an increase in pulse pressure and mean arterial pressure. The increase in mean arterial pressure is necessary so that organ systems of high priority can continue to be perfused.[1,2,4]

The respiratory system has the role of exchanging oxygen and carbon dioxide. During exercise, the respiratory system must increase the rate of gas exchange. This takes place through a series of physiologic responses. With the increase in cardiac output, a greater volume of blood under slightly increased pressure is delivered to the pulmonary vessels in the lungs. This results in opening of additional pulmonary capillary beds, producing better alveolar perfusion and a more efficient exchange of oxygen and carbon dioxide.[2]

In addition to pulmonary perfusion being enhanced during exercise, pulmonary ventilation is also increased. The respiratory rate and tidal volume increase, resulting in an increase in minute ventilation. This response is controlled by chemoreceptors, located in the medulla and aorta and carotid arteries, that monitor blood gases and pH. During exercise, decreases in blood oxygen and pH and increases in carbon dioxide stimulate an increase in the rate and depth of respiration.[5]

Neuromuscular Responses. The integration of the neurologic and musculoskeletal systems is essential for the body to have movement and participate in activity. To initiate and sustain increased activity, muscle strength, flexibility, and endurance are needed. *Muscle strength* is defined as the ability of muscle groups to produce force against resistance. *Flexibility* involves the range of movement of joints; whereas, muscle *endurance* refers to the ability of the body or muscle groups to perform increased activity for an extended period.

Skeletal muscles are adapted by heredity and activity for the type of work they predominately perform. Skeletal muscle consists of two types of muscle fibers: slow-twitch (type I) and fast-twitch (type II) muscle fibers. Major muscle groups are classified according to how fast a muscle contraction is produced in response to an electrical stimulus. Each muscle group is characterized as type I or type II muscle.

The slow-twitch fibers, which are smaller than the fast-twitch fibers, tend to produce less overall force but are more energy efficient than the fast-twitch fibers. They are better suited biochemically to perform lower-intensity work for prolonged periods of time. These fibers have a high oxidative capacity as a result of high concentrations of mitochondria and myoglobin. Slow-twitch fibers predominate in the large muscle groups such as the leg muscles and therefore play a major role in sustaining activity during prolonged exercise or endurance activities. During periods of sustained inactivity, such as prolonged immobility or bed rest, it is the slow-twitch fibers that are primarily affected and quickly deconditioned.[3,4]

In contrast to slow-twitch fibers, fast-twitch fibers are larger and better suited for high intensity work, but fatigue more easily. These fibers have high myosin adenosine triphosphatase (ATPase) activity, few mitochondria, low myoglobin concentration, and high glycolytic capacity, resulting in the need to depend on anaerobic metabolism to supply ATP for energy. Fast-twitch muscle fibers are most common in smaller muscle groups, such as those found in the arms and eye. Fast-twitch fibers predominate during activities in which short bursts of intense energy are required, such as sprinting or weight-lifting activities. Anabolic steroids enhance fast-twitch fiber activity.[3,4]

During aerobic activity, working muscles use oxygen 10 to 20 times faster than nonworking muscles. This increased oxygen demand is met by an increase in cardiac output and an increase in muscle blood flow. At rest, skeletal muscles receive 15% to 20% of the cardiac output, compared with the 85% to 95% that they receive during aerobic activities. This increased blood flow, which does not begin at the onset of exercise, is achieved through two mechanisms: dilation of blood vessels in working muscles and constriction of blood vessels in organs of low priority.[4]

Dilation of blood vessels in the working muscles is a result of increased blood flow to the muscles and increased venous return from the working muscles. Increased blood flow to working muscles is achieved by relaxation of the arterioles and the precapillary sphincters. Chemical changes such as decreased oxygen and pH and increased levels of potassium, adenosine, carbon dioxide, and phosphate also contribute to the local control of muscle blood flow during prolonged exercise and during recovery from exercise.[1] Increased venous flow is enhanced by the alternate contraction and relaxation of working muscles.

The second mechanism that increases blood flow to the working muscles is the diversion of blood from the visceral organs. The amount of blood diverted from the visceral organs is proportional to the level of exercise, and as exercise is increased, more blood is diverted to working muscles. This redistribution of blood flow results from selective vasoconstriction within organs such as the kidneys and gastrointestinal structures, which are less active than the working muscles.[1]

Skeletal muscles hypertrophy and undergo other anatomic changes in response to exercise training. "Trained muscles" have an increased number of capillaries and enhanced permeability of capillaries that surround each muscle fiber. Trained skeletal muscles are able to use oxygen more efficiently, probably because of enhanced enzymatic activity that increases oxidative capacity. Mitochondria appear to adapt by increasing the transport of oxygen and other substances to the inner regions of the muscle fiber for more efficient use of oxygen.[1,6]

Metabolic and Thermal Responses. To perform physical activities, the body requires increased energy sources. Energy is obtained from creatine phosphate (a stored form of muscle energy), glucose, glycogen, and fatty acids. As the activity begins, especially aerobic activity, the body uses its energy sources in a characteristic pattern. The first sources to be used are stored ATP, creatine phosphate, and muscle glycogen. These energy sources are used for short, intense periods of activity of 1 to 2 minutes. These fuels are used for energy through anaerobic metabolism.[7] If the activity is to be performed for a period of 3 to 40 minutes, muscle glycogen and creatine phosphate are used to meet the energy requirements through both anaerobic and aerobic metabolism. For intense, prolonged periods of activity that last more than 40 minutes, aerobic metabolism is essential. Muscle glycogen, glucose, and fatty acids are used for energy sources during prolonged activity.[3]

In order to supply the energy needed for increased activity, the person must consume a balanced diet that is high in carbohydrate. General recommendations for a balanced diet include 55% carbohydrate sources, 30% fat sources (mainly polyunsaturated fats), and 15% protein. Although proteins are not used as energy sources during increased activity, they have an essential role in the building and rebuilding of tissues and organs. During increased activity and exercise, it is essential that the person maintain adequate hydration. Increased activity can result in loss of fluids from the vascular compartment. If allowed to progress, the person may experience severe dehydration that may lead to vascular collapse. Before and during vigorous activity, a person should replenish body fluids with water and electrolyte solutions.

Under normal resting conditions, the body is able to maintain its temperature within a set range. It does this by way of two mechanisms. The first mechanism used by the body to regulate temperature is to change blood flow to the skin. When the blood vessels of the skin dilate, warm blood is shunted from the core tissues of the body to the skin surface, where heat is more easily lost to the surrounding environment. The second mechanism by which the body loses heat is through sweating. The evaporation of sweat from the skin surface contributes to the loss of heat from the body. Depending on training level and environmental conditions, the body may have difficulty regulating its temperature during vigorous exercise.[8] With sufficient training, the body adapts by increasing the rate of sweat production. Temperature regulation improves with training, and the trained person begins to sweat sooner, often within 1 to 2 minutes of the start of exercise. Sweat production begins even before the core temperature rises, and a cooling effect is initiated soon after the start of exercise; the sweat produced is more dilute than sweat produced by a nontrained person. Sweat normally contains large amounts of sodium chloride; production of a dilute sweat allows evaporative cooling to take place while sodium chloride is conserved.

During exercise, plasma proteins are shifted so that there is an increase in the amount of proteins in the blood. These proteins exert an osmotic gradient effect that draws fluid from the interstitial space into the vascular compartment. This contributes to an increase in the vascular volume that can be delivered to the working muscles and contributes to more efficient heat dissipation.[9]

Gastrointestinal Function. The gastrointestinal system is affected by intense physical activity. During increased physical activity, blood is shunted away from the gastrointestinal tract toward the active skeletal muscles. Gastrointestinal motility, secretory activity, and absorption are decreased. This can result in the person experiencing reflux, vomiting, bloating, and stomach pain. Other symptoms that the person may experience include cramping, an urge to defecate, and diarrhea.[10]

Hemostasis and Immune Function. Increased physical activity affects both hemostasis and the immune system. Increased epinephrine levels stimulate increased fibrinolytic activity. Platelet function is enhanced with regular exercise. This results in increased fibrinolytic activity that is counterbalanced by coagulative activity.[11]

The immune system is affected by acute periods of exercise, with the response depending on the intensity and duration of exercise. High-intensity endurance exercise is associated with a biphasic change in the circulating leukocyte count. Immediately after exercise, there is a 50% to 100% increase in leukocyte count, demonstrated as increases in lymphocytes and neutrophils. Within 30 minutes after the exercise period, the lymphocyte count decreases by 30% to 50% of preexercise levels. Moderate-intensity exercise is associated with leukocytosis, lymphocytosis, neutrophilia, and lymphocytopenia.[12] The transient changes in the immune system after periods of exercise are thought to be related to increased levels of catecholamines and cortisol.[13]

Psychological Responses

There is a mental component to the performance of increased activity and exercise. The mental aspect entails the motivation to initiate an activity or exercise program and the dedication to incorporate the regimen into one's lifestyle. Positive effects of regularly performed exercise include increased energy and motivation, positive self-image and self-esteem, decreased anxiety, better management of life stresses, and increased perceived locus of control.

Assessment of Activity Tolerance

The assessment of a person's ability to tolerate exercise and perform work can be conducted in several ways. One method is to administer a paper and pencil test that enables persons to describe their normal activities, their perceived level of activity tolerance, or their level of fatigue. One example of a paper and pencil test is the Human Activity Profile (HAP).[14] The HAP was originally developed to assess the quality of life for persons participating in a rehabilitation program for chronic obstructive pulmonary disease. After investigating numerous physiologic and psychological measures, it was found that the most important aspect of quality of life was the amount of daily activity the person was able to perform. The HAP consists of 94 items that represent common activities that require known amounts of energy expenditure. The person marks each item based on whether he or she is still able to perform the activity or has stopped performing the activity.

Another paper and pencil test is the Fatigue Severity Scale (Chart 55–1).[15] This tool consists of nine state-

CHART **55-1**
*Fatigue Severity Scale**

1. My motivation is lower when I am fatigued.
2. Exercise brings on my fatigue.
3. I am easily fatigued.
4. Fatigue interferes with my physical functioning.
5. Fatigue causes frequent problems for me.
6. My fatigue prevents sustained physical functioning.
7. Fatigue interferes with carrying out certain duties and responsibilities.
8. Fatigue is among my three disabling symptoms.
9. Fatigue interferes with my work, family, or social life.

*Patients are instructed to choose a number from 1 to 7 that indicates their degree of agreement with each statement; 1 indicates strongly disagree, and 7 indicates strongly agree.
(Krupp L.B., LaRocca N.G., Muire-Nash J., Steinberg A.D. [1989]. The fatigue severity scale: Application to patients with multiple sclerosis and systemic lupus erythematosus. *Archives of Neurology 46*, 1122)

ments that describe symptoms of fatigue. Persons are instructed to choose a number from 1 to 7 that best indicates their agreement with each statement. The tool is brief, easy to administer, and easily interpreted. Paper and pencil tests provide an objective way to assess a person's activity tolerance.

Another method used to assess activity tolerance is ergometry. Ergometry is a procedure for determining physical performance capacity. The ergometer is a specific tool that imposes a constant level of work. A specified workload, expressed in terms of watts or joules per second, is imposed while the person performs the task. During the performance of the work, the person's physiologic status is monitored, as is his or her subjective assessment of the work.[16]

Two examples of ergometers include the bicycle ergometer and the treadmill ergometer. A bicycle ergometer is a stationary bicycle that has a friction belt attached. The front wheel of the bicycle is rotated, and the braking force of the belt can be adjusted to alter the workload. A treadmill ergometer is more frequently used to assess workload performance, especially cardiac function. During treadmill testing, the person walks or runs on a moving belt. The workload can be altered by changing the speed and incline of the treadmill. This change is usually done in predetermined stages. During treadmill testing, the electrocardiogram (ECG) is monitored continuously, and the blood pressure is checked intermittently. Usually, the person being tested continues to exercise, completing successive stages of the test, until exhaustion or a predetermined heart rate or maximal heart rate is reached.[16]

Maximal heart rate is estimated by age. Tables of maximal heart rate by age are available, but as a general rule, the predicted maximal heart rate can be estimated by subtracting the age from 220 (*e.g.*, the target heart rate for a 40-year-old person would be 180 beats/minute). The person may continue to exercise until the predicted maximal heart rate is achieved or until a percentage (*i.e.*, 85% to 90%) of the predicted maximal rate is reached.[16]

Metabolic equivalents (METs) are commonly used to express workload at various stages of work. One MET is equivalent to the energy expended in a resting position. METs are multiples of the basal metabolic rate, and as the type of activity performed (*i.e.*, walking, running) is changed, the MET requirement also changes. For example, walking at 4 miles per hour (mph), cycling at 11 mph, playing tennis (singles), or doing carpentry requires 5 to 6 METs. Running 6 mph requires 10 METs, and running 10 mph requires 17 METs. Physically trained persons are able to achieve workloads beyond 16 METs. Healthy sedentary persons are seldom able to exercise beyond 10 or 11 METs. In persons with coronary artery disease, workloads of 8 METs often produce angina.[17]

During exercise stress testing, persons often are asked to rate their subjective feelings of the exercise experience. A commonly used tool to measure the person's feelings of the amount of work being performed is the Borg Rating of Perceived Exertion (RPE) Scale.[18] The RPE Scale is based on research that correlates heart rate to feelings of perceived exertion. The scale values range from 6 through 20. As the person is performing the exercise, he or she is asked to select a number that best corresponds to his or her feelings of exertion for the work being performed. The numbers and expressions describing perceived levels of exertion are often posted on the wall where the exercise is being performed. Number 7 represents very, very light exertion; number 9, very light exertion; number 11, fairly light exertion; number 13, somewhat hard exertion; number 15, hard exertion; number 17, very hard exertion; and number 19, very, very hard exertion.[18] The numeric values on the RPE Scale increase linearly with workload, and the total scale reflects a 10-fold increase in heart rate. As the person begins to exercise, he or she is asked to rate the intensity of the work being performed. The person selects a number from the RPE Scale, and this number should approximate the heart rate when that number is multiplied by 10 (*e.g.*, if the person rates the exercise experience as a 7, the heart rate should be 70 beats/minute).

A newer category scale with ratio properties has been developed. The numbers on this scale range from 0 to 10, with 0 representing nothing at all; 0.5, very, very weak; and 10, very, very strong. With this method, the expressions and the numbers they represent are placed in the correct position for a ratio scale. For example, because 1 represents very weak, 0.5 represents very, very weak, or one half of that intensity.[19]

Activity Intolerance and Fatigue

Activity intolerance can be defined as "a state in which a person has insufficient physical or psychological energy to endure or complete required or desired daily activity."[20,21] How frequently, intensely, and long persons are able to carry out their activities depends on a balance between available energy sources (*i.e.*, oxygen and energy substrates) and the energy that is required to complete the desired task. Factors that influence this balance of energy include overall physical condition (*e.g.*, level of fatigue, deconditioning, disease, and pain), psychosocial factors (*e.g.*, depression and anxiety), and lifestyle factors (*e.g.*, obesity, smoking, lack of regular exercise).[21] This section of the chapter focuses on acute fatigue and the chronic fatigue syndrome.

Mechanisms of Fatigue

Fatigue is a state that is experienced by everyone at some time. Fatigue can be physical, as in the case of extreme exercise by healthy persons, or it can be a normal symptom that is experienced by persons with limited exercise reserve, such as persons with impaired cardiorespiratory function, anemia, malnutrition, or those on certain types of drug therapy. Fatigue may also be related to a lack of sleep or mental stress. Like dyspnea and pain, fatigue is a subjective symptom. Fatigue is often described as a subjective feeling of tiredness that varies in terms of pleasantness, intensity, and duration and is often influenced by the time of day and a person's biorhythms.[22] It is different from the normal tiredness that most persons experience at the end of the day. Tiredness is relieved by a good night's sleep, but fatigue persists despite sufficient or adequate sleep. Fatigue is one of the most common symptoms reported to physicians, but it is one of the least understood health care problems.

Fatigue is often categorized as central or peripheral. Central fatigue is fatigue that has its origin in the central nervous system (CNS). It refers to the perception of effort or impairments in the central processing of somatic or physiologic stimuli originating in working muscles. Peripheral fatigue refers to the exhaustion of muscles during exertion and occurs because of impairments that are located in the contracting muscles and peripheral nerves. If a healthy person is fatigued during exercise, he or she may be able to force or push themselves to complete the necessary tasks or exercise. In contrast, a weak person cannot perform the necessary activity.[23]

According to Piper,[22,24] fatigue may be related to two major types of stressors: situational and developmental. Situational stressors are situation specific and can be associated with five factors: the environment (*e.g.*, excessive noise, temperature extremes, changes in weather); drug-related incidents (*e.g.*, use of tranquilizers, alcohol, toxic chemical exposure); treatment-related therapies (*e.g.*, chemotherapy, radiation therapy, surgery, anesthesia, diagnostic testing); physical exertion (*e.g.*, exercise); and nonphysical exertion (*e.g.*, monotony). Developmental stressors are associated with physical factors related to a disease process and emotional factors.

The factors contributing to fatigue are numerous and interrelated, making assessment complex and identification difficult. This is also true of the physiologic explanation of fatigue. For example, fatigue that is related to mental factors or emotional stress is often attributed to the function of the reticular activating system (RAS). The RAS, which is located in the reticular formation of the pons and midbrain, is responsible for maintaining wakefulness. A feedback system between the RAS and the cerebral cortex exists. Stimulation of this system results in wakefulness; conversely, inhibition results in fatigue.[22]

Acute Physical Fatigue

Acute fatigue has a rapid onset, is perceived to be a normal response to the activity being performed, has a short duration in which the fatigue is relieved when the activity ceases, and serves as a protective mechanism. Although acute physical fatigue can develop when insufficient oxygen or nutrients are delivered to the muscle, for the purpose of this chapter, *acute fatigue* is defined as muscle fatigue associated with increased activity or exercise that is carried out to the point of exhaustion.

Physical conditioning can influence the onset of acute fatigue. Persons who engage in regular exercise are able to perform an activity for longer periods before acute fatigue develops than sedentary persons. They are probably able to do so because their muscles use oxygen and nutrients more efficiently and because their circulatory and respiratory systems are better able to deliver oxygen and nutrients to the exercising muscles.[3]

Acute physical fatigue occurs more rapidly in deconditioned muscle. For example, acute fatigue is often seen in persons who have been on bed rest because of a surgical procedure or in persons who have had their activity curtailed because of chronic illnesses such as heart and respiratory diseases. In such cases, the acute fatigue is often out of proportion to the activity that is being performed (*e.g.*, dangling at the bedside, sitting in a chair for the first time). When resuming activity for the first time after a prolonged period of bed rest or inactivity, the person may experience tachycardia and hypotension that is greater than was expected because of the period of inactivity. Unless these parameters are changed by medications such as β-adrenergic blocking drugs, heart rate and blood pressure become particularly sensitive indicators of activity tolerance or intolerance.

Persons who require the use of assistive devices also experience acute physical fatigue. This is true of persons in wheelchairs and those using assistive devices after losing a limb. The upper arm muscles are less well adapted to prolonged exercise than the leg muscles, because arm muscles are primarily composed of type II muscle fibers, which are best suited for short bursts of activity and fatigue quickly. Persons who use wheelchairs or a pair of crutches may quickly experience fatigue until their arms become conditioned to the increased activity.

Chronic Fatigue

A second type of activity intolerance is chronic fatigue. Chronic fatigue differs from acute fatigue in terms of onset, intensity, perception, duration, and relief. In contrast to acute fatigue, chronic fatigue has a more gradual and insidious onset, is typically perceived as being unusually intense for the amount of activity performed, lasts longer than 1 month, and is not relieved by cessation of activity. Although acute fatigue often serves a protective function, chronic fatigue is not protective. Chronic fatigue may even lead to aversion of activity and be accompanied by a desire to escape certain activities. Many diseases and chronic health conditions cause persons to experience chronic fatigue. When associated with a specific disease, there often exists a physiologic basis for the fatigue. When the physiologic problem is corrected, the fatigue may be relieved.[22,24]

Chronic fatigue is one of the more common problems experienced by persons with chronic health problems (Table 55–1). It limits the amount of activity that a person can perform and may interfere with employment, the performance of activities of daily living, and the quality of life in general. Although fatigue is often viewed as a symptom of anxiety and depression, it is important to recognize that these psychological manifestations may be a symptom of the fatigue. For example, persons with persistent fatigue from a chronic illness may have to curtail their work schedules, decrease social activities, and limit their usual family responsibilities. These lifestyle changes may be the reasons for the depression rather than the depression being a cause of the fatigue.

Chronic fatigue is a common problem in persons with cancer, particularly persons who are undergoing chemotherapy or radiation therapy. Studies involving patients receiving chemotherapy for a variety of different types of cancers report incidences of fatigue ranging from 59% to 82%.[25] In all of these studies, fatigue was the most common and distressing side effect of the treatment. Among persons receiving radiation therapy, the incidence of fatigue ranged from 65% to 100% and was rated as the most severe effect of the treatment, especially during the last week of the treatment.[25] A possible explanation for the fatigue that occurs in persons with cancer involves a chemical mediator called tumor necrosis factor (TNF). TNF is secreted by activated macro-

TABLE 55–1

Chronic Illnesses and Causes of Chronic Fatigue

Chronic Illness	Cause of Fatigue
Acquired immunodeficiency syndrome	Impaired immune function, anorexia, muscle weakness, and psychosocial factors associated with the disease
Anemia	Decreased oxygen-carrying capacity of blood
Arthritis	Pain and joint dysfunction leads to impaired mobility, loss of sleep, and emotional factors
Cancer	Presence of chemical products and catabolic processes associated with tumor growth; anorexia and difficulty eating; effects of chemotherapy and radiation therapy; and psychosocial factors such as depression, grieving, hopelessness, and fear
Cardiac disease	
Myocardial infarction	Death of myocardial tissue results in decreased cardiac output, poor tissue perfusion, and impaired delivery of oxygen and nutrients to vital organs
Congestive heart failure	Impaired pumping ability of the heart results in poor perfusion of muscle tissue and vital organs
Neurologic disorders	
Multiple sclerosis	Demyelinating disease of CNS characterized by slowing of nerve conduction, resulting in lower extremity weakness and fatigue
Myasthenia gravis	Disorder of postsynaptic acetylcholine receptors of the myoneural junction, resulting in muscle weakness and fatigue
Chronic lung disease	Increased work of breathing and impaired gas exchange
Chronic renal failure	Accumulation of metabolic wastes; fluid, electrolyte, and acid-base disorders; decreased red blood cell count and oxygen-carrying capacity due to impaired erythropoietin production
Metabolic disorders	
Hypothyroidism	Decrease in basal metabolic rate manifested by fatigue
Diabetes mellitus	Impaired cellular use of glucose by muscle cells
Obesity	Imbalance in nutritional intake and energy expenditure; increased workload due to excess weight
Steroid myopathy	Glucocorticosteroids interfere with protein and glycogen synthesis, which leads to muscle wasting

phages, some tumor cells, and some T lymphocytes (see Chapter 11). It causes depletion of the protein stores of skeletal muscle. As a result, muscle wasting occurs, and persons have to expend more energy to perform simple activities such as sitting and standing.[26]

Chronic Fatigue Syndrome

Chronic fatigue syndrome (CFS) is an illness that can affect the entire body. It is described as disabling fatigue of at least 6 months' duration that is often preceded by flulike symptoms. CFS is the chief complaint of 10% to 34% of patients seen in primary care clinics.[27,28] Reports of CFS have emerged from the United States, Canada, Australia, Europe, and Asia.

In the United States, CFS first came to prominence in 1985 at Lake Tahoe, Nevada. At the Incline Village resort, approximately 200 residents (1% of the population) reported a mononucleosis-like illness to their primary care physicians. The physicians examining these patients were aware of the medical literature that described the possible association of the Epstein-Barr virus (EBV) with chronic mononucleosis. Because such a large number of the population reported the same symptoms, the Centers for Disease Control and Prevention (CDC) was asked to investigate the "epidemic." The CDC declared that this reported epidemic resulted from the attitude or activity of the physician in the area and discounted the link between EBV infection and the chronic fatigue syndrome. This incident brought national prominence to CFS and caused other persons with similar complaints to organize and request that this syndrome be further investigated.[29]

Definition. CFS may be described as a disorder that lasts 6 months or longer and is characterized by profound fatigue and by disorders of higher cerebral functioning. Other common descriptions include a state of abnormal exhaustion that follows normal activities; a decrease in energy for tasks that require sustained attention; and a global disturbance in the ability to act.[27] In 1988, a working case definition for CFS was developed by the CDC. This definition describes CFS as a complex syndrome of debilitating fatigue that is often accompanied by various other complaints, including sore throat, lymph node pain and tenderness, headache, myalgia, and arthralgia.[30]

Figure 55–1 outlines the criteria for diagnosis of CFS.[31] For a case definition of CFS to be made, criteria 1 and 2 must be present, along with six or more symptoms criteria and two or more physical criteria or eight or more of the symptoms criteria. All symptoms must be present for at least 6 months.[32]

Pathophysiology of Chronic Fatigue Syndrome. Despite much research and the development of several theories, the pathophysiology of CFS is unknown. It is known that the fatigue experienced in CFS is similar to the fatigue associated with therapeutic doses of interferon-α, suggesting a possible link to an underlying viral infection. Most theories have identified infectious agents such as EBV, human herpesvirus 6, enterovirus, human retrovirus, *Mycobacterium tuberculosis, Borrelia burgdorferi, Brucella,* and *Candida* as associated with the syndrome. However, none of these agents has conclu-

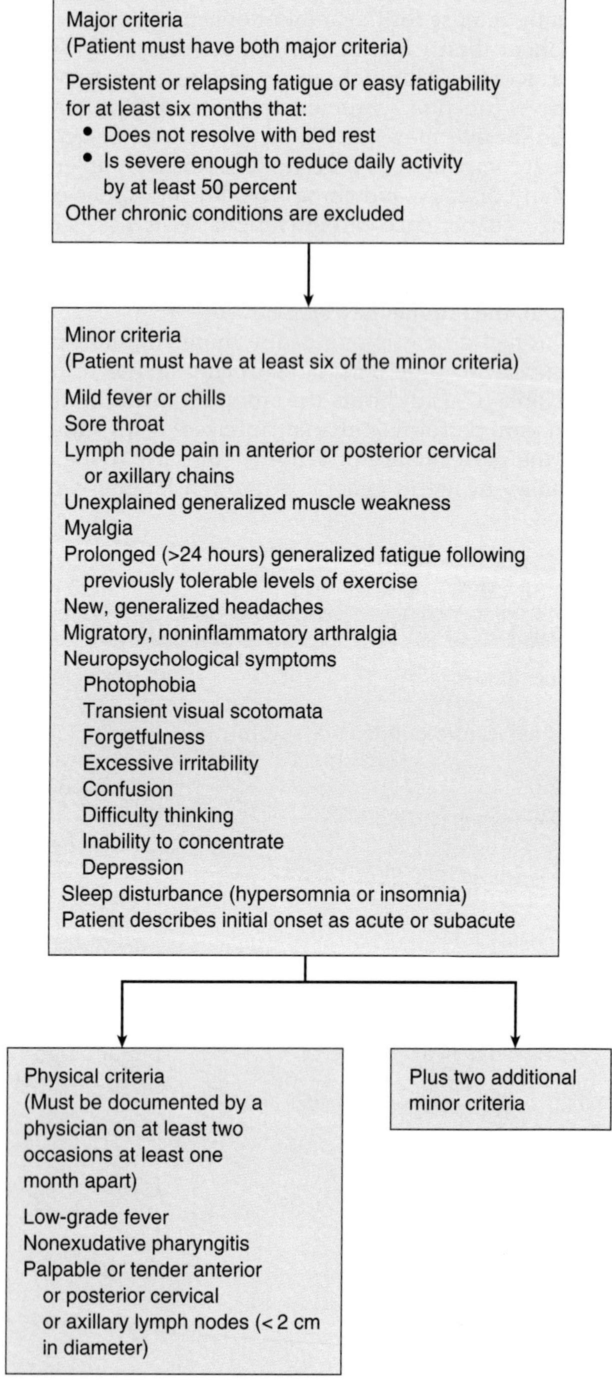

Figure 55–1
Criteria for chronic fatigue syndrome. To meet the diagnosis of chronic fatigue syndrome, the patient must have two major criteria plus eight minor criteria (for a total of 10) or two major criteria plus six minor criteria plus two physical criteria (for a total of 10). (Developed from Holmes G.P. Defining the chronic fatigue syndrome. *Reviews of Infectious Disease* 13 (Suppl. 1), S53–55)

sively been associated with the development of CFS. Associated with CFS are neuropsychologic factors and a primary immunodysregulatory phenomenon. Other theories of CFS pathogenesis identify a genetic predisposition, dysfunction in the hypothalamus-pituitary-adrenal axis, and an as yet unidentified infectious organism.[31,32] The association between psychological disorders, especially anxiety and depression, and CFS is difficult to evaluate.[33] There is considerable overlap between psychological disorders and the reactive depression of CFS. Persons with CFS have an increased occurrence and lifetime prevalence of depression that is greater than the depression associated with other chronic diseases. In 40% to 50% of the cases of CFS, depression preceded the development of CFS.[34]

A number of immunologic abnormalities have been described in persons with CFS.[31] It is hypothesized that the immune system may overreact to an environmental agent (most likely an infectious agent) or internal stimuli and be unable to self-regulate after the infectious insult is over. Another possibility is that a viral infection may produce continued suppression of the immune system. Mononuclear cells from persons with CFS have a decreased response to antigenic stimulation and proliferate at one half of the normal rate. A deficiency in natural killer cells has been proposed to explain many of these abnormalities. These lymphocytes participate in the transfer of delayed hypersensitivity and the production of interleukin-2 and interferon-γ.[31,34]

Manifestations. One of the most important findings is the person's subjective complaint of fatigue. The person reports feeling well one day and experiencing an insidious onset of overwhelming fatigue the next day. Often, the symptom of fatigue is preceded by a cold or flulike illness. Frequently, the person describes the illness as recurring. With each subsequent episode of the illness, the fatigue increases.

Physical assessment findings include low-grade fever. The fever is intermittent and occurs only when the illness recurs. Other assessment findings include nonexudative pharyngitis, palpable and tender cervical lymph nodes, a mildly enlarged thyroid gland, wheezing, splenomegaly, myalgias, arthralgias, and heme-positive stool with subsequent negative sigmoidoscopies.

Psychological problems include impaired cognition that the person describes as an inability to concentrate and to perform previously mundane tasks. Mood and sleep disturbances, balance problems, visual disturbances, and various degrees of anxiety and depression are reported. The presence of depression in approximately 50% of the cases of CFS has generated much discussion regarding whether depression is a cause of CFS or a comorbid condition.[29,31,35]

Before making the diagnosis of CFS, laboratory values to monitor include a complete blood count; serum levels of electrolytes, glucose, calcium, phosphorus, and total protein; Lyme disease titers, and renal, liver, and thyroid function tests, along with a urinalysis and stool guaiac analysis. Laboratory and other diagnostic test results often demonstrate minor abnormalities, although not of sufficient magnitude to be reflective of the degree of fatigue present. Common laboratory abnormalities include atypical lymphocytosis, mild anemia, elevation of the sedimentation rate, decreased serum phosphorus, iron deficiency, and elevated liver function tests. Chest radiographs are normal.[30]

The diagnosis of CFS is made by the physician integrating the entire clinical picture of the patient's symptoms, physical assessment findings, laboratory results, and any other diagnostic test results. The patient's symptoms must be present for at least 6 months. In some cases, the symptoms have been present for as long as 1 to 2 years before the diagnosis of CFS is made. CFS is often a diagnosis of exclusion. The physician must first exclude any infectious processes and psychological diagnoses.

Treatment. The treatment of CFS tends to be nonspecific. It centers on patient education, emotional support, treatment of symptoms, and overall management of general health. During the diagnostic workup, persons need to be supported and reassured that their symptoms are real. Local and national support groups are available for persons who experience CFS.

Symptom treatment consists of developing an exercise program that helps the person regain strength. Persons with CFS have a decreased aerobic capacity. An activity program that gradually increases in intensity is recommended. Initially, the activity program should be short—3 to 5 minutes—and gradually increased in intensity by 20% every 2 to 3 weeks.[32,33] Along with a structured activity program, persons should be encouraged to be as active as possible as they resume their activities of daily living.

Nutritional support is important. A low-fat, low-to-moderate protein, high–complex-carbohydrate diet is recommended along with a multivitamin and multimineral supplement. For overweight persons, weight loss is recommended. Alcohol should be avoided, because it exacerbates the symptoms of CFS.[35]

Analgesics and antiinflammatory nonsteroidal medications are beneficial in treating the symptoms of myalgia and arthralgia. Antidepressants may be used to treat symptoms of depression, but the medication should not be used in isolation, and appropriate supportive treatment and counseling should be provided to the person.[34]

A holistic approach to the treatment of CFS is essential. With proper treatment and support, most persons with CFS demonstrate improvement.[34] Relapses can occur. Persons diagnosed with CFS must continue to receive follow-up care and treatment on a regular basis.

In summary, the response of the body to increased activity and exercise assumes that a healthy, normal person is performing the increased activity. In disease states, especially diseases of the cardiovascular, pulmonary, or musculoskeletal systems, the body's response to increased activity is compromised. The normal physiologic responses cannot be elicited. When a person experiences disease, activities of daily living and an exercise regimen must be adapted to the physiologic limitations.

The body reacts to the increased activity of exercise by a series of physiologic responses that increase its level of performance. Heart rate, cardiac output, and stroke volume increase to deliver more blood to working muscles. Minute ventilation and diffusion of oxygen and carbon dioxide increase to provide oxygen more efficiently to meet the rising metabolic demands. Local changes in the arterioles and capillaries contribute to enhanced perfusion of the working muscles. Over time and with training, temperature regulation is altered so the body is able to perform activity without increasing its core temperature. Activity tolerance is assessed by use of paper and pencil tests or with bicycle or treadmill ergometry. Persons are required to perform a prescribed amount of work. While performing this work, they are monitored for their cardiovascular response and their subjective feelings of exertion for the specified amount of work being performed.

Fatigue is a nonspecific, self-recognized state of physical and psychological exhaustion. It results in the person not being able to perform routine activities, and it is not relieved with sleep or rest. Acute fatigue results from excessive use of the body or a specific muscle group and is often related to depletion of energy sources. Chronic fatigue is often associated with a specific disease or chronic illness and may be relieved when the effects of the disease are corrected. CFS is a complex illness that has physiologic and psychological manifestations. It is characterized by debilitating fatigue. The diagnosis is often made by a process of elimination, and treatment requires a holistic approach.

Bed Rest and Immobility

After you have completed this section of the chapter, you should be able to meet the following objectives:

- Describe the effects of gravity on the body
- Describe the effects of immobility and prolonged bed rest on the cardiovascular, pulmonary, renal, musculoskeletal, metabolic, and gastrointestinal systems
- Discuss changes in fluid and electrolyte balance associated with immobility and prolonged bed rest
- Identify alterations in serum electrolyte and hematologic values that are related to immobility and prolonged bed rest
- Discuss changes in sensory perception that are consequences of immobility and prolonged bed rest
- Identify alterations in physical assessment findings that are related to the effects of immobility and prolonged bed rest
- Describe treatment interventions that counteract the negative effects of immobility and prolonged bed rest

Immobility and bed rest are two common forms of inactivity. Immobility may be dictated by injury that requires stabilization to facilitate the healing process, or it may result from conditions that limit physical reserve. The effects of immobility can be restricted to a single extremity that is encased in a plaster cast; involve both legs, as in a person confined to a wheelchair; or involve the entire body, as in a person confined to bed rest. Bed rest and immobility are associated with various complications that include generalized weakness, orthostatic intolerance, atelectasis, pneumonia, pulmonary emboli, thrombophlebitis, muscle atrophy, osteoporosis, urinary retention, constipation, and impairment in sensory perception (Table 55–2). This section of the chapter describes the physiologic changes that occur with bed rest and immobility and treatment interventions to counteract their effects.

Bed rest is one of the oldest and most commonly used methods of treatment for various medical conditions. Before the 1940s, bed rest was prescribed for 2 weeks after childbirth, 3 weeks after herniorrhaphy, and 4 to 6 weeks after myocardial infarction. It was believed that the complex biochemical and physical demands of physical activity diverted energy from the restorative and reparative processes of healing. Rest in bed was regarded as tantamount to optimal rest of the heart and entire body.

During World War II, the shortage of hospital beds and medical personnel forced early mobilization of many patients. As often happens with this kind of action, it was soon discovered that early mobilization lessened complications and improved patient outcome. The National Aeronautics and Space Administration (NASA) conducted research that described the damaging effects of prolonged inactivity and weightlessness. These studies indicate that weightlessness and the antigravity effects of bed rest produce similar responses.

Antigravity Effects of Bed Rest

The supine position that often accompanies immobility and bed rest interferes with the effects of gravity. The force of gravity exerts beneficial effects on the body. As the body maintains a supine position, the absence of the force of gravity leads to many of the deconditioning effects associated with immobility and bed rest.

While upright, the body compensates for the effects of gravity in a variety of ways. The skeletal muscles contract and exert pressure against veins and lymph vessels. This contraction counteracts the force of gravity that would cause blood and fluid to pool in the lower extremities. Blood is kept moving through the circulatory system. Bones remain stronger because the longitudinal stress of weight bearing keeps essential minerals, such as calcium, inside the structure of the bone.

TABLE 55-2

Complications of Bedrest and Immobility

System	Complication
Cardiovascular	Decreased cardiac output, contributing to decreased aerobic capacity; orthostatic intolerance; venous thrombophlebitis
Pulmonary	Atelectasis; relative hypoxemia; pneumonia
Musculoskeletal	Muscle atrophy and loss of strength; decreased muscle oxidative capacity contributing to decreased aerobic capacity; osteoporosis (bone loss); contractures; osteoarthritis
Gastrointestinal	Constipation
Genitourinary	Incontinence; renal calculi
Skin	Pressure ulcers
Functional	Impaired ambulation and activity tolerance
Psychological	Sensory deprivation; altered sensory perception

(Harper C.M., Lyles Y.M. [1988]. Physiology and complications of bed rest. *Journal of the American Geriatric Society 36* [11], 1048)

Physiologic Responses

Cardiovascular Responses

After a period of bed rest, the cardiovascular system exhibits changes that reflect the loss of gravitational and exercise stimuli. In effect, the cardiovascular system becomes becomes deconditioned, resulting in an exaggeration of the hemodynamic changes normally seen with standing after brief bed rest. This deconditioning is manifested in three major alterations: postural hypotension, increased cardiac workload, and venous stasis and the potential for deep venous thrombosis. Bed rest also causes a negative fluid balance.

One of the most striking responses to assumption of the supine position during bed rest is the alteration of blood flow. There is a shift of fluid from the lower to the upper part of the body. In the supine position, approximately 500 ml of blood is redistributed from the lower extremities to the central circulation. Most of this blood is diverted to the lungs; a small portion is diverted to the arms and head. The increase in central blood volume results in an increase in stroke volume, which results in an increase in cardiac output. In the supine position, the normal cardiac output is 7 to 8 L/minute, compared with a cardiac output of 5 to 6 L/minute for a person in the standing position. The increase in stroke volume and cardiac output is accompanied by a slight decrease in heart rate and systemic vascular resistance and the maintenance in blood pressure. With increased fluid shifted to the head and thoracic cavity, the person may experience headache, swelling of the nasal sinuses, nasal congestion, and puffiness of the eyelids.[37]

The increase in plasma volume in the central circulation stimulates baroreceptors. The stimulation of the baroreceptors results in an inhibition of antidiuretic hormone and aldosterone, with a resultant water and sodium (*i.e.,* natriuresis) diuresis. In the supine position, diuresis begins on the first day with the shift of blood from the lower extremities to the thoracic cavity. The accompanying loss of water and sodium results in an increase in hematocrit, hemoglobin, and red blood cell mass, probably because of the loss of plasma volume. Also seen at this time are the isotonic losses of chloride, potassium, protein, albumin, creatinine, and glucose.[37–39]

After about 4 days of bed rest, fluid losses reach an equilibrium. One theory suggests that the loss of fluid from the vascular compartment is accompanied by an iso-osmotic shift of fluids from the extravascular to the intravascular compartment. Extravascular hydration is sacrificed to maintain adequate isotonic vascular volume. With a decrease in the extravascular volume and the reestablishment of intravascular volume, the osmolar receptors inhibit diuresis and natriuresis. Despite the reestablishment of intravascular volume, the extravascular spaces remain dehydrated.[37]

Orthostatic Hypotension. During bed rest, the forces of gravity and hydrostatic pressure are removed from the cardiovascular system. After 3 to 4 days of bed rest, the resumption of the upright position results in orthostatic or postural intolerance. Standing after prolonged bed rest results in a decrease in central blood volume as blood is displaced to the lower extremities and dependent parts of the body. Decreases in stroke volume and cardiac output occur along with increases in heart rate and systemic vascular resistance. The signs and symptoms of postural intolerance include tachycardia, nausea, diaphoresis, and sometimes syncope or fainting. This response probably results from β-adrenergic and sympathetic vagal stimulation. The reason for this is not completely understood, because catecholamine levels and adrenergic receptor sensitivity do not change significantly with bed rest.

Cardiac Workload and Exercise Tolerance. The major cardiovascular manifestation of deconditioning associated with bed rest is an increased workload on the heart. Initially, when a person assumes the supine position, venous return to the heart increases along with an increase in stroke volume and cardiac output, which is accompanied by a slight decrease in heart rate. Over time, cardiac output and stroke volume stabilize, but the heart rate increases. During periods of tachycardia, the time the heart spends in diastole is decreased. With decreased time spent in diastole, the heart does not have sufficient time to fill with blood, and it has to work harder to perfuse the vital organs and meet the metabolic demands of the body. This response is exaggerated when a person has to assume the upright position and begin activity after a prolonged period of bed rest. When persons begin submaximal exercise after prolonged bed rest, the heart rate increases while stroke volume and cardiac output decrease. Between 5 and 10 weeks of reconditioning exercise are required for return of heart rate, stroke volume, and cardiac output parameters to the levels before bed rest.[40,41]

Venous Stasis and Increased Blood Coagulability. Venous stasis in the legs results from lack of skeletal muscle pump function that promotes venous return to the heart. The skeletal muscle pump function is removed after assumption of the supine position, and there is mechanical compression of the veins from the position of the lower extremities against the bed. This increased pressure damages the intima of the vessel and causes platelets to adhere easily to the damaged vessel. Over time, this may be the basis for clot formation.

The development of deep vein thrombosis (DVT) is a major complication of bed rest. It is believed that three possible factors of immobility combine to predispose a person to thrombus formation: venous stasis, application of external pressure from the mattress against the veins, and hypercoagulability of the blood. However, most persons who develop DVT have risk factors in addition to bed rest.[39] The development of DVT also predisposes to the development of pulmonary emboli. As persons begin to resume activity patterns, the risk that large thrombi may dislodge and work their way through the circulatory system and lodge in a pulmonary blood vessel increases.

Various theories describe the possible causes of hypercoagulability and clot formation that occurs with bed rest. One theory cites the development of dehydration, which often occurs with bed rest, as responsible. Dehydration leads to an increased number of formed elements in the blood and contributes to increased blood viscosity. Increased viscosity contributes to clotting. Another theory cites the role of calcium. During bed rest, demineralization of bone occurs, and calcium and other minerals are released into the bloodstream. Calcium activates the conversion of prothrombin to thrombin, and thrombin becomes the activating enzyme that converts fibrinogen to fibrin. Fibrin initiates the process for clot formation.[42]

Pulmonary Responses

Bed rest and assumption of the supine position produce changes in both lung volumes and the mechanics of breathing. When a person is supine, the diaphragm moves upwards, causing a decrease in the size of the thoracic compartment. Chest expansion is limited because of the resistance of the bed. These limitations to the thoracic cavity hinder normal lung expansion. A decrease in lung compliance and in elastic recoil of the lungs also occurs, causing limitations in lung expansion. In the supine position, normal tidal volume breathing is a function of the abdominal muscles, in contrast to breathing in the upright position, in which normal breathing is primarily a function of rib cage movement. Tidal volume and functional residual capacity are decreased, and the efficiency and effectiveness of ventilation are hindered. Persons must work harder to breathe and take fewer deep breaths. Alveoli tend to collapse, resulting in areas of atelectasis and a decrease in the surface for gas exchange. These changes in function contribute to respiratory complications associated with bed rest: atelectasis, accumulation of secretions, hypoxemia, and pulmonary emboli.

Atelectasis is characterized by localized areas of lung collapse (see Chapter 23). It is caused by impaired mucociliary clearance of the airway resulting in pooling of secretions. Poor fluid intake and dehydration may cause secretions to become thick and tenacious. Stasis of secretions provides an ideal medium for bacterial growth, especially pneumococcal, staphylococcal, and streptococcal organisms. To prevent the complication of pneumonia from developing, persons must perform coughing and deep-breathing exercises. However, with the combined need of overcoming resistance to chest and lung expansion and obstructed airways, more energy is required to breathe. More oxygen is used, and more carbon dioxide is produced, causing the person to expend more energy to get less air.

Urinary Tract Responses

The kidneys are designed to function optimally with the body in the erect position. The anatomy of the kidney is such that urine flows from the kidney pelvis by gravity, whereas the action of peristalsis moves urine through the ureters to the bladder. Prolonged bed rest affects the renal system by altering the composition of body fluids and predisposing to the development of kidney stones. In the supine position, urine is not readily drained from the renal pelvis. Bed rest may also predispose to urinary tract infections and urinary incontinence because of positional changes and difficulty emptying the bladder.

A major complication of prolonged bed rest is the increased risk of developing kidney stones. Prolonged bed rest causes muscle atrophy, protein breakdown, decalcification of bone, hypercalcemia and hyperphosphatemia, and increased risk of developing calcium-containing kidney stones.[43] The urine becomes saturated with calcium salts (*i.e.*, calcium oxalate and calcium phosphate) as a result of the hypercalcemia and hyperphosphatemia, and stasis of urine resulting from the supine position favors crystallization of the stone-forming calcium salts. Moreover, urine levels of citrate, a prominent inhibitor of calcium stone formation, do not increase during bed rest.[42,43] Dehydration further increases urine concentration of stone-forming elements and risk of kidney stone formation. The pathogenesis and manifestations of kidney stones are discussed in Chapter 28.

Urinary tract infections and incontinence may also occur. The cause of incontinence is inadequate emptying of the bladder while the person is in the supine position. This position contributes to stagnation of urine in the bladder and may predispose the person to bladder and urinary tract infections.

Musculoskeletal Responses

Muscles are only as strong as they need to be to perform the work at hand. Bed rest leads to loss of about one eighth of the muscle's strength with each week of disuse.[39,44] Even normal, healthy persons lose weight when they are subjected to periods of prolonged bed rest. The weight loss occurs whether they are placed on controlled diets or allowed to eat ad libitum.[44] The reduction in weight is associated with the loss of lean muscle mass and loss of fat content. The larger the muscle, and the better trained the muscle, the faster the loss of muscle strength and the quicker the deconditioning occurs. This is best illustrated by the example that leg muscles lose strength and mass more quickly than muscles of the arms when persons are placed on prolonged bed rest.

In addition to loss of strength, muscles atrophy, change shape and appearance, and shorten when immobilized. The oxidative capacity of the muscle mitochondria decreases. These changes affect individual muscle fibers and total muscle mass.[39] Atrophy of muscles is reflected as an increase in urinary nitrogen excretion and a decrease in muscle weight. Because of the decreased oxidative capacity of the mitochondria, muscles fatigue more easily.

Muscle atrophy contributes to wasting and weakening of muscle tissue, and it plays a role in the development of contractures. A contracture is the abnormal shortening of muscle tissue, rendering the muscle highly resistant to stretch. Muscles weaken and shorten with disuse. Contractures occur when muscles do not have the necessary strength to maintain their integrity (*i.e.*, their proper function and full range of motion). Contractures mainly develop over joints when there is an imbalance in the muscle strength of the antagonistic muscle groups. If allowed to progress, the contracture eventually involves the muscle groups, tendons, ligaments, and joint capsule. The joint becomes limited in its full use and range of motion. Proper body alignment decreases the risk for the development of contractures.[39,42]

Another consequence of prolonged immobility and bed rest on the musculoskeletal system is the loss of bone mass and the development of disuse osteoporosis. Bone is a dynamic tissue that undergoes continual deposition and replacement of minerals in response to the dual stimuli of weight bearing and muscle pull. With immobility and bed rest, calcium loss from the bone begins almost immediately.

The maintenance of normal bone function depends on two types of cells: osteoblasts and osteoclasts. Osteoblasts function in building the osseous matrix of bone, and osteoclasts function in the breakdown of the bone matrix. Through their opposing forces, the bone matrix is continually turned over, and new bone is regenerated. Osteoblasts depend on the stress of mobility and weight bearing to perform their function. During immobility and bed rest, the process of building new bone stops, but the osteoclast cells continue to perform their function. This results in structural changes in the bone as the bone decalcifies. There is also an increase in the excretion of bone phosphorus and nitrogen. Despite the calcium loss from the bone, serum calcium remains normal because the excess calcium is excreted in the urine and feces.

Persons who experience disuse osteoporosis from prolonged immobility and bed rest develop soft, spongy bones. The bones may easily compress and become deformed. Because of lack of structural firmness, the bones may easily fracture. Persons with osteoporosis encounter much pain when they begin weight-bearing activities. Despite the lack of calcium in the bone, a diet high in calcium does not enhance bone uptake of calcium. Unneeded calcium is added to the excess calcium that is already being excreted in the urine. This may precipitate the formation of calcium-containing renal stones. The best measure to prevent the occurrence of osteoporosis is to begin weight bearing as soon as possible.

Skin Responses

Except for the soles of the feet, the skin is not designed for weight bearing. However, during bed rest, the large surface area of the skin bears weight and is in constant contact with the surface of the bed. Constant pressure is transmitted to the skin, subcutaneous tissue, and muscle, especially to those tissues over bony prominences. This constant contact causes increased pressure and impairs normal capillary blood flow, which interferes with the exchange of nutrients and waste products. Tissue ischemia and necrosis may result and lead to the development of pressure ulcers. Also contributing to the development of pressure ulcers is moisture from the skin being in constant contact with bed linens and affected by the forces of friction and shear.

Metabolic and Endocrine Responses

When a person is placed on bed rest, the basal metabolic rate falls in response to the decreased energy requirements of the body. Anabolic processes are slowed, and catabolic processes become accelerated. Protein breakdown occurs and leads to a protein deficiency and a negative nitrogen balance.[45] Persons in a negative nitrogen balance experience nausea and anorexia, which contribute to the catabolic state. Insulin plays a role in regulating protein metabolism and glucose use. It does this primarily by inhibiting protein breakdown.

With bed rest, persons experience an impaired responsiveness to the actions of insulin. During bed rest, it takes more insulin to maintain serum glucose. After 10 days of bed rest, there is a 100% increase in basal insulin concentration to maintain normal glucose control.[46,47] There also appears to be an induced insulin resistance that helps explain the negative nitrogen balance seen in patients who experience prolonged bed rest.

Possible reasons for the glucose unresponsiveness to the hyperinsulinemia include a change in the action of insulin because of the release of a substance that acts as an insulin inhibitor (this substance is believed to act at cell membrane binding sites); a change in some aspect of the cell membrane glucose transport system; or inhibition of the function of a second factor that has insulin-like activity. Research suggests that a factor or factors are activated with physical exercise. These factors respond to the quantity of energy expenditure and are necessary for insulin, and possibly glucose, to function normally. In the absence of activity, the action of these factors may be suppressed. A final explanation to describe glucose unresponsiveness to hyperinsulinemia is a combination of the previously mentioned causes.[46,48]

Persons who experience prolonged periods of bed rest have changes in the circadian release of various hormones. Normally, insulin and growth hormone peak twice a day. In subjects who experienced 30 days of bed rest, a single daily peak of these hormones occurred. Other hormonal changes include an afternoon peak of epinephrine rather than the normal early morning peak, and an early morning peak of aldosterone rather than the usual noonday peak that is seen in normally active persons.[49]

Gastrointestinal Responses

Gastrointestinal responses to bed rest vary. Constipation and fecal impaction are frequent complications that occur when persons experience prolonged periods of immobility and bed rest. With inactivity, there is slowed movement of feces through the colon. The act of defecation requires the integration of the abdominal muscles, the diaphragm, and the levator ani. Muscle atrophy and loss of tone occur in the immobilized person and interfere with the normal act of defecation. Lack of privacy and the supine position may compound abnormal defecation.[38,42,45]

Sensory Responses

Immobility reduces the quality and quantity of sensory information available from kinesthetic, visual, auditory, and tactile sensation. It also reduces the ability of the person to interact with the environment. Decreased kinesthetic stimulation occurs from immobilization and assumption of the supine or recumbent position. Responses to decreased kinesthetic stimulation include an impaired functioning of thought processes and decreased sensory perception. Prolonged immobility and bed rest have been associated with a number of impaired sensory responses. Common occurrences include visual and auditory hallucinations, vivid dreams, inefficient thought processes, loss of contact with reality, and alteration in tactile stimulation.

In addition to sensory deprivation related to prolonged bed rest and immobility, persons may experience a sensory monotony from the hospital environment. Repetitious and meaningless sounds from cardiac monitors, respirators, and hospital personnel, along with an environment that may be void of natural light and a normal day-night cycle, also contribute to impaired sensory perception.

Psychosocial Responses

Immobility often sets the stage for changes in a person's response to illness. Persons adapt to prolonged bed rest and immobility through a series of physiologic responses and through changes in affect, perception, and cognition. Affective changes include increased anxiety, fear, depression, hostility, rapid mood changes, and alterations in normal sleep patterns. These changes in mood occur in hospitalized patients who are subjected to periods of prolonged bed rest and immobility and in persons in confinement, such as astronauts and prisoners.

Research of immobilized or isolated persons has demonstrated that the motivation to learn decreases with periods of prolonged immobility as does the ability to learn and retain new material and transfer newly learned material to a different situation. Persons are less able and less motivated to perform problem-solving activities; they are less able to concentrate and discriminate information.[49] These studies present major implications for the timing of patient education and the preparation of education materials. Prolonged bed rest and immobility also contribute to the social isolation of the hospitalized person. Confined to a hospital bed, the person is not able to assume certain societal roles. The roles of spouse, parent, sibling, worker, friend are altered temporarily or permanently while the person is hospitalized. Persons may respond to this isolation by exhibiting various effective and ineffective coping behaviors, which include increased anxiety, depression, restlessness, fear, and rapid mood changes.

Time Course of Physiologic Responses

The deconditioning responses to the inactivity of immobility and bed rest affect all body systems. One of the important factors to keep in mind is the rapidity with which the changes occur, and the length of time required to overcome these effects. The body responds in a characteristic pattern to the effects of the supine position and bed rest. During the first 3 days of bed rest, one of the first changes to occur is a massive diuresis. Accompanying the diuresis are increases in serum osmolality, hematocrit, venous compliance, and an increase of urinary sodium and chloride excretion (Table 55–3). Fluid losses stabilize by about the fourth day. By days 4 to 7, there are changes in the hemolytic system. Fibrinogen increases along with increases in fibrinolytic activity and prolonged clotting time. The cardiovascular system responds with a decrease in cardiac output and stroke volume. No change is seen in heart rate and blood pressure. The basal metabolic rate decreases and the person begins to develop an insulin intolerance and a negative nitrogen balance.

Days 8 to 14 are characterized by additional effects on the hemolytic system. Decreases are seen in the number of red blood cells, and the phagocytic ability of leukocytes. Persons begin to experience a decrease in lean body mass. After 15 days of bed rest, osteoporosis and hypercalcuria occur. Aerobic power decreases, the cyclic excretion of some hormones is changed, and the person's thought pattern and sensory perception are altered.[47]

Interventions

A holistic approach should be initiated when caring for persons who are immobile or require prolonged periods of bed rest. Interventions and treatment should include actions that address the person's physical and psychosocial needs. The goals of care for the immobilized person include structuring a safe environment in which the person is not at risk to incur any nosocomial complications, providing diversional activities to offset problems with sensory deprivation, and preventing complications of bed rest by implementing a multidisciplinary plan of care.

In summary, during the last 75 years, the use of bed rest has been reversed as a standard of treatment for a variety of medical conditions. Over time, research findings have described the deleterious consequences of inactivity. All body systems are affected by complications of immobility and prolonged bed rest.

The responses to bed rest and immobility affect all body systems. One of the important factors is the rapidity with which the changes occur, and the long time required to overcome the effects of prolonged bed rest and immobility. Adverse effects of prolonged immobility and bed rest include a decreased cardiac output, orthostatic intolerance, dehydration, potential for thrombophlebitis, pneumonia, formation of renal calculi, development of pressure ulcers, sensory deprivation, and impaired thought processes.

TABLE 55-3

Physiologic Changes During Bedrest

0–3 Days	4–7 Days	8–14 Days	Over 15 Days
Increases in	**Increases in**	**Increases in**	**Increases in**
Urine volume Urine Na, Cl, Ca, and osmol excretion Plasma osmolality Hematocrit Venous compliance	Urine creatinine, hydroxyproline, PO_4, N, and K excretion Plasma globulin, phosphate and glucose levels Blood fibrinogen Fibrinolytic activity and clotting time Visual focal point Hyperthermia of eye conjunctiva, dilation of retinal arteries and veins Auditory threshold	Urine pyrophosphate Sweating sensitivity Exercise hyperthermia Exercise maximal heart rate	Peak hypercalciuria Sensitivity to thermal threshold Auditory threshold (secondary)
Decreases in	**Decreases in**	**Decreases in**	**Decreases in**
Total fluid intake Extracellular and intracellular fluid Calf blood flow Resting heart rate Secretion of gastric acid Glucose tolerance	Near point of visual acuity Orthostatic tolerance Nitrogen balance	Red blood cell mass Leukocyte phagocytosis Tissue heat conductance Lean body mass	Bone density

(Greenleaf J.E. [1984]. Physiological responses to prolonged bedrest and fluid immersion in humans. *Journal of Applied Physiology: Respiratory, Environmental and Exercise Physiology* 57 [3], 619–633)

REFERENCES

1. Oka R.K. (1990). Cardiovascular response to exercise. *Cardiovascular Nursing* 26 (6), 31–36.
2. Wingate S. (1991) Acute effects of exercise on the cardiovascular system. *Journal of Cardiovascular Nursing* 5 (4), 27–38.
3. Brooks G.A., Fahey T.D., White T.P. (1996). *Exercise physiology: Human bioenergetics and its applications.* Mountain View, CA: Mayfield Publishing Company.
4. Crawford M.H. (1992). Physiologic consequences of systematic training. *Cardiology Clinics* 10 (2), 209–218.
5. Casaburi R. (1994). Physiologic responses to training. *Clinics in Chest Medicine* 15 (2), 215–227.
6. Simoneau J.A. (1995). Adaptation of human skeletal muscle to exercise-training. *International Journal of Obesity* 19 (Suppl. 4), S9–S13.
7. Spurway N.C. (1992). Aerobic exercise, anaerobic exercise and the lactate threshold. *British Medical Bulletin* 48 (3), 569–591.
8. Kenney W.L., Johnson J.M. (1992). Control of skin blood flow during exercise. *Medicine and Science in Sports and Exercise* 24 (3), 303–312.
9. Nielsen B. (1994). Heat stress and acclimation. *Ergonomics* 37 (1), 49–58.
10. Brouns F., Beckers E. (1993). Is the gut an athletic organ? Digestion, absorption and exercise. *Sports Medicine* 15 (4), 242–257.
11. Streiff M., Bell W.R. (1994). Exercise and hemostasis in humans. *Seminars in Hematology* 31 (2), 155–165.
12. Nieman D.C. (1994). The effect of exercise on immune function. *Bulletin on the Rheumatic Diseases* 43 (8), 5–8.
13. Katz P. (1994). Exercise and the immune response. *Baillière's Clinical Rheumatology* 8 (1), 53–61.
14. Daughton D.M., Fix A.J. (1986). *Human Activity Profile (HAP) Manual.* Omaha, NE: Psychological Assessment Resources.
15. Krupp L.B., LaRocca N.G., Muir-Nash J., Steinberg A.D. (1989). The fatigue severity scale: Application to patients with multiple sclerosis and systemic lupus erythematosus. *Archives of Neurology* 46, 1121–1123.
16. Ulmer H.V. (1983). Work Physiology; Environmental physiology. In Schmidt R.F., Thews G. (Eds.). *Human physiology* (pp. 548–564). New York: Springer-Verlag.
17. Cantwell J.D. (1984). Exercise and coronary heart disease: Role of primary prevention. *Heart and Lung* 13, 6–13.
18. Borg G.A.V. (1973). Perceived exertion: A note on "history" and methods. *Medicine and Science in Sports* 5 (2), 90–93.
19. Borg G.A.V. (1982). Psychophysical bases of perceived exertion. *Medicine and Science in Sports* 14 (5), 377–381.
20. Carroll-Johnson R. (Ed.). (1989). *Classification of nursing diagnoses: Proceedings of the eighth conference.* Philadelphia: J.B. Lippincott.
21. MacLean S.(1991). Activity intolerance. In Maas M., Buckwalter K., Hardy M.A. (Eds.). *Nursing diagnoses and interventions for the elderly* (pp. 252–262). Redwood City, CA: Addison-Wesley Nursing.
22. Piper B.F. (1986). Fatigue. In Carrieri V.K., Lindsey A.M., West C.W. (Eds.). *Pathophysiological phenomena in nursing: Human responses to illness.* Philadelphia: W.B. Saunders.
23. Belza B. (1994). The impact of fatigue on exercise performance. *Arthritis Care and Research* 7 (4), 176–180.
24. Piper B.F. (1989). Fatigue: Current bases for practice. In Funk S.G., Tornquist E.M., Champagne M.T., Copp L.A., Wiese R.A. (Eds.). *Key aspects of comfort: Management of pain, fatigue, and nausea* (pp. 187–198). New York: Springer.
25. Nail L.M., King K.B. (1987). Fatigue. *Seminars in Oncology Nursing* 3 (4), 257–262.
26. St. Pierre B.A., Kasper C.E., Lindsey A.M. (1992). Fatigue mechanisms in patients with cancer: Effects of tumor necrosis factor and exercise on skeletal muscle. *Oncology Nursing Forum* 19 (3), 419–425.
27. Matthews D.A., Manu P., Lane T.J. (1991). Evaluation and management of patients with chronic fatigue. *The American Journal of Medical Sciences* 302 (5), 269–277.
28. Shafran S.D. (1991). The chronic fatigue syndrome. *The American Journal of Medicine* 90 (6), 730–739.
29. Gorensek M.J. (1991). Chronic fatigue and depression in the ambulatory patient. *Primary Care* 18 (2), 397–419.
30. Holmes G.P., Kaplan J.E., Gantz N.M., et al. (1988). Chronic fatigue syndrome: A working case definition. *Annals of Internal Medicine* 108, 387–389.
31. Cho W.K., Stollerman G.H. (1992). Chronic fatigue syndrome. *Hospital Practice* 27 (9), 221–245.
32. Demitrack M.A., Engleberg N.C. (1994). Chronic fatigue syndrome. *Current Therapy in Endocrinology and Metabolism* 5, 135–142.
33. Wessely S. (1995). The epidemiology of chronic fatigue syndrome. *Epidemiologic Reviews* 17 (1), 139–151.
34. Calabrese L., Danao T., Camara E., Wilke W. (1992). Chronic fatigue syndrome. *American Family Physician* 45 (3), 1205–1213.
35. Portwood M.F. (1988). Chronic fatigue syndrome: A diagnosis for consideration. *Nurse Practitioner* 13 (2), 11–23.
36. Fukuda K., Straus S.E., Hickie I., Sharpe M.C., Dobbins J.G., Komaroff A., and the International Chronic Fatigue Syndrome Study Group. (1994). The chronic fatigue syndrome: A comprehensive approach to its definition and study. *Annals of Internal Medicine* 121 (4), 953–959.
37. Dean E. (1993). Bedrest and deconditioning. *Neurology Report* 17 (1), 6–9.
38. Coletta E.M., Murphy J.B. (1992). The complications of immobility in the elderly stroke patient. *Journal of the American Board of Family Practice* 5(4), 389–397.
39. Dittmer D.K., Teasell R. (1993). Complications of immobilization and bed rest. Part 1: Musculoskeletal and cardiovascular complications. *Canadian Family Physician* 39, 1428–1437.
40. Taylor H.L., Henschel A., Brzek J., Keys A. (1949). Effects of bed rest on cardiovascular function and work performance. *Journal of Applied Physiology* 2 (5), 223–239.
41. Saltin B., Blomquist G., Mitchell J.H., Johnson R.L., Wildenthal K., Chapman C.B.. (1968). Responses to exercise after bed rest and after training: A longitudinal study of adaptive changes in oxygen transport and body composition. *Circulation* 38 (5 Suppl. 7), VII1–VII55.
42. Olson E.V., Thompson L.F., McCarthy J., et al. (1967). The hazards of immobility. *American Journal of Nursing* 67 (4), 780–797.
43. Twang T.S., Hill D., Schneider V., et al. (1988). Effect of bedrest on the propensity for renal stone formation. *Journal of Endocrinology and Metabolism* 66, 109–112.
44. Corcoran P.J. (1991). Use it or lose it: The hazards of bed rest and inactivity. *Western Journal of Medicine* 154(5), 536–538.
45. Teasell R., Dittmer D.K. (1993). Complications of immobilization and bed rest. Part 2: Other complications. *Canadian Family Physician* 39, 1440–1446.
46. Greenleaf J.E., Kozlowski S. (1982). Physiological consequences of reduced physical activity during bed rest. In Terjung R.L. (Ed.). *Exercise and sport sciences reviews* (pp. 84–119). Syracuse, NY: American College of Sports Medicine.

47. Shangraw R.E., Stuart C.A., Prince M.J., Peters E.J., Wolfe R.R. (1988). Insulin responsiveness of protein metabolism in vivo following bed rest in humans. *American Journal of Physiology* 255, E548–E558.
48. Dolkas C.B., Greenleaf J.E. (1977). Insulin and glucose responses during bed rest with isotonic and isometric exercise. *Journal of Applied Physiology* 43 (6), 1033–1038.
49. Rubin M. (1988). The physiology of bed rest. *American Journal of Nursing* 88 (1), 50–58.
50. Greenleaf J.E. (1984). Physiological responses to prolonged bed rest and fluid immersion in humans. *Journal of Applied Physiology* 57 (3), 619–633.

ADDITIONAL READINGS

Appell H.J., Soares J.M.C., Duarte J.A. (1992). Exercise, muscle damage and fatigue. *Sports Medicine* 13 (2), 108–115.

Arner P. (1995). Impact of exercise on adipose tissue metabolism in humans. *International Journal of Obesity* 19 (Suppl. 4), S18–S21.

Bearn J., Wessely S. (1994). Neurobiological aspects of the chronic fatigue syndrome. *European Journal of Clinical Investigation* 24, 79–90.

Behan P.O., Bakheit A.M.O. (1991). Clinical spectrum of postviral fatigue syndrome. *British Medical Bulletin* 47 (4), 793–808.

Belza B.L., Henke C.J., Yelin E., Epstein W.V., Gilliss C. (1993). Correlates of fatigue in older adults with rheumatoid arthritis. *Nursing Research* 42 (2), 93–99.

Berne K.H. (1992). *Running on empty*. Alameda, CA: Hunter House.

Bonde-Petersen F., Suzuki Y., Kawakubo K., Gunji A. (1994). Effects of 20 days' bed rest upon peripheral capillary filtration rate, venous compliance and blood flow in arms and legs. *Acta Physiology Scandinavica* 150 (Suppl. 616), 65–69.

Chobanian A.V., Lille R.D., Tercyak A., Blevines P. (1974). The metabolic and hemodynamic effects of prolonged bed rest in normal subjects. *Circulation* 49, 551–559.

Christensen T., Kehlet H. (1993). Postoperative fatigue. *World Journal of Surgery* 17 (2), 220–225.

Dishman R.K. (1994). Prescribing exercise intensity for healthy adults using perceived exertion. *Medicine and Science in Sports and Exercise* 26 (9), 1087–1094.

Donoghue P.J., Siegel M.E. (1992). *Sick and tired of feeling sick and tired: Living with invisible chronic illness*. New York: W.W. Norton.

Duffin J. (1994). Neural drives to breathing during exercise. *Canadian Journal of Applied Physiology* 19 (3), 289–304.

Elashoff J.D., Jacknow A.D., Shain S.G., Braunstein G.D. (1991). Effects of anabolic-androgenic steroids on muscular strength. *Annals of Internal Medicine* 115, 387–393.

Fukuoka H., Kiriyama M., Nishimura Y., Higurashi M., Suzuki Y., Gunji A. (1994). Metabolic turnover of bone and peripheral monocyte release of cytokines during short-term bed rest. *Acta Physiology Scandinavia* 150 (Suppl. 616), 37–41.

Funk S.G., Tornquist E.M., Champagne M.T., Copp L.A., Weise R.A. (Eds.). (1990). *Key aspects of recovery: Improving nutrition, rest, and mobility*. New York: Springer.

Gift A.G., Pugh L.C. (1993). Dyspnea and fatigue. *Nursing Clinics of North America* 28 (2), 373–384.

Glick O.J. (1992). Interventions related to activity and movement. *Nursing Clinics of North America* 27 (2), 541–568.

Gordon M. (1976). Assessing activity tolerance. *American Journal of Nursing* 76 (1), 72–75.

Graydon J.E., Bubela N., Irvine D., Vincent L. (1995). Fatigue-reducing strategies used by patients receiving treatment for cancer. *Cancer Nursing* 18 (1), 23–28.

Nieman D.C. (1994). Exercise, infection, and immunity. *International Journal of Sports Medicine* 15 (Suppl. 3), S131–S141.

Nieman D.C., Nehisen-Cannarella S.L. (1994). The immune response to exercise. *Seminars in Hematology* 31 (2), 166–179.

Nishimura Y., Fukuoka H., Kiriyama M., et al. (1994). Bone turnover and calcium metabolism during 20 days' bed rest in young healthy males and females. *Acta Physiology Scandinavica* 150 (Suppl. 616), 27–35.

CHAPTER 56

Alterations in Temperature Regulation

Body heat is generated in the core tissues of the body. It is transferred to the skin surface by the blood and then released into the environment surrounding the body. Body temperature rises during fever and hyperthermia due to excessive heat production or exposure to a hot environment, and it falls during hypothermia caused by exposure to cold. This chapter is organized in three sections: regulation of body temperature, fever and hyperthermia, and hypothermia.

Body Temperature Regulation

After you have completed this section of the chapter, you should be able to meet the following objectives:

- Differentiate between body core temperature and skin temperature and relate the differences to methods used for measuring body temperature
- Describe the mechanisms of heat production in the body
- Define *conduction*, *radiation*, *convection*, and *evaporation* and relate them to the mechanisms for heat loss from the body

Virtually all biochemical processes in the body are affected by changes in temperature. Metabolic processes speed up or slow down depending on whether body temperature is rising or falling. Body temperature is normally maintained within a range of 36.0°C to 37.5°C (97.0°F to 99.5°F).[1] Within this range, there are individual differences and diurnal variations; internal core temperatures reach their highest point in late afternoon and evening and their lowest point in the early morning hours (Fig. 56–1).

Body temperature reflects the difference between heat production and heat loss and varies with exercise and extremes of environmental temperature. Properly protected, the body can function in environmental conditions that range from −50°C (−48°F) to +50°C (122°F). Individual body cells, however, cannot tolerate such a wide range of temperatures—at −1°C (32°F), ice crystals form, and at +45°C (113°F), cell proteins coagulate.[2]

Most of the body's heat is produced by the deeper core tissues (*i.e.*, muscles and viscera), which are insulated from the environment and protected against heat loss by the subcutaneous tissues and skin (Fig. 56–2). Adipose tissue is a particularly good insulator, conducting heat only one third as effectively as other tissues. Heat loss occurs when the heat from the body's inner core is transferred to the skin surface by the circulating blood. If no heat were lost by the body at rest, the temperature of the body would rise 1°C (1.8°F)/ hour; with light work, the temperature would rise 2°C / hour.

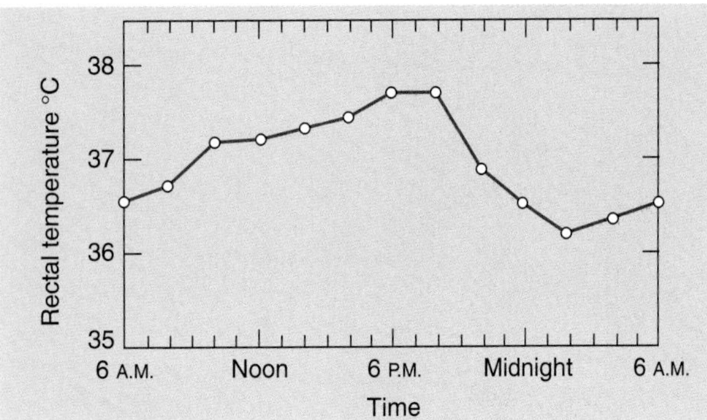

Figure 56–1
Normal diurnal variations in body temperature.

Temperatures differ in various parts of the body, with core temperatures being higher than those at the skin surface. Generally, the rectal temperature is used as a measure of core temperature. Core temperatures may also be obtained from the esophagus using a flexible thermometer, from a pulmonary artery catheter that is used for thermodilution measurement of cardiac output, or from a urinary catheter with thermosensor that measures the temperature of urine in the bladder. Because of location, pulmonary artery and esophageal temperatures closely reflect the temperature of the heart and thoracic organs. The oral temperature, taken sublingually, is usually 0.2°C (0.36°F) to 0.51°C (0.9°F) lower than the rectal temperature. The

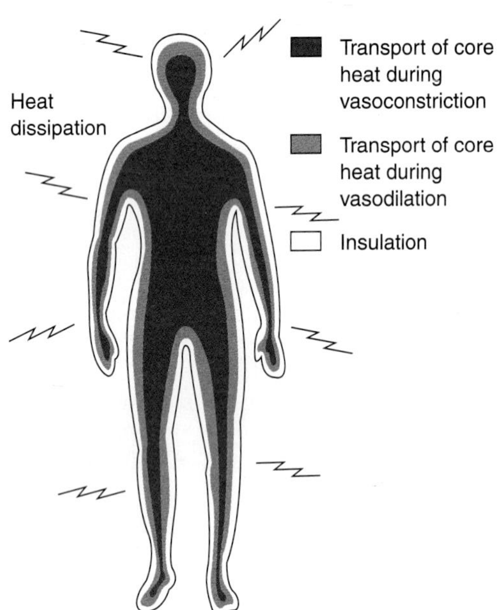

Figure 56–2
Control of heat loss. Body heat is produced in the deeper core tissues of the body, which is insulated by the subcutaneous tissues and skin to protect against heat loss. During vasodilatation, circulating blood transports heat to the skin surface, where it dissipates into the surrounding environment. Vasoconstriction decreases the transport of core heat to the skin surface, and vasodilatation increases transport.

axillary temperature can also be used as an estimate of core temperature. However, the parts of the axillary fossa must be pressed closely together because this method requires considerable heat to accumulate before the final temperature is reached.

Tympanic membrane thermometry has been introduced as a method of measuring body temperature. The method uses an infrared sensor to measure the flow of heat from the tympanic membrane and ear canal. The method is easy to use and has been reported to correlate well with rectal temperatures. It has become popular in the pediatric setting because of its ease and speed of measurement, acceptability to parents and children, and cost savings in personnel time required to take a child's temperature.[3]

Body temperature is regulated by the thermoregulatory center in the hypothalamus. This center integrates input from various thermal receptors located throughout the body with output responses that conserve body heat or increase its dissipation. It is the temperature of the body core rather than surface temperature that is regulated. The thermostatic set point of the thermoregulatory center is set so that the temperature of the body is regulated within the normal range of 36.0° to 37.5°C. When body temperature begins to rise above the normal range, heat-dissipating behaviors are initiated; when the temperature falls below the normal range, heat production is increased. Core temperatures above 41°C (105.8°F) or below 34°C (93.2°F) usually mean that the body's ability to thermoregulate is impaired (Fig. 56–3). Body responses that produce, conserve, and dissipate heat are described in Table 56–1. Spinal cord injuries that transect the cord at T6 or above can seriously impair temperature regulation, because the hypothalamus can no longer control skin blood flow or sweating.

In addition to the body's thermoregulatory mechanism, humans engage in voluntary behaviors to help regulate body temperature. These behaviors include the selection of proper clothing and regulation of environmental temperature through heating systems and air conditioning. Body positions that hold the extremities close to the body prevent heat loss and are commonly assumed in cold weather.

Mechanisms of Heat Production

The body's main source of heat production is metabolism. There is a 0.56°C (1°F) increase in body temperature for every 7% increase in metabolism. The sympathetic neurotransmitters, epinephrine and norepinephrine, which are released when an increase in body temperature is needed, act at the cellular level to shift metabolism so energy production is reduced and heat production is increased. This may be one of the reasons fever tends to produce feelings of weakness and fatigue. Thyroid hormone increases cellular metabolism, but this response usually requires several weeks to reach maximal effectiveness.

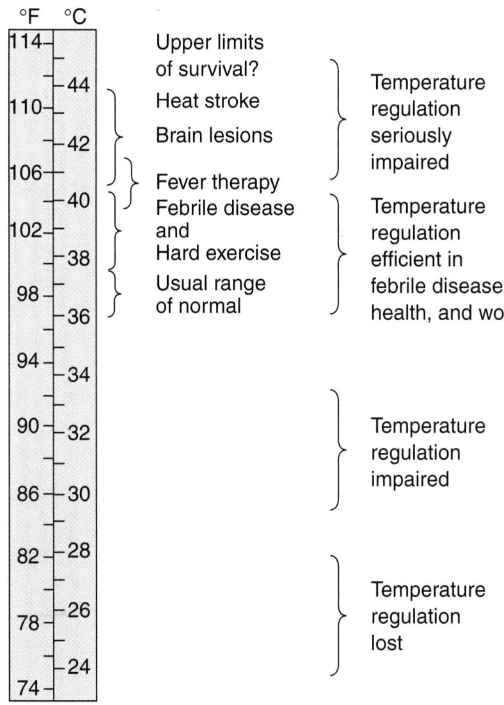

Figure 56–3
Body temperatures under different conditions. (Dubois, E.F. [1948]. *Fever and the regulation of body temperature.* Springfield, IL: Charles C. Thomas)

Fine involuntary actions such as shivering and chattering of the teeth can produce a threefold to fivefold increase in body temperature. Shivering is initiated by impulses from the hypothalamus. The first muscle change that occurs with shivering is a general increase in muscle tone, followed by an oscillating rhythmic tremor involving the spinal-level reflex that controls muscle tone. Because no external work is performed, all the energy liberated by the metabolic processes from shivering is in the form of heat.

Physical exertion increases body temperature. With strenuous exercise, more than three quarters of the increased metabolism resulting from muscle activity appears as heat within the body, and the remainder appears as external work.

Mechanisms of Heat Loss

Most of the body's heat losses occur at the skin surface as heat from the blood moves to the skin and from there into the surrounding environment. There are numerous arteriovenous (AV) shunts under the skin surface that allow blood to move directly from the arterial to the venous system. These AV shunts are much like the radiators in a heating system. When the shunts are open, body heat is freely dissipated to the skin and surrounding environment; when the shunts are closed, heat is retained in the body. The blood flow in the AV shunts is controlled almost exclusively by the sympathetic nervous system in response to changes in core temperature and environmental temperature. Contraction of the pilomotor muscles of the skin, which raises skin hairs and produces goose bumps, reduces the surface area available for heat loss.

TABLE 56-1
Heat Loss and Heat Gain Responses Used in Regulation of Body Temperature

Heat Gain		Heat Loss	
Body Response	*Mechanism of Action*	*Body Response*	*Mechanism of Action*
Vasoconstriction of the superficial blood vessels	Confines blood flow to the inner core of the body, with the skin and subcutaneous tissues acting as insulation to prevent loss of core heat	Dilatation of the superficial blood vessels	Delivers blood containing core heat to the periphery where it is dissipated through radiation, conduction, and convection
Contraction of the pilomotor muscles that surround the hairs on the skin	Reduces the heat loss surface of the skin	Sweating	Increases heat loss through evaporation
Assumption of the huddle position with the extremities held close to the body	Reduces the area for heat loss		
Shivering	Increases heat production by the muscles		
Increased production of epinephrine	Increases the heat production associated with metabolism		
Increased production of thyroid hormone	Is a long-term mechanism that increases metabolism and heat production		

Heat is lost from the body through radiation, conduction, and convection from the skin surface; through the evaporation of sweat and insensible perspiration; through the exhalation of air that has been warmed and humidified; and through heat lost in urine and feces. Of these mechanisms, only heat losses that occur at the skin surface are directly under hypothalamic control.

Conduction

Conduction is the direct transfer of heat from one molecule to another. Blood carries, or conducts, heat from the inner core of the body to the skin surface. Normally, only a small amount of body heat is lost through conduction to a cooler surface. Cooling blankets or mattresses that are used for reducing fever rely on conduction of heat from the skin to the cool surface of the mattress. Heat can also be conducted in the opposite direction—from the external environment to the body surface. For instance, body temperature may rise slightly after a hot bath.

Water has a specific heat several times greater than air, so water absorbs far greater amounts of heat than air. The loss of body heat can be excessive and life-threatening in situations of cold water immersion or cold exposure in damp or wet clothing.

The conduction of heat to the body's surface is influenced by blood volume. In hot weather, the body compensates by increasing blood volume as a means of dissipating heat. Persons who are not acclimated to a hot environment can increase their total blood volume by 10% within 2 to 4 hours of heat exposure. A mild swelling of the ankles during hot weather provides evidence of blood volume expansion. Exposure to cold produces a cold diuresis and a reduction in blood volume as a means of controlling the transfer of heat to the body's surface.

Radiation

Radiation is the transfer of heat through the air or a vacuum. Heat from the sun is carried by radiation. Heat loss by radiation varies with the temperature of the environment. Environmental temperature must be less than that of the body for heat loss to occur. Normally, about 60% to 70% of body heat is dissipated by radiation.

Convection

Convection refers to heat transfer through the circulation of air currents. Normally, a layer of warm air tends to remain near the body's surface; convection causes continual removal of the warm layer and replacement with air from the surrounding environment. The windchill factor that is often included in the weather report combines the effect of convection due to wind with the still-air temperature.

Evaporation

Evaporation involves the use of body heat to convert water on the skin to water vapor. Water that diffuses through the skin independent of sweating is called *insensible perspiration*. Insensible perspiration losses are greatest in a dry environment. Sweating occurs through the sweat glands and is controlled by the sympathetic nervous system. Unlike other sympathetically mediated functions, in which the catecholamines serve as neuromediators, sweating is mediated by acetylcholine. This means that anticholinergic drugs, such as atropine, can interfere with heat loss by interrupting sweating.

Evaporative heat losses involve insensible perspiration and sweating, with 0.58 calories being lost for each gram of water that is evaporated.[1] As long as body temperature is greater than the atmospheric temperature, heat is lost through radiation. However, when the temperature of the surrounding environment becomes greater than skin temperature, evaporation is the only way the body can rid itself of heat. Any condition that prevents evaporative heat losses causes the body temperature to rise.

In summary, body temperature is normally maintained within a range of 36.0°C to 37.4°C (97.0°F to 99.5°F). Most of the body's heat is produced by metabolic processes that occur within deeper core structures (*i.e.*, muscles and viscera) of the body. Heat loss occurs at the body's surface when heat from core structures is transported to the skin by the circulating blood. Heat is lost from the body through radiation, conduction, convection, and evaporation. The thermoregulatory center in the hypothalamus functions to modify heat production and heat losses as a means of regulating body temperature.

Increased Body Temperature

After you have completed this section of the chapter, you should be able to meet the following objectives:

- Characterize the mechanisms involved in body heat production and heat loss
- Describe the four stages of fever
- Explain what is meant by intermittent, remittent, sustained, and relapsing fevers
- State the relation between body temperature and heart rate
- Differentiate between the physiologic mechanisms involved in fever and hyperthermia
- State the criteria for high-risk status of children 0 to 36 months of age
- State the definition for fever in the elderly and cite possible mechanisms for altered febrile response in the elderly
- Compare the characteristics of fevers caused by infectious agents and drug-related fevers
- Compare the mechanisms of malignant hyperthermia and neuroleptic malignant syndrome

Fever and hyperthermia describe an increase in body temperature that is higher than the normal range. True fever is a disorder of thermoregulation in which there is upward displacement of the hypothalamic set point for temperature control. In hyperthermia, the set point is unchanged, but the mechanisms that control body temperature are ineffective in meeting the challenge of maintaining body temperature during exposure to high ambient temperature or the excess heat production that occurs with strenuous exertion.

Fever

The literature on fever dates back to the writings of Hippocrates, which contain many descriptions of febrile-course diseases, such as typhoid fever.[4] However, it was not until the development of the thermometer that measurements of body temperature became possible. One of the first studies of body temperature was reported in 1868 by the German physician Carl Wunderlich, who, during a 20-year period, studied the body temperature of 25,000 patients with observations made twice daily with a foot-long thermometer held in the axilla for 20 minutes.[5] Wunderlich observed that the thermometer was a useful instrument for providing insight into the condition of the sick. Today, temperature is one of the most frequent physiologic responses to be monitored during illness.

Mechanisms

Fever, or pyrexia, describes an elevation in body temperature that is caused by an upward displacement of the set point of the hypothalamic thermoregulatory center. When the fever has broken, the set point returns to its prefever setting. Fevers that are regulated by the hypothalamus usually do not rise above 41°C (105.8°F), suggesting a built-in thermostatic safety mechanism. Temperatures above that level are usually the result of superimposed activity, such as convulsions, hyperthermic states, or direct involvement of the temperature control center.

The mechanisms for controlling temperature are not well developed in the infant. In infants younger than 3 months, a mild elevation in temperature (*i.e.,* rectal temperature of 38°C (100.4°F]) can indicate serious infection that requires immediate medical attention.[6] Fever in elderly persons is also more likely to indicate serious infection or disease. This is because the elderly often have a lower baseline temperature, and although they increase their temperature during an infection, it may fail to reach a level that is equated with significant fever.[7–9]

Fever can be caused by a number of microorganisms and substances that are collectively called *exogenous pyrogens*. Exogenous pyrogens induce host cells to produce a fever-producing mediator called *endogenous pyrogen*. Research has identified at least three chemical substances that act as endogenous pyrogens: interleukin-1, interleukin-6, and tumor necrosis factor.[10,11] These chemical mediators, also known as *cytokines*, are synthesized by a number of body cell types, including endothelial cells, epithelial cells, lymphocytes, fibroblasts, and macrophages. The endogenous pyrogens produce fever by increasing the set point of the hypothalamic thermoregulatory center, probably through the action of prostaglandin E. In addition to their fever-producing actions, the endogenous pyrogens mediate a number of other responses. For example, interleukin-1 is an inflammatory mediator that produces other signs of inflammation such as leukocytosis, anorexia, and malaise (see Chapter 11).

Many noninfectious disorders, such as myocardial infarction, pulmonary emboli, and neoplasms, produce fever. In these conditions, the injured or abnormal cells incite the production of endogenous pyrogen. For example, trauma and surgery can be associated with up to 3 days of fever. Some malignant cells, such as those of leukemia and Hodgkin's disease, secrete endogenous pyrogen.

A fever that has its origin in the central nervous system is sometimes referred to as a *neurogenic fever*. It is usually caused by damage to the hypothalamus caused by central nervous system trauma, intracerebral bleeding, or an increase in intracranial pressure. Neurogenic fevers are characterized by a high temperature that is resistant to antipyretic therapy and is not associated with sweating.

Purpose

The purpose of fever is not completely understood. However, from a purely practical standpoint, fever is a valuable index to health status. For many, fever signals the presence of an infection and may legitimize the need for medical treatment. In ancient times, fever was thought to "cook" the poisons that caused the illness. With the availability of antipyretic drugs in the late 19th century, the belief that fever was useful began to wane, probably because most antipyretic drugs also had analgesic effects.

There is little research to support the belief that fever is harmful unless the temperature rises above 40°C (104°F). Animal studies have demonstrated a clear survival advantage in infected members with fever compared with animals that were unable to develop a fever. It has been shown that small elevations in temperature such as those that occur with fever enhance immune function. There is increased motility and activity of the white blood cells, stimulation of interferon production, and activation of T cells.[12] Many of the microbial agents that cause infection grow best at normal body temperatures, and their growth is inhibited by temperatures within the fever range. For example, the rhinoviruses responsible for the common cold are cultured best at 33°C (91.4°F), which is close to the temperature in the nasopharynx; temperature-sensitive mutants of virus that cannot grow at temperatures above 37.5°C (99.5°F) produce fewer signs and symptoms.[13]

Patterns

The patterns of temperature change in persons with fever vary and may provide information about the nature of the causative agent.[14–16] These patterns can be described as intermittent, remittent, sustained, or relapsing. An *intermittent* fever is one in which temperature returns to normal at least once every 24 hours. In a *remittent* fever, the temperature does not return to normal and varies a few degrees in either direction. In a *sustained* or *continuous* fever, the temperature remains above normal with minimal variations (usually less than 0.55°C or 1°F). A *recurrent* or *relapsing* fever is one in which there is one or more episodes of fever, each as long as several days, with one or more days of normal temperature between episodes.

Critical to the analysis of a fever pattern is the relation of heart rate to the level of temperature elevation. Normally, a 1°C rise in temperature produces a 15-beat/minute increase in heart rate (1°F, 10 beats/minute).[14] Most persons respond to an increase in temperature with an appropriate increase in heart rate. The observation that a rise in temperature is not accompanied by the anticipated change in heart rate can provide useful information about the cause of the fever. For example, a heart rate that is slower than would be anticipated can occur with Legionnaires' disease and drug fever, and a heart rate that is more rapid than anticipated can be symptomatic of hyperthyroidism and pulmonary emboli.

Manifestations

The physiologic behaviors that occur during the development of fever can be divided into four stages: a prodrome; a chill, during which the temperature rises; a flush; and defervescence. During the first or prodromal period, there are nonspecific complaints such as mild headache and fatigue, general malaise, and fleeting aches and pains. Vasoconstriction and piloerection usually precede the onset of shivering. At this point the skin is pale and covered with goose flesh. There is a feeling of being cold and an urgency to put on more clothing or covering and to curl up in a position that conserves body heat. The prodromal stage is followed by the second stage—the onset of a generalized shaking chill. Even as the temperature rises, there is the uncomfortable sensation of being chilled. When the shivering has caused the body temperature to reach the new set point of the temperature control center, the shivering ceases, and a sensation of warmth develops. At this point, the third stage begins, during which cutaneous vasodilation occurs and the skin becomes warm and flushed. The fourth, or defervescence, stage of the febrile response is marked by the initiation of sweating. Not all persons proceed through the four stages of fever development. Sweating may be absent, and fever may develop gradually with no indication of a chill or shivering.

Common manifestations of fever are anorexia, myalgia, arthralgia, and fatigue. These discomforts are worse when the temperature rises rapidly or exceeds 39.5°C (103.1°F). Respiration is increased, and the heart rate is usually elevated. Dehydration occurs because of sweating and the rapid respiratory rate that results in increased vapor losses. The occurrence of chills commonly coincides with the introduction of pyrogen into the circulation. Many of the manifestations of fever are related to the increases in the metabolic rate, increased need for oxygen, and use of body proteins as an energy source. During fever, the body switches from using glucose (an excellent medium for bacterial growth) to metabolism based on protein and fat breakdown.[11] With prolonged fever, there is increased breakdown of endogenous fat stores. If fat breakdown is rapid, metabolic acidosis may result.

Headache is a common accompaniment of fever and is thought to result from the vasodilation of cerebral vessels occurring with fever. Delirium is possible when the temperature exceeds 40°C (104°F). In the elderly, confusion and delirium may follow moderate elevations in temperature. Owing to increasingly poor oxygen uptake by the aging lung, pulmonary function may prove to be a limiting factor in the hypermetabolism that accompanies fever in older persons. Confusion, incoordination, and agitation commonly reflect cerebral hypoxemia. Febrile convulsions can occur in some children.[17] They usually occur with rapidly rising temperatures or at a threshold temperature that differs with each child.

Herpetic lesions, or fever blisters, that develop in some persons during fever are caused by a separate infection by the type I herpes simplex virus that established latency in the regional ganglia and that is reactivated by a rise in body temperature.

Diagnosis and Treatment

Fever is usually a manifestation of a disease state, and as such, determining the cause of a fever is an important aspect of its treatment. For example, fevers from infectious diseases are usually treated with antibiotics, whereas other fevers, such as those resulting from a noninfectious inflammatory condition, may be treated symptomatically.

Sometimes it is difficult to establish the cause of a fever. A prolonged fever for which the cause is difficult to ascertain is often referred to as *fever of unknown origin* (FUO). FUO is defined a temperature elevation of 38.3°C (101°F) or higher that is present for 3 weeks or longer.[18] Among the causes of FUO are malignancies (*i.e.*, lymphomas, metastases to the liver, and central nervous system); infections such as human immunodeficiency virus, tuberculosis, or abscessed infections; and drug fever. Malignancies, particularly non-Hodgkin's lymphoma, are important causes of FUO in the elderly. Cirrhosis of the liver is another cause of FUO.

The methods of fever treatment focus on modification of the external environment as a means of increasing heat transfer from the internal to the external environment, support of the hypermetabolic state that accompanies fever, protection of vulnerable body organs and systems, and treatment of the infection or condition causing the fever. Because fever is a disease symptom, its manifestation suggests the need for treatment of the primary cause.

Modification of the environment ensures that the environmental temperature facilitates heat transfer away from the body. Sponge baths with cool water or an alcohol solution can be used to increase evaporative heat losses. More profound cooling can be accomplished through the use of a cooling mattress, which facilitates the conduction of heat from the body into the coolant solution that circulates through the mattress. Care must be taken so that cooling methods do not produce vasoconstriction and shivering that decrease heat loss and increase heat production.

Adequate fluids and sufficient amounts of simple carbohydrates are needed to support the hypermetabolic state and to prevent the tissue breakdown that is characteristic of fever. Additional fluids are needed for sweating and to balance the insensible water losses from the lungs that accompany an increase in respiratory rate. Fluids are also needed to maintain an adequate vascular volume for heat transport to the skin surface.

Antipyretic drugs, such as aspirin and acetaminophen, are often used to alleviate the discomforts of fever and protect vulnerable organs, such as the brain, from extreme elevations in body temperature. These drugs act by resetting the hypothalamic temperature control center to a lower level.

Fever in Children

Fever without a source occurs frequently in infants and children and is common reason for visits to the clinic or emergency room. Approximately two thirds of children visit their health care providers with an acute febrile illness before they reach the age of 3 years.[19]

Both minor and life-threatening infections are common in the infant to 3-year age group.[19] The most common causes of fever in children are minor and more serious infections of the respiratory system, urinary system, gastrointestinal tract, or central nervous system. Occult bacteremia and meningitis also occurs in this age group and should be excluded. The Agency for Health Care Policy and Research Expert Panel has developed clinical guidelines for use in the treatment of infants and children 0 to 36 months of age with fever without a source.[20] The guidelines define fever in this age group as an elevation in rectal temperature equal to or greater than 38°C (100.4°F). The guidelines also pointed out that fever may result from overbundling or a vaccine reaction. When overbundling is suspected, it is suggested that the infant be unbundled and the temperature retaken after a period of 15 to 30 minutes.

Fever in infants and children can be classified as low risk or high risk, depending on the probability of progressing to bacteremia or meningitis. Signs of toxicity include lethargy, poor feeding, signs hypoventilation and poor tissue oxygen, and cyanosis. Infants can be considered low risk if they were delivered at term and sent home with their mother without complications and have been healthy with no previous hospitalizations or previous antimicrobial therapy. A white blood cell count and urinalysis are recommended as a means of confirming low-risk status. Blood and urine cultures, chest radiographs, and lumbar puncture are usually done in high-risk infants and children to determine the cause of fever.

The mean probability of serious bacterial infection in infants less than 3 months old is 8.6%, and in children between 3 and 36 months, it is 4.5%.[20] Infants with fever who are considered to low risk are usually managed on an outpatient basis providing the parents or caregiver are deemed reliable. Older children with fever without source may also be treated on an outpatient basis. Parents or caregivers require full instructions, preferably in writing, regarding assessment of the febrile child. They should be instructed to contact their health care provider should their child develop signs suggesting sepsis. High-risk infants and infants younger than 28 days are usually hospitalized for evaluation of their fever and treatment. Parenteral antimicrobial therapy is usually initiated after samples for blood, urine, and spinal fluid cultures have been taken.

Fever in the Elderly

Normal body temperature and the circadian pattern of temperature variation are often altered in the elderly. Elderly persons are reported to have a lower basal temperature (<36.4°C [97.6°F] in one study) than younger persons.[21] It has been recommended that the definition of fever in the elderly be expanded to include an elevation of temperature of at least 1.1°C (2°F) above baseline values.[9]

It has been suggested that 20% to 30% of elders with serious infections present with an absent or blunted febrile response.[9] When fever is present in the elderly, it generally indicates the presence of serious infection, most often caused by bacteria. The absence of fever may delay diagnosis and initiation of antimicrobial treatment. Unexplained change in functional capacity, worsening of mental status, weakness and fatigue, and weight loss are signs of infection in the elderly. They should be viewed as possible signs of infection and sepsis when fever is absent. The probable mechanisms for the blunted fever response include a disturbance in sensing of temperature by the thermoregulatory center in the hypothalamus, alterations in release of endogenous pyrogens, and the failure to elicit responses such as vasoconstriction of the skin vessels, increased heat production, and shivering that increase body temperature during a febrile response.

A factor that may delay recognition of fever in the elderly is the method of temperature measurement. Oral temperature remains the most commonly used method for measuring temperature in the elderly. It has been suggested that rectal and tympanic membrane are more effective in detecting fever in the elderly. This is because conditions such as mouth breathing, tongue tremors, and agitation often make it difficult to obtain accurate oral temperatures in the elderly.

Hyperthermia

Hyperthermia describes an increase in body temperature that occurs without a change in the set point of the hypothalamic thermoregulatory center. It occurs when the thermoregulatory mechanisms are overwhelmed by heat production, excessive environmental heat, or impaired dissipation of heat.[22,23] It includes (in order of increasing severity) heat cramps, heat syncope, heat exhaustion, and heatstroke. Malignant hyperthermia describes a rare genetic disorder of anesthetic-related hyperthermia. Fever and hyperthermia may also occur as the result of a drug reaction.

A number of factors predispose to hyperthermia. If muscle exertion is continued for long periods in warm weather, as often happens with athletes, military recruits, and laborers, excessive heat loads are generated.[24] Adequate circulatory function is essential for heat dissipation. Elderly persons and those with cardiovascular disease are at increased risk for hyperthermia. Drugs that increase muscle tone and metabolism or reduce heat loss (*e.g.*, diuretics, neuroleptics, drugs with anticholinergic action) can impair thermoregulation. Infants and small children who are left in a closed car for even short periods in hot weather are potential victims of hyperthermia. Florence Nightingale in *Notes on Nursing* observed that an excess of blankets is the commonest cause of fever in the hospital.[25]

Heat Cramps

Heat cramps are slow, painful, skeletal muscle cramps and spasms, usually in the muscles that are most heavily used, that last for 1 to 3 minutes. Cramping results from salt depletion that occurs when fluid losses from heavy sweating are replaced by water alone. The muscles are tender, and the skin is usually moist. Body temperature may be normal or slightly elevated. There is almost always a history of vigorous activity preceding the onset of symptoms.

Treatment consists of drinking an oral saline solution and resting in a cool environment. Because absorption is slow and unpredictable, salt tablets are not recommended. Salt tablets can also cause gastric irritation, vomiting, and cerebral edema. Strenuous physical activity should be avoided for several days, while dietary sodium replacement is continued.

Heat Syncope

Heat syncope is characterized by a sudden episode of unconsciousness resulting from cutaneous vasodilation and subsequent hypotension. Usually the episode follows vigorous exercise. The systolic blood pressure is usually less than 100 mm Hg, the pulse is weak, and the skin is cool and moist. The treatment consists of recumbency and rest in a cool place and administration of fluids orally or intravenously.

Heat Exhaustion

Heat exhaustion is related to a gradual loss of salt and water, usually after prolonged and heavy exertion in a hot environment. The symptoms include thirst, fatigue, nausea, oliguria, giddiness, and finally delirium. Gastrointestinal flulike symptoms are common. Hyperventilation in association with heat exhaustion may contribute to heat cramps and tetany by causing respiratory alkalosis. The skin is moist, the rectal temperature is usually higher than 37.8°C (100°F), and the heart rate is elevated, usually by more than half again the normal resting rate. Signs of heat syncope and heat cramps may accompany heat exhaustion.

Like heat cramps, heat exhaustion is treated by rest in a cool environment, the provision of adequate hydration, and salt replacement. Intravenous fluids are administered when adequate oral intake cannot be achieved.

Heatstroke

Heatstroke is a severe, life-threatening failure of thermoregulatory mechanisms resulting in an excessive rise in body temperature—a core temperature greater than 40°C (104°F), absence of sweating, and loss of consciousness. Evaporation serves as the major mechanism for heat dissipation in a warm environment, and conditions that interrupt this mechanism predispose to increased body temperature and heatstroke.

Heatstroke is seen most commonly in the elderly and disabled. Mortality may be as high as 80% among persons older than 65 years of age. In the United States, approximately 5000 deaths occur each year from heatstroke, with two thirds of these are persons older than 60 years.[26] In the elderly, the problem is often one of impaired heat loss and failure of homeostatic mechanisms, such that body temperature rises with any increase in environmental temperature. Elderly persons with decreased perception of environmental temperature changes and decreased mobility are at particular risk, because they may also be unable to take appropriate measures such as removing clothing, moving to a cooler environment, and increasing fluid intake. This is particularly true of elderly persons who live alone in small and poorly ventilated housing units and who may be too confused or weak to complain or seek help at the onset of symptoms.

The symptoms of heatstroke include dizziness, weakness, emotional lability, nausea and vomiting, confusion, delirium, blurred vision, convulsions, collapse, and coma. The skin is hot and usually dry, and the pulse is typically strong initially. The blood pressure may be elevated at first, but hypotension develops as the condition progresses. As vascular collapse occurs, the skin becomes cool. Associated abnormalities include electrocardiographic changes consistent with heart damage, blood coagulation disorders, potassium and sodium depletion, and signs of liver damage.

Treatment consists of rapidly reducing the core temperature. Care must be taken that the cooling methods used do not produce vasoconstriction or shivering and thereby decrease the cooling rate or induce heat production. Two general methods of cooling are used. One method involves submersion in cold water or application of ice packs, and the other involves spraying the body with tepid water while a fan is used to enhance heat dissipation through convection. Whatever method is used, it is important that the temperature of vital structures, such as the brain, heart, and liver, be reduced rapidly, because tissue damage ensues when core temperatures rise above 43°C (109.4°F). Selective brain cooling has been achieved by fanning the face during hyperthermia.[27] Blood flows from the emissary venous pathways of the skin on the head through the bones of the skull to the brain. In hyperthermia, face fanning is thought to cool the venous blood that flows through these emissary veins and thereby produce brain cooling by enhancing heat exchange between the hot arterial blood and the surface-cooled venous blood within the intracranial venous spaces.

Drug Fever

Drug fever has been defined as fever coinciding with the administration of a drug and disappearing after the drug has been discontinued.[28–30] Drugs can induce fever by several mechanisms. They can interfere with heat dissipation; they can alter temperature regulation by the hypothalamic centers; they can act as direct pyrogens;

they can injure tissues directly; or they can induce an immune response.[31]

Exogenous thyroid hormone increases metabolic rate and can increase heat production and body temperature. Peripheral heat dissipation can be impaired by atropine, antihistamines, phenothiazines, and tricyclic antidepressants, which decrease sweating, or by sympathomimetic drugs, which produce peripheral vasoconstriction. Cimetidine, a histamine$_2$ (H_2)–blocking drug that decreases gastric acid production, also blocks H_2 receptors in the hypothalamus and has been known to cause fever. Bleomycin (an anticancer drug), amphotericin B (an antifungal drug), and allergic extracts and vaccines that contain bacterial and viral products can all act to induce the release of pyrogens. Intravenously administered drugs can lead to infusion-related phlebitis with production of cellular pyrogens that produce fever. Treatment with anticancer drugs can cause the release of endogenous pyrogen from the cancer cells that are destroyed.

The most common cause of drug fever is a hypersensitivity reaction. Hypersensitivity drug fevers develop after several weeks of exposure to the drug, cannot be explained in terms of the drug's pharmacologic action, are not related to drug dose, disappear when the drug is stopped, and reappear when the drug is readministered. The fever pattern is typically spiking in nature and exhibits a normal diurnal rhythm. Persons with drug fevers often experience other signs of hypersensitivity reactions, such as arthralgias, urticaria, myalgias, gastrointestinal discomfort, and rashes.

Temperatures of 38.8°C to 40.0°C (102°F to 104°F) are common in drug fever. The person may be unaware of the fever and appear to be well for the degree of fever that is present. The absence of an appropriate increase in heart rate for the degree of temperature elevation is an important clue to the diagnosis of drug fever. A fever often precedes other, more serious effects of a drug reaction; for this reason, the early recognition of drug fever is important. Drug fever should be suspected whenever the temperature elevation is unexpected and occurs despite improvement in the condition for which the drug was prescribed.

Malignant Hyperthermia

Malignant hyperthermia is an autosomal dominant metabolic disorder in which heat generated by uncontrolled skeletal muscle contraction can produce severe and potentially fatal hyperthermia. The muscle contraction is caused by an abnormal release of intracellular calcium from the mitochondria and sarcoplasmic reticulum (see Chapter 1).

In affected persons, an episode of malignant hyperthermia is triggered by exposure to certain stresses or general anesthetic agents. The syndrome is most frequently associated with the halogenated anesthetic agents and the depolarizing muscle relaxant succinylcholine.[32] There are also various nonoperative precipitating factors, including trauma, exercise, environmental heat stress, and infection. The condition is particularly dangerous in a young person who has a large muscle mass to generate heat.

During malignant hyperthermia, the body temperature can rise as high as 43°C (109.4°F) at a rate of 1°C every 5 minutes. An initial sign of the disorder, when the condition occurs during anesthesia, is skeletal muscle rigidity. Cardiac arrhythmias and a hypermetabolic state follow in rapid sequence unless the triggering event is immediately discontinued. In addition to discontinuing the triggering agents, treatment includes measures to cool the body and the administration of dantrolene, a muscle relaxant drug. There is no accurate screening test for the condition. A family history of malignant hyperthermia should be considered when general anesthesia is needed, because there are anesthetic agents available that do not trigger the hyperthermic response.

Neuroleptic Malignant Syndrome

Neuroleptic malignant syndrome, which is usually explosive in onset, and consists of hyperthermia, muscle rigidity, alterations in consciousness, and autonomic nervous system dysfunction. The hyperthermia is accompanied by tachycardia (120 to 180 beats/minute) and cardiac dysrhythmias, labile blood pressure (70/50 mm Hg to 180/130 mm Hg), postural instability, dyspnea, and tachypnea (18 to 40 breaths/minute).[33] Permanent brain damage may result, and the mortality rate is nearly 30%.[34]

The disorder is associated with neuroleptic (psychotropic) medications and may occur in as many as 1% of persons taking such drugs. Some of the most commonly implicated drugs are haloperidol, chlorpromazine, thioridazine, and thiothixene. All of these drugs block dopamine receptors in the basal ganglia and hypothalamus. Hyperthermia is thought to result from alterations in the function of the hypothalamic thermoregulatory center caused by decreased dopamine levels or from uncontrolled muscle contraction like that occurring with anesthetic-induced malignant hyperthermia. Many of the neuroleptic drugs increase muscle contraction, suggesting that this mechanism may contribute to the neuroleptic malignant syndrome.

Treatment for neuroleptic malignant syndrome includes the immediate discontinuance of the neuroleptic drug, measures to decrease body temperature, and treatment of dysrhythmias and other complications of the disorder. Bromocriptine (a dopamine agonist) and dantrolene (a muscle relaxant) may be used as part of the treatment regimen.

In summary, fever and hyperthermia refer to an increase in body temperature outside the normal range. True fever is a disorder of thermoregulation in which there is an upward displacement of the set point for temperature control. In hyperthermia, the set point is unchanged, but the challenge to temperature regulation exceeds the thermoregulatory center's ability to control body temperature. Fever can be caused by a number of factors, including microorganisms, trauma, and drugs or chemicals, all of which incite the release of interleukin (formerly called endogenous pyrogen).

The reactions that occur during fever consist of four stages: a prodrome, a chill, a flush, and defervescence. A fever can follow an intermittent, remittent, sustained, or recurrent pattern. The manifestations of fever are largely related to dehydration and an increased metabolic rate. Even a low-grade fever in high-risk infants or in the elderly can indicate serious infection.

The treatment of fever focuses on modifying the external environment as a means of increasing heat transfer to the external environment; supporting the hypermetabolic state that accompanies fever; protecting vulnerable body tissues; and treating the infection or condition causing the fever.

Hyperthermia includes heat syncope, heat cramps, heat exhaustion, and heatstroke. Among the factors that contribute to the development of hyperthermia are prolonged muscular exertion in a hot environment, disorders that compromise heat dissipation, and hypersensitivity drug reactions. Malignant hyperthermia is an autosomal dominant disorder that can produce a severe and potentially fatal increase in body temperature. The condition is commonly triggered by general anesthetic agents and muscle relaxants used during surgery. The neuroleptic malignant syndrome is associated with neuroleptic drug therapy and is thought to result from alterations in the function of the thermoregulatory center or from uncontrolled muscle contraction.

Decreased Body Temperature

After you have completed this section of the chapter, you should be able to meet the following objectives:

- Define *hypothermia*
- Compare the manifestations of mild, moderate, and severe hypothermia and relate to changes in physiologic functioning that occur with decreased body temperature

Hypothermia

Hypothermia is defined as a core (*i.e.*, rectal, esophageal, or tympanic) temperature less than 35°C.[35,36] Core body temperatures in the range of 34°C to 35°C (93.2°F to 95°F) are considered mildly hypothermic; 30°C to 34°C (86°F to 93.2°F), moderately hypothermic; and less than 30°C (86°F), severely hypothermic.[37,38]

Accidental hypothermia may be defined as a spontaneous decrease in core temperature, usually in a cold environment and associated with an acute problem but without primary pathology of the temperature-regulating center. The term *submersion hypothermia* is used when cooling follows acute asphyxia, as occurs in drowning.[39] In children, the rapid cooling process, in addition to the diving reflex that triggers apnea and circulatory shunting to establish a heart-brain circulation (see Chapter 22), may account for the surprisingly high survival rate after submersion. The diving reflex is greatly diminished in adults. Children have been reported to survive 10 to 40 minutes of submersion asphyxia.[40,41] Controlled hypothermia may be used during certain types of surgeries to decrease brain metabolism.

Oral temperatures are markedly inaccurate during hypothermia because of severe vasoconstriction and sluggish blood flow. Electronic thermometers with flexible probes are available for measuring rectal, bladder, and esophageal temperatures. Rectal and bladder temperatures often lag behind fluctuations in core temperature, and esophageal temperatures may be elevated during inhalation of heated air.[35] Most clinical thermometers measure temperature only in the range of 35°C to 42°C (95°F to 107.6°F); a special thermometer that registers as low as 25°C (77°F) or an electrical thermistor probe is needed for monitoring temperatures in persons with hypothermia.[38]

Systemic hypothermia may result from exposure to prolonged cold (atmospheric or submersion). The condition may develop in otherwise healthy persons in the course of accidental exposure. Because water conducts heat more readily than air, body temperature drops rapidly when the body is submerged in cold water or when clothing becomes wet. In persons with altered homeostasis due to debility or disease, hypothermia may follow exposure to relatively small decreases in atmospheric temperature.

Elderly and inactive persons living in inadequately heated quarters are particularly vulnerable to hypothermia. Acute alcoholism is a common predisposing factor. Persons with cardiovascular disease, cerebrovascular disease, malnutrition, and hypothyroidism are also predisposed to hypothermia. The use of sedatives and tranquilizing drugs may be a contributing factor.

Manifestations

The signs and symptoms of hypothermia include poor coordination, stumbling, slurred speech, irrationality and poor judgment, amnesia, hallucinations, blueness and puffiness of the skin, dilation of the pupils, decreased respiratory rate, weak and irregular pulse, and stupor. With mild hypothermia, intense shivering generates heat and sympathetic nervous system activity is raised to resist lowering of temperature. Vasoconstriction can be profound, heart rate is accelerated, and stroke volume is increased. Blood pressure increases slightly, and hyperventilation is common. Exposure to cold augments urinary flow (*i.e.*, cold diuresis) before there is any fall in temperature. Dehydration and increased hematocrit may develop within a few hours of even mild hypothermia, augmented by an extracellular-to-intracellular water shift.

With moderate hypothermia, shivering gradually decreases, and the muscles become rigid. Shivering usually ceases at 27°C (80.6°F). Heart rate and stroke volume are reduced, and blood pressure falls. The greatest effect of hypothermia is exerted through a decrease in the metabolic rate, which falls to 50% of normal at 28°C (82.4°F).[42] Associated with this decrease in metabolic rate is a decrease in oxygen consumption and carbon dioxide production. There is roughly a 6% decrease in oxygen consumption per degree Celsius decrease in temperature. A decrease in carbon dioxide production leads to a decrease in respiratory rate. Respirations decrease as temperatures drop below 32.2°C (90°F). Decreases in mentation, the cough reflex, and respiratory tract secretions may lead to difficulty in clearing secretions and aspiration. Consciousness is usually lost at 30°C (86°F).[42]

In terms of cardiovascular function, a gradual decline in heart rate and cardiac output occurs as hypothermia progresses. Blood pressure initially rises and then gradually falls. There is increased risk of dysrhythmia developing, probably from myocardial hypoxia and autonomic nervous system imbalance. Ventricular fibrillation is a major cause of death in hypothermia.

Carbohydrate metabolism and insulin activity are decreased, resulting in a hyperglycemia that is proportional to the level of cooling. A cold-induced loss of cell membrane integrity allows intravascular fluids to move into the skin, giving the skin a puffy appearance. Acid-base disorders occur with increased frequency at temperatures below 25°C (77°F) unless adequate ventilation is maintained. Extracellular sodium and potassium concentrations decrease, and chloride levels increase. There is a temporary loss of plasma from the circulation along with sludging of red blood cells and increased blood viscosity as the result of trapping in the small vessels and skin.

Treatment

The treatment of hypothermia consists of rewarming, support of vital functions, and the prevention and treatment of complications. There are three methods of rewarming: passive rewarming, active total rewarming, and active core rewarming. Passive rewarming is done by removing the person from the cold environment, covering with a blanket, supplying warm fluids (oral or intravenous), and allowing rewarming to occur at the person's own pace. Active total rewarming involves immersing the person in warm water or placing heating pads or hot water bottles on the surface of the body, including the extremities. Active core rewarming places major emphasis on rewarming the trunk, leaving the extremities, containing the major metabolic mass, cold until the heart rewarms. Active rewarming can be done by instilling warmed fluids into the gastrointestinal tract; peritoneal dialysis; extracorporeal blood warming, in which blood is removed from the body and passed through a heat exchanger and then returned to the body; or warming by inhalation of an oxygen mixture warmed to 42°C to 46°C (107.6°F to 114.8°F).

Persons with mild hypothermia usually respond well to passive rewarming in a warm bed. Persons with moderate or severe hypothermia do not have the thermoregulatory shivering mechanism and require active rewarming. During rewarming, the cold acidotic blood from the peripheral tissues is returned to the heart and central circulation. If this is done too rapidly or before cardiopulmonary function has been adequately reestablished, the hypothermic heart cannot respond to the increased metabolic demands of warm peripheral tissues.

In summary, hypothermia is a potentially life-threatening disorder in which the body's core temperature drops below 35°C (95°F). Accidental hypothermia can develop in otherwise healthy persons in the course of accidental exposure and in elderly or disabled persons with impaired perception or response to cold. Alcoholism, cardiovascular disease, malnutrition, and hypothyroidism contribute to the risk of hypothermia. The greatest effect of hypothermia is a decrease in the metabolic rate, leading to a decrease in carbon dioxide production and respiratory rate. The signs and symptoms of hypothermia include poor coordination, stumbling, slurred speech, irrationality, poor judgment, amnesia, hallucinations, blueness and puffiness of the skin, dilation of the pupils, decreased respiratory rate, weak and irregular pulse, stupor, and coma. The treatment for moderate and severe hypothermia includes active rewarming.

REFERENCES

1. Guyton A.C., Hall J.E. (1996). *Textbook of medical physiology* (9th ed., pp. 911–922). Philadelphia: W.B. Saunders.
2. Vick R. (1984). *Contemporary medical physiology* (p. 886). Menlo Park, CA: Addison Wesley.
3. Beach P.S., McCormick D.P. (1991). Clinical applications of ear thermometry [editorial]. *Clinical Pediatrics* (Suppl), 3–4.
4. Atkins L. (1984). Fever: The old and new. *Journal of Infectious Diseases* 149, 339–348.
5. Stein M.T. (1991). Historical perspectives in fever and thermometry. *Clinical Pediatrics* (Suppl), 5–7.
6. Kruse J. (1988). Fever in children. *American Family Practice* 37 (2), 127–135.
7. Castle S.C., Norman D.C., Yeh M., et al. (1991). Fever response in elderly nursing home residents: Are the older truly colder? *Journal of the American Geriatric Society* 39, 853–857.
8. Yoshikawa T.T., Norman D.C. (1996). Approach to fever and infections in the nursing home. *Journal of American Geriatrics Society* 44, 74–82.
9. Norman D.C., Yoshikawa T.T. (1996). Fever in the elderly. *Infectious Disease Clinics of North America* 10 (1), 93–99.
10. Dinarellos C.A. (1989). The endogenous pyrogens. *Hospital Practice* 24 (11A), 111–128.
11. Saper C.B., Breder C.D. (1994). The neurologic basis of fever. *New England Journal of Medicine* 330 (26), 1880–1886.
12. Kluger M.J. (1986). Fever: A hot topic. *News of Physiologic Science* 1, 25–28.
13. Rodbard D. (1981). The role of regional temperature in the pathogenesis of disease. *New England Journal of Medicine* 305, 808–814.
14. McGee Z.A., Gorby G.L. (1987). The diagnostic value of fever patterns. *Hospital Practice* 22 (10), 103–110.
15. Cunha B.A. (1984). Implications of fever in the critical care setting. *Heart and Lung* 13, 460–465.

16. Cunha B.A. (1996). The clinical significance of fever patterns. *Infectious Disease Clinics of North America* 10 (1), 33–43.
17. Freeman JM., Vinning EPG. (1995). Febrile seizures: A decision-making analysis. *American Family Physician* 52 (5), 1401–1406.
18. Cunha B.A. (1996). Fever without source. *Infectious Disease Clinics of North America* 10 (1), 111–127.
19. Daaleman T.P. (1996). Fever without source in infants and young children. *American Family Physician* 54 (8), 2503–2512.
20. Baraff L.J., Bass J.W., Fleisher G.R., et al. (1993). Practice guidelines for the management of infants and children 0 to 36 months of age with fever without source. *Pediatrics* 82 (1), 1–12.
21. Castle S.C., Yeh M., Toledo S., et al. (1993). Lowering the temperature criterion improves detection of infections in nursing home residents. *Aging Immunology and Infectious Disease* 4, 67–76.
22. Simon HB (1993). Hyperthermia. *New England Journal of Medicine* 329 (7), 483–488.
23. Simon H.B. (1994). Hyperthermia and heatstroke. *Hospital Practice* 29 (8), 65–80.
24. Danzl D.F. (1988). Hyperthermic syndromes. *American Family Practice* 37 (6), 157.
25. Nightingale F. (1970). *Notes on nursing* (p. 45). London: Brandon Systems Press.
26. Halle A., Repasy A. (1987). Classic heatstroke: A serious challenge for the elderly. *Hospital Practice* 22 (5), 26–35.
27. Brinnel H., Nagasaka T., Cabanac M. (1987). Enhanced brain protection during passive hyperthermia in humans. *European Journal of Applied Physiology* 56, 540–545.
28. Tabor P.A. (1986). Drug-induced fever. *Drug Intelligence and Clinical Pharmacy* 20, 413–420.
29. Mackowiak P.A., LeMaistre C.F. (1986). Drug fever: A critical appraisal of conventional concepts. *Annals of Internal Medicine* 106, 728–733.
30. Hofland S.L. (1985). Drug fever: Is your patient's fever drug-related. *Critical Care Nurse* 5, 29–34.
31. Johnson D.H., Cunha B.A. (1996). Drug fever. *Infectious Disease Clinics of North America* 10 (1), 85–99.
32. Nelson T.E., Flewellen E.H. (1983). The malignant hyperthermia syndrome. *New England Journal of Medicine* 309, 416–418.
33. Parker W.A. (1987). Neuroleptic malignant syndrome. *Critical Care Nurse* 7, 40–46.
34. Goldwasser H.D., Hooper J.F. (1988). Neuroleptic malignant syndrome. *American Family Practice* 38 (5), 211–216.
35. Danzl D.F., Pozos R.S. (1994). Accidental hypothermia. *New England Journal of Medicine* 331 (26), 1756–1760.
36. Celestina F.S., Van Noord G.R., Miraglia C.P. (1988). Accidental hypothermia in the elderly. *Journal of Family Practice* 26, 259–267.
37. Lønning P.E., Skulberg A., Abyholm F. (1986). Accidental hypothermia. *Acta Anaesthesiologica Scandinavica* 30, 601–613.
38. Division of Environmental Hazards and Health Effects. (1985). Hypothermia-associated death—United States, 1968–1980. *Morbidity and Mortality Weekly Report* 34, 48.
39. Conn A.W. (1979). Near drowning and hypothermia. *Canadian Medical Association Journal* 120, 397–400.
40. Siebke H., Beivik H., Rod T. (1975). Survival after 40 minutes submersion with cerebral sequelae. *Lancet* 1, 1275–1277.
41. Moss J.F. (1988). The management of accidental severe hypothermia. *New York Journal of Medicine* 88, 411–413.
42. Wong K.C. (1983). Physiology and pharmacology of hypothermia. *Western Journal of Medicine* 138, 227–232.

ADDITIONAL READINGS

Alexander D., Kelly B. (1991). Responses of children, parents, and nurses to tympanic thermometry in the pediatric office. *Clinical Pediatrics* (Suppl), 53–59.

Bruce J.L., Grove S.K. (1992). Fever: Pathology and treatment. *Critical Care Nurse* 12 (1), 40–49.

Enright T., Hill M.G. (1989). Treatment of fever. *Focus on Critical Care* 16 (2), 96–102.

Hanson M.A. (1991). Drug fever. *Postgraduate Medicine* 89 (5), 167–173.

Kimmel S., Gemmill D.W. (1988). The young child with fever. *American Family Practice* 37, 196.

Keating H.J., Klimek J.J., Levine D.S., et al. (1984). Effect of age on the clinical significance of fever in ambulatory adult patients. *Journal of the American Geriatric Society* 32, 282–287.

Kellerman A.L., Todd K.H. (1996). Killing heat. *New England Journal of Medicine* 335 (2), 126–127.

Klein N.C., Cunha B.A. (1994). Treatment of fever. *Infectious Disease Clinics of North America* 10 (1), 211–216.

Kluger M.J., Kozak W., Conn C.A., Leon L.R., Soszynski D. (1996). The adaptive value of fever. *Infectious Disease Clinics of North America* 10 (1), 1–19.

Musher D.M., Fainstein V., Young E.J., et al. (1979). Fever patterns: Their lack of clinical significance. *Archives of Internal Medicine* 139, 1225.

Newman J. (1985). Evaluation of sponging to reduce body temperature in febrile children. *Canadian Medical Association Journal* 132, 641.

Pizzo P.A. (1993). Management of fever in patients with cancer and treatment-induced neutropenia. *New England Journal of Medicine* 328 (18), 1323–1332.

Powers J.H., Scheid W.M. (1996). Fever in neurologic diseases. *Infectious Disease Clinics of North America* 10 (1), 45–66.

Sarwari A.R., Mackowiak P.A. (1996). The pharmacologic consequences of fever. *Infectious Disease Clinics of North America* 10 (1), 21–32.

Styrt B., Sugarman B. (1990). Antipyresis and fever. *Archives of Internal Medicine* 150, 1589–1597.

Developmental Aspects of Altered Health

Early peoples were considered long-lived if they reached 30 years of age—that is, if they survived infancy. For many centuries, infant mortality was so great that large families became the tradition; many children in a family ensured that at least some would survive. Life expectancy has increased over the centuries, and today an individual in a developed country can expect to live about 71 to 79 years. Although life expectancy has increased radically since ancient times, human longevity has remained fundamentally unchanged.

The quest to solve the mystery of human longevity, which appears to be genetically programmed, began with Gregor Mendel (1822–1884), an Augustinian monk. Mendel laid the foundation of modern genetics with the pea experiments he performed in a monastery garden. Today, geneticists search for the determinant, or determinants, of the human life span. Up to this time, scientists have failed to identify an aging gene that would account for a limited life span. However, they have found that cells have a finite reproductive capacity. As they age, genes are increasingly unable to perform their functions. The cells become poorer and poorer at making the substances they need for their own special tasks or even for their own maintenance. Free radicals, mutation in a cell's DNA, and the process of programmed cell death are some of the factors that work together to affect a cell's functioning.

UNIT XV

CHAPTER 57

Concepts of Altered Health in Children

Marianne Sigda and Judy Wright Lott

Children are not merely small adults. Their level of maturity in terms of physical and psychologic development strongly influences the type of illnesses they experience and their responses to these illnesses. Although many signs and symptoms are the same in persons of all ages, some diseases and complications are more likely to occur in the child. This chapter provides an overview of the developmental stages of childhood and their relationship to the health care needs of children. Specific diseases are presented throughout other sections of the book.

At the beginning of the 20th century, a child's chances of obtaining adulthood in the United States were limited. The infant mortality rate was 200 infant deaths per 1000 live births. Infectious diseases were rampant, and children were especially vulnerable. With the introduction of antibiotics, infectious disease control, and nutritional and technologic advances, infant mortality decreased dramatically. In 1991, the infant mortality rate for the United States, 8.9 deaths per 1000 live births, was the lowest ever recorded. However, when this infant mortality rate is compared with the rates of other developed countries, the United States is ranked number 24 out of 37 countries.[1] Also of great concern is the difference in mortality rates for white and African-American infants. In 1989, the mortality rates for white and African-American infants were 8.4 and 16.5 deaths per 1000 live births, respectively, with the leading cause of death in African-American infants being prematurity and low birth weight. For white infants, the leading cause of death is congenital anomalies.[1–3]

Although the efforts to improve these rates are aimed at improving access to prenatal care, two underlying causes of neonatal (*i.e.*, infants younger than 28 days of age) mortality, congenital anomalies and preterm delivery, are still poorly understood despite continuing research. Many of the major causes of death during the postneonatal period (*i.e.*, age 28 days to 1 year), deaths from infectious diseases (*e.g.*, pneumonia, influenza), and accidents are preventable through health promotion efforts such as well-baby care, immunizations, and teaching of parenting skills.

Growth and Development

After you have completed this section of the chapter, you should be able to meet the following objectives:

- Characterize the use of percentiles to describe growth and development during infancy and childhood
- Describe the major events that occur during prenatal development from fertilization to birth
- Define the terms *low birth weight, small for gestational age,* and *large for gestational age*
- Identify reasons for abnormal uterine growth
- Describe assessment methods for determination of gestational age

The term *growth and development* describes a process whereby a fertilized ovum becomes an adult person.[4]

Physical growth describes changes in the body as a whole or in its individual parts. Development, on the other hand, embraces other aspects of differentiation such as changes in body function and psychosocial behaviors.

Physical growth occurs in a cephalocaudal direction. Relative body proportions change over the lifespan. In early fetal development, the head is the largest part of the body, but this changes as the individual grows (Fig. 57–1).

The average newborn weighs approximately 3000 to 4000 g and is 50 to 53 cm long. The first year is a period of rapid growth demonstrated by lengthening of the trunk and accumulation of subcutaneous fat. After the first year and entering into puberty, the legs grow more rapidly than any other part of the body.

The onset of puberty is marked by a significant alteration in body proportions because of the effects of the pubertal growth spurt. The feet and hands are the first to increase. Because the trunk grows faster than the legs, at adolescence a large portion of the increase in height is a result of trunk growth. The brain is another organ that undergoes a period of rapid growth. At birth, the brain is 25% of adult size; at 1 year, it is 50% of adult size; and at 5 years, it is 90% of adult size. The size of the head reflects brain growth.[2] Linear growth is a result of skeletal growth. After maturation of the skeleton is complete, linear growth is complete. By 2 years of age, the length is 50% of the adult height. Beginning with the third year, the growth rate is 5 to 6 cm for the next 9 years. During the adolescent period, there is a growth spurt. Males may add approximately 20 cm and females 16 cm to height during this time. Terminal height is reached by 16.5 years in females and 17.75 years in males. Weight is rapidly increased after birth. By 6 months of age, the birth weight is doubled, and by 1 year, it is tripled. The average weight increase is 2 to 2.75 kg per year until the adolescent growth spurt begins.[2]

Growth and development encompass a complex interaction between genetic and environmental influences. The experience of each child is unique, and the patterns of growth and development may be profoundly different for individual children within the context of what is called normal. Because of the wide variability, these norms can often be expressed only in statistical terms.

Evaluation of growth and development requires comparison of an individual's growth and development to a standard of growth and development. Statistics are calculations derived from measurements that are used to describe the sample measured or to make (infer) predictions about the rest of the population that the sample represented. Because all individuals grow and develop at different rates, the standard for growth and development must somehow take this individual variation into account. The standard is typically derived from measurements made on a sample of individuals deemed representative of the total population. When multiple measurements of biologic variables such as height, weight, head circumference, and blood pressure are made, most values fall around the center or middle of all the values. Plotting the data on a graph yields a bell-shaped curve, which depicts the normal distribution of these continuously variable values (Fig. 57–2).

The mean and standard deviation are common statistics used in describing the characteristics of a population. The *mean* represents the average of the measurements. It is the sum of the values divided by the number of values. A normal bell-shaped curve is symmetric, with the mean falling in the center of the curve and with one half of the values falling on either side of the mean. The *standard deviation* determines how far a value varies or deviates from the mean. The points one standard deviation above and below the mean include 68% of all values, two standard deviations 95% of all values, and three standard deviations 99.7% of all values. If a child's height is within one standard deviation of the mean, he or she is as tall as 68% of children in the population. If a child's height is greater than three standard deviations, he or she is taller than 99.7% of children in the population.[5]

The bell-shaped curve can also be marked by percentiles, which are useful for comparison of an individual's values to other values. When quantitative data are arranged in ascending and descending order, a middle value called the *median* can be described with one half (50%) of the values falling on either side. The values can be further divided into percentiles. A percentile is a number that indicates the percentage of values for the population that are equal to or below the number. Percentiles are most often used to compare an individual's value with a set of norms. They are used extensively to

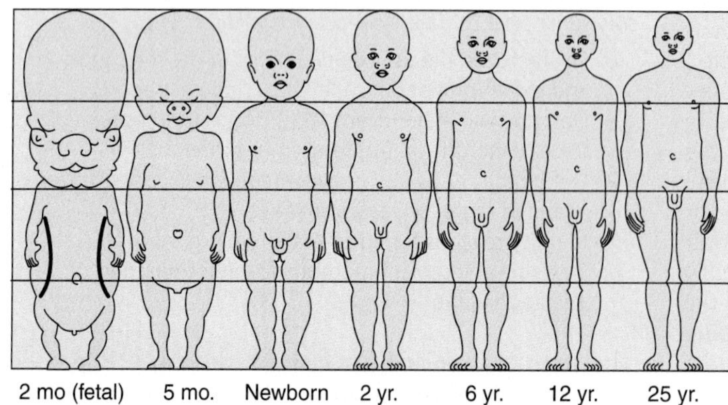

Figure 57–1 Changes in body proportions from the 2nd fetal month to adulthood. (Robbins W.J., Brody S., Hogan A.G., et al. [1928]. *Growth.* New Haven: Yale University Press. By permission of publisher)

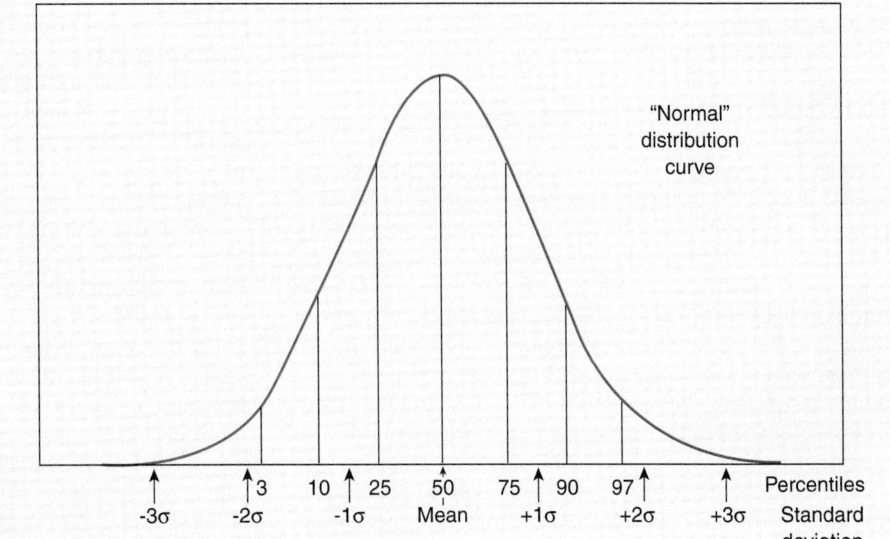

Figure 57–2 "Normal" (gaussian) distribution curve. This curve represents the theoretical distribution of values for many biologic measurements. The percentiles indicate certain positions within this distribution, as do the standard deviations from the mean. (Nelson W.E. [Ed.][1959]: *Textbook of pediatrics* [7th ed., p. 18]. Philadelphia: W.B. Saunders)

develop and interpret physical growth charts and measurements of ability and intelligence.

Prenatal Growth and Development

Human development is considered to begin with fertilization, the union of sperm and ovum resulting in a zygote. The process begins with the intermingling of a haploid number of paternal (23, X or Y) and maternal (23, X) chromosomes in the ampulla of the oviduct that fuse to form a zygote. Within 24 hours, the unicellular organism becomes a two-cell organism and, within 72 hours, a 16-cell organism, called a *morula*. This series of mitotic divisions is called *cleavage*. During cleavage, the rapidly developing cell mass travels down the oviduct to the uterus by a series of peristaltic movements. The morula enters the uterus about 3 days after fertilization. On the fourth day, the morula is separated into two parts by fluid from the uterus. The outer layer gives rise to the placenta (trophoblast), and the inner layer gives rise to the embryo (embryoblast). The structure is now called a *blastocyte*. By the sixth day, the blastocyte attaches to the endometrium. This is the beginning of implantation, and it is completed during the second week of development.[6]

Prenatal development is divided into two main periods. The first period, or *embryonic*, period, begins during the second week and continues through the eighth week after fertilization. During the embryonic period, the main organ systems are developed and many function at a minimal level (see Chapter 4). The second, or *fetal*, period begins during the ninth week. During the fetal period, the growth and differentiation of the body and organ systems occur.

Embryonic Development

With the onset of embryonic development, which begins during the second week of gestation, the trophoblast continues its rapid proliferation and differentiation, and the embryoblast evolves into a bilaminar embryonic disk. This flattened, circular plate of cells gives rise to all three germ layers of the embryo (*i.e.*, ectoderm, mesoderm, endoderm). The third week is a period of rapid development, noted for the conversion of the bilaminar embryonic disk into a trilaminar embryonic disk through a process called *gastrulation*.[6] The ectoderm differentiates into the epidermis and nervous system, and the endoderm gives rise to the epithelial linings of the respiratory passages, digestive tract, and glandular cells of organs such as the liver and pancreas. The mesoderm becomes smooth muscle tissue, connective tissue, blood vessels, blood cells, bone marrow, skeletal tissue, striated muscle tissue, and reproductive and excretory organs.

The notochord, which is the primitive axis about which the axial skeleton forms, is also formed during the third week (see Chapter 37). The neurologic system begins its development during this period. *Neurulation*, a process that involves formation of the neural plate, neural folds, and their closure, is completed by the fourth week. Disturbances during this period can result in brain and spinal defects such as spina bifida. The cardiovascular system is the first functional organ system to develop. The primitive heart, which beats and circulates blood, develops during this period (see Chapter 19).

By the fourth week, the neural tube is formed.[6] The embryo begins to curve and fold into a characteristic C-shaped structure. The limb buds are visible, as are the otic pits (*i.e.*, primordia of the internal ears) and the lens placodes (primordia of the lens of the eyes). The fifth week is notable for the rapid growth of the head secondary to brain growth.

During the sixth week, the upper limbs are formed by fusion of the swellings around the branchial groove. In the seventh week, there is the beginning of the digits, and the intestines enter the umbilical cord (umbilical herniation).[6] By the eighth week, the embryo is human-like in appearance; eyes are open, eyelids and ear auricles are easily identified.

Fetal Development

During the 9th to 12th weeks, fetal head growth slows, whereas body length growth is greatly accelerated. By the 11th week, the intestines in the proximal portion of the cord have returned to the abdomen. The primary ossification centers are present in the skull and long bones, and maturation of the fetal external genitalia is established by the 12th week. During the fetal period, the liver is the major site of red blood cell formation (*i.e.*, erythropoiesis); at 12 weeks, this activity has decreased and erythropoiesis begins in the spleen. Urine begins to form during the 9th to 12th week and is excreted into the amniotic fluid.[6]

The 13th through 16th weeks are notable for ossification of the skeleton, scalp hair patterning, and differentiation of the ovaries in female fetuses. By the 17th through 20th week, growth has slowed. The fetal skin is covered with a fine hair called *lanugo* and a white cheeselike material called *vernix caseosa*. Eyebrows and head hair are visible. In male fetuses, the testes begin to descend, and in female fetuses, the uterus is formed. Brown fat also forms during this period. Brown fat is a specialized type of adipose tissue that produces heat by oxidizing fatty acids. It is similar to white fat but has larger and more numerous mitochondria, which provide its brown color. Brown fat is found near the heart and blood vessels that supply the brain and kidneys and is thought to play a role in maintaining the temperature of these organs during exposure to environmental changes that occur after birth.

During the 25th through 26th weeks, there is a significant fetal weight gain. The type II alveolar cells of the lung begin to secrete surfactant (see Chapter 23). The pulmonary system becomes more mature and able to support respiration during the 26th through 29th weeks. Breathing movements are present secondary to central nervous system (CNS) maturation. There is also an increasing amount of subcutaneous fat, with white fat making up 3.3% of body weight.

The 30th through 34th weeks are significant for an increasing amount of white fat (8% of body weight), which gives the fetal limbs an almost chubby appearance.[6] During the 35th week, grasp and the pupillary light reflex are present.

Expected time of birth is 264 days or 38 weeks after fertilization or 40 weeks after the last menstrual period (LMP).[6] At this time, the neurologic, cardiovascular, and pulmonary systems are developed enough for the baby to make the transition to extrauterine life. The survival of the newborn depends on this adaptation after the placenta is removed.

Fetal Growth and Weight Gain. Normal growth progresses through three phases. During the first stage of embryonic and early fetal life, there is growth through cell multiplication or hyperplasia. During this phase, new cells are formed through mitosis, which is the basis for organ and tissue development and growth.[7–9] During the second stage of growth, the middle of gestation, hyperplasia continues, although at a slower rate, and growth is through enlargement of existing cells by addition of cytoplasm or hypertrophy. The last phase of growth, or the end of gestation, is primarily hypertrophy (*i.e.*, cell enlargement), although some hyperplasia is ongoing. As cells enlarge, cellular differentiation is occurring and hyperplasia is decreasing. This occurs after a few weeks of rapid hyperplasia. The process of growth is ongoing, and hypertrophy and hyperplasia continue after birth.

Fetal weight gain is linear beginning at 20 weeks' gestation, until 38 weeks' gestation. In the last half of pregnancy, the fetus gains 85% of birth weight. After 38 weeks of gestation, the rate of growth declines, probably related to the constraint of uterine size and decreased placental function. After birth, weight gain again increases similar to intrauterine rates. Birth weight can be affected by a variety of factors, including maternal nutrition, genetic factors, maternal chronic diseases, placental abnormalities, sex, socioeconomic factors, multiple births, chromosomal abnormalities, and infectious diseases.

Birth Weight and Gestational Age

At birth, the average weight of the full-term newborn is 3000 to 4000 g. In the past, infants weighing less than 2500 g were classified as premature. In 1961, infants weighing less than 2500 g were classified as low birth weight (LBW). Lubchenco and Battagila established standards for birth weight, gestational age, and intrauterine growth in the United States in the 1960s (Fig. 57–3).[10,11] With these standards, gestational age can be assessed and normal and abnormal growth can be identified. The *Colorado Growth Curve* places newborns into percentiles.[10] The 10th through 90th percentiles of intrauterine growth encompass 80% of births.[12] Growth is considered abnormal when a newborn falls above or below the 90th and 10th percentiles, respectively.

An infant is considered term when born between the beginning of the 38th week and completion of the 41st week. An infant is considered premature when born before the end of the 37th week and postmature when born at the end of the 41st week. The lowest rates of mortality occurs among newborns with weight between 3000 and 4000 g with gestational ages 38 to 42 weeks.[7–9]

Abnormal Intrauterine Growth

Growth of the fetus in the uterus depends on a multitude of intrinsic and extrinsic factors. Optimal fetal growth depends on efficient placental function, adequate provision of energy and growth substrates, appropriate hormonal environment, and adequate room in the uterus. Birth weight variability in a population is primarily determined by maternal heredity, intrinsic fetal growth potential, and environmental factors. Abnormal growth, which can occur at any time during fetal devel-

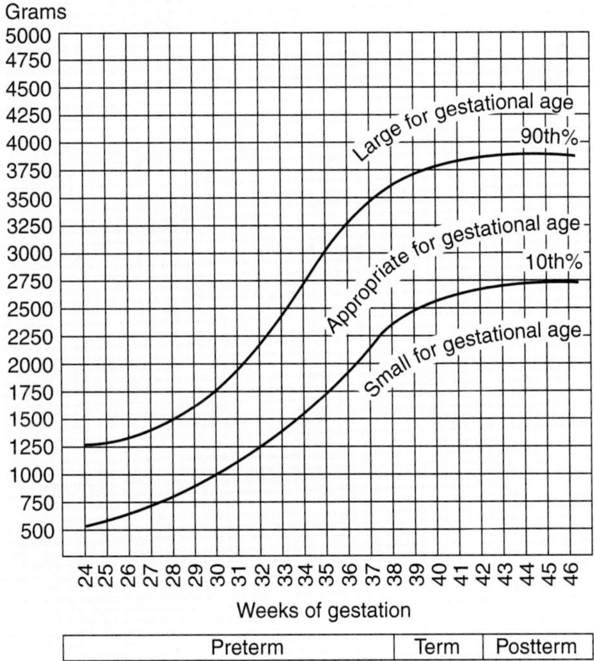

Figure 57–3
Classification of newborns by birth weight and gestational age. (Redrawn from Battaglia F.C., & Lubchenco L.O. [1967]. A practical classification of newborn infants by weight and gestational age. *Journal of Pediatrics, 71,* 159)

opment, can have immediate and long-term consequences for the infant.

Small for Gestational Age. Small for gestational age (SGA) is a term that denotes fetal undergrowth. SGA is defined as birth weight less than two standard deviations below the mean for gestational age or below the 10th percentile. It is often used interchangeably with intrauterine growth retardation (IUGR). Worldwide, between 30% and 40% of infants born at weights less than 2500 g are SGA. Mortality rates of severely affected SGA infants are five to six times that of normally grown infants of comparable gestational age.

Fetal growth retardation can occur anytime during fetal development. Depending on the time of insult, the infant can have symmetric or proportional growth retardation or asymmetric or disproportional growth retardation. Impaired growth that occurs early in pregnancy during the hyperplastic phase of growth results in a symmetric growth retardation. Because mitosis is affected, organ and tissues are smaller because of decreased cell number. Head circumference, length, and weight usually are represented within similar percentile grids, although the head may be smaller, as in microcephaly.[13] This is irreversible postnatally. Causes of proportional IUGR include chromosomal abnormalities, congenital infections, and exposure to environmental toxins.

Impaired growth that occurs later in pregnancy during the hypertrophic phase of growth results in asymmetric growth retardation.[7–9] Infants with IUGR due to intrauterine malnutrition often have weight reduction out of proportion to length or head circumference but are spared impairment of head and brain growth.[2,14] Tissues and organs are small because of decreased cell size, not decreased cell numbers. Postnatally, the impairment may be partially corrected with good nutrition.

Maternal, placental, and environmental factors affect fetal growth. Because of the effects on the placenta (it is also undergrown), the risk for perinatal complications is higher. These include birth asphyxia, hyperglycemia, polycythemia, meconium (*i.e.,* dark green, mucilaginous newborn stool) aspiration, and hypothermia. The long-term effects of growth retardation depend on the timing and severity of the insult. Many of these infants have been found to have developmental disabilities on follow-up examination, especially if the growth retardation was symmetric. They may remain small, especially if the insult occurs early. If the insult occurs later because of placental insufficiency or uterine restraint, with good nutrition catch-up growth can occur and the infant may attain appropriate growth.

Large for Gestational Age. Large for gestational age (LGA) is a term that denotes fetal overgrowth. The definition of LGA is birth weight greater than two standard deviations above the mean for gestation or above the 90th percentile. The excessive growth may result from a genetic predisposition or stimulated by abnormal conditions in utero. Infants of diabetic mothers may be LGA, especially if the diabetes was poorly controlled during pregnancy. Maternal hyperglycemia exposes the fetus to increased levels of glucose, which stimulates fetal secretion of insulin. Insulin increases fat disposition, and the result is a macrosomic infant. Babies with macrosomia have enlarged viscera and are large and plump because of an increase in body fat. Complications when an infant is LGA include birth asphyxia and trauma due to mechanical difficulties during the birth process, hypoglycemia, and polycythemia.[7]

Assessment Methods

The methods of assessing gestation can be divided into two categories: prenatal assessment and postnatal assessment. Prenatal assessment of gestational age most commonly includes careful menstrual history, physical milestones during pregnancy (*e.g.,* uterine size, detection of fetal heart rate and movements), and prenatal tests for maturity (*e.g.,* ultrasound, amniotic fluid studies). Nägele's rule uses the first day of the LMP to calculate the day of labor by adding 7 days to the LMP and counting back 3 months.[7] This method can often be inaccurate if the mother is not a good historian or has a history of irregular menses, which interferes with identification of a normal cycle.

Postnatal assessment of gestational age is most commonly done by examination of external physical and neuromuscular characteristics alone or in combination. The most common methods used in nurseries today were developed by Dubowitz or Ballard. The Dubowitz

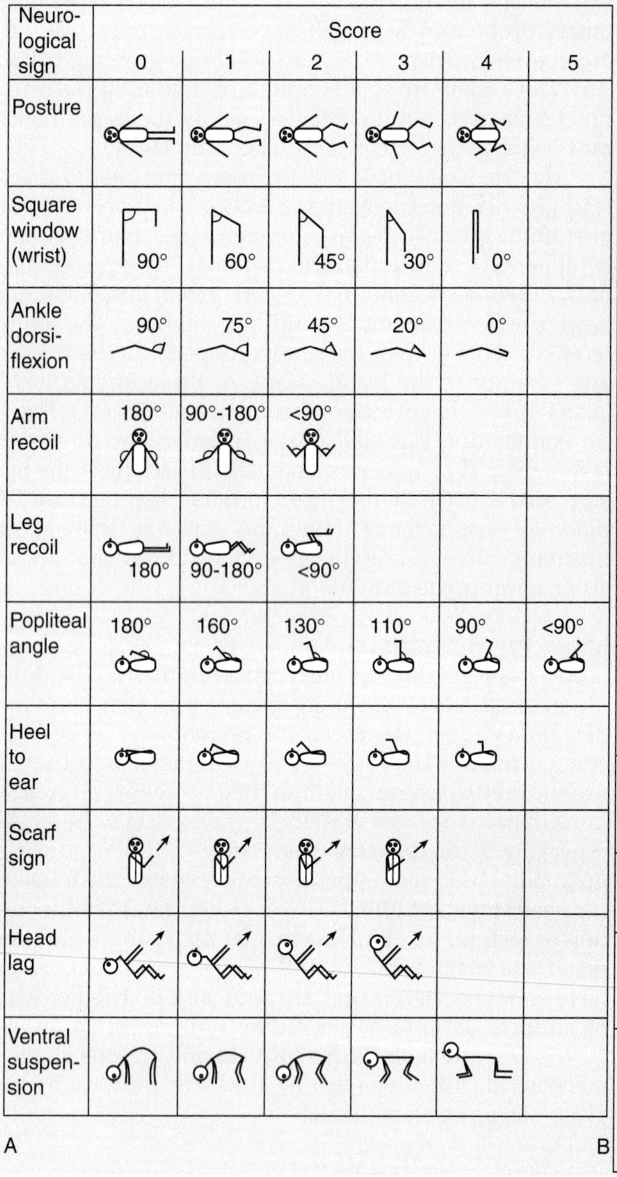

Neurological sign	Score 0	1	2	3	4	5
Posture						
Square window (wrist)	90°	60°	45°	30°	0°	
Ankle dorsiflexion	90°	75°	45°	20°	0°	
Arm recoil	180°	90°-180°	<90°			
Leg recoil	180°	90-180°	<90°			
Popliteal angle	180°	160°	130°	110°	90°	<90°
Heel to ear						
Scarf sign						
Head lag						
Ventral suspension						

A

External sign	Score 0	1	2	3	4
Oedema	Obvious oedema hands and feet pitting over tibia	No obvious oedema hands and feet, pitting over tibia	No oedema		
Skin texture	Very thin, gelatinous	Thin and smooth	Smooth medium, thickness Rash or superficial peeling	Slight thickening Superficial cracking and peeling esp. hands & feet	Thick and parchment-like, superficial or deep cracking
Skin color (infant not crying)	Dark red	Uniformly pink	Pale pink variable over body	Pale. Only pink over ears, lips, palms or soles	
Skin opacity (trunk)	Numerous veins and venules clearly seen, esp over abdomen	Veins and tributaries seen	A few large vessels seen over abdomen	A few large vessels indistinctly seen over abdomen	No blood vessels seen
Lanugo (ove back)	No lanugo	Abundant, long and thick over whole back	Hair thinning especially over lower back	Small amount of lanugo and bald areas	At least half of back devoid of lanugo
Plantar creases	No skin creases	Faint red marks over anterior half of sole	Definite red marks over more than anterior half, indentations over less than anterior third	Indentations over more than anterior third	Definite deep indentations over more than anterior third
Nipple formation	Nipple barely visible, no areola	Nipple well defined, areola smooth and flat, diameter <0.75 cm	Areola stippled, edge not raised, diameter <0.75 cm	Areola stippled, edge raised, diameter >0.75 cm	
Breast size	No breast tissue palpable	Breast tissue on one or both sides 0.5 cm diameter	Breast tissue both sides, one or both 0.5-1.0 cm	Breast tissue both sides, one or both 1 cm	
Ear form	Pinna flat and shapeless, little or no incurving of edge	Incurving of part of edge of pinna	Partial incurving whole of upper pinna	Well-defined incurving whole of upper pinna	
Ear firmness	Pinna soft, easily folded, no recoil	Pinna soft, easily folded, slow recoil	Cartilage to edge of pinna, but soft in places, ready recoil	Pinna firm, cartilage to edge, instant recoil	
Genetalia Males	Neither testis in scrotum	At least one testis high in scrotum	At least one testis right down		
Females (with hips half abducted)	Labia majora widely separated, labia minora protruding	Labia majora almost cover labia minora	Labia majora completely cover labia minora		

B

Figure 57–4 ■ ■ ■
(**A**) Neurologic characteristics of the Dubowitz examination. Neurologic criteria are recorded and added to a final score as performed for the physical assessment. (**B**) External characteristics of the Dubowitz examination. Physical criteria are recorded and a final score is obtained following the addition of each category's score. (Dubowitz L., & Dubowitz V. [1977]. *Gestational age of the newborn.* Reading, MA: Addison-Wesley)

method is comprehensive and includes 21 criteria using external physical (11) and neuromuscular (10) signs (Fig. 57–4).[15] The estimate of gestational age is best done within 48 hours of birth and is accurate within 2 weeks. The method is less accurate for infants born at gestational age less than 30 weeks. The Ballard method is an abbreviated Dubowitz method that includes 12 criteria, using 6 external physical and 6 neuromuscular signs.[12] This method is accurate for gestational ages 26 to 44 weeks.

In summary, growth and development begin with union of ovum and sperm and is ongoing throughout a child's life to adulthood. Abnormalities during this process can have profound effects on the infant. Perinatal development is composed of two periods—the embryonic period and the fetal period. During these periods, the zygote becomes the newborn with the organ maturity to make the adjustments necessary for extrauterine life. Infants born before this process is completed are called premature and can have major problems with extrauterine adjustments. Postnatal growth is rapid and ongoing and proceeds in an orderly and predictable manner.

Infancy

After you have completed this section of the chapter, you should be able to meet the following objectives:

- Describe the use of the Apgar score in evaluating infant well-being at birth
- List three injuries that can occur during the birth process
- Describe physical growth and organ development during the first year of life
- Explain how the common health care needs of the premature infant differ from the health care needs of the term newborn or infant
- Differentiate between organic and nonorganic failure to thrive syndrome

Infancy is defined as that time from birth to about 18 months of age. This is a period of rapid physical growth and maturation. The infant begins life as a relatively helpless organism and, through a process of progressive development, gains the skills to interact and cope with the environment. The infant begins life with a number of primitive reflexes and little body control. By 18 months, a child is able to run, grasp, and manipulate objects; feed self; play with toys; and communicate with others.

Growth and Development

Physical growth is rapid during infancy. After birth, there is a period of relative starvation as the infant adjusts to enteral feeding. Infants lose about 5% to 10% of their birth weight, but within days, they begin to gain weight, and by 2 weeks, they are back to birth weight. Average birth weight for a term newborn is 3000 to 4000 g, and this weight is usually doubled by 6 months and tripled by about 1 year after birth.

The median height at birth is 49.9 cm for girls and 50.5 cm for boys. During the first 6 months, height increases by 2.5 cm per month. By 1 year, the increase in length is 50% of the birth length. This increase is primarily in trunk growth. Median head circumference at birth is 34.5 cm for girls and 34.8 cm for boys. There is rapid increase in head circumference the first year, which is a good indicator of brain growth. Head circumference increases by 1.5 cm per month the first 6 months and 0.5 cm per month the second 6 months. Chest circumference at birth is smaller than head circumference. By 1 year, the head and chest are approximately equal in circumference. After 1 year, chest circumference exceeds head circumference.[2] After birth, most organ systems continue to grow and mature in an orderly fashion. Variations in growth and development are responsible for the differences in body proportions. For example, during the fetal period, the head is the predominant part because of the rapidly growing brain, whereas during infancy, the trunk predominates, and in childhood, the legs predominate. The patterns of growth are cephalocaudal, proximodistal, and mass to specific.

Organ systems must continue to grow and mature after delivery. Many are at a minimal level of functioning at birth. This often places them at risk for health problems. One example is the nervous system. Neurologic development and maturation continue after birth. At birth, the average brain weighs about 325 g. By 1 year, the weight has tripled, and the brain weighs about 1000 g. The maturation process includes an increase in neuron size, in size and number of glial cells, in myelinization, and in interneural connections and branching of axons and dendrites. As this maturation progresses, the level of functioning of the infant increases from simple to complex, from primitive reflexes to purposeful movement. The development of fine and gross motor skills follows the principles of cephalocaudal and proximodistal maturation.[2]

The respiratory system must make the transition from an intrauterine to an extrauterine existence. Onset of respiration must begin at birth for survival. The first breaths expand the alveoli and initiate gas exchange. The infant's respiratory rate is initially rapid and primarily abdominal, but with maturation, it gradually slows. Maturation of the respiratory system includes increases in the number of alveoli and the growth of the airways. Infants are obligatory nose breathers until 3 to 4 months of age; any upper airway obstruction may cause respiratory distress.[2] The trachea is small and close to the bronchi, and its branching structures enable infectious agents to be easily transmitted throughout the lungs. The softness of the supporting cartilage in the trachea, along with its small diameter, places the infant at risk for airway obstruction. The auditory (eustachian) tube is short and straight and closely communicates with the ear, putting the infant at risk for middle ear infections (see Chapter 43).

Birth initiates major changes in the cardiovascular system. The fetal shunts, the foramen ovale and ductus arteriosus, begin to close, and the circulation of blood changes from a series to a parallel circuit (see Chapter 23). At birth, the size of the heart is large in relation to the chest cavity. The size and weight of the heart double the first year. Initially, the right ventricle is more muscular than the left ventricle, but this reverses in infancy. The heart rate gradually slows, and systolic blood pressure rises.

The gastrointestinal system is immature, and most digestive processes are poorly functioning until approximately 3 months of age. Solid food may pass incompletely digested and be evident in the stool. At birth, sucking may be poor and require several days to become effective. The tongue thrust reflex is present and aids in sucking, but it disappears around 6 months of age. Stomach capacity increases rapidly in the first months, but because of the limited capacity and rapid emptying, infants require frequent feeding.[2] The infant's genitourinary system is functionally immature at birth. There is difficulty in concentrating urine, and the ability to adjust to a restricted fluid intake is limited. The small bladder capacity causes frequent voiding.

By 24 weeks' gestation age, all the nerve cells are present, and growth primarily results from an increase in cytoplasm. The most rapid period of brain growth is between 15 to 20 weeks of postnatal age, at which time there is a significant increase in neurons.

Another period of significant growth is between 30 weeks and 1 year of age. Neurologic growth and maturation continue into adolescence. The best indicator of brain growth is head circumference. Head circumference increases six times during the first year of life. At birth, the cerebral cortex is one half adult thickness. The brain surface is initially smooth, but with the advancing development that continues throughout childhood, the sulci deepen. Brain maturation includes increased interconnections between neurons and myelination of nerves. In a cephalocaudal and proximodistal sequence, myelination begins at the spinal cord and cranial nerves, followed by myelination of the brain stem and corticospinal tracts.[2,6]

The first year of life is also filled with psychosocial developmental milestones for the infant. Basic needs must be met before the infant can accomplish these developmental tasks. Erikson described the development of a sense of trust as the task of the first stage.[16] If trust is not acquired, the infant develops mistrust of others and frustration with its inability to control the surrounding environment.

Common Health Problems

The birth process is a critical event. Prenatal influences, birth trauma, and prematurity have an immediate impact on survival and health. The common health problems in this section have been divided into three sections: health problems of the newborn, special needs of the premature infant, and health problems of the infant.

Health Problems of the Newborn

Apgar Score. The Apgar score, devised by Dr. Virginia Apgar, is a scoring system that evaluates infant well-being at birth.[16] The system is composed of five categories (*i.e.,* heart rate, respiratory effort, muscle tone, reflex irritability, color) with a total score ranging from 0 to 10, depending on the degree to which these functions are presented (Table 57–1). Evaluations are performed at 1 minute and 5 minutes after delivery. A score of 0 to 3 is indicative of severe distress; 4 to 6 of moderate distress; and 7 to 10 of mild to no distress. Most infants score 6 to 7 at 1 minute and 8 to 9 at 5 minutes. If the score is 7 or less, the evaluation should be repeated every 5 minutes until a score of 7 or greater is obtained. An abnormal score at 5 minutes is more predictive of survival and neurologic outcome than at 1 minute.[7]

Birth Injuries. Injuries sustained during the birth process are responsible for a significant amount of neonatal mortality and morbidity. In 1991, birth injuries ranked as the eighth cause of infant death in the United States. Predisposing factors for birth injuries include macrosomia, prematurity, cephalopelvic disproportion, and dystocia (*i.e.,* abnormal labor or childbirth).[7,17,18]

Caput succedaneum is a localized area of scalp edema caused by sustained pressure of the presenting part against the cervix. There is an accumulation of serum or blood above the periosteum from the high pressure caused from the obstruction. The caput succedaneum may extend across suture lines and have overlying petechiae, purpura, or ecchymosis. No treatment is needed, and it usually resolves over the first week of life.[7,18]

Cephalohematoma is a subperiosteal collection of blood from ruptured blood vessels. The margins are sharply delineated and do not cross suture lines. It is usually unilateral, but it may be bilateral, and it usually occurs over the parietal area. The swelling may not be apparent for 24 to 48 hours because subperiosteal bleeding is slow. The overlying skin is not discolored. An underlying skull fracture may be present. Treatment is not needed unless the

TABLE 57–1
Apgar Score Assessment

Criterion	Score*		
	0	*1*	*2*
Heart rate	Absent	<100	>100
Respiratory effort	Absent	Weak, irregular	Crying
Muscle tone	Limp	Some flexion	Well flexed
Reflex irritability	No response	Grimace	Cry, gag
Color	Pale	Cyanotic	Pink
Total	0	5	10

*The Apgar score should be assigned at 1 minute and 5 minutes after birth, using a timer. Each criterion is assessed and assigned a 0, 1, or 2. The total score is the assigned Apgar score. If resuscitation is required beyond the 5 minutes, additional Apgar scores may also be assigned as a method to document the response of the newborn to the resuscitation.

cephalohematoma is large and results in severe blood loss or significant hyperbilirubinemia. Skull fracture and intracranial hemorrhage are associated complications. An uncomplicated cephalohematoma usually resolves within 2 weeks to 3 months.[7,18]

Skull fractures are uncommon because the infant's compressible skull is able to mold to fit the contours of the birth canal. However, fractures can occur and more often follow a forceps delivery or severe contraction of the pelvis associated with prolonged, difficult labor. Skull fractures may be linear or depressed. Uncomplicated linear fractures are often asymptomatic and do not require treatment. Depressed skull fractures are observable by the palpable indentation of the infant's head. They require surgical intervention if there is compression of underlying brain tissue. A simple linear fracture usually heals within several months.[7,18]

The *clavicle* is the most frequently fractured bone during the birth process. It is more common in LGA infants and occurs when delivery of the shoulders is difficult in vertex (*i.e.,* head) or breech presentations. The infant may or may not demonstrate restricted motion of the upper extremity, but passive motion elicits pain. There may be discoloration or deformity and, on palpation, crepitus (*i.e.,* crackling sound from bones rubbing together), and irregularity may be found. Treatment consists of immobilizing the affected arm and shoulder and providing pain relief.[7,18]

The *brachial plexuses* are situated above the clavicles in the anterolateral bases of the neck. They are composed of the spinal roots of the fifth cervical nerves through the first thoracic nerves. During vertex deliveries, excessive lateral traction of the head and neck away from the shoulders may cause a stretch injury to the brachial plexus on that side. In a breech presentation, excessive lateral traction on the trunk before delivery of the head may tear the lower roots of the cervical cord. If the breech presentation includes delivery with the arms overhead, an injury to the fifth and sixth cervical roots may result. When injury to the brachial plexus occurs, it causes paralysis of the upper extremity. The paralysis is often incomplete.

Brachial plexus injuries include three types: Erb-Duchenne paralysis (*i.e.,* upper arm); Klumpke's paralysis (*i.e.,* lower arm); and paralysis of the entire arm. Risk factors include an LGA infant and a difficult, traumatic delivery. Erb-Duchenne paralysis occurs with injury to the fifth and sixth cervical roots. It is the most common type of brachial plexus injury and manifests with variable degrees of paralysis of the shoulder and arm. The position of the affected arm is adducted and internally rotated, with extension at the elbow, pronation of the forearm, and flexion of the wrist. When the infant is lifted, the affected extremity is limp. The Moro reflex is impaired or absent, but the grasp reflex is present.[7,18]

Klumpke's paralysis results from injury to the eighth cervical and first thoracic roots. It is rare and presents with paralysis of the hand. The infant has wrist drop, the fingers are relaxed, and the grasp reflex is absent. The Moro reflex is impaired, with the upper extremity extending and abducting normally while the wrist and fingers remain flaccid.

Treatment of brachial plexus injuries includes immobilization, appropriate positioning, and an exercise program. Most infants recover in 3 to 6 months. Recovery from lower arm paralysis is less successful, and the infant may develop a claw deformity.[7,18]

Congenital Malformations. Congenital malformations are anatomic or structural abnormalities present at birth (see Chapter 4). They are a major cause of morbidity and mortality in children. In the perinatal period, 20% of deaths are attributed to congenital malformations. The malformations may be minor or major, detectable at birth or not detectable for years. Some stages of embryonic development are more at risk than others for development of congenital malformations after teratogen exposure. The causes of congenital malformations may be divided into genetic, environmental, or multifactorial.

Special Needs of the Premature Infant

Infants born before 37 weeks' gestation are considered premature. They often fall into the LBW category. The health of the LBW infant is directly related to its gestational age. Mortality and morbidity are increased in the premature population and are inversely proportional to the length of gestation. The shorter is the time of gestation, the more risk of death or disability. This is because of the immaturity of the organ systems, which interferes with the successful transition to an extrauterine life. Immaturity predisposes this population to the complications of prematurity. Also within this group are those premature infants who have grown abnormally during their shortened gestation (*i.e.,* LGA or SGA). Abnormal growth places an added stress on their transition to extrauterine life.

Despite the advances in obstetric management in the past 30 years, the rate of premature delivery has not significantly changed. In the United States, over 9% of infants are born before 37 weeks' gestation. LBW and prematurity often go hand in hand. Most infants weighing less than 2500 g, and almost all weighing less than 1500 g are premature. In the United States, LBW is responsible for two thirds of the neonatal deaths despite an increase in survival of the LBW infant. The birth rate of LBW infants was approximately 6.8% in 1985, and LBW accounted for 20% of all postnatal deaths. Contributing risk factors for prematurity are also associated with LBW. Risk factors associated with prematurity and LBW include maternal age (*i.e.,* younger than 16, older than 35), race (*i.e.,* African-American more than white), socioeconomic status, marital status (*i.e.,* single more than married), smoking, substance abuse, malnutrition, poor or no prenatal care, medical risks predating pregnancy, and medical risks in current pregnancy.[7]

The premature infant is poorly equipped to withstand the rigors of extrauterine transition. The organ systems are immature and may not be able to sustain life. The respiratory system may not be able to support gas exchange; the skin may be thin and gelatinous and easily damaged; the immune system is compromised and may not effectively fight infection; and the lack of subcutaneous fat puts the infant at risk for temperature instability. Complications of prematurity include respiratory distress syndrome (RDS), pulmonary hemorrhage, transient tachypnea, congenital pneumonia, pulmonary air leaks, bronchopulmonary dysplasia, recurrent apnea, glucose instability, hypocalcemia, hyperbilirubinemia, anemia, intraventricular hemorrhage, necrotizing enterocolitis (NEC), circulatory instability, hypothermia, bacterial or viral infection, retinopathy of prematurity, and disseminated intravascular coagulopathies.

Respiratory Problems. RDS, frequently referred to as hyaline membrane disease, is the most common complication of prematurity. In the United States, approximately 10% to 15% of infants less than 2500 g and 60% of infants at 29 weeks' gestation develop RDS. The incidence of RDS is lower in African-American infants than in white infants and lower in female infants than in male infants.

The primary problem is the lack of surfactant in the lungs. Surfactant is produced by type II alveolar cells in the lungs. It is a combination of several phospholipids that lowers the alveolar surface tension and facilitates lung expansion (see Chapters 22 and 23). At 24 weeks' gestation, there are small amounts of surfactant and few terminal air sacs (*i.e.*, primitive alveoli) with underdeveloped pulmonary vascularity. If an infant is born at this time, there is little chance of survival. By 26 to 28 weeks, there is usually sufficient surfactant and lung development to permit survival.

The availability of exogenous surfactant replacement therapy has improved the outcome of RDS and has been recognized as the main factor responsible for the 6.2% fall in the 1989 to 1990 infant mortality rate in the United States. However, because the survival of the sickest infants has improved and because their management is more complex, the incidence of complications has increased. These include air leak syndromes, bronchopulmonary dysplasia, and intracranial hemorrhage.[7,19]

Apnea and periodic breathing are common problems in premature infants. Because the respiratory center in the medulla oblongata is underdeveloped in the premature infant, the ability for sustained ventilatory drive is often impaired. *Apnea* is defined as cessation of breathing; it is characterized by failure to breath for 20 seconds or more and is often accompanied by bradycardia or cyanosis. Among infants weighing less than 1.5 kg, 50% require intervention for significant apneic spells. Apnea may be caused by an underlying disease process such as infection. This is not apnea of prematurity and should not be treated as such. *Periodic breathing* commonly occurs in those infants weighing less than 1.8 kg. It is intermittent failure to breathe in durations of less than 10 to 15 seconds. Management of apnea and periodic breathing includes use of medications or ventilatory support until the CNS is developed and able to sustain adequate ventilatory drive.[7,19]

Intraventricular Hemorrhage. Intraventricular hemorrhage (IVH) is a common problem almost exclusive to premature infants. It is a problem, second only to RDS as the major cause of death in the premature infant. For infants born after less than 35 weeks' gestation or weighing less than 1400 g, the incidence is 40% to 50% with the most immature at the highest risk of IVH. The hemorrhage often occurs in a subependymal germinal matrix layer. This is a periventricular structure located between the caudate nucleus and the thalamus at the level of or slightly posterior to the foramen of Monro. The germinal matrix is an early developmental structure that contains a fragile vascular area that is poorly supported by connective tissue. By term, this structure is gone.

Risk factors for IVH include pneumothorax, hypotension, acidosis, coagulopathy, transport, volume expansion, and bicarbonate infusion. The proposed mechanisms for IVH include an hypoxic-ischemic insult resulting in cerebral hyperperfusion of the germinal matrix area that causes vessel rupture. Another proposed mechanism is disruption of vascular integrity in the germinal matrix caused by hypotension. Four grades of hemorrhage have been identified.[7,20] Most hemorrhages resolve, but the more severe hemorrhages may obstruct the flow of cerebrospinal fluid, causing a progressive hydrocephalus.

Necrotizing Enterocolitis. NEC is an acquired gastrointestinal disease process that is a major problem in preterm infants. The incidence is 1% to 5% of admissions to the neonatal intensive care unit. Although approximately 90% of infants affected are preterm infants weighing less than 1500 g, 10% of infants affected are term infants. Mortality varies from 20% to 40%.

The exact cause of NEC is unknown but is thought to be multifactorial. Risk factors for NEC include birth asphyxia, umbilical artery catheterization, patent ductus arteriosus, polycythemia, enteral feeding, and medications such as indomethacin, vitamin E, and xanthines.[21] There is agreement that the process begins with diminished perfusion of the intestinal wall, which results in ischemia and hypoxia that leads to necrosis and gangrene. Although bacterial infection plays a role in the disease, it is not thought to be the initiating event. Milk feeding has been implicated. Approximately 93% of infants who develop NEC have been fed enterally.[13] Human milk and commercial formulas serve as substrates for bacterial growth in the gut.

The ileum is most commonly affected, followed by the ascending colon, cecum, transverse colon, and rectosigmoid. The necrosis of the intestine may be superficial, affecting only the mucosa or submucosa, or may extend through the entire intestinal wall. Perforation can occur and lead to peritonitis.

The manifestations of NEC are variable, but the usual presentation includes abdominal distention, gastric aspirates, bilious stools, lethargy, apnea, and hypoperfusion. The infant often appears septic. Laboratory examination may reveal leukocytosis or leukopenia, neutropenia, thrombocytopenia, glucose instability, electrolyte imbalance, metabolic acidosis, hypoxia, hypercapnia, and disseminated intravascular coagulation. Blood cultures are positive for only about 30% of these patients. Microorganisms reported in NEC include *Escherichia coli, Klebsiella, Enterobacter, Pseudomonas, Salmonella, Clostridium difficile,* and *Clostridium perfringens*.[21]

Clinical diagnosis is primarily radiographic. The radiographic hallmark of NEC is pneumatosis intestinalis or intramural air. Pneumoperitoneum is indicative of intestinal perforation. A large, stationary, distended loop of intestine on repeated radiographs may indicate gangrene, and a gasless abdomen may indicate peritonitis.[21]

Treatment includes cessation of feedings, stomach decompression, broad-spectrum antibiotic coverage, and supportive treatment. Intestinal perforation requires surgical intervention. Intestinal resection of dead intestine with a diverting ostomy is the procedure of choice.[21]

Health Problems of the Infant

Infants are prone to numerous health problems during the first year of life. They may become serious if not recognized and treated appropriately. A significant amount may be precipitated by the relative immaturity of the organ systems. Infants are prone to have nutritional disturbances, feeding difficulties, problems with food allergies, gastroesophageal reflux, and colic. Injuries, the major cause of death during infancy, are caused by events such as aspiration of foreign objects, suffocation, motor vehicle accidents, falls, poisoning, burns, and drowning. Childhood diseases may be a problem if the infant is not adequately immunized.

Nutrition. Good nutrition is important during infancy because of rapid growth. Human milk or commercial infant formulas form the basis for the early nutritional needs of the newborn and young infant. The American Academy of Pediatrics recommends breast-feeding for the first 12 months of life. Human milk from a well-nourished mother is easily digested and typically provides sufficient nutrients and calories for normal growth and development. Human milk also has the added benefit of offering some immune protection to the infant in most cases. Fluoride is added from birth, and iron is added at approximately 6 months of age, when the fetal iron stores are depleted.

Mothers who do not choose to breast-feed their child or who are unable to breast-feed may choose a commercial formula. Several companies produce infant formulas that contain the essential nutrients for infants. Although there are some minor differences, most infant formulas are similar, regardless of which company produces the formula.

Some infants may experience difficulties in consuming mother's milk or infant formulas that are based on cow's milk because of lactase deficiency. Lactase is an enzyme that breaks down lactose, the carbohydrate found in human milk and cow's milk. Some infant formulas contain carbohydrates other than lactose. These formulas are made from soy beans. Other feeding intolerances may also occur. Treatment of any milk or formula intolerance depends on identification of the specific offender and elimination of it from the diet. Newborns and infants frequently exhibit "spitting up" or regurgitation of formula, despite the absence of a formula intolerance. Generally, cow's milk-based formulas are preferable to soy-based formulas, and changing to a soy-based formula should only be undertaken when there is a proven case of intolerance. It is important that all claims of formula intolerance be thoroughly investigated before an infant is changed to a soy-based formula. Education of the parents about the signs and symptoms of intolerance and reassurance that spitting up formulas is normal may be all that is required. An infant who is gaining weight, appears alert and well-nourished, has adequate stools, and demonstrates normal hunger is unlikely to have a formula intolerance.

One area of infant nutrition that is still subject to much controversy is the introduction of solid foods. There is great variation regarding when to start solid foods and what solid foods to introduce. Generally, human milk or iron-fortified infant formulas should supply most infant nutrition during the first year of life. However, solid foods are usually introduced beginning at 6 months. When solid foods are being introduced, they should be considered as supplemental to the total nutrition and not as the main component of nutrition. Solid foods should be introduced only by spoon feeding. The addition of cereal to formula in a bottle or in "infant feeders" is not recommended. It has never been shown that early introduction of solid foods causes the infant to sleep longer at night.

Bland infant cereals, such as rice cereal, are usually introduced first. Slow progression to the addition of individual vegetables, fruits, and finally, meats occurs as the infant learns to chew and swallow food. Infants also become able to drink from a cup rather than a bottle during this time. The addition of desserts is not recommended because these add calories without adding substantial nutrition.

Sometime between 9 months and 12 months, the infant's intake of solid foods and formula increases, and the infant can be weaned from the breast or bottle. Much anxiety can accompany weaning, so it should be done gradually. Mothers may need reassurance that their infant is progressing normally at that time.

Irritable Infant Syndrome or Colic. Colic is generally defined as paroxysmal abdominal pain or cramping in an infant and is usually manifested by loud crying, drawing up of the legs to the abdomen, and extreme irritability. Episodes of colic may last from several minutes to several hours a day. During this time, most efforts to soothe the infant or relieve the distress are not successful. Colic is most common in infants younger than 3 months of age but can persist for up to 9 months.

Caring for an infant with colic can be frustrating. There is no one single etiologic factor that causes colic; therefore, the treatment of colic is not precise. Many nonmedical techniques and pharmacologic preparations such as antispasmodics, sedatives, and antiflatulents have been tried. Nonpharmacologic interventions should be attempted before administration of drugs. Support of the parents is probably the single most important factor in the treatment of colic. Many times the mother (or primary care provider) may be afraid to state just how frustrated she is with her inability to console the infant. An open discussion of this frustration can help the mothers or care providers recognize that their feelings of frustration are normal; frequently, this gives them the added support needed to deal with their infant.

Failure to Thrive. Failure to thrive is a term that refers to inadequate growth of the child from the inability to obtain or use essential nutrients. Failure to thrive may be organic or nonorganic. Organic failure to thrive is the result of a physiologic cause that prevents the infant from obtaining or using nutrients appropriately. An example of organic failure to thrive is inadequate growth of an infant with deficient energy reserve because of a congenital defect that makes sucking and feeding difficult. Inorganic failure to thrive is the result of psychologic factors that prevent adequate intake of nutrition. An example of nonorganic failure to thrive is inadequate weight gain caused by inadequate intake of nutrients because of parental neglect.

Diagnosis of the type of failure to thrive depends on careful examination and history of the infant and serial follow-up evaluations. An individual infant's growth can be compared with the standards for normal growth and development. Cases of organic failure to thrive are usually easier to diagnose than cases of nonorganic failure to thrive. Diagnosis of nonorganic failure to thrive requires extensive investigation of history, family situation, relationship of the care provider to the infant, and evaluation of feeding practices. The nonorganic basis should be considered early in every case of failure to thrive.

Therapy for failure to thrive depends on the cause. Because long-term nutritional deficiencies can result in impaired physical and intellectual growth, provision of optimal nutrition is essential. Methods to increase nutritional intake by adjusting caloric density of the formula or by parenteral nutrition may be required in cases of organic failure to thrive.

Sudden Infant Death Syndrome. Sudden infant death syndrome (SIDS) or crib death refers to the sudden death of an infant under 1 year of age that remains unexplained after autopsy, investigation of the death scene, and review of the history. SIDS is the leading cause of death in infants between 1 month and 1 year of age. Approximately 7000 infants succumb to SIDS each year.[22,23,25] The prone sleeping position is a significant risk factor in SIDS. The frequency of SIDS is more than threefold greater when infants sleep on their stomachs compared with sleeping on their backs.[4] Population-based education programs to decrease the practice of having babies sleep on their stomachs has resulted in a substantial decrease in SIDS.

The exact cause of SIDS is unknown. Theories center on brain stem abnormality, which prevents effective control of cardiorespiratory control. Features of SIDS include prolonged sleep apnea, increased frequency of brief inspiratory pauses, excessive periodic breathing, and impaired response to increased carbon dioxide or decreased oxygen. A diagnosis of SIDS can only be made if an autopsy is performed to exclude other causes of death. Differentiation of child abuse from SIDS is an important consideration, and each case of SIDS must be subjected to careful examination.

Support of the family of an infant with SIDS is crucial. Parents frequently feel guilty or inadequate as parents. The fact that there must be close scrutiny to differentiate a SIDS death from a death by child abuse adds to the guilt and disappointment felt by the family. After a diagnosis of SIDS is made, it is important that the parents and other family members receive information about SIDS. Health care providers need to be fully aware of resources available to families with a SIDS death. The siblings of the child who died should not be overlooked. Children also need information and support to get through the grief process. Children may blame themselves for the death or fear that they, too, may die of SIDS. Too many times, they are not given information because the adults are trying to protect them.

Injuries. Injuries are the major cause of death in infants between 6 and 12 months of age. Aspiration of foreign objects, suffocation, falls, poisonings, drowning, burns, and other bodily damage may occur because of the infant's increasing ability to investigate the environment. Childproofing the environment can be an important precaution to prevent injuries. No home or environment can be completely childproofed, but close supervision of the child by a competent care provider is essential to prevent injury.

Motor vehicle accidents are responsible for a significant number of infant deaths. After 1 year of age, motor vehicle accidents become the number one cause of accidental death. Most states require that infants be placed in an approved infant safety restraint while riding in a vehicle. The middle of the back seat is considered the safest place for the infant to ride. Many hospitals do not discharge a baby unless there is a safety restraint system in the car. If a family cannot afford a restraint system, programs are available that donate or loan the family a restraint. Health care providers must be involved in educating the public about the dangers of carrying infants in vehicles without taking proper precautions to protect them.

Immunizations. One of the most dramatic improvements in infant health has been related to widespread immunization of infants and children to the major childhood communicable diseases, including diphtheria, pertussis, tetanus, polio, measles, mumps, rubella, hepatitis, and *Haemophilus influenzae* type B. Immunizations to these infectious diseases have greatly reduced morbidity and mortality of infants and young children. These immunizations are given at standard times as part of health promotion in infants and children. However, these immunization programs have not completely eradicated these diseases but have only lowered their prevalence. Immunization programs are only effective if all children receive the immunizations. Although most immunizations can be received through local health departments at no or low cost, many infants or young children do not routinely receive immunizations or do not receive the full regimen of immunizations. Methods to improve compliance and access to immunizations continue to be needed.

In summary, infancy is defined as that period from birth to 18 months. During this time, growth and development are ongoing. The relative immaturity of many of the organ systems places the infant at risk for a variety of illnesses. Birth initiates many changes in the organ systems as a means of adjusting to postnatal life. The birth process is a critical event, and maladjustments and injuries during the birth process are a major cause of death or disability. Premature delivery is a significant health problem in the United States. The premature infant is at risk for numerous health problems because of the interruption of intrauterine growth and immaturity of organ systems.

Early Childhood

After you have completed this section of the chapter, you should be able to meet the following objectives:

- Define early childhood
- Describe the growth and development of early childhood
- Discuss the common health problems of early childhood

Early childhood is considered the period of 18 months through 5 years of age. During this time, the child passes through the stages of toddler (*i.e.*, 18 months to 3 years) and preschooler (*i.e.*, 3 years through 5 years). There are many changes as the child moves from infancy through the toddler and preschool years. The major achievements are the development and refinement of locomotion and language, which take place as children progress from dependence to independence.[7,19]

Growth and Development

Early childhood is a period of continued physical growth and maturation. Compared with infancy, physical growth is not as dramatic. Weight gain during the toddler stage is 1.8 to 2.7 kg per year (an average of 2.3 kg per year). At 2 years, the average weight is 12 kg, and by 2.5 years the birth weight has quadrupled. By the preschool years, growth slows considerably. The average weight gain is approximately 2.3 kg per year, and almost all organ systems have reached full maturity. At 3 years, the average weight is 14.5 kg, and by 6 years, it has increased to 21 kg. During early childhood, height increases an average 7.5 cm per year and is primarily through increase in leg length. At 2 years of age, the average height is 86.6 cm, and by 6 years, it has reached 116 cm. In the first 2 years of life, head circumference increases by 2.5 cm per year. After 2 years of age, head circumference growth slows, and by 5 years, the average increase in head circumference is 1.25 cm per year.[2,14]

The maturation of organ systems is ongoing during early childhood. The respiratory system continues its growth and maturation, but because of the relative immaturity of the airway structures, otitis media and respiratory infections are common. The barrel-shaped chest that is characteristic of infancy has begun to change to a more adult shape. The respiratory rate of infancy has slowed and averages 20 to 30 beats/minute. Respirations remain abdominal until 7 years of age.[2]

Neural growth remains rapid during early childhood. All brain cells are present by 12 months of age. Growth is primarily hypertrophic. The brain is 90% of adult size by 2 years of age. The cephalocaudal, proximodistal principle is followed as myelinization of the cortex, brain stem, and spinal cord is completed. The spinal cord is completely myelinated by 2 years of age. At that time, the control of anal and urethral sphincter and the motor skills of locomotion can be achieved and mastered. The continuing maturation of the neuromuscular system is increasingly evident as complex gross and fine motor skills are acquired throughout early childhood.

Growth and maturation in the musculoskeletal system continue with ossification of the skeletal system, growth of the legs, and changes in muscle and fat proportions. Legs grow faster than the trunk in early childhood; after the first year of life, about two thirds of the increase in height is leg growth. Muscle growth is balanced by a corresponding decrease in adipose tissue accumulation.

During early childhood, many important psychosocial tasks are mastered by the child. Independence begins to develop, and the child is on the way to becoming a social being in control of the environment. Development and refinement of gross and fine motor abilities allow involvement with an infinite amount of tasks and activities. Learning is ongoing and progressive and includes interactions with others, appropriate social behavior, and sex-role functions. Erikson described the tasks that must be accomplished in early childhood.[16] The toddler must acquire a sense of autonomy while overcoming a sense of doubt and shame. The preschooler must acquire a sense of initiative and develop a conscience.[2]

Common Health Problems

Early childhood years can pose significant health risks to the growing and maturing child. Injuries are the leading cause of death in children between the ages of 1 and

4 years. Only adolescents have more. Locomotion, together with a lack of awareness of danger, places toddlers and preschoolers at special risk for injuries. Motor vehicle accidents are responsible for almost 50% of all accidental deaths in this group. Many of the injuries and deaths can be prevented by appropriate restraints in car seats and seat belts. Other major causes of injuries include drowning, burns, poisoning, falls, aspiration and suffocation, and bodily damage.[2]

Infectious diseases can be a problem for children during early childhood because of their susceptibility. This may also be the time when children first enter day care, which increases their exposure to other children and infectious diseases. The major disorders include the communicable childhood diseases (*e.g.*, chickenpox, measles, roseola, mumps, pertussis, rubella, scarlet fever), conjunctivitis, and intestinal parasitic infections.[2]

Child maltreatment is an increasing problem in the United States. Although the numbers vary according to the methods and definitions used, the best estimates indicate that about 1.4 million children in the United States undergo some form of abuse.[14] Child maltreatment includes physical and emotional neglect, physical abuse, and sexual abuse. Neglect is the most common type of maltreatment and can take the form of deprivation of basic necessities or failure to meet the child's emotional needs. It is often attributed to poor parenting skills. Physical abuse is the deliberate infliction of injury. The cause is probably multifactorial with predisposing factors that include the parent, child, and environment. Sexual abuse is on the rise and includes a spectrum of types. The typical abuser is male. Children often do not report the abuse because they are afraid of not being believed.[2]

In summary, early childhood is defined as the period from 18 months to 5 years of age—the toddler and preschool years. Growth and development continue but are not as dramatic as during the prenatal and infancy periods. Early childhood is a time when the most organ systems reach maturity and the child becomes an independent, mobile being. There continue to be significant health risks during this period, especially in regards to infectious diseases and injuries. Injuries are the leading cause of death during this period. Child abuse is rapidly increasing as a major health problem.

Early School Years to Late Childhood

After you have completed this section of the chapter, you should be able to meet the following objectives:

- Define early school years
- Characterize the growth and development that occurs during the early school years
- Discuss common health problems of the child in early to late school age

In this text, early school years or late childhood is defined as the period in which a child begins school through the beginning of adolescence. These 6 years involve a great deal of change, but when one recollects "childhood," these are the years most often remembered. The experiences of this period have a profound effect on the physical, cognitive, and psychosocial development of the child, which influence the adult that the child will become.

Growth and Development

Although physical growth is steady throughout the early school years, it is slower than the previous periods and the adolescent period to follow. During late childhood, children typically gain approximately 3 to 3.5 kg and grow an average of 6 cm per year.[4] The average 6-year-old child is 116 cm tall and weighs about 21 kg. By 12 years of age, the same child may weigh 40 kg and be 150 cm tall. There is only a slight difference in the body sizes of males and females during this period, with boys being just a little taller and heavier than girls.[2]

During late childhood, a child's legs grow longer, posture improves, and their center of gravity descends to a lower point. These changes make children more graceful and help them be successful at climbing, bike riding, roller skating, and other physical activities. Body fat distribution decreases and, in combination with the lengthening skeleton, gives the child a thinner appearance. As the body fat decreases, lean muscle mass increases. By age 12, boys and girls have doubled their body strength and physical capabilities. Although muscular strength increases, the muscles are still relatively immature and injury from overstrenuous activities, such as difficult sports, can occur. With the gains in length, the head circumference decreases in relation to the height, waist circumference decreases in relation to height, and leg length increases in relation to height.

Facial proportions change as the face grows faster in relation to the rest of the cranium. The brain and skull grow very little during late childhood. Primary teeth are lost and replaced by permanent teeth. When the permanent teeth first appear, they may appear to be too big for the mouth and face. This is a temporary imbalance that is alleviated as the face grows. Caloric requirements usually are lower compared with previous periods and with the adolescent period to follow. Cardiac growth is slow. Heart rate and respiratory rates continue to decrease, and blood pressure gradually rises. Growth of the eye continues, and the normal farsightedness of the preschool child is gradually converted to 20/20 vision by about 11 to 12 years. Frequent vision assessment is recommended during late childhood as part of normal routine health screenings.[2]

Bone ossification and mineralization continues. Bones cannot resist muscle pressure and pull as well as mature bones. Precautions should be taken to prevent alterations in bone structure, such as providing properly fitting shoes and adequate desks to prevent poor posture. Children should be routinely checked for scoliosis (see Chapter 46) often during this period.

Toward the end of late childhood, the physical differences between the two sexes become apparent. Females usually enter pubescence about 2 years before males, resulting in noticeable differences in height, weight, and development of secondary sex characteristics. There is much individual variation among children of the same sex. These differences can be extremely difficult for children to cope with.

Entry into the school setting has a major impact on the psychosocial development of the child at this age. The child begins to form relationships with other children, forming groups. Peers become more important as the child moves out of the security of the family and into the bigger world. Usually during this period, children begin to form closer bonds with individual "best friends." However, the best friend relationships may frequently change. The personality of the person begins to appear. Although the personality is still developing, the basic temperament and approach to life become apparent. Although changes in personality occur with maturity, the basic elements may not change. The major task of this stage, as identified by Erikson, is the development of industry or accomplishment.[25] Failure to meet this task results in a sense of inferiority or incompetence, which can impede further progress.

Common Health Problems

Because of the high level of immune system competence in late childhood, children have an immunologic advantage over earlier years. Respiratory infections are the leading cause of illness at this time, followed by gastrointestinal disorders. The chief cause of mortality is accidents, primarily motor vehicle accidents. Immunization against the major communicable diseases of childhood has greatly improved the health of children in their early childhood years.

Health promotion includes appropriate dental care. The incidence of dental caries has decreased since the addition of fluoride to most water systems in the United States. However, there is still a high incidence of dental caries during late childhood that is related to inadequate dental care and a high amount of dietary sugar. Children at the early part of this stage may not be as effective in brushing their teeth and may require adult assistance, but they may be reluctant to allow parental help.

Infections with bacterial and fungal agents are a common problem in childhood. These infections commonly occur as respiratory, gastrointestinal, or skin diseases. Infections of the skin occur more frequently in this age group than in any other age group, probably related to increased exposure to skin lesions. Other acute or chronic health problems may surface for the first time. Asthma, caused by allergic reactions, frequently manifests for the first time during the early school years. Epilepsy may also first be diagnosed during this period. Many childhood cancers also may appear. Developmental disabilities or specific learning disabilities may initially become apparent as the child enters school.

In summary, early school years to late childhood are defined as that period from beginning school through adolescence. During these 6 years, growth is steady but much slower than in the previous periods. Entry into school begins the formation of relationships with peers and has a major impact on psychologic development. This is a wonderful period of relatively good health secondary to an immunologic advantage, but respiratory disease poses a leading cause of illness and motor vehicle accidents are the major cause of death. Several chronic health problems such as asthma, epilepsy, and childhood cancers may surface during this time.

Adolescence

After you have completed this section of the chapter, you should be able to meet the following objectives:

- Define what is meant by the period known as adolescence
- Characterize the physical and psychosocial changes that occur during adolescence
- Cite the developmental tasks that adolescents need to fulfill
- Describe common concerns of parents regarding their adolescent child
- Discuss how the changes that occur during adolescence can influence the health care needs of the adolescent

Adolescence is a transitional period between childhood and adulthood. During adolescence, there are significant physical, social, psychologic, and cognitive changes. The changes of adolescence do not occur on a strict timeline; instead, the changes occur at different times according to a unique internal calendar known only to the person. For definition's sake, adolescence is considered to begin with the development of secondary sex characteristics, around 11 or 12 years of age, and to end with the completion of somatic growth from about 18 to 20 years of age. Females generally begin and end adolescence earlier than males. The adolescent period is conveniently referred to as the "teen-aged years," from 13 through 19 years of age.

Growth and Development

Adolescence is influenced by hormonal activity that is influenced by the CNS. Physical growth occurs simultaneously with sexual maturation.

Adolescents typically experience gains of 20% to 25% in linear growth. An adolescent growth spurt, which lasts approximately 24 to 36 months, accounts for most of this somatic growth. The age at onset, the duration, and the extent of the growth vary between males and females and among individuals. In females, the growth spurt usually begins around 10 to 14 years of age. It begins earlier in females than in males and ends earlier, with less dramatic changes in weight and height. Females generally gain about 5 to 20 cm in height and 7 to 25 kg in weight. Most females have completed their growth spurt by age 16 or 17 years. Males begin their growth spurt later, but it is usually more pronounced, with an increase in height of from 10 to 30 cm and an increase in weight from 7 to 30 kg. Males may continue to gain in height until age 18 to 20 years. Increases in height are possible until about 25 years of age.[26]

The changes in physical body size are not random but have a characteristic pattern. Growth in arms, legs, hands, feet, and neck appear first, then increases in hip and chest sizes occur, followed in several months by increases in shoulder width and depth and increases in trunk length. These changes may be difficult for the adolescent and parents. Adolescents may change shoe sizes several times over several months. Although brain size is not significantly increased during adolescence, the size and shape of the skull and facial bones change. The features of the face may appear to be out of proportion until full adult growth is attained.[2,26] Muscle mass and strength also increase during adolescence. Sometimes, there may be a discrepancy between the growth of bone and muscle mass, creating a temporary dysfunction with slower or less smooth movements resulting from the mismatch of bone and muscle. Body proportions undergo typical changes during adolescence. In males, the thorax becomes broader, and the pelvis remains narrow. In females, the opposite occurs: the thorax remains narrow, and the pelvis widens.

Organ systems also undergo changes in function, and some have changes in structure. The heart increases in size as the result of increased muscle cell size. Heart rate decreases to normal adult rates, whereas blood pressure increases rapidly to adult rates. Circulating blood volume and hemoglobin concentration increase. Males demonstrate greater changes in blood volume and higher hemoglobin concentrations because of the influence of testosterone and the relatively higher muscle mass.

With adolescence, skin becomes thicker, and additional hair growth occurs in both sexes. Sebaceous and sweat gland activity increases. Plugged sebaceous glands frequently result in acne (see Chapter 15). Increased sweat gland activity results in perspiration and body odor. The eyes undergo changes that may contribute to increased myopia. Auditory acuity peaks in adolescence and begins to decline after about age 13.

Voice changes are of significant importance during adolescence for both sexes; however, the change is more pronounced in males. The voice change results from the growth of the larynx. There is more growth of the larynx of males than females. The paranasal sinuses reach adult proportion, which increases the resonance of the voice, adding to the adult sound of the voice.[2,26]

Changes in the endocrine system are of great importance in the initiation and continuation of the adolescent growth spurt. The hormones involved include growth hormone (GH), thyroid hormones, adrenal hormones, insulin, and the gonadotropic hormones. GH regulates growth in childhood but is essentially replaced by sex hormones as the primary impetus for growth during adolescence. The exact role of GH in the adolescent growth spurt is unclear. Thyroid hormone, a significant hormone in the regulation of metabolism during childhood, continues to be important during adolescence. The relation of thyroid hormone to the other hormones and its role in the adolescent growth spurt is unclear. The thyroid gland becomes larger during adolescence, and it is believed that production of thyroid hormones is increased during this period. Insulin is necessary for appropriate growth at all stages, including adolescence. Insulin must be present for GH to be effective. The pancreatic islets of Langerhans increase in size during adolescence.[2,26]

The anterior pituitary gland produces the gonadotropic hormones, follicle-stimulating hormone and luteinizing hormone. These hormones influence target organs to secrete sex hormones. The ovaries respond by secreting estrogens and progesterone, and the testes respond by producing androgens, resulting in the maturation of the primary sex characteristics and the appearance of secondary sex characteristics. Primary sex characteristics are those involved in reproductive function (*i.e.*, internal and external genitalia). The secondary sex characteristics are the physical signs that signal the presence of sexual maturity but are not directly involved in reproduction (*i.e.*, pubic and axillary hair). Androgens initiate the beginning of the growth spurt. Sex hormones, including androgens, also conclude height growth by causing bone age maturity, epiphyseal closure of bones, and discontinuation of skeletal growth.

The dramatic and extensive physical changes that occur during the transition from child to adult are matched only by the psychosocial changes that occur during the adolescent period. It is not possible to develop one guide that adequately describes and explains the tremendous changes that occur during adolescence because the experience is unique for each adolescent. There are, fortunately, some commonalities within the process, which can be used to facilitate understanding these changes. The transition from child to adult is not a smooth, continuous, or uniform process. There are frequent periods of rapid change, followed by brief plateaus. These periods can change with little or no warning, which makes living with an adolescent difficult at times.

One thing that persons who deal with adolescents must remember is that, no matter how rocky the transition from child to adult, adolescence is not a permanent disability! Eighty percent of adolescents go through adolescence with little or no lasting difficulties. Health care professionals who care for adolescents may need to offer support to worried parents that the difficulties their adolescent is experiencing and that the entire family is experiencing as a result may be normal. The adolescent may also need reassurance that his or her feelings are not abnormal.[2,26]

Common concerns identified by adolescents include conflicts with parents, conflicts with siblings, concerns about school, and concerns about peers and peer relationships. Personal identity is an overwhelming concern expressed by adolescents. Common health problems experienced by adolescents are headache, stomachache, and insomnia. These disorders may be psychosomatic in origin. Adolescents also may exhibit situational anxiety and mild depression. The health care worker may need to refer adolescents for specialized counseling or medical care if any of the health care concerns are exaggerated.

Parents of adolescents may also have concerns about their child during the adolescent period. Common concerns related to the adolescent's behavior include rebelliousness, wasting time, risk-taking behaviors, mood swings, drug experimentation, school problems, psychosomatic complaints, and sexual activity. Several "tasks" that adolescents need to fulfill have been identified. These tasks include achieving independence from parents, adopting peer codes and making personal lifestyle choices, forming or revising individual body image and coming to terms with one's body image if it is not "perfect,"and establishing sexual, ego, vocational, and moral identities.[26] The period of adolescence is one of transition from childhood to adulthood. It is filled with conflicts as the adolescent attempts to take on an adult role. Communication with the adolescent and family can help make the transition less stressful.

Common Health Problems

Adolescence is considered to be a relatively healthy period; however, significant morbidity and mortality do occur. Health promotion is of extreme importance during the adolescent period. There are fewer actual physical health problems during this period, but there is a greater risk of morbidity and mortality from other causes, such as accidents, homicide, or suicide.

Several factors contribute to the risk for injury during adolescence. The adolescent is unable to predict potentially dangerous situations, possibly because of a discrepancy between physical maturity and cognitive and emotional development. Certain behavioral and developmental characteristics of the adolescent exaggerate this problem. Adolescents may feel the need to challenge parental or other authority. They also have a strong desire to "fit in" with the peer group. Adolescents exhibit a type of magical thinking and have a need to experiment with potentially dangerous situations or behaviors.

More than 80% of deaths during adolescence are attributed to injuries. Leading causes of nonintentional injuries are automobile accidents (number 1), motorcycle accidents, and drowning (number 2). Other accidental injuries include falls, striking objects, firearm mishaps (number 3), and sports. Accidental injuries kill more adolescents every year than all other causes of death combined, with males accounting for four of five injury victims. Automobile accidents account for 50% of all deaths of adolescents from ages 16 through 19 years.[2,26] Drowning, which is more common in males than females, decreases in prevalence after 18 years of age. Most drownings occur on weekends from May through August, are associated with alcohol use, and occur in fresh water rather than in the ocean. Firearm injuries are the third leading cause of nonintentional mortality in adolescents. Firearm accidents occur much more frequently to males between the ages of 15 to 24 years than to males of any other age.[2] Many of these accidents occur in the adolescent's home while cleaning or playing with the gun.

Other nonintentional causes of death include poisoning, skateboard injuries, all-terrain vehicle accidents, and participation in sports. However, most sports injuries are not fatal. Approximately one third to one half of all injuries occur in the school. Falls are the most common cause of injury in high schools, with contusions, abrasions, swelling, sprains, strains, and dislocations being the most common injuries.[2,26] Cancer is the fourth leading cause of death in adolescents, but it is the leading cause of death from nonviolent sources. There is an increased incidence of certain types of cancer during adolescence, including lymphomas, Hodgkin's disease, and bone and genital tumors. Leukemia is the leading cause of cancer mortality in persons between the ages of 15 and 24 years.[26]

Adolescents also are subject to intentional injuries, such as homicide and suicide. Suicide rates have risen dramatically for adolescents since the 1950s, to approximately 13 to 14 per 100,000. Most of the increase can be attributed to the greater number of suicides committed by white males. It is also thought that the rate of adolescent suicide may be higher than what is reported because of underreporting on death certificates.[26] Almost 60% of suicides involve firearms.

The increasing prevalence of sexual activity among adolescents has created unique health problems. These include adolescent pregnancy, sexually transmitted diseases, and human immunodeficiency virus (HIV) transmission. Associated problems include substance abuse, such as alcohol, tobacco, inhalants, and other illicit drugs. Health care providers must not neglect discussing sexual activity with the adolescent. Nonjudgmental, open, factual communication is essential for dealing with an adolescent's sexual practices. Discussion of sexual activity is frequently difficult for the adolescent and the adolescent's family. If a relationship exists between the adolescent and the health care provider, this may provide a valuable forum for the adolescent to get accurate information about safe sex, including contraception and avoidance of high-risk behaviors for acquiring sexually transmitted diseases or acquired immunodeficiency syndrome (AIDS).[26]

Substance abuse among adolescents increased rapidly in the 1960s and 1970s but has declined since that time. However, substance abuse is still prevalent in the adolescent age group. Health care workers must be knowledgeable about the symptoms of drug abuse, the consequences of drug abuse, and the appropriate management of adolescents with substance abuse problems. Substance abuse among adolescents includes tobacco products, cigarettes and "smokeless" tobacco (*e.g.*, snuff, chewing tobacco). Other substances include alcohol, marijuana, stimulants, inhalants, cocaine, hallucinogens, tranquilizers, and sedatives. Adolescents are at high risk for succumbing to the peer pressure to participate in substance abuse. They have a strong desire to "fit in" and be accepted by their peer group. It is difficult for them to "just say no." Magical thinking leads adolescents to believe that they will not get "hooked" or that the bad consequences will not happen to them. Adolescents and the rest of society are constantly bombarded with the glamorous side of substance use. Television shows, movies, and magazine advertisements are filled with beautiful, healthy, successful, happy, and popular persons who are smoking cigarettes or drinking beer or other alcoholic beverages. Adolescents are trying to achieve the lifestyle depicted in those ads, and it takes tremendous willpower to resist that temptation. It is important that adolescents be provided with "the rest of the story" through education and constant communication.[2,26]

Pregnancy has become a major problem of the teen years. Approximately, 1 million adolescents in the United States become pregnant annually.[2] Four of every 10 teenage females become pregnant before reaching age 20. One fifth of all pregnancies occur within the first month after beginning sexual activity; one half occur within the first 6 months of sexual activity. Of the slightly more than 1 million adolescent pregnancies, 47% delivered, 40% had therapeutic abortions, and 13% had spontaneous abortions.[2]

Adolescent pregnancy carries significant risks to the mother and to the fetus or newborn. The topic of adolescent pregnancy involves issues related to physical and biologic maturity of the adolescent, growth requirements of the adolescent and fetus, and unique prenatal care requirements of the pregnant adolescent. Emotional responses and psychologic issues regarding relationships of the adolescent within her family and with the father of the baby, as well as how the pregnancy will affect the future of the adolescent, must be considered.

In summary, adolescence is a transitional period between childhood and adulthood. It begins with development of secondary sex characteristics (11 to 12 years) and ends with cessation of somatic growth (18 to 20 years). This is a period of major growth spurt, which is more pronounced in males. The endocrine system is of great importance with its numerous hormonal changes and their initiation and continuation of the growth spurt. Psychosocial changes are equally dramatic during this period and often place tremendous pressure on relationships between adults and the adolescent. Adolescence is a relatively healthy period, but significant morbidity and mortalitity exists as a result of accidents, homicide, and suicide. The increasing prevalence of sexual activity and substance abuse places the adolescent at risk for HIV infection; alcohol, tobacco, and other drug abuse; and adolescent pregnancy.

REFERENCES

1. National Center for Health Statistics. (1996). March of Dimes www.modimes.org/stats/stats.htm.
2. Whaley L.F., Wong D.L. (1995). *Nursing care of infants and children* (5th ed., pp. 2–28, 106–154, 337–363). St. Louis: Mosby–Year Book.
3. Center for Disease Control. (1993). Infant Mortality—United States, 1991. *Morbidity and Mortality Weekly Report* 42, 926.
4. Behrman R.E. (Ed.). (1992). *Nelson textbook of pediatrics* (14th ed., pp. 13–43). Philadelphia: W.B. Saunders.
5. Hermanson M. (1990). *Biostatistics: Some basic concepts*. Patterson, NY: Caduceus Medical Publishers.
6. Moore K.L. (1988). *The developing human* (4th ed.). Philadelphia: W.B. Saunders.
7. Korones S.B. (1986). Significance of the relationship of birth weight to gestational age. In Korones S.B. (Ed.). *High risk newborn infants: The basis for intensive nursing care* (pp. 38–85, 205–287, 364–392, 111–150). St. Louis: C.V. Mosby.
8. Kliegman R.M. (1992). Intrauterine growth retardation: Determinants of aberrant fetal growth. In Fanaroff A.A., Martin R.J. (Eds.). *Neonatal–perinatal medicine: Diseases of the fetus and infant* (pp. 149–185). St. Louis: Mosby–Year Book.
9. Nagey D.A., Viscardi R.M. (1993). Retarded intrauterine growth. In Jeffrey J., Pomerance C., Richardson J. (Eds.). *Neonatology for the clinician*. Norwalk, CT: Appleton & Lange.
10. Luchenco L.O., Hansman C., Dressler M., et al. (1963). Intrauterine growth as estimated from liveborn birthweight data at 24 to 42 weeks of gestation. *Pediatrics* 32, 793–800.
11. Battaglia F.C., Luchenco L.O. (1967). A practical classification of newborn infants by weight and gestational age. *Journal of Pediatrics* 71, 159.
12. Ballard J.L., Novak K., Driver M. (1979). A simplified score on assessment of fetal maturation in newly born infants. *Journal of Pediatrics* 95 (5), 769.
13. Oski F.A., DeAngelis C.D., Feign R.D., McMillan J.A., Warshaw J.B. (1994). *Principles and practice of pediatrics* (2nd ed., pp. 344, 437). Philadelphia: J.B. Lippincott.
14. Wissow L.S. (1995). Child abuse and neglect. *New England Journal of Medicine* 332 (21), 1425–1431
15. Dubowitz L.M., Dubowitz V., Goldberg C. (1970). Clinical assessment of gestational age in the newborn infant. *Journal of Pediatrics* 77, 1.
16. Apgar V. (1953). A proposal for a new method of evaluation of the newborn infant. *Current Research in Anesthesia and Analgesia* 32, 260.
17. Blackburn S.T. (1993). Assessment and management of neurologic dysfunction. In Kenner C. *Comprehensive neonatal nursing: A physiologic persepctive* (pp. 673–678). Philadelphia: W.B. Saunders.
18. Mangurten H.H. (1992). Birth injuries. In Fanaroff A.A., R.J. Martin (Eds.). *Neonatal–perinatal medicine: Diseases of the fetus and infant* (pp. 346–371). St. Louis: Mosby–Year Book.
19. Fanaroff A.A., Martin R.J. (1992). The respiratory distress syndrome and its management. In Fanaroff A.A., Martin R.J. (Eds.). *Neonatal–perinatal medicine: Diseases of the fetus and infant* (pp. 810–819). St. Louis: Mosby–Year Book.

20. Papile L. (1992). Periventricular–intraventricular hemorrhage. In Fanaroff A.A., Martin R.J. (Eds.). *Neonatal–perinatal medicine: Diseases of the fetus and infant* (pp. 719–728). St. Louis: Mosby–Year Book.
21. Byrne W.J. (1991). Disorders of the intestines and pancreas. In Tauesch W.H., Ballard R.A., Avery M.E. (Eds.). *Diseases of the newborn* (pp. 681–693). Philadelphia: W.B. Saunders.
22. Valdes-Dopena M. (1992). The sudden infant death syndrome: Pathologic findings. *Clinical Perinatology* 19, 701–716.
23. Hunt C. (1996). Sudden infant death syndrome. In Nelson W.E. (Ed.). *Nelson textbook of pediatrics* (15th ed., pp. 1991–1996). Philadelphia, W.B. Saunders.
24. Hoffman H.J., Hellman L.S. (1992). Epidemiology of the sudden death infant syndrome: Maternal, neonatal, and postnatal risk factors. *Clinical Perinatology* 19, 717–738.
25. Erikson E. (1963). *Childhood and society*. New York: W.W. Norton.
26. Neinstein L.S., Kaufman F.R. (1991). *Adolescent health care: A practical guide* (pp. 3–37, 561–575). Baltimore: Urban & Schwarzenberg.

ADDITIONAL READINGS

Castiglia P.T. (1992). Alcohol use by children. *Journal of Pediatric Health Care* 6 (5), 271.

Crawford T.O. (1992). Clinical evaluation of the floppy infant. *Pediatric Annals* 21 (6), 348–354.

D'Apolito K. (1991). What is an organized infant? *Neonatal Network* 10 (1), 23–29.

Dine M.S., Gartside P.S., Glueck C.J., et al. (1981). Relationship of head circumference to length in the first 400 days of life: A mnemonic. *Pediatrics* 67, 506–507.

Emans S.J. (1997). Menarche and beyond–Do eating and exercise make a difference. *Pediatric Annals* 26 (Suppl 2), S137–S141.

Faigel H.C.(1996). Primary care of the adolescent patient. *Hospital Practice* 31 (4), 127–148.

Gluckman P.D., Cutfield W., Harding J.E., et al. (1996). Metabolic consequences of intrauterine growth retardation. *Acta Paedriatric* 417 (Suppl), 3–6.

Lobo M.L., Barnard K.E., Coombs J.B. (1992). Failure to thrive: A parent–infant interaction. *Journal of Pediatric Nursing* 7 (4), 251.

Mathew O.P., Thoppil C.K., Belan M. (1991). Motor activity and apnea in preterm infants. *American Review of Respiratory Disease* 144, 842–844.

Neerhof M.G. (1995). Causes of intrauterine growth restriction. *Clinics in Pernatology* 22 (2), 375—386.

Robinson P. (1997). Puberty–Am I normal? *Pediatric Annals* 26 (Suppl 2), S133–S136.

Schanler R.J. (1995). Suitability of human milk for the low-birthweight infant. *Clinics in Pernatology* 22 (1), 207–222.

Wright K. (1997). Anticipatory guidance: Developing healthy sexuality. *Pediatric Annals*. 26 (Suppl 2), S143–S144.

CHAPTER 58

Concepts of Altered Health in Older Adults

Janice Kuiper Pikna

For age is opportunity no less than youth, itself, though in another dress. And as the evening twilight fades away the sky is filled with stars, invisible by day.

Henry Wadsworth Longfellow

Aging is a natural, lifelong process that brings with it unique biopsychosocial changes. These changes create special health care needs for the older adult population that merit consideration. Because the prediction for the future is a continuous rise in the older adult population, there is a need to focus on the special health care needs of this group. *Gerontology* is the discipline that studies aging and the aged from biologic, psychologic, and sociologic perspectives. It explores the dynamic processes of complex physical changes, adjustments in psychologic functioning, and alterations in social identities. Through a holistic approach, health care providers specializing in gerontology seek to assist the older adult in maximizing functional abilities while attempting to prevent and minimize illness and disability.

An important first distinction is that aging and disease are not synonymous. Unfortunately, a common assumption is that growing older is inevitably accompanied by illness, disability, and overall decline in function. The fact is that the aging body can accomplish most, if not all, of the functions of its youth; the difference is that it may take longer, require greater motivation, and be less precise. But as in youth, maintenance of physiologic function occurs through continued use.

The Elderly and Theories of Aging

After you have completed this section of the chapter, you should be able to meet the following objectives:

- State a definition for young-old, middle-old, and old-old and characterize the changing trend in the elderly population
- State a philosophy of aging that incorporates the positive aspects of the aging process
- Compare the focus of programmed change and stochastic theories of aging

Who are the Elderly?

The older adult population is typically defined in chronologic terms and includes individuals 65 years of age and older. This age was chosen somewhat arbitrarily, and historically it is linked to the Social Security Act of 1935. With this Act, the first national pension system in the United States, which designated 65 years as the pensionable age, was developed. Since then, the expression "old age" has been understood to apply to anyone older than 65 years. Because there is considerable heterogeneity among this group, older adults are often subgrouped into young-old (65 to 74 years), middle-old (75

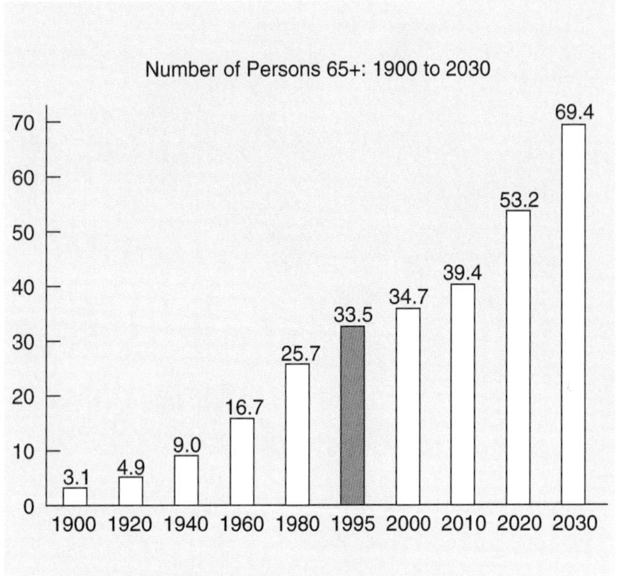

Figure 58-1 ■ ■ ■
Number of people 65 years and older, 1990 to 2030 (in millions) (American Association of Retired Persons. [1996]. A profile of older Americans, Washington, DC: AARP)

to 84 years), and old-old (85+ years) to more accurately reflect changes in function that occur. Age parameters, however, are somewhat irrelevant, because chronologic age is a poor predictor of biologic function. However, chronologic age does help to quantify the number of individuals in a group and allows predictions to be made for the future.

In 1995, 12.8% of the total United States population (approximately 33.5 million) was 65 years of age or older, and the proportion has increased yearly. This older adult population is expected to grow to 70 million by the year 2030 (Fig. 58–1). The older adult population itself is getting older. Average life expectancy has increased as a result of overall advances in health care technology, improved nutrition, and improved sanitation. Women who are now 65 years of age can expect to live an additional 18.6 years (83.6 years old), and men an additional 15.6 years (80.6 years old).[1]

Aging can be thought of somewhat as a women's issue because women tend to outlive men. In 1995, there was a sex ratio of 145 women for every 100 men older than 65 years in the United States. This ratio increases in the old-old age group, with a high of 257 women for every 100 men for individuals 85 years of age or older. Marital status also changes with advancing age. In 1994, one half of all older women living in the community were widows, and there were five times as many widows (8.5 million) as there were widowers (1.7 million).[1]

Although 3.8 million older adults were in the work force in 1995 (*i.e.*, working or actively seeking work), most were retired.[1] Retirement presents a significant role change for older adults. Attitudes and adjustment to retirement are influenced by preretirement lifestyles and values. Individuals with leisure pursuits during their work life seem to adjust better to retirement than those whose lives were dominated by work. For many of today's cohort of older adults, the work ethic of the Great Depression remains profoundly ingrained as the central purpose in life. When work is gone, a significant loss is felt, and something must be substituted in its place. Because leisure has not always been a highly valued activity, older adults may have difficulty learning to engage in meaningful leisure pursuits.

Loss of productive work is just one of many losses that can accompany the aging process. Loss of a spouse is a highly significant life event that commonly has negative implications for the survivor. Experts cite an increased mortality among recently bereaved older adults (especially men), an increased incidence of depression, psychologic distress and loneliness, and higher rates of chronic illness. Loss of physical health and loss of independence are other changes that can affect the psychosocial aspects of aging, as can relocation, loss of friends and relatives, and changes in the family structure.

Poverty is common among the elderly population. In 1995, about 3.7 million (10.5%) persons of those 65 years of age and older lived below the poverty line, with a median income of $16,484 for men and $9,355 for women. The income for African-American elderly was even lower. Social Security was the primary source of income (42%), followed by public and private pensions (19%), asset income (18%), earnings (18%), and all other sources (3%) (data reported for noninstitutionalized elderly only).[1]

Contrary to popular belief, most older adults live in community settings. Most live in some type of family setting, with a spouse, their children, or other relatives, and about 30% live alone. Only 5.0% of all individuals 65 years of age and older reside in long-term care facilities or nursing homes. However, this number increases to 24% for persons 85 years of age or older.[1]

Older adults are the largest consumers of health care. In 1994, total national health spending was $832 billion; Medicare accounted for 20% of this amount. Almost one half of all adult hospital beds are filled with patients age 65 years and older.[2]

Theories of Aging

The lifestyle changes that occur with aging have been described in various developmental theories. Probably the most widely known is Erikson's eight stages of development. According to his theory, the first seven developmental stages span the period from childbirth through middle adulthood. The eighth stage focuses on "ego integrity versus despair" of older adulthood. Ego integrity is the acceptance of one's life in relation to humanity and one's place in history. Lack of ego integrity leads to despair, signified by a nonacceptance of one's lifestyle and a fear of death. Despair may be manifested as apathy, depression, or decreased life satisfaction.[3,4]

The stages of physical change that occur as part of the aging process are less well articulated. Several theories attempt to explain the biology of aging through a variety of scientific observations at the molecular, cellular, organ, and system levels. No one theory explains all of the aging processes, but each holds some clues. In reality, it is reasonable to suppose that there are multiple influences that affect the aging process. The various theories of aging can be categorized as programmed change theories and as stochastic theories. *Programmed change theories* propose that the changes that occur with aging are genetically programmed; *stochastic theories* maintain that the changes result from an accumulation of random events or damage from environmental hazards.

One programmed change theory involves alterations in the immune system. The theory postulates that the involution of the thymus gland, a process that begins during adolescence, affects the integrity of the immune system. Specifically, it is the T-cell–dependent immune functions that become progressively impaired with aging, reducing resistance to infections and increasing the incidence of autoimmune disease.[5] At the cellular level, Moorhead and Hayflick observed more than 25 years ago that cultured human fibroblasts have a limited ability to replicate (about 50 population doublings) and then die.[6,7] This finding suggested that cell deterioration did not depend solely on environmental influences, but was intrinsic to the cell.

The free radical theory is a stochastic idea in which aging is thought to partially result from the effects of free radical damage. When paired electrons are transiently separated, they produce free radicals that may cause cellular damage (see Chapter 2). Over time, the cumulative effects of free radical damage are theorized to cause cellular dysfunction and may result in aging.[8] Another damage theory, the wear and tear theory, proposes that accumulated damage to vital parts of the cell leads to aging and death. Cellular DNA is cited as an example. If repair to damaged DNA is incomplete or defective, as is thought to occur with aging, declines in cellular function might occur.[9]

These theories help to explain some of the biologic phenomenon of aging. Scientists continue to study these processes in pursuit of a better understanding of the aging process.

In summary, aging is a natural, lifelong process that brings with it unique biopsychosocial changes. Aging is not synonymous with disease or ill health. The aging body can accomplish most or all of the functions of its youth, although they may take longer, require greater motivation, and be less precise.

The older adult population is typically defined in chronologic terms as individuals 65 years of age and older and can be further defined as young-old (65–74 years), middle-old (75–84 years), and old-old (85+ years). The number of older persons has increased and is expected to continue to grow in the future, with an anticipated 70 million Americans over age 65 by the year 2030.

There are two main types of theories used to explain the biologic changes that occur with aging: programmed change theories, which propose that aging changes are genetically programmed, and stochastic theories, which maintain that aging changes result from an accumulation of random events or damage from environmental hazards.

Physiologic Changes of Aging

After you have completed this section of the chapter, you should be able to meet the following objectives:

- Describe common skin changes that occur with aging
- Explain how muscle changes that occur with aging affect high-speed performance and endurance
- Describe the process of bone loss that occurs with aging
- State the common changes in blood pressure regulation that occur with aging
- List the changes in respiratory function that occur with aging
- Relate aging changes in neural function to the overall function of the body
- Briefly discuss the effects of aging on vision, hearing, taste, and smell
- Describe three changes that occur in the gastrointestinal tract with aging
- State the significance of decreased lean body mass on interpretation of the glomerular filtration rate using serum creatinine levels

The physiologic changes seen in the elderly reflect not only the aging process, but also the effects of years of exposure to environmental agents such as sunlight and cigarette smoke, and disease processes such as diabetes mellitus. Overall, there is a general decline in the structure and function of the body with advancing age. The decline results in a decreased reserve capacity of the various organ systems that consequently produces reduced homeostatic capabilities, making the older adult more vulnerable to stressors such as illness, trauma, surgery, medications, and environmental changes.

Research to identify true age-related changes as opposed to disease states is difficult. Studies using cross-sectional methodologies are the easiest to perform; however, mortality can confound the results. Although longitudinal studies tend to be more precise, they require years to perform and may not be able to account for numerous variables that enter into the aging equation, such as environment, occupation, and diet. However, it is important to differentiate, as much as possible, those changes that occur in the body as a result of aging from those that occur from disease. This distinction allows for more accurate diagnosis and treatment of disease conditions and helps to avoid inappropriate labeling of aging changes.

Skin

Changes in the skin more obviously reflect the aging process than do changes in other organ systems (see Chapter 15). Aging can impinge on the primary functions of the skin: protection from the environment, temperature regulation, maintenance of fluid and electrolyte balance, sensory regulation, and excretion of metabolic wastes. Exposure to sunlight and harsh weather accelerate aging of the skin.

With aging, the skin becomes wrinkled and dry and develops uneven pigmentation. The thickness of the dermis, or middle layer of skin, decreases by approximately 20%, which gives the skin an overall thin and transparent quality. This is especially true for areas exposed to sunlight. Dermal collagen fibers rearrange and degenerate, resulting in decreased skin strength and elasticity. Cellularity and vascularity of the dermis decrease with advancing age and can cause vascular fragility, leading to senile purpura (*i.e.*, skin hemorrhages) and slow skin healing. Delayed wound healing may be influenced by other factors such as poor nutrition and circulation and by changes in immune function.[10,11] The function of the sebaceous glands diminishes with age and leads to a decrease in sebum secretion. The decrease in size, number, and function of the eccrine sweat glands causes a decrease in their capacity to produce sweat.

Fingernails and toenails become dull, brittle, and thick, mostly as a result of decreased vascularity of the nail beds. Age-related changes in hair occur as well. Owing to a decline in melanin production by the hair follicle, about one half of the population over 50 years of age has at least 50% gray hair, regardless of sex or original hair color. Changes in hair growth and distribution are also seen.[10,11] Hairs on the scalp, axillae, and pubis become fewer, and the hairs of the ears and nostril coarsen. Skin disorders are common among the older adult population and can include skin cancers, keratoses (*i.e.*, warty lesions), xerosis (*i.e.*, excessive dryness), dermatitis, and pruritus (*i.e.*, generalized itching).

Stature and Musculoskeletal Function

Aging is accompanied by a a progressive decline in height, especially among older women. This decline in height is mainly attributed to compression of the spinal column. Body composition changes as well. The amount of fat increases, and lean body mass and total body water decreases with advancing age.

With aging, there is a reduction in muscle size and strength that is related to a loss of muscle fibers and a reduction in the size of the existing fibers. Although the decline in strength that occurs with aging cannot be halted, its progress can be slowed with exercise.[12] There is a decline in high-speed performance and reaction time because of a decrease in type II muscle fibers.[13] Impairments in the nervous system can also cause movements to slow. However, type I muscle fibers, which offer endurance, are thought to remain consistent with age.

Numerous studies have reported a loss of bone mass with aging, regardless of gender, race, or body size. With aging the process of bone formation (*i.e.*, renewal) is slowed in relation to bone resorption (*i.e.*, breakdown), resulting in a loss of bone mass and weakened bone structure. This is especially true for postmenopausal women. By age 65, most women have lost two thirds of their skeletal mass owing to a decrease in estrogen production.[14] Skeletal bone loss is not a uniform process. Beginning around age 30, bone loss begins predominantly in the trabecular bone (*i.e.*, fine network of bony struts and braces in the medullary cavity) of the heads of the femora and radii and in the vertebral bodies.[13,14] By age 80, women have lost nearly 43% of their trabecular bone, and men have lost 27%. This process becomes pathologic (*i.e.*, osteoporosis) when it significantly increases the predisposition to fracture and associated complications (see Chapter 46).

The prevalence of joint disease is increased among the elderly. By age 65, 80% of the population has some articular disease. Osteoarthritis is so common among the elderly that it is often incorrectly assumed to be a normal age-related change rather than a disease. The synovial joints are ultimately affected by osteoarthritis, most commonly the joints of the hands, feet, knees, hips, and shoulders. It is characterized by cartilage loss and new bone formation, accounting for a distortion in articulation, limited range of motion, and joint instability (see Chapter 47). Age is the single greatest risk factor for developing osteoarthritis, in part because of the mechanical impact on joints over time, but it is also related to injury, altered physical condition of the articular cartilage, obesity (*e.g.*, knee), congenital deformity (*e.g.*, hip), crystal deposition in articular cartilage (*e.g.*, knee), and heredity. Pain, immobility, and joint inflammation often ensue. Treatment is aimed at minimizing risk factors, weight loss if indicated, exercise to increase muscle strength, and pain relief measures.[12,14]

Cardiovascular Function

Cardiovascular disease remains the leading cause of morbidity and mortality in older adults. It is often difficult to separate true age-related changes in the cardiovascular system from disease processes. The aorta and arteries tend to become stiffer and less distensible with age, the heart becomes less responsive to the catecholamines, the maximal exercise heart rate declines, and there is a decreased rate of diastolic relaxation.

Although approximately 30% to 50% of older adults suffer from hypertension, the disorder is not considered a normal age-related process.[15] The elevation in blood pressure is more pronounced for the systolic blood pressure than for the diastolic blood pressure, probably as a result of increased aortic stiffness. In the elderly, compensatory cardiovascular mechanisms are often delayed or insufficient, so that a drop in blood pressure due to position change or consumption of a meal is common.[16] Orthostatic hypotension, or a significant drop in systolic blood pressure on assumption of the upright position, is more common among the elderly (see Chapter 18). Even in the absence of orthostatic hypotension, the elderly respond to postural stress with diminished changes in heart rate and diastolic pressure. This altered response to orthostatic stress is thought to result from changes in autonomic nervous system function, inadequate functioning of the circulatory system, or both.[17]

Senescent cardiac muscle typically displays a decreased response to β-adrenergic stimulation and circulating catecholamines, and there is increased diastolic stiffness of the ventricles that impedes filling, probably because of a slower rate of diastolic relaxation. Although early diastolic filling decreases by approximately 50% between ages 20 and 80 years, filling volumes are maintained, most likely as a result of an enhanced atrial contraction and its contribution to ventricular filling. The afterload (*i.e.,* opposition to left ventricular ejection) rises steadily with age as the ascending aorta becomes more rigid and as the resistance in peripheral arterial vessels increases. Although the overall size of the heart does not increase, the thickness of the left ventricular wall may increase with age, in part responding to the increased afterload that develops because of blood vessel changes.[18] The resting heart rate remains unchanged or decreases only slightly with age; however, the maximum heart rate than can be achieved during maximal exercise is decreased.

Despite aging changes and cardiovascular disease, overall cardiovascular function at rest in most healthy elderly persons is considered adequate to meet the body's needs. Earlier studies suggested that the resting cardiac output declines with age.[19] However, later studies in which subjects were carefully screened to exclude cardiovascular disease showed that resting cardiac output is unaffected by age. Cardiac output is essentially maintained in healthy older adults (men more than women) during exercise despite the decreased heart rate response, apparently because of a greater stroke volume resulting from increased end-diastolic volume (*i.e.,* Frank-Starling mechanism) during exercise.[20,21]

Respiratory Function

As lung function changes with age, it is often difficult to differentiate the effects of age from those of environmental and disease factors. Maximal oxygen consumption (Vo_2max), a measure used to determine overall cardiopulmonary function, declines with age. Numerous studies have indicated that Vo_2max can improve significantly with exercise and that the Vo_2max of older adult master athletes can meet and exceed that of their younger counterparts.

A progressive loss of elastic recoil within the lung is caused by changes in amount of elastin and composition of collagen fibers. Calcification of the soft tissues of the chest wall causes increased stiffness and thus increases the workload of the respiratory muscles. There is a loss of alveolar structure that decreases the surface area of gas exchange. Although the total lung capacity remains constant, the consequences of these changes result in an increased residual lung volume, a decreased functional reserve capacity, and a decline in vital capacity. There is a linear fall in arterial oxygen tension (Po_2) of about 20 mm Hg from 20 to 70 years of age. This is thought to result primarily from the ventilation-perfusion mismatching of the aging lung.[10,22]

Neurologic Function

Changes at the structural, chemical, and functional levels of the nervous system occur with normal aging, but overall they do not interfere with day-to-day routines unless specific neurologic diseases come into play. The weight of the brain decreases with age, and there is a loss of neurons in the brain and spinal cord. Neuron loss is most pronounced in the cerebral cortex, especially in the superior temporal area. Additional changes take place within the neurons and supporting cells. Atrophy of the neuronal dendrites results in impaired synaptic connections, diminished electrochemical reactions, and neural dysfunction. Synaptic transmissions are also affected by changes in the chemical neurotransmitters dopamine, acetylcholine, and serotonin. As a result, many neural processes slow. Lipofuscin deposits (*i.e.,* yellow, insoluble intracellular material) are found in greater amounts in the aged brain.[23]

Sensorimotor changes show a decline in motor strength, slowed reaction time, diminished reflexes (especially in the ankles), and proprioception changes. These changes can cause the balance problems and slow, more deliberate movements that are frequently seen in older individuals.[24]

Even though changes in the brain are associated with aging, overall cognitive abilities remain intact. Although language skills and attention are not altered with advanced age, performance and constructional task abilities can decline, as can short-term memory and immediate recall. A change in personality or significant cognitive deficits is considered unusual with normal aging, and if either occur, evaluation is in order. Dementia and / or depression can frequently be the cause.

Special Senses

Sensory changes with aging can greatly affect the older adult's level of functioning and quality of life. Vision and hearing impairments due to disease states, for example, can interfere with written and verbal communication and may lead to social isolation and depression.

Vision

There is a general decline in visual acuity with age, and nearly all individuals older than 55 years of age require vision correction for reading or distance. The decline occurs as a result of a smaller pupil diameter, loss of refractive power of the lens, and an increase in the scattering of light. The most common visual problem among older adults is presbyopia, or difficulty focusing on near objects. It is mainly caused by decreased elasticity of the lens and atrophy of the ciliary muscle (see Chapter 41).[25]

Glare and abrupt changes in light pose particular problems for older adults. Both are reasons why the elderly frequently give up night driving; they also increase their risk for falls and injury. Color discrimination changes also take place with aging. In particular, older adults have more difficulty identifying blues and greens. This is thought to be related to problems associated with filtering short wavelengths of light (*i.e.*, violet, blue, green) through a yellowed, opaque lens. Corneal sensitivity may also diminish with age, so that older adults may be less aware of injury or infection.[25]

Ophthalmologic diseases and disorders are common in the elderly. Cataracts, glaucoma, and macular degeneration are seen frequently and can greatly impair vision and function. Low-vision aids, such as special magnifiers and high-intensity lighting that mimics sunlight, can assist in optimizing vision in otherwise uncorrectable ophthalmologic problems.

Hearing

Hearing loss is common among older adults, and some degree of impairment is almost inevitable with advancing age. It has been reported that 24% of independent individuals 65 to 74 years of age and 39% of those 75 years of age and older have a hearing impairment, whereas as many as 70% of institutionalized older adults have difficulty hearing.[26]

Presbycusis, or the hearing loss of old age, is characterized by a gradual, progressive onset of bilateral and symmetric sensorineural hearing loss of high-frequency tones (see Chapter 43). Speech discrimination, or the ability to understand the spoken word, is often impaired. Accelerated speech and shouting can increase distortion and further compound the problem. When speaking to hearing-impaired older adults, it is helpful to face them directly so they can observe lip movements and facial expressions. Speech should be slow and direct. Loudness can be irritating. Rephrasing misunderstood messages can also improve understanding of the spoken word. Hearing aids can be effective for various levels of hearing loss and may greatly improve the ability to hear and communicate.

Cerumen (*i.e.*, ear wax) impaction in the external auditory canal is also commonly seen in older adults and can impair hearing. The cerumen glands, which are modified apocrine sweat glands, atrophy and produce drier cerumen. This may be partially responsible for more frequent cerumen impactions in the older adult population.

Taste and Smell

Olfaction, or the sense of smell, declines with aging possibly as a result of generalized atrophy of the olfactory bulbs and a moderate loss of olfactory neurons. A decreased sense of taste occurs with aging, but it is believed to be less affected than olfaction. Because taste and smell are necessary for the enjoyment of food flavor, older adults may not enjoy eating as much as in their youth. Drugs and disease also may affect taste. Alterations in taste and smell, along with other factors such as eating alone, decreased ability to purchase and prepare food, and the high cost of some foods, may account for poor nutritional intake in some older adults.

Immune Function

An overall decline in immune system capabilities with aging can pose an increased risk for some infections (see Chapter 11). Involution of the thymus gland is complete by about age 45 to 50, and although the total number of T cells remains unchanged, there are changes in the function of helper T cells that alter the cellular immune response of older adults. There is also evidence of an increase in various autoantibodies (*e.g.*, rheumatoid factor) as a person ages, increasing the risk of autoimmune disorders. Older adults are more susceptible to urinary tract infections, respiratory tract infections, wound infections, and nosocomial infections. The mortality rate from influenza and bronchopneumonia is increased for the older adult population. Local organ factors and coincident diseases probably play a bigger role in the acquisition of these infections than age-related changes in immunity.[10,27]

Gastrointestinal Function

The gastrointestinal tract shows less age-associated change in function than many other organ systems. Although tooth loss is common and about 40% of the older adult population is edentulous, it is not considered part of the normal aging process. Poor dental hygiene with associated caries and periodontal disease is the main reason for the loss. Toothlessness can lead to dietary changes and can be associated with malnutrition. Use of dentures can enhance mastication; however, taste sensation is inhibited. Because of improved dental technology and the fluoridated water supply, more persons are able to keep their teeth into their later years. Xerostomia (*i.e.*, dry mouth) is also common, but it is not universal among older adults, and typically occurs as a result of decreased salivary secretions. Other causes of dry mouth can include medications, such as anticholinergics and tranquilizers, radiation therapy, and obstructive nasal diseases that induce mouth breathing.

Soergel and his colleagues (1964) coined the term *presbyesophagus* to denote changes in esophageal function such as decreased motility and inadequate relaxation of the lower esophageal sphincter that occur with aging.[28] However, in studies that controlled for disease states such as diabetes mellitus and neuropathies, no increase in abnormal motility was observed. Generally, the physiologic function of the esophagus appears to remain intact with advancing age.

Atrophy of the gastric mucosa and a decrease in gastric secretions can occur in older adults. Achlorhydria (*i.e.,* decrease in hydrochloric acid secretion) occurs, probably as a result of a loss of parietal cells. Although not universal, achlorhydria is more prevalent among older adults and can cause impaired gastric absorption of substances requiring an acid environment.

Atrophic gastritis and decreased secretion of intrinsic factor are more common with aging and result in a malabsorption of vitamin B_{12}. Because vitamin B_{12} is necessary for the maturation of red blood cells, a deficiency can lead to a type of macrocytic anemia called *pernicious anemia*. Vitamin B_{12} deficiency can also cause neurologic abnormalities such as peripheral neuropathy, ataxia, and even dementia. Treatment consists of regular periodic vitamin B_{12} replacement therapy through injection, because the oral form is not absorbed because of a lack of intrinsic factor.[29]

The small intestine shows some age-related morphologic changes, such as mucosal atrophy; however, absorption of most nutrients and other functions appears to remain intact. Absorption of calcium, however, decreases with aging and may reflect decreased intestinal absorption along with other factors, such as reduced intake of vitamin D, decreased formation of vitamin D_3 by the skin because of reduced sun exposure, and decreased activation of vitamin D_3 by the liver and kidney.

Diverticula of the colon are common among older adults; more than 50% of individuals older than 80 years have diverticular disease. The high incidence appears to result mainly from a low-fiber diet. Constipation, or infrequent passage of hard stool, is another frequently occurring phenomenon. It is often attributed to immobility and decreased physical activity, a low-fiber diet, decreased fluid intake, and medications; malignancies and other disease states can also be responsible. Complications of constipation can include fecal impaction or obstruction, megacolon, rectal prolapse, hemorrhoids, and laxative abuse.

Renal Function

Although age-related anatomic and physiologic changes occur, the aging kidney remains capable of maintaining fluid and electrolyte balance remarkably well. Aging changes result in a decreased reserve capacity, which may alter the kidney's ability to maintain homeostasis in the face of illnesses or stressors. Overall, there is a general decline in kidney mass with aging, predominantly in the renal cortex. The number of functional glomeruli decreases by 30% to 50%, with an increased percentage of sclerotic or abnormal glomeruli.

Numerous cross-sectional and longitudinal studies have documented a steady, age-related decline in total renal blood flow of about 10% per decade after age 20, so that the renal blood flow of an 80-year-old person averages approximately 300 ml/minute, compared with 600 ml/minute in a younger adult. The major decline in blood flow occurs in the cortical area of the kidney, causing a progressive, age-related decrease in the *glomerular filtration rate* (GFR). Serum creatinine, a byproduct of muscle metabolism, is often used as a measure of GFR. The decline in GFR that occurs with aging is not accompanied by an equivalent increase in serum creatinine levels, because the production of creatinine is reduced as muscle mass declines with age. Serum creatinine levels are often used as an index of kidney function when prescribing and calculating drug doses for medications that are eliminated through the kidneys; this has important implications for older adults. If not carefully addressed, improper drug dosing can lead to an excess accumulation of circulating drugs and result in toxicity. A formula that adjusts for age-related changes in serum creatinine for individuals 40 through 80 years of age is available (see Chapter 29).

Renal tubular function declines with advancing age, and the ability to concentrate and dilute urine in response to fluid and electrolyte impairments is diminished. The aging kidney's ability to conserve sodium in response to sodium depletion is impaired and can result in hyponatremia. A decreased ability to concentrate urine, an age-related decrease in responsiveness to antidiuretic hormone, and an impaired thirst mechanism may account for the older adult's easier predisposition to dehydration during periods of stress and illness. Older adults are also more prone to hyperkalemia and hypokalemia when stressed than are younger individuals. An elevated serum potassium may result from a decreased GFR, lower renin and aldosterone levels, and changes in tubular function. Low potassium levels, on the other hand, are more commonly caused by gastrointestinal disorders or diuretic use. Neither is the result of aging.[30]

Genitourinary Function

Changes in the bladder occur with the aging process, resulting in a possible decline in function. Overall, the smooth muscle and supportive elastic tissue are replaced with fibrous connective tissue. This can cause incomplete bladder emptying and a diminished force of urine stream. Bladder capacity also decreases with age, whereas the frequency of urination increases. As elastic tissue and muscles weaken, stress incontinence becomes more prevalent.

In aging women, atrophy of perineal structures can cause the urethral meatus to recede along the vaginal wall. Atrophy of other pelvic organs occurs in the aging woman because of diminished estrogen production after menopause: vaginal secretions diminish; the vaginal lining is thinner, drier, less elastic, and more easily traumatized; and normal flora are altered. These changes can result in vaginal infections, pruritus, and painful intercourse.[10]

In aging men, benign prostatic hyperplasia (BPH) is very common. Incidence progressively increases to about 90% of men who are 80 years old. The condition is often asymptomatic until about age 50. Thereafter, the incidence and severity of symptoms increase with age. BPH can cause obstructive symptoms such as urinary hesitancy, diminished force of stream, retention, and postvoid dribbling; it can also cause irritative symptoms such as frequency, nocturia, urgency, and even urge incontinence (see Chapter 49).[31]

Sexual activity remains possible into late life for men and women. Generally, the duration and intensity of the sexual response cycle is diminished in both sexes. Penile erection takes longer to develop because of changes in neural innervation and vascular supply. Women take longer to experience the physiologic changes of vaginal expansion and lubrication during the excitement phase. Social factors affecting sexual behavior include the desire to remain sexually active, access to a sexually functioning partner, and availability of a conducive environment.[32]

In summary, there is a general decline in the structure and function of the body with advancing age, resulting in a decreased reserve capacity of the various organ systems, including the dermatologic, musculoskeletal, cardiorespiratory, nervous, sensory, immune, gastrointestinal, and genitourinary systems. This results in a reduction of homeostatic capabilities, making the older adult more vulnerable to stressors such as illness, trauma, surgery, medication administration, and environmental changes.

Functional Problems of Aging

After you have completed this section of the chapter, you should be able to meet the following objectives:

- Compare information obtained from functional assessment with that obtained from a physical examination used to arrive at a medical diagnosis
- Cite the differences between chronic and transient urinary incontinence
- State four risk factors for falls in older individuals
- List five symptoms of depression in older adults
- Define the term "talking therapy"
- Name a tool that can be used for assessing cognitive function
- State the difference between delirium and dementia

Although aging is not synonymous with disease, the aging process does lend itself to an increased incidence of illness. As chronologic age increases, so does the probability of having multiple chronic diseases. It has been estimated that 86% of older adults have at least one chronic condition, and most actually suffer from more than one. The extent of these problems is described in Table 58–1. Older adults are more likely to experience a decline in overall health and function due to the increased incidence of chronic illness that occurs with advancing age. Because aging also brings with it a decreased ability to maintain homeostasis, illnesses often manifest in an atypical manner.

In addition to chronic illnesses, older adults suffer disproportionately from functional disabilities, or the inability to perform the necessary activities of daily living. It is most likely that the decrements in health that can accompany the aging process are responsible for these functional disabilities. Among the more common functional problems of the older adult are urinary incontinence, falls, depression, dementia, and delirium.

Functional Assessment

Evaluation of the older adult's functional abilities is a key component in gerontologic health care. Medical diagnoses alone are incomplete without an assessment of function. Two older adults with similar medical diagnoses of arthritis, hypertension, and osteoporosis, for example, can be at opposite ends of the spectrum of functional abilities.

Assessing functional status can be done in many different ways using a variety of methods. Measures of function should attempt to systematically and objectively evaluate the level at which an individual is functioning in a variety of areas, including biologic, psychologic, and social health.

Selection of a screening tool to measure function depends on the purpose of data collection, the individual or target population to be assessed, availability and applicability of the instruments, reliability and validity of the screening tools, and the setting or environment. An issue that arises when assessing function is the question of capability versus performance. For example, an older adult may be able to bathe without supervision; however, the long-term care facility where the person resides may discourage it for safety reasons. Among the more commonly used assessment tools are those that measure the ability to perform activities of daily living and the patient's cognitive function.

When evaluating levels of function, determination of the older adult's ability to perform *activities of daily living* (ADL) and *instrumental activities of daily living*

TABLE **58-1**

Common Health Problems in the Elderly

Health Problems	Percentage With Problems
Arthritis	50
Hypertension	36
Heart disease	32
Hearing impairment	29
Cataracts	17
Orthopedic impairments	16
Sinusitis	15
Diabetes	10

(Data from American Association of Retired Persons. [1996]. *A profile of older Americans.* Washington, DC: AARP)

(IADL) should be included. Activities of daily living are basic self-care tasks, such as bathing, dressing, grooming, ambulating, transferring (*e.g.*, from a chair to bed), feeding, and communicating. Instrumental activities of daily living are more complex tasks that are necessary to function in society, such as writing, reading, cooking, cleaning, shopping, laundering, climbing stairs, using the telephone, managing money, managing medications, and using transportation. The IADL tasks indirectly examine cognitive abilities as well, because they require a certain level of cognitive skills to complete.

Several tools are available for measuring functional status. One of the more commonly used tools is the Index of Activities of Daily Living. Developed by Katz in 1963 and revised in 1970, it summarizes performance in six functions: bathing, dressing, toileting, transferring, continence, and feeding. It is used as an assessment tool to determine the need for care and the appropriateness of treatment and as a teaching aid in rehabilitation settings. Through questioning and observation, the rater forms a mental picture of the older adult's functional status as it existed during a 2-week period preceding the evaluation, using the most dependent degree of performance.[33,34] Numerous studies using the Katz Index tool show significant validity and reliability. The advantage of the tool is that it is easy to administer and provides a "snapshot" of the older adult's level of physical functioning. The disadvantage is that it does not include IADL categories that are of equal importance, especially for older adults living in the community.

Urinary Incontinence

Urinary incontinence, or involuntary loss of urine, plagues over 30% of community-living individuals over age 60, 50% of hospitalized older adults, and 60% of residents in long-term care facilities. These estimates may be low because individuals often fail to report symptoms of urinary incontinence, perhaps owing to the attached social stigma. Health care professionals often neglect to elicit such information as well.

Incontinence is an expensive problem. A conservative estimate of cost for direct care of adults with incontinence is over $15 billion annually.[35] Urinary incontinence can have deleterious consequences, such as social isolation and embarrassment, depression and dependency, skin rashes and pressure sores, and financial hardship. Although urinary incontinence is a common disorder, it is not considered a normal aspect of aging. Studies reveal that 60% to 70% of community-dwelling older adults with urinary incontinence can be successfully treated and even cured.

Changes in the micturition cycle that accompany the aging process make the older adult prone to urinary incontinence. A decrease in bladder capacity, in bladder and sphincter tone, and in the ability to inhibit detrusor (*i.e.*, bladder muscle) contractions, combined with the nervous system's increased variability to interpret bladder signals, can cause incontinence (see Chapter 30). Impaired mobility and a slower reaction time can also aggravate incontinence problems.

The causes of incontinence can be divided into two categories: transient and chronic. Of particular importance is the role of pharmaceuticals as a cause of transient urinary incontinence. Numerous medications, such as long-acting sedatives and hypnotics, psychotropics, and diuretics, can induce incontinence. Treatment of transient urinary incontinence is aimed at ameliorating or relieving the cause on the assumption that the incontinence will resolve.

Chronic, or established, urinary incontinence occurs as a failure of the bladder to store urine or a failure to empty urine. Failure to store urine can occur as a result of detrusor muscle overactivity with inappropriate bladder contractions (*i.e., urge incontinence*). There is an inability to delay voiding after the sensation of bladder fullness is perceived. Urge incontinence is typically characterized by large volume leakage episodes occurring at various times of day. Urethral incompetence (*i.e., stress incontinence*) also causes a bladder storage problem. The bladder pressure overcomes the resistance of the urethra and results in urine leakage. Stress incontinence causes an involuntary loss of small amounts of urine with activities that increase intra-abdominal pressure, such as coughing, sneezing, laughing or exercising.

Failure of the bladder to empty urine can occur because of detrusor instability, resulting in urine retention and *overflow incontinence*. Also called neurogenic incontinence, this type of incontinence can be seen with neurologic damage from conditions such as diabetes mellitus and spinal cord injury. Outlet obstruction, as with prostate enlargement and urethral stricture, can also cause urinary retention with overflow incontinence. *Functional incontinence*, or urine leakage due to toileting problems, occurs because cognitive, physical, or environmental barriers impair appropriate use of the toilet.[35,36]

After a specific diagnosis of urinary incontinence is established, treatment is aimed at correcting or ameliorating the problem. Probably the most effective interventions for older adults with incontinence are behavioral techniques. These strategies involve educating the individual and providing reinforcement for effort and progress. Techniques include bladder training, timed voiding or habit training, prompted voiding, pelvic floor muscle (*i.e.*, Kegel) exercises, and dietary modifications. Biofeedback, a training technique to teach pelvic floor muscle exercises, uses computerized instruments to relay information to individuals about their physiologic functions. Biofeedback can be helpful when used in conjunction with other behavioral treatment techniques.[35,36] Use of pads or other absorbent products should be seen as a temporary help measure and not as a cure. Numerous types of products are available to meet many different consumer needs.

Pharmacologic intervention may be helpful for some individuals. Estrogen replacement therapy in postmenopausal women, for example, may help to relieve stress incontinence. Drugs with anticholinergic and bladder smooth muscle relaxant properties (*e.g.*, oxybutynin) may help with urge incontinence. These medications are not without side effects, however, and these must be carefully weighed against the possible benefits.

Surgical intervention may help to relieve urinary incontinence symptoms in appropriate patients. Bladder neck suspension may assist with stress incontinence unrelieved by other interventions, and prostatectomy is appropriate for men with overflow incontinence due to enlarged prostate. Older adults may have medical conditions that preclude surgery. Other treatments include intermittent self-catheterization for some types of overflow incontinence.

Falls

Falls are a common source of concern for the older adult population. The literature reveals that 30% of community-dwelling individuals older than 65 years of age and 50% of nursing home residents fall each year. Most falls do not result in serious injury, but the potential for serious complications and even death is real. Accidents are the sixth leading cause of death among older adults, with falls ranking first in this category. Hip fractures are one of the most feared complications from a fall. More than 250,000 individuals fracture a hip each year; most of these are elderly women. Significant morbidity occurs as a result of a hip fracture. The literature varies, but as many as 50% of older adults who sustain a hip fracture are reported to require nursing home care for at least 1 year, and up to 20% die in the year after a hip fracture. Other bones frequently fractured by older adults who fall are the humerus, wrist, and pelvis. These bones bear the brunt of osteoporotic changes and, as a result, are more vulnerable to injury. Soft tissue injuries such as sprains and strains can also result from falls.[37,38]

Restrictions on an individual's activity may occur because of a fear by the individual or caregiver about possible falling. These anxieties may lead to unnecessary restrictions in independence and mobility and are commonly mentioned as a reason for institutionalization.

Although some falls have a single, obvious cause, such as a slip on a wet or icy surface, most are the result of several factors. Risk factors that predispose to falling include a combination of age-related biopsychosocial changes, chronic illnesses, and situational and environmental hazards. Gait and stability require the integration of information from the special senses, the nervous system, and the musculoskeletal system. Changes in gait and posture that occur in healthy aged individuals also contribute to the problem of falls. The older person's stride shortens; the elbows, trunk, and knees become more flexed; toe and heel lift decreases while walking; and sway while standing increases. Muscle strength and postural control of balance decrease, proprioception input diminishes, and righting reflexes slow. All these factors predispose the older adult to the possibility of falling.[39]

Because the central nervous system integrates sensory input and sends signals to the effector components of the musculoskeletal system, any alteration in neural function can predispose to falls. For this reason, falls have been associated with strokes, Parkinson's disease, and normal pressure hydrocephalus. Similarly, diseases or disabilities that affect the musculoskeletal system, such as arthritis, muscle weakness, or foot deformities, are associated with an increase in the incidence of falls. Age- and disease-related alterations in vision and hearing impair sensory input and can contribute to falls. Vestibular system alterations such as benign positional vertigo or Meniere's disease cause balance problems that can result in falls. Cognitive impairments such as dementia have been associated with an increased risk of falling, most likely because of impaired judgment and problem-solving abilities.

Input from the cardiovascular and respiratory systems influences function and ambulation. Cardiovascular diseases, especially postural hypotension, can cause recurrent falls, solely or in association with the previously mentioned factors. The dramatic drop in blood pressure on rising that is seen in postural hypotension can cause falls because of syncope and dizziness.

Medications are an important and potentially correctable cause of instability and falls. Centrally acting medications, such as sedatives and hypnotics, have been associated with an increase in the risk of falling and injury. Diuretics can cause volume depletion, electrolyte disturbances, and fatigue, predisposing to falls. Antihypertensive drugs can cause fatigue, orthostatic hypotension, and impaired alertness, contributing to the risk of falls.

Environmental hazards play a significant role in falling. More than 70% of falls occur in the home and often involve objects that are tripped over, such as cords, scatter rugs, and small items left on the floor. Poor lighting, ill-fitting shoes, surfaces with glare, and improper use of ambulatory devices such as canes or walkers also contribute to the problem.[37,38] Table 58–2 summarizes the possible causes of falls.

Preventing falls is the key to controlling the potential complications that can result. Because falling is generally multifactorial, the aim of the clinical evaluation is to identify risk factors that can be modified. Assessment of sensory, neurologic, and musculoskeletal systems; direct observation of gait and balance; and a careful medication inventory can help identify possible causes. Treatment can include a variety of interventions, such as surgery for cataracts or cerumen removal for hearing impairment related to excessive ear wax accumulation. Other interventions may include podiatric care, discontinuation or alteration of the medication regimen, exercise programs, physical therapy, and appropriate adaptive devices. The home should also be assessed by an appropriate health care professional (*e.g.*, occupational therapist) and recommendations made regarding modifications to promote safety. Simple changes such as removing scatter rugs, improving the lighting, and installing grab bars in the bathtub can help prevent

TABLE 58-2

Causes of Falls

Accidents
- True accidents (*e.g.*, trips, slips, etc.)
- Interactions between environmental hazards and factors increasing susceptibility

Syncope (sudden loss of consciousness)

Drop attacks (sudden leg weaknesses, without loss of consciousness)

Dizziness and/or vertigo
- Vestibular disease
- CNS disease

Orthostatic hypotension
- Hypovolemia or low cardiac output
- Autonomic dysfunction
- Impaired venous return
- Prolonged bed rest
- Drug-induced hypotension

Drug-related causes
- Diuretics
- Antihypertensives
- Tricyclic antidepressants
- Sedatives
- Antipsychotics
- Hypoglycemics
- Alcohol

Specific disease processes
- Acute illness of any kind ("premonitory fall")
- Cardiovascular
  - Arrhythmias
  - Valvular heart disease (aortic stenosis)
  - Carotid sinus syncope

Neurologic causes
- Transient ischemic attack (TIA)
- Stroke (acute)
- Seizure disorder
- Parkinson's disease
- Cervical or lumbar spondylosis (with spinal cord or nerve root compression)
- Cerebellar disease
- Normal-pressure hydrocephalus (gait disorder)
- CNS lesions (*e.g.*, tumor, subdural hematoma)

Idiopathic (no specific cause identifiable)

(Kane R.L., Ouslander J.G., Abrass I.B. [1994]. *Essentials of geriatrics* [3rd ed.]. New York: McGraw-Hill)

falling. These interventions can maximize the older adult's independence and prevent the morbidity and mortality that can occur as a result of a fall.[37,38]

Depression

Depression is a significant health problem that affects the older adult population. Estimates of depression in the elderly vary widely; however, there is a consensus that the size of the problem is underestimated owing to misdiagnosis and mistreatment. Approximately 15% of community-dwelling older adults are thought to have depressive symptoms. The estimate drops to about 3% when diagnosis is restricted to major depression. Depressive symptoms are seen in about 15% to 25% of nursing home residents.[40]

The term *depression* is used to describe a symptom, syndrome, or disease. As listed in the 1994 *American Psychiatric Association Diagnostic and Statistical Manual* (DSM-IVR), the criteria for the diagnosis and treatment of a major depression include at least five of the following symptoms during the same 2-week period, with at least one of the symptoms being depressed mood or anhedonia (*i.e.*, loss of interest or pleasure): depressed or irritable mood; loss of interest or pleasure in usual activities; appetite and weight changes; sleep disturbance; psychomotor agitation or retardation; fatigue and loss of energy; feelings of worthlessness, self-reproach, or excessive guilt; diminished ability to think or concentrate; and suicidal ideation, plan, or attempt.[41]

Depressive symptomatology can be incorrectly attributed to the aging process, making recognition and diagnosis difficult. Depressed mood, the signature symptom of depression, may be less prominent in the older adult, and more somatic complaints and increased anxiety are reported, confusing the diagnosis. Symptoms of cognitive impairment can be seen in the depressed older adult. Because it can be misdiagnosed as dementia, a thorough medical evaluation is in order. Unlike true dementia, pseudodementia of depression generally improves with treatment for depression. Although similar in clinical presentation, there are some subtle distinctions (Table 58–3). Physical illnesses can complicate the diagnosis as well. Depression can be a symptom of a medical condition, such as pancreatic cancer, hypothyroidism or hyperthyroidism, pneumonia and other infections, congestive heart failure, dementia, and stroke. Medications such as sedatives, hypnotics, steroids, antihypertensives, and analgesics can also induce a depressive state. Numerous confounding social problems, such as bereavement, loss of job or income, and loss of social support, can obscure or complicate the diagnosis.[42,43]

The course of depression in older adults is similar to that in younger persons. As many as 40% experience recurrences. Suicide rates are the highest among the elderly. There is a linear increase in suicide with age, most notably among white men older than 60 years of age. Although the exact reasons are unclear, it may be caused by the emotional alienation that can accompany the aging process, combined with complex biopsychosocial losses.[43,44]

Because diagnosis of depression can be difficult, use of a screening tool may help to objectively measure affective functioning. The Geriatric Depression Scale, an instrument of known reliability and validity, was developed to measure depression specifically in the noninstitutionalized older adult population. The 30-item dichotomous scale elicits information on topics relevant to symptoms of depression among older adults, such as memory loss and anxiety. Many other screening tools, each with its own advantages and disadvantages, exist to evaluate the older adult's level of psychologic functioning, in its entirety or as specific, separate components of function.[45]

TABLE 58-3

Characteristics That Distinguish Dementia From Pseudodementia of Depression

Dementia	Pseudodementia of Depression
Insidious onset	Rapid onset
Symptoms present for long duration	Symptoms present for relatively short time
Inaccurate in answering orientation questions; attempts to cover up inaccuracies	May show disinterest in answering questions; frequent "don't know" or "don't care" response
May try to conceal deficits	May tend to emphasize deficits; highlight disabilities
Consistently performs poorly on tasks of similar difficulty	May display marked variability in performing tasks of similar difficulty
Mood and behavior tend to be labile	Mood consistently depressed; may have superimposed agitation or anxiety
May have neurologic symptoms of dyphasia, apraxia, or agnosia	Neurologic symptoms not present

Treatment goals for older adults with depression are to decrease the symptoms of depression, improve the quality of life, reduce the risk of recurrences, improve health status, decrease health care costs, and decrease mortality. Pharmacotherapy (*i.e.*, use of antidepressants) is an effective treatment approach for the depressed older adult. The selection of a particular medication depends on a variety of factors, such as a prior positive or negative response, history of first-degree relatives responding to medication, concurrent nonpsychotropic medical illnesses that may interfere with medication use, concomitant use of nonpsychiatric medications that may alter the metabolism or increase side-effect profile, likelihood of adherence, patient preference, and cost.

Selective serotonin reuptake inhibitors (SSRIs), a relatively new class of antidepressants (*e.g.*, sertraline, paroxetine) provide high specificity by blocking or slowing serotonin reuptake without the antagonism of neurotransmitter receptors or direct cardiac effects. Because of this, they are an attractive first choice for pharmacotherapy. Dosing is generally once per day, creating ease of administration. They are also less lethal in overdose, an important consideration because of the high suicide rate among older adults. The anticholinergic and cardiovascular side effects that can be problematic with tricyclic antidepressants (*e.g.*, nortriptyline, desipramine, amitriptyline) are minimal with SSRIs. Regardless of the classification, psychotropic medications should be given in low doses initially and gradually titrated according to response and side effects. Response to antidepressants usually requires 4 to 6 weeks at a therapeutic dose levels. For a single episode of major depression, drug therapy usually should continue for a minimum of 6 months and 2 to 5 years for recurrent depression to prevent relapse.[40,42–44]

Electroconvulsive therapy (ECT) may be the treatment of choice for older adults with severe, pharmacologically resistant major depressive episodes. Studies indicate that individuals older than 60 years of age are the largest group of patients who receive ECT. Despite the negative publicity that has been associated with ECT, the evidence for its efficacy in the treatment of depression is strong. Unfortunately, relapse after ECT is common, and alternative treatment strategies, including maintenance ECT or maintenance antidepressants after ECT, are being used.[42,46]

"Talking therapy," such as supportive counseling or psychotherapy, is considered to be an important part of the treatment regimen, alone or in combination with pharmacotherapy or ECT. Alterations in life roles, lack of social support, and chronic medical illnesses are just a few examples of life event changes that may require psychosocial support and new coping skills. Counseling in the older adult population requires special considerations. Individuals with significant vision, hearing, or cognitive impairments may require special approaches. Many elderly persons do not see themselves as depressed and reject referrals to mental health professionals. Special efforts are needed to engage these individuals in treatment. Family therapy can be beneficial as a way to help the family understand more about depression and its complexities and as an important source of support for the older adult. Although depression can impose great risks for older adults, it is thought to be the most treatable psychiatric disorder in late life and therefore warrants aggressive case finding and intervention.

Dementia

Dementia is a complex and devastating problem that is a major cause of disability in the older adult population. Although the actual prevalence of dementia is unknown, estimates range from 2.5% to 24.6% of those older than 65 years of age, with the number increasing with advanced age. A community-based study in East Boston by Evans and colleagues (1989) indicated that 47.2% of those over 85 years of age had dementia.[47] In long-term care facilities, up to 50% of residents have cognitive impairments.

Although there can be a decline in intellectual function with aging, dementia, sometimes called senility, is not a normal aging process. Dementia is a syndrome of acquired, persistent impairment in several domains of intellectual function, including memory, language, visuospatial ability, and cognition (*i.e.*, abstraction, calculation, judgment, and problem solving). Mood disturbances and changes in personality and behavior often accompany the intellectual deterioration.

Dementia can result from a wide variety of conditions, including degenerative, vascular, neoplastic, demyelinating, infectious, inflammatory, toxic, metabolic, and psychiatric disorders. Up to 70% of older adults with dementia (4 million Americans) are thought to have Alzheimer's disease, a chronic, progressive neurologic disorder of unknown cause. Multi-infarct dementia is the second most common disorder, with 10% to 20% of dementias attributed to this vascular disorder in which multiple emboli disseminate throughout the brain, causing infarctions.[48]

Much work is being done in the diagnosis and treatment of dementia, in particular of Alzheimer's disease. Because there are no specific diagnostic tests to determine the presence of Alzheimer's disease, the diagnosis is essentially made by excluding other possible causes of the dementia symptoms.

A commonly used measure of cognitive function is the Mini-Mental State Examination (MMSE) developed by Folstein and colleagues in 1975. This tool provides a brief, objective measure of cognitive functioning and has been widely used. The MMSE, which can be administered in 5 to 10 minutes, consists of a variety of questions that cover memory, orientation, attention, and constructional abilities.[49] The test has been studied and found to fulfill its original goal of providing a brief screening tool that quantifies cognitive impairments and documents cognitive changes over time. However, it has been cautioned that this examination should not be used by itself as a diagnostic tool to identify dementia.

There is no cure for Alzheimer's disease. Experimental medications to halt further cognitive decline are being evaluated. Tacrine hydrochloride has been released as the first in a new therapeutic category of cognitive-enhancing drugs. Tacrine is an acetylcholinesterase inhibitor whose action elevates the acetylcholine concentrations in the cerebral cortex by slowing the degradation of acetylcholine released by still-intact cholinergic neurons. Unfortunately, the magnitude of tacrine's cognitive-enhancing effects is modest, and its use is associated with significant side effects; about 40% of persons in clinical trials experienced elevated levels of liver enzymes, which returned to normal after discontinuation of the drug.[50,51]

Donepezil has recently been released for treatment of Alzheimer's disease. Donepezil is also a cholinesterase inhibitor that increases acetylcholine concentrations by inhibiting acetylcholinesterase. Donepezil has been shown in preclinical studies to be a potent, specific inhibitor of acetylcholinesterase with minimal side effects. Clinical studies are underway to determine the drug's effectiveness.

A recent study suggests that the use of alpha-tocopherol (vitamin E) may help to slow the progression of Alzheimer's disease. The pathology of Alzheimer's disease may involve oxidative stress and the accumulation of free radicals, leading to neuronal degeneration in the brain. Vitamin E, a fat-soluble vitamin, interacts with cell membranes, traps free radicals, and may interrupt chain reactions that damage cells.

Management of older adults with Alzheimer's disease and other dementias generally involves assuming increasing responsibility for and supplying increasing care to individuals as the illness renders them incapable. Impaired judgment and cognition can prevent the older adult from making reasonable decisions and choices and eventually threatens their overall well-being. Family members often assume the monumental task of caring for older adults with dementia until the burden becomes too great, at which time many older adults may be relocated to long-term care facilities.

Some specific behavioral problems are commonly seen in older adults with dementia, including agitation, depression, hallucinations, aggressiveness, and wandering. It may be necessary to use low doses of pharmacologic agents such as neuroleptics, antidepressants, and antipsychotics. Nonpharmacologic interventions can help control behavioral problems and may preclude the need for medications. Ensuring that the individual's physical needs, such as hygiene, bowel and bladder elimination, safety, and nutrition, are met can help prevent catastrophic reactions. Providing a consistent routine in familiar surroundings also helps to alleviate stress. Matching the cognitive needs of the older adult by avoiding understimulation and overstimulation assists in preventing behavior problems.

The work of Hall has shown positive results in the care of older adults with Alzheimer's disease.[52] Hall's conceptual model, progressively lowered stress threshold (PLST), proposes that the demented individual's ability to tolerate any type of stress progressively declines as the disease advances. Interventions for the older adult with dementia therefore center on eliminating and avoiding stressors as a way to prevent dysfunctional behaviors. These stressors include fatigue, change of routine, excessive demands, overwhelming stimuli, and physical stressors. Hall's work with the PLST model has shown that individuals tend to awaken less at night, use less sedatives and hypnotics, eat better, socialize more, function at a higher level, and experience fewer episodes of anxiety, agitation, and other dysfunctional behaviors.[53,54]

Delirium

It is important to differentiate dementia from *delirium*, also referred to as acute confusional state. The demented older adult is far more likely to become delirious. The onset of delirium in the demented individual may be mistaken as an exacerbation of the dementia and consequently not treated.[54,55]

Delirium is an acute disorder developing over a period of hours to days and is frequently seen in hospitalized elderly patients. Prevalence rates range from

14% to 56% of hospitalized and up to 90% of older adults admitted to psychiatric hospitals. Delirium is defined by the 1994 DSM-IVR as an organic mental syndrome featuring a global cognitive impairment, disturbances of attention, reduced level of consciousness, increased or decreased psychomotor activity, and a disorganized sleep-wake cycle. The severity of the symptoms tends to fluctuate unpredictably but is often more pronounced at night.[41]

Delirium can be a presenting feature of a physical illness and may be seen with disorders such as myocardial infarction, pneumonia and other infections, cancer, and hypothyroidism. Patients suffering from drug toxicities may present with delirium. Malnutrition, use of physical restraints, and iatrogenic events can also precipitate delirium.

The exact reason that delirium occurs is unclear. It is speculated that the decreased central nervous system capacity in older adults may precipitate delirium. Other possible contributing factors include vision and hearing impairments, psychologic stress, and diseases of other organ systems. Delirium has a high mortality rate, ranging between 20% and 40%. Agitation, disorientation, and fearfulness—the key symptoms of delirium—place the individual at high risk for injuries such as a fracture from a fall.[55,56]

Diagnosis of delirium involves recognition of the syndrome and identification of its causes. Management involves treatment of the underlying disease condition and symptomatic relief through supportive therapy, including good nutrition and hydration, rest, comfort measures, and emotional support. Prevention of delirium is the overall goal; avoidance of the devastating and life-threatening acute confusional state is the key to successful management and treatment.

In summary, health care for older adults requires unique considerations, taking into account age-related physiologic changes and specific disease states common in this population. Although aging is not synonymous with disease, the aging process does lend itself to an increased incidence of illness. The overall goal is to assist the older adult in maximizing independence and functional capabilities and minimizing disabilities that can result from various acute and chronic illnesses.

The evaluation of the older adult's functional abilities is a key component in gerontologic health care. Medical diagnoses alone are incomplete without an assessment of function. When evaluating levels of function, determination of the older adult's ability to perform activities of daily living (ADL) and instrumental activities of daily living (IADL) should be included.

Among the functional disorders that are common in the older population are urinary incontinence, falls, depression, dementia, and delirium. The older adult is especially prone to urinary incontinence because of changes in the micturition cycle that accompany the aging process. Behavioral techniques can be an effective way to treat incontinence problems in the older adult population. Falls are a common source of concern for the older adult population; although most falls do not result in serious injury, the potential for serious complications and even death is real. Most falls are the result of several risk factors, including age-related biopsychosocial changes, chronic illness, and situational and environmental hazards. Depression is a significant but treatable health problem that is often misdiagnosed and mistreated in the older adult population. Dementia is a syndrome of acquired, persistent impairment in several domains of intellectual function, including memory, language, visuospatial ability, and cognition (*i.e.*, abstraction, calculation, judgment, and problem solving). Although there can be a slight decline in intellectual function with aging, dementia is not a normal aging process. Delirium is an acute confusional disorder developing over a period of hours to days and is often seen as a presenting feature of a physical illness or drug toxicity.

Drug Therapy in the Older Adult

After you have completed this section of the chapter, you should be able to meet the following objectives:

- Characterize drug therapy in the older adult population
- List five factors that contribute to adverse drug reactions in the elderly
- Cite cautions to be used in prescribing medications for the elderly

Drug therapy in the older adult population is a complex phenomenon influenced by numerous biopsychosocial factors. The elderly are the largest group of consumers of prescription and over-the-counter (OTC) drugs. The average older adult uses 4.5 prescription and 2.1 OTC medications and fills between 12 to 17 prescriptions yearly.[10] The incidence of adverse drug reactions in the elderly is two to three times that found in young adults. This is considered to be a conservative estimate, because drug reactions are less well recognized in older adults and because reactions can often mimic symptoms of specific disease states.

Errors in the administration of medications and in compliance are common among the older adult population, estimated by several authorities to be between 25% and 50% for community-dwelling elderly. Reasons for this high volume of errors are numerous. Poor manual dexterity, failing eyesight, lack of understanding about the treatment regimen, attitudes and beliefs about medication use, mistrust of health care providers, and forgetfulness or confusion are but a few factors that can affect the adherence to medication regimens. The role of the health care provider can also contribute to improper medication use. There can be a tendency to treat symptoms with drugs rather than fully investigate the cause of those symptoms. To compound matters, accurate diagnosis of specific disease states can be difficult, because older adults tend to underreport symptoms and because presenting symptoms are often atypical.[56,57]

Age-related physiologic changes also account for adverse effects of medications. Generally, the absorption of orally ingested drugs remains essentially unchanged with age, even though the gastric pH is known to elevate and gastric emptying time can be delayed. Changes in drug distribution, however, are clinically significant. Because lean body mass and total body water decreases with advancing age, water-soluble drugs such as digoxin and propranolol tend to have a smaller volume of distribution, resulting in higher plasma concentrations for a given dose and increased likelihood of a toxic reaction. Conversely, fat-soluble drugs such as diazepam are more widely distributed and accumulate in fatty tissue owing to an increase in adipose tissue with aging. This can cause a delay in elimination and accumulation of the drug over time (*i.e.*, prolonged half-life) with multiple doses of the same drug. Drug metabolism through the liver is thought to be altered owing to the decrease in hepatic blood flow seen in the older adult. Renal excretion controls the elimination of drugs from the body, and because kidney function declines with age, the rate of drug excretion decreases. This can result in an increased half-life of drugs and is why estimates of creatinine clearance are recommended to determine drug dosing.[57,59]

Drug use for older adults warrants a cautious approach. "Start low and go slow" is the adage governing drug prescribing in geriatric pharmacology. Older adults often can achieve therapeutic results on small doses of medications. If necessary, dosing can then be titrated slowly according to response.

Further complicating matters is the issue of polypharmacy in older adults, because they often have multiple disorders that may require multiple drug therapies. Polypharmacy increases the risk of drug interactions and adverse drug reactions and decreases compliance. Drugs and disease states can also interact, causing adverse effects. For example, psychotropic drugs administered to older adults with dementia may cause a worsening of confusion; β-blocking agents administered to an individual with chronic obstructive pulmonary disease may induce bronchoconstriction; and nonsteroidal antiinflammatory medications given to an older adult with hypertension can raise blood pressure further.

The use of certain types of medications carries a high risk for older adults and should be avoided if possible. Generally, long-acting drugs or drugs with prolonged half-lives can be problematic. Many sedatives and hypnotics fit into this category, and drugs such as diazepam and flurazepam should be avoided. Other classes of drugs, such as antidepressants and anxiolytics, may provide the necessary symptomatic relief and may be more appropriate for older adults than sedatives and hypnotics. Use of these agents warrants caution, however, with consideration for the unique pharmacokinetic changes that accompany aging. Drugs that possess anticholinergic properties should also be used with caution. Anticholinergics are used for a variety of conditions; however, side effects such as dry mouth and eyes, blurred vision, and constipation are common. These drugs can also cause more serious side effects, such as confusion, urinary retention, and orthostatic hypotension. Agents that enter the central nervous system, including narcotics and alcohol, can cause a variety of problems, most notably delirium. These problems most likely occur as a result of a decreased central nervous system reserve capacity.[10,56,58]

Because of the serious implications of medication use in the elderly, strategies need to be used to enhance therapeutic effects and prevent harm. Careful evaluation of the need for the medication by the health care provider is the first step. Once decided, analysis of the individual's current medication regimen and disease states is necessary to prevent drug-drug interactions, drug-disease interactions, and adverse responses. Dosing should be at the low end, and frequency of drug administration should be kept to a minimum to simplify the routine and enhance compliance. Timing the dose to a specific activity of daily living (*e.g.*, "take with breakfast") can also improve compliance, as can special packaging devices such as pill boxes and blister packs. The cost of medications is another important factor for older adults on reduced, fixed incomes. Choosing less expensive products of equal efficacy can increase compliance. The importance of educating the individual about the medication cannot be overemphasized. Health care professionals need to provide verbal and written information on the principles of medication use and on the specific medications being used. This facilitates active, involved participation by the older adult and enhances the individual's ability to make informed decisions.

In summary, drug therapy in the older adult population is a complex phenomenon influenced by numerous biopsychosocial factors. Alterations in pharmacokinetics occur with advancing age and increases the likelihood of toxic reactions. "Start low and go slow" is the adage governing geriatric pharmacology. Centrally acting drugs and drugs with long half-lives should be avoided when possible. Drug-drug interactions, drug-disease interactions, and adverse reactions increase in the elderly population. Educating the older adult about drug use is an important factor in ensuring compliance and accurate medication administration.

REFERENCES

1. American Association of Retired Persons. (1996). *A profile of older Americans.* Washington DC: AARP.
2. U.S. Department of Health and Human Services. (1996). *Profile of Medicare–30th Anniversary.* Health Care Financing Administration.

3. Erikson E. (1963). *Childhood and society*. New York: W.W. Norton.
4. Erikson E.H., Erikson J.M., Kivirck H.Q. (1986). *Vital involvement in old age*. New York: W.W. Norton.
5. Cristofalo V.J. (1994). Biological mechanisms of aging: An overview. In Hazzard W.R., Bierman E.L., Blass J.P., Ettinger Jr. W.H., Halter J.B. (Eds.). *Principles of geriatric medicine and gerontology* (3rd ed., pp. 3–14). New York: McGraw-Hill.
6. Hayflick L. (1985). Theories of biological aging. *Experimental Gerontology* 10, 145–159.
7. Hayflick L. (1979). Cell biology of aging. *Federation Proceedings* 38, 1847–1850.
8. Harmon D. (1983). Free radicals and the orientation, evolution, and present status of free radical theory of aging. In Armstrong D., et al. (Eds.). *Aging: Free radicals in molecular biology* (vol. 27, pp. 1–12). New York: Raven Press.
9. Blass J.P., Cherniack E.P., Weksler M.E. (1992). Theories of aging. In Calkins E., Ford A.B., Kratz P.R. (Eds.). *Practice of geriatrics* (2nd ed., pp. 10–18). Philadelphia: W.B. Saunders.
10. Abrams W.B., Beers M.H., Berkow R., Fletcher A.J. (1995). *Merck manual of geriatrics* (2nd ed.). Whitehouse Station, NJ: Merck Research Laboratories.
11. Dalziel K.L., Bickers D.R. (1992). Skin Aging. In Brocklehurst J.C., Tallis R.C., Fillet H.M. (Eds.). *Textbook of medicine and gerontology* (4th ed., pp. 898–921). Edinburgh: Churchill Livingstone.
12. Hamerman D. (1993). Aging and osteoarthritis: Basic mechanisms. *Journal of American Geriatrics Society* 41, 760–770.
13. Wilmore J.H. (1991). The aging of bone and muscle. *Clinics in Sports Medicine* 10, 231–244.
14. Timiras P.S. (1994). Aging of the skeleton, joints, and muscles. In Timiras P.S. (Ed.). *Physiological basis of aging and geriatrics* (2nd ed., pp. 259–272). Boca Raton, FL: CRC Press.
15. Applegate W.B. (1994). Hypertension. In Hazzard W.R., Bierman E.L., Blass J.P., Ettinger Jr. W.H, Halter J.B. (Eds.). *Principles of geriatric medicine and gerontology* (3rd ed., pp. 541–554). New York: McGraw-Hill.
16. Wei J.Y. (1992). Age and the cardiovascular system. *New England Journal of Medicine* 327, 1735–1739.
17. Smith J.J., Porth C.J.M. (1990). Age and the response to orthostatic stress. In Smith J.J. (Ed.). *Circulatory response to the upright position* (p. 136). Boca Raton, FL: CRC Press.
18. Lakatta E.G. (1990). Changes in cardiovascular function with aging. *European Heart Journal* 11 (Suppl C), 22–29.
19. Branfronbrener M., Landowne M., Shock N.W. (1955). Changes in cardiac output with age. *Circulation* 12, 557–566.
20. Rodeheffer R.J., Gerstenblith G., Becker L.C., et al. (1984). Exercise cardiac output is maintained with advancing age in healthy human subjects: Cardiac dilatation and increased stroke volume compensate for diminished heart rate. *Circulation* 69, 203–213.
21. Fleg J.L., O'Connor F., Gerstenblith G., et al. (1995). Impact of age on the cardiovascular response to dynamic upright exercise in healthy men and women. *Journal of Applied Physiology* 78 (3), 890–900.
22. Timiras P.S. (1994). Aging of respiration, erythrocytes and the hematopoietic system. In Timiras P.S. (Ed.). *Physiological basis of aging and geriatrics* (2nd ed., pp. 89–102). Boca Raton, FL: CRC Press.
23. Timiras P.S. (1994). Aging of the nervous system: Structural and biochemical changes. In Timiras P.S. (Ed.). *Physiological basis of aging and geriatrics* (2nd ed., pp. 89–102). Boca Raton, FL: CRC Press.
24. Morris J.C., McManus D.Q. (1991). The neurology of aging: Normal and pathological change. *Geriatrics* 46 (8), 47–54.
25. Werner J.S., Peterzell D.H., Scheetz A.J. (1990). Light, vision, and aging. *Optometry and Vision Science* 67, 214–229.
26. Rees T.S., Duckert L.G., Milezuk H.A. (1994). Auditory and vestibular dysfunction. In Hazzard W.R., Bierman E.L., Blass J.P., Ettinger Jr. W.H., Halter J.B. (Eds.). *Principles of geriatric medicine and gerontology* (3rd ed., pp. 457–472). New York: McGraw-Hill.
27. Timiras P.S. (1994). Aging of the immune system. In Timiras P.S. (Ed.). *Physiological Basis of Aging and Geriatrics.* (2nd ed, pp 75–87). Boca Raton, FL: CRC Press.
28. Soergel K.H., Zboralske F.E., Amberg J.R. (1964). Presbyesophagus: Esophageal motility in nonagenarians. *Journal of Clinical Investigation* 43, 1472.
29. Baime M.J., Nelson J.B., Castell D.O. (1994). Aging of the gastrointestinal system. In Hazzard W.R., Bierman E.L., Blass J.P., Ettinger Jr. W.H., Halter J.B. (Eds.). *Principles of geriatric medicine and gerontology* (3rd ed., pp. 665–681). New York: McGraw-Hill.
30. Beck L.M. (1994). Aging changes in renal function. In Hazzard W.R., Bierman E.L., Blass J.P., Ettinger Jr. W.H., Halter J.B. (Eds.). *Principles of geriatric medicine and gerontology* (3rd ed., pp. 615–624). New York: McGraw-Hill.
31. Brendler CB. (1994). Disorders of the prostate. In Hazzard W.R., Bierman E.L., Blass J.P., Ettinger Jr. W.H., Halter J.B. (Eds.). *Principles of geriatric medicine and gerontology* (3rd ed., pp. 657–664). New York: McGraw-Hill.
32. Levy J.A. (1994). Sexuality and aging. In Hazzard W.R., Bierman E.L., Blass J.P., Ettinger Jr. W.H., Halter J.B. (Eds.). *Principles of geriatric medicine and gerontology* (3rd ed., pp. 115–124). New York: McGraw-Hill.
33. Katz S., Ford A.B., Moskowitz R.W., et al. (1963). Studies of illness in the aged: The Index of ADL. *Journal of the American Medical Association* 185, 914–919.
34. Katz S., Downs T.D., Cash H.R., et al. (1970). Progress in development of the Index of ADL. *Gerontologist* 10, 20–30.
35. Fantl J.A., Neuman D.F., Colling J., et al. (1996). *Urinary incontinence in adults: Acute and chronic management.* Clinical practice guideline no. 2, 1996 update. Publication no. 96–06. Rockville, MD: Agency for Health Care Policy and Research.
36. Jeter K., Fuller N., Norton C. (1990). *Nursing for continence.* Philadelphia: W.B. Saunders.
37. Tinetti M.E. (1994). Falls. In Hazzard W.R., Bierman E.L., Blass J.P., Ettinger Jr. W.H., Halter J.B. (Eds.). *Principles of geriatric medicine and gerontology* (3rd ed., pp. 1313–1320). New York: McGraw-Hill.
38. King M.B., Tinnetti M.E. (1994). Falls in community-dwelling older persons. *Journal of American Geriatrics Society* 43, 1146–1154.
39. Surdarsky L. (1990). Geriatrics: Gait disorders in the elderly. *New England Journal of Medicine* 322, 1441–1446.
40. NIH Consensus Development Panel. (1995). Diagnosis and treatment of depression in late life. *JAMA* 268, 1018–1024.
41. American Psychiatric Association. (1994). *Diagnostic and statistical manual of mental disorders* (4th ed., rev.). Washington, DC: American Psychiatric Association.
42. Reynold C.F. (1995). Recognition and differentiation of elderly depression in the clinical setting. *Geriatrics* 50 (Suppl 1), S6–S15.

43. Depression Guideline Panel. (1993). *Depression in primary care: Treatment of major depression* (vol. 2). Clinical practice guideline no. 5, 1993. Publication No. 93–0551. Rockville, MD: Agency for Health Care Policy and Research.
44. Reynolds III C.F., Frank E., Kupfer D., et al. (1996). Treatment outcome in recurrent major depression: A post hoc comparison of elderly ("young old") and midlife patients. *American Journal of Psychiatry* 15 (10), 1288–1292.
45. Yesavage J.A., Brink T.L., Rose T.L., et al. (1983). Development and validation of a geriatric depression scale: A preliminary report. *Journal of Psychiatric Research* 17, 37–49.
46. Hay D.P. (1990). Electroconvulsive therapy, mental health and aging. *International Journal of Technology and Aging* 3 (1), 39–45.
47. Evans D.A., Funkenstein H., Albert M.S., et al. (1989). Prevalence of Alzheimer's disease in a community population of older persons: Higher than previously reported. *Journal of the American Medical Association* 262, 2551–2556.
48. Geldmacher D.S., Whitehouse P.J. (1996). Evaluation of dementia. *New England Journal of Medicine* 335 (5), 330–336.
49. Folstein M.F., Folstein B.E., McHugh P.R. (1975). "Mini-mental state": A practical method for grading the cognitive state of patients for the clinician. *Journal of Psychiatric Research* 12, 189–198.
50. Owens N.J. (1993). Focus on tacrine HCL. *Hospital Formulary* 28, 679–691.
51. Miller C.A. (1994). How much breakthrough is Cognex for Alzheimer's disease. *Geriatric Nursing* 55, 53–54.
52. Sono M., Ernesto M.S., Thomas R.G., et al. (1997). A controlled trial of Selegiline, alpha-tocopherol, or both as treatment for Alzheimer's disease. *New England Journal of Medicine* 336, 1216–1222.
53. Hall G.R., Buckwalter K.C. (1987). Progressively lowered stress threshold: A conceptual model for care of adults with Alzheimer's disease. *Archives of Psychiatric Nursing* 1, 399–406.
54. Richards B.S. (1990). Alzheimer's disease: A disabling neurophysiological disorder with complex nursing implications. *Archives of Psychiatric Nursing* 4 (1), 39–42.
55. Lipowski Z.J. (1990). Delirium in older patients. *Journal of the American Medical Association* 40, 829–838.
56. Inouye S.K., Chorpentier P.A. (1996). Precipitating factors in delirium in hospitalized elderly persons. *JAMA* 275 (11), 852–857.
57. Woodhouse K.W., Wynne H.A. (1992). The pharmacology of aging. In Brocklehurst J.C., Tallis R.C., Fillet H.M. (Eds.). *Textbook of medicine and gerontology* (4th ed., pp. 129–142). Edinburgh: Churchill Livingstone.
58. Wilcox S.M., Himmelsteind D.U., Woodhandler S. (1994). Inappropriate drug prescribing for the community-dwelling elderly. *JAMA* 272 (4), 292–296.
59. Beers M.H. (1992). Medication use in the elderly. In Calkins E., Ford A.B., Katz P.R. (Eds.). *Practice of geriatrics* (2nd ed., pp. 33–49). Philadelphia: W.B. Saunders.

ADDITIONAL READINGS

Blazer D.G., Bachar J.R., Manton K.G. (1986). Suicide in late life: Review and commentary. *Journal of the American Geriatric Society* 34, 519–525.

Calkins E., Ford A.B., Katz P.R. (Eds.). (1992). *Practice of geriatrics*. Philadelphia: W.B. Saunders.

Cummings J.L., Benson D.F. (1992). *Dementia: A clinical approach* (2nd ed.). Boston: Butterworth-Heinemann.

Duthie Jr. E.H. (1990). Geriatric medicine. In Kochar M.S., Kutty K. (Eds.). *Concise textbook of medicine* (2nd ed., pp. 359–380). New York: Elsevier.

Gerdner L.A., Hall G.R., Buckwalter K.C. (1996). Caregiving training for people with Alzheimer's disease based on the stress threshold model. *Image* 28 (3), 241–246.

Hazzard W.R., Bierman E.L., Blass J.P., Ettinger Jr. W.H., Halter J.B. (Eds.). (1994). *Principles of geriatric medicine and gerontology* (3rd ed.). New York: McGraw-Hill.

Kane R.A., Kane R.L. (1981). *Assessing the elderly: A practical guide to measurement*. Lexington, MA: Lexington Books.

Kane R.L., Ouslander J.G., Abrass I.B. (1994). *Essentials of geriatrics* (3rd ed.). New York: McGraw-Hill.

Ouslander J.G., Schnelle J.F. (1995). Incontinence in the nursing home. *Annals of Internal Medicine* 122 (6), 438–449.

Piraino A.J. (1995). Managing medication in the elderly. *Hospital Practice* 30 (6), 59–64.

Rubenstein L.Z., Josephson K.R., Robbins A.S. (1994). Falls in the nursing home. *Annals of Internal Medicine* 121 (6), 442–451.

Schrier R.W. (Ed.). (1990). *Geriatric medicine* (pp. 376–398). Philadelphia: W.B. Saunders.

Timiras P.S. (ED). (1994). *Physiological basis of aging and geriatrics* (2nd ed.). Boca Raton, FL: CRC Press.

Tombough T.N., McIntyre N.J. (1992). The "mini-mental state examination": A comprehensive review. *Journal of the American Geriatric Society* 40, 922–935.

Glossary

Abduct To move or spread away from a position near the midline of the body or the axial line of a limb.

Abduction The act of abducting or state of being abducted.

Abrasion The wearing or scraping away of a substance or structure, such as the skin, through an unusual or abnormal mechanical process.

Abscess A collection of pus that is restricted to a specific area in tissues, organs, or confined spaces.

Accommodation The adjustment of the lens (eye) to variations in distance.

Acromion The lateral extension of the spine of the scapula, forming the highest point of the shoulder.

Acromial Of or pertaining to the acromion.

Acuity The clearness or sharpness of perception, especially of vision.

Adaptation The adjustment of an organism to its environment, physical or psychological, through changes and responses to stress of any kind.

Adduct To move or draw toward a position near the midline of the body or the axial line of a limb.

Adduction The act of adducting or state of being adducted.

Adrenergic Activated by or characteristic of the sympathetic nervous system or its neurotransmitters (*i.e.,* epinephrine and norepinephrine).

Aerobic Growing, living, or occurring only in the presence of air or oxygen.

Afferent Bearing or conducting inward or toward a center, as an afferent neuron.

Agglutination The clumping together of particles, microorganisms, or blood cells in response to an antigen-antibody reaction.

Agonist A muscle whose action is opposed by another muscle (antagonist) with which it is paired; *or* a drug or other chemical substance that has affinity for or stimulates a predictable physiologic function.

Akinesia An abnormal state in which there is an absence or poverty of movement.

Allele One of two or more different forms of a gene that can occupy a particular locus on a chromosome.

Alveolus A small saclike structure, as in the alveolus of the lung.

Amine An organic compound containing nitrogen.

Amblyopia A condition of vision impairment without a detectable organic lesion of the eye.

Amorphous Without a definite form; shapeless.

Ampulla A saclike dilatation of a duct, canal, or any other tubular structure.

Anabolism A constructive metabolic process characterized by the conversion of simple substances into larger, complex molecules.

Anaerobic Growing, living, or occurring only in the absence of air or oxygen.

Analog A part, organ, or chemical having the same function or appearance but differing in respect to a certain component, such as origin or development.

Anaplasia A change in the structure of cells and in their orientation to each other that is characterized by a loss of cell differentiation, as in cancerous cell growth.

Anastomosis The connection or joining between two vessels; *or* an opening created by surgical, traumatic, or pathologic means.

Androgen Any substance, such as a male sex hormone, that increases male characteristics.

Anergy A state of absent or diminished reaction to an antigen or group of antigens.

Aneuploidy A variation in the number of chromosomes within a cell involving one or more missing chromosomes rather than entire sets.

Aneurysm An outpouching or dilation in the wall of a blood vessel or the heart.

Ankylose To fuse or obliterate through ankylosis, as in a joint.

Ankylosis Stiffness or fixation of separate bones or hard parts, resulting from disease, injury, or surgical procedure.

Anorexia Lack or loss of appetite for food. (Adjective: anorexic)

Anoxia An abnormal condition characterized by the total lack of oxygen.

Antagonist A muscle whose action directly opposes that of another muscle (agonist) with which it is paired; *or* a drug or other chemical substance that can diminish or nullify the action of a neuromediator or body function.

Anterior Pertaining to a surface or part that is situated near or toward the front.

Antigen A substance that generates an immune response by causing the formation of an antibody or reacting with antibodies or T cell receptors.

Apex The uppermost point, the narrowed or pointed end, or the highest point of a structure, such as an organ.

Aphagia A condition characterized by the refusal or the loss of ability to swallow.

Aplasia The absence of an organ or tissue due to a developmental failure.

Apnea The absence of spontaneous respiration.

Apophysis A projection or swelling, especially a bony outgrowth that has never entirely separated from the bone of which it forms a part.

Apraxia Loss of the ability to carry out familiar, purposeful acts or to manipulate objects in the absence of paralysis or other motor or sensory impairment.

Arrector pili muscle Smooth muscle in the skin associated with the hair follicle.

Articulation The place of connection or junction between two or more bones of the skeleton.

Ascites An abnormal accumulation of serous fluid in the peritoneal cavity.

Asepsis The condition of being free or freed from pathogenic microorganisms.

Astereognosis A neurologic disorder characterized by an inability to identify objects by touch.

Asterixis A motor disturbance characterized by a hand-flapping tremor, which results when the prolonged contraction of groups of muscles lapses intermittently.

Ataxia An abnormal condition characterized by an inability to coordinate voluntary muscular movement.

Athetosis A neuromuscular condition characterized by the continuous occurrence of slow, sinuous, writhing movements that are performed involuntarily. (Adjective: athetoid)

Atopy Genetic predisposition toward the development of a hypersensitivity or an allergic reaction to common environmental allergens.

Atresia The absence or closure of a normal body orifice or tubular organ, such as the esophagus.

Atrophy A wasting or diminution of size or physiologic activity of a cell, tissue, or organ.

Autocrine A mode of hormone action in which a hormone acts on the same type of cell that secretes it.

Autosome Any chromosome other than a sex chromosome.

Axillary Of or pertaining to the axilla, or armpit.

Bacteremia The presence of bacteria in the blood.

Ballismus An abnormal condition charcterized by violent flailing motions of the arms and, occasionally, the head, resulting from injury to or destruction of the subthalamic nucleus or its fiber connections.

Baroreceptor A type of sensory nerve ending found in the walls of the atria of the heart, the vena cava, the aortic arch, and the carotid sinus that is stimulated by changes in pressure.

Basal Pertaining to, situated at, or forming the base; *or* the fundamental or the basic.

Basophil A granulocytic white blood cell with an irregularly shaped, segmented nucleus containing granules that stain blue when exposed to a basic dye.

Benign Not malignant; *or* of the character that does not threaten health or life.

Biogenesis The doctrine that living material always arises only from preexisting life and not from inanimate matter.

Bipolar neuron A nerve cell that has a process at each end—an afferent process and an efferent process.

Bolus A rounded mass of food ready to swallow or such a mass passing through the gastrointestinal tract; *or* a concentrated mass of medicinal material or other pharmaceutic preparation injected all at once intravenously for diagnostic purposes.

Borborygmus The rumbling, gurgling, or tinkling noise produced by the propulsion of gas through the intestine.

Bruit A sound or murmur heard while auscultating an organ or gland, especially an abnormal one.

Buccal Pertaining to or directed toward the inside of the cheek.

Buffer A substance or group of substances that prevents change in the concentration of another chemical substance.

Bulla A thin-walled blister of the skin or mucous membranes greater than 5 mm in diameter containing serous or seropurulent fluid.

Bursa A fluid-filled sac or saclike cavity situated in places in the tissues at which friction would otherwise develop, such as between certain tendons and the bones beneath them.

Cachexia A condtion of general ill health and malnutrition, marked by weakness and emaciation.

Calculus A stony mass formed within body tissues, usually composed of mineral salts.

Capsid The protein shell that envelops and protects the nucleic acid of a virus.

Carcinogen Any substance or agent that causes the development or increases the incidence of cancer.

Carpal Of or pertaining to the carpus, or wrist.

Caseation A form of tissue necrosis in which the tissue is changed into a dry, amorphous mass resembling crumbly cheese.

Catabolism A metabolic process through which living organisms break down complex substances to simple compounds, liberating energy for use in work, energy storage, or heat production.

Catalyst A substance that increases the velocity of a chemical reaction without being consumed by the process.

Catecholamines Any one of a group of biogenic amines having a sympathomimetic action and composed of a catechol molecule and the aliphatic portion of an amine.

Caudal Signifying an inferior position, toward the distal end of the spine.

Cellulitis An acute, diffuse, spreading, edematous inflammation of the deep subcutaneous tissues and sometimes muscle, characterized most commonly by an area of heat, redness, pain, and swelling, and occasionally by fever, malaise, chills, and headache.

Cephalic Of or pertaining to the head, or to the head end of the body.

Cerumen The waxlike secretion produced by vestigial apocrine sweat glands in the external ear canal.

Cheilosis A noninflammatory disorder of the lips and mouth characterized by chapping and fissuring.

Chelate A chemical compound composed of a central metal ion and an organic molecule with multiple bonds, arranged in ring formation, used especially in chemotherapeutic treatments for metal poisoning.

Chemoreceptor A sensory nerve cell activated by chemical stimuli, as a chemoreceptor in the carotid that is sensitive to changes in the oxygen content in the bloodstream and reflexly increases or decreases respiration and blood pressure.

Chemotaxis A response involving cell orientation or cell movement that is either toward (positive chemotaxis) or away from (negative chemotaxis) a chemical stimulus.

Chondrocyte Any one of the mature polymorphic cells that form the cartilage of the body.

Chromatid One of the paired threadlike chromosome filaments, joined at the centromere, that make up a metaphase chromosome.

Chromosome Any one of the structures in the nucleus of a cell containing a linear thread of DNA, which functions in the transmission of genetic information.

Chyme The creamy, viscous, semifluid material produced during digestion of a meal that is expelled by the stomach into the duodenum.

Cilia The eyelid or its outer edge; *or* the small hairs growing on the edges of the eyelids. (Singular: cilium)

Circadian Being, having, pertaining to, or occurring in a period or cycle of approximately 24 hours.

Circumduction The active or passive circular movement of a limb or of the eye.

Cisterna An enclosed space, such as a cavity, that serves as a reservoir for lymph or other body fluids.

Clone One or a group of genetically identical cells or organisms derived from a single parent.

Coagulation The process of transforming a liquid into a semisolid mass, especially of blood clot formation.

Coarctation A condition of stricture or contraction of the walls of a vessel.

Coenzyme A nonprotein substance that binds with a protein molecule (apoenzyme) to form an active enzyme (holoenzyme).

Cofactor A substance that must unite with another substance in order to function.

Colic Sharp, intermittent abdominal pain localized in a hollow or tubular organ, resulting from torsion, obstruction, or smooth muscle spasm. (Adjective: colicky)

Collagen The protein substance of the white, glistening, inelastic fibers of the skin, tendons, bone, cartilage, and all other connective tissue.

Collateral Secondary or accessory rather than direct or immediate; *or* a small branch, as of a blood vessel or nerve.

Complement Any one of the complex, enzymatic serum proteins that are involved in physiologic reactions, including antigen-antibdoy reaction and anaphylaxis.

Confluent Flowing or coming together; not discrete.

Congenital Present at, and usually before, birth.

Conjugate To pair and fuse in conjugation; *or* a form of sexual reproduction seen in unicellular organisms in which genetic material is exchanged during the temporary fusion of two cells.

Contiguous In contact or nearly so in an unbroken sequence along a boundary or at a point.

Contralateral Affecting, pertaining to, or originating in the opposite side of a point or reference.

Contusion An injury of a part without a break in the skin, characterized by swelling, discoloration, and pain.

Convolution An elevation or tortuous winding, such as one of the irregular ridges on the surface of the brain, formed by a structure being infolded upon itself.

Corpuscle Any small mass, cell, or body, such as a red or white blood cell.

Coruscate To give off or reflect light in bright beams or flashes.

Costal Pertaining to a rib or ribs.

Crepitus Flatulence or the noisy discharge of fetid gas from the bowels; *or* a sound that resembles a crackling noise.

Cutaneous Pertining to the skin.

Cyanosis A bluish discoloration, especially of the skin and mucous membranes, caused by an excess of deoxygenated hemoglobin in the blood.

Cytokine Any of a class of polypeptide immunoregulatory substances that are secreted by cells of the immune system on contact with a specific antigen.

Cytology The study of cells, including their origin, structure, function, and pathology.

Decomposition The separation of a compound substance into simpler chemical forms by whatever process.

Defecation The evacuation of feces from the digestive tract through the rectum.

Deformation The process of adapting in form or shape; also the product of such alteration.

Degeneration The deterioration of a normal cell, tissue, or organ to a less functionally active form. (Adjective: degenerative)

Deglutition The act or process of swallowing.

Degradation The reduction of a chemical compound to a compound less complex, usually by splitting off one or more groups.

Dehydration The condition that results from excessive loss of water from the body tissues.

Delirium An acute, reversible organic mental syndrome characterized by confusion, disorientation, restlessness, incoherence, fear, anxiety, excitement, often illusions and hallucinations, and at times delusions.

Dendrite One of the branching processes that extends from the cell body of a neuron. (Adjective: dendritic)

Depolarization The reduction of a cell membrane potential to a less negative value than that of the potential outside the cell.

Dermatome The area of the skin supplied with afferent nerve fibers by a single posterior spinal root.

Desmosome A small, circular, dense area within the intercellular bridge that forms the site of adhesion between intermediate filaments and cell membranes.

Desquamation A normal process in which the cornified layer of the epidermis is shed in fine scales or sheets.

Dialysis The process of separating colloids and crystalline substances in solution, which involves the two distinct physical processes of diffusion and ultrafiltration; *or* a medical procedure for the removal of urea and other elements from the blood or lymph.

Diapedesis The outward passage of red or white blood corpuscles through the intact walls of the vessels.

Diaphoresis Perspiration, especially the profuse perspiration associated with an elevated body temperature, physical exertion, exposure to heat, and mental or emotional stress.

Diarthrosis A specialized articulation that permits, to some extent, free movement. (Adjective: diarthrodial)

Diastole The dilatation of the heart; *or* the period of dilatation, which is the interval between the second and the first heart sound and is the time during which blood enters the relaxed chambers of the heart from the systemic circulation and the lungs.

Differentiation The act or process in development in which unspecialized cells or tissues acquire completely individual character, including that of physical form, physiologic function, and chemical properties.

Diffusion The process of becoming widely spread, as in the spontaneous movement of molecules or other particles in solution from an area of higher concentration to an area of lower concentration, resulting in an even distribution of the particles in the fluid.

Diopter A unit of measurement of the refractive power of lenses equal to the reciprocal of the focal length in meters.

Diploid Pertaining to an individual, organism, strain, or cell that has two full sets of homologuous chromosomes.

Disarticulate To amputate or separate at a joint.

Disseminate To scatter or distribute over a considerable area.

Distal Away from or being the farthest from a point of reference.

Diurnal Of, relating to, or occurring in the daytime.

Diverticulum A pouch or sac of variable size occurring naturally or through herniation of the muscular wall of a tubular organ.

Dorsum The back or posterior. (Adjective: dorsal)

Dyslexia A disturbance in the ability to read, spell, and write words.

Dyspepsia The impairment of the power or function of digestion, especially epigastric discomfort following eating.

Dysphagia A difficulty in swallowing.

Dysphonia Any impairment of the voice that is experienced as a difficulty in speaking.

Dysplasia The alteration in size, shape, and organization of adult cells.

Eburnation The conversion of bone in which a thinning and loss of the articular cartilage occurs, resulting in exposure of the subchondral bone, which becomes denser and ivory-like in appearance.

Ecchymosis A small hemorrhagic spot, larger than a petechia, in the skin or mucous membrane caused by the extravasation of blood into the subcutaneous tissues.

Ectopic Relating to or characterized by an object or organ being situated in an unusual place, away from its normal location.

Edema The presence of an abnormal accumulation of fluid in interstitial spaces of tissues. (Adjective: edematous)

Efferent Conveyed or directed away from a center.

Effusion The escape of fluid from blood vessels into a part or tissue, as an exudation or a transudation.

Embolus A mass of clotted blood or other formed elements, such as bubbles of air, calcium fragments, or a bit of tissue or tumor, that circulates in the bloodstream until it becomes lodged in a vessel, obstructing the circulation.

Empyema An accumulation of pus in a cavity of the body, especially the pleural space.

Emulsify To disperse one liquid throughout the body of another liquid, making a colloidal suspension, or emulsion.

Endocytosis The uptake or incorporation of substances into a cell by invagination of its plasma membrane, as in the processes of phagocytosis and pinocytosis.

Endoderm The innermost of the three primary germ layers of the embryo, and from which epithelium arises.

Endogenous Growing within the body; *or* developing or originating from within the body or produced from internal causes.

Endoscopy The visualization of any cavity of the body with an endoscope.

Enteropathic Relating to any disease of the intestinal tract.

Epiphysis The expanded articular end of a long bone (head) that is separated from the shaft of the bone by the epiphyseal plate until the bone stops growing, the plate is obliterated, and the shaft and the head become united.

Epithelium The covering of the internal and the external surfaces of the body, including the lining of vessels and other small cavities.

Erectile Capable of being erected or raised to an erect position.

Erythema The redness or inflammation of the skin or mucous membranes produced by the congestion of superficial capillaries. (Adjective: erythematous)

Etiology The study or theory of all factors that may be involved in the development of a disease, including susceptibility of an individual, the nature of the disease agent, and the way in which an individual's body is invaded by the agent; *or* the cause of a disease.

Euploid Pertaining to an individual, organism, strain, or cell with a balanced set or sets of chromosomes, in any number, that is an exact multiple of the normal, basic haploid number characteristic of the species; *or* such an individual, organism, strain, or cell.

Evisceration The removal of the viscera from the abdominal cavity, or disembowelment; *or* the extrusion of an internal organ through a wound or surgical incision.

Exacerbation An increase in the severity of a disease as marked by greater intensity in any of its signs and symptoms.

Exfoliation Peeling and sloughing off of tissue cells in scales or layers. (Adjective: exfolliative)

Exocrine gland A gland that releases its secretion outwardly via a duct.

Exocytosis The discharge of cell particles, which are packaged in membrane-bound vesicles, by fusion of the vesicular membrane with the plasma membrane and subsequent release of the particles to the exterior of the cell.

Exogenous Developed or originating outside the body, as a disease caused by a bacterial or viral agent foreign to the body.

Exophthalmos A marked or abnormal protusion of the eyeball.

Extension A movement that allows the two elements of any jointed part to be drawn apart, increasing the angle between them, as extending the leg increases the angle between the femur and the tibia.

Extrapyramidal Pertaining to the tissues and structures outside the pyramidal tracts of the brain.

Extravasation A discharge or escape, usually of blood, serum, or lymph, from a vessel into the tissues.

Extubation The process of withdrawing a previously inserted tube from an orifice or cavity of the body.

Exudate Fluid, cells, or other substances that have been slowly exuded or have escaped from blood vessels and have been deposited in tissues or on tissue surfaces.

Fascia A sheet or band of fibrous connective tissue that may be separated from other specifically organized structures, as the tendons, the aponeuroses, and the ligaments.

Febrile Pertaining to or characterized by an elevated body temperature, or fever.

Fibrillation A small, local, involuntary contraction of muscle, resulting from spontaneous activation of a single muscle fiber or of an isolated bundle of nerve fibers.

Fibrin A stringy, insoluble protein formed by the action of thrombin on fibrinogen during the clotting process.

Fibrosis The formation of fibrous connective tissue, as in the repair or replacement of parenchymatous elements.

Filtration The process of passing a liquid through or as if through a filter, which is accomplished by gravity, pressure, or vacuum.

Fimbria Any structure that forms a fringe, border, or edge or that resembles such a structure.

Fissure A cleft or a groove, normal or otherwise, on the surface of an organ or a bony structure.

Fistula An abnormal passage or communication from an internal organ to the body surface or between two internal organs.

Flaccid Weak, soft, and lax; lacking normal muscle tone.

Flatus Air or gas in the intestinal tract that is expelled through the anus.

Flexion A movement that allows the two elements of any jointed part to be brought together, decreasing the angle between them, as bending the elbow.

Flora The microorganisms, such as bacteria and fungi, both normally occurring and pathological, found in or on an organ.

Focal Relating to, having, or occupying a focus.

Follicle A sac or pouchlike depression or cavity.

Fontanel A membrane-covered opening in bones or between bones, such as the soft spot covered by tough membranes between the bones of an infant's incompletely ossified skull.

Foramen A natural opening or aperture in a membranous structure or bone.

Fossa A hollow or depressed area, especially on the surface of the end of a bone.

Fovea A small pit or depression in the surface of a structure or an organ.

Fundus The base or bottom of an organ or the portion farthest from the mouth of an organ.

Ganglion One of the nerve cell bodies, chiefly collected in groups outside the central nervous system. (Plural: ganglia)

Genotype The entire genetic constitution of an individual, as determined by the particular combination and location of the genes on the chromosomes; *or* the alleles present at one or more sites on homologous chromosomes.

Glia The neuroglia, or supporting structure of nervous tissue.

Globulin One of a broad group of proteins classified by solubility, electrophoretic mobility, and size.

Gluconeogenesis The formation of glucose from any of the substances of glycolysis other than carbohydrates.

Glycolysis A series of enzymatically catalyzed reactions, occurring within cells, by which glucose and other sugars are converted to the simpler compounds lactate or pyruvate, resulting in energy stored in the form of adenosine triphosphate (ATP).

Gonad A gamete-producing gland, as an ovary or a testis.

Gradient The rate of increase or decrease of a measurable phenomenon expressed as a function of a second; ***or*** the visual representation of such a change.

Granuloma A small mass of nodular granulation tissue resulting from chronic inflammation, injury, or infection. (Adjective: granulomatous)

Hapten A small, nonproteinaceous substance that is not antigenic by itself but that can act as an antigen by combining with particular bonding sites on an antibody.

Haustrum A structure resembling a recess or sacculation. (Plural: haustra)

Hematoma A localized collection of extravasated blood trapped in an organ, space, or tissue, resulting from a break in the wall of a blood vessel.

Hematopoiesis The normal formation and development of blood cells.

Hemianopia Defective vision or blindness in half of the visual field of one or both eyes.

Heterozygous Having two different alleles at corresponding loci on homologous chromosomes.

Heterogeneous Consisting of or composed of dissimilar elements or parts; *or* not having a uniform quality throughout. (Noun: heterogeneity)

Histology The branch of anatomy that deals with the minute structure, composition, and function of cells and tissue. (Adjective: histologic)

Homolog Any organ or part corresponding in function, position, origin, and structure to another organ or part, as the flippers of a seal that correspond to human hands. (Adjective: homologous)

Homozygous Having two identical alleles at corresponding loci on homologous chromosomes.

Humoral Relating to elements dissolved in the blood or body fluids.

Hydrolysis The chemical alteration or decomposition of a compound into fragments by the addition of water.

Hyperemia An excess or engorgement of blood in a part of the body.

Hyperesthesia An unusual or pathologic increase in sensitivity of a part, especially the skin, or of a particular sense.

Hyperplasia An abnormal multiplication or increase in the number of normal cells of a body part.

Hypertonic A solution having a greater concentration of solute than another solution with which it is compared, hence exerting more osmotic pressure than that solution.

Hypertrophy The enlargement or overgrowth of an organ that is due to an increase in the size of its cells rather than the number of its cells.

Hypesthesia An abnormal decrease of sensation in response to stimulation of the sensory nerves. (Also called hypoesthesia.)

Hypotonic A solution having a lesser concentration of solute than another solution with which it is compared, hence exerting less osmotic pressure than that solution.

Hypoxia An inadequate supply of oxygen to tissue that is below physiologic levels despite adequate perfusion of the tissue by blood.

Iatrogenic Induced inadvertently through the activity of a physician or by medical treatment or diagnostic procedures.

Idiopathic Arising spontaneously or from an unknown cause.

Idiosyncrasy A physical or behavioral characteristic or manner that is unique to an individual or to a group. (Adjective: idiosyncratic)

Inclusion The act of enclosing or the condition of being enclosed; *or* anything that is enclosed.

Infarction The development and formation of an infarct; *or* an infarct.

In situ In the natural or normal place; *or* something, such as cancer, that is confined to its place of origin and has not invaded neighboring tissues.

Interferon Any one of a group of small glycoproteins prduced in response to viral infection and which inhibit viral multiplication.

Interstitial Relating to or situated between parts or in the interspaces of a tissue.

Intramural Situated or occurring within the wall of an organ.

Intrinsic Pertaining exclusively to a part or situated entirely within an organ or tissue.

In vitro A biologic reaction occurring in an artificial environment, such as a test tube.

In vivo A biologic reaction occurring within the living body.

Involution The act or instance of enfolding, entangling, or turning inward.

Ionize To separate or change into ions.

Ipsilateral Situated on, pertaining to, or affecting the same side of the body.

Ischemia Decreased blood supply to a body organ or part, usually due to functional constriction or actual obstruction of a blood vessel.

Juxtaarticular Situated near a joint or in the region of a joint.

Juxtaglomerular Near to or adjoining a glomerulus of the kidney.

Karyotype The total chromosomal characteristics of a cell; *or* the micrograph of chromosomes arranged in pairs in descending order of size.

Keratin A fibrous, sulfur-containing protein that is the primary component of the epidermis, hair, and horny tissues.

Keratinization The development or conversion into keratin or keratinous tissue.

Keratosis Any skin condition in which there is overgrowth and thickening of the cornified epithelium.

Ketone Any of a large class of organic compounds, such as acetoacetate and acetone, with a carboxyl group attached to two carbon atoms.

Ketosis A condition characterized by the abnormal accumulation of ketones in the body tissues and fluid.

Kinesthesia The sense of movement, weight, tension, and position of body parts mediated by input from joint and muscle receptors and hair cells. (Adjective: kinesthetic)

Kyphosis An abnormal condition of the vertebral column, characterized by increased convexity in the curvature of the thoracic spine as viewed from the side.

Lacuna A small pit or cavity within a structure, especially bony tissue; *or* a defect or gap, as in the field of vision.

Lateral A position farther from the median plane or midline of the body or a structure; *or* situated on, coming from, or directed towards the side.
Lethargy The lowered level of consciousness characterized by listlessness, drowsiness, and apathy; *or* a state of indifference.
Ligament One of many predominantly white, shiny, flexible bands of fibrous tissue that binds joints together and connects bones or cartilages.
Lipid Any of the group of fats and fatlike substances characterized by being insoluble in water and soluble in nonpolar organic solvents, such as chloroform and ether.
Lipoprotein Any one of the conjugated proteins that is a complex of protein and lipid.
Lobule A small lobe.
Lordosis The anterior concavity in the curvature of the lumbar and cervical spine as observed from the side.
Lumen A cavity or the channel within a tube or tubular organ of the body.
Luteal Of or pertaining to or having the properties of the corpus luteum.
Lysis Destruction or dissolution of a cell or molecule through the action of a specific agent.

Macerate To soften something solid by wetting or soaking.
Macroscopic Large enough to be visible with the unaided eye or without the microscope.
Macula A small, flat blemish, thickening, or discoloration that is flush with the skin surface. (Adjective: macular)
Malaise A vague feeling of bodily fatigue and discomfort.
Manometer A device for measuring the tension or pressure of a liquid or gas.
Manometry The measurement of pressure using a manometer.
Marasmus A condition of extreme protein-calorie malnutrition that is characterized by growth retardation and progressive wasting of subcutaneous tissue and muscle and occurs chiefly during the first year of life.
Matrix The intracellular substance of a tissue or the basic substance from which a specific organ or kind of tissue develops.
Meatus An opening or passage through any body part.
Medial Pertaining to the middle; *or* situated or oriented toward the midline of the body.
Mediastinum The mass of tissues and organs in the middle of the thorax, separating the pleural sacs containing the two lungs.
Meiosis The division of a sex cell as it matures, so that each daughter nucleus receives one half of the number of chromosomes characteristic of the somatic cells of the species.
Mesoderm The middle layer of the three primary germ layers of the developing embryo, lying between the ectoderm and the endoderm.
Metabolism The sum of all the physical and chemical processes by which living organisms are produced and maintained, and also the transformation by which energy is provided for vital processes and activities.
Metaplasis The stage in which the organism has attained completed growth.
Metastasis The transfer of disease from one organ or part to another not directly connected with it. (Adjective: metastatic)
Mitosis A type of indirect cell division that occurs in somatic cells and results in the formation of two daughter nuclei containing the identical complements of the number of chromosomes characteristic of the somatic cells of the species.
Molecule The smallest mass of matter that exhibits the properties of an element or compound.
Morphology The study of the physical form and structure of an organism; *or* the form and structure of a particular organism. (Adjective: morphologic)
Mutagen Any chemical or physical agent that induces a genetic mutation or increases the mutation rate by causing changes in DNA.
Mutation An unusual change in form, quality, or some other characteristic; *or* a permanent transmissible change in genetic material occurring spontaneously or by induction.
Mycoplasma A genus of bacteria of the family Mycoplasmataceae lacking rigid cell walls and considered to be the smallest free-living organisms.
Myoclonus A spasm of a portion of a muscle, an entire muscle, or a group of muscles.
Myoglobin The oxygen-transporting pigment of muscle consisting of one heme molecule containing one iron molecule attached to a single globin chain.
Myopathy Any disease or abnormal condition of skeletal muscle, usually characterized by muscle weakness, wasting, and histologic changes within muscle tissue.
Myotome The muscle plate or portion of an embryonic somite that develops into a voluntary muscle; *or* a group of muscles innervated by a single spinal segment.

Necrosis Localized tissue death that occurs in groups of cells or part of a structure or an organ in response to disease or injury.
Neutropenia An abnormal decrease in the number of neutrophilic leukocytes in the blood.
Nidus The point where a morbid process originates, develops, or is located.
Nociceptor A receptor, usually found in either the skin or the walls of viscera, that responds to pain caused by injury to body tissues.
Nosocomial Pertaining to or originating in a hospital, such as a nosocomial infection; an infection acquired during hospitalization.
Nystagmus Involuntary, rapid, rhythmic movements of the eyeball.

Oncogene A gene that is capable of causing the initial and continuing conversion of normal cells into cancer cells.

Oocyte A primordial or incompletely developed ovum.

Oogenesis The process of the growth and maturation of the female gametes, or ova.

Organelle Any one of the various membrane-bound particles of distinctive morphology and function present within most cells, as the mitochondria, the Golgi complex, and the lysosomes.

Orthopnea An abnormal condition in which a person must be in an upright position in order to breathe deeply or comfortably.

Osmolality The concentration of osmotically active particles in solution expressed in osmols or milliosmols per kilogram of solvent.

Osmolarity The concentration of osmotically active particles in solution expressed in osmols or milliosmols per liter of solution.

Osmosis The movement or passage of a pure solvent, such as water, through a semipermeable membrane from a solution that has a lower solute concentration to one that has a higher solute concentration.

Osteophyte A bony project or outgrowth.

Palpable Perceptible by touch.

Papilla A small nipple-shaped projection, elevation, or structure, as the conoid papillae of the tongue.

Papule A small circumscribed, solid elevation of the skin less than one centimeter in diameter. (Adjective: papular)

Paralysis An abnormal condition characterized by the impairment or loss of motor function or the loss of sensation, or both, due to a lesion of the neural or muscular mechanism.

Paraneoplastic Relating to alterations produced in tissue remote from a tumor or its metastases.

Parenchyma The basic tissue or elements of an organ as distinguished from supporting or connective tissue or elements. (Adjective: parenchymal)

Paresis Slight or partial paralysis.

Paresthesia Any abnormal touch sensation, which can be experienced as numbness, tingling, or a "pins and needles" feeling, often in the absence of external stimuli.

Parietal Pertaining to the outer wall of a cavity or organ; *or* pertaining to the parietal bone of the skull or the parietal lobe of the brain.

Parous Having borne one or more viable offspring.

Pathogen Any microorganism capable of producing disease.

Pedigree A systematic presentation, such as in a table, chart, or list, of an individual's ancestors that is used in human genetics in the analysis of inheritance.

Peptide Any of a class of molecular chain compounds composed of two or more amino acids joined by peptide bonds.

Perfusion The process or act of pouring over or through, especially the passage of a fluid through a specific organ or an area of the body.

Peripheral Pertaining to the outside, surface, or surrounding area of an organ or other structure; *or* located away from a center or central structure.

Permeable A condition of being pervious, or permitting passage, so that fluids and certain other substances can pass through, as a permeable membrane.

Pervasive Pertaining to something that becomes diffused throughout every part.

Petechia A tiny, perfectly round purplish red spot that appears on the skin as a result of minute intradermal or submucous hemorrhage. (Plural: petechiae)

Phagocytosis The process by which certain cells engulf and consume foreign material and cell debris.

Phalanx Any one of the bones composing the fingers of each hand and the toes of each foot.

Phenotype The complete physical, biochemical, and physiologic makeup of an individual, as determined by the interaction of both genetic makeup and environmental factors.

Plexus A network of intersecting nerves, blood vessels, or lymphatic vessels.

Polygene Any of a group of nonallelic genes that interact to influence the same character in the same way so that the effect is cumulative, usually of a quantitative nature, as size, weight, or skin pigmentation. (Adjective: polygenic)

Polymorph One of several, or many, forms of an organism or cell. (Adjective: polymorphic)

Polyp A small, tumor-like growth that protrudes from a mucous membrane surface.

Prodrome An early symptom indicating the onset of a condition or disease. (Adjective: prodromal)

Prolapse The falling down, sinking, or sliding of an organ from its normal position or location in the body.

Proliferation The reproduction or multiplication of similar forms, especially cells.

Pronation Assumption of a prone position; *or* the state of being prone.

Prone The position in which the ventral, or front, surface of the body faces downward.

Propagation The act or action of reproduction.

Proprioceptor Any of the sensory nerve endings, found in muscles, tendons, joints, and the vestibular apparatus, that respond to stimuli originating from within the body regarding movement and body position.

Proprioception The reception of stimuli originating from within the body regarding body position and muscular activity.

Prosthesis An artificial replacement for a missing body part; *or* a device designed and applied to improve function, such as a hearing aid.

Protagonist An agent, such as a substance or drug, that causes or supports the action of a neuromediator or body function; ***or*** a muscle that by its contraction causes a particular movement.

Proteoglycans Any one of a group of polysaccharide-protein conjugates occurring primarily in the matrix of connective tissue and cartilage.

Protooncogene A normal cellular gene that with alteration, such as by mutation, becomes an active oncogene.

Proximal Closer to a point of refercence, usually the trunk of the body, than other parts of the body.

Pruritus The symptom of itching, an uncomfortable sensation leading to the urge to rub or scratch the skin to obtain relief. (Adjective: pruritic)

Purpura A small hemorrhage, up to about 1 cm in diameter, in the skin, mucous membrane, or serosal surface; *or* any of several bleeding disorders characterized by the presence of purpuric lesions.

Purulent Producing or containing pus.

Quiescent Causing no disturbance, activity, or symptoms.

Reflux An abnormal backward or return flow of a fluid, such as stomach contents, blood, or urine.

Regurgitation A flow of material that is in the opposite direction from normal, as in the return of swallowed food into the mouth or the backward flow of blood through a defective heart valve.

Remission The partial or complete disappearance of the symptoms of a chronic or malignant disease; *or* the period of time during which the abatement of symptoms occurs.

Resorption The loss of substance or bone by physiologic or pathologic means, for example, the loss of dentin and cementum of a tooth.

Retroversion A condition in which an entire organ is tipped backward or in a posterior direction, usually wihout flexion or other distortion.

Riboflavin Vitamin B_2.

Rostral Pertaining to or resembling a beak.

Sacroiliitis Inflammation in the sacroiliac joint.

Sclerosis A condition characterized by induration or hardening of tissue resulting from any of several causes, including inflammation, diseases of the interstitial substance, and increased formation of connective tissues.

Semipermeable Partially but not wholly permeable, especially a membrane that permits the passage of some (usually small) molecules but not of other (usually larger) particles.

Senescence The process or condition of aging or growing old.

Sepsis The presence in the blood or other tissues of pathogenic microorganisms or their toxins; *or* the condition resulting from the spread of microorganisms or their products. (Adjective: septic)

Serous Relating to or resembling serum; *or* containing or producing serum, such as a serous gland.

Spastic Pertaining to or characterized by spasms or other uncontrolled contractions of the skeletal muscles.

Spasticity The condition characterized by spasms.

Spatial Relating to, having the character of, or occupying space.

Sphincter A ringlike band of muscle fibers that constricts a passage or closes a natural orifice of the body.

Stenosis An abnormal condition characterized by the narrowing or stricture of a duct or canal.

Stria A streak or a linear scarlike lesion that often results from rapidly developing tension in the skin; *or* a narrow bandlike structure, especially the longitudinal collections of nerve fibers in the brain.

Stricture An abnormal temporary or permanent narrowing of the lumen of a duct, canal, or other passage, as the esophagus, because of inflammation, external pressure, or scarring.

Stroma The supporting tissue or the matrix of an organ as distinguished from its functional element, or parenchyma.

Stupor A lowered level of consciousness characterized by lethergy and unresponsiveness in which a person seems unaware of his or her surroundings.

Subchondral Beneath a cartilage.

Subcutaneous Beneath the skin.

Sulcus A shallow groove, depression, or furrow on the surface of an organ, as a sulcus on the surface of the brain, separating the gyri.

Supination Assumption of a supine position; *or* the state of being supine.

Supine Lying horizontally on the back, or with the face upward.

Suppuration The formation of pus, or purulent matter.

Symbiosis Mode of living characterized by close association between organisms of different species, usually in a mutually beneficial relationship.

Sympathomimetic An agent or substance that produces stimulating effects on organs and structures similar to those produced by the sympathetic nervous system.

Syncope A brief lapse of consciousness due to generalized cerebral ischemia.

Syncytium A multinucleate mass of protoplasm produced by the merging of a group of cells.

Syndrome A complex of signs and symptoms that occur together to present a clinical picture of a disease or inherited abnormality.

Synergist An organ, agent, or substance that aids or cooperates with another organ, agent, or substance.

Synthesis An integration or combination of various parts or elements to create a unified whole.

Systemic Pertaining to the whole body rather than to a localized area or regional portion of the body.

Tamponade Stoppage of the flow of blood to an organ or a part of the body by pathologic compression, such as the compression of the heart by an accumulation of pericardial fluid.

Tetratogen Any agent or factor that induces or increases the incidence of developmental abnormalities in the fetus.

Tinnitus A tinkling, buzzing, or ringing noise heard in one or both ears.

Tophus A chalky deposit containing sodium urate that most often develops in periarticular fibrous tissue, typically in individuals with gout. (Plural: tophi)

Torsion The act or process of twisting in either a positive (clockwise) or negative (counterclockwise) direction.

Trabecula A supporting or anchoring stand of connective tissue, such as the delicate fibrous threads connecting the inner surface of the arachnoid to the pia mater.

Transmural Situated or occurring through the wall of an organ.

Transudate A fluid substance passed through a membrane or extruded from the blood.

Tremor Involuntary quivering or trembling movements caused by the alternating contraction and relaxation of opposing groups of skeletal muscles.

Trigone A triangular-shaped area.

Ubiquitous The condition or state of existing or being everywhere at the same time.

Ulcer A circumscribed excavation of the surface of an organ or tissue, which results from necrosis that accompanies some inflammatory, infectious, or malignant processes. (Adjective: ulcerative)

Urticaria A pruritic skin eruption of the upper dermis, usually transient, characterized by wheals of various shapes and sizes.

Uveitis An inflammation of all or part of the uveal tract of the eye.

Ventral Pertaining to a position toward the belly of the body; *or* situated or oriented toward the front or anterior of the body.

Vertigo An illusory sensation that the environment or one's own body is revolving.

Vesicle A small bladder or sac, as a small, thin-walled, raised skin lesion, containing liquid.

Visceral Pertaining to the viscera, or internal organs of the body.

Viscosity Pertaining to the physical property of fluids, caused by the adhesion of adjacent molecules, that determines the internal resistance to shear forces.

APPENDIX

Lab Values

Prefixes Denoting Decimel Factors

Prefix	Symbol	Factor
mega	M	10^{6}
kilo	k	10^{3}
hecto	h	10^{2}
deci	d	10^{-1}
centi	c	10^{-2}
milli	m	10^{-3}
micro	μ	10^{-6}
nano	n	10^{-9}
pico	p	10^{-12}
femto	f	10^{-15}

Hematology

Test	Conventional Units	SI Units
Erythrocyte count (RBC count)	M. 4.2–5.4 × 10^{6}/μL F. 3.5–5.0 × 10^{6}/μL	M. 4.2–5.4 × 10^{12}/L F. 3.6–5.0 × 10^{12}/L
Hematocrit (Hct)	M. 40–50% F. 37–47%	M. 0.40–0.50 F. 0.37–0.47
Hemoglobin (Hb)	M. 14.0–16.5 g/dL F. 12.0–15.0 g/dL	M. 140–165 g/L F. 120–150 g/L
Mean corpuscular hemoglobin (MHC)	27-34 pg/cell	0.40–0.53 fmol/cell
Mean corpuscular hemoglobin concentration (MCHC)	31-35 g/dL	310–350 g/L
Mean corpuscular volume (MCV)	80–100 fL	
Reticulocyte count	1.0–1.5% total RBC	
Leukocyte count (WBC count)	3.4–10 × 10^{3}/μL	3.4–10 × 10^{9}/L
Basophils	0-2%	
Eosinophils	0-3%	
Lymphocytes	24-40%	
Monocytes	4–9%	
Neutrophils (segmented [Segs])	47–63%	
Neutrophils (bands)	0–4%	

Blood Chemistry*

Test	Conventional Units	SI Units
Alanine aminotransferase (ALT, SGPT)	0–35 U/L	0–0.58 µkat/L
Alkaline phosphatase	41–133 U/L	0.7–2.2 µkat/L
Ammonia	18–16 µg/dL	11–35 µmol/L
Amylase	20–110 U/L†	0.33–1.83 µkat/L†
Aspartase amino transferase (AST, SGOT)	0–35 U/L†	0–0.58 µkat/L†
Bilibrubin (total)	0.1–1.2 mg/dL	2–21 µmol/L
Direct	0.1–0.4 mg/dL	< 7 µmol/L
Indirect	0.1–0.7 mg/dL	< 12 µmol/L
Blood urea nitrogen (BUN)	8-20 mg/dL	2.9–7.1 mmol/L
Calcium	8.5–10.5 mg/dL	2.1–2.6 mmol/L
Chloride	98–106 mEq/L	98–106 mmol/L
Creatine kinase (CK, CPK)	32–267 U/L†	0.53–4.45 µkat/L†
Creatine kinase (MB)	< 16 IU/L† or 4% of total CK	< 0.27 µkat/L†
Creatinine (serum)	0.6–1.2 mg/dL‡	50–100 µmol/L‡
Gamma-glutamyl-transpeptidase (GGT)	9–85 U/L†	0.15–1.42 µkat/L†
Glucose (blood)	60–115 mg/dL	3.3–6.3 mmol/L
Glycosylated hemoglobin (HbA_{1c})	3.9–6.9%	
Lactate dehydrogenase (LDH)	88–230 U/L†	1.46–3.82 µkat/L†
Lipids		
Cholesterol	< 200 mg/dL (desirable)	< 5.2 mmol/L
Triglycerides	< 165 mg/dL	< 1.65 g/L
Lipase	0-160 U/L†	0.266 µkat/L†
Magnesium	1.84–2.4 mg/dL	0.99–0.75 mmol/L
Osmolality	275–295 mOsm/kg H_2O	275–295 mmol/kg H20
Phosphorus (inorganic)	2.4–4.5 mg/dL	0.77–1.45 mmol/L
Potassium	3.5–5.0 mEq/L	3.5–5.0 mmol/L
Prostate specific antigen (PSA)	0-4 ng/mL	0-4 µg/L
Protein total	6.0–8.6 g/dL	60–86 g/L
Albumin	3.8–5.6 g/dL	38–56 g/L
Globulin	2.3–3.5 g/dL	23–35 g/L
A/G ratio	1.0–2.2	1.0–2.2
Thyroid Tests		
Thyroxine (T_4) total	5.0–11.0 µg/dL	64–142 nmol/L
Thyroxine, free (FT_4)	9-24 pmol/L†	
Triiodothyronine (T_3) total	95–190 ng/dL	1.5–2.9 nmol/L
Thyroid stimulating hormone (TSH)	0.5–6.0 µU/mL	0.4–6.0 mU/L
Thyroglobin	3–42 ng/mL	3–42 µg/L
Sodium	135–148 mEq/L	135–148 mmol/L
Uric acid	M. 2.4–7.4 mg/dL F. 1.4–5.8 mg/dL	M. 140–440 µmol/L F. 80–350 µmol/L

*Values may vary with laboratory. The values supplied by the laboratory performing the test should always be used since the ranges may be method specific.
†Laboratory and/or method specific
‡Varies with age and muscle mass
(Values obtained from Tierney LM., McPhee S.J., Papadakis M.A. [1997]. *Current medical diagnosis and treatment* [36th ed.]. Stamford, CT. Appleton & Lange, pp. 1495–1501; Fischbach F. [1995]. *Quick reference to common diagnostic and laboratory tests.* Philadelphia: Lippincott-Raven, and other sources.)

INDEX

Page numbers followed by *f* indicate figures; those followed by *t* indicate tables; those followed by *c* indicate charts.

D

E

H

J

M

S

T

W

X

Y

Z

LIPPINCOTT CREDITS

CHAPTER 1

Fig. 1–13: Chaffee, E.E., Gersheimer, E.M. (1974). *Basic Physiology and Anatomy* (3rd ed.). Philadelphia: J.B. Lippincott

Figs. 1–2, 1–3, 1–9, 1–24, 1–28: Cormack, D.H. (1993). *Essential Histology.* Philadelphia: J.B. Lippincott

Fig. 1–23: Cormack, D.H. (1987). *Ham's Histology* (9th ed.). Philadelphia: J.B. Lippincott

CHAPTER 3

Figs. 3–7, 3–8: Cormack, D.H. (1993). *Essential Histology.* Philadelphia: J.B. Lippinott

CHAPTER 4

Figs. 4–2, 4–3: Sauer, G.C., Hall, J.C. (1996). *Manual of Skin Diseases.* Philadelphia: Lippincott-Raven

CHAPTER 6

Fig. 6–3: Cormack, D.H. (1987). *Ham's Histology* (9th ed.). Philadelphia: J.B. Lippincott

CHAPTER 12

Figs. 12–2, 12–3: Oski, F.A. (Ed.). (1990). *Principles and Practice of Pediatrics.* Philadelphia: J.B. Lippincott

CHAPTER 14

Fig. 14–1: Chaffee, E.E., Lytle, I.M. (1980). *Basic Physiology and Pathology* (4th ed.). Philadelphia: J.B. Lippincott

Figs. 14–5, 14–6: Cormack, D.H. (1993). *Essential Histology.* Philadelphia: J.B. Lippincott

CHAPTER 15

Fig. 15–1: Bates, B.B. (1995). *A Guide to Physical Examination and History Taking* (6th ed.). Philadelphia: J.B. Lippincott

Figs. 15–2, 15–3, 15–4, 15–5, 15–6, 15–7, 15–8, 15–9, 15–11, 15–12, 15–13, 15–16, 15–17, 15–18, 15–19, 15–20, 15–21, 15–22, 15–23, 15–24, 15–25, 15–26, 15–27, 15–28, 15–29, 15–31, 15–32, 15–36, 15–37, 15–38: Sauer, G.C., Hall, J.C. (1996). *Manual of Skin Diseases.* Philadelphia: Lippincott-Raven

CHAPTER 16

Figs. 16–8, 16–13, 16–26, 16–28, 16–29, 16–32: Chaffee, E.E., Lytle, I.M. (1980). *Basic Physiology and Pathology* (4th ed.). Philadelphia: J.B. Lippincott

Figs. 16–6, 16–9: Cormack, D.H. (1987). *Ham's Histology* (9th ed.). Philadelphia: J.B. Lippincott

CHAPTER 17

Figs. 17–3, 17–4, 17–7: Rubin, E., Farber, J.L. (1994). *Pathology* (2nd ed.). Philadelphia: J.B. Lippincott

CHAPTER 19

Fig. 19–5: Horowitz, L.D., Groves, B.M. (1985). *Signs and Symptoms in Cardiology.* Philadelphia: J.B. Lippincott

Figs. 19–10, 19–15, 19–17: Rubin, E., Farber, J.L. (1994). *Pathology* (2nd ed.). Philadelphia, J.B. Lippincott

Fig. 19–12: Chaffee, E.E., Lytle, I.M. (1980). *Basic Physiology and Pathology* (4th ed.). Philadelphia: J.B. Lippincott

CHAPTER 20

Fig. 20–9: Hudak, C.M., Gallo, B.M. (1994). *Critical Care Nursing* (6th ed.). Philadelphia: J.B. Lippincott

CHAPTER 22

Figs. 22–3, 22–11, 22–20: Chaffee, E.E., Lytle, I.M. (1980). *Basic Physiology and Pathology* (4th ed.). Philadelphia: J.B. Lippincott

CHAPTER 23

Figs. 22–3, 23–4: Rubin, E., Farber, J.L. (1994). *Pathology* (2nd ed.). Philadelphia: J.B. Lippincott

CHAPTER 24

Figs. 24–3, 24–8: Rubin, E., Farber, J.L. (1994). *Pathology* (2nd ed.). Philadelphia: J.B. Lippincott

Fig. 24–11: Burton, G.G., Hodgkin, G.E., Ward, J.J. (1991). *Respiratory Care: A Guide to Clinical Practice* (3rd ed.). Philadelphia: J.B. Lippincott

CHAPTER 25

Figs. 25–2, 25–4: Chaffee, E.E., Lytle, I.M. (1980). *Basic Physiology and Pathology* (4th ed.). Philadelphia: J.B. Lippincott

Fig. 25–3: Cormack, D.H. (1987). *Ham's Histology* (9th ed.). Philadelphia: J.B. Lippincott

CHAPTER 26

Fig. 26–4: Chaffee, E.E., Lytle, I.M. (1980). *Basic Physiology and Pathology* (4th ed.). Philadelphia: J.B. Lippincott

CHAPTER 28

Figs. 28–1, 28–2, 28–5, 28–6, 28–9, 28–10, 28–11: Rubin, E., Farber, J.L. (1994). *Pathology* (2nd ed.). Philadelphia: J.B. Lippincott

CHAPTER 30

Figs. 30–1, 30–2: Chaffee, E.E., Lytle, I.M. (1980). *Basic Physiology and Pathology* (4th ed.). Philadelphia: J.B. Lippincott

CHAPTER 31

Figs. 31–1, 31–6, 31–7, 31–9, 31–11, 31–12: Chaffee, E.E., Lytle, I.M. (1980). *Basic Physiology and Pathology* (4th ed.). Philadelphia: J.B. Lippincott

Figs. 31–3, 31–4, 31–5: Thomson, J.S. (1977). *Core Textbook of Anatomy.* Philadelphia: J.B. Lippincott

CHAPTER 32

Figs. 32–1, 32–2, 32–3, 32–4, 32–5: Rubin, E., Farber, J.L. (1994). *Pathology* (2nd ed.). Philadelphia: J.B. Lippincott

CHAPTER 33

Figs. 33–1, 33–2, 33–3: Chaffee, E.E., Lytle, I.M. (1980). *Basic Physiology and Pathology* (4th ed.). Philadelphia: J.B. Lippincott

Fig. 33–9: Rubin, E., Farber, J.L. (1994). *Pathology* (2nd ed.). Philadelphia: J.B. Lippincott

Fig. 33–10: Schiff, L. (1982). *Diseases of the Liver.* Philadelphia: J.B. Lippincott

CHAPTER 34

Fig. 34–4: Chaffee, E.E., Lytle, I.M. (1980). *Basic Physiology and Pathology* (4th ed.). Philadelphia: J.B. Lippincott

CHAPTER 35

Figs. 35–1, 35–2: Chaffee, E.E., Lytle, I.M. (1980). *Basic Physiology and Pathology* (4th ed.). Philadelphia: J.B. Lippincott

Fig. 35–6: Rubin, E., Farber, J.L. (1994). *Pathology* (2nd ed.). Philadelphia: J.B. Lippincott

CHAPTER 36

Fig. 36–10: Bates, B.B. (1995). *A Guide to Physical Examination and History Taking* (6th ed.). Philadelphia: J.B. Lippincott

CHAPTER 37

Fig. 37–18: Barr, M.L., Kiernan, J.A. (1988). *The Human Nervous System: An Anatomical Viewpoint.* Philadelphia: J.B. Lippincott

Figs. 37–8, 37–16, 37–17, 37–20, 37–24, 37–26, 37–28, 37–29, 37–31, 37–32: Chaffee, E.E., Lytle, I.M. (1980). *Basic Physiology and Pathology* (4th ed.). Philadelphia: J.B. Lippincott

Fig. 37–19: Conn, P.M. (1995). *Neuroscience in Medicine.* Philadelphia: J.B. Lippincott

Fig. 37–30: Cormack, D.H. (1984). *Introduction to Histology.* Philadelphia: J.B. Lippincott

CHAPTER 38

Fig. 38–4: Bates, B.B. (1995). *A Guide to Physical Examination and History Taking* (6th ed.). Philadelphia: J.B. Lippincott

Figs. 38–7, 38–8: Chaffee, E.E., Lytle, I.M. (1980). *Basic Physiology and Pathology* (4th ed.). Philadelphia: J.B. Lippincott

Fig. 38–2: Hickey, J.V. (1992). *The Clinical Practice of Neurological and Neurosurgical Nursing* (3rd ed.). Philadelphia: J.B. Lippincott

Figs. 38–1, 38–5, 38–11, 38–14: Rubin, E., Farber, J.L. (1994). *Pathology* (2nd ed.). Philadelphia: J.B. Lippincott

Fig. 38–10: Smith, R.R. (1980). *Essentials of Neurosurgery.* Philadelphia: J.B. Lippincott

CHAPTER 39

Figs. 39–8, 39–12: Chaffee, E.E., Lytle, I.M. (1980). *Basic Physiology and Pathology* (4th ed.). Philadelphia: J.B. Lippincott

Figs. 39–5, 39–14, 39–15, 39–16: Hickey, J.V. (1992). *The Clinical Practice of Neurological and Neurosurgical Nursing* (3rd ed.). Philadelphia: J.B. Lippincott

Fig. 39–13: Rockwood, C.A., Green, D.P. (1977). *Fractures.* Philadelphia: J.B. Lippincott

Fig. 39–1: Wiener, W.J., Goetz, C.G. (1989). *Neurology for the Non-neurologist* (2nd ed.). Philadelphia: J.B. Lippincott

CHAPTER 40

Fig. 40–10: Chaffee, E.E., Lytle, I.M. (1980). *Basic Physiology and Pathology* (4th ed.). Philadelphia: J.B. Lippincott

Fig. 40–9: Conn, P.M. (1995). *Neuroscience in Medicine.* Philadelphia: J.B. Lippincott

Fig. 40–4: Rodman, M.J. (1979). *Pharmacologica Drug Therapy in Nursing.* Philadelphia: J.B. Lippincott

CHAPTER 41

Fig. 41–4: Akesson, A.J., Loeb, J.A., Wilson-Pauwels, L. (1990). *Thompson's Core Textbook of Anatomy* (2nd ed.). Philadelphia: J.B. Lippincott

Fig. 41–3: Bates, B.B. (1995). *A Guide to Physical Examination and History Taking* (6th ed.). Philadelphia: J.B. Lippincott

Figs. 41–1, 41–2, 41–5, 41–6, 41–9, 41–12, 41–15, 41–17: Chaffee, E.E., Lytle, I.M. (1980). *Basic Physiology and Pathology* (4th ed.). Philadelphia: J.B. Lippincott

Fig. 41–22: Conn, P.M. (1995). *Neuroscience in Medicine.* Philadelphia: J.B. Lippincott

Fig. 41–16: Cormack, D.H. (1993). *Essential Histology.* Philadelphia: J.B. Lippincott

CHAPTER 42

Figs. 42–7, 42–11: Bates, B.B. (1995). *A Guide to Physical Examination and History Taking* (6th ed.). Philadelphia: J.B. Lippincott

Figs. 42–5, 42–8: Chaffee, E.E., Lytle, I.M. (1980). *Basic Physiology and Pathology* (4th ed.). Philadelphia: J.B. Lippincott

CHAPTER 44

Figs. 44–1, 44–2, 44–5, 44–6, 44–7: Chaffee, E.E., Lytle, I.M. (1980). *Basic Physiology and Pathology* (4th ed.). Philadelphia: J.B. Lippincott

CHAPTER 45

Fig. 45–5: Farrell, J. (1986). *Illustrated Guide to Orthopedic Nursing* (3rd ed.). Philadelphia: J.B. Lippincott

CHAPTER 46

Fig. 46–1: Cormack, D.H. (1987). *Ham's Histology* (9th ed.). Philadelphia: J.B. Lippincott

Figs. 46–6, 46–7, 46–8, 46–10, 46–12, 46–13, 46–16, 46–19: Weinstein, S.L., Buckwalter, J.A. (1994). *Turek's Orthopaedics* (5th ed.). Philadelphia: J.B. Lippincott

CHAPTER 48

Figs. 48–1, 48–2, 48–3, 48–5: Chaffee, E.E., Lytle, I.M. (1980). *Basic Physiology and Pathology* (4th ed.). Philadelphia: J.B. Lippincott

CHAPTER 49

Fig. 49–2: Bates, B. (1995). *A Guide to Physical Examination and History Taking* (6th ed.). Philadelphia: J.B. Lippincott

CHAPTER 50

Figs. 50–1, 50–2, 50–3, 50–8: Chaffee, E.E., Lytle, I.M. (1980). *Basic Physiology and Pathology* (4th ed.). Philadelphia: J.B. Lippincott

CHAPTER 51

Fig. 51–7: Chaffee, E.E., Lytle, I.M. (1980). *Basic Physiology and Pathology* (4th ed.). Philadelphia: J.B. Lippincott

Figs. 51–6, 51–8: Rock, J.A., Thompson, J.D. (1992). *TeLinde's Operative Gynecology* (7th ed.). Philadelphia: J.B. Lippincott

Figs. 51–1, 51–2, 51–3, 51–4, 51–5, 51–10, 51–11: Rubin, E., Farber, J.L. (1994). *Pathology* (2nd ed.). Philadelphia: J.B. Lippincott

This electronic self-study program has been designed for use with an IBM or IBM-compatible computer and requires Windows version 3.0 or higher, 512KB RAM, a 3.5-inch disk drive, and a CGA graphics card or better.

To start the program, insert the diskette in your disk drive and type "a:" or the appropriate letter for your disk drive, then select Start, Run and type "a:/setup" at the command line.

This self-study program enables you to answer approximately 350 questions in a manner similar to the way you will take the NCLEX examination. As in the NCLEX, all questions in this program are multiple choice. To answer the questions, you will need to use only the up and down arrow keys and the <Enter> key. Use the arrow keys to highlight the answer you wish to select, and press <Enter> to make the selection. Instructions are provided as prompts at the bottom of the screen.

The Main Menu of the program looks like this:

1. Instructions
2. Choose a Test
3. Review Results
4. Quit

As in the Tests, highlight your choice using the arrow keys, and press <Enter> to select it.

Selecting the **Instructions** option displays this screen.

Selecting the **Choose a Test** option will provide you with a list of 15 tests, each corresponding to a unit in ***Pathophysiology.*** To begin taking a test, use the arrow keys to highlight the name of the Test you wish to take, and press the <Enter> key.

After you have selected a topic, you will be asked if you wish to take the test in ***Study Mode*** or ***Test Mode.*** To select a mode, press the <Alt> key at the same time as the underlined letter in your choice (<Alt>S for ***Study Mode,*** <Alt>T for ***Test Mode***).

Study Mode lets you know immediately if the answer you selected was correct and provides you with feedback for correct and incorrect choices. If you select an incorrect answer, try again until you find the correct answer.

If you select ***Test Mode,*** you will be given the option of having the test timed (press <Alt>I), having the screen display the time remaining (press <Alt>R), and having the screen display the number of questions remaining in the test (press <Alt>Q). While in ***Test Mode,*** you will not receive immediate feedback on your answers. When you have answered all the questions, or when time has expired, you will be shown how many questions you have answered correctly.

After seeing your test results in ***Test Mode,*** you will have the option of printing the results of the test (press <Alt>P), reviewing the question again in ***Study Mode*** (press <Alt>S), or returning to the main menu (press <Alt>M).

If you choose to review the questions in ***Study Mode,*** you will see all the questions in that particular test again. The questions you answered correctly will be indicated with a check mark in front of the question number. All questions without a check mark were either answered incorrectly or not answered. In this mode, you will receive instant feedback on the answers you select.

The results for each test taken in a single session are temporarily stored in memory. Choosing the **Review Results** option from the Main Menu will show you the results for any test you have taken during this session.

Selecting the **Quit** option from the Main Menu will end the session and return you to DOS.